D0854628

Library (MEC), Queens Hospital Burton
library.bur@burtonh-tr.wmids.nhs.uk
01283 511511 x2104

CLINICAL PRACTICE OF

Gastroenterology

VOLUME TWO

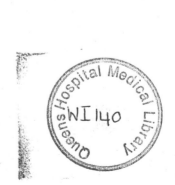

Queens Hospital Medical Library
WI 140

CLINICAL PRACTICE OF

Gastroenterology

VOLUME TWO

EDITOR-IN-CHIEF

LAWRENCE J. BRANDT, MD

Professor of Medicine
Albert Einstein College of Medicine
Director, Division of Gastroenterology
Moses Campus of Montefiore Medical Center
Bronx, New York

SECTION EDITORS

FREDRIC DAUM, MD
Chief, Division of Pediatric Gastroenterology
North Shore University Hospital
Manhasset, New York

LAWRENCE S. FRIEDMAN, MD
Associate Professor of Medicine
Harvard Medical School
Chief
Walter Sauer Firm
Physician
Gastrointestinal Unit
Massachusetts General Hospital
Boston, Massachusetts

DAVID A. PEURA, MD
Professor
Department of Medicine
Associate Chief
Gastroenterology and Hepatology
University of Virginia Medical School
Charlottesville, Virginia

C.S. PITCHUMONI, MD
Professor of Medicine
Professor of Community and
  Preventive Medicine
New York Medical College
Director of Medicine
Our Lady of Mercy Medical Center
Bronx, New York

JOHN F. REINUS, MD
Associate Professor
Department of Medicine
Albert Einstein College of Medicine
Attending Physician
Department of Gastroenterology
Montefiore Medical Center
Bronx, New York

JOEL E. RICHTER, MD
Professor of Medicine
Cleveland Clinic Health Science Center
Ohio State University
Chairman
Department of Gastroenterology
Cleveland Clinic Foundation
Cleveland, Ohio

ARVEY I. ROGERS, MD
Professor
Department of Medicine
University of Miami School of Medicine
Chief
Division of Gastroenterology
Miami Veteran's Affairs Medical Center
Gastroenterologist
University of Miami Hospital and
  Clinics
Jackson Memorial Hospital
Miami, Florida

LAWRENCE R. SCHILLER, MD
Clinical Assistant Professor
  of Internal Medicine
Department of Internal Medicine
University of Texas Southwestern
  Medical Center
Program Director
Gastroenterology Fellowship
Attending Physician
Baylor University Medical Center
Dallas, Texas

JACQUES VAN DAM, MD
Associate Director
Gastrointestinal Endoscopy
Brigham and Women's Hospital
Boston, Massachusetts

WITH 281 CONTRIBUTORS

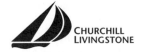
CHURCHILL
LIVINGSTONE

Developed by Current Medicine, Inc., Philadelphia

Current Medicine, Inc.
400 Market Street
Suite 700
Philadelphia, PA 19106

Director of Product Development: ...... *Lori J. Bainbridge*
Developmental Editors: .... *Joe Rusko, Paul Arthur, Shirley Claypool*
Assistant Editor: .... *Deborah Singer*
Editorial Assistants: .... *Natalie Mykysey, Erin Ritter, Leslie Sell*
Art Director: .... *Paul Fennessy*
Cover and Interior Design: .... *Patrick Ward*
Layout: .... *Christoper Allan, Robert LeBrun,*
                                                 Erika Mangan, Patrick Whelan
Illustration Director: .... *Wiesia Langenfeld*
Illustrators: .... *Marie Dean, Wiesia Langenfeld,*
                                                 Debra Wertz, Beth Starkey
Typesetting: .... *Ryan Walsh*
Production Manager: .... *Lori Holland*
Production Assistant: .... *Amy Watts*
Indexer: .... *Maria Coughlin*

Clinical practice of gastroenterology / editor-in-chief, Lawrence J. Brandt;
    section editors, Fredric Daum...[et al.].
        p. cm.
    Includes bibliographical references and index.
    ISBN 0-443-06520-9 (set). - ISBN 0-443-06521-7 (v.1). - ISBN 0-443-06522-5 (v.2)
    1. Gastrointestinal system-Diseases-Treatment. I. Brandt, Lawrence J.
    [DNLM: 1. Gastrointestinal Diseases. WI 140C6407 1999]
    RC801.C567 1999
    616.3'3-dc21
    DNLM/DLC
    for Library of Congress   98-22058
                                          CIP

Library of Congress Cataloging-in-Publication Data
ISBN 0-443-06520-9 (Set)
ISBN 0-443-06521-7 (Volume 1)
ISBN 0-443-06522-5 (Volume 2)

©Copyright 1999 by Current Medicine, Inc. All rights reserved. No part of this publication may
be reproduced, stored in a retrieval system or transmitted in any form or by any means electronic,
mechanical, photocopying, recording, or otherwise, without prior written consent of the publisher.

Although every effort has been made to ensure that drug doses and other information are presented
accurately in this publication, the ultimate responsibility rests with the prescribing physician. Neither
the publishers nor the authors can be held responsible for errors or for any consequences arising from
the use of information contained herein. Products mentioned in this publication should be used in
accordance with the prescribing information prepared by the manufacturers. No claims or endorse-
ments are made for any drug or compound at present under clinical investigation.

Prepress by Trinity Graphics.
Printed in the United States of America by Quebecor.
10 9 8 7 6 5 4 3 2 1

Contributors

NANAKRAM AGARWAL, MD, MPH, FRCSC
Professor
Department of Surgery
New York Medical College
Valhalla, New York;
Chief
Surgical Intensive Care Unit
Our Lady of Mercy Medical Center
Bronx, New York

HARVEY W. AIGES, MD
Professor of Clinical Pediatrics
Department of Pediatrics
New York University Medical School
New York City, New York;
Associate Chairman
Department of Pediatrics
North Shore University Hospital
Manhasset, New York

ESTELLA M. ALONSO, MD
Associate Professor
Department of Pediatrics
Northwestern University
Director
Hepatology and Liver Transplantation
Children's Memorial Hospital
Chicago, Illinois

DAVID F. ALTMAN, MD
Clinical Professor
Department of Medicine
University of California, San Francisco,
    School of Medicine
Vice President
The Lewin Group
San Francisco, California

R. PETER ALTMAN, MD
Professor of Surgery
Department of Surgery
Columbia-Presbyterian College of
    Physicians and Surgeons
Surgeon-in-Chief
Director
Pediatric Surgery
Babies and Children's Hospital of New York
New York City, New York

MICHAEL D. APSTEIN, MD
Assistant Professor
Department of Medicine
Harvard Medical School
Chief, Clinical Gastroenterology
Brockton/West Roxbury Veteran's Affairs
    Medical Center
Associate Physician
Division of Gastroenterology
Brigham and Women's Hospital
Boston, Massachusetts

JAIME ARANDA-MICHEL, MD
Fellow
Department of Digestive Diseases
University of Cincinnati College of Medicine
Cincinnati, Ohio

MASSIMO ARCERITO, MD
Postdoctoral Fellow
Department of Surgery
University of California, San Francisco,
    School of Medicine
San Francisco, California

BRUCE R. BACON, MD
Professor of Internal Medicine
Department of Internal Medicine
Director
Division of Gastroenterology and Hepatology
St. Louis University School of Medicine
St. Louis, Missouri

SIMMY BANK, MD, FRCP
Professor
Department of Medicine
Albert Einstein College of Medicine
Bronx, New York;
Chief
Division of Gastroenterology
Long Island Jewish Medical Center
New Hyde Park, New York

JAMIE S. BARKIN, MD
Professor of Medicine
Department of Medicine
University of Miami School of Medicine
Chief
Division of Gastroenterology
Mt. Sinai Medical Center
Miami Beach, Florida

GRAHAM F. BARNARD, MD, PhD
Assistant Professor
Department of Medicine and Biochemistry
    and Molecular Biology
Staff Physician
University of Massachusetts Medical Center
Worcester, Massachusetts

EMILY H. BATTLE, MD
Fellow
Department of Gastroenterology and
    Hepatology
University of Virginia Medical School
Fellow
Department of Gastroenterology and
    Hepatology
University of Virginia Health Sciences Center
Charlottesville, Virginia

JAMES M. BECKER, MD
James Utley Professor
Chairman
Department of Surgery
Boston University School of Medicine
Surgeon-in-Chief
Boston Medical Center
Boston, Massachusetts

STANLEY B. BENJAMIN, MD
Brick Professor of Medicine
Department of Medicine
Georgetown School of Medicine
Washington, DC

CHRISTOPHER C. BENSON, MD
Senior Fellow
Department of Gastroenterology
University of Southern Alabama
Mobile, Alabama

LESLIE H. BERNSTEIN, MD
Professor of Medicine
Department of Medicine/Gastroenterology
Albert Einstein College of Medicine
Division of Gastroenterology
Montefiore Medical Center
Bronx, New York

STEPHEN J. BICKSTON, MD
Assistant Professor of Medicine
Department of Internal Medicine
University of Virginia Health Sciences Center
Charlottesville, Virginia

DAVID J. BJORKMAN, MD
Associate Professor
Division of Gastroenterology
University of Utah School of Medicine
University of Utah Health Sciences Center
Salt Lake City, Utah

SCOTT J. BOLEY, MD
Professor of Surgery and Pediatric Surgery
Department of Surgery and Pediatric Surgery
Albert Einstein College of Medicine
Chief
Pediatric Surgical Services
Montefiore Medical Center
Bronx, New York

EUGENE S. BONAPACE, Jr, MD
Instructor of Medicine
Department of Medicine
Temple University School of Medicine
Gastroenterology Section
Temple University Hospital
Philadelphia, Pennsylvania

JOHN H. BOND, MD
Professor
Department of Medicine
University of Minnesota
Chief
Gastroenterology Section
Minneapolis Veteran's Affairs Medical Center
Minneapolis, Minnesota

HERBERT L. BONKOVSKY, MD
Professor
Department of Medicine and Biochemistry
    and Molecular Biology
Director
Division of Digestive Disease and Nutrition
    and Liver Center
University of Massachusetts Medical Center
Worcester, Massachusetts

STEPHEN M. BOROWITZ, MD
Associate Professor
Department of Pediatrics
University of Virginia Health Sciences Center
Charlottesville, Virginia

ROBERT F. BOYNTON, MD
Assistant Professor
Department of Medicine
Allegheny University of the Health Sciences
MCP – Hahnemann School of Medicine
Allegheny University Hospitals
Philadelphia, Pennsylvania

LAWRENCE J. BRANDT, MD
Professor of Medicine
Albert Einstein College of Medicine
Director
Division of Gastroenterology
Moses Campus of Montefiore Medical Center
Bronx, New York

STEVEN L. BRANDWEIN, MD
Research Fellow in Medicine
Harvard Medical School
Clinical and Research Fellow in Medicine
Gastrointestinal Unit
Massachusetts General Hospital
Boston, Massachusetts

DAVID C. BROOKS, MD
Associate Professor
Department of Surgery
Harvard University
Senior Surgeon
Division of Gastrointestinal Surgery
Brigham and Women's Hospital
Boston, Massachusetts

RUSSELL D. BROWN, MD
Assistant Professor of Medicine
Department of Medicine
University of Illinois at Chicago
    School of Medicine
Director
Gastrointestinal Laboratory
University of Illinois Hospital
Chicago, Illinois

WILLIAM R. BRUGGE, MD
Assistant Professor of Medicine
Department of Medicine
Gastrointestinal Unit
Harvard Medical School
Massachusetts General Hospital
Department of Gastroenterology
Boston, Massachusetts

ROBERT BURAKOFF, MD
Professor of Medicine
Department of Medicine
State University of New York at
    Stony Brook Health Sciences Center
Stony Brook, New York;
Chief
Division of Gastroenterology, Hepatology,
    and Nutrition
Winthrop University Hospital
Mineola, New York

WILLIAM J. BYRNE, MD
Clinical Professor of Pediatrics
Department of Pediatrics
University of California, San Francisco
San Francisco, California;
Medical Director
Senior Vice President for Medical Affairs
Children's Hospital Oakland
Oakland, California

MAURO CASSARO, MD
Department of Pathology
Cittadella Hospital
University of Padua
Padua, Italy

DAVID R. CAVE, MD, PhD
Associate Professor
Department of Medicine
Tufts University School of Medicine
Boston, Massachusetts;
Chief
Department of Gastroenterology
St. Elizabeth's Medical Center of Boston
Brighton, Massachusetts

AMITABH CHAK, MD
Assistant Professor
Department of Medicine
Case Western Reserve University
Head
Section of Gastrointestinal Endoscopy
University Hospitals of Cleveland
Cleveland, Ohio

ANUPAMA CHAWLA, MD, DCH
Assistant Professor of Pediatrics
Department of Pediatrics
New York University
New York City, New York;
Pediatric Gastroenterologist
North Shore University Hospital
Manhasset, New York

WILLIAM D. CHEY, MD
Assistant Professor
Department of Internal Medicine
Director
Gastrointestinal Physiology Laboratory
University of Michigan
Ann Arbor, Michigan

JAYANTA ROY CHOWDHURY, MD
Professor of Medicine and Molecular Genetics
Department of Medicine and Molecular Genetics
Director
Gastroenterology and Liver Diseases
Liver Research Center
Albert Einstein College of Medicine
Bronx, New York

NAMITA ROY CHOWDHURY, PhD
Professor of Medicine and Molecular Genetics
Department of Medicine and Molecular Genetics
Liver Research Center
Albert Einstein College of Medicine
Bronx, New York

MARY H. CLENCH, PhD
Retired
Gainesville, Florida

RAY E. CLOUSE, MD
Professor of Medicine
Department of Medicine
Washington University School of Medicine
Physician
Barnes-Jewish Hospital
St. Louis, Missouri

DAVID COHEN, MD
Physician
Physicians Group of South Florida
Miami Beach, Florida

MITCHELL B. COHEN, MD
Associate Professor
Department of Pediatrics
University of Cincinnati
Attending Physician
Division of Pediatric Gastroenterology
    and Nutrition
Children's Hospital Medical Center
Cincinnati, Ohio

ROGER B. COHEN, MD
Associate Professor of Medicine
Department of Internal Medicine
Division of Hematology-Oncology
University of Virginia
Cancer Center
Charlottesville, Virginia

FRANCIS P. COLIZZO, MD
Instructor
Department of Medicine
Harvard Medical School
Harvard Pilgrim Healthcare
Boston, Massachusetts

RICHARD B. COLLETTI, MD
Associate Professor
Department of Pediatrics
University of Vermont College of Medicine
Burlington, Vermont

CAROLYN C. COMPTON, MD, PhD
Professor
Department of Pathology
Harvard Medical School
Massachusetts General Hospital
Boston, Massachusetts

ARNOLD G. CORAN
Professor
Department of Surgery
University of Michigan
Surgeon-in-Chief
C.S. Mott Children's Hospital
Ann Arbor, Michigan

CHRISTINA M. COYLE, MD
Assistant Professor
Department of Medicine
Albert Einstein College of Medicine
Assistant Director of Medicine
Jacobi Hospital
Bronx, New York

JEFFREY W. CRONK, MD
Fellow
Department of Hematology and Oncology
University of Virginia Medical School
Resident Physician
University of Virginia Hospitals
Charlottesville, Virginia

KIMBERLY A. CUSATO, MD
Senior Fellow
Department of Medicine
Stanford University Medical Center
Stanford, California

ALAN F. CUTLER, MD
Assistant Professor of Medicine
Department of Medicine
Wayne State University
Director of Research
Department of Medicine
Sinai Hospital
Gastroenterology Section
Detroit, Michigan

MARK H. DELEGGE, MD
Associate Clinical Professor of Medicine
Department of Internal Medicine
University of North Carolina - Chapel Hill
Chapel Hill, North Carolina;
Charlotte Clinic for Gastrointestinal
  and Liver Disease
Charlotte, North Carolina

REBECCA COPHENHAVER DELEGGE, MS
Consultant
GI Technologies
Cornelius, North Carolina

CHRISTOPHER D. DERBY, MD
Resident in Surgery
Department of Surgery
University of Virginia Medical School
Charlottesville, Virginia

ADRIAN M. DI BISCEGLIE, MD
Professor of Internal Medicine
Department of Internal Medicine
St. Louis University School of Medicine
St. Louis, Missouri

ANNA MAE DIEHL, MD
Professor
Department of Medicine
Staff Gastroenterologist
Johns Hopkins University
Baltimore, Maryland

R. D. DIGNAN, MD
Chief
Department of Colon and Rectal Surgery
Baylor University Medical Center
Dallas, Texas

ANTHONY J. DIMARINO, JR, MD
William Rorer Professor of Medicine
Department of Medicine
Chief
Division of Gastroenterology and Hepatology
Thomas Jefferson University
Philadelphia, Pennsylvania

JACK A. DiPALMA, MD
Professor
Department of Internal Medicine
University of South Alabama
Mobile, Alabama

LORRAINE M. DOWDY, DO
Assistant Professor of Clinical Medicine
Department of Medicine
Division of Infectious Diseases
University of Miami
Attending Physician
University of Miami/JMH Medical Center
Miami, Florida

ANDRE DUBOIS, MD, PhD
Research Professor
Department of Medicine and Surgery
Uniformed Services University
Bethesda, Maryland

ERVIN Y. EAKER, MD
Associate Professor
Department of Medicine
Kansas University Medical Center
Kansas City, Kansas

DAVID E. ELLIOTT, MD, PhD
Assistant Professor
Department of Internal Medicine
University of Iowa
Physician
Division of Gastroenterology and Hepatology
University of Iowa Hospital and Clinics
Iowa City, Iowa

GREGORY T. EVERSON, MD
Professor of Medicine
Division of Gastroenterology and Hepatology
University of Colorado Health Sciences Center
Director
Section of Hepatology
University Hospital
Denver, Colorado

NABIL FAHMY, MD
Fellow in Advanced Therapeutic Endoscopy
Department of Gastroenterology
Medical College of Virginia
Richmond, Virginia

DOUGLAS O. FAIGEL, MD
Assistant Professor
Department of Medicine
Oregon Health Sciences University
Director
Gastrointestinal Endoscopy
Portland Veteran's Affairs Medical Center
Portland, Oregon

GARY W. FALK, MD
Staff Gastroenterologist
Department of Gastroenterology
Cleveland Clinic Foundation
Cleveland, Ohio

JOHN C. FANG, MD
Assistant Professor
Department of Gastroenterology
University of Utah
Attending
University of Utah Hospital
Salt Lake City, Utah

GEORGE T. FANTRY, MD
Associate Professor
Department of Medicine
Director
Clinical Gastroenterology
University of Maryland
Baltimore, Maryland

FRANCIS A. FARRAYE, MD
Assistant Professor
Department of Medicine
Harvard Medical School
Brigham and Women's Hospital
Division of Gastroenterology
Boston, Massachusetts;
Harvard Vanguard Medical Associates
West Roxbury, Massachusetts

M. BRIAN FENNERTY, MD
Associate Professor
Department of Medicine
Section Chief
Division of Gastroenterology
Oregon Health Sciences University
Portland, Oregon

STANLEY E. FISHER, MD
Professor and Chairman
Department of Pediatrics
State University of New York Health Science
  Center, Brooklyn College of Medicine
Physician-in-Chief
Children's Medical Center of Brooklyn
Brooklyn, New York

JOSEPH F. FITZGERALD, MD
Professor of Pediatrics
Department of Pediatric
  Gastroenterology/Hepatology/Nutrition
Indiana University
Director
Department of Gastroenterology
J. Whitcomb Riley Hospital for Children
Indianapolis, Indiana

PAUL FOCKENS, MD, PhD
Assistant Professor
Department of Gastroenterology
Director
Endoscopic Ultrasonography
Academic Medical Center
University of Amsterdam
Amsterdam, The Netherlands

CHARLES F. FREY, MD
Professor
Department of Surgery
University of California Davis Medical Center
Sacramento, California

LAWRENCE S. FRIEDMAN, MD
Associate Professor of Medicine
Harvard Medical School
Chief
Walter Sauer Firm
Physician
Gastrointestinal Unit
Massachusetts General Hospital
Boston, Massachusetts

GABRIEL GARCIA, MD
Associate Professor
Department of Medicine
Stanford University Medical Center
Stanford, California

ROBERT M. GENTA, MD
Professor of Pathology, Medicine and
    Microbiology and Immunology
Baylor College of Medicine
Chief
Pathology and Laboratory Service
Department of Pathology
Veteran's Affairs Medical Center
Houston, Texas

DONALD E. GEORGE, MD
Clinical Associate Professor
Department of Gastroenterology
University of Florida
President of Medical Staff
Nemours Children's Clinic
Jacksonville, Florida

MARTHA S. GHOSH, MD
Department of Gastroenterology
University of Pennsylvania School of Medicine
Chief
Gastroenterology and Hepatology Service
Philadelphia Veteran's Affairs Medical Center
Philadelphia, Pennsylvania

RALPH A. GIANNELLA, MD
Mark Brown Professor
Department of Medicine
Director
Division of Digestive Diseases
University of Cincinnati College of Medicine
Cincinnati, Ohio

MARK S. GLASSMAN, MS, MD
Professor
Department of Pediatrics
New York Medical College
Valhalla, New York
Director
Department of Pediatrics
Sound Shore Medical Center
New Rochelle, New York

JAMES S. GOFF, MD, MSPH
Fellow
Division of Gastroenterology
University of Colorado Health Sciences Center
Denver, Colorado

GEORGE F. GOLDIN, MD
Gastroenterologist/Hepatologist
Department of Gastroenterology
The Harbin Clinic
Rome, Georgia

SHERWOOD L. GORBACH, MD
Professor
Departments of Family Medicine and
    Community Health
Tufts University School of Medicine
Staff Physician
Infectious Disease Clinic
New England Medical Center Hospital
Boston, Massachusetts

CHRISTOPHER J. GOSTOUT, MD
Associate Professor of Medicine
Department of Gastroenterology
    and Hepatology
Mayo Medical School
Director
Department of Endoscopy
Mayo Clinic
Rochester, Minnesota

DAVID A. GREENWALD, MD
Assistant Professor
Department of Medicine
Albert Einstein College of Medicine
Assistant Attending
Division of Gastroenterology
Montefiore Medical Center
Bronx, New York

IAN GRIMM, MD
Assistant Professor of Medicine
Department of Digestive Diseases and Nutrition
University of North Carolina School of Medicine
Chapel Hill, North Carolina

MARIA GUIDO, MD
Cattedra di Istochimica and
    Immunohistochimica Patologica
Universita' di Padova – Anatomia Patologica
Ospedale di Cittadella
Regione Veneto, Italy

VIVEK V. GUMASTE, MD, MRCP
Associate Professor
Department of Medicine
Mount Sinai School of Medicine
New York City, New York;
Chief
Division of Gastroenterology
Mt. Sinai Services
Elmhurst General Hospital
Elmhurst, New York

DAVIDSON H. HAMER, MD
Assistant Professor of Medicine
Department of Medicine
Tufts University School of Medicine
Director
Traveler's Health Service
New England Medical Center
Boston, Massachusetts

RONALD J. HAPKE, MD
Fellow
Department of Gastroenterology
Oregon Health Sciences University
Portland, Oregon;
Hillsboro Gastroenterology Associates
Hillsboro, Oregon

WILLIAM L. HASLER, MD
Associate Professor
Department of Internal Medicine
University of Michigan
Ann Arbor, Michigan

ERIC HASSALL, MBCHB, FRCPC
Associate Professor
Department of Pediatrics
University of British Columbia
Division of Gastroenterology
British Columbia Children's Hospital
Vancouver, British Columbia, Canada

J. MICHAEL HENDERSON, MD
Chairman of General Surgery
Cleveland Clinic Foundation
Cleveland, Ohio

JAMES E. HEUBI, MD
Professor
Department of Pediatrics
University of Cincinnati
Director
Clinical Research Center
Children's Hospital Medical Center
Cincinnati, Ohio

DONALD J. HILLEBRAND, MD
Assistant Professor
Department of Medicine
Division of Gastroenterology/Hepatology
Associate Medical Director
Department of Liver Transplantation
Loma Linda University Medical Center
Loma Linda, California

JAY A. HOCHMAN, MD
Attending
Division of Pediatric Gastroenterology,
    Hepatology, and Nutrition
Egelston Children's Hospital
Atlanta, Georgia

JEFFREY S. HYAMS, MD
Professor
Department of Pediatrics
University of Connecticut School of Medicine
Farmington, Connecticut;
Head
Division of Digestive Diseases
Connecticut Children's Medical Center
Hartford, Connecticut

GERARD ISENBERG, MD
Assistant Professor of Medicine
Department of Medicine
Case Western Reserve University
Advanced Endoscopy Fellow
Division of Gastroenterology
University Hospitals of Cleveland
Cleveland, Ohio

ESTHER JACOBOWITZ ISRAEL, MD
Assistant Professor
Department of Pediatrics
Harvard Medical School
Associate Chief
Pediatric Gastroenterology and Nutrition
Massachusetts General Hospital
Boston, Massachusetts

IRA M. JACOBSON, MD
Clinical Associate Professor
Department of Medicine
Cornell Medical College
Attending Physician
New York Hospital
Lenox Hill Hospital
New York City, New York

AMINAH JATOI, MD
Assistant Professor
Department of Medicine
Divisions of Hematology/Oncology
    and Clinical Nutrition
Tufts University School of Medicine
Division of Hematology/Oncology
New England Medical Center
Boston, Massachusetts

DAVID A. JOHNSON, MD
Professor
Department of Internal Medicine
Eastern Virginia School of Medicine
Norfolk, Virginia

DENNIE V. JONES, Jr, MD
Clinical Scientist
Genentech, Inc.
South San Francisco, California

ELLEN KAHN, MD
Clinical Professor of Pathology and Pediatrics
Department of Pathology and Pediatrics
New York University School of Medicine
New York City, New York;
Attending Pathologist
Department of Pathology
Associate Attending
Department of Pediatrics
North Shore University Hospital
Manhasset, New York

MARTIN H. KALSER, MD
Professor
Department of Medicine
Gastroenterologist
Division of Gastroenterology
University of Miami School of Medicine
Miami, Florida

JEFFREY B. KANER, MD
Senior Gastrointestinal Fellow
Department of Medicine
University of Miami School of Medicine
Miami, Florida

MARSHALL M. KAPLAN, MD
Professor
Department of Medicine
Tufts University School of Medicine
Chief
Division of Gastroenterology
New England Medical Center Hospital
Boston, Massachusetts

WILLIAM V. KASTRINAKIS, MD
Instructor in Surgery
Department of Surgery
Harvard Medical School
Assistant to the Surgeon-in-Chief
Division of Gastrointestinal Surgery
Brigham and Women's Hospital
Boston, Massachusetts

PHILIP O. KATZ, MD
Associate Professor
Department of Medicine
Allegheny University of the Health Sciences
Vice Chairman
Department of Medicine
Allegheny University Hospitals, Graduate
Philadelphia, Pennsylvania

DAVID A. KATZKA, MD
Associate Professor of Medicine
Chief of Gastroenterology
Allegheny University Hospitals, Graduate
Philadelphia, Pennsylvania

GORDON L. KAUFFMAN, Jr, MD
Chief
Section of General Surgery
Department of Surgery
The Pennsylvania State University
    College of Medicine
Penn State Geisinger Health System
The Milton S. Hershey Medical Center
Hershey, Pennsylvania

EMMET B. KEEFFE, MD
Professor of Medicine
School of Medicine
Stanford University
Medical Director
Liver Transplant Program
Stanford University Medical Center
Stanford, California

KENNETH KENIGSBERG, MD
Clinical Assistant Professor of Surgery
Department of Surgery
Harvard Medical School
Boston, Massachusetts;
Chief
Pediatric Surgery Department
North Shore University Hospital
Manhasset, New York

JAMES WALTER KIKENDALL, MD
Associate Professor
Department of Medicine
Uniformed Services University of
    the Health Sciences
Bethesda, Maryland;
Director
Clinical Gastroenterology Services
Gastroenterology Service
Walter Reed Army Medical Center
Washington, DC

CHRISTOPHER Y. KIM, MD
Assistant Professor of Medicine
Department of Gastroenterology
    and Hepatology
Medical University of South Carolina
Charleston, South Carolina

MICHAEL B. KIMMEY, MD
Professor
Department of Medicine
University of Washington
Director
Gastrointestinal Endoscopy
University of Washington Medical Center
Seattle, Washington

WILLIAM J. KLISH, MD
Professor of Pediatrics
Department of Pediatrics
Baylor College of Medicine
Head
Pediatric Gastroenterology and Nutrition
Texas Children's Hospital
Houston, Texas

KENNETH L. KOCH, MD
Professor of Medicine
Department of Gastroenterology
    and Hepatology
The Pennsylvania State University
College of Medicine
Attending Physician
Gastroenterology and Hepatology
The Penn State Geisinger Health System
The Milton S. Hershey Medical Center
Hershey, Pennsylvania

RAYMOND S. KOFF, MD
Professor of Medicine
Department of Medicine
University of Massachusetts Medical School
Worcester, Massachusetts;
Chairman
Department of Medicine
Metrowest Medical Center
Framingham, Massachusetts

RABIA KÖKSAL, MD
Harbor–University of California, Los Angeles
    Medical Center
Torrance Memorial Medical Center
Torrance, California

KRIS V. KOWDLEY, MD
Associate Professor
Department of Medicine and Gastroenterology
University of Washington School of Medicine
University of Washington Medical Center
Seattle, Washington

RICHARD A. KOZAREK, MD
Clinical Professor of Medicine
University of Washington School of Medicine
Chief
Department of Gastroenterology
Virginia Mason Medical Center
Seattle, Washington

ERIC J. KRAUT, MD
Staff Physician
Department of Surgery
University of California Davis Medical Center
Sacramento, California

EDWARD L. KRAWITT, MD
Professor of Medicine
College of Medicine
University of Vermont
Burlington, Vermont;
Adjunct Professor of Medicine
Dartmouth Medical School
Hanover, New Hampshire

HOWARD S. KROOP, MD
Clinical Associate Professor
Department of Medicine
Thomas Jefferson University
Philadelphia, Pennsylvania

NEIL D. KUTIN, MD
Assistant Professor of Surgery
Department of Surgery
New York University School of Medicine
New York City, New York;
BSK Pediatric Surgical Associates
New Hyde Park, New York

ANNE M. LARSON, MD
Acting Instructor
Department of Medicine
Division of Gastroenterology
University of Washington School of Medicine
University of Washington Medical Center
Seattle, Washington

JEAN-FRANÇOIS LATULIPPE, MD, FRCSC
Clinical Fellow
Cleveland Clinic Florida
Fort Lauderdale, Florida

ERIC L. LAZAR, MD
Assistant Professor
Department of Pediatric Surgery
Columbia-Presbyterian College of
    Physicians and Surgeons
New York City, New York

GLEN A. LEHMAN, MD
Professor of Medicine and Radiology
Department of Medicine
Indiana University Medical School
University Hospital
Indianapolis, Indiana

TONY LEMBO, MD
Instructor of Medicine
Department of Medicine
Harvard University
Boston, Massachusetts

JOEL S. LEVINE, MD
Professor of Medicine
Division of Gastroenterology
University of Colorado Health Sciences Center
Denver, Colorado

JAMES H. LEWIS, MD
Associate Professor
Department of Medicine
Georgetown University
Director of Hepatology
Georgetown University Hospital
Washington, DC

ERIC D. LIBBY, MD
Assistant Professor
Department of Medicine
Tufts University School of Medicine
Attending Physician
New England Medical Center
Boston, Massachusetts

HARVEY LICHT, MD
Associate Professor of Medicine
Division of Gastroenterology and Hepatology
Allegheny University of the Health Sciences
Allegheny University Hospitals, MCP
Philadelphia, Pennsylvania

CARLOS H. LIFSCHITZ, MD
Associate Professor
Department of Pediatrics
Baylor College of Medicine
Attending Pediatric Gastroenterologist
Texas Children's Hospital
Houston, Texas

SIMON K. LO, MD
Associate Clinical Professor
Department of Medicine
University of California, Los Angeles,
    School of Medicine
Los Angeles, California
Southern California Gastroenterology Institute
Torrance Memorial Medical Center
Torrance, California

ANNA S. F. LOK, MD, FRCP
Professor
Department of Internal Medicine
University of Michigan Medical Center
Ann Arbor, Michigan

KATHLEEN M. LOOMES, MD
Fellow
Division of Gastroenterology and Nutrition
Children's Hospital of Philadelphia
Philadelphia, Pennsylvania

GORDON D. LUK, MD
Staff Physician
Dallas Veteran's Affairs Medical Center
Dallas, Texas

ERIC S. MALLER, MD
Assistant Professor
Department of Pediatrics
University of Pennsylvania School of Medicine
Medical Director
Liver Transplant Program
Attending Physician
Division of Gastroenterology and Nutrition
Children's Hospital of Philadelphia
Philadelphia, Pennsylvania

HOWARD D. MANTEN, MD
Associate Professor
Department of Medicine
Division of Pediatrics
University of Miami School of Medicine
Jackson Memorial Hospital, Veteran's Affairs
    Medical Center
Miami, Florida

JAMES F. MARKOWITZ, MD
Associate Professor
Department of Pediatrics
New York University School of Medicine
New York City, New York;
Pediatric Gastroenterologist
Division of Pediatric Gastroenterology
North Shore University Hospital
Manhasset, New York

PAUL MARTIN, MD
Associate Professor
Department of Medicine
University of California, Los Angeles,
    School of Medicine
Director
Hepatology, Division of Digestive Diseases
Dumont-University of California, Los Angeles,
    Transplant Center
Los Angeles, California

JOEL B. MASON, MD
Associate Professor of Medicine and Nutrition
Tufts University Medical Center
Acting Chief
Division of Clinical Nutrition
Staff
Department of Gastroenterology
New England Medical Center
Boston, Massachusetts

JOHN R. MATHIAS, MD
Director of the Institutional Review Board
The Woman's Hospital of Texas
Gastrointestinal Consultants of Houston
    Professional Associates
Houston, Texas

PAUL N. MATON, MD, FRCP
Clinical Professor of Medicine
Department of Medicine
College of Medicine
Digestive Disease Research Institute
Digestive Disease Specialists, Inc.
Oklahoma City, Oklahoma

CHESTER J. MAXSON, MD
Assistant Professor
Department of Medicine
MCP - The Hahnemann School of Medicine
Philadelphia, Pennsylvania
Koerner, Taub and Flaxman, MD,
    Professional Association
Jupiter, Florida

EMERAN A. MAYER, MD
Professor
Department of Medicine and Physiology
University of California, Los Angeles,
    School of Medicine
Los Angeles, California

KARAN E. McBRIDE, MD
Fellow
Department of Gastroenterology and Nutrition
University of Pennsylvania School of Medicine
Fellow
Division of Gastroenterology and Nutrition
Children's Hospital of Philadelphia
Philadelphia, Pennsylvania

ROBERT P. McCABE, JR, MD
Clinical Assistant Professor
Department of Medicine
University of Minnesota
Gastroenterologist
Minnesota Gastroenterology
Minneapolis, Minnesota

JAMES E. McGUIGAN, MD
Professor
Department of Medicine
Division of Gastroenterology
University of Florida College of Medicine
Gainesville, Florida

JOHN D. McKEE, MD
Clinical Instructor of Medicine
Harvard Medical School
Interventional Fellow
Division of Gastroenterology
Beth Israel Deaconess Medical Center
Boston, Massachusetts

MARVIN S. MEDOW, PhD
Associate Professor
Department of Pediatrics and Physiology
Division of Pediatric Gastroenterology and
   Nutrition
New York Medical College
Valhalla, New York

CLIFFORD MELNYK, MD
Professor of Medicine
Department of Medicine
Oregon Health Sciences University
Portland, Oregon

DAVID C. METZ, MD
Associate Professor
Department of Medicine
University of Pennsylvania School of Medicine
Attending Physician
Hospital of University of Pennsylvania
Philadelphia, Pennsylvania

ADAM G. MEZOFF, MD
Associate Professor
Department of Pediatrics
Department of Medicine
Wright State School of Medicine
Director
Gastroenterology and Nutrition
Children's Medical Center
Dayton, Ohio

JOHN S. MINASI, MD
Assistant Professor of Surgery
Department of Surgery
University of Virginia Medical School
Charlottesville, Virginia

IRVIN M. MODLIN, MD, PhD, FRCS
Professor
Department of Surgery
Yale University School of Medicine
New Haven, Connecticut

PARVATHI MOHAN, MD
Assistant Professor
Department of Pediatrics
George Washington University
Attending Physician
Department of Gastroenterology and Nutrition
Children's National Medical Center
Washington, DC

ENRIQUE G. MOLINA, MD, BM
Assistant Professor of Medicine
Department of Hepatology
Universidad del Zulia
Zulia, Venezuela;
Assistant Professor of Clinical Medicine
Center for Liver Diseases
Miami, Florida

CHRISTOPHER A. MOSKALUK, MD, PhD
Assistant Professor
Department of Pathology, Biochemistry
   and Molecular Genetics
University of Virginia Health Sciences Center
Charlottesville, Virginia

ANDREW E. MULBERG, MD
Assistant Professor of Pediatrics
Department of Pediatrics
University of Pennsylvania School of Medicine
Attending Physician
Division of Pediatric Gastroenterology
   and Nutrition
Children's Hospital of Philadelphia
Philadelphia, Pennsylvania

DARREN E. MULLINS, MD
Hematologist/Oncologist
Piedmont Cancer Institute
Greensboro, North Carolina

FRANCESCO NEGRO, MD
Gastroenterologist
Division of Hepatology and Gastroenterology
University of Geneva
Hôpital Cantonal
Geneva, Switzerland

BRETT R. NEUSTATER, MD
Attending Physician
Ornstein, Silverman and Roman, MD
North Miami Beach, Florida

CHARLES M. NOYER, MD
Assistant Professor
Department of Medicine
Albert Einstein College of Medicine
Director
Department of Endoscopy
Jacobi Medical Center
Bronx, New York

KEVIN OLDEN, MD
Consultant
Division of Gastroenterology
Mayo Clinic
Scottsdale, Arizona

MARIA M. OLIVA-HEMKER, MD
Assistant Professor
Department of Pediatrics
The Johns Hopkins School of Medicine
Attending Physician
Division of Pediatric Gastroenterology
   and Nutrition
The Johns Hopkins Hospital
Baltimore, Maryland

JOSÉE PARENT, MD, FRCPC
Assistant Professor
Department of Medicine
Division of Gastroenterology
McGill University
Montreal General Hospital
Montreal, Quebec, Canada

HENRY P. PARKMAN, MD
Associate Professor
Department of Medicine
Temple University School of Medicine
Director
Gastrointestinal Motility Laboratory
Gastrointestinal Section
Temple University Hospital
Philadelphia, Pennsylvania

DILIP G. PATEL, MD, FRCPC
Associate Professor
Department of Medicine
Faculty of Medicine Ottawa
Acting Chief
Gastroenterology
Ottawa Civic Hospital
Ottawa, Ontario, Canada

MARCO G. PATTI, MD
Assistant Professor of Surgery
Department of General Surgery
University of California, San Francisco,
   School of Medicine
Director
University of California San Francisco
   Swallowing Center
Attending Surgeon
Moffit Long Hospital
San Francisco, California

S. KIRK PAYNE, MD
Associate
Department of Internal Medicine
Program in Biomedical Ethics and Medical
   Humanities
University of Iowa College of Medicine
Iowa City, Iowa

CARLOS A. PELLEGRINI, MD
The Henry N. Harkins Professor and Chairman
Department of Surgery
University of Washington Medical Center
Seattle, Washington

JEAN PERRAULT, MD, MSC
Associate Professor
Department of Medicine and Pediatrics
Mayo Medical School
Division of Gastroenterology
Mayo Clinic
Rochester, Minnesota

DAVID A. PEURA, MD
Professor
Department of Medicine
Associate Chief
Gastroenterology and Hepatology
University of Virginia Medical School
Charlottesville, Virginia

DAVID A. PICCOLI, MD
Associate Professor
Department of Pediatrics
University of Pennsylvania School of Medicine
Acting Chief
Division of Gastroenterology and Nutrition
Children's Hospital of Philadelphia
Philadelphia, Pennsylvania

C. S. PITCHUMONI, MD, FRCPC, MPH
Professor of Medicine
Professor of Community and
   Preventive Medicine
New York Medical College
Director of Medicine
Our Lady of Mercy Medical Center
Bronx, New York

MARK B. POCHAPIN, MD
Assistant Professor
Department of Medicine
Division of Digestive Diseases
Cornell University
Associate Chairman
Educational Affairs
New York Hospital
New York City, New York

STEPHEN M. POWELL, MD
Assistant Professor of Medicine
Department of Medicine
University of Virginia Health Sciences Center
Charlottesville, Virginia

ROY PROUJANSKY, MD
Associate Professor of Pediatrics
Vice Chairman for Research
Department of Pediatrics
Thomas Jefferson University
Philadelphia, Pennsylvania;
Chief
Division of Gastroenterology and Nutrition
Alfred I. DuPont Hospital for Children
Wilmington, Delaware

GOTTUMUKKALA S. RAJU, MD, MRCP
Assistant Professor of Medicine
Department of Gastroenterology
University of Kansas Medical Center
Kansas City, Kansas

NIZAR N. RAMZAN, MD
Senior Associate Consultant
Department of Medicine
Division of Gastroenterology
Mayo Medical School
Mayo Clinic Scottsdale
Scottsdale, Arizona

JEFFREY B. RASKIN, MD
Professor of Medicine
Division of Gastroenterology
Chief of Endoscopy
University of Miami School of Medicine
Medical Director
Gastrointestinal Diagnostic Unit
Jackson Memorial Medical Center
Miami, Florida

HOWARD A. REBER, MD
Professor
Department of Surgery
Chief
Gastrointestinal Surgery
University of California, Los Angeles,
    School of Medicine
Los Angeles, California

K. RAJENDER REDDY, MD
Professor of Medicine
Department of Hepatology
Osmania University
Hyderbod, India;
Professor of Medicine
Department of Medicine
Division of Hepatology
Center for Liver Diseases
Miami, Florida

MIGUEL D. REGUEIRO, MD
Assistant Professor of Medicine
Department of Internal Medicine
Allegheny University Hospitals
Director
Inflammatory Bowel Disease Center
Allegheny Center for Digestive Health
Pittsburgh, Pennsylvania

JOHN F. REINUS, MD
Associate Professor
Department of Medicine
Albert Einstein College of Medicine
Attending Physician
Department of Gastroenterology
Montefiore Medical Center
Bronx, New York

DOUGLAS K. REX, MD
Professor of Medicine
Department of Medicine
Indiana University School of Medicine
Director
Department of Endoscopy
Indiana University Hospital
Indianapolis, Indiana

JAMES C. REYNOLDS, MD
Professor of Medicine
Department of Medicine
Chair
Division of Gastroenterology and Hepatology
Allegheny University of the Health Sciences
Allegheny University Center for Digestive
    Health
Philadelphia, Pennsylvania

THOMAS W. RICE, MD
Head
Section of General Thoracic Surgery
Cleveland Clinic Foundation
Cleveland, Ohio

JOEL E. RICHTER, MD
Professor of Medicine
Cleveland Clinic Health Science Center
Ohio State University
Chairman
Department of Gastroenterology
Cleveland Clinic Foundation
Cleveland, Ohio

ARVEY I. ROGERS, MD
Professor
Department of Medicine
University of Miami School of Medicine
Chief
Division of Gastroenterology
Miami Veteran's Affairs Medical Center
Gastroenterologist
University of Miami Hospital and Clinics
Jackson Memorial Hospital
Miami, Florida

CHARLES M. ROSEN, MD
Clinical Professor of Medicine
Department of Medicine
University of Miami School of Medicine
Associate
Division of Gastroenterology
Mt. Sinai Medical Center
Miami Beach, Florida

HUGO R. ROSEN, MD
Assistant Professor
Department of Medicine, Molecular
    Microbiology, and Immunology
Staff Physician
Department of Gastroenterology and
    Hepatology
Oregon Health Sciences University
Portland, Oregon

PHILIP ROSENTHAL, MD
Professor of Pediatrics and Surgery
Department of Pediatrics
Department of Surgery
Director
Liver Transplant Service
University of California, San Francisco
    Medical Center
San Francisco, California

THOMAS M. ROSSI, MD
Associate Professor
Department of Pediatrics
State University of New York
Chief
Division of Gastroenterology and Nutrition
Director
Nutrition Support Service
Children's Hospital of Buffalo
Buffalo, New York

ALLA M. ROZENBLIT, MD
Associate Professor
Department of Radiology
Albert Einstein College of Medicine
Director
Body Imaging
Montefiore Medical Center
Bronx, New York

WALTER RUBIN, MD
Professor
Department of Medicine
Allegheny University of the Health Sciences
MCP – Hahnemann School of Medicine
Chief
Section of Gastroenterology
Allegheny University Hospitals, MCP
Philadelphia, Pennsylvania

BRUCE A. RUNYON, MD
Professor
Department of Medicine
Loma Linda University School of Medicine
Director
Liver Service
Medical Director of Liver Transplantation
Loma Linda University Medical Center
Loma Linda, California

MARK W. RUSSO, MD, MPH
Clinical Instructor
Department of Medicine
University of North Carolina School of Medicine
Fellow
Department of Gastroenterology
University of North Carolina Hospitals
Chapel Hill, North Carolina

JOSÉ M. SAAVEDRA, MD
Associate Professor
Department of Pediatrics
Johns Hopkins University School of Medicine
Director
Pediatric Nutrition
Johns Hopkins University Hospital
Baltimore, Maryland

ARUN J. SANYAL, MBBS, MD
Associate Professor
Department of Internal Medicine
School of Medicine/Gastrointestinal Hepatology
Medical College of Virginia at Virginia
    Commonwealth University
Richmond, Virginia

MICHAEL D. SAUNDERS, MD
Fellow
Department of Gastroenterology
University of Washington School of Medicine
Seattle, Washington

BERNHARD V. SAUTER, MD
Research Asssociate
Department of Medicine
Albert Einstein College of Medicine
Liver Research Center
Bronx, New York

LAWRENCE R. SCHILLER, MD
Clinical Assistant Professor of Internal
    Medicine
Department of Internal Medicine
University of Texas Southwestern
    Medical Center
Program Director
Gastroenterology Fellowship
Attending Physician
Baylor University Medical Center
Dallas, Texas

MICHAEL L. SCHILSKY, MD
Associate Professor
Department of Medicine
Albert Einstein College of Medicine
Member
Division of Gastroenterology and
    Liver Research Center
Marion Bessin Liver Research Center
Bronx, New York

STEFAN W. SCHMID, MD
Department of Visceral and
    Transplantation Surgery
Inselspital
University of Bern
Bern, Switzerland

SARAH JANE SCHWARZENBERG, MD
Associate Professor
Department of Pediatrics
University of Minnesota Medical School
Minneapolis, Minnesota

JOSEPH SELLIN, MD
Professor of Medicine and Integrative Biology
Department of Internal Medicine
University of Texas at Houston
Chief
Department of Gastroenterology
Hermann Hospital
Houston, Texas

REZA SHAKER, MD
Professor
Department of Medicine, Radiology, Surgery
    (Otolaryngology)
Medical College of Wisconsin
Chief
Froedtert Memorial Lutheran Hospital
Division of Gastroenterology and Hepatology
Milwaukee, Wisconsin

LINDA SHALON, MD
Assistant Professor of Pediatrics
Department of Pediatrics
Brown University School of Medicine
Attending Physician in Pediatrics
Division of Pediatric Gastroenterology
    and Nutrition
Rhode Island Hospital/Hasbro Children's
    Hospital
Providence, Rhode Island

HARVEY L. SHARP, MD
Professor
Department of Pediatrics
University of Minnesota Medical Center
Professor in Chief
Division of Pediatric Gastroenterology
    and Nutrition
Fairview University Medical Center
Minneapolis, Minnesota

STUART SHERMAN, MD
Associate Professor of Medicine and Radiology
Department of Medicine
Indiana University School of Medicine
Director
Endoscopic Retrograde
    Colangiopancreatography Service
Indiana University Medical Center
Indianapolis, Indiana

STEVEN J. SHIELDS, MD
Instructor of Medicine
Harvard Medical School
Assistant Director of Endoscopy
Associate Physician
Brigham and Women's Hospital
Boston, Massachusetts

MITCHELL L. SHIFFMAN, MD
Associate Professor
Department of Medicine
Hepatology Section
Medical College of Virginia of Virginia
    Commonwealth University
Richmond, Virginia

ROSHAN SHRESTHA, MD
Assistant Professor of Medicine
Division of Gastroenterology and Hepatology
University of Colorado Health Science Center
Associate Director
Medical Liver Transplantation
University Hospital
Denver, Colorado

DOUGLAS SIMON, MD
Associate Professor
Department of Medicine
Albert Einstein College of Medicine
Chief
Division of Gastroenterology
Jacobi Hospital
Bronx, New York

EDWIN SIMPSER, MD
Assistant Professor of Pediatrics
Department of Pediatrics
New York University School of Medicine
New York City, New York;
Chief
Division of Pediatric Nutrition
North Shore University Hospital
Manhasset, New York

ANDREA J. SINGER, MD
Assistant Professor
Department of Medicine
Georgetown University Medical Center
Washington, DC

ADAM SLIVKA, MD, PhD
Assistant Professor
Department of Medicine
University of Pittsburgh
Chief
Department of Endoscopy
University of Pittsburgh Medical Center
Presbyterian University Hospital
Pittsburgh, Pennsylvania

AMY E. SMITHLINE, MD
Assistant Professor of Medicine
Department of Medicine
Division of Gastroenterology
Albert Einstein College of Medicine
Gastrointestinal Division
Montefiore Medical Center
Bronx, New York

CHARLES A. SNINSKY, MD
Professor of Medicine
Division of Gastroenterology, Hepatology,
    and Nutrition
University of Florida College of Medicine
Joint Associate Professor
Pharmacodynamics
University of Florida College of Pharmacy
Physiological Sciences
University of Florida
Chief
Gastroenterology Section
Veteran's Affairs Medical Center
Gainesville, Florida

ROY SOETIKNO, MD, MS
Clinical Instructor
Department of Medicine
Stanford University
Stanford, California;
Chief of Endoscopy
Veterans Affairs Palo Alto Health Care System
Palo Alto, California

STEPHEN J. SONTAG, MD
Associate Professor of Medicine
Department of Medicine
Loyola University Stritch School of Medicine
Maywood, Illinois
Staff Physician
Hines Veterans Affairs Hospital
Hines, Illinois

MICHAEL SOSSENHEIMER, MD
Advanced Therapeutic Endoscopy Fellow
Department of Gastroenterology
Harvard Medical School
Brigham and Women's Hospital
Boston, Massachusetts

ASSAAD M. SOWEID, MD
Clinical Instructor
Division of Gastroenterology
Case Western Reserve University
Physician
University Hospitals of Cleveland
Cleveland, Ohio

STUART JON SPECHLER, MD
Professor
Department of Medicine
University of Texas Southwestern Medical
    Center at Dallas
Chief
Division of Gastroenterology
Dallas Veteran's Affairs Medical Center
Dallas, Texas

MITCHELL K. SPINNELL, MD
Fellow
Department of Gastroenterology
Albert Einstein College of Medicine
Fellow
Montefiore Medical Center
Bronx, New York

JULIE SPIVACK, MD
Assistant Professor
Department of Medicine
New York Medical College
Valhalla, New York;
Program Director
Gastroenterology and Hepatology
St. Vincent's Medical Center
Bridgeport, Connecticut

ROBERT H. SQUIRES, Jr, MD
Associate Professor
Department of Pediatrics
University of Texas Southwestern Medical Center
Attending Physician
Pediatric Gastroenterology-Children's Medical
    Center
Dallas, Texas

DAVID M. STAFF, MD
Assistant Professor
Department of Medicine
Division of Gastroenterology
Medical College of Wisconsin
Froedtert Memorial Lutheran Hospital
Milwaukee, Wisconsin

ANDREAS M. STEFAN, MD
Fellow
Division of Gastroenterology
University of Toronto
Fellow
The Wellesley Hospital
Toronto, Ontario, Canada

RICHARD K. STERLING, MD
Assistant Professor of Medicine
Section of Hepatology
Medical College of Virginia of Virginia
    Commonwealth University
Richmond, Virginia

MARK E. STOKER, MD
Assistant Clinical Professor
Department of Surgery
University of Massachusetts Medical School
Chief
General and Vascular Surgery
The Fallon Clinic
Worcester, Massachusetts

NEIL H. STOLLMAN, MD
Assistant Professor
Department of Medicine
University of Miami School of Medicine
Veteran's Affairs Medical Center
Miami, Florida

RISË STRIBLING, MD
Clinical Instructor
Division of Digestive Diseases
University of California, Los Angeles,
    School of Medicine
Los Angeles, California

FRANCIS P. SUNARYO, MD
Clinical Assistant Professor of Pediatrics
Department of Pediatrics
University of Medicine and Dentistry
    of New Jersey
Director
Pediatric Gastroenterology
Children's Hospital of New Jersey at Newark
    Beth Israel Medical Center
Newark, New Jersey

CHRISTINA M. SURAWICZ, MD
Professor
Department of Medicine
University of Washington School of Medicine
Section Chief
Gastroenterology
Harborview Medical Center
Seattle, Washington

TONY THAM, MD, MRCP
Consultant Gastroenterologist
Department of Medicine
Ulster Hospital, Dundonald
Belfast, Northern Ireland

W. GRANT THOMPSON, MD, FRCPC
Professor
Department of Medicine
University of Ottawa
Gastroenterology Division
Ottawa Civic Hospital
Ottawa, Ontario, Canada

SWAN N. THUNG, MD
Professor
Department of Pathology
Mount Sinai School of Medicine
The Mount Sinai Hospital
New York City, New York

RICHARD W. TOBIN, MD
Assistant Professor
Department of Medicine
Division of Gastroenterology
University of Washington School of Medicine
Seattle, Washington

KAREN E. TODD, MD
Surgery Resident
Department of Surgery
University of California, Los Angeles,
    School of Medicine
Los Angeles, California

VASUNDHARA TOLIA, MD
Professor
Department of Pediatrics
Wayne State University
Director
Division of Gastroenterology
Children's Hospital of Michigan
Detroit, Michigan

KEITH G. TOLMAN, MD
Professor
Department of Internal Medicine
Division of Gastroenterology
University of Utah School of Medicine
Gastroenterologist
University of Utah Medical Center
Salt Lake City, Utah

EDMUND C. TRAMONT, MD
Professor
Department of Infectious Diseases
University of Maryland, Baltimore
Director
Medical Biotechnology Center
Baltimore, Maryland

L. W. TRAVERSO, MD
Clinical Associate Professor of Surgery
Department of Surgery
University of Washington School of Medicine
Staff Surgeon
Director
The Hepatobiliary Fellowship
Virginia Mason Medical Center
Seattle, Washington

WILLIAM R. TREEM, MD
Professor
Department of Pediatrics
Duke University Medical Center
Chief
Division of Pediatric Gastroenterology
    and Nutrition
Duke Children's Hospital
Durham, North Carolina

WILLIAM J. TREMAINE, MD
Associate Professor
Department of Medicine
Mayo Medical School
Mayo Clinic
Rochester, Minnesota

JOSEPH TRIPODI, DO
Assistant Professor of Clinical Medicine
Department of Gastroenterology
State University of New York at Stony Brook
    Health Sciences Center
Stony Brook, New York

JORGE E. VALENZUELA, MD
Emeritus Professor
Department of Medicine
University of Southern California
Los Angeles, California
Clinica Las Condes
Las Condes, Chile

JON A. VANDERHOOF, MD
Professor of Pediatrics
Department of Pediatrics
Section of Gastroenterology and Nutrition
University of Nebraska/Creighton University
Director
Joint Section Gastroenterology and Nutrition
Creighton University
Omaha, Nebraska

JO VANDERVOORT, MD
Staff Physician
Department of Gastroenterology
Onze-Lieve-Vrouw Ziekenhuis
Aalst, Belgium

DIRK J. van LEEUWEN, MD, PhD
Associate Professor of Medicine
Department of Medicine
Division of Gastroenterology and Hepatology
    (Liver Center), and Scientist Cancer Center
University of Alabama at Birmingham
Attending Physician
Birmingham Veterans Medical Center
Birmingham, Alabama

RAMA P. VENU, MD
Clinical Professor of Medicine
Section of Digestive and Liver Disease
University of Illinois at Chicago
Director
Biliary Endoscopy Services
University of Illinois Hospital
Chicago, Illinois

DAVID P. VOGT, MD
General and Liver Transplant Surgeon
Cleveland Clinic Foundation
Cleveland, Ohio

ARNOLD WALD, MD
Professor
Department of Medicine
Associate Chief
Division of Gastroenterology and Hepatology
Director
Fellowship Training Program in
    Gastroenterology and Hepatology
University of Pittsburgh
Pittsburgh, Pennsylvania

IRVING WAXMAN, MD
Associate Professor of Medicine
Director of Endoscopy
Division of Gastroenterology
University of Texas Medical Branch
    at Galveston
Galveston, Texas

FRANCIS R. WEINER, MD
Associate Professor of Medicine
Department of Gastroenterology
Mt. Sinai School of Medicine
Montefiore Medical Center
Attending Physician
Department of Gastroenterology
Weiler Hospital
Bronx, New York

JOEL V. WEINSTOCK, MD, PhD
Professor
Department of Internal Medicine
University of Iowa
Director
Gastroenterology Division
Department of Internal Medicine
University of Iowa Hospitals and Clinics
Iowa City, Iowa

REBECCA G. WELLS, MD
Assistant Professor of Medicine
Department of Medicine
Yale University School of Medicine
New Haven, Connecticut

STEVEN D. WEXNER, MD
Professor of Surgery
Cleveland Clinic Foundation Health Sciences
    Center of Ohio State University
Columbus, Ohio;
Chairman and Residency Program Director
Department of Colorectal Surgery
Chief of Staff
Cleveland Clinic Florida
Fort Lauderdale, Florida

MUNSEY S. WHEBY, MD
Professor
Department of Internal Medicine
Division of Hematology and Oncology
University of Virginia Health Sciences Center
Charlottesville, Virginia

GARY J. WHITMAN, MD
Assistant Professor of Radiology
Department of Diagnostic Imaging
The University of Texas
MD Anderson Cancer Center
Houston, Texas

C. MEL WILCOX, MD
Associate Professor
Department of Medicine
University of Alabama, Birmingham
Chief of Endoscopy
University Hospital
Birmingham, Alabama

MURRAY WITTNER, MD, PhD
Professor
Department of Pathology (Parasitology)
Albert Einstein College of Medicine
Attending Physician
Director
Tropical Medicine Clinic
Parasitology and Tropical Medicine Laboratory
Jacobi Medical Center
Bronx, New York

JACQUELINE L. WOLF, MD
Associate Professor of Clinical Medicine
Department of Medicine
Harvard Medical School
Physician
Brigham and Women's Hospital
Gastroenterology Division
Boston, Massachusetts

M. MICHAEL WOLFE, MD
Professor of Medicine
Chief
Section of Gastroenterology
Boston University School of Medicine
Chief
Department of Gastroenterology
Boston Medical Center
Boston, Massachusetts

ALLAN W. WOLKOFF, MD
Professor
Department of Medicine and Anatomy and
    Structural Biology
Albert Einstein College of Medicine
Bronx, New York

RICHARD C. K. WONG, MBBS
Assistant Professor of Medicine
Department of Medicine
Case Western Reserve University
Attending Physician
Division of Gastroenterology
University Hospitals of Cleveland
Cleveland, Ohio

MARK T. WORTHINGTON, MD
Assistant Professor
Department of Internal Medicine
Department of Gastroenterology and
    Hepatology
Associate Program Director
Attending Physician
Division of Gastroenterology
University of Virginia Health Sciences Center
Charlottesville, Virginia

PAUL YEATON, MD
Assistant Professor of Clinical Medicine
Department of Internal Medicine
Division of Gastroenterology
University of Virginia Medical School
Director
Endoscopic Services
University of Virginia Health Sciences Center
Charlottesville, Virginia

CYNTHIA M. YOSHIDA, MD
Assistant Professor
Department of Internal Medicine
University of Virginia Health Sciences Center
Charlottesville, Virginia

STEVEN ZACKS, MD, MPH
Research Fellow
Division of Digestive Diseases and Nutrition
Department of Medicine
University of North Carolina – Chapel Hill
    School of Medicine
Chapel Hill, North Carolina

WISAM F. ZAKKO, MD
Head
Section of Hepatology
Department of Gastroenterology
Cleveland Clinic Florida
Fort Lauderdale, Florida

GREGORY ZUCCARO, Jr, MD
Head
Section of Gastrointestinal Endoscopy
Department of Gastroenterology
Cleveland Clinic Foundation
Cleveland, Ohio

Preface

The practice of medicine has become exceedingly complex during the past few decades, with increasing reliance on applied advances in molecular biology, immunology, and a variety of sophisticated imaging techniques. It is with this recognition that *Clinical Practice of Gastroenterology* was conceived, its purpose to offer the latest clinical information in an easy-to-read format, thereby aiding the busy practitioner to care for his or her patients. To help achieve this goal, the reader will find more than 2200 figures in this text, including algorithms, charts, graphs, radiographs, endoscopic pictures, intraoperative photographs, photomicrographs, and tables.

In addition to the usual topics covered in standard textbooks, *Clinical Practice of Gastroenterology* contains a complete section on liver disease and 41 chapters on pediatric gastrointestinal and liver disorders.

In recognition of the difficulties and time constraints of clinical practice today, the nine section editors and I have labored to limit chapter content to the essentials of patient care.

This book is dedicated to our fellow practitioners in appreciation of their daily contributions and sacrifices and to our patients whom we serve and from whom we learn each day.

Lawrence J. Brandt, MD

Contents

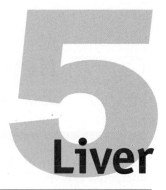

5
Liver

Edited by John F. Reinus

Contributors

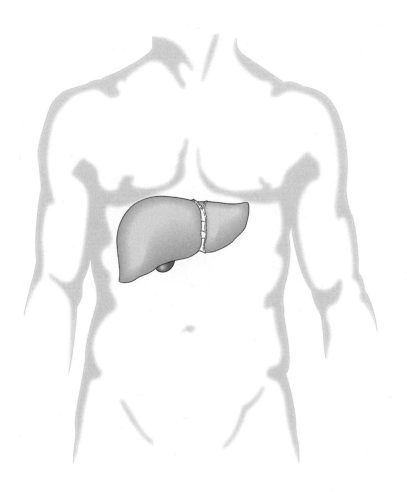

Bruce R. Bacon

Graham F. Barnard

Herbert L. Bonkovsky

Jayanta Roy Chowdhury

Namita Roy Chowdhury

Christina M. Coyle

Kimberly A. Cusato

Adrian M. Di Bisceglie

Anna Mae Diehl

Gregory T. Everson

Nabil Fahmy

Gabriel Garcia

Maria Guido

J. Michael Henderson

Donald J. Hillebrand

Marshall M. Kaplan

Emmet B. Keeffe

Raymond S. Koff

Edward L. Krawitt

James H. Lewis

Eric D. Libby

Anna S. F. Lok

Paul Martin

Enrique G. Molina

Francesco Negro

Charles M. Noyer

K. Rajender Reddy

John F. Reinus

Hugo R. Rosen

Alla M. Rozenblit

Bruce A. Runyon

Arun J. Sanyal

Bernhard V. Sauter

Mitchell L. Shiffman

Michael L. Schilsky

Sarah Jane Schwarzenberg

Harvey L. Sharp

Mitchell L. Shiffman

Roshan Shrestha

Douglas Simon

Andrea J. Singer

Richard K. Sterling

Risë Stribling

Swan N. Thung

David P. Vogt

Francis R. Weiner

Murray Wittner

Allan W. Wolkoff

87 Hepatic Structure and Function

John F. Reinus

It is useful to think of the liver as a metabolically active filter interposed between the splanchnic and systemic circulations. Splanchnic blood entering the liver contains nutrients and foreign antigens, whereas systemic blood leaving the liver must have a stable composition capable of supporting the life and well-being of body tissues. Thus, the function of the liver is to regulate the composition of the blood, a role to which the liver's gross and microscopic structures are perfectly adapted [1•,2•].

GROSS ANATOMY

The normal liver weighs approximately 1500 g and consists of a continuous mass of cells incompletely divided by connective tissue septae. Within this continuous cell mass, the subdivisions of the bile ducts and the hepatic vasculature make numerous connections.

The Lobes of the Liver

The liver is arbitrarily considered to be composed of lobes. The right and left lobes are divided by the line of insertion of the falciform ligament, the right lobe comprising five sixths, and the left lobe one sixth, of the hepatic mass. The caudate lobe is on the posterior surface of the liver between the fissure of the ligamentum venosum (the obliterated ductus venosus) and the deep groove containing the inferior vena cava (Fig. 87-1). The quadrate lobe is on the inferior surface of the liver between the gallbladder fossa and the ligamentum teres (the obliterated umbilical vein). Some persons have a downward projection of the right lobe called Riedel's lobe, and accessory liver lobes sometimes are found in the mesentery, spleen, or adrenals.

The Segments of the Liver

Hepatic segments are defined as the regions of the liver served by the main subdivisions of the portal vein, hepatic artery, and common hepatic duct, all of which branch and travel together through the hepatic parenchyma (Fig. 87-2). Thus, the right lobe may be divided into anterior and posterior segments and the left lobe may be divided into medial and lateral segments. These segments, in turn, sometimes are subdivided into superior and inferior portions. In this system, the quadrate and most of the caudate lobe together make up the left medial hepatic segment.

Although numerous connections exist between small branches of the bile ducts and afferent blood vessels in one liver segment and corresponding structures in adjacent segments, the main bile ducts and afferent blood vessels within a liver segment do not cross its boundaries. Thus, the concept of hepatic segments is useful in planning liver surgery. It should be noted, however, that the hepatic veins do not branch in a segmental fashion, and may show considerable anatomic variation from

Figure 87-1

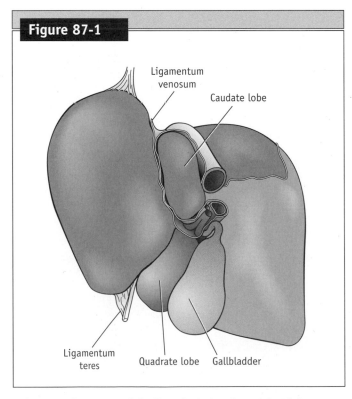

The posterior aspect of the liver depicting the caudate lobe between the inferior vena cava and ligamentum venosum and the quadrate lobe between the gallbladder and the ligamentum teres.

Figure 87-2

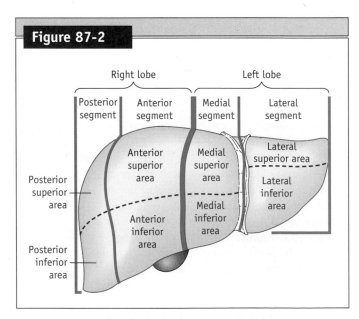

The anterior aspect of the liver depicting the liver segments.

person to person. Tributaries of the hepatic vein are intersegmental, usually coalescing into right, middle, and left hepatic veins, which each receive blood from more than one hepatic segment.

Glisson's Capsule

The liver is completely covered by a thin connective tissue membrane (Glisson's capsule) and, except for bare areas over the posterior diaphragmatic portion and the gallbladder bed, by the parietal peritoneum. At the porta hepatis, the capsule thickens and extends into the parenchyma, where it merges with the connective tissue surrounding the major vascular structures and, ultimately, their small branches within the portal areas.

▓▓▓ MICROSCOPIC ANATOMY

The Liver Lobule

The liver parenchyma is composed of epithelial cells (hepatocytes) arranged in plates, or laminae, that interconnect, forming a three-dimensional latticework that converges on small branches of the hepatic vein (central veins) (Fig. 87-3). The location of the central vein at the hub of a convergent array of liver cell plates is the basis for the concept of the liver lobule, proposed by Malpighi in 1666 (Fig. 87-5). The liver lobule is a hexagonal array of liver cell plates with a primary branch of the hepatic vein at its center and portal areas at its periphery.

The structure of the Malpighian lobule is inconsistent with the lobular architecture of most glands, which centers on exiting ducts, not on blood vessels. For this reason Mall proposed an alternative scheme of organization, the portal lobule, that places the portal area with its small bile duct at the center of the lobule, and the hepatic veins at the periphery (Fig. 87-5). This concept allows the draining duct and the blood supply to be central, as they are in other glands.

The Liver Acinus and Its Zones

In 1954, Rappaport revised the concept of the portal lobule to make interpretation of microscopic liver structure correspond more closely to the smallest complete unit of liver function, which he called the liver acinus (Fig. 87-5). The liver acinus is a globular array of liver cells surrounding a bile ductule and small terminal branches of the portal vein and the hepatic artery. These branches leave the portal areas at intervals, traveling a path perpendicular to that of the portal vessels as well as the central vein, and parallel to the surface of a section through the classic hexagonal liver lobule. The surrounding hepatocytes that form the liver acinus, therefore, come from adjacent Malpighian liver lobules.

The liver acinus is the basis for differentiation of hepatic parenchymal zones (Fig. 87-4). Zone one represents the area of liver tissue immediately surrounding a bile ductule and associated terminal branches of the portal vein and the hepatic artery. Zone three includes the parenchyma farthest removed from these structures, the region surrounding the central vein where adjacent acini merge. Zone two is formed by liver tissue lying between the other two zones. In keeping with the functional basis for this concept, liver cells in each successive zone are farther away from the draining bile ductule and also from the supply of oxygen and nutrients carried to the liver by the afferent vascular structures.

The Portal Area and the Hepatic Microcirculation

The portal area (space, tract, triad, canal) contains small branches of the hepatic artery and the portal vein, a small interlobular bile duct, and fine lymphatics (Fig. 87-6). These structures are surrounded by connective tissue from Glisson's capsule that extends into the liver through the porta hepatis, accompa-

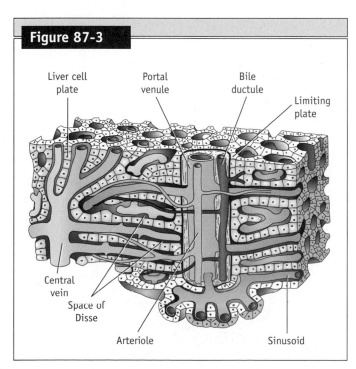

Figure 87-3

The liver parenchyma. The hepatocytes are arranged in plates that converge on the central vein.

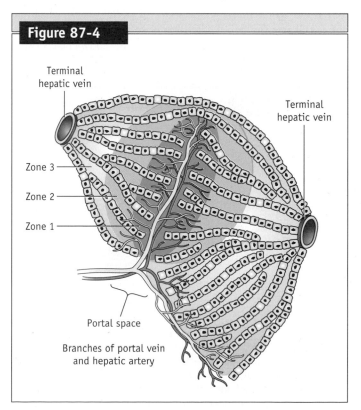

Figure 87-4

The liver acinus and its three zones: the periportal zone (*zone 1*), the intermediate zone (*zone 2*), and the perivenous zone (*zone 3*).

nying and dividing with the hepatic vasculature to the level of the liver lobule. The connective tissue from Glisson's capsule forms the perivascular fibrous capsule that provides an internal supporting framework for the hepatic parenchyma. The size of a portal tract and its component structures decreases as the portal tract branches within the hepatic parenchyma.

Hepatic arterioles within the portal area are recognized on light microscopy by the presence of an endothelial lining, smooth muscle, and an elastic layer. Hepatic arterioles give off numerous branches to a dense capillary network called the peribiliary or periductal plexus that surrounds the bile ductules and drains into the hepatic sinusoids. The existence of the periductal plexus suggests the possibility of an exchange mechanism between arterial blood and bile ductules.

The portal venule is the largest structure in the portal canal, and appears under the light microscope as an empty space, possibly containing some red blood cells, surrounded by a thin endothelium. The interlobular bile duct forms the third element of the portal triad and can be identified on light microscopy as a ring of cuboidal cells approximately the same size as its accompanying hepatic arteriole.

None of these vessels is in direct communication with the hepatic parenchyma. The portal space is surrounded by a continuous barrier of liver cells, the limiting plate, that contains openings through which pass the smallest branches of the hepatic artery and portal vein. It is these small vessels that lie at the center of the liver acinus and that perfuse the hepatic sinusoids. The hepatic parenchyma immediately surrounding the portal space is referred to as the periportal area.

The Hepatic Sinusoid

Blood from the terminal branches of the portal vessels, which exit the portal area through the limiting plate, perfuses a complex network of vascular spaces, the hepatic sinusoids, sandwiched between adjacent liver cell plates (Figs. 87-6 and 87-7). The hepatic

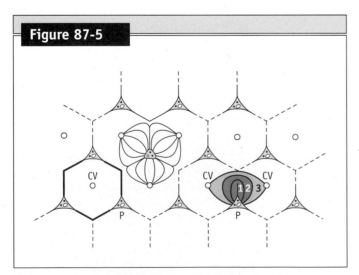

Figure 87-5

Schematic drawing of (*left*) the classic hexagonal liver lobule surrounded by portal areas (P) and centered on a central vein (CV); (*middle*) the portal lobule with a portal area at its center and central veins at its periphery; (*right*) the liver acinus with terminal afferent vessels at its center and central veins at its periphery; the acinar zones (zones 1,2,3) are shown.

sinusoid is composed of four cell types: 1) endothelial, 2) Kupffer, 3) pit, and 4) stellate (fat-storing cells, lipocytes, Ito) cells [3,4].

Sinusoidal endothelial cells are flat, characterized by the absence of a basement membrane and by the presence of fenestrations, or pores, clustered in small patches called sieve plates. Thus, fenestrations form a direct communication between the intrasinusoidal space and the space of Disse, which overlies the liver cell plate and contains an ultrafiltrate of blood.

Kupffer cells are tissue macrophages located in the sinusoidal lumen and attached to endothelial cells. They are difficult to distinguish from endothelial cells with the light microscope. In response to various stimuli, Kupffer cells proliferate through mitosis, and marrow progenitor cells are recruited to the liver to form new Kupffer cells. Monocyte-derived macrophages also are found in the liver in inflammatory diseases.

Pit cells are a special hepatic population of large granular lymphocytes anchored to the sinusoidal endothelium by pseudopodia. Pit cells also circulate in the blood and are found in other nonlymphoid organs. They are named *pit cells* because of their characteristic cytoplasmic granules, or pits, that contain cytotoxic factors.

Stellate cells are mesenchymal cells normally located in the space of Disse, but also are found in proximity to hepatocytes damaged by chronic inflammation. Under the latter circumstances,

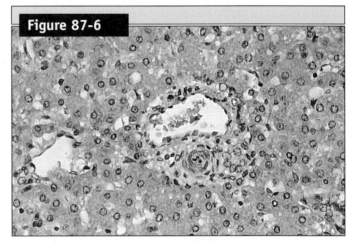

Figure 87-6

Micrograph of the portal area showing the portal venule, hepatic arteriole, bile ductule, and limiting plate.

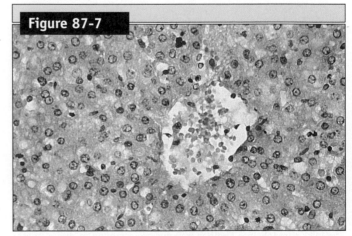

Figure 87-7

Micrograph of the central vein and hepatic sinusoids.

stellate cells loose their characteristic cytoplasmic fat droplets and undergo metaplasia into myofibroblasts [5••].

The Liver Cell Plate and the Hepatocyte

The bulk of the hepatic parenchyma is comprised of an interconnecting network of liver cell plates (Fig. 87-3). These plates are usually one, but occasionally two cells thick, so that each hepatocyte is in direct contact with another liver cell, an intervening bile canniliculus, and the space of Disse. The liver cell plates are supported by a reticulin network that forms the skeleton of the hepatic parenchyma and that is continuous with the extension of the perivascular fibrous capsule surrounding the vessels at the center of the acinus. The reticulin fibers are not associated with fibroblasts and probably are made by sinusoidal lining cells.

Sixty percent of the cells that constitute the human liver are hepatocytes. They are polyhedral cells, 20 to 30 μm across, with round, central, or eccentric nuclei, 6 to 9 μm in diameter. The nuclei contain scattered clumps of chromatin and one or two nucleoli. As many as 25% of hepatocytes are binucleate, but mitotic figures rarely are seen. The cytoplasm of liver cells is variable in appearance, probably reflecting their complexity and functional diversity. Much of this variation is due to stored glycogen and small amounts of fat, which ordinarily are removed in the preparation of histologic sections. Irregular, empty spaces dispersed uniformly throughout the cell indicate the former presence of glycogen; scattered, round, colorless vacuoles indicate the former presence of lipid. In adults, the cytoplasm of centrilobular hepatocytes may contain fine, yellow-brown lipofuscin granules. Otherwise, liver cells stained with hematoxylin and eosin have an eosinophilic cytoplasm faintly stippled with fine basophilic granules.

Hepatocytes of the different acinar zones display structural heterogeneity, reflecting their functional diversity. This diversity is believed to be a response to the microenvironment of the liver cell, rather than an expression of fundamental developmental differences.

The Space of Disse and the Hepatic Lymph

Liver cells are separated from the sinusoids by the space of Disse (Fig. 87-3). Because there are fenestrations in the sinusoidal endothelium, plasma can pass freely from the sinusoidal lumen into the space of Disse and come into direct contact with the hepatocyte surface. The liver cell membranes facing the space of Disse have a large number of microvilli, some of which penetrate the openings of the sieve plate.

Plasma circulates through the space of Disse and returns to the portal area through the interstitial space surrounding the small branches of the portal vessels at the center of the acinus. This tissue fluid is drained by lymphatics that originate in the portal space; no lymphatics have been demonstrated within the liver lobule. The liver produces 25% to 50% of the lymph passing through the thoracic duct. Hepatic lymph contains more protein than does lymph from other parts of the body.

The Bile Canaliculus

A bile canaliculus is located between each adjacent pair of hepatocytes (Fig. 87-3); the canalicular wall consists of a specialized portion of the liver cell membrane covered by microvilli. The canaliculi form an uninterrupted network of interconnected channels extending throughout the hepatic parenchyma. The lumen of the bile canaliculus is completely isolated from the intercellular space, including the space of Disse, by junctional complexes. Bile canaliculi are too small to be seen with the light microscope.

Bile flows from the canaliculi through openings in the limiting plate called canals of Hering, into the smallest biliary radicals, the portal bile ductules (also called cholangioles). The bile ductules and the larger bile ducts are lined by cholangiocytes. Bile ductules join together to form interlobular and then septal bile ducts; several generations of septal bile ducts ultimately merge into the right and left hepatic ducts, which, in turn, join to form the common hepatic duct near the liver hilus. Bile ductules, interlobular bile ducts, and first- and second-generation septal bile ducts constitute the small duct biliary system. Larger septal bile ducts, segmental bile ducts, the hepatic ducts, and the common bile duct form the large duct biliary system.

The Central Vein

Sinusoidal blood flows into central veins located at the periphery of the liver acinus (Fig. 87-7). These vessels originally were named *central veins* because they were at the center of the Malpighian liver lobule (see previous discussion). Small central veins collect into larger intersegmental branches of the right, left, and middle hepatic veins, which, in turn, coalesce into the hepatic vein proper. The walls of central veins have many openings that connect their lumens with those of the hepatic sinusoids. Central veins, therefore, are not isolated from the hepatic parenchyma, as are the afferent vessels of portal areas, which are surrounded by limiting plates.

■ PHYSIOLOGY

To regulate the composition of the blood, the liver must perform a large and diverse group of functions (Table 87-1). The normal liver filters splanchnic blood flow and, in so doing, both adds substances to and removes substances from the circulation. The liver acts as an endocrine gland, as an exocrine gland, as part of the mononuclear phagocyte system, and as a complex metabolic factory. It plays a central role in the intermediate metabolism of absorbed nutrients, synthesizes essential blood factors, shields the body from exposure to foreign antigens, neutralizes toxic compounds, and forms and excretes bile.

Portal Perfusion and Blood Pressure

The liver receives 20% of the cardiac output: three fourths through the portal vein and one fourth through the hepatic artery. The hepatic artery, nevertheless, provides half of the oxygen consumed by the liver in the resting state and more during periods of increased metabolic demand. Much of the hepatic arterial blood flow perfuses the connective tissue stroma of the liver. Portal venous blood contains growth factors, including insulin, that influence liver size and the quality of liver function. The presence of hepatotropic factors in portal blood explains liver atrophy in persons with portal hypertension who develop hepatofugal portal venous blood flow, as well as the necessity of connecting hepatic allografts to the portal vein.

Portal blood pressure, like that of systemic circulation, is related to both vascular resistance and blood flow, according to the equation

$$P = R \times Q$$

In the case of the portal circulation, P is portal blood pressure, R portal vascular resistance, and Q portal blood flow.

The flow of blood through the portal circulation is determined entirely by the venous return from the splanchnic organs. Splanchnic venous outflow, in turn, depends on the diameter of the splanchnic arterioles, which is influenced by numerous complex local and systemic factors, *eg*, the presence of nutrients within the intestinal lumen and cardiac function. These factors act through neural reflexes and the release of vasoactive hormones.

Normal portal blood vessels are highly compliant, allowing the vascular space to accommodate physiologic increases in flow volume by passively enlarging. Sinusoidal compliance may be influenced by relaxation of stellate cells in response to local formation of nitric oxide (see later discussion). Many liver diseases, however, cause a reduction in vascular compliance as well as an increase in portal vascular resistance and blood flow, contributing to the development of portal hypertension.

Sinusoidal Function

The hepatic sinusoid is not merely a passive conduit; sinusoidal cells perform a number of important physiologic functions. They are active in both receptor- and non-receptor–mediated endocytosis; they secrete bioactive lipids and cytokines; they have cytotoxic activity; they produce collagen; and they are the gatekeepers for the intrahepatic filtration of portal blood.

The hepatic sinusoidal endothelium is highly permeable to plasma solutes. Because of the fenestrations in the sinusoidal endothelial cells and the absence of covering diaphragms or a basement membrane, there is no hepatic barrier to filtration of macromolecules up to 250,000 D in weight, or of particles up to 0.2 μm in diameter. Chylomicron remnants and very low-density lipoprotein particles can traverse the sinusoidal endothelium freely and enter the space of Disse. Direct contact between plasma solutes and the absorptive surface of hepatocytes facilitates exchange of materials between blood and the hepatic parenchyma.

Movement of fluid and solutes out of the sinusoidal lumen is primarily dependent on the pressure gradient between the intravascular space and the space of Disse. The elevation of intrasinusoidal pressure in many forms of portal hypertension tends to force more fluid and solute out of the hepatic sinusoid. When this volume of material is too great to be returned to the systemic circulation by the lymphatics, it weeps off the surface of the liver and may accumulate in the peritoneal cavity as ascites.

Sinusoidal endothelial cells also secrete bioactive compounds, including prostaglandin E_2, prostacyclin, and cytokines, and are involved in the secretion of the extracellular matrix. Sinusoidal endothelial cells also are actively engaged in endocytosis, making them a part of the reticuloendothelial system along with Kupffer and pit cells.

Kupffer cells, the largest population of tissue macrophages in the mononuclear phagocyte system, are strategically located within the hepatic sinusoid to survey the filtered portal blood for the presence of a variety of foreign substances. Kupffer cells engage in endocytosis of microbes, enzymes, tumor cells, antigens, and immune complexes. Kupffer cells are the principal site for clearance of endotoxin from portal blood and display the highest capacity for detoxifying endotoxin of any tissue macrophage. Kupffer cells act as antigen-processing cells: they sequester some antigens, *eg*, dietary proteins, to prevent initiation of an immune response, and act as antigen-presenting cells to induce an immune response to other antigens. When activated by the proper stimuli, Kupffer cells release bioactive lipids (prostaglandins and leukotrienes) and peptides (interleukins, interferon, and tumor necrosis factor) which play a central role in immune and inflammatory reactions. Kupffer cells also participate in these reactions by killing tumor cells and intracellular protozoan parasites. Finally, Kupffer cells are responsible for the clearance of senescent erythrocytes and the degradation of hemoglobin. There is evidence suggesting functional heterogeneity of Kupffer cells; periportal

Table 87-1. Functions of the Liver

Metabolic functions	Exocrine functions	Endocrine functions	Defensive functions	Circulatory functions
Energy and nitrogen balance	Bile formation and excretion	Elimination of hormones and mediators	Detoxification of xenobiotic compounds	Active and passive blood storage
Glucose uptake and release		Synthesis of (pro)hormones and mediators	Elimination of foreign macromolecules	Mechanical filtration of portal blood
Ketone body production			Elimination of tumor cells	
Urea production				
Amino acid uptake and release				
Lipid processing				
Biosynthesis and biodegradation				
Plasma protein synthesis and degradation				

(Adapted from Jungermann [1•].)

Kupffer cells are more numerous, larger, have more lysosomes, and display more phagocytic activity but less tumor cytotoxic potential than do Kupffer cells in acinar zones 2 and 3.

Pit cells are another group of immune-effector cells resident in the hepatic sinusoid. Pit cells are non-T, non-B cells of natural killer lineage, responsible for killing tumor cells and cells infected with virus particles.

The stellate cell participates with hepatocytes in the storage and metabolism of retinoids. Stellate cells also normally take part in the secretion of extracellular matrix, and, when stimulated by inflammatory mediators, change into myofibroblasts that synthesize a diverse array of connective tissue components, including collagen types I, III, and IV; fibronectin; laminin; chondroitin sulfate; and others. In addition, stellate cells secrete a variety of growth factors, *eg*, hepatocyte growth factor, which stimulates parenchymal cell proliferation; and transforming growth factor (TGF)-β, which inhibits parenchymal cell proliferation and stimulates connective tissue synthesis. Stellate cells are the primary effectors of fibrogenesis in hepatic injury. There is strong evidence that stellate cells also are contractile and regulate sinusoidal blood flow in response to stimulation by endothelins and nitric oxide. Stellate cells are most numerous in the periportal area.

Hepatocyte Function

Hepatocytes account for 80% of the cytoplasmic mass of the liver and are the site of most liver functions, including nutrient metabolism, synthesis and degradation of plasma proteins, detoxification of xenobiotic compounds, and bile formation. Variations exist in the ability of hepatocytes in different hepatic zones to perform some of these functions (functional heterogeneity).

Hepatocytes play a pivotal role in nutrient metabolism and regulation of energy and nitrogen balance by uptake and release of glucose and amino acids; by glycogen synthesis and storage; by processing lipids; and by production of ketone bodies and urea. Hepatocytes differ in the amounts and activities of the rate-limiting enzymes of carbohydrate and oxidative metabolism which they possess, and, therefore, in their metabolic capacities. Periportal hepatocytes are mainly responsible for oxidative catabolism of fatty and amino acids and also for glucose release and glycogen formation through gluconeogenesis. Perivenous hepatocytes primarily use glucose to synthesize glycogen and for glycolysis coupled to liponeogenesis. Similar differences exist between periportal and perivenous hepatocytes with respect to their capacities for ammonia and amino acid metabolism. Hepatocytes in the periportal zone have a high capacity for uptake and catabolism of most amino acids and also for urea synthesis. Perivenous cells are mainly active in glutamine synthesis and remove ammonia that has escaped urea synthesis in the periportal area from the sinusoidal blood. This form of functional heterogeneity allows the liver to play an important role in acid-base homeostasis.

Another major hepatocyte function is the synthesis and degradation of plasma proteins, including those that maintain plasma oncotic pressure (albumin); serve as carrier molecules (albumin, transferrin, ceruloplasmin, haptoglobin, lipoproteins); inhibit proteases (albumin, α_1-antitrypsin, α_2-macroglobulin); act as intercellular messengers (hormones, prohormones); and

participate in hemostasis (coagulation factors, regulatory proteins, fibrinolytic proteins). The coagulopathy that may complicate acute or chronic liver disease is caused not only by impaired synthesis of clotting factors (II, V, VII, IX, X, XIII), but also by decreased synthesis of contact activation factors (XI, XII, prekallikrein, high molecular weight kininogen), fibrinolytic factors (plasminogen) and regulatory proteins (α_2-antiplasmin, α_2-macroglobulin, antithrombin III), and by decreased hepatic clearance and degradation of activated factors. All hepatocytes are engaged in protein metabolism; it is unclear whether different areas of the liver display functional heterogeneity in the synthesis and degradation of plasma proteins.

Hepatocytes are the cells responsible for detoxification of xenobiotic compounds, most notably drugs. The hepatocyte contains a heterogeneous group of proteins, the cytochrome P-450 enzymes, which catalyze the oxidation and reduction reactions of the first step in the biotransformation of drugs (phase one metabolism). After completion of phase one metabolism, drug metabolites are conjugated by the hepatocyte to glucuronic acid, sulfate, or glutathione (phase two metabolism) making them water-soluble so that they can be excreted in the bile or the urine.

Bile formation and excretion is one of the most important functions of the hepatocyte (see Chapter 88).

▮▮ TESTS OF LIVER FUNCTION

Given the number and complexity of the tasks performed by the liver, it is not surprising that there is no single reliable test of liver function. Instead, the functional integrity of the liver must be assessed using multiple tests of specific functions and serum markers of hepatobiliary disease in conjunction with clinical information obtained by interviewing and examining the patient.

Serum Markers of Hepatobiliary Disease (Liver Tests)

Serum markers of hepatobiliary disease measured in clinical chemistry laboratories by automated analyzers are commonly referred to as *liver function tests* (Table 87-2). This is a misnomer, inasmuch as many of these tests identify enzymes and other substances released into the blood as a result of liver cell damage, but do not assess liver function per se. Thus, the aminotransferases, aspartate aminotransferase (AST) and alanine aminotransferase (ALT) are liver enzymes released into the blood as a result of hepatocyte injury or death.

Other serum markers of hepatobiliary disease provide broad or indirect information about liver functions. Results of measurements of serum bilirubin, alkaline phosphatase, and cholesterol may indicate the presence of cholestasis, but they do not test the adequacy of a specific physiologic liver function. Similarly, abnormalities of serum albumin, cholesterol, and prothrombin time reflect derangements of processes involving multiple liver functions. Finally, measurements of serum globulin may suggest derangements of the immune surveillance activities of the hepatic sinusoidal cells but do not provide information concerning the specific abnormalities responsible for the finding. All of these tests must be interpreted with the awareness that their results are reflections of multiple interrelated physiologic and pathologic processes and not quantitative tests of *liver function* predictive of the overall health of the liver (see Chapter 91).

Table 87-2. Serum and Hematologic Markers of Hepatobiliary Disease (Liver Tests)

Tests of hepatocellular injury or death
Aspartate aminotransferase
Alanine aminotransferase

Tests of cholestasis
Bilirubin
Alkaline phosphatase
γ-Glutamyltransferase
5'-Nucleotidase
Cholesterol

Tests of biosynthesis and biodegradation
Prothrombin time
Albumin
Cholesterol
Mean corpuscular red cell volume

Tests of immune surveillance
Globulin

Tests of Specific Liver Functions

Organic anion transport tests measure the ability of hepatocytes to remove lipophilic molecules from plasma and excrete them into bile. This process depends on selective, charge-dependent, carrier-mediated mechanisms for excreting organic molecules. Thus, there is a mechanism for excretion of neutral compounds and another for excretion of compounds with a net positive charge. Compounds with a net negative charge are handled by two mechanisms, one of which is reserved exclusively for bile acids. Several quantitative tests of the two latter hepatocyte functions have been developed. These include determination of the fractional disappearance, plasma half-life and clearance of indocyanine green or sulfobromophthalein, and measurement by radioimmunoassay, enzymatic assay, or gas chromatography of serum bile acids in the fasting state, postprandially, or after administration of cholecystokinin.

Tests of the metabolic capacity of the liver rely on administration and measurement of test substances selectively eliminated by the liver in proportion to its functional mass. Commonly used tests are those of hepatic drug metabolism, notably the clearance of plasma antipyrine and the [14C]-aminopyrine breath test, the maximum rate of urea synthesis, and the galactose tolerance test. Although quantitative liver function tests of these types have been used extensively to evaluate patients with a variety of liver diseases, the clinical utility of the information they provide has not justified their difficulty and expense.

REFERENCES

1.• Jungermann K: Zonal liver cell heterogeneity. *Enzyme* 1992, 46:5–7.
This article, part of an entire issue devoted to the structure and function of the liver, explains the concept of liver cell heterogeneity and how it applies to different liver functions.

2.• Sasse D, Spornitz UM, Maly IP: Liver architecture. *Enzyme* 1992, 46:8–32.
This article, part of an entire issue devoted to the structure and function of the liver, offers a well-illustrated description of liver architecture.

3. *The Role of Hepatic Sinusoidal Cells in Liver Disease.* Edited by Rothschild MA, Berk PD, Bioulac-Sage P, Balabaud C. *Seminars in Liver Disease* 1993, Vol 13, No 1.

4. Bouwens L, De Bleser P, Vanderkerken K, Geerts B, Wisse E: Liver cell heterogeneity: functions of non-parenchymal cells. *Enzyme* 1992, 46:155–168.

5.•• Rockey D: The cellular pathogenesis of portal hypertension: stellate cell contractility, endothelin, and nitric oxide. *Hepatology* 1997, 25:2–5.
This review explains the function of the stellate cell and its role in the pathogenesis of portal hypertension. This articles is of particular interest because it emphasizes the effects of some important biologically active compounds on liver physiology.

Bile Formation and Excretion

Allan W. Wolkoff

Removal of relatively small hydrophobic molecules (*ie*, molecular weight of 400–1000 D) from the circulation is an important liver function. These molecules, which are protein-bound, include endogenous compounds, such as bilirubin and bile acids, and xenobiotics such as sulfobromophthalein. After uptake into the hepatocyte, these compounds typically are metabolized to more water-soluble derivatives that are excreted across the apical plasma membrane into the bile canaliculus. This chapter examines these transport mechanisms and their relationship to bile formation.

FUNCTIONAL ANATOMY OF THE HEPATOCYTE

The liver is constructed to optimize its ability to remove highly protein-bound substances from the circulation (see Chapter 87). Albumin-bound molecules, such as bilirubin, enter the space of Disse and interact directly with specific transporters on the hepatocyte sinusoidal (basolateral) surface.

Entry of compounds into the bile canaliculus is regulated by canalicular (apical) membrane-specific transporters. These transporters appear to use energy (*ie*, ATP) to pump solutes against a concentration gradient. Movement of compounds back into the cell is prevented by the unidirectionality of transporters and by tight junctions, which close off the intercellular space. Under pathologic circumstances, such as in cholestasis, the functional integrity of tight junctions may be compromised, allowing excreted compounds such as bile acids to return to the circulation.

▣ TRANSPORTERS OF THE SINUSOIDAL MEMBRANE OF THE HEPATOCYTE

The hepatocyte removes many compounds with a wide range of physical properties from the blood [1•,2•,3]. A brief review of what is known about hepatocellular uptake of organic anions and cations follows.

Uptake of Organic Anions by the Hepatocyte

Figure 88-1 shows the structures of three anionic organic compounds excreted by the hepatocyte. Although these compounds have little obvious structural homology, they bind avidly to albumin and appear to share, at least in part, specific transporters that facilitate their entry into the liver cell.

The uptake mechanism for bilirubin and sulfobromophthalein is very efficient; as much as 50% of these compounds is removed from portal blood during a single pass through the liver. Despite the fact that these compounds are bound avidly to albumin, it is the free organic anion rather than the albumin-bound fraction that enters the hepatocyte. Albumin is not likely to mediate organic anion uptake through a previously postulated albumin receptor. Rather, experimental evidence suggests that there is a specific sodium-independent organic anion transporter for bilirubin and sulfobromophthalein on the hepatocyte sinusoidal surface.

In contrast, hepatocellular uptake of bile acids such as taurocholic acid is primarily sodium-dependent, although there is also a significant sodium-independent component [2•]. Similar to sulfobromophthalein and bilirubin, plasma disappearance of bile acids is rapid and highly efficient. A major driving force for sodium-dependent bile acid uptake is probably the large sodium ion gradient between plasma and the inside of the liver cell that is established by cellular sodium-potassium ATPase.

Uptake of Organic Cations by the Hepatocyte

Many of the drugs used in clinical practice, as well as endogenously synthesized compounds, are organic cations that are eliminated by the liver. Examples of three such cationic compounds are shown in Figure 88-2. The mechanisms by which the hepatocyte transports these compounds have been the subject of investigation, but identification and characterization of these transport processes are still incomplete.

At least four sinusoidal organic cation transporters exist. Transporters for choline and tetraethylammonium are electrogenic and are driven by membrane potential. Transporters for thiamine and N′-methylnicotinamide mediate organic cation–H+ exchange.

Figure 88-1

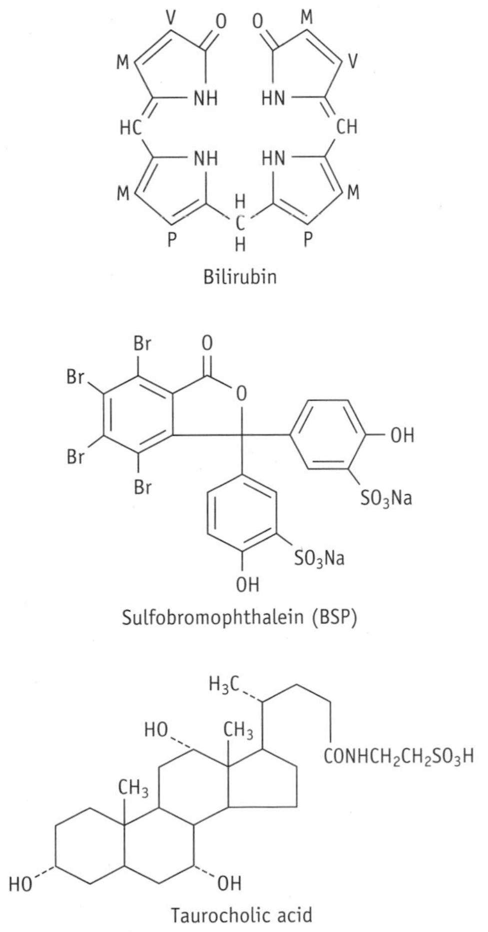

Bilirubin

Sulfobromophthalein (BSP)

Taurocholic acid

Structures of three typical organic anions that are removed from the circulation by the hepatocyte.

Figure 88-2

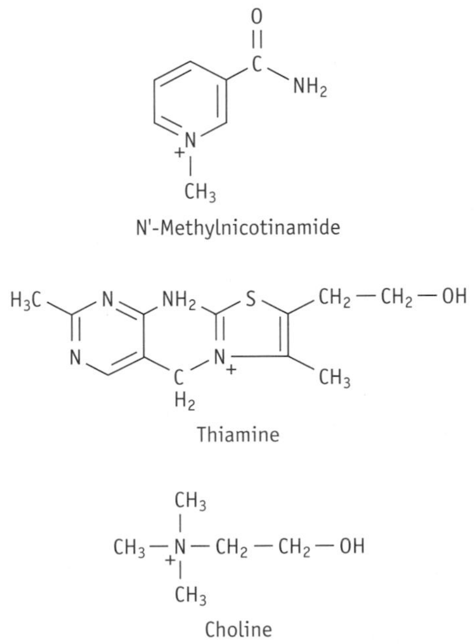

N′-Methylnicotinamide

Thiamine

Choline

Structures of three typical organic cations that are removed from the circulation by the hepatocyte.

CANALICULAR SECRETION AND BILE FORMATION

After uptake by the hepatocyte, many compounds interact with intracellular proteins and undergo biotransformation to more polar (water-soluble) derivatives. For example, bilirubin is converted to a glucuronide conjugate, sulfobromophthalein to a glutathione conjugate, and cholic acid to taurine and glycine conjugates. For the most part, these derivatives then interact with specific transporters, often ATP-dependent, located on the canalicular plasma membrane, resulting in their excretion into bile.

Composition and Formation of Bile

Bile may be thought of as the hepatic counterpart of urine. Hepatic bile is isosmotic with plasma and is secreted at a rate of 500 to 600 mL each day. It contains electrolytes, including sodium chloride and sodium bicarbonate, bile acids, bilirubin glucuronides, phospholipids, cholesterol, some proteins, and the tripeptide glutathione [4].

The major determinant of bile formation appears to be active secretion of bile acids into the bile canaliculus with passive diffusion of water down its osmotic gradient. A smaller fraction of bile results from secretion of compounds other than bile acids. These compounds include glutathione, which is secreted into bile in substantial amounts [3,4].

Bile Acids and the Enterohepatic Circulation

Bile acids are a family of detergent-like cholesterol metabolites formed in the liver (ie, primary bile acids) and modified by intestinal bacteria (ie, secondary bile acids) (Fig. 88-3). After initial hepatic synthesis, they are conjugated with glycine or taurine and then are excreted in the bile. Bile salts stimulate biliary cholesterol and phospholipid secretion, solubilize cholesterol in bile, and play a role in intestinal lipid digestion and fat-soluble vitamin absorption. The metabolic cost of performing these functions is reduced by intestinal absorption and reuse of bile acids.

Mechanism for Secretion of Solutes Into Bile

The canalicular membrane of the hepatocyte contains a number of ATP-dependent transporters that act as pumps that secrete their substrates against large concentration gradients [5••]. These substrates include glycine- and taurine-conjugated bile acids, bilirubin glucuronides, and glutathione. Most of these ATP-dependent transporters appear to be members of a transporter family known as the ATP-binding cassette transporters, which include the multidrug resistance (MDR) protein 1, which excretes lipophilic cations; MDR2, which excretes phospholipids; and the canalicular multispecific organic anion transporter (cMOAT), also known as multidrug resistance-associated protein 2 (MRP2), which helps to excrete compounds such as bilirubin

Figure 88-3

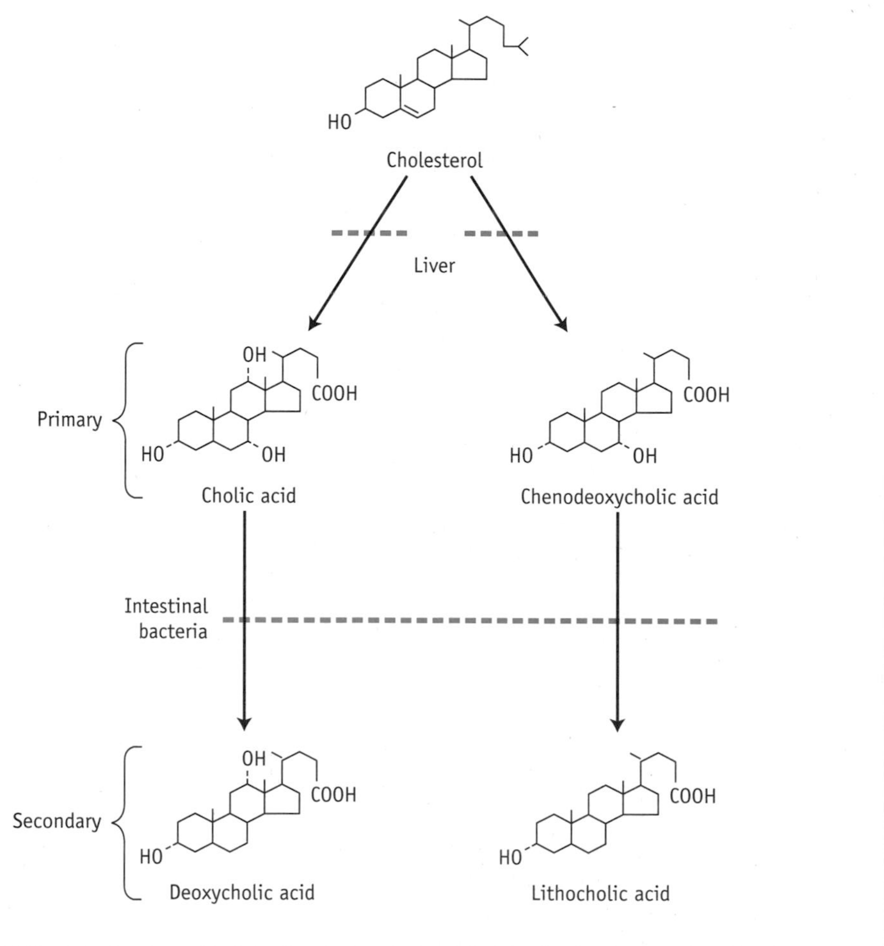

Synthesis and modification of bile acids. (*From* Carey and Duane [6]; with permission.)

glucuronides and sulfobromophthalein-glutathione. The latter protein is deficient in patients with the Dubin-Johnson syndrome, a benign disorder characterized by mild, chronic conjugated hyperbilirubinemia. There is also strong evidence for existence of a canalicular, ATP-dependent bile acid transporter and for a canalicular glutathione transporter.

Cholestasis

Reduced canalicular bile formation may lead to intrahepatic cholestasis (see Chapters 105 and 106), characterized by retention of compounds such as bile acids and bilirubin glucuronides that normally would be excreted into bile [4]. Pathogenetic factors responsible for intrahepatic cholestasis include primary alterations in bile acid and lipid transporters and disordered cellular cytoskeleton and canalicular membrane structures.

▮▮ REFERENCES

Recently published papers of particular interest have been highlighted as follows:
- •   Of interest
- •• Of outstanding interest

1.• Wolkoff AW: Hepatocellular sinusoidal membrane organic anion transport and transporters. *Semin Liver Dis* 1996, 16:121–127.

2.• Hagenbuch B, Meier PJ: Sinusoidal (basolateral) bile salt uptake systems of hepatocytes. *Semin Liver Dis* 1996, 16:129–136.
This article reviews advances in cloning and the characterization of important hepatocyte sinusoidal membrane transporters.

3.   Fernandez-Checa JC, Yi JR, Garcia Ruiz C, *et al.*: Plasma membrane and mitochondrial transport of hepatic reduced glutathione. *Semin Liver Dis* 1996, 16:147–158.

4.   Moseley RH: Bile secretion and cholestasis. In *Liver and Biliary Diseases*, edn 2. Edited by Kaplowitz N. Baltimore: Williams & Wilkins; 1996:185–204.

5.•• Keppler D, Arias IM: Transport across the hepatocyte canalicular membrane. *FASEB J* 1997, 11:199–205.
This is an outstanding review of ATP-dependent transport pumps at the hepatocyte canalicular membrane.

6.   Carey MC, Duane WC: Enterohepatic circulation. In *The Liver: Biology and Pathobiology*. Edited by Arias IM, Boyer JL, Fausto N, *et al.* New York: Raven Press; 1994:719–767.

Bilirubin Metabolism and Jaundice

Bernhard V. Sauter, Namita Roy Chowdhury, and Jayanta Roy Chowdhury

Bilirubin is formed by the breakdown of heme present in hemoglobin, myoglobin, cytochromes, catalase, peroxidase, and tryptophan pyrrolase. Because bilirubin is potentially toxic, elaborate physiologic mechanisms exist for its detoxification and disposition.

▮▮ FORMATION AND CHEMISTRY OF BILIRUBIN

Eighty percent of the bilirubin produced daily (250 to 400 mg) is derived from hemoglobin; the remaining 20% is contributed by other hemoproteins such as the cytochromes, catalase, and peroxidase and by a small pool of free heme. Formation of bilirubin is catalyzed by two groups of enzymes. The first group consists of microsomal heme oxygenases that open the heme ring, forming biliverdin. Iron and one molecule of carbon monoxide are released in the process. Heme oxygenase activity is rate-limiting in bilirubin formation. The second group consists of cytosolic reductases that reduce biliverdin to bilirubin.

Increased bilirubin formation is found in diseases associated with increased red cell turnover, for example, intramedullar or intravascular hemolysis (*eg*, hemolytic, dyserythropoietic, megaloblastic, iron deficiency anemias; lead poisoning).

Structure and measurement. Bilirubin is insoluble in water at physiologic pH because of internal hydrogen bonding. Water-insoluble, unconjugated bilirubin causes all the known toxic effects of bilirubin. Conversion of bilirubin to a water-soluble form by disruption of the hydrogen bonds is essential for its elimination by the liver and kidney and for its detoxification. This conversion occurs physiologically by glucuronic acid conjugation mediated by a specific enzyme, bilirubin-UDP-glucuronosyltransferase (bilirubin-UGT). The hydrogen bonds also can be disrupted by exposure to light, resulting in more water-soluble photoproducts that can be excreted in bile without conjugation. This mechanism is the rationale for phototherapy, which is used to reduce serum bilirubin levels in neonatal jaundice and Crigler-Najjar syndrome type I [1].

Bilirubin that is internally hydrogen bonded and unconjugated reacts very slowly with diazo reagents. Disrupting the hydrogen bonds by adding accelerators makes the diazo reaction rapid and complete (total bilirubin). Conjugated bilirubin is not hydrogen bonded; therefore, the diazo reaction occurs without accelerators (direct-reacting fraction). Unconjugated bilirubin concentration is calculated by subtracting the direct-reacting fraction from the total serum bilirubin. This assay, used commonly in clinical practice, is called the van den Bergh reaction. In prolonged, conjugated hyperbilirubinemia, covalently bound albumin-bilirubin complexes are formed (delta bilirubin), which also produce a direct diazo reaction. More accurate and sensitive quantification of bilirubin can be achieved with high-pressure liquid chromatography [2••].

Distribution in body fluids. In normal plasma, only up to 4% of bilirubin is conjugated. In hemolytic jaundice, total plasma bilirubin increases, but the proportion of unconjugated and conjugated fractions remains unchanged. In inherited disorders of bilirubin conjugation, total serum bilirubin concentration increases, but the absolute concentration of conjugated bilirubin may remain normal or may be reduced, thereby increasing the proportion of unconjugated bilirubin. In biliary obstruction or hepatocellular diseases, both conjugated and unconjugated bilirubin accumulate in plasma, and their proportion changes in favor of conjugated bilirubin. Bilirubin in normal human bile is predominantly the diglucuronide conjugate (>80%). Unconjugated bilirubin accounts for only 1% to 4% of biliary pigments. Tight binding of unconjugated bilirubin to albumin precludes glomerular filtration [3•]. Conjugated bilirubin is less tightly bound to albumin than is unconjugated bilirubin and, therefore, appears in urine. In the severely jaundiced patient, bilirubin is found in virtually all tissue fluids, especially those with high albumin content. Thus, bilirubin concentration in cerebrospinal fluid is normally much lower than that in serum. Binding of bilirubin to the elastic tissue of skin and conjunctiva causes their yellow discoloration in hyperbilirubinemia, which may persist for some time after the resolution of hyperbilirubinemia.

Toxicity. High serum levels of unconjugated bilirubin (usually >20 mg/dL) in the newborn may result in clinical evidence of brain damage, ranging from subtle neurologic abnormalities to severe encephalopathy or fully developed kernicterus. The brain, particularly the basal ganglia, hippocampus, thalamus, nuclei of the cerebellum, pons, and medulla, are grossly pigmented in infants dying of acute bilirubin encephalopathy [4]. In premature babies, or in those whom acidosis, hypoxia or sepsis is present, or in whom drugs are used which compete with bilirubin for albumin binding, encephalopathy is manifested at lower bilirubin concentrations. Immaturity of the blood-brain barrier conventionally has been implicated in the vulnerability of neonates to bilirubin encephalopathy; however, little evidence supports the theory that neonates have an immature blood-brain barrier. Kernicterus most commonly occurs between 3 and 6 days of life and is characterized by loss of the Moro reflex, truncal hypertonicity, and opisthotonus after a startling stimulus. Survivors may have no residual brain damage or may develop irreversible hearing loss, muscle spasticity, paralysis of upward gaze, athetosis, and mental retardation in various combinations [5•].

▇▇ DISPOSITION OF BILIRUBIN

Unconjugated bilirubin, like many other water-insoluble compounds, remains in solution by binding to plasma albumin. Albumin binding prevents bilirubin deposition in extrahepatic tissues, thereby protecting sensitive tissues such as the brain. At the sinusoidal surface of the hepatocyte, the pigment dissociates from albumin and enters the liver cell, whereas albumin remains in the plasma. Other ligands that bind to albumin (eg, sulfonamides, coumadin, anti-inflammatory drugs, cholecystographic contrast media) may displace bilirubin from albumin, thereby precipitating bilirubin

encephalopathy in newborns, without altering serum bilirubin levels.

Normally, albumin binding of bilirubin is reversible; however, irreversible binding can occur in prolonged conjugated hyperbilirubinemia (eg, during biliary obstruction). The bilirubin fraction irreversibly bound to albumin (*delta bilirubin*) is not cleared by the liver or kidney, and because of the long half-life of albumin, it lingers in the plasma. This persistence may result in prolonged hyperbilirubinemia after endoscopic or surgical relief of biliary obstruction. Because delta bilirubin produces a direct diazo reaction, this test may give the false impression of persistent bile duct obstruction [2••].

Uptake and storage by hepatocytes. In liver sinusoids, the albumin-bilirubin complex comes in direct contact with the sinusoidal surface of hepatocytes because of the fenestrated structure of sinusoidal endothelial cells (Fig. 89-1). Bilirubin is then taken up by the hepatocyte by facilitated diffusion. Bilirubin transport at the sinusoidal membrane is bidirectional; binding to cytosolic ligandins (also termed glutathion-*S*-transferases) reduces the efflux component, thereby increasing net uptake.

Bilirubin uptake is reduced in some, but not all, patients with Gilbert syndrome (see later in this chapter). Some drugs (eg, flavaspidic acid, rifampicin, and cholecystographic dyes) inhibit the uptake process. In cirrhosis, a portion of the bilirubin produced in the spleen may bypass the liver by way of the portosystemic collaterals, resulting in an increase in serum levels of unconjugated bilirubin.

Bilirubin Conjugation

Glucuronidation of bilirubin and a large variety of endogenous compounds (eg, steroid hormones, thyroid hormones, catecholamines, bile salts) and a wide array of exogenous substrates (eg, drugs, toxins, carcinogens, laboratory xenobiotics) is mediated by a family of UDPglucuronosyltransferase (UGT) enzymes.

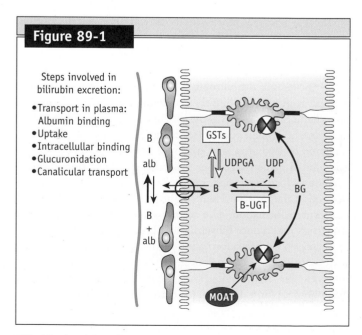

Figure 89-1

Steps involved in bilirubin excretion:

- Transport in plasma: Albumin binding
- Uptake
- Intracellular binding
- Glucuronidation
- Canalicular transport

Bilirubin throughput by the liver.

Glucuronides are more water soluble and generally are less biologically reactive than are the nonglucuronidated substrates, and are readily excreted in bile and urine. Enzyme-catalyzed glucuronidation is an important detoxification mechanism that is critical for excretion of bilirubin in the bile. One specific form of UGT, called bilirubin-UGT$_1$, is responsible for bilirubin glucuronidation in the human liver. Reduction of this enzyme activity results in accumulation of unconjugated bilirubin in plasma [6•].

Bilirubin diglucuronide is the predominant pigment (>80%) in normal adult human bile. In persons with reduced bilirubin-UGT activity, the proportion of bilirubin monoglucuronide in bile increases (see Gilbert syndrome and Crigler-Najjar syndrome, type II, later in this chapter). Reduction of conjugating enzyme activity to approximately 30% of normal results in a mild but discernible increase in serum bilirubin levels.

Various degrees of bilirubin-UGT are found in inherited disorders, for example, Gilbert syndrome and Crigler-Najjar syndrome, types I and II. Inhibitors of hepatic bilirubin-UGT are secreted in the breast milk of some mothers (maternal milk jaundice). In other cases, an inhibitory factor in maternal plasma may be transplacentally transferred to the fetus (Lucey-Driscoll syndrome). The antibiotic novobiocin inhibits bilirubin conjugation and may cause unconjugated hyperbilirubinemia.

Bilirubin Excretion

Conjugated bilirubin is secreted across the hepatocyte's bile-canalicular membrane by an active transport mechanism. A multispecific organic-anion transporter mediates the active canalicular secretion of bilirubin and many other organic anions, with the notable exception of bile acids (see Chapter 88). Abnormalities of excretion of conjugated bilirubin occur in specific transport disorders (*eg*, Dubin-Johnson syndrome), or in hepatic storage abnormalities (*eg*, Rotor's syndrome). Reduced canalicular excretion also may complicate alcoholic or viral hepatitis. Canalicular excretion defect also underlies cholestasis of pregnancy and cholestasis caused by a variety of drugs (*eg*, alkylated steroids, chlorpromazine) [7].

Bilirubin excreted in bile is mostly conjugated. Conjugated bilirubin is absorbed in the intestine, but the unconjugated bilirubin fraction (0.5% to 2%) is only partly reabsorbed. In the colon, bilirubin is reduced by bacterial enzymes to urobilinogens, which are oxidized to urobilins that impart a yellow color to urine and stool. In complete biliary obstruction (*eg*, some cases of pancreatic carcinoma) or severe intrahepatic cholestasis (*eg*, the early phase of acute viral hepatitis), lack of urobilinogen may give the feces the appearance of china clay. Urobilinogens and their derivatives are partly absorbed from the bowel, undergo enterohepatic recycling, and are eventually excreted in urine and feces [8].

Unconjugated bilirubin is tightly bound to albumin and therefore not filtered by the glomerulus. Conjugated bilirubin is less tightly bound to albumin; therefore, in disorders associated with elevated plasma levels of conjugated bilirubin (*eg*, intrahepatic or extrahepatic cholestasis), renal elimination is the major pathway of bilirubin excretion.

■ CLINICAL CLASSIFICATION OF JAUNDICE

For purposes of clinical evaluation, jaundice may be classified according to the predominant type of bile pigments that accumulate in plasma (Fig. 89-2).

Disorders Associated with Unconjugated Hyperbilirubinemia
Neonatal Jaundice

All newborns have higher serum bilirubin levels (mainly unconjugated bilirubin) than do adults (physiologic jaundice). Jaundice is clinically obvious in about 50% of neonates during the first 5 days of life. In approximately 16% of newborns, maximum serum bilirubin concentrations reach or exceed 10 mg/dL. Physiologic jaundice of the newborn may result from a combination of increased bilirubin production and decreased elimination of bilirubin as compared with that in adults. Any disorder leading to enhanced bilirubin formation or impaired bilirubin disposition may exaggerate hyperbilirubinemia and potentially result in kernicterus (Fig. 89-3).

Increased bilirubin load. Bilirubin production ordinarily is greater during the neonatal period. ABO blood group or Rh incompatibility, inherited disorders (*eg*, sickle cell disease and hereditary spherocytosis), and drug reactions are common causes of hemolytic jaundice in the newborn. Ineffective erythropoiesis occurs in people with thalassemia, vitamin B$_{12}$ deficiency, and congenital dyserythropoietic anemias. In some cases, the rate of bilirubin production may exceed the bile canalicular-excretory capacity, resulting in accumulation of conjugated bilirubin in serum [2••].

Immaturity of hepatic bilirubin clearance. Hepatic bilirubin uptake is low at birth compared with levels in the adult. Reduced caloric intake, as in gastric outlet obstruction, also may contribute to hyperbilirubinemia by reducing hepatic bilirubin clearance. Bilirubin-UGT activity, which is at only 1% of normal adult levels at birth, regardless of gestational age, progressively increases to adult levels by the 14th week of life.

Maternal milk jaundice. Breast-fed infants have higher mean serum bilirubin levels than do formula-fed babies. Occasionally, serum bilirubin levels in breast-fed babies reach 15 to 24 mg/dL by 10 to 19 days of life. The unconjugated hyperbilirubinemia may continue for 4 weeks but promptly resolves when breast-feeding is discontinued. Neurologic damage has not been reported in babies

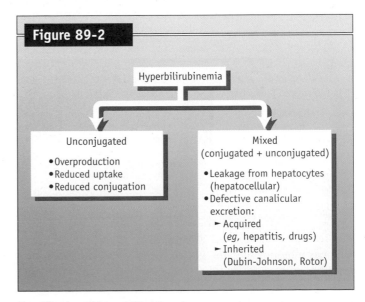

Figure 89-2

Hyperbilirubinemia

Unconjugated
• Overproduction
• Reduced uptake
• Reduced conjugation

Mixed (conjugated + unconjugated)
• Leakage from hepatocytes (hepatocellular)
• Defective canalicular excretion:
  ► Acquired (*eg*, hepatitis, drugs)
  ► Inherited (Dubin-Johnson, Rotor)

Classification of hyperbilirubinemia.

with this syndrome, which is caused by an inhibitor of bilirubin-UGT in maternal milk.

Maternal serum jaundice. Jaundice during the first 4 days of life with peak serum bilirubin concentrations of 8.9 to 65 mg/dL reached within 7 days may result from the presence of an unidentified inhibitor of UGT, which entered the fetus from maternal serum. In this disorder, known as Lucey-Driscoll syndrome, jaundice begins earlier than in maternal milk jaundice, is more severe, can persist for several weeks, and occasionally is associated with kernicterus.

Inherited disorders of bilirubin glucuronidation. Inherited bilirubin-UGT syndromes, for example, Crigler-Najjar syndromes type I and II, may present with severe unconjugated hyperbilirubinemia in the newborn period. These disorders are discussed later in this review.

The differential diagnosis of neonatal jaundice also includes conditions common to newborns and adults (eg, viral hepatitis, total parenteral nutrition, cholelithiasis, septic cholestasis, tumors); a wide variety of metabolic disorders of amino acids, lipids, and carbohydrates; and finally, idiopathic congenital syndromes of intrahepatic and extrahepatic cholestasis that give rise to elevated levels of conjugated bilirubin (neonatal cholestasis, see later in this chapter).

Jaundice due to Overproduction of Bilirubin

Excessive heme catabolism occurs with extravascular or intravascular hemolysis, extravasation of blood into tissues, or dyserythropoiesis. In most hemolytic disorders, there is an increase in the normal extravascular destruction of erythrocytes in the reticuloendothelial cells of the spleen, bone marrow, and liver. In contrast to extravascular hemolysis, in cases of intravascular hemolysis, liver and kidney are major sites of bilirubin formation. In some blood diseases, collectively termed dyserythropoiesis, a large fraction of hemoglobin heme is degraded without incorporation into erythrocytes. These disorders include megaloblastic and sideroblastic anemias, severe iron deficiency anemia, erythropoietic porphyria, erythroleukemia, lead poisoning, and a rare disorder of unknown pathogenesis, primary shunt hyperbilirubinemia. At a steady-state blood hemoglobin level, in the presence of normal liver function, sustained plasma bilirubin concentrations do not exceed 4 mg/dL despite maximum bilirubin production. In conjunction with even mild liver disease, hemolysis may result in marked hyperbilirubinemia. The increased bilirubin excretion in bile results in increased urobilinogen excretion in stool and urine. Conversion of bilirubin to urobilinogen, however, is not quantitative, and measurement of urobilinogen does not provide clinically reliable information about the severity of the underlying disorder. Chronically increased bile pigment excretion may result in the precipitation of monoconjugated and unconjugated bile pigments, leading to formation of brown or black pigment stones!

Impaired Hepatic Bilirubin Uptake

Reduced hepatic blood flow due to congestive cardiac failure or naturally occurring or surgically created portosystemic shunts may compromise the delivery of bilirubin to hepatocytes and result in predominantly unconjugated hyperbilirubinemia. Further reduction of bilirubin uptake may result from loss of sinusoidal endothelial cell fenestrae (capillarization of the sinusoidal endothelium) as occurs in cirrhosis. Rifamycin antibiotics, probenecid, flavaspidic acid, and bunamiodyl, a cholecystographic agent, interfere with bilirubin uptake. Hyperbilirubinemia due to these agents resolves within 48 hours of discontinuing the drug.

Impaired Bilirubin Conjugation

Decreased or absent–bilirubin-UDP-glucuronosyltransferase activity may occur in several inherited or acquired disorders.

Acquired disorders. The most ubiquitous form of acquired decrease in bilirubin conjugation occurs in neonates (described previously).

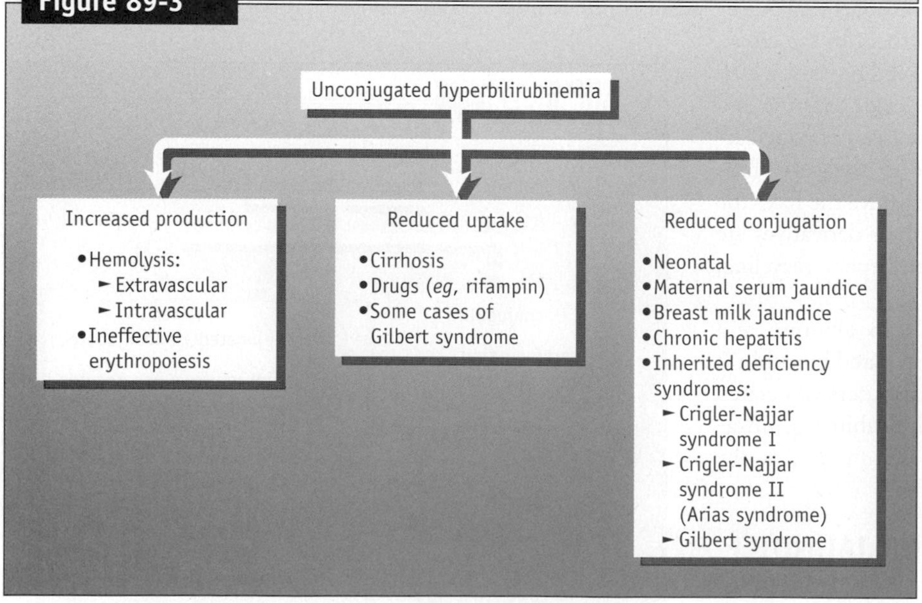

Types of unconjugated hyperbilirubinemia.

Figure 89-3

Unconjugated hyperbilirubinemia

Increased production
- Hemolysis:
  - ► Extravascular
  - ► Intravascular
- Ineffective erythropoiesis

Reduced uptake
- Cirrhosis
- Drugs (eg, rifampin)
- Some cases of Gilbert syndrome

Reduced conjugation
- Neonatal
- Maternal serum jaundice
- Breast milk jaundice
- Chronic hepatitis
- Inherited deficiency syndromes:
  - ► Crigler-Najjar syndrome I
  - ► Crigler-Najjar syndrome II (Arias syndrome)
  - ► Gilbert syndrome

Bilirubin-UGT activity also is decreased in hyperthyroidism and is inhibited by ethynylestradiol, but not by other contraceptive agents. Novobiocin and gentamycin, at higher than therapeutic blood levels, inhibit bilirubin glucuronidation. Decreased hepatic bilirubin-UGT activity has been reported in patients with chronic persistent hepatitis, advanced cirrhosis, and Wilson's disease.

Inherited disorders. Three degrees of inherited defects of bilirubin conjugation are known to exist in humans. Of these, Crigler-Najjar syndrome type I is the most severe, followed by Crigler-Najjar syndrome type II (Arias syndrome), and Gilbert syndrome. An overview of their main characteristics is presented in Table 89-1 [2••].

Crigler-Najjar syndrome type I. This rare disorder is characterized by severe life-long unconjugated hyperbilirubinemia with undetectable hepatic bilirubin-UGT [9]. The syndrome occurs in all ethnic groups, is inherited as an autosomal recessive trait, and presents in the first days of life. Unless vigorously treated, most affected patients die by 15 months of life. Some others remain icteric until puberty, when they succumb to kernicterus precipitated by unknown causes. In recent years, with advances in the management of hyperbilirubinemia, more patients with Crigler-Najjar syndrome type I are surviving to adulthood. Liver tests other than high serum unconjugated bilirubin levels are normal. Serum bilirubin concentrations usually range from 20 to 40 mg/dL, but may be as high as 50 mg/dL. Phenobarbital therapy does not reduce serum bilirubin levels significantly. Conjugated bilirubin is absent from serum, and bilirubin is not present in urine. The gallbladder is visualized by oral cholecystography despite very high serum bilirubin levels because excretion of nonglucuronidated organic anions is normal. Bile collected by duodenal aspiration is light yellow because of small amounts of unconjugated bilirubin. Bilirubin monoconjugates and diconjugates are nearly absent from the bile. Analysis of pigments excreted in bile is the most reliable method of differentiating between Crigler-Najjar syndrome type I and type II (see the following discussion). Liver histology is normal in affected individuals, and hepatic bilirubin-UGT activity is undetectable [10].

Conventional treatment of Crigler-Najjar syndrome type I, is aimed at reducing serum bilirubin concentrations. Phototherapy is the most common routinely used measure; it results in the forma-tion of bilirubin photoisomers that can be excreted in bile without conjugation. The effectiveness of phototherapy decreases after the age of 3 to 4 years because the ratio of skin surface area to body mass is reduced and because of thickening and pigmentation of the skin. During a crisis, faster removal of bilirubin from the body can be accomplished by plasmapheresis. Orthotopic liver transplantation or transplantation of a liver segment almost instantly normalizes serum bilirubin levels. Liver transplantation is the only definitive treatment for Crigler-Najjar syndrome type I. Because liver architecture is normal in Crigler-Najjar syndrome type I and because a small fraction of the normal bilirubin activity is sufficient to reduce serum bilirubin concentrations to safe levels, transplantation of hepatocytes would be an attractive alternative to orthotopic liver transplant. At the time of this writing, one patient has been treated successfully by transplantation of allogeneic hepatocytes.

Crigler-Najjar syndrome type II (Arias syndrome). This disorder is characterized by a severe, incomplete reduction of hepatic bilirubin-UGT activity, with serum bilirubin levels ranging from 7 to 20 mg/dL. During surgery or intercurrent illnesses, the level in affected people may increase to as much as 40 mg/dL. Induction of residual enzyme activity by phenobarbital administration reduces serum bilirubin levels significantly in most cases, which distinguishes this syndrome from Crigler-Najjar syndrome type I. This syndrome runs a more benign clinical course than does Crigler-Najjar syndrome type I, although several cases of bilirubin-induced brain damage in people with Arias syndrome have been reported. The most effective way of distinguishing this disorder from Crigler-Najjar type I is chromatographic analysis of pigments excreted in bile. In Crigler-Najjar syndrome type II, but not in type I, bile contains significant amounts of conjugated bilirubin, although the proportion of bilirubin monoglucuronide in bile is increased.

Gilbert syndrome. Gilbert syndrome, also called constitutional hepatic dysfunction or familial nonhemolytic jaundice, is the mildest form of inherited nonhemolytic unconjugated hyperbilirubinemia and is among the most common inherited disorders [11]. Serum bilirubin concentrations in persons with Gilbert syndrome generally range from 1 to 5 mg/dL. The serum bilirubin level of affected persons fluctuates with time and increases during fasting,

Table 89-1. Characteristics of BUGT Deficiency Syndromes

Parameters	Crigler-Najjar syndrome, type I	Crigler-Najjar syndrome, type II	Gilbert syndrome
Serum bilirubin	20–50 mg/dL	7–20 mg/dL (fluctuating)	1–5 mg/dL (fluctuating)
Routine LTs	Normal	Normal	Normal
Histology	Normal	Normal	Normal
BUGT activity	Absent	Markedly reduced	Reduced to 30% to 50%
Bile pigments	Traces of BMG and BDG	Increased BMG:BDG ratio	Increased BMG:BDG ratio
Phenobarbital	No effect	Reduces bilirubin by >25%	Jaundice disappears
Prevalence	Rare	Uncommon	Common (<5% of the population)
Age at diagnosis	1–3 d postnatal	Usually during first year	Usually early adulthood
Prognosis	Kernicterus, unless OLT	Kernicterus unusual	No neuropathy, benign

BMG/BDG—bilirubin mono/di glucuronides; LT—liver function test; OLT—orthotopic liver transplantation.

intercurrent illness, or emotional stress. A relationship to the menstrual cycle has also been reported. Gilbert syndrome affects 4% to 7% of the population, but because bilirubin levels fluctuate, its precise incidence is difficult to determine. Apart from mild jaundice, physical examination of people with Gilbert syndrome is normal. Hyperbilirubinemia is the only serum biochemical abnormality. Hepatic bilirubin-UGT activity is consistently decreased to approximately 30% of normal in individuals with Gilbert syndrome. Reduced transferase activity is reflected by an increased proportion of bilirubin monoconjugates in bile. Gilbert syndrome is more commonly diagnosed in boys after puberty than in girls. The apparent gender difference is probably due to the fact that daily bilirubin production is lower in women, and the residual bilirubin-UGT activity may be sufficient for excreting the daily bilirubin load. Gilbert syndrome is conventionally diagnosed in individuals with mild unconjugated hyperbilirubinemia without evidence of hemolysis or structural liver disease. Coexistent mild, compensated hemolysis, however, may increase serum bilirubin levels, thereby bringing affected people to the attention of the physician. Gilbert syndrome needs to be differentiated from other disorders associated with mild chronic hyperbilirubinemia. Mild acquired liver diseases (*eg*, mild chronic hepatitis), may cause predominantly unconjugated hyperbilirubinemia. Fasting and postprandial serum bile acid levels are increased in most acquired liver diseases, but not in inherited disorders of bilirubin metabolism. In some cases, liver biopsy may be required to rule out chronic hepatitis in people with unconjugated hyperbilirubinemia. In people with only a minimal elevation of serum bilirubin levels, differentiation from normal may be difficult. For these cases, two provocative tests, caloric deprivation and nicotinic acid administration, have been used. A significant number of false-positive and false-negative results, however, limits the value of these tests in patients with marginal elevation of serum bilirubin concentration. Recently, a promoter abnormality of the bilirubin-UGT$_1$ gene has been found to be associated with Gilbert syndrome [12•]. Although all subjects with this promoter abnormality do not have overt hyperbilirubinemia, this genetic analysis may be used as a screening test for Gilbert syndrome. Gilbert syndrome is thought to be harmless. Therefore, once the diagnosis is made, only reassurance is necessary.

Disorders Associated With Conjugated Hyperbilirubinemia

Acquired Disorders

Biliary obstruction. The differential diagnosis of biliary obstruction includes a wide spectrum of diseases, including cholelithiasis, intrinsic and extrinsic tumors, primary sclerosing cholangitis, parasitic infections, AIDS cholangiopathy, acute and chronic pancreatitis, and strictures after invasive procedures. In hepatobiliary obstruction, conjugated bile pigments and other contents of bile, including bile salts and alkaline phosphatase, regurgitate into the circulation through the junctions of hepatocyte plasma membranes that enclose bile canaliculi. Obstruction to outflow may cause some unconjugated bilirubin to leak from hepatocytes back into plasma. Thus, both unconjugated and conjugated bilirubin accumulate in serum in people with biliary obstruction.

Intrahepatic cholestasis. Cholestasis is the predominant manifestation of primary biliary cirrhosis and occasionally, viral hepatitis may present as a predominant cholestatic syndrome. Cholestasis also may be the outstanding feature of alcoholic hepatitis (see Chapters 96, 105, and 106).

Some drugs, including alkylated steroids (*eg*, methyltestosterone and ethynylestradiol) cause cholestasis in a dose-related fashion, while others, for example, chlorpromazine, cause idiosyncratic cholestasis in a minority of recipients. Cholestasis in patients with bacterial sepsis is multifactorial, resulting from hypotension, drugs, and bacterial endotoxins that may inhibit organic anion uptake. Granulomatous diseases (*eg*, sarcoidosis, tuberculosis) may lead to a mainly cholestatic picture. Steatosis, lipidosis, and cholestasis are frequently observed in patients receiving total parenteral nutrition (TPN), usually after 2 to 3 weeks of therapy. In certain circumstances, infiltrative liver diseases (*eg*, lymphoma) precipitate intrahepatic cholestasis and heart failure or hypotension. Thyrotoxicosis rarely is accompanied by intrahepatic cholestasis.

Cholestasis is common after bone marrow or liver transplantation not only because these patients are generally ill, receiving multiple drugs and possibly TPN, and are susceptible to infections, but also because of graft-versus-host disease and veno-occlusive disease of the liver as sequelae of intensive pretransplant radiotherapy and chemotherapy of the bone marrow recipients. After orthotopic liver transplantation, cholestasis may result from preservation injury of the donor liver or acute or chronic allograft rejection ("vanishing bile duct syndrome").

Cholestasis of pregnancy typically starts with pruritus in the third trimester or earlier, may result in clinical jaundice and may increase the risk of stillbirth. Delivery resolves all the pathologic changes.

The jaundice frequently observed in postoperative patients may result from increased bilirubin production (*eg*, from blood transfusions, hematoma resorption, hemolysis after heart surgery), or cholestasis resulting from infections, TPN, drugs (including general anesthetics), hypoxia, hypotension, or viral hepatitis. Concomitant renal failure will increase hyperbilirubinemia, as will Gilbert syndrome or a preexisting hemolytic disease.

Hepatocellular injury. There is a considerable overlap between disorders associated with predominant hepatocellular injury and cholestatic syndromes. Many of the latter can be accompanied by hepatocellular damage, and many of the former are associated with hyperbilirubinemia.

Inherited and Congenital Disorders

Neonatal cholestasis. Although neonatal cholestasis usually runs a benign course and is self-limited, some potentially life-threatening disorders may present as cholestasis during this period (see Chapter 173). Biliary obstruction may result from a choledochal cyst or biliary atresia. Early diagnosis and operation in the first few weeks of life are crucial to avoid the necessity of orthotopic liver transplantation. Sepsis and idiopathic neonatal hepatitis are important causes of prolonged intrahepatic cholestasis in the newborn. Byler's syndrome (progressive familial intrahepatic cholestasis), hereditary cholestasis with lymphedema, and cholestasis of North American Indians are familial and associated with giant cell formation in the livers of infants. Decrease of interlobular bile ducts as solitary lesions or in association with congenital malformations (Alagille syndrome) can cause intrahepatic cholestasis in neonates and infants.

A number of diseases affecting amino acid (*eg*, tyrosinemia), lipid (*eg*, Niemann-Pick, Gaucher, Wolman), or carbohydrate (*eg*, galactosemia, fructosemia, glycogenosis type IV) metabolism can cause neonatal cholestasis (see Chapter 178). The presentation of neonatal jaundice in cystic fibrosis may be similar to that of biliary atresia and often is associated with meconium ileus and bowel obstruction. Liver histology may resemble that seen in neonatal hepatitis (giant cells) or biliary atresia (bile plugs, bile duct proliferation, portal fibrosis). The classic amorphous eosinophilic material in the bile ductules is usually absent in neonates.

Dubin-Johnson syndrome and Rotor syndrome. In contrast to cholestasis, in which canalicular excretion of all organic anions, including bile salts, is decreased, inherited disorders of hepatic organic anion excretion cause an excretory abnormality that is limited to organic anions other than bile salts (Table 89-2). Other liver tests are normal in affected individuals. Because accumulation of conjugated bilirubin in plasma usually is associated with liver disease, correct diagnosis of these benign disorders is important from both a prognostic and management point of view [2••].

Dubin-Johnson syndrome is characterized by mild, predominantly conjugated hyperbilirubinemia and a black liver [13]. Dubin-Johnson syndrome is common (1 in 1300) in Persian Jews in whom it is associated with clotting factor VII deficiency, but it occurs in people of all races and both genders. This syndrome is inherited as an autosomal recessive trait. Affected individuals usually are asymptomatic, although mild complaints, for example, vague abdominal pain and weakness, occur occasionally. Because plasma bile salt levels are normal, pruritus is absent. Serum bilirubin levels usually range from 2 to 5 mg/dL. The syndrome may be initially detected during intercurrent illness, pregnancy, or use of oral contraceptives, which increase mild hyperbilirubinemia to a level at which jaundice becomes apparent. Except for jaundice, physical examination is normal, although hepatosplenomegaly rarely has been reported. Dubin-Johnson syndrome usually is detected after puberty, although cases have been reported in neonates. Macroscopically, the liver is black. Liver histology is

normal except for accumulation of a melanin-related pigment; the degree of hepatic pigmentation varies. During attacks of coincidental diseases, such as acute viral hepatitis, the pigment is cleared from the liver and reaccumulates slowly after recovery.

The mutation in Dubin-Johnson syndrome affects canalicular excretion of many organic anions, except bile salts, probably because of an abnormality of the multispecific organic anion transporter. Therefore, plasma bile salt levels are normal in affected individuals and there is no pruritus. Lack of excretion of cholecystographic contrast agents results in nonopacification of the gallbladder. Because the uptake of organic anions is normal, plasma bromosulphophthalein levels 45 minutes after an intravenous injection are normal, but a second peak appears after 90 minutes because of regurgitation of the dye initially taken up by hepatocytes.

Another curious abnormality found in people with Dubin-Johnson syndrome involves urinary porphyrin excretion. Total urinary coproporphyrinogen excretion is normal, but the proportion of isomer I is over 80% (normally isomer III is the predominant form in urine). This pattern is highly characteristic of Dubin-Johnson syndrome and is useful in its diagnosis.

Rotor syndrome also is characterized by chronic, mild, predominantly conjugated hyperbilirubinemia; physical examination and routine liver tests in affected people are otherwise normal [14]. This rare benign disorder is recessively inherited and is distinct from Dubin-Johnson syndrome. Rotor syndrome is thought to result from an abnormality of hepatic storage, rather than one of canalicular excretion. Unlike Dubin-Johnson syndrome, the liver in Rotor syndrome is not hyperpigmented, and there is no secondary rise in plasma bromosulphophthalein levels after an intravenous injection of the dye. Oral cholecystography usually opacifies the gallbladder. Total urinary coproporphyrin excretion is increased by 250% to 500% over normal in patients with Rotor syndrome, and the proportion of coproporphyrin I in urine is approximately 65% of the total. These features differentiate this disorder from Dubin-Johnson syndrome.

Benign recurrent intrahepatic cholestasis. Usually after a preicteric phase of 2 to 4 weeks with malaise, anorexia, and

Table 89-2. Characteristics of Inherited Disorders of Organic Anion Excretion

Parameters	Dubin-Johnson syndrome	Rotor syndrome
Serum bilirubin	2–5 (-20) mg/dL (~60% conjugated)	2–5 (-20) mg/dL (~60% conjugated)
Routine LFTs	Normal	Normal
Histology	Dark pigment, centrilobular	Normal
Plasma BSP retention (45 min)	Normal or slightly elevated, secondary rise at 90 min	Elevated, no secondary rise at 90 min
BSP infusion studies	T_{max} reduced to 10% S normal	T_{max} reduced to 50%, S reduced to 10% to 25%
Oral cholecystogram	Gallbladder usually not visualized	Gallbladder usually visualized
Urinary coproporphyrin	Normal total > 80% as coproporphyrin I	Elevated total Elevated coproporphyrin I, but < 80%
Mode of inheritance	Autosomal recessive	Autosomal recessive
Prevalence	Uncommon (1:1300) in Persian Jews)	Rare
Prognosis	Benign (occasionally hepatosplenomegaly)	Benign

BSP—bromsulphalein; LFT—liver function test; S—hepatic storage capacity; T_{max}—transport maximum.

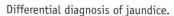

Differential diagnosis of jaundice.

Figure 89-4

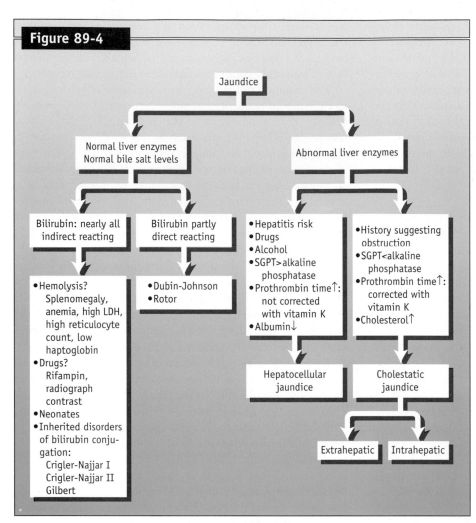

pruritus, affected patients become jaundiced and may have tender hepatomegaly without fever. The attacks, clinically suggestive of biliary obstruction, last from several weeks to several months, accompanied by malabsorption and weight loss secondary to steatorrhea, which may require parenteral administration of fat-soluble vitamins. Episodes in a given patient resemble each other in duration and symptoms. Intervals between attacks range from months to years; there are no abnormalities in these patients between episodes. The onset of symptoms is usually in adolescence or early adulthood, although earlier and later presentations have been described. This disorder clearly is familial, but its mode of inheritance has not yet been documented [15].

Laboratory tests. Serum bile acids, alkaline phosphatase, and conjugated bilirubin all increase to abnormal levels in people with benign recurrent intrahepatic cholestasis. Serum aminotransferases may be mildly elevated. Malabsorption of vitamin K can result in an abnormal prothrombin time. During cholestatic attacks, unconjugated serum bilirubin concentration is normal, whereas serum conjugated bilirubin levels are elevated due to reflux from the hepatocyte. Light and electron microscopy reveal features typical of intrahepatic cholestasis during acute episodes, and are normal between attacks. The pathogenesis of this disorder is unknown. A specific treatment to prevent or shorten cholestatic episodes is currently not available.

DIFFERENTIAL DIAGNOSIS OF JAUNDICE

The initial clinical approach to the icteric patient is outlined in Figure 89-4. It must be emphasized that in many cases jaundice is caused by a variety of coexisting factors. As briefly discussed previously, especially after general surgery, organ transplantation, during TPN, and in AIDS patients, jaundice frequently can only be explained as a result of multiple concomitant disorders. The underlying illness, the type of therapy administered (drugs, surgery), and the possible resulting complications must be taken in account when evaluating these patients.

REFERENCES

Recently published papers of particular interest have been highlighted as follows:
•   Of interest
••   Of outstanding interest

1.   Itho S, Onishi S: Kinetic study of the photochemical changes of (ZZ)-bilirubin IXa bound to human serum albumin: demonstration of (EZ)-bilirubin IXa as an intermediate in photochemical changes from (ZZ)-bilirubin IXa to (EZ)-cyclobilirubin Ixa. *Biochem J* 1985, 226:251.

2.••   Roy Chowdhury J, Jansen PLM: Metabolism of bilirubin. In *Hepatology: A Textbook of Liver Disease*, edn 3. Edited by Zakim D, Boyer TD. Philadelphia: W.B. Saunders; 1996:323–347.
This is a comprehensive review of bilirubin metabolism, and the molecular basis and clinical manifestations of its disorders.

3.•   Weiss JS, Gautam AJJ, Lauff MW, *et al.*: The clinical importance of a protein-bound fraction of serum bilirubin in patients with hyperbilirubinemia. *N Engl J Med* 1983, 309:147–150.
This paper describes the bilirubin-albumin adduct (delta-bilirubin) and its clinical importance.

4. Turkel SB, Miller CA, Guttenberg ME, *et al.*: A clinical pathologic reappraisal of kernicterus. *Pediatrics* 1982, 69:267.

5.• Lee KS, Gartner LM: Management of unconjugated hyperbilirubinemia in the newborn. *Semin Liver Dis* 1983, 3:52.
Unconjugated hyperbilirubinemia occurs very frequently in the newborn. This paper describes the management of unconjugated hyperbilirubinemia in pathologic conditions.

6.• Jansen PLM, Bosma PJ, Roy Chowdhury J: Molecular biology of bilirubin metabolism. *In Progress in Liver Diseases*, vol XIII. Edited by Boyer JL, Ockner RK. Philadelphia: W.B. Saunders; 1995:125–150.
This is a review of bilirubin glucuronidation and molecular bases of its disorders.

7. Crawford JM, Gollan JL: Bilirubin metabolism and the pathophysiology of jaundice. In *Diseases of the Liver*, edn 7. Edited by Schiff L, Schiff E. Philadelphia: J.B. Lippincott; 1993:53.

8. Roy Chowdhury J, Roy Chowdhury N: Physiology and disorders of bilirubin metabolism. In *Liver and Biliary Diseases*, edn 2. Edited by Kaplowitz N. Baltimore: Williams and Wilkins; 1995:153–170.

9. Crigler JF, Najjar VA: Congenital familial non-hemolytic jaundice with kernicterus. *Pediatrics* 1952, 10:169.

10. Bosma PJ, Roy Chowdhury N, Goldhoorn BG, *et al.*: Sequence of exons and the flanking regions of human bilirubin-UDP-glucuronosyl-transferase gene complex and identification of a genetic mutation in a patient with Crigler-Najjar syndrome, Type I. *Hepatology* 1992, 15:941.

11. Gilbert A, Lereboullet P: La cholamae simple familiale. *Semin Med* 1901, 21:241.

12.• Bosma PJ, Roy Chowdhury J, Bakker C, *et al.*: A sequence abnormality in the promoter region results in reduced expression of bilirubin UGT1 in Gilbert's syndrome. *N Engl J Med* 1995, 333:1171.
This paper sheds light for the first time on the possible molecular basis of one of the most common inherited disorders.

13. Dubin IN, Johnson FB: Chronic idiopathic jaundice with unidentified pigment in liver cells: a new clinocopathologic entity with a report of 12 cases. *Medicine* 1954, 33:155.

14. Rotor AB, Manahan L, Florentin A: Familial nonhemolytic jaundice with direct van den Bergh reaction. *Acta Med Phil* 1948, 5:37.

15. Summerskill WHJ, Walshe JM: Benign recurrent intrahepatic obstructive jaundice. *Lancet* 1959, 2:686.

90 Morphologic Patterns of Liver Injury
Maria Guido and Swan N. Thung

The work of pathologists and clinicians is closely intertwined, and the importance of cooperation between these two groups of physicians has been frequently emphasized in patient care. One of the most important aspects of cooperation between clinicians and pathologists is a shared terminology. For this purpose, a description of the morphologic changes seen in the most common liver diseases is provided in this chapter, which should be considered a tool box in which internists, gastroenterologists, and pathologists may find appropriate instruments to do their daily work. Readers may refer to other chapters in this section for other examples of histopathologic illustrations of liver disorders.

ACUTE HEPATITIS

Parenchymal changes seen in acute hepatitis are damage to the hepatocytes and infiltration by mononuclear inflammatory cells, predominantly lymphocytes, plasma cells, and macrophages [1]. Hepatocellular injury in patients with acute hepatitis takes two forms: ballooning and acidophilic degeneration or apoptosis.

Hepatocytes with ballooning degeneration are swollen (Fig. 90-1); their cytoplasm is enlarged and pale staining. Cells that undergo ballooning degeneration rupture easily and trigger an inflammatory response. The term focal necrosis describes this inflammatory response in an area where a single or small number of hepatocytes have been lost. Kupffer cells are enlarged and form clusters containing periodic acid–Schiff (PAS)–positive, diastase-resistant cellular debris.

Hepatocytes undergoing *acidophilic degeneration* are shrunken and have deeply acidophilic cytoplasm (Fig. 90-2). The nuclei are often pyknotic or show margination of chromatin along the nuclear membrane. These cells, called *acidophilic* or *apoptotic bodies*, eventually are rounded up and extruded from the liver cell plates into the sinusoids. *Apoptosis* in hepatitis is cell death mediated by cytotoxic T lymphocytes. The cytotoxic T lymphocytes kill hepatocytes by injecting them with proteases that induce apoptosis or through induction of cytokines, including tumor necrosis factor-α and interferon-γ. Syncytial giant hepatocytes often are observed in infants with neonatal hepatitis and are less commonly seen in adults. Characteristically, the necroinflammatory lesions in acute hepatitis are spotty throughout the lobules (*ie*, spotty necrosis). In more severe disease, the area of necrosis may bridge central to central or portal to central regions (*ie*, bridging necrosis) (Fig. 90-3), may involve large portions of the

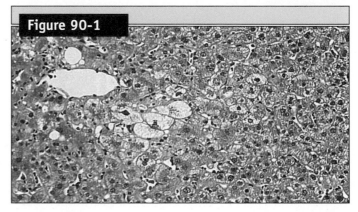

Figure 90-1

Enlarged, ballooned hepatocytes with pale cytoplasm (hematoxylin and eosin stain × 100).

lobules (*ie*, submassive necrosis), or may involve several adjacent lobules (*ie*, massive necrosis) (Fig. 90-4).

Surviving hepatocytes regenerate. These regenerating cells are seen as small hepatocytes arranged in two-cell-thick plates. In massive necrosis, regeneration occurs in the form of ductular hepatocytes. Although the parenchymal lesions are the most characteristic changes in acute hepatitis, portal tract involvement by inflammation, predominantly of lymphocytes and macrophages, always is seen.

The morphologic features of acute hepatitis caused by hepatotropic viruses A, B, C, D, and E are indistinguishable, except for cholestasis, which is seen more frequently in acute hepatitis A and E [2].

CHRONIC HEPATITIS

The parenchymal lesions in chronic hepatitis are usually less severe than those in acute hepatitis, but portal and periportal inflammation and fibrosis are more prominent [3]. There is a predominantly mononuclear inflammatory cell infiltrate in portal tracts, which may be associated with various degrees of piecemeal necrosis, bile duct damage, and portal fibrosis. Dense lymphocytic aggregates or lymphoid follicles may form. Hepatocellular damage and necrosis may involve individual hepatocytes or small or large groups of hepatocytes. The degree of inflammatory cell infiltration in the lobules varies. The sinusoidal lining cells are usually prominent (*ie*, sinusoidal activation). Marked piecemeal necrosis and bridging necrosis, defined as confluent necrosis linking vascular structures in the hepatic parenchyma, are features of severe disease that may progress to cirrhosis.

Portal fibrosis and formation of fibrous septa indicate disease progression. Erosion of the limiting plate, called *piecemeal necrosis* (*ie*, interface hepatitis), is followed by the formation of tonguelike septa extending into the lobular parenchyma or connecting adjacent portal tracts. Fibrosis in areas of bridging necrosis produces septa that link centrolobular region and portal tracts. The ongoing necroinflammatory activity, fibrosis, and hepatocellular regeneration produce gradual architectural distortion, resulting first in incomplete nodular transformation (*ie*, transition to cirrhosis) and, later, in cirrhosis.

In most cases, the cause of chronic hepatitis cannot be deduced with certainty from the histologic findings. The identification of "ground-glass" hepatocytes denotes chronic hepatitis B. The characteristic appearance of these cells results from cytoplasmic accumulation of hepatitis B surface antigen (HBsAg) in smooth endoplasmic reticulum. "Sanded nuclei" in hepatocytes suggest the presence of hepatitis B core antigen (HBcAg). HBsAg can be demonstrated with histochemical (*eg*, Shikata's orcein, Victoria blue) or with immunohistochemical staining methods. HBcAg also can be detected by immunohistochemistry. Routine application of immunohistochemical stains [4••] to determine the viral replicative state is advocated for biopsy specimens from patients with hepatitis B virus infection.

The triad of dense lymphoid aggregates or lymphoid follicles in portal tracts, bile duct damage, and mild steatosis strongly suggests hepatitis C virus infection [5,6]. Autoimmune hepatitis often is associated with severe necroinflammatory activity, marked piecemeal necrosis (*ie*, interface hepatitis) and bridging necrosis, and a prominent plasma cellular component in the inflammatory infiltrate [7].

A new classification of chronic hepatitis employs all clinical, etiologic, and histologic information available and recommends that the final diagnosis include the cause, grade, and stage of disease [8••]. Grading is a measure of necroinflammatory activity, and staging is a measure of the extent of fibrosis and disease progression.

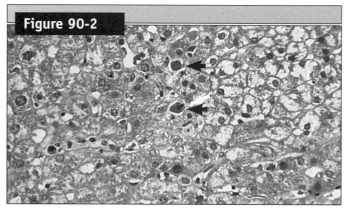

Figure 90-2

Acute viral hepatitis. Scattered hepatocytes are undergoing acidophilic degeneration (*arrows*) (hematoxylin and eosin stain × 250).

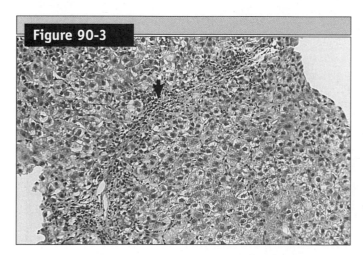

Figure 90-3

Hepatitis with linear, bridging necrosis (*arrow*) (hematoxylin and eosin stain × 100).

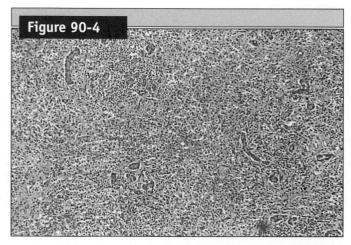

Figure 90-4

Massive necrosis involves several adjacent lobules (hematoxylin and eosin stain ×40).

HEPATITIS CAUSED BY NONHEPATOTROPIC VIRUSES

The characteristic features of hepatitis caused by nonhepatotropic viruses are areas of *"punched-out" focal necrosis* that are nonzonal. The inflammatory cells in the necrotic areas consist predominantly of polymorphonuclear cells. Unlike acute hepatitis caused by hepatotropic viruses, diffuse hepatocellular damage is mild or absent, and hepatocytes usually appear normal; sinusoidal lining cells are enlarged, and mononuclear inflammatory cells infiltrate the portal tracts and sinusoidal lumen but usually are not in contact with hepatocytes. Viral inclusions may be observed in the nucleus or cytoplasm of adjacent hepatocytes. Cytomegalic cells with characteristic nuclear or cytoplasmic inclusions in hepatocytes, bile duct cells, and Kupffer cells or endothelial cells are characteristic of cytomegalovirus hepatitis [9].

Microabscesses, which represent well-circumscribed clusters of polymorphonuclear cells replacing necrotic hepatocytes, also are characteristic of cytomegalovirus hepatitis. In adenovirus infections, the typical "blueberry" basophilic intranuclear inclusions may be seen, and in herpes simplex, varicella, and varicella-zoster virus infections, the intranuclear inclusions (*ie*, Cowdry type A and B) may be observed. Punched-out focal necrosis may become confluent, leading to massive hepatic necrosis.

ALCOHOLIC HEPATITIS AND STEATOHEPATITIS

Alcoholic hepatitis is defined as alcohol-induced hepatocellular injury and inflammation, usually accompanied by fibrosis. Hepatocytes in this area are ballooned, and some of them contain *Mallory hyalin* in their cytoplasm and are surrounded by polymorphonuclear leukocytes, forming classic Mallory bodies (Fig. 90-5). Alcoholic hyalin represents eosinophilic clumped or skeinlike perinuclear material composed largely of intermediate filaments of cytokeratin type. Steatosis, which is often present, is predominantly macrovesicular. The severity of alcoholic hepatitis ranges from a few foci of hepatocellular injury and inflammation with rare Mallory bodies to extensive hepatocellular necrosis. Characteristically, the pathologic changes predominate in the centrolobular areas (zone 3). This centrolobular hepatocyte injury gives rise to central hyalin sclerosis and chicken-wire–like pericellular fibrosis (Fig. 90-6). Progressive sclerosis may lead to compression of central venules or complete obliteration of their lumens by intimal fibrosis, so-called phlebitis, or veno-occlusive lesions. In more advanced cases, broad and fibrous septa extend from centrolobular areas to adjacent venules or portal tracts. This pattern contrasts with that of chronic hepatitis, in which fibrosis starts in portal and periportal regions. *Steatosis* of various degrees that is predominantly macrovesicular may be observed in alcoholic liver injury in the absence of alcoholic hepatitis.

Similar changes in the absence of a history of alcoholism can be seen in patients with adult-onset diabetes mellitus, obesity (which is usually truncal and may be mild), jejunoileal bypass, gastrointestinal and pancreatic disorders, extensive bowel resection, total parenteral nutrition, Wilson's disease, and with exposure to certain drugs, such as amiodarone, nifedipine, perhexiline maleate, glucocorticoids, and estrogens. This condition is called *nonalcoholic steatohepatitis* [10•]. Steatosis varies from mild to severe and is mainly macrovesicular. Overall, there is more fat and less hepatocellular damage, hyalin, inflammation, and fibrosis than in alcoholic hepatitis. Typical Mallory hyalin is often difficult to find, except in Wilson's disease and with liver damage from exposure to antiarrhythmic drugs such as amiodarone and perhexiline maleate.

HEPATIC GRANULOMAS

A granuloma is a focal accumulation of epithelioid cells, which are modified cells of the mononuclear phagocyte system. A number of lymphocytes usually is associated with the granuloma, and other cells, including eosinophils, plasma cells, and fibroblasts, may be found. Giant cells (probably derived from the fusion of epithelioid cells) may be present. A wide range of diseases may be associated with the presence of hepatic granulomas [11]. Granulomas are found in portal tracts and in lobular parenchyma, often in the perivenular zone.

The morphology of the granuloma helps little in determining the cause. Giant cells of the Langerhans type and of caseous necrosis are typical of tuberculosis. Tuberculosis granulomas typ-

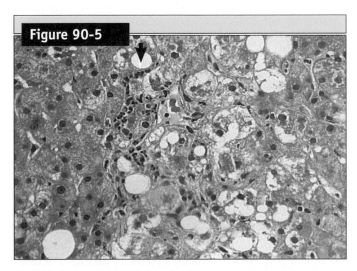

Figure 90-5

Alcoholic hepatitis with Mallory hyalins (*arrow*) in centrolobular hepatocytes (hematoxylin and eosin stain × 250).

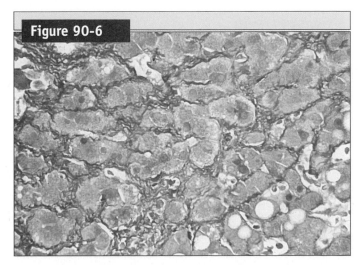

Figure 90-6

Central hyalin sclerosis and chicken-wire–like pericellular fibrosis in chronic alcoholic liver injury (trichrome stain × 250).

ically are located in portal tracts and parenchyma. Exogenous material in the cytoplasm of giant cells is seen in a foreign body reaction. Calcified intracytoplasmic inclusions, known as Schaumann bodies, have been described in sarcoidosis, but they are not pathognomonic. Sarcoid granulomas are typically non-caseating, multiple, and coalescent and show a preferential localization in the portal tracts. Lipogranulomas are seen in steatosis and consist of accumulation of fat droplets, macrophages, a few lymphocytes, and rare eosinophils. The cause of hepatic granulomas is unknown in approximately 30% of cases.

LIVER CIRRHOSIS

Cirrhosis is the irreversible end stage of most chronic liver diseases. Regardless the cause, cirrhosis is defined as transformation of the normal architecture of the entire liver into parenchymal nodules consisting of regenerating hepatocytes surrounded by fibrous septa (Fig. 90-7). This architectural disturbance is responsible for vascular anomalies that lead to portal hypertension and to metabolic abnormalities that characterize the clinical picture of cirrhosis.

Fibrosis and nodules are not always indicative of cirrhosis, because they may occur in other diseases. *Congenital hepatic fibrosis* is characterized by fibrous septa formation associated with some nodules, which lack regeneration, in a context of otherwise normal parenchyma. In *regenerative nodular hyperplasia*, regenerating nodular transformation of liver tissue is not accompanied by fibrous septa. *Nodular focal hyperplasia* is a benign, usually focal, process that can be misinterpreted as cirrhosis if only small samples are histologically examined.

Grossly, cirrhosis is classified as micronodular or macronodular, according to whether parenchymal nodules are smaller or larger than 3 mm in diameter, respectively. Nodules more than 8 to 10 mm in diameter are defined as macroregenerative nodules. Micronodular cirrhosis often is related to alcohol abuse, and macronodular disease is related to chronic viral hepatitis.

Histologically, fibrous septa may be of various thicknesses and may contain any number of inflammatory cells, proliferating ductules, and vascular structures. Patterns of inflammation reflect the cause of the cirrhosis. Parenchymal nodules are formed by regenerating hepatocytes, usually arranged in plates. Nodular

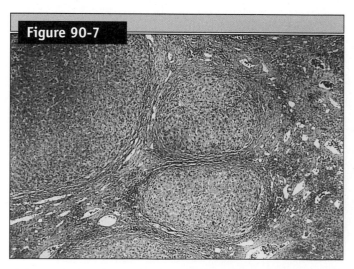

Figure 90-7

Cirrhosis with nodules separated by fibrous septa (hematoxylin and eosin stain × 40).

parenchyma may demonstrate degenerative, necrotic, and inflammatory changes, which reflect the cause of the cirrhosis. Active cirrhosis is identified by necroinflammatory lesions at the septal-parenchymal interface and in the nodules. Fully established, inactive cirrhosis usually lacks histologic findings indicative of the cause, which can only be inferred from the clinical background.

The pathogenesis of cirrhosis is incompletely understood. Hepatocellular degeneration and necrosis are the stimulus for fibrogenesis and regeneration in most cases. Regardless of the type of underlying diseases, hepatic stellate cells (*ie*, fat-storing cells or Ito cells) are the most important cell type producing collagen [12].

CHOLESTASIS

Cholestasis is defined morphologically as the microscopic accumulation of bile and its components in liver tissue, which is caused by anomalies of bile flow. According to its pathogenesis, cholestasis is classified as extrahepatic or intrahepatic.

Several findings are characteristic of cholestasis. *Bilirubinostasis* consists of fine granules of bilirubin in the hepatocyte cytoplasm and of coarse granules or plugs in the intercellular spaces, typically in acinar zone 3. Bilirubin appears dark green or brownish on hematoxylin-eosin–stained sections. Extension of bilirubinostasis to zones 2 and 1 is observed only in severe or chronic forms of cholestasis. The association between bilirubinostasis and clinical and biochemical signs of cholestasis is not constant, particularly in the early phase of incomplete bile duct obstruction. Ultrastructural examination may be useful in such cases, showing a typical pattern of canalicular changes even in the absence of bile deposition.

Cholate stasis is hydropic swelling of periportal hepatocytes, which appear as large, pale cells containing coarse, perinuclear granules of remaining cytoplasm or Mallory bodies. Cholate stasis is a sign of cholestasis of longer duration.

Feathery degeneration typically is observed in hepatocytes adjacent to bile thrombi or concretions. It consists of rarefaction of the cytoplasm that precedes lytic necrosis of the cells, which eventually are replaced by inflammatory cells. When feathery degeneration and subsequent necrosis occur in a large group of adjacent hepatocytes, the lesion is called *bile infarction*. Large bile infarcts typically are observed in mechanical obstruction of extrahepatic bile ducts.

Extrahepatic Cholestasis

Extrahepatic cholestasis is caused by complete or partial mechanical obstruction of large bile ducts outside the liver or at the porta hepatis. The main causes of extrahepatic cholestasis include lithiasis, tumors of the bile duct system, atresia or choledochal cyst, and strictures after surgery.

The histologic picture of extrahepatic cholestasis is related to the duration of obstruction. The earliest lesion is represented by zone 3 bilirubinostasis, which may be associated with focal liver cell necrosis. When cholestasis continues, bilirubinostasis extends through all three acinar zones, and mononuclear intrasinusoidal inflammation associated with pigment-laden macrophages develops in the acinar parenchyma and portal tracts. The pigment is bilirubin, lipofuscin, and lipid derived from phagocytosis of necrotic cells. Portal tracts appear edematous, causing a concentric appearance of connective tissue fibers around bile ducts. At the periphery of portal tracts, an increasing number of bile ductules becomes evident, associated with an inflammatory infiltrate of polymorphonuclear cells, an appearance called *ductular reaction*, that reflects a response to the irritative action of bile [13].

In long-standing cholestasis, feathery degeneration, biliary infarcts, and xanthomatous cells (*ie*, foamy histiocytes), single or in small groups, may be seen. Cholate stasis is usually evident in periportal zones. The association of cholate stasis with ductular proliferation and polymorphonuclear cells gives the appearance of limiting plate disruption, called *biliary piecemeal necrosis*. The tubular arrangement of hepatocytes around dilated bile canaliculi (*ie*, pseudorosette) also may be a prominent aspect of chronic cholestasis. If the cause of obstruction is not removed, portal fibrosis develops with fibrous septa formation (*ie*, biliary fibrosis), eventually progressing to cirrhosis (*ie*, secondary biliary cirrhosis).

Large bile duct obstruction must be differentiated from sepsis, drug reactions, cholestatic viral hepatitis, and acute transplant rejection. These distinctions may be histologically difficult and impossible in some cases, such as drug-induced cholestasis and viral cholestatic hepatitis.

Intrahepatic Cholestasis

Intrahepatic cholestasis usually is regarded as synonymous with functional or metabolic cholestasis and is related to alterations of hepatocytes and bile canaliculi (*ie*, intrahepatic, intra-acinar cholestasis) or to damage of intrahepatic bile ducts (*ie*, intrahepatic, extra-acinar cholestasis) [14•]. This distinction is not rigorous, because both mechanisms may be recognized in some cholestatic diseases. In some disorders, distinction between extrahepatic and intrahepatic cholestasis is impossible, because the entire biliary tree may be involved in the pathologic process.

Intrahepatic cholestasis is characterized pathologically by different combinations of the classic cholestatic changes, with bilirubinostasis of acinar zone 3 representing the earliest lesions. In some infantile forms, giant cell transformation of hepatocytes is a prominent aspect (*eg*, Byler's disease, North American Indian cholestasis). Cirrhosis represents the end stage of disease in some cases (*eg*, Byler's disease). The histologic appearance of intrahepatic obstruction may be indistinguishable from that observed in extrahepatic obstruction.

■ PRIMARY BILIARY CIRRHOSIS AND SCLEROSING CHOLANGITIS

Primary Biliary Cirrhosis

Primary biliary cirrhosis (PBC) is a nonsuppurative, destructive cholangitis of small intrahepatic bile ducts that leads to parenchymal changes and fibrous septum formation, eventually evolving into cirrhosis. The name is correctly applied only to the late, terminal stage of the disease. Morphologically, PBC progresses through four stages that reflect sequential portal tract changes. Because of the focal and segmental character of damage, there is considerable overlap between stages, and lesions characteristic of different stages may be observed in the same biopsy. Histologic stages correlate poorly with clinical and biochemical symptoms.

The change typical of stage 1 PBC, "florid" duct lesion, is a mixed inflammatory or granulomatous infiltrate of portal tracts around small and medium-sized bile ducts whose epithelia

appears irregular and multistratified. Inflammatory cells, mostly CD4 and CD8 T lymphocytes, infiltrate the epithelium, with focal breaks in the basement membrane [15•]. Biliary epithelial cells show degenerative changes and necrosis (Fig. 90-8). With progression of disease, there is bile duct loss. At this stage, parenchymal changes are usually mild and consist of small epithelioid granulomas (about 25% of cases), focal lymphocytic infiltration, and Kupffer cell hyperplasia, with no or minimal necrosis. Because of the segmental nature of disease, pathologists and clinicians should be aware that early-stage lesions of the small ducts may be missed by needle biopsy, but this does not exclude the diagnosis of PBC.

Stage 2 PBC is the stage of ductular proliferation at the periphery of portal tracts, which appear widened. Proliferating ductules are accompanied by polymorphonuclear cells. Bile ducts are reduced in number.

In stage 3, the scarring stage, there is fibrous expansion of portal tracts with fibrous septum formation. Most small bile ducts are no longer identifiable.

Stage 4 PBC is the true cirrhotic stage. Cirrhosis is predominantly micronodular, and fibrous septa usually are hypocellular. Erosion of the limiting plate damage usually is observed in the late stages of PBC and appears as *biliary piecemeal necrosis*, characterized by disruption of the limiting plate from ductular reaction, cholate stasis, and inflammation (in which polymorphonuclear cells predominate), or as *fibrous piecemeal necrosis*, observed at the edge of fibrous septa and characterized by loose connective tissue extending into the disrupted limiting plate. *Lymphocytic piecemeal necrosis*, mediated by immune mechanisms, similar to that observed in chronic active hepatitis, also may be detected.

In its earlier stages, PBC must be morphologically differentiated from chronic hepatitis, Wilson's disease, drug-induced hepatitis, and primary sclerosing cholangitis (PSC). Differentiation from chronic hepatitis and PSC may be extremely difficult on the basis of histology alone.

The term *autoimmune cholangitis* defines cases with the pathologic picture of PBC in antimitochondrial antibody (AMA)–negative patients with high titers of serum antinuclear

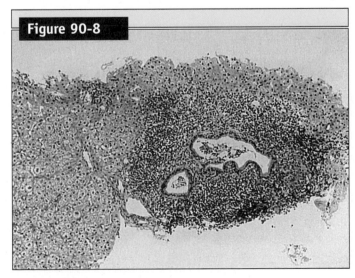

Figure 90-8

Florid duct lesion in primary biliary cirrhosis, stage 1 (hematoxylin and eosin stain × 40).

antibodies (ANA). These cases are regarded as variants of PBC [16••].

Primary Sclerosing Cholangitis

The basic pathology of PSC is represented by a fibroinflammation of biliary ducts. The extrahepatic biliary tree primarily is affected, but as the disease progresses, all segments become involved. When only the intrahepatic bile ducts are affected, the condition is called *small duct primary sclerosing cholangitis*. Differentiation from secondary sclerosing cholangitis is based on the exclusion of known causes of biliary obstruction, including choledocholithiasis, cholangiocarcinoma, and biliary surgery.

The histologic lesion diagnostic of PSC is a periductal, concentric, "onion-skin," fibrosis of medium- and large-sized ducts associated with degeneration of the epithelial lining, eventually progressing to complete obliteration and disappearance of the ducts (Fig. 90-9). Similar to PBC, four progressive morphologic stages are described for PSC.

Histologically, PSC must be differentiated from large bile duct obstruction, chronic hepatitis, cholangiopathy of acquired immunodeficiency syndrome (AIDS), and PBC. Differentiation from PBC may be impossible on morphologic grounds alone.

■ IRON OVERLOAD

Liver is the major storage site of excess iron [17]. With hematoxylin and eosin stain, iron appears as refractile, coarse, brownish granules predominately located in zone 1. Reliable and easy identification of iron is accomplished using the Perls' method. With this stain, ferritin iron appears as a diffuse bluish stain in the cytoplasm or as coarser, intense blue granules when ferritin and hemosiderin are stored together in pericanalicular siderosomes. When assessing hepatic iron content on liver biopsy, the amount and cellular distribution must be considered.

Hepatic iron content is graded from 0 to 4, according to the ease with which iron is seen at different magnifications. This method has shown good interobserver reproducibility and correlates with tissue iron levels evaluated by chemical methods. It is useful for routine diagnostic purposes. Grade 0 or 1 corresponds to a normal iron value (about 5 to 40 mmol/g dry

weight); grade 2 reflects a mild increase, and grades 3 and 4 correspond to severe iron deposition (about 130 to 850 mmol/g dry weight) [18]. For special studies, a finer grading system may be used that semiquantitatively scores iron deposition in Kupffer cells, hepatocytes, and connective tissue separately [19].

Genetic Hemochromatosis

Morphologic examination of the liver in genetic hemochromatosis reveals iron accumulation in hepatocytes, Kupffer cells, and biliary epithelium. In the early stages of genetic hemochromatosis, only periportal hepatocytes are involved, and in later stages, all zones are involved along with nonparenchymal cells. When iron deposition increases, portal tract fibrosis occurs, followed by fibrous septum formation that evolves into micronodular cirrhosis. Necrotic or inflammatory changes are not observed in patients with this disease [20].

Early-stage genetic hemochromatosis in a young homozygotic person must be differentiated from a similar pattern of siderosis observed in about 25% of heterozygotes. In heterozygotes, iron deposition does not increase with age, and massive deposition is not observed.

The pathogenic mechanism of iron toxicity is not clear [21]. It has been suggested that fibrosis occurs after deposition of iron in Kupffer cells because of phagocytosis of necrotic iron-loaded hepatocytes. This process has been called *sideronecrosis*. Cellular necrosis is a rare event in hemochromatosis.

Other Causes of Iron Overload

Iron overload in patients with chronic anemia is a consequence of repeated transfusions. Hepatic abnormalities in such cases may resemble those of genetic hemochromatosis, but a large amount of iron is evident in Kupffer cells, and clusters of iron-loaded macrophages are easily identified in parenchyma and in portal tracts. There is heavy deposition of iron in Kupffer cells in zone 3. Cirrhosis is rare in these patients.

Severe hepatic iron overload with prevalent hepatocytic localization and associated with fibrosis or cirrhosis rarely has been observed in cases of β-thalassemia minor, hereditary spherocytosis, and sideroblastic anemia. Other disorders in which stainable hepatic iron may be detected include alcoholic liver disease, viral hepatitis, porphyria cutanea tarda, portocaval shunts, and ceruloplasmin deficiency. The pathogenesis and clinical significance of these deposits are unclear. Iron deposition is usually mild in these cases, and excessive siderosis should raise a suspicion of genetic hemochromatosis. In chronic hepatitis C, stainable iron may be observed in hepatocytes and in reticuloendothelial cells.

■ VASCULAR DISORDERS

Vascular disorders of the liver are described according to the main site of the circulatory defect.

Portal Veins

The morphologic consequences of portal vein occlusion are related to the type of obstruction. When the portal trunk or large portal veins are completely and rapidly obstructed, there is passive congestion of the abdominal organs, and death occurs. When obstruction is incomplete or occurs slowly with collateral

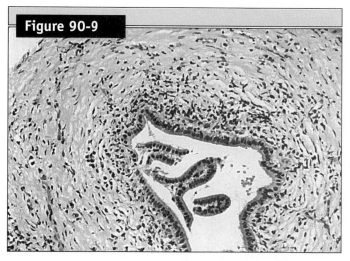

Figure 90-9

Periductal fibroinflammatory lesion in primary sclerosing cholangitis (hematoxylin and eosin stain × 100).

channel formation, the liver may appear morphologically normal. Acute occlusion of small intrahepatic portal veins, as seen in neoplastic thrombosis, leads to a *pseudo-infarct of Zahn*, a clinically silent lesion often discovered at autopsy [27]. Macroscopic examination of the liver in these cases reveals a dark red, triangular area below the capsule, and it is histologically characterized by severe centrilobular sinusoidal congestion.

Hepatic Arteries

Ischemic necrosis [22] is the pathologic consequence of arterial obstruction. Lesions may be focal or involve the entire organ, according to the site and the rapidity of arterial obstruction. Because of the double hepatic supply and the wide collateral circulation provided by multiple branches of the hepatic artery, zone 3 necrosis is more common than infarction. Histologically, zone 3 necrosis appears as a sharp centrilobular area of coagulated hepatocytes that retains its normal lobular architecture (Fig. 90-10). Inflammation is not present in earlier lesions. In advanced lesions, there is lysis of hepatocytes and phagocytosis by macrophages. Neutrophils also are seen, and portal tracts may contain polymorphic inflammation. If the damage is not extensive and the patient survives, it may lead to centrilobular and sinusoidal scarring or, more commonly, complete resolution. Infarction is characterized by confluent areas of ischemic, coagulative necrosis [22].

Hepatic Veins

Hepatic venous outflow obstruction is responsible for *hepatic congestion*. Budd-Chiari syndrome is the classic example of this abnormality. The liver appears macroscopically enlarged and dark red. Histologically, there is marked congestion and dilation of sinusoids in zones 3 and 2, with erythrocytes infiltrating the spaces of Disse. As a consequence, hepatocyte compression and loss may occur with formation of blood lakes. In long-standing obstruction, central fibrosis develops and may progress to central-central fibrous septum formation. True cirrhosis is rarely observed.

Veno-occlusive disease (VOD) is characterized by fibrosis occlusion of small hepatic veins resulting from endothelial damage by toxic agents or hepatic irradiation. Cholestasis may be seen in cases of VOD induced by chemotherapeutic agents.

Cardiac disorders (*eg*, congestive heart failure, mitral stenosis, tricuspid incompetence, constrictive pericarditis), pulmonary disorders (*eg*, pulmonary hypertension), and mediastinal disorders (*eg*, tumors, mediastinal fibrosis) are responsible for *chronic passive congestion* of the liver. Terminal hepatic venules appear dilated. Similar to Budd-Chiari and VOD, there is centrilobular sinusoidal congestion with compression of hepatocytes. Fibrosis may occur with central to central fibrous septum formation in severe cases. Cardiac cirrhosis lacking hepatocyte regeneration and complex vascular alterations of true cirrhosis may develop.

Hepatic Sinusoids

Pathologic changes responsible for abnormal sinusoidal blood flow include hepatocyte degeneration, such as hydropic swelling and panacinar steatosis; Kupffer and hepatic stellate cell hyperplasia or hypertrophy; fibrosis in the space of Disse; fibrin thrombus deposition; and severe inflammation.

Hepatic peliosis is a peculiar disorder characterized by severe sinusoidal dilation with formation of blood-filled cystic spaces. The cystic spaces do not show preferential topographical localization and are separated by cords of normal or compressed hepatocytes (Fig. 90-11). The cavity walls may or may not have an endothelial lining. Peliosis hepatis may be drug induced (*eg*, oral contraceptives, anabolic steroids), and it has been described in AIDS patients with *Rochalimaea* infection.

▰▰▰ DRUG- AND TOXIN-INDUCED LESIONS

Morphologic changes in the liver induced by drugs and toxins vary and may mimic those observed in other pathologic disorders. In many cases, it is possible to identify a main cellular compartment that is involved, and this helps to identify the responsible agent.

Parenchymal Changes

Macrovesicular and microvesicular steatoses are frequently observed in patients with toxic liver injury. Steatosis caused by methotrexate therapy usually is associated with portal and acinar

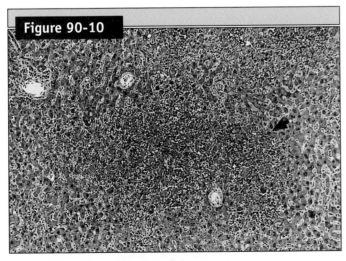

Figure 90-10

Centrolobular coagulative necrosis resulting from ischemia (*arrow*) (hematoxylin and eosin stain × 40).

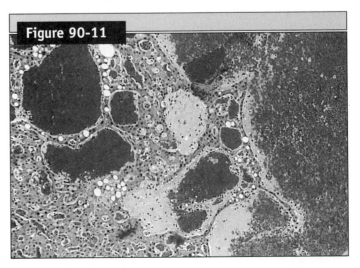

Figure 90-11

Hepatic peliosis with blood-filled cystic spaces (hematoxylin and eosin stain × 40).

fibrosis, which rarely may evolve into cirrhosis. Microvesicular steatosis has been related to valproic acid therapy. The pathogenesis of this form of steatosis is unclear; mitochondrial lesions are sometimes observed in infected persons. Granulomatous reaction is a frequent finding in cases of drug toxicity. *Induced cytoplasm* is a lesion characterized by the ground-glass hepatocyte cytoplasm resulting from hypertrophic and hyperplastic smooth endoplasmic reticulum (*ie*, induction cells). It represents cellular adaptation to chronic exposure to some toxins, including alcohol. Orcein staining is negative in these cases, which differentiates induction cells from ground-glass cells in hepatitis B infection.

A hepatocyte change called *phospholipidosis* has been observed in patients receiving 4,4'-diethylamino-ethoxyhexoestrol, perhexiline maleate, or amiodarone. It is characterized by hepatocyte swelling and a foamy and granular cytoplasm caused by the presence of abnormal laminated lysosomes.

In toxic liver injury, necrosis shows a preferential zone 3 localization, while periportal zones usually are spared. A few agents cause zone 1 necrosis. Lytic necrosis leads to cellular drop out and substitution by inflammatory and phagocytic cells. In some cases, it extends through all acinar zones, giving the appearance of "spotty necrosis," typically observed in viral hepatitis. Diffuse necrosis is characteristic of idiosyncratic agents. Necrosis may be associated with ballooning degeneration, eosinophilic degeneration with apoptotic body formation, and portal tract inflammation. In these cases, differentiation from viral hepatitis may be extremely difficult. Chronic hepatitis with heavy portal inflammation and piecemeal necrosis is a consequence of α-methyldopa, isoniazid, nitrofurantoin, dantrolene, or sulfamide administration. If the drugs are continued, portal fibrosis and cirrhosis may develop.

Biliary Changes

Some drugs cause "pure" cholestasis, characterized by the presence of bile thrombi in zone 3 canaliculi, or cholestatic hepatitis with inflammatory reaction. Cholestasis has been related to the use of contraceptive and anabolic steroids and to phenothiazine. Paraquat poisoning causes bile duct injury and cholangiodestructive cholestasis.

Vascular Changes

Drugs and toxins may be responsible for some forms of vascular changes; examples include contraceptive steroids in Budd-Chiari syndrome, androgenic and estrogenic steroids in hepatic peliosis, chemotherapeutic drugs in VOD, and corticosteroids in nodular regenerative hyperplasia.

Tumors

The carcinogenic actions of toxins and drugs have been well documented in experimental models. In humans, the association between thorotrast and hepatocellular and biliary carcinoma is well known. Steroid therapy increases the risk for the development of hepatocellular adenoma and carcinoma.

Metabolic Disorders

Pathologic abnormalities in metabolic disorders result from accumulation of abnormal metabolites in parenchymal and nonparenchymal liver cells. The histopathologic changes range from minimal and nonspecific changes to severe, including cirrhosis and hepatic carcinoma. Lesions may be pathognomonic at a microscopic or ultrastructural level or nonspecific [23]. Routine fixation of liver samples in 10% buffered formalin is adequate for diagnosis in most cases. Different fixatives may be necessary in special cases to preserve the metabolite, as in cystinosis. When a metabolic disease is suspected, glutaraldehyde fixation of a small part of the specimen for ultrastructural examination is recommended.

Disorders of bilirubin metabolism are sometimes characterized by bile (*eg*, Crigler-Najjar syndrome) or dark pigment deposition (*eg*, Dubin-Johnson syndrome) (Fig. 90-12). In Gilbert syndrome and Rotor syndrome, the liver appears normal. Typical birefringent hepatocyte inclusions may be observed in some disorders of porphyrin metabolism (*eg*, porphyria cutanea tarda, erythropoietic protoporphyria).

Glycogen inclusions are observed in the glycogen storage diseases. *Disorders of lipid metabolism* are morphologically characterized by enlarged foamy hepatocytes or Kupffer cells. Swollen hepatocytes and Kupffer cells with vacuolated cytoplasm also are seen in disorders of glycoprotein and protein metabolism.

α_1-Antitrypsin deficiency is characterized by the presence of PAS-diastase–positive globular inclusions in the cytoplasm of periportal hepatocytes (Fig. 90-13). The globules contain α_1-antitripsin that is stainable by immunohistochemical methods.

Liver changes in Wilson's disease are nonspecific. They may resemble chronic active hepatitis, with or without cirrhosis. Diffuse steatosis, glycogenated nuclei, copper deposition, and Mallory hyalin in zone 1 are helpful in making the diagnosis [24••]. Cystic fibrosis is characterized by inspissated PAS-positive mucus in dilated bile ducts and proliferating ductules surrounded by inflammatory cells and fibrosis.

■ PATHOLOGY OF HEPATIC ALLOGRAFTS
Rejection

Changes of *hyperacute rejection* consist of large areas of coagulative and hemorrhagic liver necrosis with fibrin thrombi in arteries, veins, and sinusoids. Numerous erythrocytes and neu-

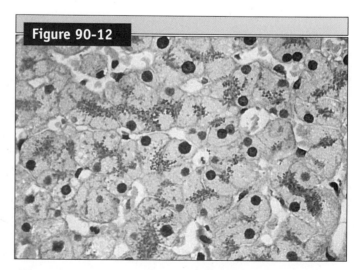

Figure 90-12

Course, brown pigmentation along the bile canaliculi in a patient with Dubin-Johnson syndrome (hematoxylin and eosin stain × 250).

trophils are trapped in sinusoids and in portal tracts. Hyperacute rejection represents an antibody-mediated reaction in presensitized recipients and occurs within few hours of the orthotopic liver transplantation (OLT) [25].

Histologic lesions of *acute rejection* are easily identified early after transplantation, before antirejection treatment is started, and predominantly represent manifestations of cell-mediated immunity. They consist of a characteristic triad: portal tract enlargement and infiltration by mixed inflammatory cells; endotheliitis of portal veins and often of central venules; and bile duct degeneration and inflammation. Inflammatory cells infiltrating the biliary epithelium are usually lymphocytes, but neutrophils also may be seen, and this feature should not be confused with suppurative cholangitis. Parenchymal lesions may be associated and include sinusoidal cell activation and sinusoidal infiltration by inflammatory cells. Cholestasis is usually present. Parenchymal necrosis with hepatocellular drop out, mostly in centrilobular areas, is seen when rejection is severe [26]. Acute rejection occurs as early as a few days after transplantation.

Chronic rejection more frequently occurs 3 to 4 months after OLT, but it may be observed years after transplantation. Typical findings consist of mild portal inflammation, predominantly lymphocytic and around damaged bile ducts, and loss of small bile ducts. Centrolobular cholestasis is usually more severe than it is in acute rejection. Occlusion of branches of the hepatic artery by lipid-laden macrophages may be seen in chronic rejection, probably resulting from immunologic damage to arterial endothelium. This process usually affects large branches of hepatic arteries and therefore is not seen in needle biopsy specimens. Centrilobular hepatocyte swelling and necrosis and centrilobular fibrosis suggest arterial obstruction by these lipid-laden cells. The term *vascular rejection* is used to define a type of chronic rejection characterized by foam cells or rejection arteritis [27].

Changes in Hepatic Allografts Other Than Rejection

Harvesting or preservation injury is a term used to describe lesions resulting from ischemic injury during organ retrieval, storage, and implantation. Histologic examination reveals various degrees of

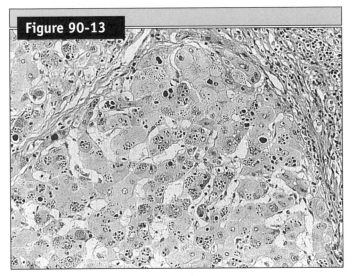

Figure 90-13

Periodic acid–Schiff (PAS) reactive, diastase-resistant globules and granules, representing α_1-antitrypsin deposits (D-PAS stain × 100).

parenchymal involvement, ranging from focal accumulation of lymphocytes and polymorphonuclear cells mimicking surgical hepatitis to more severe centrilobular necrosis. Cholestasis may be present.

Other conditions that may affect allografts include changes resulting from technical problems, such as biliary or vascular obstruction; infections, particularly by opportunistic agents [28]; reaction to immunosuppressive drugs or to antibiotics [29]; and recurrence of the primary disease, particularly viral hepatitis. The pathologic pattern of liver allografts is complex, because two or more different disorders may affect grafts simultaneously. In some cases, clinical correlation with laboratory and radiologic data are needed before a correct diagnosis can be reached.

▆ REFERENCES

Recently published papers of particular interest have been highlighted as follows:
- •   Of interest
- ••   Of outstanding interest

1.   Thung SN, Gerber MA, Popper H: Acute hepatitis: histopathology and ultrastructural features. In *Modern Concepts of Acute and Chronic Hepatitis*. Edited by Gitnick G. New York: Plenum Publishing; 1989:19–34.

2.   Farber E: Programmed cell death: necrosis versus apoptosis. *Mod Pathol* 1994, 5:605–609.

3.   Ishak KG: Chronic hepatitis: morphology and nomenclature. *Mod Pathol* 1994, 7:690–712.

4.•• Gerber MA, Thung SN: The localization of hepatitis virus in tissues. *Int Rev Exp Pathol* 1979, 29:49–76.

5.   Gerber MA, Krawczynski K, Alter MJ, *et al.*: Histopathology of community acquired chronic hepatitis C. *Mod Pathol* 1992, 5:483–486.

6.   Scheuer PJ, Ashrafzadeh P, Sherlock S, *et al.*: The pathology of hepatitis C. *Hepatology* 1992, 15:567–571.

7.   Bach N, Thung SN, Schaffner F: The histological features of chronic hepatitis C and autoimmune chronic active hepatitis: a comparative analysis. *Hepatology* 1992, 572–577.

8.•• Desmet VJ, Gerber M, Hoofnagle JH, *et al.*: Classification of chronic hepatitis: diagnosis, grading and staging. *Hepatology* 1994, 19:1513–1520.
This article offers guidelines for a revised system of classifying chronic hepatitis, emphasizing cause as the most important factor affecting the course of the disease. The concepts of grading and staging of chronic hepatitis are clarified.

9.   Thung SN, Gerber M: *Differential Diagnosis in Pathology: Liver Disorders*. Edited by Epstein JI. New York: Igaku-Shoin; 1995.

10.• Bacon BR, Farahvash MJ, Janney CG, Neuschwander-Tetri BA: Nonalcoholic steatohepatitis: an expanded clinical entity. *Gastroenterology* 1994, 107:1103–1109.
This study describes 33 patients with nonalcoholic steatohepatitis, providing evidence of the progression of this disease.

11.   Denk H, Scheuer PJ, Baptista A, *et al.*: Guidelines for the diagnosis and interpretation of hepatic granulomas. *Histopathology* 1994, 25:209–218.

12.   Pinzani M: Hepatic stellate (ItO) cells: expanding roles for a liver-specific pericyte [review]. *J Hepatol* 1995, 22:700–706.

13.   Desmet VJ: Cholestasis: extrahepatic obstruction and secondary biliary cirrhosis. In *Pathology of the Liver*. Edited by Mc Sween TNM, Anthony PP, Scheuer PJ, *et al.* Edinburgh: Churchill Livingstone; 1994:349–396.

14.• Scheuer PJ, Lefkowitch JH: *Liver Biopsy Interpretation*, edn 5. London: WB Saunders; 1994.

15.   Nakanuma Y, Tsuneyama K, Gershwin ME, Yasoshima M: Pathology and immunopathology of primary biliary cirrhosis with emphasis on bile duct lesions: recent progress. *Semin Liver Dis* 1995, 4:313–328.

16.•• Goodman ZD, McNally PR, Davis DR, Ishak KG: Autoimmune cholangitis: a variant of primary biliary cirrhosis. Clinicopathologic and serologic correlations in 200 cases. *Dig Dis Sci* 1995, 6:1232–1242.
Two hundred patients with morphologic diagnoses consistent with primary biliary cirrhosis were reevaluated in the light of their AMA and ANA status. Clinical, biochemical, and histopathologic profiles did not show any significant differences, regardless the presence or absence of AMA. On this basis, autoimmune cholangitis (AMA negative and ANA positive) can be considered an AMA-negative variant of primary biliary cirrhosis.

17. Searle J, Kerr JFR, Halliday JW, Powell LW: Iron storage disease. In *Pathology of the Liver*. Edited by Mc Sween TNM, Anthony PP, Scheuer PJ, *et al*. Edinburgh: Churchill Livingstone; 1994:349–396.

18. Brissot P, Bourel M, Herry D, *et al*.: Assessment of liver iron content in 271 patients: a reevaluation of direct and indirect methods. *Gastroenterology* 1981, 80:557–565.

19. Deugnier YM, Loreal O, Turlin B, *et al*.: Liver pathology in genetic hemochromatosis: a review of 135 homozygous cases and their bioclinical correlations. *Gastroenterology* 1992, 102:2050–2059.

20. Summers KM, Halliday JW, Powell LW: Identification of homozygous hemochromatosis subjects by measurement of hepatic iron index. *Hepatology* 1990, 12:20–25.

21. Powell LW, Burt MJ, Halliday JW, Jazwinska EC: Hemochromatosis: genetics and pathogenesis. *Semin Liver Dis* 1996, 16:55–63.

22. Gitlin N, Serio KM: Ischemic hepatitis: widening horizons. *Am J Gastroenterol* 1992, 87:831–836.

23. Ishak KG: Pathology of inherited metabolic disorders. In *Pediatric Hepatology*. Edited by Balistreri WF, Stocker JT. New York: Hemisphere Publishing; 1990:77–181.

24.•• Ludwig J, Moyer TP, Rakela J: The liver biopsy diagnosis of Wilson's disease. *Am J Clin Pathol* 1994, 102:443–446.
This study provides guidelines for the diagnosis of Wilson's disease based on routine histologic examination and chemical tissue copper analysis of the paraffin-embedded specimen.

25. Thung SN, Gerber MA: Histopathology of liver transplantation. In *Guide to Liver Transplantation*. Edited by Fabry TL, Klion FM. New York: Igaku-Shoin; 1992:265–298.

26. Demetris AJ, Batts KP, Dhillon AP, *et al*.: Banff schema for grading liver allograft rejection: an international consensus document. *Hepatology* 1997, 25:658–663.

27. Vierling JM, Fennel RH: Histopathology of early and late human hepatic allograft rejection: evidence of progressive destruction of interlobular bile ducts. *Hepatology* 1985, 4:1076–1082.

28. Markin RS, Langnas AN, Donovan JP, *et al*.: Opportunistic viral hepatitis in liver transplant recipients. *Transplant Proc* 1991, 23:1520–1521.

29. Thung SN, Shim KS, Shieh YS, *et al*.: Hepatitis C in liver allografts. *Arch Pathol Lab Med* 1993, 117:145–149.

Laboratory Evaluation of the Patient with Signs and Symptoms of Liver Disease

Hugo R. Rosen and Emmet B. Keeffe

The large number and wide variety of tasks performed by the liver make it impossible to evaluate liver function with a single laboratory test. However, panels of serum "liver chemistry" tests, performed serially and interpreted in the context of a person's medical history, physical examination, and other laboratory test results, are very useful in the evaluation of the patient with signs and symptoms of liver disease. Although the serum biochemical test pattern may suggest a diagnosis in such a patient, confirmation of the diagnosis usually requires further investigation with specific serologic or imaging studies and, possibly, liver biopsy.

Many serum biochemical tests provide indirect evidence for the presence of hepatobiliary disease and, therefore, are used to evaluate persons with potential asymptomatic liver disease, to confirm the presence of suspected liver disease in symptomatic patients, and to monitor disease progression and response to therapy in patients already diagnosed as having a specific liver disease. These tests are commonly referred to as *liver function tests*, although such usage is inaccurate and misleading. Two of the tests most commonly used for these purposes, measurements of serum alanine aminotransferase (ALT) and aspartate aminotransferase (AST), become abnormal when liver cells are damaged or die, and consequently are *liver injury tests*. Although abnormalities of serum alkaline phosphatase are seen in patients with liver disease, they have little to do with abnormalities of liver function, and although bile formation and excretion are liver functions, serum bilirubin levels may be elevated in patients with a perfectly normal liver. Even the results of laboratory tests that directly or indirectly measure substances produced by hepatocytes, for example serum albumin and coagulation factors (prothrombin time), often are abnormal in situations in which there is no liver damage. Thus, the general descriptive term *liver test* is more appropriate for this type of biochemical laboratory study.

Asymptomatic persons who have an abnormal result for one or more liver tests often present a diagnostic challenge, especially when the test results are almost within the normal range. Up to 6% of apparently healthy, asymptomatic persons have abnormal serum ALT, AST, or alkaline phosphatase levels; however, the prevalence of liver disease in the general population is significantly lower (1% to 2%) [1]. Therefore, it is important to develop a rational, cost-effective approach to the evaluation of asymptomatic persons with liver test results outside the normal range. The physician also must be alert to the fact that "mild" liver test abnormalities may be an early clue to the presence of potentially significant liver disease. For example, persons with chronic hepatitis C virus (HCV) infection are almost always asymptomatic unless they have end-stage liver disease and usually have "mild" serum ALT elevations; nevertheless, liver disease resulting from HCV is the most common indication for liver transplantation in adults.

The use of liver tests is limited by their lack of sensitivity (the likelihood of an abnormal test result in a patient with liver disease) in some clinical settings: patients with cirrhosis may have serum aminotransferase levels near or within the normal range. These tests also lack specificity (the likelihood of liver disease in a patient with an abnormal test result): AST levels may rise as a result of damage to nonhepatic tissues. As indicated previously, even the results of tests that superficially seem to measure specific hepatic functions, such as serum albumin and bilirubin concentrations and prothrombin time, are affected by numerous extrahepatic factors (Table 91-1) [2]. This chapter describes laboratory tests that may produce abnormal results in persons with liver disease and discusses their use in patient evaluation.

■ HEPATOCELLULAR INJURY
Aminotransferases
Abnormal serum aminotransferase levels signify the presence of hepatocellular injury and necrosis. These enzymes—ALT

(formerly serum glutamic-pyruvic transaminase) and AST (formerly serum glutamic-oxaloacetic transaminase)—catalyze the transfer of the α-amino groups of alanine and aspartate, respectively, to the α-keto group of ketoglutaric acid (Fig. 91-1). ALT is found almost exclusively in hepatocytes, but AST is present in many tissues, including cardiac and skeletal muscle, kidney, brain, pancreas, lung, red blood cells, and liver. Whereas AST is present in the mitochondria and the cytosol of hepatocytes, ALT is found only in the cytosol [3]. The evaluation of an asymptomatic person with an isolated elevation of the serum ALT level is outlined in Figure 91-2.

Although there are no standard, accepted definitions of *minimal*, *moderate*, and *severe* liver test abnormalities, working definitions of these terms have been proposed and are presented in Table 91-2 [4]. The degree to which these test results are abnormal in a given patient is often an important clue to the cause of the abnormality. Minimal aminotransferase elevations typically are found in patients with hepatic steatosis (fatty liver), nonalcoholic steatohepatitis, or chronic viral hepatitis. Fluctuations of the serum ALT level, including periods when the test result is normal or near normal, characterize chronic hepatitis C. The highest elevations of serum ALT occur in patients with acute viral hepatitis, drug- or toxin-induced hepatic necrosis, or hepatic ischemia. The degree of aminotransferase elevation does not correlate with the amount of necrosis as demonstrated on liver biopsy in cross-sectional studies (studies of large numbers of people with liver disease). Because the ALT level is not a reliable measure of the severity of liver disease, liver biopsy remains a clinically important diagnostic tool. ALT levels, however, do correlate well with histologic assessments of hepatic inflammation in longitudinal studies (studies of individual patients over time) and may be used to monitor the progression of liver disease once its cause and

Table 91-1. Nonhepatic Causes of Abnormal Liver Tests

Test	Nonhepatic causes	Discriminating Tests
Decreased albumin	Protein-losing enteropathy	Serum globulins, α_1-antitrypsin clearance
Increased alkaline phosphatase	Nephrotic syndrome	Urinalysis, 24-h urinary protein
	Congestive heart failure	Clinical setting
	Bone disease	GGT, SLAP, 5'-NT
	Pregnancy	GGT, 5'-NT
	Malignancy	Alkaline phosphatase electrophoresis
	Myocardial infarction	MB-CK
	Muscle disorders	Creatine kinase
	Hemolysis	Reticulocyte count, peripheral smear, urine bilirubin
Increased bilirubin	Sepsis	Clinical setting, cultures
	Ineffective erythropoiesis	Peripheral smear, urine bilirubin, hemoglobin electrophoresis, bone marrow examination
Increased prothrombin time	Shunt hyperbilirubinemia	Clinical setting
	Antibiotic and anticoagulant use, steatorrhea, dietary deficiency of vitamin K (rare)	Response to vitamin K, clinical setting

AST—aspartate aminotransferase; GGT—γ-glutamyl transpeptidase; 5'-NT—5'-nucleotidase; SLAP—serum leucine aminopeptidase.
Adapted from Moseley [2].

severity have been established. A notable exception is fulminant hepatic failure; a rapidly declining aminotransferase level in a patient with fulminant hepatic failure, regardless of the cause, may reflect a decreased number of hepatocytes, indicating a poor prognosis. The clinician's task in evaluating a patient for the presence of liver disease is complicated by the fact that patients who have normal aminotransferase levels may have significant liver damage; liver biopsies of persons infected with HCV may demonstrate chronic hepatitis and even cirrhosis, despite their having repeatedly normal serum ALT levels [5].

The AST/ALT ratio may be helpful in the diagnosis of alcoholic hepatitis. Patients with alcoholic hepatitis rarely have an

Figure 91-1

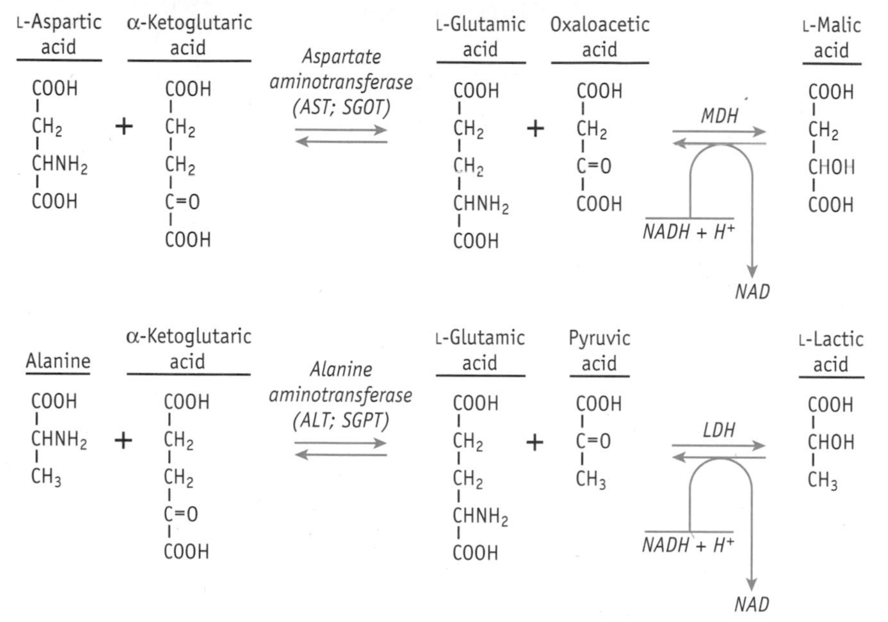

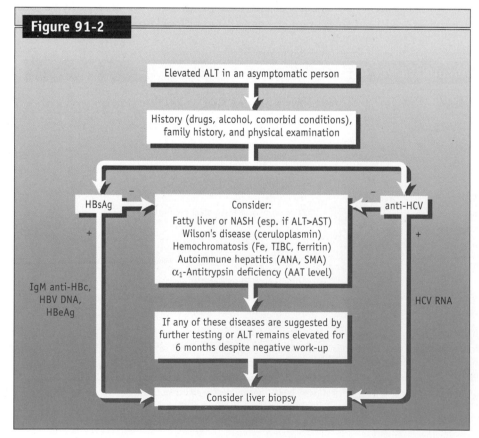

Enzymatic assay of aspartate aminotransferase (AST) and alanine aminotransferase (ALT). LDH—lactic dehydrogenase; MDH—malic dehydrogenase; NAD—nicotinamide-adenine dinucleotide; NADH—reduced nicotinamide-adenine dinucleotide; SGOT—serum glutamate oxalacetate transaminase; SGPT—serum glutamate pyruvate transaminase. (*Adapted from* Schiff and Schiff [22]; with permission.)

Figure 91-2

Evaluation of an elevated serum alanine aminotransferase (ALT) level in an asymptomatic person. AAT—α antitrypsin; ANA—antinuclear antibody; AST—aspartate aminotransferase; Fe—iron; HBV—hepatitis B virus; HBc—hepatitis B core; HBsAg—hepatitis B surface antigen; HCV—hepatitis C virus; IgM—immunoglobulin M; NASH—nonalcoholic steatohepatitis; SMA—smooth muscle antibody; TIBC—total iron binding capacity.

AST level greater than 300 U/L, and the ratio of AST to ALT approaches 3:1 as the severity of the disease increases (Fig. 91-3). The reason for the relatively greater increase in serum AST compared with serum ALT levels in these patients may be a deficiency in alcoholics of pyridoxine-5-phosphate, a co-factor in ALT production. Oral pyridoxine-5-phosphate supplements have been reported to increase the serum ALT levels in alcoholics with hepatitis. Although an AST/ALT ratio of greater than 2 strongly suggests a diagnosis of alcoholic hepatitis [6], it does not preclude the possibility that a patient with this finding has another liver disease. Conversely, the serum ALT level may actually be greater than the serum AST level in some patients with alcoholic hepatitis, a finding more typical of nonalcoholic steatohepatitis. In viral hepatitis, the AST/ALT ratio is usually less than 1 but may increase as cirrhosis develops [3].

It is important to note that end-stage renal disease frequently is associated with a decrease in serum aminotransferase levels. Yasuda and colleagues have shown that in patients undergoing dialysis, aminotransferase levels greater than 20 may be abnormal [7]. Also, many of these patients have HCV infection, although their aminotransferase levels are normal [8]. Figure 91-4 depicts a strategy for evaluating abnormal aminotransferases in patients with end-stage renal disease.

Lactate Dehydrogenase

Lactate dehydrogenase (LDH) is a cytosolic enzyme present in tissues throughout the body. Of the five LDH isoenzymes, the one with the slowest elecrophoretic mobility is found predominantly in the liver. However, abnormal serum levels of the hepatic isoenzyme are neither sensitive nor specific in predicting the presence of liver disease. Rather, an abnormal serum LDH level in a patient with other signs of liver disease suggests that the cause of the disorder is an entity also affecting nonhepatic tissues (eg, ischemia).

■ TESTS OF CHOLESTASIS

Alkaline Phosphatase

Abnormal serum alkaline phosphatase (ALP) levels are seen primarily in patients with cholestasis, but they also occur in persons with infiltrative liver disease and in some persons without hepatic disorders.

Alkaline phosphatase is the name for a group of enzymes that catalyze the hydrolysis of phosphate esters at alkaline pH. These enzymes are found in bone, intestine, placenta, and even in some malignant neoplasms (eg, Regan variety), as well as the liver. As a result of active bone growth, a normal serum ALP level in children and adolescents may be up to three times as great as the upper limit of normal levels in adults. The half-life of ALP in serum is 7 days. In persons with cholestasis, de novo production of ALP by the hepatocyte and the cholangiocyte increases, possibly in response to a rise in canalicular pressure or bile acid stasis, and ALP is released into the circulation. Extra- and intrahepatic cholestasis cannot be differentiated based on the degree of ALP elevation. Figure 91-5 outlines a method for evaluating an isolated or predominant mild ALP elevation. Markedly elevated serum ALP levels suggest a diagnosis of extrahepatic biliary obstruction, primary biliary cirrhosis, primary sclerosing cholangitis, or drug-induced cholestasis. Mild to moderate ALP abnormalities are typical of infiltrative processes, notably amyloidosis, granulomatous diseases, and neoplasms. Some patients with Hodgkin's disease or renal cell carcinoma have abnormal ALP levels without liver or bone involvement (Stauffer's syndrome). A two- to fourfold increase in serum ALP, unassociated with any detectable liver or bone disease, also has been reported as an isolated genetic disorder

Table 91-2. Characteristics of Elevated Concentrations of Liver Enzymes

Test	Normal*	Mild†	Moderate†	Marked†
AST	11–32	< 2–3	2–3 to 20	> 20
ALT	3–30	< 2–3	2–3 to 20	> 20
ALP	35–105	< 1.5–2	1.5–2 to 5	> 5
GGT	2–65	< 2–3	2–3 to 10	> 10

*Units for normal are U/L; normal ranges vary with the assay used and should be obtained from the laboratory performing the test.
†Numbers in table refer to multiples of the upper limits of normal.
Adapted from Keeffe [4].

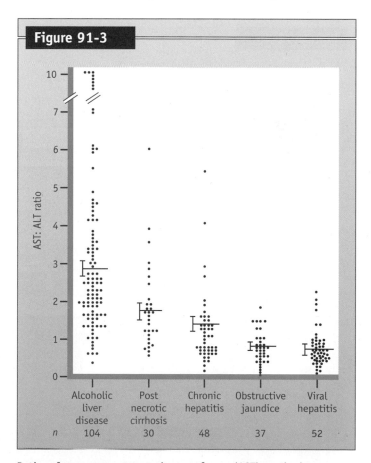

Figure 91-3

Ratios of serum aspartate aminotransferase (AST) to alanine aminotransferase (ALT) in patients with biopsy-proven liver disease. Of patients with alcoholic liver disease, 70% had ratios greater than two, compared with 26% of patients with postnecrotic cirrhosis, 8% with chronic active hepatitis, 4% with viral hepatitis, and none with obstructive jaundice. (*Adapted from* Cohen and Kaplan [6].)

with an autosomal dominant inheritance pattern. In contrast, normal ALP levels occasionally are seen in patients with liver metastases or complete bile duct obstruction. Low serum levels of ALP may be associated with congenital hypophosphatasia, hypothyroidism, pernicious anemia, or zinc deficiency, and patients with fulminant Wilson's disease may have undetectable serum ALP levels [3].

γ-Glutamyltransferase

γ-Glutamyltransferase (GGT) is an enzyme found in the cell membranes of many organs, including the pancreas, kidney, heart, and brain, as well as the liver, but importantly, not bone. Thus, the serum GGT level is used clinically to confirm that an abnormal ALP test result is caused by hepatobiliary, and not bone, disease. GGT levels do not rise during pregnancy. However, GGT test results often are abnormal in persons who drink even small amounts of alcohol or who take barbiturates, phenytoin, or some other drugs (Fig. 91-6) [9]. In addition, familial elevations of serum GGT have been reported.

5'-Nucleotidase

The serum level of 5'-nucleotidase, another enzyme that has the same hepatic location as ALP, also rises in hepatobiliary disease. Like GGT, 5'-nucleotidase is not found in bone, and con-

sequently its serum levels do not become abnormal in diseases affecting the skeletal system. Therefore, 5'-nucleotidase also is used clinically to confirm that an abnormal serum ALP level is caused by hepatobiliary disease, and it has the advantage of not increasing in response to ethanol ingestion and medication use. Serum 5'-nucleotidase levels may be elevated in pregnancy, and are substantially lower in children than in adults. A normal 5'-nucleotidase test result in a patient with an elevated serum ALP does not exclude the presence of hepatobiliary disease [10].

Bilirubin

Bilirubin is an endogenous organic anion derived primarily from the catabolism of red blood cell heme and, to a lesser extent, from the degradation of myoglobin, cytochromes, catalase, and peroxidase. Bilirubin binds reversibly to albumin and is transported to the liver where it is conjugated to glucuronic acid and excreted in the bile (see Chapters 88 and 89). Thus, healthy persons have a small amount of unconjugated bilirubin in their blood but no conjugated bilirubin. Commonly used laboratory tests, however, mistakenly identify some serum bilirubin in healthy persons as being conjugated to glucuronic acid, explaining the reported "normal" range for conjugated ("direct") bilirubin.

When the conjugated, or direct-reacting, fraction of total bilirubin exceeds the upper limit of normal, even if the total

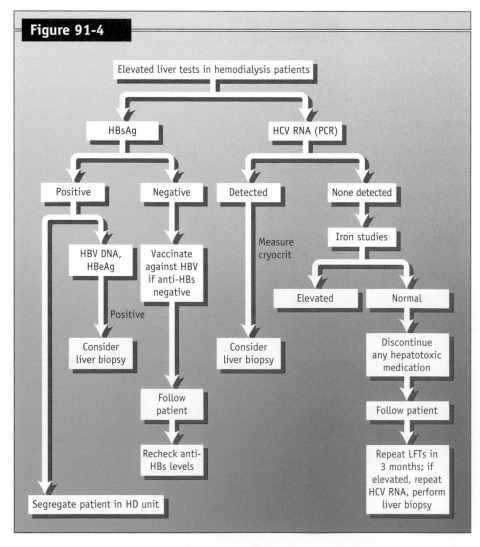

Figure 91-4

Algorithm for evaluating elevated liver function tests (LFTs) in a hemodialysis (HD) patient. Anti-HBs—antibody to hepatitis B surface antigen; HBsAg—hepatitis B surface antigen; HBV—hepatitis B virus; PCR—polymerase chain reaction. (*Adapted from* Rosen and coworkers [9]; with permission.)

serum bilirubin concentration is normal or near normal, the patient has hepatobiliary disease. Similarly, the appearance of water-soluble, conjugated bilirubin in urine (bilirubinuria) always signifies the presence of hepatobiliary disease. A few common pathophysiologic states, most notably hemolysis and Gilbert's syndrome, produce a pure, unconjugated hyperbilirubinemia; in these disorders, the total serum bilirubin concentration is virtually always less than 5 mg/dL. In almost every other situation in which the serum bilirubin is elevated, conjugated as well as unconjugated bilirubin is in the blood. It is impossible to determine whether the site of a defect in bilirubin excretion is intrahepatic or extrahepatic based on the ratio of conjugated to unconjugated serum bilirubin.

When the common bile duct is completely obstructed, the total serum bilirubin concentration rises to approximately 30 mg/dL, the point at which equilibrium is established between bilirubin production and renal excretion of water-soluble bilirubin glucuronide formed in the liver. Serum bilirubin levels greatly exceeding 30 mg/dL are seen in some patients who have common bile duct obstruction as well as either impaired bilirubin conjugation resulting from hepatic dysfunction or impaired renal bilirubin excretion as a result of renal insufficiency. Similarly, persons with severe hepatocellular dysfunction as well as renal insufficiency may have serum bilirubin concentrations greater than 30 mg/dL. The clinical approach to the patient with jaundice is outlined in Table 91-3 [11].

The serum bilirubin level has been used to predict the natural history of specific liver diseases. Shapiro and others [12] have reported that patients with primary biliary cirrhosis typically have a long, stable course followed by an accelerated preterminal phase. The preterminal phase is characterized in part by the development of hyperbilirubinemia, with a mean survival of only 1.4 years in patients with a serum bilirubin concentration greater than 10 mg/dL [12]. The degree of hyperbilirubinemia and prothrombin time (PT) are used in patients with alcoholic hepatitis to predict acute mortality (discriminant function of Maddrey) [13]. Recent studies of liver transplant recipients have suggested that marked and transient hyperbilirubinemia is common after HCV reinfection of an allograft, and that the level of hyperbilirubinemia may provide prognostic information beyond that derived from the histologic score [14].

■ TESTS OF SYNTHETIC DYSFUNCTION
Serum Albumin

Albumin is quantitatively the most important serum protein made by the liver, accounting for three quarters of the plasma colloid oncotic pressure. The liver is the only organ that synthesizes albumin; it normally produces 12 to 15 g of this protein each day. Plasma albumin concentration is decreased in severe acute or chronic liver disease and is one of the criteria of the Child-Pugh classification, which commonly is used to grade the

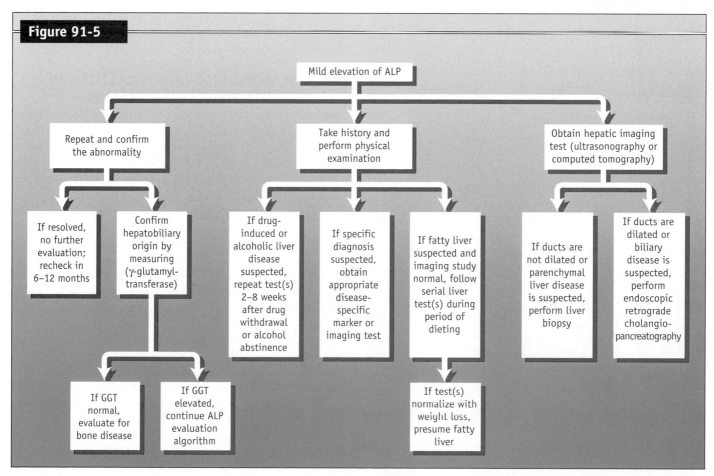

Figure 91-5

Algorithm for evaluation of isolated (or predominant) mild elevation of alkaline phosphatase (ALP) concentration.

Diagnostic approach to mild elevation of liver enzyme levels. GGT— γ-glutamyltransferase. (*Adapted from* Keeffe [4]; with permission.)

degree of liver dysfunction in patients with cirrhosis (Table 91-4). Originally this classification was developed to predict survival of cirrhotic patients after portosystemic shunt surgery. Hypoalbuminemia also may result from gastrointestinal or renal protein loss, infectious or inflammatory processes, and hypergammaglobulinemia, which may produce feedback inhibition of albumin synthesis [15,16]. Pre-albumin (half-life, 2 d) appears to be more sensitive than albumin (half-life, 20 d) as an index of hepatic protein synthesis, particularly in patients with acute liver failure.

Prothrombin Time

With the exception of factor VIII, which is made by vascular endothelium and reticuloendothelial cells, all of the clotting factors are synthesized by the liver. The clotting factors that determine PT have half-lives of only a few hours; therefore, PT is a useful test for evaluating hepatocellular function in cases of acute liver injury. PT has been used in a number of settings to predict outcome in patients with liver disease, for example, as part of the discriminant function of Maddrey (see earlier discussion) in patients with alcoholic hepatitis [17]. Unfortunately, PT is not a sensitive index of global liver function in chronic liver disease, as it may be normal in patients with cirrhosis.

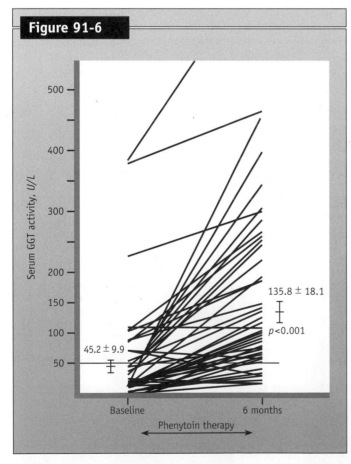

Figure 91-6

Individual and mean changes in serum γ-glutamyltransferase (GGT) activity from baseline to 6 months of phenytoin therapy in 58 patients. Of the total group, 52 patients demonstrated a rise and six patients a fall in GGT activity. (*Adapted from* Keeffe and coworkers [11]; with permission.)

Cholesterol

The liver is the principal site of cholesterol synthesis; serum cholesterol has been used, along with serum albumin and bilirubin, as a prognostic indicator in patients with compensated cirrhosis [18]. The typical serum lipoprotein pattern in persons with cirrhosis is characterized by normal levels of low-density lipoprotein (LDL) cholesterol, but decreased levels of very low-density lipoprotein (VLDL) and total serum cholesterol. In contrast to this pattern, patients with chronic cholestatic liver disease, for example primary biliary cirrhosis, have elevated LDL, high-density lipoprotein (HDL), and total cholesterol levels. Hypercholesterolemia also may be seen as a result of increased synthesis in patients with hepatocellular carcinoma.

Quantitative Liver Function Tests

Patients with normal liver test results of the type described earlier may have significantly impaired liver function; conversely, hepatic function may be well-preserved in persons with abnormal aminotransferase levels and abnormal results on other routine tests. Although quantitation of hepatic functional reserve is not performed often in clinical practice, a number of quantitative liver function tests have been devised (Table 91-5).

Use of these tests has been limited because some are difficult to perform and because their results often are not that helpful in patient management. Development of one or more simple, non-invasive, reliable measures of liver function would be a major advance with many important clinical applications. For example, a true liver function test would be invaluable in managing patients with chronic hepatitis and selecting candidates for liver transplantation.

■■■ HEMATOPOIETIC ABNORMALITIES IN PATIENTS WITH LIVER DISEASE

Liver disease has numerous effects on the production, distribution, and survival of the formed elements of the blood; anemia, thrombocytopenia, and neutropenia frequently occur in patients with severe hepatic dysfunction. Liver disease *per se* causes anemia by shortening red blood cell (RBC) survival, increasing plasma volume, and impairing bone marrow response to reduced hemoglobin levels. The mean corpuscular volume (MCV) rises in many patients with chronic liver disease as a result of an increase in RBC membrane lipids; abnormal RBC membrane lipid composition may cause hemolysis and spur cell anemia in these patients. In addition, patients with severe chronic liver disease often develop anemia from bone marrow suppression by ethanol, gastrointestinal bleeding, and hypersplenism (see Chapter 112). About two thirds of patients with other signs of hypersplenism also have leukopenia; these individuals usually have a normal differential white blood cell count. Most patients with hypersplenism have secondary thrombocytopenia, with platelet counts of 140,000 to 50,000/mm³. Thrombocytopenia in persons with liver disease is associated with an increased risk of bleeding, although the bleeding time usually is normal. Splenic sequestration and expansion of plasma volume are the most important factors contributing to development of cytopenias in patients with liver disease, but levels of thrombopoietin, which is produced mainly by the liver, also are low in this setting.

OTHER TESTS USED IN THE EVALUATION OF LIVER DISEASE

Many other laboratory tests are used to evaluate patients suspected of having specific liver diseases; the use of these tests is reviewed in the chapters addressing these disorders.

Immunoglobulins and Markers of Autoimmunity

The liver is an important organ of the reticuloendothelial system, and liver cells play a role in the removal of foreign antigens from portal blood. When liver tissue is damaged by disease and when hepatic blood flow is distorted by remodel-

---

Table 91-3. Clinical Approach to the Patient With Jaundice

Diagnostic factors	Type of jaundice			
	Hemolytic	**Hepatocellular**	**Intrahepatic cholestatic**	**Extrahepatic cholestatic**
Symptoms	May be asymptomatic or backache, joint pain	Nausea, vomiting, fever, anorexia	Deep jaundice, dark-colored urine, light-colored stools, pruritus	Deep jaundice, dark-colored urine, light-colored stools, pruritus, cholangitis, biliary colic
Physical findings	Splenomegaly	Tender hepatomegaly, splenomegaly*	Tender hepatomegaly	Hepatomegaly, palpable gall-bladder
Liver tests				
Bilirubin				
Total	< 6 mg/dL	Variable	Variable, may be > 30 mg/dL	< 30 mg/dL
Direct	< 20%	> 50%	> 50%	> 50%
Alanine aminotransferase	Normal	> Fivefold increase	Two- to fivefold increase	< Two- to threefold increase, higher with cholangitis
Alkaline phosphatase	Normal	< Two- to threefold increase	> Three- to fivefold increase	> Three- to fivefold increase
Prothrombin time	Normal	Prolonged	Prolonged	Prolonged
Corrected by vitamin K	—	No	Variable	Yes
Ultrasonography of liver				
Biliary dilation	No	No	No	Yes
ERCP	Not necessary	Not necessary	Usually not necessary	Usually necessary

*May or may not be present.
ERCP—endoscopic retrograde cholangiopancreatography.
Adapted from Kamath [13]; with permission.

Table 91-4. Child-Turcotte Prognostic Classification (Pugh's Modification)*

Specific scores

	Points		
Factor	**1**	**2**	**3**
Encephalopathy, *grade*	0	1–2	3–4
Ascites	None	Slight	Moderate
Bilirubin, *mg/dL*	1–2	2–3	> 3
Albumin, *g/dL*	≥ 3.5	2.8–3.5	< 2.8
Prothrombin time, *s*	1–4	5–6	> 6

Summary scores

Grade	Total score, *points*
A	5–6
B	7–9
C	10–15

*Original classification used malnutrition in place of prothrombin time.
Data from Pugh and coworkers [21]; with permission.

Table 91-5. Quantitative Liver Tests

Test	Estimates
Galactose elimination capacity Maximal removal of indocyanine green	Metabolic capacity
Aminopyrine demethylation Caffeine clearance Antipyrine clearance	Microsomal enzyme function
Galactose clearance Sorbitol clearance Indocyanine green clearance Sulfobromophthalein clearance	Functional hepatic perfusion
Formation of monoethylglycine xylidide from lignocaine	Microsomal enzyme function and hepatic perfusion

Adapted from Hawker [14].

ing in response to liver injury (cirrhosis), antigenic material escapes removal and reaches the systemic circulation, where it stimulates polyclonal Ig production by lymphocytes. For unclear reasons, in alcoholic liver disease there is a tendency for IgA to be increased out of proportion to other Igs. Patients with primary biliary cirrhosis have a predominant increase in IgM that is explained by the pathophysiology of this particular disease (see Chapter 106). Similarly, hyperglobulinemia is a specific feature of autoimmune hepatitis that is probably directly related to the disease process itself (see Chapter 97). Autoimmune hepatitis is associated with the presence in serum of high titers ($\geq$ 1:160) of antinuclear antibodies (ANA) and anti–smooth muscle antibodies (SMA); these autoantibodies also often are detected in lower titers in the sera of patients with other chronic liver diseases (*eg*, HCV infection).

Tumor Markers

α-Fetoprotein (AFP), carcinoembryonic antigen (CEA), and CA 19-19 are often found in the blood of patients with chronic liver disease. AFP is a unique globulin normally synthesized by embryonic and regenerating liver cells. Patients with acute viral hepatitis and chronic liver disease frequently have serum AFP concentrations of up to 500 ng/mL. AFP levels of greater than 1000 ng/mL are seen in many patients with primary hepatocellular carcinoma (HCC). However, no correlation exists between serum AFP concentration and the clinical features of the disease, including the size and stage of the tumor and survival time following diagnosis. Less marked elevations of serum AFP may occur in patients with hepatic metastases.

Serum CEA concentrations are increased in approximately 50% of patients with HCC, although the elevation is only mild or moderate in the vast majority of patients. In a Mayo Clinic study of patients with primary sclerosing cholangitis (PSC), CEA concentrations were significantly higher in persons with cholangiocarcinoma than in individuals with only PSC. Initial enthusiasm related to use of CA 19-19 in the diagnosis of cholangiocarcinoma in patients with PSC has been tempered by problems with the specificity and positive predictive value of the test when it is used for this purpose [19].

Iron Indices

Measurement of serum iron, total iron binding capacity (TIBC), transferrin, and ferritin levels may be useful in the evaluation of patients with suspected liver disease. Serum iron levels vary diurnally and are affected by eating; therefore, the most accurate serum iron test results are obtained when these tests are performed on fasting patients. Serum iron concentration alone is not an accurate screening test for iron overload states, and serum transferrin saturation and serum ferritin levels are more sensitive and specific for diagnosing hemochromatosis (see Chapter 108). Inflammation, malignancy, and chronic liver disease without significant iron overload may affect the results of serum iron tests. For example, up to 40% of patients with chronic viral hepatitis and nonalcoholic steatohepatitis have elevated serum ferritin levels. Liver biopsy with histologic assessment of iron load and determination of the hepatic iron concentration and hepatic iron index is essential for differentiating between hemochromatosis and other causes of abnormal serum iron test results.

Ammonia

Blood ammonia levels usually are elevated in patients with hepatic encephalopathy, although the relationship between the ammonia level and the presence of hepatic encephalopathy is not sufficiently reliable to allow this diagnosis to be made strictly on the basis of an abnormal ammonia test result (see Chapter 115). Once the diagnosis of hepatic encephalopathy has been made, the progress of therapy can be documented by measurement of blood ammonia level.

New Tests

A number of promising research tests eventually may be added to the armamentarium of clinical laboratory studies. The serum level of desialylated transferrin (dTf) may distinguish alcoholic hepatitis from other forms of liver disease [20]. Plasma levels of Gc protein, a liver cell product that sequesters actin released into the circulation after massive hepatocyte necrosis, have been shown to compare favorably with multivariate predictive models of survival in fulminant hepatic failure [21].

▉ REFERENCES

1. Flora KD, Keeffe EB: Evaluation of mildly abnormal liver tests in asymptomatic patients. *J Insur Med* 1990, 22:264–267.

2. Mosely RH: Evaluation of abnormal liver function tests. *Med Clin N Am* 1996, 80:887–906.

3. Friedman LS, Martin P, Munoz SJ: Liver function tests and the objective evaluation of the patient with liver disease. In *Hepatology: A Textbook of Liver Disease.* Edited by Zakim D, Boyer TD. Philadelphia: WB Saunders; 1996:791–833.

4. Keeffe EB: Diagnostic approach to mild elevation of liver enzyme levels. *Gastrointestinal Dis Today* 1994, 3:1–9.

5. Healey CJ, Chapman RWG, Fleming KA: Liver histology in hepatitis C infection: a comparison between patients with persistently normal or abnormal transaminases. *Gut* 1995, 37:274–278.

6. Cohen JA, Kaplan MM: The SGOT/SGPT ratio: an indicator of alcoholic liver disease. *Dig Dis Sci* 1979, 24:835–838.

7. Yasuda K, Kunio O, Endo N, *et al.*: Hypoaminotransferasemia in patients undergoing long-term hemodialysis: clinical and biochemical appraisal. *Gastroenterology* 1995, 109:1295–1300.

8. Rosen HR, Friedman LS, Martin P: Hepatitis C in renal dialysis and transplant patients. *Viral Hepatitis Reviews* 1996, 2:91–110.

9. Keeffe EB, Sunderland MC, Gabourel JD: Serum gamma-glutamyl transpeptidase activity in patients receiving chronic phenytoin therapy. *Dig Dis Sci* 1986, 31:1056–1061.

10. Bacq Y, Zarka O, Brechot J-F, *et al.*: Liver function tests in normal pregnancy: a prospective study of 103 pregnant women and 103 matched controls. *Hepatology* 1996, 23:1030–1034.

11. Kamath PS: Clinical approach to the patient with abnormal liver test results. *Mayo Clinic Proc* 1996, 71:1089–1095.

12. Shapiro JM, Smith H, Schaffner F: Serum bilirubin. A prognostic factor in primary biliary cirrhosis. *Gut* 1979, 20:137–141.

13. Maddrey C: Alcoholic hepatitis: clinicopathologic features and therapy. *Semin Liver Dis* 1988, 8:91–102.

14. Rosen HR, Oehlke M, Benner KG, *et al.*: Timing and severity of hepatitis C recurrence following liver transplantation as predictors of long-term allograft injury. *Transplantation* 1998, 65:1178–1182.

15. Pietrangelo A, Pandura A, Roy Chowdhury J, Shafritz DA: Albumin gene expression is down-regulated by albumin or macromolecule infusion in the rat. *J Clin Invest* 1992, 89:1755–1760.

16. Rothschild MA, Oratz M, Schreiber SS: Serum albumin. *Hepatology* 1988, 8:385–401.

17. Christensen E, Bremmelgaard A, Bahnsen M, *et al.*: Prediction of fatality in fulminant hepatic failure. *Scan J Gastroenterol* 1984, 19:90.

18. Zoli M, Cordiani RM, Marchesini G, *et al.*: Prognostic indicators in compensated cirrhosis. *Am J Gastroenterol* 1991, 86:1508–1513.

19. Nichols JC, Gores GJ, LaRusso NF, *et al.*: Diagnostic role of serum CA 19-9 for cholangiocarcinoma in patients with primary sclerosing cholangitis. *Mayo Clinic Proc* 1993, 68:874–879.

20. Magarian GJ, Lucas LM, Kumar KL: Clinical significance in alcoholic patients of commonly encountered laboratory test results. *West J Med* 1992, 156:287–294.

21. Lee WM, Galbraith RM, Watt GH, *et al.*: Predicting survival in fulminant hepatic failure using serum Gc protein concentrations. *Hepatology* 1995, 21:101–105.

22. Schiff, Schiff: *Disease of the Liver*, edn 6. Philadelphia: JB Lippincott; 234.

92 Radiologic Evaluation of Patients With Liver Disease

Alla M. Rozenblit

Radiologic evaluation of the liver is performed routinely for patients with known primary extrahepatic malignancies and for those at high risk for developing hepatocellular carcinoma (HCC). Other common clinical problems that may require hepatic imaging include hepatomegaly, right upper quadrant pain, a palpable abdominal mass, jaundice, ascites, abnormal liver test results, unexplained abdominal infection, and abdominal trauma. Diffuse hepatic processes, including cirrhosis, hemochromatosis, steatosis, and storage diseases, are less common indications for liver imaging. In addition, liver imaging often is performed for persons without overt clinical abnormalities to characterize hepatic lesions that are discovered incidentally during tests done to evaluate other problems. Most patients in the latter group have benign disease, such as cavernous hemangioma, hepatic cyst, or focal nodular hyperplasia (FNH), although a silent primary or metastatic liver neoplasm sometimes is discovered.

Various imaging modalities can be employed for evaluation of liver pathology. Different methods have their specific advantages and limitations. They are often used in combination to provide complimentary diagnostic information regarding focal and diffuse liver disease (Tables 92-1 and 92-2).

▇ IMAGING TESTS
Ultrasonography

Ultrasonography is the most commonly used imaging test and often is employed as the first step in evaluation of the liver. The main advantages include wide availability, excellent patient compliance, absence of side effects, and relatively low cost. Ultrasonography is highly sensitive and specific for detection of cholelithiasis and biliary ductal dilation. It therefore is commonly performed to exclude or confirm biliary disease and to screen for parenchymal involvement in patients with a confusing clinical presentation and laboratory data that are difficult to interpret. Parenchymal liver masses are well depicted and accurately localized to specific anatomic segments by ultrasonography, which also is effective in differentiating cystic from solid hepatic lesions and highly accurate for diagnosis of simple cysts. However, the echo pattern of solid liver masses is generally nonspecific, with a wide overlap between benign and malignant tumors [1]. Further investigation of such sonographic findings with other imaging tests or biopsy is often warranted.

Duplex and color Doppler ultrasonography allow noninvasive characterization of blood flow in major hepatic vessels and parenchymal lesions [2] (Fig. 92-1, see also **Color Plate**). Color Doppler ultrasonography can differentiate a vascular mass from a hypovascular or avascular structure. Spectral analysis may be more specific for malignancy when imaging demonstrates arteriovenous shunting, a sign of malignant neovascularity. Power Doppler ultrasonography, relatively new for hepatic imaging, is more sensitive than color Doppler ultrasonography for displaying organ perfusion, and it is free of some artifacts and limitations of the conventional color setting [2].

Technical limitations of Doppler ultrasonography include image-degrading artifacts, particularly in the left hepatic lobe from respiratory and cardiac motion. Overall limitations of transcutaneous ultrasonography include difficulties in imaging liver overlaid by bowel gas or bone and liver lesions located in the dome or near the right lateral hepatic border [1]. In general, patients with a large body habitus are difficult to study with ultrasonography. The lower-frequency transducers, needed for these patients because of better penetration, have inferior spatial resolution. Because the overall sensitivity of ultrasonography for detection of focal lesions is lower than that of computed tomography (CT) and magnetic resonance (MR) imaging, ultrasonography is not recommended as a screening imaging test for oncology patients [3].

Intraoperative ultrasonography is an accurate and increasingly popular technique used to localize primary and secondary hepatic tumors. With this method, the liver is evaluated with high-frequency sonographic transducers during laparotomy or laparoscopy. The technique is highly sensitive for diagnosis of small (<1 cm) liver lesions [4].

Computed Tomography

Because of its versatility for evaluation of the entire body, CT commonly is used to study the liver in oncology patients. Nononcologic indications for CT of the liver include abdominal trauma, suspicion of biliary obstruction or liver abscess, postoperative complications, evaluation of a liver allograft, and some hepatic vascular abnormalities. The major drawbacks of CT are the need to use intravenous iodinated contrast media and the

associated ionizing radiation. Contraindications to evaluation with contrast-enhanced CT include hypersensitivity to iodinated contrast media, abnormal renal function, and concurrent treatment with metformin hydrochloride (Glucophage), an oral hypoglycemic agent. Because contrast studies with iodinated materials in patients on Glucophage can lead to renal failure and lactic acidosis, this drug should be withheld for 48 hours before such a procedure and reinstituted only after renal function is shown to be normal.

Noncontrast CT alone may be useful for assessment of some diffuse hepatic abnormalities, such as fatty infiltration and iron overload, but it is not accurate for detecting liver tumors. Contrast-enhanced CT therefore is routinely used for evaluation of the liver. Hepatic lesions are classified as hypervascular or hypovascular, depending on when they enhance with intravenous contrast (Fig. 92-2). Hypervascular lesions enhance greater than normal liver in the early arterial phase. During the

Table 92-1 Application of Noninvasive Imaging Tests in Patients With Liver Disease

Applications	US	CT	MRI	Nuclear medicine
Optimal	Thin patients Biliary disease Cystic vs solid lesion Liver abscess, cyst Hepatic and portal venous flow in cirrhotic liver Hepatic and portal venous thrombosis Flow in TIPS (best noninvasive test) Guidance for biopsies	Metastases* Follow-up of oncologic patients* Extrahepatic tumor Liver transplant* Trauma* Acute hematoma Cystic vs solid lesion* Abscess Advanced cirrhosis Collateral veins in portal hypertension* Extent of venous thrombosis* Guidance for abscess drainage and biopsies	Metastases if iodinated intravenous contrast cannot be used† Oncologic patients with fatty liver† Hepatoma in cirrhotic liver† Hemangioma < 2 cm† Tumor vs focal fat vs typical regenerative nodule vs FNH† Hemochromatosis and iron overload† Subacute and chronic hematoma Microabscesses Cystic vs solid lesion† Venous thrombosis†	Hepatobiliary scan for biliary dynamics Blood pool scan for hemangioma > 2 cm PET scan for metastases
Often helpful	Typical incidental hemangioma Focal lesions > 2 cm Blood flow in focal masses Diffuse fatty liver Advanced cirrhosis Guidance for simple drainage procedures	Typical hemangioma, FNH, focal fat* Diffuse fatty liver Extent of abscess, primary tumor, biliary disease* Flow in TIPS*	Acute hematoma Extrahepatic tumor Cirrhosis†	Sulfur colloid scan for cirrhosis and FNH Gallium scan for hepatoma
Rarely helpful	Obese patients Focal lesions in fatty liver FNH Extrahepatic tumor Iron deposition	Direction of blood flow in hepatic vessels Iron deposition Hepatoma vs adenoma vs regenerative nodule Chronic hematoma	Hepatoma vs adenoma Flow in TIPS Guidance for biopsies	Sulfur colloid scan for metastases

*Intravenous contrast is required.
†Intravenous Gadolinium is often required.
MRI—magnetic resonance imaging; US—ultrasonography.

later portal venous phase they may become isoattenuating, and therefore, undetectable. This enhancement pattern is observed in most primary liver tumors, although only in the minority of metastases. Hypovascular lesions, which represent most hepatic metastases and some HCC enhance less than normal hepatic parenchyma. These are seen during the portal venous phase of blood flow as areas of low attenuation compared with normal liver [3]. Detection of hypovascular lesions using conventional CT scanners with relatively slow image acquisition may be improved by the bolus-dynamic technique, but hypervascular masses often are missed this way. With helical CT scanners, high-quality images are made much faster during the optimal scanning time and with superior detection of small hepatic masses. Moreover, with helical CT, the liver can be scanned

twice, during the hepatic arterial phase of blood flow and then during the portal venous phase. This technique of dual-phase helical scanning maximizes detection of hypervascular hepatic lesions and has been advocated for evaluation of primary hepatic tumors and potential hypervascular metastases [5••].

CT arteriography is an invasive technique that encompasses CT arterial portography (CTAP) and CT hepatic arteriography (CTHA). These techniques maximize detection of focal liver lesions and are used before hepatic resection. These methods require intra-arterial injection of iodinated contrast media through a catheter placed in the superior mesenteric or splenic artery (CTAP) or in the hepatic artery (CTHA). Of all preoperative imaging tests, CTAP has the highest sensitivity for detection of small (≤1 cm) liver lesions. Limitations of CTAP

Table 92-2. Diagnostic Strategies With Liver Imaging

Disease	Screening test	Alternative test	Addtional tests
Suspected metastases	CT → biopsy	MRI	Preoperative CTAP, or MRI with ferrumoxides, or PET-FDG scintigraphy
Suspected hepatoma	US → biopsy	CT or MRI → biopsy	Preoperative MRI with ferrumoxides, or CTAP
Elevated LFTs RUQ pain	US	Negative US → CT or MRI	Variable, depending on findings
Cirrhosis	US	CT or MRI	Hepatic vein wedge pressure Biopsy
Incidental lesion > 2 cm by US or CT	Blood pool scintigraphy for hemangioma	MRI for both hemangioma and FNH → biopsy of indeterminate lesions	Sulfur-colloid scintigraphy for FNH
Incidental lesion < 2 cm by US or CT	MRI	CT	Biopsy or follow-up MRI for indeterminate lesions
Abscess	US	CT or MRI	Aspiration or drainage
Budd-Chiari syndrome	US	CT or MRI	Hepatic venography and wedge pressure Biopsy for venoocclusive disease
Hemochromatosis and iron overload	MRI	Biopsy	Follow-up MRI

CTAP—CT arterial portography; FNH—focal nodular hyperplasia; MRI—magnetic resonance imaging; PET-FDG—positron emission topography-fluorodeoxyglucose; US—ultrasonography.

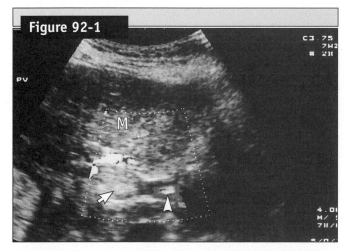

Figure 92-1

The sagittal sonogram demonstrates hyperechoic liver metastases (M) in a patient with melanoma. A thrombus in the main portal vein (*arrow*) with some flow caudally (*arrowhead*) is demonstrated by color Doppler ultrasonography. See also **Color Plate**.

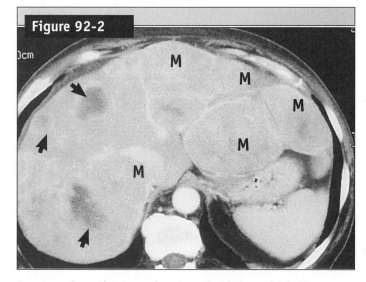

Figure 92-2

Contrast-enhanced computed tomography shows multiple liver metastases in a patient with breast cancer. Lesions of low attenuation are hypovascular (*arrows*); others are hypervascular (*M*).

and CTHA include invasiveness, inability to characterize small lesions, and flow artifacts [6].

Magnetic Resonance Imaging

Inherent tissue contrast between liver and a focal lesion is superior with MR imaging to that with any other imaging technique. There is no exposure to ionizing radiation and no need for intravenous iodinated contrast medium. Compared with CT, however, MR imaging plays a relatively small clinical role in evaluation of the liver. The high cost, inability to reliably image extrahepatic disease, and relatively long examination time of MR imaging limit its application. MR imaging is contraindicated for patients with cardiac pacemakers, implanted defibrillators and other electronic devices, metallic foreign bodies in the orbit, some ocular implants, and ferromagnetic aneurysm clips.

MR imaging is used as a problem-solving tool when CT or ultrasonography is unable to detect or characterize a lesion. MR is indicated as a primary imaging test in patients with suspected or known cancer when there is contraindication to the use of iodinated contrast material, poor intravenous access, a failed contrast CT study, or hepatic steatosis identified on a good-quality CT scan [3]. The most common indication for MR imaging of the liver is the necessity to characterize an indeterminate lesion incidentally discovered by CT or ultrasonography. Hemangiomas, cysts, focal fat, and some regenerative nodules can be diagnosed accurately and differentiated from tumor with MR imaging (Fig. 92-3). MR imaging also is useful for diagnosis of some diffuse processes, such as iron overload, and can be used to monitor treatment of patients with hemochromatosis.

To image the liver optimally, most investigators recommend at least two sequences, T1- and T2-weighted, for every examination [7].

At the time of preparing this manuscript, two types of intravenous contrast have been approved in the United States for use in MR imaging: gadolinium chelates and ferumoxides [7]. The former are extracellular agents that have a distribution and clearance similar to that of the iodinated compounds used in CT. Similar enhancement patterns for hypovascular and hyper-

vascular lesions are observed in contrast CT and MR imaging with gadolinium chelates. These agents improve detection and characterization of liver lesions and have excellent safety records without evidence of nephrotoxicity [7,8••].

Ferumoxides are a recently introduced colloid containing iron oxide particles that undergo phagocytosis by reticuloendothelial cells and markedly decrease signal intensity for normal liver. Focal liver lesions that do not contain Kupffer cells are identified by their bright signal on a T2-weighted scan [7,8••].

Nuclear Scintigraphy

A liver-spleen scan with [99m]technetium-sulfur–labeled colloid is based on uptake of sulfur colloid by reticuloendothelial cells. This technique plays almost no role in lesion detection, because it has relatively low spatial resolution compared with cross-sectional imaging. Even with the improved sensitivity of single-photon emission computed tomography (SPECT), detection of lesions smaller than 2 cm remains problematic [9]. In addition, detected cold defects are nonspecific. Sulfur colloid scintigraphy is useful in characterization of FNH. It also is performed in conjunction with blood-pool imaging for assessment of hemangiomas.

Hepatobiliary scintigraphy with ^{99m}Tc-labeled iminodiacetic acid (IDA) analogues frequently is used to asses the patency of the cystic duct in patients suspected of having cholecystitis. This technique also may be used to evaluate the function of hepatocytes in focal liver lesions [10].

Hepatic blood-pool imaging with 99m Tc-labeled red blood cells is the most reliable and cost-effective method of confirming that an incidentally discovered liver lesion is a hemangioma [2,10]. Labeled red blood cells allow imaging of the large blood vessels and blood-pool activity in the liver, revealing the typical flow pattern of a hemangioma.

Immunoscintigraphy with monoclonal antibodies and positron emission tomography (PET) can be obtained for modern oncologic imaging. The degree of tracer uptake by the liver in the former technique varies from increased to none, depending on the tumor size and presence of necrosis, allowing a significant number of liver metastases to be missed [9,11]. With PET scanning, tumor detection is based on increased glucose metabolism by malignant cells; PET scanning can identify very small tumor foci as areas of increased uptake. The most common positron-emitting radiopharmaceutical used for these studies is [18]fluorine-labeled deoxyglucose (FDG). PET-FDG scanning is highly accurate in detecting recurrent malignant disease and liver metastases, with reported sensitivities and specificities considerably higher than those of CT [12]. The major limitation of PET is its high cost and the necessity to correlate the findings with CT to localize the foci of increased uptake in the liver [11]. Nevertheless, the technique may prove to be cost-effective, if unnecessary surgery is avoided.

[67]Gallium citrate-labeled and [111]indium-labeled leukocyte scintigraphy can be employed to evaluate focal liver infections. These tracers are used infrequently, because CT and ultrasonography are superior in diagnosing liver abscesses and can guide percutaneous drainage of infection. These tests are not specific for hepatic infection, and the radionuclides accumulate in areas of inflammation and in some neoplasms, including HCC.

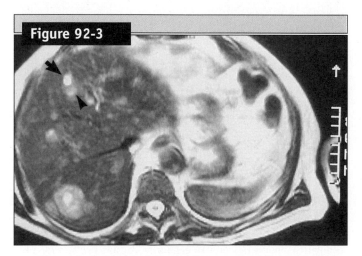

Figure 92-3

Metastases of colon cancer (*arrowhead*) are moderately hyperintense on T2-weighted magnetic resonance images. The small, very bright lesion (*arrow*) represents a cyst adjacent to a metastasis.

■ MALIGNANT HEPATIC LESIONS
Metastases

The goals of liver imaging in oncologic patients include detection of hepatic lesions, characterization of each lesion as benign or malignant, and assessment of resectability in candidates for curative hepatic resection. Patients with less than 30% estimated residual liver volume after resection, involvement of the right and left lobes, or more than four metastatic lesions are considered poor surgical candidates; additional superficial liver lesions, however may be removed by wedge resection [13].

Unfortunately, routine CT scanning, MR imaging, and ultrasonography have poor sensitivity for detecting liver lesions, with overall reported sensitivities of less than 80% and considerably lower detection rates for lesions smaller than 1 cm [6,13]. The highest tumor detection rates, between 81% and 93%, have been achieved with CTAP [13,14], and this technique often is used to evaluate patients before resection of hepatic metastases. Comparable results have been reported with two noninvasive tests: PET-FDG scintigraphy [10] and MR imaging with ferumoxides [14].

CT is considered the initial imaging test of choice for detection of liver metastases [3,6]. Noncontrast CT can identify approximately 50% of metastatic liver lesions, which typically are multiple. Mucin-producing tumors from the colon, stomach, or ovary may contain fine calcifications. Cystic metastases are rare [3] and must be differentiated from hepatic cysts and abscesses. After intravenous injection of contrast medium, the features of metastases seen depend on the timing of the scan and the vascularity of the tumor. Peripheral rim enhancement may be observed during the arterial phase, and inhomogeneous hypoattenuated masses, sometimes with a target appearance, are typically seen during the portal venous phase (Fig. 92-2) [11]. Some hypervascular metastases, usually originating from primary endocrine, renal cell, and breast tumors, may be identified only during the arterial phase of dual-phase helical CT scanning [5••].

The ability of CT to detect metastases is limited by decreased attenuation of the liver caused by steatosis or hepatic dysfunction associated with chronic portal venous or biliary obstruction. Tumors in such hypodense areas may be difficult to detect because of low liver-to-lesion contrast [3].

Most investigators agree that unenhanced MR is as sensitive as enhanced CT for detection of liver metastases and is superior to CT for lesion characterization [6]. Tumor deposits often are inhomogeneous, with irregular contours. MR signal intensity is typically low on unenhanced T1-weighted images and moderately high on T2-weighted scans (Fig. 92-3). Changes in the typical signal intensities of metastatic tumors may occur with hemorrhage or necrosis. T2-weighted images enhanced with ferumoxides have shown improved detection of metastases [14]. Chemical shift sequences allow differentiation of metastases from focal or diffuse fatty infiltration. The use of intravenous gadolinium chelates helps differentiate most hepatic metastases from hemangiomas.

Most metastatic lesions are hypoechoic on transcutaneous ultrasonography, but hyperechoic (Fig. 92-1), isoechoic, target-like, calcified, and cystic metastases also may be observed. Color-flow Doppler patterns of metastases are nonspecific.

Hepatocellular Carcinoma

The imaging features of HCC depend on whether the tumor is expansile, infiltrating, multifocal, or diffuse [4] (see Chapter 102). Although infiltrating and diffuse lesions may be indistinguishable from metastases, many expansile and some multifocal tumors have features that are considered to be typical of HCC: encapsulation, intratumoral steatosis, and mosaic internal morphology attributed to the differential growth of multiple nodules. Daughter nodules, portal or hepatic venous invasion, and cirrhotic changes in the liver are common associated findings [4]. These features of HCC are detected by all cross-sectional imaging tests. Regardless of the specific imaging features of a focal lesion in a cirrhotic liver, it should be considered to be HCC until proved otherwise.

Ultrasonography is the test most commonly used to screen for HCC, but its reported sensitivity for detecting primary cancer in a cirrhotic liver is less than 50%. The diffuse type of HCC is particularly difficult to diagnose by ultrasonography.

Dual-phase helical CT scanning is preferable to conventional CT for detection of HCC in cirrhotic patients [4]. It typically shows hyperattenuating tumors during the arterial phase and rapidly decreasing attenuation during the portal venous phase. A capsule may be seen as an enhancing rim (Fig. 92-4). Larger tumors may have a mosaic appearance [4]. Invasive tumors are poorly defined and heterogeneous. Arterioportal shunting may be identified during the arterial phase of contrast enhancement. CT is the best technique for evaluation of extrahepatic spread of hepatoma, including distant metastases.

Most HCC tumors are hypointense on T1-weighted MR sequences. T1-hyperintense lesions are seen in approximately 40% of cases [4]. With T2-weighting, HCC tumors usually are hyperintensive. Larger lesions are often heterogeneous [4]. The mosaic appearance of some tumors is identified as multiple nodules of different signal intensity (Fig. 92-5). Enhancement of HCC with intravenous gadolinium shows changes similar to those described with contrast-enhanced CT. Intravenous ferumoxides improve detection of small satellite lesions [8]. MR angiography may be performed to evaluate the patency of the portal vein, hepatic veins, and inferior vena cava.

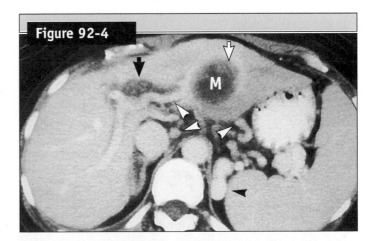

Figure 92-4

Contrast-enhanced computed tomography (CT) shows a hepatocellular carcinoma (*M*) with an enhancing capsule (*white arrow*) in a patient with cirrhosis. The CT scan also demonstrates a thrombus in the left portal vein (*arrow*), collateral veins (*white arrowheads*), splenomegaly, and perisplenic varices (*black arrowhead*).

HCC tumors accumulate gallium on scintigraphic studies in 90% to 95% of cases. They are cold on sulfur colloid scans. Well-differentiated tumors may show increased uptake on hepatobiliary scintigraphy in up to 50% of cases [15].

Fibrolamellar Carcinoma

Fibrolamellar carcinoma is a disease that affects young adults without underlying cirrhosis [15] (see Chapter 102). Some of the imaging features of this malignant tumor are remarkably similar to those of FNH, a benign lesion (see Chapter 101). This similarity is caused by the characteristics common to both lesions: a central scar and hypervascularity [8••].

A preoperative diagnosis of fibrolamellar carcinoma can be made by nuclear scintigraphy. Sulfur colloid scanning often shows a cold defect and no evidence of cirrhosis in patients with fibrolamellar carcinoma, but gallium scanning typically demonstrates increased uptake in these persons. Fibrolamellar carcinoma usually is isointense on T1- and T2-weighted MR sequences. However, it may be slightly hyperintense and slightly hypointense on T2-weighted scans. A central fibrous scar of FLC is hypointense on both T1- and T2-weighted sequences [8••]. Ultrasonography usually shows a large well-defined mass of mixed echogenicity, sometimes with acoustic shadowing due to calcification [15]. On CT, fibrolamellar carcinoma may be heterogeneous with a hypodense, occasionally calcified scar and have marked contrast enhancement [15].

■ BENIGN HEPATIC LESIONS
Cavernous Hemangioma

Cavernous hemangiomas are the most common benign liver lesions, occurring in 0.5% to 20% of persons [6,8••] (see Chapter 101). Most hemangiomas are clinically insignificant, but their appearance is frequently atypical and may prompt an extensive investigation. Most hemangiomas are smaller than 4 cm, but larger lesions occur rarely. They are multiple in about 10% to 20% of cases.

On ultrasonography, about 70% of hemangiomas appear as well-defined, homogeneous hyperechoic masses with posterior acoustic enhancement. The remaining 30% are nonspecific solid lesions that may have hypoechoic, isoechoic or mixed echogenicity [16]. The very slow blood flow in hemangiomas usually is not detected by color or duplex Doppler ultrasonography but can be demonstrated by power Doppler ultrasonography, which is more sensitive to slow flow [2].

A dedicated CT protocol used in the 1980s to confirm the diagnosis of hemangioma, is now uncommonly used, because it is only 54% sensitive and 86% specific for hemangioma in oncology patients [2,6,9]. Some studies indicate that hemangioma can be diagnosed reliably with routine contrast-enhanced CT; typical is a focal nodular pattern of peripheral enhancement, which is isodense with the vascular compartment and reflects filling of vascular lakes of the lesion (Fig. 92-6) [19].

On MR imaging, a hemangioma is a sharply delineated and usually homogeneous mass, although heterogeneity may be caused by fibrosis. On T1-weighted images, these lesions are hypointense; marked hyperintensity on T2-weighted and heavily T2-wieghted sequences differentiates hemangiomas from most solid lesions (Fig. 92-7A), the so-called light bulb sign [2]. Unfortunately, hypervascular metastases may have identical signal characteristics. For more accurate diagnosis of hemangioma, serial gadolinium-enhanced imaging is required [17]; nodular peripheral enhancement with progressive fill-in is characteristic of this lesion (Fig. 92-7B). Very small hemangiomas may still be difficult to differentiate from hypervascular metastases.

The diagnosis of hemangioma is made on blood-pool scintigraphy by identification of a "perfusion and blood-pool mismatch." This is done by comparing immediate flow to later static images. On early blood-pool images, hemangiomas are usually photon deficient, or cold. They show progressive increased uptake (ie, blood pooling) on delayed images (Fig. 92-7C and 92-7D). The technique is cost-effective and highly specific; its sensitivity has been improved by application of SPECT systems [10]. False-positive results rarely occur for atypical primary or metastatic tumors. Most false-negative results were found with small hemangiomas (<2 to 2.5 cm) and those adjacent to the heart, large vessels, or diaphragm [10].

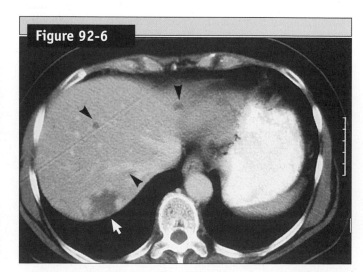

Figure 92-5

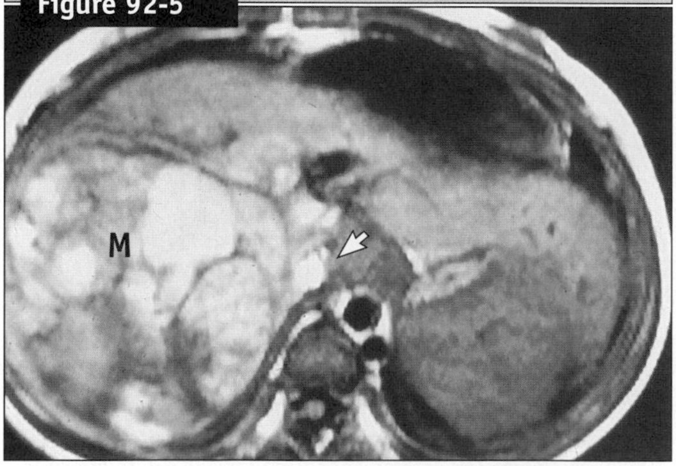

An encapsulated hepatocellular carcinoma (*M*) with a mosaic pattern is demonstrated on T1-weighted magnetic resonance imaging. The inferior vena cava (*arrow*) is occluded.

Figure 92-6

Contrast-enhanced computed tomography shows an incidental hemangioma (*arrow*) with characteristic nodular peripheral enhancement and very small hepatic cysts (*arrowheads*).

When a typical hemangioma is detected by ultrasonography or CT in an asymptomatic patient without a known primary tumor, most investigators recommend no further studies or follow-up assessment [2], but some believe that follow-up sonography in 3 to 6 months later is justified to confirm stability of the lesion [16]. Other physicians recommend confirmation of the diagnosis with SPECT blood-pool scintigraphy for lesions larger than 2.5 cm and with MR imaging for smaller masses. In patients who are at risk for developing HCC or have a history of cancer, at least one of these techniques is required to confirm that a lesion is a hemangioma. Atypical lesions are evaluated with biopsy [16].

Focal Steatosis

Unlike diffuse steatosis, which can be recognized easily by increased hepatic echogenicity on ultrasonography and hypoattenuation on CT, the appearance of focal steatosis may be confusing. On sonography, zones of focal fat may appear as hyperechoic masses in some patients, whereas in others, areas of focal sparing resemble hypoechoic tumors. On CT, a typical case of focal steatosis can be diagnosed by characteristic peripheral locations, lack of mass-effect, nonspherical geo-

graphical shapes, and interdigitation or straight interface with normal liver. Unfortunately, in many instances both focal fat and focally spared normal parenchyma may stimulate tumors on CT. Additionally, focal as well as diffuse steatosis can obscure true metastases.

MR imaging is the method of choice to diagnose focal steatosis using chemical shift imaging technique. Areas of focal fat become hypointense on opposed phase sequences compared with in-phase images. True malignancy can be detected by hyperintensity on T2-weighted images.

Focal Nodular Hyperplasia

FNH is the second most common benign liver mass after hemangioma and usually is detected incidentally in an asymptomatic person (see Chapter 101) [8••]. Lesions typically are smaller than 5 cm in diameter, solitary, unencapsulated, well-circumscribed, and homogeneous, with a central scar that contains an arteriovenous malformation [2,8••]. Multiple lesions may occur in as many as 20% of cases [16].

On ultrasonography, FNH is often a subtle mass with variable echogenicity; it commonly is hyperechoic to normal liver tissue. The central scar is often hypoechoic, but it may be poor-

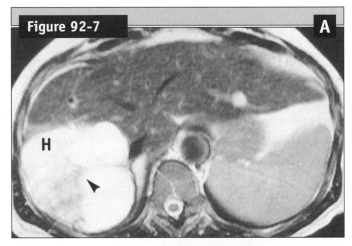

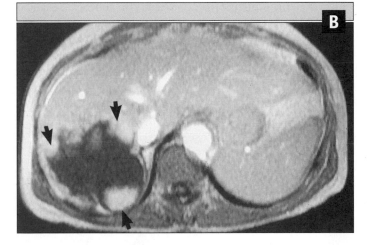

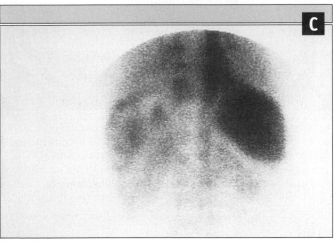

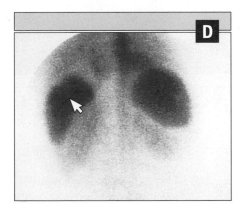

A, T2-weighted magnetic resonance (MR) imaging shows a markedly hyperintense incidental hemangioma (*H*) with dark central fibrosis (*arrowhead*) in the right hepatic lobe. A second tiny hemangioma (*arrow*) is located in the left lobe. **B**, Enhanced T1-weighted MR sequences shows peripheral nodular enhancement (*arrows*) of the large lesion, which is typical for a hemangioma. A small, left lobe lesion is completely enhanced and no longer visualized. **C**, Blood pool scintigraphy shows minimal accumulation of the tracer on an early static scan. **D**, Increased uptake on a delayed scan (*arrow*) is characteristic of a hemangioma.

ly visible [1]. Characteristic Doppler ultrasonographic features include a predominantly arterial signal in the central scar with well-developed peripheral vessels [2].

Nuclear scintigraphy is diagnostic of FNH when it shows focal increased uptake of sulfur colloid (*ie*, hot lesions), a feature found in approximately 10% of these lesions [9]. A cold defect is seen on scintigraphy in 40% of patients with FNH, while the remaining 50% of affected persons have uptake by the lesion similar to that of normal liver (*ie*, warm lesions) [16] (Fig. 92-8). Contrary to previous belief, warm lesions are not always FNH; they may be adenomas, focal fatty infiltration, or regenerative nodules [10].

On CT with intravenous contrast, there is strong enhancement of FNH during the arterial phase and a rapid decrease in attenuation in the portal venous phase (Fig. 92-8). FNH usually is homogeneous and isointense to liver on T1- and T2-weighted MR images. However, these lesions may be slightly hypo- or hyperintense on T2-weighted images, mimicking other solid tumors. The central scar is usually hypointense on T1-weighted and hyperintense on T2-weighted images. The latter helps differentiate an FNH scar from others that are typically T2-hypointense [8] (Fig. 92-8*B*). With gadolinium chelates, FNH shows marked enhancement, similar to its appearance on contrast-enhanced CT. Delayed enhancement of the central scar may be observed [17]. In general, central scars are not specific to FNH and have been shown with other benign and malignant liver tumors. However, a T2-hyperintense and enhancing scar suggests an FNH.

Hepatocellular Adenoma

Hepatocellular adenoma is an uncommon lesion associated with use of oral contraceptives (see Chapter 101). Hepatocellular adenomas are typically large, well-defined, encapsulated lesions that are cold on sulfur colloid scintigraphy. Some lesions, however, may show normal sulfur colloid uptake similar to that of FNH [9].

The cross-sectional appearance of an adenoma depends on the amount and chronicity of associated hemorrhage, necrosis, and fibrosis. On ultrasonography, the lesion may have variable echogenicity. Acute hemorrhage within the adenoma may be detected by unenhanced CT scanning as a zone of high attenuation; in a symptomatic young woman without a history of trauma, this suggests the diagnosis [2]. Contrast-enhanced CT of a person with hepatocellular adenoma typically shows an otherwise nonspecific mass to be hypervascular. On MR imaging, the variable signal intensity of hepatocellular adenoma often overlaps with that of HCC. No specific features of hepatocellular adenoma have been reported on contrast-enhanced MR imaging [8••].

Hepatic Cysts

Benign hepatic cysts are found in approximately 2.5% of all persons [1,16]. Cysts appear as sharply defined, thin-walled lesions with occasional thin septations on cross-sectional imaging. Wall thickening, excessive septation, and internal debris should suggest that the lesion is not a simple cyst, but another type of cystic process, such as a cystic metastasis, abscess, hydatid cyst, or biliary cystadenoma.

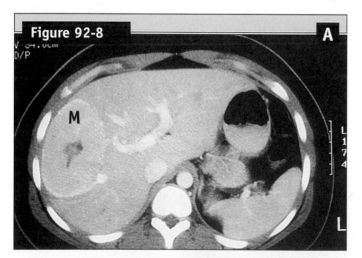

Figure 92-8

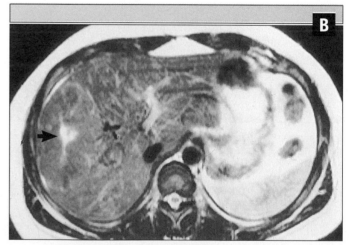

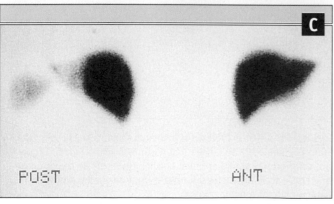

A, Computed tomography demonstrates a hypervascular mass (*M*) with a central scar in a patient with focal nodular hyperplasia and right lower quadrant pain. **B**, The mass is isointense with a hyperintense central scar (*arrow*) seen on T2-weighted magnetic resonance imaging. **C**, Sulfur colloid scintigraphy shows no corresponding defect, indicating the reticuloendothelial function of the lesion.

On ultrasonography, cysts are anechoic, with acoustic enhancement. On CT scans, they have the attenuation of water and do not enhance. On MR imaging, cysts are hypointense on T1-weighted images and markedly hyperintense on T2- and heavily T2-weighted images, similar to hemangioma. Unlike hemangiomas, cysts do not enhance with gadolinium chelates [16]. Cysts smaller than 1 cm in diameter may be difficult to characterize with CT and MR scanning because of volume averaging.

Abscess

The most common hepatic abscesses, pyogenic and amebic, have similar appearances: well-defined, thick-walled, oval or round, and usually solitary masses. Amebic abscesses tend to be subcapsular. Multiple microabscesses may be seen in immuno-compromised patients and are sometimes difficult to detect.

Ultrasonography can detect 80% of hepatic abscesses [16]. Pyogenic and amebic collections may have fluid levels, debris, and overall variable echogenicity with or without acoustic enhancement [1]. A pyogenic abscess often has internal septations and may contain gas.

On CT, abscesses have attenuation greater than that of water and have rim enhancement with intravenous contrast [16]. On MR, they have a fluid-like signal intensity and peripheral enhancement with gadolinium [17]. On gallium scintigraphy, pyogenic abscesses have diffusely increased uptake, and amebic collections concentrate the tracer at the periphery [9].

◼ DIFFUSE LIVER DISEASE
Cirrhosis

Regardless of cause, cirrhosis is characterized by fibrosis and nodular regeneration [16,18]. Late in the disease, this typically results in atrophy of the right lobe and the medial segment of the left lobe, while the caudate lobe and the lateral segment of the left lobe undergo hypertrophy; there is an overall decrease in liver volume. These morphologic changes are detected by cross-sectional imaging; a caudate lobe to right lobe ratio of 0.65 or greater allows diagnosis of cirrhosis with 96% confidence [18].

Parenchymal abnormalities are not detected by imaging tests early in the course of disease, with the exception of steatosis that is commonly associated with alcoholic cirrhosis [16]. Later, a heterogeneous hepatic texture and nodular contour can be seen on CT and T2-weighted MR (Fig. 92-9). Contour irregularity also may be identified on ultrasonography. Sonographically, cirrhotic liver is characterized by increased echogenicity with coarse texture and decreased sound transmission [16]. These findings, however, are not specific and overlap with those of hepatic steatosis.

Regenerative nodules usually are hypoechoic on ultrasonography. On CT, nodules with increased iron content show high attenuation on unenhanced scans and isoattenuation on enhanced images. On MR imaging, regenerative nodules with an increased iron content can be more definitively identified by low signal intensity on T2-weighted images combined with low signal intensity on T1-weighted images (Fig. 92-9). Any other combination of signal is nonspecific for a regenerative nodule, and in a cirrhotic liver it may represent an HCC [9]. Most commonly, an HCC is hyperintense on T2-weighted images [4,8••,17].

Evidence of portal hypertension, including splenomegaly, ascites, varices, and enlargement of the portal, splenic, superior mesenteric, and coronary veins, can be documented with all cross-sectional imaging. A portal vein larger than 1.3 cm in diameter is 100% specific for portal hypertension, but it is only 75% sensitive [18]. CT and MR imaging can detect periesophageal, azygos, and retroperitoneal varices that are not seen on ultrasonography. MR angiographic sequences can be used to evaluate portal venous flow. However, Doppler ultrasonography is considered the test of choice for detection of portal hypertension and evaluation of some portosystemic collaterals [18].

Sulfur colloid scintigraphy during the early stages of cirrhosis is nonspecific, showing hepatomegaly with patchy hepatic uptake and redistribution of tracer to the spleen and bone marrow. Similar findings are seen in patient with hepatitis or diffuse metastatic disease. Later, when liver size is decreased, extrahepatic tracer uptake correlates well with the presence of portal hypertension [18].

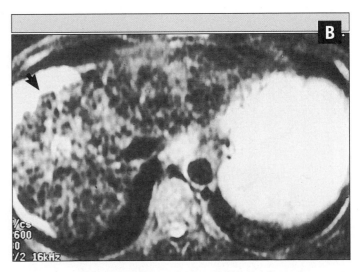

A, In a patient with cirrhosis, T1-weighted magnetic resonance (MR) imaging shows a nodular liver contour (*arrowheads*) and multiple, small, hypointense regenerative nodules, as well as splenomegaly and large gastric varices (*arrows*). **B,** In the same patient, the regenerative nodules are hypointense on T2-weighted MR sequence. Ascites (*arrow*) is also demonstrated.

Budd-Chiari Syndrome

Budd-Chiari syndrome is caused by obstruction of the main hepatic veins or inferior vena cava (see Chapter 14). Associated findings including ascites, hepatomegaly, and caudate lobe enlargement, which can be identified by all imaging tests.

Ultrasonography can demonstrate morphologic abnormalities in the main hepatic veins, including congenital webs, stenosis, wall thickening, and thrombosis. Flow abnormalities can be assessed with Doppler ultrasonography [16].

CT and MR imaging can show the level of thrombosis, narrowing of the vena cava, and nonvisualization of the venous confluence. With intravenous contrast, the liver parenchyma is inhomogeneous, with decreased enhancement around the hepatic veins. Intrahepatic venous collaterals also are seen (*ie*, the comma sign). On MR imaging, comma-shaped intrahepatic collaterals can be seen without contrast [16].

Hemochromatosis

Hemochromatosis can be diagnosed accurately by MR imaging, because iron deposited in hepatocytes causes a marked decrease of hepatic signal intensity on T2-weighted images (see Chapter 108). Associated findings in patients with hemochromatosis include similarly decreased signal intensity in the pancreas and myocardium, additional sites of parenchymal iron accumulation (Fig. 92-10). Primary hemochromatosis may be differentiated from hemosiderosis by MR scans. Hemochromatosis and hemosiderosis are characterized by low hepatic signal intensity, but in hemosiderosis, the spleen and bone marrow also have low signal intensity, while the pancreas and myocardium retain their normal signals.

Hemochromatosis causes increased attenuation of the liver on noncontrast CT [16], but it is less sensitive than MR imaging for making the diagnosis, because associated fatty infiltration often diminishes liver density to within the normal range. CT also is less specific than MR imaging because increased liver attenuation may occur in other diseases, such as glycogen storage disease, shock liver, amiodarone toxicity, and Wilson's disease [16,18]. Ultrasonography is not useful in the diagnosis of hemochromatosis.

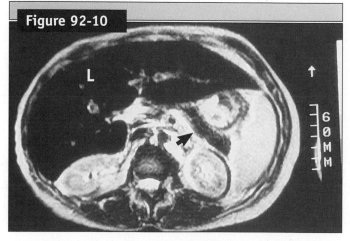

Figure 92-10

T2-weighted magnetic resonance imaging demonstrates the decreased signal intensity of the liver (*L*) and pancreas (*arrow*), which is characteristic for hemochromatosis.

REFERENCES

Recently published papers of particular interest have been highlighted as follows:
•   Of interest
••   Of outstanding interest

1. Nisenbaum HL, Rowling SE: Ultrasound of focal hepatic lesions. *Semin Roentgenol* 1995, 30:324–346.

2. Wilson SR: Hepatic tumors: part 2. Imaging of benign hepatic lesions. In *Radiology of the Liver, Biliary Tract, and Pancreas: Categorical Course Syllabus.* Edited by Freeny PC, Dodd GD II, Cooperberg PL, Ros PR. Reston, VA: ARRS; 1996:17–25.

3. Nelson RC: Hepatic metastases: detection and staging. In *Radiology of the Liver, Biliary Tract, and Pancreas: Categorical Course Syllabus.* Edited by Freeny PC, Dodd GD III, Cooperberg PL, Ros PR. Reston, VA: ARRS; 1996:47–53.

4. Johnson CD: Imaging of hepatocellular carcinoma. In *Radiology of the Liver, Biliary Tract, and Pancreas: Categorical Course Syllabus.* Edited by Freeny PC, Dodd GD III, Cooperberg PL, Ros PR. Reston, VA: ARRS; 1996:41–46.

5.•• Oliver JH, Baron RL: Helical biphasic contrast-enhanced CT of the liver: technique, indications, interpretation, and pitfalls. *Radiology* 1996, 201:1–14.
In this report, the authors discuss the value of a duel-phase helical CT for improved detection and differentiation of various liver lesions. They provide readers with the understanding of normal enhancement patterns of the liver as well as the appearance of tumors, benign lesions, and artifacts.

6. Ferrucci JT: Liver tumor imaging: current concepts. *Radiol Clin North Am* 1994, 32:39–54.

7. Weinreb JC: Hepatobiliary MR imaging. In *Practical MR Imaging: Categorical Course Syllabus.* Edited by McCarthy SM, Ramsey RG, Weinreb JC. Reston, VA: ARRS; 1997:107–115.

8.•• Powers C, Ros PR, Stoupis C, *et al.*: Primary liver neoplasms: MR imaging with pathologic correlation. *Radiographics* 1994, 14:459–482.
In this report, the authors correlate pathologic features of benign and malignant primary liver tumors with MR imaging findings. The powerful potential of MR imaging for tissue characterization and determination of tumor extent is well-illustrated.

9. Kinnard MF, Alavi A, Rubin RA, Lichtenstein GR: Nuclear imaging of solid hepatic masses. *Semin Roentgenol* 1995, 30:375–395.

10. Middleton ML: Scintigraphic evaluation of hepatic mass lesions: emphasis on hemangioma detection. *Semin Nucl Med* 1996, 26:4–15.

11. Thoeni RF: Colorectal cancer: radiologic staging. *Radiol Clin North Am* 1997, 35:457–485.

12. Gupta N, Bradfield H: Role of positron emission tomography scanning in evaluating gastrointestinal neoplasms. *Semin Nucl Med* 1996, 26:65–73.

13. Soyer P, Bluemke DA, Fishman EK: CT during arterial portography for the preoperative evaluation of hepatic tumors: how, when, and why? *AJR* 1994, 163:1325–1331.

14. Seneterre E, Taourel P, Bouvier Y, *et al.*: Detection of hepatic metastases: ferumoxide-enhanced MR imaging versus unenhanced MR imaging and CT during arterial portography. *Radiology* 1996, 200:7895–792.

15. Ros PR: Malignant liver tumors. In *Textbook of Gastrointestinal Radiology.* Edited by Gore RM, Levine MS, Laufer I. Philadelphia: WB Saunders; 1994.

16. Vassiliades VG, Bree RL, Korobkin M: Focal and diffuse benign hepatic disease: correlative imaging. *Semin Ultrasound CT MR* 1992, 13:313–335.

17. Larson RE, Semelka R: Magnetic resonance imaging of the liver. *Top Magn Reson Imaging* 1995, 7:71–81.

18. Gore RM: Diffuse liver disease. In *Textbook of Gastrointestinal Radiology.* Edited by Gore RM, Levine MS, Laufer I. Philadelphia: WB Saunders; 1994.

19. Quinn SF, Benjamin GG: Hepatic cavernous hemangioma: simple diagnostic sign with dynamic belus CT. *Radiology* 1992; 182:545–548.

93 Acute Viral Hepatitis

Raymond S. Koff

Viral infection is the most common cause of acute and chronic liver disease in the world. Acute liver failure, end-stage chronic liver disease, and hepatocellular carcinoma related to hepatitis virus infection are responsible for more than 1 million deaths annually and extensive morbidity. The spectrum of clinical illness due to hepatitis infection is extraordinarily broad. In many patients, infection is asymptomatic, anicteric, and entirely subclinical; in others, acute, life-threatening liver failure may occur. At present, there is no specific, effective treatment for acute viral hepatitis with the exception of liver transplant for patients with acute irreversible liver failure.

Hepatitis viruses may be classified into two distinct groups: the enterically transmitted, nonenveloped agents, including hepatitis A virus (HAV) and hepatitis E virus (HEV), and the bloodborne, enveloped agents, including hepatitis B virus (HBV), hepatitis D virus (HDV), and hepatitis C virus (HCV) [1]. A fourth bloodborne agent, the hepatitis G virus (HGV) also has been described, but it appears unlikely to be a true hepatitis virus and will not be discussed further here. The enterically transmitted hepatitis viruses survive exposure to bile, are shed in feces, and produce infections that are generally self-limited although they may cause severe hepatitis and acute liver failure; neither a viremic nor an intestinal carrier state occurs and chronic liver disease is not seen. In contrast, the bloodborne, enveloped hepatitis viruses are disrupted by exposure to bile or detergents, are not shed in feces, and may be associated with prolonged viremia, persistent infectivity, and progression to chronic liver disease.

Superbly effective and safe vaccines are available for immunoprophylaxis against HAV and HBV infections. HBV vaccine also prevents HDV infection but a specific HDV vaccine is not available. Immunoprophylaxis against infection with other hepatitis viruses is not currently available [2••] (Table 93-1).

ETIOLOGIC AGENTS OF ACUTE VIRAL HEPATITIS

Hepatitis A Virus

Hepatitis A virus is a small (27 to 28 nm in diameter), spherical RNA virus that is a member of the genus *Hepatovirus*, in the family Picornaviridae. It replicates in the cytoplasm of infected hepatocytes; replication in extrahepatic sites, *eg*, the intestine, has not been documented [1]. The HAV genome is a single-stranded, linear RNA molecule of 7.5 kb. Only one HAV serotype has been recognized in humans, although other serotypes exist in nonhuman primates. Seven HAV genotypes have been identified. HAV is thought to contain a single immunodominant neutralization site against which specific protective antibody is directed. HAV has been propagated in tissue culture, permitting the development of an inactivated HAV vaccine [2••].

Hepatitis E Virus

Hepatitis E virus also is a small (27 to 34 nm in diameter), spherical, RNA virus with a linear 7.5 kb RNA genome. It has been classified in the α-like supergroup of positive-stranded RNA viruses [1]. Only one HEV serotype has been identified. HEV structural proteins and nonstructural proteins are encoded in three overlapping open-reading frames. An immunodominant neutralization site has been localized to the structural protein encoded by the second open-reading frame. Nonstructural proteins involved in viral replication include an RNA-dependent RNA polymerase and a helicase. In vivo replication appears to take place only in hepatocytes. Although in vitro viral culture has

Table 93-1. Overview of the Five Established Hepatitis Viruses

Agent	Nucleic acid	Enveloped	Fecal shedding	Acute liver failure	Prolonged infectivity	Chronic hepatitis	Vaccine available
HAV	RNA	No	Yes	Rare	No	No	Yes
HEV	RNA	No	Yes	10% to 20% in pregnancy	No	No	Trials
HBV	DNA	HBsAg	No	Uncommon	Yes	Yes	Yes
HDV	RNA	HBsAg	No	More common than HBV	Yes	Yes	No
HCV	RNA	Yes	No	Rare	Yes	Yes	Prototype

HAV–hepatitis A virus; HBsAg–hepatitis B surface antigen.

been reported, it has not yet provided an adequate model for study or sufficient antigenic material for vaccine development.

Hepatitis B Virus

Hepatitis B virus is an enveloped, spherical particle 42 nm in diameter with a DNA genome. It is the only member of the hepatotropic family of DNA viruses, the Hepadnaviridae, capable of infecting humans [1]. The HBV particle is composed of an electron-dense nucleocapsid core and an outer lipoprotein envelope. The nucleocapsid core contains a circular, mostly double-stranded and partially single-stranded DNA molecule, a DNA polymerase protein with reverse transcriptase activity, and the hepatitis B core antigen (HBcAg), a structural protein. A nonstructural protein, the hepatitis B early antigen (HBeAg), is a derivative of the HBcAg. The presence of HBeAg in serum correlates with that of HBV DNA and active HBV replication.

The lipoprotein envelope of intact HBV virions also forms smaller, 22 nm spherical and filamentous noninfectious particles. These antigenic particles are present in the blood of infected individuals far in excess of intact HBV. The envelope lipoprotein is termed the *hepatitis B surface antigen* (HBsAg). Three distinct envelope proteins, the major-, large-, and middle-sized, have been characterized. HBV subtypes are recognized based on differences in HBsAg proteins.

HBV replicates in the liver and also in a number of extrahepatic tissues. Replication occurs through reverse transcription, ie, the long strand of HBV DNA is transcribed from an RNA molecule. As a consequence of the poor proofreading ability of the HBV reverse transcriptase, a number of HBV mutations occur. These include an HBeAg-negative precore mutant, and a so-called HBV vaccine-induced escape mutant, both rare in the United States.

Hepatitis D Virus

Hepatitis D virus is a spherical particle 35 to 37 nm in diameter, enveloped by the HBsAg of HBV, and containing single-stranded, covalently closed, circular RNA, with a length of 1.6 kb [3]. HDV requires the helper function of HBV for its expression and pathogenicity. The small RNA genome and its close relationship to HBV have suggested that HDV may be a satellite virus, analogous to the plant satellite viruses. HDV replication is limited to the hepatocyte. There appears to be but one HDV serotype, however, at least three genotypes have been recognized. Although culture of HDV has been difficult to achieve, cell lines have been transfected and express HDV RNA and HDV proteins.

Hepatitis C Virus

This enveloped, single-stranded RNA virus has been reported to be approximately 55 nm in diameter. It has been classified as a distinct genus in the family Flaviviridae. The HCV RNA genome is 9.4 kb in length and encodes a large polyprotein of about 3000 amino acids. About one-third of the polyprotein is cleaved into a series of structural proteins, including a nucleocapsid or core protein, and two glycosylated envelope proteins. The envelope proteins may elicit the production of neutralizing antibodies [2••]. The remainder of the polyprotein consists of a group of nonstructural proteins including a serine protease, a helicase and an RNA-dependent RNA polymerase that participate in HCV replication. Multiple HCV genotypes with variable geographic distribution

have been identified and slightly heterogeneous HCV viruses with only minor amino acid differences, called *quasispecies*, are commonly found in infected individuals. Whether the site of replication of HCV is limited to the liver or to the liver and lymphocytes remains uncertain. Despite numerous reports of culture of HCV, available information suggests that replication in vitro is inefficient.

▇ EPIDEMIOLOGY OF ACUTE VIRAL HEPATITIS

Hepatitis A

The incubation period of HAV is from 15 to 50 days, with a mean of approximately 30 days. HAV infection has a wide geographic distribution, with areas of high endemicity in developing countries and in some native populations of the United States. The overall prevalence of serologic markers of past HAV infection in the United States is about 33%. Fecal excretion of viral particles begins a few weeks before and lasts for at least 1 week after the onset of clinical illness. Although fecal HAV excretion for months has been reported in infected neonates [4•], the epidemiologic importance of this observation remains to be determined. In general, the period of viremia is short, and a carrier state does not exist.

Person-to-person fecal-oral household spread is the predominant mode of HAV transmission and is correlated with household size and sanitary standards. Young children, in whom the infection is difficult to recognize, often play a key role in community outbreaks. Case clusters have been linked to specific fomites, *eg*, contaminated food and water, or inadequately cooked bivalve mollusks. Sporadic cases and clusters of cases have been seen in daycare centers, in institutions for the retarded, and among those sharing drug paraphernalia. Travelers to developing countries and individuals who engage in oral-anal sex are at risk for HAV infection. Maternal-neonatal transmission is epidemiologically unimportant. Rarely, recipients of clotting factors have been infected. No risk factor for HAV infection can be identified in approximately 50% of cases (Fig. 93-1).

Hepatitis E

The incubation period of HEV infection is approximately 40 days. It is the most common form of sporadic hepatitis among young adults in the developing world, but waterborne outbreaks

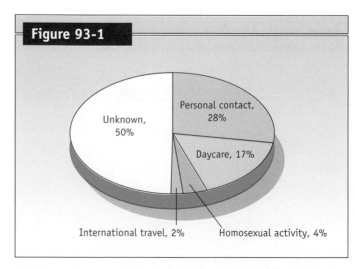

Figure 93-1

Risk factors for hepatitis A virus infection in the United States.

in countries in which the disease is endemic may affect persons of any age. The virus is shed in feces during the acute phase of illness; viremia also is present during this period. Prolonged viremia and fecal shedding are highly unusual but have been reported. Although initially thought to be uncommon, intrafamilial—and household—secondary case attack rates may approach 20%. No endemic foci of HEV infection have been identified in the United States. Hence, hepatitis E is considered an imported infection, limited to returning travelers and visitors from endemic regions. Maternal-neonatal transmission of HEV has been reported [5], but its epidemiologic significance is uncertain. Percutaneous transmission is not an established route of spread.

Hepatitis B

The incubation period of this infection, the most common global cause of persistent viremia, is approximately 60 to 90 days, although an even wider range, 15 to 180 days, often is cited [1]. In self-limited acute HBV infections, viremia may last for weeks to months. Only 1% to 5% of infected adults develop chronic infection with prolonged viremia. In contrast, as many as 90% of neonatal infections and about 50% of infections acquired during infancy result in persistent viremia. Persistent infection may lead to an asymptomatic carrier state, chronic hepatitis (see Chapter 94), cirrhosis, and hepatocellular carcinoma. In the United States, the overall HBV carrier rate is under 1%. In sub-Saharan Africa and parts of Asia, carrier rates of 9% to 12% are reported (Fig. 93-2).

Hepatitis B virus is present in the blood, lymph, semen, cervicovaginal secretions, saliva, and other body fluids of infected individuals. There is no evidence of fecal-oral spread. Major modes of transmission include bloodborne, percutaneous, and sexual routes (Fig. 93-3).

In the past, persons in the United States who were most likely to develop HBV infection were individuals who injected drugs, recipients of high-risk blood products, hemodialysis patients, and health care workers exposed to blood and body fluids. Today, drug injection continues to be a particular risk factor for HBV infection in the United States. Sexual transmission between heterosexual and homosexual partners accounts for nearly 50% of reported cases of hepatitis B [6]. Percutaneous or permucosal transfer of HBV via shared razor blades and toothbrushes, tattooing, body-piercing, and acupuncture may occur, but the overall importance of these modes of transmission in the epidemiology of HBV infection is ill-defined. No risk factor can be identified in as many as 25% of infected patients. Maternal-neonatal and maternal-infant transmission from infected mothers are responsible for high carrier rates observed in many parts of the world [1].

Hepatitis D

The incubation period of this variably distributed infection has been estimated to be 4 to 7 weeks. Because hepatitis D cannot occur in the absence of HBV infection, it is not surprising that there is a considerable degree of concordance in the prevalence of serologic markers of infection with these two viruses. Nonetheless, hepatitis D is not invariably present in areas in which hepatitis B

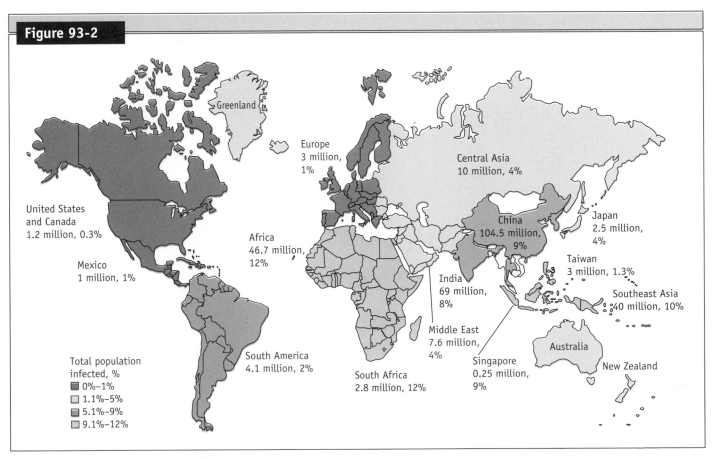

Figure 93-2

Estimates of hepatitis B virus carriers and frequency of the carrier state.

is endemic. Regions of the world where HDV is endemic include the southern Mediterranean and Balkan countries, some Eastern European nations and former Soviet republics, parts of the Middle East, and the countries of the Amazon basin [3] (Fig. 93-4).

In most instances of coinfection with HBV and HDV, the period of HDV viremia is short-lived; in contrast, prolonged infection is more common when HDV occurs as a superinfection in an individual with established HBV infection. Modes of HDV transmission parallel those of HBV.

Hepatitis C

The incubation period of hepatitis C is approximately 50 days, with a very wide range of 15 to 120 days or more [1]. The infec-

tion occurs with variable seroprevalence rates throughout the world. In the United States, just under 2% of the general population has been infected. Higher infection rates are found in specific populations, *eg*, persons who inject illicit drugs, hemophilia patients, and individuals on hemodialysis. In some parts of the world infection rates approach 20%. In contrast to the other bloodborne hepatitis viruses, HCV causes prolonged viremia and persistent hepatitis in as many as 85% of infections. Use of shared drug paraphernalia is currently the predominant mode of spread of HCV in the United States [7]. Before 1989, blood transfusion also was a significant risk factor for infection, but donor screening has nearly eliminated the risk of transfusion-associated hepatitis C [8]. Sexual spread [9] and maternal-neonatal transmission occur but do so far less frequently than in HBV. A variable proportion of infections cannot be attributed to any specific risk factor during the 6 months before onset of illness [6] (Fig. 93-5).

■ PATHOPHYSIOLOGY

The mechanisms responsible for the development of liver injury in acute viral hepatitis remain ill-defined. A direct cytopathic effect of hepatotropic viruses generally is believed to be unlikely. Under specific circumstances, however, it has been postulated that HDV and HCV may directly injure infected liver cells. Whether such a cytopathic effect is related to the replication rate of the virus or the expression of a cytotoxic viral gene product is unknown. A large body of circumstantial and immunologic data support the theory that a T-lymphocyte cell-mediated attack on infected hepatocytes is the predominant mechanism for acute liver injury in viral hepatitis [10]. The specific steps in the pathogenesis of hepatocyte necrosis remain to be determined.

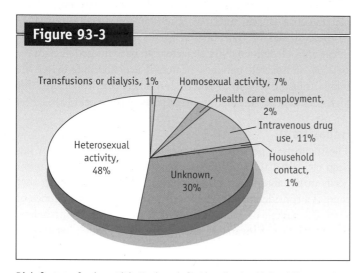

Figure 93-3

Risk factors for hepatitis B virus infection in the United States.

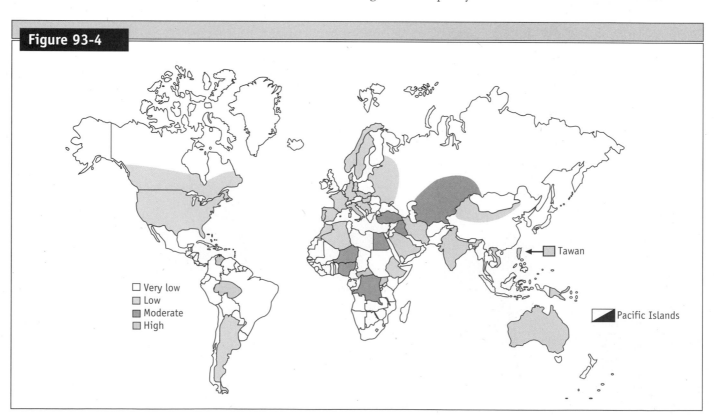

Figure 93-4

Estimates of hepatitis D virus infection rates.

CLINICAL, LABORATORY, AND HISTOLOGIC FEATURES

Self-limited Disease

Each of the etiologic forms of viral hepatitis may cause self-limited disease [1]. Ultimate resolution rates vary widely, however, from nearly 100% in hepatitis A to only about 15% in hepatitis C. Although jaundice is often considered a cardinal feature of acute disease, most viral hepatitis is anicteric, asymptomatic, and unrecognized. Patients with self-limited hepatitis may present with nonspecific prodromal symptoms, followed by constitutional and gastrointestinal complaints and jaundice. Malaise, nausea, vomiting, and anorexia often are present. A serum-sickness syndrome occurs during the prodrome of HBV infection in less than 10% of affected patients. Mild hepatomegaly and slight liver tenderness are common in persons with acute hepatitis, and minimal splenomegaly may be present. Histologic changes in acute viral hepatitis typically include focal hepatocyte necrosis, drop-out, and ballooning degeneration, and Councilman-like bodies, accompanied by central vein endophlebitis, and a round cell infiltrate in the portal tracts and within the hepatic parenchyma (Table 93-2).

Marked elevation of serum alanine and aspartate aminotransferase (ALT and AST) levels with peaks of 500 to 5000 U/mL or higher are typical of the acute phase of viral hepatitis. Serum bilirubin levels are variable, but uncommonly exceed 10 mg/dL. Tests of synthetic function usually are normal or only minimally abnormal. Mild leukopenia with or without atypical lymphocytes and a relative lymphocytosis may be seen. The illness usually peaks within a few weeks of onset and then wanes over a period of weeks, with a marked reduction in symptoms and resolution of biochemical abnormalities.

Fulminant Hepatitis (Acute Liver Failure)

Although unusual, acute liver failure (ALF) may complicate any etiologic form of acute viral hepatitis [1]. ALF is seen most commonly in pregnant women infected with HEV during the third trimester; as many as 20% of such women develop ALF. ALF complicates approximately 1% of HBV and combined HBV and HDV infections. In persons under age 40 with hepatitis A, ALF is even rarer, although it may be seen in 1% to 2.5% of affected patients over age 40. Development of ALF is characterized by alterations in mental status and by coagulopathy with marked hypoprothrombinemia (see Chapter 116). Laboratory features include progressive jaundice with high aminotransferases levels that may decline and approach normal despite clinical deterioration. The course of ALF often includes development of renal failure, gastrointestinal bleeding, and sepsis. Adult respiratory distress syndrome, central hypotension, and arrhythmias also are seen in many affected patients. In the absence of emergency liver transplantation, case-fatality rates approach 90%.

Cholestatic Hepatitis

A very small proportion of patients with acute viral hepatitis, most commonly adults with acute hepatitis A, have severe associated cholestasis. In these individuals, serum bilirubin levels may exceed 20 mg/dL and remain elevated for many weeks to months. Pruritus often is prominent and may be the most distressing feature of this syndrome. Histologic features of cholestatic hepatitis include those of self-limited hepatitis accompanied by prominent bile plugging of dilated hepatocyte canaliculi and pseudoglandular transformation of hepatocytes. In many affected patients, the serum alkaline phosphatase level is normal or only mildly elevated; serum aminotransferase levels decline despite persistent jaundice and synthetic function usually remains normal. The prognosis of cholestatic hepatitis is excellent and complete resolution is to be expected.

Relapsing Hepatitis

Occasionally symptoms of hepatitis and abnormal laboratory tests may recur a few weeks to months after apparent clinical and laboratory recovery from typical acute disease [11]. Such relapses more frequently complicate hepatitis A than other forms of viral hepatitis. Relapsing hepatitis has no specific histologic features. During relapse, peak serum bilirubin and aminotransferases levels may be higher or lower than those seen initially. Arthritis, vasculitis, and cryoglobulinemia have been described in a few patients with relapsing hepatitis A. Despite one or more relapses, the prognosis for complete recovery still is excellent.

DIAGNOSIS

Differential Diagnosis

The differential diagnosis of acute hepatitis includes drug-induced hepatotoxicity and toxin-induced liver disease (see Chapter 96). Shock liver also should be considered in the

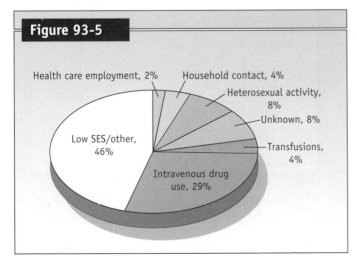

Figure 93-5

Health care employment, 2%   Household contact, 4%

Heterosexual activity, 8%

Unknown, 8%

Low SES/other, 46%

Transfusions, 4%

Intravenous drug use, 29%

Risk factors for hepatitis C virus infection in the United States; SES—socioeconomic status.

Table 93-2. Major Histopathologic Features of Acute Viral Hepatitis

Focal hepatocyte necrosis, drop-out, and ballooning degeneration

Councilman-like/apoptotic bodies

Lobular disarray

Round cell infiltration of portal triads and parenchyma

Central vein endophlebitis

Kupffer cell hypertrophy

Variable cholestasis

Evidence of hepatocyte regeneration

appropriate clinical setting. Infrequently, autoimmune liver disease may present as an acute hepatitis, and early in the course of biliary obstruction due to gallstones, aminotransferase levels may approach those seen in acute hepatitis (see Chapter 97). Alcoholic hepatitis usually is distinguished readily by history and laboratory features (see Chapter 95). Liver biopsy rarely is necessary to diagnose acute viral hepatitis.

Serologic Diagnosis

The diagnosis of hepatitis A requires detection of serum immunoglobulin M (IgM) antibody to HAV (IgM anti-HAV) in a patient with signs or symptoms of acute hepatitis. This antibody persists for approximately 3 to 6 months and then disappears (Fig. 93-6).

A serum test positive for total antibody (IgM and IgG) to HAV, but negative for IgM anti-HAV, indicates previous HAV infection. Research assays for detection of antibodies to HEV are available but should be reserved for those patients at risk because of recent travel to endemic regions (Fig. 93-7).

Serologic diagnosis of acute hepatitis B is made by detection of serum HBsAg and IgM antibody to hepatitis B core antigen (IgM anti-HBc) in a patient with acute hepatitis (Fig. 93-8).

HBsAg appears in serum first and usually is present at the onset of clinical symptoms but may disappear shortly thereafter. The presence of IgM anti-HBc is then diagnostic. HBeAg and HBV DNA are detectable in serum in patients with acute and chronic hepatitis; disappearance of serum HBeAg during the course of acute HBV infection usually indicates viral clearance and recovery. Serum IgG anti-HBc is found in patients with past or continuing HBV infection; it is not induced by administration of HBV vaccine. Antibody to HBsAg (anti-HBs) is the last antibody to appear in the serum of patients with acute hepatitis B and is thought to be responsible for viral clearance and immunity to re-infection. Serum anti-HBs also develops in response to HBV vaccination.

In the HBsAg-positive patient with acute hepatitis, the presence of antibody to HDV (anti-HDV) and circulating HDV RNA are diagnostic of HDV infection. In coinfections, the IgM anti-HBc is markedly positive; in superinfections, anti-HBc is largely of the IgG class (Fig. 93-9).

Serologic diagnosis of HCV is dependent on detection of serum antibodies (anti-HCV) to recombinant HCV antigens. Serum anti-HCV is detected in approximately 60% of patients during the early acute phase of illness (Fig. 93-10).

In the remainder of acutely infected individuals, serum anti-HCV appears weeks to months later.

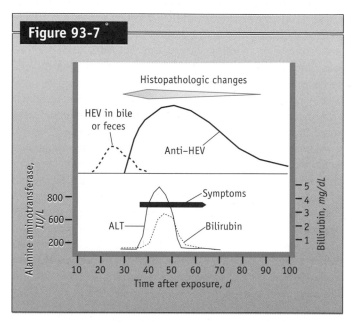

Figure 93-7

Virologic, serologic, biochemical, histopathologic, and clinical changes in acute hepatitis E virus (HEV) infection. (*From* Brown et al [21]; with permission.)

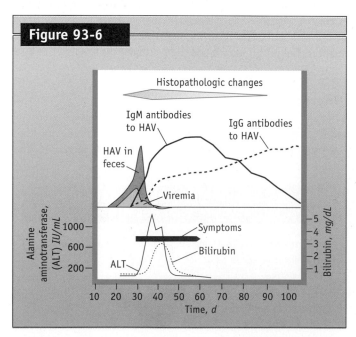

Figure 93-6

Typical serologic, biochemical, clinical, and histopathologic changes in acute hepatitis A virus (HAV) infection; Ig—immunoglobulin. (*From* Brown et al [21]; with permission.)

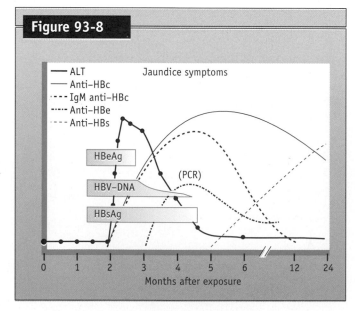

Figure 93-8

Typical clinical, serologic, and virologic time course of hepatitis B. ALT— alanine aminotransferase; HBc—hepatitis B core; HBeAg—hepatitis B early antigen; HBsAg—hepatitis B surface antigen; HBV—hepatitis B virus; PCR—polymerase chain reaction. (*From* Rabin [19].)

Current anti-HCV assays are positive in greater than 95% of infected patients. Unfortunately, serum anti-HCV generally persists for prolonged periods. Hence a positive serum anti-HCV test does not differentiate acute or ongoing infection from previous infection with recovery; HCV RNA, the earliest marker of acute HCV infection, may be used for this purpose.

TREATMENT
Self-limited Infection
Individuals with self-limited acute viral hepatitis ordinarily do not require hospitalization or intravenous fluids and parenteral nutrition unless they have persistent vomiting or severe anorexia. Affected patients should be encouraged to eat a large breakfast, because this meal usually is well tolerated. Unless essential, all drugs, including alcohol, should be discontinued during the acute phase of illness. No specific limitation is placed on activity, but patients are asked to avoid extremely vigorous or prolonged physical exertion. Antiviral therapy for acute hepatitis is not available; limited data suggest that treatment of patients with acute hepatitis C with α-interferon may reduce, but not eliminate, the risk of developing chronic infection.

Fulminant Hepatitis
Management of ALF requires continuous monitoring and support in the intensive care facility of a medical center with a liver transplantation program (see Chapter 116). Although no specific therapy for ALF is currently available, early liver transplantation has improved survival rates dramatically.

Cholestatic Hepatitis
The course of cholestatic hepatitis A appears to be shortened by treatment with prednisone or ursodeoxycholic acid, although this has not been proven by controlled trials. Severe pruritus, unresponsive to these therapies, may be ameliorated by treatment with cholestyramine.

Relapsing Hepatitis
Management of relapses is identical to that of the original episode.

PREVENTION
Hepatitis A
Pre-exposure immunoprophylaxis is achieved best by administration of safe, well-tolerated, and highly effective inactivated HAV vaccines [2••,12]. Vaccination induces development of protective antibodies in more than 85% of vaccinees by 2 weeks after inoculation and in nearly 100% by 4 weeks. Both commercially available vaccines usually are given in a two-dose regimen: an initial dose followed by a second dose 6 to 12 months later. The first dose is likely to provide protective levels of antibody for at least 1 or 2 years. Pre-exposure immunoprophylaxis is offered to travelers to HAV-endemic regions, to homosexual men, to parenteral drug users, to hemophilia patients, and to native peoples of the Americas and Alaska, all with high attack rates of HAV infection. HAV vaccine has been recommended for susceptible patients with chronic liver disease and for children and young adults in communities experiencing community-wide outbreaks. Combined HAV and HBV vaccines have been developed and are likely to be available in the future [13].

Although HAV vaccines may have efficacy in the postexposure setting, immune globulin is the only proven form of immunoprophylaxis for persons exposed to HAV. Immune globulin should be administered to all household and intimate contacts of index cases as early as possible after exposure. Immune globulin also may be given to persons who plan to travel in endemic areas but do not have sufficient time to develop vaccine-induced immunity (Table 93-3).

Hepatitis E
No form of immunoprophylaxis is available for HEV infection. A prototype, recombinant HEV vaccine is under study. Avoidance of unboiled water in endemic regions may reduce the risk of infection until a vaccine is available.

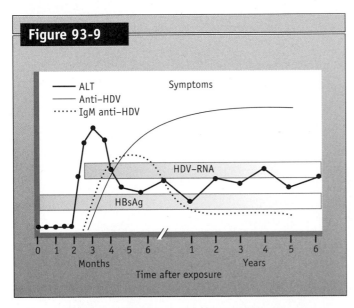

Figure 93-9

Clinical, virologic, and serologic courses of a typical case of acute hepatitis D superinfection in a patient with chronic hepatitis B, leading to chronic hepatitis D virus (HDV) infection. ALT—alanine aminotransferase; HBsAg—hepatitis B surface antigen; Ig—immunoglobulin. (*From* Rabin [19].)

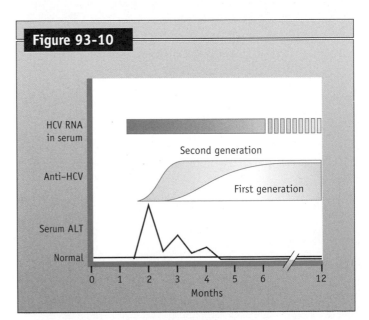

Figure 93-10

Virologic, serologic, and biochemical changes in acute hepatitis C virus (HCV) infection. ALT—alanine aminotransferase.

Hepatitis B

Prevention of HBV infection is best achieved by pre-exposure immunoprophylaxis with HBV vaccine [2••,14••]. The recombinant HBV vaccines currently available in the United States are highly immunogenic, safe, and well tolerated [15]. Seroprotective levels of anti-HBs are achieved in 95% to 100% of infants, children, and young adults inoculated with three doses of HBsAg-containing vaccines. The second dose is usually given 1 to 2 months after the first; the third dose may be given 6 to 12 months later. Boosters are not recommended, except in immunocompromised individuals, because protection appears to last 10 years or longer [16]. Injection into the deltoid muscle of adults and the anterolateral muscle of the thigh in infants is preferred. Universal infant immunization, catch-up vaccination of previously unvaccinated adolescents; and vaccination of members of high-risk groups, *eg*, family contacts of HBV carriers, health care workers, male homosexuals, and parenteral drug users, is recommended (Table 93-4).

Postexposure immunoprophylaxis with HBV vaccine and hepatitis B immune globulin (HBIG), an immune globulin preparation containing high titers of anti-HBs, is appropriate for the nonimmune sexual contacts of patients with acute or chronic hepatitis B and the infants of HBsAg-positive mothers identified by testing during pregnancy. In the latter circumstance, both HBIG and the first dose of HBV vaccine should be given within 12 hours of birth. The protective efficacy of neonatal vaccination and HBIG administration exceeds 95%. The protective efficacy of the recommended postsexual exposure immunoprophylaxis regimen is ill-defined.

Hepatitis D

Unfortunately, neither an HDV vaccine nor an HDV immune globulin is available. Prevention of HDV infection is entirely dependent on prevention of HBV infection; immunity to hepatitis B provides immunity to hepatitis D.

Hepatitis C

Prevention of HCV infection is a subject of current study. Neutralizing antibodies to HCV have been identified, and a prototype, recombinant vaccine is being investigated [17]. Currently available immune globulin preparations are not protective and a hyperimmune HCV globulin is not available. Better blood donor selection and screening of donors for anti-HCV has dramatically reduced the risk of posttransfusion HCV infection [8]. Safe sexual practices may reduce that risk; similarly, needle exchange programs may reduce the risk of HCV infection among parenteral drug users.

◼◼◼ REFERENCES

Recently published papers of particular interest have been highlighted as follows:
- • Of interest
- •• Of outstanding interest

1. Koff RS: Viral hepatitis. Solving the mysteries of viral hepatitis. *Sci Am Sci Med* 1994, 1:24–33.
2.•• Lemon SM, Thomas DL: Vaccines to prevent viral hepatitis. *N Engl J Med* 1997, 336:196–204.
This is an outstanding review of the current status of the HAV and HBV vaccines.
3. Polish LB, Gallagher M, Fields HA, Hadler SC: Delta hepatitis: molecular biology and clinical and epidemiological features. *Clin Microbiol Rev* 1993, 6:211–229.
4.• Yotsuyanagi H, Koike K, Yasuda K, *et al.*: Prolonged fecal excretion of hepatitis A virus in adult patients with hepatitis A as determined by polymerase chain reaction. *Hepatology* 1996, 24:10–13.
In this study, fecal HAV was detectable by polymerase chain reaction (PCR) for more than 1 month after the onset of clinical symptoms in adult patients. In one instance HAV remained detectable for up to 3 months. Whether fecal shedding detected by PCR is epidemiologically important remains to be determined.

Table 93-3. Immunoprophylaxis of Hepatitis A: Immune Globulin Vs Inactivated HAV Vaccine

Feature	Immune Globulin	Inactivated HAV vaccine
Derived from blood	Yes	No
Acquisition of Anti-HAV	Passive	Active
Preferred injection site	Deltoid	Deltoid
Peak Anti-HAV level	Low	High, approaching level in natural infection
Preexposure efficacy	Yes	Yes
Duration of protection	2–3 months	> 10 years
Postexposure efficacy	Yes, if given within 2 weeks of exposure	Possibly, but limited data
Cost	$	$

Adapted from Koff [20]; with permission

Table 93-4. Groups With Increased Risk of Hepatitis B Virus Infection

Medical, dental, and laboratory workers and others with exposure to human blood

Homosexual men

Heterosexuals with multiple sex partners or with sexually transmitted diseases

Highly hepatitis B virus-endemic populations, (eg, Alaskan natives)

Household contacts of HBsAg-positive individuals

Parenteral drug users who share needles

Hemophilia patients

Hemodialysis patients

Patients for whom multiple blood or blood product infusions are anticipated

Prison inmates and staff

Staff and patients of institutions for mentally disabled

Travelers to highly hepatitis B virus-endemic areas with anticipated exposure to human blood, sexual contacts with locals, or prolonged living in households with locals

Newborn infants of serum HBsAg-positive mothers

5. Khuroo MS, Kamili S, Jameel S: Vertical transmission of hepatitis E virus. _Lancet_ 1995, 345:1025–1026.

6. McQuillan G, Alter MJ, Everhart JE: Viral hepatitis. In _Digestive Diseases in the United States_, edited by J.E. Everhart. NIH Publication No.94-1447 Bethesda MD: National Institute of Health; 1994:127–156.

7. Garfein RS, Vlahov D, Galai N, _et al._: Viral infections in short-term injection drug users: the prevalence of the hepatitis C, hepatitis B, human immunodeficiency, and human T-lymphotropic viruses. _Am J Publ Health_ 1996, 86:655–661.

8. Schreiber GB, Busch MP, Kleinman SH, _et al._: The risk of transfusion-transmitted viral infections. _N Engl J Med_ 1996, 334:1685–1690.

9. Thomas DL, Zenilman JM, Alter HJ, _et al._: Sexual transmission of hepatitis C virus among patients attending sexually transmitted diseases clinics in Baltimore—an analysis of 309 sex partnerships. _J Infect Dis_ 1995, 171:768–775.

10. Pham B-N, Mosnier J-F, Durand F, _et al._: Immunostaining for membrane attack complex of complement is related to cell necrosis in fulminant and acute hepatitis. _Gastroenterology_ 1995, 108:495–504.

11. Glikson M, Galun E, Oren R, _et al._: Relapsing hepatitis A: review of 14 cases and literature survey. _Medicine_ 1992, 71:14–23.

12. Innis BL, Snitbhan R, Kunasol P, _et al._: Protection against hepatitis A by an inactivated vaccine. _JAMA_ 1994, 271:1328–1334.

13. LeRoux-Roels G, Moreau E, Desombere I, Safary A: Safety and immunogenicity of a combined hepatitis A and B vaccine in young healthy adults. _Scand J Gastroenterol_ 1996, 31:1027–1031.

14.•• Chen H-L, Chang M-H, Ni Y-H, _et al._: Seroepidemiology of hepatitis B virus infection in children. Ten years of mass vaccination in Taiwan. _JAMA_ 1996, 276:906–908.

A universal newborn HBV vaccination program in Taiwan, begun for infants of HBsAg-positive mothers in 1984 and extended to all infants in 1986, resulted in a striking decline in HBV infections in children under age 12 years studied in 1989 and 1994. HBsAg prevalence in 1984 was 9.8%, falling to 4.8% in 1989, and to 1.3% in 1994. These data prove the effectiveness of mass HBV vaccination in reducing HBV infection and the development of the carrier state in a hyperendemic region.

15. Treadwell TL, Keeffe EB, Lake J, _et al._: Immunogenicity of two recombinant hepatitis B vaccines in older individuals. _Am J Med_ 1993, 95:584–588.

16. Wainwright RB, Bulkow LR, Parkinson AJ, _et al._: Protection provided by hepatitis B vaccine in a Yupik Eskimo population: results of a 10-year study. _J Infect Dis_ 1997, 175:674–677.

17. Choo QL, Kuo G, Ralston R, _et al._: Vaccination of chimpanzees against infection by the hepatitis C virus. _PNAS USA_ 1994, 91:1294–1298.

18. Rabin L: Hepatitis. In _Atlas of Infectious Diseases: Infections, Hepatitis, and Gastroenteritis_, vol. 7. Edited by Lorber B. Philadelphia: Current Medicine; 1996:2.1–2.54.

19. Koff RS: Acute viral hepatitis. In _Gastroenterology and Hepatology: The Comprehensive Visual Reference, The Liver_, vol. 1. Edited by Maddrey WC. Philadelphia: Current Medicine; 1996:2.1–2.21.

20. Robinson WS: Hepatitis B virus and hepatitis D virus. In _Principles and Practice of Infectious Diseases_, edn 4. Edited by Mandell GL, Bennett JE, Dolin R. New York: Churchill Livingstone; 1995:1406–1439.

21. Brown EA, Ticehurst J, Lemon SM: Immunopathogenesis of hepatitis A and E virus infections. In _Immunology of Liver Disease_. Edited by Thomas HC, Waters J. Dordrecht: Kluwer Academic Publishers; 1994: 361–372.

⑨④ Chronic Viral Hepatitis
Francesco Negro and Anna S. F. Lok

Chronic viral hepatitis is defined as more than 6 months of clinical, biochemical, or histologic evidence of liver damage in a patient with serologic markers of infection with a hepatitis virus known to cause chronic liver disease (Table 94-1). Chronic infection with hepatitis virus B, C, D, or G (HBV, HCV, HDV, or HGV) may produce an asymptomatic carrier state or active liver disease, including chronic hepatitis, cirrhosis, and hepatocellular carcinoma (HCC). This chapter reviews the epidemiology, diagnosis, natural history, treatment, and prevention of chronic HBV, HCV, HDV, and HGV infections.

■ CHRONIC HEPATITIS B VIRUS INFECTION
Epidemiology and Transmission

HBV infection is a public health problem of global significance. Of the estimated 350 million HBV carriers in the world, approximately 1 to 1.25 million live in the United States. The prevalence of chronic HBV infection in different regions of the world depends on the predominant mode of transmission and age at time of infection. Chronic infection occurs in approximately 90% of infants infected at birth, in 20% to 50% of children infected between the ages of 1 and 5 years, and in fewer than 5% of immunocompetent adults.

In regions where the rate of chronic infection is high (_eg_, Southeast Asia), most transmission occurs perinatally or during early childhood. In regions where the rate of chronic infection is intermediate (_eg_, Mediterranean basin), infection occurs in all age groups, although the high rate of chronic infection is maintained primarily by transmission during early childhood. In regions where the rate of chronic infection is low (_eg_, North America), most infection occurs among adults, especially those who belong to high-risk groups. In the United States, heterosexual transmission is the most common mode of HBV spread.

Diagnosis

Diagnosis of HBV infection is facilitated by a large number of serologic and molecular virologic tests (Table 94-2). The sera of patients with chronic HBV infection are positive for hepatitis B surface antigen (HBsAg) and hepatitis B core antibody (anti-HBc). In most cases, the anti-HBc is predominantly immunoglobulin G (IgG), but during acute exacerbations of chronic hepatitis, IgM anti-HBc may be present in titers equivalent to those seen in patients with acute infection. Initial evaluation of persons with chronic HBV infection should include testing for hepatitis B early antigen (HBeAg); patients who are HBeAg seropositive should be tested for serum HBV DNA by hybridization assay or branched DNA (bDNA) assay. Persons with detectable serum HBV DNA and active liver disease are candidates for therapy. Patients who are HBeAg negative and HBe antibody (anti-HBe) seropositive usually do not have detectable serum HBV DNA by hybridizations assays, although most of them have detectable HBV DNA when tested by polymerase chain reaction (PCR) assays.

The pathogenic significance of low levels of HBV DNA detectable by PCR but not by hybridization and bDNA assays is uncertain. For clinical purposes, tests for serum HBV DNA should only be performed using hybridization or bDNA assays. A small proportion of anti-HBe–seropositive patients continue to have active liver disease. These patients should be tested for HBV DNA by hybridization assay to determine whether the liver disease results from replicative HBV infection (ie, wild-type or precore mutant) or another cause of liver disease, such as superinfection with HCV and HDV.

Clinical Manifestations

Patients with chronic HBV infection may be asymptomatic carriers with normal alanine aminotransferase (ALT) levels and minimal changes evident on liver biopsy, or they may have chronic hepatitis with progression to cirrhosis and HCC. These two clinical courses are not mutually exclusive; carriers can develop chronic hepatitis and cirrhosis, and patients with chronic hepatitis can have spontaneous or treatment-induced remissions.

Symptoms of chronic hepatitis B usually are nonspecific, mild, and intermittent. The history and physical examination findings are unreliable in assessing the severity of liver disease, except for patients with decompensated cirrhosis. Although ALT levels correlate well with histologic assessment of inflammatory activity in longitudinal studies, biochemical test results are less accurate in predicting the activity or stage of liver disease in cross-sectional studies. Liver biopsies are important for assessing the severity of liver disease and for diagnosing well-compensated cirrhosis. Extrahepatic manifestations, including glomerulonephritis and polyarteritis nodosa, have been reported with chronic HBV infection in fewer than 5% of patients.

Natural History

The natural course of perinatally acquired chronic HBV infection has three phases [1•] (Fig. 94-1). In the first phase (ie, immune tolerance), patients are HBeAg positive and have high serum levels of HBV DNA but have no symptoms, normal ALT levels, and minimal changes on liver biopsy. The reason immune tolerance develops is unclear. Experiments using mice suggest that transplacental transfer of maternal HBeAg may impair T-cell responses to HBeAg and HBcAg.

Transition from the immune-tolerant phase to the second phase (ie, immune clearance) of perinatally acquired chronic HBV infection usually occurs between 15 and 35 years of age. During this phase, the level of HBV replication declines, and spontaneous HBeAg to anti-HBe seroconversion is observed, frequently preceded by an increase in the ALT level, which is thought to represent immune-mediated lysis of infected hepatocytes. These exacerbations may be asymptomatic or clinically apparent, simulating acute hepatitis. In the latter case, patients with previously unrecognized chronic HBV infection may be misdiagnosed as having acute hepatitis B, because IgM anti-HBc may reach titers comparable to those seen in acute infection. Not all exacerbations, however, are accompanied by successful elimination of replicating virus. Some patients experience recurrent exacerbations with intermittent disappearance of serum HBV DNA, with or without transient loss of HBeAg.

Table 94-1. Definition of Chronic Viral Hepatitis

Duration	More than 6 mo
Clinical features	Stigmata of chronic liver disease
Biochemical features	Elevated ALT levels
Histologic features	Periportal necroinflammation, fibrosis, or cirrhosis
Virologic features	
HBV	HBsAg+, IgG anti-HBc+, HBeAg or anti-HBe+, HBV DNA+
HDV	HBsAg+, anti-HDV+
HCV	Anti-HCV+, HCV RNA+
HGV	HGV RNA+

ALT—alanine aminotranferase; anti-HBc—hepatitis B core antibody; anti-HBe—hepatitis B early antibody; anti-HCV—hepatitis C virus antibody; anti-HDV—hepatitis D virus antibody; HBeAg—hepatitis B early antigen; HBsAg—hepatitis B surface antigen; HBV, HCV, HDV, HGV—hepatitis B,C,D,G virus, respectively; Ig—immunoglobulin; plus sign—positive status.

Table 94-2. Serologic Markers of Hepatitis B Viral Infection

Marker	Implication
HBsAg+	Acute or chronic HBV infection
Anti-HBs+	Immunity to HBV infection
Anti-HBc (IgM)+	Recent HBV infection
HBeAg+	Active virus replication, high infectivity
Anti-HBe+	Inactive (low level) virus replication, low infectivity
HBV DNA+	Marker of virus replication and infectivity
HBsAg+, IgG anti-HBc+	Chronic HBV infection
Anti-HBs+, IgG anti-HBc+	Past HBV infection

anti-HBC—hepatitis B core antibody; anti-HBe—hepatitis B early antibody; anti-HBs—hepatitis B surface antibody; HBeAg—hepatitis B early antigen; HBsAg—hepatitis B surface antigen; HBV—hepatitis B virus; Ig—immunoglobulin; plus sign—positive status.

The third phase of perinatally acquired HBV infection is that of nonreplicative infection. In this phase, conventional serologic markers of HBV replication (*ie*, HBeAg and HBV DNA detected by hybridization assay) are no longer detectable, but HBsAg

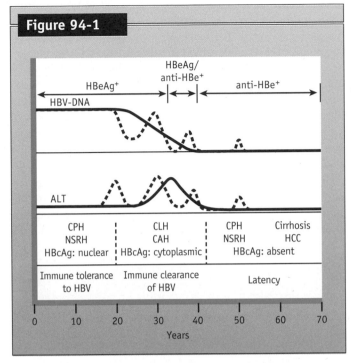

Figure 94-1

Proposed scheme for the natural history of perinatally acquired hepatitis B virus (HBV) infection. During the immune tolerance phase, liver disease is inactive despite high levels of HBV replication. During the immune clearance phase, liver disease is active, possibly because of lysis of infected hepatocytes, and the virus load is reduced. During the latent phase, liver disease is in remission, and virus replication is undetectable by hybridization assays, although HBV DNA is usually detectable by polymerase chain reaction assays. ALT—alanine aminotransferase; anti-HBe—hepatitis B early antibody; CAH—chronic active hepatitis; CLH—chronic lobular hepatitis; CPH—chronic persistent hepatitis; HBcAg—hepatitis B core antigen; HBeAg—hepatitis B early antigen; HCC—hepatocellular carcinoma; NSRH—nonspecific reactive hepatitis; plus sign—positive status.

persists, and serum HBV DNA is usually detectable by PCR assay. The disease should be considered to be in a low-replicative rather than a nonreplicative phase. Reactivation of HBV replication with a flare in the ALT level and reappearance of HBeAg and serum HBV DNA is possible, especially in immunocompromised patients. During the low-replicative phase, patients are usually asymptomatic, and liver disease is inactive; the disease of some patients, however, may progress to cirrhosis and HCC. The ultimate outcome of chronic HBV infection appears to depend on the severity of liver injury after HBV replication is arrested. Patients with recurrent exacerbations caused by prolonged and fluctuating transitions between replicative and nonreplicative infection are more likely to develop cirrhosis and HCC.

In chronic HBV infection acquired during adulthood, there is no initial immune tolerance phase. In general, the clinical course consists of a replicative phase with active liver disease and a low-replicative or nonreplicative phase with remission of liver disease.

Several studies have shown that patients with a prolonged replicative phase are more likely to develop exacerbations, cirrhosis, hepatic decompensation, and death from liver failure [2••,3]. Among untreated patients, the average rates of spontaneous HBeAg and HBsAg seroconversion have been reported to be 10% and 1% per year, respectively. Progression from chronic hepatitis to cirrhosis and from compensated cirrhosis to hepatic decompensation and to HCC have been estimated to be 12% to 20%, 20% to 23%, and 6% to 15% at 5 years, respectively. Survival after development of compensated cirrhosis is favorable initially (85% at 5 years) but decreases dramatically after the onset of hepatic decompensation to 55% to 70% at 1 year and 14% to 35% at 5 years.

Hepatitis B Virus Mutants

Because the reverse transcriptase of the virus lacks a proofreading mechanism, HBV mutants may be generated during the course of chronic HBV infection. Mutants may be selected because they increase viral replication efficiency or help the virus to evade immune clearance. Naturally occurring mutations have been detected in all regions of the HBV genome [4]; those in the precore region have been most extensively studied.

The most important mutation creates a premature stop codon (Fig. 94-2) that prevents the production of HBeAg, but

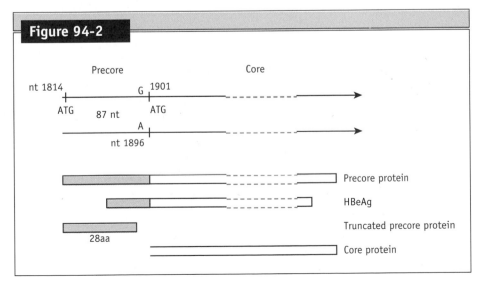

Figure 94-2

Molecular basis for the hepatitis B early antigen (HBeAg)–negative mutant. Translation from the start codon of the precore-core region produces a precursor protein that is cleaved at the N- and C-terminal ends to a smaller protein, HBeAg, which is secreted. The most common mutation involves a guanine (G) to adenine (A) change at nucleotide (nt) 1896, creating a premature stop codon in the precore region and preventing translation of the precore protein and HBeAg secretion. Translation from the start codon of the core region produces a smaller protein, hepatitis B core antigen (HBcAg), which is an intracellular protein.

virus replication and HBcAg expression persist. Failure to produce HBeAg may help the virus to evade immune clearance. Initial studies suggested that these mutants might cause more severe liver disease because they were predominantly found in anti-HBe–positive patients with chronic active hepatitis orfulminant hepatitis. Recent studies reported that the precore mutants can be found in asymptomatic carriers. Longitudinal studies showed that precore mutants tended to appear around the time of HBeAg seroconversion. The precore stop codon mutation only occurs in some HBV genotypes, and its prevalence varies among different regions of the world.

Treatment

The main aim of treatment of chronic HBV infection is tosuppress replication of the virus before there is significant, irreversible liver damage. The initial end points of therapy are sustained clearance of HBeAg and HBV DNA in the serum (assessed by hybridization assay) and improvement in liver disease, as indicated by normalization of ALT and a decrease in necroinflammation determined on liver biopsy (Table 94-3). The ultimate end points of treatment are sustained clearance of serum HBsAg and HBV DNA (by PCR assay), decreased incidence of cirrhosis and HCC, and prolonged survival.

Interferon-α

Interferon-α (IFN-α) is the only approved treatment for chronic HBV infection in most countries. Interferons have antiviral, antiproliferative, and immunomodulatory effects. A meta-analysis of 16 randomized, controlled trials concluded that IFN-α was beneficial for HBeAg-positive patients who were treated for 3 to 6 months [5•]. When treated patients were compared with untreated controls after 6 to 12 months of posttreatment follow-up, treated patients more frequently had a loss of HBeAg (33% vs 12%), serum HBV DNA (37% vs 17%), and HBsAg (7.8% vs 1.8%). Long-term follow-up studies found that more than 80% of successfully treated patients maintained their response. An increasing proportion of North American and European, but not Asian, responders eventually lost HBsAg [6••]. Between 50% and 100% of patients who lost HBsAg did not have detectable serum HBV DNA when tested by PCR assay. A long-term follow-up report found that responders had improved overall survival and survival free of hepatic decompensation [7]. These findings are encouraging, but more

data are needed to substantiate the hypothesis that sustained antiviral response can decrease the risks of cirrhosis and HCC and improve survival in patients with chronic HBV infection.

IFN-α therapy should be considered for patients with chronic HBV infection (ie, HBsAg positive for more than 6 months), who have evidence of active virus replication (ie, HBeAg and serum HBV DNA positive by hybridization assay), and active liver disease (ie, abnormal ALT and chronic hepatitis on liver biopsy) [6••] (Table 94-4). IFN should be administered as subcutaneous or intramuscular injections in doses of 5 million units daily or 10 million units three times weekly for 3 to 6 months. Several factors associated with a favorable response to IFN treatment have been identified: a high pretreatment serum ALT level, low pretreatment serum HBV DNA level, adult-acquired HBV infection, liver histology indicating active disease, female gender, and no concomitant HIV or HDV infection.

The benefit of IFN therapy in several clinical settings has not been established [6••] (Table 94-4). Although pilot studies suggested that pretreatment with prednisone may enhance the effect of IFN therapy, large-scale, randomized, controlled trials

Table 94-3. End-Points for Treatment of Chronic Viral Hepatitis

Features	Chronic hepatitis B	Chronic hepatitis C	Chronic hepatitis D
Biochemical	Normal ALT	Normal ALT	Normal ALT
Virologic	HBV DNA neg. by hybridization assay	HCV RNA neg. by PCR assay	HDV RNA neg. by hybridization assay

ALT—alanine aminotransferase; PCR—polymerase chain reaction.

Table 94-4. Treatment Strategies for Patients With Chronic Hepatitis B Virus Infection

Profile	Comment
Normal ALT, HBeAg+, HBV DNA+	This profile is frequently found in Asian patients, especially children who were infected at birth. Interferon treatment is not warranted for these patients, because the response rate is less than 10%. Persons with this clinical profile should be monitored regularly because immune tolerance may break down later, rendering them more responsive to treatment.
Decompensated cirrhosis, HBV DNA+	A small proportion of patients with cirrhosis remain HBV DNA positive. Interferon can inhibit HBV replication in this setting, resulting in clinical improvement. However, there is a high risk of serious infection and hepatic failure even with low doses of interferon. These patients are best managed in specialized centers.
Children, abnormal ALT, HBeAg+, HBV DNA+	These children should be referred to specialized centers.
Abnormal ALT, HBeAg-	Patients with this clinical profile should be tested for HBV DNA. Those who are HBV DNA positive and have no other cause of liver disease may be infected with a precore HBV mutant. Interferon treatment of these patients usually is associated with decreased serum HBV DNA and ALT levels, but posttreatment relapse is common. These patients are best managed in specialized centers.

ALT—alanine aminotransferase; HBeAg—hepatitis B early antigen; HBV—hepatitis B virus; minus sign—negative status; plus sign—positive status.

of therapy with prednisone followed by IFN have reported conflicting results [8]. Based on current data, prednisone priming should not be used as primary therapy. Its role in treating nonresponders and patients who relapse after IFN therapy has not been determined.

IFN therapy is associated with a wide range of adverse effects (Tables 94-5 and 94-6). During the first 1 to 2 weeks of treatment, influenza-like symptoms, including chills, fever, headache, malaise, muscle aches, nausea, and anorexia, are common. These symptoms can be reduced by increased fluid intake, administering IFN at bedtime, and pretreatment with acetaminophen. Other possible adverse effects during the course of treatment include fatigue, low-grade fever, mild weight loss, hair loss, and emotional lability or depression. Although emotional problems are more common in patients with a history of neuropsychiatric illness, they also have been reported for previously asymptomatic patients. Careful monitoring is imperative, because any patient receiving IFN may experience severe depression, frank psychosis, and suicide attempts. Mild myelosuppression is common, and cell counts should be checked during treatment, but dose reduction rarely is needed in patients who have normal counts before therapy. IFN has been reported to induce formation of a wide range of autoantibodies and to exacerbate previously undiagnosed autoimmune hepatitis, but induction of clinically overt autoimmune disorders requiring treatment is uncommon, except for hypothyroidism or hyperthyroidism. Other less common adverse effects include worsening of diabetes, psoriasis, and retinopathy (usually subclinical).

Alternative Therapy

Many antiviral agents have been evaluated for the treatment of chronic HBV infection. Unfortunately, most have been ineffective or too toxic. Of the antiviral agents that are being evaluated in clinical trials, lamivudine and famciclovir are the most promising [9]. Lamivudine (3TC, Epivir) inhibits HBV reverse transcriptase and DNA polymerase activities. Clinical trials have shown that 4- to 12-week courses of lamivudine are well tolerated and produce a rapid and profound decrease in serum HBV DNA levels in patients with chronic HBV infection [10•]. However, the beneficial effect was not sustained after treatment was discontinued, and few (0% to 12%) patients lost HBeAg. Increasing the duration of treatment appears to induce a higher sustained response rate; in a report of 24 patients with chronic HBV infection who received lamivudine for a median of 52 weeks, 39% lost HBeAg, and 9% lost HBsAg. Unfortunately, two (8%) patients developed drug-resistant mutants. The ease of oral administration and the absence of serious adverse effects (particularly the lack of myelotoxicity and significant ALT flares) have led to clinical trials of lamivudine for patients with decompensated cirrhosis or recurrent HBV infection after liver transplantation, conditions in which IFN is ineffective and contraindicated. Preliminary reports indicate that lamivudine is well tolerated and effective in inhibiting HBV replication and improving liver disease in these patients [11]. Nevertheless, drug-resistant mutants also have been reported in these settings.

Famciclovir is the oral prodrug of penciclovir that can inhibit HBV DNA polymerase activity and priming of HBV reverse transcription. Two clinical studies showed that famciclovir was well tolerated and effective in inhibiting HBV replication in patients with chronic HBV infection. Famciclovir decreases HBV replication and improves liver function in patients with decompensated cirrhosis or recurrent HBV infection after liver transplantation. As with lamivudine, a sustained effect was rarely achieved after short courses of famciclovir treatment. Unfortunately, drug-resistant mutants have been reported in patients who have been on long-term treatment. Lamivudine and famciclovir remain experimental therapies and should only be used in clinical trials.

Several HBV-specific immunomodulatory therapies have been developed, including DNA vaccination, immunization with vaccines containing pre-S and S antigens, autologous lymphocyte transfer, and inoculation with synthetic peptide vaccines that contain the cytotoxic T lymphocyte epitope of HBcAg. Some of these therapies are undergoing phase I and phase II clinical trials. Future treatment of chronic HBV infection may involve combination therapy of two or more antiviral agents or an antiviral agent plus immunomodulation.

Prevention

Safe and effective vaccines are available for the prevention of HBV infection. Vaccination of newborns is the most effective prophylaxis because of the high acceptance rate (especially if incorporated with other childhood vaccinations) and its effect on reducing chronic infection. Routine vaccination of all

---

Table 94-5. Adverse Effects of Interferon Therapy

Initial influenza-like illness

Fatigue

Anorexia and nausea

Weight loss

Hair loss

Emotional lability and depression

Bone marrow suppression

Induction of autoantibodies, unmasking or exacerbation of autoimmune disease

---

Table 94-6. Monitoring Adverse Effects of Interferon Therapy

Pretreatment
Complete blood cell count (CBC); levels of thyroid-stimulating hormone (TSH), fasting glucose, blood urea nitrogen, creatinine, antinuclear antibody, smooth muscle antibody

During treatment
CBC at week 2, week 4, and monthly thereafter; TSH every 12 weeks; fasting glucose every 12 weeks

Posttreatment
TSH 3 months after cessation of therapy

newborns has resulted in significant reduction in carrier rates in countries where HBV infection is endemic.

The United States has adopted a broad approach to eliminate HBV transmission, including prenatal screening of all pregnant women for HBsAg; providing hepatitis B immune globulin (HBIG) and HBV vaccine to infants born to infected mothers; routine hepatitis B vaccination of all infants; catch-up vaccination of children at high risk for the disease; vaccination of adolescents 11 to 12 years of age who have not previously been vaccinated; and vaccination of high-risk adults.

■ CHRONIC HEPATITIS D VIRUS INFECTION

Hepatitis D is caused by a defective virus. Although HDV can replicate autonomously, the simultaneous presence of HBV is required for complete virion assembly and secretion [12]. Persons with HDV infection are always dually infected with HDV and HBV.

Epidemiology

Approximately 5% of HBV carriers worldwide are infected with HDV. However, the geographic distribution of HDV infection does not parallel that of HBV; HDV is almost completely absent from some areas where chronic HBV infection is prevalent, such as the Far East. HDV infection is endemic in Mediterranean countries, where infection tends to occur early, affecting mainly children and young adults.

The main route of transmission is inapparent mucosal or percutaneous spread; intrafamilial transmission also is common. HDV infection is rare in Western countries, where it is predominantly confined to high-risk groups: intravenous drug addicts and multiply transfused persons such as hemophiliacs. A significant decline in the incidence of HDV infection has been observed during the past 10 years, notably in Italy, possibly as a result of improvement in socioeconomic conditions, changes in lifestyle that decrease the risk of parenteral and sexual transmission, and aggressive HBV vaccination policies.

Diagnosis

The diagnosis of chronic hepatitis D depends on the detection of serologic markers of HDV and HBV infections [13•]. In the United States, the only commercially available test for the diagnosis of hepatitis D is the total HDV antibody (anti-HDV) test. The diagnosis of chronic HDV infection relies on demonstrating the presence of anti-HDV and HBsAg. In patients with acute HDV infection, anti-HDV appears late, and repeated testing may be necessary to document seroconversion. Persons with chronic HDV infection have persistent high titers of anti-HDV in their sera and intrahepatic expression of hepatitis D antigen (HDAg). In these patients, HBeAg usually is absent, and HBV DNA is undetectable in serum because of suppression of HBV replication by the simultaneous presence of HDV.

Clinical Manifestations

The clinical manifestations and course of HDV infection depend on the timing of infection [12]. *Coinfection* with HBV and HDV is usually transient and self-limited. HDV *superinfection* may present as an unusually severe, acute hepatitis in a previously undiagnosed HBV carrier or as an exacerbation of preexisting chronic hepatitis B. Subsequent progression to chronic HDV infection occurs in almost all of the latter patients. Chronic HDV infection may produce an asymptomatic carrier state or severe and rapidly progressive liver disease.

Treatment and Prevention

The goals of treatment of chronic HDV infection are to suppress HDV replication and to induce remission of liver disease (Table 94-3). IFN-α is the only therapy that has been shown to suppress HDV replication and decrease aminotransferase levels. However, even when used in high doses (9 million units three times weekly) and for long periods (48 weeks), the effects of IFN tend to be transient [14]. Because the worldwide experience of treating chronic HDV infection is limited, therapy should be restricted to clinical trials in referral centers.

Prevention of HDV infection is best achieved by vaccination against its helper virus, HBV, because persons who are immune to HBV infection also are immune to HDV infection.

■ CHRONIC HEPATITIS C VIRUS INFECTION

HCV is the predominant cause of parenterally transmitted non-A, non-B hepatitis and is one of the most common causes of chronic liver disease in the United States. Scientists from the Centers for Disease Control (CDC) estimate there are approximately 35,000 new HCV infections each year in the United States and 3.9 million persons chronically infected with HCV in this country.

Epidemiology

HCV is predominantly transmitted parenterally. Many investigators have observed that 40% to 50% of patients with chronic HCV infection have no identifiable risk factors. Studies found that "covert" intravenous drug use and possibly straw sharing during intranasal cocaine use may account for many cases of community-acquired HCV infection [15]. Nonpercutaneous routes such as sexual and perinatal transmission are inefficient modes of spread, possibly because of the low levels of viremia in most HCV-infected individuals.

Diagnosis

The diagnosis of chronic hepatitis C involves confirmation of the presence of HCV infection and assessment of the severity of liver disease. Enzyme immunoassays (EIA-3) for HCV antibody (anti-HCV) are the most practical screening tests for the diagnosis of HCV infection. Recombinant immunoblot assay (RIBA) is a supplementary, but not confirmatory, test for the diagnosis of HCV infection because it tests for the same HCV antibodies as do EIAs. Confirmation of ongoing HCV infection relies on detection of viremia. PCR assays are preferred to bDNA assays because of their increased sensitivities. Between 10% and 30% of patients with chronic hepatitis C who are HCV RNA positive by PCR assays may have undetectable HCV RNA if tested by bDNA assay.

The need for and the choice of supplementary or confirmatory tests for HCV infection depend on the clinical setting and the likelihood of a true-positive EIA result [16••] (Fig. 94-3). Confirmatory tests usually are unnecessary for anti-HCV–positive patients who present with chronic liver disease, especially for those who have risk factors for HCV infection, because more than 90% have detectable HCV RNA when their sera are tested using PCR assays. Although qualitative PCR assays can confirm the diagnosis, quantitative tests should be considered if treatment is contemplated, because patients with low HCV RNA levels are more likely to respond to therapy than those with high HCV RNA levels.

Unlike results for patients with chronic liver disease, EIA has a high false-positive rate for low-risk populations such as blood donors. Only 30% to 40% anti-HCV–positive blood donors (by EIA-2) are RIBA positive, and only 35% to 45% have detectable HCV RNA when sera are tested by PCR assay. Anti-HCV–positive blood donors (by EIA) should be retested for anti-HCV using RIBA; those who are positive by RIBA or indeterminate should then be tested for HCV RNA using a PCR assay. The same diagnostic algorithm should be used for persons who are incidentally found to be anti-HCV positive and have normal ALT levels. Although it is possible that they may have a false-positive EIA test result or resolved HCV infection, many (especially those who are positive by RIBA) are viremic, and up to 70% of those who are viremic are found to have chronic hepatitis on liver biopsy. False-negative EIA-2 results have been reported for 2.5% to 10.5% of immunocom-promised patients, including hemodialysis patients and transplant recipients, because of impaired antibody response to HCV antigens. Tests for HCV RNA should be performed in immunocompromised patients who are anti-HCV negative when there is clinical suspicion of HCV infection.

Screening for HCV with an EIA should be performed for persons with risk factors for HCV infection: history of transfusions of blood or blood products before 1990, hemodialysis, injection drug use, multiple sex partners, and spouses or sexual partners of patients with hepatitis C. Anti-HCV testing with an EIA should be part of the diagnostic evaluation for all patients who present with chronic liver disease or elevated ALT levels, with or without risk factors for hepatitis C.

Although anti-HCV–positive patients who have abnormal ALT levels are more likely to have significant liver disease found on liver biopsy than those who have persistently normal ALT levels, histologic evidence of chronic hepatitis can be found in 30% to 70% of persons identified positive by RIBA-2 and PCR despite persistently normal ALT levels [17]. Among patients with elevated ALT levels, there is little correlation between the ALT level and histologic diagnosis. Liver histology remains the gold standard for assessing the severity of chronic liver disease. Liver biopsy is the only means of diagnosing well-compensated cirrhosis. It is useful in determining inflammatory activity and the extent of fibrosis in patients with chronic hepatitis. Histologic grading and staging can help in predicting the risk of progression to cirrhosis. Cirrhosis is one of the most important independent factors associated with a poor response to IFN treatment.

Clinical Manifestations

Eighty-five percent of HCV infections are likely to progress to chronic infections. Symptoms of chronic HCV infection usually are nonspecific, mild, and intermittent: fatigue, nausea, anorexia, muscle aches, and arthralgias. Clinical manifestations are more persistent and significant in patients with cirrhosis. History and physical examination findings are unreliable in assessing the severity of liver disease, except for persons with decompensated cirrhosis. Although most patients with chronic HCV infection have abnormal ALT levels, ALT test results are only intermittently abnormal for many affected persons and are persistently normal for approximately 20% to 30% of patients.

A plethora of extrahepatic syndromes are associated with chronic HCV infection, including lichen planus, glomerulonephritis, essential mixed cryoglobulinemia (EMC), and porphyria cutanea tarda. EMC is a syndrome characterized by various combinations of fatigue, muscle and joint aches, arthritis, rash, neuropathy, and glomerulonephritis. Cryoglobulins are detectable in up to 30% of patients with chronic HCV infection, but the clinical syndrome of EMC occurs in only 1% to 2% of affected persons. Treatment of chronic HCV infection leads to resolution of the symptoms of EMC [18], but the benefit of therapy is rarely sustained. Glomerulonephritis usually represents the renal involvement of HCV-related EMC.

Natural History

Data on the natural history of chronic HCV infection are limited because most patients have subclinical illness during the

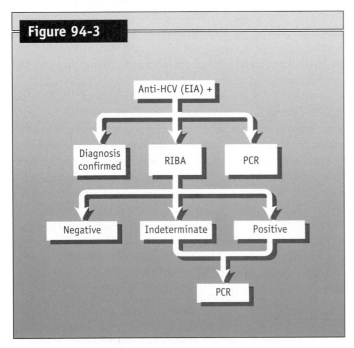

Figure 94-3

Diagnostic algorithm for hepatitis C virus (HCV) infection. Most anti-HCV–positive patients (determined by enzyme immunoassay-3 [EIA-3]) with chronic liver disease have ongoing HCV infection. Confirmatory tests may not be necessary. When indicated, polymerase chain reaction (PCR) assay for HCV RNA is more appropriate than recombinant immunoblot assay (RIBA). Confirmatory tests always should be performed for anti-HCV-positive blood donors (determined by EIA-2 or EIA-3) and persons with normal alanine aminotransferase (ALT) levels. The most appropriate approach is to retest for anti-HCV using RIBA and, for persons who are RIBA positive or indeterminate, to test for HCV RNA using a PCR assay. Direct confirmation using a PCR assay is not recommended for persons with normal ALT levels because of poor standardization of the assays.

acute infection. It is often impossible to determine the onset or duration of infection. Another confounding factor is the indolent and protracted course of the disease. Long-term follow-up studies of patients with defined onsets suggest that chronic HCV infection is a slowly progressive disease [19••]. Most patients remain asymptomatic, with no obvious increase in morbidity and mortality during the first 2 decades of chronic HCV infection [20•]. Follow-up evaluations of patients who presented with chronic liver disease, however, suggest that approximately 20% patients developed cirrhosis after 20 years of infection. The intervals between the onset of infection and development of chronic hepatitis, cirrhosis, and HCC have been estimated to be 10, 20, and 30 years, respectively [21], but cirrhosis has been reported as early as 5 and as late as 50 years after the initial infection. Several factors may contribute to the increased severity and rate of progression of liver disease in some patients with chronic HCV infection: male sex, alcohol use, older age at the time of infection, HCV genotype 1b, and coinfection with other viruses such as HBV and HIV [22•].

The consensus is that symptomatic liver disease, morbidity, and mortality are largely confined to patients who have developed cirrhosis and that this is rare during the first 2 decades of infection [19••]. Even for patients who have developed cirrhosis, the prognosis is good as long as there is no clinical decompensation. A European study reported survival rates for patients with compensated cirrhosis of 91% at 5 years and 79% at 10 years. However, survival decreased rapidly after the first episode of decompensation to 50% at 5 years [23••].

Treatment

The goals of treatment of patients with chronic hepatitis C are to eradicate HCV, to induce remission of liver disease, and to prevent the development of cirrhosis and HCC. IFN-α remains the mainstay of treatment for chronic hepatitis C. During therapy, ALT levels follow one of three patterns: ALT levels normalize and remain normal until the end of treatment (ie, response), ALT levels remain abnormal throughout treatment (ie, nonresponse), or ALT levels temporarily normalize but become abnormal again sometime during treatment (ie, breakthrough) (Fig. 94-4).

Among the responders, ALT levels may remain normal (ie, sustained response) or become abnormal again after discontinuation of treatment (ie, relapse). In most patients, there is a parallel response in serum ALT and HCV RNA levels during IFN therapy. However, serum HCV RNA levels may remain detectable in some responders. These patients are more likely to relapse after cessation of treatment, but posttreatment relapse also may occur for patients who become serum HCV RNA negative at the end of therapy. *Response* is defined as biochemical (ie, normalization in ALT level), virologic (ie, undetectable HCV RNA by PCR assay), and histologic (ie, improvement of histology activity index by ≥2 points) based on assessment at the end of treatment (ie, end of treatment response [ETR]) and during posttreatment follow-up (ie, sustained response [SR]) [24••] (Table 94-3).

Short-Term Efficacy

When used in doses of 3 million units three times weekly, a 6-month course of IFN-α treatment is associated with a biochemical ETR rate of 40% to 50% and a biochemical SR rate of 15% to 20%, and the virologic ETR and SR rates are 30% to 40% and 10% to 20%, respectively [23••,24••]. Response is only marginally improved by initiating treatment at higher doses. Although prolonging the duration of treatment to 12 or 18 months does not increase the ETR rate, longer duration of treatment significantly reduces relapse rates, increasing the SR rate (biochemical and virologic) from 20% to 30% [24••,25].

Factors That Influence Response

Several factors are associated with higher rates of response to IFN therapy [26•]. The most important are young age, absence of cirrhosis, low serum HCV RNA level, and HCV genotypes 2 and 3. Other factors that may influence response include heterogeneity in HCV RNA quasispecies and hepatic iron concentration.

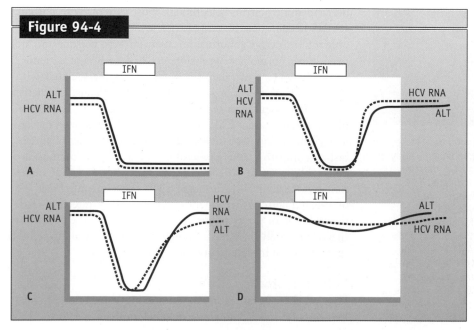

Figure 94-4

Patterns of response to interferon (IFN) therapy in patients with hepatitis C virus (HCV) infection. The end of treatment response (ETR) is defined as normalization in alanine aminotransferase (ALT) levels and HCV RNA levels that are undetectable by polymerase chain reaction (PCR) assay at the end of treatment. **A**, A sustained response is defined as persistent normalization in ALT levels and undetectable HCV RNA by PCR at the end of treatment and during posttreatment follow-up. **B**, Patients who have an ETR but who have elevated ALT levels or detectable HCV RNA after treatment are considered to have relapsed. **C**, Patients who have elevated ALT levels and reappearance of HCV RNA during treatment after an initial response are considered to have breakthroughs. **D**, Patients who have persistently elevated ALT levels and detectable HCV RNA during treatment are considered to be nonresponders.

Long-Term Response

Relapse after treatment usually occurs within 6 months of cessation of therapy, predominantly in patients who had detectable HCV RNA despite normal ALT levels at the conclusion of treatment. Long-term follow-up of responders who maintained normal ALT and had no detectable HCV RNA 1 year after discontinuation of treatment showed that most remained in remission with improvement in liver histology. The impact of IFN therapy on the long-term clinical outcome of patients with chronic HCV infection is unknown.

Alternative and Combination Therapies

Alternative treatments that have been evaluated include ribavirin, phlebotomy, ursodeoxycholic acid, amantadine, and nonsteroidal anti-inflammatory agents. Experience with these agents is limited, and they should be used only in clinical trials.

Ribavirin is the most extensively studied [27•]. It is an orally administered compound with broad-spectrum activity against DNA and RNA viruses, and it has immunomodulatory effects. When used alone, ribavirin decreased ALT levels in most treated patients, but this effect was usually transient; few patients had normal ALT levels at the end of therapy, and serum HCV RNA levels were usually unchanged. The most common side effect of ribavirin is mild hemolysis. Several studies have reported that combination therapy with IFN and ribavirin appears to have increased efficacy, resulting in higher rates of sustained response in previously untreated patients compared with treatment with IFN alone [27•].

Phlebotomy has been evaluated as a treatment for chronic HCV infection because of the observation that nonresponders tended to have increased hepatic iron concentrations. Preliminary studies found that phlebotomy alone decreased ALT levels but had little effect on HCV RNA levels. Combination therapy with phlebotomy and IFN is being tested in ongoing multicenter trials.

Improving Responses at the End of Treatment

The ETR rate can be greatly improved by restricting treatment to young, precirrhotic patients with low serum HCV RNA levels and infection with HCV genotypes 2 and 3. However, few patients fulfill all of these criteria. Moreover, a small percentage of patients with one or more unfavorable features may still respond to therapy. These data should not be used to exclude patients from treatment.

Treatment with higher doses (5 or 6 million units) of IFN is associated with a small increase in the overall response rate, but side effects occur more frequently, and the cost of therapy is higher [25,28]. Most patients who respond have normal ALT levels by the end of the third month of therapy. Continuing IFN therapy at the same dose is unlikely to achieve a response in patients who have persistently abnormal ALT levels after 3 months of treatment. Dose escalation to 5 or 10 million units may result in normalization in ALT levels in 10% to 15% of patients, but a sustained response is seldom achieved [28]. Preliminary studies suggest that the ETR rate may be improved by therapy with a combination of IFN and ribavirin. These observations need to be confirmed in larger, randomized, controlled trials.

Management of Patients Who Relapse and Nonresponders

Approximately 50% of patients who respond during a 6-month course of treatment relapse after therapy. Retreatment with IFN alone at the same dose for 12 to 18 months may induce a sustained response in up to 50% of these persons [29•]. Pilot studies suggest that retreatment with the combination of IFN and ribavirin can induce a higher rate of sustained remission than retreatment with IFN alone, but these data need to be confirmed [27•].

There is no effective treatment for patients who have not responded to a course of IFN at the standard dose of 3 million units. Retreatment with IFN at higher doses or for longer durations may induce responses in approximately 15% of patients during treatment, but fewer than 5% of these persons have sustained responses [29•]. Pilot studies on combination therapy with IFN and ribavirin have reported limited successes [27•].

Current Treatment Strategies

The decision to treat a patient with IFN depends on several factors: the patient's age, presence of symptoms, severity of liver disease, likelihood of response to treatment, concomitant medical problems, and contraindications to the use of IFN (Fig. 94-5). The decision should be made jointly by the physician and the patient after a discussion of the nature, purpose, potential risks and benefits, and alternatives to therapy. Patients who are anti-HCV positive with detectable serum HCV RNA, abnormal ALT levels, and moderate to severe chronic hepatitis on liver biopsy should be considered for treatment (Fig. 94-5). Those with decompensated cirrhosis, significant medical or neuropsychiatric disorders, or recent substance abuse should not receive IFN.

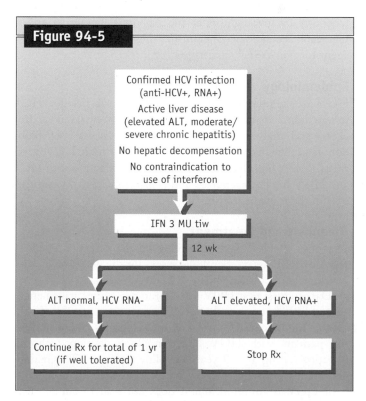

Figure 94-5

Strategy for treatment of chronic hepatitis C virus (HCV) infection. ALT—alanine aminotransferase; IFN—interferon; Rx—treatment.

Therapy should be initiated with 3 million units of IFN-α administered three times weekly. Patients who fail to respond after 3 months of therapy should have treatment discontinued. When possible, responders should continue treatment for a total of 12 to 18 months. Patients who relapse after 6 months of therapy may be retreated with a longer course of IFN at the same dose or referred to specialized centers for experimental therapy. There is no effective treatment for nonresponders.

Treatment is not recommended for patients with normal ALT levels. Although therapy may reduce HCV RNA levels, sustained virus clearance is rare, and some patients have developed abnormal ALT levels during or shortly after treatment with IFN [17]. Although the abnormal ALT levels may represent spontaneous fluctuations rather than IFN-induced worsening of liver disease, there is no evidence that treatment is beneficial.

Prevention

Neutralizing antibodies against HCV envelope proteins have been detected, but they usually are present in low titers and are specific for individual isolates or variants [30]. In view of the high mutation rate of HCV and the presence of viral quasispecies, these antibodies are insufficient to clear the virus, accounting for the high rate of chronic infection and reports of recurrent HCV infection in patients who are repeatedly exposed to the virus. The genetic diversity of HCV and the high mutation rate also hamper development of vaccines that can protect against all prevalent HCV genotypes and those that may emerge in the future.

■ CHRONIC HEPATITIS G VIRUS INFECTION

HGV (*ie*, GBV-C) is a virus that was discovered nearly simultaneously by investigators at the Abbott Laboratories and at Genelabs Technologies Inc. during their search for an etiologic agent for non-A–E hepatitis [31,32•].

Epidemiology

HGV is parenterally transmitted. Persons at risk for HGV infection include blood transfusion recipients, intravenous drug users, and dialysis patients. Approximately 1.5% of blood donors in the United States appear to have chronic HGV infection [32•]. A high frequency of chronic coinfection with HCV and HGV has been reported and is probably related to similarities in the route of transmission.

Diagnosis and Treatment

Diagnosis of HGV infection relies on the detection of HGV RNA by PCR assays. Serologic assays for the detection of anti-envelope antibodies are being evaluated.

Data suggest that HGV infection rarely causes acute hepatitis and little or no liver disease during chronic infection. In the Center for Disease Control Sentinel Counties Study, none of the patients with HGV infection alone developed chronic hepatitis during 1 to 9 years of follow-up, but 75% remained persistently positive for HGV RNA [33•]. Persistent infection with HGV is common, but it does not lead to chronic liver disease. Studies of patients with chronic liver disease also found that coinfection with HGV does not worsen the clinical course

of HCV infection [34]. In view of the low pathogenicity of HGV, treatment of HGV infection probably is unnecessary.

■ REFERENCES

Recently published papers of particular interest have been highlighted as follows:
•   Of interest
••   Of outstanding interest

1.• Lok ASF: Natural history and control of perinatally acquired hepatitis B virus infection. *Dig Dis Sci* 1992, 10:46–52.

2.•• Fattovich G, Giustina G, Schalm SW, *et al*., and the EUROHEP Study Group on Hepatitis B Virus and Cirrhosis: Occurrence of hepatocellular carcinoma and decompensation in western European patients with cirrhosis type B. *Hepatology* 1995, 21:77–82.

3. Liaw YF, Lin DY, Chen TJ, Chu CM: Natural course after the development of cirrhosis in patients with chronic type B hepatitis: a prospective study. *Liver* 1989, 9:235–241.

4. Carman WF, Thomas HC: Implications of genetic variation on the pathogenesis of hepatitis B virus infection. *Arch Virol* 1993, 8(suppl):143–154.

5.• Wong DKH, Cheung AM, O'Rourke K, *et al*.: Effect of α interferon treatment in patients with hepatitis Be antigen positive chronic hepatitis B. *Ann Intern Med* 1993, 119:312–323.

6.•• Lok ASF: Treatment of chronic hepatitis B. *J Viral Hepatitis* 1994, 1:105–124.

7. Niederau C, Heintges T, Lange S, *et el*.: Long-term follow-up of HBeAg-positive patients treated with interferon α for chronic hepatitis B. *N Engl J Med* 1996, 334:1422–1427.

8. Cohard M, Poynard T, Mathurin P, Zarski JP: Prednisone-interferon combination in the treatment of chronic hepatitis B: direct and indirect metanalysis. *Hepatology* 1994, 20:1390–1398.

9. Fontana RJ, Lok ASF: Combination therapy for chronic hepatitis B. *Hepatology* 1997, 26:234–237.

10.• Dienstag JL, Perrillo RP, Schiff ER, *et al*.: A preliminary trial of lamivudine for chronic hepatitis B infection. *N Engl J Med* 1995, 333:1657–1661.

11. Bartholomew MM, Jansen RW, Jeffries LJ, *et al*.: Hepatitis B virus resistance to lamivudine given for recurrent infection after orthotopic liver transplantation. *Lancet* 1997, 349:20–22.

12. Taylor J, Negro F, Rizzetto M: Hepatitis Δ virus: from structure to disease expression. *Rev Med Virol* 1992, 2:161.

13.• DiBisceglie AM, Negro F: Diagnosis of hepatitis Δ virus infection. *Hepatology* 1989, 10:1014–1016.

14. Farci P, Mandas A, Coiana A, *et al*.: Treatment of chronic hepatitis D with interferon α-2a. *N Engl J Med* 1994, 330:88–94.

15. Conry-Cantilena C, Vanraden M, Gibble J, *et al*.: Routes of infection, viremia and liver disease in blood donors found to have hepatitis C virus infection. *N Engl J Med* 1996, 334:1691–1696.

16.•• Lok ASF, Gunaratnam NT: Diagnosis of hepatitis CL. NIH Consensus Development Conference on Management of Hepatitis C. *Hepatology* 1997, 26(suppl 1):48s–56s.

17. Marcellin P, Levy S, Erlinger S: Treatment of patients with normal ALT levels. NIH Consensus Development Conference on Management of Hepatitis C. *Hepatology* 1997, 26(suppl 1):133S–136S.

18. Agnello V, Chung RT, Kaplan LM: A role of hepatitis C virus infection in type II cryoglobulinemia. *N Engl J Med*, 1992, 327:1490–1495.

19.•• Seeff LB: Natural history of hepatitis C. NIH Consensus Development Conference on Management of Hepatitis C. *Hepatology* 1997, 26(suppl 1):21s–28s.

20.• Seeff LB, Buskell-Bales Z, Wright EC, *et al*.: Long-term mortality after transfusion non-A, non-B hepatitis. *N Engl J Med* 1992, 327:1906–1911.

21. Tong MJ, El-Farra NS, Reikes AR, *et al.*: Clinical outcomes after transfusion-associated hepatitis C. *N Engl J Med* 1995, 332:1463–1466.

22.• Poynard T, Bedossa P, Opolon R: Natural history of liver fibrosis progression in patients with chronic hepatitis C. *Lancet* 1997, 349:825–832.

23.•• Fattovich G, Giustina G, Degos F, *et al.*: Morbidity and mortality in compensated cirrhosis type C: a retrospective follow-up study of 384 patients. *Gastroenterology* 1997, 112:463–472.

24.•• Lindsay KL: Therapy of hepatitis C: overview. NIH Consensus Development Conference on Management of Hepatitis C. *Hepatology* 1997, 26(suppl 1):71s–77s.

25. Poynard T, Leroy V, Cohard M, *et al.*: Meta-analysis of interferon randomized trials in the treatment of viral hepatitis C: effects of dose and duration. *Hepatology* 1996, 24:778–789.

26.• Davis GL, Lan JYN: Predictive factors for a beneficial response. NIH Consensus Development Conference on Management of Hepatitis C. *Hepatology* 1997, 26(suppl 1):122s–127s.

27.• Reichard O, Schuarez R, Weiland O: Ribavirin treatment alone or in combination with interferon. NIH Consensus Development Conference on Management of Hepatitis C. *Hepatology* 1997, 26 (suppl 1):108s–111s.

28. Lindsay KL, Davis GL, Schiff ER, *et al.*: Response to higher doses of interferon α-2b in patients with chronic hepatitis C: a randomized multicenter study. *Hepatology* 1996, 24:1034–1040.

29.• Alberti A, Chemello L, Noventa F, *et al.*: Retreatment with interferon. NIH Consensus Development Conference on Management of Hepatitis C. *Hepatology* 1997, 26(suppl 1):137s–142s.

30. Farci P, Alter HJ, Govindarajan S, *et al.*: Lack of protective immunity against reinfection with hepatitis C virus. *Science* 1992, 258:135–140.

31. Simons JN, Leary TP, Dawson GJ, *et al.*: Isolation of novel virus-like sequences associated with human hepatitis. *Nat Med* 1995, 6:564–569.

32.• Linnen J, Wages JJ, Zhang-Keck Z-Y, *et al.*: Molecular cloning and disease association of hepatitis G virus: a transfusion-transmissible agent. *Science* 1996, 271:505–508.

33.• Alter MJ, Gallagher M, Morris TT, *et al.*: Acute non-A–E hepatitis in the United States and the role of hepatitis G virus infection. *N Engl J Med* 1997, 336:741–746.

34. Tanaka E, Alter HJ, Nakatsuji Y, *et al.*: Effect of hepatitis G virus infection on chronic hepatitis C. *Ann Intern Med* 1996, 125:740–743.

Alcoholic Liver Injury, Steatosis, and Steatohepatitis

Anna Mae Diehl

ALCOHOLIC LIVER INJURY

Alcohol has been suspected to cause liver disease for centuries; in the 19th century, Laennec emphasized an increased prevalence of cirrhosis among alcoholics. Modern epidemiologic data from many societies corroborate the association between per capita alcohol consumption and deaths from cirrhosis [1]. Animal studies further demonstrate that chronic consumption of alcohol results in liver disease. For example, hepatic steatosis, steatohepatitis, and fibrosis are more common in baboons that are fed ethanol-containing diets than in control animals fed isocaloric amounts of a similar diet in which carbohydrate has been substituted for ethanol [2].

ALCOHOLIC STEATOSIS AND STEATOHEPATITIS

Alcohol consumption produces a spectrum of histologic abnormalities in the liver, including steatosis (fatty liver), steatohepatitis (alcoholic hepatitis), and cirrhosis. In patients with steatosis, lipid accumulates in large (*ie*, macrovesicular) and small (*ie*, microvesicular) droplets within hepatocytes (Fig. 95-1*A*). Although infiltration of the liver with inflammatory cells is not conspicuous in patients with steatosis, some affected persons may demonstrate fibrosis around terminal hepatic venules

(*ie*, perivenular fibrosis) and/or hepatocytes (*ie*, pericellular fibrosis). Steatohepatitis generally is considered to be a more histologically advanced stage of alcohol-induced liver injury than steatosis, because in patients with steatohepatitis, steatosis is associated with hepatocellular injury, acute and chronic inflammation, and various degrees of fibrosis (Fig. 95-1*B*). Some injured hepatocytes may contain eosinophilic fibrillar material (*ie*, Mallory's hyalin). Lobular infiltration with polymorphonuclear leukocytes distinguishes steatohepatitis from most other forms of hepatitis (in which the inflammatory infiltrate is predominantly periportal and mononuclear). Steatohepatitis eventually progresses to cirrhosis (Fig. 95-1*C*) in some patients.

NONALCOHOLIC STEATOSIS AND STEATOHEPATITIS

Although alcohol is a widely acknowledged cause of steatosis and steatohepatitis, other conditions also have been associated with this histologic pattern of liver injury; these are listed in Table 95-1. Many groups have reported an increased prevalence of nonalcoholic steatohepatitis (NASH) in obese women with adult onset diabetes and/or hyperlipidemia [3•]. The condition also occurs commonly in men who are as little as 10% above ideal body weight.

▌▌ PATHOGENESIS

Steatosis

Alcohol-induced steatosis is a reproducible consequence of ethanol oxidation. Steatosis results from the redox imbalance that follows metabolism of ethanol to acetate and is seen in all humans and animals after consumption of large amounts of ethanol. Excessive reducing equivalents (NADH) generated by the oxidation of ethanol favor lipid synthesis and accumulation relative to lipid degradation. With abstinence, the normal redox state is restored; lipid is mobilized and steatosis resolves [2].

The pathogenesis of nonalcoholic steatosis is poorly understood, but presumably resembles that of alcoholic steatosis, such as the creation of intracellular conditions that favor net accumulation of lipid.

Steatohepatitis

The precise mechanisms responsible for alcohol-induced steatohepatitis are unknown. Evidence suggests that ethanol metabolism generates toxic intermediates (*eg*, acetaldehyde) and results in "oxidative stress." The latter triggers local release of proinflammatory cytokines that attract inflammatory cells, injure hepatocytes, and promote fibrogenesis. Recently, gut-derived bacterial products, including lipopolysaccharide (LPS) or endotoxin, also have been implicated in the pathogenesis of

alcoholic liver disease. Chronic alcohol consumption increases intestinal permeability and is associated with endotoxemia, which is known to induce production of proinflammatory and profibrogenic cytokines.

The pathogenesis of nonalcoholic steatohepatitis is much less certain than that of alcohol-induced steatohepatitis. Recent work in the experimental model of obese rodents that develop steatosis and steatohepatitis suggest that similar pathogenetic mechanisms may be involved in both entities. The obese mice demonstrate increased sensitivity to the hepatotoxic actions of endotoxin. This observation is particularly intriguing because endotoxin is thought to contribute to the liver disease that occurs after jejunoileal bypass surgery for obesity [4]. Defective macrophage phagocytosis and abnormal cytokine production also have been noted in obese mice. If confirmed in humans, these findings could have important implications for the pathogenesis of this type of liver injury.

The development of steatohepatitis appears to be a major rate-limiting step in the pathogenesis of cirrhosis. Although cirrhosis rarely develops in patients with simple steatosis, 40% to 50% of patients with steatohepatitis due to alcohol or obesity develop cirrhosis within 5 years [5•,6•]. Clarification of the mechanisms that lead to steatohepatitis may suggest strategies that can abort the evolution of cirrhosis.

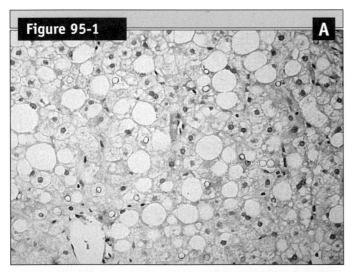

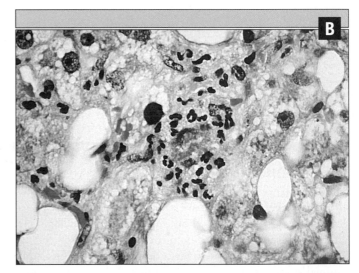

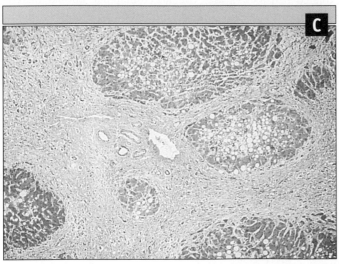

Histology of alcoholic liver disease. **A**, Steatosis. Lipid accumulates in macrovesicular and microvesicular droplets within hepatocytes, but hepatocyte necrosis and infiltration with inflammatory cells are not conspicuous. **B**, Steatohepatitis. Foci of hepatocyte necrosis and infiltration of the liver with acute and chronic inflammatory cells differentiate steatohepatitis from simple steatosis. Some cells may also develop eosinophilic bodies (*ie*, Mallory bodies) that represent condensations of cytoskeletal elements. **C**, Cirrhosis. Broad bands of connective tissue distort the hepatic architecture, leaving islands of regenerating hepatocytes.

DIAGNOSIS

Clinical Signs and Symptoms

Alcohol-induced steatosis usually is asymptomatic in ambulatory patients. Hepatomegaly is common in hospitalized patients, occurring in over 70% of persons with biopsy-proven steatosis. Although this histologic lesion is completely reversible, occasional fatal outcomes have been reported, although the cause of death in these patients is uncertain.

Alcoholic steatohepatitis also may be asymptomatic or present as isolated hepatomegaly, but jaundice, fever, splenomegaly, and encephalopathy are found in 10% to 70% of hospitalized patients. The classic clinical syndrome associated with alcoholic hepatitis includes fever, malaise, jaundice, and tender hepatomegaly. This syndrome, however, occurs in only a minority of patients. Cirrhosis may coexist with alcoholic steatohepatitis. Hence, complications of portal hypertension (eg, ascites or variceal bleeding) may bring patients to the doctor.

The spectrum of physical findings is less well-defined in nonalcoholic patients with steatosis or steatohepatitis. Most patients in reported series have been asymptomatic or have isolated hepatomegaly [3•]. However, under certain circumstances, patients with nonalcoholic steatosis may be quite symptomatic. This is illustrated by reports of severe lactic acidosis, liver failure, and occasional fatality in patients who develop microvesicular steatosis after taking nucleoside analogs for more than 4 months.

Laboratory Abnormalities

Liver Enzymes and Bilirubin

Abnormal aminotransferases and bilirubin are found in about one third of hospitalized patients with alcohol-induced steatosis. In such patients, elevated bilirubin levels largely result from increases in the indirect-reacting fraction and may reflect alcohol-associated hemolysis. Direct-reacting hyperbilirubinemia is common in hospitalized patients with steatohepatitis. In such patients, total bilirubin levels provide a crude estimate of disease severity, because the 1-month mortality correlates roughly with the degree of bilirubin elevation. The pattern of aminotransferase abnormalities provides a useful clue to the diagnosis of alcohol-induced steatohepatitis in hospitalized patients. Typically, the aspartate aminotransferase (AST) is elevated two to three times greater than alanine aminotransferase (ALT) and neither enzyme activity exceeds 300 IU/L. In several series, more than 80% of hospitalized patients with alcoholic steatohepatitis had an AST-to-ALT ratio of 2 or more. The explanation for this pattern of enzyme abnormality is not entirely known. It may be secondary to decreased cytosolic concentration of these enzymes in alcoholics, increased release of AST from nonhepatic sources (muscle, erythrocytes), or due to decreased concentrations of co-enzymes, such as pyridoxal phosphate, that lead to inadvertent underestimation of serum ALT activity. Serum alkaline phosphatase may be increased twofold to threefold in hospitalized patients with alcoholic steatohepatitis, and alkaline phosphatase elevation is occasionally the predominant liver enzyme abnormality. It is important to rule out bile duct obstruction in alcoholic patients with a cholestatic pattern of liver test abnormalities, particularly when cholestasis occurs in the setting of fever, right upper quadrant (RUQ) tenderness, leukocytosis, and elevated serum amylase values.

Modest aminotransferase elevations with normal to mildly increased alkaline phosphatase values are typical of patients with nonalcoholic steatosis and steatohepatitis. AST-to-ALT ratios are typically less than 1. Hyperbilirubinemia is rare in persons with nonalcoholic steatohepatitis, even after the disease has progressed to cirrhosis. Interestingly, a study of ambulatory (ie, nonhospitalized) persons with alcoholic steatosis and steatohepatitis demonstrated that they had liver enzyme and bilirubin abnormalities that mimicked those noted in patients with nonalcoholic steatosis and steatohepatitis. That is, AST-to-ALT ratios were less than 1, and bilirubin levels were generally within the normal range [7•]. The pattern of liver enzyme abnormalities is probably not helpful in differentiating alcohol from other causes of steatohepatitis in ambulatory patients.

Other Blood Tests

Chronic consumption of large amounts of alcohol commonly results in derangements in serum electrolyte and trace element levels. Decreased K, Mg^{2+}, and PO_4 levels are common in hospitalized alcoholics. These electrolyte abnormalities should alert the clinician to the possibility of chronic alcohol abuse and potential alcohol-induced liver injury. Various other laboratory

Table 95-1. Conditions Associated With Nonalcoholic Steatosis and Steatohepatitis

Drugs and toxins	Hereditary metabolic disorders	Acquired metabolic disorders
Amiodarone	Abetalipoproteinemia	Cachexia and starvation
Azaserine	Familial hepatosteatosis	Diabetes
Bleomycin	Galactosemia	Hyperlipidemia
Estrogens	Glycogen storage disease	Inflammatory bowel disease
L-Asparaginase	Hereditary fructose intolerance	Jejunoileal bypass
Methotrexate	Homocystinuria	Obesity
Perhexiline	Lipodystrophy	Total parenteral nutrition
Puromycin	Systemic carnitine deficiency	
Steroids	Tyrosinemia	
Tetracycline	Refsum's disease	
Warfarin	Schwachman's syndrome	
	Wilson's disease	

tests, including mitochondrial AST, γ-glutamyl transpeptidase, mean corpuscular volume, and carbohydrate deficient transferrin have been used as surrogate markers of alcohol abuse. Unfortunately, with the possible exception of carbohydrate deficient transferrin, the sensitivity and specificity of individual tests are relatively poor for this purpose. Nonetheless, abnormalities of several of these tests may suggest chronic alcohol consumption and therefore implicate alcohol as a potential cause of liver disease. It is equally important to recognize that none of these tests, alone or in combination, can reliably distinguish alcohol-induced liver injury from other causes of liver injury in an alcoholic person. Hence, a careful search for other causes of liver disease is mandatory before concluding the liver problem is caused by alcohol. This is particularly important because hepatitis B and C infections are more prevalent in alcoholics, with and without liver disease, than in the general population [8]. Furthermore, alcoholism is not known to decrease the incidence of hemochromatosis or other congenital liver diseases. There is little to suggest that the prevalence of hepatitis B or C infections is increased in nonalcoholics with steatosis or steatohepatitis [9].

Hyperglycemia and hyperlipidemia (hypercholesterolemia, hypertriglyceridemia) have been associated with nonalcoholic steatosis-steatohepatitis [3•]. At present, it is not clear if diabetes and hyperlipidemia are causes or consequences of the liver disease. In any case, these laboratory test abnormalities do not distinguish nonalcoholic from alcoholic steatosis-steatohepatitis, because they are also noted in alcoholics. Dramatic hypertriglyceridemia and hemolysis (Zieve's syndrome) have long been recognized as manifestations of florid alcohol abuse [2].

Although the degree of abnormality in aminotransferase, other enzymes, and electrolyte levels correlates poorly with the severity of histologic injury and with the clinical prognosis in patients with steatosis-steatohepatitis, abnormalities in prothrombin time, albumin, bilirubin, and ammonia levels convey some prognostic information. Similarly, serum concentrations of certain proinflammatory cytokines, including tumor necrosis factor-α, interleukin-6, and interleukin-8, may correlate with mortality in hospitalized patients with alcohol-induced steatohepatitis.

Imaging Test Abnormalities

Sonography, computed tomography (CT) and magnetic resonance imaging (MRI) are useful in suggesting steatosis, but these tests can neither define its cause nor exclude associated steatohepatitis. These tests can detect evidence of portal hypertension (eg, collateral vessels, ascites, splenomegaly) before it becomes clinically apparent and, therefore, are useful in suggesting the existence of "subclinical" cirrhosis. These imaging tests are also helpful in detecting bile duct dilation and can be used to exclude bile duct obstruction in patients with a cholestatic pattern of liver test abnormalities. Patients rarely require adjunctive endoscopic retrograde cholangiopancreatography (ERCP) for further diagnostic clarification. Scintigraphy is seldom helpful in the evaluation of the biliary tree in jaundiced patients because hepatic uptake and concentration of tracer are impaired.

Liver Biopsy

Biopsy is the most sensitive and specific means of evaluating the degree of liver cell injury and hepatic fibrosis. Hence, liver biopsy remains the only way to reliably detect steatohepatitis and cirrhosis in asymptomatic persons. Once clinical evidence of portal hypertension is apparent, biopsy is less critical for that purpose. Given evidence that many alcoholics and most nonalcoholics with steatohepatitis are relatively asymptomatic, biopsy can provide unique insights into which persons within these large populations are developing cirrhosis.

Histology is also useful in distinguishing the cause of liver injury in persons who have more than one potential cause of liver disease. For example, biopsy findings indicate whether there is significant hepatic iron accumulation in patients with increased transferrin saturations and serum ferritins. Similarly, histology can suggest if chronic viral infection or steatohepatitis is the major cause of liver disease in patients with positive viral serologies. Because biopsy results assist in the identification of patients with potentially progressive liver disease and help establish the cause of that disease, it should be considered a useful diagnostic test in the evaluation of suspected steatohepatitis.

▣ PROGNOSIS

Steatosis

Although rare fatal cases have been reported, alcoholic steatosis is considered a benign lesion because it is reversible with discontinuation of alcohol consumption. Cirrhosis, however, may develop in persons with fibrosis around terminal hepatic venules (perivenular fibrosis). The prognosis of nonalcoholic steatosis may not be as good as that of alcohol-induced steatosis.

There are a few, well-documented cases of this lesion progressing to cirrhosis in obese patients despite weight loss [3•,6•]. Some nonalcoholic persons with steatosis associated with nucleoside analogs have a high risk of acute, liver-related mortality.

Steatohepatitis

Early Prognosis

The early prognosis of hospitalized patients with alcohol-induced steatohepatitis is highly variable, with 1-month mortality rates between 0% and almost 50%. Outcome is best predicted by combinations of clinical findings and laboratory abnormalities that reflect potentially reversible, metabolic toxicities associated with alcohol use and the severity of injury to vital organs, including the liver. Two formulas (the Composite Clinical Laboratory Index [CCLI] and the discriminant function [DF]) have been developed to estimate the short-term (1 month) mortality of hospitalized patients with alcohol-induced steatohepatitis.

A group of Canadian investigators have identified clinical and laboratory variables that predict a poor 1-month survival in alcoholic patients hospitalized with decompensated liver disease [9] (Table 95-2). These variables are assigned a numerical value based on their importance as predictors of outcome. The sum of values gives the CCLI. Patients with a low CCLI are likely to survive, whereas those with a high CCLI are at risk of dying before discharge from the hospital (Fig. 95-2). Calculation of the CCLI is useful because it permits a linear estimate of acute mortality in patients with alcoholic liver disease. The disadvantage of this approach is the large number of variables that must be scored and the complexity of the calculation itself.

Maddrey and colleagues simplified assessment of outcome in alcoholic liver disease by developing a DF [10]. According to their formula, patients in whom the equation (4.6 × [difference between the patient's and control's prothrombin times] + bilirubin) exceeds 32 have a greater than 50% chance of dying in the hospital. The utility of the DF has been prospectively validated and offers the advantage of few variables and simple computation. It is, however, important to recognize the relative imprecision of the DF. At best, it provides a crude (50:50) estimate of mortality.

Evidence that serum concentrations of tumor necrosis factor (TNF)-α and certain TNF-inducible cytokines (interleukins 6 and 8) correlate with mortality in hospitalized patients with alcoholic liver disease suggests that these parameters also may provide useful prognostic information. These tests, however, are not available for general clinical use and their utility has not been compared with that of the CCLI or DF.

Although it has not been systematically evaluated, the short-term prognosis of nonalcoholic steatohepatitis appears to be excellent because there are few reports of patients with this lesion requiring hospitalization for liver disease.

Late Prognosis

The long-term prognosis of patients with alcohol-induced steatohepatitis is dictated by the degree of irreversible injury sustained by the liver (*eg*, whether cirrhosis has developed) and whether superimposed acute liver injury occurs (*eg*, continued alcohol toxicity, associated viral infection, drug toxicity). At least two studies suggest that progression to cirrhosis correlates with continued alcohol use and with the severity of the initial acute liver injury. Female gender also appears to convey an independent risk for progression to cirrhosis. Studies in which patients with alcohol-induced steatohepatitis have been re-biopsied after 5 years indicate that almost 50% of these persons develop cirrhosis during this time period and very few (<10%) have restoration of normal hepatic architecture [5•].

Once cirrhosis has developed, clinical outcome is dictated by the development of complications of portal hypertension and parenchymal failure. This is estimated using the Child's-Pugh criteria. It is important to recognize that alcohol consumption continues to influence prognosis even after cirrhosis has developed. Clinically compensated cirrhotic patients who become abstinent have a 90% chance of surviving for 5 years. In contrast, if these same patients continue to drink, their chance of survival falls to about 70%. Once signs of clinical decompensation develop in patients with alcohol-induced cirrhosis, patients who stop drinking can expect a 5-year survival of about 60% versus only 30% if they continue to drink alcohol.

The long-term prognosis of nonalcoholic steatohepatitis has not been defined. Several series, however, indicate that at least a third to perhaps one half of patients with this lesion ultimately become cirrhotic. Although this has not been systematically studied, the bulk of patients with histologic cirrhosis appear to

Table 95-2. Scoring System for the Composite Clinical Laboratory Index

Sign or symptom	Score
Hepatomegaly	1
Splenomegaly	1
Ascites	
1+	1
2+	2
3+	3
Encephalopathy	
Grade 1	1
Grade 2	2
Grade 3	3
Clinical bleeding	1
Spider nevi	1
Palmar erythema	1
Collateral circulation	1
Peripheral edema	1
Anorexia	1
Weakness	1
AST > 200	1
ALT	
> 100 IU/L	1
> 200 IU/L	2
Alkaline phosphatase > 80 U/L	1
Albumin < 2.59%	1
Prothrombin time	
< 3	1
3–5	2
> 5	3
Bilirubin (mg/dL)	
1.2–2	1
2.1–5	2
> 5	3

ALT—alanine aminotransferase; AST—aspartate aminotransferase.

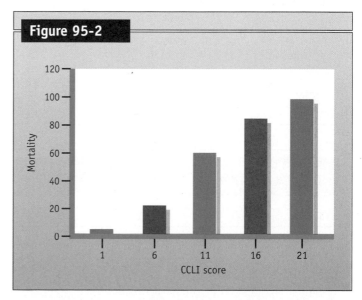

Figure 95-2

Short-term mortality rates for alcoholic liver disease as estimated by the Composite Clinical Laboratory Index (CCLI). The CCLI is calculated as described in Table 95-2.

remain well-compensated clinically and, hence, appear to have an excellent chance of surviving for at least 5 years [3•,7•]. Obese patients who develop cirrhosis after jejunoileal bypass surgery are notable exceptions to this general rule, because a relatively high percentage of these persons experience complications of liver failure and portal hypertension within a few years of their surgery. At least some patients with cirrhosis due to nonalcoholic steatohepatitis have required liver transplantation [11].

■ THERAPY

Steatosis

Steatosis resolves within 2 weeks of discontinuing alcohol. Abstinence is the therapy for alcohol-induced steatosis. Observations that weight reduction results in normalization of aminotransferases in obese patients with steatosis suggest that weight reduction is a useful treatment for obese patients with nonalcoholic steatosis.

Steatohepatitis

Much attention has been directed toward treating alcoholic patients with acutely decompensated liver disease. As shown in Table 95-3, a number of different agents have been tested as therapies for acute alcohol-induced steatohepatitis. Unfortunately, only one has proven beneficial. Corticosteroids improve the 1-month mortality of a subset of severely decompensated patients (defined as patients with a DF >32) with acutely decompensated alcoholic steatohepatitis [12,13•,14]. It is not clear if the beneficial effects of prednisone reflect treatment-related improvements in hepatic injury, because posttreatment

Table 95-3. Putative Therapies for Acute Alcoholic Liver Disease

Therapy	Benefit
Corticosteroids	Yes*
Amino acids	No
Anabolic steroids	No
Insulin/glucagon	No
Cytoprotectants	No
Antifibrotics	No

* Selected patients only.

Table 95-4. Putative Therapies for Nonalcoholic Steatohepatitis

Therapy	Benefit
Jejunoileal bypass reversal	Yes*
Weight loss	?
Antibiotics	?
Ursodiol	?

* In some obese patients with jejunoileal bypass.

liver biopsies were rarely performed. Prednisone has not been tested in patients with coincident gastrointestinal bleeding, serious infections, or acute pancreatitis. Furthermore, it is uncertain if the drug benefits such patients when it is introduced after these comorbid conditions have been treated. The impact of a short course of prednisone on the ultimate prognosis of patients who survive hospitalization is also unknown.

Chronic treatment of alcoholic patients with steatohepatitis has rarely been attempted. Two studies suggest that long-term therapy may be beneficial.

Chronic treatment with colchicine [15•] or propylthiouracil [16•] was reported to decrease the 5- to 10-year mortality in actively drinking alcoholic patients with cirrhosis. Because both studies were plagued by high rates of noncompliance and drop-out, their conclusions may be inadvertently misleading. Abstinence from alcohol definitely improves the morbidity and mortality of patients with alcohol-induced steatohepatitis and cirrhosis. There is also no question that orthotopic liver transplantation improves the survival of patients with alcohol-induced cirrhosis. This therapy, however, is generally reserved for patients who have decompensated liver disease despite documented sobriety for at least 6 months. For such patients, posttransplant survival is equal to, or better than, adult patients who undergo transplantation for other types of liver disease [17•].

Little is known about the impact of therapy on the outcome of nonalcoholic steatohepatitis. Some of the treatments that have been used for this condition are listed in Table 95-4. In obese patients, weight reduction clearly improves some of the associated laboratory abnormalities, but it is unclear if this reduces the risk of progression to cirrhosis [18•]. Some anecdotal evidence suggests that it may not [3•]. If the liver lesion is thought to be drug-induced or provoked by jejunoileal bypass surgery, discontinuation of the presumed toxin or reversal of the bypass improve liver disease in some, but not in all, patients [4]. Selective gut-decontamination (with metronidazole) and supplemental nutrition have been reported to convey some short-term benefit in patients with jejunoileal bypass-associated liver disease [3•,19•]. One suggested that steatosis and steatohepatitis can recur after liver transplantation in patients with intact intestinal bypass loops [20•]. A few patients with total parenteral nutrition (TPN)–induced steatohepatitis may have been helped by ursodiol therapy [3•]. Until we have a better understanding of the mechanisms responsible for development of nonalcoholic steatohepatitis, the odds of stumbling on generally effective therapy are poor.

■ REFERENCES

Recently published papers of particular interest have been highlighted as follows:
•   Of interest
••   Of outstanding interest

1.   Dufour M, Stinson FS, FeCaces M: Trends in cirrhosis morbidity and mortality: United States, 1979–1988. *Semin Liver Dis* 1993, 13:109–116.

2.   Lieber CS: Biochemical factors in alcoholic liver disease. *Semin Liver Dis* 1993, 13:136–147.

3.• Sheth SG, Gordon FD, Chopra S: Nonalcoholic steatohepatitis. *Ann Intern Med*. 1997, 126:137–145.
     The article summarizes the literature about nonalcoholic steatohepatitis.

4. Vyberg M, Ravn V, Andersen B: Patterns of progression of liver injury following jejunoileal bypass for morbid obesity. *Liver* 1987, 7:271–276.

5.• Pares A, Caballeria J, Brugera M: Histologic course of alcoholic hepatitis: influence of abstinence, sex, and extent of hepatic damage. *J Hepatol* 1986, 2:33–38.
The paper assesses the parameters that influence liver disease progression in alcoholics.

6.• Powell EE, Cooksley GE, Hanson R, *et al.*: The natural history of nonalcoholic steatohepatitis: a follow-up study of 42 patients followed for up to 21 years. *Hepatology* 1990, 11:74–80.
This is one of the few studies to follow the natural history of patients with nonalcoholic steatohepatitis.

7.• Pinto HC, Babtista A, Camilo ME, *et al.*: Nonalcoholic steatohepatitis: clinicopathological comparison with alcoholic hepatitis in ambulatory and hospitalized patients. *Dig Dis Sci* 1996, 41:172–179.
The paper provides important recognition that ambulatory patients with nonalcoholic steatohepatitis and alcoholic liver disease are indistinguishable on clinical or histopathologic grounds.

8. Mendenhall CL, Seeff L, Diehl AM, *et al.*: Antibodies to hepatitis B virus and hepatitis C virus in alcoholic hepatitis and cirrhosis: their prevalence and clinical relevance. *Hepatology* 1991, 14:581–585.

9. Rogers DW, Lee CH, Pound DC, *et al.*: Hepatitis C virus does not cause nonalcoholic steatohepatitis. *Dig Dis Sci* 1992, 37:1644–1486.

10. Maddrey WC, Boitnott J, Bedine MS, *et al.*: Corticosteroid therapy of alcoholic hepatitis. *Gastroenterology* 1978, 75:193–199.

11. Requarth JA, Burchard KW, Colacchio TA, *et al.*: Long-term morbidity following jejunoileal bypass: the continuing potential need for surgical reversal. *Arch Surg* 1995, 130:318–325.

12. Carithers RL, Herlong HF, Diehl AM, *et al.*: Methylprednisolone therapy in patients with severe alcoholic hepatitis: a randomized multi-center trial. *Ann Intern Med* 1989, 110:685–688.

13.• Imperiale TF, McCullough AJ: Do corticosteroids reduce mortality from alcoholic hepatitis? A meta-analysis of the randomized trials. *Ann Intern Med* 1990, 113:299–303.
This often-cited meta-analysis confirms that corticosteroids reduce the mortality of selected patients with alcoholic hepatitis.

14. Ramond MJ, Poynard T, Rueff B, *et al.*: A randomized trial of pred-nisolone in patients with severe alcoholic hepatitis. *N Engl J Med* 1992, 326:507–510.

15.• Kershenobich D, Vargas R, Garcia-Tsao G, *et al.*: Colchicine in the treatment of cirrhosis of the liver. *N Engl J Med* 1988, 318:1709–1711.
This is one of the two long-term treatment trials for patients with alcoholic liver disease.

16.• Orrego H, Blade JE, Blendis LM, *et al.*: Long-term treatment of alcoholic liver disease with propylthiouracil. *N Engl J Med* 1987, 317:1421–1425.
This is the only other long-term treatment trial for patients with alcoholic liver disease.

17.• Osorio RW, Friese CE, Ascher NL, *et al.*: Orthotopic liver transplan-tation for end-stage alcoholic liver disease. *Transplant Proc* 1993, 25:1139–1142.
This landmark study documented the benefit of liver transplantation for patients with decompensated alcoholic liver disease.

18.• Palmer M, Schaffner F: Effect of weight reduction on hepatic abnor-malities in overweight patients. *Gastroenterology* 1990, 99:1408–1411.
The article addresses a much-asked question: does weight reduction improve liver disease associated with obesity?

19.• Freund HR, Muggia-Sullam M, Lafrance R, *et al.*: A possible benefi-cial effect of metronidazole in reducing TPN-associated liver function derangements. *J Surg* 1985, 38:356–360.
This article provided one of the first clues that gut-derived bacterial prod-ucts might play a role in the pathogenesis of steatohepatitis.

20.• D'Souze-Gburek S, Batts KP, Nikias GA, *et al.*: Liver transplantation for jejunoileal bypass-associated cirrhosis: allograft histology in the setting of an intact bypassed limb. *Liver Transplant Surg* 1997, 3:23–27.
The article suggests that persistent metabolic derangements in transplant recipients are responsible for the recurrence of steatohepatitis after liver transplantation for that disease.

96 Medication-Related and Other Forms of Toxic Liver Injury

James H. Lewis

More than 600 medications and toxins have been reported to cause drug-induced liver disease (DILD). DILD is responsible for an estimated 2% to 5% of cases of jaundice in hospitalized patients and for approximately 10% of all cases of acute hepati-tis. More importantly, drugs and toxins are the cause of 20% to 40% of cases of fulminant hepatic failure.

Each component of the liver is the target of one or more drugs and toxins. Knowledge about the characteristic microscopic and biochemical patterns of injury from these agents is important in ascribing causation in suspected cases of DILD. As a result of important differences in physiologic function between the hepa-tocytes of periportal zone 1 and those of centrilobular zone 3 (see

Chapter 87), the zonal injury patterns of specific agents vary. Because the centrilobular area of the liver is rich in enzymes responsible for much of the metabolism and detoxification of drugs, it is also the area most prone to DILD. Examples of zonal patterns of DILD and other hepatic targets of drugs and chemi-cals are given in Table 96-1.

■ EPIDEMIOLOGY AND RISK FACTORS

Drug-induced liver disease accounts for an estimated 3% to 9% of all adverse drug reactions, and the incidence of DILD appears to be rising. Table 96-2 lists the estimated frequency of asymp-tomatic (subclinical) biochemical abnormalities from the use of various medicines. For example, as many as 50% of persons who receive tacrine for Alzheimer's disease develop elevations of their serum aminotransferase levels. Other drugs associated with relatively high rates of abnormal liver test results but not overt or clinically significant hepatic injury include chlorpromazine (25%), amiodarone (up to 25%), isoniazid (10% to 30%), phenytoin (10%), and erythromycin estolate (10% to 20%).

Table 96-3 lists the estimated frequency of clinically overt hepatocellular or cholestatic hepatic injury caused by various drugs. Liver disease associated with the use of some medicines is well documented, whereas only anecdotal case reports of injury from other agents exist. Use of antibiotics such as penicillin, although associated with a high incidence of allergic reactions, rarely causes DILD. Other medications, such as isoniazid, amiodarone, and chlorpromazine, cause significant clinical liver injury in 1% to 2% of patients receiving them. In many instances, asymptomatic enzyme abnormalities caused by med-

ications resolve spontaneously or do not progress to clinical liver disease; as a result, clinically overt DILD is less common.

Drug-induced liver disease may result from intentional overdose, accidental ingestion, or "therapeutic misadventure," in which a drug used in its recommended dose nevertheless causes injury. Factors associated with enhanced susceptibility to DILD are listed in Table 96-4. Certain drug formulations have been associated with

Table 96-1. Anatomic Targets of Drug-Induced Liver Disease

Anatomic target	Example
Zone 3 (centrilobular)	Carbon tetrachloride, acetaminophen, halothane
Zone 2 (midzone)	Beryllium, chloroform, furosemide
Zone 1 (periportal)	Iron, phosphorous, allyl formate trinitrotoluene
Larger bile ducts	Paraquat, rapeseed oil
Bile ductules (cholangioles)	Benoxaprofen
Central veins	Pyrrolizidine, alkaloids, azathioprine, antineoplastic agents
Hepatic veins	Contraceptive steroids
Hepatic artery	Floxuridine, phenytoin, contraceptive steroids
Lipocytes	Vitamin A
Canalicular membrane	Chlorpromazine, erythromycin estolate
Sinusoidal membrane	Ethinylestradiol
Mitochondria	Fialuridine

Table 96-2. Estimated Prevalence of Subclinical Hepatic Enzyme Elevations with Various Drugs

Prevalence, %	Examples
25–50	Tacrine
20–25	Chlorpromazine, triacetyloleandomycin, phenytoin, amiodarone, perhexiline, papaverine, cisplatin, nicotinic acid, valproate, 6-mercaptopurine
10–20	Isoniazid, ketoconazole, androgens, erythromycin estolate, etretinate
5–10	Penicillamine, chenodeoxycholate, flucytosine, disulfiram, tienilic acid
< 5	Salicylates, gold salts, sulfonamides, dantrolene, sulfonylureas, quinidine, thiabendazole, ticarcillin, tricyclic antidepressants, ethionamide

Table 96-3. Estimated Frequency of Clinically Overt Hepatitis or Jaundice From Medicinal Agents

Incidence, %	Examples
> 2	Para-aminosalicylate, triacetyloleandomycin, dapsone, chenodeoxycholate
1–2	Lovastatin, cyclosporine, dantrolene
1	Isoniazid, amiodarone
0.5–1	Phenytoin, sulfonamides, chlorpromazine
0.1–0.5	Gold salts, salicylates, methyldopa, chlorpropamide, erythromycin estolate, tienilic acid
< 0.01	Ketoconazole, contraceptive steroids
< 0.001	Hydralazine, halothane
< 0.0001	Penicillin, enflurane, cimetidine, ranitidine

Table 96-4. Host Factors Enhancing Susceptibility to Drug-Induced Liver Disease

Factor	Example
Age	
Older	Acetaminophen, halothane, isoniazid, amoxicillin and potassium clavulanate
Younger	Salicylates, valproate, mushroom toxicity
Fasting or malnutrition (reduced glutathione)	Acetaminophen
Obesity	Halothane
Diabetes mellitus	Methotrexate, niacin
Renal failure	Tetracycline (IV), allopurinol
HLA-DR4 phenotype	Hydralazine
Rheumatoid arthritis, lupus	Aspirin
Gender	
Female	Halothane, nitrofurantoin, sulindac, oxyphenisatin, methyldopa
Male	Amoxicillin and potassium clavulanate
Drug formulation	IV tetracycline, sustained-release nicotinic acid
AIDS	Dapsone, trimethoprim-sulfamethoxazole
Preexisting liver disease	Niacin, tetracycline, methotrexate
Alcohol	Acetaminophen, isoniazid, methotrexate, vitamin A

IV—intravenous.

toxicity. For example, it is rare to see hepatic injury from the oral form of tetracycline, whereas the intravenous preparation was associated with clinically significant steatosis. The sustained-release formulation of nicotinic acid is more likely to produce hepatic injury than the crystalline type, and continuous daily administration of methotrexate is more likely to cause chronic hepatic injury than intermittent therapy. Renal failure increases the risk of DILD from tetracycline and allopurinol, obesity does so for halothane, and diabetes has been linked to methotrexate hepatotoxicity. In general, patients with preexisting liver disease are not considered to be at greater risk for DILD than persons who do not have underlying liver damage, although patients with liver disease receiving niacin, tetracycline, and methotrexate should be closely monitored.

Concomitant use of alcohol plays an important role in enhancing susceptibility to many agents through induction of the cytochrome P450 (CYP) system and through depletion of glutathione (Fig. 96-1). Most notably, this is seen with acetaminophen ingestion, which may cause serious or even fatal hepatic injury when taken in recommended doses by chronic alcohol users. Other hepatotoxic agents whose toxicity is enhanced by alcohol include isoniazid, cocaine, vitamin A, methotrexate, carbon tetrachloride, vinyl chloride, trichloroethylene, dimethylnitrosamine, 1,2–trichloroethane, bromobenzene, and galactosamine.

Genetic defects in metabolism that predispose to liver injury have been identified for a few drugs (Table 96-5). Persons who metabolize the antiarrhythmic debrisoquine slowly are at increased risk for injury from perhexiline maleate; an inherited defect in epoxide hydrolase activity is associated with an increased risk for injury from phenytoin and halothane; and a defect in the detoxification of arene oxides has led to DILD from phenytoin. A genetic susceptibility to contraceptive steroid-induced cholestasis also appears to exist.

PHYSIOLOGY

Drug detoxification and metabolism are predominantly hepatic processes, facilitated by absorption of drugs and other compounds from the intestine into portal blood. Most medicines undergo a two-phase biotransformation that makes them pharmacologically inactive and allows them to be excreted. Phase I reactions convert the parent compound to metabolites through oxidation, reduction, or hydrolysis, alone or in combination. Phase I reactions are catalyzed by hepatic microsomal enzymes (ie, mixed function oxidases), especially the CYP proteins of the endoplasmic reticulum. Some drugs are converted through immunologic and nonimmunologic mechanisms into reactive metabolites that are potentially toxic to hepatocytes. Certain drugs have the potential to cause DILD because they are substrates for specific CYP enzymes. For example, the cytochrome induced by metabolism of ethanol (CYP2E1) also produces the toxic metabolite of acetaminophen (Fig. 96-1). Phase II reactions couple the drug or its metabolites to glucuronide, sulfate, or other substrates to create water-soluble products that are excreted in the urine or bile.

Figure 96-1

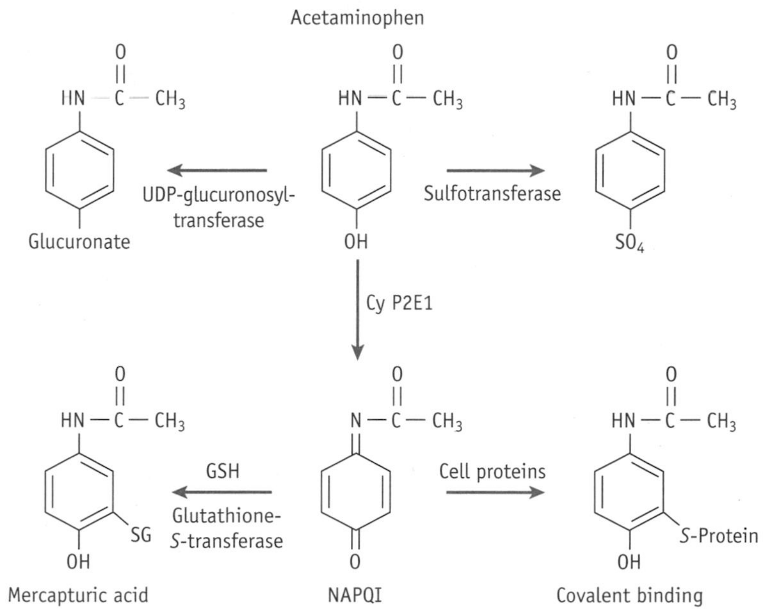

Metabolic pathway of acetaminophen. Acetaminophen primarily undergoes sulfation and glucuronidation (phase 2 reactions) but is metabolized by cytochrome P450-2E1 (CYP2E1) in a phase 1 reaction to N-acetyl-p-benzoquinoneimine (NAPQI) if the capacity of phase 2 reactions is exceeded or if cytochrome CYP2E1 synthesis is induced. Glutathione-S-transferase is capable of detoxifying NAPQI to yield mercapturic acid and its derivatives if glutathione is available. In the absence of glutathione substrate, covalent binding to cell proteins occurs. N-acetylcysteine is an excellent source of glutathione substrate. UDP—uridine diphosphate; GSH—reduced glutathione. (From Farrell [2•].)

Table 96-5. Genetic Predisposition to Drug-Induced Liver Disease

Drug	Genetic defect of polymorphism
Perhexiline maleate	Deficiency of debrisoquine hydroxylase (lack of CYP2D6)
Hydralazine	Slow acetylator status
Halothane	Familial tendency, enhanced sensitivity to phenytoin metabolites
Contraceptive steroids	Familial tendency
Phenytoin	Deficiency of epoxide hydrolase

ETIOLOGY

Hundreds of medicines and other chemical compounds have been reported to produce DILD. Table 96-6 provides an overview of the various classes of drugs, including examples and the types of acute injury they are most likely to produce (*ie*, hepatocellular, cholestatic, or mixed). Drugs that cause fulminant hepatic failure include acetaminophen, isoniazid, valproic acid, halothane, enflurane, phenytoin, sulfonamides, propylthiouracil, dapsone, ketoconazole, ticrynafen,

Table 96-6. Types of Hepatic Injury Caused by Drugs in Various Therapeutic Classes

Class	Predominantly hepatocellular	Predominantly cholestatic	Mixed	Trivial or no injury
Anesthetics	Halothane, Methoxyflurane, Enflurane, Isoflurane (rare)	—	—	Cyclopropane, Divinyl ether, Diethyl ether, Nitrous oxide
Anticonvulsants	Phenytoin, Valproate, Paramethadione, Progabide, Phenacemide, Felbamate	—	Carbamazepine, Phenobarbital	—
Psychotropics				
Phenothiazines	—	Chlorpromazine, Prochlorperazine, Promazine, Thioridazine	—	—
Butyrophenones	—	Haloperidol	—	
Anxiolytics	—	—	Chlordiazepoxide, Diazepam, Alprazolam	—
Alzheimer treatment	Tacrine	—	—	—
Tricyclic antidepressants	Most	Trimipramine	Amitriptyline, Imipramine, Desipramine	—
Serotonin-reuptake inhibitors		Trazodone	Fluoxetine	—
MAO inhibitors	Phenelzine, Most hydrazines, Tranylcypromine	—	—	Buspirone
CNS stimulants	Pemoline	—	—	—
Analgesic/anti-inflammatory antigout agents	Acetaminophen, Salicylates, Diclofenac, Fenbufen, Fenoprofen, Ibuprofen (rare), Indomethacin, Oxaprozin, Piroxicam, Pirprofen, Tolmetin, Probenecid (rare), Dantrolene, Flurbiprofen (rare)	Sulindac, Diflunisal, Naproxen, Benoxaprofen, Propoxyphene	Phenylbutazone, Gold, Allopurinol	Ritalin, Ketoprofen
Oral hypoglycemics	Acetohexamide, Carbutamide, Metahexamide	Chlorpropamide, Glibenclamide, Tolazamide, Tolbutamide	—	Metformin
Antithyroid	Propylthiouracil	Carbimazole, Methimazole	Thiouracil	
Steroids or hormonal agents	Glucocorticoids (fat), Diethylstilbestrol, Tamoxifen	Anabolic-androgenic, Oral contraceptive, Danazol	—	—
Cardiovascular agents				
Antihypertensives	Methyldopa, Hydralazine, Enalapril, Lisinopril, Verapamil, Atenolol, Labetalol, Metoprolol (rare)	Captopril, Nifedipine	Diltiazem	Propranolol, Nitroglycerine
Antiarrhythmics	Quinidine, Amiodarone, Procainamide	Propafenone, Ajmaline, Disopyramide	Aprindine	—
Anticoagulants	Streptokinase (rare),	Ticlopidine, Warfarin	Phenindione	Heparin
Lipid lowering	Lovastatin, Pravastatin, Simvastatin, Fluvastatin, Nicotinic acid	—	—	Clofibrate, Gemfibrozil, Cholestyramine

CNS—central nervous system; MAO—monoamine oxidase.

Table 96-6. Types of Hepatic Injury Caused by Drugs in Various Therapeutic Classes (continued)

Class	Predominantly hepatocellular	Predominantly cholestatic	Mixed	Trivial or no injury
Diuretics	Furosemide (rare), Ticrynafen	Chlorthalidone, Thiazides	—	—
Antibiotics	Chloramphenicol, Clindamycin, Tetracycline, Nitrofurantoin, Sulfonamides, Amphotericin, Ketoconazole, Fluconazole (rare), Isoniazid, p-aminosalicylate, Pyrazinamide, Amodiaquine, Rifampicin, Ethionamide, Dapsone, Minocycline	Cephalosporins (rare), Erythromycins, Augmentin, 5-Fluorocytosine, Thiabendazole, Oxacillin, Cloxacillin, Arsenicals, Griseofulvin, Ciprofloxacin	Penicillin (rare), Clarithromycin, Sulfamethoxazole, Pyrimethamine	Amoxicillin, Cycloserine, Ethambutol, Streptomycin, Metronidazole, Carbenicillin
Antivirals	Fialuridine, Zidovudine, Didanosine	—	—	Ribavirin, Lamivudine, Stavudine, Amantadine, Acyclovir, Ganciclovir, Famciclovir, Foscarnet, Interferon
Antineoplastics	Actinomycin D, Asparaginase, Bleomycin, Carmustine, Chlorambucil, Cisplatin, Cyclophosphamide, Dacarbazine, Etoposide, Fluorouracil, Hydroxyurea, Methotrexate, Mithramycin, Mitomycin, Nitrosoureas, Procarbazine, Streptozotocin, Thiotepa, Thioguanine, Vincristine	Aminoglutethimide, Busulfan, Floxuridine, Cyclosporine, Interleukin-2, Tamoxifen	Azathioprine, Mercaptopurine	Interferons, Lomustine, Melphalan, Semustine
Miscellaneous agents	Disulfiram, Iodide ion, Oxyphenisatin, Loratadine, Tannic acid, Vitamin A, p-aminobenzoic acid, Ranitidine (rare), Etretinate, Nizatidine (rare), Famotidine (rare), Olsalazine (rare), Sulfasalazine, Omeprazole (rare), Ondansetron, Granisetron	Cimetidine (rare), Propoxyphene, Rapeseed oil aniline, Methylene dianiline, Penicillamine, Terfenadine	—	Misoprostol, Sucralfate, Antacids, Bismuth, Metoclopramide, Cisapride, Ursodiol, Octreotide, Loperamide

diclofenac, sulindac, disulfiram, carbamazepine, nicotinic acid, labetalol, flutamide, and etodolac. Table 96-7 lists herbal therapies that have been associated with hepatotoxicity. Important occupational, environmental, and domestic chemical hepatotoxins and the types of injury they produce are given in Tables 96-8 and 96-9.

■ PATHOPHYSIOLOGY

Few predictably hepatotoxic medicines are in use. The one major exception is acetaminophen, which is converted to a toxic metabolite (N-acetyl-p-benzoquinoneimine) by CYP enzymes when more than the recommended dose is taken or when glutathione is depleted and the cytochrome system is induced by chronic alcohol use.

Most drugs that cause liver injury do so in an unpredictable manner and only in susceptible persons. DILD also may be produced by a toxic metabolite that binds to cell proteins, leading to necrosis (ie, metabolic idiosyncrasy), or that acts as an antigen (ie, drug-hapten) to stimulate T lymphocytes, leading to an immune reaction that causes hepatic injury (ie, hypersensitivity or drug allergy). Tables 96-10 and 96-11 describe these mechanisms and provide examples of drugs responsible for such injuries. Hypersensitivity often is associated with fever, rash, and eosinophilia; has a fixed latency period; and promptly recurs when the responsible medicine is given a second time (ie, rechallenge). In contrast, aberrant drug metabolism with formation of toxic metabolites generally does not produce a systemic allergic reaction and has a long or variable latency period; patients often have a delayed response to rechallenge. Toxic drug metabolites injure or kill hepatocytes by damaging cellular membranes or binding to liver macromolecules (Fig. 96-2).

PATHOLOGY

A variety of changes in liver morphology is seen in patients with DILD, including lesions that resemble those seen in other types of liver disease (Table 96-12). It is useful to divide acute hepatocellular injury into three categories: predominantly cytotoxic (*ie*, hepatocellular necrosis), predominantly cholestatic, or mixed, with components of hepatocellular necrosis and cholestasis (Table 96-13).

Besides hepatocellular necrosis and cholestasis, several other types of liver DILD occur. For example, many drugs lead to accumulation of fat within liver cells (*ie*, steatosis). Microvesicular hepatic steatosis can be caused by acetylsalicylic acid, aflatoxin, alcohol (*ie*, "alcohol foamy degeneration"), amiodarone, camphor, cocaine, desferrioxamine, fialuridine, hypoglycin A, Margosa oil, methyl salicylate, piroxicam, tetracyclines, tol-metin, or valproic acid. Macrovesicular hepatic steatosis can be caused by alcohol, asparaginase, chromium toxicity, corticosteroids, mercury poisoning, methotrexate, minocycline, nifedipine, parenteral nutrition, perhexiline maleate, or phosphorous poisoning.

Mallory bodies are eosinophilic structures, originally described as alcoholic hyaline, that are thought to represent clumping of microtubules. Mallory bodies can be caused by drugs such as alcohol, griseofulvin, amiodarone, perhexiline maleate, and nifedipine. They are also seen in Wilson's disease, Indian childhood cirrhosis, primary biliary cirrhosis, and jejunoileal bypass performed for obesity. Many drugs can cause hepatic granuloma formation (Table 96-14), some of which are associated with granulomatous hepatitis (*eg*, carbamazepine).

Drugs can cause chronic liver injury, such as chronic hepatitis, fibrosis, or cirrhosis. Chronic hepatitis can be caused by oxyphenisatin, methyldopa, benzarone, isoniazid, nitrofurantoin, dantrolene, or clometacin. Fibrosis can result from exposure to vinyl chloride, thorotrast, heroin, methotrexate, or combination chemotherapy for metastatic breast cancer. Cirrhosis can be caused by isoniazid, methotrexate, or methyldopa.

Table 96-7. Herbal Preparations Indicated as Possible Hepatotoxins*

Common names	Scientific names	Folk uses	Possible toxic component	Hepatic disorder
Chaparral (creosote bush, greasewood, governadora)	*Larrea tridentata* *Larrea divaricata*	Cancer, arthritis, bruises, diarrhea, eczema, colds, bronchitis, menstrual cramps, amenorrhea, veneral disease, "blood purifier," emetic, antiseptic, diuretic	Nordihydroquaiaretic acid (DNGA) and other related compounds	Acute and subacute hepatitis
Chinese herbs				
Chuen-Lin (Huang-Lien, Ma Huang)	*Coptis senesia* *Coptis japonicum*	Tonic, to remove "toxic products of pregnancy" in neonates	Unknown	Unconjugated hyperbilirubinemia
Yin-Chen	*Antemesia scoparia*	Neonatal jaundice	Unknown	Potential kernicterus
Comfrey	*Symphytum officinate*	Fatigue, abdominal pain, allergy	Pyrrolizidine alkaloids	Veno-occlusive disease
Germander	*Teucrium chamaedrys*	Weight control, bitter tonic, appetizer, choleretic, antiseptic	Furano neoclerodane deterpenoids	Reversible acute hepatitis, fatal massive hepatic necrosis
Gordolobo	*Verbascum thaprus,* *Senecio longilobus,* *Gnaphalium macounii*	—	Pyrrolizidine alkaloids	Potential for veno-occlusive disease
Mistletoe	*Viscum album,* *Phoradendron flavescens*	Infertility, asthma, epilepsy, aphrodisiac	β-Phenylethylamine, tyramine, acetylcholine, propionylcholine	Hepatitis with piecemeal necrosis and distortion of lobular architecture
Senna	*Cassia angustifolia,* *Cassia acutifolia*	Laxative or cathartic	Sennosides, rhein anthron	Hepatitis
Skullcap	*Scuttelaria galericulata*	Sedative, anticonvulsant	—	Hepatitis with centrilobular and bridging necrosis
Valerian (garden heliotrope)	*Valerian officinalis*	Sedative, hypnotic, spasmolytic, hypotensive	—	Hepatitis with piecemeal necrosis, chronic aggressive hepatitis with fibrosis

* Herbal teas vary widely in composition and may contain several potential toxins, often containing pyrrolizidine alkaloids from Senecio, Symphytum, Crotalaria, or Heliotropum. Intrauterine damage may also result from maternal consumption of these concoctions. Babies may develop toxic liver disease from consuming herbal beverages or milk from mothers taking toxin-containing herbal drinks.

There are two types of drug-induced chronic cholestatic injury. The primary biliary cirrhosis–like form can be caused by chlorpromazine, prochlorperazine, thiabendazole, tolbutamide, ajmaline sulfamethoxazole, trimethoprim, haloperidol, troleandomycin, benoxaprofen, and chlorpropamide plus erythromycin. The primary sclerosing cholangitis–like form can be caused by arterial infusion with floxuridine, formalin injection into hydatid cyst, or hepatic artery embolization (eg, Gelfoam, alcohol).

Toxic causes of vascular liver damage are given in Table 96-15. Several other drugs interrupt hepatocyte lipid metabolism by inhibiting phospholipases: amiodarone, perhexiline maleate, hexestrol (diethylamino ethoxyhexestrol), thioridazine, and chlorphentermine. This leads to cellular deposition of phospholipids, giving a characteristic foamy texture to the cytoplasm (ie, phospholipidosis).

Some drugs and toxins have been associated with hepatic neoplasia; benign adenomas of the liver were virtually unheard of before introduction of oral contraceptive steroids (see Chapter 101), and regression often occurs when the oral contraceptive is discontinued. The causes of other benign and malignant hepatic tumors are given in Table 96-16. The pathologic spectrum of liver injury resulting from exposure to chemicals and environmental toxins is given in Table 96-17.

CLINICAL PRESENTATIONS

The clinical manifestations of DILD are as varied as the morphologic patterns of injury hepatotoxins produce. Many drugs cause asymptomatic (subclinical) elevations in hepatic enzymes that do not progress to clinical liver disease despite continued use of the medication. This "tolerance" is characteristic of drugs such as tacrine, isoniazid, and phenytoin. In contrast, some patients develop persistent biochemical abnormalities while taking a medication

Table 96-8. Occupational Agents Causing Hepatic Injury

Class	Major forms of hepatic injury
Chlorinated aliphatic hydrocarbons	
Carbon tetrachloride	Acute zone 3 necrosis, steatosis
Trichloroethane	Subacute necrosis
Chloroform	Zone 3 necrosis
Methylchloroform	Zone 3 necrosis, cirrhosis ?
Chlorinated ethylenes	
Vinyl chloride	Nodular subcapsular fibrosis, sinusoidal dilation, periportal fibrosis, angiosarcoma
Polyvinyl chloride	Elevated LAE
Trichloroethylene	Zone 3 necrosis
Tetrachloroethylene	Zone 3 necrosis
Nonhalogenated organic compounds	
Toluene	Steatosis
Xylene	Steatosis
Styrene	Elevated LAE
Nitroaromatic compounds	
Trinitrotoluene	Acute and subacute necrosis, cirrhosis
Dinitrobenzene	Necrosis
Nitrobenzene	Necrosis
Dinitrophenol	Necrosis, cholestasis
Nitroaliphatic compounds	
Nitromethane, nitroethane	Minor zone 3 necrosis, steatosis
Nitropropane	Necrosis, steatosis
Halogenated aromatic compounds	
Polychlorinated biphenyls*	Acute, subacute necrosis, cirrhosis
Polybrominated biphenyls	Hepatomegaly, elevated LAE
Miscellaneous agents	
Hydrazine	Focal necrosis, steatosis
Dimethylformamide	Necrosis, microvesicular steatosis

* In combination with chloronaphthalene.

LAE—Liver-associated enzymes (usually aspartate aminotransferase, alanine aminotransferase).

Table 96-9. Environmental and Domestic Hepatotoxins

Agent	Major forms of hepatic injury
Metals	
Phosphorus	Acute zone 1 steatosis, necrosis
Iron	Zone 1 necrosis
Copper salts	Zone 3 necrosis
Thorium dioxide	Angiosarcoma, veno-occlusive disease
Pesticides or fungicides	
DDT	Necrosis
Chlordane	Necrosis
Paraquat	Cholestasis, steatosis, zone 3 necrosis
Dioxin	Porphyria cutanea tarda
Chlordecone	Steatosis
Arsenic	Veno-occlusive disease, cirrhosis, angiosarcoma
Monochlorobenzene	Necrosis
Adulterated cooking products	
Epping jaundice (methylene dianiline)	Cholestasis
Toxic oil syndrome (aniline)	Necrosis, cholestasis, nodular regenerative hyperplasia
Yusho oil disease (polychlorinated biphenyls)	Acute, subacute necrosis
Drug abuse	
Cocaine	Acute zone 3 necrosis, midzone steatosis
Trichloroethylene ("glue sniffing")	Zone 3 necrosis
Toluene ("glue sniffing")	Necrosis, steatosis
Methylenedioxymethamphetamine ("ecstasy")	Necrosis
Phencyclidine ("angel dust")	Zone 3 necrosis, congestion
Botanicals	
Poisonous mushrooms	Steatosis, acute zone 3 necrosis
Cycasin	Zone 3 necrosis, carcinoma?
Akee (hypoglycin)	Microvesicular steatosis
Pennyroyal	Necrosis
Margosa oil	Microvesicular steatosis
Tannic acid	Necrosis
Aflatoxins	Zone 3 necrosis, cholestasis, giant cells, hepatocellular carcinoma
Pyrrolizidine alkaloids	Veno-occlusive disease, cirrhosis

Table 96-10. Intrinsic and Idiosyncratic Reactions to Hepatotoxins

Characteristics	Intrinsic	Idiosyncratic
Incidence	High	Low
Predictability	Yes	No
Dose dependence	Yes	No
Reproducibility in animals	Yes	No
Host dependence	No	Yes
Morphologic expression	Usually necrosis	Broad spectrum
Mechanism of injury	Metabolic	Metabolic or immunologic
Examples	Acetaminophen	Valproic acid, phenytoin, halothane, sulfonamides, isoniazid

that may worsen and result in clinically overt or fatal hepatic injury if use of the drug continues. Certain drugs are associated with specific clinical syndromes or organ toxicity (Table 96-18). The biochemical patterns and clinical correlates of DILD are given in Table 96-19. Drug-induced hepatocellular necrosis often mimics acute viral hepatitis, with markedly elevated aminotransferase levels. Cholestatic injury is characterized by a greater than threefold elevation of the serum alkaline phosphatase level (usually with parallel elevations of γ-glutamyltransferase and 5′-nucleotidase levels) and is caused by inflammation or destruction of bile ductules or ducts. Certain drugs produce a mixed pattern of injury with elements of hepatocellular necrosis and cholestasis.

Jaundice may result from hepatocellular injury or cholestasis but often is not seen with DILD. Chronic cholestasis has been reported with a number of agents and may mimic sclerosing cholangitis or primary biliary cirrhosis. Many medications have been associated with fulminant hepatic failure, as previously described. Fulminant liver failure caused by medications or toxins, such as acetaminophen or carbon tetrachloride, often progresses through three distinct phases of injury (Table 96-20).

Table 96-11. Types of Idiosyncratic Hepatic Injury

Type	Latency	Clinical features	Examples	Rechallenge
Hypersensitivity (immune mediated)	1–5 wk (fixed)	Systemic reaction, rash, fever, eosinophilia	Sulindac, halothane, phenytoin, carbamazepine, valproate, sulfonamides, tienilic acid	Prompt
Aberrant metabolism (metabolic idiosyncrasy)	Weeks to months (variable)	Liver only	Diclofenac, isoniazid, ketoconazole	Delayed
Mixed	Variable	Both	Phenylbutazone	Prompt

Figure 96-2

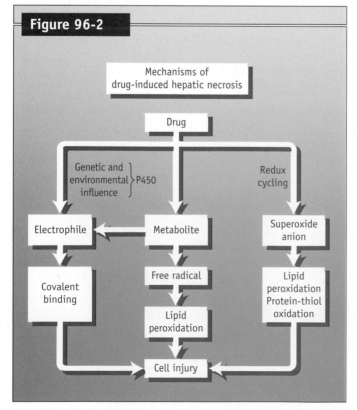

Hepatocellular injury usually is caused by the metabolic products of a drug, not by the drug itself. Under genetic and environmental influences, the drug metabolizing enzymes (cytochrome P450 system) generate electrophilic substances, which seek and accept electrons from other compounds by forming covalent bonds. Electrophiles may form bonds with thiol groups, as occurs in acetaminophen toxicity, or with amino groups, as occurs in halothane toxicity. Covalent binding of alkylating, arylating, or acylating agents to hepatic molecules adversely affects normal cell function, and cell necrosis ensues. This condition is potentiated by depletion of cytoprotective substances such as glutathione, which preferentially combine with toxic metabolites. Cell necrosis also results from damage caused by free radicals produced in the course of oxidative drug metabolism. Free radicals can bind the proteins and fatty acids of the cell membrane, resulting in lipid peroxidation and in disruption of membrane and mitochondrial functions. Redox cycling can produce superoxide anions, which cause lipid peroxidation. The leading free radical scavenger is tocopherol, but uric acid, bilirubin, ascorbic acid, and vitamin A may also be important in preventing lipid peroxidation.

◼ DRUG-INDUCED LIVER DISEASE FROM SPECIFIC AGENTS

Asymptomatic Hepatocellular Injury

Tacrine, a medication used in the treatment of Alzheimer's disease, is an example of a drug that produces asymptomatic aminotransferase abnormalities. Increased serum alanine aminotransferase (ALT) levels have been observed in as many as 50% of patients treated with tacrine; the ALT level usually returns to normal. Serum alkaline phosphatase and bilirubin levels are rarely elevated in these patients. Severe injury is rare.

Table 96-12. Clinical-Morphologic Spectrum of Drug-Induced Liver Disease

Pathology	Resembles
Acute hepatocellular injury	Acute viral hepatitis
Massive necrosis	Fulminant hepatic failure
Steatosis	Acute fatty liver of pregnancy or Reye's syndrome
Acute cholestatic injury	Obstructive jaundice
Chronic cholestatic injury	Primary biliary cirrhosis
Granulomatous hepatitis	Sarcoidosis
Chronic hepatocellular injury	Chronic autoimmune hepatitis cirrhosis
Vascular injury	Budd-Chiari syndrome, veno-occlusive disease
Neoplasia	Hepatic tumors
Phospholipidosis	Inborn errors such as Niemann-Pick disease

Table 96-13. Pathologic Spectrum of Drugs Causing Acute Cytotoxic Liver Injury

Type of injury	Examples
Predominantly hepatocellular injury	
Spotty pan-acinar injury	
Resembling "classic" viral hepatitis	Methyldopa, isoniazid, papaverine
Mononucleosis-like	Phenytoin, sulfonamides, dapsone
Submassive necrosis	
Acinar zone 3	Acetaminophen, halothane, dihydralazine, mushroom poisoning, aflatoxin poisoning, piroxicam
Acinar zone 1	Phosphorous or iron poisoning, cocaine
Massive necrosis	Halothane, enflurane, ticrynafen, phenelzine, naproxen, diclofenac
Mixed hepatocellular necrosis	Isoniazid, ethambutol, phenytoin, phenylbutazone, enflurane

When ALT values rise above five to six times the upper limit of normal, the dose of the drug should be reduced, or the drug should be discontinued until the ALT level returns to within the normal range. It is appropriate to rechallenge a patient with this medication; in more than 80% of persons treated in this fashion, the ALT abnormalities do not recur.

Symptomatic Hepatocellular Injury

Acute hepatocellular necrosis resembling acute viral hepatitis is seen with isoniazid in about 1% of treated patients. The risk is greater than 2% for persons older than 50 years of age; persons younger than 20 years of age rarely develop severe liver injury. Between 10% and 30% of patients receiving isoniazid develop asymptomatic ALT elevations, usually during the first 2 months of therapy. In most patients, the ALT level returns to normal while isoniazid is continued, but when it rises, especially when it is greater than 200 IU/L, severe liver injury may exist. The mortality rate is 10% for patients taking isoniazid who develop symptoms, notably jaundice, although clinical and biochemical recovery is rapid in nonfatal cases when the drug is discontinued promptly. Histologically, there is focal and sometimes massive liver cell necrosis.

Injury appears to be idiosyncratic, independent of the dose or blood level, and probably involves production of a toxic metabolite. Combined use of isoniazid and rifampicin appears to be more hepatotoxic than use of either drug alone, with an incidence of DILD of up to 8%. In general, rifampicin injury occurs within the first 4 weeks of therapy, and isoniazid injury is seen in the second or third month of treatment. Similarly, an

Table 96-14. Drugs Associated With Hepatic Granulomatous Reactions

Allopurinol	Oral contraceptives
α-Methyldopa	Oxacillin
Amiodarone	Oxyphenbutazone
Amoxicillin and clavulanic acid	Papaverine
Aprindine	Penicillin
Aspirin	Phenazone
BCG therapy or vaccination	Phenylbutazone
Cephalexin	Phenytoin
Chlorpromazine	Procainamide
Dapsone	Procarbazine
Diazepam	Pronestyl
Diltiazem	Quinidine
Disopyramide	Sulfadiazine
Gold (fine black granules in reticulo endothelial cells)	Sulfanilamide
	Sulfasalazine
Halothane	Talc (needle-shaped birefringent crystals)
Hydralazine	
Isoniazid	Tetrahydroaminoacridine (tacrine)
Methimazole	
Methotrexate	Thorium dioxide (coarse, pink-brown granules)
Metolazone	
Mineral oil (lipogranuloma)	Tocainide
Nitrofurantoin	Tolbutamide

increased risk of DILD from isoniazid and pyrazinamide exists. Frequent monitoring of ALT levels during the first several months of isoniazid therapy is recommended for persons older than 35 years of age, because clinical signs of hepatic injury generally occur well after the development of biochemical abnormalities. Those receiving isoniazid plus pyrazinamide should be monitered as frequently as every 1 to 2 weeks for the first 2 months.

Fulminant hepatic failure caused by acetaminophen is seen when this drug is taken in large amounts, although there is no precise dose threshold for fatal injury. Hepatotoxicity results from accumulation of toxic metabolites (Fig. 96-1) that cause centrilobular necrosis. The injury typically occurs in three clinical phases. During the first phase, several hours after ingestion, anorexia, nausea, and vomiting develop. These gastrointestinal symptoms often abate for 24 to 48 hours during what is called the second or latent phase of injury. In the third phase (3 to 5 days after ingestion), symptoms of overt hepatic injury, including jaundice, develop and often are associated with renal failure and other organ toxicity. Case-fatality rates are in the range of 15%, despite the availability of medical treatment with acetylcysteine.

Chronic alcohol use may lower the threshold for development of acetaminophen hepatotoxicity by inducing CYP2E1 and depleting glutathione (Fig. 96-1). Although the amount of acetaminophen that may cause DILD in alcoholics is unknown, it is advisable to warn patients about this potential alcohol-acetaminophen interaction. Acetaminophen toxicity is associated with towering levels of aspartate aminotransferase (AST) and ALT, often exceeding 10,000 IU/L. Levels this high are almost never seen in patients with uncomplicated viral hepatitis or most other forms of acute liver injury, although patients with hepatic ischemia, another form of zone 3 liver damage, also may have very high aminotransferase levels.

Acute Cholestasis

Amoxicillin plus clavulanic acid (Augmentin) is an important cause of drug-induced cholestasis. This form of cholestasis is slightly more common in men than in women, and most affected persons are middle-aged or older. Children do not appear to be susceptible to injury from this drug. Affected persons may present with nausea, vomiting, fatigue, malaise, abdominal discomfort, fever, pruritus, and jaundice.

Acute interstitial nephritis and acute lacrimal gland inflammation occasionally are seen. The interval between the start of therapy with amoxicillin plus clavulanic acid and the onset of jaundice is usually less than 4 weeks, but it may be as long as 6 to 7 weeks. Fever, rash, and eosinophilia are seen in 30% to 60% of persons with this form of DILD, suggesting a hypersensitivity reaction. Jaundice with bilirubin levels of greater than 20 mg/dL is often seen, and serum levels of alkaline phosphatase, AST, and ALT may be elevated. Most patients recover within 1 to 8 weeks of discontinuing treatment, although prolonged jaundice after completion of therapy has been described. Histologically, centrizonal cholestasis without a severe inflammatory component is seen, along with lymphocytic infiltration of the portal tract with destruction of biliary epithelium. In some cases, the acute cholestatic injury can mimic acute cholecystitis or extrahepatic biliary obstruction.

Chronic Cholestasis

Chlorpromazine, a major tranquilizer and antiemetic, produces cholestatic hepatitis in about 1% of treated patients. The drug is concentrated in bile and affects membrane fluidity, reducing bile flow. An influenza-like prodrome is seen in up to 80% of patients who develop hepatic injury from chlorpromazine, and pruritus

Table 96-15. Drug-Induced Vascular Injury of the Liver

Injury site	Examples
Sinusoids	
Sinusoidal dilation	Contraceptive steroids, azathioprine, heroin
Peliosis hepatis	Anabolic steroids, danazol, tamoxifen, thorotrast, arsenics, trioxide
Hepatic veins	
Phlebosclerosis	Alcohol, heroin
Veno-occlusive disease	Pyrrolizidine alkaloids, azathioprine, dacarbazine, cyclophosphamide, busulfan, oral contraceptive steroids, urethane
Hepatic vein thrombosis	Contraceptive steroids; total parenteral nutrition
Portal vein	
Thrombosis or pylephlebitis	Umbilical vein catheterization, dihydroergotamine
Hepatoportal sclerosis	Arsenic, azathioprine
Hepatic artery	
Intimal hyperplasia	Oral contraceptives
Drug-induced vasculitis	Phenytoin, penicillin, methyl amphetamine
Necrotizing angitis	Phenytoin, sulfonamides, allopurinol
Granulomatous vasculitis	Phenytoin, allopurinol
Thrombosis with infarction	Oral contraceptives

Table 96-16. Drug and Chemical-Induced Hepatic Neoplasia

Neoplasm type	Cause
Nodular transformation	Spanish toxic oil Contraceptive steroids Anabolic steroids Anticonvulsants Azathioprine
Hepatic adenoma	Contraceptive steroids Anabolic steroids
Angiosarcoma	Vinyl chloride Thorotrast (thorium dioxide) Inorganic arsenicals
Epithelioid hemangioendothelioma	Vinyl chloride
Cholangiocarcinoma	Arsenicals
Hepatocellular carcinoma	Contraceptive steroids ? Anabolic steroids Aflatoxin Vinyl chloride Thorotrast (thorium dioxide) Arsenic
Focal nodular hyperplasia	Contraceptive steroids ?

occurs in approximately 20%. Hypersensitivity is suggested by eosinophilia and fever in 10% to 40% of affected patients. Although most patients recover within 8 weeks of discontinuing therapy, 5% to 10% develop chronic cholestasis with jaundice, pruritus, and serum alkaline phosphatase elevations that may persist for several months or years. Although chronic cholestasis due to chlorpromazine may mimic primary biliary cirrhosis, it has a benign prognosis; nearly all affected patients eventually recover. In contrast to primary biliary cirrhosis, affected persons do not have antimitochondrial antibodies and do not develop progressive bile duct injury.

Granulomatous Hepatitis

Carbamazepine is the most common cause of drug-induced granulomatous hepatitis; it occurs in approximately 75% of patients who develop DILD from therapy with this agent. Clinical features include fever, night sweats, chills, anorexia, malaise, jaundice, right upper quadrant discomfort, nausea, and vomiting. Patients occasionally develop an exfoliative rash and fever as part of a Stevens-Johnson syndrome. Histologically, granulomas and chronic inflammation are seen along with a vari-

able degree of cholestatic injury. Affected persons may also develop a vanishing bile duct syndrome. Mild to moderate ALT elevations occur in up to 20% of patients treated with carbamazepine, usually during the first 6 to 8 weeks of therapy. Clinical liver injury may be caused by a mechanism similar to that responsible for DILD due to phenytoin, which suggests an inherited deficiency of epoxide hydrolase activity. Fatal hepatitis is rare; most patients recover after the drug has been discontinued.

▣ CHRONIC AUTOIMMUNE HEPATITIS

Nitrofurantoin produces both cholestatic and hepatocellular injury. It is also one of several drugs that may cause chronic active hepatitis especially after long-term use. Ninety percent of persons with chronic liver injury have been women older than 40 years of age who were exposed for longer than 6 months. Pulmonary disease with cough and dyspnea develops in approximately 20% to 30% of persons with liver disease.

The features of chronic hepatitis due to nitrofurantoin resemble those of autoimmune hepatitis, with a gradual onset of malaise, jaundice, and hepatomegaly, and a biopsy that shows a striking periportal inflammatory response with plasma cells. Cirrhosis has been reported to develop in up to 20% of persons with nitrofurantoin hepatitis. Between 70% and 80% of patients have antinuclear antibodies, anti–smooth muscle antibodies, or both.

The prognosis for this form of DILD generally is good, provided the drug is withdrawn before advanced liver disease develops. After the drug is discontinued, gradual improvement occurs over 1 to 3 months. Autoantibody levels usually decline after the drug is withdrawn but may still be detectable for more than 1 year, and immunologic "memory" may last for many years.

Table 96-17. Pathologic Spectrum of Chemical and Environmental Hepatotoxins

Type of injury	Agent
Acute	Carbon tetrachloride
Cytotoxic (hepatocellular necrosis, steatosis, or both)	Toxic mushrooms Aflatoxins, mycotoxins Poisons: phosphorus, arsenicals, copper salts, pesticides Drugs: acetaminophen, iron salts, other toxic agents
Cholestasis	Methylene dianiline* Paraquat Rapeseed oil aniline†
Subacute hepatic necrosis, degeneration	Trinitrotoluene, tetrachloroethane, dimethylnitrosamine, dimethylformamide PCBs-chloronaphthalenes, dioxins Hexachlorobenzene‡
Veno-occlusive disease	Pyrrolizidine alkaloids
Cirrhosis	Carbon tetrachloride and other haloaliphatics Trinitrotoluene, tetrachloroethane Polychlorinated biphenyls (chloronaphthalenes), dioxin Arsenicals Mycotoxins, cyasin Pyrrolizidine alkaloids
Hepatoportal sclerosis	Arsenic, vinyl chloride
Carcinoma	Aflatoxin, alcohol, arsenic, carcinogenic chemicals
Angiosarcoma	Arsenic, vinyl chloride, thorium dioxide

PCBs—polychlorinated biphenyls
* 4,4'-diaminodiphenylmethane; cause of "Epping jaundice."
† Toxic oil syndrome of Spain.
‡ Led to epidemic of porphyria cutanea tarda.

Table 96-18. Clinical Syndromes Caused by Acute Hepatotoxins

Fever, rash, eosinophilia	Chlorpromazine, phenylbutazone, halogenated anesthetics, sulindac, dapsone
Acute viral hepatitis	Isoniazid, halothane
Obstructive jaundice	Chlorpromazine, erythromycin estolate, amoxicillin plus potassium clavulanate
Pseudomononucleosis*	Diphenylhydantoin (phenytoin)
Serum sickness syndrome	Para-aminosalicylate, diphenylhydantoin, sulfonamides
Autoimmune hemolysis	Methyldopa, oxyphenisatin
Muscular syndrome†	Clofibrate
Antinuclear antibodies	Procainamide
Associated marrow injury	Anticonvulsants, gold salts, propylthiouracil, phenylbutazone, chloramphenicol
Associated pulmonary injury	Amiodarone, nitrofurantoin
Associated renal injury	Methoxyflurane, gold salts, penicillamine, paraquat
Fatty liver of pregnancy	Tetracycline
Bland jaundice	C-17 steroids, rifampicin

* Atypical lymphocytosis, lymphadenopathy.
† Myalgia, stiffness, weakness, elevated creatine phosphokinase.

Table 96-19. Clinicopathologic Correlations of Drug-Induced Liver Disease

Category	Mechanisms	AST/ALT levels	Alk phos	Histology	Clinical aspects	Mortality	Examples
Intrinsic toxicity							
Direct	Direct physico-chemical destruction or distortion of cells	8–500×	1–2×	Necrosis or steatosis	Hepatic, renal failure	High	Carbon tetrachloride, trichloroethylene, phosphorus
Indirect							
Cytotoxic	Interference with specific metabolic pathways leading to structural injury	8–500×	1–2×	Necrosis	Severe viral hepatitis-like illness	10%–50%	Isoniazid, phenytoin, acetaminophen, ketoconazole, methyldopa, dantrolene ticrynafen, 6-mercaptopurine
		5–20×	1–2×	Steatosis (microvesicular)	Fatty liver of pregnancy, Reye's syndrome	High	Valproate, ethionine, tetracycline
		1–3×	1–2×	Steatosis (microvesicular)	Few manifestations	—	Methotrexate, ethanol
Cholestatic	Interference with hepatic excretory pathways						
Canalicular	—	1–5×	1–3×	Bile casts	Bland jaundice	0%	Anabolic, contraceptive steroids
Hepato canalicular	—	1–8×	3–10	Portal infiltrates	Resembles extrahepatic obstruction	10%	Chlorpromazine, erythromycin estolate
Ductal		1–5×	3–10×	—	—	—	—
	Ductules	—	—	Inspissated bile	Jaundice	High*	Benoxaprofen
	Interlobular ducts	—	—	Destruction of portal area ducts	Primary biliary cirrhosis	High	Paraquat, Margosa oil
	Septal ducts	—	—	Fibrosis of septal ducts	Sclerosing cholangitis	Increased	5-Floxuridine
Mixed injury	Variable	Variable	Variable	Variable cholestatic and hepatocellular injury	May resemble viral hepatitis or obstructive jaundice	Variable	Phenylbutazone, sulfonamides
Host idiosyncrasy							
Hypersensitivity	Drug allergy	Variable	Variable	Necrosis or cholestasis	Variable	—	Phenytoin, chlorpromazine, sulfonamides, erythromycin estolate
Metabolic abnormality	Production of hepatotoxic metabolites	Variable	Variable	Necrosis or cholestasis	Variable	—	Isoniazid, halothane, hydralazine, valproate, ticrynafen, ketoconazole, methyldopa, acetaminophen

AST—aspartate aminotransferase; ALT—alanine aminotransferase; Alk phos—alkaline phosphate.
*Mortality from other factors.

VENO-OCCLUSIVE DISEASE

Treatment with azathioprine has been associated with development of hepatic veno-occlusive disease in renal allograft recipients, bone marrow transplant patients, and patients with inflammatory bowel disease. Clinically, these patients may have a hypersensitivity syndrome with rash, fever, and nausea, but affected persons more commonly develop subclinical liver test abnormalities 3 weeks to 6 months after starting therapy. Hepatotoxicity appears to be idiosyncratic, with features of cholestasis and hepatocellular injury. Veno-occlusive disease should be suspected in patients who develop jaundice followed by the rapid appearance of ascites and portal hypertension. In general, veno-occlusive disease occurs within the first 20 days after bone marrow transplantation, differentiating it from other causes of hepatic dysfunction in transplant recipients. The initial liver lesion is zone 3 necrosis, followed by a progressive decrease in the caliber of the central hepatic venules leading to congestion and eventually to cirrhosis.

Acute veno-occlusive disease from exposure to high doses of toxic alkaloids found in some herbal teas (eg, comfrey) leads to abrupt onset of abdominal pain, ascites, and hepatomegaly, which may be reversible but is sometimes fatal. In persons exposed to small doses of these alkaloids over a long period, a chronic form of veno-occlusive disease develops with the insidious onset of ascites and portal hypertension due to progressive cirrhosis.

DIAGNOSIS

The physician should consider a diagnosis of DILD for any patient with clinical liver disease who is taking medicine. Physicians must be aware that commonly prescribed drugs may cause asymptomatic liver test abnormalities. Patterns of liver injury caused by medicines and toxins are important, as is the dose, duration of therapy, and time between initiation of therapy and development of disease.

Several diagnostic criteria are used to evaluate patients with suspected DILD. These include a high index of suspicion; exclusion of viral hepatitis, alcoholic liver disease, and metabolic or other causes of injury; presence or absence of hypersensitivity features, liver biopsy revealing a morphologic pattern and features of injury, exclusion of extrahepatic biliary obstruction in cases of cholestasis, response to dechallenge, and response to rechallenge.

Radiographic and ultrasonographic imaging studies are useful predominantly to exclude extrahepatic biliary obstruction and mass lesions. Liver biopsy may confirm the presence of a specific histologic pattern of injury. The wide clinical and pathologic spectrums of injury that can be seen with many different agents, however, often make ascribing causation to a specific drug difficult.

Perhaps the most important indication that a patient has DILD is the response to discontinuation of therapy, or following

Table 96-20. Clinical Phases of Acute Fulminant Hepatic Injury From Drugs or Chemical Toxins

Phase	Acetaminophen	Toxic mushrooms	Phosphorus	Carbon tetrachloride
Phase I (1st 24 h)				
Onset (h) after intake	1–4	6–15	<1	1–4
Manifestations				
Central nervous system	+	+	+	+
Gastrointestinal tract				
Diarrhea	-	-	+	+
Vomiting	±	+	+	±
Pain	-	-	+	±
Hemorrhage	-	-	+	-
Shock	±	±	+	-
Phase II (24–72 h)				
"Asymptomatic" period	Yes	Yes	Yes	No
Jaundice	-	-	-	+
Renal	-	+	±	±
Central nervous system	±	+	-	-
Phase III (48–72 h)				
Hepatic failure†	+	+	+	+
Jaundice	+	4+	4+	4+
Renal failure	±	+	+	+
Hemorrhagic phenomena	+	+	+	+
Hepatic steatosis	±	4+	4+	+
Necrosis	Zone 3	Zone 3	Zone 1	Zone 3
Case-fatality rate	15%	25%–50%	30%–40%	10%–20%

Four plus—prominent; minus sign—absent; plus sign—present; plus/minus sign—may be present.

rechallenge with the suspected offending drug. Liver test abnormalities and symptoms usually resolve promptly after the drug is stopped, if it was the cause. Although it may be appropriate to rechallenge a patient with the suspected drug to confirm that it was the cause of DILD, this usually is not done with drugs that cause jaundice because of the risk of precipitating more serious or even fatal hepatic injury. Rechallenge with drugs that cause only subclinical liver test abnormalities may be performed safely if alternative drugs are not available. Persons who are rechallenged should be monitored closely for the reappearance of any sign or symptom of liver damage.

Excluding other causes of hepatic injury in patients suspected of having DILD is of paramount importance. In this situation, the evaluation should be tailored to the injury pattern. Persons with abnormal serum aminotransferase levels should be tested for infection with viruses that cause acute or chronic hepatitis. The availability of a test for hepatitis C virus infection has been helpful in the evaluation of the latter type of patient. Imaging studies are used to exclude extrahepatic causes of jaundice. The peak serum AST level and the ratio of serum AST to ALT levels are useful in diagnosing alcoholic hepatitis; the serum AST level in alcoholic liver injury is almost always less than 300 IU/L, the serum ALT level is almost always less than 100 IU/L, and the ratio of serum AST to ALT levels is usually 2 to 1 or 3 to 1. In contrast, the serum AST and ALT levels are usually much higher in persons with viral or DILD and the ratio is often closer to 1 to 1.

■■ PREVENTION AND TREATMENT

Early diagnosis of DILD is essential to minimize injury. Monitoring hepatic enzymes is appropriate in patients being treated with some medicines, especially those such as isoniazid that may cause significant liver damage. For drugs that produce liver injury unpredictably, surveillance liver tests are less useful. Serum ALT levels that are initially normal but then rise twofold or threefold are reason for enhanced vigilance by the physician. Serum ALT levels rising four or five times the upper limit of normal should lead to prompt discontinuation of the drug. Alcoholics risk liver injury from certain medicines and should be cautioned about their use (Fig. 96-1). In particular, fasting patients with a history of regular alcohol use or abuse who take acetaminophen with therapeutic intent may be at increased risk for liver injury.

In the future, CYP profiling may be available to identify persons who are predisposed to develop DILD from certain medicines and toxins. Decreased use of aspirin in children with viral diseases has nearly eliminated this agent as a cause of Reye's syndrome.

Specific therapy for DILD is limited almost exclusively to the use of *N*-acetylcysteine to treat acetaminophen toxicity. *N*-acetylcysteine substitutes for glutathione as a sulfhydryl donor for conjugation of the toxic metabolite. It is the treatment of choice for acetaminophen overdose, but to be optimally effective, it must be given less than 24 hours and preferably less than 16 hours after acetaminophen ingestion.

The treatment for most other causes of DILD is supportive. Patients who develop drug-induced fulminant hepatic failure may be candidates for liver transplantation, and in this setting, appropriate arrangements should be made for this lifesaving procedure.

■■ PROGNOSIS

Drug-induced hepatitis with jaundice usually had a mortality rate of 10% to 50% before liver transplantation was available. Although fatalities from acetaminophen poisoning have been dramatically reduced by use of *N*-acetylcysteine, there is still a 15% to 20% mortality rate from therapeutic misadventure with acetaminophen, because affected persons often present later in the course with liver failure. Drug-induced cholestatic liver injury is seldom fatal. The mixed pattern of DILD has a variable mortality rate; the hepatocellular component is largely responsible for reported deaths. Table 96-19 gives the mortality of DILD associated with the various biochemical injury patterns.

Complete biochemical and histologic recovery is the rule after withdrawal of a medicine responsible for DILD, even after near-fatal hepatic injury; residual hepatic damage seems to be rare when drug use is discontinued. Relative exceptions include some medicines that produce chronic cholestatic injury, including chlorpromazine and amoxicillin-clavulanic acid. Jaundice and other abnormalities caused by these agents may take a year or longer to fully resolve, but eventual recovery is usual even in these cases.

Patients with underlying liver disease generally are no more likely to develop DILD than are normal persons. Persons with chronic liver disease, however, may have altered drug metabolism and should be monitored closely when receiving potentially hepatotoxic medications. In these patients, the physician must distinguish between the abnormalities of underlying liver disease and those from drugs. Use of some medicines is contraindicated in patients who have severe underlying liver disease. Methotrexate, for example, should be avoided in persons with chronic hepatitis or cirrhosis, because it may worsen liver injury.

■■ REFERENCES

Recently published papers of particular interest have been highlighted as follows:
- •   Of interest
- ••   Of outstanding interest

1.• Lewis JH, ed: Drug-induced liver disease. *Gastroenterol Clin North Am* 1995, 24:739–1094.
This monograph provides an overview of the morphologic spectrum of injury, mechanisms of injury, and types of injury for all of the major classes of medicinal and chemical agents.

2.• Farrell GC: *Drug-Induced Liver Disease*. Edinburgh: Churchill Livingstone; 1994.
The textbook covers all aspects of drug-induced liver disease based on their morphologic pattern of injury. An excellent reference list is provided.

3. Zimmerman HJ: Hepatotoxicity. In *The Adverse Effects of Drugs and Other Chemicals on the Liver*. New York: Appleton-Century-Crofts; 1978.

4. Zimmerman HJ, Lewis JH: Drug-induced cholestasis. *Med Toxicol* 1987, 2:112–160.

5.• Zimmerman HJ, Maddrey WC: Acetaminophen (Paracetamol) hepatotoxicity with regular intake of alcohol: analysis of instances of therapeutic misadventure. *Hepatology* 1995, 22:767–773.
The authors review the general literature and cases collected in a registry, summarizing the phenomenon known as *therapeutic misadventure* with acetaminophen, in which recommended daily doses have led to severe hepatic injury in patients who regularly consume alcohol. Although many persons took less than 4 g of acetaminophen, the mortality rate was nearly 20% in this case series. By depleting hepatic glutathione and inducing production of the toxic metabolite through the enzyme CYP2E1, alcohol renders these persons more susceptible to the hepatic toxicity of acetaminophen. The syndrome of acetaminophen toxicity is characterized by towering elevations in AST and ALT, which sets it apart from alcohol injury alone and from most other causes.

6. Watkins PB: Role of cytochromes P-450 in drug metabolism and hepatotoxicity. *Semin Liver Dis* 1990, 10:235–250.

7. Larrey D, Pageaux GP: Hepatotoxicity of herbal remedies and mushrooms. *Semin Liver Dis* 1995, 15:183–188.

8. Van Pelt FNAM, Straub P, Manns MP: Molecular basis of drug-induced immunological liver injury. *Semin Liver Dis* 1995, 15:283–300.

97 Autoimmune Hepatitis
Edward L. Krawitt

Autoimmune hepatitis is a chronic, progressive, and sometimes fluctuating necroinflammatory liver disorder of unknown origin. It is characterized by immunologic and autoimmune features, including the presence of circulating autoantibodies and elevated serum globulin levels, a heterogeneous clinical picture, and a response to therapeutic immunosuppression. The distinction between autoimmune hepatitis and other autoimmune liver diseases (*eg*, primary biliary cirrhosis, primary sclerosing cholangitis) is primarily based on characteristic histologic, clinical, and immunologic features [1]. Overlap syndromes of autoimmune liver diseases may obscure the classic clinical and seroimmunologic boundaries of these disorders.

It is important to differentiate autoimmune hepatitis from other forms of liver disease, because a high percentage of patients respond to treatment. Early diagnosis with appropriate management can improve quality of life, prolong survival, and defer liver transplantation.

PATHOGENESIS

Genetic factors in autoimmune hepatitis appear to play a major role in determining disease susceptibility and disease severity, although the associations among genes and the cirrhosis-producing autoimmune processes remain largely undefined [2]. The search for genetic predisposing factors mostly has been directed at genes of the immunoglobulin superfamily that includes those encoding the human leukocyte antigens (HLA) located in the major histocompatibility complex, the immunoglobulins, and the T-cell receptor molecules. Classic (type 1) autoimmune hepatitis is associated with the HLA-DR3 serotype (found in linkage disequilibrium with HLA-B8 and HLA-A1) and with HLA-DR4. HLA-DR3–associated disease is found more commonly in the early-onset, severe form of disease (often affecting girls and young women), and HLA-DR4 is more common among patients with the late-onset form of the disease and appears to be associated with a higher incidence of extrahepatic manifestations. In Japan, where HLA-DR3 is rare, the primary association of hepatitis is with HLA-DR4. No association with HLA-DR3 exists in type 2 autoimmune hepatitis, and in children with type 1 or type 2 disease, HLA-DR4 appears to be protective. Other loci, which appear to encode complement factors, immunoglobulins, and T-cell receptors, appear to play a role in the genetic predisposition to autoimmune hepatitis.

The presumed environmental triggering agents important in autoimmune hepatitis are unknown. It has been proposed that autoimmune hepatitis represents a sequel of viral infection, and some evidence has implicated the measles virus, hepatitis viruses, and Epstein-Barr virus as initiators of disease. Hepatocellular injury that mimics autoimmune hepatitis can be caused by a few drugs, including nitrofurantoin, α-methyldopa, diclofenac, and minocycline [3••]. Although autoantibodies and hyperglobulinemia frequently are associated with administration of these agents and severe liver disease may be produced by them, the underlying pathogenic mechanisms are not well understood, and unambiguous evidence that self-perpetuating injury occurs on discontinuation of the drug does not exist. It is possible that interferon treatment for chronic viral hepatitis may induce autoimmunity or uncover latent autoimmune hepatitis [4].

Despite extensive investigation into humoral and cell-mediated aspects of the immunopathogenesis of autoimmune hepatitis, the relevant antigens and the mechanisms underlying the chronicity of necrosis and inflammation remain largely undefined. In contrast to some autoimmune diseases in which circulating antibodies have been found to play a pathogenetic role, the commonly observed circulating autoantibodies found in autoimmune hepatitis probably serve only as markers of disease. Other autoantibodies directed at a liver-specific antigen, such as the asialoglycoprotein receptor, may be involved in the pathogenesis [5]. Hepatocyte damage may be mediated in part by antibody-dependent cellular cytotoxicity.

Studies of experimental animals and of patients suggest that the pathogenesis involves altered immune regulation of T-cell and B-cell functions. Early studies of immune regulation primarily based on in vitro observations supported this concept by demonstrating that suppressor cell dysfunction could be reversed with glucocorticosteroid treatment [6]. Based on observations of a murine model and of patients with autoimmune hepatitis, it has been postulated that spontaneous remission and long-lasting remission after discontinuance of immunosuppressive therapy may represent spontaneous immunosuppression [7].

CLINICAL FEATURES
Classification

Classification of autoimmune hepatitis can be based on a number of features, including histology, genetics, pathogenesis, and clinical manifestations. One system, which uses circulating autoantibody status, is helpful in differentiating different types of autoimmune hepatitis from overlap syndromes (Table 97-1), but the usefulness and validity of this approach remain a matter of debate [8].

Type 1 Autoimmune Hepatitis

The form of autoimmune hepatitis identified as type 1, or classic autoimmune hepatitis, was originally known as active chronic hepatitis and subsequently as lupoid, plasma cell, or autoimmune chronic active hepatitis; the preferred designation is autoimmune hepatitis [1]. It is characterized by circulating antinuclear antibodies (ANA) or smooth muscle antibodies (SMA); the latter are thought to reflect more specific antibodies to actin [9]. Antibodies to soluble liver antigens (cytokeratins 8 and 18) occur in approximately 10% of patients with type 1 autoimmune hepatitis. Antibodies to neutrophil cytoplasmic antigens (ANCA), to a liver pancreas protein, to nuclear envelope proteins (lamins A and C), and to a variety of anticytoskeleton antibodies have been described. Circulating antibodies to the liver-specific asialoglycoprotein receptor [5] and other membrane proteins also may be seen in classic autoimmune hepatitis.

Type 2 Autoimmune Hepatitis

A second type of autoimmune hepatitis, usually seen in children and characterized by antibodies to cytochrome P450 IID6 (anti–liver/kidney microsome antibodies [ALKM-1]), is referred to as type 2 or ALKM-1 autoimmune hepatitis [10,11•]. Patients with this type of autoimmune hepatitis frequently also possess anti–liver cytosol antibodies (ALC-1) or occasionally have only ALC-1. ALKM-2 antibodies, present in ticrynafen-induced hepatitis, and ALKM-3 antibodies, present in chronic delta hepatitis, are not thought to be characteristic of type 2 autoimmune hepatitis. ALKM-1 antibodies also occur in patients with chronic hepatitis C, although rarely in North America [12].

Overlap Conditions

In addition to type 1 and type 2 autoimmune hepatitis, there are two conditions that exhibit features of autoimmune hepatitis and primary biliary cirrhosis occur. In the *overlap syndrome*, serologic findings are those of primary biliary cirrhosis, characterized by antimitochondrial antibodies directed toward enzymes in the 2-oxoacid dehydrogenase family but with the histologic findings of autoimmune hepatitis [13]. These patients generally respond to glucocorticosteroid therapy. *Immune cholangiopathy*, also called immune cholangitis and autoimmune cholangitis, has the histopathologic features of primary biliary cirrhosis, but circulating ANA and/or SMA are present [14]. This condition also may respond to glucocorticosteroid treatment. Another overlap between autoimmune hepatitis and primary sclerosing cholangitis has been proposed.

Histology

Autoimmune hepatitis cannot be differentiated histologically from other forms of chronic hepatitis. Portal and periportal infiltrates of mononuclear cells, which may be accompanied by cirrhosis [15], is characteristic. Although rosettes of hepatocytes, multinucleated cells, and an exuberant plasma cell infiltrate frequently are present (Fig. 97-1), the clinical presentation does not necessarily correlate with the histopathologic appearance. Although patients with severe clinical presentations often have advanced histopathologic findings, asymptomatic patients also may have severe disease, even established cirrhosis. The histologic picture of patients with a spontaneous or pharmacologically induced remission may revert to that of strictly portal inflammation or, if cirrhosis has already ensued, to that of an inactive cirrhosis.

Differential Diagnosis

The differential diagnosis of autoimmune hepatitis includes other conditions in which there is a chronic necroinflammatory process, often accompanied by fibrosis or cirrhosis (Table 97-2). The distinction between autoimmune hepatitis and other autoimmune liver diseases generally is based on clinical, histologic, and immunologic features. Many of the features seen in autoimmune hepatitis may occur in acute or chronic viral hepatitis, drug-associated chronic hepatitis, and a variety of other conditions. The presence of hyperglobulinemia, autoan-

Table 97-1. Classification of Autoimmune Hepatitis

Disorder	Autoantibody
Type 1 (classic)	Antinuclear antibody*
	Smooth muscle antibody*
	Antiactin antibody*
	Antineutrophil cytoplasmic antibody*
	Antisoluble liver antigen*†
Type 2	Antiliver/kidney microsome-1 antibody*
	Antiliver cytosol-1 antibody
Overlap syndrome	Antimitochondrial antibody*
Immune cholangiopathy	Antinuclear antibody*
	Smooth muscle antibody*

Commercially available.
†*Also known as anticytokeratin antibody.*

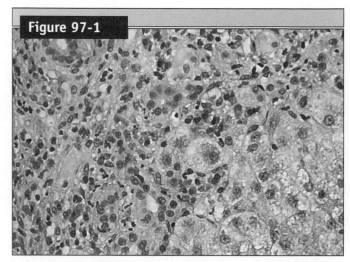

Figure 97-1

Plasma cell infiltration in autoimmune hepatitis (hematoxylin and eosin stain; original magnification × 400).

tibodies, or both in chronic viral hepatitis, for which clinical and histologic findings may be identical to those of autoimmune hepatitis, presents a diagnostic dilemma for physicians.

Approximately 5% of patients with chronic hepatitis C have circulating ANA or SMA, and a similar prevalence for ALKM-1 has been observed in some parts of Europe [12]. In the acute setting, it is necessary to differentiate autoimmune hepatitis from acute viral hepatitis caused by hepatitis viruses A, B, C, or D; hepatitis E in certain parts of the world; and acute hepatocellular damage caused by a variety of agents. Because antibodies to hepatitis C may not appear until up to 12 months after the onset of infection, it may be necessary in the acute setting to measure circulating hepatitis C virus by polymerase chain reaction or a branched DNA method to identify hepatitis C masquerading as autoimmune hepatitis (see Chapter 94).

A raised serum ferritin level, sometimes accompanied by an elevated transferrin saturation value, sometimes occurs in autoimmune or chronic viral hepatitis. Idiopathic genetic hemochromatosis can be excluded in this situation by measuring the hepatic iron concentration and calculating the hepatic iron index (see Chapter 108).

Differentiating autoimmune hepatitis from nonalcoholic steatohepatitis, especially when the ANA result is positive, may be difficult. In addition to clinical features, the magnitude of fatty infiltration and the presence of polymorphonuclear leukocytes and central fibrosis point to a diagnosis of nonalcoholic steatohepatitis.

Presentation

Autoimmune hepatitis most commonly affects girls and premenopausal women, but it occurs also in postmenopausal women and in men of all ages. Type 2 autoimmune hepatitis is predominantly a disease of girls and young women. It is often a fluctuating disease, and its clinical presentation is variable (Table 97-3). Classic autoimmune hepatitis may occur in a variety of persons, including asymptomatic patients, in whom it may be discovered when abnormal laboratory values are obtained during a screening examination; persons who present with insidious, mild, nonspecific symptoms; and those who present with acute or fulminant disease. In the latter group, presentation is characterized by profound symptoms, jaundice, and laboratory test result abnormalities identical to those of severe viral hepatitis. Autoimmune hepatitis sometimes manifests as decompensated cirrhosis, with ascites or bleeding from portal hypertension as the first indication of a serious hepatic disease. Not infrequently, complications of hypersplenism, such as leukopenia and thrombocytopenia, bring patients with autoimmune hepatitis to medical attention.

Some patients with autoimmune hepatitis present with clinically advanced cirrhosis but without evidence of circulating autoantibodies; their disease usually is called cryptogenic chronic hepatitis or cirrhosis. A therapeutic response to glucocorticosteroid therapy may be the only indication that their underlying disease is autoimmune hepatitis.

Laboratory Features

Elevation of serum aminotransferase levels is the most common laboratory abnormality encountered. Alkaline phosphatase usually is only mildly increased, and bilirubin levels depend on disease severity. A variety of autoantibodies is commonly seen (Table 97-1). One striking laboratory feature of autoimmune hepatitis is hyperglobulinemia. Although not specific, marked elevations of serum globulins, particularly IgG, are characteristic of autoimmune hepatitis. This nonspecific response also may manifest as circulating antibodies to non–organ-specific cellular constituents and to a variety of viruses, a feature that may cause diagnostic uncertainty for clinicians trying to differentiate autoimmune hepatitis from viral illness.

Associated Disorders

Autoimmune hepatitis occurs in families that have a variety of autoimmune diseases and may affect isolated persons with other diseases in which immune or autoimmune features play a role (Table 97-4). Although nonspecific ulcerative colitis most frequently is associated with primary sclerosing cholangitis, it can occur in patients with autoimmune hepatitis. Autoimmune hepatitis sometimes is associated with autoimmune endocrinopathies, which may occur as a single disease or in the setting of polyendocrinopathy syndromes.

Table 97-2. Differential Diagnosis of Autoimmune Hepatitis

Other autoimmune liver disease
  Primary biliary cirrhosis
  Primary sclerosing cholangitis
  Overlap syndromes
Chronic viral hepatitis
  Chronic hepatitis B (± delta hepatitis)
  Chronic hepatitis C
Alcoholic liver disease
Nonalcoholic steatohepatitis
Drug-induced liver disease
α_1-Antitrypsin deficiency
Wilson's disease
Hemochromatosis
Systemic lupus erythematosus
Granulomatous hepatitis
AIDS cholangiopathy

Table 97-3. Clinical Presentations of Autoimmune Hepatitis

Asymptomatic
Acute
Insidious
Fluctuating clinical course, sometimes with subclinical periods
Abnormal liver biochemistry profile
Hyperglobulinemia
Circulating autoantibodies
Hematologic abnormalities
Decompensated cirrhosis
Association with other autoimmune diseases

Complications

The complications of autoimmune hepatitis are those of any progressive liver disease and occur in patients with untreated or unresponsive disease. Primary hepatocellular carcinoma is thought to be a natural consequence of the chronic hepatitis to cirrhosis disease progression. Autoimmune hepatitis is not an exception to this hypothesis, although progression to carcinoma occurs less frequently than in chronic viral hepatitis. Some patients with autoimmune hepatitis and hepatocellular carcinoma have hepatitis C as a complicating condition, making the relation to autoimmune hepatitis uncertain [16]. Azathioprine may play a role in the development of malignancy in patients chronically treated with this drug [17•].

Table 97-4. Disorders Associated With Autoimmune Hepatitis
Ulcerative colitis
Hemolytic anemia
Idiopathic thrombocytopenia purpura
Thyroiditis
Hyperthyroidism
Diabetes mellitus
Diabetes insipidus
Polyendocrinopathy syndromes
Celiac sprue
Polymyositis
Mixed connective tissue disease
Pulmonary fibrosis
Glomerulonephritis
Pityriasis lichenoides et variola
Febrile panniculitis
Sweet's syndrome

TREATMENT

Despite the striking heterogeneity of autoimmune hepatitis and our incomplete understanding of its pathogenesis, it usually is a steroid-responsive condition. The response rate is probably better than that indicated in early controlled trials that involved more patients with severe disease and that antedated our ability to test for hepatitis B and C markers. The 10-year survival rate for treated patients is higher than 90% [18]. The remission rate induced by initial therapy is approximately 80% [19], and approximately one half of the patients remain in remission or have only mild disease after drugs are withdrawn. A biochemical response, which is indicated by reductions in serum enzyme and globulin levels, usually is seen within a few months, but in a small percentage of patients, it may happen only after years of treatment (Fig. 97-2). A histologic response occurs after the biochemical response.

Remission does not necessarily mean resolution. Although some patients remain in remission after drugs are withdrawn, most require long-term maintenance therapy. In general, the response is better for patients with milder disease. Patients whose initial biopsy indicates cirrhosis rarely stay in remission when treatment is withdrawn and usually require maintenance therapy.

Initial treatment with prednisone, alone or in combination with azathioprine (Table 97-5), should be instituted for all patients with autoimmune hepatitis in whom the histologic appearance is that of a severe hepatitis with or without fibrosis or cirrhosis. For patients with mild hepatitis on biopsy, the decision to treat often is determined by symptoms. Asymptomatic persons and those with mild changes may be observed without treatment, but their clinical status and liver biopsy appearance should be monitored carefully for evidence of disease progression, keeping in mind the sometimes fluctuating nature of this disease. To avoid the effects of steroid treatment, particularly in

Probabilities of remission during glucocorticosteroid treatment.

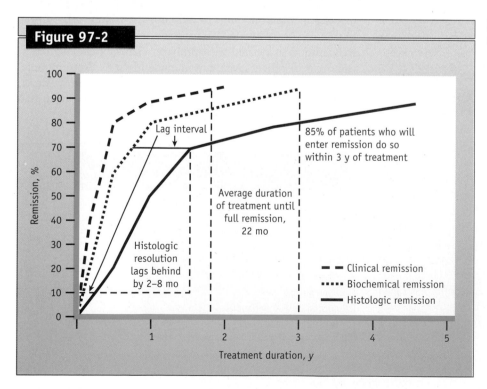

Figure 97-2

Lag interval

85% of patients who will enter remission do so within 3 y of treatment

Average duration of treatment until full remission, 22 mo

Histologic resolution lags behind by 2–8 mo

- - - Clinical remission
····· Biochemical remission
—— Histologic remission

Remission, %

Treatment duration, y

Table 97-5. Treatment of Autoimmune Hepatitis

Rejection	Single-drug therapy	Combination therapy
Initial	Prednisone, 20–30 mg daily*	Prednisone, 10–20 mg daily, and azathioprine, 50–100 mg daily
Maintenance	Prednisone, 7.5–15 mg daily, or azathioprine, 100–200 mg daily	Prednisone, 5–10 mg daily, and azathioprine, 50–150 mg daily

Prednisolone may be substituted for prednisone.

postmenopausal women, some physicians elect to treat initially with a combination of prednisone and azathioprine (Table 97-5). Others wait until a remission is induced before adding azathioprine and reducing steroids. However, all initial treatment regimens should include prednisone or prednisolone. Azathioprine as monotherapy should be used only in maintenance of remission achieved by prednisone or prednisolone, alone or in combination with azathioprine.

Many patients can be maintained on low-dose prednisone or on combination regimens of 5 to 10 mg of prednisone and 50 to 150 mg of azathioprine. Patients who can be maintained on azathioprine alone generally require approximately 2 mg/kg body weight [17•]. Using azathioprine as a steroid-sparing agent or alone involves weighing the long-term side effects of glucocorticosteroids against those of azathioprine. In patients intolerant of or unresponsive to azathioprine, 6-mercaptopurine sometimes can be successfully substituted [20].

Some patients stay in remission for months to years before their disease flares. These patients may enjoy long periods during which they do not require anti-inflammatory therapy, but therapy should be reinstated when the disease reactivates. Because glucocorticosteroids have severe side effects, partial immunosuppression using low doses of corticosteroids may benefit patients who suffer multiple relapses. This approach results in a significant reduction in side effects without increasing the rates of development of cirrhosis or mortality [21•]. Less strict control of this type seems particularly appropriate for postmenopausal women (in whom osteoporosis is of great concern), for patients with diabetes mellitus, and for those intolerant of glucocorticosteroid side effects.

No firm guidelines exist for withdrawal or reduction of medication, especially because histologic changes may occur after biochemical changes, levels of autoantibodies do not parallel disease activity, and a quiescent histologic appearance while patients are still on therapy does not necessarily predict remission will be maintained after treatment is discontinued. Traditionally, the histologic end points of response have been normal aminotransferase levels and histologic inactivity or mild activity with confinement of inflammatory changes to the portal areas.

Despite anti-inflammatory therapy, treatment failures occur. The role of cyclosporine or tacrolimus in patients unresponsive to standard therapy is not established. Only preliminary studies of other drugs and approaches have been completed. Sustained activity results in the development or worsening of cirrhosis, with eventual complications and death without orthotopic liver transplantation. Patient and graft survival rates after transplantation are comparable to those seen with other autoimmune diseases [19]. Disease recurrence has been reported after transplantation, but it may not appear until levels of immunosuppression have been reduced.

REFERENCES

Recently published papers of particular interest have been highlighted as follows:
• Of interest
•• Of outstanding interest

1. Johnson PJ, McFarlane IG: Meeting report: international autoimmune hepatitis group. *Hepatology* 1993, 18:998–1005.

2. Donaldson P, Albertini RJ, Krawitt EL: Immunogenetic studies of autoimmune hepatitis and primary sclerosing cholangitis. In *Autoimmune Liver Diseases*, edn 2. Edited by Krawitt EL, Wiesner RH, Nishioka M. Amsterdam: Elsevier Science Publishers, 1998:in press.

3.•• Gough A, Chapman S, Wagstaff K, *et al.*: Minocycline induced autoimmune hepatitis and systemic lupus erythematosus-like syndrome. *Br Med J* 1996, 312:169–172.
The article discusses a drug-induced form of hepatitis.

4. Ruiz-Moreno M, Rua JM, Carreño V, *et al.*: Autoimmune chronic hepatitis type 1 manifested during interferon therapy in children. *J Hepatol* 1991, 12:265–266.

5. Treichel U, McFarlane BM, Seki T, *et al.*: Demographics of anti-asialoglycoprotein receptor autoantibodies in autoimmune hepatitis. *Gastroenterology* 1994, 107:799–804.

6. Nouri-Aria KT, Hegarty JE, Alexander GJM *et al.*: Effect of corticosteroids on suppressor-cell activity in "autoimmune" and viral chronic active hepatitis. *N Engl J Med* 1982, 307:1301–1304.

7. Lohse AW, Kogel M, zum Büschenfelde M: Evidence for spontaneous immunosuppression in autoimmune hepatitis. *Hepatology* 1995, 22:381–388.

8. Czaja AJ, Manns MP: The validity and importance of subtypes in autoimmune hepatitis: a point of view. *Am J Gastroenterol* 1995, 90:1206.

9. Czaja AJ, Cassani F, Cataleta M, *et al.*: Frequency and significance of antibodies to actin in type 1 autoimmune hepatitis. *Hepatology* 1996, 24:1068–1073.

10. Homberg J-C, Abuaf N, Benard O, *et al.*: Chronic active hepatitis associated with anti liver/kidney microsome antibody type 1: a second type of "autoimmune" hepatitis. *Hepatology* 1987, 7:1333–1339.

11.• Gregorio GV, Portmann B, Reid F, *et al.*: Autoimmune hepatitis in childhood: a 20-year experience. *Hepatology* 1997, 25:541–547.
The article reviews an extensive series in children with type 1 and type 2 disease.

12. Reddy KR, Krawitt EL, Homberg J-C, *et al.*: Absence of anti-LKM-1 antibody in hepatitis C viral infection in the United States of America. *J Viral Hepatitis* 1995, 2:175–179.

13. Davis PA, Leung P, Manns M, *et al.*: M4 and M9 antibodies in the overlap syndrome of primary biliary cirrhosis and chronic active hepatitis: epitopes of epiphenomena? *Hepatology* 1992, 16:1128–1136.

14. Ben-Ari Z, Dhillon AP, Sherlock S: Autoimmune cholangiopathy: part of the spectrum of autoimmune chronic active hepatitis. *Hepatology* 1993, 18:10–15.

15. Ludwig J, Batts KP: Histopathology of autoimmune liver disease. In *Autoimmune Liver Diseases*, edn 2. Edited by Krawitt EL, Wiesner RH, Nishioka M. Amsterdam: Elsevier Science Publishers, 1998:in press.

16. Ryder SD, Koskinas J, Rizzi PM, *et al.*: Hepatocellular carcinoma complicating autoimmune hepatitis: role of hepatitis C virus. *Hepatology* 1995, 22:718–722.

17.• Johnson PJ, McFarlane IG, Williams R: Azathioprine for long-term maintenance of remission in autoimmune hepatitis. *N Engl J Med* 1995, 333:958–963.

This is the classic reference on azathioprine maintenance.

18. Roberts SK, Therneau TM, Czaja AJ: Prognosis of histological cirrhosis in type 1 autoimmune hepatitis. *Gastroenterology* 1996, 110:848–857.

19. Sanchez-Urdazpal LS, Czaja AJ, van Hoek B, *et al.*: Prognostic features and role of liver transplantation in severe corticosteroid-treated autoimmune chronic active hepatitis. *Hepatology* 1992, 15:215–221.

20. Pratt DS, Flavin DP, Kaplan MM: The successful treatment of autoimmune hepatitis with 6-mercaptopurine after failure with azathioprine. *Gastroenterology* 1996, 110:271–274.

21.• Czaja AJ: Low-dose corticosteroid therapy after multiple releases of severe HBsAg-negative chronic active hepatitis. *Hepatology* 1992, 11:1044–1049.

This important paper substantiates the value of partial immunosuppression in certain patients.

Hepatic Granulomas

Kimberly A. Cusato and Gabriel Garcia

Granulomata are found in 3% to 10% of liver biopsy specimens (Fig. 98-1). The term *granuloma* is used to describe a variety of lesions characterized by a localized cellular reaction involving inflammatory cells (predominantly macrophages but also lymphocytes), plasma cells, and eosinophils. Granulomata are often distinguished using the following nomenclature:

An *epithelioid granuloma* consists of modified or transformed cells of the mononuclear phagocyte system (Fig. 98-2) [1•].

A *giant cell* may form as the result of epithelioid cell fusion, as pseudopods of the individual cells intertwine and cell-to-cell borders become blurred (Fig. 98-3, see also *Color Plate*).

A *foreign-body giant cell* has randomly dispersed organelles and nuclei.

A *Langhans giant cell* has extensively organized organelles and nuclei as a result of microtubule-mediated reorga-

nization [2]. The nuclei of the Langhans giant cell may be arranged in a complete or incomplete ring at the periphery of the cell [1•].

A *lipogranuloma* is a granuloma surrounding or containing lipid. It is comprised of macrophages or epithelioid cells just as with epithelioid granulomas (Fig. 98-4) and can be found in patients with fatty livers (*eg*, alcoholics, diabetics, obese patients). Ingestion of mineral oil also can stimulate the formation of lipogranulomas [1•].

A *fibrin ring granuloma* is characterized by a central fat vacuole surrounded by a fibrinous ring mixed with inflammatory cells (Fig. 98-5). This type of granuloma is most readily associated with *Coxiella burnetii* infection (*ie*, Q fever) but has also been found in patients with Hodgkin's disease; allopurinol hypersensitivity; visceral leishmaniasis (*ie*, kala-azar); giant-cell (tempo-

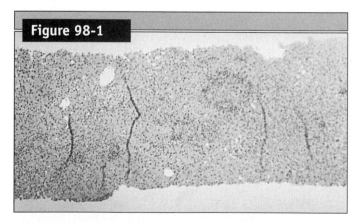

Figure 98-1

Multiple granulomata of various sizes in a percutaneous liver biopsy specimen from a patient with disseminated histoplasmosis. (Original magnification × 4; hematoxylin and eosin stain). (*Courtesy of* C.M. Knauer, MD.)

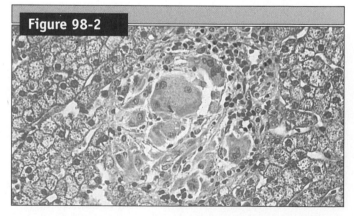

Figure 98-2

An epithelioid granuloma from a patient with sarcoidosis and hepatic involvement contains a large epithelioid cell with two nuclei (*center*). (Original magnification × 40; hematoxylin and eosin stain).

ral) arteritis; viral infections, including hepatitis A virus, cytomegalovirus, and Epstein-Barr virus [3–5]; and possibly in staphylococcal sepsis and systemic lupus erythematosus [5].

A *caseating granuloma* has a necrotic center (Fig. 98-6, see also *Color Plate*). The term "caseous" originates from the macroscopic appearance of these lesions, which resembles soft cheese. Microscopically, the necrotic region is devoid of cellular structure and may contain debris from dead hepatocytes [1•,6•]. Although this type of granuloma is closely associated with tuberculosis, it can be found with mycotic infections, syphilis, and, very rarely, in sarcoidosis [1•,7].

PATHOGENESIS

Granulomata develop as a result of the host's immune response to a variety of antigenic stimuli when the acute inflammatory processes cannot destroy a foreign agent [6•]. During this process, cytokines transform macrophages into epithelioid or giant cells.

There are a wide variety of infectious and noninfectious causes of hepatic granulomas; some are encountered frequently, others are noted only in single case reports. The most common etiologies of granuloma formation are discussed.

Noninfectious Causes

A list of noninfectious causes (excluding drug-related causes) for hepatic granulomas is presented in Table 98-1.

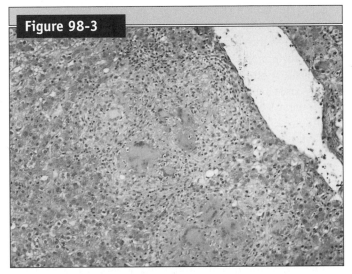

Figure 98-3

Two large granulomata near a central vein. Each granuloma contains multiple giant cells, some with peripherally positioned nuclei (*ie,* Langhans giant cells). This patient had tuberculosis, and caseating granulomata were seen in other sections of the biopsy specimen (see Fig. 98-6). (Original magnification × 10; trichrome stain). See also *Color Plate*. (*Courtesy of* C.M. Knauer, MD.)

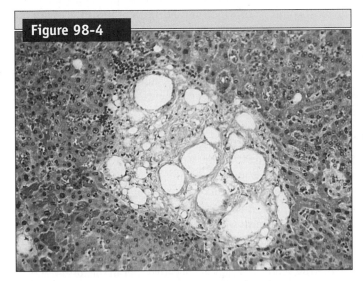

Figure 98-4

Large hepatic lipogranuloma with surrounding lymphocytes. (Original magnification × 10; hematoxylin and eosin stain). (*Courtesy of* K. Ishak, MD.)

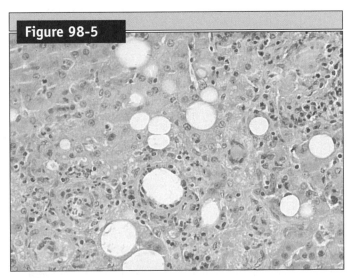

Figure 98-5

Hepatic fibrin ring granuloma from a patient with Q fever. (Original magnification × 100; hematoxylin and eosin stain). (*Courtesy of* K. Ishak, MD.)

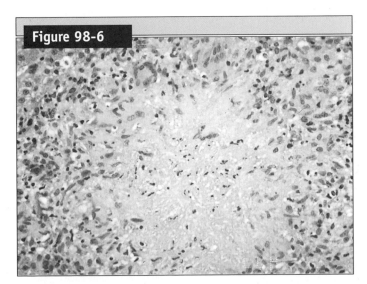

Figure 98-6

A caseating granuloma from the patient in Figure 98-3 shows necrotic debris and a lack of distinct cellular elements (*center*). (Original magnification × 40; trichrome stain). See also *Color Plate*. (*Courtesy of* C.M. Knauer, MD.)

Sarcoidosis

Sarcoidosis is a multisystem granulomatous disease of unknown etiology. It is one of the leading causes of hepatic granulomata, accounting for 12% to 55% of all cases. Liver involvement is seen in 60% to 90% of patients diagnosed with sarcoidosis. Symptoms and signs referable to the liver are uncommon in this disease; when symptoms do occur, patients may present with fever and abdominal pain. Hepatomegaly with serum aminotransferase and alkaline phosphatase elevations also may be seen. If hepatic involvement is extensive, jaundice and portal hypertension can result.

Diagnosis of sarcoidosis depends on a combination of physical, radiologic, biochemical, and pathologic findings. Patients may present with a wide range of signs and symptoms, the most common of which are shortness of breath, dyspnea on exertion, and cough due to pulmonary involvement. Chest radiographs may show hilar lymphadenopathy and evidence of pulmonary fibrosis. Skin manifestations of sarcoidosis include erythema nodosum, facial skin plaques, and maculopapular eruptions. About one in four patients have eye involvement, including uveitis, iritis, and choroiditis.

Laboratory abnormalities that aid in diagnosis of sarcoidosis include an elevated serum angiotensin-converting enzyme level, which is present in 50% to 60% of patients, and, rarely, an elevated serum calcium concentration. The Kveim-Siltzbach test, (rarely performed today due to inavailability of reagents and lag time for results), is performed by intradermal injection of a heat-treated suspension of a sarcoidosis-spleen extract, followed 4 to 6 weeks later by biopsy of the injection site. Sarcoid granulomata are present in 50% to 80% of tested individuals with sarcoidosis; results typically are negative later in the disease and in patients without hilar adenopathy. It is important to distinguish sarcoidosis from primary biliary cirrhosis (PBC), another cause of hepatic granulomata (see Chapter 106). The Kveim-Siltzbach test also may be positive in patients with PBC however, and the two diseases may coexist on rare occasions.

Radiographic findings in persons with hepatic sarcoidosis are nonspecific at best. Hepatomegaly, focal calcifications, and multiple heterogeneous low-density lesions may be seen on computed tomography; however, the liver may appear completely normal, even in patients with biopsy-proven hepatic involvement. Ultrasonography may show heterogeneity and increased echogenicity with organ enlargement. On magnetic resonance imaging the liver may appear heterogeneous and may show discrete nodules, contour irregularity, and spiculation of intrahepatic vessels. These findings are similar to those seen in cirrhosis and therefore are not diagnostic.

Histologically, sarcoid hepatic granulomata are located predominantly in the periportal regions and portal tracts, but they may be found anywhere in the hepatic parenchyma, especially in persons with extensive disease. They are noncaseating and often contain multinucleated giant cells (Fig. 98-2). Calcified intracytoplasmic inclusions known as Schaumann bodies rarely may be seen, but in general, the appearance of the granulomata is nonspecific.

Corticosteroids are the initial treatment for symptomatic sarcoidosis, regardless of the organ involved. The decision to treat is based on the severity of the patient's symptoms. Fever and systemic symptoms attributed to liver involvement respond rapidly to high-dose prednisone (0.5 to 1.0 mg/kg daily) and less predictably to lower doses. Fever and constitutional symptoms may recur after treatment is discontinued, necessitating additional therapy for several months. Hepatic sarcoidosis rarely progresses to fibrosis, and it has not been proven that corticosteroids reduce the incidence of this complication.

Primary Biliary Cirrhosis

Primary biliary cirrhosis is the second most common noninfectious cause of hepatic granulomata (see Chapter 106). PBC is a chronic, progressive, nonsuppurative, cholestatic disease that results in the destruction of intralobular bile ducts and ultimately leads to cirrhosis. The majority of granulomata in patients with PBC are epithelioid and are associated with bile ducts. The granulomata usually are seen in the initial stages of the disease, when bile duct damage occurs (Fig. 98-7).

Table 98-1. Noninfectious Causes of Hepatic Granulomata	
Sarcoidosis	Malignancies
Primary hepatic disease	Hodgkin's lymphoma
Primary biliary cirrhosis	Carcinoma
Fatty infiltration	Leukemia
Alcoholic liver disease	Other
Idiopathic	Crohn's disease
Collagen vascular disease	Ulcerative colitis
Wegener's granulomatosis	Post–jejunoileal bypass
Polymyalgia rheumatica	Hemodialysis
Giant cell (temporal) arteritis	Celiac disease
Allergic granulomatosis	Foreign body
Systemic lupus erythematosus	(intravenous drug use)
	Hypogammaglobulinemia
	Familial granulomatous
	arthritis (Blau syndrome)
	Drugs (see Table 98-2)

Figure 98-7

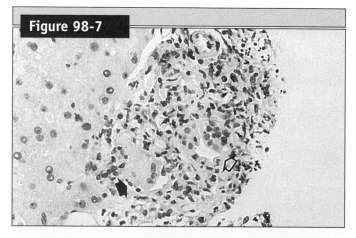

Granulomatous elements within the portal tract of a patient with primary biliary cirrhosis. A multinucleated giant cell is present (*closed arrow*), as well as bile duct destruction with lymphocyte infiltration (*open arrow*), which is typical for this disease. (Original magnification × 40; hematoxylin and eosin stain.)

Hodgkin's Disease

Hodgkin's lymphoma is the most common neoplasm associated with the development of hepatic granulomata. These lesions, however, do not indicate the presence of hepatic tumor and can be found in all stages of the disease. The pathogenesis of granulomata in patients with Hodgkin's disease is unknown, but it is hypothesized that an altered immune state with abnormal or defective antigen processing may play a role.

The histologic appearance of granulomata associated with Hodgkin's disease is nonspecific, closely resembling that of sarcoid granulomata. The granulomata are noncaseating, with solid epithelioid aggregates and giant cells. Lipogranulomas also may be found; these are thought to be caused by use of an oily contrast medium in staging lymphangiography.

A small subset of patients with hepatic granulomata are later found to have Hodgkin's disease. Liver biopsy alone may be diagnostic if Reed-Sternberg cells are found within a granuloma (Fig. 98-8); however, biopsy findings are more often nonspecific, and affected patients may be labeled as having "idiopathic hepatic granulomatosis"(discussed later) until other manifestations of Hodgkin's disease become apparent.

Drug-Induced Causes

It is estimated that drugs and other exogenous agents are responsible for 5% to 25% of cases of hepatic granulomata (Table 98-2). Most of these are thought to be caused by delayed hypersensitivity reactions (see Chapter 96). The presentation of persons with hepatic granulomata is varied; patients may be asymptomatic with mild liver test abnormalities, or they may have a severe reaction with elevated serum aminotransferase and alkaline phosphatase levels, clinical cholestasis, fever, hepatomegaly, and peripheral eosinophilia. The onset of symptoms typically occurs 2 to 6 weeks after exposure to the causative agent.

The granulomata caused by a hypersensitivity reaction are similar in appearance to those seen in other diseases; they are noncaseating and are located predominantly in portal-lobular and pericentral regions of the liver; their size is quite variable, and giant cells are prominent. The occasional abundance of eosinophils within the granuloma may aid in the diagnosis. Patients with talc granulomata have diagnostic birefringent crystals within their portal triads (Fig. 98-9).

Certain drugs may cause more severe injury. In addition to granulomata, certain drugs such as phenylbutazone, allopurinol, and quinidine may also cause significant hepatocellular injury, with ballooning degeneration and focal necrosis. Chlorpromazine, allopurinol, and methyldopa may cause cholangitis, and phenytoin, penicillin, and sulfonamides may cause systemic vasculitis.

The treatment of granulomatous hypersensitivity reactions requires identification and cessation of the causative agent and supportive care. Fatalities as a result of acute granulomatous liver injury are rare, but they can occur in patients with associated systemic vasculitis.

Infectious Causes

Tuberculosis

Mycobacterium tuberculosis is the leading infectious cause of hepatic granulomata, accounting for 10% to 55% of all cases (Table 98-3). The majority of patients with primary acute

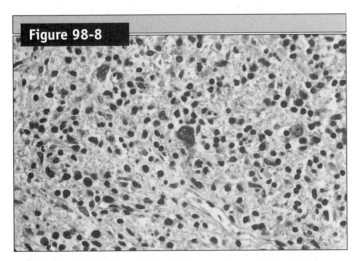

Figure 98-8

Poorly formed hepatic granuloma from a patient with Hodgkin's disease and liver involvement. Several multinucleated Reed-Sternberg cells are surrounded by granulomatous hyalin. (Original magnification × 40; hematoxylin and eosin stain.) (*Courtesy of* K. Ishak, MD.)

Table 98-2. Drugs and Other Exogenous Agents That Cause Hepatic Granulomata
Most common
Phenytoin
Allopurinol
Methyldopa
Procainamide
Carbamazepine
Phenylbutazone
Bacille Calmette-Guérin vaccine
Sulfonamides
Penicillin
Aspirin
Less common individual case reports
Dapsone
Halothane
Hydrochlorothiazide
Oxyphenbutazone
Metolazone
Isoniazid
Glyburide
Clofibrate
Cromolyn sodium
Estrogen/progesterone contraceptive
Propylthiouracil
Amoxicillin-clavulanate
Gold
Cephalosporins
Diltiazem
Interferon α2b
Exogenous agents
Berylliosis
Thorium dioxide (contrast medium)
Barium
Copper (vineyard sprays)
Silicone (dialysis, ball valve prosthesis)
Talc

pulmonary tuberculosis have hepatic granulomata, which are usually asymptomatic [2]. Tuberculosis of the liver is rare but does occur and is thought to be the result of reactivation of bacilli disseminated during primary infection. Patients with extensive liver involvement may present with fever, weight loss, anorexia, abdominal pain, hepatomegaly, and, rarely, jaundice and ascites.

Laboratory abnormalities in patients with granulomatous tuberculous hepatitis include hypoalbuminemia, elevated serum aminotransferase levels, anemia, and elevated erythrocyte sedimentation rate. Chest radiographs may show findings typical of active pulmonary tuberculosis, but results of imaging studies of the liver in affected patients usually are nonspecific.

Classically, patients with granulomatous tuberculous hepatitis have caseating granulomata on liver biopsy (Fig. 98-6). Although identification of acid-fast bacilli is diagnostic of mycobacterial disease (Fig. 98-10, see also *Color Plate*), organisms are found in liver biopsy specimens in less than 35% of affected immunocompetent patients. Culture of biopsy tissue is the gold standard for diagnosis, but this method is time-consuming. A report evaluating the sensitivity and specificity of detection of *M. tuberculosis* DNA using polymerase chain reaction (PCR) suggests that this test may be a useful additional diagnostic tool. The PCR method is more rapid than culture and may help distinguish between infection with *M. tuberculosis* and

infection with *M. avium intracellulare* in the immunocompromised host (see Chapter 91).

Therapy of tuberculosis with liver involvement is the same as that for other active forms of the disease. In most cases, symptoms resolve 2 to 3 months after initiating treatment.

Brucellosis

Brucellosis is a multisystem granulomatous disorder caused by gram-negative coccobacilli of the *Brucella* species, usually *B. melitensis*, *B. abortus*, or *B. suis*. The organism's intracellular location and preference for organs of the reticuloendothelial system often results in disease that persists for months or years. Unpasteurized dairy products are a common mode of transmission of this infection. Hepatic involvement is common; in one study, 70% of brucellosis patients had liver granulomata.

Patients may present with fever, hepatomegaly, and elevated serum aminotransferase levels. Jaundice is rare. Blood cultures are diagnostic but the yield is low. Serology is quite useful, and a serum PCR test appears promising as an aid to early diagnosis.

Histologically, hepatic granulomata in patients with brucellosis are lobular and contain epithelioid cells, lymphocytes, and occasional giant cells. Caseous necrosis is rare but has been reported in persons with *B. suis* infection.

Brucellosis is treated with tetracycline and streptomycin in combination for 3 to 6 weeks. Liver test abnormalities begin to resolve after approximately 2 weeks of therapy.

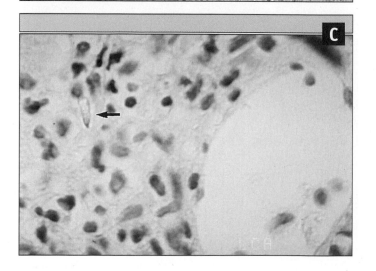

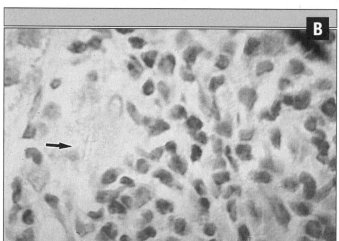

Figure 98-9

Talc crystals in the liver are barely identifiable on low-power magnification, but become easily apparent at higher-power magnification. **A**, Small granuloma (*arrow*) within the portal tract seen at low-power magnification. (Original magnification × 40; hematoxylin and eosin stain). **B**, At higher-power magnification, the talc crystals (*arrow*) can be seen. (Original magnification × 100; hematoxylin and eosin stain). **C**, Talc crystal (*arrow*) located near the central vein. (Original magnification × 100; hematoxylin and eosin stain). (*Courtesy of* C.M. Knauer, MD.)

Schistosomiasis

Schistosomiasis is caused by infection with parasitic trematode blood flukes of the genus *Schistosoma* (see Chapters 61 and 104). Affected individuals may have portal granulomata, consisting of eggs containing viable larvae (Fig. 98-11, see also ***Color Plate***) surrounded by multinucleated giant cells, macrophages, lymphocyte aggregates, and eosinophils. This granulomatous reaction to eggs deposited in portal vein radicles often is the cause of symptomatic portal hypertension.

Q Fever

Q fever is caused by *Coxiella burnetii*, a rickettsia-like organism thought to be transmitted to humans from domesticated animals through respiratory spread, by insect bites, and by ingestion of unpasteurized milk. Infected individuals develop an acute febrile illness characterized by headache, malaise, and respiratory symptoms. The acute disease is usually mild and self-limited, but with extensive hepatic involvement, presentation and liver tests may be identical to those found in persons with acute viral hepatitis. Diagnosis of Q fever may be made by culture or serum PCR, but is most often made serologically and histologically. Liver biopsy specimens from affected patients show fibrin ring granulomata (Fig. 98-5). Choice of treatment depends on presentation; pneumonia typically resolves within 15 days without therapy, although a course of antibiotics is recommended. Doxycycline, 200 mg orally for 15 days, is appropriate initial treatment, but this regimen may not cure symptoms related to hepatic involvement. In this instance, prednisone, 40 mg daily, in conjunction with antibiotics, may be of clinical benefit. Tetracycline, erythromycin, chloramphenicol, and quinolones also have been used to treat patients with Q fever.

Fungal Infections

Hepatic granulomata have been reported in patients infected with a variety of fungal species (Table 98-3). Histoplasmosis may mimic sarcoidosis pathologically and clinically, but the disease may be distinguished histologically from sarcoid by identification of thin-walled yeast forms in liver tissue using special stains. Coccidioidomycosis is transmitted by inhalation of spores and disseminates on rare occasions. Thick-walled, nonbudding spherules release endospores which stimulate a granulomatous response. *Candida albicans* has been reported to be a possible cause of hepatic granulomata in patients with leukemia. Negative fungal blood cultures in these cases suggest direct infection of the liver from the gastrointestinal tract through the portal circulation.

Idiopathic Hepatic Granulomatosis

Despite extensive evaluation, a clear cause of hepatic granulomata cannot be found in 5% to 36% of cases. Fever is the most common symptom in patients with idiopathic granulomatous disease of this type and often is the reason liver biopsy is performed. Accompanying signs and symptoms are nonspecific and may include rigors, night sweats, abdominal pain, weight

Table 98-3. Infectious Causes of Hepatic Granulomata

Bacterial	Viral
Mycobacterial	Cytomegalovirus
Tuberculosis	Epstein-Barr virus
Leprosy	Hepatitis A virus
Mycobacterium avium complex	Influenza B
Brucellosis	Parasitic
Tularemia	Schistosomiasis
Listeriosis	Strongyloidosis
Typhoid	Ascariasis
Nocardiosis	Toxoplasmosis
Melioidosis	Pinworm
Syphilis	Linguatula serrata
Cat-scratch disease	Amebiasis
(*B. henselae*)	Malaria
Q fever (*C. burnetii*)	Visceral larva migrans
Fungal	Fascioliasis
Histoplasmosis	Ancylostomiasis
Cryptococcosis	Capillariasis
Blastomycosis	Other
Candidiasis	Granuloma inguinale
Aspergillosis	
Torulopsosis	

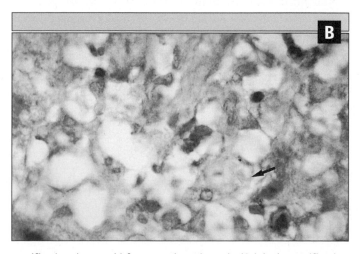

Figure 98-10

Hepatic granuloma in a patient with leprosy. **A**, Whole granuloma with giant cell. (Original magnification × 40; Fite stain). **B**, Higher-power magnification shows acid-fast organisms (*arrow*). (Original magnification × 100; Fite stain). See also ***Color Plate***. (*Courtesy of* C.M. Knauer, MD.)

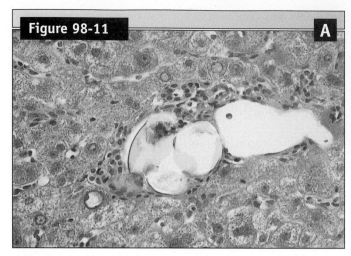

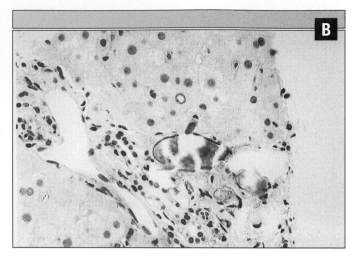

Schistosoma-induced granulomatous changes in the portal tract. Partially destroyed organisms and egg fragments are clearly seen. **A**, Original magnification × 40; hematoxylin and eosin stain.

B, Original magnification × 40; trichrome stain. See also **Color Plate**. (*Courtesy of* C.M. Knauer, MD.)

loss, fatigue, nausea, and arthralgias. Cultures are, by definition, negative, and patients often have an elevated erythrocyte sedimentation rate and mild anemia. Hepatomegaly is demonstrated in about one half of affected patients. The diagnosis is made by exclusion of all other causes and should not be made in haste. A significant percentage of patients thought to have idiopathic hepatic granulomatosis ultimately are found to have infection, sarcoid, or malignancy. One study suggests that if a patient has no hepatosplenomegaly or peripheral eosinophilia and has a spontaneously remitting fever, the course is likely to be benign.

If the diagnosis of idiopathic hepatic granulomatosis is made after careful investigation, therapy with oral corticosteroids may be initiated. Treatment with nonsteroidal anti-inflammatory drugs also may be useful, and a large percentage of patients improve spontaneously.

Hepatic Granulomata in Patients With Acquired Immunodeficiency Syndrome

Hepatic disorders are common in patients infected with human immunodeficiency virus (HIV) (see Chapter 111). The most common cause of hepatic granulomata in patients with acquired immunodeficiency syndrome (AIDS) is *Mycobacterium avium intracellulare* infection. Other etiologies include cytomegalovirus infection, fungal infections, and chronic viral hepatitis.

■ REFERENCES

Recently published papers of particular interest have been highlighted as follows:
- Of interest
- •• Of outstanding interest

1.• Denk H, Scheuer PJ, Baptista A, *et al.*: Guidelines for the diagnosis and interpretation of hepatic granulomas. *Histopathology* 1994, 25:209–218.
In this paper, the authors distinguish the different classifications of granuloma histologically, with excellent photomicrographs. This paper contains 32 references.

2. Adams DO: The granulomatous inflammatory response. *Am J Pathol* 1976, 84:164–191.

3. Rice PS, Kudesia G, McKendrick MW, Cullen DR: *Coxiella burnetii* serology in granulomatous hepatitis. *J Infect* 1993, 27:63–66.

4. Hofmann CE, Heaton JW: Q fever hepatitis. *Gastroenterology* 1982, 83:474–479.

5. Murphy E, Griffiths MR, Hunter JA, Burt AD: Fibrin-ring granulomas: a non-specific reaction to liver injury? *Histopathology* 1991, 19:91–93.

6.• Zumla A, James DG: Granulomatous infections: etiology and classification. *Clin Infect Dis* 1996, 23:146–158.
This paper details the proposed mechanism of granuloma formation as mediated by infectious agents. It contains 133 references.

7. Devaney K, Goodman ZD, Epstein MS, *et al.*: Hepatic sarcoidosis. *Am J Surg Pathol* 1993, 17:1272–1280.

α_1-Antitrypsin Deficiency

Harvey L. Sharp and Sarah Jane Schwarzenberg

Homozygous α_1-antitrypsin deficiency predisposes adults to develop emphysema and cirrhosis, which may be complicated by primary hepatocellular carcinoma. Liver disease related to α_1-antitrypsin deficiency progresses with age, particularly in male patients. The interval between clinical detection of liver disease and death usually is 2 to 5 years. There are a few asymptomatic adolescents with documented liver disease, often with splenomegaly, who must be monitored during young adulthood. The prognosis is unknown for the 10% of α_1-antitrypsin–deficient patients, aged 18 years, who have no signs of liver disease except an abnormal liver test [1••]. Liver transplantation remains the only curative therapy for cirrhosis; lung transplant is offered for those with end-stage emphysema.

The α_1-antitrypsin gene is located on the long arm of chromosome 14. The product of this gene, a circulating glycoprotein serum protease inhibitor (serpin), is synthesized in the hepatocyte. The major substrate in it activates elastase.

The most common deficiency mutation of the α_1-antitrypsin gene encodes a product which is retained by the endoplasmic reticulum of the hepatocyte, resulting in only 10% to 20% of normal α_1-antitrypsin secretion by the liver (Fig. 99-1, see also **Color Plate**). It is presumed that events associated with accumulation of α_1-antitrypsin in the liver predispose the patient to develop cirrhosis. This chapter reviews α_1-antitrypsin deficiency in adults and is intended to complement the discussion of α_1-antitrypsin deficiency in children in Chapter 174.

CLINICAL FEATURES OF LIVER DISEASE IN ADULTS

In contrast to emphysema, which develops in α_1-antitrypsin–deficient young adults, adult α_1-antitrypsin–related liver disease becomes apparent with aging. Both disease processes may be present in a single individual, but it is uncommon for both to be clinically significant. There are five characteristic features of α_1-antitrypsin deficiency.

1) Emphysema
2) Family history of liver or lung disease
3) Glomerulonephritis
4) Periodic acid–Schiff (PAS)-positive, diastase-resistant eosinophilic globules in periportal hepatocytes
5) Undiagnosed childhood liver disease

Adults with liver disease due to α_1-antitrypsin deficiency may present with asymptomatic liver test abnormalities, hepatosplenomegaly, ascites, variceal hemorrhage, or sepsis from subacute bacterial peritonitis. The incidence of liver disease is 2% in α_1-antitrypsin–deficient persons 20 to 40 years of age and increases to 5% in affected individuals 41 to 50 years of age. For unexplained reasons, male preponderance is evident in patients between 51 and 60 years of age, when the incidence of liver disease increases to 15%. In an autopsy series of 246 α_1-antitrypsin–deficient patients in Sweden, the incidence of cirrhosis was 12%; this incidence increased to 19% in individuals older than 50 years of age. Neither viral nor alcoholic hepatitis has been shown to be a predisposing factor; toxic liver injury may cause rapid development of cirrhosis. It is extremely rare for liver cancer to occur in women with α_1-antitrypsin deficiency but an increased incidence is reported in men. No serum test, including α-fetoprotein level, indicates development of hepatocellular carcinoma in persons with this disorder.

DIAGNOSIS AND PROTEASE INHIBITOR TYPING

The name of each α_1-antitrypsin variant is determined by its relative electrophoretic mobility in gels (Table 99-1) [3•]. Allelic variants are named by a letter of the alphabet from A (anode-migrating) to Z (cathode-migrating), preceded by the letters PI (protease inhibitor). Most α_1-antitrypsin variants are the result of a single amino acid substitution; more than 75 alleles of the α_1-antitrypsin gene have been described. The names of investigators or, alternatively, the cities where specific variants were discovered, or subclassification numbers, are used to designate comigrating PI subtypes. For example, liver disease has been reported in persons with PI* Malton and PI M Duarte, which comigrate with normal PI M_{1-5} variants. Similar to the Z mutation, these variants demonstrate intrahepatic aggregation of α_1-antitrypsin and extremely low serum α_1-antitrypsin levels. Null alleles (*ie*, alleles

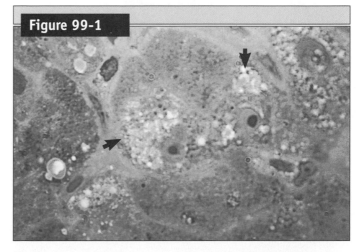

Figure 99-1

Thick section of the hepatocyte ultrastructure of a PI ZZ adult man who was the father of a PI ZZ cirrhotic child. The patient had an otherwise normal liver biopsy specimen and normal liver tests. He subsequently developed gangrenous cholecystitis and bile duct compromise, and became cirrhotic 6 months later. Arrows designate some of the retained A1AT. See also **Color Plate**.

that do not produce α_1-antitrypsin) are designated PI*QO. A null allele is not detected by routine PI typing because it does not encode an α_1-antitrypsin protein that can be measured in gels or by serum assay. Although intracellular α_1-antitrypsin has been detected in the livers of persons with three distinct null alleles, there is no evidence for liver pathologic relevance. Liver disease has only been reported in one patient with null allelles.

Phenotypic expression of α_1-antitrypsin reflects contributions of both alleles (*ie*, codominant transmission; Fig. 99-2). Liver disease usually is associated with the PIZZ genotype (Table 99-2). Serum α_1-antitrypsin levels in persons with this genotype are 10% to 15% of normal (Table 99-3). The PI*Z mutation occurs in 1% to 2% of white persons of Northern European ancestry. The highest incidence of this genotype is found in Scandinavian countries; it is virtually absent in black and Asian populations.

Two percent of adults with emphysema and 1% of adult cirrhotics have a very low circulating α_1-antitrypsin level. Unfortunately, the normal serum α_1-antitrypsin concentration range varies depending on the technique used by the testing laboratory. An individual with the most common normal genotype (PIMM) has a serum α_1-antitrypsin level of 130 mg/dL,

although normal results from various laboratories usually range from 100 to 360 mg/dL. A serum α_1-antitrypsin concentration below 100 mg/dL is abnormal; levels 40% of normal or less require further investigation by PI typing. Low levels of α_1-antitrypsin may be found in individuals who have a normal PI type in end-stage acute liver failure and severe protein-losing enteropathy or nephrotic syndrome.

■ PATHOLOGY OF THE LIVER IN ADULTS

Diastase-resistant PAS-positive globules in periportal (zone 1) hepatocytes are the hallmark of α_1-antitrypsin deficiency (Figs. 99-3 and 99-4). Rarely, these eosinophilic globules are present in liver biopsy specimens from persons with a normal α_1-antitrypsin phenotype who are overwhelmed by an acute inflammatory process. α_1-Antitrypsin globules also may be seen within hepatocellular carcinoma cells in patients with normal α_1-antitrypsin phenotypes. See Table 99-4 for a complete list of α_1-antitrypsin PI types with documented hepatocyte globules.

Cirrhosis in persons with α_1-antitrypsin deficiency usually is a mixed macronodular and micronodular type. Other than the globules, the histopathologic appearance is nonspecific and con-

Table 99-1. Identity of Phenotype

PI*M$_{1-5}$

PI*Z, PI*S, PI*QO

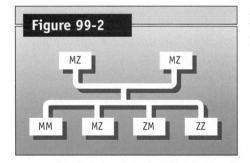

Figure 99-2

A typical inheritance pattern.

Table 99-2. Identity of Genotype

PIM$_1$, PIM$_2$

Homozygote PIM$_1$M$_1$, PIZZ, PIQOQO

Heterozyote PIM$_1$Z, PISZ, PIMQO

Table 99-3. α_1-Antitrypsin Levels in Serum

Normal 100–200 mg/dL (varies with technique)

PI*M: 50%

PI*S: 30%

PI*Z: 5%–10%

PI*QO: 0%

Predisposition to disease: ≤ 40%

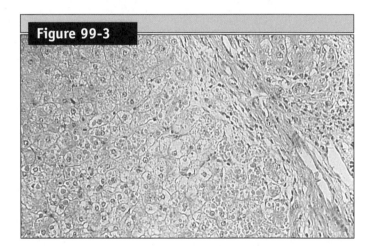

Figure 99-3

Hematoxylin and eosin stain reveals hepatocyte cytoplasmic globules in an α_1-antitrypsin–deficient patient.

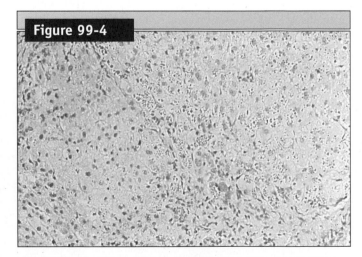

Figure 99-4

Hepatocyte cytoplasmic globules shown by periodic acid–Schiff staining with or after diastase in an α_1-antitrypsin–deficient patient.

sistent with cryptogenic cirrhosis or, rarely, chronic active hepatitis. Mild fat accumulation is also usually seen; iron accumulation is variable. Mild lymphocytic portal infiltration may occur. α_1-Antitrypsin globules may be detected in heterozygotes, but in these individuals other etiologies for liver disease are found, including hepatitis B and C infections, autoimmune hepatitis, and alcoholic liver disease [5]. Whether or not heterozygosity predisposes individuals to a worse prognosis from these other forms of liver disease is unclear.

PATHOPHYSIOLOGY

α_1-Antitrypsin is a glycoprotein formed by a single polypeptide chain with a carbohydrate side chain that allows it to circulate for 5 to 7 days, in contrast to recombinant α_1-antitrypsin with no carbohydrate, which only circulates for minutes. An exposed polypeptide loop containing the PI reactive site on the globular surface of α_1-antitrypsin forms a one-to one complex with elastase. Complexes also may form less efficiently with other serine proteases.

Aggregation of normal α_1-antitrypsin occurs within the lumen of the endoplasmic reticulum of the hepatocyte during extreme inflammatory conditions. The Z mutation, however, allows aggregation to occur more readily. Aggregated α_1-antitrypsin normally is degraded within the endoplasmic reticulum of the hepatocyte (Fig. 99-5). Perlmutter *et al.* have proposed that individuals with α_1-antitrypsin deficiency and liver disease have defects in the degradation of α-antitrypsin [6•].

OTHER ORGAN INVOLVEMENT

In addition to liver and lung disease, individuals with α_1-antitrypsin deficiency also may develop renal disease and cutaneous and subcutaneous fat necrosis.

Table 99-4. α_1-Antitrypsin Globules
PI Z, MZ
PI M Malton
PI M Duarte
PI M Leuven acquired
PI Elemberg M
PI MM

Kidney Disease

Membranoglomerulonephritis occurs in up to 12% of children with α_1-antitrypsin deficiency and is found only in persons with liver disease. Its clinical presentation is subtle, with minimal proteinuria and a serum albumin concentration lower than 2 gm/dL. Immunofluorescent antibody studies reveal Z-α_1-antitrypsin, immunoglobulins, and complement in the subendothelial portion of the renal glomerular basement membrane (Figs. 99-6 [see also **Color Plate**] and 99-7). This lesion is presumed to be caused by an immunologic reaction to α_1-antitrypsin released from injured hepatocytes. The natural history of this renal disease is unknown; in particular it is not known whether the glomerular lesion normalizes following liver transplant.

Pulmonary Disease

Emphysema rarely occurs before 18 years of age, although there appears to be a higher incidence of reactive airway disease in α_1-antitrypsin–deficient individuals even before adulthood. The mean age at which clinical symptoms appear is 35 years in smokers and 45 to 50 years in nonsmokers. Men are more often affected than women, presumably because of gender-associated smoking habits. Reduced expiratory air flow is attributed to loss of elastic recoil caused by the alteration of lung elastin by uninhibited elastase.

Cigarette smoking is the major risk factor for lung disease and also the major determinant of disease progression. Smokers have increased neutrophils in their airways which produce excess elastase, have the potential to produce damaging oxidants, and also can inactivate α_1-antitrypsin; occupational exposure to airway irritants is another independent risk factor. Nonsmoking α_1-antitrypsin heterozygotes are not at increased risk for emphysema with the possible exception of PI SZ and PI FM individuals. Median life expectancy may be shortened by as much as 20 years in these individuals.

Skin Disease and Vasculitis

The association of systemic nodular panniculitis with α_1-antitrypsin deficiency is well documented, especially with PI ZZ, MZ, and SS genotypes. Lesions begin as erythematous cutaneous and subcutaneous nodules and progress to deep, painless ulcers. Dermal and subcutaneous fat necrosis is accompanied by vasculitis. α_1-Antitrypsin is a natural inhibitor of proteinase-3, a target for antineutrophil cytoplasmic antibody in some vasculi-

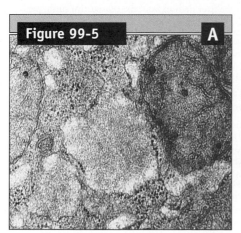
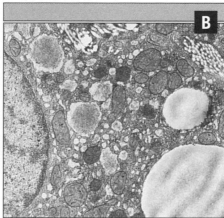

Figure 99-5   **A**   **B**

Ultrastructure study demonstrating α_1-antitrypsin aggregation in the transition zone of the rough endoplasmic reticulum within the cytoplasm of a hepatocyte.

Figure 99-6

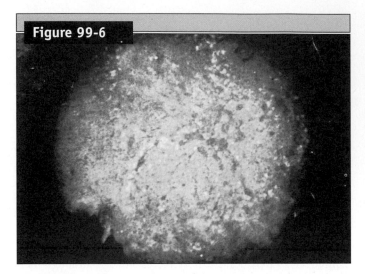

Immunofluorescence of a nodule with α_1-antitrypsin antibody in an α_1-antitrypsin–deficient patient. See also **Color Plate**.

Figure 99-7

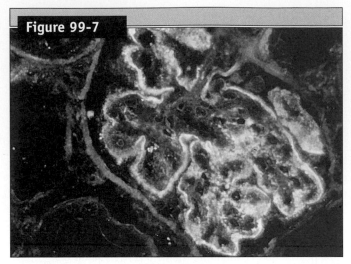

Immunofluorescence of α_1-antitrypsin on glomeruli in a patient with α_1-antitrypsin–deficient glomerulonephritis.

tides whose manifestations resemble Wegener's granulomatosis. The incidence of α_1-antitrypsin deficiency is higher in such individuals. Skin lesions respond occasionally to dapsone and rarely to α_1-antitrypsin replacement therapy, and there is recent evidence that they may respond to liver transplant.

Pancreatitis

One of the mysteries of α_1-antitrypsin deficiency is the rarity of pancreatitis, because α_1-antitrypsin complexes with pancreatic elastase more efficiently than it does with any other serine protease. Pancreatitis may complicate α_1-antitrypsin deficiency in patients with cirrhosis who have a higher incidence of biliary sludge and gallstones.

■ THERAPY

The only proven therapy for α_1-antitrypsin deficiency, regardless of clinical manifestations, is liver transplantation (see Chapter 117). After liver transplant, donor hepatocytes provide normal serum α_1-antitrypsin, and patients with early pulmonary symptoms become asymptomatic. Theoretically, renal disease in patients with mild glomerular damage will not progress and may improve after transplant; thus, combined liver-kidney transplantation is recommended only for patients with systemic hypertension or evidence of significant proteinuria and a decrease in glomerular filtration rate. Liver donors are not screened for α_1-antitrypsin deficiency, so it is possible that an asymptomatic heterozygote or even a homozygote may be a donor; however, there is no known reason why an otherwise normal heterozygote should not be an organ donor except if the donor or recipient has hepatitis B or C infection.

Medical treatment for liver disease due to abnormal α_1-antitrypsin is supportive and includes vitamin A, D, E, and K supplementation; ascites management; control of bleeding varices; and pneumococcal vaccination (see Chapters 112 and 113). Antibiotic prophylaxis should be considered for patients who have had pneumococcal sepsis or subacute bacterial peritonitis.

Lung transplantation has been used to treat patients with α_1-antitrypsin deficiency and respiratory failure, with improve-

ments in lung function and survival. Infusions of plasma-derived α_1-antitrypsin also have been reported to slow disease progression. Discontinuance of smoking is critical.

■ PROGNOSIS

The prognosis for asymptomatic adults with homozygous α_1-antitrypsin deficiency is good except for those persons with null defects. Although α_1-antitrypsin gene defects are relatively common (roughly 1 in 2000 in white North European populations), the disease incidence has never come close to this figure. Not only is this true with respect to chronic liver disease, but it is also true for chronic lung disease. In fact, there are no good data on the incidence of chronic lung disease in this population. The possibility that this defect only predisposes to disease complicates evaluations of medical therapy, which is successful only if given prior to development of irreversible changes (*eg*, cirrhosis).

■ REFERENCES

Recently published papers of particular interest have been highlighted as follows:
•   Of interest
•• Of outstanding interest

1.•• Sveger T, Eriksson S: The liver in adolescents with α_1-antitrypsin deficiency. *Hepatology* 1995, 22(2):514–517.
The definitive report on the liver derived from the prospective study, performed in Sweden, of the first 18 years of life.

2.   Elzouki A-NY, Eriksson S: Risk of hepatobiliary disease in adults with severe α_1-antitrypsin deficiency (PiZZ): is chronic viral hepatitis B or C an additional risk factor for cirrhosis and hepatocellular carcinoma? *Eur J Gastroenterol Hepatol* 1996, 8(10):989–994.
No increase in hepatitis B, C, or gallbladder disease was detected in patients with cirrhosis or hepatocellular carcinoma.

3.• Cox DW: α_1-Antitrypsin deficiency. In *The Metabolic and Molecular Bases of Inherited Disease*, vol 3. Edited by Scriver CR, Beaudet AL, Sly WS, Valle D. New York: McGraw-Hill: 1995:4125–4158.
Contains descriptions of PI typing and prenatal diagnosis.

4.   Elzouki AN, Hultcrantz R, Stål P, *et al*.: Increased PiZ gene frequency for α_1-antitrypsin in patients with genetic haemochromatosis. *Gut* 1995, 36:922–926.
PI Z and iron.

5.   Propst T, Propst A, Dietze O, *et al.*: High prevalence of viral infection in adults with homozygous and heterozygous α$_1$-antitrypsin deficiency and chronic liver disease. *Ann Intern Med* 1992, 117(7–9):641–645.
Other etiologies of liver disease can be found in heterozygotes.

6.•   Teckman JH, Qu D, Perlmutter DH: Molecular pathogenesis of liver disease in α$_1$-antitrypsin deficiency. *Hepatology* 1996, 24:1504–1516.
The best current understanding of why chronic liver disease develops in only a small percentage of α$_1$-antitrypsin–deficient individuals.

7.   McElvaney NG, Stoller JK, Buist AS, *et al.*, and The α$_1$-Antitrypsin Deficiency Registry Study Group: Baseline characteristics of enrollees in the National Heart, Lung and Blood Institute Registry of α$_1$-Antitrypsin Deficiency. *Chest* 1997, 3(2):394–403.
Contains data on more than 1000 patients enrolled between 1989 and 1992. There are many α$_1$-antitrypsin-deficient patients who are undiagnosed or not ill in the United States; it is hypothesized that only 2% had evidence of liver disease.

100 Hepatic Vascular Compromise: Budd-Chiari Syndrome, Veno-occlusive Disease, Portal Vein Thrombosis, and Hepatic Ischemia

Nabil Fahmy and Mitchell L. Shiffman

Disorders of the hepatic vasculature may affect large and small hepatic veins and the portal vein, resulting in portal hypertension and degrees of hepatic dysfunction varying from mild liver test abnormalities to frank liver failure. In contrast, arterial thrombosis rarely causes significant hepatic dysfunction because the liver has a dual blood supply. This chapter reviews the causes, evaluation, and treatment of hepatic vascular compromise.

HEPATIC VASCULAR ANATOMY

The liver has a dual blood supply (Fig. 100-1) (see Chapter 87). Approximately 75% of hepatic blood enters the liver via the portal vein, which drains the alimentary tract, spleen, pancreas, and gallbladder. The hepatic artery, most often a branch of the celiac axis, enters the liver alongside the portal vein and follows a similar course through the parenchyma. The hepatic artery supplies 25% of hepatic blood flow but 50% of the liver's oxygen supply.

Blood leaves the liver through the right and left hepatic veins, which join the intrahepatic portion of the inferior vena cava (IVC) through separate ostia located in close proximity. Blood from the caudate lobe drains directly into the IVC.

CLINICAL ASSESSMENT OF THE HEPATIC VASCULATURE

The hepatic artery and portal and hepatic veins can be evaluated noninvasively with Doppler ultrasonography, CT scans and MR images. In addition, these vessels can be evaluated invasively using angiography.

Doppler Ultrasonography

Patency of the hepatic artery and portal and hepatic veins can be assessed by duplex ultrasonography (Fig. 100-2). Flow velocity through these vessels also can be calculated using this technique. Features of vascular obstruction that may be detected by duplex ultrasonography include the presence of thrombus within the

vascular lumen (Fig. 100-3) and reduced or complete absence of blood flow. Duplex ultrasonography is the most convenient and least costly method of imaging the hepatic arterial, venous, and portal systems and should be the initial screening test in patients with suspected hepatic vascular thrombosis [1•]. Failure to detect blood flow in these vessels usually must be validated by another imaging test.

Computed Tomography

Computed tomographic imaging of the hepatic vasculature requires injection of intravenous contrast and typically is used to confirm findings on Doppler ultrasonography. CT is superior to

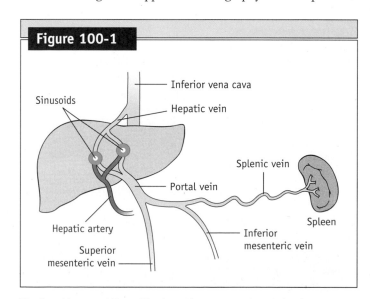

Figure 100-1

The hepatic vasculature. The hepatic artery and portal vein enter the liver at the porta hepatis. Arterial and portal venous blood mix within the hepatic sinusoids. The hepatic sinusoids drain into the hepatic veins, which empty into the inferior vena cava.

ultrasonography as a means of detecting intrahepatic lesions, which may be the cause or result of hepatic vascular occlusion, including hepatic infarcts, parenchymal changes due to hepatic vein occlusion, and intrahepatic mass lesions.

Magnetic Resonance Imaging

Magnetic resonance provides excellent images of the hepatic arterial, portal, and venous systems (Fig. 100-4) and, as with CT scanning, is used to confirm suspected vascular occlusion observed on screening ultrasonography. In addition, MRI may reveal compression of the IVC by caudate lobe hypertrophy in patients with hepatic vein thrombosis (HVT; Fig. 100-5). MRI is an excellent method of imaging the hepatic parenchyma.

Angiography

Hepatic arteriography is accomplished by direct catheterization via the celiac axis (Fig. 100-6) [2]. In contrast, portal venography requires selective catheterization of the mesenteric artery; delayed images of the portal system are obtained during the venous phase of blood flow (Fig. 100-7). Failure to see the portal vein and demonstration of collateral vessels following mesenteric arterial contrast injection are diagnostic of portal vein thrombosis (PVT). Recanalization of the portal vein also may be observed.

Hepatic venography is performed by direct cannulation of the hepatic veins with retrograde injection. Failure to cannulate these vessels does not definitively exclude hepatic vein occlusion. Free and wedged hepatic venous pressure measurements can be made during venography; wedged pressure reflects intrahepatic sinusoidal pressure (Table 100-1). Pressure measurements are useful in the evaluation of portal hypertension (see Chapter 112).

▆▆ HEPATIC VEIN THROMBOSIS (BUDD-CHIARI SYNDROME)

The clinical features of HVT were first described by Budd in 1845, and about 50 years later, Chiari described the pathologic features of obliterating endophlebitis of the hepatic veins. Decades

ago, HVT was usually considered idiopathic, but today a cause is found in most cases. HVT is seen most frequently in patients with myeloproliferative disorders. At least 33% of patients with HVT have polycythemia vera. In many cases of HVT, hematologic abnormalities characteristic of a myeloproliferative disorder are not present initially, and diagnosis is made subsequently by bone marrow biopsy and culture of marrow progenitor cells.

It is now recognized that many patients with HVT have a primary clotting abnormality, including deficiency of antithrombin III, protein C, or protein S [3••]. Recent studies have demonstrated that the most common etiology of thrombotic disorders is a defect of the Leiden factor V gene, which causes resistance to protein C activity. This gene defect has been reported to be present in approximately 20% of persons with peripheral venous thrombosis [4••] and has been identified in patients with portal and hepatic venous thrombosis.

Procoagulants (*eg*, anticardiolipin antibody) predispose individuals to develop HVT; thrombogenic antibodies typically are found in persons with immunologic disorders. These patients also may develop HVT as a result of vasculitis involving the hepatic veins.

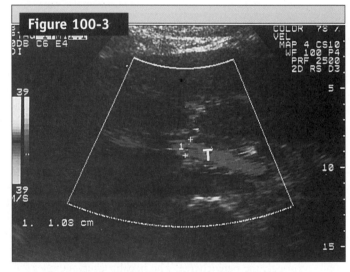

Figure 100-3

Transverse Doppler ultrasonography demonstrating portal vein thrombosis following bone marrow transplantation. Cursors (+) outline the boundaries of the right portal vein. T—thrombus.

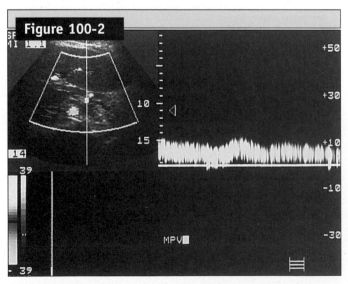

Figure 100-2

Doppler ultrasonography of a patent portal hepatic vein. Transverse ultrasound image (*left*) with Doppler wave form (*right*) of the main portal vein. Flow velocity was measured at 10 cm/second. The cursor (box) is focused on the main portal vein.

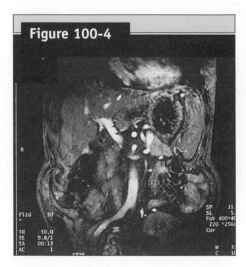

Figure 100-4

Magnetic resonance coronal image demonstrating a patent portal vein (*arrowheads*) in a patient with cirrhosis.

There is a slight but significant risk of HVT in women taking oral contraceptives and during the postpartum period [5•]. However, many affected women also have an associated thrombotic condition; HVT in this setting should initiate an evaluation for a hypercoagulable state.

Structural lesions of the suprahepatic portion of the IVC and hepatic vein ostia may cause hepatic outflow obstruction and clinical manifestations identical to those observed in patients with HVT. Membranous obstruction of the IVC typically occurs at the level of the hepatic veins and is the most common cause of hepatic vein obstruction in the Far East and South Africa [6]. Membranous lesions may be congenital or secondary to IVC thrombosis. Hepatic veins also may be occluded by intrahepatic or extrahepatic tumors. Renal cell carcinoma may grow through the renal veins into the IVC and obstruct the hepatic veins. Hepatocellular carcinoma also frequently invades and obstructs hepatic veins.

The cause of hepatic vein obstruction cannot be identified in approximately one third of affected patients. Most of these individuals are believed to have latent or undiagnosed myeloproliferative or coagulation disorders [7••].

Clinical Features

The presentation of HVT varies from asymptomatic hepatomegaly with slow accumulation of ascites to fulminant hepatic failure. The type of presentation depends on the rate of vascular occlusion, the rate of development of collateral blood flow, and the amount of hepatocyte necrosis.

Patients with acute HVT present with sudden, right upper quadrant abdominal pain and hepatomegaly. They may have ascites or develop it shortly after their initial evaluation. Serum aminotransferase levels are markedly elevated in these patients, and there may be evidence of liver failure with an abnormal prothrombin time, hyperbilirubinemia, and hepatic encephalopathy. Liver biopsy specimens in affected patients demonstrate massive necrosis and hemorrhage in zones II and III with preservation of portal areas (Fig. 100-8, see also *Color Plate*). Patients with this form of acute obstruction die of complications related to liver failure within a few days unless they receive emergent hepatic transplant.

Hepatic vein thrombosis and its complications also may develop insidiously over months to years. Persons with this chronic variant experience vague, right upper quadrant discomfort and

have hepatomegaly on physical examination. Serum aminotransferase levels are either normal or minimally elevated, and hepatic synthetic and metabolic functions typically are preserved. Preservation of hepatic function in these patients results from development of venous collaterals, which decompress the liver. Because venous outflow from the caudate lobe enters the IVC at a point separate from that of the rest of the liver, the hepatic veins often empty through collateral connections with the veins of the caudate lobe. This results in marked hypertrophy of the caudate lobe, which ultimately may compress and obstruct the IVC (Fig. 100-5). Liver biopsy specimens in patients with this indolent presentation typically demonstrate mild central venous congestion and dilation of hepatic sinusoids without hepatic necrosis (Fig. 100-9, see also *Color Plate*).

Although persons with chronic HVT appear stable and may have normal liver function when diagnosed, the associated liver injury is progressive and eventually will result in liver failure and its complications, especially ascites. Ascites in patients with HVT may have a high protein content, but it is usually transudative and often is resistant to medical therapy. In one series, 3-year survival of individuals with chronic HVT was 50%.

Evaluation

Doppler ultrasonographic examination is the imaging procedure of choice for patients suspected of having HVT [8]. The sensitivity of this procedure in diagnosing HVT is greater than 85%. Ultrasonography typically demonstrates absence of blood flow

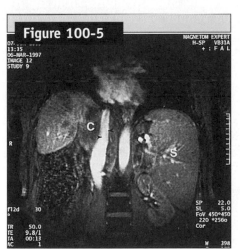

Figure 100-5

Magnetic resonance coronal image in a patient with hepatic vein thrombosis. There is marked hypertrophy of the caudate lobe (C) with compression of the inferior vena cava (*arrowheads*). Marked enlargement of the spleen (S) is also evident.

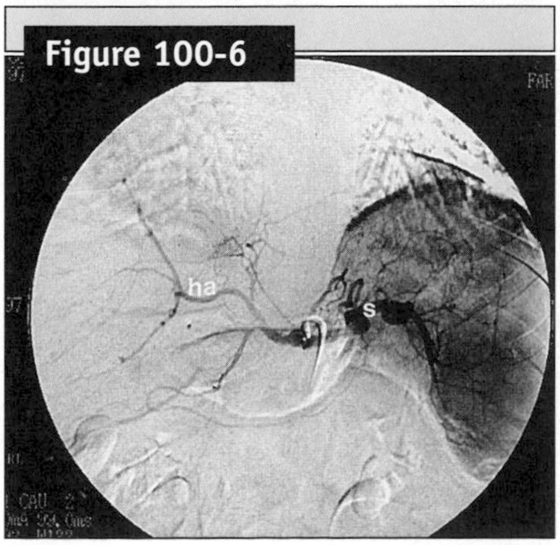

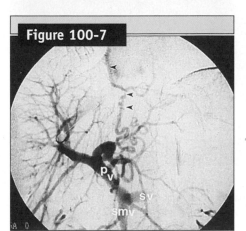

Figure 100-6

Angiogram demonstrating the hepatic artery in a patient with cirrhosis. The angiography catheter is located in the celiac axis. ha—patent hepatic artery; S—splenic artery.

Figure 100-7

Angiogram demonstrating the portal venous system in a patient with cirrhosis. Esophageal varices (*arrows*) can be seen. pv—patent portal vein; smv—superior mesenteric vein; sv—splenic vein.

through the hepatic veins; reversal of flow through the portal vein also may be observed. In severe cases, the liver may have an inhomogeneous appearance on CT (Fig. 100-10). MR typically demonstrates absence of the hepatic veins, caudate lobe hypertrophy, and an inhomogeneous liver [9] (Fig. 100-11). Hepatic venography may confirm narrowing of the IVC as a result of caudate lobe hypertrophy and also may reveal narrowing of the hepatic vein ostia and a "spider-web" appearance of intrahepatic collateral veins (Fig. 100-12). The latter finding is pathognomonic for HVT. Hepatic venous pressure measurements demonstrate either normal or elevated pressures in the IVC, depending on the level of obstruction (Table 100-1). In addition, both the free and wedged hepatic venous pressure are elevated. A diagnostic algorithm for evaluation of patients suspected of having HVT is presented in Figure 100-13.

Treatment

Treatment of patients with HVT includes medical and surgical therapies directed at the underlying disorder and relief of hepatic venous outflow obstruction and its resultant liver dysfunction.

Nearly two thirds of patients with HVT have an underlying myeloproliferative disorder or hypercoagulable state. Persons shown to have or strongly suspected of having a coagulation abnormality should be treated with long-term anticoagulation therapy.

The most common complication of HVT is ascites; this is treated in the usual manner with salt restriction and gentle diuretic agents (see Chapter 113). Ascites in patients with HVT, however, usually is refractory to standard medical therapy. Patients with liver failure are candidates for hepatic transplant.

The primary treatment for patients with HVT is relief of outflow obstruction. This is accomplished either by radiologic techniques or by creation of a surgical shunt. Treatment selection is based on the severity of liver disease and the patency of the IVC and portal vein.

For patients with preserved hepatic function, balloon angioplasty (Fig. 100-14) of the hepatic veins, with or without placement of a vascular stent (Fig. 100-15), may relieve the outflow obstruction [10]. In patients with acute onset of symptoms and recent thrombosis, direct infusion of thrombolytic agents into the hepatic vein may be attempted; however, this therapy is contraindicated in patients with liver dysfunction and coagulopathy. The main limitation of angioplasty and thrombolysis is the high rate of recurrent HVT after treatment. As a result, all patients with HVT should be placed on lifelong anticoagulation therapy following these procedures.

Creation of a surgical shunt is reserved for patients with adequate hepatic function who have not achieved successful results with medical and radiologic therapies. The shunt procedures used to treat patients with HVT are the side-to-side portocaval

Table 100-1. Pressure Measurements From the Hepatic Portal and Venous Systems and Their Interpretation

	Central venous pressure	Free hepatic vein pressure	Wedged hepatic venous pressure
Normal	<5 mm Hg	6 mm Hg	8–12 mm Hg
Portal vein thrombosis	Normal	Normal	Normal
Cirrhosis	Normal	Normal	Elevated
Hepatic vein occlusion	Normal	Elevated	Elevated
Inferior vena cava occlusion	Elevated	Elevated	Elevated

Figure 100-8

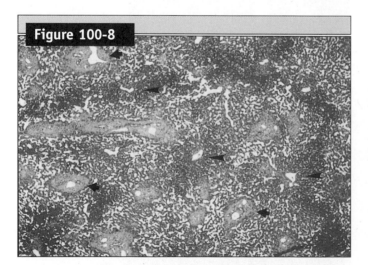

Liver biopsy specimen from a patient with severe hepatic venous thrombosis and fulminant hepatic failure. There is massive hemorrhage into zones II and III (*arrowheads*); only zone I hepatocytes and portal triads (*arrows*) are preserved. See also **Color Plate.**

Figure 100-9

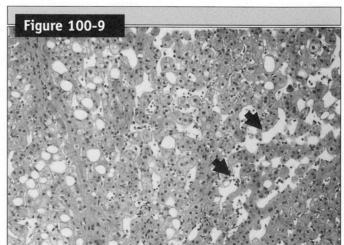

Liver biopsy specimen from a patient with hepatic vein thrombosis and hepatomegaly but preserved hepatic synthetic function and absence of ascites. There is only mild congestion and dilation of hepatic sinusoids within zone III (*arrows*). See also **Color Plate.**

shunt and the mesocaval shunt. These shunts decompress the intrahepatic vasculature by converting the portal vein from an inflow to an outflow tract. The mortality of persons undergoing shunt surgery is less than 20% as long as they do not have significant hepatic fibrosis and liver function is well preserved. Ascites resolves and the caudate lobe shrinks in nearly all patients after surgical shunting. Contraindications to shunt construction include an IVC pressure greater than 20 mm Hg and PVT. In individuals with near-total occlusion of the IVC due to caudate lobe hypertrophy, portocaval and mesocaval shunts may be impossible. These patients should receive a temporary mesoatrial shunt to decompress the liver and allow the caudate lobe to shrink prior to definitive portocaval or mesocaval shunt surgery (Fig. 100-16, see also *Color Plate*).

VENO-OCCLUSIVE DISEASE

Veno-occlusive disease (VOD) is caused by nonthrombotic occlusion of small- or medium-sized hepatic veins. This lesion results from concentric fibrosis and obliteration of central venules; large hepatic veins are unaffected and remain patent. Regardless of etiology, VOD leads to rapidly progressive liver failure. Mortality is nearly 100% within 6 to 12 months of the onset of symptoms.

Ingestion of pyrrolizidine alkaloids is a common cause of VOD in developing countries. These alkaloids are found in many plants throughout the world and especially in tropical climates, where plants containing these compounds often are used to make herbal teas. Pyrrolizidine is metabolized by the liver to highly toxic compounds that cause dose-dependent hepatotoxicity; acute liver injury may result from a single large ingestion of these alkaloids, and chronic liver injury may develop when these agents are consumed in small amounts over long periods of time.

Other common etiologies of VOD are treatment with antineoplastic drugs and hepatic irradiation; the risk is additive when patients receive both therapies, as commonly occurs during preparation for bone marrow transplant [11]. VOD develops in 15% of marrow transplant patients treated with chemotherapy and radiation, and nearly one half of affected individuals die of complications related to liver failure. Symptoms typically develop 4 to 6 weeks after transplant. Risk factors for developing VOD in this setting include conditioning with busulfan and cyclophosphamide, pretransplant fungal infection, a pretransplant Karnofsky score less than 90% of normal, prior liver disease, and age older than 20 years. In contrast, the risk of developing VOD does not appear to be affected by a history of prior chemotherapy or by the type of malignancy for which the marrow transplant is performed [12••]. Recent studies in the bone marrow transplant population demonstrated that administration of low-molecular-weight heparin following transplant is associated with a reduced incidence of VOD [13•].

Hepatic irradiation alone may cause VOD, depending on the total dose received by the patient; the disorder is uncommon in persons treated with less than 30 Gy. Signs and symptoms of VOD usually develop 4 to 6 weeks after therapy. Chemotherapeutic drugs that may cause VOD when given without accompanying radiation therapy include vincristine, mitomycin C, BCNU, Dacarbazine, and adriamycin.

Azathioprine and 6-mercaptopurine also have been associated with development of VOD in renal transplant recipients. Several features of VOD in this population are unique. The onset of the symptoms is late—anywhere from 6 months to 8 years after transplantation. In addition, affected individuals develop not only central vein sclerosis but also nodular regenerative hyperplasia and peliosis hepatitis. Rapidly progressive liver failure is common in this setting, with survival of less than 1 year from onset of symptoms.

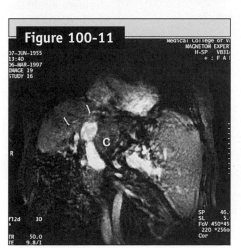

Figure 100-10 Computed tomographic image from a patient with hepatic venous thrombosis demonstrating heterogenous liver parenchyma (*arrowheads*), hypertrophy of the caudate lobe (C) and marked splenomegaly (S). I—inferior vena cava; A—aorta.

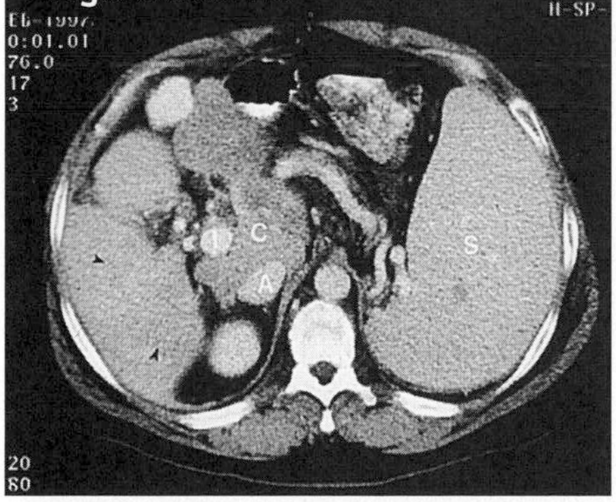

Figure 100-11 Magnetic resonance image from a patient with hepatic vein thrombosis demonstrating the absence of hepatic veins (*area between brackets*) and caudate lobe hypertrophy (C).

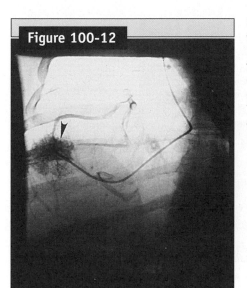

Figure 100-12 Hepatic venogram from a patient with hepatic venous thrombosis demonstrating the characteristic "spider-web" appearance (*arrowhead*).

Clinical Features and Evaluation

Patients with VOD typically have hepatomegaly with right upper quadrant tenderness and ascites and a progressive rise in serum alkaline phosphate and bilirubin levels. As the disease advances, patients develop hepatic synthetic dysfunction. Ultrasonography demonstrates normal flow through the hepatic and portal veins and absence of biliary ductal dilation. There are no specific findings on either CT or MR in patients with this disorder. The diagnosis is confirmed by examination of liver biopsy specimens, which demonstrate zone III hemorrhagic necrosis and fibrosis and obliteration of central veins [12••] (Fig. 100-17, see also *Color Plate*).

Treatment

Management of patients with VOD is difficult, and the prognosis is poor. Nearly every affected patient develops progressive liver failure and succumbs to complications of end-stage liver disease. Although it is reasonable to assume that decompressive surgical and transjugular intrahepatic portosystemic shunts are effective in treating patients with this disorder, the efficacy of shunts in this setting has not been demonstrated. Liver transplant has been performed successfully in patients with VOD without recurrence of the disorder.

▰ PORTAL VEIN THROMBOSIS

In the United States, PVT is the leading cause of prehepatic portal hypertension. PVT most commonly develops in children as a consequence of umbilical vein infection. In adults, PVT usually is associated with intra-abdominal infection, abdominal trauma or malignancy, intra-abdominal surgery, or an underlying hypercoagulable state [14•]. Patients with splenic vein thrombosis, usually secondary to pancreatitis, and patients who have undergone splenectomy also are at increased risk of developing PVT. Nearly one half of patients with PVT of unknown cause have a latent myeloproliferative disorder or other hypercoagulable state.

Approximately 15% of persons with cirrhosis develop PVT; advanced Child's class and hepatocellular carcinoma increase the risk of thrombosis. There appears to be no relation between PVT and the etiology of the underlying liver disease.

In many affected individuals, particularly those who developed PVT during childhood, the portal vein recanalizes by forming numerous small channels through the thrombosed portion, resulting in cavernous transformation. Because there is continued resistance to blood flow through the recanalize portal vein, portal hypertension usually does not resolve in these patients.

Figure 100-13

```
        Suspect hepatic
        vein thrombosis
              │
              ▼
        Duplex ultrasound
        of liver vasculature
         │      │      │
         ▼      ▼      ▼
   No flow in  Equivocal  Flow in
 hepatic veins          hepatic veins
         │      │      │
         └──────┼──────┘
                ▼
           Hepatic
           venography
           │        │
           ▼        ▼
   Hepatic vein   Hepatic vein
    occluded        patent
         │             │
         ▼             ▼
  Evaluation for    Thrombosis
  etiology and       excluded
  management, and
  assess liver function
         │
    ┌────┴────┐
    ▼         ▼
 Preserved  Hepatic
 liver      failure
 function     │
    │         ▼
    ▼      Consider
 Radiologic  hepatic
 or surgical transplanation
 management
```

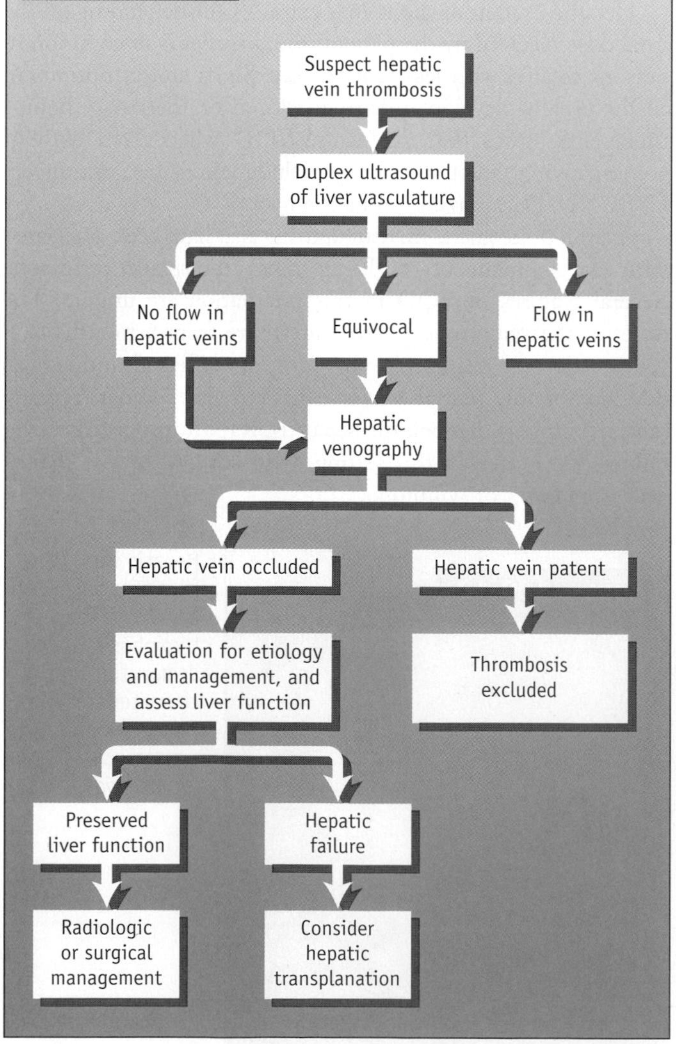

Diagnostic algorithm for evaluation of a patient with suspected hepatic vein thrombosis.

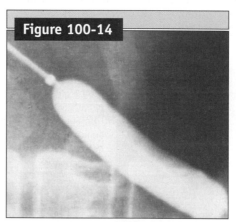

Figure 100-14

Balloon angioplasty in a patient with hepatic vein thrombosis. The balloon is fully inflated within the hepatic vein.

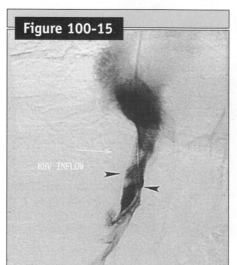

Figure 100-15

Wall stent (*between arrowheads*) deployed within the right hepatic vein following angioplasty in a patient with hepatic vein thrombosis.

RHV INFLOW

PVT does not affect hepatic function because hepatic blood flow is maintained through the hepatic artery, and because the obstruction to blood flow through the liver is presinusoidal, PVT is not associated with development of ascites.

Clinical Features and Evaluation

Many patients with PVT are asymptomatic and are found to have evidence of portal hypertension only incidentally (*eg*, splenomegaly found on routine physical examination, esophageal varices found on endoscopy) [14•]. Other patients have left upper quadrant discomfort secondary to splenomegaly, and some patients present with variceal hemorrhage. Mortality associated with variceal hemorrhage in patients with PVT in the absence of cirrhosis is less than 5%, whereas mortality is 33% in persons with portal hypertension secondary to cirrhosis.

Identification of a patient with signs and symptoms of portal hypertension should prompt a thorough medical evaluation (see Chapter 112). In patients with PVT, this vessel either cannot be identified on duplex ultrasonography or has increased echogenicity within its lumen consistent with thrombosis (Fig. 100-3). PVT may be confirmed by MR or angiography, although angiography usually is unnecessary. Liver histology is normal in patients with PVT unless they have underlying chronic liver disease.

Treatment

The management of patients with PVT in the absence of liver disease is determined by the severity of the portal hypertension, its related symptoms, and the occurrence of variceal hemorrhage. For asymptomatic patients in whom PVT is discovered incidentally, no treatment is indicated. There are no data indicating that treatment of portal hypertension with β-blockers reduces the risk of initial variceal hemorrhage in patients with isolated PVT as it does in patients with cirrhosis.

A variety of treatment options are available for symptomatic patients. Individuals with variceal hemorrhage should undergo emergent sclerotherapy or banding followed by repeated sclerotherapy or banding until varices are obliterated. If variceal hemorrhage recurs, or if varices cannot be obliterated by endoscopic therapy, patients with PVT are excellent candidates for surgical shunt procedures; effective operations include mesocaval and distal splenorenal shunts. Portocaval shunts cannot be constructed in patients with PVT. Because most persons with PVT do not have underlying liver disease, the long-term prognosis of affected patients after portal decompression is excellent. Patients with PVT and cirrhosis are potential candidates for orthotopic liver transplant. Contrary to early reports, PVT is not an absolute contraindication to this procedure. A management algorithm for patients with PVT is provided in Figure 100-18.

HEPATIC ISCHEMIA

Because 50% of the oxygen consumed by the liver is delivered by the hepatic artery, a sudden reduction in hepatic arterial blood flow may be associated with hepatic ischemia. Occlusion of both the hepatic artery and the portal vein results in liver failure and death.

Hepatic Artery Thrombosis

Sudden occlusion of the hepatic artery most commonly is associated with autoimmune disease (*eg*, vasculitis) and emboli to one or more branches of the hepatic artery [15]. Hepatic artery thrombosis (HAT) also occurs in patients taking oral contraceptives and in persons with hypercoagulable states. The most common autoimmune disorder of the hepatic arterial vasculature is polyarteritis nodosa. Affected vessels typically have multiple aneurysmal dilations that may rupture and cause intrahepatic hemorrhage. This picture is most commonly observed in patients with polyarteritis nodosa who have acute and chronic viral hepatitis B. Blind percutaneous liver biopsy in a patient with polyarteritis and multiple aneurysms of the hepatic artery is contraindicated.

Acute HAT causes acute necrosis of liver segments; the size of the liver infarct depends on the specific branch point at which the hepatic artery is occluded. Gradual occlusion of the hepatic artery from advanced atherosclerosis also has been

Figure 100-16

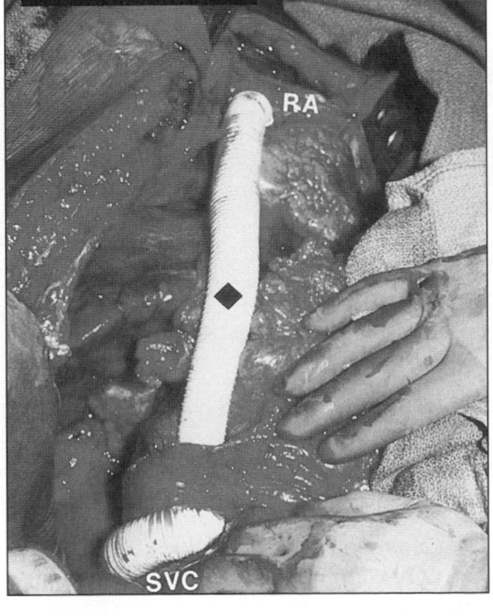

Meso-atrial shunt constructed in a patient with hepatic vein thrombosis and inferior vena cava obstruction from caudate lobe hypertrophy. The shunt is constructed using a Gortex graft (diamond) to connect the superior mesenteric vein (SVC) to the right atrium (RA), bypassing the obstruction. See also **Color Plate**.

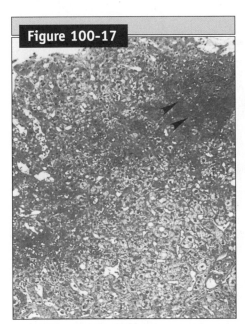

Figure 100-17

Histologic specimen of the liver from a patient with veno-occlusive disease following bone marrow transplantation. There is severe hemorrhage within zone III (*arrowheads*). See also **Color Plate**.

reported; collateral blood flow frequently develops in this setting, and hepatic ischemia from chronic hepatic arterial occlusion is relatively mild or entirely absent.

Clinical Features and Evaluation

Patients with hepatic infarction typically present with acute, severe, right upper quadrant pain and marked elevations of serum aminotransferase levels to values greater than 1000 IU/L. Serum bilirubin concentrations and prothrombin time are increased to varying degrees depending on the size of the infarct. In severe cases involving more than 50% of the liver mass, the patient also may develop hepatic encephalopathy and fulminant liver failure.

Doppler ultrasonography in patients suspected of having HAT may demonstrate an absence of hepatic arterial blood flow. Ultrasonography, CT, and MR reveal a hypodense, wedged-shaped area of infarction. In patients with polyarteritis nodosa, large aneurysmal dilations of the hepatic artery may be seen on CT, MR, and angiography [15] (Fig. 100-19).

Treatment

HAT is potentially a life-threatening disorder. Affected individuals should be monitored closely in case they develop fulminant hepatic failure. If this occurs, liver transplant should be considered. The acute management of patients with HAT usually is directed at restoration of hepatic blood flow. There are scattered case reports of selective hepatic artery infusion of thrombolytic agents, but the overall success of this treatment is unclear. Patients with a hypercoagulable state may receive anticoagulation therapy to reduce the risk of future thrombosis. In persons with polyarteritis nodosa, corticosteroids are indicated. In general, however, the treatment of patients with HAT is supportive.

Occasionally, the ischemic hepatic segment may become infected. If this occurs, surgical resection of the affected segment is indicated; however, most patients recover from HAT if the infarcted segment is of limited size and acute liver failure does not occur.

Shock Liver

Acute hepatic ischemia also may complicate an episode of hypotension. This most common complication is observed in patients with myocardial infarction and cardiogenic shock and in persons with sepsis. Affected individuals usually present with an abrupt increase in serum aminotransferase values to greater than 500 IU/L without associated abdominal pain. Following the acute injury, serum liver enzyme levels rapidly decline and usually become normal within 7 days. The serum bilirubin level also may increase and reaches a maximum value within 3 to 5 days. "Shock liver" rarely progresses to acute liver failure. Although the prothrombin time may be abnormal during the acute presentation, it rapidly returns to normal with restoration of adequate blood pressure and hepatic blood flow. Because zone III of the hepatic lobule is most sensitive to ischemic injury, liver biopsy specimens in patients with shock liver demonstrate zone III necrosis (Fig. 100-20, see also *Color Plate*). This histologic picture

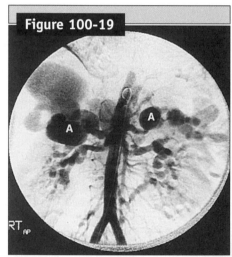

Figure 100-19

Hepatic arteriogram from a patient with polyarteritis nodosa. There are multiple aneurysmal dilations (A) of the hepatic and splenic arteries.

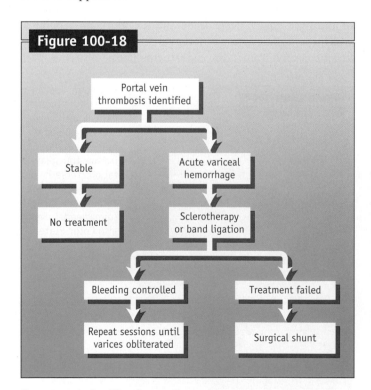

Figure 100-18

Management algorithm for a patient with portal vein thrombosis.

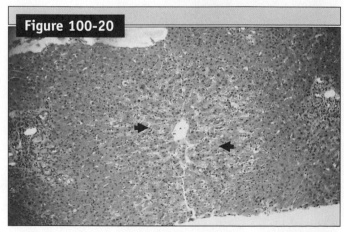

Figure 100-20

Liver biopsy specimen from a patient with "shock liver." There is necrosis of zone III hepatocytes (*arrows*) surrounding the central vein. See also **Color Plate**.

usually disappears several days after restoration of hepatic blood flow. Imaging studies of the liver in patients with shock liver generally are unremarkable. Treatment is directed at the underlying disorder; specific therapy is neither indicated nor necessary.

REFERENCES

Recently published papers of particular interest have been highlighted as follows:
* Of interest
** Of outstanding interest

1.• Parvey HR, Eisenberg RL, Giyanani V, *et al.*: Duplex sonography of the portal venous system: pitfalls and limitations. *AJR Am J Roentgenol* 1989, 152:765–770.

2. Crummy AB, McDermott JC, Starck EE: Imaging of the liver by angiographic techniques. In *Modern Imaging of the Liver.* Edited by Wilson MA, Ruzicka FF. New York: Marcel Dekker; 1989:247–264.

3.•• Bourliere M, LeTreut YP, Arnoux D, *et al.*: Acute Budd-Chiari syndrome with hepatic failure and obstruction of the inferior vena cava as presenting manifestation of hereditary protein C deficiency. *Gut* 1990, 31:949.

4.•• Simioni P, Prandoni P, Lensing AWA, *et al.*: The risk of recurrent venous thromboembolism in patients with an Arg506—Gln mutation in the gene factor V (factor V Leiden). *N Engl J Med* 1997, 336:399–403.

5.• Valla D, Le MG, Poynard T, *et al.*: Risk of hepatic vein thrombosis in relation to recent use of oral contraceptives: a case control-study. *Gastroenterology* 1986, 90:807.

6. Clinical-Pathological Conference. Aetiology of membranous obstruction of the inferior vena cava: congenital or acquired? *Gastroenterol Int* 1990, 3:70.

7.•• Dilawari JB, Bambery P, Chawla Y, *et al.*: Hepatic outflow obstruction (Budd-Chiari syndrome): experience of 177 patients and a review of the literature. *Medicine* 1993, 73:21–36.

8. Brown BP, Abu-Yousef M, Farner R, *et al.*: Doppler sonography: a noninvasive method for evaluation of hepatic venocclusive disease. *AJR Am J Roentgenol* 1990, 154:721–724.

9. Stark DD, Hahn PF, Trey C, *et al.*: MRI of the Budd-Chiari syndrome. *AJR Am J Roentgenol* 1986, 146:1141–1148.

10. Martin LG, Henderson JM, Millikan WJ, *et al.*: Angioplasty for long term treatment of patients with Budd-Chiari syndrome. *AJR Am J Roentgenol* 1990, 154:1007–1010.

11. Shulman HM, Hinterberger W: Hepatic veno-occlusive disease: liver toxicity syndrome after bone marrow transplantation. *Bone Marrow Transplant* 1992, 10:197–214.

12.•• McDonald GB, Sharma P, Mathews DE, *et al.*: Veno-occlusive disease of the liver after bone marrow transplantation: diagnosis, incidence, and predisposing factors. *Hepatology* 1984, 4:116–122.

13.• Or R, Nagler A, Shpilberg O, *et al.*: Low molecular weight heparin for the prevention of veno-occlusive disease of the liver in bone marrow transplantation patients. *Transplantation* 1996, 61:1067–1071.

14.• Webb LJ, Sherlock S: The etiology, presentation and natural history of extrahepatic portal venous obstruction. *QJM* 1979, 48:627–639.

15. Gibson PR, Dudley FJ: Ischemic hepatitis: clinical features, diagnosis, and prognosis. *Aust N Z J Med* 1984, 14:822.

101 Benign Liver Masses
Emmet B. Keeffe

Primary hepatic tumors, benign or malignant, may be epithelial and arise from hepatocytes or bile duct epithelium, may be mesenchymal and arise from supporting tissues, or may be composed of cells of both epithelial and mesenchymal origin [1•]. A number of benign, tumor-like lesions also are found in the liver. In this chapter, the most common benign mass lesions of the liver are discussed.

BENIGN MASS LESIONS OF THE LIVER

Cavernous hemangioma, focal nodular hyperplasia (FNH), and hepatocellular adenoma are the most common benign mass lesions of the liver (Table 101-1). Other benign liver masses (*eg*, infantile hemangioendothelioma, hamartoma) are rare or are diagnosed most frequently in children. In adults, benign mass lesions of the liver usually are asymptomatic and are detected incidentally by abdominal imaging. Liver tests in affected individuals may be normal, or there may be a slight elevation of the serum alkaline phosphatase and γ-glutamyl-transpeptidase levels. A history of cancer or chronic liver disease suggests that a liver mass may be a metastatic or primary malignancy; this possibility always is a major concern in patients dis-covered to have a mass lesion of the liver, regardless of the circumstances. An algorithm for the evaluation of an apparently benign liver lesion is presented in Figure 101-1 [2–4,5••].

CAVERNOUS HEMANGIOMA

Cavernous hemangioma, a hamartoma, is the most common benign liver mass and, after metastases, the second most common mass lesion of the liver [6,7•]. The prevalence of cavernous hemangiomas as reported in autopsy series varies from 0.4% to 7%, with an average of 3%. Small, asymptomatic cavernous hemangiomas are being detected with increasing frequency as a result of the widespread use of abdominal imaging. Lesions of this type with characteristic radiologic features usually are observed expectantly and do not require surgical removal. Cavernous hemangiomas are diagnosed in persons of all ages but are most often discovered during the third to fifth decades of life. They affect women more often than men, with reported male-to-female ratios of 4:1 to 6:1.

Pathology

Cavernous hemangiomas are hamartomas: malformations that resemble tumors but are not true neoplasms. These lesions usually are solitary and less than 4 cm in diameter, but they may be massive, and multiple lesions occur in approximately 10% of cases. Cavernous hemangiomas are found in all portions of the liver but are most common in the right lobe. They may be located deep within the liver or on the surface, and larger lesions may be pedunculated. Hemangiomas larger than 4 cm in diameter are arbitrarily referred to as "giant cavernous hemangiomas" and often contain areas of fibrosis and calcification. Microscopically, cavernous hemangiomas are composed of dilated vascular spaces lined by mature, flattened endothelial cells supported by fibrous septa.

Pathogenesis

Cavernous hemangiomas are believed to be congenital malformations that may slowly increase in size. The more frequent occurrence of this lesion in women and observations that hemangiomas may grow during pregnancy or with the administration of estrogens suggest that female sex hormones play some role in their pathogenesis. It is generally believed, however, that female sex hormones are promotive or permissive rather than causative in the pathogenesis of this lesion.

Clinical Presentation

As is characteristic of all benign liver masses, cavernous hemangiomas usually are found incidentally during imaging studies, on physical examination, or at autopsy. Most patients have small lesions and are asymptomatic. Giant cavernous hemangiomas may present with chronic abdominal pain caused by distension of Glisson's capsule or pressure on adjacent abdominal viscera. Episodes of more severe acute abdominal pain may be the result of the unusual occurrence of bleeding or thrombosis within the lesion. There are only rare reports of rupture of a cavernous hemangioma with hemoperitoneum. Malignant transformation of cavernous hemangiomas has not been reported because these lesions are not true neoplasms. In infants with large hemangiomas, high-output congestive heart failure, or disseminated

---

Table 101-1. Common Benign Mass Lesions of the Liver

Epithelial tumors and tumor-like masses
  Hepatocellular adenoma*
  Focal nodular hyperplasia
  Bile duct adenoma
  Hepatobiliary cystadenoma
Mesenchymal tumors and tumor-like masses
  Cavernous hemangioma*
  Infantile hemangioendothelioma
  Lipoma
  Leiomyoma
  Fibroma
Miscellaneous lesions (mixed, uncertain origin, tumor-like)
  Carcinoid
  Teratoma
  Hamartoma
  Microhamartoma (von Meyenburg complex)
  Inflammatory pseudotumor
  Focal fatty change

Most common and important benign lesions.

---

intravascular coagulation, thrombocytopenia and hypofibrinogenemia (Kasabach-Merritt syndrome) may occur.

Diagnosis

The results of liver biochemical tests are usually normal in patients with cavernous hemangiomas. Occasionally, serum alkaline phosphatase or γ-glutamyltranspeptidase levels are slightly elevated, possibly secondary to compression of intrahepatic bile ducts.

A number of imaging techniques have been used to diagnose cavernous hemangiomas [2–4,5••,6]. On ultrasonograms, these lesions are well-defined, hyperechoic masses with through transmission (Fig. 101-2). Sequential dynamic-bolus computed tomography (CT) shows a hypodense lesion initially, with subsequent peripheral contrast enhancement, followed by complete filling to isodensity or hyperdensity on delayed scans. Magnetic resonance (MR) imaging is quite sensitive in diagnosing cavernous hemangiomas, which have a low signal density on T1-weighted images and a very high signal density ("light bulb") on T2-weighted images (Fig. 101-3). Technetium-labeled red blood cell nuclear medicine studies also are quite specific. During the initial dynamic phase of the examination, low or normal blood flow is seen, but on delayed scanning the radionuclide pools ("cotton-wool") and is seen as a persistent area of radioactivity. Technetium-labeled red blood cell scanning probably is as accurate as MR in diagnosing cavernous hemangiomas and is much less expensive. Although seldom required, hepatic arteriography is the definitive test for diagnosing cavernous hemangiomas. Arteriography shows early, persistent opacification of irregular areas or lakes in affected patients; no abnormal vessels or neovascularity is seen. For practical purposes, a characteristic ultrasound appearance with confirmation by MR or bolus CT is adequate for demonstrating that an hepatic mass is a cavernous hemangioma in most situations.

Liver biopsy of cavernous hemangiomas usually can be done safely, although there is probably an increased risk of bleeding with use of standard-sized needles. Fine-needle biopsy probably is not associated with an increased risk of bleeding, but this procedure may not be diagnostic.

Prognosis

The prognosis of patients with cavernous hemangiomas is generally quite good. Smaller lesions do not cause complications, but there is some risk of thrombosis or bleeding with lesions larger than 4 to 6 cm; abdominal pain from thrombosis or bleeding responds to conservative management. Only a few cases of spontaneous rupture into the peritoneum have been reported.

Treatment

In general, small, asymptomatic lesions should be observed, and large symptomatic lesions should be resected if feasible and if the operative risk is not too great [6]. Surgical treatment is the exception rather than the rule and is used to relieve persistent abdominal pain. Alternative therapies, including hepatic artery ligation, embolization, and radiotherapy, usually are not employed. In patients with severe symptoms from giant cavernous hemangiomas involving both lobes of the liver, liver transplant has been performed.

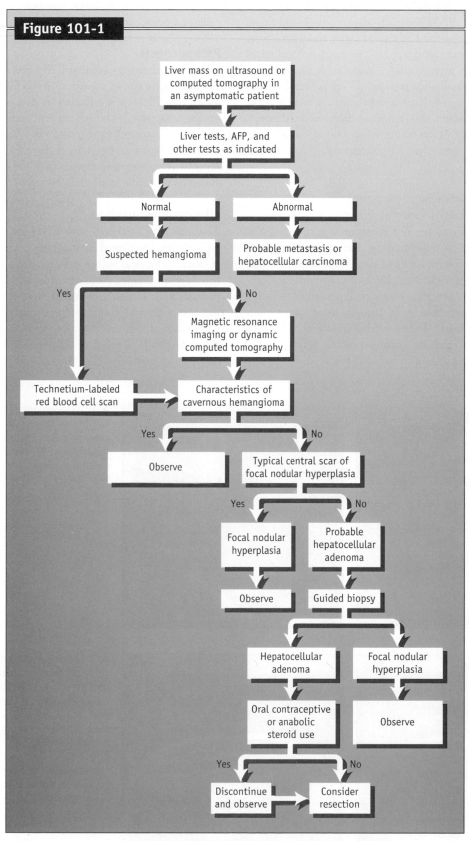

Figure 101-1

Algorithm for the differential diagnosis of an asymptomatic single tumor of the liver.

FOCAL NODULAR HYPERPLASIA

Focal nodular hyperplasia is much less common than cavernous hemangioma but more common than hepatocellular adenoma (Table 101-2) [5••,8,9]. FNH is usually asymptomatic and found incidentally, but up to one third of lesions cause abdominal pain. FNH only rarely ruptures and appears to have no malignant potential; therefore, an asymptomatic lesion with characteristic radiologic features is usually not resected. FNH is found at least twice as often in women as in men, and patients are usually in the fourth decade of life when this lesion is diagnosed. Although FNH may be hormonally dependent, studies do not support an increased incidence in users of oral contraceptives.

Pathology

Focal nodular hyperplasia typically is well circumscribed, unencapsulated, and firm. Lesions vary in size; they may be tiny or larger than 15 cm in diameter, but most are less than 5 cm in diameter. Lesions are usually solitary, but multiple nodules occur. FNH is found in both lobes of the liver, although it may be more common in the right lobe. Lesions commonly are subcapsular and frequently protrude or are pedunculated.

Focal nodular hyperplasia is a benign mass of normal-appearing hepatocytes and Kupffer cells arranged in radially oriented septa, which emanate from a central, dense, stellate scar containing bile ductules and vessels (Fig. 101-4, see also Color Plate). The hepatocytes in areas of FNH are indistinguishable from those in the rest of the liver, but they may be somewhat smaller. Variable numbers of lymphocytes, plasma cells, and histiocytes may be found within the fibrous septa.

Pathogenesis

Recent evidence suggests that FNH develops in response to arterial hyperperfusion of a portion of the liver. It is now well established that FNH is not caused by oral contraceptives, although lesions do appear to be hormone dependent. There are a number of reports documenting regression of FNH with cessation of oral contraceptive use and growth of these lesions with use of contraceptives. There are also reports of FNH becoming symptomatic and even rupturing in patients taking oral contraceptives.

Clinical Presentation

The majority of patients with FNH are asymptomatic. Lesions typically are discovered incidentally during abdominal imaging, at laparotomy, or at autopsy. A few affected individuals are identified when being evaluated for abdominal pain, and rare patients will have an abdominal mass on physical examination. Patients with symptoms are more likely to be taking oral contraceptives, which may promote growth of hyperplastic lesions associated with bleeding or necrosis or, very rarely, rupture and hemoperitoneum.

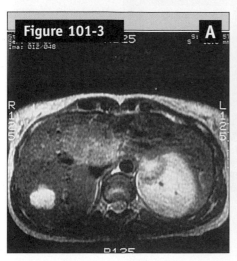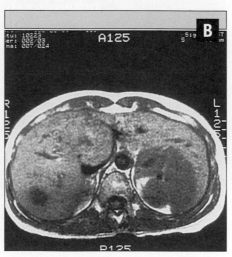

A, Ultrasonographic image of the liver shows two benign tumors in the same patient: a cavernous hemangioma and a focal nodular hyperplasia. **B**, Further images show the focal nodular hyperplasia more clearly. (*Courtesy of* R.B. Jeffrey Jr, MD.)

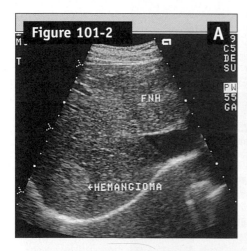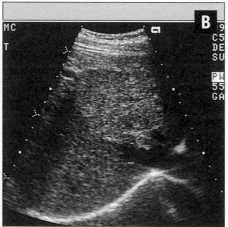

A, A T2 sequence on a magnetic resonance study shows the characteristic "light bulb" pattern of the cavernous hemangioma and the obviously vascular but not as bright focal nodular hyperplasia. **B**, A T1 sequence on the same magnetic resonance study shows a negative shadow in the area of the cavernous hemangioma and a small negative shadow compatible with a central scar in the focal nodular hyperplasia. (*Courtesy of* R.B. Jeffrey Jr, MD.)

Diagnosis

It is often difficult to distinguish FNH from hepatocellular adenoma on imaging studies [2–4,5••,8–10]. Because of the presence of Kupffer cells in FNH, approximately 50% of lesions will take up isotope on technetium-99m sulfur colloid liver scan (Fig. 101-5); however, approximately 20% of hepatocellular adenomas also have Kupffer cells and take up isotope. On ultrasonograms, FNH may be hypoechoic, hyperechoic, or mixed in appearance, and on CT, a central scar may be visible in some, but not all cases (Fig. 101-6). The lesion appears bright during the arterial phase of CT with contrast injection, and the central scar may be seen during the venous phase of the study (Fig. 101-7). MR may be the most useful imaging study for diagnosis of FNH, with a sensitivity of 70% and a specificity of 98%. The central stellate scar is detected more often by MR than by CT; MR also may show that the central portion of the lesion is vascular and thus not an area of necrosis or hemorrhage, a finding more typical of hepatocellular adenoma. On arteriography, FNH is a hypervascular mass with tortuous vessels within the lesion (Fig. 101-8).

Prognosis

Focal nodular hyperplasia is only rarely complicated by rupture in patients not taking oral contraceptives. FNH is not a tumor and does not undergo malignant degeneration. If a mass has typical features of FNH, expectant follow-up without histologic confirmation or surgical resection is appropriate, and long-term prognosis is good.

Table 101-2. Prevalence of Benign Liver Lesions in Young Women

Tumor	Prevalence, %
Cavernous hemangioma	3
Focal nodular hyperplasia	0.03
Hepatocellular adenoma	< 0.001

Adapted from Benhamou [4]; with permission.

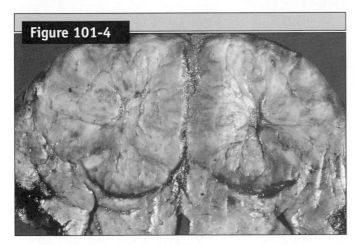

Figure 101-4

Gross liver specimen from a resected focal nodular hyperplasia shows a central scar. See also **Color Plate**.

Treatment

Incidentally discovered FNH requires no treatment [8–10]. Mass lesions of uncertain type or that cause symptoms should be biopsied. A decision regarding surgery should be based on biopsy findings and ease of resection.

HEPATOCELLULAR ADENOMA

Hepatocellular adenoma, or liver cell adenoma, occurs primarily in women taking oral contraceptives, with an estimated prevalence of one to three cases per 100,000 contraceptive users [8–10]. Of the three most common benign liver masses, hepatocellular adenoma is the most important lesion to identify because its natural history includes possible rupture with hemoperitoneum and malignant degeneration.

Pathology

Hepatocellular adenomas are solitary in three fourths of cases and are usually soft and well demarcated. These lesions may or may not have a capsule. Two thirds of tumors are found in the right lobe of the liver. Hepatocellular adenomas tend to be subcapsular and protrude from the surface of the liver. Tumors vary from 1 cm to greater than 30 cm in diameter, but most are 5 to 15 cm in diameter. The largest tumors are found in women taking oral contraceptives.

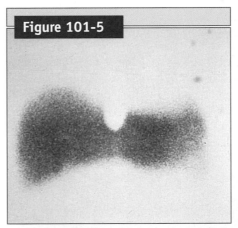

Figure 101-5

Technetium-99m sulfur colloid liver scan shows a normal liver, with filling-in of the lesion noted on computed tomographic scan (Fig. 101-6) and arteriogram (Fig. 101-8).

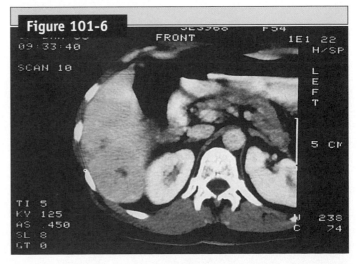

Figure 101-6

This computed tomographic image shows a 4- by 6-cm mass located inferiorly in the right lobe of the liver. A negative shadow compatible with a central scar is seen in the middle of this lesion.

Microscopically, hepatocellular adenomas consist of sheets of large, pale hepatocytes separated by compressed sinusoids lined by endothelial cells. There is an absence of portal tracts, central veins, and bile ducts, and only occasional Kupffer cells are seen. Bile stasis and canalicular thrombi may be present. The tumor contains blood vessels, especially running over its surface, and the walls of arteries and veins may be abnormally thick. Hemorrhage within tumors is not uncommon (Fig. 101-9, see also **Color Plate**).

Hepatocellular adenomatosis is a variant of hepatocellular adenoma characterized by the presence of more than four adenomas [11]. This syndrome occurs in both men and women, has no relation to oral contraceptive use, and causes elevation of serum alkaline phosphatase and γ-glutamyltranspeptidase levels. The tumors have radiologic and pathologic features similar to those of usual hepatocellular adenomas (Fig. 101-10).

Pathogenesis

A number of etiologic factors, including estrogen and anabolic steroid use, galactosemia, and glycogen storage disease type IA (von Gierke's disease), are associated with development of hepatocellular adenomas. In addition, this tumor may occur spontaneously without recognized risk factors and rarely may occur in a familial pattern. The association between oral contra-

ceptive use and hepatocellular adenoma is particularly strong with prolonged use of these agents; most affected patients have been using oral contraceptives for more than 4 years, and the risk of developing an hepatocellular adenoma increases from 5-fold to as much as 25-fold that of the general population in women taking the drug more than 9 years. Hepatocellular adenomas are less common now than they were in the past, probably due to the advent of oral contraceptive agents with lower estrogen content.

Clinical Presentation

Hepatocellular adenoma is diagnosed primarily in women in the third or fourth decades of life, although this tumor also has been described in children and men. Presentation is variable. The tumor is found incidentally in 5% to 10% of cases. Patients may note a painless abdominal mass, abdominal pain, or a tender abdominal mass; the tumor may rupture and the patient may go into shock. Abdominal pain associated with an hepatocellular adenoma typically is vague and may be accompanied by anorexia, nausea, or vomiting. Pain becomes severe with impending rupture or actual intraperitoneal bleeding, and mortality is high with this complication. The tumors that rupture usually are large and solitary and occur in patients taking oral contraceptives.

Diagnosis

A patient with a benign-appearing liver mass is more likely to have a cavernous hemangioma or FNH than a hepatocellular adenoma (Table 101-2). Patients with hepatocellular adenomas usually have normal liver tests, except when bleeding into the tumor occurs. When serum liver enzyme levels are elevated, the pattern is nonspecific and not diagnostic. The diagnosis of hepatocellular adenoma is based on clinical awareness, knowledge of the association of adenomas with use of oral contraceptives, and appropriate results of hepatic imaging studies, including ultrasonography, CT, MR, and radionuclide liver scan [2–4,5••,8–10]. Ultrasonography is usually not diagnostic, because the echogenicity of hepatocellular adenoma, like that of FNH, varies. Doppler ultrasonography may help to differentiate adenomas from FNH by showing arterial signals in the latter

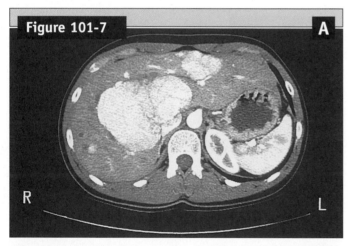

Figure 101-7

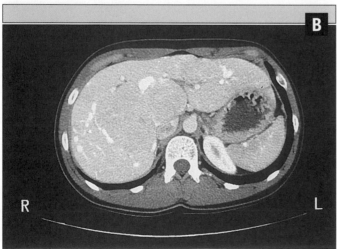

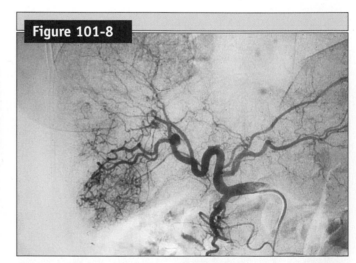

Figure 101-8

A, A computed tomographic image from arterial phase shows two bright focal nodular hyperplasia lesions. **B**, Computed tomographic image from venous phase shows a small central scar.

On this subtraction hepatic arteriogram, a 4- by 6-cm hypervascular lesion in the inferior aspect of the right lobe of the liver is seen. The vascular pattern is nonspecific.

and venous signals in the former. In patients with an apparent benign liver tumor without characteristic features of cavernous hemangioma—a central stellate scar or areas of hemorrhage or necrosis—a diagnosis of hepatocellular adenoma is likely. Hepatic arteriography appears to be the most sensitive radiologic technique for diagnosing hepatocellular adenoma. In affected patients, this test demonstrates radiating vessels entering from the periphery ("spoke-wheel" appearance) and a sharply demarcated capillary tumor stain in the late phase. Lesions may be hypovascular or hypervascular, and directed biopsy is preferred to blind percutaneous biopsy because of the potential for bleeding.

Prognosis

There is a substantial risk of bleeding from an hepatocellular adenoma, particularly in patients with tumors larger than 4 to 6 cm in diameter and in those who use oral contraceptives. Tumors may regress when oral contraceptives are discontinued, but serial imaging is necessary because new growth and rupture may occur. In addition, tumors may undergo malignant degeneration to hepatocellular carcinoma. Small lesions probably can be observed without substantial morbidity if resection is not feasible.

Treatment

Surgical resection is recommended whenever possible, particularly if the tumor is larger than 4 to 6 cm in diameter, in view of the risk of rupture and malignant degeneration [8–10]. Whether or not the lesion is resected, oral contraceptives should be discontinued; this may be associated with spontaneous regression of the tumor over many months. Unfortunately, lack of regression and even progression of hepatocellular adenoma has been reported following discontinuation of steroid contraceptives. Rarely, lesions are so large that liver transplant has been required (12).

■ FOCAL FATTY CHANGE

Focal fatty change is a tumor-like lesion often discovered incidentally on an imaging study [13,14]. Most patients with focal fatty change have an underlying disorder associated with hepatic steatosis (*eg*, obesity, diabetes, malnutrition). Diffuse macrovesicular steatosis also may be present elsewhere in the liver. The pathogenesis of focal fatty change is unknown, but regional tissue hypoxia is postulated to play a role in development of these lesions. Ultrasonograms show an area of increased echogenicity, and CT shows an area of low attenuation, characteristically with a fan-shaped or geographic profile. Focal fatty change may occur as a single lesion or multiple lesions. These tumor-like masses typically are several centimeters across but occasionally are as large as 10 cm in diameter. The lesions usually are subcapsular and often are adjacent to the falciform ligament. Focal fatty liver may be mistaken for other benign or malignant tumors, and guided liver biopsy may be required to confirm the diagnosis. The primary importance of focal fatty liver is in the differential diagnosis of benign and malignant lesions of the liver.

■ REFERENCES

Recently published papers of particular interest have been highlighted as follows:
•   Of interest
••   Of outstanding interest

1.•   Craig JR, Peters RL, Edmondson HA: *Tumors of the Liver and Intrahepatic Bile Ducts*. Washington, DC: Armed Forces Institute of Pathology, 1989.
This atlas of tumor pathology is the definitive source for pathologic and clinical correlations of all tumors affecting the liver. The authors are recognized experts who have had a long interest in tumors of the liver and a wealth of experience and material from Los Angeles County Hospital.

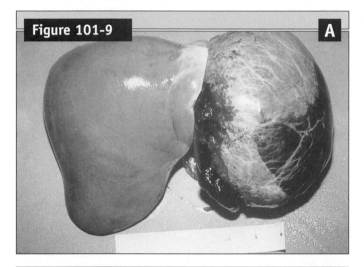

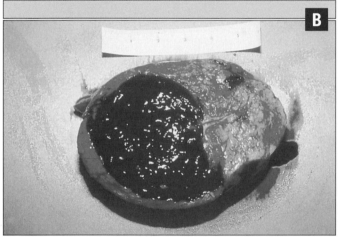

A, A gross liver specimen removed at autopsy shows a large tumor of the left lobe of the liver with subcapsular hemorrhage. **B**, Cut section of the hepatocellular adenoma shows hemorrhage with clot. See also **Color Plate**.

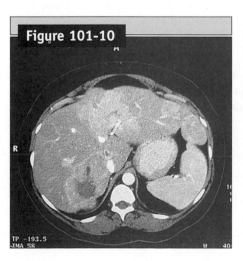

A computed tomographic scan shows multiple hepatocellular adenomas in a 50-year-old woman who had biopsy confirmation 18 years previous to this scan when she underwent cholecystectomy. The lesion in the inferior right lobe shows an area of necrosis.

2.   Reddy KR, Schiff ER: Approach to a liver mass. *Semin Liver Dis* 1993, 13:423–435.

3.   Johnson CD: Magnetic resonance imaging of the liver: current clinical applications. *Mayo Clin Proc* 1993, 68:147–156.

4.   Benhamou JP: Diagnostic approach to a liver mass: diagnosis of an asymptomatic liver tumor in a young woman. *J Hepatol* 1996, 25(suppl 1):30–34.

5.•• Cherqui D, Rahmouni A, Charlotte F, *et al.*: Management of focal nodular hyperplasia and hepatocellular adenoma in young women: a series of 41 patients with clinical, radiological, and pathological correlations. *Hepatology* 1995, 22:1674–1681.

Consecutive patients with FNH or hepatocellular adenoma seen at a single institution were retrospectively analyzed to define the role of modern imaging studies in the diagnosis of these two lesions. The authors concluded that FNH is much more common than hepatocellular adenoma; MR can allow a diagnosis of FNH in 70% of cases; and when clinical, biochemical, and radiologic findings are not typical of FNH, surgery with histologic diagnosis is mandatory and resection of hepatocellular adenomas is generally appropriate.

6.   Reading NG, Forbes A, Nunnerly HB, Williams R: Hepatic haemangioma: a critical review of diagnosis and management. *QJM* 1988, 67:431–445.

7.• Lise M, Feltrin G, Da Pian PP, *et al.*: Giant cavernous hemangiomas: diagnosis and surgical strategies. *World J Surg* 1992, 16:516–520.

Cavernous hemangiomas that are small and asymptomatic do not require surgical resection, which should be reserved for large, symptomatic tumors.

8.   Kerlin P, Davis GL, McGill DB, *et al.*: Hepatic adenoma and focal nodular hyperplasia: clinical, pathologic, and radiologic features. *Gastroenterology* 1983, 84:994–1002.

9.   Knowles DM II, Casarella WJ, Johnson PM, Wolff M: The clinical, radiologic, and pathologic characterization of benign hepatic neoplasms: alleged association with oral contraceptives. *Medicine* 1978, 57:223–237.

10. Vilgrain V, Flejou JF, Arrive L, *et al.*: Focal nodular hyperplasia of the liver: MR imaging and pathologic correlation in 37 patients. *Radiology* 1992, 184:669–703.

11. Arsenault TM, Johnson CD, Gorman B, Burgart LJ: Hepatic adenomatosis. *Mayo Clin Proc* 1996, 71:478–480.

12. Mueller J, Keeffe EB, Esquivel CO: Liver transplantation for treatment of giant hepatocellular adenomas. *Liver Transpl Surg* 1995, 1:99–102.

13. Brawer MK, Austin G, Lewin KJ: Focal fatty change of the liver, a hitherto poorly recognized entity. *Gastroenterology* 1980, 78:247–252.

14. Kester NL, Elmore SG: Focal hypoechoic regions in the liver at the porta hepatis: prevalence in ambulatory patients. *J Ultrasound Med* 1995, 14:649–652.

102 Liver Tumors

Risë Stribling, Paul Martin, and Adrian M. Di Bisceglie

There are several distinct hepatic malignancies, each with varying risk factors and unique epidemiology (Table 102-1). In addition, there are a variety of benign hepatic tumors that are being diagnosed with increasing frequency because of the widespread use of imaging studies (*eg*, abdominal ultrasound).

HEPATOCELLULAR CARCINOMA

Hepatocellular carcinoma (HCC) is one of the more common tumors worldwide. In an autopsy survey combined with a study from a large referral unit in Los Angeles county, 720 primary liver cancers were found in 96,625 postmortem examinations. Of these primary liver cancers, 642 (89.2%) were HCC, 71 (9.9%) were cholangiocarcinomas, and five (0.7%) were hepatoblastomas (HBA). There also were two carcinoid tumors [1]. Worldwide, the incidence of HCC varies from greater than 20 cases per 100,000 per year in some undeveloped countries, Japan, and South Africa, to less than five cases per 100,000 per year in the United States and Western Europe. HCC is more common in men than in women and has an important association with hepatitis B virus (HBV) infection in populations where this infection is endemic.

Etiology

A number of epidemiologic studies have helped establish significant risk factors for HCC. Although many patients who develop HCC have cirrhosis, HCC also has been found in the absence of underlying liver disease. In a review of 804 cases of HCC diagnosed at the Armed Forces Institute of Pathology (AFIP) from 1980 to 1993, only 462 (57.4%) of lesions were in cirrhotic livers [2]. Cirrhosis resulting from chronic viral hepatitis (*eg*, chronic hepatitis C virus [HCV] infection, chronic HBV infection), metabolic liver diseases (*eg*, hemochromatosis), and environmental toxins, especially alcohol, all have been implicated in HCC development. In areas of high prevalence of chronic HBV infection and HBV-related cirrhosis (*eg*, Asia, sub-Saharan Africa), the incidence of HCC is much higher than in areas where HBV infection is uncommon. Recently, HCV

Table 102-1. Risk Factors for Development of Hepatocellular Carcinoma	
Aflatoxin B	Wilson's disease (rare)
Chronic hepatitis B	Hypercitrullinemia
Chronic hepatitis C	Hereditary fructose intolerance
Thorotrast (thorium dioxide)	Hereditary tyrosinemia
α_1-Antitrypsin deficiency	Glycogen storage disease type I
Hemochromatosis	Oral contraceptives ?
Cirrhosis	

infection has been linked to HCC, with evidence of a synergistic role for alcohol; in one Japanese study of cirrhotics, 19% of alcoholics, 57% of patients with HCV infection, and 81% of patients with both alcoholism and HCV infection developed HCC during 10 years of follow-up [3]. The risk of HCC is probably no higher in alcoholic cirrhosis alone than in most other forms of cirrhosis. Other toxins linked to HCC include aflatoxin B1, a metabolite of *Aspergillus* and related fungal species that contaminate corn, rice, peanuts, and other foods stored under humid conditions, and thorium dioxide, which formerly was used as an intravenous radiographic contrast agent [4,5].

Various metabolic liver diseases have been associated with development of HCC [6••]. In patients with genetic hemachromatosis and cirrhosis, there is a 200-fold increased risk of developing HCC. Other metabolic disorders associated with HCC include α_1-antitrypsin deficiency and Wilson's disease.

Pharmacologic doses of androgens and estrogens, including oral contraceptives, are possible risk factors for HCC. Anti-estrogen and anti-androgen agents have been used to treat HCC, but the results have not been promising.

The fibrolamellar variant of HCC usually is seen in patients without liver disease. In the AFIP review of 804 cases of HCC in North America, there were 44 tumors (5.5%) classified as the fibrolamellar variant, and 37 (84%) of these were seen in non-cirrhotic livers [2]. These tumors occur in patients who are, on average, a decade younger than cirrhotics with HCC, and tumors typically are large and symptomatic at presentation. No particular risk factors for development of fibrolamellar HCC have been identified, and its prognosis is better than that of more typical HCC in cirrhotics.

Diagnosis

Particularly when small, HCC may grow slowly, with tumor-doubling times ranging from 27 to 605 days, with mean values of approximately 200 days [1]. By the time a patient presents with symptomatic HCC, however, prognosis is poor, and life expectancy is only weeks. Doubling times are much shorter for larger tumors. Presymptomatic diagnosis of small HCC is difficult, because not all affected patients have an elevated α-fetoprotein (AFP) level, and radiologic detection of lesions smaller than 2 cm in diameter is difficult. Elevated serum AFP, especially when greater than 400 ng/mL, is almost diagnostic; however, lower levels of AFP lack both sensitivity and specificity and have been associated with other conditions (*eg*, chronic hepatitis, ovarian malignancies) [7].

Ultrasonography and serial serum AFP measurements are the most commonly used screening tests for HCC. For lesions 1 to 3 cm in diameter, ultrasonography has been shown to have sensitivity rates of up to 92%, but sensitivity rates fall to less than 40% in lesions smaller than 1 cm [8]. Computed tomographic (CT) scanning and modified CT scanning (*eg*, CT portography, which requires mesenteric arterial catheterization; lipoidal-enhanced CT scanning, which requires hepatic arterial injection of iodized oil) also have sensitivity rates of 87% to 93% for lesions smaller than 3 cm in diameter (Fig. 102-1) [8,9].

Magnetic resonance (MR) imaging has been used to distinguish HCC from vascular lesions (*eg*, cavernous hemangiomas). A number of innovations have been added to MR to increase diagnostic accuracy, including fast low-angle shot (FLASH) sequences, iron oxide–enhanced imaging, and use of chondroitin sulfate iron colloid as a contrast agent. The diagnostic accuracy of MR is slightly less than that of CT portography, but the former procedure is less invasive. Many of these diagnostic modalities are not widely available. In addition, they are expensive, may be invasive, require radiation exposure, and thus are not appropriate for diagnosis of many cases of HCC. In high-risk patients with cirrhosis, a commonly recommended screening regimen is measurement of serum AFP every 2 to 4 months and ultrasonographic screening every 3 to 6 months [10].

The role of biopsy in confirming the diagnosis of HCC is controversial. In patients with cirrhosis, markedly elevated or steadily rising serum AFP levels and a mass on imaging studies, biopsy is not usually necessary and may be contraindicated if

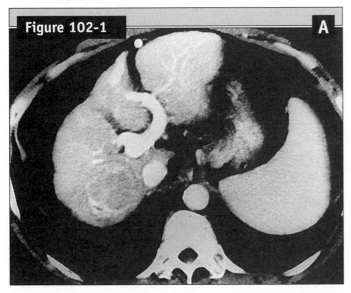

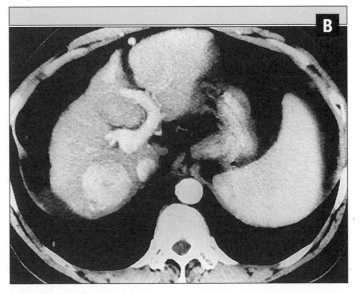

A, Hepatic phase of a dual-phase helical computed tomographic scan showing a large hepatocellular carcinoma. **B**, Arterial phase of a dual-phase helical computed tomographic scan showing a large, hypervascular hepatocellular carcinoma.

curative resection is planned due to reports of needle-track seeding with malignant cells. In patients with no obvious underlying liver disease or a normal serum AFP level with a liver mass, biopsy may be more appropriate.

Treatment

Hepatocellular carcinoma frequently is asymptomatic until the tumor is quite large; thus, many patients present with advanced and incurable disease. Resection technically may be possible in patients with adequate hepatic reserve, but only a minority of patients are candidates for a resection. In patients with impaired hepatic reserve and cirrhosis, liver transplant is the only surgical option that provides any hope of long-term survival.

In the early days of liver transplants, primary HCC was regarded as an appropriate indication for orthotopic liver transplantation (OLT); however, initial survival rates were disappointing, with both Pittsburgh and the University of California Los Angeles reporting 3-year survival rates of 25% to 30% [11]. It has become clear that with careful staging, survival rates improve dramatically. Using the TNM (tumor-node-metastasis) classification, tumors are classified based on size and extent of the primary tumor (T), presence or absence of nodal spread (N), and evidence of metastatic disease (M) (Table 102-2).

Ringe et al. [12] showed that 5-year survival rates are 10% to 20% in patients with stage IV tumors, tumors in more than one lobe of the liver, invasion of the portal vein, and evidence of metastatic spread. In a series from Pittsburgh, Selby et al. [13] showed that patients with solitary lesions smaller than 2 cm in diameter and no evidence of vascular invasion (stage I) have a 5-year survival rate of 75%, but those with stage IV tumors have a 5-year survival rate of 10.9%. Several studies have confirmed that tumors smaller than 2 cm in diameter found incidentally during liver transplant have no significant impact on overall survival.

Transarterial chemoembolization (TAE) with gelatin sponge material has been used at several centers to treat HCC. Hepatic arteriography is employed to localize the dominant arterial inflow of the tumor, and iodized oil and chemotherapeutic agents also are injected. Using this technique, Bronowicki et al. [14] reported 1- and 3-year survival rates of 64% and 27%, respectively. By comparison, in a study of 793 subjects from Japan treated with TAE [15], the 1- and 3-year survival rates were 51% and 12%, respectively. In a multicenter French study,

Bronowicki et al. [16••] retrospectively examined outcomes of patients who received no therapy (33 patients), surgical resection (30 patients), OLT (17 patients) and TAE (42 patients). In all treated groups, 3- and 5-year survival rates ranged from 43% to 54% and 43% to 48%, respectively. Recurrence rate at 3 years was 35% after TAE, 64% after surgical resection, and 76% after OLT. The TAE procedure is not without complications. Treated patients frequently develop right upper quadrant pain and high fever. Less commonly, hepatic decompensation, tumor rupture and hemorrhage, aneurysm formation, vasculitis, and cholecystitis occur.

Other therapeutic options for patients with HCC include percutaneous ethanol injection (PEI) and cryosurgery. In 1995, Livraghi et al. [17] reported a large series of 746 patients from Italy showing 1- and 3-year survival rates from 85% to 97% and 16% to 68%, respectively, in patients undergoing PEI. It has become increasingly clear that multimodal therapy is frequently needed for patients with HCC. HCC continues to be an aggressive tumor with frequent recurrence; current treatment regimens simply delay disease progression [18].

▪ HEPATOBLASTOMA

Hepatoblastoma is one of the most common primary liver tumors in children younger than 5 years of age; HBA is rare in adults. This tumor also is more frequent in males. HBA commonly presents as an abdominal mass in a patient with anorexia, fever, and weight loss [1]. Underlying liver disease or cirrhosis is uncommon. This tumor is classified according to histology as epithelial or mixed epithelial and mesenchymal, with subtypes of each major type. The fetal subtype of epithelial HBA is the most common and appears to have the best prognosis. Surgical resection is the mainstay of therapy. In patients whose lesions are deemed unresectable at the initial evaluation, neoadjuvant chemotherapy combined with surgical resection has shown promise. Liver transplant also has been performed in patients with HBA; 2-year survival after liver transplant is 50% on average, with approximately one third of the tumors recurring. Small tumors may be resected successfully with good survival rates [19,20]. In patients who are deemed inoperable at initial evaluation, a trial of chemotherapy is warranted. If there is a response, resection should be considered.

▪ METASTATIC TUMORS OF THE LIVER

Metastatic spread of malignant tumors to the liver occurs through the portal vein or hepatic artery, through the lymphatic system, and by direct extension. In the AFIP series of 94,556 autopsies, there were 19,208 malignant extrahepatic tumors, of which 7299 (38%) had spread to the liver [21]. Many different tumors metastasize to the liver (Table 102-3). Hepatic metastasies have been reported in more than 70% of patients with pancreas and gallbladder cancer and in 40% to 60% of individuals with bronchogenic, colon, breast, stomach, ovary, or testicular cancer. Colorectal carcinoma is now the second most common cancer in the United States, and hepatic metastases are reported in more than 50% of cases. Less frequently, hepatic metastases have been seen in persons with thyroid, prostate, cervical, or renal cancer. Lymphoma frequently involves the liver; up to 50% of patients with adult T-cell lymphoma have hepatic lesions [21].

Table 102-2. TNM Staging for Primary Hepatic Malignancies

| | Classification | | |
Stage	T	N	M
I	T1	N0	M0
II	T2	N0	M0
II	T1	N1	M0
	T2	N1	M0
	T3	Any N	M0
IVA	T4	Any N	M0
IVB	Any T	Any N	M1

Metastatic liver cancer has been treated with the same chemotherapeutic drugs used to treat the primary tumor. In a study [22] examining survival and recurrence rates after hepatic resection for metastatic colorectal carcinoma, the authors reported 131 hepatic resections with an overall 5-year survival of 25% and a disease-free survival of 16%; there was a significantly decreased survival associated with positive resection margins, extrahepatic disease, and noncurative resections. In the absence of better alternative therapies for metastatic colorectal cancer to the liver, resection should be considered. Hepatic resection also has been performed for patients with noncolorectal and nonneuroendocrine metastases [23]. A selective approach is recommended in patients with renal cell carcinoma, Wilms' tumor, and adrenocortical cancer; there are only isolated cases of long-term survival after resection of hepatic metastases from tumors of the esophagus, stomach, small intestine, and pancreas. Resection also should be considered for palliation in patients with symptomatic bulky tumors.

Neuroendocrine tumors (NETs) of the liver are divided into carcinoid and noncarcinoid lesions. Carcinoid tumors most frequently arise in the bronchial tree and gastrointestinal tract, where the most common sites are the ileum (35%) and the appendix (31%). The least aggressive and frequently incidentally noted carcinoid tumors were found in the appendix; none were metastatic and all were cured with appendectomy. In contrast, carcinoid tumors of the small intestine tend to be more aggressive, are frequently metastatic at time of diagnosis, and have an overall poor survival when compared with other carcinoid tumors of the gastrointestinal tract. The majority of the *noncarcinoid* lesions are pancreatic islet cell tumors. NETs frequently metastasize to the liver and mesentery and less often to bone and peritoneum [24]. Metastases to the liver usually are multifocal and involve both lobes. Hepatic metastasis are present in as many as 70% of NETs at the time of diagnosis of the primary lesion [24]. Typical carcinoid syndrome is noted in about one half of reported cases of metastatic carcinoid tumors, and diarrhea and recurrent gastroduodenal ulcers are reported in 44% of noncarcinoid lesions. In selected patients, cytoreductive surgery for debulking the primary tumor resulted in 5-year survival rates of up to 50% [25]. Palliative therapy with systemic or intra-arterial chemotherapy has been associated with 5-year survival rates of 25% to 35% [24,26]. The actuarial 5-year survival rate following OLT for carcinoid tumors is 69%, compared with 8% 4-year survival after OLT for patients with noncarcinoid lesions. OLT is recommended for patients who have not achieved results with previous resection and palliative therapy and have pain or symptoms of hormonal syndromes.

▨ REFERENCES

Recently published papers of particular interest have been highlighted as follows:
- • Of interest
- •• Of outstanding interest

1. Schiff L, Schiff ER: *Diseases of the Liver*, edn 7. Philadelphia: JB Lippincott; 1993.

2. Nzeako UC, Goodman ZD, Ishak KG: Hepatocellular carcinoma in cirrhotic and noncirrhotic livers: a clinico-histopathological study. *Am J Clin Pathol* 1996, 105:65–75.

3. Yamauchi M, Nakahara M, Maezawa Y, *et al.*: Prevalence of hepatocellular carcinoma in patients with alcoholic cirrhosis and prior exposure to hepatitis C. *Am J Gastroenterol* 1993, 88:39.

4. Kew MC, Popper H: Relationship between hepatocellular carcinoma and cirrhosis. *Semin Liver Dis* 1984, 4:136–46.

5. Columbo M: Hepatocellular carcinoma: recent progress. *J Hepatol* 1992, 15:225–236.

6.•• Khakoo S, Grellier L, Soni P, *et al*: Etiology, screening and treatment of hepatocellular carcinoma. *Med Clin North Am* 1996, 5:1121–1145.
The authors provide an excellent recent review of HCC.

7. Ramsey WH, Wu GY: Hepatocellular carcinoma: update on diagnosis and treatment. *Dig Dis* 1995, 13:81–91.

8. Takayasu K, Moriyama N, Muramatsu Y, *et al*.: The diagnosis of small hepatocellular carcinomas: efficacy of various imaging procedures in 100 patients. *AJR Am J Roentgenol* 1990, 155:49–54.

9. Nelson RC, Chezmar JL, Sugarbaker PH, Bernardino ME: Hepatic tumors: comparison of CT during arterial portography, delayed CT, and MR imaging for preoperative evaluation. *Radiology* 1989, 172:27–34.

10. Unoura M, Kaneko S, Matsushita E, *et al*.: High-risk groups and screening strategies for early detection of hepatocellular carcinoma in patients with chronic liver disease. *Hepatol Gastroenterol* 1993, 40:305–310.

11. Olthoff KM, Millis M, Rosove MH, *et al*.: Is liver transplantation justified for the treatment of hepatic malignancies? *Arch Surg* 1990, 125:1261–1268.

12. Ringe B, Pichlmayr R, Wittekind C, *et al*.: Surgical treatment of hepatocellular carcinoma: experience with liver resection and transplantation in 198 patients. *World J Surg* 1991, 15:270–285.

13. Selby R, Kadry Z, Carr B, *et al*.: Liver transplantation for hepatocellular carcinoma. *World J Surg* 1995, 19:53–58.

14. Bronowicki JP, Vetter D, Dumas F, *et al*.: Transcatheter oily chemoembolization for hepatocellular carcinoma: a 4-year study of 127 French patients. *Cancer* 1994, 74:16–24.

15. Yamada R, Kishi K, Sonomura T, *et al*.: Transcatheter arterial chemomobilization in unresectable hepatocellular carcinoma. *Cardiovasc Intervent Radiol* 1990, 13:135–139.

16.•• Bronowicki JP, Boudjema K, Chone L, *et al*.: Comparison of resection, liver transplantation and transcatheter oily chemoembolization in the treatment of hepatocellular carcinoma. *J Hepatol* 1996, 24:293–300.
This represents a retrospective multicenter French study comparing resection, OLT, and TAE treatment methods to determine 3- and 5-year survival rates.

17. Livraghi T, Giorgio A, Marin G, *et al*.: Hepatocellular carcinoma and cirrhosis in 746 patients: long-term results of percutaneous ethanol injection. *Radiology* 1995, 197:101–108.

18. Marsh JW, Dvorchik I, Subotin M, *et al*.: The prediction of risk of recurrence of hepatocellular carcinoma after orthotopic liver transplantation: a pilot study. *Hepatology* 1997, 26:444–450.

Table 102-3. Extrahepatic Malignant Tumors That Metastasize to the Liver

Lung	Melanoma
Colon	Urinary bladder and ureter
Pancreas	Esophagus
Breast	Testis
Stomach	Endometrium
Thyroid	Kidney
Ovary	Hodgkin's disease
Prostate	Sarcoma
Gallbladder	Melanoma
Cervix	Lymphoma

19. Penn I: Hepatic transplantation for primary and metastatic cancers of the liver. *Surgery* 1991, 110:726–735.

20. Koneru B, Flye MW, Busuttil RW, *et al.*: Liver transplantation for hepatoblastoma: the American experience. *Ann Surg* 1991, 213:118–121.

21. Craig JR, Peters RL, Edmondson AL: *Tumors of the Liver and Intrahepatic Bile Ducts.* Washington, DC: Armed Forces Institute of Pathology; 1989.

22. Jenkins LT, Millikan KW, Bines SD, *et al.*: Hepatic resection for metastatic colorectal cancer. *Am Surg* 1997, 63:605–610.

23. Schwartz SI: Hepatic resection for noncolorectal nonneuroendocrine metastases. *World J Surg* 1995, 19:72–75.

24. Le Treut YP, Delpero JR, Dousset B, *et al.*: Results of liver transplantation in the treatment of metastatic neuroendocrine tumors. *Ann Surg* 1997, 225:355–364.

25. Nagorney DM, Que FG: Cytoreductive hepatic surgery for metastatic gastrointestinal neuroendocrine tumors. *Front Gastrointest Res* 23:416–430.

26. Ihse I, Persson B, Tibblin S: Neuroendocrine metastasis to the liver. *World J Surg* 1995, 19:76–82.

103 Pyogenic Liver Abscess
Charles M. Noyer

The mortality rate of pyogenic liver abscess (PLA) was nearly 100% until 1938, at which time the introduction of antibiotics, in conjunction with surgical drainage, vastly improved survival. The development of the technique of percutaneous drainage, first successfully used to treat PLA in 1953, lowered mortality rates even further. Although the past few decades have witnessed an increased incidence of PLA, the mortality rate of this disorder has decreased steadily, to about 10%.

EPIDEMIOLOGY

The incidence of PLA has been reported as five to 13 cases per 100,000 patient admissions; recent figures of 22 to 30 cases per 100,000 probably reflect the use of improved imaging techniques rather than an actual increase in the incidence of disease [1••]. PLA once was reported to be more common in men, but today it is seen with equal frequency in men and women. PLA caused by biliary tract disease, however, is more common in women. Early in this century, PLA was a disease of younger men, with a peak incidence during the third and fourth decades; now it occurs most frequently during the sixth and seventh decades.

ETIOLOGY AND PATHOPHYSIOLOGY

In 1938, Ochsner *et al.* [2•] found that 34% of patients with PLA reported by other authors had underlying suppurative appendicitis, whereas only 11% of their own patients did. A large number of Ochsner's patients—60%—had "cryptogenic" PLA, in contrast to the patients reported in the literature, of whom 17% had cryptogenic PLA and 45% had pylephlebitis. Today, cryptogenic abscesses predominate in some studies, whereas in others, a biliary tract lesion is found in 31% to 70% of cases (Table 103-1). The most common benign biliary disorders associated with PLA are cholelithiasis, choledocholithiasis, sclerosing cholangitis, and biliary atresia. Malignant lesions associated with PLA include gallbladder and pancreatic carcinoma, cholangiocarcinoma, and hepatocellular carcinoma. Tumor-related PLA may occur after necrosis of a hepatic lesion, attempted ablation with arterial chemoembolization, or intralesional administration of chemotherapeutic agents. Seeding of the liver from endocarditis or omphalitis is rare, but does occur.

The pathogenesis of cryptogenic PLA remains speculative. Investigators have postulated subclinical abdominal infection with undetected seeding of the portal venous system; spontaneous infection within the liver related to microscopic thromboembolism or thrombophlebitis; and unrecognized ischemic insults with bacterial seeding.

Patients with cryptogenic PLA are likely to be men between the ages of 40 and 50 years with minimal liver test abnormalities, a single PLA, and negative blood and abscess culture results. Whether or not aggressive evaluation of the gastrointestinal tract

---

Table 103-1. Lesions Associated With PLA Grouped According to Cause

Cryptogenic

Biliary
 Choledocholithiasis
 Cholecystitis with perforation
 Biliary stricture
 Cholangiocarcinoma
 Sclerosing cholangitis
 Choledochal cysts
 Parasitic infection

Hepatic parenchyma
 Hepatoma
 Other tumors
 Metastases
 Cysts: simple, echinococcus, amebic

Trauma/invasive therapy
 Tumor ablation
 Hepatic artery embolization

Pylephlebitis
 Diverticulitis
 Appendicitis
 Inflammatory bowel disease
 Pelvic inflammatory disease
 Pancreatitis
 Perforated peptic ulcer

Systemic infection
 Endocarditis or bacteremia
 Omphalitis

Direct extension
 Subphrenic, perihepatic abscess
 Perinephric abscess

Immunodeficiency
 Job's syndrome
 Chronic granulomatous disease
 AIDS-associated perianal disease

PLA—pyogenic liver abscess.

or thorough dental examination can decrease the percentage of cryptogenic PLA diagnosed is not clear. Such evaluations are not recommended unless the patient has symptoms that point to gastrointestinal or dental involvement. Diabetes mellitus appears to be a risk factor for PLA, particularly gas-containing abscesses.

About 70% of single abscesses are located in the right lobe, whereas multiple abscesses are found in one or both lobes with equal frequency. The causes of single and multiple abscesses are similar. Classification of PLA by size, number, cause, and origin of infection enables one to perform subgroup analysis, but the frequent overlap among groups makes this system cumbersome and does not help predict outcome.

■■ MICROBIOLOGY

At least one pathogen is isolated in 90% of patients in whom both blood and abscess cultures are obtained. Slightly less than half of all patients have positive cultures of both abscess and blood. Abscess culture results are more often positive than are those of blood cultures (81% vs 50%) and, therefore, should be obtained whenever possible. Polymicrobial infections occur in about 10% of patients; isolation of different pathogens from the blood and the abscess is not unusual. Patients with cryptogenic abscesses are more likely to have negative culture results, and polymicrobial infections occur more often in patients with biliary tract lesions.

Some of the organisms that have been isolated from the blood or abscesses of patients with PLA are listed in Table 103-2. This list is not complete, but includes some of the more common and interesting organisms that have been recovered. *Escherichia coli*, *Klebsiella* spp., enterococci, and *Bacteroides* spp. are the most commonly isolated bacterial pathogens; recovering anaerobes requires careful culture technique. Some organisms are associated with specific causes of PLA. For example, *Staphylococcus aureus*–related infections occur more often in the setting of Job's syndrome and chronic granulomatous disease, especially in children. Organisms of *Klebsiella* spp. may predispose patients, particularly diabetics, to the severe complication of endophthalmitis, and should be the presumed pathogen when imaging tests demonstrate that abscesses contain gas. Organisms of *Yersinia* spp. are known to cause PLA in patients with underlying hemochromatosis.

■■ CLINICAL PICTURE

Symptoms
The classic presentation of fever, right upper quadrant pain, and tender hepatomegaly is unusual. Indeed, the frequency of any particular symptom varies widely among reports. Most patients with PLA have one or more of the following symptoms: fever, chills, anorexia, and abdominal pain; a significant number have nausea, vomiting, weight loss, cough, chest pain, and diarrhea as well (Table 103-3). The duration of symptoms does not correlate with the number of abscesses, but those patients with the longest duration of symptoms are more likely to have underlying abdominal lesions and pylephlebitis.

Physical Findings
There is no single physical finding that occurs in a majority of patients with PLA. The most common findings are fever, right upper quadrant tenderness, hepatomegaly, abnormal findings in pulmonary examination, and jaundice. Guarding, epigastric tenderness, distention, and septic shock are seen less frequently.

Laboratory Tests
Most patients with PLA have leukocytosis and mild anemia; thrombocytosis is less common (Table 103-4). Liver test abnormalities are common in persons with PLA and are not specific, although a PLA in the presence of marked hyperbilirubinemia (>5.0 mg/dL) usually denotes an underlying biliary tract lesion.

Imaging Studies
Plain Radiographs
In at least half of patients with PLA, an abnormality such as an elevated right hemidiaphragm, right lower lobe atelectasis, pleural effusion, or pneumonia is noted on a plain chest radiograph. If perforation of a PLA has occurred, there may be free

---

Table 103-2. Abbreviated List of Microbes Associated With PLA

Aerobes	Other aerobes
Escherichia coli	*Streptococcus milleri*
Klebsiella sp	*Proteus* sp
Proteus sp	*Salmonella typhi*
Enterococci	*Mycobacterium tuberculosis*
Streptococcus sanguis	Miscellaneous
Staphylococci	*Listeria monocytogenes*
Streptococci	*Schistosoma mansoni*
Brucella melitensis	*Yersinia enterocolitica*
Anaerobes	*Campylobacter jejuni*
Bacteroides sp	*Enterocytozoon (Septata)*
Peptostreptococcus sp	*intestinalis*
Actinomyces sp	Fungi
Fusobacterium sp	*Candida* sp
Eikenella corrodens	*Aspergillus* sp

PLA—pyogenic liver abscess.

Table 103-3. The Symptoms and Signs Associated With PLA Listed in Decreasing Frequency

Symptoms	Signs
Systemic	Fever
Fever	Right upper quadrant, epigastric pain
Chills	
Weight loss	Hepatomegaly
Malaise	Abnormal pulmonary findings
Nausea, vomiting	Rales
Abdominal pain	Dullness
Pulmonary	Splinting
Pleuritic, chest pain	Jaundice
Cough	Guarding, rebound
Abdominal distention	Abdominal distention
	Sepsis
	Ascites

PLA—pyogenic liver abscess.

air under the diaphragm. A plain abdominal radiograph may reveal an ileus. Because no more than one third of patients with PLA have gas in the abscess cavity, it is unusual to see gas on plain radiography (Fig. 103-1).

Ultrasound

The overall sensitivity of ultrasound for detecting PLA is about 80% but it is slightly higher in cases of multiple abscesses [3]. False-negative studies may occur when abscesses are located in the dome or right lobe of the liver if they are small or just beginning to develop. Abscesses vary in appearance from cystic anechoic lesions to hyperechoic solid lesions. Early abscesses may have a subtle appearance similar in echogenicity to adjacent parenchyma. Developed lesions may be hypoechoic and elliptic, or rounded with ill-defined margins and internal echoes.

Computed Tomography

Computed tomography (CT) has a sensitivity of at least 95% for detecting abscesses and is not limited by patient body habi-tus, bowel gas, or technician expertise, all of which can limit ultrasound [3]. PLAs appear as areas of decreased attenuation with rim enhancement after administration of intravenous contrast. It is neither useful nor necessary in most cases, however, to administer contrast once the abscess has been detected, because it does not significantly increase the sensitivity of CT in this setting and, rarely, may cause a false-negative reading. Infrequently, a diffuse low-density pattern throughout the liver (*eg*, fatty liver) may mask an abscess. With CT, gas can be detected in the abscess 7% to 30% of the time (Fig. 103-2).

Magnetic Resonance Imaging

Pyogenic liver abscesses have the following appearances on magnetic resonance (MR) imaging: hypointense on T1-weighted images; hyperintense on T2-weighted images; and rim-enhancing with intravenous gadopentetate dimeglumine. The sensitivity of MR imaging is not superior to that of CT in diagnosis of PLA.

Nuclear medicine scans using technetium sulfur colloid have about the same sensitivity as ultrasound [3]. They must be used in conjunction with gallium scans to be diagnostic and cannot detect lesions smaller than 2 cm in diameter.

■ DIFFERENTIAL DIAGNOSIS

Because the specificity of imaging studies in the diagnosis of PLA is only 15%, any lesion detected in the liver with standard imaging tests and thought to be a PLA must be evaluated in concert with the clinical presentation. Several lesions may mimic PLA, including amebic abscess, infected congenital or echinococcal cyst, primary or metastatic liver cancer, leiomyosarcoma, and subhepatic or subphrenic abscess. Serologic tests for ameba and echinococcus infection are readily available, and stool should be sent for ova and parasites when indicated. It is not uncommon for amebic abscesses to occur in patients with no history of diarrhea.

■ THERAPY

Percutaneous needle aspiration (PNA) and CT- or ultrasound-guided catheter drainage (PCD) have replaced surgery as the

Table 103-4. Frequency of Hematologic and Liver Test Abnormalities in All Patients With PLA	
Liver test abnormality	**Frequency**
Leukocytosis	64%–75%
Anemia	50%–75%
Thrombocytosis	20%
Elevated ESR	Frequent
Alkaline phosphatase	80%–90%
Bilirubin	81%
AST/ALT	66%
Albumin	66%
Prothrombin time	33%

ALT—alanine aminotransferase; AST—aspartate aminotransferase; ESR—erythrocyte sedimentation rate; PLA—pyogenic liver abscess.

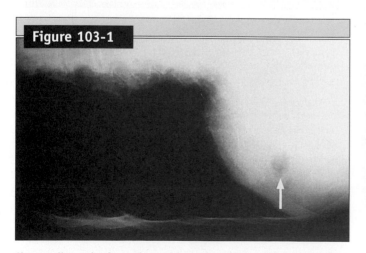

Figure 103-1

Chest radiograph of a patient with a pyogenic liver abscess shows gas (*arrow*) within the lesion. (*Courtesy of* D. Alterman, MD.)

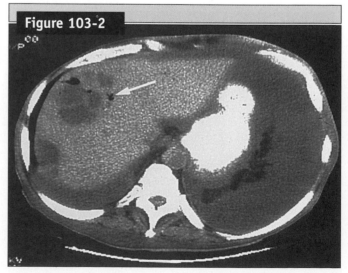

Figure 103-2

Presence of gas (*arrow*) within a pyogenic liver abscess as seen on computed tomographic scan. This patient was treated with antibiotics and percutaneous catheter drainage.

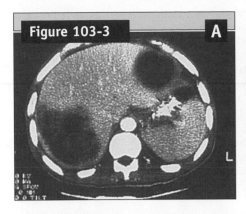

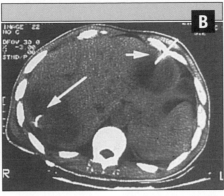

Figure 103-3

A, A patient with two large abscesses involving the right and left lobes. **B**,The same patient after insertion of a percutaneous catheter into the right lobe (*long arrow*) and undergoing catheter insertion into the left lobe (*short arrow*).

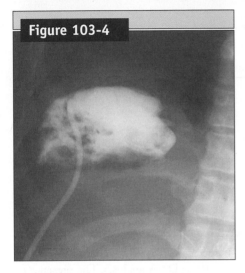

Figure 103-4

Contrast study through a catheter into an abscess to evaluate change in cavity size with drainage.

treatments of choice for PLA [4]. With PCD, a catheter remains in place for several days, allowing continued drainage and access to the abscess cavity. The radiologist usually chooses between PNA and PCD, but most large or more complicated abscesses should be treated with PCD (Fig. 103-3). Fifty percent of patients treated with PNA require more than one puncture, which should be taken into account when considering this approach (Fig. 103-4).

Administration of antibiotics that "cover" the typical gram-negative and anaerobic organisms found in PLA should be started once the diagnosis is suspected, with adjustments made when culture results and organism sensitivities are known. Metronidazole should be given if amebic liver abscess is a possibility. Many reports recommend giving intravenous antibiotics for at least 2 weeks, and oral antibiotics should be given for a short period thereafter. Fever typically resolves between 3 and 7 days after therapeutic intervention. Antibiotic therapy alone is not recommended unless percutaneous or surgical drainage is contraindicated or if the abscess is very small.

Less than 10% of all cases of PLA require surgical drainage. Surgery typically is reserved for refractory or recurrent abscesses and perhaps when cholecystitis, choledocholithiasis, biliary strictures, and obstructing tumors are present. In patients with multiple small abscesses related to biliary obstruction, endoscopic retrograde cholangiopancreatography (ERCP) with biliary drainage and intravenous antibiotics have been used successfully and should be considered in appropriate circumstances [5].

PROGNOSIS

In the early 1900s, the mortality rate of PLA, particularly when associated with pylephlebitis, rupture and peritonitis, or pleuropulmonary extension, was 51% to 100%. With the availability of percutaneous drainage and antibiotics, the mortality rate has dropped to 10%, although it is significantly higher when there are underlying pancreaticobiliary or hepatic malignancies. Recurrence rates are less than 5% for cryptogenic abscesses, but are much higher when an underlying cause, such as biliary obstruction or diverticulitis, is not corrected.

Age, gas-containing abscesses, multilobe involvement, sepsis, multiorgan failure, hyperbilirubinemia, hypoalbuminemia, and rupture are mentioned with varying frequency as prognostic indicators [6•,7]. Rupture is associated with mortality rates of up to 45%.

COMPLICATIONS

The most severe complications of PLA include sepsis; multiorgan failure; rupture into the peritoneum, lung or pericardium; and endophthalmitis [8,9]. Septic endophthalmitis occurs in 1.7% to 3% in all patients with PLA [10], but in up to 8% of patients in whom *Klebsiella pneumoniae* is the causative organism [11]. Underlying diabetes mellitus also is a risk factor for this complication, which almost always results in blindness. Visual complaints from any patient with PLA warrant emergent ophthalmologic consultation.

Pyogenic liver abscess is not uncommon, but may be missed early in its course because of nonspecific symptoms and clinical features. Earlier and more frequent diagnoses are expected to be possible with improved imaging techniques, which also can be used to guide percutaneous drainage. Antibiotic therapy should be tailored to cover the most frequent causative organisms, and the underlying cause addressed with surgical or other therapies as needed.

REFERENCES

Recently published papers of particular interest have been highlighted as follows:
•   Of interest
••   Of outstanding interest

1.••   Seeto RK, Rockey DC: Pyogenic liver abscess: changes in etiology, management, and outcome. *Medicine* 1996, 75:99–113.
A thorough review of 142 patients with pyogenic liver abscess. This article covers the causes, presentation, microbiology, diagnosis, and management of this disorder, demonstrating the rising incidence of cryptogenic abscesses, higher yields of cultures, pattern of laboratory abnormalities, and the changing management.

2.• Ochsner A, De Bakey M, Murray S: Pyogenic abscess of the liver. II. An analysis of forty-seven cases with review of the literature. *Am J Surg* 1938, 40:292–319.
This is a classic article that becomes more interesting when read along with the article by Seeto and Rockey [1]. It establishes the importance of pyle-phlebitis as a cause of PLA early in this century.

3. Halvorsen RA, Foster WL, Wilkinson RH, *et al.*: Hepatic abscess: sensitivity of imaging tests and clinical findings. *Gastrointest Radiol* 1988, 13:135–141.

4. Giorgio A, Tarantino L, Mariniello N, *et al.*: Pyogenic liver abscesses: 13 years of experience in percutaneous needle aspiration with US guidance. *Radiology* 1995, 195:122–124.

5. Edelman K: Multiple pyogenic liver abscesses communicating with the biliary tree: treatment by endoscopic stenting and stone removal. *Am J Gastroenterol* 1994, 89:2070–2072.

6.• Chou FF, Sheen-Chen SM, Chen YS, *et al.*: Prognostic factors for pyogenic abscess of the liver. *J Am Coll Surg* 1994, 179:727–732.
This paper discusses some of the dependent and independent variables that predict mortality in PLA.

7. Yang CC, Chen CY, Lin XZ, *et al.*: Pyogenic liver abscess in Taiwan: emphasis on gas-forming liver abscess in diabetics. *Am J Gastroenterol* 1993, 88:1911–1915.

8. Chou FF, Sheen Chen SM, Chen YS, Lee TY: The comparison of clinical course and results of treatment between gas-forming and non-gas-forming pyogenic liver abscess. *Arch Surg* 1995, 130:401–405.

9. Chou FF, Sheen-Chen SM, Lee TY: Rupture of pyogenic liver abscess. *Am J Gastroenterol* 1995, 90:767–770.

10. Chou FF, Kou HK: Endogenous endophthalmitis associated with pyogenic hepatic abscess. *J Am Coll Surg* 1996, 182:33–36.

11. Han SH: Review of hepatic abscess from *Klebsiella pneumoniae*. An association with diabetes mellitus and septic endophthalmitis. *West J Med* 1995, 162:220–224.

104 Parasitic Diseases of the Liver
Christina M. Coyle and Murray Wittner

■■ PROTOZOAN INFECTIONS

Amebic Liver Abscess

Several species of ameba cause human disease, but amebiasis most commonly is caused by infection with *Entamoeba histolytica*. Hepatic abscess is the most common extraintestinal complication of amebiasis. The initial ameba infection occurs through the gastrointestinal tract. Hepatic involvement may become evident when amebas no longer can be found in the bowel, or there may be no history suggestive of amebic colitis. If unrecognized and untreated, hepatic abscess results in life-threatening disease.

Epidemiology and Classification

Entamoeba histolytica has a worldwide distribution, with higher rates of infection occurring on the Indian subcontinent, in southern and western Africa, and in areas of South and Central America and Mexico. The prevalence of amebic infection is closely related to cultural habits, level of sanitation, crowding, and socioeconomic status. Less than 1% of patients with intestinal amebiasis develop hepatic disease.

The classification of *Entamoeba sp* is based on morphology, antigenic differences, DNA characterization, isozyme analysis, drug susceptibility, host specificity, in vitro growth characteristics, and in vivo virulence. The distinctions between the non-pathogenic *E. dispar* and the pathogenic zymodemes of *E. histolytica* was first defined by the mobility of 4 isozymes on starch-gel electrophoresis. The pathogenic zymodemes of *E. histolytica* also have numerous antigenic diferences from *E. dispar* which is the more widespread species and is associated with an asymptomatic carrier state. Although morphologically indis-tinguishable, these two species can be differentiated by poly-merase chain reaction (PCR) or DNA analysis. The presence of ingested erythroctyes on microscopy is highly suggestive of *E. histolytica* rather than the nonpathogenic *E. dispar*. Similarly, the so-called small race of *E. histolytica* or *E. hartmanni* is also nonpathogenic and is antigenically distinct.

Life Cycle

Entamoeba histolytica has trophozoite, precyst, cyst, and metacyst stages. The cyst, or infectious stage, is ingested and excysts in the small bowel. Almost immediately these metacysts, containing four nuclei, undergo a series of divisions, resulting in eight unin-ucleate trophozoites; these ultimately reside, feed, and multiply in the lumen of the colon. They may then invade the colonic mucosa or encyst in the colon. Cysts are excreted, after which they can remain viable for weeks to months when temperature and mois-ture conditions are favorable. Trophozoites, which may be seen in the stool during an episode of acute colitis, degenerate rapidly outside the body and, therefore, do not transmit infection. The incubation period of amebiasis ordinarily is about 1 to 2 weeks, although it may be shorter with large oral inoculums.

Pathology

Entamoeba histolytica causes clinical disease by secreting a wide variety of hydrolytic enzymes that cause extensive tissue necrosis. Hepatic infection occurs when trophozoites enter the portal blood after invading the blood vessels of the intestinal wall. Triangular areas of ischemic hepatic necrosis may be caused by obstruction of portal vessels. Trophozoites initiate lytic necrosis of the hepatic parenchyma with abscess formation. The abscess is made up of an inner necrotic area filled with viscous liquid, a middle zone of dead hepatic cells or hepatic stroma, and an outer, relatively normal, region in which invading amebas can be identified. The smallest lesions are a few millimeters in diameter, but others may extend to destroy most of the liver. Rapidly forming abscesses need not have an outer limiting capsule. Multiple microabscesses may coalesce to form a single large lesion (Fig. 104-1).

Clinical Manifestations

Patients may present acutely with fever as high as 40°C, chills, and right upper quadrant abdominal pain lasting less than 10 days. At times, pain is referred to the right shoulder or right lower quadrant of the abdomen. Abscesses usually are found in the right lobe of the liver (78%); up to 50% of patients have multiple lesions. Most patients have an enlarged liver and right upper quadrant abdominal tenderness; a mass may be palpable. Punch tenderness over the liver often is elicited. Polymorphonuclear leukocytosis of 15,000 to 20,000/mm³ is common in affected patients, who also have moderate anemia and an elevated erythrocyte sedimentation rate (ESR). The serum alkaline phosphatase level is moderately elevated in about one third of patients; jaundice is not seen as commonly as with pyogenic abscesses [2•]. Routine chest radiographs reveal abnormalities in 25% to 90% of patients with amebic liver abscess; elevation of the right hemidiaphragm, consolidation of the right lung base, or an effusion may be present. An abscess of the left lobe of the liver may present as an epigastric mass, which often is mistaken for a neoplasm. The presence of peritonitis or pericardial rub implies rupture into the peritoneum or pericardial sac, respectively, both of which are life-threatening complications [3•]. A right hepatic abscess may extend through the diaphragm into the right chest cavity or into the pulmonary parenchyma, with subsequent rupture and drainage through a bronchus.

Diagnosis

The diagnosis of amebic liver abscess is suggested by the clinical presentation and confirmed by appropriate imaging and serologic studies. Up to 30% of affected patients have no history of diarrhea. In about 30% of cases parasites are not found on stool examination. Ultrasound, computed tomography (CT), and magnetic resonance imaging (MRI) have dramatically improved the ability to make the diagnosis of amebic abscess; ultrasound is considered the imaging procedure of choice. Although CT has better resolution, it does not provide additional data unless one wishes to evaluate impending rupture through the diaphragm (Fig. 104-2) [4]. Diagnostic aspiration under CT or ultrasound guidance may yield typical reddish brown "anchovy paste" material, although the aspirate is more often yellow or gray-green. Typically, the aspirate is sterile. Amebas rarely are seen by direct examination of aspirated fluid, although often they can be isolated if the aspirate material is cultured.

Serology, an important adjunct to imaging studies, may be helpful in diagnosing extraintestinal amebiasis. Serum antibodies develop only to *E. histolytica* infection (not to *E. dispar*, a non-pathogenic species of ameba, morphologically indistinguishable from *E. histolytica*) and may remain positive for years after infection; they are present in 99% of patients with amebic liver abscess. Results of serologic tests done on patients who have recently arrived from endemic areas may be misleading. If the presentation is acute (*ie*, within the first week of infection) the serologic test results may be negative but will turn positive within 10 days. The absence of antibodies in a patient who has had symptoms for more than 1 week argues strongly against the diagnosis of amebiasis. Enzyme-linked immunosorbent assay (ELISA) and indirect hemagglutination assay cannot differentiate between acute and past infection in endemic areas. An ELISA that detects antigen in serum and stool has recently been developed; early studies suggest that this method can differentiate between intestinal infection with *E. histolytica* and *E. dispar*.

Treatment

Most hepatic abscesses respond dramatically to metronidazole, 750 mg, given orally or intravenously three times a day for 10 days. Relapses have been reported in a small number of patients. If relapse occurs, treatment with metronidazole should be reinstituted and a luminicidal drug (*eg*, iodoquinol or diloxanide furoate) should be given. In a small number of patients, it may be necessary to drain amebic abscesses surgically, especially if the lesions are

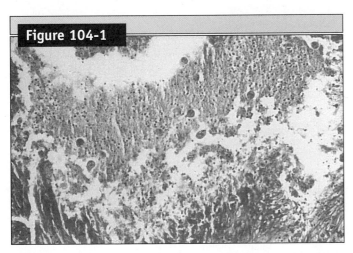

Figure 104-1

Microscopic section of an amebic liver abscess shows necrotic liver tissue. A few amebaes are present.

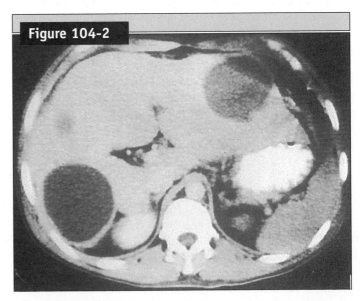

Figure 104-2

Computed tomographic scan shows right and left amebic abscesses. They were treated medically without drainage.

larger than 6 or 8 cm in diameter. Radiographic abnormalities may persist for up to 2 years, but patients should be observed until temperature and leukocyte counts have remained normal for at least 2 weeks after therapy has been completed and the ESR has returned to normal. A rising ESR suggests that the patient has had a relapse.

Prevention

Infection often is acquired by drinking contaminated water or eating fresh fruits and vegetables that were fertilized with human feces or washed with contaminated water. Food handlers should have stools examined and should be treated if *E. histolytica* is found. Human feces to be used as fertilizer should be composted; composting should eradicate cysts. Drinking water in unsafe communities, including water for brushing teeth, should be boiled or treated with Globaline tablets that contain 20 mg of tetraglycine hydroperiodide, 90 mg of sodium hydropyrophosphate, and 5 mg of talc. Fruit should be washed with Globaline-treated water or blanched at 80° to 85°C for 30 to 45 seconds.

Leishmania

Leishmaniasis is a spectrum of diseases of the viscera, mucous membranes, and skin caused by a group of obligate intracellular protozoans of the genus *Leishmania*. These infections, which are transmitted by a variety of phlebotomine sandfly species, are enzootic in feral and domestic animals, especially canines and rodents. Organisms of *Leishmania* spp. are morphologically indistinguishable but fall into several defined species complexes based on clinical and epidemiologic features; they often can be distinguished by serologic and biochemical tests.

Three major clinical forms of leishmaniasis are recognized: visceral leishmaniasis or kala-azar caused by *Leishmania donovani* and the related species *Leishmania infantum* in the Middle East and *Leishmania chagasi* in the western hemisphere; Old World cutaneous leishmaniasis caused by *Leishmania major*, *Leishmania tropica*, and *Leishmania aethiopica*; and American (or New World) cutaneous and mucocutaneous leishmaniasis caused by species complexes of *Leishmania mexicana* and *Leishmania braziliensis*, respectively. *Leishmania donovani* invades and multiplies in visceral reticuloendothelial cells, resulting in enlargement of these organs, fever, and profound anemia; untreated disease is fatal in 90% to 95% of cases. Hepatic manifestations occur almost exclusively in visceralizing disease. Visceral leishmaniasis or kala-azar is found widely from the Straits of Gibraltar across the Mediterranean through Asia to the east coast of China. In the western hemisphere, it occurs in Brazil, northern Argentina, Paraguay, Venezuela, Colombia, Guatemala, and Mexico [5].

Life Cycle

Amastigotes, the obligate intracellular form of leishmania, are round or oval bodies about 2 to 4 mm in diameter that have a single nucleus and a rod-shaped kinetoplast with a flagellar rudiment. Amastigotes are engulfed by macrophages, in which they multiply repeatedly by binary fission, and which they eventually destroy. Released parasites are again phagocytized, and the process is repeated. A sandfly feeding on an infected host ingests amastigote-infected macrophages, which are liberated in the midgut, develop into promastigotes, multiply, and then gradually move to the buccal cavity for deposit in the bite wound during the next blood meal.

Pathology

The principal pathologic lesions in leishmaniasis are a result of reticuloendothelial cell hyperplasia, especially in the liver and spleen. Later, marrow and lymph nodes become crowded with infected macrophages and myelophthisic anemia, and leukopenia may result. The Kupffer cells of the liver, filled with amastigotes, are swollen and hyperplastic, and centrilobular necrosis and fatty infiltration often are observed (Fig. 104-3). In late-stage or chronic disease, fibrosis may give a nodular cirrhotic appearance. The liver in subclinical cases may contain noncaseating granulomas with a few scattered parasites.

Seroepidemiologic studies have shown that subclinical visceral leishmaniasis is much more common than is clinical disease. Evidently, individuals who are able to develop a suitable cell-mediated immune reaction (Th1) can control the infection, whereas those who have defective cell-mediated immunity (Th2) have low levels of interferon-γ, interleukin-1, and interleukin-2 and exhibit clinical disease until they are able to mount a suitable cell-mediated immune reaction, such as is seen following successful clinical therapy.

Clinical Manifestations

At the bite wound, a small pea-sized dermal lesion may form, and parasites, initially localized in dermal macrophages, disseminate within macrophages to the spleen, liver, bone marrow, and lymph nodes, predominantly. Within these organs, lymphocytogenesis and histiocytogenesis occur, resulting in hepatosplenomegaly and lymphadenopathy. Massive splenomegaly (about 1500 to 2000 g) occurs often. The dark gray appearance of the skin seen in Indian visceral leishmaniasis has given rise to the name *kala-azar* (black sickness). Progressive disease is marked by weight loss, canker sores, and fever; a bleeding diathesis often develops shortly before death. Hyperglobulinemia (>10 g/dL), polyclonal B-cell activation, leukopenia, eosinopenia, and anemia are typical. As a patient becomes debilitated and the immune system is compromised, bacterial superinfection or malaria supervenes and often is the imme-

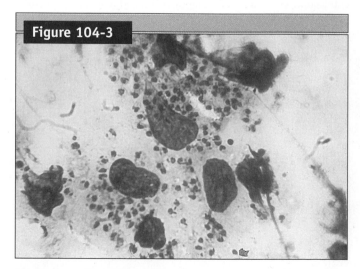

Figure 104-3

Touch preparation of liver biopsy shows numerous amastigotes in Kupffer's cells.

diate cause of death. Visceral leishmaniasis has become recognized as an important opportunistic infection in patients with AIDS.

Diagnosis

Visceral leishmaniasis is diagnosed by detection of organisms in stained smears of splenic aspirate, bone marrow, liver biopsy, or the buffy coat. Splenic puncture and liver biopsy usually are diagnostic in infected people, but the former is hazardous in individuals with a bleeding diathesis. ELISA and indirect fluorescent antibody (IFA) test results usually are positive in patients with visceral leishmaniasis. The IFA is highly specific, as are the indirect hemagglutination and gel diffusion tests. The complement fixation test results, however, are positive in only 65% to 70% of affected individuals. Sera from patients with visceral leishmaniasis are known to give false-positive results with antibodies to *Trypanosoma cruzi*; thus, in the western hemisphere, these antibodies may have to be absorbed out. It is important to recognize that IFA titers usually drop after cure so that a negative titer is often regarded as a sign of successful therapy.

Treatment

Pentavalent antimonials have been the standard therapy for visceral leishmaniasis for many years. These compounds are available in the form of sodium stibogluconate (Pentostam; Wellcome, United Kingdom, available from The Centers for Disease Control and Prevention [CDC]) and meglumine antimoniate (Glucantime; France). Alternative treatments for visceral leishmaniasis include amphotericin B and pentamidine, but these drugs usually are reserved for therapy of cases unresponsive to antimony or patients who relapse [6].

Other Protozoan Infections

Other protozoan infections also have been associated with hepatitis syndromes. *Toxoplasma gondii* may cause hepatitis with granulomatous changes, as has been described in congenital toxoplasmosis associated with the TORCH syndrome (toxoplasma, rubella, cytomegalovirus, herpes virus). In other hosts, both immunocompromised and immunocompetent, hepatitis is associated with fever and disseminated infection. In infants and immunocompromised persons these infections have responded to pyrimethamine and sulfadiazine.

Microsporidia also are associated with granulomatous hepatitis. Microsporidia belonging to the families *Encephalitozoonidae* and *Trachipleistophora* cause a disseminated infection in immunocompromised persons and are primarily described in AIDS patients with granulomatous hepatitis. Response to albendazole has been noted in various case reports. A microsporidian of the genus *Nosema* was associated with disseminated disease and hepatitis in an athymic child.

▬ TREMATODE INFECTIONS
Schistosomiasis

Schistosomiasis is caused by infection with human blood flukes. Human disease is most commonly associated with the granulomatous response of the host to eggs deposited in tissues by worms. Five schistosome species cause human infection; they differ in global distribution, morphology, location in the host, and pathogenic mechanism. *Schistosoma mansoni* infects the inferior mesenteric veins and is found in the Middle East, Africa, the Caribbean, and South America. *Schistosoma japonicum* infects the superior mesenteric veins; its endemic areas include China, the Philippines, and a few areas of Southeastern Asia. *Schistosoma haematobium* infects the vesicle venous plexus and is found principally in Africa and the Middle East. *Schistosoma intercalatum* infects the inferior mesenteric veins and is endemic to West and Central Africa. *Schistosoma mekongi* infects the mesenteric veins and is found in Southeast Asia.

Life Cycle

Schistosomes have two distinct hosts: humans are the definitive host, and snails of particular species are the intermediate hosts. Sexual maturation and mating occur in the human host, whereas the asexual stage and reproduction occur in the snail. The longer female resides within a fold or schist (*ie*, the gynecophoric canal) of the male and deposits eggs into the small veins of the intestine or urinary bladder of the host. About half the eggs (Fig. 104-4, see also **Color Plate**) make their way through the tissues to the lumen of the intestine or urinary bladder, from which they are deposited in fresh water, where they hatch, releasing a free-swimming ciliated embryo, or *miracidium*. The latter find and penetrate a susceptible snail and undergo asexual reproduction, leading to the shedding of thousands of free-swimming larvae, termed *cercariae*. These fork-tailed cercariae penetrate human skin, and, in doing so, lose their tails and develop into schistosomula. Schistosomula migrate through the venous system to the lungs and then the liver, where they mature, pair, and mate. The paired worms leave the liver through the portal veins and migrate to their final destination. Oviposition usually begins about 3 to 12 weeks after cercarial penetration. Eggs are released into the superior or inferior mesenteric or vesicle plexus of veins. About half of the eggs lodge locally in the tissue (intestinal submucosa or mucosa or bladder wall) or are swept back by the portal or systemic blood flow, ultimately lodging in the portal triads of the liver and the small vessels of the lung. The location of the eggs determines the clinical presentation.

Pathology

Many of the pathologic findings in chronic schistosomiasis are caused by the delayed hypersensitivity reaction of the host to the

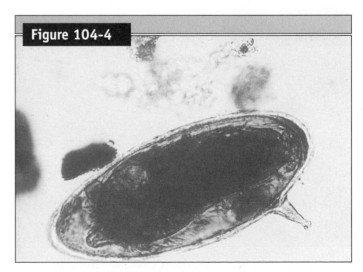

Figure 104-4

Ovum of *Schistosoma mansoni* in the stool (iodine stain). See also **Color Plate**.

eggs and the granulomata that form in the tissue surrounding them. Granulomata consist of macrophages, lymphocytes, and eosinophils, and ultimately heal by fibrosis. Disease occurs if granulomata and the fibrosis they stimulate are situated in crucial anatomic sites.

Eggs that lodge in the portal triads cause periportal fibrosis that may lead to severe "pipe-stem" portal fibrosis (*ie*, Symmers fibrosis) resulting in presinusoidal portal hypertension (Fig. 104-5). Liver involvement is primarily mesenchymal rather than parenchymal; therefore, liver function usually is preserved until late in the disease. Splenomegaly (Banti's splenopathy) and hypersplenism may cause severe pancytopenia requiring splenectomy. Eggs may reach the pulmonary vasculature through portosystemic anastomoses and elicit a fibrotic granulomatous reaction resulting in chronic obliterative arteritis, pulmonary hypertension, and, eventually, cor pulmonale.

Clinical Presentation

Cercarial penetration of the skin causes a transient, pruritic, papular rash known as *Kabure itch*. Katayama fever or acute schistosomiasis may occur with maturation of the worms and the onset of egg production. This is a serum sickness–like syndrome that includes fever, eosinophilia, urticaria, melena, lymphadenopathy, and hepatosplenomegaly. Symptoms may persist for months before abating gradually, although very severe cases may result in death.

Hepatomegaly is an early sign of liver involvement. True cirrhosis does not occur unless there is coinfection with hepatitis B (HBV) or C (HCV) virus. Splenic enlargement and a large left hepatic lobe are seen in compensated hepatosplenic schistosomiasis. Serum aminotransferase levels usually are normal, and a mildly elevated serum alkaline phosphatase level often is observed. Severe hematemesis secondary to esophageal varices may be the presenting symptom in chronic hepatosplenic schistosomiasis. Because hepatocellular function is preserved in affected individuals, their prognosis after a variceal bleed is better than that of patients with diffuse hepatocellular disease. Ascites, commonly seen in Egypt, is rarely reported in Brazil. End-stage liver disease usually is heralded by liver failure, encephalopathy, ascites, and hypoalbuminemia.

Schistosomiasis is associated with recurrent salmonella bacteremia. It has been suggested that the schistosome tegument binds salmonella. Concurrent hepatosplenic schistosomiasis and HBV infection are associated with severe liver disease that may be caused by the simultaneous presence of two hepatic pathogens; affected patients often develop jaundice, intractable ascites, and hepatic failure. As mentioned, significant comorbidity with HBV and HCV infections has been well described. Patients with hepatitis C and schistosomiasis have decreased response to interferon therapy [7]. The clinical management of hepatitis is more complicated in these patients, and the prognosis is worse than that for hepatosplenic schistosomiasis alone. Patients chronically infected with schistosomiasis (most commonly those with *S. mansoni* and *S. japonicum* infection) also may develop proteinuria and nephrotic syndrome leading to chronic renal failure.

Diagnosis

A definitive diagnosis is made by detection of schistosome eggs in stool, urine, or biopsy specimens. Because of limited sampling ability, liver biopsy is not a sensitive method for diagnosis (Fig. 104-6, see also **Color Plate**), but it is an important tool when evaluating comorbid conditions such as hepatitis. Rectal biopsy is useful in making the diagnosis. The Kato-Katz thick smear is used to detect and quantitate eggs in the stool. This method makes use of glycerol, which traps the eggs and makes them visible to the observer. The CDC offers a screening enzyme-linked immunosorbent assay (FAST-ELISA) and a confirmatory Western blot assay to detect antibodies against adult worm antigens. Serologic abnormalities may remain positive long after infection has resolved, limiting the usefulness of these tests in patients indigenous to endemic areas.

Treatment

Praziquantal, a broad-spectrum antihelminthic agent, is well-tolerated and is effective against all species of schistosomiasis. Praziquantal is given for *S. haematobium* and *S. mansoni* orally in two doses of 20 mg/kg for 1 day. *S. japonicum* and *S. mekongi* are treated with 20 mg/kg in three doses for 1 day. The medication

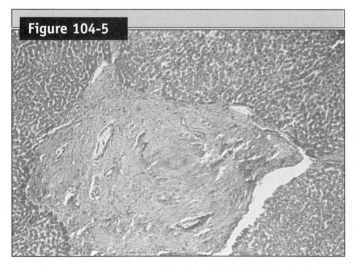

Figure 104-5

Extensive periportal fibrosis (Symmer's pipestem fibrosis) in hepatosplenic schistosomiasis. Bile capillary proliferation is evident.

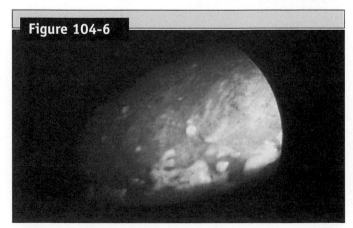

Figure 104-6

Laparoscopic photograph of the liver shows multiple granulomata in a Surinamese woman. See also **Color Plate**.

may produce transient mild side effects, including nausea, anorexia, abdominal discomfort, headache, dizziness, drowsiness, and itching. Cure rates range from 60% to 98%.

In patients with hepatosplenic schistosomiasis, treatment halts the progression of disease by decreasing worm burden and egg deposition; periportal fibrosis often slowly regresses. Patients with severe portal hypertension and extensive fibrosis are less likely to respond to treatment [8].

Patients with hepatosplenic schistosomiasis complicated by varices may benefit from prophylaxis with propanolol. Sclerotherapy has been shown to control variceal bleeding effectively. Long-term portal decompression with transjugular intrahepatic portosystemic stent shunts (TIPSS) may be complicated by shunt stenosis from pseudointimal hyperplasia. Decompressive shunt surgery, particularly with nonselective shunts, may lead to hepatic encephalopathy; distal splenorenal shunts, therefore, are recommended. Esophagogastric devascularization, when performed correctly, may have the highest survival and lowest encephalopathy rates.

Fasciola hepatica

Fasciola hepatica, the sheep liver fluke, a large (2 to 3 cm), leaf-shaped trematode of herbivores parasite, is found most commonly in underdeveloped countries but also is reported in Europe (Fig. 104-7). This flatworm resides in the bile ducts, where it produces eggs that pass into bile, the intestine, and, ultimately, freshwater streams. The egg matures in water and ciliated larva (miracidium) develop, which, upon hatching, penetrate particular species of snails (Fig. 104-8). After 1 or 2 months, free-swimming cercariae emerge from the snail and encyst on the leaves of aquatic vegetation, forming metacercariae. Human disease usually occurs after ingestion of watercress or contaminated water. The ingested larvae excyst, penetrate the gut wall, enter the peritoneal cavity, pass into the liver through Glisson's capsule, and eventually invade the intrahepatic bile ducts.

Clinical Manifestations

There are acute and chronic forms of fascioliasis. Acute disease can present with the classic triad of prolonged fever, hepatomegaly, and abdominal pain localized to the hypochondrium or epigastrium [9••]. Asthenia, anorexia, wasting, and urticaria are common, and marked eosinophilia is almost universally present. Intraductal bleeding may occur during the invasion of the liver, giving rise to hemobilia [10], hemoperitoneum, subcapsular hematoma, or a hepatic mass. Infrequently, affected patients may complain of respiratory symptoms, with chest radiographs revealing parenchymal infiltrates resembling Löffler's syndrome. Some patients may have a more prolonged course and present with painful hepatomegaly suggestive of a malignancy; in these cases the eosinophilia should be a clue to the diagnosis.

After a few months, young flukes migrate into the bile ducts, mature, and begin to oviposit. Periductal fibrosis and bile duct epithelial hyperplasia often develop. Adult worms may persist in the bile ducts for years, leading to chronic fascioliasis, which usu-

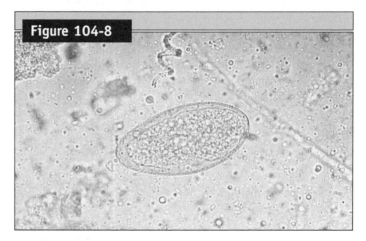

Figure 104-8

Egg of *Fasciola hepatica*. Eggs that pass into the duodenum can be found by stool examination. These eggs must be differentiated from those of *Fasciolopsis buski*.

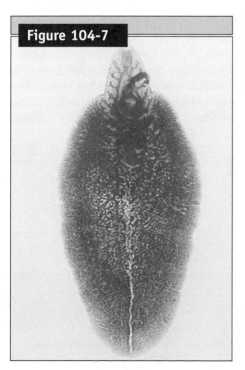

Figure 104-7

Fasciola hepatica, the sheep liver fluke. These organisms are found in the biliary ducts and may cause obstruction.

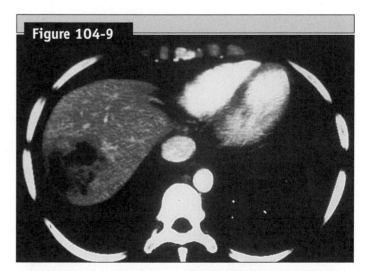

Figure 104-9

Computed tomographic scan of the liver shows acute fascioliasis with 45% eosinophilia in a woman 29 years of age from the Dominican Republic. Diagnosis was suggested by a history of eating fresh watercress and confirmed by serologic studies.

ally manifests as episodic biliary pain or cholangitis. Worms or their egg masses trapped in mucus may serve as a nidus for stone formation and bile duct obstruction. Patients often are incorrectly diagnosed as having cholelithiasis [11].

Diagnosis

Imaging studies are important for establishing the diagnosis and for following patients on therapy (Fig. 104-9). CT scans may show small areas of attenuation in the periphery of the liver in acute fasciola infections; these resolve spontaneously or with treatment [12••]. Thickening of the liver capsule secondary to inflammation or subcapsular hematoma also may be seen. In chronic fascioliasis, ultrasound is useful for evaluating the biliary tree. Findings on ultrasound include irregular linear echogenic images in the gallbladder, biliary dilation, and thickening of the bile duct. Percutaneous cholangiography and endoscopic retrograde cholangiopancreatography (ERCP) may reveal filling defects in the chronic stage, which may be misinterpreted as sclerosing cholangitis. Flukes have been extracted from the pancreatic and bile ducts using an endoscope.

The method most widely used for immunodiagnosis of *Fasciola hepatica* is ELISA. The ELISA rapidly detects antibody to the excretory–secretory (E-S) antigen products of adult *F. hepatica* and is 100% sensitive and 97.8% specific for detection of antigen product. Cross-reactivity with schistosome, however, has been observed. Antibodies develop as early as 2 to 4 weeks after infection in the animal model. Antibody levels to E-S antigen remain elevated for years and decline with successful therapy. These tests are not currently available in the United States.

Treatment

The therapies currently available for fascioliasis have been disappointing. Emetine hydrochloride, for acute and chronic disease, must be given intramuscularly and can be cardiotoxic, although it has been successful in clearing stools in patients with chronic fasciola infection. Side effects include hypotension, tachycardia, and electrocardiographic changes. Dehydroemetine is tolerated better, with fewer cardiac side effects, and may be an alternative.

Although initially encouraging, praziquantal has proven to be ineffective as treatment of this disease. Albendazole, used against fasciola infections in animals, has a high failure rate in humans. Bithionol (2,2′-thiobis-(4,6-dichlorophenol) is given on alternate days (50 mg/kg/d) for 15 days; the cure rate is approximately 50%. Triclabendazole, a thiobenzimidazole, has good fasciolicide activity against acute and chronic infections in animals. Data on the efficacy and ease of administration of triclabendazole are encouraging. Ninety percent of patients (19 of 24) with chronic fasciola had no eggs in their stools 2 months after treatment with a single dose of triclabendazole. At 12 months, 91.3% of patients had negative ELISA serology. Patients with persistently positive ELISA titers were retreated, and their ELISA serology reverted to normal. This treatment for fasciola is promising, given the single dose required, few adverse side effects, and efficacy [13].

Prevention

Avoiding consumption of raw watercress is the most effective means of preventing fascioliasis. Eradication of this disease, however, probably depends on eliminating the infection in herbivores by suitable therapy. Because the infection rate of sheep in Europe and the United States is extremely high, this infection is a constant threat unless veterinary control is exercised.

Clonorchis

Clonorchis sinensis infection is endemic to China, Hong Kong, Japan, Taiwan, and Vietnam, with dogs and cats as reservoir hosts and humans and other fish-eating mammals as definitive hosts. The moderate-sized (1 to 2.5 cm) adult worms may live in the biliary tract for years and occasionally invade the pancreatic duct (Fig. 104-10, see also **Color Plate**). They produce small brownish eggs with a distinctive operculum (lid) which are released into the bile and pass into fresh water with the feces (Fig. 104-11) [14]; snails ingest the eggs, and sporocysts and rediae develop. In 4 to 6 weeks cercariae escape from the snails and encyst under the scales or in the flesh of many species of freshwater fish, especially members of the carp family, to develop into metacercariae. If the uncooked infected fish is eaten, the metacercariae excyst in the duodenum of the host, enter the common bile duct through the ampulla of Vater, and migrate to intrahepatic biliary radicals, where they mature in about 3 to 5 weeks. Consumption of raw infected fish causes infection in the definitive hosts including humans and other fish-eating mammals. Disease most often is the result of cumulative infection

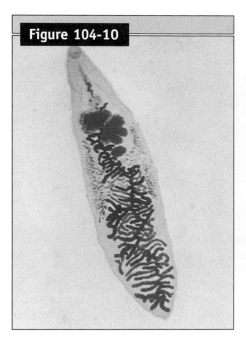

Figure 104-10

Adult *Clonorchis sinensis*, the Chinese liver fluke. This organism, which is found in the biliary ducts, can be present in very large numbers, causing the signs and symptoms of bile duct obstruction. See also **Color Plate**.

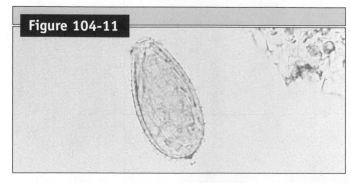

Figure 104-11

Egg of *Clonorchis sinensis*. These small, characteristic eggs pass into the duodenum from the biliary ducts and can be recognized on examination of the stool.

during a lifetime of eating raw fish. Metacercariae are resistant to refrigeration, brine, vinegar, and spices. Because raw fish is rarely consumed by young children, the incidence of disease is low in those under 5 years of age. Many immigrants from Asia to the United States are infected with *C. sinensis*.

Pathology

Worms in the bile ducts provoke ductal epithelial and goblet cell hyperplasia, fibroblastic proliferation of the wall, and periductal fibrosis, with infiltration of neutrophils, eosinophils, lymphocytes, and plasma cells (Fig. 104-12). In heavy infections, there may be extensive periportal fibrosis. Dead worms and egg masses trapped in mucus also serve as a nidus for stone formation [15].

Clinical Manifestations

Depending on the number of worms present in the bile ducts, disease may be asymptomatic or may present as complete biliary obstruction. In acute clonorchiasis following initial exposure to infected fish, patients may have chills and fever to 40°C. The liver may enlarge and become tender, and an eosinophilia of 10% to 40% may be seen. Serum liver enzyme and bilirubin levels may increase. Eggs may be found in the stool 3 to 5 weeks after the acute episode (Fig. 104-11). In later years, signs of recurrent cholelithiasis, cholecystitis, and biliary obstruction may appear. It is not uncommon for an infection with hundreds of worms to be active for 20 or more years, with few or no serious side effects.

The most common complication of clonorchiasis is recurrent pyogenic cholangitis, or "oriental" cholangiohepatitis, typified by cholestasis and secondary bacterial infection with *Escherichia coli*. The eggs, excess mucous, and bacteria furnish a nidus for formation of pigment gallstones. Repeated episodes of abdominal pain, fever, jaundice, and hepatomegaly occur secondary to partial biliary obstruction. Cholangiography demonstrates markedly dilated intrahepatic ducts and defects representing stones or a mass of flukes. Pericholangitis, multiple hepatic abscesses, and a postnecrotic or biliary cirrhosis have been reported, as has stricture of the left hepatic duct. Severe infections are associated with pancreatitis and cholangiocarcinoma. Recovery of eggs from stools or duodenal aspirate fluid is diagnostic (Fig. 104-11).

Treatment

Clonorchiasis can be treated successfully with praziquantal, 25 mg/kg, three times in 1 day. Because praziquantal has not been approved for this use, informed consent should be obtained from patients before treatment. Secondary suppurative cholangitis should be treated with appropriate antibiotics, and surgical intervention may be indicated for biliary obstruction. In light infections the outlook usually is good. Avoiding raw fish probably is the best means of reducing infection. Human feces are used in China as a source of nitrogen for ponds in which carp are being raised; composting feces before use decreases the spread of clonorchiasis (Fig. 104-13).

Opisthorchiasis

Opisthorchiasis is caused by *Opisthorchis felineus* and *Opisthorchis viverrini*. The former is common in southern, central, and especially eastern Europe; central Asia; India; Japan; the Philippines; and Vietnam. The latter is reported in northeastern Thailand and Laos, where the prevalence of infection can reach nearly 95%. The life cycle, pathology, clinical presentation, and treatment of these disorders are similar to those of clonorchiasis.

Metorchiasis

The North American liver fluke, *Metorchis conjunctus*, regularly infects many fish-eating mammals in North America. It also has been reported to infect humans, although infrequently.

Metorchis conjunctus (Fig. 104-14*A*, see also **Color Plate**) is widely reported in carnivores from the Atlantic coast of the United States extending westward to the prairie states, and as far south as South Carolina. *M. conjunctus* has also been reported in carnivores from the Atlantic coast of Canada and the Canadian provinces, to the northern territories of Canada. This fluke is closey related to *Clonorchis sinensis*, *Opisthorchis viverrini* and *O. felineus*. The first intermediate host is the aquatic snail *Amnicola limosa* and several species of fresh water fish serve as the second intermediate hosts; most commonly the white sucker *Catostomus commersoni*. The life history of *Metorchis* is similar to that of *Clonorchis*.

In a clinical outbreak of 19 individuals who ate raw fish (sashimi), 17 developed symptoms consisting of fatigue (79%), persis-

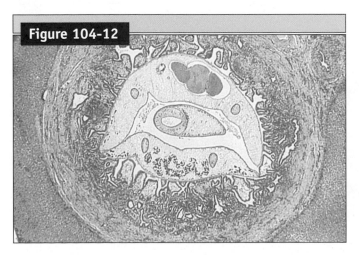

Figure 104-12

Two flukes (*Clonorchis sinensis*) in a bile duct. There is bile duct epithelial hyperplasia and periductal fibrosis.

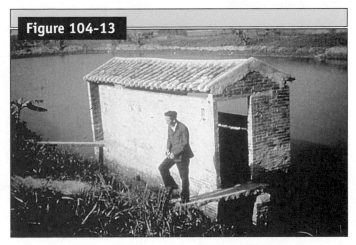

Figure 104-13

This fish pond in southern China is fertilized with human waste, ensuring the growth of large, nutritious, but infectious, carp.

tent upper abdominal pain (68%), low grade fever (63%), headache (63%), weight loss (58%), and diarrhea (26%). Abnormal liver function was found in most patients; leukocytosis and eosinophilia were also noted, the latter to return to normal levels in about a month after treatment with praziquantel [16]. Asymptomatic human infections have been occasionally reported, diagnosed by finding metorchis eggs on fecal examination (Fig. 104-14B). Because the metacercaria (Fig. 104-14C) of this fluke is found in yellow perch, brook trout, longnose sucker, and fallfish, as well as the white sucker, the extent of this infection in humans in North America remains to be determined. No chronic cases have been recognized.

Dicrocoeliasis and Eurytremiasis

Dicrocoeliasis and eurytremiasis are trematode diseases of the biliary tree and pancreatic duct in herbivores caused by the trematodes *Dicrocoelium dendriticum* and *Eurytrema pancreaticum*. *D. dendriticum* is found in the bile ducts of sheep, deer, water buffalo, and cattle and occurs in Europe, Turkey, northern Africa, and parts of the Far East. *E. pancreaticum*, a parasite of the pancreatic duct of herbivores, has been reported to cause human disease in Hong Kong, Kiangsu province in China, and Japan [17].

Life Cycle

The life cycles of these organisms are similar, requiring two intermediate hosts, a snail and an insect. Eggs of the adult fluke, which lives in the biliary tree of herbivores, pass into feces and are ingested by land snails. In the snail, cercariae develop and are released in slime shed by the snail on vegetation. Cercariae develop into infective metacercariae when ingested by various insects, the second intermediate host. Various species of ants are the second intermediate hosts of *D. dendriticum*; *E. pancreaticum* infects grasshoppers in Malaysia and tree crickets in central Asia. The life cycle is completed when the insect is ingested by a grazing herbivore. Humans become infected after accidental ingestion of infected insects or, more commonly, after ingestion of infected animal livers. Disease in humans is unusual.

Clinical Manifestations

Symptoms usually are mild, although with heavy infection there may be biliary colic, vomiting, and diarrhea. Hepatomegaly, jaundice, and eosinophilia are rare.

Diagnosis and Treatment

Diagnosis is made by finding the characteristic eggs in the stool. The eggs of *E. pancreaticum* and *D. dendriticum* are indistinguishable. Spurious infection or false dicrocoeliasis, caused by eating infected raw sheep liver, must be ruled out by repeated examinations of the stool.

Treatment is praziquantal, using the same dosage employed for opisthorchiasis and clonorchiasis.

Visceral Larva Migrans

Visceral larva migrans occurs when a zoonotic larval nematode, unable to finish its life cycle, migrates through tissue and incites an inflammatory reaction in the host. The roundworms of the dog (*Toxocara canis*) and cat (*T. cati*) are most often implicated as the cause of this disease. In humans, most infections have been reported in children 1 to 4 years of age with a history of either contact with puppies or pica, especially geophagy. Serologic surveys in children in the United States suggest that the prevalence of human toxocara infection ranges from 2% to 10%.

Life Cycle

The adult worm, which is 8 to 12 cm long, lives in the small intestine of the adult dog or cat. The ova are deposited with the feces and become infective within 2 weeks. Because of their thick shells, they may remain viable for months to years (Fig. 104-15). If they are swallowed by young dogs, second stage larvae hatch in the small intestine, penetrate the intestinal wall, migrate to the lungs, and finally reach the small intestine, where they mature. In older dogs, larvae may undergo somatic migration and encyst in the tissues. Encystment occurs more often in bitches than in males, and the encysted larvae serve as the source of perinatal infection in puppies. The infection also can be transmitted via colostrum [18].

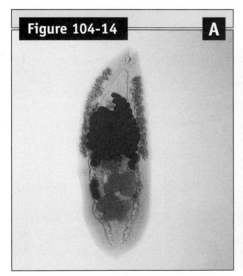
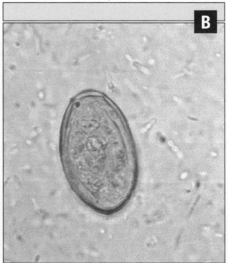
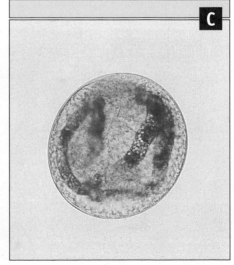

Figure 104-14   **A**   **B**   **C**

A, Adult *Metorchis conjunctus*. See also **Color Plate**. **B**, Egg of *Metorchis conjunctus*. **C**, Metacercaria of *Metorchis conjunctus* from fish flesh. (**A** to **C** *Courtesy of* J.D. MacLean, MD.)

In human hosts, following ingestion of an embryonated egg, a second-stage larva emerges and penetrates the intestinal wall, initiating somatic migration that may last for weeks or months, with a predilection for the liver, lungs, heart, central nervous system, and eyes; other organs also may be invaded. Once in the tissues, the larvae fail to develop, and they incite an inflammatory reaction; thus, diagnostic eggs are never found in stool. Another syndrome, ocular larva migrans (OLM), has been recognized; it occurs most often in older children, in whom pica is uncommon.

Pathology

The liver is the organ most often involved in toxocariasis, probably because of the mesenteric venous portal drainage. Lesions are typically small, gray-white, elevated nodules about 2 to 4 mm in diameter. The liver has irregular areas of focal necrosis and inflammatory reaction around necrotic foci in the portal spaces. Necrotic liver cells are replaced either by amorphous acidophilic material or eosinophilic leukocytes and occasional foreign body giant cells. Larvae occasionally can be recognized in biopsy specimens.

Clinical Presentation

Clinical presentation ranges from asymptomatic eosinophilia to fever, hepatomegaly, hyperglobulinemia, and marked eosinophilia. Patients may complain of wheezing and have pulmonary infiltrates, signs of myocarditis, or evidence of central nervous system involvement. In moderate to heavy toxocara infections, larval invasion of the liver may cause right upper quadrant pain and hepatomegaly. Most infections, however, are subclinical.

Diagnosis

Diagnosis usually is made clinically. Close association with a dog or cat and a history of pica commonly are elicited in cases of visceral larva migrans. Persistent eosinophilia, markedly elevated anti-A or anti-B isohemagglutinin antibody titers in patients who are not blood type AB, a moderate to high increase in serum γ globulin levels, and an elevated ESR all help to confirm the diagnosis. A highly specific and sensitive serologic test employing second-stage secretory antigen in an ELISA appears to be diagnostic and is associated with elevated serum IgM and IgG, but not IgA levels. Hepatic capillariasis must be distinguished from toxocariasis. Liver biopsy may demonstrate characteristic eggs of Capillaria in hepatic granulomata, as discussed later in this chapter.

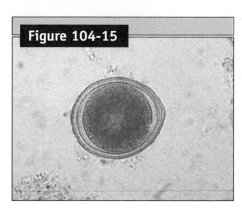

Figure 104-15 Egg of the dog ascarid, *Toxocara canis*. This worm is one of the many causes of visceral larva migrans.

Treatment

Most infections resolve spontaneously, but symptomatic visceral larva migrans appears to respond to oral diethylcarbamazine, 6 mg/kg/d, three doses per day for 7 to 10 days. Albendazole, 400 mg bid for 3 days, and mebendazole, 100 to 200 mg bid for 5 days, also have been used successfully.

Baylisascariasis

Baylisascariasis procyonis is a North American raccoon parasite and also has been reported in Japan and Germany. Humans become infected after accidentally ingesting eggs from areas or objects contaminated with raccoon feces. Bayliascarid eggs may remain infective for years in the soil, posing a long-term health threat. Migrating larvae cause mechanical damage, release toxic enzymes, and incite a vigorous host inflammatory response. Patients may present with visceral, ocular, or neural larva migrans. Signs of visceral larva migrans include hepatomegaly, eosinophilia, and elevation of serum isohemagglutinin titers similar to those in toxocariasis. Severe or fatal baylisascariasis has been reported in children [19]. Neural larva migrans is characterized by cerebrospinal fluid and peripheral eosinophilia. The diagnosis is made on clinical and epidemiologic grounds with supportive serologic testing. Antihelminthics with the greatest promise for therapy include albendazole, mebendazole, fenbendazole, thiabendazole, and levamisole. Clinical neural larva migrans caused by organisms of *Baylisacaris* spp. has a high mortality rate. This infection is largely unrecognized by the medical community.

Capillaria hepatica

Capillaria hepatica is a common cause of hepatic infection in rats and other mammals. It has been found in mice, gerbils, squirrels, muskrats, hares, dogs, pigs, beavers, and some species of monkeys, as well as rats. A single host is required for the life cycle, and the liver contains both the adult parasite and eggs. After the death of the host, the animal decomposes, releasing eggs into the soil; alternatively, the host is eaten by a carnivorous animal and eggs are passed with feces. Eggs are infectious upon embryonization, which occurs after 30 days. Humans are accidentally infected by ingesting soil or food contaminated with eggs. Following ingestion, larvae are released in the intestine and migrate through the intestinal wall to the liver, where they mature, mate, and then disintegrate, releasing numerous eggs, which elicit an intense inflammatory response in the liver parenchyma (Fig. 104-16, see also **Color Plate**). Granulomata that contain eggs and fragments of parasites surrounded by a heavy infiltrate of eosinophils, neutrophils, lymphocytes, and plasma cells are formed, leading to widespread hepatic necrosis, massive hepatomegaly, and fever. Laboratory tests may reveal a leukocytosis of 30,000 to 80,000 leukocytes/mm^3 and eosinophilia of up to 85%. The diagnosis is made by observation of characteristic eggs on liver biopsy. Mortality in this disease is high; patients often die of liver failure. Mebendazole, 200 mg twice a day for 20 days, is the therapy of choice. Albendazole and thiabendazole are considered investigational drugs for this indication by the US Food and Drug Administration. Killing adult worms in the liver may result in an intense inflammatory response further aggravating the disease process.

Hydatid Disease

Hydatid disease is the result of human infection with the larval stage of the dog tapeworm *Echinococcus granulosus*. Sheep- and cattle-raising areas throughout the world are the most heavily endemic regions. In the United States most infections are found in immigrants from endemic areas, including Italy, Greece, and Syria. Canines are the definitive host, and sheep (herbivores) are the intermediate host. A sylvatic cycle in which wolves and coyotes are the definitive hosts and caribou and moose are the intermediate hosts has been reported in the north central United States, Canada, and Alaska and has been responsible for sporadic disease. In the southwestern United States, Navajo, Zuni, and Santo Domingan Indians are infected, as are Basque sheep farmers in the central valley of California and Mormon sheep farmers in Utah.

Life Cycle

The adult worm (0.2 to 1.0 cm long) possesses an armed scolex with one or two immature, one or two mature, and one gravid proglottid (Fig. 104-17). Numerous adult worms may infect the dog's small intestine, passing proglottids or eggs into the stool and, ultimately, the environment. Once the egg is ingest-

ed, it hatches in the duodenum, releasing a hexacanth embryo. This embryo penetrates the duodenal wall and gains access to the lymphatics and blood vessels, then lodges in the liver and at other sites. The surviving larvae develop into cysts that have an inner germinal layer and an outer, noncellular, laminated wall surrounded by fibrosis. The germinal layer proliferates inwardly, forming brood capsules, daughter cysts, and protoscolices (Fig. 104-18). Together, these are termed *hydatid sand*. An individual cyst may contain several million protoscolices (*ie*, hydatid sand), each of which upon ingestion by a canine is capable of becoming a tapeworm. Cyst growth is slow—for example, at 5 to 6 months after infection, the cyst may measure approximately 10 mm.

Pathology

The cysts trigger an encapsulating inflammatory and fibroblastic reaction. These expanding cysts compress and destroy hepatic and

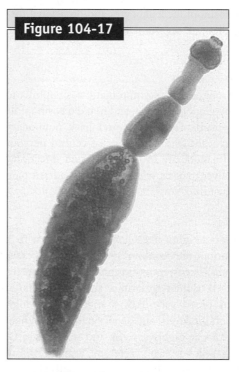

Figure 104-17

Adult *Echinococcus granulosis* from the intestine of a dog. This tapeworm consists of a scolex, an immature, mature and a gravid proglottid.

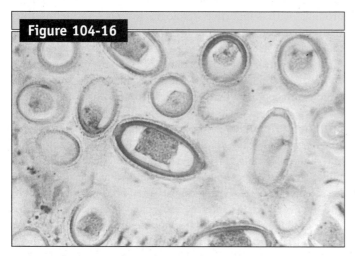

Figure 104-16

Capillariasis caused by *Capillaria hepatica*. Numerous eggs are present in the hepatic parenchyma, causing granulomatous hepatitis. See also **Color Plate**.

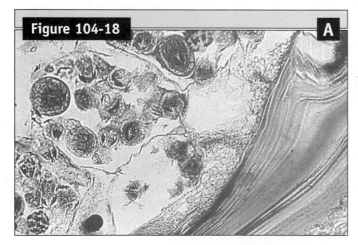

Figure 104-18   **A**

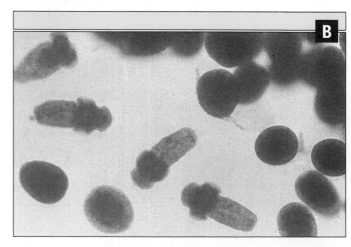

B

A, The wall of a hydatid cyst shows the outer acellular laminar membrane, the inner germinal membrane, and several brood capsules budding from the germinal membrane. Protoscolices are present within the brood capsules. **B,** Protoscolices aspirated from a hydatid cyst.

pulmonary tissues. The fluid within the friable cyst may leak into surrounding tissue, causing a severe hypersensitivity reaction and sometimes fatal anaphylactic shock. At other times, the leaking cyst may seed adjacent tissue with hydatid sand or leak into the peritoneum or lung, resulting in development of multiple daughter cysts. Cysts may develop in any tissue or organ. Seventy percent of cysts occur in the liver (75% of them in the right lobe), and 20% to 30% involve the lung. Other common sites are the kidneys, bones, and brain. When a cyst filled with protoscolices is ingested by the definitive host, *eg*, a dog, large numbers of adult tapeworms develop in the small intestine.

Clinical Presentation

Cysts may grow slowly and silently, and, if they do not impinge on a vital or sensitive area, may be detected incidentally only at autopsy as calcified cysts. Commonly, hepatic cysts present as a tender mass in the right upper quadrant. Patients may complain of early satiety or reflux symptoms if the cyst presses on the stomach. Recognition of complications is vital when caring for a patient with hydatid disease. Minute fissure-like communications between the cyst and the biliary system develop during evolution of the disease in as many as 80% to 90% of patients. Intermittent leakage of hydatid fluid into bile ducts may cause episodes of acute upper abdominal colicky pain with or without allergic manifestations. Some patients develop signs and symptoms of biliary tract disease; in 5% to 8% of patients the cyst ruptures directly into the biliary tree, with partial drainage into the duodenum. Biliary obstruction may occur secondary to impacted parasitic membranes, and ascending cholangitis and pyogenic infection of the cyst cavity may occur (Fig. 104-19, see also **Color Plate**). Affected individuals may present initially with right upper quadrant pain, acholic stools, elevation of serum liver enzyme levels, and fever. Stools may reveal hydatid membranes if partial drainage has occurred. Acalculous gangrenous cholecystitis occurs, although not commonly, secondary to cyst rupture into the gallbladder with obstruction of the gallbladder neck and cystic duct by parasitic membranes acting as a ball valve. Pancreatitis has also been reported. A dreaded complication is rupture of a cyst into the abdominal cavity spontaneously or after trauma. Such rupture causes severe peritonitis and spreads hydatid sand, which may develop into new cysts, throughout the peritoneum. Cysts may rupture through the dome of the liver and diaphragm into the lung or pleural cavity. Development of a persistent cough may herald rupture of a cyst as it impinges on the diaphragm. These patients should be considered for surgical rather than medical therapy. If rupture occurs, the cough may increase, with the appearance of hydatid fluid and membranes in the mouth.

Figure 104-19

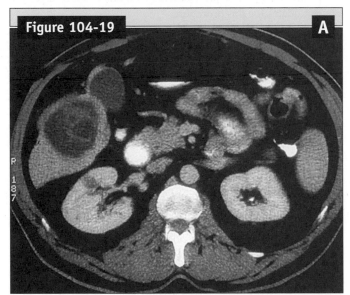

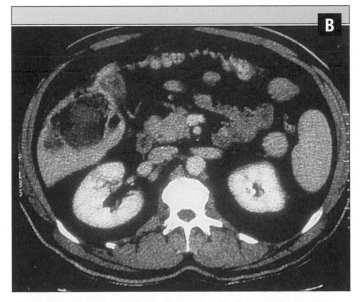

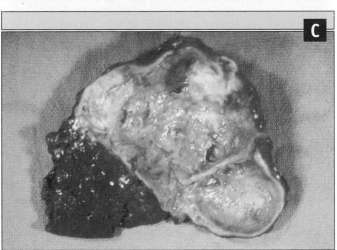

A, A person 52 years of age with right upper quadrant pain, fever, and acholic stools. Computed tomographic scan reveals a hydatid cyst; intracystic membranes are evident. **B,** Ascending cholangitis and superinfection of cyst were seen in the same patient. The cyst ruptured into the hepatic parenchyma. **C,** Surgical specimen from a partial right hepatectomy performed on the same patient. See also **Color Plate**.

Leakage of hydatid fluid often causes allergic symptoms, including urticaria, pruritus, eosinophilia, and respiratory distress. Sudden release of cyst fluid has been reported to cause nearly instantaneous, fatal anaphylactic shock.

Diagnosis

A cystic liver lesion must be differentiated from tumor and bacterial and amebic abscess. A diagnosis of hepatic hydatid disease usually is considered after imaging, and reveals a cystic liver lesion. An epidemiologic history consistent with the diagnosis is an important, if not an essential confirmatory consideration in making the diagnosis.

The principal CT findings in hepatic involvement by *E. granulosus* consist of one or more spherical or oval, sharply defined lesions of water density. This appearance, although consistent with hydatid cyst, is not pathognomonic, because CT images of abscesses, cystic metastases, and congenital cysts may be identical. Findings suggestive of hydatid disease include imaging of the cyst wall on plain CT scan, imaging of daughter cysts within the main lesions, signs of membrane detachment from the inner cyst wall, and intracystic septations. Calcification of the cyst wall is suggestive but not pathognomonic of a hydatid cyst.

Once the diagnosis has been suggested by imaging studies, serologic tests should be done to confirm the diagnosis. Invasive diagnostic studies, including liver biopsy and aspiration, are contraindicated to avoid leaking and spilling. To achieve the highest sensitivity and specificity in serologic diagnosis, more than one test procedure should be performed. An ELISA test using standardized hydatid fluid as antigen, which has high sensitivity but low specificity, and a Western blot (immunoblot) test, which is highly sensitive and specific, should be done concurrently.

Endoscopic retrograde cholangiopancreatography is the diagnostic procedure of choice for identifying a cyst–biliary communication and is indicated in any patient who presents with an echinococcal cyst and jaundice [20]. Patients may have frank intrabiliary rupture with obstruction from impacted membranes; small cyst–biliary communications may be present, or the cyst may cause compression and displacement of the major bile ducts [21]. Cholangiography may be helpful in delineating compression and displacement of the bile ducts before surgery in jaundiced patients. Membranes may be distinguished from stone disease in a patient with biliary obstruction, and an endoscopic approach may be used to evaluate bile duct membranes. Small cyst–biliary communications may be missed because they are usually kept closed by high intracystic pressure. In postsurgical patients with biliary obstruction, cholangiography can distinguish among residual hydatid material, stones, and damage to the duct.

Therapy

The mainstay of therapy for hydatid disease is surgery; this requires careful assessment of the lesion and a skilled surgeon. Techniques include enucleation of small cysts and lobectomy for large or multiple cysts. Just before or at the time of surgery, the cyst should be aspirated to determine whether it is viable and to reduce intracystic pressure [22]. Every patient should receive a 10- to 14-day course of medical therapy with albendazole or praziquantal, which are cysticidal and scolicidal agents.

Ultrasound- and CT-guided percutaneous drainage of hydatid cysts with injection of scolicidal agents have been demonstrated to be safe and effective alternatives to surgery in patients with uncomplicated disease [23•]. A full 28-day course of albendazole should precede percutaneous drainage. Before draining the cyst it is reasonable to perform a cholangiogram to look for biliary communications, which contraindicate percutaneous therapy. Guided drainage consists of aspiration of cyst contents under ultrasound or CT guidance, followed by sclerosing of the cavity. A pigtail catheter is placed within the cavity, which is then completely drained and filled with contrast material to image communications or areas of multiloculation. Sclerosing of the lumen is performed with 95% ethanol, hypertonic saline, or cetrimide in a volume of 20 % to 30% of the cystic fluid aspirated. The fluid is left in the cavity for 20 to 30 minutes while the patient changes position. Hypertonic saline is recommended for inactivating cysts because it is effective and probably safer than alcohol or other scolicidal agents. Albendazole should be given before the procedure and continued for 10 days afterward. Intracystic injection of a scolicidal agent has been performed successfully with a low complication rate. Reported complications include bacterial infection of the punctured cyst, biliary rupture of the cyst, fever, and urticaria. To date there have been no reports of anaphylaxis or spread to the peritoneum. Patients with one or a few large cysts are candidates for this procedure.

Mebendazole has been used extensively to treat this disease, with mixed results, possibly because of poor intestinal absorption. Albendazole, a related benzimidazole with similar activity, has largely replaced mebendazole and appears to be better absorbed [24]. The drug is well-tolerated, with few side effects at 400 mg twice a day for 28 days, although it is reported to be teratogenic and embryotoxic in animals. A reversible elevation of serum aminotransferase levels has been reported after prolonged therapy. Absorption of albendazole is increased when it is taken with a high-fat meal. Surgery may not be feasible in some patients with extensive hydatid disease or in patients with severe underlying medical disorders. During the past few years, patients have been treated successfully with albendazole alone for hydatid disease. In addition, as stated earlier, albendazole has been used in conjunction with surgery and percutaneous drainage. Complete regression of extensive intraabdominal hydatid cystic disease with a prolonged course of albendazole over several years has been reported. Medical treatment of hydatid disease is indicated before surgery and percutaneous drainage and in patients in whom surgery is contraindicated or not possible. Unless otherwise contraindicated, uncomplicated cysts should be treated medically with albendazole. Multiple courses of therapy may be used inasmuch as albendazole is relatively nontoxic and well-tolerated. Postsurgical or post-drainage patients should receive 14 days of praziquantal or 28 days of albendazole therapy to kill larval forms that may have spilled during these procedures.

Alveolar Hydatid Disease

Echinococcus multilocularis is a small tapeworm of foxes, cats, and dogs in which the intermediate hosts are various rodents. The cyst stage consists of multiple small cystic cavities into which protoscolices bud. This parasite originally was described in southern Germany, the republics of the former Soviet Union, and Alaska, and has been reported in foxes in Iowa, Montana, Minnesota, and North Dakota. Humans acquire this infection by ingesting food contaminated with fox and sled dog feces containing eggs. The human liver lesion often is difficult to recognize as being of parasitic origin. The parasite causes a marked inflammatory necrotic lesion that resembles an undifferentiated, locally spreading tumor that has undergone cystic necrosis. Eosinophils and other inflammatory cells are present. Protoscolices usually are not formed. The parasite has been reported to metastasize to other organs, although multiorgan involvement may represent multiple sites of infection [25].

Surgery has been the usual treatment for alveolar hydatid cyst disease. Usually, wide excision of liver is required, because there is no clear demarcation between diseased and normal tissue. If partial hepatectomy is possible, cures often are effected, as indicated by a sharp decline in antibody titer. Recently, long-term high-dose mebendazole therapy (40 mg/kg/d) in inoperable patients appears to have arrested cyst growth or even to have caused cyst regression. Specific antibody levels, however, have remained elevated, suggesting that the infection has not been cured.

Coenurus Infection

Coenuriasis is a relatively unusual zoonotic disease of humans caused by the larval stage (*coenurus*) of a dog tapeworm, *Taenia multiceps*. This parasite has a wide distribution in temperate areas, where it usually circulates in a domestic cycle between dogs and herbivores (sheep). Human infection occurs if eggs are accidentally ingested after being shed in dog feces. After ingestion of the egg, larvae hatch, penetrate the intestinal wall, and migrate to various tissues, where they develop into large cystic larvae. Symptoms are caused by the presence of a cyst in a vital structure. Lymphadenopathy, fever, and malaise may occur, raising the suspicion of lymphoma; eosinophilia is rare [26]. Cysts are found in liver, muscle, and brain. The cysticercus scrology on Western blot is reported to be negative in this infection. Definitive diagnosis depends on surgical removal, which is also therapeutic; benzimidazoles (albendazole) may have some therapeutic efficacy.

▆▆ REFERENCES

Recently published papers of particular interest have been highlighted as follows:
* • Of interest
* •• Of outstanding interest

1. Petri WA, Jackson TFHG, Gathiram V, *et al.*: Pathogenic and non-pathogenic strains of *E. histolytica* can be differentiated by monoclonal antibodies to galactose specific adherence lectin. *Infect Immun* 1990, 581:1802–1806.
2.• Barnes PF, De Cock KM, Reynolds TN: A comparison of amebic and pyogenic abscess of the liver. *Medicine* 1987, 66:472–483.
This is a review and comparison of 96 cases of amebic liver abscess and 48 cases of pyogenic hepatic abscess. The article covers the presentation, diagnosis, and management of each disease.
3.• Adams EB, MacLeod IN: Invasive amebiasis. II. Amebic liver abscess and its complications. *Medicine* 1977, 56:325–334.
This is an excellent review of the complications of amebic liver abscess.
4. Katzenstein D, Rickerson V, Braude M: New concepts of amebic liver abscess derived from hepatic imaging, serodiagnosis, and hepatic enzymes in 67 consecutive cases in San Diego. *Medicine* 1982, 61:237–246.
5. Magill AJ, Grogl M, Gasser RA Jr, *et al.*: Visceral infection caused by *Leishmania tropica* in veterans of Operation Desert Storm. *N Engl J Med* 1993, 328:1383–1387.

6. Chulay JD: Leishmaniasis. In *Hunter's Tropical Medicine*, edn 7. Edited by Strickland GT. Philadelphia: WB Saunders; 1991:638–655.
7. el-Sazly Y, Abdel-Salam AF, Abdel-Ghaffar A, *et al.*: Schistosomiasis as an important determining factor for the response of Egyptian patients with chronic hepatitis C to therapy with recombinant human alpha-2 interferon. *Trans R Soc Trop Med Hyg* 1994, 88:229–231.
8. Homeida MA, el Tom I, Nash T, *et al.*: Association of therapeutic activity of praziquantal with the reversal of Symmers' fibrosis induced by *Schistosoma mansoni*. *Am J Trop Med Hyg* 1991, 45:360–365.
9.•• Arjona R, Riancho JA, Aguado JM, *et al.*: Fascioliasis in developing countries: a review of classic and aberrant forms of the disease. *Medicine* 1995, 74:13–23.
This is a classic review of the varied presentations of fascioliasis.
10. Acuna-Soto R, Braum-Roth G: Bleeding ulcer in the common bile duct due to *Fasciola hepatica*. *Am J Gastro* 1987, 82:560–562.
11. Faiguenbaum J, Feres A, Dunckastea R *et al.*: Fascioliasis (distomiasis) hépatica humana. *Parasitol* 1962, 17:7–12.
12.•• Price TA, Tuazon Cu, Simon GL: Fascioliasis: case reports and review. *Clin Infect Dis* 1993, 17:426–430.
The authors report two cases of fascioliasis, with an excellent discussion of the clinical features, emphasizing serologic, radiographic, and histopathologic studies.
13. Apt W, Aguilera X, Vega F, *et al.*: Treatment of human chronic fascioliasis with triclabendazole: drug efficacy and serologic response. *Am J Trop Med Hyg* 1995, 52:532–535.
14. Lin AC, Chapman SW, Turner HR, Wofford JD: Clonorchiasis: an update. *South Med J* 1987, 80:919–922.
15. Sun Tsieh MD: Pathology and immunology of *Clonorchis sinensis* infection of the liver. *Ann Clin Lab Sci* 1984, 14:208–209.
16. MacLean JD, Arthur JR, Ward BJ, *et al.*: Common-source outbreak of acute infection due to the North American liver fluke *Metorchis conjunctus*. *Lancet* 1996, 347:154–158.
17. Bunnag D, Bunnag T, Goldsmith R: Dicrocoeliasis and eurytremiasis. In *Hunter's Tropical Medicine*, edn 7. Edited by Strickland GT. Philadelphia: WB Saunders; 1991:826–827.
18. Wittner M: Toxocariasis (visceral and ocular larva migrans). In *Rudolph's Pediatrics*, edn 20. Edited by Rudolph AM, Hoffman JIE, Rudolph CD. Stamford, CT: Appleton & Lange; 1996:715–716.
19. Fox AS, Kazacos KR, Gould NS, *et al.*: Fatal eosinophilic meningoencephalitis and visceral larva migrans caused by raccoon ascarid *Baylisascaris procyonis*. *N Engl J Med* 1985, 312:1619–1623.
20. Al Karawi MA, Yasawi MI, el Shiekh Mohamed AR: Endoscopic management of biliary hydatid disease: report on six cases. *Endoscopy* 1991, 23:278.
21. Van Steenbergen W, Fevery J, Broeckaert L, *et al.*: Hepatic echinococcosis ruptured into the biliary tract: clinical, radiological therapeutic features during five episodes of spontaneous biliary rupture in three patients with hepatic hydatidosis. *J Hepatol* 1987, 4:13.
22. Barros JL: Hydatid disease of the liver. *Am J Surg* 1978, 135:597.
23.• Salama H, Farid Abdel-Wahab M, Strickland GT: Diagnosis and treatment of hepatic hydatid cysts with the aid of echo-guided percutaneous cyst puncture. *Clin Infect Dis* 1995, 21:1372–1376.
In this report, the procedure and 3-year follow-up are described for 45 patients with hepatic hydatid cyst who were treated with percutaneous cyst puncture.
24. Gil-Grande LA, Rodriquez-Caabeiro F, Prieto J, *et al.*: Randomised controlled trial of efficacy of albendazole in intraabdominal hydatid disease. *Lancet* 1992, 342:1269
25. Wilson JF, Rausch RL: Alveolar hydatid disease: a review of clinical features of 33 indigenous cases of *Echinococcus multilocularis* in Alaskan Eskimos. *Am J Trop Med Hyg* 1980, 29:1340.
26. Benger A, Rennie RP, Roberts JT, *et al.*: A human Coenurus infection in Canada. *Am J Trop Med Hyg* 1981, 30:638–644.

105 Acute Cholestatic Diseases

Eric D. Libby and Marshall M. Kaplan

Cholestasis is characterized by the accumulation in blood of substances normally secreted in bile. Patients with acute cholestasis may have jaundice, pruritus, dark urine, and acholic stools, although the diagnosis frequently is first suggested by abnormal blood test results. Liver tests are said to have a cholestatic pattern when serum alkaline phosphatase (SAP) and γ-glutamyl transpeptidase (GGT) levels are more abnormal than are serum aminotransferase levels. Serum bilirubin and cholesterol levels sometimes also increase in patients with acute cholestasis. Although rarely measured, serum bile acid levels typically also are elevated.

Acute cholestasis develops in response to a specific insult (*eg*, sepsis, choledocholithiasis, and drug reactions) and almost always resolves when the cause is eliminated. Chronic cholestatic disorders are discussed in Chapter 106, including primary biliary cirrhosis, primary sclerosing cholangitis, vanishing bile duct syndrome, and secondary biliary cirrhosis.

ANATOMY

One of the functions of the liver is the production of bile (see Chapter 87). Bilirubin, bile acids, and other constituents of bile are secreted by hepatocytes into an anastomosing network of canaliculi that lies between each pair of adjacent liver cells (see Chapter 88). The cell membrane of the hepatocytes is the wall of the bile canaliculus. Bile flows from the canaliculi through the canals (or openings) of Hering into the smallest biliary radicals, the portal bile ductules, that are lined by cholangiocytes. These bile ductules then join to form interlobular and then septal bile ducts. Several generations of septal bile ducts ultimately coalesce into the right and left hepatic ducts that, in turn, join to form the common hepatic duct near the hilum of the liver. Interruption of bile flow at any point from the hepatocytes to the large extrahepatic bile ducts may be responsible for cholestasis (Fig. 105-1).

PHYSIOLOGY

Hepatocytes form bile by actively transporting fluid, electrolytes, bilirubin, lipids, bile salts, and other substances to the bile canaliculi. Bilirubin, formed by catabolism of heme, is transported to the liver. There, bilirubin is conjugated with glucuronic acid within the hepatocytes and secreted into the bile canaliculi against a concentration gradient by a carrier-mediated process. Similarly, bile salts are transported into bile against a concentration gradient in a process that depends on electrolyte exchange. Although hepatocytes transport most fluid and electrolytes into the bile, the biliary ductular epithelia also contribute to transportation of bicarbonate and water "downstream" from the hepatocytes. The details of bile secretion and bilirubin metabolism are discussed in greater detail in Chapters 88 and 89.

Production and excretion of bile are essential to normal physiology (Fig. 105-2). In the duodenum, bile salts emulsify dietary fat and facilitate digestion by lipases. Bilirubin is eliminated in bile, as are many toxins and micronutrients, especially copper. Numerous macromolecules synthesized by the liver, including bile salts and lipids, are maintained at normal levels by hepatic elimination. Most of the constituents of bile are excreted in feces. Some bile acids, drugs, and drug metabolites, however, are reabsorbed from the intestine and reenter the bloodstream. This process is called *enterohepatic circulation.*

PATHOPHYSIOLOGY

Most liver diseases are characterized by hepatocellular injury with predominant abnormalities of the serum aminotransferases. In these disorders, massive hepatocyte damage must occur before the liver loses its ability to secrete bile. In contrast, cholestatic liver disease is characterized by injury to the secretory apparatus downstream from the hepatocytes. Typically, SAP levels initially are elevated and serum aminotransferase levels are normal, or near normal. Problems related to failure of bile secretion occur early, whereas hepatic synthetic and immunologic functions remain intact until late in the disease. Thus, a patient with cholestatic liver disease may develop itching or jaundice but have a normal serum albumin level and prothrombin time.

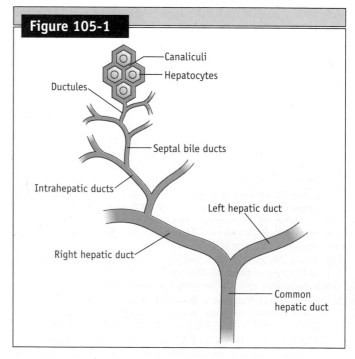

Figure 105-1

Course of bile from hepatocytes to common hepatic duct.

Acute cholestasis may be caused by a defect anywhere in the path of bile secretion, from the hepatocytes to the distal bile duct. Disease affecting the extrahepatic bile ducts typically produces cholestasis due to direct obstruction of bile flow. In contrast, intrahepatic disease may cause either ductular obstruction or secretory failure. Hepatocytes may lose their normal polarity and return substances from the cytosol to the hepatic sinusoids. Alternatively, some substances may return flow from canalicular bile directly into the sinusoids by passing between the hepatocytes across damaged junctional complexes.

Cholestatic disease may progress to liver cell destruction and ultimately to cirrhosis. Damage to hepatocytes caused by cholestasis appears to be mediated partly by accumulation of bile acids and copper in the liver. Because the regenerative capacity of the bile ducts is much less than that of the hepatocytes, cholestasis may not be reversible once significant parenchymal injury occurs.

CLINICAL FEATURES

Incidental discovery of one or more abnormal liver test results is the most common means of detecting cholestasis. In patients with cholestasis, SAP levels are nearly always elevated, often to a high degree. Serum GGT and 5'-nucleotidase levels parallel those of SAP. Serum aminotransferase levels may be normal early in the course of the disease but may become somewhat abnormal later. Typically, serum bilirubin levels also are normal in the early asymptomatic phase of cholestasis (Table 105-3).

Fatigue is the most common symptom of acute cholestasis but is nonspecific (Table 105-1). The earliest specific symptom of cholestasis is pruritus, often developing long before the appearance of jaundice. The occurrence of pruritus correlates closely with elevations of serum bile acid levels, although bile salts themselves do not appear to be the cause of itching. Instead, endogenous opioids may cause pruritus. Opiate antagonists have been shown to ameliorate the itching associated with cholestasis [1••].

Jaundice develops as bilirubin accumulates in serum and diffuses into extracellular fluid. Jaundice usually is observed when the serum bilirubin concentration is 3 mg/dL or more (see Chapters 89 and 91). With progression of cholestasis, serum lipid levels may increase. The hyperlipidemia of cholestasis does not predispose patients to develop atherosclerosis but may lead to lipid deposition in the skin (xanthoma), particularly around the eyelids (xanthelasma). Malabsorption of fats and fat-soluble vitamins with associated steatorrhea, weight loss, and coagulopathy may result from inadequate delivery of bile salts to the duodenum. Persistent cholestasis ultimately will cause cirrhosis and liver failure.

DIAGNOSIS

The patient's medical history often reveals the cause of acute cholestasis. Patients should be questioned about alcohol consumption and use of prescription and nonprescription medications. Previous episodes of jaundice may indicate that the patient has a metabolic abnormality. Abdominal pain, nausea, weight loss, or steatorrhea may suggest extrahepatic biliary obstruction. Some potential causes of cholestasis are obvious, including sepsis, total parenteral nutrition (TPN), pregnancy, and recent surgery (Table 105-2). Others, including hemolysis, may not be immediately apparent.

Evaluation of patients with cholestasis should include laboratory studies measuring the levels of direct and indirect serum bilirubin, SAP, aspartate aminotransferase (AST), and

Figure 105-2

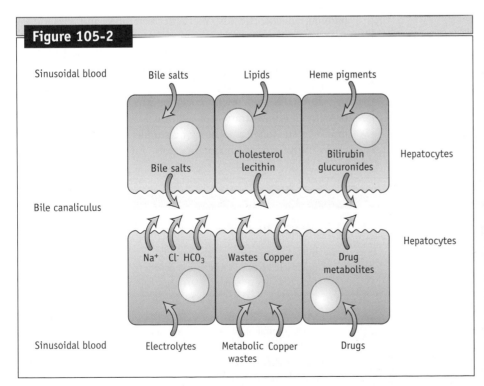

Formation of bile. Bile salts, electrolytes, lipids, and various wastes are transported from hepatic sinusoidal blood into the hepatocytes. These substances are processed and then transported out of the hepatocytes and into the canaliculi for excretion as bile.

Table 105-1. Clinical Features of Cholestasis

Fatigue
Pruritus
Jaundice
Malabsorption of fat-soluble vitamins
Steatorrhea
Hyperlipidemia, xanthomas, xanthelasmas
Cirrhosis

Table 105-2. Common Causes of Acute Cholestasis

Drug reaction
Biliary obstruction
Benign postoperative jaundice
Sepsis
Total parenteral nutrition
Viral hepatitis
Alcoholic hepatitis
Inherited bilirubin metabolic abnormalities (Gilbert's, Rotor's, Dubin-Johnson)
Cholestasis of pregnancy

alanine aminotransferase (ALT). Tests for serum GGT or 5'-nucleotidase levels may be used to confirm a hepatic source of an isolated elevation of SAP. Levels of serum ceruloplasmin and copper frequently are elevated; however, these findings do not help establish the cause of cholestatic disorders. Measurement of serum antimitochondrial antibody titers is appropriate for patients with chronic cholestatic disorders but seldom is useful in evaluating acute cholestasis.

Occasionally, patients with viral hepatitis exhibit severe persistent jaundice. All of the hepatotropic viruses have been reported to cause cholestatic hepatitis; however, it is seen most commonly in persons with hepatitis A virus infection. This diagnosis should be considered when cholestasis occurs as part of an illness consistent with acute viral hepatitis. Similarly, serologic evaluation for Epstein-Barr virus infection is indicated in an otherwise healthy patient exhibiting a viral syndrome and cholestasis.

Most patients with acute cholestasis require ultrasound examination of the biliary tract to exclude extrahepatic biliary obstruction. Occasionally, computed tomography (CT) imaging is indicated in the evaluation of patients with cholestasis to look for lymphadenopathy and pancreatic or intrahepatic tumors. Although abdominal CT imaging is a less sensitive means for detecting bile duct dilation and gallstones, it has better resolu-tion than does ultrasonography for tumor imaging. Depending on the differential diagnosis, invasive tests such as liver biopsy, endoscopic retrograde cholangiopancreatography, and percutaneous transhepatic cholangiography may be indicated. Recently, magnetic resonance imaging of the pancreatobiliary system has emerged as a potential noninvasive alternative to direct cholangiography [2].

■ TREATMENT

Most patients with acute cholestatic disorders do not require specific treatment. Cholestasis occurring postoperatively or resulting from sepsis, hemolysis, and heart failure rarely contributes to morbidity and generally resolves with appropriate therapy. Drug-induced cholestasis usually resolves on discontinuation of the responsible agent. Extrahepatic obstruction caused by gallstones, bile duct injury, or tumors, however, requires active intervention to prevent infection, halt progressive liver injury, and restore hepatic function.

Occasionally, acute cholestasis causes symptoms that require palliation. Although not clearly caused by bile acids, pruritus frequently responds to treatment with bile acid–binding resins (eg, cholestyramine and colestipol). Antihistamines usually are not helpful in the treatment of pruritus caused by cholestasis, and their sedative effects are undesirable. Rifampin relieves pruritus in some patients. Recently, opiate antagonists also have been used to treat the pruritus of cholestasis. Naloxone has a short half-life, requiring frequent subcutaneous injections; naltrexone, an oral opioid antagonist, has been suggested as an alternative [3]. Ursodeoxycholic acid is effective therapy in some patients with cholestasis; however, pruritus may worsen for several weeks before relief is obtained. Other helpful treatments for intractable pruritus include exposure to ultraviolet light, phenobarbital, glucocorticoids, methyltestosterone, and cimetidine. Although expensive and impractical, large-volume plasmapheresis almost always palliates incapacitating pruritus (Table 105-4).

Malabsorption of fat-soluble vitamins can be corrected by oral replacement of vitamins A, D, E, and K. Rapid correction of vitamin K–dependent coagulopathy can be achieved by parenteral administration of vitamin K. A low-fat diet usually improves steatorrhea and may be supplemented with medium-chain triglycerides to maintain caloric intake.

Table 105-3. Laboratory Findings Typical for Acute Cholestasis

Type	Findings	Comments
Aspartate aminotransferase	1–3 times normal	
Alanine aminotransferase	1–3 times normal	
Alkaline phosphatase	2–10 times normal	
Bilirubin	Normal or elevated	
γ-Glutamyl transpeptidase	Elevated	Confirms hepatic source of alkaline phosphatase
Bile acids	Elevated	Rarely used clinically

Table 105-4. Agents Used to Treat Pruritus

Treatment	Dosage	Putative Mechanism of Action
Cholestyramine	4 g bid–qid	Binds bile acids and related compounds
Colestipol	5 g bid–qid	Binds bile acids and related compounds
Rifampin	150–300 mg bid	Increases detoxification of bile salts
Phenobarbital	60–120 mg/d	Induces hepatic microsomal enzymes
Naloxone	3 mg q3–24 h, sc or IV	Blocks central opioidergic tone (short acting)
Naltrexone	25 mg bid	Blocks central opioidergic tone (long acting)
Ursodiol	10–20 mg/kg/d	Modifies composition of bile salt pool
Ultraviolet B light	2 treatments/wk	Alters cutaneous bile salts or skin sensitivity
Plasmapheresis		Removes pruritogens from serum

bid—two times a day; IV—intravenously; qid—four times a day; sc—subcutaneously.

DISEASES AND CONDITIONS RELATED TO CHOLESTASIS

Extrahepatic Obstruction

Choledocholithiasis is a common cause of acute cholestasis accompanied by abdominal pain, nausea, and fever. In patients with choledocholithiasis, abnormal serum AST and ALT levels often are the first indication of liver disease followed shortly by an increase in SAP levels. Abdominal ultrasonography usually suffices to identify gallstones within the gallbladder. Intrahepatic or common bile duct dilation on ultrasonography suggests large duct obstruction but is not found in every patient with bile duct stones. Gallstones within the common bile duct are difficult to image using ultrasonography, with normal results seen in as many as one third of patients ultimately found to have choledocholithiasis. Cholangiography often is required to confirm or exclude a diagnosis of choledocholithiasis.

Neoplastic causes of biliary obstruction include pancreatic cancer, ampullary tumors, cholangiocarcinoma, lymphoma, and hepatic metastases. Patients may exhibit painless jaundice, nausea, abdominal pain, or weight loss. Certain malignancies, including renal cell carcinoma and non-Hodgkin's lymphoma, may cause cholestasis in the absence of direct hepatobiliary involvement, a paraneoplastic phenomenon that usually resolves with treatment of the extrabiliary malignancy [4,5].

In the United States, infestation of the biliary tree by parasites or protozoa is an uncommon cause of acute cholestasis and occurs in patients in certain high-risk groups. Patients from Southeast Asia may exhibit biliary obstruction caused by liver fluke infestations by *Clonorchis sinensis*, *Opisthorchis viverrini*, or *Opisthorchis felineus*. The nematode *Ascaris lumbricoides* also can invade the biliary tree and cause acute obstruction [6]. Liver fluke infestation appears to be restricted to persons from Asia. *A. lumbricoides* is found throughout much of the Third World.

Patients with AIDS may develop cholestasis resulting from papillary stenosis or segmental sclerosis of the intrahepatic or extrahepatic bile ducts. The cholangiopathy associated with AIDS is related to biliary infection by *Cryptosporidium*, *Microsporidium*, or cytomegalovirus.

Drug Reactions

As a group, drug reactions may be the most common cause of abnormal cholestatic liver test results (see Chapter 96) [7•]. Cholestatic drug reactions usually are the result of an idiosyncratic response to the agent or one of its metabolites. Although almost any medication may produce a cholestatic reaction, those most often implicated are listed in Table 105-5.

Patients with drug-induced cholestasis may exhibit pure cholestasis, a combination of cholestasis and hepatitis, or an acute cholangitis-like syndrome with bile duct injury. Hepatotoxicity may not develop until the patient has taken a drug for several weeks, and occasionally, cholestasis occurs only on repeated exposure to a drug over several years. Often, abnormal liver test results are unaccompanied by symptoms; however, patients may have anorexia, nausea, abdominal pain, pruritus, and jaundice. Rash and fever, although rare, are particularly suggestive of drug hypersensitivity.

The diagnosis of drug-induced cholestasis is suggested primarily by the patient's medical history. In those who have begun taking a new drug within the preceding 3 months a drug reaction is particularly likely to be the cause of acute cholestasis, especially if the medication is known to cause drug-induced liver disease. Patients over 60 years of age are most susceptible to developing drug-induced cholestasis.

When present, eosinophilia suggests that a patient with acute cholestasis is having a drug reaction. Laboratory tests rarely are diagnostic in this setting and are used primarily to exclude other causes of cholestasis, including viral hepatitis, primary biliary cirrhosis, and idiopathic autoimmune hepatitis. Liver biopsy findings also rarely are diagnostic but may suggest that cholestasis is due to a drug reaction. Liver biopsy and cholangiography are particularly helpful in excluding viral hepatitis and extrahepatic biliary obstruction as the causes of cholestasis.

Drug-induced cholestasis resolves in most patients once the drug therapy is discontinued. Normalization of liver test results after the drug is discontinued strengthens the diagnosis. Some patients may experience relief with the use of glucocorticoids.

Table 105-5. Drugs Associated With Cholestatic Liver Injury

Cholestasis without hepatitis	Cholestatic hepatitis		Cholestasis with bile duct injury
Amoxicillin and clavulanic acid	Angiotensin-converting enzyme inhibitors	Haloperidol and other butyrophenones	Penicillin derivatives
Androgenic steroids	Allopurinol	Ketoconazole	Phenothiazines
Cyclosporin A	Arsenic compounds	Nitrofurantoin	Propoxyphene
Estrogens	Azathioprine	Nonsteroidal anti-inflammatory drugs	
Glyburide	Barbiturates	Oral hypoglycemic agents	
Oral contraceptives	Benzodiazepines	Penicillamine	
Tamoxifen	Chlorpromazine and other phenothiazines	Phenytoin	
Warfarin	Clavulanic acid	Prochlorperazine	
	Erythromycin	Propothiouracil and other antithyroid drugs	
	Flucloxacillin and other penicillin derivatives	Sulfonamides	
	Fluoxetine	Thiabendazole	
	H_2-receptor antagonists	Tricyclic antidepressants	

Because drug reactions are uncommon and unpredictable, however, steroid therapy of drug-induced cholestasis has not been evaluated in formal trials. Ursodeoxycholic acid also has been recommended for treatment of severe drug-induced cholestasis Evidence of the effectiveness of this drug is anecdotal. A patient should not resume taking a drug thought to have caused a cholestatic reaction and should avoid taking similar drugs (*eg*, substitution of one phenothiazine for another or one penicillin derivative for another).

Hyperbilirubinemia of Sepsis

When a patient who has a fever develops jaundice, it may be the result of a phenomenon known as hyperbilirubinemia of sepsis [8]. Patients usually are quite ill and have had evidence of infection for several days before the jaundice became apparent. Serum levels of conjugated bilirubin may be highly elevated, with only minimal increases in SAP and serum aminotransferase levels.

Although gram-negative enteric infections and toxic shock syndrome have been particularly associated with the hyperbilirubinemia of sepsis, this syndrome also has been described in persons with pneumococcal pneumonia, staphylococcal endocarditis, and pyelonephritis. Endotoxins and gram-positive exotoxins have been implicated in the pathogenesis of cholestasis [9]. These bacterial products appear to directly impair the function of organic ion transporters in cell membranes, leading to cholestasis at the level of the hepatocytes.

Extrahepatic biliary obstruction should be excluded by ultrasonography in most patients suspected of having hyperbilirubinemia of sepsis. The finding of disproportionately elevated serum bilirubin levels in the appropriate clinical setting, however, is generally sufficient to make the diagnosis. Rarely, liver biopsy or additional tests are needed to exclude other causes of jaundice. Although hyperbilirubinemia has been associated with increased mortality in patients with bacteremia, hepatic dysfunction rarely contributes to overall morbidity; therapy is directed toward control of sepsis [10].

Postoperative Jaundice

Postoperative jaundice can be a distressing complication of an otherwise uneventful surgical procedure. Approximately 1% of patients develop clinical jaundice after surgery requiring anesthesia, whereas after major surgery (*eg*, cardiac bypass surgery) the incidence may be considerably higher [11]. As with cholestasis in other settings, the differential diagnosis of jaundice in the postoperative period includes biliary obstruction and hepatocellular dysfunction. In addition, increased pigment load from hemolysis or reabsorption of hematoma may cause jaundice (Table 105-6).

The temporal relationship between surgery and the onset of jaundice is perhaps the most helpful factor in making a diagnosis. Jaundice that develops within a few days of surgery suggests such causes as hepatic ischemia and hemolysis. Anesthetic-related cholestatic hepatitis rarely develops before the seventh postoperative day. Viral hepatitis from transfused blood is not seen until several weeks after surgery. Similarly, drug-induced hepatitis may not be noted until the patient has been taking a newly prescribed medication for weeks or months. Most postoperative jaundice is self-limited, and thus a conservative diagnostic approach usually is appropriate.

A careful review of the patient's medical history is crucial to evaluate patients with postoperative jaundice [12,13••], with special attention to a history of hypotension or respiratory failure. Perioperative hypotension and hypoxia frequently result in postoperative hepatic ischemia, with patients having high serum aminotransferase levels and sometimes jaundice. Multiple transfusions and absorption of hematomas may result in transient production of more bilirubin than the liver can conjugate and excrete. Drugs administered intraoperatively or postoperatively may cause hemolysis, particularly in patients with glucose-6-phosphate dehydrogenase deficiency. The stresses of surgery occasionally unmask undiagnosed previously well-compensated chronic liver disease, an important risk factor for development of postoperative jaundice. Although patients with Child's class A tolerate surgery without excessive risk, patients with Child's class C may exhibit decompensation after even relatively minor surgical procedures, developing jaundice, worsening ascites, deterioration of hepatic synthetic function, and hepatic encephalopathy.

Anesthetic hepatotoxicity is now uncommon as a result of the decreased use of halothane and other volatile agents known to cause liver injury, including methoxyflurane and enflurane. Patients with anesthetic-induced liver injury exhibit acute hepatitis, having serum aminotransferase levels of 500 to over 1000. Typically, jaundice develops a week after exposure. Liver injury is thought to result from hypersensitivity to anesthetic metabolites incorporated into hepatocyte proteins. Repeated exposure to volatile anesthetics usually is required for development of fulminant hepatitis; mortality from fulminant disease approaches 30% [14•]. Treatment in most cases is supportive.

Postoperative pancreatitis occasionally complicates cardiac or abdominal surgery and may cause obstructive jaundice in up to one third of patients. Bile duct injury may complicate abdominal surgery and should be suspected in patients with jaundice after cholecystectomy, other biliary tract surgery, or gastrectomy. Ultrasonography is performed to exclude this diagnosis in certain patients, and occasionally cholangiography is also required.

Table 105-6. Common Causes of Postoperative Jaundice

Cause	Mechanism
Drugs	Idiosyncratic hypersensitivity reaction
Multiple drug transfusions	Excess bilirubin load
Resorption of hematomas	Excess bilirubin load
Infection	Hyperbilirubinemia of sepsis
Hepatic ischemia	Systemic hypotension or hypoxia
Acute viral hepatitis	Hepatocellular injury, hepatitis A or C
Decompensation of subclinical liver disease	Demand outstrips limited reserve
Abnormalities of bilirubin metabolism (Gilbert's)	Unmasked by fasting
Choledocholithiasis, pancreatitis	Direct biliary obstruction
Anesthetic hepatotoxicity	Hypersensitivity, rare, primarily halothane

The term *benign postoperative jaundice* has been used to describe a nonspecific cholestatic syndrome that may occur in the postoperative period [13••]. Patients typically have had lengthy and extensive surgery with multiple complications, including hypotension, hemorrhage, hypoxia, sepsis, cardiac decompensation, and renal failure. Any of these factors alone or in combination may cause postoperative jaundice. Patients with this syndrome have marked hyperbilirubinemia, with peak serum levels of 10 to 40 mg/dL noted 2 to 10 days after surgery. Usually, SAP levels also are elevated significantly; however, serum aminotransferase levels are seldom more than twice that of normal. Benign postoperative jaundice often is diagnosed clinically; however, care must be taken to distinguish postoperative cholestasis from extrahepatic biliary obstruction. Occasionally, patients with an unusually complicated course of the disease may require liver biopsy or cholangiography.

Total Parenteral Nutrition

Total parenteral nutrition is a common iatrogenic cause of acute nonobstructive cholestasis. Possible mechanisms for TPN-induced cholestasis include hepatotoxicity of TPN solutions, nutrient deficiencies, endotoxemia, alterations in bile acid pools, and lack of appropriate hormonal stimulation from the inactive gut [15]. The actual etiology is likely to be multifactorial.

Patients typically develop serum liver enzyme abnormalities 1 to 4 weeks after initiation of TPN, which usually resolve despite continued parenteral feeding. Steatohepatitis is the most common hepatic complication of TPN in adults; cholestasis usually develops only in patients receiving long-term hyperalimentation. In patients with cholestasis, extrahepatic bile duct obstruction should be excluded by ultrasonography. Liver biopsy, although rarely required, may show steatosis and canalicular fibrosis in addition to cholestasis.

There is no established treatment for TPN-induced cholestasis. Metronidazole, cholecystokinin, and choline have been reported to improve jaundice; however, their efficacy is unproven. Administration of oral ursodeoxycholic acid has been shown to improve laboratory values in patients treated with TPN; however, the clinical value of this therapy is unknown [16,17]. In adults, TPN-induced cholestasis rarely progresses to cirrhosis and usually can be tolerated by patients. Liver test results usually return to normal when enteral feeding resumes.

Alcoholic Liver Disease

Alcohol, a common cause of hepatitis, is an uncommon cause of acute cholestasis. Patients with acute alcoholic hepatitis are often febrile and typically have tender hepatomegaly. In most cases, the diagnosis is apparent from a history of alcohol abuse. However, it is important to exclude extrahepatic biliary obstruction in patients who have a fever and leukocytosis. A liver biopsy rarely is required, but usually is diagnostic; in addition to cholestasis, characteristic histologic changes of alcoholic hepatitis are seen.

Viral Hepatitis

Acute viral hepatitis is a hepatocellular disease; however, patients may exhibit predominant cholestatic features. All hepatotropic viruses have been reported to cause cholestatic hepatitis, although it is most common in patients with hepatitis A. Epstein-Barr virus and cytomegalovirus also may cause hepatitis with cholestatic features. Symptoms of acute viral hepatitis, including fever, anorexia, and right upper quadrant discomfort, usually precede the onset of jaundice, which is often accompanied by pruritus. Serum aminotransferase levels are usually in the thousands during the hepatic phase of the illness but generally decrease to less than 200 by the time cholestasis becomes apparent. Serologic tests are usually sufficient to diagnose the cause of the infection. Cholestatic viral hepatitis A may be slow to resolve, with jaundice and pruritus persisting for many months.

Granulomatous Liver Disease

Patients with granulomatous liver disease typically exhibit a cholestatic liver test pattern characterized by a predominant increase in SAP and serum GGT levels. Cholestasis may be produced by any cause of hepatic granulomata, including infection, sarcoidosis, lymphoma, Crohn's disease, primary biliary cirrhosis, drug hypersensitivity, and idiopathic hepatic granulomatous disease. The diagnosis is made by liver biopsy; when granulomata are found, further evaluation is required to exclude an infectious agent. A diagnosis of idiopathic granulomatous liver disease is not made until other potential causes are excluded. Glucocorticoids or immunosuppressive agents are used to treat idiopathic granulomatous hepatitis (see Chapter 98).

Cholestasis of Pregnancy

High SAP levels during pregnancy are normal, particularly in the third trimester, and are due to leakage of placental alkaline phosphatase into maternal serum. In *cholestasis of pregnancy*, however, elevations of SAP are paralleled by abnormalities in serum GGT levels, and often by serum aminotransferase and bilirubin levels (see Chapter 110). The pathogenesis appears to be related to an inherited sensitivity to estrogens. This syndrome is particularly common among women from Scandinavia or Chile. Cholestasis also may develop in women who are taking birth control pills.

Patients with cholestasis of pregnancy develop anorexia, fatigue, and pruritus during the third trimester. Jaundice is uncommon, and serum bilirubin levels rarely exceed four times the upper limit of normal. Serum bile acid concentrations, however, may be markedly elevated. Ultrasonography of the biliary tree is indicated to exclude choledocholithiasis, and serologic testing should be done to exclude viral hepatitis. The disease itself requires no treatment; however, the associated pruritus may require therapy. Patients with cholestasis of pregnancy should be treated at centers that specialize in high-risk obstetrics [18•].

Benign Recurrent Intrahepatic Cholestasis

Benign recurrent intrahepatic cholestasis (BRIC) is a rare syndrome characterized by recurrent episodes of severe acute cholestasis in otherwise healthy persons. BRIC often begins in childhood or adolescence, and both familial and sporadic forms have been described. During an attack, patients develop anorexia, jaundice, and pruritus. The results of liver tests have a typical cholestatic pattern. Liver biopsy demonstrates bile plugging while cholangiography is normal. After several weeks to months, the attack subsides spontaneously, the patient becomes completely asymptomatic, and results of liver tests and histology return to normal.

Patients may have abnormal bile salt pools, with decreased levels of primary bile acids and elevated concentrations of the secondary bile acids lithocholate and deoxycholate. Similar abnormalities produce cholestasis in experimental animals, and high lithocholate levels have been observed in patients with TPN-related cholestasis [19]. No clear underlying defect of bile acid metabolism has been identified, however, and the cause of this disorder remains obscure.

Over years of follow-up, some patients develop cirrhosis but most do not [20]. Proposed treatments for BRIC have included cholestyramine, steroids, phenobarbital, S-adenosylmethionine, and ursodeoxycholate; none has convincingly been proven effective.

Isolated Abnormalities of Bilirubin Metabolism

Some metabolic abnormalities that cause hyperbilirubinemia and that may be confused with cholestatic liver disease are briefly described here. A more extensive discussion of these disorders is found in Chapter 89.

Gilbert's, Dubin-Johnson, and Rotor's syndromes are inherited metabolic disorders in which mild hyperbilirubinemia exists in the absence of true liver disease. Patients with these syndromes usually are asymptomatic but may become jaundiced intermittently, particularly when fasting or stressed by illness. Other liver test results are normal, including prothrombin time and SAP, serum aminotransferase, and albumin levels.

Of the US population, 5% to 10% have Gilbert's syndrome, which is characterized by a mild increase in serum unconjugated bilirubin concentration. Baseline serum bilirubin levels are normal or slightly elevated in these patients but often will double after an overnight fast. Most patients have a slight but measurable defect in their ability to conjugate bilirubin to form glucuronic acid within liver cells. Recent studies suggest that Gilbert's syndrome is caused by a recessive abnormality in the promoter region of the bilirubin uridine-diphosphate glucuronosyltransferase gene [21].

Dubin-Johnson and Rotor's syndromes are characterized by similarly benign elevations of conjugated serum bilirubin. In these disorders the defect appears to reside at the level of transport proteins near or at the bile canalicular side of the hepatocytes. In Dubin-Johnson syndrome the liver is black because of retention of lipofuscin pigment in hepatocytes. In contrast, the liver is of normal color in Rotor's syndrome. Neither disorder requires therapy.

PROGNOSIS

The overall prognosis for patients with acute cholestasis depends on the underlying cause but generally is good. Patients with postoperative jaundice, BRIC, or cholestasis of pregnancy have an excellent prognosis. Almost all patients with cholestatic reactions to drugs or TPN will recover completely. Those with choledocholithiasis or hyperbilirubinemia of sepsis also will recover completely if the underlying disease responds to treatment. Patients with malignant causes of jaundice or cholangiopathy associated with AIDS have a much poorer prognosis that is directly attributable to their underlying diseases.

REFERENCES

Recently published papers of particular interest have been highlighted as follows:
•   Of interest
••   Of outstanding interest

1.•• Gilliespie DA, Vickers CR: Pruritus and cholestasis: therapeutic options. *Gastroenterol Hepatology* 1993, 8:168–173.

2. Soto JA, Barish MA, Yucel EK, *et al.*: Magnetic resonance cholangiography: comparison with endoscopic retrograde cholangiopancreatography. *Gastroenterology* 1996, 110:589–597.

3. Carson KL, Tran TT, Cotton P, *et al.*: Pilot study of the use of naltrexone to treat the severe pruritus of cholestatic liver disease. *Am J Gastroenterol* 1996, 91:1022–1023.

4. Jakobovits AW, Crimmins FB, Sherlock S, Erlinger S: Cholestasis as a paraneoplastic manifestation of carcinoma of the kidney. *Aust NZ J Med* 1981, 11:65–67.

5. Warncr AS, Whitcomb FF: Extrahepatic Hodgkin's disease and cholestasis. *Am J Gastroenterol* 1994, 89:940–941.

6. Khuroo MA: Ascariasis. *Gastroenterol Clin North Am* 1996, 25:553–577.

7.• Farrell GC: Drug-induced cholestasis. In *Drug-Induced Liver Disease.* Edited by Farrell GC. New York: Churchill Livingstone; 1994:319–370.

8. Banks JG, Foulis AK, Ledingham IM, Macsween RNM: Liver function in septic shock. *J Clin Pathol* 1982, 35:1249–1252.

9. Quale JM, Mandel LJ, Bergasa NV, Straus EW: Clinical significance and pathogenesis of hyperbilirubinemia associated with *Staphylococcus aureus* septicemia. *Am J Med* 1988, 85:615–618.

10. Moseley RH: Sepsis-associated cholestasis. *Gastroenterology* 1997, 112:302–305.

11. Chu C-M, Chang C-H, Liaw Y-F, Hsiesh M-J: Jaundice after open heart surgery: a prospective study. *Thorax* 1984, 39:52–56.

12. Matloff DS, Kaplan MM: Postoperative jaundice. *Orthop Clin North Am* 1978, 9:799–810.

13.•• Becker SD, Lamont JT: Postoperative jaundice. *Sem Liver Dis* 1988, 8:183–190.

14.• Elliott RH, Strunin L: Hepatotoxicity of volatile anesthetics. *Br J Anesthesiology* 1993, 70:339–348.

15. Quigley EM, Marsh MN, Shaffer JL, Markin RS: Hepatobiliary complications of total parenteral nutrition. *Gastroenterology* 1993, 104:286–301.

16. Spagnuolo MI, Iorio R, Vegnente A, Guarino A: Ursodeoxycholic acid for treatment of cholestasis in children on long-term parenteral nutrition: a pilot study. *Gastroenterology* 1996, 111:716–719.

17. Beau P, Labat-Labourdette J, Ingrand P, Beauchant M: Is ursodeoxycholic acid an effective therapy for total parenteral nutrition-related liver disease? *J Hepatology* 1994, 20:240–244.

18.• Knox TA, Olans LB: Liver disease in pregnancy. *N Engl J Med* 1996, 335:569–576.

19. Crosignani A, Podda M, Bertolini E, *et al.*: Failure of ursodeoxycholic acid to prevent a cholestatic episode in a patient with benign recurrent intrahepatic cholestasis: a study of bile acid metabolism. *Hepatology* 1991, 13:1076–1083.

20. Brenard R, Geubel AP, Benhamou JP: Benign recurrent intrahepatic cholestasis: a report of 26 cases. *J Clin Gastroenterol* 1989, 11:546–551.

21. Bosma PJ, Chowdhury JR, Bakker C, *et al.*: The genetic basis of the reduced expression of bilirubin UDP-glucuronosyltransferase 1 in Gilbert's syndrome. *N Engl J Med* 1995, 333:1171–1175.

106 Chronic Cholestatic Disorders

Eric D. Libby and Marshall M. Kaplan

Once thought to have only a few causes, chronic liver disease now is known to have many. In Western countries, the most common causes are alcohol use and viral infection. Cholestatic liver disease is less common but not rare, occurring in approximately 1 per 10,000 persons.

DEFINITION

Cholestasis is a syndrome of decreased bile excretion in which the substances normally found in bile accumulate in the blood. This syndrome may result from obstruction of either the extrahepatic or intrahepatic bile ducts. Cholestasis also may occur at the hepatocellular level, as seen in certain drug reactions, or as a complication of sepsis, total parenteral nutrition, or pregnancy. Chronic cholestatic liver diseases most often result from bile duct obstruction, as exemplified by primary biliary cirrhosis (PBC), primary sclerosing cholangitis (PSC), chronic graft-versus-host disease (GVHD), and ductopenic liver transplantation rejection.

ANATOMY AND PHYSIOLOGY

Hepatocytes and bile duct epithelia produce bile by active transport of water, electrolytes, bile salts, bilirubin, and other substances across cell membranes into the canaliculi and ducts (see Chapters 88 and 89). Bile flows through the canaliculi between hepatocytes into ductules and then into the intralobular, intrahepatic, and ultimately, extrahepatic bile ducts before emptying through the ampulla of Vater into the duodenum (see Chapter 87).

PATHOPHYSIOLOGY

Most liver diseases result from direct injury to hepatocytes. Hepatocellular damage from alcohol or viral infection leads to loss of hepatocellular mass, and synthetic function often deteriorates before bile secretion is significantly impaired. In chronic cholestatic liver diseases, however, the bile ducts appear to be the primary targets of disease activity, with hepatocellular injury a secondary phenomenon. Manifestation of problems related to failure of biliary secretion occur early, whereas hepatic synthetic and immunologic functions remain intact until late in the disease. Because the regenerative capacity of the bile ducts is much less than that of hepatocytes, liver disease owing to obstructive cholestasis often is irreversible once it has progressed to the point of hepatocellular loss.

The process causing bile duct damage is primarily immunologically mediated. Thus, diseases as diverse as PBC, GVHD, and drug-induced *vanishing bile duct syndrome* (see the subsequent section on "Chronic Liver Transplantation Rejection") are characterized by bile duct destruction via activated T lymphocytes targeted against biliary epithelial cells. Although the initiating events appear to be unrelated, in each instance immune-mediated duct destruction leads to accumulation of toxic bile acids in the microenvironment of the liver and bile ductules. In addition, the resulting cholestasis appears to cause aberrant expression of HLA class II antigens on biliary epithelia, potentiating ductular damage.

Retention within the liver of toxic substances normally excreted in bile leads to hepatocellular damage (Fig. 106-1). Bile salts, including chenodiol and deoxycholate, are detergents that may dissolve cell membranes. In obstructive cholestasis, bile leakage into the hepatic parenchyma leads to accumulation of toxic levels of bile acids and copper, ultimately causing secondary hepatocellular injury. Hepatocytes respond to cholestasis by increasing expression of HLA class I antigens on their surfaces, thereby augmenting the potential for immunologic injury. Ultimately, this process leads to scarring and irreversible parenchymal destruction.

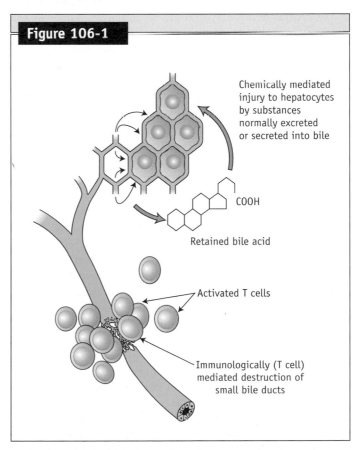

Figure 106-1

Chemically mediated injury to hepatocytes by substances normally excreted or secreted into bile

COOH

Retained bile acid

Activated T cells

Immunologically (T cell) mediated destruction of small bile ducts

The pathogenesis of primary biliary cirrhosis. The immunologically mediated bile duct injury contributes to the accumulation of toxic agents normally excreted in bile, which then causes chemically mediated hepatocyte injury. (*From* Kaplan [21]; with permission).

EXTRAHEPATIC EFFECTS

Fatigue is the most common and frequently the earliest symptom of chronic cholestatic disease. The cause of this nonspecific symptom is unclear. Some studies in animals have implicated secondary abnormalities in the hypothalamic-pituitary-adrenal axis; other studies have pointed to alterations in serotonin and opioid neurotransmission [1].

The earliest specific symptom of cholestasis is pruritus. It is assumed that substances normally excreted in bile such as bilirubin, bile acids, and lipids are pruritogenic when they accumulate in blood or tissues. Bile acids long have been thought to be the mediators of pruritus, particularly because the bile salt binding agents cholestyramine and colestipol are effective in treating this symptom (see Table 105-4). Tissue levels of bile acids, however, do not correlate with the severity of pruritus. Tissue histamine levels are elevated in patients with PSC and PBC who have pruritus; however, antihistamine therapy is remarkably ineffective in these patients. It has been assumed that a pruritogenic agent acts locally at the skin or in peripheral nerves. This theory recently has been challenged, and the possibility of a central nervous system origin of cholestatic pruritus has emerged. Patients with cholestasis have high levels of endogenous opioids and may exhibit transient symptoms resembling those seen in drug withdrawal when opiate antagonists are given. Treatment with the narcotic antagonist naloxone has been demonstrated to relieve pruritus in patients with cholestasis [2•]. This result supports the theory that elevated levels of endogenous opioids in the central nervous system are an important factor in the cause of pruritus in cholestasis.

Jaundice is the result of the failure of the liver to excrete bilirubin. As bilirubin accumulates in serum and tissues, icterus becomes apparent. As a result of renal excretion, serum bilirubin concentrations typically plateau at 20 to 30 mg/dL and seldom exceed this level in the absence of hemolysis or renal insufficiency. In general, hyperbilirubinemia does not affect other organ systems in adults; however, obstructive jaundice is associated with an increased incidence of acute renal failure and impaired cardiac function.

Patients with cholestasis may develop high serum lipid levels owing to decreased biliary lipid excretion. Serum cholesterol levels often are very high; however, atherosclerosis is not accelerated. The phenomenon is attributed to the relatively high levels of high-density lipoproteins and disproportionate increase in lipoprotein X, which is devoid of apoB. Lipids are deposited in the skin around the eyes (xanthelasma) and around the elbows, knees, ankles, and hands (xanthomas). The deleterious effects of lipid deposition are primarily cosmetic, but may include painful neuropathy. Xanthomatous lesions may be seen in various types of chronic cholestasis, especially PBC [3].

Decreased bile salt concentrations in the small intestine may result in inadequate emulsification, digestion, and absorption of dietary fats, leading to steatorrhea and subsequent deficiencies of vitamins A, D, E, and K. Deficiencies of vitamins A and D are particularly common in patients with chronic cholestasis; however, the incidence of clinical manifestations is low. Although osteopenia is common in patients with cholestasis, it appears to be unrelated to vitamin D deficiency. Coagulopathy caused by vitamin K malabsorption may be clinically important but usually is seen only in patients with jaundice who are taking cholestyramine. Symptomatic vitamin E deficiency is rare.

Hepatic osteodystrophy is a common extrahepatic manifestation of cholestatic liver disease, particularly in patients with PBC. These patients develop osteopenia and secondary fractures, particularly of the spine. Because of the frequency of vitamin D deficiency owing to fat malabsorption in patients with cholestasis, it originally was assumed that the characteristic lesion was osteomalacia. Histologic analysis of bone biopsy specimens, however, demonstrates that the predominant lesion is osteoporosis, not osteomalacia. Furthermore, vitamin D replacement therapy has not been shown to improve bone mineral density or prevent fractures in these patients [4]. The underlying cause of osteoporosis in cholestasis remains unknown. Low rates of new bone formation have been implicated in some studies, whereas other studies have found increased bone reabsorption [5].

As in any liver disease that progresses to cirrhosis, cholestatic disease may result in development of portal hypertension, with splenomegaly, varices, and ascites. In contrast to primary hepatocellular disease, however, patients with cholestatic disorders may develop symptomatic portal hypertension at an early phase while hepatic synthetic function remains intact. The portal hypertension may be presinusoidal owing to nodular regenerative hyperplasia and thus may occur even in the absence of true cirrhosis.

CLINICAL MANIFESTATIONS

Patients with chronic cholestasis most commonly experience fatigue; however, because it is nonspecific, fatigue is not always recognized as a symptom of liver disease. Most often, pruritus is the symptom that leads the physician to search for underlying liver disease, and jaundice is a relatively late phenomenon. With progression of cholestatic disease, hyperlipidemia, xanthomas, and xanthelasmas become increasingly common. Despite fat malabsorption, symptomatic steatorrhea and fat-soluble vitamin deficiency are relatively uncommon.

The most common presentation in persons with cholestatic liver disease is the incidental discovery of abnormal liver test results. As a result of widespread biochemical screening, a patient often is asymptomatic when a laboratory abnormality first is noted. The serum alkaline phosphatase (SAP) level is nearly always elevated. Elevations of serum γ-glutamyl transpeptidase (GGT) and 5'-nucleotidase levels parallel that of SAP. The serum aminotransferase levels also are elevated slightly but may be normal early in the course of the disease. The serum bilirubin concentration typically is normal in the early, asymptomatic phase of chronic cholestasis.

DIAGNOSTIC APPROACH
History

Patient demographics and details of the medical history are particularly important in distinguishing the different types of chronic cholestatic liver disease. Thus, a woman aged 50 years with a history of thyroiditis is most likely to have PBC, whereas a man aged 35 years with ulcerative colitis is most likely to have PSC. Patients should be questioned carefully about medication use, possible substance abuse, and a history of blood transfusion, liver disease, biliary tract surgery, inflammatory bowel disease, and other immunologic disorders.

Laboratory Evaluation

Suspicion of cholestatic liver disease is raised by finding an SAP level increased out of proportion to those of the serum aminotransferases. When serum aminotransferase levels are normal, it may be prudent to confirm the hepatic source of SAP with testing for either a serum GGT or a 5′-nucleotidase level.

Serum antimitochondrial antibodies (AMAs) are present in 95% of patients with PBC. AMAs are highly specific for this disorder, although occasionally they are seen in patients with idiopathic autoimmune hepatitis or other diseases. Levels of serum antineutrophil cytoplasm antibodies and anti–smooth muscle antibodies often are present in patients with PBC; however, these levels are neither sensitive nor specific for diagnosis. Marked elevations of serum antinuclear antibodies often are seen in persons with idiopathic autoimmune hepatitis. These elevations, however, may also be found in numerous other disorders and are nonspecific.

Viral hepatitis generally causes elevations in serum liver enzymes with a hepatocellular pattern, *ie*, serum aminotransferase levels greater than those of SAP. Occasionally, patients with hepatitis B or C exhibit a cholestatic picture. Thus, appropriate serologic studies should be obtained to exclude these causes. Rarely, hepatitis A may have a prolonged cholestatic phase. When cholestasis occurs after an illness consistent with acute hepatitis, serum immunoglobulin M antibody to hepatitis A should be measured.

Radiologic Evaluation

Ultrasonography of the liver should be performed to exclude extrahepatic biliary obstruction and gallstones in patients with cholestasis. If a tumor is suspected, abdominal computed tomography (CT) imaging is appropriate. Direct cholangiography often is required to establish definitively whether extrahepatic bile duct obstruction is present, particularly when other tests leave the diagnosis in doubt. Endoscopic retrograde cholangiopancreatography (ERCP) is generally the preferred approach; however, percutaneous transhepatic cholangiography may be required when ERCP is unsuccessful or technically impossible. Magnetic resonance cholangiographic imaging appears to offer a less invasive alternative to direct cholangiography. Additional experience with this technique, however, is required before its accuracy can be compared with that of conventional cholangiography.

Liver Biopsy

Percutaneous liver biopsy frequently helps establish the diagnosis in patients with cholestatic liver disease. Histologic examination of biopsy specimens usually is diagnostic in PBC and alcoholic hepatitis, and often it is helpful in the diagnosis of PSC and viral and drug-induced hepatitis. In addition, biopsy specimens are useful in evaluating the stage or severity of liver disease. Thus, they aid in planning therapy and predicting prognosis.

▄▄▄ TREATMENT

The appropriate treatment of cholestatic liver diseases depends on the underlying cause. Specific therapy is discussed along with the individual diseases. A general approach to treatment of cholestasis is reviewed subsequently.

Pruritus

One of the most disturbing problems for patients with cholestasis is pruritus. It may lead to severe skin excoriation and frequently interferes with sleep. Although bile acid retention does not appear to cause pruritus directly, itching usually responds to treatment with bile acid sequestering agents. Oral cholestyramine, 4 g given four times daily, relieves pruritus in most cases. The dose of this nonabsorbable resin must be adjusted for each patient, and it may take up to a week after treatment initiation before symptoms respond. By increasing fecal elimination of bile acids, therapy with cholestyramine results in a reduction in the total bile salt pool. This drug, however, may act by binding as yet uncharacterized pruritogenic agents in addition to bile salts [6••]. Cholestyramine therapy is nearly always effective if the patient can tolerate the drug. Unfortunately, the accompanying side effects of constipation or diarrhea and bloating (depending on the formulation) may be dose-limiting. The bile acid sequestering agent colestipol is an equally effective alternative to cholestyramine.

Antihistamines are surprisingly ineffective in treating pruritus caused by cholestasis. They appear useful only for mild itching, and their sedative effects may be quite debilitating. In patients with advanced liver disease, antihistamines may exacerbate or trigger encephalopathy. Therefore their use is not recommended.

Opiate antagonists, including naloxone and naltrexone, may relieve pruritus by blocking the central effects of endogenous opioids in patients with cholestasis. Naloxone has been shown convincingly to reduce pruritus and excoriation; however, its short half-life and subcutaneous route of administration render it relatively impractical as therapy [2•]. The oral opiate antagonist naltrexone may be a more practical alternative. Ursodeoxycholic acid is effective in some patients but results are variable. By inducing various hepatic enzymes, the drugs rifampin and phenobarbital alter the bile salt pool and alleviate pruritus in some patients. However, these drugs also may be toxic in patients with liver disease. Therefore, careful monitoring of patients is essential. Other helpful approaches in patients with intractable pruritus include exposure to ultraviolet light and treatment with glucocorticoids, methyltestosterone, and cimetidine. Large-volume plasmapheresis relieves pruritus in the rare patient who does not respond to any of the previously mentioned treatments but is invasive, expensive, and impractical (see Table 105-4).

Malabsorption

Malabsorption of fat-soluble vitamins occurs primarily in patients with advanced long-standing cholestasis or steatorrhea. Lipid malabsorption most often results from decreased intestinal bile salt concentrations, with poor emulsification leading to incomplete digestion of triglycerides. Pancreatic insufficiency owing to the sicca syndrome in patients with PBC or pancreatic duct involvement in PSC also may cause fat malabsorption. Concomitant therapy with cholestyramine further worsens fat malabsorption. Levels of lipid-soluble vitamins should be determined twice a year in patients with chronic cholestatic liver disease, and vitamin supplements should be given to those whose blood levels suggest deficiency. Supplements should be continued indefinitely unless improvement occurs in the underlying disease. Although uptake of fat-soluble vitamins is less efficient in the setting of cholestasis, deficiencies of vitamins A, D, E and K usually can be corrected by oral replacement therapy. In severe cases, parenteral injections may be required.

Improvement usually occurs in symptomatic steatorrhea when patients follow a low-fat diet. Caloric intake may be increased by oral administration of medium-chain triglycerides, which do not require emulsification for intestinal absorption. Patients with exocrine pancreatic insufficiency should be given oral pancreatic enzyme supplements.

Osteopenia

Metabolic bone disease with associated vertebral fractures is one of the most disabling manifestations of cholestatic liver disease. The cause of osteoporosis in these patients remains unknown, and no specific therapy has been proved effective. Correction of vitamin D deficiency is reasonable; however, studies have found routine vitamin D supplementation to be ineffective in preventing and treating hepatic osteodystrophy. Dietary calcium supplementation is safe, and patients should be encouraged to eat a diet high in calcium. Estrogen replacement therapy holds promise for preventing bone loss, particularly among postmenopausal women. Recent experience indicates that estrogen replacement therapy is safe in cholestatic syndromes and neither induces nor worsens cholestasis. Calcitonin and bisphosphonates are of potential benefit in therapy of cholestatic osteopenia; however, the efficacy of these relatively expensive medications is uncertain at present. In patients with cholestasis who are at risk for developing osteopenia corticosteroid therapy should be avoided, if possible. Patients should be instructed to exercise and avoid smoking cigarettes.

▮ PRIMARY BILIARY CIRRHOSIS

Primary biliary cirrhosis (PBC) is a chronic progressive liver disease characterized by destruction of the small intrahepatic bile ducts. PBC is predominantly a disease of middle-aged women. It often is discovered on routine liver screening tests when abnormal SAP levels are found. PBC may remain quiescent for long periods; however, if not treated, progression to cirrhosis and liver failure ultimately will occur. Results of treatment with ursodeoxycholic acid, colchicine, and methotrexate are promising. However, an insufficient number of patients have been followed up for long enough to be certain that these drugs alter the natural history of PBC.

Epidemiology

Although uncommon, PBC is not rare. Its estimated prevalence is 19 to 151 cases per million persons [7••], and it occurs in members of all races. Worldwide, PBC accounts for up to 2% of deaths from cirrhosis. In the United States, PBC is the third most common cause of liver disease leading to liver transplantation, behind only alcoholic liver disease and viral hepatitis C.

Even though genetic factors play a role in a patient's susceptibility to PBC, the disease is not inherited in a simple Mendelian fashion. The prevalence of PBC in families with one affected member is estimated to be a thousand times higher than that in the general population. Certain HLA haplotypes, particularly HLA-DR8, occur with increased frequency in patients with PBC; however, these associations are relatively weak.

Pathophysiology

Primary biliary cirrhosis is characterized by a T-cell–mediated attack on the small intralobular bile ducts that leads to their gradual destruction and disappearance. The exact cause of ductular damage in PBC remains unclear; however, an autoimmune mechanism is thought to be responsible. Numerous abnormalities of the immune system are associated with PBC, including elevated serum immunoglobulin levels, circulating autoantibodies, granuloma in the liver and regional lymph nodes, and impaired T-lymphocyte regulation. The gender distribution of affected patients is similar to that found in other autoimmune disorders. Most women with PBC have at least one other autoimmune disease, for example, CREST syndrome (calcinosis, Raynaud's phenomenon, esophageal involvement, sclerodactyly, and telangiectasia); Sjögren's syndrome; Hashimoto's thyroiditis; and rheumatoid arthritis.

Current data suggest there are two distinct requirements for the development of PBC. The first is genetic and is characterized by an inherited abnormality of immune regulation, with the inability to suppress an inflammatory attack on the bile ducts once it is initiated. The second is environmental, a triggering event that sets the inflammatory process in motion. Theoretically, any factor that damages bile ducts (including chlorpromazine and α-interferon, each of which has been reported to initiate the development of PBC) may serve as a trigger in a susceptible host. Other potential triggers include choledocholithiasis and bile duct infections. Once the disease process begins, the susceptible host lacks the ability to shut down the inflammatory process.

Antimitochondrial antibodies are found in the serum of nearly every patient with PBC. The antigens against which these antibodies are directed are the E2 subunits of a family of mitochondrial enzymes. The target antigens are located on the inner surfaces of the mitochondria and are not exposed to circulating antibodies. A molecule that shares antigenic determinants with these subunits is found on the luminal surface of biliary epithelial cells in patients with early PBC. It has been suggested that damage to bile duct epithelial cells in PBC may unmask an antigen that is recognized by both hepatic and peripheral T lymphocytes in the blood. Expression of this autoantigen on the luminal surface of biliary epithelial cells may then provoke immunoglobulin A antibody– or T-cell–mediated attack [8].

Patients with high serum AMA titers are no more likely to have aggressive disease than those with low titers. Thus, AMAs may have no direct role in the pathogenesis of PBC. Laboratory animals immunized against antimitochondrial antigen do not develop either bile duct lesions or liver disease.

Once the bile duct disease has been set in motion, there is continued immunologically mediated destruction of ductal epithelial cells. In addition, chronic progressive hepatic injury occurs as a result of hepatic retention of toxic bile acids. This chemically mediated injury leads to hepatocyte destruction and eventually to cirrhosis.

Diagnosis

The diagnosis of PBC most often is suggested by the finding of an elevated SAP level in an asymptomatic or minimally symptomatic middle-aged woman. Elevated AMA titers are found in 95% of patients with a specificity of 98%. Characteristic liver histologic findings confirm the diagnosis and are quite helpful in staging the disease.

Primary biliary cirrhosis is divided into four histologic stages. The stage I lesion is the earliest and is characterized by damage to epithelial cells in the small intrahepatic bile ducts, often with surrounding lymphocytic inflammation. Classically, a "florid bile duct lesion" is seen with a granuloma-like structure containing histiocytes, lymphocytes, plasma cells, and eosinophils surrounding a necrotic bile duct (Fig. 106-2*A*). In stage I, inflammation is confined to the portal triads but is spotty. Thus, it can be missed on needle biopsy of the liver. As the disease progresses to stage II, the portal triads become more scarred, and inflammatory cells spill into the surrounding parenchyma with piecemeal necrosis (Fig. 106-2*B*). Many triads lack bile ducts, whereas others contain numerous atypical bile ducts that do not have lumens. In stage III, portal inflammation and scar tissue link the portal triads (Fig. 106-2*C*). In stage IV, frank cirrhosis exists (Fig. 106-2*D*).

Clinically, the combination of cholestatic liver tests, the presence of serum AMAs, and characteristic liver histologic findings makes for a firm diagnosis of PBC. Because PBC affects small intralobular bile ducts beyond the resolution of conventional radiology, the results on cholangiography are normal. When biopsy results are equivocal or serum AMAs are absent, ERCP may be required to exclude PSC or other causes of extrahepatic bile duct obstruction.

Complications

Complications of PBC are those typical of any chronic cholestatic liver disease. Fatigue is a nonspecific symptom found in many otherwise healthy individuals. Nevertheless, it is reported as a significant problem in two thirds of all patients with PBC and can be quite severe and frustrating [3]. Pruritus may occur with or without jaundice. Xanthomas or xanthelasmas are particularly characteristic of PBC, although they are seen in a minority of patients. Metabolic bone disease is common; however, spontaneous fractures of the spine or pelvis now occur in less than 5% of patients with PBC.

Portal hypertension frequently appears before other signs of cirrhosis appear. The disparity between hepatic synthetic function and portal pressure appears to be the result of nodular regenerative hyperplasia in some patients; large regenerative nodules may compress the portal veins. In this setting, symptomatic portal hypertension, even when complicated by variceal bleeding, does not mandate preparation for liver transplanta-

Figure 106-2

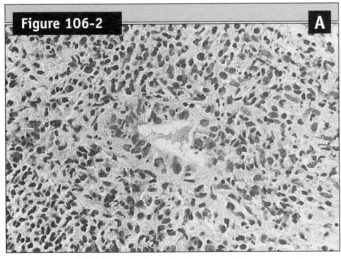 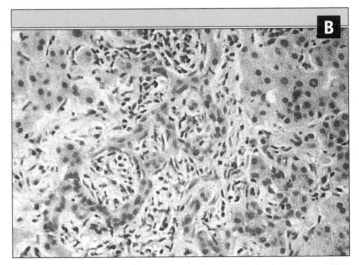

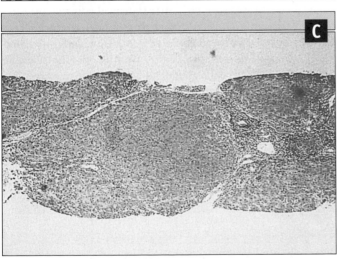 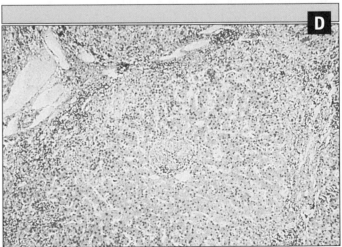

Histologic staging of primary biliary cirrhosis. **A**, Stage 1. Bile duct at center shows epithelial damage and lymphocyte infiltration. **B**, Stage 2. Atypical, tortuous bile ducts are hyperplastic and there is lymphocytic inflammation. **C**, Stage 3. Adjacent portal triads are connected by septa with dense infiltrates of mononuclear cells and strands of connective tissue. **D**, Stage 4. Cirrhosis is present with bands of connective tissue and inflammatory cells. A noncaseating granuloma is present at the center of a nodule. (*From* Kaplan [7•]; with permission.)

tion. A decompressive procedure such as a distal splenorenal shunt or a transjugular intrahepatic portosystemic shunt may provide many years of relief in patients who have preserved synthetic function. When other signs of cirrhosis (eg, low serum albumin levels, coagulopathy, muscle wasting, and encephalopathy) indicate hepatic deterioration, the patient has entered a phase of end-stage liver disease. Referral for transplantation is then appropriate.

Treatment

Symptomatic therapy for patients with PBC is similar to that for patients with other cholestatic liver diseases. No generally accepted treatment exists for the underlying disease process. Encouraging results have been obtained with ursodeoxycholic acid, colchicine, and methotrexate; however, the long-term utility of these agents remains controversial. The goals of therapy include halting progression of damage to biliary epithelia and minimizing hepatocellular damage that results from the obstructive cholestasis (Table 106-1).

Ursodeoxycholic acid. Ursodeoxycholic acid is a naturally occurring bile acid that normally accounts for 1% of the bile acid pool [9•]. When ursodiol is given in pharmacologic doses, 10 to 15 mg/kg/d, bile ursodiol concentration increases to approximately 40% of total bile acids and intestinal reabsorption of endogenous bile acids is inhibited. The net result is a decrease in the amount of toxic bile acids, for example, cholic acid and deoxycholic acid. This change in bile acid composition appears to reduce the cytotoxic effects of cholestasis. Some evidence suggests that ursodeoxycholic acid also reduces the cholestasis-mediated overexpression of HLA class I antigens on hepatocytes, an action that may make hepatocytes less vulnerable to lymphocytic attack. Although these effects appear to ameliorate hepatocyte injury in PBC, no evidence indicates that ursodiol prevents progression of bile duct damage.

Clinically, ursodiol is remarkably safe and well tolerated in PBC patients, the most common side effect being mild diarrhea. Randomized prospective double-blind trials have shown that ursodiol therapy results in a significant improvement in liver test results [10,11•,12]. Improvement in liver histologic findings was noted in some studies; however, symptoms did not appear to be significantly affected. In three of the four studies, patients initially randomized to placebo were switched to ursodiol after 2 years. Thus, it has been difficult to determine the effects on patient survival and the need for transplantation. Nevertheless, ursodeoxycholic acid appears to extend the time before a patient requires liver transplantation or succumbs to liver disease. Ursodiol is most effective in patients with early

PBC and is ineffective in patients with advanced disease. Its use is recommended for all PBC patients with pre-cirrhotic disease.

Colchicine. Colchicine is an immunomodulatory drug with a well-established safety profile. Three double-blind studies of colchicine therapy for PBC have suggested modest efficacy with little toxicity. In only one study was the improvement in liver test results and survival statistically significant [13]. No studies have documented improvement in symptoms or histology.

Colchicine appears to slow progression of PBC but does not prevent the ultimate development of end-stage disease. Colchicine may have a role when used in addition to ursodeoxycholic acid [14•]; however, its long-term efficacy in patients with PBC appears to be modest. Colchicine is relatively well tolerated when given in doses of 0.6 mg twice daily. The only common side effect is diarrhea, which rapidly abates when the dose is lowered or the drug is discontinued. Colchicine is recommended for patients in early-stage disease.

Immunosuppressive drugs. Because PBC is assumed to be mediated by autoimmune bile duct destruction, a number of immunosuppressive agents have been proposed as treatments. Corticosteroids have been used to treat patients with PBC for many years, and improvements in pruritus and fatigue have been reported. This modest benefit, however, is offset by accelerated osteoporosis. A controlled trial of prednisolone found unimpressive improvement in liver test results without changes in serum bilirubin concentration or liver histology. Owing to a lack of significant efficacy and the risk of side effects, use of corticosteroids cannot be recommended. Azathioprine has been found to be relatively ineffective, and chlorambucil has been associated with significant bone marrow toxicity. Therapy with D-penicillamine also was found to be without benefit, and toxicity occurred in more than 20% of patients with PBC.

Cyclosporine. Cyclosporine has been evaluated in three randomized trials and found to have modest positive effects on liver histology and, perhaps, a beneficial effect on survival [15]. Survival benefit was seen only after statistical adjustment using a multiple-hazards model. Although these results seem encouraging, they must be balanced against the known toxicity associated with long-term use of cyclosporine. Considering the available data, it is difficult to recommend cyclosporine as the sole treatment of PBC.

Methotrexate. Methotrexate is usually classified as an antimetabolite because of its effect on folic acid metabolism. Unlike high-dose therapy, low doses of methotrexate, 0.25 mg/kg

Table 106-1. Potential Treatments for Primary Biliary Cirrhosis

Agent	Dosage	Comments
Ursodiol	12–15 mg/kg/d	Retards progression, seldom halts it, well-tolerated
Colchicine	0.6 mg bid	Improves liver function tests, modest effect on natural history, diarrhea, rare bone marrow suppression
Methotrexate	12.5–15 mg/wk	Efficacy uncertain, sustained remission in some, pneumonitis, rare bone marrow suppression
Cyclosporin A	3 mg/kg/d	Efficacy remains uncertain, significant renal toxicity, hypertension; frequent monitoring required

body weight weekly, used to treat PBC rarely suppress bone marrow function. Studies of low-dose methotrexate in patients with rheumatoid arthritis have shown that neither folate supplementation nor rescue with leucovorin reduces the therapeutic effect of methotrexate on inflammation. Clearly, mechanisms other than inhibition of dihydrofolate reductase are responsible for the immunomodulatory effects of low-dose methotrexate.

In a pilot study, methotrexate improved liver test results and symptoms in nine patients followed up for 2 years. Liver histologic findings improved in five patients and stabilized in four. Response to treatment with methotrexate was slower than was response to treatment with ursodiol, occurring over several years. Most patients exhibited a transient increase in serum aminotransferase levels after beginning therapy with methotrexate, which appeared to predict a favorable response [16•]. Interim analysis of a larger randomized double-blind trial comparing methotrexate with colchicine confirmed improvements in liver test results, pruritus, and findings on liver histology in patients treated with methotrexate.

Recently, we have described sustained remission of well-established PBC in five women with stages II to IV disease. These women were treated with methotrexate for 6 to 8 years and have been monitored for 8 to 16 years [17]. In all patients, liver test results returned to normal, and relief of pruritus and fatigue occurred. Most importantly, examination of serial liver biopsy specimens demonstrated progressive improvement. Such striking efficacy, however, is not noted in all patients. Some patients have shown neither clinical nor biochemical improvement while taking methotrexate. This finding raises the possibility that different types of PBC exist; some may be particularly responsive to immunosuppressive therapy, whereas others may be recalcitrant. This situation may be analogous to our experience with autoimmune hepatitis.

Because ursodiol and methotrexate have different mechanisms of action, it is believed that their effects on PBC will be complementary. Such an additive effect has been reported by some authors [18] but not others [19]. Currently, methotrexate is a potentially promising therapy for PBC; however, its long-term efficacy has not been determined. It should be noted that methotrexate may cause a serious, but reversible, interstitial pneumonitis in up to 15% of patients. Today, methotrexate is best used in clinical studies or cautiously in individuals with pre-cirrhotic PBC who do not respond to more conventional therapy with ursodiol and colchicine. No therapy is likely to be helpful once cirrhosis and signs of liver failure develop.

Liver Transplantation

When cirrhosis is advanced, liver transplantation is the only therapeutic option available for patients with PBC (see Chapter 117). Survival curves at 1 year after successful hepatic transplantation for PBC resemble those of healthy persons matched for age and sex. Some patients develop minor histologic lesions in the new liver that resemble changes seen in early PBC. These lesions appear to be distributed inconsistently, however, and they are not specifically associated with symptoms or serum biochemical abnormalities. Whether these histologic findings represent recurrence of PBC in the allograft or merely mild transplantation rejection remains controversial.

General Treatment Approach

Primary biliary cirrhosis is a progressive disease, and we believe that it is best to treat every patient with this disorder. Initial treatment is based on the combination of symptoms, liver test results, and histologic findings. We begin with ursodiol alone in asymptomatic patients with histologic stage I or II disease and monitor blood test results every 3 months. If test results normalize within 6 months, ursodiol is continued and liver biopsy repeated in 2 years. For patients in whom the histologic appearance remains stable, ursodiol is continued indefinitely, with repeat liver biopsy obtained every 2 to 3 years. The AMA titer is not useful in assessing response to therapy in patients with PBC. Antibody titers tend to be stable over time in certain patients and do not correlate with disease severity or rate of progression.

When the initial liver biopsy shows florid bile duct lesions with active bile duct necrosis or when liver test results do not normalize with ursodeoxycholic acid therapy, colchicine is added. Liver biopsy is then repeated after a year of treatment. If the disease stabilizes, treatment with colchicine and ursodiol is continued with surveillance as described previously. For patients with progressive disease, incapacitating fatigue or pruritus despite treatment, or stage III or IV disease revealed on examination of liver biopsy specimens, we recommend addition of more aggressive therapy such as methotrexate. Until the efficacy of these treatments is established, they ought to be administered in the setting of clinical studies.

Prognosis

The natural history of PBC is one of progressive loss of bile ducts accompanied by deterioration in liver function. Patients who are asymptomatic have a better prognosis than do those who are symptomatic at presentation; however, their life expectancies are shorter than those of age-matched controls. Furthermore, given enough time, patients who are asymptomatic can be expected to develop symptoms.

Once patients become symptomatic, median survival is estimated to be 5 to 7 years. The course of the disease may vary considerably from patient to patient, and statistical models have been developed to predict survival more accurately [20•]. Unfortunately, these models are quite cumbersome and do not take into account the effects of potentially beneficial therapies. Elevation of the serum bilirubin concentration is the single most important prognosticator in each of the statistical models. The appearance of significant hyperbilirubinemia or symptoms of cirrhosis portends short survival and is often followed by rapid clinical deterioration.

▰▰▰ PRIMARY SCLEROSING CHOLANGITIS

Primary sclerosing cholangitis is characterized by inflammatory destruction and fibrosis of the extrahepatic and intrahepatic bile ducts (see Chapter 128).

▰▰▰ GRAFT-VERSUS-HOST DISEASE

Graft-versus-host disease (GVHD) develops when transplanted immune cells react against the histocompatability antigens of the recipient. This phenomenon occurs most commonly after allogeneic bone marrow transplantation. It also may be seen after blood transfusion in an immunocompromized host and, rarely, in patients after liver transplantation. GVHD is a multiorgan illness with liver involvement in most cases. Donor immune cells, predominantly T lymphocytes, initially attack bile duct cells and blood vessel endothelia. Eventually hepatocytes may be damaged. The usual consequence of hepatic involvement is bile duct destruction and cholestasis.

Acute GVHD occurs within 6 weeks of bone marrow transplantation, with patients exhibiting rash, enteritis, and cholestasis. The diagnosis is established clinically when the presentation is typical and can be confirmed readily by skin biopsy. Liver biopsy is required only in atypical cases. Damage to the small bile ducts is seen in all cases. Treatment is aggressive immunosuppression with supportive care of enteritis but frequently is ineffective.

Chronic GVHD develops more than 6 weeks after bone marrow transplantation and may be a sequel to acute disease. Clinically, there is a disproportionate elevation in SAP levels as compared with those of serum aminotransferases. Disruption of the small intrahepatic bile ducts is the predominant liver lesion, with histology resembling that of PBC. Despite increased immunosuppressive therapy, a clinical picture identical to that of advanced PBC may develop. Clinical cholestasis is prominent, often with striking pruritus and jaundice. Treatment with Ursodiol in patients with early GVHD has been associated with improved liver test results. No evidence exits that Ursodiol affects the long-term course of this disease.

◼ CHRONIC LIVER TRANSPLANTATION REJECTION

A syndrome of chronic cellular rejection affecting recipients of liver transplantation has been called *vanishing bile duct syndrome* because of a characteristic progressive loss of the small bile ducts (see Chapter 117). The interlobular bile ducts are attacked by recipient lymphocytes, with additional ischemic injury resulting from damage to endothelial cells in the hepatic arterioles. This form of rejection typically follows an earlier episode of acute cellular rejection, although it is unclear whether the pathogenic mechanisms are similar. As in PBC, PSC, and chronic GVHD, the biliary epithelia in ductopenic transplantation rejection aberrantly express HLA class II antigens on cell surfaces. Infection with cytomegalovirus has been proposed as a possible triggering event.

Patients are asymptomatic during most of the course of chronic allograft rejection, with the only signs being elevations of SAP and GGT levels. Jaundice appears subsequently, with hepatic synthetic function remaining intact until late in the course of rejection. Liver biopsy reveals cholestasis, arteritis, and loss of interlobular and septal bile ducts with lymphocytic infiltration. The differential diagnosis includes extrahepatic biliary obstruction and ischemic injury. With improvements in posttransplant immunosuppressive regimens, and perhaps because of routine prophylaxis for cytomegalovirus infection, the incidence of ductopenic rejection is decreasing. Nevertheless, treatment of established cases of chronic allograft rejection remains unsatisfactory, with most patients ultimately requiring repeat transplantation.

◼ CYSTIC FIBROSIS

Advances in the management of pulmonary complications of cystic fibrosis have allowed many patients to survive well into adulthood. It is estimated that 5% to 20% of these adults will go on to develop chronic cholestatic liver disease. Owing to the absence of a specific transmembrane chloride channel on the biliary epithelial cells, bile produced by patients with cystic fibrosis is particularly viscous. The large and small bile ducts may become plugged by inspissated secretions. Localized strictures similar in appearance to those in PSC have been described in the intrahepatic and extrahepatic ducts, and liver biopsy specimens may show periportal inflammation and fibrosis. Secondary biliary cirrhosis results from prolonged cholestasis. Treatment with ursodiol has been associated with improvements in results of liver tests and hepatic scintigraphy and with stabilization of global health-performance scores. The long-term effects on progression of liver disease, however, are unknown.

◼ EXTRAHEPATIC CHOLESTASIS

Occasionally, chronic cholestatic liver disease is caused by abnormalities completely extrinsic to the liver. Extrahepatic cholestasis occurs when there is mechanical obstruction of the large bile ducts outside the liver. Numerous potential causes of extrahepatic biliary obstruction exist, including gallstones, tumors, benign strictures, congenital anomalies, and infections.

Extrinsic obstruction of bile flow has consequences similar to those of intrahepatic obstruction. In most cases, because extrinsic lesions are more amenable to surgical or endoscopic treatment, the duration of biliary obstruction is less prolonged. Hence, chronic cholestatic liver disease is less likely to be seen in diseases confined to the extrahepatic bile ducts.

The initial hepatic effect of obstruction is failure to secrete bile. Eventually, bilirubin, bile salts, and various toxins accumulate in the blood. The first indicator of early partial obstruction of the bile ducts is an isolated elevation in SAP levels. The typical presenting symptom is pruritus. Nausea and pain may occur from distention of the large bile ducts. Jaundice is a later sign or implies almost complete bile duct obstruction. If obstruction continues for weeks or months in the absence of infection, progressive liver damage may develop. Reflux of bile components into the hepatic parenchyma occurs with accumulation of toxins and reactive inflammation. Direct chemical damage and subsequent immunologic reaction result in destruction of hepatocytes. If this process continues over months or years, irreversible liver damage with scarring, called *secondary biliary cirrhosis*, may ensue.

The treatment for extrahepatic cholestasis is relief of biliary obstruction. Because the responsible lesions are located in the large extrahepatic ducts, therapy frequently is successful and may be achieved by surgical, percutaneous, or endoscopic means. It is unclear whether cirrhosis reverses or improves after relief of bile duct obstruction. We have followed up several patients with cirrhosis whose course over many years suggests that such reversal may occur. After relief of biliary obstruction, blood test results return to normal and the results of subsequent liver biopsies suggest a diminution of scarring. It should be noted that sampling variations in liver biopsy specimens make it impossible to be certain that the cirrhosis has truly reversed or remitted. It is clear, however, that hepatocytes can recover and regenerate. The prognosis in extrahepatic cholestasis is primarily related to the cause of biliary obstruction.

REFERENCES

Recently published papers of particular interest have been highlighted as follows:
- Of interest
- Of outstanding interest

1. Jones EA, Yurdaydin C: Is fatigue associated with cholestasis mediated by altered central neurotransmission? *Hepatology* 1997, 25:492–494.

2.• Bergasa NV, Alling DW, Talbot TL, *et al.*: Effects of naloxone infusions in patients with the pruritus of cholestasis. A double-blind, randomized, controlled trial. *Ann Intern Med* 1995, 123:161–167.

3. Heathcote J: The clinical expression of primary biliary cirrhosis. *Sem Liver Dis* 1996, 17:23–33.

4. Matloff DS, Kaplan MM, Neer RM, *et al.*: Osteoporosis in primary biliary cirrhosis: effects of 25-hydroxyvitamin D_3 treatment. *Gastroenterology* 1982, 83:97–102.

5. Hay JE: Bone disease in cholestatic liver disease. *Gastroenterology* 1995, 108:276–283.

6.•• Gilliespie DA, Vickers CR: Pruritus and cholestasis: therapeutic options. *Gastroenterol Hepatology* 1993, 8:168–173.

7.• Kaplan MM: Primary biliary cirrhosis. *N Engl J Med* 1996, 335:1570–1580.

8. Van de Water J, Turchany L, Leung PS, *et al.*: Molecular mimicry in primary biliary cirrhosis. Evidence for biliary epithelial expression of a molecular cross-reactive with pyruvate dehydrogenase complex-E2. *J Clin Invest* 1993, 91:2653–2664.

9.• Rubin RA, Kowalski TE, Khandelwal M, Malet PF. Ursodiol for hepatobiliary disorders. *Ann Intern Med* 1994, 121:207–218.

10. Heathcote EJ, Cauch-Dudek K, Walker V, *et al.*: The Canadian multicenter double-blind randomized controlled trial of ursodeoxycholic acid in primary biliary cirrhosis. *Hepatology* 1994, 19:1149–1156.

11.• Lindor KD, Dickson ER, Baldus WP, *et al.*: Ursodeoxycholic acid in the treatment of primary biliary cirrhosis. *Gastroenterology* 1994, 106:1284–1290.

12. Combes B, Carithers RLJ, Maddrey WC, *et al.*: A randomized, double-blind, placebo-controlled trial of ursodeoxycholic acid in primary biliary cirrhosis. *Hepatology* 1995, 22:759–766.

13. Kaplan MM, Alling DW, Zimmerman HW, *et al.*: A prospective trial of colchicine for primary biliary cirrhosis. *New Engl J Med* 1986, 315:1448–1454.

14.• Poupon RE, Huet PM, Poupon R, *et al.*: A randomized trial comparing colchicine and ursodeoxycholic acid combination to ursodeoxycholic acid in primary biliary cirrhosis. UDCA-PBC Study Group. *Hepatology* 1996, 24:1098 1103.

15. Lombard M, Portmann B, Neuberger J, *et al.*: Cyclosporin A treatment in primary biliary cirrhosis: results of a long-term placebo controlled trial. *Gastroenterology* 1993, 104:519–526.

16.• Kaplan MM, Knox TA: Treatment of primary biliary cirrhosis with low-dose weekly methotrexate. *Gastroenterol* 1991, 101:1332–1338.

17. Kaplan MM, DeLellis RA, Wolfe HJ: Sustained biochemical and histologic remission of primary biliary cirrhosis in response to medical treatment. *Ann Intern Med* 1997, 126:682–688.

18. Buscher HP, Zietzschmann Y, Gerok W: Positive responses to methotrexate and ursodeoxycholic acid in patients with primary biliary cirrhosis responding insufficiently to ursodeoxycholic acid alone. *Hepatology* 1993, 18:9–14.

19. Lindor KD, Dickson ER, Jorgensen RA, *et al.*: The combination of ursodeoxycholic acid and methotrexate for patients with primary biliary cirrhosis: the results of a pilot study. *Hepatology* 1995, 22:1158–1162.

20.• Dickson ER, Grambsch PM, Fleming TR, *et al.*: Prognosis in primary biliary cirrhosis: model for decision making. *Hepatology* 1989, 10:1–7.

21. Kaplan MM: The use of methotrexate, colchicine, and other immunomodulatory drugs in the treatment of primary biliary cirrhosis. *Semin Liver Dis* 1997, 17:130.

107 Wilson's Disease
Michael L. Schilsky

Wilson's disease is an autosomal recessive genetic disorder of copper metabolism that affects about one in 30,000 people. The gene for Wilson's disease is located on chromosome 13 and encodes a copper-transporting ATPase, ATP7B, which is highly expressed in liver. Individuals who inherit disease-specific mutations of both ATP7B alleles express the disease, whereas individuals with a mutation of only one ATP7B allele are heterozygotes who do not develop Wilson's disease and do not require treatment. The diagnosis of Wilson's disease is made on the basis of a combination of physical and biochemical findings, most notably a decrease in circulating levels of ceruloplasmin, the presence of Kayser-Fleischer rings, and a hepatic copper content of greater than 250 µg per gram of liver (dry weight). If left untreated, patients develop hepatic insufficiency, neurologic or psychiatric symptoms, and, ultimately, liver failure. Treatment with metal-chelating agents effectively reverses or stabilizes the disease in most symptomatic people. Lifelong treatment with metal-chelating agents or, alternatively, with zinc salts results in excellent survival. Fulminant hepatic failure and hepatic insufficiency unresponsive to medical therapy resulting from Wilson's disease are treated best by orthotopic liver transplantation, which is curative.

GENETICS

Recognition that Wilson's disease is a genetic disorder dates to Wilson's original description in 1912 [1]; Bearn and Kunkel are credited with the discovery that the gene defect is inherited in an autosomal recessive fashion. The Wilson's disease gene, located on chromosome 13 and designated ATP7B, is highly expressed in liver. Proof that this gene is responsible for Wilson's disease followed identification of disease-specific mutations [2]; more than 60 individual mutations of the

ATP7B gene have been described to date. Most affected individuals have two different mutations, one on each allele of chromosome 13, which makes molecular genetic diagnosis by direct mutation analysis difficult, as discussed later in this chapter.

PATHOPHYSIOLOGY

Copper is an essential cofactor for many enzymes and proteins and also plays a role in iron metabolism. The hepatocyte is responsible for extraction of ingested copper from the portal circulation, incorporation of the copper into the secretory glycoprotein ceruloplasmin, and its biliary excretion. Biliary copper excretion is critical to normal copper homeostasis, because excreted copper undergoes minimal enterohepatic recirculation. Reduced biliary excretion of copper is responsible for hepatic accumulation of this metal in persons with Wilson's disease. Figure 107-1 provides a brief summary of copper metabolism and the pathophysiology of Wilson's disease.

Reduced or absent function of the ATP7B gene product is thought to be responsible for decreased biliary copper excretion and reduced incorporation of copper into ceruloplasmin. The transported copper is subsequently incorporated into ceruloplasmin as well as transferred to lysosomes for export in bile.

In people with Wilson's disease, the accumulation of copper that results from decreased copper excretion causes hepatocellular injury. Toxic effects of excess copper include generation of free radicals, lipid peroxidation of cell membranes and DNA, inhibition of protein synthesis, and altered levels of cellular antioxidants [3]. The final result of unchecked hepatocyte damage is cell death, and the balance among injury, cell death, and hepatocyte regeneration determines the status of liver function.

The saturation of hepatocellular storage sites for copper and copper-induced liver injury result in release of stored metal and an increase in circulating non–ceruloplasmin-bound copper. This process is thought to be responsible for extrahepatic copper deposition, the most important site of which is the brain. Copper-induced brain injury is responsible for the neurologic and psychiatric manifestations of Wilson's disease.

PATHOLOGY

A diagnosis of Wilson's disease is suggested by characteristic histologic and histochemical features discovered on liver biopsy. The most common associated biopsy findings in the early stages of disease are microvesicular and macrovesicular steatosis, glycogen nuclei, and cytoplasmic nuclear invaginations (Fig. 107-2, see **Color Plate**). Common late findings include active inflammation with piecemeal necrosis, fibrosis, and cirrhosis. Patients presenting with fulminant hepatic failure may have severe hepatocellular injury with parenchymal loss as well as fibrosis or cirrhosis [4].

Histochemical staining of liver biopsy specimens for copper-binding protein using rhodanine may assist in recognition of this disorder, but a negative result does not exclude the diagnosis. The livers of patients with Wilson's disease typically have some nodules that contain excess copper-binding protein and others that do not (Fig. 107-2C, see **Color Plate**) [5]. Rhodanine also may stain some periportal cells in liver biopsy specimens from patients with cholestatic liver disease and hepatic copper accumulation not due to Wilson's disease.

CLINICAL FEATURES

Although Wilson's disease may affect many different organs as it progresses, patients with this disorder most commonly present with liver disease, or with neurologic or psychiatric symptoms (Table 107-1). Affected individuals found by family screening, however, often are asymptomatic. Failure to begin

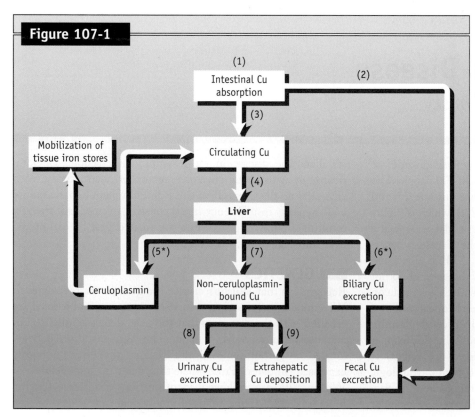

Figure 107-1

Copper metabolism and pathophysiology of Wilson's disease. Copper ingested in the diet is absorbed in the proximal small intestine [1], whereas nonabsorbed copper or copper bound within shed enterocytes passes into the feces [2]. Absorbed copper is bound mainly to albumin in the portal circulation [3] and is avidly extracted by hepatocytes [4]. Hepatocellular copper is utilized directly for metabolic needs, bound to endogenous chelators, incorporated into ceruloplasmin for secretion [5], or excreted into bile [6], where it does not undergo enterohepatic recycling and, therefore, is excreted in the feces. In Wilson's disease, biliary copper excretion is reduced [5*], and copper accumulates within hepatocytes. Incorporation of copper into ceruloplasmin also is impaired [6*], leading to decreased circulating levels of this protein in most patients. When cellular stores are overloaded or following hepatocellular injury caused by excess copper, there is an increase in the release of non–ceruloplasmin-bound copper [7], leading to an increase in urinary copper excretion [8] and extrahepatic deposition of this metal [9].

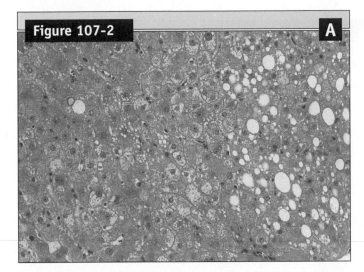

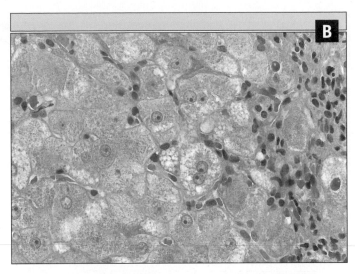

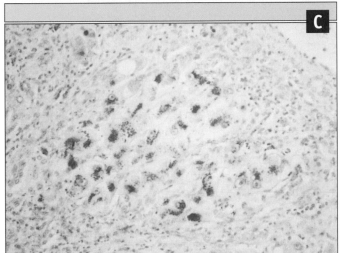

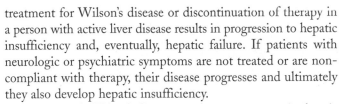

Light microscopic findings in the liver in Wilson's disease. **A,** Prominent microvesicular and macrovesicular steatosis and some inflammatory cells in a specimen from an asymptomatic patient with Wilson's disease. **B,** Hepatocellular ballooning and degeneration in a biopsy specimen from a patient with fulminant Wilsonian hepatitis. **C,** Rhodamine-positive nodule in a patient with Wilson's disease. See **Color Plate.**

Table 107-1. Clinical Presentations of Wilson's Disease

Asymptomatic

Liver disease

Neurologic signs and symptoms

Psychiatric symptoms

Renal disease

---

treatment for Wilson's disease or discontinuation of therapy in a person with active liver disease results in progression to hepatic insufficiency and, eventually, hepatic failure. If patients with neurologic or psychiatric symptoms are not treated or are non-compliant with therapy, their disease progresses and ultimately they also develop hepatic insufficiency.

Patients with Wilson's disease may have asymptomatic chronic hepatitis with liver test abnormalities and histologic evidence of hepatic injury, fulminant hepatic failure, or cirrhosis with or without hepatic insufficiency. Fulminant hepatic failure resulting from Wilson's disease probably represents a combination of acute and chronic liver injury. People with Wilson's disease nearly always develop liver disease before the age of 20 years.

Patients who present with neurologic or psychiatric manifestations of Wilson's disease do so at a later age than those who present with hepatic symptoms [4]. Most of these patients already have asymptomatic liver disease when their neurologic disease becomes evident. The neurologic disease often is characterized by motor abnormalities with parkinsonian characteristics. Patients with dysarthria also may have transfer dysphagia.

Rare clinical manifestations of Wilson's disease include nephrocalcinosis, hematuria, and aminoaciduria [4]. Patients also may experience arthralgias and develop premature osteoarthrosis [6]. Accumulation of copper in the myocardium has been reported to cause cardiomyopathy and arrhythmias [7].

▮▮▮ DIAGNOSIS

The diagnosis of Wilson's disease is based on a combination of clinical and biochemical findings (Table 107-2).

Ophthalmologic features of Wilson's disease, best seen on slit-lamp examination, include characteristic corneal deposition of copper in Descemet's membrane (*ie*, Kayser-Fleischer rings; Fig. 107-3, see **Color Plate**), and, rarely, sunflower cataracts [8]. There is a low circulating ceruloplasmin level in 95% of patients with Wilson's disease, but also in 20% of heterozygotes. Because approximately 90% of serum copper is incorporated in ceruloplasmin, total serum copper is low in most individuals, except in the presence of fulminant hepatitis with associated hemolysis, in which case it often is markedly elevated. People with Wilson's disease also may have other biochemical evidence of liver disease, including abnormal serum aminotransferase, bilirubin, and albumin levels, and a prolonged prothrombin time. Heterozygotes do not develop liver disease; individuals with a low serum ceruloplasmin, no Kayser-Fleischer rings, and abnormal liver tests must have a liver biopsy to exclude the diagnosis.

The presence of Kayser-Fleischer rings and a low serum ceruloplasmin level, liver disease, or neurologic or psychiatric symptoms establishes the diagnosis of Wilson's disease. Only rarely do patients with long-standing cholestasis caused by other types of liver disease have Kayser-Fleischer rings [9].

Table 107-2. Diagnostic Testing for Wilson's Disease

Diagnostic test	Normal	Wilson's disease	Comment
Slit-lamp examination	Normal	Kayser-Fleischer rings	Absent early in the disease
Ceruloplasmin	20–40 mg/dL	<20 mg/dL	Normal in 5% of patients; decreased in 20% of heterozygotes; decreased in newborns and people with congenital hypoceruloplasminemia, severe protein-losing enteropathy, or nephropathy, and in severe hepatic insufficiency
Serum copper	70–150 µg/dL	<100 µg/dL	Proportional to ceruloplasmin concentration except in fulminant Wilsonian hepatitis, where it is markedly elevated
24-hour urine copper	<50 µg	>100 µg	Abnormal in most symptomatic patients; often normal or intermediate in asymptomatic patients
Hepatic copper	<100 µg/g dry wt	>250 µg/g dry wt	Can be intermediate in heterozygotes; elevated in disorders with chronic cholestasis
Histopathology	Normal	Abnormal	Steatosis, glycogen nuclei, fibrosis, chronic active hepatitis, cirrhosis
Histochemistry for copper	Negative	Positive	In some but not all nodules; useful only if positive
Electron microscopy of liver	Normal	Abnormal	Stage-specific alterations in mitochondrial and lysosomal ultrastructure
MRI of brain	Normal	Abnormal	T_2-weighted scans best highlight abnormalities of the basal ganglia, subcortical white matter, midbrain, and pons in most patients with neurologic or psychiatric symptoms and in some asymptomatic patients

Figure 107-3

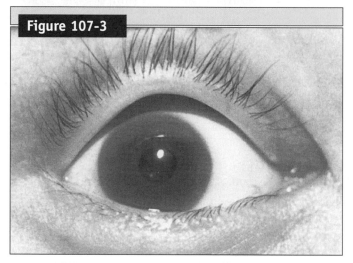

Kayser-Fleischer ring in a patient 17 years of age with neurologic symptoms caused by Wilson's disease. See **Color Plate**.

Figure 107-4

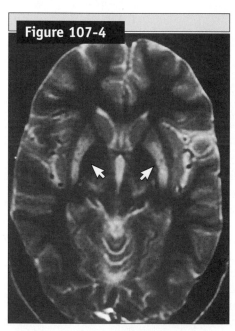

Magnetic resonance image of the brain of a woman 21 years of age with dysarthria, dysphagia, slurring of speech, and tremors caused by Wilson's disease. Note the hyperintensity in the region of the basal ganglia (*arrows*).

When Kayser-Fleischer rings are absent, a liver biopsy almost always is necessary to look for histologic features of Wilson's disease and to determine hepatic copper content. If a percutaneous liver biopsy is contraindicated, and a transjugular liver biopsy cannot be performed, a combination of a low serum ceruloplasmin and a high 24-hour urinary copper excretion may be used to make the diagnosis. Measurement of urinary copper alone is not reliable for excluding a diagnosis of Wilson's disease because values often are normal in asymptomatic subjects and may be somewhat high in heterozygotes and in persons with other severe liver diseases. Martins da Costa *et al*. [10] have proposed use of a penicillamine-stimulation test for urinary copper excretion in children with liver disease, but this test has not been evaluated in adults. Screening of first-degree relatives of patients with Wilson's disease is mandatory.

Wilson's disease may present as fulminant hepatic failure, often associated with nonimmune hemolytic anemia, low serum alkaline phosphatase, and high serum and urinary copper levels [11–13]. Kayser-Fleischer rings, if present in a patient with fulminant hepatic failure, confirm the diagnosis. The ratio of serum alkaline phosphatase to serum bilirubin is often, but not always, less than 2 to 1 in affected individuals, whereas it is usually greater than 2 to 1 in people with fulminant hepatic failure from other causes.

Characteristic brain abnormalities seen on magnetic resonance imaging (MRI) may suggest that a patient with neurologic symptoms has Wilson's disease (Fig. 107-4) [14•]; these abnormalities have been detected before the onset of clinical symptoms and in the absence of Kayser-Fleischer rings. In contrast, persons with neurologic or psychiatric symptoms almost invariably have Kayser-Fleischer rings [4].

First-degree relatives of patients with Wilson's disease should have a slit-lamp examination and a clinical evaluation for neurologic and hepatic disease, and biochemical studies including liver tests and a serum ceruloplasmin level. If this evaluation is negative, then the individual is either a normal homozygote or heterozygous for the Wilson's disease gene mutation; usually, no further testing is required. Urinary copper excretion has been used by some experts to screen family members of patients with Wilson's disease, but results of this test often are ambiguous in asymptomatic individuals and abnormal in some patients with other types of liver disease. If the diagnosis remains in question, a liver biopsy for quantitative copper and histology should be performed.

The discovery of the Wilson's disease gene has made family screening for disease-specific mutations possible. Only 15% to 30% of patients have the most common mutation; the rest have numerous different mutations of the ATP7B gene. Detection of these mutations currently is not commercially available and possible only at specialized centers, but it should become available in the future.

■ TREATMENT AND FOLLOW-UP MANAGEMENT

In Wilson's disease, the major goal of therapy is to reverse accumulation of copper and thereby prevent progression of disease. Treatment may be categorized into care of symptomatic patients, care of asymptomatic patients, and maintenance therapy.

The drugs used to treat Wilson's disease include chelating agents and zinc salts (Table 107-3). Chelating agents (eg, penicillamine, trientine, British antilewisite [BAL], and tetrathiomolybdate) remove and detoxify copper from within cells. Zinc salts primarily block absorption of dietary copper, but also stimulate hepatic synthesis of endogenous chelators, which detoxify remaining metal [15].

Treatment of asymptomatic patients (a group that does not include those with abnormal liver tests or histologic hepatitis) is the same as maintenance therapy. The largest maintenance experience has been with penicillamine; however, availability of alternative drugs with fewer potential side effects, including trientine and zinc salts, suggests that these agents, previously used only to treat penicillamine-intolerant patients, should be considered as primary therapy and for long-term use. Although any of these medications may be used effectively, monitoring for efficacy and patient compliance is critical.

The best treatment for symptomatic patients is controversial. A chelating agent as initial therapy for patients with hepatic or neuropsychiatric symptoms is recommended. Penicillamine is the chelating agent with which the largest number of patients have been treated; there are great variations in the reported incidence of side effects from this drug [4,16]. Regression of neurologic symptoms may occur during initiation of penicillamine therapy in about 10% of treated patients. Whether or not this regression would have occurred with other chelating agents is uncertain. Trientine has proven to be effective in treating penicillamine-intolerant patients [17]; there is growing experience with this drug as first-line therapy for hepatic and neurologic disease, although most reports of its use as primary treatment are limited to just a few cases [18]. For patients who cannot tolerate penicillamine and trientine, zinc salts may be used as initial therapy. Another chelating agent, tetrathiomolybdate, currently is being evaluated as an initial treatment for patients with neurologic symptoms.

British antilewisite was the first therapy for Wilson's disease; currently it is used only to treat patients with neurologic or psychiatric symptoms that are refractory to oral chelation therapy [4]. This intramuscularly administered drug may be given with either penicillamine or trientine, and has some theoretical advantage in patients with central nervous system involvement because it is lipophilic and able to cross the blood-brain barrier. Its main drawbacks are the difficulty and discomfort associated with intramuscular injection.

Patients with severe hepatic insufficiency unresponsive to medical therapy and those with fulminant hepatic failure are candidates for orthotopic liver transplantation. Approximately 80% of patients who receive liver transplants for treatment of hepatic Wilson's disease survive [19]; liver transplant cures the disease and may improve neurologic symptoms.

Treatment of Wilson's disease in pregnant women is modified to maintain adequate disease control and reduce teratogenicity and problems with wound healing. Patients treated with penicillamine, trientine, and zinc have had successful pregnancies [4,20]. The doses of chelating agents should be lowered during the second trimester and the first 2 months of the third trimester to 500 mg/d; they should be lowered further to 250 mg/d for the 6 weeks before delivery and during wound healing

---

Table 107-3. Therapy for Wilson's Disease

Penicillamine

Trientine

Zinc salts (zinc sulfate, gluconate, acetate)

British antiLewisite (BAL, dimercaptopropanol)

Tetrathiomolybdate

Orthotopic liver transplantation

Table 107-4. Maintenance Therapy for Wilson's Disease

Agent	Oral maintenance dosage (adult)	Comments
Penicillamine	750–1000 mg in 3 or 4 divided doses	Monitor for lupus-like reactions, and marrow suppression; requires supplemental pyridoxine; dosage reduction for surgery and pregnancy
Trientine	750–1000 mg in 3 or 4 divided doses	Monitor for sideroblastic anemia; dosage reduction for surgery and pregnancy
Zinc salts	150 mg elemental zinc in 3 divided doses	Occasional gastric intolerance

if the baby is delivered by cesarean section. Zinc therapy need not be modified during pregnancy.

If they require surgery, patients with Wilson's disease who are treated with a chelating agent should have the dose reduced perioperatively to avoid problems with wound healing. Doses of penicillamine and trientine can be reduced to 250 to 500 mg daily during this time and increased rapidly after the wound has healed (Table 107-4).

Patient compliance with treatment is extremely important to the long-term success of pharmacotherapy of Wilson's disease. Compliance may be monitored by clinical evaluation for changes in symptoms and signs of liver and neurologic disease, screening for laboratory evidence of hepatitis, periodic slit-lamp examination, and testing for non–ceruloplasmin-bound copper. The level of non–ceruloplasmin-bound copper is the difference between total serum copper and total ceruloplasmin copper as derived from its oxidase activity (bioactive ceruloplasmin contains 0.47 μmol copper per mg protein). In healthy individuals and appropriately treated patients, non–ceruloplasmin-bound copper should be no more than 10 μg. In untreated, inadequately treated, and noncompliant patients, this value often is greater than 25 μg. Urinary copper excretion also may be used to monitor compliance with chelation therapy. During early treatment, values often are more than 1000 μg per day; they decline to about 250 to 500 μg per day over time. Lower values suggest either noncompliance with therapy or possible misdiagnosis. Urinary zinc excretion and plasma zinc levels also may be used to monitor compliance with zinc therapy. Patients on zinc therapy do not have significantly elevated 24-hour urinary copper excretions because zinc prevents copper absorption. Urinary copper absorption greater than 150 to 250 μg per day in a patient treated with zinc may indicate noncompliance or inadequate therapy.

▇ PROGNOSIS

The prognosis for treated patients with Wilson's disease is excellent, even if they have cirrhosis or chronic hepatitis at the time of diagnosis [21]. Many patients with neurologic or psychiatric symptoms improve in the months or years following initiation of therapy. Some patients have persistent neurologic symptoms but stable liver disease. At present, there is no way to predict the degree to which symptomatic patients with Wilson's disease will respond to treatment. Approximately 80% of individuals who undergo orthotopic liver transplantation for Wilson's disease survive, and, with rare exceptions, require no further treatment for Wilson's disease [19].

▇ REFERENCES

Recently published papers of particular interest have been highlighted as follows:
- Of interest
- •• Of outstanding interest

1. Wilson SAK: Progressive lenticular degeneration: a familial nervous disease associated with cirrhosis of the liver. *Brain* 1912, 34:295–507.

2. Tanzi RE, Petrukhin K, Chernov I, *et al*.: The Wilson's disease gene is a copper transporting ATPase with homology to the Menkes disease gene. *Nature Genet* 1993, 5:344–350.

3. Sternlieb I: Copper and zinc. In *The Liver: Biology and Pathobiology*, vol 3. Edited by Arias IM, Boyer JL, Fausto N, *et al*. New York: Raven Press; 1994:585–596.

4. Scheinberg IH, Sternlieb I: *Wilson's disease*. Philadelphia: WB Saunders; 1984.

5. Alt E, Sternlieb I, Goldfischer S: The cytopathology of metal overload [review]. *Int Rev Exp Pathol* 1990, 31:165–188.

6. Mindelzun R, Elkin M, Scheinberg IH, *et al*.: Skeletal changes in Wilson's disease: a radiologic study. *Radiology* 1970, 94:127–132.

7. Kuan P: Fatal cardiac complications of Wilson's disease. *Am Heart J* 1982, 104:314–316.

8. Cairns JE, Williams HP, Walshe JM: Sunflower cataract in Wilson's disease. *Br Med J* 1969, 3:95–96.

9. Tauber J, Steinert RF: Pseudo-Kayser-Fleischer ring of the cornea associated with non-Wilsonian liver disease: a case report and literature review [review]. *Cornea* 1993, 12:74–77.

10. Martins da Costa C, Baldwin D, Portmann B, *et al*.: Value of urinary copper excretion after penicillamine challenge in the diagnosis of Wilson's disease. *Hepatology* 1992, 15:609–615.

11. McCullough AJ, Fleming CR, Thistle JL, *et al*.: Diagnosis of Wilson's disease presenting as fulminant hepatic failure. *Gastroenterology* 1983, 84:161–167.

12. Shaver WA, Bhatt H, Combes B: Low serum alkaline phosphatase activity in Wilson's disease. *Hepatology* 1986, 6:859–863.

13. Berman DH, Leventhal RI, Gavaler JS, *et al*.: Clinical differentiation of fulminant Wilsonian hepatitis for other causes of hepatic failure. *Gastroenterology* 1991, 100:1129–1134.

14.• Van Wassenaer-van Hall HN, van den Huewel AG, Algra A, *et al*.: Wilson's disease: findings at MR imaging and CT of the brain with clinical correlation. *Radiology* 1996, 198:531–536.

This report provides a recent comparison of the use of brain MRI and computed tomography (CT) in Wilson's disease and its correlation with patients neurologic status.

15. Danks DM: Disorders of copper metabolism, vol 1. In *The Metabolic Basis of Inherited Disease*. Edited by Scriver CR, Beaudet AL, Sly WS, Valle D. New York: McGraw-Hill; 1989:1411–1431.

16. Brewer GJ, Terry CA, Aisen AM, Hall GM: Worsening of neurologic syndrome in patients with Wilson's disease with metal penicillamine therapy. *Arch Neurol* 1987, 44:490–493.

17. Scheinberg IH, Jaffe ME, Sternlieb I: The use of trientine in preventing the effects of interrupting penicillamine therapy in Wilson's disease. *N Engl J Med* 1987, 317:209–213.

18. Santos-Silva EE, Sarles J, Buts JP, Sokol EM: Successful medical treatment of severely decompensated Wilson disease. *J Pediatr* 1996, 128:285–287.

19.• Schilsky ML, Scheinberg IH, Sternlieb I: Hepatic transplantation for Wilson's disease: indication and outcome. *Hepatology* 1994, 19:583–587.

Overall transplant survival was 80%. Fulminant hepatitis and severe hepatic insufficiency unresponsive to pharmacotherapy remain appropiate indications for orthotopic liver transplantation.

20. Brewer JB, Yuzbasiyan-Gurkan V: Wilson's disease. *Medicine* 1992, 71:139–163.

21. Schilsky ML, Scheinberg IH, Sternlieb I: Prognosis of Wilsonian chronic active hepatitis. *Gastroenterology* 1991, 100:762–767.

108 Hemochromatosis

Bruce R. Bacon

Hemochromatosis is an HLA-linked inherited disease caused by inappropriate iron absorption and pathologic iron deposition in parenchymal cells of the liver, heart, pancreas, and other organs. Excessive tissue iron eventually results in cell damage, fibrosis, and functional insufficiency. Other clinically distinct syndromes of iron overload that should be distinguished from hereditary hemochromatosis include secondary iron overload caused by ineffective erythropoiesis, primary liver disease, excessive iron ingestion, and congenital atransferrinemia (Table 108-1). Iatrogenic parenteral iron overload may be caused by red blood cell (RBC) transfusions or iron dextran injections. Patients with hematologic disorders treated with RBC transfusions may have both secondary and parenteral iron overload. Neonatal iron overload is a rare disorder that has been recognized only during the past 15 years; no relationship between neonatal iron overload and hereditary hemochromatosis has been identified. African iron overload is presumed to be caused by a genetic abnormality that is not HLA-linked in addition to ingestion of iron-enriched home-brewed beer [1,2].

Table 108-1. Classification of Iron Overload Syndromes

Hereditary hemochromatosis (inherited, HLA linked)
Secondary iron overload
  Anemia caused by ineffective erythropoiesis
    β-Thalassemia
    Sideroblastic anemia
    Aplastic anemia
    Pyruvate kinase deficiency
    Pyridoxine-responsive anemia
    X-linked iron-loading anemia
  Liver disease
    Alcoholic cirrhosis
    Chronic viral hepatitis
    After portocaval shunt
    Porphyria cutanea tarda
  Other
    Excessive iron ingestion
    Congenital atransferrinemia (rare)
Parenteral iron overload
  Red blood cell transfusions
  Iron dextran injections
  Associated with long-term hemodialysis
Neonatal iron overload
African iron overload (inherited, non–HLA linked)

INHERITANCE AND PATHOPHYSIOLOGY

Hereditary hemochromatosis is a common autosomal recessive disorder of iron metabolism that affects about one in 300 persons. Prospective screening studies of predominately white populations have shown that as many as one in 300 persons are homozygotes and between one in eight and one in 12 persons are heterozygotes, making hereditary hemochromatosis the most common inherited disease. It now is possible to detect hereditary hemochromatosis in asymptomatic probands and in presymptomatic relatives of patients, which allows diagnosis of this disease in persons who have not yet developed organ damage. Accordingly, the diagnosis no longer is confined to symptomatic patients and persons with cirrhosis, diabetes, or skin pigmentation; rather, every person with both alleles of the hemochromatosis gene and direct or indirect markers of iron overload should be regarded as having hereditary hemochromatosis. It still is not known whether every homozygote with hereditary hemochromatosis develops iron overload.

A candidate hereditary hemochromatosis gene has been identified on the short arm of chromosome 6 and named *HFE*. Studies have shown that 64% to 100% of persons with phenotypic hereditary hemochromatosis have a tyrosine molecule substituted for a cysteine molecule at position 282 (C282Y) of both *HFE* genes. An additional 5% of patients with hereditary hemochromatosis have this mutation in one *HFE* gene and an aspartate molecule substituted for a histidine molecule at position 63 (H63D) of the other *HFE* gene (compound heterozygotes). More studies are necessary to determine the clinical significance of the compound heterozygous condition. Of patients with a clinical syndrome resembling hereditary hemochromatosis, 10% to 15% do not have the C282Y mutation. Some of these patients may have another *HFE* mutation, whereas others may have secondary iron overload.

The *HFE* gene encodes a cell-membrane protein that interacts with β_2-microglobulin, which plays a role in normal cellular iron uptake and distribution. The mechanisms by which the HFE protein regulates the iron absorption and the ways in which the C282Y mutation impair normal HFE protein function are not yet understood.

PATHOLOGIC FEATURES

In uncomplicated hereditary hemochromatosis, the most iron is deposited in periportal hepatocytes, and decreasing amounts of iron are found in lobular hepatocytes closer to the central vein. Iron deposition is predominantly hepatocellular, with little, if any, in Kupffer's cells or macrophages (Fig. 108-1, see **Color Plate**). Fibrosis and cirrhosis usually develop when the hepatic iron concentration (HIC) is greater than 20,000 μg of iron per 1 g of liver (dry weight), although such changes may occur when the HIC is much lower in patients with other liver diseases, such as chronic viral hepatitis or alcoholic liver disease. When the diagnosis of hereditary hemochromatosis is considered, a portion of the liver biopsy sample should be reserved for determination of the HIC; patients with symptomatic hereditary hemochromatosis usually have HICs of greater than 10,000 μg/g, and levels may be as high as 40,000 μg/g in some individuals. In younger patients who do not have symptoms, hepatic iron levels are increased but commonly are less than 10,000 μg/g. In addition to iron, other findings on liver biopsy in patients with hereditary hemochromatosis include steatosis, which usually is seen in patients who also are diabetic or obese. Distinct histopathologic changes also are found in the heart, skin, joints, brain, pancreas, and other endocrine organs of patients with hereditary hemochromatosis, depending on the extent of disease.

■ CLINICAL FEATURES

Patients with hereditary hemochromatosis may have numerous symptoms and findings on physical examination (Tables 108-2 and 108-3), but many affected patients, including relatives of

persons with hereditary hemochromatosis, are identified by screening only serum iron studies [4,5]. More than 75% of patients identified by screening do not have symptoms, with a low incidence (<25%) of cirrhosis, diabetes, and skin pigmentation. In older series of patients diagnosed by symptoms and signs of the disease, women typically are described as presenting about 10 years later than men, presumably because of the protective effect of menstrual blood loss and iron loss during pregnancy. Recently, more patients with hereditary hemochromatosis have been identified on the basis of blood tests done before symptoms developed; therefore, age at diagnosis is roughly equivalent for women and men. When confronted with abnormal iron studies, physicians should not wait for typical symptoms or signs of hereditary hemochromatosis to develop before considering the diagnosis and should be aware that young, multiparous women can be iron-loaded and, thus, should not be excluded from further evaluation. The most common symptoms of hereditary hemochromatosis are weakness, fatigue, and

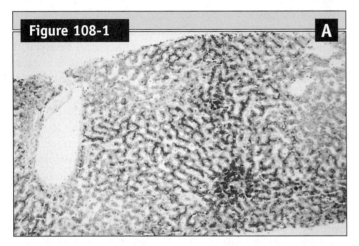 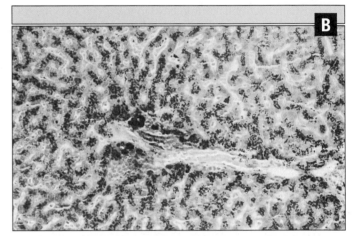

Figure 108-1

Liver histology in hereditary hemochromatosis. **A**, At low power, increased iron deposition can be seen in a periportal distribution (Perls' Prussian blue stain, original magnification × 40). **B**, At higher power, the iron deposits can be seen predominantly in hepatocytes in a pericanalicular distribution (Perls' Prussian blue stain, original magnification × 200). See **Color Plate**.

Table 108-2. Symptoms of Hereditary Hemochromatosis

Nonspecific, systemic symptoms
  Weakness
  Lethargy
  Fatigue
  Apathy
  Weight loss
Specific, organ-related symptoms
  Abdominal pain (hepatomegaly)
  Arthralgias (arthritis)
  Loss of libido, impotence (pituitary, liver)
  Amenorrhea (cirrhosis)
  Congestive heart failure (heart)
  Diabetes (endocrine, pancreas)
Asymptomatic
  Abnormal serum iron studies on routine screening
  Workup of abnormal liver tests
  Identified by family screening
  Identified by population screening

Table 108-3. Physical Findings in Patients With Hereditary Hemochromatosis

Liver
  Hepatomegaly
  Stigmata of chronic liver disease
  Splenomegaly
  Hepatic failure
Joints
  Arthritis
  Joint swelling
Heart
  Dilated cardiomyopathy
  Congestive heart failure
Skin
  Increased pigmentation
Endocrine organs
  Testicular atrophy
  Hypogonadism
  Hypothyroidism

arthralgia. The full clinical expression of hereditary hemochromatosis is influenced by gender, age, environment, and other unknown factors, and the disease may not be expressed fully in all homozygotes.

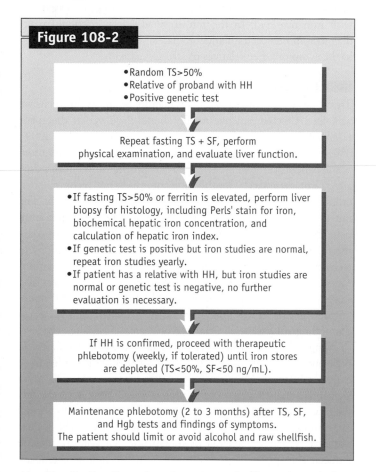

Figure 108-2

- Random TS>50%
- Relative of proband with HH
- Positive genetic test

↓

Repeat fasting TS + SF, perform physical examination, and evaluate liver function.

↓

- If fasting TS>50% or ferritin is elevated, perform liver biopsy for histology, including Perls' stain for iron, biochemical hepatic iron concentration, and calculation of hepatic iron index.
- If genetic test is positive but iron studies are normal, repeat iron studies yearly.
- If patient has a relative with HH, but iron studies are normal or genetic test is negative, no further evaluation is necessary.

↓

If HH is confirmed, proceed with therapeutic phlebotomy (weekly, if tolerated) until iron stores are depleted (TS<50%, SF<50 ng/mL).

↓

Maintenance phlebotomy (2 to 3 months) after TS, SF, and Hgb tests and findings of symptoms. The patient should limit or avoid alcohol and raw shellfish.

Algorithm for the diagnosis and management of hemochromatosis. Hgb—hemoglobin; HH—hereditary hemochromatosis; SF—serum transferrin; TS—transferrin saturation.

DIAGNOSIS

When a relative of a person with hereditary hemochromatosis or when a person with an abnormal serum iron level or signs or symptoms compatible with hemochromatosis is suspected of having hereditary hemochromatosis, definitive diagnosis is relatively straightforward (Fig. 108-2). Fasting serum iron and total iron-binding capacity or serum transferrin should be measured and the transferrin saturation calculated. The serum ferritin level also should be determined (Table 108-4). Both the transferrin saturation and the serum ferritin level are elevated in symptomatic patients, but these tests are neither sensitive nor specific for the diagnosis of hereditary hemochromatosis in young persons without symptoms or in patients with other chronic liver diseases. As many as half of women younger than 30 years of age with hereditary hemochromatosis have normal transferrin saturation levels [6], and serum iron studies (predominantly ferritin) are abnormal in about 40% to 50% of patients with chronic viral hepatitis [7], nonalcoholic steatohepatitis [8], and alcoholic liver disease [9], in the absence of hereditary hemochromatosis. Thus, serum iron studies alone have many false-positive and false-negative results in predicting iron stores, and reliance on these studies for the diagnosis of hereditary hemochromatosis can result in error.

If either the fasting serum transferrin saturation or the ferritin level is elevated, regardless of the reason for the test, a liver biopsy should be performed to establish or refute a diagnosis of hereditary hemochromatosis by histology, determine the HIC, and calculate the hepatic iron index. The hepatic iron index is helpful in establishing a diagnosis of hereditary hemochromatosis and in distinguishing heterozygotes and patients with alcoholic liver disease with secondary iron overload from homozygotes. The hepatic iron index is based on the concept that persons who have hereditary hemochromatosis, but not heterozygotes for hereditary hemochromatosis, and persons with various forms of secondary iron overload experience a progressive increase in HIC with age [10]. The hepatic iron index is calculated by dividing the HIC in micromoles of iron per 1 g of dry liver by the patient's age in

Table 108-4. Representative Iron Measurements in Patients With Overt Hereditary Hemochromatosis

Measurements	Normal subjects	Patients with hereditary hemochromatosis
Blood (fasting)		
Serum iron level (μg/dL)	60–180	180–300
Serum transferrin level (mg/dL)	220–410	200–300
Transferrin saturation (%)	20–50	80–100
Serum ferritin level (ng/mL)		
Men	20–200	500–6000
Women	15–150	500–6000
Liver		
Hepatic iron concentration:		
μg/g, dry weight	300–1500	10,000–30,000*
μmol/g, dry weight	5–27	175–550
Hepatic iron index †	< 1.5	> 1.9
Liver histology:	0–1+	2+–4+
Perls' Prussian blue stain		

*Lower degrees of hepatic iron overload can be seen in asymptomatic young homozygotes.

†This index is calculated by dividing the hepatic iron concentration (in μmol/g, dry weight) by the age of the patient (in years).

years. Numerous studies from around the world have shown that a hepatic iron index of greater than 1.9 is consistent with the diagnosis of homozygous hereditary hemochromatosis (Table 108-5). The index, however, is not meant to be used in persons with parenteral (or transfusional) iron overload. Recent studies have shown that as many as 10% of subjects with hereditary hemochromatosis (identified by either HLA typing or genotyping) have a hepatic iron index of less than 1.9. As additional experience with genotyping is obtained, it is anticipated that many people will be found who have a hepatic iron index of less than 1.9 and are homozygous for the genetic defect (Table 108-5).

Liver biopsy is considered necessary to make a definitive diagnosis of hereditary hemochromatosis. An exception may be made for young persons identified as a result of family studies or genetic screening. For example, in a patient who is younger than 35 years, who was identified by genetic testing as part of a screening survey or is a relative of a proband, and has an elevated serum transferrin saturation or ferritin level but no clinical liver disease, it might be appropriate to proceed with therapeutic phlebotomy without doing a liver biopsy. In this setting, it is unlikely that the patient will have cirrhosis or a significant increase in hepatic fibrosis, and with a positive genetic test and appropriate blood studies, the accuracy of the diagnosis is high. Prospective studies evaluating all of the parameters used for diagnosis (transferrin saturation, ferritin, genetic tests, HIC, hepatic iron index, liver biopsy findings) should be performed during the next several years to delineate the relative predictive power of each diagnostic test.

Dual-energy CT scanning, magnetic resonance imaging (MRI), and magnetic susceptibility testing are three noninvasive methods of estimating the HIC. Magnetic susceptibility is not widely available, and special MRI and CT techniques are required to estimate the HIC; however, it is unclear whether these imaging techniques are sensitive enough to detect low levels of hepatic iron overload. Also, imaging studies do not provide information about the presence of fibrosis or cirrhosis.

When patients have abnormal serum iron studies and liver enzyme levels, it may be unclear whether the liver test results are caused by hereditary hemochromatosis or by another liver disease. About 40% to 50% of patients with alcoholic liver disease, chronic viral hepatitis, and nonalcoholic steatohepatitis

have abnormal serum iron studies; 10% of these patients may have a mild increase in HIC, but not to the degree seen in hereditary hemochromatosis. Liver biopsy and measurement of HIC with calculation of the hepatic iron index is necessary to distinguish hereditary hemochromatosis from other liver diseases associated with iron overload. In the future, genetic testing should make diagnosis of hereditary hemochromatosis easier in this setting and in the symptom-free relatives of affected patients.

■ TREATMENT

Treatment of hereditary hemochromatosis is simple, inexpensive, and safe. Affected patients initially should have weekly therapeutic phlebotomy of 500 mL of whole blood, which contains 200 to 250 mg of iron, depending on the hemoglobin concentration. Some patients can tolerate twice-weekly phlebotomy, but this usually is not necessary. Monthly phlebotomy is not recommended unless patients cannot tolerate phlebotomy more frequently. The initial weekly therapeutic phlebotomy should be performed until patients develop iron-limited erythropoiesis, which is identified by the failure of the hemoglobin and hematocrit concentrations to recover before the next phlebotomy. It is reasonable to monitor transferrin saturation and ferritin levels periodically to assess iron stores. Therapeutic phlebotomy should be continued until transferrin saturation is less than 50% and serum ferritin levels are less than 50 ng/mL; some clinicians favor decreasing the ferritin level to 20 ng/mL. It is not necessary to make patients anemic or iron deficient; rather, the desired end point of therapy is depletion of excess iron stores. Most patients tolerate therapeutic phlebotomy well and actually have a sense of improved well-being after the initial procedures. Abnormal liver enzymes typically return to normal after iron stores have been depleted, but established cirrhosis does not reverse. Other benefits of therapeutic phlebotomy include reduced skin pigmentation, improved cardiac function, reduced insulin requirements in diabetic subjects, lessened abdominal pain, and improved sense of well-being. Unfortunately, testicular atrophy, cirrhosis, and arthropathy do not reverse with phlebotomy.

Once the initial therapeutic phlebotomy has been completed and excess iron stores have been depleted, most patients require maintenance phlebotomy of 1 unit of blood every 2 to 3 months. Patients with hereditary hemochromatosis absorb about 3 mg/d of iron in excess of their daily requirements and, therefore, accumulate an excess of about 270 mg of iron every 3 months. This is balanced by the 250 mg of iron removed by therapeutic phlebotomy of 500 mL of whole blood; thus, maintenance phlebotomy every 3 months usually maintains patients in normal iron balance. Some patients absorb more than 3 mg/d of iron and require maintenance phlebotomy more often; it is unusual for patients to require phlebotomy more frequently than once every 2 months. Occasionally, for reasons that are unclear, patients in whom hereditary hemochromatosis has been diagnosed accurately do not reaccumulate iron. These usually are older persons who are presumed to absorb iron less efficiently than they did when younger.

The survival of patients with hereditary hemochromatosis that was diagnosed before the development of cirrhosis is equivalent to that of age- and gender-matched controls [3]. If patients are diagnosed after they have cirrhosis, then their expected survival may be reduced. Thirty percent of patients with cirrhosis caused by hemochromatosis develop hepatocellular cancer, and compli-

Table 108-5. Hepatic Iron Index* in Hereditary Hemochromatosis

Normal subjects	Alcoholic liver disease patients	Hemochromatosis	
		Heterozygotes	Homozygotes
< 0.7–1.1	< 1.1–1.6	< 1.5–1.8	> 1.9†

*The hepatic iron index is calculated by dividing the hepatic iron concentration (in μmol/g, dry weight) by the age of the patient (in years). Usually, hepatic iron concentrations are reported as μg/g dry weight. Therefore, to convert to μmol/g, the result should first be divided by 56, the molecular weight of iron.

†In one study, four of 45 homozygotes had hepatic iron index levels between 1.5 and 1.9, a range in which genotyping would be useful to confirm a diagnosis of hereditary hemochromatosis.

cations of chronic liver disease and hepatocellular cancer are the most common causes of premature death in these patients.

SCREENING

It is recommended that all first-degree relatives of affected patients be screened for hereditary hemochromatosis; recommendations are for siblings, parents, and children but certainly could be extended to aunts, uncles, and cousins. These persons should undergo, at minimum, a fasting serum transferrin saturation level. Phenotypic expression of hereditary hemochromatosis is present in most homozygous patients older than 35 years of age, although the accuracy of transferrin saturation tests has never been evaluated using the genetic test as a gold standard. In the past, HLA studies of first-degree relatives of patients with hereditary hemochromatosis were used as "surrogate" genetic tests; relatives with an HLA haplotype at the A and B loci identical to that of the proband were thought to be homozygous for the disease. With increased availability of the genetic test, it is expected that HLA typing will no longer be used.

Elevated serum transferrin saturation and ferritin levels in a family member of a patient with hereditary hemochromatosis warrants further evaluation with either a genetic test, if available, or a liver biopsy for histology and measurement of hepatic iron stores. Whether the genetic test (C282Y mutation in *HFE* gene) should be used as a population screening test has yet to be determined and will depend on studies demonstrating its utility and cost-effectiveness. It has been predicted that general population screening using a genetic test would be cost-effective if the test cost less than $20. When patients without a family history of hereditary hemochromatosis are diagnosed by genetic testing, a liver biopsy should be performed to confirm the diagnosis if they have elevated serum transferrin saturation or ferritin levels. As experience with the genetic test increases, treatment decisions may be made on the basis of the genetic test and serum iron studies alone, without liver biopsy.

SUMMARY

Hereditary hemochromatosis is a common disorder of iron metabolism that increasingly is diagnosed and treated before development of cirrhosis and diabetes. It is estimated that 1 million Americans have hereditary hemochromatosis. The discovery of a candidate hereditary hemochromatosis gene undoubtedly will result in improved diagnosis of hereditary hemochromatosis and, ultimately, a better understanding of iron absorption, hepatic iron uptake and release, and whole-body iron metabolism.

REFERENCES

Recently published papers of particular interest have been highlighted as follows:
- • Of interest
- •• Of outstanding interest

1. Gordeuk VR, Mukiibi J, Haastedt SJ, *et al.*: Iron overload in Africa: interaction between a gene and dietary iron content. *N Engl J Med* 1992, 326:95–100.
2. Bacon BR: Causes of iron overload. *N Engl J Med* 1992, 326:126–127.
3. Niederau C, Fischer R, Purschel A, *et al.*: Long-term survival in patients with hereditary hemochromatosis. *Gastroenterology* 1996, 110:1107–1119.
4.• Bacon BR, Sadiq S: Hereditary hemochromatosis: diagnosis in the 1990's. *Am J Gastroenterol* 1997, 92:784–789.

This study demonstrates that most patients newly diagnosed in the 1990s come to medical attention because of screening iron studies or routine chemistry panels. When this is the case most are asymptomatic without significant organ involvement.

5.• Adams PC, Kertesz AE, Valberg LS: Clinical presentation of hemochromatosis: a changing scene. *Am J Med* 1991, 90:445–449.

These two studies demonstrate that when patients are identified by family screening, complications of hemochromatosis (*eg*, cirrhosis, diabetes) are seen infrequently.

6. Edwards CQ, Griffen LM, Goldgar D, *et al.*: Prevalence of hemochromatosis among 11,065 presumably healthy blood donors. *N Engl J Med* 1988, 318:1355–1362.
7. Di Bisceglie AM, Axiotis CA, Hoofnagle JH, *et al.*: Measurement of iron status in patients with chronic hepatitis. *Gastroenterology* 1992, 102:2108–2113.
8. Bacon BR, Faravesh MJ, Janney CG, *et al.*: Nonalcoholic steatohepatitis: an expanded clinical entity. *Gastroenterology* 1994, 107:1103–1109.
9. Chapman RW, Morgan MY, Laulicht M, *et al.*: Hepatic iron stores and markers of iron overload in alcoholics and patients with idiopathic hemochromatosis. *Dig Dis Sci* 1982, 27:909–916.
10. Bassett ML, Halliday JW, Powell LW: Value of hepatic iron measurements in early hemochromatosis and determination of the critical iron level associated with fibrosis. *Hepatology* 1986, 6:24–29.

109 The Hepatic Porphyrias

Herbert L. Bonkovsky and Graham F. Barnard

The word *porphyria* comes from the Greek *porphyra,* which means purple. This derivation is apt because the biochemical hallmark of the porphyrias is overproduction and excretion of compounds called *porphyrins,* which have a deep red or purple color. The porphyrias are a group of metabolic disorders in which there are defects in the synthetic pathway for heme, the critical moiety for numerous hemoproteins, such as hemoglobin, myoglobin, catalase, and microsomal cytochromes b_5 and P-450. The clinical manifestations of these disorders are varied, and as a result, patients may be referred to a wide variety of subspecialists for evaluation. The two major clinical forms of porphyria are the *acute porphyrias,* in which patients suffer recurrent bouts of pain, especially abdominal pain, and the *cutaneous porphyrias,* in which patients have painful skin lesions.

Elucidation of the heme biosynthetic pathway provided the basis for exploring the abnormal accumulation of metabolic intermediates in patients with porphyrias. Characterization of these intermediates and the enzymes responsible for their formation, together with observed patterns of metabolite excretion in patients with porphyria, suggested the enzyme deficiency that causes each type of porphyria (Fig. 109-1). Knowledge of the regulation of heme synthesis as well as the physical and chemical properties of porphyrias helped to explain how drugs and other factors produce the clinical manifestations of these diseases. Thus, to understand the porphyrias, one must understand the properties of porphyrins and heme and the control of their biosynthesis.

NORMAL PHYSIOLOGY AND BIOCHEMISTRY OF PORPHYRIN AND HEME METABOLISM

Structures and Properties of Porphyrins and Heme

Porphyrins are cyclic tetrapyrroles in which the four pyrrole rings are linked by methene bridges (-CH=) (Fig. 109-2). All naturally occurring porphyrins have side chains attached to the carbon atoms of the pyrrole rings. For uroporphyrins, these side chains are acetate and propionate; for coproporphyrins, they are methyl and propionate; and for protoporphyrins, they are methyl, propionate, and vinyl groups (Fig. 109-2). Naturally occurring uroporphyrin and coproporphyrin are two of four possible isomer types. In the case of protoporphyrin, 15 isomers are possible, but only one isomer (called protoporphyrin IX) occurs in nature.

Porphyrins are planar, highly stable compounds that are strongly fluorescent, emitting intense red light when excited by light of the Soret-band (~ 400 nm) wavelength. These properties are a result of the system of conjugated double bonds and facilitate detection of porphyrins, even at low concentrations. In contrast, the porphyrinogens, which are reduced porphyrins, and intermediates for most steps of heme synthesis (Fig. 109-1) lack this resonance structure, do not absorb light of 400 nm wavelength, are colorless, and do not fluoresce. They are, however, readily oxidized to the corresponding porphyrins, a process that may occur within cells as well as in excreted urine or stool. Heme differs from protoporphyrin only in that its tetrapyrrole ring contains an iron atom, which increases its stability and causes it to lose its fluorescent properties.

Heme Biosynthesis and Regulation of Hepatic Heme Metabolism

The enzymes of heme biosynthesis are compartmentalized within the cell. The first and last three steps of the pathway take place in mitochondria, whereas intermediate steps take place in the cell cytoplasm. Under normal conditions, the first enzyme of the pathway (5-aminolevulinate [ALA] synthase) is the rate-controlling enzyme. ALA synthase in the liver has a short life span (half-life about 1 hour), as does the mRNA coding for it (half-life about 3 hours). Therefore, agents that decrease or increase the rate of synthesis of ALA synthase mRNA or the rate of mRNA translation have a dramatic effect within minutes on the amount of intracellular ALA synthase and, thus, on the rate of synthesis of porphyrins and heme.

Chemicals that cause porphyria also profoundly affect sites other than ALA synthase and are believed to decrease the size

---

Figure 109-1

Step	Enzyme defect	Type of porphyria	Urine	Stool	Plasma	RBCs
Glycine + Succinyl-CoA	ALA synthase					
↓						
5-Aminolevulinate (ALA)	ALA dehydratase	ALA dehydratase deficiency (ADP)	ALA	—	ALA	Zn PROTO
↓						
Porphobilinogen (PBG) / Hydroxymethyl bilane	PBG deaminase	Acute intermittent porphyria (AIP)	ALA, PBG	—	ALA, PBG	—
↓	Uroporphyrinogen III Synthase (cosynthase)	Congenital erythropoietic porphyria (CEP)	URO, COPRO	COPRO	URO	URO, COPRO
Uroporphyrinogen III	Uroporphyrinogen III Decarboxylase	Porphyria cutanea tarda (PCT)	URO	ISOCOPRO	URO	—
↓		Hepatoerythropoietic porphyria (HEP)	URO	ISOCOPRO	URO	Zn PROTO
Coproporphyrinogen III	Coproporphyrinogen III Oxidase	Hereditary coproporphyria (HCP)	ALA, PBG, COPRO	COPRO (PROTO)	COPRO	—
↓						
Protoporphyrinogen IX	Protoporphyrinogen Oxidase	Variegate porphyria (VP)	ALA, PBG, COPRO	PROTO (COPRO)	PROTO (COPRO)	—
↓						
Protoporphyrin IX Fe^{2+}↓	Ferrochelatase	(Erythropoietic) Protoporphyria ([E]PP)	—	PROTO	PROTO	PROTO
Heme						

Nonenzymatic branch: → UROGEN I → COPROGEN I

Heme biosynthetic pathway showing the sites of enzyme defects in the porphyrias and the major biochemical abnormalities in biochemically active disease. Only the major increases in the urine, stool, plasma, and erythrocyte (RBC) values are shown. The dashes represent no abnormalities. For several of the diseases, many patients are biochemically silent ("latent") carriers of the enzymatic defects for most of their lives (see text). COPRO—coproporphyrin; COPROGEN—coproporphyrinogen; ISOCOPRO—isocoproporphyrin; PROTO—protoporphyrin; URO—uroporphyrin; UROGEN—uroporphyrinogen; Zn—zinc.

of a small but critical (regulatory) heme pool in liver cells. Heme depletion is thought to lead to a secondary increase in ALA synthase activity. The most porphyrogenic chemicals, such as allylisopropylacetamide, produce a rapid and profound reduction of cytochromes P-450 heme, leading to induction of ALA synthase. Heme in hepatocytes down-regulates ALA synthase activity, although its site of action is still somewhat controversial. There is consensus that heme blocks the uptake of ALA synthase into mitochrondria. Some chemicals that are capable of producing experimental porphyria (eg,, barbiturates or hydantoins), do not deplete liver heme but rather induce both ALA synthase and cytochromes P-450. The overall regulation of the heme pathway is summarized in Figure 109-3.

Figure 109-2

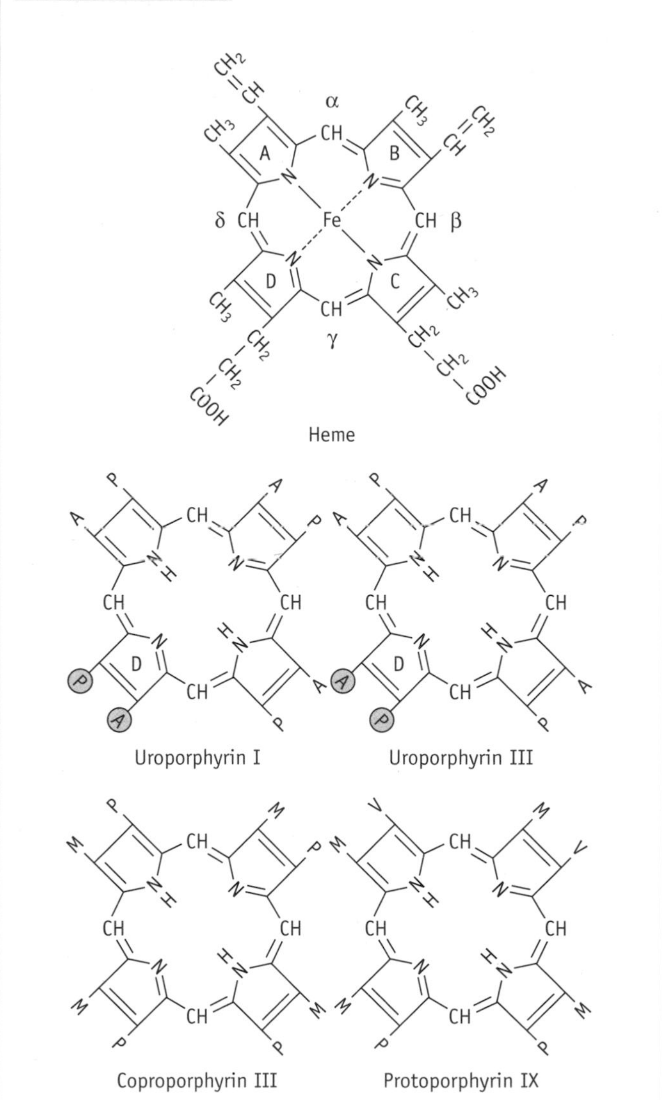

Structures of heme and selected porphyrins. All porphyrins have the same basic ring structure but differ in the side chains that are attached to the pyrrole rings. Porphyrinogens are reduced (hexahydro) forms in which the methene bridges linking the pyrroles are replaced by methylene (-CH$_2$-) groups, and all four nitrogens are linked to hydrogens. A—acetate; P—propionate; M—methyl; V—vinyl. (*Modified from* Bloomer and Straka [9]; with permission.)

Nutritional status plays an important role in regulation of heme synthesis. The activity of hepatic ALA synthase is increased by fasting or starvation, whereas carbohydrate feeding decreases basal enzyme activity and markedly diminishes enzyme induction by porphyrogenic chemicals. Dietary proteins exert similar effects. The exact mechanism for the glucose effect on ALA synthase is still not understood but is of considerable clinical significance; a mainstay of therapy of the acute porphyrias is administration of large amounts of glucose.

The previous discussion refers only to regulation of hepatic heme metabolism. In the bone marrow, the tissue in which the largest amount of heme is formed, the regulation of ALA synthase activity differs from that in the liver. Developing red blood cells contain an erythroid form of ALA synthase different from the "housekeeping" form found in the liver and other organs. Activity of erythroid ALA synthase is down-regulated, not by heme, but rather by a deficiency of iron in the developing red blood cell. Conversely, an adequate supply of iron leads to an increased rate of enzyme synthesis.

■ OVERVIEW OF THE PORPHYRIAS

The porphyrias are a group of metabolic disorders characterized by excessive accumulation and excretion of porphyrins and their precursors and result from specific inherited or acquired enzyme defects in the heme synthetic pathway. Their main clinical manifestations are cutaneous photosensitivity and neurologic dysfunction, most often presenting as abdominal pain. Many patients with enzyme defects of this type do not have clinical manifestations. Porphyric attacks can be fatal, however, so diagnosis of carriers and affected persons is important; these persons should be advised to avoid drug and alcohol use and fasting, activities that can precipitate an acute attack. If neurovisceral symptoms suggest an acute porphyric attack, a rapid screening test for porphobilinogen (PBG) should be performed. If a cutaneous porphyria is suspected, screening tests for increased plasma and/or erythrocytic porphyrins should be done. Positive screening test results should be confirmed by specific quantitative tests.

Enzymatic assays and DNA-based tests are useful for kindred evaluation, genetic diagnosis, and pinpointing a mutation but are not needed for rapid diagnosis of symptomatic disease. Prevention is central to management of patients with porphyria. Intravenous hematin, high carbohydrate intake, and pain control are used to treat acute neurovisceral attacks. Limitation of exposure to sunlight and use of skin protection are important to reduce cutaneous complications.

■ CLASSIFICATION

The porphyrias are classified based on the principal site of expression of the enzymatic defect (hepatic or erythroid; Table 109-1), and on the dominant clinical presentation (cutaneous manifestations only or neurovisceral features with or without cutaneous manifestations; Table 109-2).

For the most part, the hereditary porphyrias are autosomal dominant disorders (acute intermittent porphyria [AIP], hereditary coproporphyria [HCP], variegate porphyria [VP], and the familial form of porphyria cutanea tarda [PCT]), although some are recessive (ALA dehydratase porphyria [ADP], hepatoerythropoietic porphyria [HEP], and congenital erythropoietic porphyria

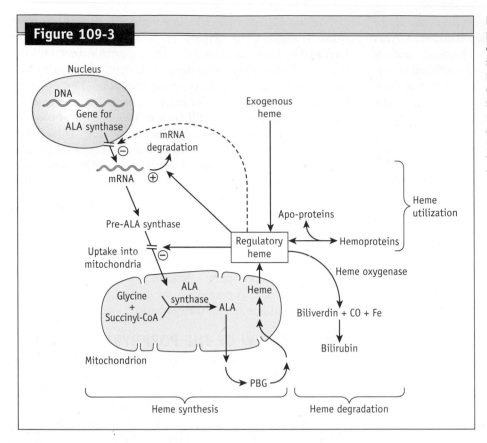

Figure 109-3

Regulation of the hepatic heme biosynthetic pathway and subcellular localization of the enzymes of the pathway, including the synthesis of heme and its regulation. The regulatory heme pool acts to stimulate (+) or down-regulate (-) the indicated steps. Those steps indicated as not within the nucleus or mitochondrion take place in the cytosol. The dashed line indicates a still controversial regulatory effect of heme to decrease transcription of the gene for 5-aminolevulinate (ALA) synthase. CO—carbon monoxide; CoA—coenzyme A; PBG—porphobilinogen.

Table 109-1. Classification of the Porphyrias

Hepatic	Acute inducible hepatic	Erythropoietic
ALA dehydrate porphyria	ALA dehydratase porphyria	Hepatoerythropoietic porphyria
Acute intermittent porphyria	Acute intermittent porphyria	Congenital erythropoietic porphyria
Hereditary coproporphyria	Hereditary copro- porphyria	(Erythropoietic) protoporphyrla
Variegate porphyria	Variegate porphyria	
Porphyria cutanea tarda		
Hepatoerythropoietic porphyria		

[CEP]). Most patients with PCT, however, have acquired disease, perhaps with a genetic predisposition. The inheritance of (erthropoietic) protoporphyria [(E)PP] in somewhat unsettled. In most instances, active (E)PP probably requires a heterozygous defect in the ferrochelatase gene plus another defect in some other gene. An overview of the porphyrias is provided in Figure 109-1.

Pathophysiology

The dominant symptom of the acute porphyrias is abdominal pain, which has been attributed to an autonomic neuropathy affecting the gut. This neurologic dysfunction may occur in all of the porphyrias that cause acute attacks (ADP, AIP, HCP, and VP) and probably is related to excess ALA or PBG. Acute attacks usually are precipitated by an increase in hepatic ALA

synthase activity or by a deficiency of heme within neurons or other tissues (Fig. 109-4). ALA or PBG also may be directly neurotoxic, or ALA may adversely affect neuronal function.

Plasma porphyrins are increased in all of the porphyrias characterized by photosensitivity. Photocutaneous lesions are caused by excess skin porphyrins and may occur in most of the porphyrias except ADP and AIP because the enzyme deficiencies in these two disorders precede porphyrin formation (Fig. 109-1). Skin exposed to light may manifest porphyrin-induced photosensitivity either by bulla formation and injury from mild trauma (PCT, HCP, VP) or acute erythema, burning, and itching (EPP). The Soret-band light, which excites porphyrins and results in skin damage, passes through ordinary window glass; therefore, porphyric patients are not protected simply by remaining indoors.

Mild hepatic abnormalities are not uncommon in the acute porphyrias. Recent data from Scandinavia and France suggest an increased risk of hepatocellular carcinoma in patients with acute porphyria. Liver damage may be most apparent in PCT and (E)PP, and apparent to a lesser degree in HEP, even though (E)PP is not usually classified as one of the "hepatic" porphyrias. Liver biopsy specimens from patients with PCT show red fluorescence, hemosiderosis, fatty infiltration, and variable fibrosis and necrosis. Chronic injury may result in cirrhosis and hepatocellular carcinoma. There is a high incidence of alcohol abuse, hepatitis C virus infection, iron overload, and heterozygosity for hereditary hemochromatosis in PCT patients. Patients with protoporphyria are at increased risk of developing pigment gallstones. A few patients with protoporphyria have developed pigmentary cirrhosis and fatal liver damage; their liver biopsy results have shown birefringent crystalline protoporphyrin.

Enzymatic Defects

The enzymatic defects responsible for the porphyrias are outlined in Figure 109-1. Many of these enzymes can be assayed only in a research setting. The enzyme abnormality may not itself be sufficient to cause disease; many patients with deficient enzyme activity do not have clinical or biochemical manifestations of porphyria. Induction of hepatic ALA synthase by any means can enhance production of porphyrin precursors and exacerbate porphyria. Because most of the porphyrias are genetic disorders, the enzyme defects can be detected in several tissues, including liver, bone marrow, peripheral blood mononuclear cells, and skin fibroblasts. Much progress had been made in recent years in defining the genetic defects responsible for the porphyrias.

Traditional methods of diagnosing porphyria, based on urine, serum, and stool levels of porphyrins or porphyrin precursors, or on liver and erythrocyte enzyme assays, still are probably best when the specific mutation is not known. The method of diagnosing each of the porphyrias is shown in Figure 109-1. When a specific mutation is suspected in a family or geographic cluster of patients, then a variety of molecular methods may simplify diagnosis.

■ CLINICAL FEATURES

General Comments on Diagnosis

A diagnosis of porphyria is made on the basis of an appropriate clinical history in a patient with increased amounts of porphyrin or porphyrin precursors in the urine, feces, and blood [1,2,3•].

Rapid screening tests are useful in the initial evaluation. The Watson-Schwartz and Hoesch tests detect urinary PBG because it reacts with Ehrlich's reagent to produce a red color. Urinary PBG is increased in most acute porphyric attacks with neurologic abnormalities. A positive screening test result should be confirmed by specific quantitative tests for urinary ALA and PBG. If clinical features suggest a cutaneous porphyria with solar urticaria and acute photosensitivity (suggesting [E]PP), screening tests for increased erythrocyte porphyrins should be done; if the patient has vesiculobullous formation (suggesting PCT, HCP, or VP), a screening test for urinary porphyrins should be done. A strategy for diagnosis of the porphyrias is given in Figure 109-5; diagnostic essentials are shown in Figure 109-1; fecal, urine, erythrocytic, and plasma levels of porphyrins and their precursors are shown in Table 109-3.

The porphyrin precursors ALA and PBG are excreted in the urine; during acute porphyric attacks, their levels are markedly increased. The porphyrinogens spontaneously, or after the addition of oxidizing agents, are converted to their corresponding porphyrins, which then can be measured.

The Acute Porphyrias

Episodic acute attacks of neurologic dysfunction, rather than any acute hepatic involvement, give the acute porphyrias their name. AIP is the most common acute hepatic porphyria in the United States and probably the most common "genetic" porphyria; it is a paradigm of all the acute hepatic porphyrias.

Table 109-2. Major Clinical Features of the Porphyrias

Type of porphyria	Clinical manifestations		
	Neurovisceral	Cutaneous	Hepatic damage
ALA dehydratase porphyria	Yes	No	No
Acute intermittent porphyria	Yes	No	No
Hereditary coproporphyria	Yes	Yes (bullae, fragility)	No
Variegate porphyria	Yes	Yes (bullae, fragility)	No
Porphyria cutanea tarda	No	Yes (bullae, fragility)	Yes
Hepatoerythropoietic porphyria	No	Yes (bullae, fragility)	Yes
Congenital erythropoietic porphyria	No	Yes (bullae, fragility)	Occasional
(Erythropoietic) protoporphyria	Rarely*	Yes (urticaria, erythema)	Yes (10%)

*(E)PP with end-stage liver disease, especially just after liver transplantation, rarely is associated with neurovisceral manifestations.

Figure 109-4

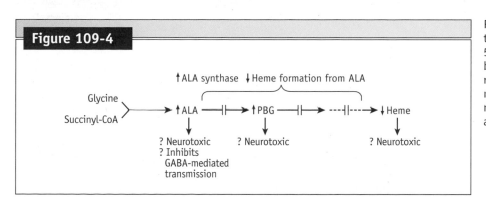

Pathogenesis of the neurovisceral features of the acute porphyrias. An increase in 5-aminolevulinate (ALA) and porpho-bilinogen (PBG) levels, accompanied by reduced heme concentrations in the liver and nervous system, likely causes the neurovisceral features. GABA—gamma-aminobutyric acid.

Figure 109-5

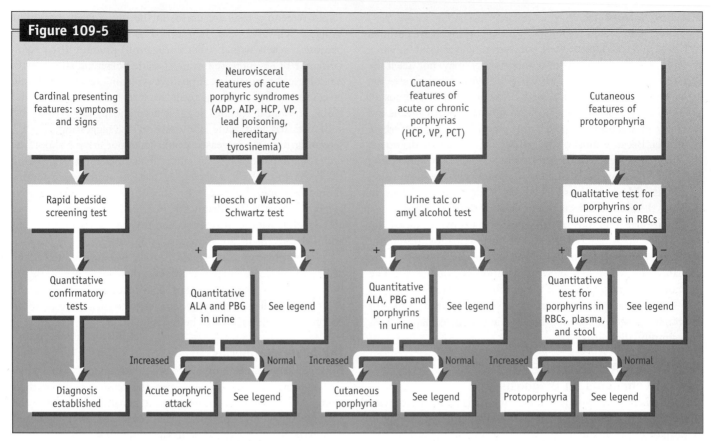

Algorithm for the use of laboratory tests in the evaluation of patients with possible porphyric syndromes. If the rapid screening tests are negative but there is a high index of suspicion, then proceed to the indicated quantitative tests. If these are normal or if there is only a low index of suspicion, then continue searching for the correct diagnosis, not a porphyria. After the diagnosis of a porphyria has been established, additional tests should be used for the specific differential diagnosis: quantitative fecal and urinary total porphyrin; separation of porphyrin types; assay of enzymatic activities in erythrocytes and lymphocytes. For cutaneous porphyrias, plasma total porphyrin and fluorescence pattern may be helpful. ADP—ALA dehydratase porphyria; AIP—acute intermittent porphyria; ALA—5-aminolevulinate; HCP—hereditary coproporphyria; PBG—porphobilinogen; PCT—porphyria cutanea tarda; VP—variegate porphyria.

Table 109-3. Normal Urinary, Fecal, and Blood Levels of Porphyrins and Precursors*

Analyte	Urine		Feces	Erythrocytes	Plasma
	µg/g Cr†	µg/24 h	µg/g dry wt	µg/100 mL packed RBCs	µg/100 mL
5-Aminolevulinate	< 3000	< 4000	—	—	15–23
Porphobilinogen	< 2500	< 3500	—	—	—
Uroporphyrin	10–60	< 80	< 5	< 2	< 2
Coproporphyrin	50–250	< 280	< 50	< 2	< 1
Protoporphyrin	—	—	< 120	< 90	< 2
Isocoproporphyrin	—	—	—	—	—
Porphyrins (total)	35–300	50–400	< 175	—	< 2

*Typical normal values for adults are tabulated; there is some variability in normal levels, depending on the laboratory performing the tests and the methods used.

†Normal urine creatinine (Cr) = 0.8–2.0 g per 24 h.

Dashes indicate no detectable levels or not routinely tested.

Acute Intermittent Porphyria

Epidemiology. Acute intermittent porphyria is an autosomal dominant disorder with variable penetrance. The prevalence of the defective gene is about 5 to 10 per 100,000 persons in the United States and may be three times higher in hospitalized psychiatric patients. AIP is most prevalent in Scandinavia, especially in Lapland, where it occurs in 1 in 1500 persons. The United Kingdom is another country with high prevalence.

Clinical features. Symptoms of AIP are more common in women than in men; they typically develop in women in their 20s and in men in their 30s. Attacks usually are precipitated by a factor that most likely induces ALA synthase, such as drug use (especially barbiturates, sulfonamides, and hydantoins), hormonal changes (especially those accompanying menstruation), heavy alcohol use, and fasting (Tables 109-4 and 109-5).

The four most common symptoms of AIP are abdominal pain, extremity pain and paresthesias, constipation, and vomiting (Table 109-6). The disease has no cutaneous manifestations. The abdominal pain of AIP usually is colicky, typically occurs in the lower abdomen, and may last for hours or days. It may be severe, mimicking that of a surgical abdomen, but the abdomen is soft. Autonomic neuropathy may manifest as tachycardia, systemic arterial hypertension, postural hypotension, vomiting, constipation, diarrhea, diaphoresis, and abnormal bladder function. The other neuropathic features are equally diverse; virtually any type of neuropathy can occur in patients with AIP (Table 109-7),

but motor neuropathies are more common than are sensory neuropathies [4••]. Back, chest, and extremity pain and paresthesias are common and can occur in the absence of abdominal pain. Patients may have urinary symptoms, including retention, incontinence, dysuria, and increased frequency. Severely affected

Table 109-4. Factors That May Precipitate a Porphyric Attack

Porphyrogenic drugs and chemicals (see Table 109-5)

Ethanol

Fasting or a low-calorie diet

Steroids (gonadal, endogenous, exogenous)

Infections

Intercurrent illness

Surgery (including dental extraction)

Table 109-5. Drugs and Chemicals in Acute Hepatic Porphyrias*

Reported to exacerbate disease		Theoretically risky		Believed to be safe	
Aminoglutethimide	Imipramine	Alcuronium	Methyclothiazide	Acetaminophen	Meperidine
Antipyrine	Isopropylmeprobamate	Alfadolone acetate†	Metoclopramide	Amitriptyline	Methadone
Aminopyrine	Mephenytoin	Alfaxalone†	Metyrapone	Aspirin	Methylphenidate
Barbiturates	*Meprobamate*	Allyl-containing	Mitotane	Atropine	Morphine
Bemegride	Methyldopa	compounds	(o,p'-DDD)	Bromides	Naproxen
N-Butylscopolammonium	Methyprylon	Amphetamines	Nalidixic acid	Calcium salts	Narcotic
bromide	Methsuximide	Bupivacaine	Nefazadine	Captopril	analgesics
Carbamazepine	Nikethamide	Bupropion	Nifedepine	Chloral hydrate	Neostigmine
Carbromal	Novobiocin	Camphor	Nitrazepam	Chlorpromazine	Nitrofurantoin
Chloramphenicol	*Oral contraceptives*	Chloroform	Nortriptyline	Colchicine	Nitrous oxide
Chlordiazepoxide	Pentazocine	Clonazepam	o,p'-DDD	Corticosteroids	Oxazepam
Chloroquine	Phensuximide	(large doses)	Pargyline	Cyclopropane	Oxylate/sodium
Chlorpropamide	Phenylbutazone	Clonidine	Pentylenetetrazol	Dezocine	Pancuronium
Danazol	*Phenytoin*	Colistin	Phenoxybenzamine	Dicumarol	Paraldehyde
Dapsone	Primidone	Diazepam	Prilocaine	Diltiazem	Paroxetine
Diazepam	*Progestogens*	Dramamine	Pyrrocaine	Digoxin	Penicillamine
Diclofenac	Pyrazinamide	Enalapril	Rifampicin	Diphenhydramine	Penicillin
Enflurane	Pyrazolone derivatives	Etidocaine	Sulfonylureas	Droperidol	Pentamethonium†
Ergot preparations	Succinimides	Etomidate	Spironolactone	EDTA	Pentazocine
Estrogens	*Sulfonamides*	Erythromycin	Terpenes	Epinephrine	Phenothiazines
Ethanol excess	Sulfonethylmethane†	Felbamate	Tiagabine	Ether	Procaine
Ethchlorvynol	Theophylline and its	Fluroxene†	Tramadol	Fentanyl	Promazine
Ethinamate	derivatives	Food additives	Tranylcypromine	Fluoxetine	Promethazine
Eucalyptol	Tolazamide	(selected)	Triazolam	Gabapentin	Propanidid†
(in mouthwash)	Tolbutamide	Furosemide	All agents known to	Gallamine	Propoxyphene
Glutethimide	Trimethadione	Heavy metals	induce cytochromes	Guanethidine	Propanolol
Griseofulvin	Troxidone	Hydralazine	P-450 or to increase	Heparin	Rauwolfia
Halothane	Valproate	Lamotrigine	hepatic heme	Hyoscine	alkaloids
Hydantoins		Lidocaine	turnover	Ibuprofen	Reserpine
		Mepivacaine		Indomethacin	Streptomycin
				Insulin	Succinylcholine
				Labetalol	Tetracycline
				Lisinopril	Thiouracil
				Lithium	Thyroxine
				Losartan	Vigabatrin
				Mandelamine	Vitamins A, B, C,
				Mefenamic acid	D, and E

*Among agents reported to exacerbate disease, those in italics have been incriminated most often. Those listed as theoretically risky have not been reported to exacerbate human porphyria, but they are prophyrogenic in experimental systems and probably in humans too. Those believed to be safe have been used in human acute prophyria without apparent ill effects and are not theoretically risky.

†Agents not available in the United States.

Adapted from Bonkovsky [11]; with permission.

patients also may have central nervous system symptoms; depression and anxiety may be reactive, secondary to the illness rather than a direct consequence of it. Seizures, delirium, and coma can occur from porphyria itself or secondary to hyponatremia attributed to salt loss and to hypothalamic antidiuretic hormone release. Fatal attacks often are characterized by prolonged flaccid and respiratory paralysis and secondary infectious complications.

The four most common presenting signs in patients hospitalized for AIP are tachycardia, dark urine, confusion, and a peripheral motor deficit (Table 109-6). The leukocyte count may be elevated because of stress or intercurrent infection. Serum sodium and magnesium concentrations may be decreased. Other abnormalities noted include increased serum thyroxine, thyroxine-binding globulin (AIP patients rarely are thyrotoxic), cholesterol, and low-density lipoprotein levels, which simulate exaggerated estrogen effect.

A presumed deficiency of hepatic cytochrome P-450 may account for altered metabolism of some drugs, such as salicylamide, antipyrine, and aminopyrine, in patients with AIP, although other drugs metabolized by cytochrome P-450 (eg, phenylbutazone) are eliminated normally. An increased incidence of hepatocellular carcinoma was found in European series of deceased patients with AIP, but this has not yet been observed in the United States.

Metabolic defect. Acute intermittent porphyria is caused by a deficiency of PBG deaminase, resulting in accumulation of PBG and ALA; attacks are precipitated by inducers of ALA synthase. AIP is associated with half-normal activity of hepatic PBG deaminase, consistent with a heterozygous state. Most carriers (80%) have no symptoms throughout their lives and are considered to have latent AIP. The diagnosis of asymptomatic disease in heterozygotes is crucial for prevention of potentially life-threatening acute attacks by avoidance of known precipitating factors (Table 109-4). AIP is the most virulent of the acute porphyrias because PBG deaminase activity normally is only marginally greater than the rate-limiting step catalyzed by ALA synthase. The other acute porphyrias are expressed less often clinically and are less severe. The primary defect in AIP is metabolic; resultant histologic lesions occur late. The major pathologic findings in AIP are in muscle and nerve. Electromyography studies may be consistent with muscle denervation. There is reduced motor nerve conduction velocity, edema and irregularity of the myelin sheaths, and thinned axons with vacuolization and degeneration. Central nervous system findings include vacuolization of neurons and focal demyelination. There are few morphologic abnormalities in the liver, even though the underlying defect in classic AIP is expressed in the liver.

Diagnosis. Latent gene carriers of AIP gene defects may not have abnormal urinary ALA or PBG excretion. All patients with true signs and symptoms of AIP, however, have increased urinary ALA and PBG, often as much as 25 to 100 mg/d of ALA and 50 to 200 mg/d of PBG during an acute attack. This is the *sine qua non* for the diagnosis of AIP. In AIP, the milligram amount of urinary PBG is greater than that of ALA; if this is not the case, another diagnosis is more likely. In other porphyrias, lead poisoning, and hereditary tyrosinemia, the amount of ALA usually exceeds that of PBG, even though the clinical manifestations of these disorders may resemble those of AIP. Urinary PBG may be converted nonenzymatically to uroporphyrin; therefore, even though AIP patients have insufficient PBG deaminase, they may have increased uroporphyrin and coproporphyrin in their urine. The urine of patients with AIP may turn red or black when exposed to air and light.

Table 109-6. Symptoms and Signs of Attacks of Acute Intermittent Porphyria: Clinical Features in Hospitalized Patients

Symptom or sign*	Percentage of patients, %
Symptoms	
Abdominal pain	87
Nausea and vomiting	60
Extremity pain or paresthesia	50
Constipation	50
Back or chest pain	41
Diarrhea	7
Signs	
Tachycardia	90 (38)[†]
Dark urine	74
Mental confusion	53
Peripheral motor deficit	47
Bulbar involvement	46
Hypertension	40
Absent reflexes	29
Peripheral sensory deficit	26
Postural hypotension	21
Palpable dilated bowel loops	21
Seizures	20
Fever	9 (31)[†]

*The symptoms and signs refer to patients with AIP based on reported large series of AIP patients.

[†]Numbers in parentheses refer to percentages from individual large series with discrepant frequencies.

Table 109-7. Neurologic Manifestations of the Acute Porphyrias*

Autonomic neuropathy (cardiovascular, bladder, bowel)
Peripheral neuropathy (predominantly motor)
Sensory loss over the trunk
Neuropsychiatric manifestations (anxiety, depression, insomnia, disorientation, hallucinations, paranoia)
Cranial neuropathy (mostly lower cranial nerves VII and X)
Seizures or coma
Rarely, cerebellar, optic nerve, basal ganglion, or pyramidal tract involvement

*Manifestations are listed in descending order of frequency.

The diagnosis of classic AIP (about 85% of cases) can made by measuring erythrocyte PBG deaminase levels. In the so-called variant, or type II AIP (about 15% of AIP patients), PBG deaminase deficiency is demonstrated only in nonerythroid cells (eg, lymphocytes or cultured fibroblasts); alternatively, diagnosis of type II AIP may be made by DNA hybridization using oligonucleotides specific for the mutated allele. There is significant overlap of erythrocyte PBG deaminase activity values between normal controls and latent carriers, which can result in ambiguous assay results (Fig. 109-6). For this reason, erythrocyte PBG deaminase assays cannot be depended on to diagnose AIP. Because erythrocyte PBG deaminase activity is higher in young than in old red blood cells, erythrocyte PBG deaminase is increased in hemolytic diseases, hepatic diseases, and neonates; it is decreased in uremia.

A variety of molecular methods have been used to assist in the diagnosis of the porphyrias, but these are not commercially available.

Management. Prevention is the key to managing AIP. Affected persons should wear a medical alert bracelet. Carriers of the gene defect should be counseled to avoid situations that can precipitate acute attacks. AIP patients should be advised to use as few drugs as possible, and only those drugs judged to be safe on the basis of experimental and clinical experience should be prescribed (Table 109-5). Oral carbohydrate intake always should be adequate, and starvation and fad diets should be avoided. Polycose (Abbott Laboratories, North Chicago, IL) supplementation may be used to increase oral carbohydrate intake. Infections should be treated promptly, and other stresses should be avoided, if possible. Relatives should be screened for the disease at centers with special expertise in the diagnosis and management of porphyria.

The treatment aim is to reduce the activity of hepatic ALA synthase. The essentials of treatment of acute porphyric attacks are given in Table 109-8. If possible, the patient should discontinue all drugs that might precipitate an acute attack and should have at least 300 g/d of enteral or parenteral carbohydrate as glucose or other readily metabolized carbohydrate. Fluid replacement is important, particularly in patients with poor oral intake or vomiting. Patients should be monitored for development of hyponatremia and hypomagnesemia and treated appropriately. Pain control can be achieved with regular and frequent doses of meperidine, but narcotics may exacerbate urinary retention and constipation. The intermittent nature of symptoms or attacks means that narcotic addiction is unusual. Agitation and anxiety can be treated with chlorpromazine (50–400 mg/d) and sympathetic hyperactivity with propranolol (in the absence of contraindications); tachycardia and hypertension may be labile.

If there is no clear improvement after 2 or 3 days of therapy or if there is progressive neurologic dysfunction, intravenous

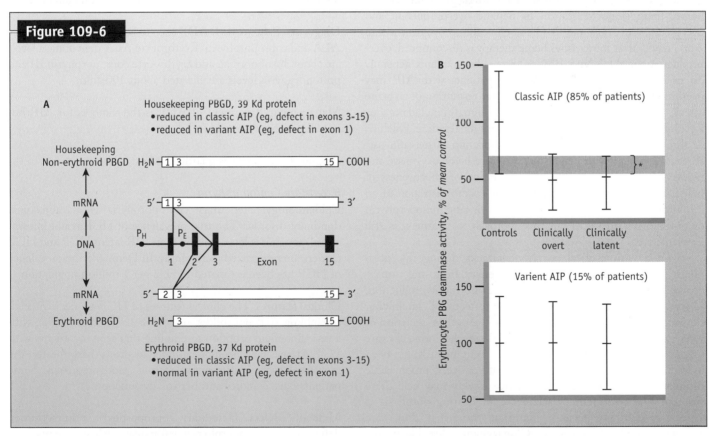

Figure 109-6

The enzymatic defects in acute intermittent porphyria (AIP): the two forms of porphobilinogen (PBG) deaminase and how the diagnosis of variant AIP is missed by measuring erythrocyte PBG deaminase activity. The PBC deaminase gene with 15 exons is illustrated. When erythroid PBC deminase is measured in classic AIP, there is about a 50% reduction, as compared with controls. An indeterminate zone of PBG deaminase activity (*) overlaps the lower range of control values and those seen in some AIP patients. In variant AIP, there is no reduction in erythrocytic PBG deaminase levels. The graphs illustrate the mean and range of measurements anticipated for hypothetical groups of patients with classic and variant AIP.

Table 109-8. Essentials of Treatment of Acute Porphyric Attacks

Discontinue all known or potentially harmful drugs (Table 109-5)

Include 300 g of carbohydrate intake per day in diet

Institute fluid replacement (fluid restriction in patients with the syndrome of inappropriate secretion of antidiuretic hormone)

Monitor for potential hyponatremia with or without hypomagnesemia

Administer meperidine (400–1600 mg/d) or morphine (32–128 mg/d) for pain control

Administer chlorpromazine (50–400 mg/d) for agitation and anxiety

Administer propranolol (40–200 mg/d) for sympathetic hyperactivity

Administer heme intravenously (3–5 mg/kg/d)

Treat infection promptly

Treat intercurrent disease

heme should be given. The only preparation available for use in the United States is Panhematin (Abbott Laboratories, North Chicago Hematin Hot Line 1-800-622-2688); 3 to 5 mg/kg/d of hematin is the usual dose. Resuspension of lyophilized hematin powder in human serum albumin prolongs its limited stability (one vial of panhematin, 313 mg of heme, is dissolved in 132 mL of 25% human serum albumin and administered over 1 hour). In most patients with acute porphyria given intravenous heme, there is normalization of hepatic overproduction and overexcretion of ALA and PBG and clinical improvement within 2 or 3 days. After intravenous heme therapy is discontinued, overproduction of ALA and PBG resumes, but patients generally do not redevelop symptoms. Indeed, patients with AIP may overexcrete ALA and PBG for years after resolution of an acute attack. Risks associated with intravenous hematin include coagulopathy, vasculitis, hemolysis, and transient renal failure. Phlebitis or thrombophlebitis is a frequent complication of hematin use. Repeated therapy with hematin may induce heme oxygenase and reduce its therapeutic benefit. The duration of effectiveness of heme may be increased significantly by coadministration of an inhibitor of heme oxygenase, such as tin or zinc mesoporphyrin or protoporphyrin [5•,6] but this approach to treatment is still experimental.

Women with cyclical porphyric attacks during the luteal phase of their menstrual cycles may benefit from oral contraceptives to block endogenous cyclical sex hormone production. Hormone analogues that block the effects of luteinizing hormone–releasing hormone and, thus, the cyclical secretion of luteinizing hormone and follicle-stimulating hormone also are useful. Leuprolide, 1 to 2 mg/d given subcutaneously, has been used most widely for this purpose. Alternatively, prophylactic intravenous heme given once or twice weekly may help these women. The treatment of seizures complicating porphyria is especially difficult because many of the usual drugs are contraindicated in this disease. Clonazepam is less likely than hydantoins or barbiturates to worsen porphyric attacks. Bromides can be used safely, but they have a narrow therapeutic range. Parenteral magnesium may be useful acutely. Among the newer anticonvulsants, gabapentin and vigabatrin appear to be safe, whereas felbamate, lamotrigine, and tigabine are not.

Prognosis. The clinical course of an acute attack is variable. Attacks may last for a few days or for months; in some patients, a chronic porphyriac syndrome develops, but most patients do not have symptoms between attacks. The prognosis of AIP generally is good, especially for patients with gene defects who are counseled to avoid drugs and other precipitants of acute attacks; attacks must be treated promptly with intravenous hematin when required. Patients with long-standing pareses may be left with a residual deficit when the attack resolves, usually a foot or wrist drop, or wasting of the intrinsic hand muscles. Chronic renal failure, perhaps partly secondary to sustained hypertension or analgesic nephropathy, occurs in patients with AIP. The mortality rate of 136 AIP patients hospitalized in the United States between 1940 and 1988 was 3.2 times that of age-matched controls. There has been an improved survival rate since the introduction of hematin therapy in 1976.

Five-Aminolevulinate Dehydratase Deficiency Porphyria

Epidemiology. Only about six homozygotes with ALA dehydratase porphyria have been described.

Clinical features. Symptoms of ADP are similar to those of AIP.

Metabolic defect. This type of porphyria results from a severe deficiency of ALA dehydratase (<10% of normal) with secondary induction of ALA synthase and overproduction of ALA.

Diagnosis. Patients with ADP excrete large amounts of urinary ALA and coproporphyrin. Erythrocyte ALA dehydratase levels are about 3% of normal, and erythrocyte coproporphyrin III and protoporphyrin levels are elevated about 100-fold.

Management. Treatment of ADP is the same as for AIP, but not all patients respond [7••].

Prognosis. Prognosis is guarded, at best.

Hereditary Coproporphyria

Epidemiology. Hereditary coproporphyria is an autosomal dominant disorder. The true prevalence of HCP is not known, and although it is less common than AIP, latent HCP and HCP carriers are recognized increasingly. In Denmark, the prevalence of HCP has been estimated to be 2 per 1 million population.

Clinical features. The clinical features of HCP are neurovisceral, resembling AIP, but milder, or cutaneous (in about 30%), with a vesiculobullous eruption resembling that seen in patients with PCT. Attacks have been precipitated by drugs (barbiturates) the menstrual cycle, contraceptive steroids, and pregnancy. Some patients have jaundice and hepatic dysfunction.

Metabolic defect. Hereditary coproporphyria results from a deficiency of coproporphyrinogen oxidase. Most patients have about half the normal enzyme activity. Coproporphyrin is deposited in the livers of patients with active HCP, and liver biopsy specimens fluoresce red when exposed to Soret-band light. A variant of HCP with 10% of control enzymatic activity produces *harderoporphyria*, with a clinically severe phenotype;

harderoporphyrinogen is a normal heme intermediate that usually does not accumulate to any measurable degree.

Diagnosis. Patients with HCP have a moderate to marked increase in fecal and to some extent urinary coproporphyrin III levels during and between attacks. During acute attacks, urinary ALA and, in lesser amounts, urinary PBG levels also are increased, but in contrast to AIP, these levels usually normalize between attacks. PBG deaminase levels are normal. Just as in AIP, there are silent carriers with a mutation who excrete normal amounts of porphyrins and their precursors. Patients with harderoporphyria have increased red blood cell protoporphyrin and fecal harderoporphyrin.

Management. Avoidance of precipitating factors is crucial to the management of HCP. Acute attacks of HCP are treated in the same way as are those of AIP. Opaque sunscreens and avoidance of sunlight are recommended in the treatment and prevention of cutaneous manifestations. β-carotene may be of some benefit in reducing photosensitivity.

Prognosis. Death from respiratory paralysis has been reported, although the disease usually is relatively mild.

Variegate Porphyria

Epidemiology. Variegate porphyria is inherited as an autosomal dominant disorder of low penetrance. Synonyms for VP include the *royal malady, protocoporporphyria,* and *South African porphyria.* The prevalence of VP is much higher in South Africa, especially among Afrikaners (about 3 per 1000 population) than it is elsewhere.

Clinical features. The presentation of VP is variable, hence its name. Photosensitivity and photodermatitis may develop, as in HCP and PCT, but at an earlier age than in PCT with bullae, erosions, or ulcers following mild trauma of light-exposed skin and with similar chronic skin changes. Acute neuropsychiatric attacks occur, as in AIP, with abdominal pain, vomiting, constipation, tachycardia, hypertension, psychiatric symptoms, and occasionally quadriplegia. The liver usually is not involved in the disease.

Metabolic defect. Variegate porphyria usually results from a heterozygous deficiency of protoporphyrinogen oxidase activity, which is about half the normal activity. If hepatic ALA synthase is induced, there is a marked overproduction of ALA, PBG, coproporphyrin, and protoporphyrin associated with acute attacks and cutaneous manifestations. During attacks, urinary ALA and PBG are increased but return to normal when attacks resolve.

Diagnosis. Variegate porphyria is characterized by increased levels of fecal protoporphyrin and coproporphyrin. There is increased ALA, PBG, and coproporphyrin in urine.

Management. Avoidance of precipitating factors similar to those that exacerbate AIP is key. Therapy for acute attacks is the same as that for attacks of AIP. Opaque sunscreens and avoidance of sunlight are recommended to prevent cutaneous manifestations; protective clothing is important, canthraxanthrin (a β-carotene analogue) may be helpful.

Prognosis. The prognosis of VP is good, although the disease has life-threatening potential.

Other Hepatic Porphyrias

Porphyria Cutanea Tarda

Epidemiology. Porphyria cutanea tarda is synonymous with *symptomatic porphyria, idiosyncratic porphyria, chemical porphyria,* and *acquired hepatic porphyria.* PCT is the most common form of porphyria in the United States. The sporadic form (s-PCT) may be purely acquired, although a genetic predisposition likely is present in many affected patients. The familial form (f-PCT) is inherited in most families as an autosomal dominant disorder with low clinical penetrance.

Clinical features. Sporadic and familial PCT usually become symptomatic in adults. PCT patients do not present with acute neurologic attacks; symptoms are limited mainly to the skin. Increased skin fragility affects the backs of the hands and forearms, resulting in bullae, vesicles, blisters, and sores (Fig. 109-7*A*, see **Color Plate**). These lesions are not caused by acute photosensitivity but result instead from mild trauma to sun-exposed areas; the acute photosensitivity of the erythropoietic porphyrias is rare in patients with PCT. Milia may develop, particularly on the hands and fingers; these typically are 1- to 5-mm, pearly-white subepidermal inclusions seen in patients with PCT, HCP, and VP. Lesions also may be seen on the forehead, ears, neck, and other sun-exposed areas. The lesions often become infected and tend to heal slowly and to leave residual areas of hypopigmentation, hyperpigmentation, sclerodermatous changes. Increased facial hair occurs in patients with PCT (Fig. 109-7*B*, see **Color Plate**) and is more noticeable in women. Alopecia may develop at sites of repeated skin damage. The characteristic histopathologic finding of PCT in the skin is subepidermal bullae with minimal inflammation.

The typical patient with PCT is a middle-aged man who consumes excessive alcohol and has evidence of hepatic disease, with elevated serum aminotransferases and gamma-glutamyl transpeptidase. Alcohol induces hepatic ALA synthase in patients with PCT and reduces erythrocyte uroporphyrinogen decarboxylase (UROD) activity. Alcohol also inhibits other heme pathway enzymes, and chronic alcoholism suppresses erythropoiesis and increases dietary iron absorption. Other patient groups with a relatively high incidence of PCT are those with diabetes mellitus, young women who use oral contraceptives, and chronic hemodialysis patients; the latter often have chronic hepatitis C infection or iron overload from multiple blood transfusions. The livers of patients with PCT contain high concentrations of uroporphyrins and hepta-carboxyl porphyrins, which fluoresce an intense red; fat deposition, inflammation, and variable amounts of necrosis and fibrosis often are present. Some degree of siderosis is apparent on liver biopsy in 80% of PCT patients, and most have increased ferritin, serum iron, and iron-binding saturation. Iron loading is associated with HLA-linked hereditary hemochromatosis; in recent studies from Northern Europe and the United States, about 75% of patients with PCT have had one of the mutations in the HFE gene associated with hemochromatosis. Iron in the liver plays an important role in the pathogenesis of PCT. Cirrhosis develops in 30% to 40% of patients with PCT, and the incidence of hepatocellular carcinoma in these persons is greater than normal. In some countries, including the United States, there is a high prevalence of positive tests for serum hepatitis C virus (HCV) antibody and HCV RNA in PCT patients. Liver damage in some patients with PCT, therefore, may be caused by chronic HCV virus infection.

Metabolic defect. Porphyria cutanea tarda is caused by an inherited or acquired reduction in hepatic UROD activity. The pathogenesis of PCT is complex, involving increased oxidative stress in the liver. This stress may be mediated by multiple exogenous or endogenous factors, including alcohol, iron, estrogen, porphyrins, chronic HCV infections, and polychlorinated organic compounds. Inheritance of one or more hemochromatosis genes may be an important factor contributing to development of sporadic PCT.

Diagnosis. Patients with PCT have a marked increase in urinary uroporphyrins and hepta-carboxyl porphyrins. Urinary ALA levels often are slightly elevated, but PBG levels usually are normal. A variety of fecal porphyrins are found in patients with PCT; an elevated ratio of stool isocoproporphyrin to coproporphyria is almost diagnostic of PCT. Urinary uroporphyrin levels greater than coproporphyrin levels favor a diagnosis of PCT, whereas urinary coproporphyrin levels greater than uroporphyrin levels favor a diagnosis of VP or HCP. Measurement of UROD is a research procedure.

Management. Cutaneous symptoms of PCT are treated by eliminating precipitating factors, such as alcohol and estrogens. Patients should be advised to wear protective clothing, avoid strong sunlight, and apply opaque sunscreens, such as zinc oxide paste. Sunscreens that protect against sunburn are not adequate because they do not screen the Soret band of light.

Phlebotomy to remove hepatic iron cures sporadic PCT and results in normalization of hepatic UROD activity. Initially, 450 mL of blood are removed one to two times per week, and then at increasing intervals, to produce a mild degree of iron deficiency (hemat ocrit <35% and serum ferritin <10 ng/mL). Iron deficiency usually develops after removal of 12 to 16 U of blood (3–4 g of iron). Phlebotomy may induce clinical remission, reduce urinary porphyrins, and be associated with regression of scleroderma-like skin changes, but it has not been proved to improve liver histology. About 10% to 20% of patients relapse within 1 year but are likely to respond again to phlebotomy if there are no other causative factors. Hydroxy-chloroquine and other antimalarials form water-soluble complexes with octa- and hepta-carboxyl porphyrins and facilitate their excretion in urine. This treatment may be appropriate if phlebotomy is contraindicated or ineffective. Treatment should be initiated at a low dose (125 mg two to three times per week) to reduce the likelihood of acute hepatic injury (fever, right upper quadrant pain related to massive uroporphyrin removal from the liver) and retinopathy. Improvement or remission typically takes 6 to 9 months. Patients with chronic hepatitis C should be treated with interferon in an attempt to eradicate this virus. Such treatment is probably best used after initial iron depletion.

Prognosis. The prognosis of PCT is good for patients who avoid alcohol; the overall prognosis depends on the nature and severity of the underlying liver disease.

Hepatoerythropoietic Porphyria

Epidemiology. Hepatoerythropoietic porphyria, also called *hepatoerythrocytic porphyria*, is the homozygous form of familial PCT or UROD deficiency and is extremely rare; only about 25 patients have been identified.

Clinical features. The clinical manifestations of HEP are similar to those of CEP and develop within the first year of life. Patients have severe photosensitivity with skin fragility and subepidermal bullae, resulting in scarring of the hands and face, sclerodermatous changes, and acrosclerosis. There is excess facial hair, and erythrodontia has been noted. Hepatosplenomegaly also has been described, and liver disease develops later; the photosensitivity may improve over time. Liver biopsy specimens

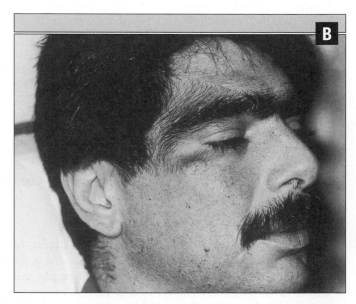

Figure 109-7

Manifestations of porphyria cutanea tarda. **A**, Cutaneous lesions with bullae, vesicles, and erosions on the dorsal hands. **B**, Hypertrichosis of the lateral forehead. (*From* Werth and McKinley-Grant [10]; with permission.) See **Color Plate.**

demonstrate portal inflammation and fluoresce red; serum aminotransferase may be mildly elevated. Serum iron levels usually are normal. Adults with HEP have mild normocytic anemia, and erythroid precursors in the bone marrow fluoresce.

Metabolic defect. Hepatoerythropoietic porphyria is the result of homozygous (or compound heterozygous) and severe UROD deficiency in familial PCT (type II PCT). As the name implies, excess porphyrins are synthesized both in the liver and bone marrow.

Diagnosis. The clinical diagnosis of HEP is based chiefly on detection of elevated urinary uroporphyrins and hepta-carboxyl porphyrins; erythrocyte zinc protoporphyrin levels also are elevated.

Management. Management of HEP is the same as that of PCT and includes avoidance of sunlight. Phlebotomy is unlikely to be beneficial. Gene therapy may prove effective in the future.

Prognosis. The prognosis of HEP is poor because of the severity of the defect in UROD activity.

Erythropoietic Porphyrias
Congenital Erythropoietic Porphyria
Congenital erythropoietic porphyria, also known as *Günther's disease* and *hereditary erythropoietic uroporphyria*, is caused by a homozygous deficiency of uroporphyrinogen III cosynthase. The bone marrow is the predominant site of the metabolic abnormality. CEP is uncommon, and only about 200 cases have been reported. Photosensitivity is the major clinical feature of CEP and usually begins in infancy. Hepatomegaly may be present with increased iron, and cirrhosis occurs occasionally. Splenomegaly is common and results from hemolysis. Porphyrin-rich gallstones have been reported. The urine contains a large quantity of uroporphyrin I because uroporphyrin III cannot be formed. Urinary ALA and PBG levels usually are normal. Increases of both urinary and erythrocyte porphyrins are highly suggestive of CEP. Treatment is based on avoidance of sun exposure and skin trauma, treatment of skin infections, and prolonged treatment with activated charcoal. Several patients have been treated successfully with bone marrow transplantation.

Erythopoietic Protoporphyria
Epidemiology. Protoporphyria, also called *erythropoietic protoporphyria* and *erythrohepatic protoporphyria*, is relatively common, probably second only to PCT among the porphyrias in prevalence. (E)PP has no sex predominance and affects members of all ethnic groups.

Clinical features. The clinical expression of (E)PP is highly variable, but photosensitivity is its major clinical manifestation. Cutaneous symptoms develop in childhood, usually in infancy (Table 109-9). Some persons with increased erythrocytic protoporphyrins, however, have no symptoms. Conversely, skin discomfort may be disproportionate to the severity of visible lesions, and (E)PP has been confused with psychoneurosis.

Less than 10% of patients with (E)PP develop severe liver disease with cirrhosis and acute cholestasis. Some patients have died of hepatic failure and were found to have black, nodular, cirrhotic livers. Polarization microscopy of liver specimens shows birefringence caused by crystals of protoporphyrin in hepatocytes, Küpffer cells, and bile canaliculi. In patients with liver disease, erythrocyte protoporphyrin levels have exceeded 2,000 µg/dL, higher than is usually seen in patients with (E)PP. Only rarely do patients recover after jaundice develops. Usually, liver failure is not thought to be related to alcohol-, virus-, or drug-induced hepatitis. Cholelithiasis may be prominent.

Metabolic defect. (Erythropoietic) protoporphyria results from a deficiency of ferrochelatase in all heme-forming tissues. Although inheritance of (E)PP is thought to be autosomal dominant, the activity of ferrochelatase in affected persons is only 15% to 25% of normal; the parents of many patients are phenotypically normal and do not have symptoms, although about one half of them demonstrate decreases in ferrochelatase activity. Rare compound heterozygotes with severe phenotypes, causing liver failure in adolescence, have been reported [8].

In patients with (E)PP, massive amounts of excess protoporphyrin, mostly from the bone marrow, accumulate in tissues and feces. Patients do not have abnormal urinary porphyrins or porphyrin precursors; protoporphyrin is excreted unaltered by the liver into bile and, subsequently, feces; the rate-limiting step is canalicular excretion. If the hepatic load exceeds the excretion

Table 109-9. Causes of Secondary Porphyrinurias*

Anemias	Hereditary conjugated
Dyserythropoietic	hyperbilirubinemias
Aplastic	Dubin-Johnson syndromes
Hemolytic	Rotor's syndrome
Pernicious	Liver diseases
Leukemias and lymphomas	Alcoholic
Acute myelogenous leukemia	Cholestatic
Chronic myelogenous leukemia	Chronic hepatitis
Acute lymphocytic leukemia	Cirrhosis
Chronic lymphocytic leukemia	Viral hepatitis
Hodgkin's disease	(especially hepatitis C)
Chemicals and drugs	Miscellaneous causes
Barbiturates	Bronze-baby syndrome
Benzene	Diabetes mellitus
Estrogen	Infectious diseases
Ethanol	Myocardial infarction
Carbamazepine	Pregnancy
Carbon tetrachloride	Starvation
Halogenated aromatic	
hydrocarbons	
Heavy metal exposure	
(As, Hg, Pb)	
Phenytoin	
Progestogens	

Secondary porphyrinurias are the most common causes of increased porphyrins in the urine. These increases are mild-to-moderate in degree (less than threefold above the upper limit of normal), usually caused mainly by coproporphyrins. Stool porphyrins generally are normal.

capacity, protoporphyrin accumulates in the liver and causes liver damage, initiating a vicious cycle of worsening cholestasis and worsening protoporphyrin accumulation, which may result in pigmentary cirrhosis.

Diagnosis. Erythrocytes, feces, and plasma have increased protoporphyrin levels, but urinary porphyrins and porphyrin precursors are normal. The erythrocytic protoporphyrin is free and not the zinc chelate (as in lead poisoning and iron deficiency anemia).

Management. Patients must be protected from sunlight. Patients should be followed for development of liver disease; routine liver tests, however, are not reliable indicators of liver damage. Liver biopsy may be indicated in patients with very high protoporphyrin levels (greater than 1500 µg/dL in erythrocytes or 50 µg/dL in plasma) or unexplained liver test abnormalities; those with necrosis or fibrosis should be referred to specialized centers for therapy. Liver transplantation does not correct the underlying defect in bone marrow and other nonhepatic tissues.

Prognosis. The prognosis of (E)PP for most patients is good.

Secondary Porphyrinurias

The secondary porphyrinurias, sometimes called *porphyrinopathies*, are a large group of conditions in which mild to moderate increases in urinary porphyrin excretion occur in the absence of clinical or biochemical evidence of true porphyria. They constitute the most common causes of increased urinary porphyrins (Table 109-9). These include anemias, leukemias, lymphomas, disorders of the liver, exposures to a variety of chemicals and drugs, and a group of miscellaneous causes. Ethanol is responsible for secondary porphyrinuria more often than any other toxin. When such chemical changes are detected in patients with abdominal pain (caused, eg, by alcoholic gastropathy, alcohol withdrawal, irritable bowel syndrome), patients may be misdiagnosed as having acute porphyria. This diagnostic pitfall is best avoided by measurement of urinary ALA and PBG levels, which are the *sine qua non* for establishing the diagnosis of true symptomatic acute porphyria. The presence of mild to moderate increases in urinary porphyrin levels (less than three times the upper limit of normal), without definite increases in urinary ALA or PBG levels, is not diagnostic of acute porphyria. Stool porphyrin concentrations are normal or minimally increased in secondary porphyrinuria, which helps to exclude HCP and VP.

Multiple Chemical Sensitivity Syndrome and Porphyria

The diagnosis of multiple chemical sensitivity syndrome is popular despite the lack of consensus on the criteria for making this diagnosis. There is no known pathogenic link between the diverse symptoms reported by patients who believe that they have multiple chemical sensitivity syndrome and HCP or, for that matter, any other known disorder of porphyrin metabolism.

Pathogenesis of Secondary Porphyrinurias

In most instances, the nature of the defect that gives rise to secondary porphyrinuria is unknown. Probably, the abnormalities are different in different conditions.

Secondary porphyrinurias are important mainly because they may be confused with true porphyrias, leading to inappropriate treatment. In fact, mild increases in coproporphyrin levels in the urine alone do not require any treatment. Rather, the underlying disease should be treated in accordance with usual good standards of medical practice. The prognosis for patients with secondary porphyrinurias depends on the prognosis of the underlying disease and is not influenced by the urinary porphyrin excretion.

◾ ACKNOWLEDGMENTS

This work was supported by grants from the US National Institutes of Health (R01 DK38825 to Dr. Bonkovsky and R29 CA68479 to Dr. Barnard). The opinions expressed in this paper are those of the authors; they do not necessarily reflect the official views of the US Public Health Service or the National Institutes of Health.

◾ REFERENCES

Recently published papers of particular interest have been highlighted as follows:
•   Of interest
••   Of outstanding interest

1.   Bonkovsky HL: The porphyrias. In *Current Diagnosis*. Edited by Conn RB. Philadelphia: WB Saunders; 1985:799–809.

2.   Bonkovsky HL: The porphyrias. In *Conn's Current Therapy*. Edited by Rakel RE. Philadelphia: WB Saunders; 1993:427–433.

3.• Hahn M, Bonkovsky HL: Disorders of porphyrin metabolism. In *Disease of the Liver and Bile Ducts: A Practical Guide to Diagnosis and Treatment*. Edited by Wu G, Israel J. Philadelphia: WB Saunders; 1998, in press.
This is an up-to-date review of hepatic porphyrias.

4.•• Windebank AJ, Bonkovsky HL: Porphyric neuropathy. In *Peripheral Neuropathy*, edn 3. Edited by Dyck PJ, Thomas PK, Griffin JW, *et al.* Philadelphia: WB Saunders; 1992:1161–1168.
This is a complete review of the neurological manifestation of the porphyrias.

5.   Bonkovsky HL: Advances in understanding and treating the "little imitator," acute porphyria. *Gastroenterology* 1993, 105.590–594.
This is a review of the current status of management of acute porphyria.

6.   Dover SB, Moore MR, Fitzsimmons EJ, *et al.*: Tin protoporphyrin prolongs the biochemical remission produced by heme arginate in acute hepatic porphyria. *Gastroenterology* 1993, 105:500–506.

7.•• Kappas A, Sassa S, Galbraith RA, *et al.*: The porphyrias. In *The Metabolic and Molecular Bases of Inherited Disease*, edn 7, vol 2. Edited by Schriver CP, Beaudet AL, Sly WA, *et al.* New York: McGraw-Hill; 1995:2103–2161.
This is a detailed account, including enzymology and molecular biology.

8.   Serkany RPE, Cox: Autosomal recessive erythropoietic protoporphyria: a syndrome of severe photosensitivity and liver failure. *Q J Med* 1995, 88:541–549.

9.   Bloomer JR, Straka JG: Porphyrin metabolism. In *The Liver: Biology and Pathobiology*. Edited by Arias IM, Jakoby WB, Popper H, *et al.* New York: Raven Press; 1988:451–466.

10. Werth VP, McKinley-Grant L: Cutaneous manifestations of endocrine and metabolic disorders. In *Current Practice of Medicine*, vol 2. Edited by Bone RC. Philadelphia: Current Medicine; 1996:V.21.1–V.21.12.

11. Bonkovsky, HL: Porphyrin and heme metabolism and the porphyrias. In *Hepatology: A Textbook of Liver Disease*, edn 2. Edited by Zalkin D and Boyer TD. Philadelphia: WB Saunders, 1990:399.

110 The Pregnant Patient With Liver Disease
Andrea J. Singer

Liver diseases encountered in pregnant patients include those present before conception, those that occur coincident with pregnancy, and those that are unique to pregnancy. This chapter describes the features of liver diseases unique to pregnancy and also contains a brief discussion of the pregnant patient with viral hepatitis.

EFFECTS OF PREGNANCY ON LIVER TEST RESULTS

De novo liver test abnormalities in pregnant patients are uncommon, occurring in 5% or fewer of pregnancies in the United States [1]. Recognition of liver test abnormalities in pregnant women and identification of the cause is essential, however, because of potential morbidity and mortality associated with undiagnosed pregnancy-induced hypertension, acute fatty liver of pregnancy, and hepatic rupture.

The range of normal liver test results in pregnant women differs from that in nonpregnant persons (Table 110-1). Total serum protein and serum albumin concentrations decrease in midpregnancy as a result of dilution caused by an increase in maternal blood volume. In contrast, serum alkaline phosphatase levels rise gradually during the first two trimesters of pregnancy, then more rapidly during the third trimester, reaching a peak of about two to four times the value in nonpregnant persons at term [1–3]. This elevation is accounted for largely by alkaline phosphatase of placental origin. Serum aminotransferase levels are only slightly altered by normal pregnancy and usually remain within the normal range. Abnormalities in serum aspartate aminotransferase and alanine aminotransferase levels during pregnancy thus remain sensitive indicators of hepatocellular damage. Similarly, serum bilirubin levels are largely unaltered by pregnancy, and abnormal values may signify the presence of hepatobiliary disease.

APPROACH TO THE PREGNANT PATIENT WITH ABNORMAL LIVER TEST RESULTS

In the evaluation of the pregnant patient with abnormal liver test results, the physician should note the stage of gestation during which symptoms, if any, developed. Some liver diseases may present at any time during pregnancy, whereas others are much more likely to occur during the second half of gestation (Table 110-2). In addition, because the likelihood of developing some liver diseases seen exclusively during pregnancy depends on the clinical features of the pregnancy, and because some of these disorders may recur during subsequent pregnancies, a thorough obstetric history should be obtained. Pertinent information includes parity, number of fetuses (single or multiple), history of similar symptoms during previous pregnancies, outcomes of

Table 110-1. Liver Tests Related to Normal Pregnancy*

Test	Range during pregnancy
Blood volume	Increased 40%–50%
Plasma volume	Increased 50%
Total protein	Decreased 20%
Albumin	Decreased 10%–60%
Transaminases	
AST	Unchanged
ALT	Unchanged or slightly increased to upper limits of normal
Bilirubin	Unchanged or slightly decreased
GGTP	Unchanged or slightly decreased
Alkaline phosphatase	Increased two- to fourfold
Cholesterol	Increased twofold
Triglycerides	Increased two- to threefold
Total bile acids	Unchanged or slightly increased to upper limits of normal
Fibrinogen	Increased 50%
Prothrombin time	Unchanged

*Data from Wolf [1], Fallon and Riely [2], Bacq et al. [3], and Fagan [4]; with permission.
ALT—alanine aminotransferase; AST—aspartate aminotransferase; GGTP—γ-glutamyl transpeptidase.

Table 110-2. Differential Diagnosis of Abnormal Liver Tests and Jaundice in Pregnancy*

Disorder	Onset
Hyperemesis gravidarum	Usually 1st trimester; 4–20 wk
Intrahepatic cholestasis of pregnancy	2nd or 3rd Trimester; usually > 30 wk
Preeclampsia or eclampsia	Late 2nd or 3rd trimester; > 20 wk
HELLP syndrome	Usually 3rd trimester; 27 wk to immediate postpartum
Acute fatty liver of pregnancy	3rd Trimester; 26 wk to immediate postpartum
Hepatic rupture	Usually 3rd trimester
Viral hepatitis	All trimesters
Gallstones	All trimesters

*Modified from Olans and Wolf JL [12]; with permission.
HELLP—hemolysis, elevated liver tests, low platelets.

prior pregnancies, and history of oral contraceptive intolerance. A family history of pregnancy-induced hypertension, intrahepatic cholestasis of pregnancy, oral contraceptive intolerance, or cholelithiasis also is important.

Although the physical examination rarely is diagnostic, the physician should search for stigmata of liver disease in pregnant patients with abnormal liver test results. Spider angiomas and palmar erythema are common in healthy pregnant women; if prominent during early pregnancy, however, the patient may have pre-existing liver disease. Jaundice, ascites, splenomegaly, and Murphy's sign are not normal features of pregnancy. Other abnormal physical findings that may be found in the pregnant patient with liver disease include fever, hypertension, orthostatic hypotension, peripheral edema, excoriations, petechiae, and neurologic abnormalities.

Evaluation of pregnant patients with abnormal liver test results is similar to that of nonpregnant patients suspected of having liver disease. A complete blood count, coagulation studies including prothrombin time, and blood chemistries including liver tests and serum glucose and electrolyte concentrations should be performed. The serum uric acid level may be elevated in pregnancy-induced hypertension and related liver disorders. Serologic tests for viral hepatitis should be done in most patients with abnormal liver tests; hepatitis B surface antigen testing is part of the routine prenatal evaluation, but hepatitis C antibody testing and serum aminotransferase levels often are not.

HYPEREMESIS GRAVIDARUM

Nausea and vomiting are normal features of early pregnancy. Hyperemesis gravidarum is characterized by persistent vomiting, which threatens to cause dehydration, electrolyte disturbances, and nutritional deficiencies with accompanying weight loss. Also known as pernicious vomiting of pregnancy, hyperemesis gravidarum occurs in about 3.5 per 1000 pregnancies. It is more common in primigravidas, younger women (especially those younger than 20 years), women with less than 12 years of education, obese women, and nonsmokers. Multiple gestations and trophoblastic disease also appear to predispose to this disorder.

Although usually self-limited, the natural history of hyperemesis gravidarum is one of slow recovery with frequent relapses. Fluid, electrolyte, and nutritional derangements may be associated with liver test abnormalities (Table 110-3). Minor serum aminotransferase level elevations occur in 15% to 25% of women with hyperemesis gravidarum and reverse promptly with restoration of fluid balance, improved nutrition, and cessation of vomiting [4]. Synthetic liver function, as reflected by the prothrombin time, remains intact except in patients with marked cholestasis and vitamin K deficiency.

Hyperemesis gravidarum usually is not a cause of excess maternal and fetal morbidity and mortality. There is no associated increase in the frequency of premature delivery, and the risk of miscarriage and stillbirth in affected women is less than half that in normal pregnant women [5].

Treatment of hyperemesis gravidarum is supportive and includes reassurance, small frequent meals, dietary fat restriction, and, in severe or refractory cases, intravenous hydration and sometimes enteral or parenteral alimentation [6]. Patients with severe hyperemesis gravidarum should be treated by specialists in maternal-fetal medicine (perinatology).

INTRAHEPATIC CHOLESTASIS OF PREGNANCY

Intrahepatic cholestasis of pregnancy is a cholestatic liver disorder characterized by development of pruritus with or without associated jaundice in the second and third trimesters of pregnancy.

Epidemiology and Risk Factors

The incidence of intrahepatic cholestasis of pregnancy varies with geography and ethnicity. It is most common in Chile among Araucanian Indians and also is seen commonly in Bolivia and Sweden [1,7], but rarely is diagnosed in African-American women. Seasonal variations in occurrence have been observed; for example, there is a higher incidence of intrahepatic cholestasis of pregnancy during winter than during summer in Finland [7]. Intrahepatic cholestasis of pregnancy is more common in women with a family history of the disease and in those who have had cholestasis while taking oral contraceptives. The disorder also tends to recur during subsequent pregnancies.

Pathogenesis

The physiologic defect responsible for intrahepatic cholestasis of pregnancy is unknown. It is clear, however, that genetic and hormonal factors play a role in its development. Women with intrahepatic cholestasis of pregnancy are more likely to have histocompatibility haplotypes HLA-B8 and HLA-Bw16 than are controls, suggesting a genetic predisposition to this disorder. As mentioned previously, intrahepatic cholestasis of pregnancy is more common in women with a family history of the disease, and family studies have suggested a dominant mode of inheritance; fathers can transmit susceptibility to intrahepatic cholestasis of pregnancy to their daughters.

Table 110-3. Hyperemesis Gravidarum

Clinical features	Associations	Abnormal laboratory values
Nausea, vomiting	Primigravidas	Bilirubin (increases to < 4–5 mg/dL)
Ptyalism	Young age	Transaminases (increase 1–2×)
Weight loss	Obesity	Alkaline phosphatase (increase 1–2×)
Possible mild jaundice	Trophoblastic disease	Urine ketones (present)
Malnutrition, dehydration if severe	Hyperthyroidism	
	Multiple gestation	

Estrogens are thought to be involved in the pathogenesis of intrahepatic cholestasis of pregnancy because the features of this disorder may be reproduced in previously affected women by use of oral contraceptives containing estrogen. Furthermore, women with a history of intrahepatic cholestasis of pregnancy, nulliparous women, and also men with a family history of intrahepatic cholestasis of pregnancy have been shown to have an exaggerated hepatic metabolic response to estrogens [7].

Clinical Features

Intrahepatic cholestasis of pregnancy typically occurs during the third trimester and is characterized by generalized pruritus, which may be severe and often is worse at night (see Table 110-4). Pruritus typically is associated with insomnia, mood changes, anorexia, and malaise. Twenty to 60% of affected women may develop jaundice, dark urine, and light stools 2 to 4 weeks after the onset of pruritus. Both pruritus and jaundice usually persist throughout the remainder of gestation and improve rapidly after parturition. Patients with intrahepatic cholestasis of pregnancy may develop steatorrhea, which can affect maternal nutrition and absorption of fat-soluble vitamins.

Results of physical examination of patients with intrahepatic cholestasis of pregnancy usually are unremarkable, with the possible exception of excoriations secondary to pruritus. Affected women may have elevated serum bilirubin concentrations, which typically are below 6 mg/dL, and possibly a mild to moderate increase in serum aminotransferase levels. The serum concentration of total bile acids may increase as much as 100-fold; this may be the first and only laboratory abnormality in patients with intrahepatic cholestasis of pregnancy. Serum cholesterol and triglyceride levels also may be elevated. Liver biopsy in affected women reveals cholestasis without hepatocellular necrosis but usually is not needed for diagnosis.

Maternal and Fetal Outcome

Despite the fact that intrahepatic cholestasis of pregnancy also has been called "benign" cholestasis of pregnancy, there are potential complications, especially for the fetus. Intrahepatic cholestasis of pregnancy has been associated with an increased incidence of stillbirth, fetal distress, and preterm labor. Steatorrhea-induced vitamin K deficiency, exacerbated by use of cholestyramine, may cause maternal postpartum hemorrhage [2,7,8]. Women with a history of intrahepatic cholestasis of pregnancy also are prone to develop cholelithiasis.

Management

Treatment of the mother is symptomatic and directed at relieving pruritus. Rest, low-fat diet, sleeping in a cool room, and topical alcohol may be beneficial for pruritus. Phenobarbital and antihistamines provide only partial and unpredictable relief from pruritus and may contribute to respiratory depression in the newborn if used near term. Cholestyramine, a bile salt–binding resin, given orally in a dose of 4 g four or five times a day, improves pruritus within 1 to 2 weeks in many women with intrahepatic cholestasis of pregnancy. Side effects are common, however, and include constipation, bloating, mild nausea, and anorexia. Cholestyramine may cause or exacerbate malabsorption of fat and fat-soluble vitamins; prophylactic parenteral vitamin K, therefore, is recommended in patients treated with this medicine.

S-adenosyl-L-methionine, a molecule thought to inactivate estrogen metabolites and alter bile acid metabolism, initially was shown to improve clinical and laboratory findings in patients with intrahepatic cholestasis of pregnancy, but a subsequent double-blind placebo-controlled trial failed to confirm any benefit [9]. In several small, uncontrolled studies, ursodeoxycholic acid, a hydrophilic bile salt, has been shown to reduce pruritus and laboratory abnormalities in women with intrahepatic cholestasis of pregnancy without adversely affecting the fetus [9,10]. Ursodeoxycholic acid is thought to act by replacing other, more hydrophobic and cytotoxic bile salts in the bile acid pool.

Careful preterm monitoring by experts in maternal-fetal medicine is recommended for pregnant women with intrahepatic cholestasis of pregnancy.

PREGNANCY-INDUCED HYPERTENSION

Pregnancy-induced hypertension, formerly called *pre-eclampsia*, is a multisystem disorder that often involves the liver and that is defined by the presence of maternal hypertension, proteinuria, and edema during the third trimester of pregnancy. Eclampsia is the development of seizures in a patient with pregnancy-induced hypertension.

Epidemiology and Risk Factors

Pregnancy-induced hypertension occurs in 4% to 10% of pregnancies that progress beyond the first trimester [1,2,11], and eclampsia occurs in 0.1% to 0.2% of pregnancies [1]. Pregnancy-induced hypertension is primarily a disease of first pregnancies; about two-thirds to three-fourths of cases occur in primiparous women [11]. Extremes of maternal age, a family history of pregnancy-induced hypertension, a history of

Table 110-4. Intrahepatic Cholestasis of Pregnancy		
Clinical features	**Associations**	**Abnormal laboratory values**
Pruritus	Oral contraceptive–induced cholestasis	Bilirubin (increases to < 6 mg/dL) Transaminases
Jaundice in 20%–60%	Family history of intrahepatic cholestasis of pregnancy	Alkaline phosphatase Serum bile acids (increase 30- to 100-fold) Prothrombin time Cholesterol Triglycerides

Table 110-5. Pregnancy-Induced Hypertension (Preeclampsia)

Hypertension	Proteinuria	Edema
Increase of ≥ 30 mm Hg in systolic blood pressure relative to readings before 20 weeks' gestation, *or*	Excretion of ≥ 300 mg of protein in 24 h	Clinically evident swelling, especially of hands, face, or both
Increase of ≥ 15 mm Hg in diastolic blood pressure relative to readings before 20 weeks' gestation, *or*		Rapid weight gain
Blood pressure ≥ 140/90 mm Hg after 20 weeks' gestation		

pregnancy-induced hypertension complicating a previous pregnancy, diabetes, renal or vascular disease, and hypertension that antedates pregnancy all predispose a pregnant patient to develop pregnancy-induced hypertension. Furthermore, the incidence of pregnancy-induced hypertension is significantly increased in women with multiple fetuses or a hydatidiform mole as compared with controls.

Pathogenesis

The cause of pregnancy-induced hypertension is unknown, and various etiologies have been proposed to explain its development. Studies indicate that poor tissue perfusion secondary to severe vasospasm and endothelial cell injury is an important pathogenic factor in the development of pregnancy-induced hypertension. Explanations for vasospasm include a greater than normal response to endogenous pressors, particularly angiotensin II, and increased production of the vasoconstrictor, endothelin-1, in pregnant women with pregnancy-induced hypertension as compared with normal pregnant women [11].

A growing body of literature suggests that altered eicosanoid production may lead to pregnancy-induced hypertension [2,11]. Synthesis of thromboxane A2, a potent vasoconstrictor, is increased in this disorder, whereas production of prostacyclin, a potent vasodilator, is decreased. In addition, the synthesis and release of endothelium-derived relaxing factor, another important vasodilator, are impaired in patients with pregnancy-induced hypertension [2]. Finally, there has been some speculation that immunologic factors may contribute to development of pregnancy-induced hypertension.

Clinical Features

Pregnancy-induced hypertension may occur after 20 weeks' gestation and before the seventh postpartum day but is most common during the third trimester. Diagnosis is based on the presence of hypertension, often accompanied by proteinuria and edema (Table 110-5). Although edema is a common early sign of pregnancy-induced hypertension, it is not invariably present. Furthermore, edema occurs in 30% of normal pregnancies. It is clinically useful to separate pregnancy-induced hypertension into mild and severe disease (Table 110-6).

Most women with early pregnancy-induced hypertension do not have symptoms, but numerous signs and a multitude of symptoms may develop in affected women; many are indicative of the severity of the disease. Symptoms and signs of hepatic capsular distention, including abdominal pain, nausea, hepatomegaly, and hepatic tenderness, are particularly ominous because they may be associated with intrahepatic hemorrhage and may precede

Table 110-6. Features of Severe Pregnancy-Induced Hypertension (Preeclampsia)

Blood pressure ≥ 160 mm Hg systolic or 110 mm Hg diastolic

Dense proteinuria (> 5 g/24 h or 3+ to 4+ as determined by dipstick)

Oliguria (≤ 500 mL urine/24 h) or elevated serum creatinine (> 1.2 mg/dL) in a patient with previously normal creatinine

Cerebral or visual disturbances

Epigastric pain, right upper quadrant pain, or evidence of hepatocellular damage

Pulmonary edema

Retinal hemorrhages, exudates, or papilledema

Coagulation abnormalities

hepatic rupture. Women with pregnancy-induced hypertension and abdominal complaints also may have the HELLP syndrome and acute fatty liver of pregnancy (see later).

Laboratory evaluation of patients with severe pregnancy-induced hypertension may reveal elevated serum aminotransferase levels, thrombocytopenia, microangiopathic hemolytic anemia, and disseminated intravascular coagulation.

The diagnosis of pregnancy-induced hypertension with liver involvement is primarily a clinical one. Although almost never necessary for diagnosis, when performed, liver biopsy may reveal periportal deposition of fibrin and fibrinogen with associated hemorrhage and sometimes necrosis.

Management

In the past, pregnancy-induced hypertension was a major cause of mortality. Today, however, routine prenatal care, physician awareness, and effective therapies have made maternal and fetal death caused by pregnancy-induced hypertension a rarity. When death does occur, it is primarily the result of complications, including liver disease. Care by physicians experienced in the management of pregnancy-induced hypertension is recommended for patients with this disorder; women with severe or complicated disease should be managed by experts in maternal-fetal medicine.

■ HELLP SYNDROME
Epidemiology and Risk Factors

About 4% to 12% of women with pregnancy-induced hypertension develop hemolysis (H), elevated liver tests (EL), and low platelets (LP): the HELLP syndrome [1,9,12,13•]. HELLP also may occur independently [1,8,12]. It is more common in white women of older maternal age. The risk of recurrent HELLP in subsequent pregnancies is low [13•].

Pathogenesis

The cause of HELLP is unknown, but it likely is part of the spectrum of manifestations of pregnancy-induced hypertension. As such, a vascular cause, with abnormal vascular tone, vasospasm, and endothelial cell injury, is favored. It is postulated that vasospasm leads to endothelial cell injury, which in turn causes platelet adherence and aggregation and deposition of fibrin. Obstruction of blood flow and increased intraluminal pressure may result in distention and hemorrhage. Circulating immune complexes and a genetic predisposition also have been proposed as factors contributing to HELLP.

Clinical Features

Most cases of HELLP occur between 27 and 36 weeks' gestation, but about one third occur postpartum. Presenting symptoms include right upper quadrant or epigastric pain, malaise, nausea and vomiting, and headache. Jaundice develops in only about 5% of patients [8]. Physical examination may reveal right upper quadrant tenderness, edema, and weight gain, but elevated blood pressure may be absent.

The HELLP syndrome is marked by a host of abnormal laboratory findings that peak on the first or second day after delivery. A microangiopathic, hemolytic anemia occurs with Burr's cells and schistocytes seen on peripheral smear. There may be low serum haptoglobin, increased serum lactate dehydrogenase levels, and indirect hyperbilirubinemia. Serum aminotransferase levels are elevated 2 to 10 times above the upper limit of normal, and low platelet counts are found. Increased serum uric acid and creatinine concentrations also are common. Liver histology, although not usually obtained, may demonstrate periportal or focal necrosis with hyaline deposits in sinusoids (Fig. 110-1, see also **Color Plate**).

The differential diagnosis of HELLP syndrome includes other liver diseases specific to pregnancy and pregnancy-induced hypertension as well as thrombotic thrombocytopenic purpura and hemolytic uremia syndrome (Table 110-7).

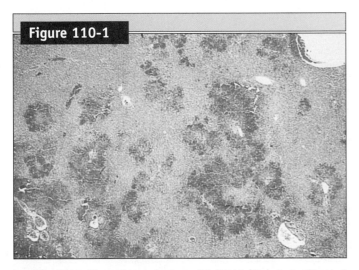

Figure 110-1

Section of liver biopsy from a patient with HELLP (Hemolysis, Elevated Liver enzymes, amd Low Platelets) syndrome. See also **Color Plate**.

Maternal and Fetal Outcome

The maternal mortality rate associated with HELLP syndrome is about 1% to 3% in tertiary care settings, but rates as high as 25% have been reported in community hospitals [8]. Maternal complications of HELLP syndrome resemble those of severe pregnancy-induced hypertension and include disseminated intravascular coagulation, abruptio placenta, acute renal failure, pulmonary edema, and hepatic hematoma and rupture. The infant mortality rate in the perinatal period is 10% to 60%, depending on the severity of the disease at the time of diagnosis and delivery [1,8,12]. Infants are at increased risk of prematurity, intrauterine growth restriction, and thrombocytopenia.

Management

Delivery is the definitive treatment for HELLP syndrome. If HELLP or associated pregnancy-induced hypertension is severe or develops after about 36 weeks' gestation, and if there is evidence of fetal lung maturity, delivery is recommended. Controversy still exists about the appropriate treatment of patients with HELLP syndrome at less than 34 weeks' gestation.

ACUTE FATTY LIVER OF PREGNANCY
Epidemiology and Risk Factors

Acute fatty liver of pregnancy is an uncommon but potentially fatal disease of late gestation. Before 1980, the estimated incidence of acute fatty liver of pregnancy was 1 case per 1 million pregnancies [1,12,14]; more recently, the incidence has been estimated to be about 1 case per 15,000 deliveries, the increase attributed to heightened awareness of the disorder, recognition of milder cases, and generally improved prenatal care.

The incidence of acute fatty liver of pregnancy is highest in primiparas and in women with multiple and male fetuses. Acute fatty liver of pregnancy usually does not recur, although there are now three case reports of recurrent disease in subsequent pregnancies.

Pathogenesis

Despite its characteristic clinical features and distinct histologic appearance, the pathogenesis of acute fatty liver of pregnancy is unknown. Many mechanisms for development of this disorder have been proposed, including nutritional deficiencies, alterations in lipoprotein synthesis, and mitochondrial dysfunction, but none has been confirmed by clinical investigations. Many authors believe that acute fatty liver of pregnancy, HELLP syndrome, and pregnancy-induced hypertension are features of the same fundamental disorder, namely systemic alteration in vascular endothelial function. Reports of the recurrence of acute fatty liver of pregnancy in multiparas and the possible association of acute fatty liver of pregnancy with deficiency of long chain 3-hydroxyacyl–coenzyme A dehydrogenase, raise the possibility of a genetic or metabolic defect [15].

Clinical Features

Acute fatty liver of pregnancy presents during the third trimester, with a mean gestational age at onset of 36 weeks. It has been reported to occur as early as 26 weeks and as late as immediately postpartum. Initial manifestations are nonspecific, often resemble those of pregnancy-induced hypertension, and include headache, fatigue, malaise, anorexia, nausea, and vomiting. Abdominal pain, usually in the right upper quadrant or epigastrium, is described by most patients with acute fatty liver of pregnancy. Jaundice often follows these symptoms. If untreated, acute fatty liver of pregnancy often progresses to hepatic failure, renal failure, disseminated intravascular coagulation, gastrointestinal or uterine bleeding, pancreatitis, seizures, coma, and death. The obstetric history of a patient with acute fatty liver of pregnancy commonly resembles that of a patient with pregnancy-induced hypertension, and affected women often have peripheral edema, proteinuria, and modest elevations in blood pressure.

Serum aminotransferase levels usually are 300 to 500 U/mL. Levels above 1000 U/mL suggest viral hepatitis. Serum bilirubin concentrations may be normal early in the course of acute fatty liver of pregnancy but rise if pregnancy is not terminated. Hematologic abnormalities in severe acute fatty liver of pregnancy are similar to those in severe pregnancy-induced hypertension and include leukocytosis, microangiopathic hemolytic anemia, and thrombocytopenia. The prothrombin time and partial thromboplastin time may be prolonged. If disseminated intravascular coagulation is present, fibrinogen concentration may be decreased, with an increase in fibrin degradation products. Hypoglycemia is a common complication of severe acute fatty liver of pregnancy and may be profound. Hyperuricemia also is common in these patients, and as hepatic failure progresses, serum ammonia levels increase.

Ultrasonography and computed tomography (CT) of the liver have been suggested as possible diagnostic tools because they are noninvasive and safe in patients with coagulation abnormalities. Ultrasound reveals increased hepatic echogenicity in acute fatty liver of pregnancy, whereas CT shows decreased attenuation. Neither test is sufficiently sensitive to exclude a diagnosis of acute fatty liver of pregnancy, and the principal use

Table 110-7. Differential Diagnosis of Liver Failure in Pregnancy

	PIH (Preeclampsia eclampsia)	HELLP	AFLP	Hepatic rupture	Viral hepatitis
Trimester	2 or 3	3	3	3	Any
Risk factors	Nulliparity Extremes of maternal age Chronic hypertension, diabetes, or renal disease Multiple gestation Trophoblastic disease	Older maternal age White women	Primigravidas Multiple gestation Male fetus	Multigravidas Older maternal age	Coinfection with HIV
Associations	HELLP Hepatic rupture AFLP	PIH Hepatic rupture	PIH Long-chain 3-hydroxyacyl-coenzyme A dehydrogenase deficiency	PIH HELLP	Vertical transmission
Clinical manifestations	Hypertension Proteinuria Edema Nausea, vomiting Abdominal pain Seizures None	Abdominal pain Nausea, vomiting Malaise	Abdominal pain Nausea, vomiting Jaundice Altered sensorium	Acute abdominal pain Nausea, vomiting Hypotension	Nausea, vomiting Abdominal pain Jaundice Altered sensorium in presence of hepatic encephalopathy
Laboratory findings	Aminotransferases increase (< 500 U) Bilirubin increases mildly Uric acid increases Proteinuria Thrombocytopenia DIC	Aminotransferases increase (< 500 U) Bilirubin increases mildly Uric acid increases LDH increases Hemolytic anemia Thrombocytopenia DIC	Aminotransferases increase (< 500 U) Uric acid increases Low glucose Leukocytosis Thrombocytopenia DIC	Aminotransferases increase Anemia Thrombocytopenia DIC	Aminotransferases increase (> 500 U) Bilirubin increases Hepatic serologies positive
Liver biopsy	Fibrin thrombi Periportal hemorrhage Some necrosis	Periportal or focal necrosis Hyaline deposits in sinusoids	Microvesicular fat	—	Marked inflammation and necrosis

AFLP—acute fatty liver of pregnancy; DIC—disseminated intravascular coagulation; HELLP—hemolysis, elevated liver tests, low platelets.

of abdominal imaging in this setting is to diagnose intrahepatic hemorrhage and rare instances of common bile duct obstruction.

Liver biopsy is diagnostic and is characterized by accumulation of microvesicular fat within hepatocytes; liver biopsy, however, rarely is necessary in patients with suspected acute fatty liver of pregnancy (Fig. 110-2, see also **Color Plate**).

Maternal and Fetal Outcome

In the past, maternal and fetal mortality rates in acute fatty liver of pregnancy were as high as 85%. Early detection, rapid delivery after diagnosis, and aggressive supportive care have reduced maternal and fetal mortality rates to much less than 25%, even in more severe cases [1,8,14]. Despite appropriate care, however, the patient's condition may deteriorate immediately after delivery, and if aggressive action is not taken, fulminant hepatic failure and death may ensue. Survivors have no long-term sequelae, and liver histology returns to normal.

Management

Acute fatty liver of pregnancy is managed by expeditious delivery and intensive medical support by experts in maternal-fetal medicine. The route of delivery should be guided by obstetric indications. Interim therapeutic goals include maintenance of adequate oxygenation and perfusion of both mother and fetus; correction of electrolyte abnormalities and metabolic disturbances, such as hypoglycemia and acidosis; correction of hematologic and coagulation abnormalities to the degree possible; and continuous fetal surveillance. Insertion of a Swan-Ganz catheter to assist in fluid management, mechanical ventilation, and hemodialysis may be required. Liver transplantation has been successful in women with fulminant acute fatty liver of pregnancy.

▬ HEPATIC RUPTURE
Epidemiology and Risk Factors

Hepatic rupture is one of the rarest but most lethal hepatic complications of pregnancy. The incidence of hepatic rupture varies from one case in 40,000 to 250,000 deliveries [16]. Hepatic rupture has been reported to occur in 1% to 2% of patients with pregnancy-induced hypertension or HELLP

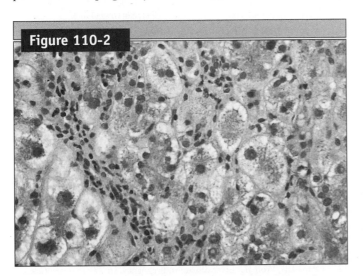

Figure 110-2

Section of liver biopsy from a patient with acute fatty liver of pregnancy showing microvesicular fat. See also **Color Plate**.

syndrome [2,16]; more than 80% of cases of hepatic rupture in pregnancy occur in women with pregnancy-induced hypertension [1,16]. Affected women are more likely to be multigravidas and older. Only one case of recurrent hepatic rupture during pregnancy has been reported [16].

Pathogenesis

The cause of hepatic rupture in pregnancy is unknown, but it likely is related to the pathophysiologic abnormality responsible for pregnancy-induced hypertension. In cases associated with pregnancy-induced hypertension or HELLP syndrome, disseminated intravascular coagulation has been implicated, with fibrin deposition in hepatic sinusoids as the initiating event [16]. Hepatic rupture has been reported, however, in pregnant patients with only minimal or early signs of disseminated intravascular coagulation. Another proposed mechanism for hepatic rupture is microangiopathy or a toxic vasculopathy causing ischemic injury and intrahepatic bleeding [16].

Clinical Features

Hepatic hemorrhage and rupture occur most often during the third trimester but may occur from late in the second trimester to immediately after delivery; affected women usually have signs and symptoms of pregnancy-induced hypertension. The initial symptoms often are related to stretching or irritation of the liver capsule from hemorrhage, with pain in the right upper quadrant or right lower chest and associated nausea and vomiting. With rupture of the capsule and hemorrhage into the peritoneum, abdominal distention and hypovolemic shock ensue. Rupture is most common in the right lobe of the liver, although the left or both lobes may be involved [1].

Affected women have elevated serum aminotransferase levels, thrombocytopenia, and profound anemia and may have laboratory evidence of disseminated intravascular coagulation. Diagnostic tests used to evaluate suspected hepatic rupture include abdominal ultrasound, CT, magnetic resonance imaging, and angiography.

Maternal and Fetal Outcome

Maternal and fetal mortality rates are greater than 50% in this disorder [1,16]. The most frequent cause of maternal death after rupture is uncontrolled hemorrhage; thus, the mortality rate is lower in women with contained hematomas. Maternal survival depends on early recognition and prompt intervention. If the mother survives, the liver returns to normal. Fetal survival depends, in large part, on the degree of prematurity and the outcome of the mother.

Management

Management of hepatic rupture must be aggressive, with emergent delivery and surgical intervention, including evacuation of the hematoma, packing or hemostatic wrapping, oversewing defects, hepatic artery ligation, and lobectomy. Angiographic embolization of the ruptured vessel may be effective, particularly if rupture is limited to one lobe of the liver. If the patient has an intrahepatic or subcapsular hematoma alone, without free rupture, expectant management with close observation and maximal support in an intensive care unit may be appropriate.

VIRAL HEPATITIS

The most common cause of jaundice in pregnant women in the United States is viral hepatitis. With the exception of hepatitis E, the clinical course and histologic findings in hepatitis A, B, and C and delta hepatitis in pregnant women do not differ from those in nonpregnant persons.

Acute Hepatitis A

Pregnant women with hepatitis A generally do not transmit the infection to their offspring. Presumably, the risk of transmission is limited by the brief viremic period, passive antibody transfer, and lack of fecal contamination during delivery. Diagnosis and management do not differ from those in nonpregnant patients (see Chapter 93). Immune globulin is effective prophylaxis against infection after exposure to hepatitis A and should be offered to pregnant women with household or sexual contacts who have acute disease.

Acute Hepatitis B

Infection with hepatitis B virus is a major cause of acute and chronic hepatitis, cirrhosis, and primary hepatocellular carcinoma throughout the world (see Chapters 93 and 94). Although pregnancy does not affect the course of hepatitis B, and hepatitis B does not appear to affect pregnancy adversely, concern centers around vertical transmission of this virus from mother to child, which almost always occurs at the time of birth. Certain features appear to determine the likelihood and rate of perinatal transmission of hepatitis B virus, including the period in pregnancy during which infection occurs, the mother's infectivity as reflected by amount of replication and viremia, and the mother's racial and geographic background. Women who have acute hepatitis B during the first or second trimester rarely transmit the infection to their neonates and only do so if they become chronic carriers. On the other hand, women who contract the disease during the third trimester or near the time of delivery have a high probability of transmitting the virus to their offspring. Mothers positive for both hepatitis B virus surface and E antigens (HBsAg and HBeAg) infect more than 80% of untreated infants. Transmission by symptom-free mothers is much higher in African and Asian countries (30% to 70%) than it is in the United States (5% to 20%) and most other Western countries [17•].

The most common outcome of infection in the newborn is persistent antigenemia; as many as 90% of infants infected with hepatitis B virus at birth become carriers. Many ultimately develop chronic active hepatitis, cirrhosis, and primary hepatocellular carcinoma. In addition, female carriers subsequently may perpetuate the cycle of perinatal transmission when, as adults, they become pregnant. Because of the high prevalence of infection with hepatitis B virus, routine HbsAg screening is recommended for all pregnant women. All infants of HBsAg-positive mothers should receive hepatitis B immune globulin (0.5 mL) in the delivery room and should be immunized with hepatitis B vaccine immediately, 1 month later, and again at about 6 months of age, a practice that is now standard in the United States.

Hepatitis C

Infection with hepatitis C virus is a serious health problem. Despite the relatively benign nature of acute infection, there is a high frequency of chronic infection (85%), chronic hepatitis (as many as 60%), cirrhosis (20%), and hepatocellular carcinoma. Vertical transmission of hepatitis C virus is far less common than that of hepatitis B virus. Coinfection with human immunodeficiency virus in the mother and active viral replication may enhance transmission of hepatitis C virus to the neonate. Routine screening of pregnant women for hepatitis C virus infection has been recommended by some authorities to identify symptom-free persons with hepatitis C who may be treated before they develop complicated liver disease.

Delta Hepatitis

Delta hepatitis is caused by a defective RNA virus that is dependent on hepatitis B virus for replication (see Chapter 93). Perinatal transmission of delta hepatitis is rare. Delta infection in the neonate can occur only if delta hepatitis is transmitted along with hepatitis B virus.

Hepatitis E

Hepatitis E is a serious disease in pregnant women but is not endemic to the United States. It is responsible for a high frequency of fatal, fulminant hepatitis in pregnant women in areas of the world, such as India, where infection occurs (see Chapter 93).

REFERENCES

Recently published papers of particular interest have been highlighted as follows:
• 	Of interest
•• 	Of outstanding interest

1. 	Wolf JL: Liver disease in pregnancy. *Med Clin North Am* 1996, 80:1167–1187.

2. 	Fallon HJ, Riely CA: Liver diseases. In *Medical Complications During Pregnancy*. Edited by Burrow GN, Ferris TF. Philadelphia: WB Saunders; 1995:307–342.

3. 	Bacq Y, Zarka O, Brechot JF, *et al.*: Liver function test in normal pregnancy: a prospective study of 103 pregnant women and 103 matched controls. *Hepatology* 1996, 23:1030–1034.

4. 	Fagan EA: Diseases of liver, biliary system, and pancreas. In *Maternal-Fetal Medicine, Principles and Practice*. Edited by Creasy RK, Resnik R. Philadelphia: WB Saunders; 1994:1040–1061.

5. 	Singer AJ, Brandt LJ: Pathophysiology of the gastrointestinal tract during pregnancy. *Am J Gastroenterol* 1991, 86:1695–1712.

6. 	van Stuijvenberg ME, Schabort I, Labadarios D, *et al.*: The nutritional status and treatment of patients with hyperemesis gravidarum. *Am J Obstet Gynecol* 1995, 172:1585–1591.

7. 	Reyes H: The spectrum of liver and gastrointestinal disease seen in cholestasis of pregnancy. *Gastroenterol Clin North Am* 1992, 21:905–921.

8. 	Knox TA, Olans LB: Liver disease in pregnancy. *N Engl J Med* 1996, 335:569–576.

9. 	Davies MH, da Silva RCMA, Jones SR, *et al.*: Fetal mortality associated with cholestasis of pregnancy and the potential benefit of therapy with ursodeoxycholic acid. *Gut* 1995, 37:580–584.

10. 	Palma J, Reyes H, Riblata J, *et al.*: Effects of ursodeoxycholic acid in patients with intrahepatic cholestasis of pregnancy. *Hepatology* 1992, 15:1043–1047.

11. 	Roberts JM: Pregnancy-related hypertension. In *Maternal-Fetal Medicine, Principles and Practice*. Edited by Creasy RK, Resnik R. Philadelphia: WB Saunders; 1994:804–829.

12. 	Olans LB, Wolf JL: Liver disease in pregnancy. In *The Primary Care of Women*. Edited by Carlson KJ, Eisenstat SA. St Louis: Mosby-Year Book; 1995:360–367.

13.• Sibai BM, Ramadan MK, Chari RS, *et al.*: Pregnancies complicated by HELLP syndrome (hemolysis, elevated liver enzymes, and low platelets): subsequent pregnancy outcome and long-term prognosis. *Am J Obstet Gynecol* 1995, 172:125–129.
This descriptive and analytical study of 341 women with HELLP syndrome identifies increased risk for obstetric complications in future pregnancies.

14. Mabie WC: Acute fatty liver of pregnancy. *Gastroenterol Clin North Am* 1992, 21:951–960.

15. Treem WR, Rinalso P, Hale DE, *et al.*: Acute fatty liver of pregnancy and long-chain 3-hydroxyacyl-coenzyme A dehydrogenase deficiency. *Hepatology* 1994, 19:339–345.

16. Greenstein D, Henderson JM, Boyer TD: Liver hemorrhage: recurrent episodes during pregnancy complicated by preeclampsia. *Gastroenterology* 1994, 106:1668–1671.

17.• Mishra L, Seeff LB: Viral hepatitis, A through E, complicating pregnancy. *Gastroenterol Clin North Am* 1992, 21:873.
This comprehensive review of viral hepatitis includes a general discussion of the disease followed by examination of the issues that have particular relevance to pregnancy and the newborn.

111 Liver Disease in Patients With Acquired Immunodeficiency Syndrome

Francis R. Weiner and Douglas Simon

It is estimated that by the year 2000, more than 1 million people in the United States will be infected with human immunodeficiency virus (HIV). Gastrointestinal complications are common in patients with the acquired immunodeficiency syndrome (AIDS), and the liver commonly is involved. Hepatomegaly has been reported in two-thirds of AIDS patients, and an abnormality of at least one serum liver test occurs in more than 70% of infected persons [1••].

Liver disease complicating AIDS results in large part from HIV-induced immunosuppression, which permits AIDS-related diseases to involve the liver. In addition, previous intravenous drug use and sexual promiscuity in some AIDS patients predisposes them to hepatotrophic virus infection. Liver disease complicating AIDS usually is caused by opportunistic infections, neoplasms, or drugs. Non-HIV associated disorders, such as viral hepatitis, alcoholism, and malnutrition, also can result in liver dysfunction.

EPIDEMIOLOGY

Hepatomegaly has been detected clinically in 60% and at autopsy in 72% of AIDS patients. Abnormal liver tests have been reported in 78% of AIDS patients; serum aminotransaminase levels are elevated in 61% and serum alkaline phosphatase (SAP) levels are elevated in 51% of cases [1••]. Jaundice has been reported less commonly, occurring in 11% of persons with AIDS [1••].

Opportunistic infections are the most common causes of parenchymal liver disease in AIDS patients (Fig. 111-1); they are reported in 34% of patients who undergo liver biopsy and in 38% of autopsy cases [1••]. AIDS patients with homosexual contact as their HIV risk factor usually have liver involvement with cytomegalovirus (CMV), whereas acid-fast bacilli are more commonly found in the livers of intravenous drug users [1••]. The overall prevalence of opportunistic infection, however, does not differ in these two risk groups. Hepatic neoplasms occur less often than does hepatic infection and usually are diagnosed at autopsy. The prevalence of hepatic non-Hodgkin's lymphoma (NHL) in AIDS patients appears to be increasing, and this disorder now may be more common than hepatic Kaposi's sarcoma in persons with AIDS; Kaposi's sarcoma still is more common in HIV-infected homosexuals [2••]. Finally, parenchymal liver disease, either cirrhosis or chronic active hepatitis, is more frequent in HIV-infected drug addicts than in HIV-infected homosexuals [1••], most likely reflecting the more frequent exposure of drug addicts to hepatotrophic viruses.

ETIOLOGY

Infections

Mycobacteria

The most common hepatic pathogen in AIDS patients is *Mycobacterium avium–intracellulare* complex (MAC) [3]. In one series, MAC was found on liver biopsy or at autopsy in 42% of cases [4••]. MAC generally is found in the more severely immunosuppressed patients, and the liver usually is involved as part of disseminated MAC infection. Clinically, hepatic infection with MAC usually is silent except for the presence of abnormal liver tests, but patients may present with fever, weight loss, night sweats, anorexia, and diarrhea [3]. Rare presentations include biliary obstruction secondary to enlarged porta hepatis lymph nodes or granulomatous obstruction of terminal intrahepatic bile ducts [3].

Histologically, hepatic MAC infiltrates the portal tracts or the hepatic parenchyma. Granulomas, found in 76% of MAC liver infections (Fig. 111-2), are poorly formed and noncaseating (Fig. 111-3); they also may be absent. Large numbers of acid-fast bacilli generally are seen (Fig. 111-4) [3]. Liver biopsy is more sensitive than bone marrow biopsy (75% vs 25%) in diagnosing MAC [2••].

In contrast, *Mycobacterium tuberculosis* generally is found in AIDS patients who are less immunosuppressed (*ie*, with CD4 counts > 200/mL) and occurs more commonly in parenteral

Figure 111-1

Hepatic parenchymal disease
  More common
    Mycobacterium avium–intracellulare
    Drug induced, especially zidovudine, sulfa drugs
    Cytomegalovirus
    Bacillary peliosis hepatis
    Lymphoma
    Mycobacterium tuberculosis
    Cryptococcus species
    Kaposi's sarcoma
    Hepatitis C
    Pneumocystis carinii
    Hepatitis B, D
    Microsporidia
  Less common
Biliary tract disease

Differential diagnosis of abnormal liver tests and hepatomegaly in patients with AIDS. (*From* Friedman [30]; with permission.)

Figure 111-2

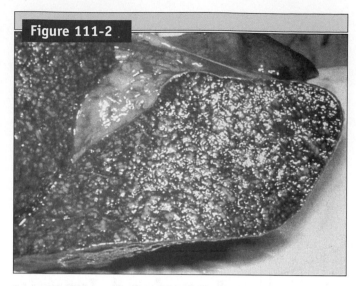

Gross pathologic section demonstrating extensive granulomatous infiltration of the liver due to disseminated *Mycobacterium avium–intracellulare* in a patient with AIDS.

Figure 111-3

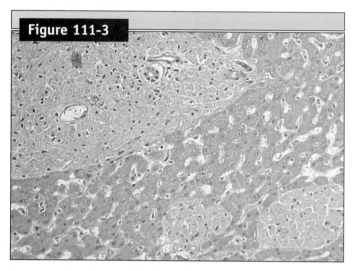

Granuloma-like clusters of Kupffer's cells and "foamy" portal macrophages are seen throughout the liver in this HIV-positive patient with *Mycobacterium avium–intracellulare*. (Hematoxylin and eosin stain.)

Figure 111-4

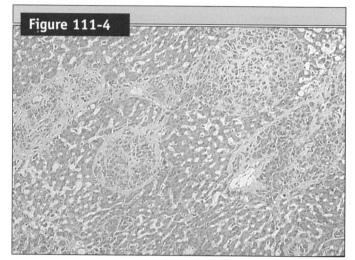

Ziehl-Neelsen stain demonstrating numerous acid-fast bacilli in macrophages in the liver of an HIV-positive patient with *Mycobacterium avium–intracellulare*.

drug users [1••]. Defects in T-helper cell function, impaired lymphokine production, and impaired macrophage function may predispose AIDS patients to developing mycobacterial infections with atypical manifestations [5]. Sixty percent of AIDS patients with tuberculosis present with extrapulmonic disease, of which 7.5% have hepatic tuberculosis. Disease is more likely a result of reactivation than of primary infection [2••]. As in MAC, clinical signs or symptoms of intrahepatic tuberculosis are unusual. Tuberculous abscess and biliary obstruction secondary to a bile duct tuberculoma are rare complications. Histologically, well-formed caseous granulomas with few acid-fast bacilli are seen [2••].

In 6% of AIDS patients, other acid-fast bacilli have been associated with intrahepatic infection [1••]. These organisms include *Mycobacterium xenopi*, *Mycobacterium kansasii*, and other unspecified acid-fast bacilli. Other bacteria, including *Salmonella typhimurium*, *Staphylococcus aureus*, and *Mycoplasma*

incognitus, also have been implicated in AIDS-associated liver infections [1••,3,6].

Bacillary Peliosis Hepatis

The rickettsial organisms, *Rochalimaea (Bartonella) quintana* and *Rochalimaea henselae* are considered responsible for bacillary peliosis hepatis [2••], systemic infection associated with dilated vascular lakes or spaces in the liver (Fig. 111-5). Using silver-based stains (*eg*, Warthin-Starry stain), organisms can be identified in and around dilated hepatic sinusoids and in sinusoidal endothelial cells (Figs. 111-6 and 111-7) [2••,7•]. This systemic infection commonly is found in AIDS patients with advanced disease (*eg*, with CD4 counts less than 200/mL). Associated symptoms include fever, lymphadenopathy, hepatosplenomegaly, cutaneous angiomatous lesions, and painful bony lytic lesions. Treatment with appropriate antibiotics (*eg*, erythromycin) may result in resolution of macroscopic and micro-

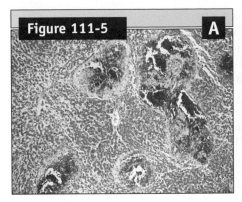

Figure 111-5 **A**

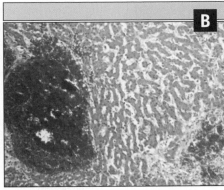

B

Bacillary peliosis hepatis. **A,** "Punched-out" hemorrhagic areas in the liver of a patient with AIDS. **B,** "Blood lakes" and degenerating granuloma-like areas and spotty hemorrhage. (*Both panels,* hematoxylin-eosin stain. Original magnification: *panel A,* X 10; *panel B,* X 25.)

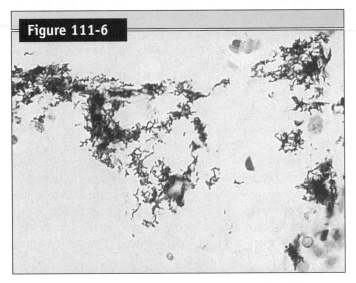

Figure 111-6

Warthin-Starry silver stain demonstrating clusters of bacilli consisting of *Rochalimaea* species in peliotic areas.

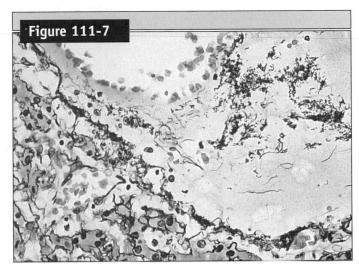

Figure 111-7

Modified Manuel's reticulum stain showing clusters of entangled bacilli at the periphery of a peliotic lesion in the liver of an HIV-positive patient with bacillary peliosis hepatis.

scopic peliotic spaces [2••]. *R. henselae* also can cause hepatic necrosis and intrahepatic lymphohistocytic collections in the absence of peliosis in AIDS patients [8].

Fungi

A number of fungi have been found to infect the livers of AIDS patients. Hepatic fungal infections generally occur in patients with advanced disease and are associated with systemic fungemia [2••]. *Cryptococcus neoformans* has been reported to involve the liver in 18% of AIDS patients with extraneural disease. Histologically, cryptococci incite a weak inflammatory response, and hepatic granuloma formation is poor. Liver infection with *C. neoformans* usually is asymptomatic [1••].

Histoplasma capsulatum infection involves the liver in 16% of AIDS patients with disseminated histoplasmosis [1••]. Patients may or may not come from endemic areas. The hepatic inflammatory response to *H. capsulatum* is weak, but granulomas sometimes are found. Liver involvement usually is asymptomatic. Systemic histoplasmosis (*eg,* pulmonary involvement found in half of cases) generally allows initial isolation of this organism from other tissues [2••].

Other intrahepatic fungal pathogens associated with AIDS include *Coccidioides immitis, Sporothrix schenckii, Blastomyces dermatitidis, Aspergillus fumigatus,* and *Candida albicans* [1••]. Coccidioidomycosis should be suspected in AIDS patients

coming from the Southwestern United States, where it is endemic. Aspergilli have been isolated from liver abscesses, and *C. albicans* has been associated with intrahepatic microabscess and macroabscess formation in neutropenic AIDS patients.

Hepatotrophic Viruses

Patients infected with HIV commonly also are infected, or show evidence of past infection, with hepatotrophic viruses, including hepatitis B virus (HBV), hepatitis C virus (HCV), and hepatitis A virus (HAV). This occurs because of common risk factors (*eg,* unprotected and high-risk sex, parenteral drug use, blood or blood product transfusion) for infection with these viruses and HIV. It also is possible that these viruses influence each other's behavior during co-infection. This may be especially true of HIV because it suppresses host immunity. Although several clinical studies have attempted to address this issue, results of such investigations have been confusing and contradictory.

There is no clinical evidence that HBV has any effect on HIV replication or AIDS [9••]. In contrast, there is good evidence to suggest that HIV does influence the clinical behavior of HBV (Table 111-1) [9••]. Although serologic evidence of past or active HBV infection is found in 90% of AIDS patients, seropositivity for HBV in these patients is no greater than that in a similar group of high-risk patients who are HIV negative.

Table 111-1. Effects of HIV on Hepatitis B Virus Infection

Decreased response to vaccination

Decreased response to α-interferon therapy

Increased risk of HBV reactivation after HIV infection

Elevated HBV levels and replication

Increased risk of developing chronic HBV infection after acute infection

Decreased liver damage in patients with chronic HBV infection

Therefore, HIV does not alter HBV seropositivity but does affect the clinical behavior of HBV infection [9••]. For example, the HBV carrier rate is higher in HIV-positive patients than in HIV-negative patients (20% vs 6%) [10]. Reactivation of HBV infection in HIV-infected patients has been associated with severe clinical disease. The response of HIV-positive patients with chronic HBV to interferon has been reported to be lower than that of HIV-negative patients [10]. HIV-positive patients receiving either plasma-derived or recombinant HBV vaccine have a lower response rate, lower antibody titers when they do respond, and a shorter duration of response than do HIV-negative persons [10]. Nonetheless, evidence exists that clinical hepatitis may be less severe in vaccinated patients and, therefore, that HIV-infected patients should be vaccinated. Finally, co-infected patients have high rates of HBV replication [10]. In contrast, serum aminotransferase levels are lower and histologic liver disease is less severe in these patients [2••,10,11]. Other investigations, however, have found no effect of HIV infection on HBV replication and HBV-induced liver disease [2••,12].

Studies of HCV-induced liver disease in HIV-infected patients also have yielded conflicting results [11]. There is no effect of HCV on HIV-associated disease [9••]. Studies of HCV- and HIV-infected patients have reported increased, decreased, and no difference in HCV-associated liver disease and response to interferon compared with HCV-positive, HIV-negative patients [11]. There is good evidence that HIV infection increases neonatal transmission of HCV from mother to infant.

Hepatitis D has no known adverse effect in AIDS patients, nor is the prevalence of HDV disease increased in HIV-infected patients [10,12]. HIV may alter the suppressive effects of HDV on HBV replication and increase HDV replication and HDV-induced liver disease. After infection with HIV, reactivation of HDV and development of clinical liver disease have been reported [10]. HAV has no effect on HIV, nor does HIV increase the severity of HAV [10]. HIV also does not cause loss of immunity to HAV [10].

Nonhepatrophic Viruses

Human immunodeficiency virus infects the liver, although the significance of this infection is unknown [2••]. The liver is not a primary target organ of HIV, and HIV is not known to cause clinically significant liver disease [10]. The significance of hepatic HIV infection is that the liver may serve as a major reservoir of virus [2••]. In addition, infection of Kupffer's cells,

the largest macrophage population in the body, may interfere with their phagocytic function and contribute to the increased rate of enteric bacteremia reported in AIDS patients [2••].

Cytomegalovirus is the most common infection in AIDS patients and is known to infect the liver; 5% to 25% of AIDS patients infected with CMV have hepatic involvement, usually in the later stages of the disease [2••]. Infection usually is asymptomatic, which partially may explain its uncommon antemortem diagnosis [1••,2••]. SAP and serum aminotransferase levels may be elevated in persons with hepatic CMV infection [11]. Histologically, intranuclear and intracytoplasmic inclusion bodies, often surrounded by a clear halo ("owl-eye" appearance); giant cell formation; and granulomas are seen [1••,2••,11]. Hepatocytes, Kupffer's cells, endothelial cells, and biliary epithelial cells may be infected [1••]. Other AIDS-associated disseminated viral infections capable of causing hepatitis include herpes simplex virus, adenovirus, Epstein-Barr virus, and varicella-zoster virus infections [1••,10].

Protozoa

Pneumocystis carinii, which generally infects the lung, may disseminate and involve the liver. In one autopsy series of AIDS patients with extrapulmonic *P. carinii*, 39% had liver involvement [1••]. The use of aerosolized pentamidine to prevent *P. carinii* pneumonia is thought to facilitate its spread [1••]. Serum aminotransferase and SAP levels are moderately elevated [1••]. Histologically, acellular exudative masses resembling pulmonary lesions are seen in the liver, and organisms may be identified using silver stains [3].

Microsporida, an obligate intracellular spore-forming protozoan, also is capable of infecting the liver in AIDS patients [1••]. *Encephalitozoon cuniculi*, *Enterocytozoon bieneusi*, and *Encephalitozoon intestinalis* all have been associated with hepatic infections in AIDS patients [1••,3,13,14]. *E. cuniculi* has been reported to cause granulomatous liver necrosis and *E. intestinalis* to cause necrotizing cholangitis [13,14]. Although stool and urine examination may be helpful in identifying these organisms, electron microscopy is required to distinguish among species. A specific diagnosis is important because the various species differ in their sensitivity to albendazole [13].

Neoplasms

Non-Hodgkin's Lymphoma

Liver involvement has been reported in 14% of AIDS patients with NHL [1••]. The association between the development of NHL and AIDS has led to its acceptance as an AIDS-defining illness [14]. The prevalence of NHL in AIDS patients is increasing, leading some to suggest that it is the most common AIDS-related neoplasm [2••]. Liver involvement in NHL without evidence of extrahepatic disease has been reported to occur in 14.3% of AIDS patients [4••]. Although NHL may develop at any stage of AIDS, it usually occurs late; aggressive high-grade B-cell tumors with extranodal involvement usually are found [2••,14]. Epstein-Barr viral genome has been found in HIV-related NHL in 36% to 100% of affected patients [14]. AIDS patients with NHL commonly present with abnormal liver tests (*eg*, increased SAP levels) and hepatomegaly [2••]. B-type symptoms of weight loss, night sweats, and fever often are present [14]. Large hepatic tumors may be associated with dull right upper quadrant pain and jaundice [14]. Abdominal computed tomography (CT) may aid in the diagnosis of NHL [2••]. Tissue sent for diagnosis should be soaked in either paraformaldehyde or saline to allow immunotyping.

Hodgkin's Disease

Hepatic involvement occurs in about 25% of AIDS patients with Hodgkin's disease [1••]. Mixed cellularity and nodular sclerosis subtypes are found almost exclusively [1••]. This tumor generally is aggressive, with advanced disease noted at the time of diagnosis [1••]. Thus, systemic symptoms are common, and the prognosis generally is poor [14].

Kaposi's Sarcoma

Kaposi's sarcoma is the most common tumor in AIDS patients, although its frequency in the developed world is decreasing [14]. Kaposi's sarcoma is found most often in homosexuals, suggesting an increased risk of developing this tumor in AIDS patients who acquired HIV by a sexual rather than a parenteral route [14]. Kaposi's sarcoma is thought to arise from lymphatic endothelial cells [2••]. Recent studies have provided compelling evidence for a newly recognized herpes virus, called either *Kaposi's sarcoma–associated virus* or *human herpesvirus 8,* as the transmissible agent responsible for development of Kaposi's sarcoma. Although there are case reports of Kaposi's sarcoma diagnosed antemortem on liver biopsy, most cases are found at autopsy [2••,3,16,17]. Kaposi's sarcoma forms violaceous, hemorrhagic nodules in or on the surface of the liver (Fig. 111-8, see also **Color Plate**). Histologically, Kaposi's sarcoma consists of proliferating abnormal vascular structures lined by large endothelial cells, surrounded by proliferating spindle cells and located in portal and periportal areas (Fig. 111-8, see also **Color Plate**) [3]. Tumor involvement is multicentric, including skin and other viscera in addition to liver (Fig. 111-9, see also **Color Plate**). Kaposi's sarcoma involving the liver, before development of cutaneous or other visceral lesions, is rare but has been reported [1••,16,17]. Liver involvement rarely is symptomatic, although elevation of the SAP level is common.

Drug-Induced Hepatotoxicity

Drug-induced liver test abnormalities are common in AIDS patients because these patients usually take medications that can cause liver injury (Table 111-2; see Chapter 96). For example, in one study, it was estimated that 90% of hospitalized AIDS patients were taking at least one known hepatotoxic drug [6]. AIDS patients also may have increased sensitivity to the adverse effects of many of the medicines they are required to use [2••], variously attributed to underlying hepatic disorders that affect hepatic drug metabolism, the concurrent use of more than one hepatotoxic medication, and associated liver dysfunction secondary to hepatic infection [6]. Trimethoprim-sulfamethoxazole and pentamidine, used to treat *P. carinii* pneumonia, are associated with elevations of serum aminotransferase and SAP levels in as many as half of treated AIDS patients [1••]. Sulfa drugs have been associated with development of granulomatous and cholestatic hepatitis [1••]. Ketoconazole and fluconazole have been reported to elevate serum aminotransferase levels in 21% and 16%, respectively, of AIDS patients [1••]. The antiretroviral agents zidovudine and 2,3-dideoxyinosine are rare causes of cholestatic hepatitis and liver failure, believed to be caused by mitochondrial damage [11]. Treatment with ganciclovir has been associated with liver toxicity and a four-fold increase in serum aminotransferase levels [1••]. Antimycobacterial drugs known to produce hepatotoxicity in immunocompetent patients may be associated with severe liver disease in AIDS patients [2••]. Acetaminophen may cause severe hepatotoxicity in AIDS patients also taking zidovudine [2••]. In any AIDS patient with abnormal liver tests, drug-induced causes must be considered.

Miscellaneous Causes

Other causes of liver test abnormalities and liver disease in AIDS patients are not necessarily specific to AIDS but must be considered. Alcoholic liver disease is common in AIDS patients; as many as 29% of HIV-infected patients are heavy alcohol users [1••]. Alcoholic hepatitis and cirrhosis have been reported in 6% and 7%, respectively, of HIV-infected patients [1••]. In one series, hepatic amyloid was reported in 48% of HIV-infected

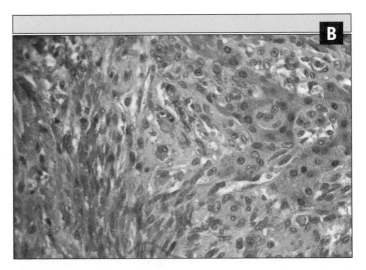

Figure 111-8

Macroscopic (*panel A*) and microscopic (*panel B*) views of Kaposi's sarcoma lesion in the liver of a patient with AIDS. See also **Color Plate**. (*Courtesy of* Dr. J. Reinus.)

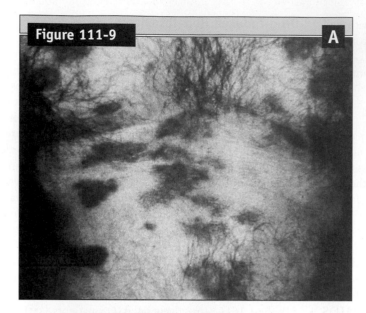

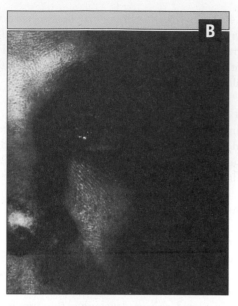

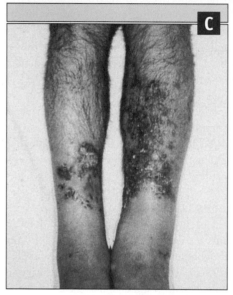

Skin lesions found with Kaposi's sarcoma in a patient with AIDS. **A,** Lesions may be few and small or widespread and large. **B,** Cosmetically disfiguring lesions of Kaposi's sarcoma. Periorbital lesions may produce swelling and interfere with vision. **C,** Lymphedema, which is common in patients with Kaposi's sarcoma. See also **Color Plate.**

patients [2••]. Other causes of liver dysfunction in AIDS patients include protein-calorie malnutrition, total parenteral nutrition–induced liver disease, hypoxia, hypotension, congestive heart failure, and postoperative liver dysfunction [6].

CLINICAL FEATURES

The clinical manifestations of AIDS-associated liver disease are variable. Most patients have asymptomatic disease, and liver involvement is suspected on the basis of either hepatomegaly or abnormal liver tests [2••]. When present, symptoms usually are nonspecific. Right upper quadrant abdominal pain has been reported in 30% of patients [4••]. Jaundice has been reported to occur in 11% of AIDS patients and, when caused by intrahepatic cholestasis, should strongly suggest a diagnosis of drug-induced liver disease [8]. AIDS patients may present with signs and symptoms of fulminant hepatic failure or of cirrhosis and portal hypertension caused by chronic viral hepatitis. Constitutional symptoms, including fever (83%), night sweats (22%), and weight loss (76%), are common, but not necessarily from liver disease [4••].

Hepatomegaly is the most common finding on physical examination, present in 60% to 80% of AIDS patients with liver disease [1••,18]. Splenomegaly has been reported in as many as 72% of persons with AIDS [18]. Common laboratory abnormalities in these patients include elevated serum aminotransferase, SAP, and, least commonly, total bilirubin levels. At least one liver test has been reported to be abnormal in 78% of HIV-infected patients [1••]; serum aminotransferase and SAP levels have been reported to be abnormal in 61% and 51%, respectively, of AIDS patients with liver dysfunction respectively [1••,8].

HISTOLOGY

Histologic abnormalities of the liver have been reported in 90% of AIDS patients (see Chapter 90). These changes are diagnostic of a specific disorder in 42% to 57% of cases [8,18]. Nonspecific abnormalities commonly are seen in livers of AIDS patients; the most common of these is macrovesicular steatosis, found in up to 42% of biopsy specimens [1••,8,10]. Whether steatosis is related to malnutrition, drugs, alcohol ingestion, or a systemic disease usually is unknown. Granulomas are found in 14% to 48% of

Table 111-2. Pattern of Liver Test Abnormalities of Drugs Commonly Used in Patients With HIV

Hepatocellular	Cholestatic	Mixed
Acetaminophen	Amitryptiline	Amitryptiline
Aminosalicylic acid	Anabolic steroids	Carbamazepine
Ciprofloxacin	Carbenicillin	Clarithromycin
Clarithromycin	Cimetidine	Diazepam
Clindamycin	Clarithromycin	Doxepin
Didanosine	Contraceptive steroids	Haldol
Dilantin	Diazepam	Naprosyn
Ethionamide	Doxepin	Phenobarbitol
Fluconazole	Erythromycin	Piroxicam
Foscarnet	Haldol	Prochlorperazine
Ganciclovir	Naprosyn	Sulfonamides
Isonicotinic acid hydrazide	Prochlorperazine	Sulfones
Itraconazole	Ranitidine	Trimethoprim-sulfa
Ketoconazole	Sulindac	**Steatosis**
Mebendazole	Thiabendazole	Glucocorticoids
Oxacillin	Zidovudine	Tetracycline
Pentamidine	**Peliosis**	Valproic acid
Pyrazinamide	Anabolic steroids	Zidovudine
Quinacrine	Estrogens	
Ranitidine	Oral contraceptives	
Rifabutin	Tamoxifen	
Sulfonamides		
Sulfones		
Tetracycline		
Trimethoprim-sulfa		
Vitamin A		
Zalcitabine		
Zidovudine		

livers of HIV-infected patients [1••,8,19]. Two types of granulomas have been described: well-formed, caseous granulomas most commonly are caused by tuberculosis; and poorly formed, noncaseous granulomas usually are seen in patients with MAC [5]. Granulomas also may be found in livers of HIV-infected patients without any identifiable cause [20]. Other nonspecific histologic findings include portal inflammation (35%), focal necrosis (12%), bile stasis (6%), Kupffer's cell hyperplasia (7%), and hypertrophy of hepatic stellate cells [4••]. Peliosis hepatis has been reported to occur in 8%, cirrhosis and hepatitis in 3% to 23%, and hemosiderosis secondary to multiple transfusions or viral infection in 26% of AIDS patients [1••,2••,6,8,10].

■ DIAGNOSIS

The differential diagnosis of abnormal liver tests or liver disease in AIDS patients is broad, and Figure 111-10 provides an algorithm for the approach to these patients. A detailed drug history should be obtained, because of the frequent use of hepatotoxic medicines by AIDS patients [1••]. A history of parenteral drug use indicates exposure to hepatotrophic viruses. Male homosexuality is associated with an increased risk of Kaposi's sarcoma [2••]. Residents of areas endemic for fungal infections may have fungal

liver disease. The physical examination also may be helpful; cutaneous Kaposi's sarcoma may suggest hepatic involvement, and splenomegaly may indicate the presence of lymphoma.

Noninvasive Tests

Although routine liver tests are not diagnostic in AIDS patients, the magnitude and pattern of liver test abnormalities may distinguish hepatocellular from cholestatic disorders and suggest a possible cause of liver injury [2••]. For example, a markedly increased SAP level in the absence of bile duct obstruction is suggestive of intrahepatic MAC, fungal infection, or lymphoma [2••,21]. Elevation of total serum bilirubin and SAP levels in the absence of ductal dilation suggests drug- or virus-induced intrahepatic cholestasis.

The CD4 count always should be obtained because it indicates the extent of immunosuppression. Certain infections (eg, MAC) and tumors (eg, Hodgkin's disease) are more likely to occur in severely immunosuppressed AIDS patients [2••,21]. In contrast, tuberculosis is found more commonly in patients who are less immunosuppressed [21]. Blood cultures for MAC, tuberculosis, and fungal disease should be obtained when these infections are suspected, although it may be several weeks

Figure 111-10

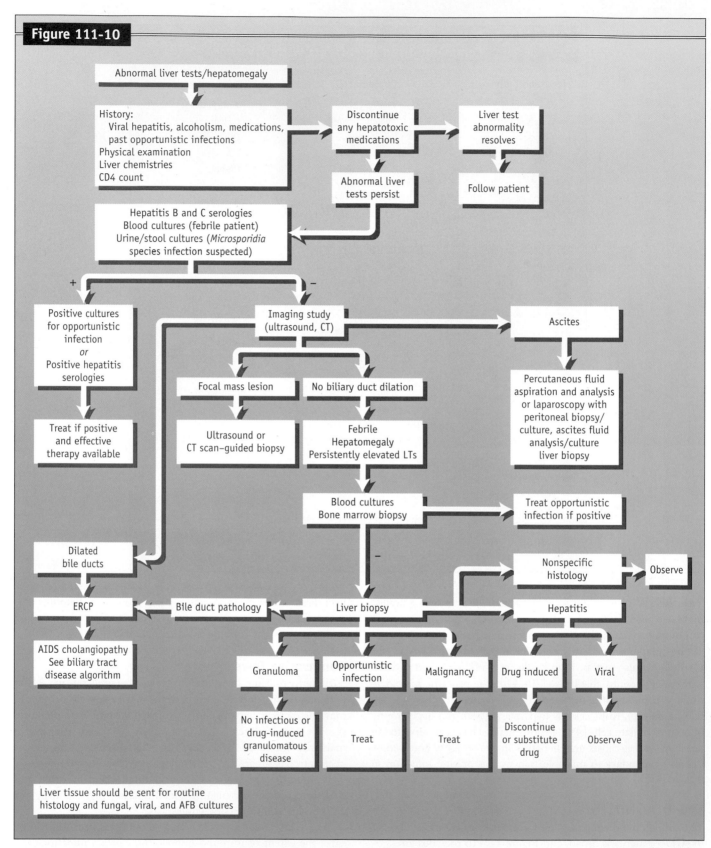

Approach to the HIV-positive patient with abnormal liver tests. AFB—acid-fast bacillus; CT—computed tomography; ERCP—endoscopic retrograde cholangiopancreatography; LT—liver tests.

before they become positive [21]. Examination of stool and urine for spores may help diagnose microsporidial infection. In AIDS patients in whom acute or chronic hepatitis is suspected, especially those with high-risk behaviors, serologic testing for HAV, HBV, HDV, and HCV infection should be done.

Routine chest radiographs may reveal abnormalities suggestive of tuberculosis, MAC, or fungal infection, but a normal chest film does not exclude the presence of these infections [21]. Abdominal ultrasound and CT are important in the noninvasive evaluation of AIDS patients with liver abnormalities. Ultrasonographic abnormalities of the hepatobiliary system have been reported in 66% of AIDS patients [2••]. These abnormalities include evidence of gallbladder or biliary disease, hepatomegaly, and splenomegaly [2••]. Ultrasound is particularly useful in the evaluation of biliary abnormalities; abdominal CT is more useful in the evaluation of hepatosplenomegaly, focal hepatic lesions, and intra-abdominal adenopathy [21]. Lymphoma and large peliotic spaces are seen well on CT [2••]. Although CT is sensitive in the diagnosis of parenchymal lesions, it lacks specificity [1••]. Both tests offer the ability to perform guided liver biopsy or needle aspiration of focal hepatic defects [21]. Liver-spleen scintigraphy adds little to the evaluation of liver dysfunction in AIDS patients [2••].

Invasive Tests

The role of percutaneous liver biopsy in the evaluation of AIDS patients with parenchymal liver disease in the absence of a focal defect on ultrasound or CT examination is controversial [8]. Liver biopsy is recommended based on its sensitivity and speed in diagnosing specific infections, such as mycobacterial infection. In addition, a specific diagnosis can be made on liver biopsy in up to half of AIDS patients with liver disease [18,22•,23]. The initial enthusiasm for percutaneous liver biopsy has been tempered recently by a greater appreciation of the nature of AIDS-associated liver disease. First, the liver is uncommonly the sole site of infection or tumor in AIDS patients, and these diseases, therefore, may be diagnosed by biopsy or culture of more accessible tissues [1••,2••]; in only 8% of cases is a diagnosis made on liver biopsy that could not be made otherwise [2••]. Second, although a specific diagnosis may be made on liver biopsy, just as commonly, findings are nonspecific [2••]. Third, therapy may be influenced little by liver biopsy findings because of the systemic nature of many of the disorders affecting the liver in AIDS patients and the advanced stage of AIDS when these disorders present. Fourth, there are reports of massive and fatal bleeding after percutaneous liver biopsy in AIDS patients with normal clotting tests [16,24,25]. Finally, it has not been shown that findings on liver biopsy result in an improved quality of life or survival in AIDS patients [2••,26]. Still, percutaneous liver biopsy is the procedure of choice in some circumstances and can be performed relatively safely in AIDS patients [2••]. Indications for liver biopsy in AIDS patients include systemic infection or neoplasm involving the liver that cannot be diagnosed by other means and persistent fever, symptomatic hepatomegaly, or abnormal liver tests for which a treatable or diagnosed cause has not been found using less invasive methods [2••,8]. In AIDS patients with systemic disease and abnormal liver tests,

however, less invasive methods of making a diagnosis (*ie*, blood cultures or bone marrow aspirate) should be tried [21]. When a liver biopsy is performed, cultures and special stains should be obtained in addition to routine histology [3]. Fixation of liver tissue in paraformaldehyde aids the diagnosis of lymphoma [15••]. Liver tissue may be obtained by ultrasound- or CT-guided biopsy or laparoscopy; laparoscopy is particularly useful when peritoneal disease or ascites is present.

■ TREATMENT

Although antiretroviral therapy has resulted in improved survival in patients with AIDS, these patients who have liver disease continue to respond poorly to therapy because of their advanced state of immunosuppression [2••]. The presence of systemic infection complicates treatment further [2••]. Alternatively, liver disease in AIDS patients seldom is symptomatic or the cause of death, so therapy directed at the liver is unnecessary in most cases.

Infections

Mycobacteria

Antituberculous drugs include isoniazid, rifampin, ethambutol, and pyrazinamide [3]. For MAC, additional drugs include clarithromycin, azithromycin, and clofazimine. The type and duration of therapy is determined by susceptibility and drug tolerance [1••]. Adverse reactions to these medicines may be more common in AIDS patients [3].

Bacillary Peliosis Hepatis

A number of different antibiotics, including erythromycin, ampicillin-sulbactam, doxycycline, and antituberculous drugs, are effective in the treatment of bacillary peliosis hepatis [1••,7•,27]. After successful treatment, lesions resolve.

Fungi

Because of systemic involvement in AIDS patients with fungal liver disease, therapy with amphotericin and flucytosine is necessary [1••,3]. Whether amphotericin is used alone or in combination with flucytosine is dependent on which organism is being treated. Because relapse is common, long-term suppressive therapy often is necessary [1••,3].

Viruses

No treatment is necessary for HAV infection. Interferon therapy in HIV-infected patients with chronic HBV infection has been disappointing [9••]. The role of interferon in the treatment of HDV-infected AIDS patients is unknown. The efficacy of interferon in HIV-infected patients with chronic HCV is controversial. Response to interferon in HCV- and HIV-infected patients appears to be greatest in the least severely immunocompromised patients [2••]. If HIV increases HCV replication in the later stages of AIDS, as has been found by some investigators, interferon should be less effective at a time when one would most like to administer it. Zidovudine also is ineffective in these patients, and whether newer antiviral medications (*eg*, ganciclovir, foscarnet, famciclovir, lamivudine) have any role in the treatment of these patients has not been determined [9••]. Ganciclovir has been shown to be effective in the treatment of

CMV infection of many organs, but no data on its use in treatment of CMV liver disease are available [1••,3,26].

Protozoa

Intravenous pentamidine therapy is required for treatment of disseminated *P. carinii*. Albendazole has been used successfully to treat some infections caused by the microsporidial species; however, experience with this infection and therapy with albendazole in AIDS patients are limited.

Neoplasms

Non-Hodgkin's Lymphoma

Combination chemotherapy has resulted in remission rates as great as 50% in HIV-infected patients with NHL; however, recurrence rates are high, and disease-free survival is short [15••]. The more aggressive the chemotherapy regimen, the higher the response rate, but greater the degree of immunosuppression and subsequent risk of opportunistic infection. In addition, central nervous system recurrences are a problem. Factors affecting response rate to chemotherapy include CD4 count, presence of other AIDS-associated diseases, and Karnofsky performance score [15••]. Radiation also has been used to treat these patients, although HIV-associated lymphoma appears to be more radioresistant [15••].

Hodgkin's Disease

Various chemotherapeutic regimens with and without radiation have been used to treat Hodgkin's disease in HIV-infected patients [1••,15••]. Even patients with liver involvement have been reported to improve with therapy [1••].

Kaposi's Sarcoma

Kaposi's sarcoma of the liver by itself does not require therapy because it rarely is symptomatic or a cause of death. Various chemotherapy regimens have been used to treat Kaposi's sarcoma; cutaneous and visceral Kaposi's sarcoma respond equally well to chemotherapy. Multidrug regimens result in higher response rates than do single agents but cause more immunosuppression and hence increase the risk of opportunistic infection [15••]. Involvement of liver does not affect response to chemotherapy [15••]. Interferon-alpha also is effective in the treatment of Kaposi's sarcoma; response is better in patients with higher CD4 counts [15••]. Kaposi's sarcoma tumors also are radiosensitive, and radiation generally is well tolerated by affected patients. Bleeding visceral lesions may require surgical resection.

Drug-Induced Hepatotoxicity

Therapy of drug-induced liver disease consists of discontinuing the offending medicine if possible. Other drugs may be substituted for the one injuring the liver. Not all drug-induced liver test abnormalities, however, require discontinuation of therapy with the causative medicine because liver test abnormalities may be transient and without significant associated liver disease [1••]; the elevation in serum aminotransferase activity with ketoconazole is illustrative. Transient drug reactions require no specific therapy. If continued use of the drug is deemed necessary, then continued observation of liver tests is required until results return to normal [1••]. In cases in which clinical liver disease may result if therapy is not stopped, prompt discontinuation is necessary to ensure complete recovery.

■ PROGNOSIS

Liver disease in AIDS patients caused by either infection or neoplasm rarely is a cause of morbidity or mortality [2••]; rather, it indicates systemic involvement with infection or tumor attributed to AIDS-associated immunosuppression. Several factors are important in determining the prognosis of AIDS patients with liver disease, including the degree of immunosuppression, whether the patient has systemic disease, and the availability of effective treatment. Of these factors, the degree of immunosuppression is most important [2••]. For example, despite effective therapy, AIDS patients with MAC have a mean survival of 3 to 5 months because they are severely immunosuppressed [1••]. The prognosis is equally poor in AIDS patients with systemic fungal infections or Hodgkin's disease. In contrast, HIV-infected patients with tuberculosis are less immunosuppressed (with CD4 counts > 200/mL) and respond well to treatment [21].

■ ASCITES

Although ascites is found in as few as 2% of HIV-infected patients, it may be underdiagnosed [29]. Lymphoma is the most common cause of ascites in AIDS patients; other causes include tuberculosis, MAC, fungal infection, and *P. carinii* infection [30]. In addition, non-HIV related causes, including alcoholic and viral cirrhosis, congestive heart failure, and hepatoma, have been reported to cause ascites in AIDS patients [29]. In one study, as many as half of AIDS patients with ascites had chronic peritonitis, for which no etiologic agent could be identified [29].

The clinical presentation of AIDS patients with ascites is similar to that of noninfected patients with ascites. Affected patients complain of abdominal distention and pain (33%), leg edema (42%), and dyspnea (38%) [29]. Fever and night sweats are more common in HIV-infected patients with ascites than in patients with ascites but not AIDS [29]. On physical examination, abdominal distention, shifting dullness, peripheral edema, and abdominal tenderness occur with similar frequencies in HIV-infected and noninfected patients with ascites, whereas splenomegaly, fever, and peripheral adenopathy occur more often in AIDS patients than in others [29]. AIDS patients commonly have high-protein, exudative ascites; transudative ascites also has been reported and is suggestive of non–HIV-associated causes, such as cirrhosis [29].

Evaluation of AIDS patients with ascites should include paracentesis and imaging studies. Ultrasound and CT confirm the presence and amount of ascites, help in assessment of the cause (*eg*, splenomegaly and adenopathy suggest lymphoma), and indicate the presence of peritoneal disease. Although imaging studies typically are abnormal, they rarely are diagnostic. Ascitic fluid analysis should consist of routine studies and cytology, acid-fast bacilli and fungal stains, and culture [29]. If peritoneal disease is suspected, then a peritoneal biopsy may be necessary. In selected cases, laparoscopic evaluation also may be useful.

The treatment of HIV-associated ascites is determined by its cause. In patients with ascites of unknown cause, treatment is primarily symptomatic. Prognosis is governed by the amount of

AIDS-induced immunosuppression at the time ascites develops and, to a lesser extent, by the cause of ascites and availability of specific therapy.

▌▌ REFERENCES

Recently published papers of particular interest have been highlighted as follows:
• Of interest
•• Of outstanding interest

1.•• Bonacini M: Hepatobiliary complications in patients with human immunodeficiency virus infection. *Am J Med* 1992, 92:404–411.
The authors provide an extensive description and epidemiology of the various types of liver disease associated with AIDS.

2.•• Mel Wilcox C, Rabeneck L, Friedman S: AGA technical review: malnutrition and cachexia, chronic diarrhea, and hepatobiliary disease in patients with human immunodeficiency virus infection. *Gastroenterology* 1996, 111:1724–1752.
This excellent series of papers outlines the official recommendations of the American Gastroenterologic Association concerning the management of AIDS patients with hepatobiliary and gastrointestinal disease. In addition, the authors provide a comprehensive discussion of the pathophysiology, clinical manifestations, and diagnostic approach to these patients.

3. Cappell MS: Hepatobiliary manifestations of the acquired immune deficiency syndrome. *Am J Gastroenterol* 1991, 86:1–14.

4.•• Schneiderman DJ, Arenson DM, Cello JP: Hepatic disease in patients with the acquired immune deficiency syndrome (AIDS). *Hepatology* 1987, 7:925–930.
This is one of the earliest and best descriptions of liver disease in AIDS patients. Histologic analysis of liver biopsy or autopsy samples from 85 patients with AIDS were analyzed. The usefulness of percutaneous liver biopsy in the evaluation of AIDS patients with liver disease also is discussed.

5. Wright RW: Hepatic mycobacterial disease and AIDS. *Hepatology* 1990, 11:506–507.

6. Dworkin BM, Stahl RE, Giardina MA: The liver in acquired immune deficiency syndrome: emphasis on patients with intravenous drug abuse. *Am J Gastroenterol* 1987, 82:321–236.

7.• Perkocha LA, Geaghan SM, Benedict Yen TS: Clinical and pathological features of bacillary peliosis hepatis in association with human immunodeficiency virus infection. *N Engl J Med* 1990, 323:1581–1586.
The is one of the first papers to identify the cause of AIDS-associated peliosis hepatis.

8. Grendell JH, Cello JP: HIV-associated hepatobiliary disease. In *Hepatology: A Textbook of Liver Disease.* Edited by Zakim D, Boyer TD. Philadelphia: WB Saunders; 1996:1699–1706.

9.•• Horvath J, Raffanti SP: Clinical aspects of the interaction between human immunodeficiency virus and the hepatotrophic viruses. *Clin Infect Dis* 1994, 18:339–347.
The authors provide an excellent review of the clinical interactions of HIV with hepatis A, B, D, and C viruses.

10. McNair ANB, Main J, Thomas HC: Interaction of the human immunodeficiency virus and the hepatotrophic viruses. *Semin Liver Dis* 1992, 12:188–196.

11. Tanowitz HB, Simon D, Weiss LM, *et al.*: Gastrointestinal manifestations of AIDS. *Clin North Am* 1996, 80:1395–1414.

12. Housset C, Pol S, Carnot F, *et al.*: Interaction between human immunodeficiency virus-1, hepatitis delta virus and hepatitis B virus infection in 260 chronic carriers of hepatitis B. *Hepatology* 1992, 15:578–583.

13. Wilson R, Harrington R, Stewart B, *et al.*: Human immunodeficiency virus 1 associated necrotizing cholangitis caused by infection with Septata intestinalis. *Gastroenterology* 1995, 108:247–251.

14. Weber R, Deplazes P, Flepp M, *et al.*: Cerebral microsporidiosis due to *Encephalitozoon cuniculi* in a patient with human immunodeficiency virus infection. *N Engl J Med* 1997, 336:474–478.

15.•• Herndier BG, Friedman SL: Neoplasms of the gastrointestinal tract and hepatobiliary system in acquired immunodeficiency syndrome. *Semin Liver Dis* 1992, 12:128–141.
This excellent paper includes an extensive description of the epidemiology, histologic and clinical features, diagnosis, therapy, and prognosis of Hodgkin's lymphoma, non-Hodgkin's lymphoma, and Kaposi's sarcoma patients with AIDS.

16. Gottesman D, Dyrszka H, Albarran J, *et al.*: AIDS-associated hepatic Kaposi's sarcoma: massive bleeding following liver biopsy. *Am J Gastroenterol* 1993, 88:762–764.

17. Hasan FA, Jeffers LJ, Welsh SW, *et al.*: Hepatic involvement as the primary manifestation of Kaposi's sarcoma in the acquired immunodeficiency syndrome. *Am J Gastroenterol* 1989, 84:1449–1451.

18. Cappell MS, Schwartz MS, Biempica L: Clinical utility of liver biopsy in patients with serum antibodies to the human immunodeficiency virus. *Am J Med* 1990, 88:123–130.

19. Glasgow BJ, Anders K, Lester J, *et al.*: Clinical and pathologic findings of the liver in the acquired immune deficiency syndrome (AIDS). *Am J Clin Pathol* 1985, 83:582–588.

20. Gordon SC, Reddy GK, Edwin EE, *et al.*: The spectrum of liver disease in the acquired immunodeficiency syndrome. *J Hepatol* 1986, 2:475–484.

21. Mel Wilcox C: Hepatic disease associated with human immunodeficiency virus infection. *Pract Gastroenterol* 1993, 26:10–19.

22. Prego V, Glatt AE, Roy V, *et al.*: Comparative yield of blood culture for fungi and mycobacteria, liver biopsy, and bone marrow biopsy in the diagnosis of fever of undetermined origin in human immunodeficiency virus-infected patients. *Arch Intern Med* 1990, 150:333–336.

23. Beale TJ, Wetton CW, Crofton ME: A sonographic-pathological correlation of liver biopsy in patients with the acquired immune deficiency syndrome (AIDS). *Clin Radiol* 1995, 50:761–764.

24. Churchill DR, Mann D, Coker RJ, *et al.*: Fatal haemorrhage following liver biopsy in patients with HIV infection. *Genitourin Med* 1996, 72:62–64.

25. Gordon SC, McFadden RF, Reddy KR, *et al.*: Major hemorrhage after percutaneous liver biopsy in patients with AIDS. *Gastroenterology* 1991, 30:1787.

26. Poles MA, Dieterich DT, Schwarz ED, *et al.*: Liver biopsy findings in 501 patients with human immunodeficiency virus (HIV). *J Acquir Immune Defic Retrovirol* 1996, 11:170–177.

27. Garcia-Tsao G, Panzini L, Yoselevitz M, *et al.*: Bacillary peliosis hepatis as a cause of acute anemia in a patients with the acquired immunodeficiency syndrome. *Gastroenterology* 1992,102:1065–1070.

28.•• Crumpacker CS: Ganciclovir. *N Engl J Med* 1996, 335:721–729.
The authors provide an excellent and extensive review of ganciclovir and other therapies for the treatment of various types of cytomegalovirus infection.

29. Cappell MS, Shetty V: A multicenter, case-controlled study of the clinical presentation and etiology of ascites and of the safety and clinical efficacy of diagnostic abdominal paracentesis in HIV seropositive patients. *Am J Gastroenterol* 1994, 89:2172–2177.

30. Friedman SL: Gastrointestinal manifestations of the acquired immunodeficiency syndrome. In *Gastrointestinal Disease: Pathophysiology/Diagnosis/Management.* Edited by Sleisenger MH, Fordtran JS. Philadelphia; WB Saunders; 1993:239–267.

112 Portal Hypertension and Variceal Bleeding

Enrique G. Molina and K. Rajender Reddy

PATHOPHYSIOLOGY

Portal hypertension is a pathologic rise in portal venous pressure. Clinically, portal pressure is determined indirectly by subtracting the free hepatic venous, or inferior vena cava, pressure from the wedged hepatic venous pressure. This gradient is known as the *hepatic venous pressure gradient* (HVPG). Portal hypertension is present when the HVPG is greater than 6 mm Hg.

The pressure in a vascular system is directly proportional to resistance and blood flow. Normally, vascular resistance in the portal system is regulated by splanchnic arterioles and not by hepatic blood vessels. In cirrhosis, intrahepatic resistance increases because of compression of vascular structures by scar tissue, regenerating nodules, and collagenization of the space of Disse (fixed component). Vascular tone also increases as a result of stellate cell contraction in response to an imbalance between endothelial vasodilators (nitric oxide) and vasoconstrictors (endothelin-1; variable component).

Portal blood flow increases with portal hypertension. Peripheral vasodilation and increased splanchnic blood flow occur in portal hypertension caused by an increased concentration of vasodilators and a decreased responsiveness to vasoconstrictors [1]. Peripheral vasodilation results in relative vascular underfilling and stimulates sodium retention and plasma volume expansion. These changes lead to a hyperdynamic state characterized by decreased systemic vascular resistance, decreased arterial pressure, increased plasma volume, elevated splanchnic blood flow, and elevated cardiac index.

Increasing portal blood flow and resistance lead to dilation of portosystemic collateral channels, which form varices in the esophagus and rectum and around the umbilicus and ovaries. Common ectopic sites of varices include the small bowel, cecum, and stomal anastomoses.

ETIOLOGY OF PORTAL HYPERTENSION

In the Western world, the most common cause of portal hypertension is cirrhosis, of either viral etiology or caused by alcohol abuse. Pathophysiologically, causes of portal hypertension are categorized in one of three groups, based on whether obstruction is at the sinusoidal level, at the portal venular level, or in the hepatic veins. Furthermore, presinusoidal and postsinusoidal obstruction may be either intrahepatic or extrahepatic. Measurements of HVPG often indicate the site of resistance in portal hypertension (Fig. 112-1).

Noncirrhotic, intrahepatic portal hypertension (NCIPH) is a consequence of increased intrahepatic vascular resistance either at the sinusoidal level or portal venular level or in the venous outflow tract. In most cases, abnormalities are on the basis of endothelial cell lesions and thrombotic obliteration or fibrosis of the intrahepatic portal or hepatic veins.

A number of different disorders cause NCIPH (Table 112-1). It is seen in patients with perisinusoidal fibrosis caused by accumulation of collagen fibers within the space of Disse; this may complicate alcoholic liver disease and, occasionally, hypervitaminosis A and myeloproliferative disorders. Other causes of NCIPH include schistosomiasis, noncirrhotic portal fibrosis, and fibrosis around central veins as seen after radiation therapy and treatment with antineoplastic drugs and in persons with alcoholic liver disease.

Generally, patients with NCIPH have better outcomes after esophageal variceal bleeding than do patients with cirrhosis. Ascites is more likely to evolve in patients who have resistance at the hepatic venular level or in the sinusoidal bed; ascites in presinusoidal portal hypertension is distinctly uncommon.

NATURAL HISTORY OF VARICES
Incidence

For varices to occur, the HPVG must be equal to or greater than 10 to 12 mm Hg [2••,3]. Portal hypertension is a necessary, but not sufficient, condition for development of esophageal varices.

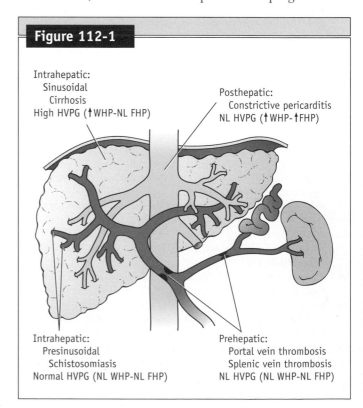

Figure 112-1

Intrahepatic:
Sinusoidal
Cirrhosis
High HVPG (↑WHP-NL FHP)

Posthepatic:
Constrictive pericarditis
NL HVPG (↑WHP-↑FHP)

Intrahepatic:
Presinusoidal
Schistosomiasis
Normal HVPG (NL WHP-NL FHP)

Prehepatic:
Portal vein thrombosis
Splenic vein thrombosis
NL HVPG (NL WHP-NL FHP)

Causes of portal hypertension and hepatic venous pressure gradients (HVPG). FHP—free hepatic pressure; NL—normal; WHP—wedged hepatic pressure. (*Adapted from* Roberts and Kamath [1].)

Varices in the distal 5 cm of the esophagus are found in about half of cirrhotic patients; patients with clinical evidence of portal hypertension (splenomegaly or ascites) are most likely to have varices. Eventually, up to 90% of cirrhotic patients develop varices; in 20%, the varices are medium to large. In view of this high prevalence of esophageal varices in cirrhotic patients, routine endoscopic evaluation is recommended for these patients. The risk of developing new varices after initial negative endoscopy findings is 8% each year. Once present, the risk of the varices enlarging is 10% to 20% per year [4]. If small varices are found at initial endoscopy, subsequent surveillance endoscopy should be performed.

Bleeding

For varices to bleed, a threshold pressure greater than 12 mm Hg must be reached [5]. The risk of bleeding from untreated varices is 25% to 30% over 2 to 8 years [6,7•]. The highest risk of bleeding is during the initial year after diagnosis; the mortality rate of an initial variceal bleeding episode is about 30% to 50% [8,9]. The larger the size of the varix, the more likely it is to bleed; bleeding probably is related to increasing wall tension and decreasing wall thickness as the vessel radius increases. Child's class, size of varices, and presence of red wale markings are each independent predictors of bleeding [10] (Table 112-2 and Fig. 112-2, see also **Color Plate**). Alcohol ingestion increases portal pressure, and continued use of alcohol by alcoholic cirrhotic patients also is a risk factor for bleeding. The level of portal hypertension correlates with bleeding and survival in alcoholic cirrhotic patients.

The presence of gastric varices and portal hypertensive gastropathy also has been reported to predict upper gastrointestinal bleeding. Gastric varices are classified according to location; gastric varices located in the fundus (isolated or gastroesophageal) have the greatest risk of bleeding. Besides location, Child's class and the size and presence of red spots also are independent predictors of gastric variceal hemorrhage. Bleeding from gastric varices tends to be more severe than esophageal variceal bleeding. Portal hypertensive gastropathy is a common endoscopic finding in patients with cirrhosis and also may be a source of bleeding. Bleeding caused by gastropathy tends to be occult or to cause melena, but hematemesis rarely may occur.

Rebleeding

Rebleeding occurs early after an initial bleeding episode and is associated with a high mortality rate. The risk of rebleeding is about 50% to 70%. Most rebleeding occurs within 48 hours of the initial presentation. The mortality rate associated with rebleeding ranges from 20% to 70%. Mortality is highest during the first 6 weeks after an initial bleeding episode [11,12]. Early mortality depends on the severity of liver dysfunction and bleeding, the presence of renal failure, and the magnitude of the portal pressure. The mortality rate based on Child's class is as follows: A, 5%; B, 25% or less; and C, 50% or more. One third of affected patients die during the initial hospitalization for an index bleed, one third have a rebleeding episode within 6 weeks, and one third survive 1 year or longer [11]. After 6 weeks the risk of bleeding is constant.

■■ PREVENTION OF INITIAL BLEEDING
Pharmacologic Prophylaxis

There is evidence that bleeding from varices may be prevented by reducing the HVPG at least by 20% and ideally to below 12 mm Hg. The HVPG decreases with beta-blockers in one third of treated patients. This reduction also may occur in up to 18% of placebo-treated patients. β-Blockers reduce variceal pressure because they decrease splanchnic blood flow by promoting splanchnic vasoconstriction and by reducing cardiac output. When HVPG measures are not available to guide the treatment, doses are adjusted to decrease the heart rate by 25% but not to less than 55 bpm.

Only therapy with nonselective β-blockers (propranolol and nadolol) and with long-acting nitrates has been evaluated in prospective randomized, controlled trials [13]. A meta-analysis of

---

Table 112-1. Causes of Noncirrhotic Intrahepatic Portal Hypertension

Sinusoidal
  Hypervitaminosis A
  Alcoholic liver disease
  Myeloproliferative disorders
  Renal transplantation
  Azathioprine, drugs
  Neoplasia, lymphoma

Portal venules
  Toxins: arsenic or vinyl chloride
  Hypercoagulable states
  Primary biliary cirrhosis
  Primary sclerosing cholangitis
  Sarcoidosis
  Schistosomiasis
  Noncirrhotic portal fibrosis
  Congenital hepatic fibrosis

Hepatic venules
  Alcoholic steatohepatitis
  Drugs, plant alkaloids
  Radiation
  Antineoplastic drugs
  Bone marrow transplantation

Table 112-2. Risk Factors for Variceal Bleeding

Endoscopic signs
  Variceal size
  Red signs (wales, cherry-red spots, hemocytic spots)

Clinical parameters
  Child's class
  Alcohol ingestion

Hemodynamic
  Hepatic venous pressure gradient

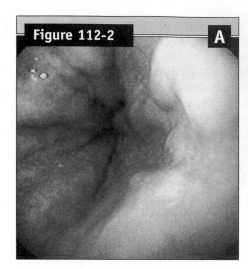
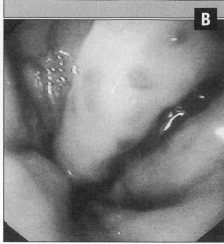
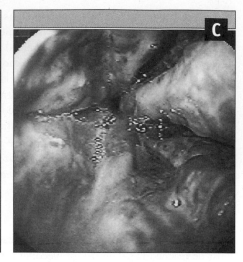

Endoscopic images of esophageal varices. **A,** Small varices with no stigmata. **B,** Large varices: red spots. **C,** Large varices: red wales. See also **Color Plate**.

seven published trials shows a significant benefit of β-blockers in this setting; β-blocker therapy reduces the bleeding rate 40%, from 27.2% to 16.3%; therefore, 11 patients need to be treated to prevent one bleeding episode. Prophylaxis with beta-blockers is most likely to benefit Child's class A and B patients with large varices, with or without ascites [14]. Side effects lead to discontinuation of treatment in 7% to 27% of patients, usually because of worsening of underlying cardiac or pulmonary disease, asthma, insulin-dependent diabetes mellitus, or other medical problems. Nadolol appears to be better tolerated than propranolol. If β-blockers are contraindicated or not tolerated, isosorbide-5-mononitrate may be substituted, with the expectation of similar results. The combination of propranolol and isosorbide-5-mononitrate reduces HVPG more than does propranolol alone and may lower HVPG in patients who fail to respond to propranolol alone; however, it may worsen ascites, requiring an adjustment of diuretic therapy.

Endoscopic Prophylaxis

Randomized trials of prophylactic sclerotherapy in the prevention of an initial variceal bleeding episode show mixed results; favorable trials have high bleeding rates in controls. The Veterans Administration cooperative study was terminated because of increased mortality in the sclerotherapy group; the mortality rate promptly declined after prophylactic sclerotherapy was stopped. Therefore, prophylactic sclerotherapy cannot be recommended. The role of endoscopic ligation in this setting has not been adequately studied.

Other Therapeutic Options

Transjugular intrahepatic portosystemic shunt (TIPS) and surgery are not indicated in the prevention of an initial variceal bleeding episode [15••]. Shunt surgery decreases the risk of bleeding but also decreases life expectancy by increasing mortality from liver failure and hepatic encephalopathy.

▇ CONTROL OF ACUTE BLEEDING

Up to half of patients die as a result of their first variceal bleeding episode. Variceal bleeding is the cause of death in 30% of all cirrhotic patients. The mortality rate increases from 20% in Child's class A or B cirrhotic patients to more than 60% in Child's class C patients.

Initial management of variceal bleeding involves fluid resuscitation; blood and fresh frozen plasma are used to stabilize the patient and to correct coagulopathy. There is no need, however, to correct an elevated prothrombin time with fresh frozen plasma if the patient is not bleeding. Overexpansion of intravascular volume should be avoided because it may reinitiate variceal bleeding. Unstable patients and those with ongoing hematemesis benefit from endotracheal intubation before endoscopy.

Any patient with suspected variceal bleeding should undergo endoscopy, even if there are no signs of active bleeding. Endoscopic therapy is superior to balloon tamponade and treatment with pharmacologic agents to control acute variceal hemorrhage, with a reported success rate of 75% to 90%.

Patients with Child's class C cirrhosis or rebleeding have a high risk of infection. The use of systemic antibiotic prophylaxis has been shown to reduce infection from 52.9% to 18.2%. Aminoglycoside therapy should be avoided because these antibiotics frequently cause nephrotoxicity in cirrhotic subjects.

Pharmacologic Therapy

Pharmacologic therapy with vasopressin and nitroglycerin may be started in the emergency room while the patient awaits endoscopy. This therapy is effective in the treatment of bleeding from esophageal and nonesophageal sites, portal hypertensive gastropathy, and gastric varices. Intravenous infusion of vasopressin causes splanchnic vasoconstriction and decreases portal blood flow and portal and variceal pressure. Although it controls bleeding, it is associated with significant cardiac and systemic complications and does not improve survival. When nitroglycerin is added, vascular resistance in the portal system decreases, further reducing portal pressure. Intravenous, sublingual, or transdermal nitroglycerin decreases the systemic hemodynamic side effects and complications of vasopressin therapy. Vasopressin, therefore, should be used only in combination with nitroglycerin; this combination controls bleeding in 55% to 83% of treated patients.

Terlipressin is a long-acting synthetic analogue of vasopressin with fewer side effects than either vasopressin alone or vasopressin in combination with nitroglycerin. Because of its longer duration of action, it may be administered as an intravenous bolus every 4 to 6 hours. Terlipressin controls bleeding in 79% of cases. Therapy may be initiated at home, as has been done by a physician on an emergency team, and has been associated with reduced mortality. Randomized, controlled trials show that it is superior to placebo and vasopressin and comparable to somatostatin and balloon tamponade in the control of acute variceal bleeding.

Somatostatin decreases portal pressure and collateral flow by its selective action on mesenteric vascular smooth muscle; somatostatin does not produce systemic vasoconstriction and does not have the same side effects as vasopressin. Somatostatin is as effective as terlipressin, balloon tamponade, and endoscopic sclerotherapy in the treatment of variceal bleeding. Octreotide is a synthetic analogue of somatostatin with a longer half-life; it decreases portal pressure by reducing portal blood flow. When given as a continuous intravenous infusion for 48 hours, octreotide is as effective as sclerotherapy in controlling variceal bleeding. When combined with endoscopic treatment, intravenous octreotide also may decrease early rebleeding [16]. Octreotide has become the most widely used pharmacologic agent in the United States for control of acute variceal bleeding [17••,18••].

Endoscopic Treatment

Endoscopy can suggest that varices are the source of bleeding and provides access for sclerotherapy or band ligation, with control of bleeding in 70% to 90% of treated patients. Endoscopic sclerotherapy is superior to balloon tamponade and vasopressin but may not be better than somatostatin in the treatment of variceal hemorrhage. In the United States, the most commonly used sclerosants are sodium tetradecyl, sodium morrhuate, ethanolamine, and alcohol. A total of less than 20 mL of sclerosant is injected in 1- to 2-mL aliquots into the varices. When bleeding has stopped, the procedure is repeated every 1 to 3 weeks until varices in the distal 5 cm of the esophagus have been eradicated. Acute bleeding is controlled in one session of endoscopic sclerotherapy in 62% of patients and in 82% of patients in two sessions [19]. If bleeding is not controlled after two sessions, alternative treatment should be considered [20]. Endoscopic

sclerotherapy is associated with serious complications, including esophageal ulceration, perforation, bleeding, and stricture formation in 10% to 20% of treated patients.

Endoscopic variceal ligation causes strangulation of the varices, mucosal sloughing, and scar formation to the level of the muscularis propria. Newer endoscopic variceal ligation devices allow multiple bands to be placed without removing the endoscope and without use of an overtube, which has been associated with complications. Compared with sclerotherapy, endoscopic variceal ligation has lower rates of rebleeding, mortality, and complications, and fewer treatments are needed to eradicate varices. For these reasons, endoscopic variceal ligation is now the treatment of choice for patients with esophageal variceal bleeding [21] (Fig. 112-3, see also **Color Plate**).

Other Treatment Options

In the 10% of patients in whom two endoscopic sessions within 24 hours do not result in control of bleeding, other treatment options must be considered, including balloon tamponade, TIPS, and surgical shunts.

In patients with massive bleeding present, balloon tamponade may be used as a temporizing measure. Balloon tamponade controls bleeding in 70% to 90% of treated patients. Compression should be limited to 24 hours, and endotracheal intubation is recommended to protect the airway and prevent aspiration. Rebleeding occurs in half of patients treated with tamponade within 24 hours of balloon deflation and is associated with fatal complications in 6% to 20% of treated patients. Balloon tamponade should be considered a heroic temporizing measure after endoscopic therapy has failed.

Transjugular intrahepatic portosystemic shunting is an intrahepatic shunt between portal and hepatic veins created using an intravascular metallic stent placed with fluoroscopic guidance by the vascular radiologist. It is effective more than 90% of the time, leaving a residual portal pressure gradient of 9 to 15 mm Hg and controlling bleeding in 81% to 94% of treated patients. When used to treat acute variceal bleeding in Child's class C patients, it is associated with a high 90-day mortality rate [22]. TIPS may control bleeding from sites inaccessible to endoscopic therapy, including small intestine

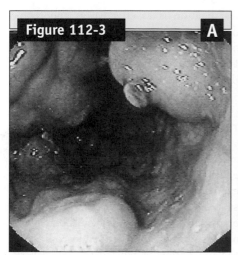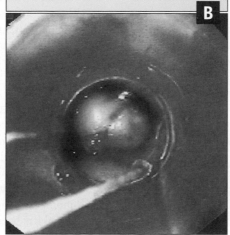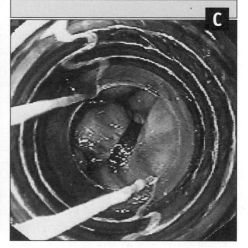

Large varices of stigmata of recent bleeding. See also **Color Plate**.

and colonic, stomal, and anorectal varices. TIPS also controls refractory anemia or bleeding from portal hypertensive gastropathy. TIPS is best used in candidates for liver transplantation [23]. Contraindications to TIPS include severe congestive heart failure and pulmonary hypertension, polycystic liver disease, and severe hepatic failure. Rebleeding occurs in about 20% of treated patients within 1 year, usually a result of stenosis or occlusion of the shunt, and routine follow-up with Doppler ultrasound and balloon dilation of occluded stents or placement of additional stents is necessary to prevent rebleeding. Patency assisted by invasive revision is 85% at 1 year, as compared with 50% to 65% without further intervention [24]. Encephalopathy occurs in 10% to 35% of treated patients and usually responds to conventional medical management. Procedure-related complications occur in 10% of treated patients and are life-threatening in 1% to 2%. Early complications include perforation of the liver capsule or portal vein wall, leading to intra-abdominal hemorrhage, hemobilia, sepsis, portal vein thrombosis, shunt occlusion, shunt migration, and cardiac failure resulting from increased venous return. Hemolysis and jaundice after TIPS usually are self-limited.

Surgical options for treatment of variceal bleeding include central, partial, or selective shunts and devascularization procedures [25]. Shunt surgery decreases the risk of rebleeding better than any other therapy but increases the risk of encephalopathy and progressive liver failure. Surgical shunts should be used to treat patients with good liver function and disease that has failed medical and endoscopic therapy, and those who live far from a tertiary care center. Central portocaval shunts (end-to-side, side-to-side, or large interposition graft) eliminate portal hypertension, control and prevent variceal bleeding, and with the exception of the end-to-side portocaval shunt, are useful in controlling ascites. They divert all portal blood flow and are associated with an increased incidence of encephalopathy and accelerated progression of the underlying liver disease. Partial shunting with an 8-mm interposition graft and ligation of collateral vessels maintains some hepatopedal blood flow, reduces portal pressure by more than 40%, and has a lower rate of encephalopathy. Early thrombosis occurs in 16% of surgical shunts but is amenable to radiologic dilation to maintain patency.

Selective surgical shunts maintain portal blood flow while decompressing esophageal and gastric varices. The splenorenal shunt controls acute variceal bleeding and prevents recurrent bleeding in more than 90% of treated patients and is associated with encephalopathy rates of less than 10%. The distal splenorenal shunt is as effective as portocaval shunts. Devascularization is effective in controlling variceal bleeding and has a low rate of encephalopathy and hepatic failure; however, outside Japan, devascularization is associated with rebleeding rates of up to 37%. Maximal benefit is obtained with esophageal transection and reanastomosis, truncal vagotomy, pyloroplasty, splenectomy, and ligation of perigastric and periesophageal vessels. Splenectomy alone may be curative in patients with bleeding gastric varices and splenic vein thrombosis but is not indicated in portal hypertension secondary to cirrhosis. Staple transection of the esophagus was found to be more effective and as safe as two sessions of sclerotherapy for emergency control of variceal bleeding after medical manage-

ment failed. Devascularization procedures are used mainly in unshuntable patients with thrombosed splenic and portal venous systems.

The distal splenorenal shunt and TIPS have not been compared in randomized, controlled trials. Based on the available data, a Child's class A cirrhotic patient who is otherwise a good surgical candidate should receive a surgical shunt after medical therapy has failed; for Child's A patients who are poor surgical candidates, TIPS is the best alternative. For patients with more advanced liver disease, TIPS is used to control bleeding until liver transplantation [26].

▮▮ PREVENTION OF RECURRENT BLEEDING

The risk of rebleeding after an acute variceal bleeding episode approaches 70%. In patients with alcoholic cirrhosis, abstinence from drinking increases longevity and decreases the risk of rebleeding. Every survivor of a bleeding episode should be treated to prevent rebleeding. If therapy decreases the HPVG more than 20%, there is a significant reduction in rebleeding; if the HPVG is less than 12 mm Hg, patients do not rebleed.

Pharmacologic Treatment

Pharmacologic treatment prevents rebleeding. A meta-analysis of 11 randomized, controlled trials comparing beta-blockers (propranolol or nadolol) to placebo or no treatment showed a 32% reduction in the risk of rebleeding. A reduction in mortality, however, was not clearly established [27•]. Propranolol also has been shown to reduce acute and chronic bleeding from portal gastropathy. If β-blockers are not tolerated, a long-acting nitrate is a reasonable alternative.

Endoscopic Treatment

Endoscopic sclerotherapy significantly reduces rebleeding from esophageal varices, as compared with placebo. After initial treatment, endoscopic sclerotherapy or variceal ligation is repeated every 1 to 3 weeks until varices are obliterated. This may take four or five endoscopic sessions during 3 to 6 months. Surveillance endoscopy should be performed at progressively longer intervals after obliteration of varices to treat recurrent varices while they are small. Bleeding recurs in 50% to 60% of patients followed for 3 to 5 years.

Endoscopic variceal ligation is as effective as endoscopic sclerotherapy in eradicating esophageal varices and preventing rebleeding. As mentioned previously, endoscopic variceal ligation may eradicate varices in fewer sessions and with fewer side effects; therefore, it is the endoscopic treatment of choice for esophageal varices.

Combination Pharmacologic and Endoscopic Treatment

Octreotide given immediately after initial sclerotherapy may prevent early rebleeding and bleeding-related mortality. Octreotide is administered as a continuous intravenous infusion of 25 μg/h for 5 days.

Combination therapy with endoscopic sclerotherapy and propranolol has been shown to be better than endoscopic sclerotherapy alone in the prevention of rebleeding but with no advantage in patient survival.

Other Therapeutic Options

If medical and endoscopic therapy fail, TIPS or surgical shunts should be considered just as for acute variceal bleeding. Surgical shunts are more effective than is endoscopic sclerotherapy in preventing recurrent variceal bleeding; however, shunt surgery increases encephalopathy without improving survival. Because survival of these patients depends primarily on the severity of the underlying liver disease, liver transplantation is the only modality that corrects liver failure and is capable of improving long-term survival in appropriate candidates.

◼◼ REFERENCES

Recently published papers of particular interest have been highlighted as follows:
* • Of interest
* •• Of outstanding interest

1. Roberts L, Kamath P: Pathophysiology and treatment of variceal hemorrhage. *Mayo Clin Proc* 1996, 71:973–983.

2.•• D'Amico G, Pagliaro L, Bosch J: The treatment of portal hypertension: a meta-analytical review. *Hepatology* 1995, 22:332–354.
The authors provide an excellent review of randomized, controlled trials, including data on available treatment options for prevention of first bleeding, treatment of acute bleeding, and prevention of rebleeding from esophageal varices.

3. Garcia-Tsao G, Groszmann R, Fisher R, *et al.*: Portal pressure, presence of gastroesophageal varices and variceal bleeding. *Hepatology* 1985, 5:419–424.

4. Cales P, Desmorat H, Vinel J, *et al.*: Incidence of large oesophageal varices in patients with cirrhosis: application to prophylaxis of first bleeding. *Gut* 1990, 31:1298–1302.

5. Groszmann R, Bosch J, Grace N, *et al.*: Hemodynamic events in a prospective randomized trial of propranolol versus placebo in the prevention of first variceal hemorrhage. *Gastroenterology* 1990, 99:1401–1407.

6. Pagliaro L, D'Amico G, Sorensen T, *et al.*: Prevention of first bleeding in cirrhosis: a meta-analysis of randomized trials of nonsurgical treatment. *Ann Intern Med* 1992, 117:59–70.

7.• Burroughs A, D'Heygere, McIntyre N: Pitfalls in studies of prophylactic therapy for variceal bleeding in cirrhotics. *Hepatology* 1986, 6:1407–1413.
This paper reviews factors associated with the risk of bleeding from esophageal varices that might modify the outcome of a study, including patient characteristics, follow-up, and statistical considerations.

8. The North Italian Endoscopic Club for the Study and Treatment of Esophageal Varices: Prediction of the first variceal hemorrhage in patients with cirrhosis of the liver and esophageal varices. *N Engl J Med* 1988, 319:983–989.

9. Zoli M, Merkel C, Magalotti D, *et al.*: Evaluation of a new endoscopic index to predict first bleeding from the upper gastrointestinal tract in patients with cirrhosis. *Hepatology* 1996, 24:1047–1052.

10. Beppu K, Inokuchi K, Koyanagi N, *et al.*: Prediction of variceal hemorrhage by esophageal endoscopy. *Gastrointest Endosc* 1981, 27:213–218.

11. Graham D, Smith L: The course of patients after variceal hemorrhage. *Gastroenterology* 1981, 80:800–809.

12. Burroughs A, Mezzanotte G, Phillips A, *et al.*: Cirrhotics with variceal hemorrhage: The importance of the time interval between admission and the start of analysis for survival and rebleeding rates. *Hepatology* 1989, 9:801–807.

13. Poynard T, Cales P, Pasta L, *et al.*: Beta-adrenergic-antagonist drugs in the prevention of gastrointestinal bleeding in patients with cirrhosis and esophageal varices. *N Engl J Med* 1991, 324:1532–1538.

14: The Italian Multicenter Project for Propranolol in Prevention of Bleeding: Propranolol for prophylaxis of bleeding in cirrhotic patients with large varices: a multicenter, randomized clinical trial. *Hepatology* 1988, 8:1–5.

15.•• Shiffman M, Jeffers L, Hoofnagle J, *et al.*: The role of transjugular intrahepatic portosystemic shunt for treatment of portal hypertension and its complications. *Hepatology* 1995, 22:1591–1597.
The organizers of a scientific conference sponsored by the National Digestive Disease Advisory Board outline the recommendations regarding safety, efficacy, and indications for TIPS in the management of portal hypertension.

16. Besson I, Ingrand P, Person B, *et al.*: Sclerotherapy with or without octreotide for acute variceal bleeding. *N Engl J Med* 1995, 333:555–560.

17.•• Grace N, Bhattacharya K: Pharmacologic therapy of portal hypertension and variceal hemorrhage. *Clin Liver Dis* 1997, 1:59–75.
This first issue of *Clinics in Liver Disease* is devoted to clinically relevant aspects of portal hypertension. It is an excellent resource for in-depth reviews of the pathophysiology and the medical, endoscopic, radiologic, and surgical treatment of portal hypertension.

18.•• Grace N: Diagnosis and treatment of gastrointestinal bleeding secondary to portal hypertension. *Am J Gastroenterol* 1997, 92:1081–1091.
These are the guidelines for clinical practice developed by the American College of Gastroenterology for the diagnosis and treatment of variceal bleeding.

19. Burroughs A, Hamilton G, Phillips A, *et al.*: A comparison of sclerotherapy with staple transection of the esophagus for the emergency control of bleeding from esophageal varices. *N Engl J Med* 1989, 321:857–862.

20. Goustout C: Evaluation and management of esophageal variceal bleeding. *ASGE Clin Update* 1996, 4:1–4.

21. Laine L, Cook D: Endoscopic ligation compared to sclerotherapy for treatment of esophageal variceal bleeding. *Ann Intern Med* 1995, 123:280–287.

22. Spiess S, Matalon T, Jensen D, *et al.*: Transjugular intrahepatic portosystemic shunt in nonliver transplant candidates: is it indicated?. *Am J Gastroenterol* 1995, 90:1238–1243.

23. Rossle M, Haag K, Ochs A, *et al.*: The transjugular intrahepatic portosystemic stent-shunt procedure for variceal bleeding. *N Engl J Med* 1994, 330:1665–1171.

24. LaBerge J, Somberg K, Lake J, *et al.*: Two-year outcome following transjugular intrahepatic portosystemic shunt for variceal bleeding. *Gastroenterology* 1995, 108:1143–1151.

25. Henderson J, Carey W, Vogt D, *et al.*: Management of variceal bleeding in the 1990's. *Cleve Clin J Med* 1993, 60:431–438.

26. Knechtle S, Kalayoglu M, D'Alessandro A, *et al.*: Portal hypertension: surgical management in the 1990's. *Surgery* 1994, 116:687–695.

27.• Bernard B, Lebrec D, Mathurin P, *et al.*: Beta-adrenergic antagonists in the prevention of gastrointestinal rebleeding in patients with cirrhosis: a meta-analysis. *Hepatology* 1997, 25:63–70.
The authors reviewed 12 selected, randomized, controlled trials to assess the efficacy of beta-adrenergic antagonists in the prevention of rebleeding and their effect on survival in patients with cirrhosis. They concluded that beta-adrenergic antagonists increase the mean percentage of patients free of rebleeding and the mean survival rate at 2 years.

113 Ascites: Physiology, Complications, and Management

Bruce A. Runyon and Donald J. Hillebrand

ANATOMY OF THE PERITONEAL CAVITY

The peritoneal cavity is a potential space, lined in its entirety by a single layer of mesothelial cells, the peritoneum. The peritoneum lines ligaments, mesenteries, intra-abdominal organs, the abdominal and pelvic walls, and the inferior surface of the diaphragm. The abdominal cavity is divided into interconnected compartments by the omentum, ligaments, and mesenteries. The nature of these interconnected compartments governs the spread of intra-abdominal infection and tumor. Mesothelial venous pores allow peritoneal fluid and solute resorption (via the portal vein); resorption of fluid, solutes, and particulate matter also occurs by way of lymphatic pores and return via the thoracic lymphatics. The diaphragmatic lymphatic pores (stomata) allow rapid and efficient clearance of particles up to the size of red blood cells and bacteria. Ascites is the term used to describe the pathologic accumulation of fluid within the peritoneal cavity.

PHYSIOLOGY OF ASCITIC FLUID FORMATION

Cirrhosis

Cirrhosis is the most common cause of ascites in the United States. There are two leading theories concerning the pathophysiology of ascitic fluid formation in cirrhosis, each of which attempts to explain how portal hypertension leads to development of ascites. In the setting of portal hypertension, increased pressure within hepatic sinusoids contributes to excess formation of fluid, overwhelming the capacity of the congested hepatic sinusoids and the intrahepatic lymphatics to return the fluid to the systemic circulation. Fluid subsequently weeps through the liver capsule, pooling within the peritoneal cavity as ascites. In addition to accounting for these findings, theories of ascites formation must explain the increased secretion of renin, angiotensin, aldosterone and vasopressin, and the stimulation of the sympathetic nervous system that occurs in patients with cirrhosis and portal hypertension.

The *Underfill Theory* is the traditional explanation of ascites formation. As proposed by this theory, ascites results in a contraction in the size of the intravascular fluid compartment. A compensating increase in renal sodium and fluid retention results from this fall in plasma volume, which is sensed by volume receptors. Despite continued renal compensation, continued formation of ascites prevents adequate refilling of the intravascular compartment. This theory has been modified by Schrier and an international group to the *Peripheral Arterial Vasodilation Hypothesis*. In this modification, peripheral arterial vasodilation and decreased peripheral vascular resistance increase vascular capacitance, and decrease "effective" plasma

volume, causing secondary renal sodium and water retention. The renal compensation attempts to return plasma volume to normal, but is unsuccessful because of ascites formation, and a continued increase in intravascular capacitance.

The *Overflow Theory*, originally proposed by Lieberman in 1970, states that an unidentified stimulus results in a primary increase in renal sodium retention and high plasma volumes. The combination of increased plasma volume and portal hypertension results in ascites formation.

Peritoneal Diseases

Peritoneal diseases may lead to ascites formation by several mechanisms (Table 113-1). *Peritoneal carcinomatosis*, infections, and connective tissue diseases (Figs. 113-1 and 113-2, see also **Color Plate**) lead to exudation of protein-rich fluid into the peritoneal cavity. Extracellular fluid follows to re-establish the oncotic pressure gradient between the peritoneal cavity and the intra-vascular space. *Massive liver metastases and major vascular involvement by tumor* (*eg*, Budd-Chiari or portal vein thrombosis) lead to development of portal hypertension and, subsequently, ascites by the same mechanisms as in cirrhotic ascites. Lastly, *lymphatic invasion* may lead to development of ascites by disruption of the intra-abdominal lymphatics with pooling of lymph fluid within the peritoneal cavity.

Cardiac Ascites

Cardiac ascites forms as a result of the same mechanisms responsible for cirrhotic ascites. Decreased effective arterial plasma volume due to either diminished peripheral vascular resistance in high-output failure or decreased cardiac output in low-output failure triggers compensatory mechanisms similar to

---

Table 113-1. Mechanisms of Ascites Development in Malignancy

Peritoneal carcinomatosis
Massive liver metastases
  Diffuse infiltration of the liver sinusoids or portal triads by tumor cells
  Replacement of the liver substance by large tumor deposits
Major vessel involvement
  Hepatic veins or suprahepatic vena cava invasion (ie, Budd-Chiari)
  Portal vein thrombosis
Lymphatic involvement
  Central lymphatic vessels
  Intra-abdominal lymphatics within mesenteries or retroperitoneum

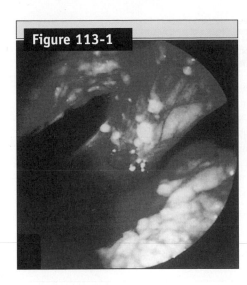

Figure 113-1 Laparoscopic appearance of peritoneal carcinomatosis with large white nodules of various sizes. (From Chu CM [Gastrointest Endosc 1994, 40:285–289.] with permission). See also **Color Plate**.

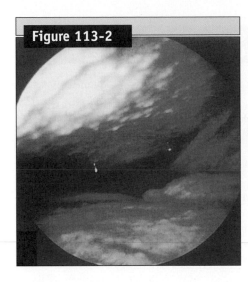

Figure 113-2 Laparoscopic appearance of tuberculous peritonitis with numerous small yellowish-white nodules present on the peritoneal surfaces. See also **Color Plate**. (From Chu CM [Gastrointest Endosc 1994, 40:285–289.] with permission).

those found in cirrhotic patients. Secondary sodium and water retention overwhelm the ability of congested hepatic sinusoids to return fluid to the systemic circulation.

EPIDEMIOLOGY

Chronic parenchymal liver diseases, including cirrhosis and alcoholic hepatitis are the most common causes of ascites in the United States (Table 113-2) [1]. Ovarian cancer is the most common cause of peritoneal carcinomatosis complicated by ascites followed by cancer of unknown primary site, uterine, pancreatic, gastric, breast and lung cancers, and lymphoma. In patients with acquired immunodeficiency syndrome (AIDS), opportunistic infections and lymphomas often are etiologies of ascites.

Ascites is the most common complication of cirrhosis; within 10 years of diagnosis, approximately half of patients with cirrhosis will develop ascites. Ascites in a cirrhotic patient is associated with a poor prognosis; affected patients have only a 50% 2-year survival.

DIAGNOSIS

Unfortunately, physical examination is a relatively insensitive method of detecting ascites. The classic finding of a fluid wave is present only in persons with a large amount of fluid. Shifting dullness is the most reliable sign of ascites, but at least 1.5 L of fluid are required for shifting dullness to be present consistently. The absence of flank dullness reliably predicts that a patient has little or no ascitic fluid. The most sensitive finding for diagnosis of ascites is the "puddle sign," which is positive in patients with as little as one deciliter of fluid. Unfortunately, patients with ascites often are unable to kneel on their hands and knees long enough for an examiner to percuss for dependent periumbilical dullness from a fluid pool. Imaging studies are much more sensitive than physical examination in diagnosing ascitic fluid; ultrasound and computerized tomography reliably detect small amounts of ascites.

Diagnostic Paracentesis

Diagnostic paracentesis is a critical step in the evaluation of new-onset ascites. Indications for diagnostic paracentesis are listed in Table 113-3. Contraindications to paracentesis primarily include

disseminated intravascular coagulation and fibrinolysis. Coagulopathy is not a contraindication to diagnostic paracentesis, and, therefore, delaying the procedure while the prothrombin time is measured and intravenous fresh frozen plasma is administered is not appropriate. Large-volume paracentesis may be associated with a higher rate of hemorrhagic complications than regular paracentesis, but still does not warrant prophylactic administration of intravenous fresh frozen plasma [2].

Diagnostic paracentesis is best performed in the left lower quadrant. Care should be taken to insert the needle at a site sufficiently lateral to avoid the inferior hypogastric veins. Paracentesis should not be performed in areas near scars, because they often form adhesions with collateral vessels or fixed loops of bowel. A 22-gauge needle is inserted through a Z-tract, 25 to 50 mL of fluid are withdrawn, and blood culture bottles are inoculated immediately with 10 mL of ascitic fluid each. The remainder of the fluid is then quickly placed in appropriate tubes for cell counts and chemistries. Abdominal wall hematoma is the most common complication of paracentesis, but occurs infrequently (0.9%).

Ascitic Fluid Appearance

Sterile ascitic fluid usually is clear and yellow. Clinical situations in which ascitic fluid is cloudy include infection (neutrophils and lymphocytes), chylous ascites (triglycerides) (Fig. 113-3, see also **Color Plate**), and peritoneal carcinomatosis (malignant cells and lymphocytes). A "traumatic" paracentesis is the most common cause of blood-tinged or frankly bloody ascites. Other causes of bloody ascites include peritoneal carcinomatosis, tuberculosis, hepatoma (Fig. 113-4, see also **Color Plate**), and rupture of intraperitoneal varices.

Laboratory Analysis of Ascitic Fluid

Analysis of ascitic fluid should include cell count, chemistries, and culture. Commonly ordered ascitic fluid tests are listed in Table 113-4.

Determination of the serum-ascites albumin gradient (SAAG) is useful in patients with ascites. According to Starling's law, ascitic fluid albumin concentration is primarily determined by portal pressure. At equilibrium, the hydrostatic pressure promoting ascites formation (portal venous pressure) is balanced by the oncotic pressure (difference between serum and

Table 113-2. Causes of Ascites in the United States

Cause	Percentage of total %*
Chronic parenchymal liver disease (includes cirrhosis and alcoholic hepatitis)	81.4
Malignancy	10.0
Congestive heart failure	3.0
Tuberculosis	1.7
Nephrogenous (dialysis ascites)	1.0
Pancreatic	0.9
Miscellaneous (includes fulminant hepatic failure, biliary, lymphatic tear, Chlamydia, and nephrotic syndrome)	each < 1.0

* Mixed ascites (ie, more than one cause of ascites) found in 4.3% of patients. Adapted from Runyon BA, Reynolds TB [ ]; with permission .

Table 113-3. Indications for Diagnostic Paracentesis

New onset of ascites

At the time of hospital admission as part of physical exam of the patient with ascites

Ascitic fluid infection is suspected clinically*

Evaluation of the response of an ascitic fluid infection to antibiotic therapy

Hepatic encephalopathy develops raising the suspicion of infection

Deterioration of renal function

* Clinical presentation of ascitic fluid infection ranges from the classical presentation of abdominal pain, fever, and leukocytosis to being asymptomatic in one third of patients.

ascitic fluid albumin concentrations), promoting ascitic fluid resorption. SAAG is determined primarily by portal pressure while total ascitic fluid protein is determined by both total serum protein concentration and portal pressure. The magnitude of the SAAG correlates directly with portal pressure [portal pressure in mm Hg = (6.2) × (SAAG) + 5.3] [3]. The SAAG is calculated by subtracting the ascitic fluid albumin concentration from the serum albumin concentration obtained on the same day; the difference in albumin concentrations (gradient) is the SAAG. A SAAG greater than or equal to 1.1 g/dL is 96.7% accurate in detecting portal hypertension [4]. By comparison, use of total ascitic fluid protein to determine whether ascites is transudative or exudative is accurate only half of the time [4]. Failure of the "exudate-transudate" concept is explained by the wide variability in total serum protein and portal pressure in cirrhotic patients with ascites. The concept of "high-gradient" (SAAG≥1.1 g/dL) and "low-gradient" (SAAG<1.1 g/dL) ascites has replaced the older "exudate-transudate" classification (Table 113-5). An elevated SAAG (≥1.1 g/dL) reliably diagnoses portal hypertension and suggests diuretic sensitivity. In contrast, a low SAAG (<1.1 g/dL) excludes portal hypertension as the cause of ascites, and should prompt further evaluation (Table 113-5). Shock and markedly increased serum globulin concentration may decrease the reliability of SAAG determination.

In patients with cirrhotic ascites, total ascitic fluid protein concentration helps estimate the risk of subsequent ascitic fluid infection (spontaneous bacterial peritonitis [SBP]) because the antibacterial properties of ascites correlate directly with this clinical variable. A total ascitic fluid protein concentration below 1.0 g/dL indicates a significantly increased risk of infection, while ascitic fluid infection is quite unusual in noncirrhotic ascites (eg, peritoneal carcinomatosis) which generally has a total ascitic fluid protein concentration greater than 2.5 g/dL. Differentiating SBP from secondary bacterial peritonitis also is aided by determination of total ascitic fluid protein. Fifteen percent to 27% of cirrhotic patients with ascites have SBP or sec-

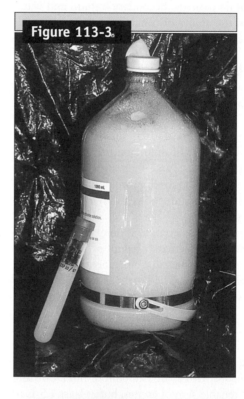

Figure 113-3.

Chylous ascitic fluid. See also **Color Plate**.

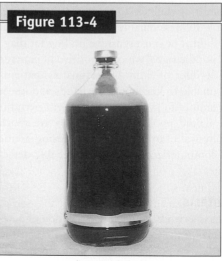

Figure 113-4

Bloody ascitic fluid from a patient with peritoneal carcinomatosis. See also **Color Plate**.

Table 113-4. Ascitic Fluid Analysis

Routine	Optional	Unusual	Unhelpful
Cell count	Glucose	Tuberulosis smear/culture	pH
Culture*	LDH	Cytology	Lactate
Albumin†	Amylase	Triglyceride	CEA
Total protein	Gram stain	Bilirubin	Cholesterol
			AFP

Immediate inoculation of two blood culture bottles at the bedside.
† *Routine on initial ascitic fluid analysis only.*
LDH—lactate dehydrogenase.
Adapted from Runyon BA [1]; with permission.

Table 113-5. Classification of Ascites by Serum-Ascites Albumin Concentration Gradient

High gradient (≥ 1.1g/dL)	Low gradient (≤1.1g/dL)
Cirrhosis	Peritoneal carcinomatosis
Alcoholic hepatitis	Tuberculosis (without cirrhosis)
Massive liver metastases	Pancreatic ascites (without cirrhosis)
Cardiac ascites	Nephrotic syndrome
Fulminant hepatic failure	Biliary ascites
Budd-Chiari syndrome	Ascites related to connective tissue diseases
Portal vein thrombosis	Ascites related to bowel obstruction
Veno-occlusive disease	
Acute fatty liver or pregnancy	
Myxedema	
"Mixed ascites"	

Adapted from Runyon BA [1]; with permission.

ondary bacterial peritonitis at the time of hospital admission. For this reason diagnostic paracentesis should be a standard part of the admitting examination of patients with cirrhosis and ascites.

Ascitic fluid cell count is the fastest way to diagnose infection in ascites. An ascitic fluid leukocyte count of greater than or equal to 250 per mm^3 with a predominance of neutrophils is consistent with a presumptive diagnosis of SBP. Antibiotic therapy most commonly is initiated on the basis of the ascitic fluid neutrophil count; any inflammatory or infectious process, or complication of ascites, however, may raise the ascitic fluid neutrophil count (neutrocytic ascites). Other causes of neutrocytic ascites include peritoneal carcinomatosis, pancreatic ascites, and connective tissue diseases. Tuberculous peritonitis, on occasion, may be associated with neutrocytic ascites. These other causes should be investigated when an atypical clinical picture accompanies the neutrocytic ascites, or when there is a lack of clinical response to antibiotic treatment. Tuberculous peritonitis most commonly results in a predominance of lymphocytes in the elevated ascitic fluid leukocyte count [5]. In the event of a traumatic paracentesis with bloody ascitic fluid, the neutrophil count is corrected by subtraction of one neutrophil for every 250 red blood cells on cell count. This allows evaluation for SBP even after a difficult and traumatic paracentesis.

Clinical studies have demonstrated that immediate inoculation of blood culture bottles each with 10 mL of ascitic fluid at the bedside is a more sensitive (90%) method of culturing ascitic fluid than the conventional method of plating a loop of fluid on agar (50%). In SBP, the bacterial load is on the order of one to two organisms per milliliter, which is similar to that found in bacteremia.

Optional ascitic fluid tests (Table 113-4) are ordered when noncirrhotic ascites or a complication is suspected clinically. Gram stain of ascitic fluid is predictably insensitive (10%) in demonstrating bacteria, in view of the low bacterial load in SBP. A positive ascitic fluid Gram stain more commonly is found in cases of secondary bacterial peritonitis. Ascitic fluid neutrophil count or clinical signs and symptoms of infection dictate empiric use of antibiotics. Ascitic fluid chemistries, including total protein, glucose, and lactate dehydrogenase concentrations may be helpful in differentiating SBP from secondary bacterial peritonitis [6]. In cases of suspected peritoneal carcinomatosis, ascitic fluid cytology may be a rapid, minimally invasive, and cost-effective method of diagnosis; cytologic examination should be performed in all cases of low-SAAG ascites. In peritoneal carcinomatosis, the yield of ascitic fluid cytology interpreted by an experienced cytopathologist is excellent (nearly 100%) when the fluid is processed properly. The yield of ascitic fluid cytology, however, predictably is poor in malignancy-related ascites that occurs in the absence of peritoneal implants and, instead, is secondary to massive liver replacement with tumor or major vascular involvement. Tuberculous peritonitis is an uncommon cause of ascites in the United States (Table 113-2). Unfortunately, the ascitic fluid mycobacterial smear rarely is helpful and mycobacterial culture has limited sensitivity. The role of measuring ascitic fluid adenosine deaminase concentration in the diagnosis of tuberculous peritonitis varies, depending on the prevalences of tuberculosis and cirrhosis in patients in the area where the test is performed [5]. In cases of suspected tuberculous peritonitis, peritoneoscopy with histopathologic examination and culturing of directed peritoneal biopsies for mycobacteria is the best method of diagnosis.

■ COMPLICATIONS OF ASCITES

Development of ascites in a patient with cirrhosis is associated with a two-year survival of 50%. In addition to signaling the end stages of cirrhosis, development of ascites may be complicated by a number of secondary disorders (Table 113-6).

Medical Deterioration Related to the Presence of Ascites

The abdominal distention which accompanies ascites may result in symptoms ranging from vague abdominal fullness or heaviness to diffuse pain. Tense ascites is characterized by a distended and firm abdomen with taut, glistening skin. Patients with tense ascites typically will note abdominal discomfort, early satiety, and dyspnea from accompanying respiratory compromise (Fig. 113-5, see also **Color Plate**). The presence of significant ascites increases resting energy expenditure, thus contributing to progressive malnutrition, weight loss, and proximal muscle wasting. In the cirrhotic patient, caloric requirements are increased at the same time that caloric intake is limited by anorexia, dysgeusia, and early satiety from abdominal distention.

Hepatic hydrothorax may occur in patients with ascites in the absence of primary pulmonary or cardiac disease [7]. Because intra-abdominal pressure is greater than intra-thoracic pressure, fluid moves from the abdomen to the chest through small diaphragmatic pores [8]. The fluid accumulates within the pleural space and may impair respiratory function. A diagnosis of hepatic hydrothorax may be confirmed by injecting an isotopic tracer into the peritoneal space and later detecting it in the thoracic cavity [9]. Management of hepatic hydrothorax involves treatment of ascites; insertion of a chest tube is contraindicated due to the potential for persistent high-volume drainage with resulting electrolyte and intravascular volume derangements. Therapeutic transjugular intrahepatic portosystemic shunt (TIPS) has been attempted with promising early results [10].

Ascites also promotes formation or worsening of umbilical and inguinal hernias. Previously trivial inguinal hernias may enlarge as they collect ascitic fluid; these hernias rarely incarcerate. As umbilical hernias enlarge, the risk of rupture increases; skin overlying the umbilical hernia typically thins and ulcerates before rupture (Fig. 113-6, see also **Color Plate**). Rupture of an umbilical hernia (Flood syndrome) has an associated mortality of 20% to 40% due to associated intravascular volume and electrolyte disturbances, and intraperitoneal infection.

Spontaneous Bacterial Peritonitis

Spontaneous Bacterial Peritonitis (SBP) is the most common form of ascitic fluid infection, and is defined as findings of a positive ascitic fluid culture (usually with a single organism) and an ascitic fluid neutrophil count of greater than or equal to 250 per ml in a patient without an intra-abdominal, surgically treatable source of infection (Table 113-7) [6]. Risk factors for development of SBP include a total ascitic fluid protein of less than 1g/dL, gastrointestinal hemorrhage, and prior SBP. Each year, cirrhotic patients with ascites have a greater than 10% risk of developing this disorder. Persons with SBP may be

---

Table 113-6. Common Complications of Ascites

Medical deterioration
    Symptomatic ascites (discomfort, early satiety, and dyspnea)
    Malnutrition and weight loss
    Proximal muscle wasting
    Respiratory compromise (restrictive lung dynamics)
Infection
    Spontaneous bacterial peritonitis and its variants
    Polymicrobial bacterascites
    Secondary bacterial peritonitis
Development of hernias with their associated complications
    Inguinal hernia
    Umbilical hernia
    Flood syndrome
Hepatic hydrothorax

Figure 113-5

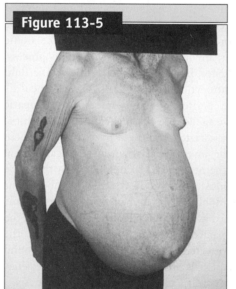

Abdominal appearance of a cirrhotic patient with tense ascites. Note the proximal muscles wasting in the setting of a hugely protuberant abdomen, prominent abdominal wall venous collaterals and small umbilical hernia. See also **Color Plate**.

Figure 113-6

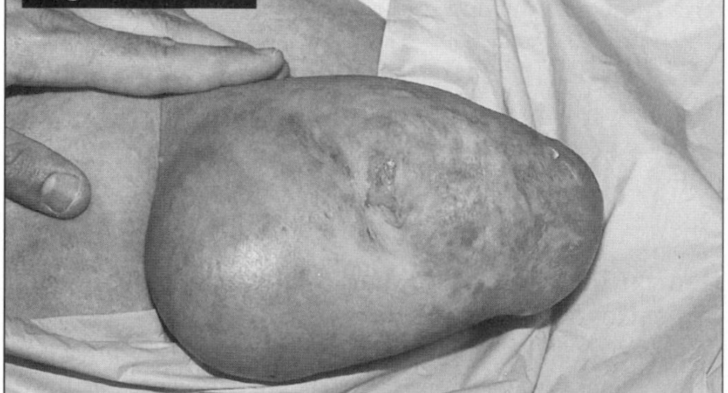

Large complicated umbilical hernia with signs of impending rupture in a patient with massive ascites. See also **Color Plate**.

Table 113-7. Spontaneous Bacterial Peritonitis and its Variants

Ascitic Fluid Infection	Definition
Spontaneous bacterial peritonitis	Single organism culture positivity
	Neutrophil count ≥ 250 per mm³
	No known or suspected surgical source
Culture-negative neutrocytic ascites	Neutrophil count ≥250 per mm³
	Negative culture
	No known or suspected surgical source

asymptomatic; have nonspecific, mild complaints; or present with classic findings of abdominal pain, fever, and hypotension. Common clinical symptoms and signs in these individuals include abdominal pain and tenderness, nausea, anorexia, fever, diarrhea, altered mental status, leukocytosis, azotemia, tachycardia, and hypotension. As many as 25% of cirrhotics with ascites have SBP on admission to the hospital [6]. Given the subtle presentation of SBP in some individuals, all cirrhotic patients with ascites should undergo diagnostic paracentesis when they enter the hospital. In addition, paracentesis should be repeated at the time of any clinical deterioration. Half of all episodes of SBP are associated with bacteremia.

Knowledge of the bacteria which cause SBP guides the choice of antibiotic therapy. *Escherichia coli* is the most common organism infecting ascites. Taken together, *E. coli, Klebsiella*, and Streptococcal species account for 77% of SBP (6). In addition, anaerobic organisms and fungal organisms rarely cause SBP.

The antibiotic treatment of choice for SBP is a third-generation cephalosporin, for example cefotaxime, 2 g intravenously every 8 hours for 5 days. Use of aminoglycosides in cirrhotic patients is associated with an unacceptably high rate of nephrotoxicity and should be avoided. Cefotaxime is adequate treatment for 94% of the bacteria that cause SBP. Superinfection is uncommon. With prompt initiation of cefotaxime therapy, mortality of SBP is minimized. Current survival (mean infection-related and hospital-related mortality rates of 29 and 43%, respectively) likely is explained by an increased ability to diagnose SBP and through more liberal use of diagnostic paracentesis, use of non-nephrotoxic antibiotics, and an overall improvement in the care of critically ill cirrhotic patients.

More than two thirds of patients who survive an initial episode of SBP experience a recurrence within 1 year, and half of these individuals die during this period [11]. Antibiotic prophylaxis has been used in an attempt to improve this prognosis. Norfloxacin (Noroxin tablets) is a poorly absorbed fluoroquinolone antibiotic active against enteric gram-negative bacteria, the principal pathogens which cause SBP. Norfloxacin, 400 mg by mouth once daily, decreases the 1-year recurrence rate of SBP from 68% to 20% [11]. There is, however, no associated increase in survival with antibiotic prophylaxis. Gram-positive organisms accounted for the recurrences in patients taking norfloxacin prophylaxis. Prophylaxis also has been used to prevent infection in hospitalized patients with low-protein ascites (total ascitic fluid protein less than 1.5 g/dL). These individuals are known to develop SBP at a 10-fold higher rate than patients with high-protein ascites. Norfloxacin, 400 mg by mouth daily, virtually eliminates gram-negative SBP but does not affect in-hospital mortality [12]. Cirrhotic patients with gastrointestinal bleeding are at high risk for developing SBP; norfloxacin 400 mg orally twice daily for 1 week following a bleeding episode decreases the overall incidence of infections and bacteremia in these individuals [13]. Although there is, again, no survival benefit, antibiotic prophylaxis results in a 62% decrease in the cost of antibiotic therapy, overall. Other antibiotics have been studied including ciprofloxacin and trimethoprim-sulfamethoxazole. Among patients with cirrhosis and ascites, trimethoprim-sulfamethoxazole reduced the incidence of SBP from 27% to 3% during a median follow-up of 90 days [14], albeit with only a

trend toward a decrease in mortality in patients receiving prophylaxis (20% mortality in those not receiving prophylaxis vs 7% mortality in those receiving trimethoprim-sulfamethoxazole).

Use of prophylactic norfloxacin has been shown to lead to appearance of quinolone-resistant organisms in the feces within 2 weeks of beginning therapy in half of treated patients (15). Antibiotic selection pressure may lead to an increase in the incidence of SBP due to antibiotic-resistant organisms (*eg, Enterococcus* and *Pseudomonas*). Short-term prophylaxis appears to be valuable, cost-effective, safe, and free of significant serious side effects, but the role of long-term primary or secondary antibiotic prophylaxis must be better defined.

Culture-Negative Neutrocytic Ascites

Culture-negative neutrocytic ascites (CNNA) is a variant of SBP in which there is an ascitic-fluid neutrophil count of greater than or equal to 250 per mL, a negative ascitic fluid culture in the absence of recent antibiotic therapy, and no identified intra-abdominal, surgically treatable source of infection. Most episodes of CNNA resolve spontaneously. When intraperitoneal defense mechanisms are deficient, continued bacterial growth may lead to SBP. Other causes of neutrocytic ascites including pancreatitis, peritoneal carcinomatosis, and tuberculous peritonitis, should be considered in patients without clinical findings of SBP. Overall, the morbidity and mortality of CNNA is comparable to that of SBP. In addition, there are no clinical factors that predict which patients with CNNA will improve without antibiotic therapy and which will develop overt infection. Affected patients, therefore, should receive empiric antibiotic therapy.

Monomicrobial-Nonneutrocytic Bacterascites

Monomicrobial, nonneutrocytic bacterascites (MNB) is diagnosed when there is a positive ascitic fluid culture with a single organism and a normal ascitic fluid neutrophil count. Patients with MNB typically have less severe liver disease than do patients with classic SBP, but do not have a different total ascitic fluid protein concentration. MNB is felt to represent transient colonization of ascitic fluid. The presence or absence of associated clinical symptoms appears to differentiate those patients destined to progress to SBP from those who will have spontaneous resolution of colonization. If clinical findings compatible with SBP are present, antibiotic therapy should be initiated and continued until repeat paracentesis demonstrates a normal ascitic fluid neutrophil count and sterile cultures.

Polymicrobial Bacterascites

Patients with polymicrobial bacterascites have an ascitic fluid culture which grows multiple organisms and a normal ascitic fluid neutrophil count (<250 neutrophils per mL). This finding signals puncture of the bowel with the paracentesis needle. An extremely difficult paracentesis, aspiration of stool or air during paracentesis, or multiple organisms on the ascitic fluid Gram stain in the setting of a normal ascitic fluid neutrophil count should alert the clinician to possible bowel puncture at paracentesis. Repeat paracentesis should be performed after a suspected needlestick puncture to evaluate the patient for development of a neutrocytic peritoneal response. Fortunately, this problem is rare. In addition, the vast majority of affected patients do not develop SBP. When repeat paracentesis demonstrates a neutrocytic response, treatment with nonnephrotoxic broad-spectrum antibiotics with coverage for gram-negative enteric, gram-positive, and anaerobic organisms is indicated.

Secondary Bacterial Peritonitis

Inherent to diagnosis of SBP and its variants is exclusion of an intra-abdominal source of infection requiring surgical treatment; such peritonitis is found in a small percentage of cirrhotic patients with ascites at the time of hospital admission. Subsequent management of these individuals differs considerably from that of patients with SBP; secondary bacterial peritonitis requires surgical as well as antibiotic treatment. In patients with secondary bacterial peritonitis, the ascitic fluid culture is positive (usually for multiple enteric organisms), the ascitic fluid neutrophil count is greater than or equal to 250 cells per mL, and there is an identifiable intra-abdominal source, for example a perforated hollow viscus or an abscess. In the absence of AIDS or malignancy, fungal infection of ascites only occurs in secondary bacterial peritonitis. In addition, if repeat paracentesis performed 48 hours after beginning appropriate antibiotic therapy for SBP demonstrates an increase in the ascitic fluid neutrophil count, SBP should be suspected, and imaging of the abdomen either by radiograph, ultrasound, or computerized tomography constitutes the next management step.

■ MANAGEMENT OF CIRRHOTIC ASCITES

Care of patients with ascites begins with a search for the cause. Many liver diseases have a reversible component, even when ascites is present. Acute alcoholic hepatitis may cause a previously stable cirrhotic to develop ascites; with abstinence, acute injury and ascites may resolve. Similarly, patients with ascites and autoimmune hepatitis or chronic active hepatitis B may improve considerably with appropriate treatment.

Evaluation of patients with new-onset or worsening ascites should include an investigation for possible aggravating factors, including dietary indiscretion with excessive salt intake, noncompliance with diuretic therapy, portal-vein thrombosis, and hepatocellular carcinoma. Use of nonsteroidal anti-inflammatory drugs (NSAIDs) may lead to decompensation through several mechanisms. NSAIDs interfere with renal prostaglandin synthesis and may impair sodium excretion and free-water clearance. Use of drugs which may cause renal dysfunction should be avoided.

Concept of Sodium Balance

Medical management of patients with cirrhotic ascites revolves around sodium balance. To achieve negative sodium balance, sodium intake must be matched by renal sodium excretion and, to a lesser extent, by insensible and fecal sodium loss. Insensible sodium loss is less than 5 mmol/d in the absence of fever, and fecal sodium loss is less than five mmol/d unless diarrhea is present. The primary route of sodium excretion is urinary and, therefore, negative sodium balance results in diuresis that leads to mobilization of edema and ascites, and a decrease in weight. Determination of sodium balance simply requires subtraction of urinary sodium excretion from dietary sodium intake. Urinary

sodium excretion is best assessed by measuring the sodium content of a 24-hour urine collection. Serial monitoring aids in determining the optimal diuretic dose. A urinary sodium excretion greater than the estimated sodium intake suggests dietary noncompliance; a urinary sodium excretion less than the estimated sodium intake indicates a need for additional diuretics, if renal function and serum electrolyte levels will allow this. A less accurate method of estimating urinary sodium excretion is the measurement of a spot urinary sodium value (U_{na+}) and multiplying this value by the measured 24-hour urine volume. However, this method assumes a steady urinary sodium excretion throughout the 24 hours. Negative sodium balance and a loss of 0.5 kg/d is the goal of therapy in patients without peripheral edema; patients with edema tolerate more aggressive diuresis. Urinary sodium excretion, weight, physical examination (abdominal distention, edema, intravascular volume, and mental status), serum electrolyte levels and renal function are followed to assess the response to therapy and look for potential complications.

Dietary sodium restriction is the initial treatment of cirrhotic ascites; reasonable sodium restriction decreases the sodium load that the kidneys must dispose of either spontaneously, or with diuretic therapy. A minority (15% to 20%) of patients achieve negative sodium balance and ascites control with dietary restriction alone; dietary sodium of 2 g (88 mmol) is an achievable goal. Further sodium restriction decreases the palatability of food and may not be reasonable in chronically ill, malnourished patients. In the minority of patients who fail to respond to moderate dietary sodium restriction and aggressive diuresis (<10%), further dietary sodium restriction may be attempted.

The role of restricting fluid intake in management of cirrhotic ascites often is misunderstood; formal fluid restriction usually is not necessary. Mild asymptomatic hyponatremia is a common finding in cirrhotic patients with ascites, and usually is not clinically significant. Hyponatremia does not mandate fluid restriction unless the serum sodium concentration falls to 120 mmol/L or less.

Diuretic Therapy

The majority of patients with cirrhotic ascites require diuretic therapy to achieve negative sodium balance; spironolactone is the agent of choice. This diuretic is potassium-sparing and antagonizes the hyperaldosteronism common among cirrhotics with ascites. Spironolactone is a relatively mild diuretic which causes excretion of less than 5% of filtered sodium. Single-agent therapy with the more potent diuretic, furosemide, is less effective than single-agent spironolactone therapy and commonly causes hypokalemia. In patients with cirrhosis, the half-life of spironolactone is 5 to 7 days. Thus, the onset of diuresis and maximal diuretic effect of spironolactone may not occur for several weeks. This long half-life, however, allows single daily dosing which enhances patient compliance. The maximum dose of spironolactone is 400 mg daily.

In the majority of patients, combination therapy with spironolactone and furosemide is the most effective regimen. The typical starting doses for the combination regimen are spironolactone 100 mg and furosemide 40 mg taken together orally once in the morning. Use of the mild potassium-sparing diuretic, spironolactone and the potent potassium-wasting diuretic, furosemide leads to fewer difficulties with serum potassium derangements and shorter hospital stays. If a patient fails to achieve a negative sodium balance and mobilization of edema or ascites after 3 days on a given regimen, then the diuretics should be sequentially increased, maintaining the same ratio of the two diuretics (*ie*, increasing spironolactone to 200 mg and furosemide to 80 mg daily). The maximum regimen includes spironolactone 400 mg and furosemide 160 mg daily. Patients with ascites treated with potent diuretics must be observed very carefully for development of complications, including, hypo- and hyperkalemia, metabolic alkalosis, volume depletion, azotemia, hyponatremia, and encephalopathy. Spironolactone also may cause sexual dysfunction and gynecomastia in males.

Refractory Ascites

Ascites that cannot be mobilized or recurs rapidly following therapeutic paracentesis despite medical therapy is deemed to be refractory [16]. Refractory ascites may be diuretic-resistant (lack of adequate response to maximum diuretics and dietary sodium restriction) or diuretic-intractable (diuretic-induced complications prevent use of an adequate diuretic dose). Development of diuretic-induced complications most commonly limits successful medical management; azotemia is the most common limiting event. The prognosis for a patient with refractory ascites who is not treated with liver transplantation is quite poor; only 25% of these individuals survive for 1 year.

Large-volume paracentesis has recently regained favor among gastroenterologists and hepatologists managing patients with cirrhotic ascites. Studies support the use of large-volume paracentesis and intravenous albumin infusion as an effective method of short-term management of tense ascites. In large-volume paracentesis, 10 to 15 L of ascitic fluid may be removed in one session offering rapid symptomatic relief. At present, periodic large-volume paracentesis may be the treatment of choice for refractory ascites, particularly in patients in whom liver transplantation is anticipated. The role of post-paracentesis plasma volume expansion using albumin or dextran remains controversial. Routine intravenous albumin infusion postparacentesis cannot be recommended, but instead, should be considered on an individual basis.

Peritoneovenous shunting of ascitic fluid with either a Denver or LeVeen shunt offers another method of managing refractory ascites. The LeVeen shunt appears to offer long-term control of ascites, but shunt occlusion is common (probability of obstruction, 40% at 1 year and 52% at 2 years) limiting its effectiveness [17]. Furthermore, peritoneovenous shunting offers no survival advantage over medical management, including intermittent large-volume paracentesis.

In addition to controlling variceal bleeding, TIPS also has been noted to improve ascites. The only published randomized trial of TIPS for treatment of refractory ascites, however, demonstrated poorer survival in the TIPS group than in medically managed patients [18]. Additional problems associated with TIPS occlusion and other complications also limit its effectiveness in treatment of refractory ascites [19].

Surgical porto-systemic shunts generally have been reserved for treatment of variceal hemorrhage in patients with cirrhosis.

Retrospective studies reveal that shunt surgery alters the natural history of cirrhosis, reducing the occurrence of ascites, SBP, and hepatorenal syndrome in treated patients [20]. Shunt surgery, however, does not improve survival in these individuals, and is more frequently associated with hepatic encephalopathy than is medical therapy.

Orthotopic liver transplantation is the treatment of choice for patients with refractory ascites (see Chapter 117). Appropriate candidates for liver transplantation should be referred for this procedure before any further decline in nutritional status and renal function. After successful liver transplantation, ascites typically resolves quickly.

▅▅ REFERENCES

Recently published papers of particular interest have been highlighted as follows:
* •   Of interest
* ••   Of outstanding interest

1.   Runyon BA: Care of Patients with Ascites. *N Engl J Med* 1994, 330:337–42.

2.   Webster ST, Brown KL, Lucey MR, Nostrant TT: Hemorrhagic complications of large volume abdominal paracentesis. *Amer J Gastroenterol* 1996, 91:366–368.

3.   Rector WG, Reynolds TB: Superiority of the serum-ascites albumin gradient over the ascites total protein concentration in separation of transudative and exudative ascites. *Amer J Med* 1984, 77:83–85.

4.•• Runyon BA, Montano AA, Akriviadis EA, *et al*: The serum-ascites albumin gradient is superior to the exudate-transudate concept in the differential diagnosis of ascites. *Ann Intern Med* 1992, 117:215–220.
A prospective collection of 901 paired serum and ascitic fluid samples from consecutive patients definitively demonstrated the high accuracy (96.7%) of the serum-ascites albumin gradient (SAAG) as a marker for portal hypertension in the classification of ascites. The exudate-transudate concept utilizing ascitic fluid total protein concentration correctly classified the ascites only 55.6% of the time.

5.   Hillebrand DJ, Runyon BA, Yasmineh WG, Rynders GP: Ascitic fluid adenosine deaminase insensitivity in detecting tuberculous peritonitis in the United States. *Hepatology* 1996, 24:1408–1412.

6.   McHutchison JG, Runyon BA: Spontaneous Bacterial Peritonitis. In *Gastrointestinal and Hepatic Infections*. Edited by Surawicz C, Owen RL. Philadelphia: Saunders; 1995:455–475.

7.   King PD, Rumbaut R, Sanchez C: Pulmonary manifestations of chronic liver disease. *Dig Dis* 1996, 14:73–82.

8.   Alberts WM, Salem AJ, Solomon DA, Boyce G: Hepatic hydrothorax clinical management. *Arch Intern Med* 1991, 151:2383–2388.

9.   Daly JJ, Potts JM, Gordon L, Buse MG: Scintigraphic diagnosis of peritoneo-pleural communication in the absence of ascites. *Clin Nuc Med* 1994, 19:892–894.

10. Strauss RM, Martin LG, Kaufman SL, Boyer TD: Transjugular intrahepatic portal systemic shunt for the management of symptomatic cirrhotic hydrothorax. *Amer J Gastroenterol* 1994, 89:1520–1522.

11. Gines P, Rimola A, Planas R, *et al*: Norfloxacin prevents spontaneous bacterial peritonitis recurrence in cirrhosis: Results of a double-blind, placebo-controlled trial. *Hepatology* 1990, 12:716–724.

12. Soriano G, Guarner C, Teixido M, *et al*: Selective intestinal decontamination prevents spontaneous bacterial peritonitis. *Gastroenterol* 1991, 100:477–481.

13. Soriano G, Guarner C, Tomas A, *et al*: Norfloxacin prevents bacterial infection in cirrhotics with gastrointestinal hemorrhage. *Gastroenterol* 1992, 103:1267–1332.

14. Singh N, Gayowski T, Yu VL, Wagener MM: Trimethoprim-sulfamethoxazole for the prevention of spontaneous bacterial peritonitis in cirrhosis: a randomized trial. *Ann Intern Med* 1995, 122:595–598.

15. Dupeyron C, Mangeney N, Sedrati L, *et al.*: Rapid emergence of quinolone resistance in cirrhotic patients treated with norfloxacin to prevent spontaneous bacterial peritonitis. *Antimicrob Agents Chemother* 1994, 38:340–344.

16. Arroyo V, Gines P, Gerbes AL, *et al.*: Definition and diagnostic criteria of refractory ascites and hepatorenal syndrome in cirrhosis. *Hepatology* 1996, 23:164–176.

17. Gines P, Arroyo V, Vargas V, *et al.*: Paracentesis with intravenous infusion of albumin as compared with peritoneovenous shunting in cirrhosis with refractory ascites. *N Engl J Med* 1991, 325:829–835.

18.• Lebrec D, Giuily N, Hadengue A, *et al.*: Transjugular intrahepatic portosystemic shunts: comparison with paracentesis in patients with cirrhosis and refractory ascites. *J Hepatology* 1996, 25:135–144.

Only randomized study of TIPS versus periodic large volume paracentesis in cirrhotic patients with diuretic-refractory ascites. Child's class B patients had improved ascites control with TIPS but without an associated improvement in survival. Overall, the two years survival was worsened with TIPS placement for diuretic-refractory ascites (TIPS group 29—13% vs 56—17% in the paracentesis group).

19. Martinet JP, Fenyves D, Legault L, *et al.*: Treatment of refractory ascites using a transjugular intrahepatic portosystemic shunt (TIPS): a caution. *Dig Dis Sci* 1997, 42:161–166.

20. Castells A, Salo J, Planas R, *et al*: Impact of shunt surgery for variceal bleeding in the natural history of ascites in cirrhosis: a retrospective study. *Hepatology* 1994, 20:584–591.

114 Hepatorenal Syndrome

Arun J. Sanyal

Hepatorenal syndrome (HRS) is defined as renal insufficiency in a patient with liver failure and no structural renal abnormality [1••]. It is associated with intense renal vasospasm, decreased renal plasma flow (RPF) and glomerular filtration rate (GFR), and severe renal sodium and water retention. Consequently, the clinical hallmarks of HRS are oliguria, azotemia, urinary concentration, and a urine sodium concentration below 10 mEq/L in the setting of severe underlying liver disease. A key aspect of the diagnosis is careful exclusion of other causes of renal failure, for example, drug-induced nephrotoxicity, urinary tract infection, and obstructive uropathy. Perhaps the clinical condition with which hepatorenal syndrome is confused most frequently is hypovolemia. HRS and hypovolemia are each associated with decreased renal perfusion, urinary concentration, marked sodium retention and a fractional sodium excretion (FENa) of less than one. Distinction between these two disorders usually requires a trial of volume expansion that produces a diuresis in patients with hypovolemia but not in those with HRS. These considerations have led to development of formal diagnostic criteria for hepatorenal syndrome (Table 114-1).

PATHOPHYSIOLOGY

The hepatorenal syndrome is often considered to represent the most severe manifestation of a continuum of pathophysiologic abnormalities that develop in patients with cirrhosis and progressive ascites. These abnormalities are primarily functional rather than structural, and the underlying kidneys of affected patients are considered to be otherwise normal and capable of functioning normally in the setting of normal liver function [2]. Indeed, kidneys from individuals with fatal HRS have been successfully transplanted into patients with chronic renal disease.

Persons with HRS have three principal physiologic abnormalities (Chapters 112, 113, and 116) (Fig. 114-1): portal hypertension and liver failure; marked alterations in systemic, splanchnic, and renal hemodynamics; and severe renal salt and water retention. In persons with portal hypertension, increased sinusoidal pressure forces salt and water into the peritoneal cavity, leading to accumulation of ascites, intravascular volume depletion, and decreased renal blood flow [2]. An intrahepatic, volume-dependent, baroreceptor pathway also has been implicated

Table 114-1. International Ascites Club Diagnostic Criteria for Hepatorenal Syndrome

Major criteria	Additional criteria
Chronic or acute liver disease with advanced hepatic failure and portal hypertension	Urine vol < 500 mL/d
Low glomerular filtration rate as indicated by a serum creatinine > 1.5 mg/dL or creatinine clearance < 40mL/min	Urine Na < 10 mEq/L
Absence of shock, ongoing bacterial infection, and recent treatment with nephrotoxic drugs	Urine red cells < 50/high power field
Absence of gastrointestinal symptoms (diarrhea or gastrointestinal bleeding) or other causes of renal failure, *eg*, obstructive uropathy (weight loss > 500 gm/d for several days for those with ascites and no peripheral edema and > 1000 gm/d for those with ascites and peripheral edema)	Serum Na < 130 mEq/L
Failure to achieve a sustained improvement in renal function (creatinine < 1.5 mg/dL) following diuretic withdrawal and expansion of plasma volume with 1.5 liters of isotonic saline	
Proteinuria < 500 gm/dL and no ultrasonographic evidence of obstructive uropathy or parenchymal renal disease	

From Arroyo V et al. [1••]; with permission.

as a cause of decreased renal blood flow. As a result, affected individuals develop volume-dependent and volume-independent renal salt and water retention, and urine output declines. Simultaneously, patients with portal hypertension frequently have a decrease in systemic vascular resistance [3•, 4,5••] associated with an increase in vascular capacitance (Table 114-2). Vascular capacitance may increase faster than total blood volume, causing relative hypovolemia and a further decrease in renal perfusion. Relative hypovolemia in these individuals is worsened by redistribution of blood flow away from the viscera to the skin and subcutaneous tissues. Clinically, these changes result in an increase in cardiac output; a decrease in mean arterial pressure; tachycardia; warm, flushed extremities; and a steady decline in urine output. This decline in urine output signals the onset of HRS. As these physiologic changes occur, the liver function of affected patients deteriorates further.

CLINICAL PRESENTATION AND NATURAL HISTORY

Two clinical patterns of functional renal failure have been described in the setting of severe liver disease [1••,2].

Type I Hepatorenal Syndrome

The features of Type I HRS are those traditionally thought to characterize renal failure secondary to liver disease. Type I HRS occurs in the setting of both chronic and acute liver failure, and often develops following hospitalization for an unrelated reason, although a precipitating cause may never be identified. Most patients with cirrhosis who develop type I HRS have moderate to severe ascites and also some degree of encephalopathy. Virtually all patients with Type I HRS have a low mean arterial pressure, even as compared with their own baseline blood pressure. Jaundice may or may not be present in these individuals.

The onset of type I HRS is manifested by the sudden occurrence of oliguria (24 hr urine volume < 500 mL) accompanied by progressive azotemia. The serum creatinine level of affected persons usually rises 1 to 1.5 mg/d. Their urine is concentrated and the urine sodium concentration typically is less than 10 mEq/L. Patients with type I HRS do not have significant proteinuria, urinary red cell casts, or microscopic hematuria. Despite an adequate fluid challenge, their urine output does not improve, and the clinical course progresses inexorably to death in more than 90% of affected individuals. Rare instances of spontaneous remission of type I HRS have been described, usually in patients with alcoholic hepatitis or acute liver injury in whom liver function may improve rapidly. For practical purposes, type I HRS is nearly always fatal unless a liver transplant is performed emergently.

Type II Hepatorenal Syndrome

Type II HRS usually occurs in patients with cirrhosis and tense ascites refractory to medical treatment. Affected individuals often have some degree of encephalopathy, and jaundice typically is mild if present at all. The serum creatinine level in these patients remains over 1.5 mg/dL and their urine volume fluctuates, although severe oliguria or anuria does not occur. Mean blood pressure in patients with type II HRS is lower than normal and treatment with medicines that raise mean blood pressure produces a temporary increase in urine volume and decrease in serum creatinine level. Azotemia, however, never resolves completely and, over time, the serum creatinine concentration increases as renal dysfunction worsens. While the median survival of patients with type II HRS is longer than that of those with type I HRS, the eventual outcome is just as grim unless a liver transplant is performed.

DIAGNOSIS

Azotemia often heralds a progressive decline in the condition of the patient with severe liver failure [10]. Besides its affect on mor-

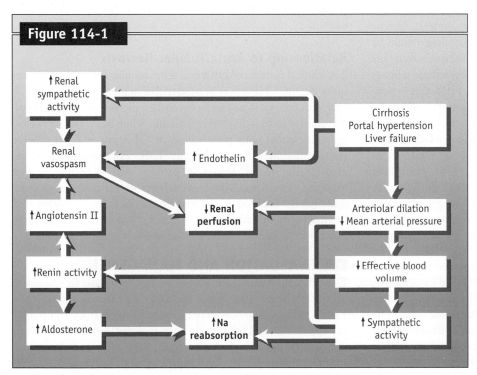

Figure 114-1

A simple outline of the key pathophysiologic events in the development of ascites and hepatorenal syndrome. Portal hypertension and liver failure cause arterial vasodilation, decreasing the effective arterial volume. This activates the renin-angiotensin system as well as sympathetic activity, causing renal sodium retention. The decrease in mean arterial pressure due to arterial vasodilation further decreases renal perfusion.

Table 114-2. Putative Mediators of the Hemodynamic Changes in Hepatorenal Syndrome

Vasodilators	Vasoconstrictors
Nitric oxide	Neurohumoral regulators
Glucagon	Systemic sympathetic activity
Prostacyclins	Renal sympathetic activity
Endotoxin	Angiotensin
Adenosine	Endothelin
	Primarily intrarenal vasoconstrictors
	Cysteinyl leukotrienes
	Thromboxane A_2
	F_2-isoprostanes

Table 114-3. Disorders Associated With Renal and Liver Failure

Congenital
  Caroli's disease and medullary sponge kidneys
  Polycystic liver and kidney disease (rare)
Vascular
  Severe congestive heart failure
  Shock
  Thrombosis of inferior vena cava
Infectious
  Sepsis
  Leptospirosis
  Yellow fever and other hemorrhagic virus infections
  Falciparum malaria
Toxic
  Acetaminophen overdose
  Phosphorus (in rat poisons)
  Methoxyflurane
  CCl_4
  Tetracycline
Vasculitides and immunologic disorders
  Polyarteritis nodosa
  Systemic lupus erythematosus
  Amyloidosis
Pregnancy-related
  Toxemia of pregnancy
  HELLP syndrome
Neoplastic
  Hepatocellular carcinoma and hypercalcemia or polycythemia
  Metastatic disease
Miscellaneous disorders
  Reye's syndrome
  Hypovolemia in a patient with cirrhosis
Hepatorenal syndrome

tality in those who are not candidates for liver transplantation, renal failure is a major risk factor for perioperative morbidity and mortality in those who do undergo liver transplantation [15••,16]. Development of renal insufficiency in a patient with severe liver disease should, therefore, be vigorously evaluated and treated.

The key to evaluation of HRS is exclusion of other causes of renal failure. A list of disorders associated with either simultaneous renal and liver failure or renal failure in the setting of liver disease is provided in Table 114-3. While most of these conditions are easily excluded, two problems which often are difficult to diagnose in patients with liver disease and which may cause diagnostic confusion are hypovolemia and sepsis.

True hypovolemia has the same clinical manifestations as does the relative hypovolemia seen in persons with HRS. The features of peripheral vasoconstriction usually associated with hypovolemia may not develop in the cirrhotic patient because of underlying vasodilation. The two most common causes of true hypovolemia in persons with liver disease are diuresis and lactulose-induced diarrhea. Therefore, when azotemia develops, diuretic therapy should be stopped or decreased. The dose of lactulose should be adjusted so that the patient has three to four bowel movements per day; appropriate fluid replacement must be provided for persons with diarrhea. Ultimately distinction between HRS and hypovolemia often requires a fluid challenge. Patients with true hypovolemia respond to a fluid challenge with an increase in urine output and correction of azotemia, whereas those with HRS do not.

Sepsis is another complication frequently encountered in patients with end-stage cirrhosis. Individuals with severe liver disease often do not have a febrile response to infection. Alternately, some patients with cirrhosis have low-grade fever in the absence of infection. Any alteration in mental status or unexplained deterioration in the clinical condition should prompt a search for infection in a cirrhotic individual. Ascitic fluid must be sampled for culture and cell count, and the presence of pneumonia, urinary tract infection, and bacteremia excluded by appropriate tests. The hemodynamic changes of septicemia are identical to those of HRS and, therefore, are not of diagnostic value. The final diagnosis of HRS requires demonstration of azotemia that does not respond to fluid challenge in the setting of severe liver failure and no other obvious cause of renal failure.

Relationship to Acute Tubular Necrosis

The clinical pictures of HRS and acute tubular necrosis usually are quite different. HRS is associated with a marked decrease in GFR and with tubular injury and a secondary increase in the fractional excretion of sodium to greater than one, while acute tubular necrosis is associated with preservation of GFR and marked tubular reabsorption of sodium and water. Laboratory indices, however, occasionally are ambiguous in patients with liver disease and azotemia, and there have been reports of HRS progressing to acute tubular necrosis. Also, recent studies have shown evidence of tubular injury in patients with HRS. It therefore is possible that HRS may progress to acute tubular necrosis in some patients.

■ EVALUATION AND MANAGEMENT

Evaluation and therapy must begin simultaneously in suspected cases of HRS because of the seriousness of the disorder (Table 114-4). Many diagnoses may be excluded by history and physical examination. Diuretic therapy worsens electrolyte abnormalities in persons with azotemia, and therefore should be stopped. In those with diarrhea, the dose of lactulose should be decreased until diarrhea resolves, and appropriate volume replacement should be provided for fluid losses. Urine electrolytes should be measured, and blood cultures, urine analysis, and a chest radiograph should be performed to rule out infection; urine analysis should include a search for crystalluria that may contribute to renal insufficiency. Ascitic fluid must be examined to exclude development of spontaneous bacterial peritonitis. Nonsteroidal anti-inflammatory drugs should be avoided and other potentially nephrotoxic drugs should be stopped. Finally, a renal ultrasound examination for evidence of obstructive uropathy should be performed.

These diagnostic measures are accompanied by therapy to optimize the volume status of the patient. This usually involves administration of an intravenous fluid challenge of 1 and 1.5 L over a 12–24-hour period. While no data exist indicating the type of intravenous fluids that should be used, a combination of colloid (albumin infusion) and crystalloid (NaCl) is recommended. Diagnosis of HRS hinges on the failure of the patient to improve after such a fluid challenge.

Many of these diagnostic maneuvers also serve as treatment of renal insufficiency in patients with cirrhosis. This is particularly true in cases of iatrogenic renal insufficiency, where discontinuation of diuretic therapy may improve renal function. In those with HRS, management is guided by the natural history of the untreated disease, which almost always ends in death within one to two weeks [15••]. Orthotopic liver transplant is the only treatment that has been consistently shown to correct HRS [16••]. The candidacy of a patient with HRS for liver transplant, therefore, must be established as early as possible (see Chapter 117).

A key aspect of the general management of a patient with HRS is optimization of hemodynamic status (Table 114-5). The aggressiveness with which this is attempted often depends on the patient's candidacy for liver transplantation. Ideally, the patient should be moved to an intensive care unit and a Swan-Ganz catheter placed to guide volume replacement. The goal of intravenous colloid and crystalloid administration is to bring the pulmonary capillary wedge pressure to values of between 13 and 17 mm Hg. The risks of invasive monitoring may be minimized by correction of coagulopathy. Life-threatening acid-base

disorders also should be corrected. During this process, the patient should be monitored closely for signs of worsening azotemia, (eg, encephalopathy, hyperphosphatemia, hypermagnesemia, and pericardial friction rub).

Systemic Vasoconstrictors

Therapy with systemic vasoconstrictors and large-volume paracentesis may be used to increase mean arterial pressure and decrease renal vein pressures respectively, thereby improving renal perfusion. A number of phamacologic agents have been used for this purpose, but the results have, in general, been disappointing.

Renal Vasodilators

After an attempt to improve systemic hemodynamics has failed to produce a diuresis, treatment with a renal vasodilator may be initiated, either alone or in combination with systemic vasoconstrictors. A single study found that intravenous infusion of "renal-dose" dopamine induced a diuresis in patients with HRS [17]. Other agents that have been used include phentolamine, and prostaglandins A1 and E; an initial study found a beneficial effect of vasodilatory prostaglandins in patients with HRS [18]. Unfortunately, other studies have failed to corroborate these data.

Splanchnic Vasoconstrictors

The rationale for use of splanchnic vasoconstrictors to treat HRS is that they will shift blood that has pooled in the splanchnic bed back into the systemic circulation, thereby correcting relative hypovolemia and decreasing the tendency for sodium retention and improving renal perfusion. There are anecdotal reports of

---

Table 114-4. Diagnostic Evaluation of Renal Insufficiency in a Patient With Cirrhosis and Ascites

Clinical evaluation
Laboratory studies
  Complete blood count
  BUN, serum creatinine, serum electrolytes, liver tests, phosphate, magnesium
  Urine analysis
  Urine Na, Fe_{Na}
Renal ultrasound
Abdominal paracentesis
Blood cultures (if indicated)
Chest radiograph
Fluid challenge

Table 114-5. Management of Hepatorenal Syndrome

Exclude hypovolemia and sepsis
  Fluid challenge
  Swan-Ganz catherization
  Antibiotics
Optimization of hemodynamics
  Steps to increase mean arterial pressure
    Correct anemia
    Colloid and crystalloid infusion
    Systemic vasoconstrictors: dopamine, norepinephrine
    Splanchnic vasoconstrictors: vasopressin
  Renal vasodilators
    Renal dose dopamine
    Prostaglandins
  Large-volume paracentesis with intravenous albumin infusion
Hemodialysis
Orthotopic liver transplant
Miscellaneous
  Peritoneovenous shunt
  Transjugular intrahepatic portasystemic shunt
General measures
  Treat encephalopathy
  Cardiopulmonary support
  Monitor for sepsis

the use of vasopressin and terlipressin for this purpose [19], although there are no data to show that these agents modify the natural history of HRS. In the patient who is not a transplant candidate, it may be reasonable to attempt a therapeutic trial of splanchnic vasoconstrictors, because there is little else to offer.

Dialysis

Perhaps the most important treatment available to support patients with HRS is hemodialysis. Hemodialysis corrects life-threatening azotemia and prolongs life, albeit with some morbidity and at considerable cost. Although evaluable data on cost-efficacy do not exist, dialysis usually is not performed on patients with terminal liver failure and HRS who are not liver transplant candidates. In the appropriate setting, (eg, a patient with acute alcoholic hepatitis and HRS but not cirrhosis), treatment with hemodialysis is not unreasonable, even though liver transplant is not being considered in the immediate future.

Peritoneovenous Shunt

Several studies have shown that a diuresis occurs following placement of a peritoneovenous shunt in patients with refractory ascites or HRS [20••,21]. This treatment, however, is associated with considerable morbidity and some mortality, and outcome after peritoneovenous shunting is not as good in patients with HRS as in those with ascites refractory to medical therapy. Shunt procedures of this type may be complicated by pulmonary edema in patients with poor myocardial function. Use of peritoneovenous shunts has declined considerably in the United States during the past 15 years.

Surgical Portal Decompression

Surgical construction of venous shunts to correct portal hypertension may be done to reverse the hemodynamic abnormalities associated with HRS. Given the very high morbidity and mortality of surgical shunting in patients with HRS, it is, however, rarely used.

Transjugular Intrahepatic Portasystemic Shunt

Transjugular intrahepatic portasystemic shunt (TIPS) achieves portal decompression without the risks of general anesthesia and major surgery. Two preliminary anecdotal studies reported improvement of azotemia and diuresis after TIPS placement in patients with HRS [22,23]. Prospective data on large numbers of patients, however, are unavailable. The use of TIPS in the therapy of HRS therefore must be considered experimental at this time. This is particularly so because TIPS may worsen renal failure due to the radiocontrast used and also worsen liver function by diverting sinusoidal blood flow away from the liver.

Orthotopic Liver Transplantation

Liver transplantation is, without a doubt, the single most effective treatment modality for patients with HRS [16••]; it corrects the underlying liver disease as well as HRS. Every patient with HRS is, by definition, a candidate for liver transplantation unless a specific contraindication exists to this procedure. It is, therefore, critically important to refer the patient to a transplant center early in the course of HRS. A quick evaluation to assess the potential risks and contraindications to transplant should be performed as soon as possible after diagnosis.

Future Therapies

There is considerable interest in development of endothelin antagonists, and thromboxane and nitric oxide inhibitors for treatment of HRS. Clinical trials of these and other agents will be necessary to define their roles in the future therapy of HRS.

Use of Specific Therapies

The numerous treatments for HRS are testimony to their limited efficacy; the precise approach to therapy used at a given institution and even for a given patient varies significantly. Evaluation of patients with HRS for liver transplantation at the time of presentation is recommended (Fig. 114-2). Potential transplantation candidates are moved to an intensive care unit if they fail to respond to an intravenous fluid challenge. Diuretics are discontinued and diarrheal fluid and electrolyte losses are corrected. A Swan-Ganz catheter is inserted to guide volume therapy in transplantation candidates. When the pulmonary wedge pressure is approximately 15 mm Hg, a large-volume paracentesis is performed, accompanied by infusion of intravenous albumin (6–8 g/L ascites removed), and a dopamine infusion is started at renal vasodilatory doses. If a diuresis does not occur within 12 hours of beginning treatment, systemic vasoconstrictive doses of dopamine are administered; prostaglandin infusion may be substituted for dopamine in selected cases. Hemodialysis may be performed to correct symptomatic azotemia, hyerphosphatemia, or hypermagnesemia. General supportive care including cardiopulmonary life support is provided until a liver transplantation can be performed or the patient dies. Either a TIPS or a peritoneovenous shunt may be attempted in patients with HRS who are not transplantation candidates although neither has been shown conclusively to improve survival.

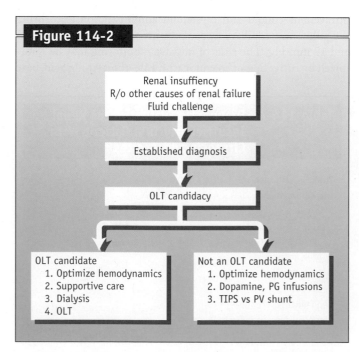

Figure 114-2

Renal insuffiency
R/o other causes of renal failure
Fluid challenge

↓

Established diagnosis

↓

OLT candidacy

OLT candidate
1. Optimize hemodynamics
2. Supportive care
3. Dialysis
4. OLT

Not an OLT candidate
1. Optimize hemodynamics
2. Dopamine, PG infusions
3. TIPS vs PV shunt

A general scheme for the management of the patient with hepatorenal syndrome.

REFERENCES

Recently published papers of particular interest have been highlighted as follows:
- • Of interest
- •• Of outstanding interest

1.•• Arroyo V, Gines P, Gerbes AL, *et al.*: Definition and diagnostic criteria of refractory ascites and hepatorenal syndrome in cirrhosis. *Hepatol* 1996, 23:(1):164–176.

2. Henriksen J: Cirrhosis: ascites and hepatorenal syndrome: recent advances in pathogenesis. *J Hepatol* 1995, 23:(suppl 1):25–30.

3.• Moore K: The hepatorenal syndrome. *Clin Science* 1997, 92:433–443.

4. Henriksen JH: Systemic hemodynamic alterations in hepatic cirrhosis. *Eur J Gastroenterol Hepatol* 1991, 3:705–713.

5.•• Groszmann RJ: Hyperdynamic state in chronic liver disease. *J Hepatol* 1993, 17:538–540.

6. Lewis FW, Adair O, Rector WG: Arterial vasodilation is not the cause of increased cardiac output in alcoholic cirrhosis. *Gastro* 1992, 102:1024–1029.

7. Benoit JN, Granger DN: Splanchnic hemodynamics in chronic portal hypertension. *Semin Liv Dis* 1986, 6:287–298.

8. Cioni G, D'Alimonte P, Zerbinati F, *et al.*: Duplex-Doppler ultrasonography in the evaluation of cirrhotic patients with portal hypertension and in the analysis of their response to drugs. *J Gastroenterol Hepatol* 1992, 7:388–392.

9. Darnault P, Bretagne JF, Raoul JL, *et al.*: Assessment of the role of portal hypertension and liver failure in lowering splanchnic vascular resistance. *Gastro International* 1988, 1:1017–1023.

10. Van Roey G, Moore K: The hepatorenal syndrome. *Pediatr Nephrol* 1996, 10:100–107.

11. Schrier RW, Arroyo V, Bernardi M, *et al.*: Peripheral arterial vasodilation hypothesis: a proposal for the initiation of renal sodium and water retention in cirrhosis. *Hepatol* 1988, 8:1151–1157.

12. Bomzon A, Blendis L: The nitric oxide hypothesis and the hyperdynamic circulation in cirrhosis. *Hepatol* 1994, 20:1343–1350.

13. Moncada S, Palmer RMJ, Higgs EA: Nitric oxide: physiology, pathophysiology and pharmacology. *Pharmacol Rev* 1991, 43:109–142.

14. Wood LJ, Massie D, Mclean AJ, Dudley FJ: Renal sodium retention in cirrhosis: tubular site and relation to hepatic dysfunction. *Hepatol* 1988, 8:831–836.

15.•• Gines A, Escorsell A, Gines P, *et al.*: Incidence, predictive factors and prognosis of the HRS in patients with liver cirrhosis and ascites with and without functional renal failure. *Gastro* 1993, 105:229–236.

16.•• Gonwa TA, Morris CA, Goldstein RM, Doe J: Long-term survival and renal function following liver transplantation in patients with and without hepatorenal syndrome-experience in 300 patients. *Transplantation* 1991, 51:428–430.

17. Bacq Y, Gaudin C, Hadengue A, *et al.*: Systemic, splanchnic and renal hemodynamic effects of a dopaminergic dose of dopamine in patients with cirrhosis. *Hepatol* 1991, 14:483–487.

18. Fevery J, Van Cutsem E, Nevens F, Doe J: Reversal of hepatorenal syndrome in four patients by peroral misoprostol and albumin infusion. *J Hepatol* 1990, 11:153–158.

19. Ganne-Carrie N, Hadengue A, Mathurin P, *et al.*: Hepatorenal syndrome: long-term treatment with terlipressin as a bridge to liver transplantation. *Dig Dis Sci* 1996, 41:1054–1056.

20.•• Stanley MM, Ochi S, Lee KK, Nemchausky BA: Peritoneovenous shunting as compared with medical treatment in patients with alcoholic cirrhosis and massive ascites. *N Engl J Med* 1989, 321:1632–1638.

21. Linas SL, Schaefer JW, Moore EE, *et al.*: Peritoneovenous shunt in the management of the HRS. *Kidney Int* 1986, 30:736–740.

22. Spahr L, Fenyves D, N'Guyen VV, *et al.*: Improvement of hepatorenal syndrome by transjugular intrahepatic portosystemic shunt. *Am J Gastroenterol* 1995, 90:1169–1171.

23. Sturgis TM: Hepatorenal syndrome: resolution after transjugular intrahepatic portosystemic shunt. *J Clin Gastroenterol* 1995, 20:241–243.

115 Hepatic Encephalopathy

Gregory T. Everson and Roshan Shrestha

DEFINITION

Hepatic encephalopathy (portal-systemic encephalopathy [PSE]) is a neuropsychiatric syndrome that occurs in patients with either severe acute liver failure, chronic liver disease, or as a consequence of surgical or radiologic portal-systemic shunts [1••]. It is characterized by personality changes, impaired mental function, motor abnormalities (asterixis, tremor, hyperventilation, hyperactive reflexes), and altered consciousness. The encephalopathy accompanying acute hepatic failure has an abrupt onset with a short prodrome, a rapid progression, and often ends in the death of the patient. Patients sequentially experience drowsiness, delirium, agitation or convulsions, decerebrate rigidity, unresponsiveness, and deep coma within a comparatively short period of time, usually hours to days (Table 115-1). Encephalopathy in the setting of acute liver failure commonly is associated with cerebral edema and increased intracranial pressure. If untreated, irreversible neurologic damage may occur as a result of brain ischemia or herniation. Patients who develop coma in the setting of acute liver failure have a grave prognosis; fewer than 20% survive without hepatic transplantation.

In patients with chronic liver disease, encephalopathy develops insidiously and often is heralded by a change in mental status or behavior. Episodes are sporadic, characterized by exacerbations and remissions, and generally are precipitated by inciting events. Although the initial manifestation of PSE usually is a subtle change in mentation, neurologic dysfunction may progress to confusion, lethargy, and even coma (Table 115-1). Neurologic signs vary and fluctuate, but usually include asterixis, hyper-reflexia, clonus, and an extensor plantar response.

Causes of chronic PSE may not always be apparent, but azotemia, sepsis, gastrointestinal bleeding, dehydration, and sedatives are frequent precipitants (Table 115-2). In some patients, encephalopathy may not be obvious clinically and only may be detectable by psychometric testing. By these tests, about two-thirds of cirrhotic patients with portal hypertension have subclinical PSE [2].

PATHOGENESIS AND MECHANISMS OF ENCEPHALOPATHY

No single abnormality of hepatic or neurologic metabolism adequately explains all of the clinical, biochemical, physiologic, and experimental findings of PSE in either patients or animals [1••]. Abnormal levels of multiple neurotransmitters, including glutamate, γ-aminobutyric acid (GABA), dopamine, serotonin, and opioids, have been described and plasma levels of a wide array of potential neurotoxins (ammonia, GABA, short-chain fatty acids, methanethiols) are increased (Table 115-3). Despite this seeming confusion, several lines of investigation continue to focus on ammonia as a key factor in the pathogenesis of PSE. Recent studies suggest a causative role for ammonia in the derangement of glutamate and glutamine metabolism in the central nervous system (CNS). Other studies suggest that GABA metabolism and its function as an inhibitory neurotransmitter are severely altered. The central benzodiazepine receptor is physically linked to the GABA receptor, providing a rationale for use of benzodiazepine antagonists in the treatment of PSE. Neuropathologic studies demonstrate marked changes in CNS glial cells. Acute encephalopathy is characterized by astrocytic swelling but chronic encephalopathy is characterized by Alzheimer type II astrocytosis. Finally, acute liver failure also is characterized by disordered cerebral blood flow, impaired cerebral vascular autoregulation, and altered cerebral metabolism.

AMMONIA HYPOTHESIS

The ammonia (NH3) hypothesis states that the major cause of PSE is excessive accumulation of NH3 and increased cerebral sensitivity to its toxic effects. Studies using positron-emission tomography (PET) have demonstrated an increase in cerebral

metabolic rate and increased permeability of the blood-brain barrier to ammonia in PSE. Blood ammonia originates mainly from four sources: intrahepatic deamination of amino acids, extrahepatic metabolism of nucleotides, gut metabolism of glutamine, and bacterial degradation of intestinal protein and urea [3•]; more than 50% of blood ammonia is derived from the latter source. Ammonia normally is metabolized by the liver to either urea or glutamine by the actions of carbamoyl-phosphate synthetase I (initiating enzyme of the urea cycle) and glutamine synthetase, respectively. Patients with hepatic failure have impaired ammonia metabolism related to a reduction in liver metabolism and an increase in portal-systemic shunting. As a result, an elevation in blood ammonia is a characteristic feature of severely impaired hepatic function [4•]. Clinical and experimental observations link an increase in blood ammonia levels to PSE.

Increased Plasma Levels of Ammonia

Hyperammonemia and elevated cerebrospinal fluid (CSF) ammonia concentrations are features of acute and chronic hepatic

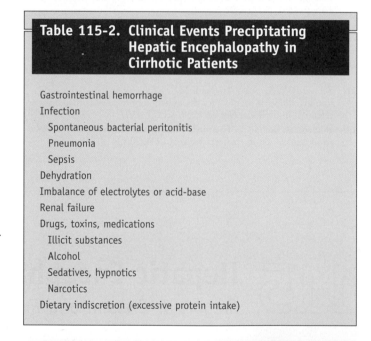

Table 115-2. Clinical Events Precipitating Hepatic Encephalopathy in Cirrhotic Patients

Gastrointestinal hemorrhage
Infection
   Spontaneous bacterial peritonitis
   Pneumonia
   Sepsis
Dehydration
Imbalance of electrolytes or acid-base
Renal failure
Drugs, toxins, medications
   Illicit substances
   Alcohol
   Sedatives, hypnotics
   Narcotics
Dietary indiscretion (excessive protein intake)

Table 115-3. Brain Neurotoxins or Neuroinhibitors That Accumulate in Hepatic Failure

Ammonia
Manganese
Glutamine
GABA
Taurine
Benzodiazepine receptor ligands
Monoamines
Opioids
Methanethiols

GABA—γ-aminobutyric acid.

Table 115-1. Stages of Encephalopathy*

Stage	Clinical signs
Stage I	Mental slowness, mild confusion, euphoria, slurred speech, and disordered sleep rhythm
Stage II	Drowsiness, inappropriate behavior, inability to control sphincter tone (incontinence of urine and stool), and agitation
Stage III	Lethargic, sleeps most of the time but arousable, speech is incoherent, marked confusion
Stage IV	Coma, patient may or may not respond to painful stimuli

* Patients with acute liver failure commonly exhibit cerebral edema by either imaging studies of the brain or by ICP monitoring when they have either Stage III or IV encephalopathy. Patients with chronic liver disease rarely demonstrate cerebral edema, regardless of the stage of encephalopathy.

encephalopathy, Reye's syndrome, deficiencies of urea cycle enzymes, and sodium valproate toxicity.

Ammonia Challenge

In cirrhotics or patients with portacaval shunts, ingestion of ammonia-generating substances (protein, amino acids, urea, ammonium salts) may precipitate PSE. In animals, chronic administration of ammonium salts results in Alzheimer type II astrocytosis, a change indistinguishable from that observed in patients with chronic PSE.

Ammonia, Glutamine, Glutamatergic Neurotransmitter System

The glutamatergic excitatory neurotransmitter system in the CNS is markedly altered in patients with both acute and chronic liver disease and in animal models of PSE. CNS astrocytes are a major regulatory cell in the glutamatergic system. Normally, the astrocyte avidly takes up excess glutamate from the synaptic cleft, an important function that terminates glutamate-induced neuroexcitation. Once glutamate is taken up by the astrocyte, it is metabolized to glutamine by glutamine synthetase, which utilizes blood-derived ammonia (Fig. 115-1). In liver failure and hyperammonemia, glutamate uptake into neurons and astrocytes is diminished and glutamate accumulates in extracellular fluid. Hyperammonemia favors formation of glutamine but also impairs release of glutamine from the astrocyte; accumulation of osmotically active glutamine in the astrocyte is associated with cell swelling. Clinically, levels of glutamine and glutamate increase in CSF in hyperammonemic states, and CSF glutamine concentrations correlate loosely with the stage of PSE. In animal models of acute PSE, blockade of glutamine production by an inhibitor of glutamine synthetase, methionine sulfoximine, decreases cerebral edema and reduces astrocyte swelling.

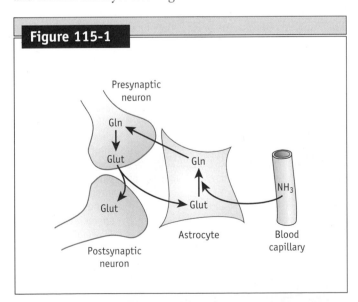

Figure 115-1

The formation of glutamine occurs predominantly in the astrocyte. Glutamine is pumped out of the astrocyte and taken up by presynaptic neurons where it is converted to glutamate. Nerve stimulation releases glutamate, which acts as an excitatory neurotransmitter. Astrocytes avidly take up glutamate from the synaptic cleft, to abolish neuronal stimulation. Gln—glutamine; Glut—glutamate; NH_3—ammonia.

Clinical Results of Reduced Intestinal Production of Ammonia

Intestinal production of ammonia is reduced by oral neomycin and nonabsorbable disaccharides, including lactulose, lactitol, and lactose in lactase-deficient patients. These treatments lower plasma ammonia and improve subjective and objective measures of PSE.

Lack of Correlation Between Blood Ammonia Level and the Degree of Encephalopathy

Other clinical and experimental observations refute the link between ammonia and hepatic encephalopathy. Blood ammonia levels are elevated in cirrhotic patients regardless of whether they have PSE. Some patients with PSE have normal blood ammonia levels. The grade of PSE does not correlate with blood ammonia concentration.

Seizures Are Not a Feature of Portal-Systemic Encephalopathy

Seizures and hyperexcitability commonly are observed in animals with ammonia intoxication and in human congenital hyperammonemias, but rarely are observed in patients with chronic PSE. Administration of ammonium chloride to cirrhotic patients induces a mild hyperkinesis but fails to exacerbate typical chronic encephalopathy.

■ γ-AMINOBUTYRIC ACID-BENZODIAZEPINE RECEPTOR HYPOTHESIS

γ-Aminobutyric acid (GABA) is an inhibitory neurotransmitter found throughout the CNS [5••]. The GABA hypothesis states that an excess of GABA, or increased sensitivity to GABA, is responsible for PSE [6]. GABA originates from the intestine, and plasma GABA levels increase in liver failure due to inadequate hepatic extraction. In patients with acute liver failure, the blood-brain barrier becomes more permeable and increased amounts of GABA enter the brain [7]. Once in the brain, GABA binds to its receptor to produce neuroinhibition and clinical encephalopathy. A key component to understanding the relationship of GABA and benzodiazepines was the recognition that the GABA receptor was tightly linked to and modulated by the benzodiazepine receptor. Binding of benzodiazepines to the benzodiazepine receptor induces a conformational change in the GABA receptor, enhancing the binding of GABA and neuroinhibition [8•]. Activation of the GABA receptor opens a chloride channel, the third component of the GABA receptor complex (Fig. 115-2).

The GABA hypothesis predicts that benzodiazepines will increase the severity of PSE and that benzodiazepine antagonists (eg, flumazenil), may ameliorate PSE. Clinical experience clearly suggests that cirrhotic patients, especially those with PSE, are particularly sensitive to the amnesic and sedative effects of benzodiazepines. Indeed, use of benzodiazepines and other sedative-hypnotics is a common reason for exacerbations of PSE. Recent studies have demonstrated that patients with PSE have increased plasma level of benzodiazepines or "natural" benzodiazepine-like compounds which then may act as "false neurotransmitters" [9,10]. Some have suggested that persons with PSE are particularly sensitive to GABA neuroinhibition, due to an increase in background benzodiazepine stimulation of the GABA receptor.

▰▰ OTHER NEUROTRANSMITTERS AND NEUROTOXINS

Dopaminergic System

Patients with chronic PSE often have abnormal motor functions, including tremor, slowness of gait, ataxia, and even rigidity. Although they typically lack other features of Parkinsonism (pill-rolling, resting tremor, masklike facies, cogwheel rigidity), their motor abnormalities prompted investigators to suggest that patients with PSE may have impairment of the dopaminergic system. It is postulated that "false" neurotransmitters occupy dopaminergic-binding sites within the CNS, and inactivate and inhibit dopaminergic activity. Clinical trials in humans, however, have failed to provide much support for this hypothesis. Both L-dopa and bromcriptine, an L-dopa agonist, are ineffective therapies for PSE (see below).

Serotonergic System

A number of alterations in CNS serotonin have been described in both humans and experimental animal models of PSE. CNS levels of serotonin, serotonin receptors, and monoamine oxidases are increased. The exact role of serotonin in PSE, however, remains undefined.

Taurine

Taurine is an inhibitory neurotransmitter that is increased in brains of animals with PSE and in the CSF of primates with PSE secondary to portacaval shunts. Plasma levels of taurine are greatest in patients with the greatest degrees of PSE, suggesting that this inhibitory neurotransmitter may be involved in PSE. Other neurotransmitters that may be altered in PSE include opioids and melatonin.

Methanethiols

Interest in methanethiol as a potential neurotoxin began with the finding of methanethiol in the urine of a patient with fetor hepaticus [9]. Subsequently, methanethiol, 4-methylthio-2-oxobutyrate, and methanethiol-mixed disulfide levels were elevated in the plasma of cirrhotic patients. It was suggested that these compounds may exacerbate the toxic effects of ammonia and short-chain fatty acids. Blood levels of methonethiols, however, are similar in deeply comatose patients and those with only mild cerebral dysfunction, and there is little correlation of grade of PSE with blood levels.

Fatty Acids

Short chain fatty acid (SCFA) levels are increased in the peripheral circulation of cirrhotic patients with PSE. Normally, the liver metabolizes these fatty acids after they are absorbed from the gut, but this function is impaired in cirrhotics. The clinical severity of PSE correlates poorly with plasma levels of acetic, propionic, butyric, valeric, and octanoic acids, and SCFAs have been administered to patients with cirrhosis without worsening of PSE. SCFAs are not likely to cause PSE.

Manganese, Zinc

The liver is responsible for manganese excretion and liver disease is associated with manganese accumulation. Magnetic resonance imaging of the brain in patients with cirrhosis reveals pallidal hyperintensity on TI-weight images (Fig. 115-3) which correlates with the presence of extrapyramidal signs and symptoms and blood levels of manganese [10]. Manganese concentrations in the globus pallidus are markedly increased in autopsy studies of cirrhotic patients who died in hepatic coma. PET scanning reveals reduced cerebral glucose utilization in these areas. These findings suggest a relationship between manganese, brain hypometabolism, and some of the neuropsychiatric and motor abnormalities of PSE. Zinc deficiency is common in patients with long-standing cirrhosis. Its importance in the pathogenesis of PSE is unknown, and three randomized, controlled trials of zinc supplementation have yielded conflicting results as regards to improvement in PSE (one positive, two negative).

▰▰ CLINICAL FEATURES

The initial manifestations of PSE may be quite subtle and include personality changes, mental slowing, euphoria, or depression. With progression, symptoms reflect global neurologic impairment

---

Figure 115-2

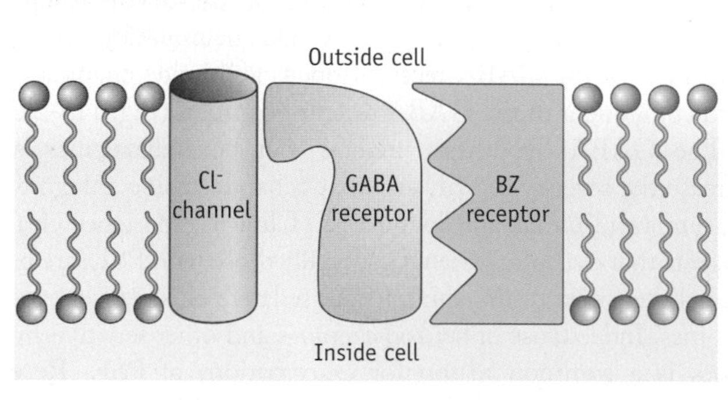

Outside cell

Cl⁻ channel | GABA receptor | BZ receptor

Inside cell

The GABA receptor complex is composed of the GABA receptor, central benzodiazepine receptor (BZ-R), and chloride channel. Binding of GABA to GABA-R opens the chloride channel, hyperpolarizes the neuronal membrane, and inhibits neurotransmission. Activation of the BZ-R by BZ or BZ-like compounds potentiates the binding of GABA to GABA-R.

Figure 115-3

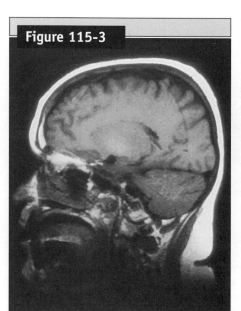

This magnetic resonance image (MRI) is a sagittal view of the brain through the region of the globus pallidus. Hyperintensity of the globus pallidus is appreciated on this T1-weighted scan (whitish area in the middle of the field).

(*eg*, confusion, and disorientation to place, time, and person). In patients with chronic liver disease, fetor hepaticus is common but not invariable. Asterixis, the "flapping tremor," is due to involuntary intermittent relaxation of sustained motor activity but is less specific than fetor hepaticus for PSE and usually is only present in the late stages of encephalopathy. Asterixis is most easily elicited with the patient's arm outstretched, fingers separated, and wrists hyperextended. As the patient recovers from PSE, asterixis usually disappears. Initially, reflexes are present; the patient will respond to noxious stimuli, and deep tendon reflexes tend to be accentuated. As encephalopathy deepens, the patient may become areflexic with absent corneal reflexes, absent caloric responses, and loss of sphincter tone. Other neurologic findings may include decorticate rigidity or even decerebrate rigidity. All of these changes are potentially reversible with either medical therapy or recovery of liver function.

■ RISK FACTORS AND PRECIPITATING EVENTS

Gastrointestinal Hemorrhage

Gastrointestinal hemorrhage, even when hemodynamically insignificant, may still be life-threatening in patients with PSE, because blood in the gastrointestinal tract will acutely increase the protein load and precipitate more severe PSE. Extreme bleeding with hemodynamic compromise (*eg*, from bleeding esophageal varices), may decrease hepatic perfusion, induce ischemic liver injury, and further impair the liver's ability to metabolize the excess protein load. Rapid diagnosis and treatment of gastrointestinal hemorrhage is essential to proper management and control of PSE. For patients who do not respond to the usual medical therapies, it may be necessary to perform a portal-systemic shunt either surgically or radiologically (transjugular intrahepatic portal-systemic shunt (TIPS). Currently, TIPS is preferred; encephalopathy may worsen after either TIPS or surgical shunts (Table 115-4) [11•,12••].

Infection

Infection, in particular sepsis, may precipitate PSE in patients with chronic liver disease. The diagnosis of spontaneous bacterial peritonitis (SBP) should always be considered in a patient with ascites and new-onset PSE even in the absence of fever and abdominal pain (see Chapter 113). Patients with cirrhosis and malnutrition are susceptible to infections due to reduced

leukocyte migration, decreased serum bactericidal activity, depressed white-cell mobilization, and impaired phagocytosis. Infection increases protein catabolism, releasing aromatic amino acids that may contribute to PSE. Primary therapy is directed against the infection.

Protein Load

The link between dietary protein and PSE was established by clinical and experimental observations. PSE may be precipitated by protein ingestion and improved by reducing dietary protein. Protein is the major source of both ammonia and methanethiols. Controlled trials have shown that protein restriction ameliorates not only subjective clinical signs but also objective psychometric tests in PSE.

Patients with chronic liver disease have increased plasma levels of the aromatic amino acids, phenylalanine, tyrosine, methionine and free tryptophan, and decreased branched-chain amino acids. Some, but not all, studies have suggested that not only total protein load but also increases in aromatic amino acids may be associated with PSE.

Medications (Sedatives)

There are no sedatives that may be administered safely to cirrhotic patients with PSE. Because liver metabolism usually is severely impaired in these patients, the clearances of benzodiazepines, barbiturates, chlorpromazine, morphine, and opioid derivatives, including methadone, meperidine, and codeine, are reduced. With repeated dosing all of these compounds tend to accumulate in cirrhotic patients, increasing the degree and prolonging the duration of sedation.

Renal Failure

A common precipitant of PSE is excessive diuresis, resulting in relative depletion of intravascular volume and prerenal azotemia. Factors contributing to PSE include: electrolyte and acid-base imbalances; reduced fluid volume; and impaired renal clearance of metabolites, drugs, and toxins. Acute decompensation of intrinsic or chronic renal disease may be another cause of PSE. Certain renal disorders tend to occur in the setting of certain liver diseases: IgA nephropathy (Laennec's cirrhosis); membranoproliferative glomerulonephritis (viral hepatitis); nephrolithiasis (primary sclerosing cholangitis with inflammatory bowel disease); medullary sponge kidney (congenital hepatic fibrosis); and autosomal dominant polycystic kidney (polycystic liver).

Fluid, Electrolyte, and Acid-Base Imbalance

Portal Systemic Encephalopathy may be precipitated by dehydration, hypokalemia, and alkalosis. Metabolic alkalosis increases serum levels of nonionic ammonia that diffuses very rapidly into the CNS. Diffusion of ammonia into the brain and enhanced glutamine production may precipitate PSE either by astrocyte swelling and dysfunction or impairment of glutamatergic neurotransmission. With hepatic impairment, kidneys produce glucose from branched-chain amino acids (gluconeogenesis) in an attempt to maintain the peripheral energy supply. This process results in a decrease in serum branched-chain amino acid levels and an increase in the levels of relatively more toxic aromatic amino acids which may diffuse into the brain.

Table 115-4. Incidence of Clinical Encephalopathy After Portal-Systemic Shunts

Type of portal-systemic shunt	% PSE
Surgical shunt	
Proximal portal-caval shunt	21–43
Distal splenorenal shunt	18–51
TIPS	14–45

PSE—portal systemic encephalopathy; TIPS—transjugular intrahepatic portal-systemic shunt.

Hepatocellular Carcinoma

Hepatocellular carcinoma commonly occurs in cirrhotic patients (estimated risk of 1% to 3% per year) and its presence may be heralded by the onset of spontaneous PSE. If all other precipitating factors for PSE are excluded, the diagnosis of hepatocellular carcinoma should be entertained and serum alpha-fetoprotein levels measured, and imaging studies of the liver (ultrasound, CT scan, MRI) performed.

Surgical Shunt Procedure or TIPS

Portal-Systemic Encephalopathy is a common complication of diversion of portal blood flow by surgical portal-systemic shunts or TIPS (Table 115-4). Predictors of post-shunt PSE include: pre-shunt PSE, severe liver disease (Child-Pugh score ≥ 10); poor hepatic clearance of indocyanine green and lidocaine; and old age. The mechanisms of PSE after placement of a portal-systemic shunt include lack of compensatory dilation of the hepatic artery, lack of portal perfusion of the liver, and reduction in hepatocyte function. Clinically apparent PSE after placement of a shunt usually responds to medical treatment (low-protein diet, lactulose, neomycin). In rare circumstances, narrowing with a flow-reducing stent or occlusion of the shunt may be necessary to control the encephalopathy [13].

Noncompliance With Therapy

One of the most common factors precipitating PSE is noncompliance with dietary protein restriction and medical treatment. A careful history focusing on adherence to medical therapy is necessary in the evaluation of the encephalopathic patient.

■ DIAGNOSIS

The diagnosis of PSE is based on clinical suspicion in a patient with chronic liver disease and the impression is confirmed by resolution of signs and symptoms with medical therapy.

In acute liver failure, PSE rapidly progresses through well-defined stages from mild confusion to coma (Table 115-1). Computerized tomography may be performed to eliminate other possible diagnoses, including intracerebral or subdural hemorrhage, tumor, or infection. The major mechanism of PSE in the setting of acute liver failure is cerebral edema (Fig. 115-4); development of cerebral edema is unique to acute liver failure and is not a feature of PSE in chronic liver disease. Intracranial pressure (ICP) is monitored, usually when the patient achieves grade III encephalopathy, to guide treatment and to establish the prognosis for neurologic recovery. The key variable is cerebral perfusion pressure (CPP), defined as the difference between mean arterial pressure (MAP) and ICP. If CPP decreases below 40 mm Hg for 2 hours or longer, then meaningful neurologic recovery is unlikely.

In patients with chronic liver failure, PSE often occurs as the result of another complication, such as gastrointestinal hemorrhage. PSE typically resolves with effective treatment of the underlying condition, (eg, resolution of hemorrhage or treatment of infection), and institution of protein restriction and therapy with either lactulose or neomycin.

Occasionally, additional tests may be necessary to confirm the diagnosis of PSE. This is particularly true when PSE is the primary clinical manifestation of otherwise unsuspected liver disease or if the manifestations of PSE are predominantly a change in behavior or an unusual neurologic syndrome (seizure, focal neurologic deficits).

Plasma Ammonia

Elevated blood ammonia levels are common in cirrhotic patients, especially those with PSE [4•]. Some studies have demonstrated a correlation between blood ammonia level and the presence and grade of PSE, while others have not. In general, blood ammonia levels may be useful as a marker of liver disease but are of little diagnostic or clinical value in managing the cirrhotic patient with PSE.

Cerebrospinal Fluid Glutamine

The chronic elevation in blood ammonia level leads to accumulation of glutamine in the CNS. Measuring CSF glutamine levels may be useful in confusing cases, where the diagnosis of high-grade (III or IV) PSE is uncertain or questionable. A normal CSF glutamine level would virtually exclude the diagnosis; increased CSF glutamine levels could provide evidence in favor of the diagnosis.

Electroencephalography

Electroencephalography (EEG) abnormalities are relatively nonspecific in PSE and are similar to changes observed in patients with other forms of metabolic encephalopathy. Two findings have some specificity as regards PSE: reduced brain-stem auditory-evoked potentials and diminished visual-evoked potentials. In various studies, the percentage of encephalopathic cirrhotics with EEG abnormalities is highly variable (14% to 78%). Nevertheless, EEG findings are objective and may be used as an endpoint in evaluating response to therapy.

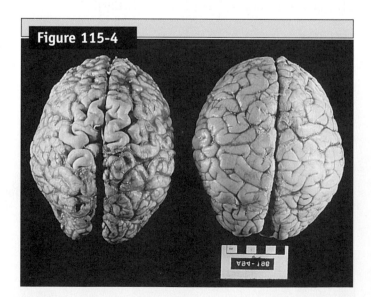

Figure 115-4

This figure shows two brain specimens which were removed at autopsy. The normal-appearing brain on the left exhibits well-spaced sulci between gyri. The brain on the right was removed from a patient with fulminant hepatic failure who died of cerebral edema with central brainstem herniation. Gyri are swollen and effaced with little remaining space remaining in the sulci.

Radiologic Imaging

Standard CT or nuclear brain scans exhibit little or no specific distinguishing features in patients with Laennec's cirrhosis and chronic PSE [14•] (Fig. 115-5), although loss of cortical volume may be common. CT may be used to document cerebral edema (Fig. 115-6) or to exclude CNS complications including tumor, infection, and hemorrhage. MRI may reveal a few relatively unique features of PSE. One feature, hyperintensity on T1-weighted images of globus pallidus (Fig. 115-3) correlates with motor disorders (extrapyramidal) and excess accumulation of manganese [15].

Neuropsychiatric Testing

In general, neuropsychiatric testing is used primarily to follow efficacy of treatment. A battery of tests is employed to distinguish

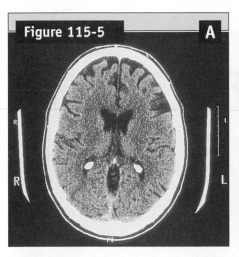
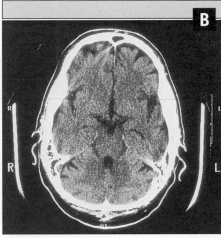

Computed tomography (CT) scans of the brain of a 42-year-old man with Laennec's cirrhosis and encephalopathy are shown. The image on the left demonstrates atrophy of the frontal cortex; the right image shows cerebellar atrophy.

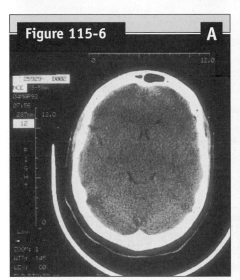
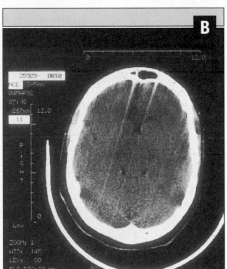
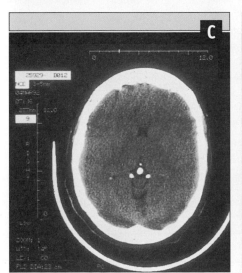
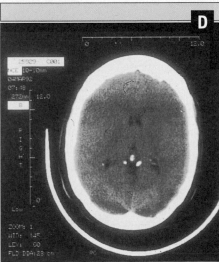

A to D Computed tomography (CT) scans of the brain of a patient with fulminant hepatic failure, stage IV hepatic coma, and cerebral edema. Note the diminished sulci and lack of distinction between white and gray matter. This patient's cerebral edema resolved with medical management and she subsequently received a liver transplant. She achieved complete neurologic recovery post-transplant.

PSE and organic brain syndrome from other causes of encephalopathy and underlying psychiatric disease. These tests are listed in Table 115-5. Poor performance on number connection tests correlates reasonably well with severity of encephalopathy and Child-Pugh classification.

THERAPY
Cerebral Edema

The management of cerebral edema in the setting of fulminant hepatic failure is a specialized topic beyond the scope of this chapter. Our general approach to treating this problem is presented in Table 115-6. Epidural or subdural placement of ICP transducers is preferred because intraparenchymal transducers are associated with a significant risk of intracerebral hemorrhage and even death. Treatment, which may include mechanical ventilation, intravenous mannitol infusion, barbiturate-induced coma, and continuous arteriovenous hemodialysis, is tailored to the clinical condition of the patient and to keep ICP pressure within the normal range.

HEPATIC ENCEPHALOPATHY (PORTAL-SYSTEMIC ENCEPHALOPATHY)
Low-Protein Diet

Traditional treatment for PSE has been to place patients on a protein-restricted diet of 40 to 70 g/d [16]. Several lines of clinical evidence support this recommendation: dietary protein is a major source of ammonia and methanethiols; an excessive ingestion of dietary protein has been documented to precipitate PSE in cirrhotic patients; restriction of dietary protein reduces the frequency and severity of attacks of PSE. Although restriction of dietary protein is recommended, patients are often noncompliant with this treatment because it requires a significant reduction in consumption of both meat and dairy products. In our experience, dietary indiscretion is a common cause of "spontaneous encephalopathy." A careful history and corroboration by family members is required to quantitate protein intake; consultation with a dietician is helpful to guide patients and their families. It is not necessary to restrict protein consumption in every cirrhotic patient; protein restriction should be limited to those with clinically evident PSE. Cirrhotic patients, especially those with advanced disease, often develop severe muscle wasting and unnecessary protein restriction may further worsen their poor nutritional state.

Branched-Chain Amino Acids

Early studies demonstrated that cirrhotic patients had an increase in aromatic amino acid levels and a decrease in branched-chain amino acid (BCAA) levels in blood samples. Subsequent clinical work suggested that patients with the greatest imbalance in plasma amino acids were more likely to be encephalopathic and to experience early and higher mortality. For this reason there have been at least 14 controlled trials of the use of BCAAs in the treatment of cirrhotic patients with chronic PSE. The results of these trials have been inconsistent and two separate meta-analyses yielded opposite conclusions regarding efficacy (one positive and one negative). In addition, BCAA preparations are much more expensive than standard amino acid supplements. Because the efficacy of therapy is unknown and its cost relatively high, we do

not currently recommend use of BCAAs in routine management of patients with chronic PSE. A trial of BCAA may be considered in a patient who is highly protein intolerant and who has severe protein-calorie malnutrition; BCAA supplements may allow adequate protein intake in this select group of individuals without increasing the frequency of PSE attacks.

Total Parenteral Nutrition

Total parenteral nutrition (TPN) often is inappropriate therapy for patients with severe chronic liver disease; it is expensive, and

---

Table 115-5. Neuropsychiatric Tests Used to Evaluate Hepatic Encephalopathy

	Test
Cerebral Function	
Learning and delayed recall	Story memory test
	Figure memory test
Concentration	Digit vigilance test
Fine motor coordination	Grooved pegboard
Sequential procedures	Trail-making test
Problem solving	Wisconsin card sorting test
Attention	WAIS-R digit symbol subtest
Vocabulary	WAIS-R vocabulary subtest
Verbal fluency skills	Controlled oral word association
	Animal naming
Auditory comprehension	Complex material
Visual-spatial analysis	WAIS-R block design subtest
Psychological function	MMPI-2

MMPI-2—Minnesota Multiphasic Personality Inventory-2; WAIS-R—Wechsler Adult Intelligence Scale-revised

---

Table 115-6. Treatment of Cerebral Edema in the Setting of Fulminant Hepatic Failure

General measures
Mechanical ventilation
  Head of bed elevation of 15° to 30°
  Hyperventilate to keep pCO_2 approximately 28–35 mmol/L
  Hyperventilate to keep PH 7.45–7.50
Monitoring of ICP
  Epidural or subdural transducers
  Maintain coagulation with FFP, cryoprecipitate, and platelets

Specific measures
Intravenous infusion of thiopental (or propofol)
Mannitol as needed to control ICP (do not exceed serum osmolarity of 310 mOsm/L)
Continuous hemodialysis for those in renal failure (mannitol is dialyzable)

ICP—intracranial pressure.

may cause complications (electrolyte imbalance, fluid overload, and infection). In most cases, TPN should be avoided and enteral feedings used in its place; care must be taken to avoid high enteral osmotic loads that may precipitate diarrhea and fluid and electrolyte imbalance. In addition, many enteral preparations have a high protein content (Table 115-7) for the amount of calories delivered. We currently use Suplena, which contains 7.1 g of protein for each 475 kcal. Enteral feeding tubes may erode esophageal varices and cause variceal hemorrhage.

Occasionally cirrhotic patients require TPN; indications include: the inability to deliver adequate calories by the enteral route; intercurrent disease (infection, diarrhea, bowel obstruction, forced purgation) which complicates the use of the enteral route for nutritional support; or a long stay in the intensive care unit. Encephalopathic patients should be restricted to 40 to 70 g of protein per day with the bulk of calories supplied as glucose and fat.

Lactulose

One of the most successful treatments for PSE is lactulose, a nonabsorbable disaccharide that is fermented by bacteria in the intestine to yield acetic, butyric, proprionic and lactic acids [17•, 18•,19]. The fermentation of lactulose produces an acidic milieu that alters the composition of the bacterial flora, lowers colonic pH, and produces an osmotic diarrhea. Each of these effects may be responsible for some of the beneficial effects of lactulose on PSE. Changing the composition of the bacterial flora may alter the metabolism of fecal contents and reduce production of ammonia, methanthiols, and other toxins that are responsible for PSE. The acidic luminal milieu creates an environment capable of trapping ammonia as ammonium ion. Ammonia (NH_3) is neutral and freely diffuses across the mucosal barrier of the colon where it then enters portal blood for delivery to the body. In contrast, the ammonium ion (NH_4^+), produced from the reaction of ammonia with hydrogen ion, is ionized, highly polar and cannot readily diffuse across the lipid bilayer of mucosal cells. NH_4^+ is "trapped" in the fecal effluent and eliminated with passage of a bowel movement. In addition to these properties, the breakdown of each molecule of lactulose produces at least four osmotically active particles. Water diffuses into the lumen, down the osmotic gradient, increasing fecal water content, and, if enough lactulose is given, a dose-dependent osmotic diarrhea results. The purgative effect of lactulose also may be responsible for altering the composition of colonic bacteria and helps to eliminate toxins and wastes that might otherwise accumulate. The usual recommendation is that enough lactulose be given to produce two to three semi-formed stools each day. Excessive lactulose will produce severe diarrhea with volume loss and electrolyte imbalance and should be avoided.

Neomycin

Neomycin is highly nephrotoxic and should never be given intravenously or parenterally. Orally administered neomycin is poorly absorbed, and is, therefore, much less nephrotoxic. The goal of oral neomycin therapy is to alter the bacterial composition of the colonic flora. The major advantage of neomycin over lactulose is that it does not cause diarrhea. The main disadvantage is that despite its poor absorption, some neomycin does enter the body and may cause nephrotoxicity. We recommend use of neomycin in patients who cannot tolerate lactulose (usually because of diarrhea). Also, we may add neomycin to lactulose to improve the efficacy of the medical regimen in controlling encephalopathy. Some have recommended that neomycin be given in short courses, lasting only 2 to 8 weeks, or only to bed-bound hospital patients [20•, 21].

Metronidazole

Studies have demonstrated that oral metronidazole 0.5 to 1.5 g/d given for one week was well tolerated, safe, and as effective as neomycin or lactulose in controlling PSE. Others have not observed similar efficacy and have shown only little effect of metronidazole on blood ammonia levels (Fig. 115-7). The advantages of metronidazole are that it does not cause diarrhea and it is not nephrotoxic. Disadvantages are that it may cause epigastric discomfort resulting in poor compliance with long-term treatment; maintenance therapy may cause peripheral neuropathy (already a problem in patients with advanced liver disease); and a "disulfiram reaction" when alcohol is consumed. The physician prescribing metronidazole to cirrhotic patients also should be aware that this drug undergoes extensive hepatic metabolism. One study of cirrhotic patients with PSE revealed a three-fold reduction in hepatic elimination of metronidazole and maintenance of therapeutic levels with as little as 500 mg given every 24 to 48 hours.

Dopaminergic Agents

One of the theories regarding the pathogenesis of PSE is that cirrhotic patients may have a relative deficiency of dopaminergic activity within the CNS. There have been three trials of the

Table 115-7.	Composition of Commonly Used Enteral Feedings				
Product	Volume, *oz*	Calories, *kcal*	Protein, *g*	Fat, *g*	CHO, *g*
Ensure	8	250	8.8	6.1	40.0
Ensure Plus	8	355	13.0	12.6	47.3
Osmolyte	8	250	8.8	8.2	35.6
Osmolyte HN Plus	8	284	13.2	9.3	37.5
Suplena*	8	475	7.1	22.7	60.6

CHO—carbohydrate.

Specifically recommended for patients who require protein, electrolyte, and fluid restriction.

use of L-dopa and bromcriptine, an L-dopa agonist that increases CNS L-dopa concentrations in the treatment of chronic PSE. Both agents were ineffective in improving clinical PSE, EEG, and encephalopathy scores. L-Dopa also was associated with impaired bowel motility and caused obstipation, an effect that counteracted the potentially beneficial CNS effects of the drug. For these reasons, dopaminergic agents have not been used in the clinical treatment of PSE.

Benzodiazepine Antagonists

There have been several randomized, controlled trials of flumazenil in the short-term treatment of PSE [22••,23-25]. In three of these studies, flumazenil was superior to placebo in improving the grade of PSE, 30% to 60% of encephalopathic patients improved after receiving flumazenil and EEGs changes paralleled this improvement. Patients in the two negative studies had milder grades of PSE. In the latter studies, flumazenil was no better than placebo in ameliorating symptoms of PSE and EEGs did not improve. In one study, brainstem acoustic-evoked responses were analyzed and again there was no effect of flumazenil. Given these somewhat contradictory results, it is unclear whether flumazenil is truly efficacious in the treatment of PSE and additional trials of larger numbers of subjects with varying grades of PSE are needed. Despite inconclusive results, however, the above studies are provocative. The striking reversal of PSE in some patients after administration of flumazenil suggests that the GABA-benzodiazepine receptor system is an important factor in the development of PSE.

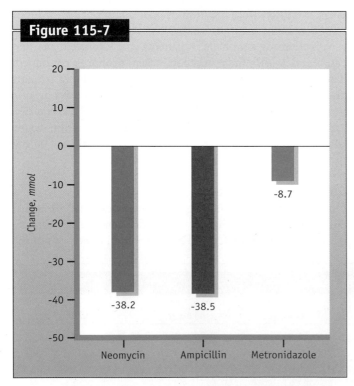

Figure 115-7

The authors observed that both neomycin and ampicillin had an equivalent effect on ammonia blood levels (*P*<0.01) but metronidazole was ineffective in lowering blood ammonia (*P* = NS). They also observed that stool pH was lower with neomycin and ampicillin and that bacterial urease and protease activity were markedly pH sensitive (inhibited by low pH).

Hepatic Transplantation

The neurologic manifestations of liver disease are listed in Table 115-8. Development of PSE in a patient with chronic liver disease indicates severe portal-systemic shunting and hepatic dysfunction [26••]. The prognosis for a patient who develops this complication is grim: 80% 1-year, 65% 2-year, and 55% 3-year survivals are reported. In addition, PSE is associated with significant morbidity including the inability to continue gainful employment, poor function at home, nursing strains on spouse or family, inability to drive a vehicle, and inability to handle personal finances. Although medical therapies may ameliorate the major symptoms of PSE, they rarely are effective enough to return the patient to full function. Often the patient with PSE is at risk for other life-threatening complications of liver disease, such as, variceal hemorrhage and SBP. In contrast, our current (University of Colorado Program in Liver Transplantation) overall 1-, 2-, and 3-year survivals after liver transplantation are 88%, 85%, and 82%, respectively (Fig. 115-8). For all of the above reasons, any patient with PSE should be considered for hepatic transplantation (Chapter 117).

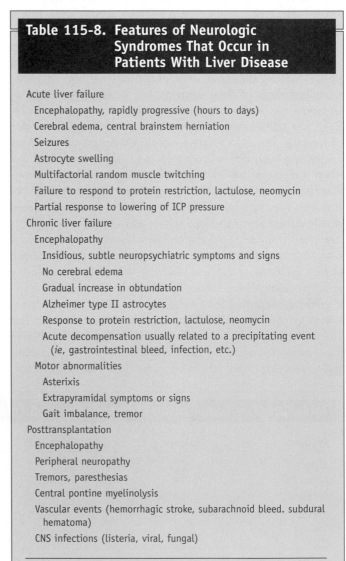

Table 115-8. Features of Neurologic Syndromes That Occur in Patients With Liver Disease

Acute liver failure
  Encephalopathy, rapidly progressive (hours to days)
  Cerebral edema, central brainstem herniation
  Seizures
  Astrocyte swelling
  Multifactorial random muscle twitching
  Failure to respond to protein restriction, lactulose, neomycin
  Partial response to lowering of ICP pressure
Chronic liver failure
  Encephalopathy
    Insidious, subtle neuropsychiatric symptoms and signs
    No cerebral edema
    Gradual increase in obtundation
    Alzheimer type II astrocytes
    Response to protein restriction, lactulose, neomycin
    Acute decompensation usually related to a precipitating event (*ie*, gastrointestinal bleed, infection, etc.)
  Motor abnormalities
    Asterixis
    Extrapyramidal symptoms or signs
    Gait imbalance, tremor
Posttransplantation
  Encephalopathy
  Peripheral neuropathy
  Tremors, paresthesias
  Central pontine myelinolysis
  Vascular events (hemorrhagic stroke, subarachnoid bleed. subdural hematoma)
  CNS infections (listeria, viral, fungal)

CNS—central nervous system; ICP—intracranial pressure.

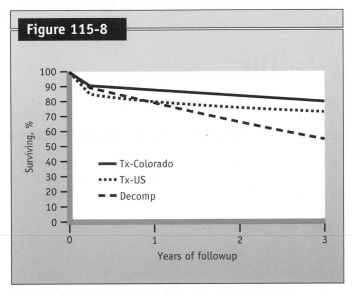

Figure 115-8

Survival of patients with HCV after onset of decompensation (encephalopathy, ascites or variceal bleed) is shown by the *dashed line* and compared with survival after transplantation in the US by the *dotted line* or in our program by the *solid line* (1996 Report of the UNOS Registry). A significant survival advantage is enjoyed by decompensated patients undergoing hepatic transplantation, without any excess early mortality.

■ REFERENCES

Recently published papers of particular interest have been highlighted as:
- • Of interest
- •• Of particular interest

1.•• Butterworth RF: The neurobiology of hepatic encephalopathy. *Seminars in Liver Disease* 1996; 16:235–244.

2. Quero JC, Schalm SW: Subclinical hepatic encephalopathy. *Seminars in Liver Disease* 1996; 16:321–328.

3.• Huizenga JR, Gips CH, Tangerman A: The contribution of various organs to ammonia formation: A review of factors determining the arterial ammonia concentration. *Annals of Clinical Biochemistry* 1996;33:23–30.

4.• Vogels BA, van Steynen B, Maas MA, Jorning GG, Chamuleau RA: The effects of ammonia and portal-systemic shunting on brain metabolism, neurotransmission and intracranial hypertension in hyperammonaemia-induced encephalopathy. *Journal of Hepatology* 1997;26:387–395.

5.•• Minuk GY: Gamma-aminobutyric acid and the liver. *Dig Dis* 1993;11(1):45–54.

6. Butterworth RF: Neuroactive amino acids in hepatic encephalopathy. *Metabolic Brain Disease* 1996;11:165–173.

7. Wilkinson SP: GABA, benzodiazepines and hepatic encephalopathy. *European Journal of Gastroenterology & Hepatology* 1995;7:323–324.

8.• MacDonald GA, Frey KA, Agranoff BW, *et al.*: Cerebral benzodiazepine receptor binding in vivo in patients with recurrent hepatic encephalopathy. *Hepatol* 1997; 26:277–282.

9. Mullen KD, Conjeevaram HS, Kaminsky-Russ K: Studies of "endogenous" benzodiazepine in human hepatic encephalopathy. *Alcohol & Alcoholism Supplement* 1993;2:187–190.

10. Jones EA, Basile AS, Yurdaydin C, Skolnich P: Do benzodiazepine ligands contribute to hepatic encephalopathy? *Advances in Experimental Medicine & Biology* 1993;341:57–69.

11.• Somberg KA, Riegler JL, LaBerge JM, *et al.*: Hepatic encephalopathy after transjugular intrahepatic portosystemic shunts: Incidence and risk factors. *Am J Gastro* 1995;90:549–555.

12.•• Pomier-Layrargues G: TIPS and hepatic encephalopathy. *Seminars in Liver Disease* 1996; 16:315–320.

13. Sakurabayashi S, Sezai S, Yamamoto Y, *et al.*: Embolization of portal-systemic shunts in cirrhotic patients with chronic recurrent hepatic encephalopathy. *Cardiovascular & Interventional Radiology* 1997;20:120–124.

14.• Morgan MY: Noninvasive neuroinvestigation in liver disease. *Seminars in Liver Disease* 1996; 16:293–313.

15. Ross BD, Danielsen ER, Bluml S: Proton magnetic resonance spectroscopy: The new gold standard for diagnosis of clinical and subclinical hepatic encephalopathy? *Dig Dis* 1996;14 Suppl 1:30–39.

16. Bianchi GP, Marchesini G, Fabbri A, *et al.*: Vegetable versus animal protein diet in cirrhotic patients with chronic encephalopathy: A randomized cross-over comparison. *Journal of Internal Medicine* 1993; 233:385–392.

17. Weber FL Jr: Lactulose and combination therapy of hepatic encephalopathy: The role of the intestinal microflora. *Dig Dis* 1996;14 Suppl 1:53–63.

18.• Ferenci P: Treatment of hepatic encephalopathy in patients with cirrhosis of the liver. *Dig Dis* 1996;14 Suppl 1:40–52.

19. Horsmans Y, Solbreux PM, Daenens C, *et al.*: Lactulose improves psychometric testing in cirrhotic patients with subclinical encephalopathy. *Alimentary Pharmacology & Therapeutics* 1997;11:165–170.

20.• Festi D, Mazzella G, Parini P, *et al.*: Treatment of hepatic encephalopathy with non-absorbable antibiotics. *Italian Journal of Gastroenterology* 1992;24(9 Suppl 2):14–16.

21. Strauss E, Tramote R, Silva EP, *et al.*: Double-blind randomized clinical trial comparing neomycin and placebo in the treatment of exogenous hepatic encephalopathy. *Hepato-Gastroenterology* 1992;39:542–545.

22.•• Pomier-Layrargues G, Giguere JF, Lavoie J, *et al.*: Flumazenil in cirrhotic patients in hepatic coma: a randomized double-blind placebo-controlled crossover trial. *Hepatol* 1994;19:32–37.

23. Howard CD, Seifert CF: Flumazenil in the treatment of hepatic encephalopathy. *Annals of Pharmacotherapy* 1993;27:46–48.

24. Gyr K, Meier R, Haussler J, *et al.*: Evaluation of the efficacy and safety of flumazenil in the treatment of portal systemic encephalopathy: A double-blind, randomised, placebo controlled multicentre study. *Gut* 1996;39:319–324.

25. Cadranel JF, el Younsi M, Pidoux B, *et al.*: Flumazenil therapy for hepatic encephalopathy in cirrhotic patients: A double-blind pragmatic randomized, placebo study. *Eur J Gastro & Hepatol* 1995;7:325–329.

26.•• Fattovich G, Giustina G, Degos F, *et al.*: Morbidity and mortality in compensated cirrhosis type C: A retrospective follow-up study of 384 patients. *Gastroenterology* 1997;112:463–472.

116 Fulminant Hepatic Failure

Richard K. Sterling and Mitchell L. Shiffman

Fulminant hepatic failure (FHF) is the most devastating sequela of acute hepatic injury. It is most commonly seen in patients with viral- or drug-induced liver disease; the cause of FHF, however, cannot be identified in many cases. Despite improvements in the diagnosis and management of this disorder, mortality continues to be between 50% and 80%. Emergent hepatic transplantation is the only effective treatment for patients with a low likelihood of spontaneous recovery from FHF. This chapter reviews the etiologies of FHF, ways in which to assess prognosis of affected individuals, and issues related to patient management.

DEFINITIONS

Most patients with acute hepatitis are asymptomatic (Fig. 116-1). The etiologic agent, either a virus, drug, or toxin, causes minor degrees of hepatocyte necrosis and variable elevations in serum aminotransferase levels. Liver function is unaffected, and many patients are unaware of their disease. As the degree of liver necrosis increases patients develop symptoms, including right upper-quadrant tenderness, fatigue, malaise, arthralgias, myalgias, and jaundice. Acute hepatitis with jaundice and coagulopathy is referred to as *severe acute hepatitis*. The prognosis for affected individuals usually is excellent, although patients with severe acute hepatitis may develop liver failure and therefore must be closely monitored until they recover.

Fulminant hepatic failure is defined as severe acute hepatitis complicated by the rapid development of hepatic encephalopathy in a patient without preexisting liver disease. This syndrome originally was described by Trey and Davidson, in 1970 [1•]. A separate classification—subfulminant hepatic failure (SFHF)—has been made for patients with more insidious liver failure [2•]. Although these disorders have overlapping etiologies and clinical manifestations, they have different prognoses. The characteristics of severe acute hepatitis, FHF, and SFHF are listed in Table 116-1.

Fulminant Hepatic Failure

In FHF, hepatic encephalopathy develops within 2 weeks of the onset of jaundice [3,4•,5•]. FHF most frequently is caused by viral hepatitis (A, B, D, or E), acetaminophen overdose, and other toxins that cause dose-dependent hepatocyte necrosis. Although many patients with FHF die, recovery is possible without the need for hepatic transplantation. Patients who survive FHF typically do not have abnormalities of hepatic architecture, including fibrosis and cirrhosis. Exceptions are patients

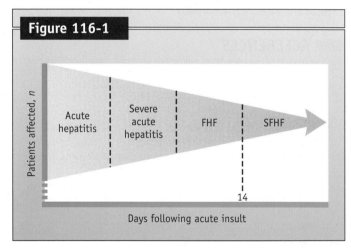

Figure 116-1

The relative number of patients with acute hepatitis who progress to severe acute hepatitis, fulminant hepatic failure (FHF), and subfulminant hepatic failure (SFHF).

Table 116-1. Comparison of Severe Actue Hepatitis, Fulminant, and Subfulminant Hepatic Failure

Clinical events	Severe acute hepatitis	Fulminant hepatic failure	Subfulminant hepatic failure
Hepatic encephalopathy (HE)	Never	Always	Always
Onset of HE after jaundice	N/A	< 2 wk	> 2 wk
Renal failure	Uncommon (except with acetaminophen)	Less common	Common
Survival	Excellent	50%–80%	< 20%
Development of chronic liver disease in patients who recover	Possible with viral etiologies	Rare	Frequent
Common etiologies	Acetaminophen Other drugs Toxins Viral hepatitis: A–E	Acetaminophen, *Amanita phalloides*, viral hepatitis: A, B, D, E	Idiosyncratic drug reactions, viral hepatitis: non-A–E, viral hepatitis B and D

with viral hepatitis B or B and D co-infection who develop chronic viral hepatitis, although this is uncommon.

Subfulminant Hepatic Failure

In SFHF, patients with severe acute hepatitis develop hepatic encephalopathy 2 weeks to 3 months after the onset of jaundice. SFHF most frequently is caused by viral infection and idiosyncratic drug reactions. It is uncommon for patients to survive SFHF without hepatic transplantation; those who do survive typically have chronic liver failure.

ETIOLOGIES

The most common etiologies of acute liver failure are listed in Table 116-2. These include viruses, drugs, toxins, and miscellaneous causes. A specific etiology often cannot be identified.

Hepatitis Viruses

Acute infection with a hepatitis virus is the most common identifiable cause of FHF and SFHF in the United States. Most cases of acute viral hepatitis in this country are due to hepatitis A virus (HAV). Epidemiologists at the Centers for Disease Control estimate that 100 of the approximately 200,000 people infected with HAV annually develop FHF, a rate of 0.05% to 0.1%.

Hepatitis B virus (HBV) causes nearly 25% of cases of FHF. In addition to acute HBV infection, reactivation of hepatitis B and spontaneous seroconversion from HBV e antigen-positive to HBV e antibody-positive may result in acute liver failure. Acute hepatitis D virus (HDV) co-infection or superinfection in patients with hepatitis B is associated with a high risk of FHF. Acute liver failure is observed in 2.5% to 6% of all cases of HDV infection; HDV infection is implicated in 15% of all cases of FHF.

Acute hepatitis E virus (HEV) infection first was reported to cause FHF in India, particularly in women during the third trimester of pregnancy. The incidence of FHF due to HEV in the United States population is unknown.

Infection with unclassified hepatitis viruses accounts for the majority of cases of acute liver failure. These cases may be due to an as yet unknown virus or an environmental immunogen or toxin. Other viruses that have been implicated as causes of acute liver failure include varicella-zoster, cytomegalovirus, Epstein-Barr syndrome, adenovirus, and paramyxovirus. Herpes simplex virus also has been associated with FHF in immunosuppressed individuals and during the third trimester of pregnancy.

Although isolated case reports have associated hepatitis C virus with acute liver injury, the overwhelming evidence suggests this virus does not cause acute liver failure [6,7]. Similarly, there are no reported cases of acute liver failure due to hepatitis G virus.

Drug-Induced Liver Failure

Drugs are the cause of 10% to 20% of cases of acute liver failure. Risk factors for development of drug-induced liver failure include very young and old age, abnormal renal function, obesity, preexisting liver disease, and concurrent use of other hepatotoxic agents. Because most medicines are metabolized by the liver, almost any drug can cause acute hepatitis. It is rare, however, for such reactions to progress to FHF or SFHF.

The hepatotoxicity of a medication is intrinsic, dose-dependent, and predictable, or the result of an idiosyncratic reaction (see Chapter 96). Idiosyncratic drug toxicity is the result of immunologic reactions to the agent or, more commonly, one of its metabolites. Most idiosyncratic drug reactions develop 4 to 6 weeks after the start of a new medication; it is exceptionally rare for an idiosyncratic reaction to develop after months or years of regular medication use. Most idiosyncratic drug reactions that progress to liver failure result in SFHF and have a

Table 116-2. Etiologies of Acute Liver Failure

	Cases, %
Viral	60–80
Hepatitis A	1–5
Acute hepatitis B	25
Hepatitis D coinfection or superinfection	15
Acute hepatitis E	
Viral hepatitis non A–G	25
Herpes simplex	
Varicella zoster	
Cytomegalovirus	
Epstein-Barr	
Adenovirus	
Paramyxovirus	
Drugs	10–30
Acetaminophen	10
Halothane	
Isoniazid	
Rifampin	
Nonsteroidal anti-inflammatory agents	
Sulfonamides	
Tetracycline	
Valproate	
Phenytoin	
Methyldopa	
Amiodarone	
Toxins	2–5
Amanita mushroom	
Carbon tetrachloride	
Industrial solvents	
Yellow phosphorus	
Some herbal remedies	
Miscellaneous	5
Wilson's disease	
Acute fatty liver of pregnancy	
Reye's syndrome	
Budd-Chiari syndrome	
Autoimmune hepatitis	
Shock liver	
Hyperthermia	
Sepsis	
Malignant infiltration	
Primary nonfunction post liver transplantation	

poor prognosis. The agents most commonly responsible for liver failure are isoniazid, phenytoin, rifampin, nonsteroidal anti-inflammatory drugs (NSAIDs), and sulfonamides.

Acetaminophen

Overdose with the intrinsically hepatotoxic drug acetaminophen is the most common cause of drug-induced liver failure in the United States and other developed countries (see Chapter 96). Acetaminophen undergoes phase I metabolism by hepatic cytochrome P-450 E2 enzymes into a toxic intermediate N-acetyl-p-benzoquinone imine (NAPQI), which is rapidly detoxified by glutathione reductase. Under normal conditions, little or no NAPQI accumulates within hepatocytes. In patients with acetaminophen overdose, however, large amounts of the toxic metabolite are produced and hepatocyte necrosis ensues. The severity of acute liver injury is related to the amount of acetaminophen ingested and NAPQI produced.

Chronic alcohol use induces synthesis of P-450 and, to a minor extent, depletes intrahepatic glutathione stores, thereby both enhancing the synthesis and reducing the degradation of the toxic metabolite (Fig. 116-2). As a result, even therapeutic doses of acetaminophen can cause accumulation of NAPQI and precipitate FHF in alcoholic patients [8].

Toxins

Various ingested and inhaled toxins account for 2% to 5% of FHF. Amanita mushroom poisoning is common in Europe, the Appalachian mountains, and the Pacific Northwest of the United States. Cases peak in autumn months, when mushrooms are plentiful. The toxin in these mushrooms, α-Amanitin, is heat stable and not destroyed by cooking. Approximately three medium-sized mushrooms contain sufficient toxin to cause FHF. Other common hepatotoxins include organic industrial solvents, yellow phosphorus (a component of pesticides), and aflatoxin. An increasing number of cases of FHF due to herbal medications such as jin bu huan are being reported.

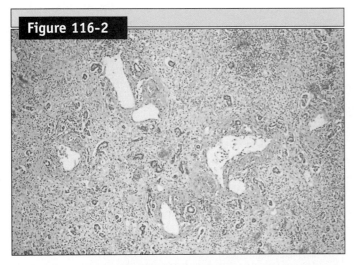

Figure 116-2

Liver biopsy from a patient with fulminant hepatic failure. There is massive necrosis of hepatocytes, loss of cell boundaries, and loss of nuclei. See also **Color Plate.**

Other Etiologies

Other less common etiologies account for up to 5% of cases of FHF and are listed in Table 116-2. These include acute fatty liver of pregnancy, "shock liver," autoimmune hepatitis, Budd-Chiari syndrome, and Wilson's disease (see Chapter 100). The latter should be suspected in a young patient who presents with a Coombs-negative hemolytic anemia, low serum alkaline phosphatase level, and hypouricemia. These abnormalities are the result of acute copper toxicity. Kayser-Fleischer rings, commonly observed by slit lamp ophthalmic examination in many patients with chronic Wilson's disease, may not be present in this setting.

■ PATHOGENESIS

Fulminant hepatic failure develops as a result of cytotoxic and cytopathic injury, alone or in combination. Cytotoxicity results from direct injury by hepatotoxic viruses (eg, HAV), drugs or their toxic metabolites, and environmental toxins. In contrast, cytopathic injury results from an immune-mediated response to hepatocytes with abnormal cell surface antigens, as is commonly observed in patients with HBV and idiosyncratic drug reactions.

Two histologic patterns are seen in patients with FHF. The most common pattern is massive hepatocellular necrosis (Fig. 116-2). This typically is observed in response to severe viral infections, drugs, and various toxins. Histologic examination demonstrates sheets of necrotic hepatocytes with or without complete loss of normal hepatic architecture and collapse of the hepatic lobule. In some patients, islands of regenerating hepatocytes can be seen. Numerous polymorphonuclear cells may be scattered throughout the liver tissue. In cases of immune-mediated liver injury, lymphocytes and plasma cells also may be seen. Eosinophils often are observed in liver tissue of patients with idiosyncratic drug reactions.

The second histologic pattern observed in patients with FHF is microvesicular steatosis (Fig. 116-3). This occurs in patients with acute fatty liver of pregnancy (AFLP), Reye's syndrome, valproate, and tetracycline toxicity, and during treatment of chronic HBV hepatitis with antinucleoside analogs. Microvesicular steatosis is associated with acquired defects in mitochondrial fatty acid and ammonia metabolism, leading to marked lipid deposition within hepatocytes and hyperammonemia.

■ CLINICAL FEATURES

The most common clinical features of acute liver failure are abnormal liver tests, hepatic encephalopathy, coagulopathy, and hypoglycemia (Table 116-3). Patients with FHF also may develop cerebral edema, a major factor contributing to mortality in these patients. In addition to these clinical features, patients with SFHF frequently develop renal failure, sepsis, cardiopulmonary collapse, adult respiratory distress syndrome, pancreatitis, and acid-base disturbances. The major cause of death in patients with SFHF is multiorgan failure.

Liver Chemistries

Patients with acute liver injury typically are recognized because they are icteric and have markedly elevated serum aminotransferase levels. Patients with FHF associated with microvesicular steatosis, however, are exceptions. The latter group of patients present with mental status changes and profound increases in

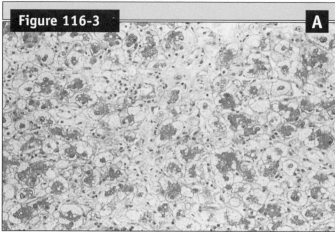

Figure 116-3

A, Liver biopsy from a patient with fulminant hepatic failure secondary to fialuridine toxicity. There is diffuse microvesicular steatosis without hepatocyte necrosis. **B**, Same patient as in **A**. The biopsy is stained with oil red O to enhance visualization of steatosis. See also **Color Plate**.

Table 116-3. Systemic Complications of Acute Liver Failure

Type	Fulminant hepatic failure	Subfulminant hepatic failure
Hepatic encephalopathy	Always	Always
Cerebral edema	+ + +	+
Acute renal failure	+ + +	+ + +
Thrombocytopenia	+ +	+ +
Gastrointestinal bleeding	+ +	+ + +
Infections	+ + +	+ + + +
Hypoglycemia	+ + + +	+ +
Acidosis	+ + +	+
Alkalosis	+	+
Pancreatitis	+	+
Cardiovascular collapse	+ + +	+ + +
Multi-organ failure	+	+ + +

+ = < 10% of cases; + + = 30%–50% of cases; + + + = 50%–75% of cases; + + + + = 75%–100% of cases.

serum ammonia levels but trivial abnormalities of serum aminotransferase and bilirubin levels and prothrombin time. The typical patient with FHF has peak serum aminotransferase values of 5000 to 10,000 IU/L, which decline rapidly to normal as the serum bilirubin concentration continues to increase (Fig. 116-4). The degree to which serum aminotransferase levels are elevated and their rate of decline in patients with FHF does not reflect prognosis. Serum bilirubin concentration declines to normal in patients who recover but continues to increase in patients who do not.

Hepatic Encephalopathy

The presence of hepatic encephalopathy for the diagnosis of FHF is an absolute requirement, and its time of onset after the appearance of jaundice is the clinical feature used to distinguish between FHF and SFHF. Criteria for grading the severity of hepatic encephalopathy are listed in Table 116-4. Alterations in the electroencephalogram commonly observed in patients with hepatic encephalopathy include diffuse slowing of cortical electrical activity and high-amplitude waveforms of five to seven cycles per second. Alterations in mental status caused by hepatic encephalopathy increase the risk of aspiration pneumonia and acute respiratory distress syndrome (ARDS).

The time at which hepatic encephalopathy first appears during the course of liver failure and the rate at which it worsens varies with the etiology of FHF. For patients with acetaminophen overdose or *Amanita* poisoning, encephalopathy develops 3 to 4 days after exposure and may progress to stage IV coma within 24 hours. In contrast, the onset of hepatic encephalopathy typically is delayed in patients with viral hepatitis and idiosyncratic drug reactions.

Cerebral Edema

Cerebral edema develops in more than 50% of patients with FHF. It is most commonly observed in patients with rapidly progressing encephalopathy and is the leading cause of death in these individuals. Cerebral edema, when severe, leads to seizures and brain stem herniation within days of onset. For patients who survive, the risk for residual neurologic deficit is great. In contrast, only 10% of patients with SFHF appear to develop cerebral edema.

Cerebral edema is not the result of severe hepatic encephalopathy. Rather, it is considered to be a separate neurologic manifestation of FHF caused by an increase in the permeability of the blood–brain barrier that allows low–molecular weight molecules to enter the cerebral space and produce neuronal swelling. High levels of circulating endotoxin and toxic metabolites may damage the integrity of the cerebral vasculature and play a role in this process. The systemic effects of cerebral edema include systolic hypertension, increased muscle tone, decerebrate posturing, hyperventilation, pupillary dilation, myoclonus, and seizures.

Coagulopathy

Most coagulation factors are synthesized by the liver. The exception is factor VIII, which is synthesized by vascular endothelium. Acute liver failure results in an abrupt and profound decrease in

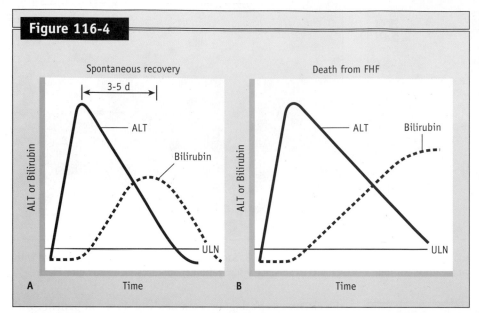

Figure 116-4

Pattern of serum alanine aminotransferase (ALT) and bilirubin for two selected patients with fulminant hepatic failure (FHF) who had, spontaneous recovery (**A**) or, death (**B**) from FHF. In both patients, serum ALT (*solid line*) gradually declines after reaching its maximum value. For those patients who recover, the peak in serum bilirubin (*dashed line*) typically occurs 3 to 5 days following the peak in serum ALT. For patients who do not survive, bilirubin continues to increase. ULN—upper limits of normal.

Table 116-4. Grading Scale for Hepatic Encephalopathy

Grade	Clinical findings
1	Confused
	Altered mood or behavior
	Psychomotor defects
	Sleep disturbance
2	Drowsy
	Inappropriate behavior
	Slow mentation
	Bowel or bladder incontinence
	Asterixis
3	Stuporous but speaking
	Ability to obey simple commands
	Inarticulate speech
	Marked confusion
	Asterixis
4	Coma with or without response to pain

the synthesis of coagulation proteins. Because factor VII has the shortest half-life of the coagulation factors (4–6 h), serial prothrombin time measurements are useful to gauge the severity of acute liver injury and recovery from this event. In addition to clotting factors, the liver also synthesizes anti-clotting proteins (proteins C and S) and clears activated clotting factors from plasma. As a result, patients with FHF typically have elevated plasma fibrin split product levels and a hematologic picture resembling that in disseminated intravascular coagulation.

Hypoglycemia
Hypoglycemia is observed in as many as 45% of patients with FHF and results from a combination of factors, including impaired gluconeogenesis, depletion of hepatic glycogen stores,

increased circulating insulin, and increased glucose utilization by peripheral tissues. Profound hypoglycemia, which is unresponsive to the intravenous infusion of concentrated glucose solutions, is a sign of impending death.

Systemic Manifestations
Systemic manifestations, including cardiovascular collapse, sepsis, renal failure, and ARDS, typically are observed in patients with SFHF (Table 116-3). Hypotension and cardiovascular collapse may result from high circulating levels of endotoxin and tumor necrosis factor. Cardiac arrhythmias are frequently the result of marked electrolyte abnormalities. Confusion secondary to hepatic encephalopathy increases the risk for aspiration. This, along with intravenous infusion of blood products to correct coagulopathy, may contribute to pulmonary edema and ARDS. Acute renal failure is seen in as many as 30% to 70% of patients with liver failure. Renal failure is produced by a combination of intravascular volume depletion, sepsis, and disseminated intravascular coagulation in patients with liver failure and/or due to direct nephrotoxicity from acetaminophen or NSAID. Pancreatitis has been reported in patients with liver failure; the cause of this condition is unclear. Patients with acute liver failure also frequently develop sepsis and gastrointestinal hemorrhage, which often are the immediate cause of death in these individuals [9,10].

▇ ASSESSING PROGNOSIS
Survival in patients with acute liver failure is 30% to 80% and is dependent on many factors, including etiology, patient age, severity of hepatic dysfunction, degree of liver necrosis, number and nature of complications, and the duration of the disease. Survival tends to be greater if FHF due to HAV infection and acetaminophen overdose (Fig. 116-5). In contrast, when acute liver failure is due to idiosyncratic drug reactions, environmental toxins, idiopathic hepatitis, and co-infection with HBV and HDV, the mortality rate approaches 80% to 90%. The severity of encephalopathy at presentation is useful in estimating prognosis; patients who do not progress past grade I encephalopathy have an excellent outcome with near universal survival (Fig. 116-6). In

contrast, survival rates of patients who progress to stage 4 coma are less than 25% without hepatic transplantation. The presence of renal failure increases mortality regardless of the cause.

Several prognostic models have been developed to assess the likelihood of spontaneous recovery from acute liver failure and the need for hepatic transplantation [11,12,13,14]. The most commonly used model was developed at King's College by retrospective analysis of data from over 580 patients with FHF [13••]. Slightly different criteria for acctaminophen- and non–acetaminophen-induced liver failure were established and applied prospectively to 175 patients with acute liver failure with a positive predictive value and predictive accuracy of 98% and 94%, respectively (Table 116-5). When estimating the prognosis of a patient with this model, it is important to understand that the value for prothrombin time is markedly affected by the type of thromboplastin reagent used in the assay. Although the international normalized ratio (INR) was developed as a way to correct for interlaboratory variation in prothrombin time, a study suggests that INR may not be an ideal way to assess coagulopathy in a patient with acute or chronic liver disease [15].

Other models developed to predict outcome in patients with acute liver failure are based on the ratio of the activity of factor VIII, which is produced by vascular endothelium, to those of coagulation factors produced by the liver. In a French study, patients with a factor V activity level less than 20% to 30% had a mortality rate from FHF that approached 90% [15a]. Factor VIII activity actually increases in patients with acute hepatitis. A factor VIII to factor V activity ratio of greater than 30 indicates a poor prognosis in acute liver failure (Table 116-5) [15b]. Factor VII activity of less than 25% of normal that fails to increase 24 hours after administration of vitamin K also is associated with a poor prognosis [14•].

Liver Biopsy

Liver biopsy may confirm the suspected etiology of liver failure and aid in assessing the degree of hepatocyte necrosis. Use of this procedure is hampered by coagulopathy and thrombocytopenia in most patients with severe liver disease. However, a study demonstrated that an adequate specimen for evaluation can be obtained by transjugular liver biopsy with very little associated morbidity [16]. Tissue obtained in this study confirmed the clinically suspected etiology of liver failure in 63% of biopsied patients but altered the diagnosis in nearly one third of patients examined. Necrosis of more than 70% of liver cells in the biopsy specimen was associated with a mortality rate approaching 90% in those patients who did not undergo emergent hepatic transplantation.

■■■ MANAGEMENT

The liver has the unique ability to regenerate following massive injury, and patients who survive FHF have restitution of normal liver architecture and function. The medical management of acute liver failure is directed at preventing life-ending complications and providing sufficient time for the liver to regenerate [17••].

Hepatic Encephalopathy

The treatment of hepatic encephalopathy associated with liver failure is directed at limiting the production of ammonia [18] (see Chapter 115), which is made primarily by intestinal bacteria.

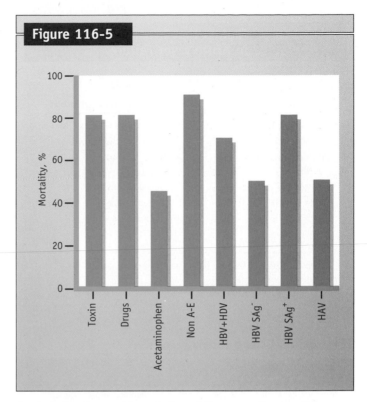

Figure 116-5

Survival of patients with acute liver failure according to etiology.

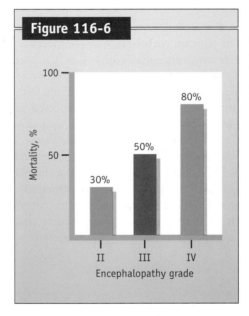

Figure 116-6

Relationship between survival in patients with fulminant hepatic failure and the grade of hepatic encephalopathy at presentation.

Lactulose may be useful in the therapy of grades 1 to 2 encephalopathy, but it has not been found to improve survival rates in patients with more severe grades of hepatic encephalopathy. Oral antibiotics directed against enteric bacteria (neomycin, flagyl) also may be administered. Neomycin is said to be nonabsorbable, but its potential for nephrotoxicity is so great that its use in patients with liver failure, who are already at high risk for development of renal insufficiency, should be avoided. Experimental treatments to reduce serum ammonia levels include exchange transfusion, charcoal hemoperfusion, and plasmaphere-sis. Although each of these therapies reduces serum ammonia levels, none improves survival rates.

Table 116-5. Factors that Predict Poor Survival in Acute Liver Failure

King's college criteria [13]

Acetaminophen overdose	Nonacetminophen etiology
Arterial pH < 7.3	Prothrombin time > 100 s (INR > 6.7)
Or *all* of the following:	Or any three of the following:
Prothrombin time > 100 s (INR > 6.7)	Age < 10 or > 40 y
Creatinine > 3.4 mg/dL	Viral hepatitis: non A–E or drug induced causes
Grade 3–4 HE	Prothrombin time > 50 s (INR > 4)
	Bilirubin > 17.4 mg/dL

Clichy criteria [15a]

Factor V < 20% in persons < 30 years of age
Or *both* of the following:
Factor V < 30%
Grade 3–4 HE

Factor VIII/factor V criteria [15b]

Factor VIII/factor V > 30

Numbers in brackets indicate references. HE—hepatic encephalopathy; INR—international normalization ratio.

Endogenous benzodiazepine-like substances have been identified in the sera of patients with FHF and contribute to the development of hepatic encephalopathy (see Chapter 115). Use of benzodiazepines for treatment of agitation worsens encephalopathy and is contraindicated in patients with acute liver failure. Intravenous flumazenil has been used to treat encephalopathy in patients with FHF with limited success [19].

Patients with hepatic encephalopathy often aspirate oral secretions and blood and subsequently develop pneumonia and ARDS. Aspiration and its complications are contraindications to hepatic transplantation and are preterminal events in many patients with FHF. Therefore, it is imperative that patients with significant encephalopathy be intubated to protect their airways.

Cerebral Edema

Cerebral edema and brain stem herniation are common causes of death in patients with FHF [20]. Significant cerebral edema is present when there is an elevation in intracranial pressure (ICP) of greater than 30 mm Hg. ICP is measured by an intradural or epidural monitoring device; ICP should be monitored in all liver failure patients with grades III to IV hepatic encephalopathy who are candidates for emergent hepatic transplantation. Two measurements are useful in evaluating the severity of cerebral edema in patients with FHF: absolute ICP and the cerebral perfusion pressure (CPP). The latter is defined as mean arterial pressure (MAP) minus ICP. Patients with an ICP greater than 30 mm Hg or a CPP less than 40 mm Hg for more than 2 hours experience irreversible brain injury. Thus, measurements of ICP and CPP are critical

to the management of these patients and useful in determining when patients with FHF and cerebral edema no longer are candidates for hepatic transplantation.

Figure 116-7 is an algorithm for treatment of encephalopathy and cerebral edema in patients with FHF. Conservative therapy of cerebral edema involves limiting those factors that raise MAP and taking measures to improve cerebral perfusion. These include elevating the head of the bed to a 30° to 40° angle, hyperventilation to reduce arterial PCO_2 to less than 35 mm Hg, and preventing overhydration. However, compensatory vascular mechanisms limit the effectiveness of these efforts. Patients with an ICP greater than 30 mm Hg and those who exhibit decerebrate posturing or other early signs of brain stem herniation should be treated with an intravenous bolus infusion of mannitol (0.5–1.0 g/kg). Side effects of mannitol therapy include hyperosmolarity and acute renal failure, both of which may limit further treatment. For patients whose ICP cannot be controlled with mannitol, intravenous thiopental or phenobarbital may be used to slow cerebral activity and limit irreversible brain injury [21]. Steroids are ineffective in the treatment of cerebral edema associated with FHF.

Coagulopathy

Although most patients with acute liver failure have a profound coagulopathy, development of spontaneous hemorrhage is uncommon. Acute liver necrosis results in the loss of vitamin K stores, and therefore, all patients with acute liver failure should receive vitamin K, 10 mg intravenously or subcutaneously, daily for 3 consecutive days. Because prothrombin time and plasma clotting factor levels (V and VII) are useful in following the clinical course of acute liver failure, routine administration of fresh frozen plasma to patients with this disorder is not recommended. In those patients who develop hemorrhage or require placement of central venous catheters or an ICP monitoring device, however, an attempt to correct coagulopathy is necessary and most efficiently accomplished by exchange plasmapheresis using fresh frozen plasma and cryoprecipitate (Fig. 116-8).

General Supportive Measures

Infection is commonly observed in patients with liver failure; sepsis is a frequent preterminal event in these individuals and is a contraindication to hepatic transplantation. Many septic patients with liver failure do not have fever or leukocytosis. Surveillance blood cultures should be obtained every 24 to 48 hours, and the threshold for starting antibiotic therapy should be low. Because patients with liver failure often develop renal failure as well, use of aminoglycosides is contraindicated. Antacid therapy should be used empirically in an attempt to reduce the incidence of gastrointestinal bleeding. Patients with acute renal failure may be treated with dialysis or hemofiltration.

Patients with an acetaminophen overdose should receive oral acetylcysteine [22••]; recent studies have demonstrated that this therapy is beneficial even when administered up to 36 hours after acetaminophen ingestion [23]. Additional studies suggest that oral acetyl cysteine may be beneficial even when the etiology of FHF is a drug or toxin other than acetaminophen.

Most patients with FHF were healthy prior to developing liver disease, and malnutrition is not an issue in their cases. However, patients with SFHF may be ill for weeks to months prior to development of encephalopathy and may have profound malnutrition. These patients should receive enteral or parenteral nutritional support. Although not proven to reduce encephalopathy, branched-chain amino acid formulations may be preferable to standard amino acid regimens in treatment of patients with liver failure. Lipid emulsions have been demonstrated to be safe in these patients. Serum glucose levels should be closely monitored because patients with liver failure often develop hypoglycemia.

Specific Therapies for Liver Failure

Over the past two decades, several treatments for acute liver failure have been evaluated. These therapies, their proposed mechanisms of action, and their general effectiveness are summarized in Table 116-6.

Medical therapies of acute liver failure that have been evaluated include insulin and glucagon infusions, corticosteroids [24], and intravenous prostaglandin E1. Controlled trials have demonstrated that none of these treatments improves survival rates in liver failure; steroid therapy is associated with an increased incidence of infection. Various treatments to remove circulating toxins include charcoal hemoperfusion, exchange transfusion, and plasmapheresis. Although these techniques may lower serum ammonia concentration and improve prothrombin time, con-

trolled trials have demonstrated that they do not improve survival in patients with acute liver failure.

During the past several years, "liver assist" devices have been developed and tested in clinical trials [25,26]. These devices are made by placing either porcine or human liver cells in a specialized canister, which is perfused with the patient's blood in a manner similar to hemodialysis. Use of these devices in selected patients with FHF has yielded promising results. Controlled clinical trials are anticipated to determine the effectiveness of these devices. Other experimental treatments for FHF include extracorporeal whole-liver perfusion and hepatocyte transplantation [27]. In the former, a human liver that could not be used for transplantation is perfused with the patient's blood outside the body. Liver cell transplantation involves injecting preserved human hepatocytes previously isolated from livers not used for transplantation into the splenic bed. Although both techniques are promising, their applicability is severely hampered by the limited availability of human liver tissue.

Liver Transplantation

The only proven treatment for acute liver failure is hepatic transplantation [28]. Survival rates of patients with liver failure after hepatic transplantation are 50% to 90%. The major impediment to transplantation in this setting is delay in obtaining an appropriate donor organ, which must be transplanted before the recipient

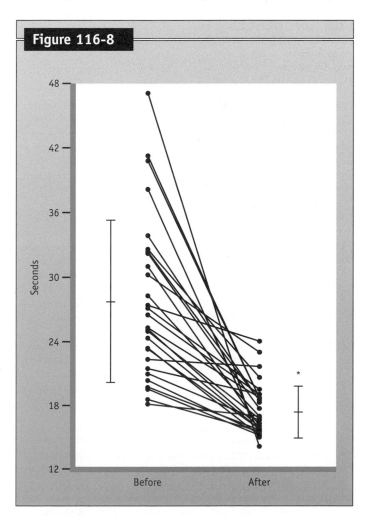

Figure 116-7

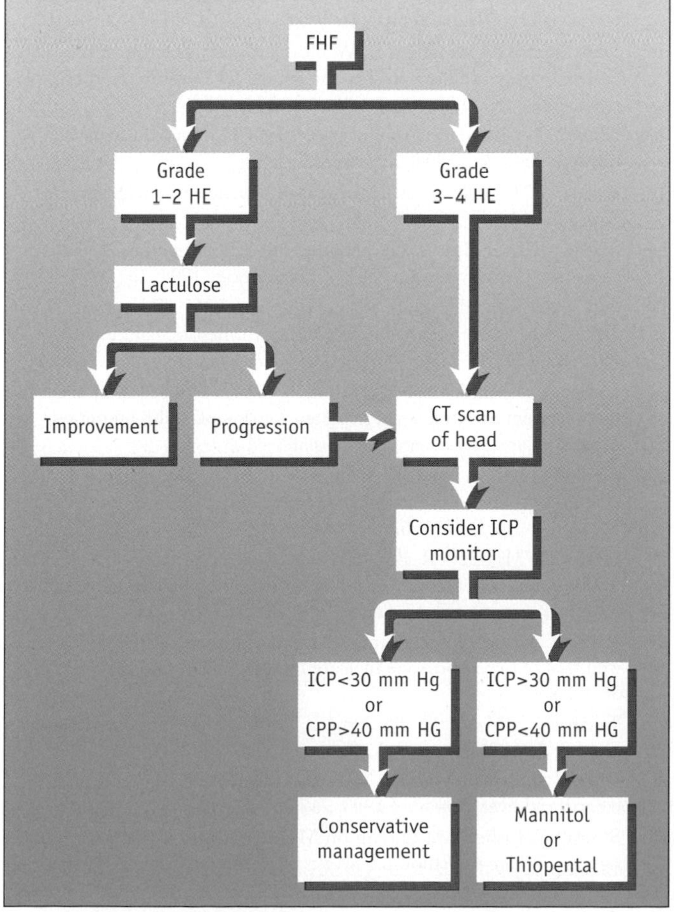

FHF → Grade 1–2 HE / Grade 3–4 HE

Grade 1–2 HE → Lactulose → Improvement / Progression

Progression → CT scan of head

Grade 3–4 HE → CT scan of head

CT scan of head → Consider ICP monitor

Consider ICP monitor → ICP<30 mm Hg or CPP>40 mm HG / ICP>30 mm Hg or CPP<40 mm HG

ICP<30 mm Hg or CPP>40 mm HG → Conservative management

ICP>30 mm Hg or CPP<40 mm HG → Mannitol or Thiopental

Algorithm for management of hepatic encephalopathy and cerebral edema in patients with fulminant hepatic failure.

Figure 116-8

Seconds (y-axis: 12, 18, 24, 30, 36, 42, 48)
Before / After
*

Effect of exchange plasmapheresis on prothrombin time in patients with acute liver failure.

Table 116-6. Proposed Treatments for Acute Liver Failure

Treatment	Proposed mechanism of action	Effect on survival
Insulin and glucagon	Enhance regeneration	Ineffective
Prostaglandin E1	Reduce hepatic necrosis	Ineffective
	Enhance regeneration	
Corticosteroids	Reduce hepatic necrosis	Ineffective
Charcoal hemoperfusion	Clear circulating toxins	Ineffective
Exchange transfusion	Clear circulating toxins	Ineffective
Plasmapheresis	Clear circulating toxins	Ineffective
Extracorporeal liver perfusion	Enhance liver function	Possibly effective
Liver assist devices	Enhance liver function	Possibly effective
Hepatocyte transplantation	Enhance liver function	Possibly effective
Orthotopic liver transplantation	Restores liver function	Proven effective

develops either irreversible neurologic impairment or multiorgan failure. The mortality rate of patients with FHF awaiting hepatic transplantation is 10- to 20-fold greater than that of patients with nonfulminant chronic liver disease. As a result, once a patient with acute liver failure is identified, it is imperative that he or she be moved to a liver transplant center as soon as possible.

■ REFERENCES

Recently published papers of particular interest have been highlighted as follows:
• Of interest
•• Of outstanding interest

1.• Trey C, Davidson LS: The management of fulminant hepatic failure. In *Progress in Liver Disease*. Edited by Popper H, Schaffner F. New York: Grune & Stratton; 1970: 3:282–298.

2.• Bernuau J, Rueff B, Benhamou J-P: Fulminant and subfulminant liver failure: definitions and causes. *Sem Liver Dis* 1986, 6:97–106.

3. Capocaccia L, Angelico M: Fulminant hepatic failure: clinical features, etiology, epidemiology, and current management. *Dig Dis Sci* 1991, 36:775–779.

4.• Lee WE: Medical progress: acute liver failure. *N Engl J Med* 1993, 329:1862–1872.

5.• Hoofnagle JH, Carithers RL, Shapiro C, Ascher N: Fulminant hepatic failure: summary of a workshop. *Hepatology* 1995, 21:240–252.

6. Wright T, Hsu H, Donegan E, *et al.*: Hepatitis C virus is not found in fulminant non-A, non-B hepatitis. *Ann Intern Med* 1991, 115:111–113.

7. Liang TJ, Jeffers L, Reddy RK, *et al.*: Fulminant or subfulminant Non-A, Non-B viral hepatitis: the role of hepatitis C and E viruses. *Gastroenterology* 1993, 104:556–562.

8. Zimmerman HJ, Maddrey WC: Acetaminophen (Paracetamol) hepatoxicity with regular intake of alcohol: analysis of instances of therapeutic misadventure. *Hepatology* 1995, 22:767–773.

9. Rolando N, Harvey F, Brahm J, *et al.*: Prospective study of bacterial infection in acute liver failure: an analysis of fifty patients. *Hepatology* 1990, 11:49–53.

10. Rolando N, Harvey F, Brahm J, *et al.*: Fungal infection: a common unrecognized complication of acute liver failure. *J Hepatology* 1991, 12:1–9.

11. Lake JR, Sussman NL: Determining prognosis in patients with fulminant hepatic failure: when you absolutely, positively have to know the answer. *Hepatology* 1995, 21:879–882

12. Bernuau J, Goudeau A, Poynard T, *et al.*: Multivariate analysis of prognostic factors in fulminant hepatitis. *Hepatology* 1986, 6:648–651.

13.•• O'Grady JG, Alexander GJM, Hallyar KM, Williams R: Early indicators of prognosis in fulminant hepatic failure. *Gastroenterology* 1989, 97:439–445.

14.• Takahashi Y, Kumada H, Shimizu M, *et al.*: A multicenter study on the prognosis of fulminant viral hepatitis: early prediction for liver transplantation. *Hepatology* 1994, 19:1065–1071.

15. Robert A, Chazouilleres O: Prothrombin time in liver failure: time, ratio, activity percentage, or international normalized ratio? *Hepatology* 1996, 24:1392–1394.

15a. Bernuau J, Samuel D, Durand F, *et al.*: Criteria for emergency liver transplantation in patients with acute viral hepatitis and factor V below 50% of normal: a prospective study. *Hepatology* 1991, 14:49A.

15b. Pereira LMMB, Langley PG, Hayllar KM, *et al.*: Coagulation factor V and VIII/V ratio as predictors of outcome in paracetamol induced fulminant hepatic failure: relation to other prognostic factors. *Gut* 1992, 33:98–102.

16. Donaldson BW, Gopinath R, Wanless IR, *et al.*: The role of transjugular liver biopsy in fulminant hepatic failure: relationship to other prognostic indicators. *Hepatology* 1993, 18:1370–1374.

17.•• Munoz SJ: Difficult management problems in fulminant hepatic failure. *Sem Liver Dis* 1993, 13:395–413.

18. Riordan SM, Williams R: Treatment of hepatic encephalopathy. *N Engl J Med* 1997, 337:473–478.

19. Sterling RK, Shiffman ML, Schubert ML: Flumazenil for hepatic coma: the elusive wake-up call? *Gastroenterology* 1994, 107:1204–1205.

20. Wijdicks EFM, Plevak DJ, Rakela J, Wiesner RH: Clinical and radiologic features of cerebral edema in fulminant hepatic failure. *Mayo Clin Proc* 1995, 70:119–124.

21. Forbes A, Alexander GJM, O'Grady JG, *et al.*: Thiopental infusion in the treatment of intracranial hypertension complication fulminant hepatic failure. *Hepatology* 1989, 10:306–310.

22.• Smilkstein MJ, Knapp GL, Kulig KW, Rumack BH: Efficacy of oral N-acetylcysteine in the treatment of acetaminophen overdose. *N Engl J Med* 1988, 319:1557–1562.

23. Harrison PM, Keays R, Bray GP, *et al.*: Late N-acetylcysteine administration improves outcome for patients developing paracetamol-induced fulminant hepatic failure. *Lancet* 1990, 335:1572–1573.

24. Rakela J, Mosley JW, Edwards VM, *et al.*: A double-blinded, randomized trial of hydrocortisone in acute hepatic failure. *Dig Dis Sci* 1991, 36:1223–1228.

25. Takahashi T, Malchesky PS, Nose Y: Artificial liver: state of the art. *Dig Dis Sci* 1991, 36:1327–1340.

26. Rozga J, Holzman MD, Ro M-S, *et al.*: Development of a hybrid bioartificial liver. *Ann Surg* 1993, 217:502–511.

27. Strom SC, Fisher RA, Thompson MT, *et al.*: Hepatocyte transplantation as a bridge to orthotopic liver transplantation in terminal liver failure. *Transplantation* 1997, 63:559–569.

28. Devlin J, Wendon J, Heaton N, *et al.*: Pretransplantation clinical status and outcome of emergency transplantation for acute liver failure. *Hepatology* 1995, 21:1018–1024.

Liver Transplantation: Patient Selection and Postoperative Management

David P. Vogt and J. Michael Henderson

Although the first orthotopic liver transplant (OLT) was performed in 1963 by Thomas Starzl, the procedure has become accepted as standard therapy for end-stage liver disease (ESLD) only during the past decade. Several factors have been responsible for the promulgation of OLT, including a better understanding of liver disease, improved immunosuppression (particularly the introduction of cyclosporine), refinements and standardization in surgical techniques, better and prolonged organ preservation, earlier recipient referral, increased donor availability, improved donor management and selection, meticulous postoperative care, and the training of new liver transplant teams.

The results of OLT have improved steadily. The overall 1-year patient survival after OLT was 83% in 1995 compared with 77% in 1988. At the end of 1996, 7467 patients were waiting for a donor organ; only 4451 cadaver livers were recovered during that same year, and 954 patients died while waiting for a transplant. As of March, 1997, 121 liver-transplant programs existed in the United States; in May of 1997, over 8300 patients were listed for OLT (United Network for Organ Sharing [UNOS] web site, July 1997). Clearly, donor organ availability has become the rate-limiting factor in OLT and will remain so in the foreseeable future.

■ INDICATIONS

Initially, OLT was performed only as a life-saving procedure. As results of OLT improved, however, it justifiably could be offered to patients earlier in their disease to improve their quality of life. The majority of patients with chronic liver disease referred for OLT have complications of cirrhosis and portal hypertension, including bleeding from gastroesophageal varices, intractable ascites, encephalopathy, spontaneous bacterial peritonitis, malnutrition, muscle wasting, clotting abnormalities, progressive fatigue, and significantly deranged synthetic function. Other symptoms related to advanced liver disease include severe pruritus, metabolic bone disease, and recurrent cholangitis.

A patient with either chronic, progressive, or fulminant liver disease for which no other effective medical or surgical therapy exists may be a transplant candidate. There must be no absolute contraindications, and the patient (or the patient's family in the case of pediatric patients) must be able to understand and accept the magnitude of the procedure, including the associated commitment, compliance, and cost.

The specific indications for OLT and their relative frequencies in adults are listed in Table 117-1 [1•]. Alcohol-induced cirrhosis is the most common indication for transplantation in the United States. Other common indications include chronic viral hepatitis, primary biliary cirrhosis, and primary sclerosing cholangitis.

Few patients with malignancy, either primary hepatocellular carcinoma or cholangiocarcinoma, are considered for OLT because of poor results and the limited supply of donor organs. Patients with malignancy who are considered for OLT must be on a protocol of both preoperative and postoperative adjuvant therapy. If extrahepatic or metastatic disease is found at the time of OLT, the operation should be terminated and the donor organ given to a patient with nonmalignant disease.

Biliary atresia accounts for at least 50% of OLTs performed in pediatric patients (Table 117-2) [2••]. Other common indications for OLT in children include metabolic diseases and autoimmune hepatitis. Several OLTs have been performed for inborn errors of metabolism in children whose livers lack an important enzyme but are otherwise normal. Liver transplantation presumably corrects the enzyme deficiency and cures diseases such as primary hereditary oxalosis, Crigler-Najjar syndrome, and various urea cycle enzyme deficiencies.

Acute hepatic failure is the indication for OLT in approximately 6% of adults and 11% of children (see Table 117-1) (see Chapter 116). This syndrome is characterized by the rapid onset of severe liver dysfunction with jaundice, coagulopathy, and encephalopathy in a patient who has no prior history of liver disease. Without OLT, fulminant liver failure leads to death in

Table 117-1. Indications for Liver Transplantation in Adults

Indications	Transplants performed, %
Cirrhosis	
Alcohol	21.6
Hepatitis C	19.5
Cryptogenic	12
Hepatitis B	6
Autoimmune	5
Cholestatic liver disease	—
Primary biliary cirrhosis	11
Primary sclerosing cholangitis	10
Fulminant hepatic failure	6
Malignancy	5
Metabolic	4
Other	2

From UNOS [5].

10% to 25% of affected individuals within 8 weeks of onset, whereas 50% to 85% of selected patients survive following liver transplantation. Because patients with acute liver failure can deteriorate within hours to days, early referral to a transplantation center is mandatory for an optimal outcome.

■ CONTRAINDICATIONS

Our understanding of the contraindications to OLT continues to evolve. Over the years, the list of absolute contraindications to OLT has become smaller.

Absolute Contraindications

Any clinical condition that virtually ensures failure of liver transplantation is defined as an absolute contraindication. The list of absolute contraindications has become smaller over the years (Table 117-3) [2••]. Human immunodeficiency virus (HIV) infection is currently considered to be an absolute contraindication to OLT by most transplant centers because of poor posttransplant survival rates. There is some controversy concerning OLT for HIV-positive patients with normal T cell counts.

Extrahepatic malignancy is an absolute contraindication to OLT. Lesions may be found by preoperative imaging or at the time of transplant surgery. Disease progression is enhanced by immunosuppression, and affected patients usually die within months of transplantation. Patients with basal cell carcinoma of the skin, however, may be considered as transplant candidates because this lesion rarely metastasizes. Patients previously treated for an extrahepatic neoplasm, such as breast or colon cancer, may be candidates for OLT depending on the type and stage of the tumor and when it was treated; a patient who is disease-free 2 years after therapy for an early carcinoma may be considered for liver transplantation.

Uncontrolled infection is another absolute contraindication to OLT. The additive affects of major surgery and immunosuppression are disastrous. Spontaneous bacterial peritonitis, cholangitis, pneumonia, and urosepsis are the most frequently encountered pretransplant infections. Antibiotics are successful in clearing most infections within 2 to 3 days, allowing the transplant to be performed.

With few exceptions, most centers will not transplant patients who are active substance abusers. A few centers will consider patients with alcoholic hepatitis for OLT because the short-term results are good. The risk of recidivism, however, is significantly higher in patients with acute alcoholic hepatitis than in those who have been through a substance abuse rehabilitation program and have been abstinent for at least 3 months.

Advanced cardiac and non–cirrhosis-related pulmonary disease, such as severe chronic obstructive pulmonary disease, are contraindications to OLT. Patients who have had coronary artery bypass surgery may be candidates for OLT if cardiac catheterization demonstrates minimal disease and if their ventricular function is good. Patients with hepatopulmonary syndrome often are good candidates for OLT [3]; intrapulmonary shunting has reversed in all of the patients with hepatopulmonary syndrome transplanted at our center. In contrast, patients with severe pulmonary hypertension usually do poorly after OLT and succumb to progressive pulmonary hypertension within months of the procedure. Carefully selected patients with cirrhosis and pulmonary hypertension may be candidates for combined lung and liver transplant.

Relative Contraindications

Several conditions which by themselves are not absolute contraindications to OLT have been associated with poor survival after liver transplantation. The list of these disorders is constantly changing and may vary among medical centers (Table 117-4). Because of a virtual 100% recurrence rate and significantly reduced survival, some centers do not perform transplants in people with hepatitis B who have a positive test for e antigen or hepatitis B virus DNA (HBV DNA). However, good results have been obtained in this group of patients with aggressive protocols employing passive immunotherapy with hepatitis B immunoglobulin (HBIG). Patients treated in this fashion become HBV DNA– and hepatitis B surface antigen–negative in the perioperative period. More recently, antiviral agents, including famciclovir, ganciclovir, and lamivudine, have been used to reduce viral load or even eliminate virus from the blood prior to OLT. Postoperatively, antiviral agents alone have not been able to prevent recurrent infection in 20% to 30% of treated patients because of viral mutations. The combination of HBIG and antiviral agents may be the best regimen to prevent recurrent hepatitis B after OLT.

Portal vein thrombosis once was considered an absolute contraindication to OLT, but with the evolution of surgical techniques it has become only a relative contraindication to the procedure. OLT is still feasible in people with portal vein thrombosis if the superior mesenteric vein (SMV) is patent. A graft of donor iliac vein is used to bridge the gap between the SMV of the recipient and the portal vein of the donor organ. If

Table 117-2. Indications for Liver Transplantation in Children	
Indications	**Transplants performed, %**
Biliary atresia	55
Metabolic	15
Other cholestatic disorders	11
Fulminant hepatic failure	11
Cryptogenic	6
Malignancy	1.5

Table 117-3. Absolute Contraindications to Liver Transplantation
HIV infection
Extrahepatic malignancy
Uncontrolled infection
Active substance abuse
Advanced cardiopulmonary disease
Severe pulmonary hypertension

an arteriogram reveals thrombosis of the entire portal venous system, OLT is not possible.

Advanced age (older than 65 years) and UNOS status 1 also are relative contraindications to OLT. The 5-year survival rate after OLT in those older than age 65 years is 57% compared with 68% for patients in other age groups. People older than 65 years may do well after OLT if they are carefully screened before the procedure for comorbid diseases and if they have no major perioperative complications [4]. Patients with the highest priority, UNOS status 1, have a lower survival than do less sick individuals. The greatest difference between members of these two groups is seen in the first year following transplant. Since status 1 has been redefined to include only patients with acute liver failure, primary nonfunction, and perioperative hepatic artery thrombosis, the survival gap between patients with the highest and those with the lowest priorities may diminish.

Individuals whose primary indication for OLT is hepatobiliary malignancy have the worst results, with 2- and 5-year survival rates of 50% and 38%, respectively [5•]. Death is almost always from recurrent cancer. Centers that continue to transplant patients with malignancy do so with protocols that use adjuvant therapy, both preoperatively and postoperatively. The outcomes for patients with large, poorly differentiated tumors with vascular invasion are poor. The results of OLT for cholangiocarcinoma are even worse than those for hepatocellular carcinoma. Consequently, most centers do not consider patients with cholangiocarcinoma for transplantation.

Extensive prior right-upper-quadrant surgery may be a relative contraindication for OLT, particularly in patients who have had a portocaval shunt. Although the operative mortality has not been shown to be significantly higher, the operative procedure is considerably more difficult and bloodier and results in more postoperative morbidity.

■ EVALUATION

A successful liver transplant program requires the expertise and collaboration of specialists in different medical disciplines and ancillary services (Table 117-5). The liver transplant evaluation involves information gathering by members of the evaluation team, the patient, and members of the patient's family. Potential OLT recipients must be informed about the evaluation, the approval and listing process, the expected waiting time for a donor organ, the operative procedure, the average length of stay following surgery, the early and late complications of OLT, the need for life-long medications after OLT and their associated

toxicities, the anticipated survival results and improvement in quality of life, and the commitment necessary from the patient and his or her support system.

The goals of the transplant team are to
• determine, if possible, the specific etiology of the patient's liver disease
• assess the severity of the liver disease and its affect on survival
• determine whether there are medical or other surgical therapies that may postpone OLT or make it unnecessary
• assess the intellectual, social, financial, and psychiatric status of the candidate.

The success of liver transplantation has resulted in earlier patient referral, which is desirable because the average waiting time for elective OLT is 1 to 2 years.

The imaging studies and other tests used to evaluate candidates for OLT are listed in Tables 117-6 and 117-7. Magnetic resonance imaging is done selectively in patients with a computed tomography scan suggesting a hepatoma. Angiograms are obtained in patients with abnormal duplex ultrasound examinations or prior portosystemic shunt. Liver biopsies are reviewed by a hepatopathologist. A recent cholangiogram with brushings for cytology is necessary in patients with primary sclerosing cholangitis (PSC). Similarly, colonoscopy is performed in patients with PSC whether they have inflammatory bowel disease or not.

Other tests performed include an echocardiogram with a bubble-shunt study for right-to-left shunt, pulmonary function testing, chest radiograph, and electrocardiogram. Patients with a history of coronary artery disease are referred to cardiology for cardiac catheterization. Patients without symptoms of cardiac disease but with typical risk factors, including age older than 55 years, smoking, male gender, and especially diabetes, receive noninvasive stress tests [6]. Cardiac catheterization is done to evaluate candidates with abnormal stress tests. Other consultations are arranged as needed.

Assessing the severity of the liver disease is an equally important part of the evaluation process because it affects the need for transplantation and the timing of the procedure. Most patients referred for a liver transplant evaluation have complications of cirrhosis, including variceal bleeding, ascites, muscle wasting, fatigue, poor liver synthetic function, encephalopathy, and spontaneous bacterial peritonitis. Test

---

Table 117-4. Relative Contraindications to Liver Transplantation

Hepatitis B
  e Antigen, DNA positive
Portal vein thrombosis
Age > 65 y
Malignancy
UNOS Status 1
Extensive prior right upper-quadrant surgery

Table 117-5. Liver Transplant Team

Evaluation team	Transplant management team
Hepatologists	Operating room and intensive care nurses
Surgeons	
Transplant coordinator	Perfusionists (management of veno-venous bypass)
Psychiatrists	
Chemical dependency experts	Dialysis technicians
Social workers	Hepatopathologists
Bioethicists	Infectious disease specialists
Financial advisors	Hematologists and blood bank technicians
Anesthesiologists	
	Neurologists

Table 117-6. Pretransplant Blood Studies

CBC with differential

SMA-16

ALT, GGTP

PT, PTT

RPR

Alpha fetoprotein

ABO blood type

Hepatitis serologies: A, B, C

HIV

Viral serologies: cytomegalovirus, herpes, Epstein-Barr virus

Transferrin

Fibrinogen

CA-19-9

HCV RNA (HCV patients)

HBV DNA (HBV patients)

Anti–smooth muscle antibody

Antimitochondrial antibody

Antinuclear antibody

α_1-antitrypsin phenotype

Ceruloplasm

*GGTP—gamma-glutamyl transpeptidase; PT—prothrombin time ;
PTT—partial thromboplastin time; RPR—rapid plasma reagin (test).*

Table 117-7. Pretransplant Imaging and Other Studies

Duplex ultrasound of the portal vein

Angiography (selectively)

Computed tomography

Magnetic resonance imaging (selectively)

Cholangiogram (primary sclerosing cholangitis)

Esophagogastroduodenoscopy

Colonoscopy

Echocardiogram

Echocardiogram with bubble-shunt study

Stress test/cardiac catheterization (selective)

Galactose elimination capacity

results helpful in assessing liver function include serum bilirubin and albumin levels, prothrombin time, platelet count, and measurements of nutritional status. The Child-Pugh classification is used to quantitate the severity of liver disease; patients with a score of C are candidates for immediate listing. Of the several survival models based on Cox regression analysis for cholestatic liver disease (particularly primary biliary cirrhosis), the Mayo Clinic model is the one used most often. One-, 3- and 5-year survival estimates are made based on age, serum albumin and bilirubin concentrations, amount of edema, and prothrombin time [7•]. The severity of liver disease also affects both quality of life and timing of OLT. Patients who can no longer work, attend school, or run a household are sufficiently ill to be listed for OLT.

Once the etiology and severity of the liver disease have been determined, alternatives to OLT must be considered. For instance, a surgical shunt (distal splenorenal shunt) or transhepatic intraparenchymal portal-systemic shunt (TIPS) procedure may be a better choice in a patient with well-preserved liver function whose major problem is recurrent variceal bleeding. Although the patient's liver disease will progress, OLT may not be necessary for several years. Neither of the decompressive procedures mentioned would preclude a subsequent transplant. In most patients, however, there are no alternatives to OLT.

A psychosocial assessment is necessary to evaluate the candidate's support system and his/her understanding of the commitment and compliance necessary for the long-term success of OLT. Assessments by the social worker and bioethicist are particularly helpful in gathering this information. If the patient is a child, the parents need to understand the magnitude of the commitment associated with OLT.

Renal dysfunction often is associated with ESLD and may affect postoperative morbidity and mortality. Hepatorenal syndrome (see Chapter 114) resolves after successful OLT, but patients who require dialysis prior to OLT, either to treat chronic renal disease or acute tubular necrosis, have more morbidity and a higher mortality following transplant than do persons with normal renal function [8•]. Because of postoperative problems and the nephrotoxicity of cyclosporine and tacrolimus, patients with chronic renal disease are better served by a combined liver-kidney transplant. Patients with acute renal injury, for example from a contrast study or a drug, should be supported and not transplanted until their renal function improves.

TIMING

When to list a patient for OLT remains a subjective decision. The two major factors to consider are the severity of the liver disease and the estimated waiting time for a donor organ. In general, a patient who has developed complications of cirrhosis and who has completed an evaluation should be listed for OLT because the waiting time for a donor organ for a nonhospitalized patient in most areas of the United States is 1 to 2 years. Individuals too ill to be evaluated as outpatients are transferred to liver transplant centers. An evaluation can be performed, and the patient can be listed within a few days of arrival. Patients with acute liver failure can be evaluated and listed for emergent OLT within 24 hours of admission.

APPROVAL AND LISTING PROCESS

Most centers hold weekly liver transplant selection committee meetings in which candidates who have been evaluated are discussed. Patients who are approved for listing are added to the UNOS waiting list based on their blood type, size, and urgency. A pager is issued to the patient so that he or she can be reached at any time. A selective bowel decontamination protocol, which consists of noroxin and mycostatin, is begun when the patient is third or fourth from the top of the list. Frequent follow-up and continued management by the transplant center's hepatology team are important for optimal care prior to OLT.

TRANSPLANT PROCEDURE

The average liver transplant procedure takes 7 to 8 hours. Hepatectomy is the most demanding part of the operation because of portal hypertension and coagulopathy. Adhesions from prior right upper-quadrant surgery increase the technical difficulty and blood requirements. Many centers routinely use venovenous bypass during the anhepatic stage of the procedure in an effort to minimize hemodynamic changes and blood loss [9](Fig. 117-1). After implantation of the donor liver, blood flow is re-established; bleeding from fibrinolysis and consumptive coagulopathy may occur at this time. After adequate hemostasis, the biliary tree is reconstructed, the gallbladder is removed, and the incision is closed [9] (Fig. 117-2).

POSTOPERATIVE MANAGEMENT

The two factors that most influence the initial postoperative course after OLT are the preoperative condition of the recipient and the ease of the transplant procedure. Surgery free of technical problems, major blood loss, and hypotension usually results in a relatively uncomplicated postoperative course. Patients who were ambulatory prior to OLT usually are discharged from the intensive care unit on the second or third postoperative day. In contrast, patients who were severely ill prior to OLT may require prolonged ventilatory support, aggressive nutritional assistance, and dialysis after the procedure under the care of experts in intensive care medicine and liver transplant management.

Indicators of early graft function include bile production; prothrombin time; serum aminotransferase levels, which peak at 2000 U/L or less and decrease in the first 24 to 48 hours after surgery; and the patient's neurologic status. T-tube drainage of 100 to 200 mL/d of dark, thick bile reflects good graft function, as does a prothrombin time of 20 seconds or less. Efforts to reduce the prothrombin time to less than 18 seconds may cause hepatic artery thrombosis, especially in very small-sized children. Patients who were encephalopathic for a long time prior to OLT may not be alert and neurologically normal until several days after OLT. The immediate postoperative elevation of the aminotransferase reflects the ischemic injury to the graft liver.

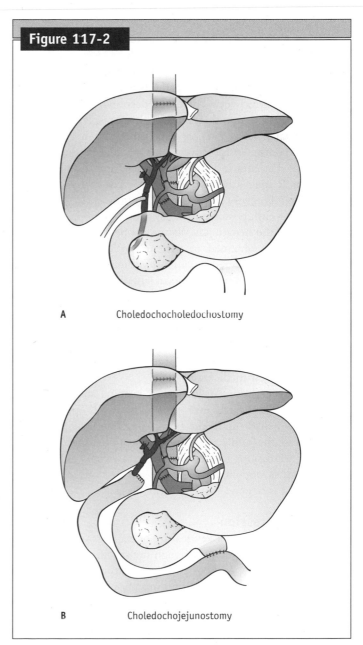

Figure 117-2

A   Choledochocholedochostomy

B   Choledochojejunostomy

Preferred anastomosis is duct-to-duct (choledochocholedochostomy). In situations where the recipient duct is diseased, absent, or too small, Roux-en-Y choledochojejunostomy provides an equally safe alternative. (*Adapted from* Starzl et al. [9].)

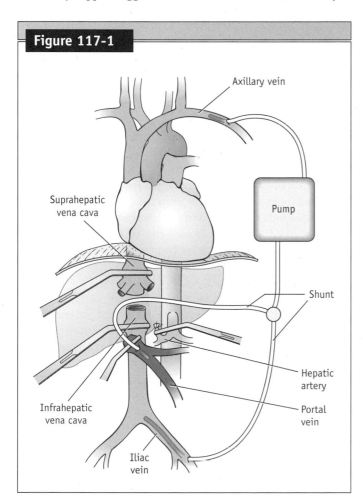

Figure 117-1

Axillary vein

Suprahepatic vena cava

Pump

Shunt

Hepatic artery

Infrahepatic vena cava

Portal vein

Iliac vein

The centrifugal pump circulates blood from the iliac and portal veins, bypassing into the axillary vein for return to the heart. (*Adapted from* Starzl et al. [9].)

Bleeding and primary graft nonfunction are two severe complications of OLT that may occur immediately following transplant. Surgical exploration may be necessary to control intra-abdominal bleeding. Primary graft nonfunction usually results in death unless another OLT is performed immediately. Primary graft nonfunction occurs in approximately 10% of post-transplant patients; its etiology is not well understood, but it is thought to be related to preservation injury of the graft sinusoidal endothelium. Clinical manifestations of primary graft nonfunction include scant bile production, encephalopathy, persistently abnormal serum aminotransferase levels, uncorrectable coagulopathy, multiorgan system failure, and ultimately, death.

Most patients are transferred to a regular nursing floor on the second or third postoperative day. Oral intake is resumed within a couple of days of the procedure except in patients who have had a choledochojejunostomy for biliary drainage. Liquids are started in these patients on the fourth or fifth postoperative day. The diet is advanced rapidly, and patients begin ambulation as soon as possible. Debilitated patients may need physical therapy during their recovery. The bowel decontamination protocol is continued for 1 month following the transplant procedure. Intravenous ganciclovir, which is started on the first postoperative day, is continued for 2 weeks for cytomegalovirus (CMV) prophylaxis. Patients at high risk for CMV infection (seropositive donor, seronegative recipient) also receive hyperimmune gamma-globulin every 2 weeks for 3 months.

On the seventh postoperative day, a liver biopsy and a duplex ultrasound of the hepatic vasculature are performed. A cholangiogram also is obtained in patients with a T-tube; biliary scintigraphy is performed in patients without a T-tube. Further evaluation is dictated by the clinical situation.

Patient education is begun as soon as the patient is transferred to a regular nursing unit. Patients and their families are instructed by nurses on the unit and the transplant coordinators. Patients learn how to take their own vital signs, which they monitor twice daily after discharge. They also must become familiar with their medications.

The mean and median lengths of hospital stay following a relatively uncomplicated liver transplant are 25 and 20 days, respectively. Follow-up in the transplant clinic is at 2 weeks, 6 weeks, 5 months, and 1 year after transplant. Additional office visits and admissions to the hospital are arranged as necessary. Blood work is obtained weekly for the first several months; eventually, it is obtained on a monthly basis.

Immunosuppression

Immunosuppression is a key feature of the postoperative management of OLT patients. Although the specific drug strategies vary among centers, corticosteroids and either cyclosporine or tacrolimus are the basis of all antirejection regimens. Several weeks after OLT, an attempt is made to wean patients off prednisone. The dose is slowly reduced, and if liver function remains stable, prednisone is stopped completely, often within 1 year of transplantation.

Cyclosporine and tacrolimus are the major immunosuppressant drugs used after liver transplantation. Neither of these medications is given during the first day or two after surgery because they are nephrotoxic. Cyclosporine is available in a microemulsion form, Neoral (Novartis Pharmaceutical Corp., East Hanover, NJ), which does not require bile for absorption from the gut. Tacrolimus (FK 506, Prograf; Fugisawa USA, Deerfield, IL) is similar to cyclosporine, but more potent. Most centers use only the oral preparation; the intravenous form has been associated with a higher incidence of toxicity. Treatment with either tacrolimus or cyclosporine results in similar patient and graft survival 6 months and 1 year after OLT [10••,11••]. Patients treated with tacrolimus, however, have fewer rejection episodes, particularly recurrent rejection and steroid resistant rejection. Other benefits of tacrolimus are less hypertension and less overall corticosteroid usage. In our experience, approximately 33% of acute rejection episodes can be reversed by simply increasing the dose of tacrolimus. The major toxicities of both tacrolimus and cyclosporine are renal and neurologic. Tacrolimus may be more diabetogenic than cyclosporine. Both drugs are administered every 12 hours; daily measurement of trough blood levels is mandatory for proper patient management.

Other immunosuppressant agents used to treat OLT patients include azathioprine, mycophenolate, antilymphocyte globulin, and OKT3 (a monoclonal anti-T cell antibody). Many centers routinely use triple therapy, with corticosteroids, either azathioprine (Imuran; Glaxo Wellcome, Research Triangle Park, NC) or mycophenolate (CellCept; Roche Pharmaceuticals, Nutley, NJ), and either cyclosporine or tacrolimus. Azathioprine and mycophenolate are both antimetabolites that inhibit T- and B-cell proliferation. Bone marrow suppression is the major toxicity of both medications. Recent trials have shown that mycophenolate is superior to azathioprine in controlling rejection. We use triple therapy selectively in patients who require three drugs to control rejection or in patients whose renal dysfunction will not allow a full dose of either cyclosporine or tacrolimus.

Antilymphocyte globulin and OKT3 are intravenous medicines used for induction therapy or to treat steroid-resistant rejection. Both agents are very powerful immunosuppressants that have been associated with an increased risk of CMV infection and development of a post-transplant lymphoproliferative disorder.

◼ POSTOPERATIVE COMPLICATIONS

Liver transplantation may be associated with significant postoperative morbidity. In fact, only 15% to 20% of patients do not develop some complication after OLT. Complications generally may be categorized as either graft-related or extrahepatic.

Graft Dysfunction

Graft dysfunction, defined as abnormal liver tests, occurs in 50% to 60% of OLT patients in the perioperative period (Table 117-8). Studies necessary to evaluate a patient with graft dysfunction include a liver biopsy, a cholangiogram or biliary scintigraphy, and a duplex ultrasound of the hepatic blood vessels; computed tomography and angiography also may be required. As discussed earlier, primary nonfunction is evident within 24 hours of OLT and results in a mortality rate of 80% without immediate retransplantation. Severe dysfunction may respond to treatment with intravenous prostaglandin E1.

Table 117-8. Postoperative Complications

Graft-related	Extrahepatic
Primary nonfunction	Pulmonary
Preservation injury	Pneumonia
Rejection	Pleural effusion
Vascular thrombosis	Gastrointestinal
Infection	Bleeding
Biliary tract complications	Pancreatitis
Hemolysis	Perforation
Drug injury	Renal dysfunction
	Neurologic
	Infection
	Cardiovascular
	Hypertension
	Myocardial
	infarction/dysfunction
	Malignancy
	Lymphoma

Rejection is the most frequent cause of graft dysfunction during the first 3 months after transplantation. The reported incidence of rejection is 40% to 100%; approximately 45% to 50% of our patients develop rejection. Although acute rejection usually does not develop until at least 7 to 10 days after OLT, it can occur as early as the fifth day after surgery. As a result, physicians at most centers perform liver biopsies on the seventh day after OLT. The pattern of liver tests most suggestive of rejection are rising serum levels of bilirubin, alkaline phosphatase, and γ-glutamyl transpeptidase. Cholestasis from preservation injury, which is treated with "benign neglect," also develops about 1 week after transplant. A liver biopsy therefore is required to make the diagnosis of rejection. The histologic hallmarks of rejection include a portal lymphoid infiltrate, bile duct injury, and endothelial inflammation of the portal and central veins. Liver tests improve without any change in therapy in 10% to 15% of patients whose biopsies exhibit histologic changes of rejection. Treatment of rejection is required, however, when liver tests continue to rise.

By definition, patients whose rejection does not respond to higher doses of tacrolimus and corticosteroids have steroid-resistant rejection, which requires treatment with monoclonal antibodies (OKT3). Because we have been using tacrolimus, few patients in our practice have required a course of OKT3. A third agent, either azathioprine or mycophenolate, is added to the immunosuppressant regimen as necessary. Retransplantation for uncontrollable acute rejection is rare, and rejection itself is responsible for only a small percentage of deaths after OLT.

Vascular complications associated with OLT include thrombosis of the hepatic artery, portal vein, or hepatic veins. Hepatic artery thrombosis (HAT) is the most common of these, occurring in 2% to 8% of adults and 3% to 20% of children [12•]. Nontechnical causes of HAT include rejection, with graft edema and reduced blood flow, and a hematocrit greater than 45%. Although some patients with HAT may not have symptoms, almost all affected patients present with fulminant hepatic necrosis, relapsing bacteremia, or biliary complications.

Fulminant hepatic necrosis usually develops in the perioperative period; approximately 25% of affected patients survive with retransplantation. Relapsing bacteremia most often develops weeks to months after OLT and present with insidious fever, leukocytosis, positive blood cultures, and mildly abnormal liver tests. Although ultrasound or computed tomography may demonstrate liver abscesses, areas of hepatic infection may be microscopic in size. Diagnosis of HAT requires a high degree of suspicion and, often, angiography. Antibiotics are temporarily effective in suppressing bacteremia, but retransplantation is the only cure. HAT causes biliary complications because the hepatic artery is the sole blood supply of the graft biliary tree. Biliary problems associated with HAT include bile duct necrosis and bile leaks as well as multiple ductular strictures radiographically similar to primary sclerosing cholangitis. A bile leak often requires operative drainage. Strictures may be temporarily managed endoscopically or percutaneously by dilation and stenting, but the only long-term solution to stricturing is retransplantation. Ultimately, 75% to 80% of patients with HAT require retransplantation, and 50% of affected individuals die.

A bile leak or an anastomotic stricture can occur in the absence of HAT. The incidence of biliary complications after OLT is 15% to 20%. Leaks usually occur within the first couple of weeks after OLT. An anastomotic leak requires surgical repair. Anastomotic strictures occur much later and are more frequent after a choledochojejunostomy. Percutaneous or endoscopic dilatation and stenting may be corrective, but surgical revision is often necessary.

Infection, hemolysis, and drug-induced injury are other causes of graft dysfunction. Bacterial and fungal sepsis can cause hyperbilirubinemia; viruses, particularly CMV, can infect the graft directly. Hepatitis B and C can recur within several weeks of OLT. Hemolysis is a manifestation of graft-versus-host disease and is self-limited, resolving without treatment in days to weeks. Cyclosporine and amphotericin can cause dose-related cholestasis.

Infection

Infection is responsible for over 50% of deaths following OLT. Sixty percent to 80% of patients develop an average of 2.5 infections each following transplant. Fifty percent of infection-related deaths occur in the first postoperative month and 90% in the first 2 postoperative months. Some of the risk factors for infection include the overall state of health of the recipient, the quality of the donor organ, the urgency of the transplant, retransplantation, a lengthy, complicated and bloody operative procedure, preexisting infection, and immunosuppression.

Infections after OLT may be classified by etiologic agent and time of occurrence. Fifty percent to 60% of infections are bacterial, 20% to 40% are viral, and 5% to 15% are fungal; less than 10% are due to *Pneumocystis carinii* or *Toxoplasma*. Bacterial and fungal infections are seen early in the postoperative course and often result from either pre-transplant conditions or surgical complications, for example HAT, bile leak, intra-abdominal abscess, central venous catheter sepsis, and gastrointestinal perforation. Both gram-positive (*Staphylococcus aureus*) and gram-negative organisms (*Pseudomonas aeruginosa*) are common pathogens. Diagnosis of a bacterial infection may be difficult because of immunosuppression, which can blunt the usual signs of fever, leukocytosis, and abnormal physical findings. In addition to obtaining cultures, imaging studies and a liver biopsy may be necessary to identify the source of sepsis.

Fungal infections, which develop in 15% to 20% of liver transplant recipients, are associated with a mortality of 50% to 80%. The incidence of fungal infections is higher in liver transplant patients than in other organ recipients because of intraoperative manipulation of the gastrointestinal tract and biliary tree. Eighty percent of fungal infections occur within the first postoperative month. Candida species, particularly *C. albicans*, are responsible for 75% to 80% of fungal infections; the remaining 15% to 20% are caused by *Aspergillus*. Patients who are severely debilitated prior to transplantation, particularly those requiring continuous hospitalization, are most likely to develop a postoperative fungal infection. Other risk factors include a lengthy operation, spillage of bowel contents or bile, recurrent bacterial infections, multiple organ dysfunction, graft dysfunction, and prolonged courses of multiple antibiotics. A high degree of suspicion is required for timely diagnosis of fungal infection. Multiple cultures of body fluids, including image-guided percutaneous drainage of intra-abdominal collections, may be necessary to make the diagnosis. Mycostatin is begun a few months prior to transplant as part of a bowel decontamination protocol to prevent or reduce the incidence of fungal infection. Colonization, as often occurs in the bladder, can be treated with fluconazole; invasive infections and candidemia require therapy with amphotericin.

Invasive aspergillosis occurs in approximately 4% of liver transplant patients and carries a mortality rate of almost 100%. Most aspergillosis infections manifest within 6 weeks of surgery; risk factors are debilitation, multiorgan dysfunction, retransplantation, OKT3 administration, and repeat laparotomies. The lungs are the most frequently affected site, but systemic infection can involve virtually any organ. The diagnosis may be elusive because cultures are not always positive; tissue biopsy may be necessary to demonstrate the organism. Amphotericin B therapy for invasive aspergillosis is frequently unsuccessful, in part because of delayed diagnosis.

Pneumocystis carinii is another organism that may cause infection weeks to months after transplantation. Pneumocystis, which has been reclassified as a fungus, infects approximately 5% to 10% of OLT patients not receiving prophylaxis. Disease due to *P. carinii* presents with fever, cough, and dyspnea. Hypoxemia may be dramatic, and the patient may require ventilatory support. Bilateral interstitial infiltrates are seen on chest radiograph. The diagnosis is established by detection of organisms in either induced sputum or bronchoalveolar lavage fluid. The therapy of choice is a 2- to 3-week course of trimethoprim-sulfamethoxazole. Pentamidine is used to treat patients who fail to improve or have a drug reaction. Prophylaxis with either trimethoprim-sulfamethoxazole three times per week or pentamidine once per month is started a few days before hospital discharge and continued indefinitely.

Viral infections are common in transplant patients. CMV infection occurs in up to 70% of OLT patients, and CMV disease, defined as symptomatic infection, with graft, pulmonary, or systemic involvement, occurs in approximately 40%. Most CMV infections occur between 3 and 8 weeks after OLT; they may be primary, transmitted either by the donor organ or a blood product, or due to reactivation of the virus. Treatment with antilymphocyte globulin or OKT3 increases the risk of CMV infection. The most common manifestation of CMV disease is graft involvement. Pulmonary and gastrointestinal infection, and a mononucleosis-like syndrome with fever, malaise, leukopenia and thrombocytopenia, also occur. Diagnosis requires cultures, and possibly, biopsy of the liver or gastrointestinal tract. A 2- to 4-week course of intravenous ganciclovir is the only effective therapy. Because of the morbidity and mortality associated with CMV infection, every OLT patient receives CMV prophylaxis with intravenous ganciclovir during the immediate postoperative period.

Herpes simplex, varicella-zoster, and Epstein-Barr viruses also may cause infection in OLT patients. Herpes simplex infections occur in as many as 40% of patients within 3 weeks of transplant as a result of viral reactivation. Diagnosis is made from cultures that are usually taken from oral or genital vesicular lesions, and affected individuals are treated with acyclovir. Herpes zoster is usually a localized cutaneous disease that occurs in 5% to 10% of OLT patients; acyclovir also is used to treat herpes zoster.

Epstein-Barr virus infection, primary or reactivated, occurs in 25% to 50% of liver transplant patients. Most of these infections present within the first 6 months of surgery. Although most patients are asymptomatic, a primary infection can result in a mononucleosis-like syndrome with fever, malaise, and lymphadenopathy. Epstein-Barr virus is also responsible for development of post-transplantation lymphoproliferative disorders (PTLD), particularly in patients who receive OKT3. Epstein-Barr virus is a B-cell lymphotrophic virus capable of inducing proliferative changes, ranging from polyclonal reactive lymphoid hyperplasia to monoclonal large-cell lymphoma. PTLD is a serious complication of OLT with a mortality of approximately 50% in patients who develop lymphoma. Therapy consists of stopping or dramatically reducing immunosuppression and adding acyclovir or ganciclovir. Chemotherapy has been used with some success to treat patients with lymphoma.

Extrahepatic Complications
Renal Dysfunction
Renal dysfunction occurs in as many as 30% of OLT patients. Manifestations include oliguria, elevated serum creatinine, hyperkalemia, and hypertension. New renal dysfunction during the first postoperative week often is caused by cyclosporine or tacrolimus toxicity. Other independent predictors of early postoperative renal dysfunction include preoperative hepatorenal syndrome and intraoperative hypotension. Immunosuppressive therapy must be modified to allow renal dysfunction to improve or resolve. Renal dysfunction after the first postoperative week may be caused by cyclosporine or tacrolimus, or by sepsis or adverse reactions to other drugs.

Hypertension
Systemic hypertension is not uncommon following OLT. Causes include cyclosporine, tacrolimus, corticosteroids, genetic

predisposition, and volume overload. Hypertension immediately after surgery is often secondary to the large volume of fluids and blood products administered during the transplant procedure and in the early perioperative period. Aggressive diuresis usually decreases the blood pressure within the first week. Hypertension that persists after diuresis and with nontoxic serum cyclosporine or tacrolimus levels requires antihypertensive therapy. In our experience, 80% of patients treated with cyclosporine and 35% of patients treated with tacrolimus require antihypertensive therapy.

Glucose Intolerance

Hyperglycemia in the early post-transplant period is common. Predisposing factors include stress and therapy with corticosteroids, cyclosporine, and tacrolimus. The incidence of glucose intolerance, approximately 15% to 20%, is similar with either cyclosporine or tacrolimus. Some patients may require long-term treatment with insulin, whereas others may need only therapy with an oral hypoglycemic agent or no therapy at all.

Neurologic Toxicity

Neurologic complications occur in 20% to 30% of liver transplant patients [13•]. These complications include headaches, seizures, tremor, coma, paresthesias, confusion, visual hallucinations, and ataxic and cerebellar syndromes. OLT patients may develop infectious meningitis as well as aseptic meningitis associated with OKT3 therapy. Brachial plexus and peroneal nerve palsies can result from improper patient positioning during the surgical procedure. Although neurologic complications occurred in liver transplant patients before the use of either cyclosporine or tacrolimus, each of these agents has been implicated as a cause of some of the toxicities listed here. Other etiologic factors include hypomagnesemia, high-dose steroids, fluid overload, hypocholesterolemia, and demyelination. Seizures usually are treated with phenytoin, which may lower serum levels of both cyclosporine and tacrolimus by increasing drug metabolism. Drug levels in patients treated with phenytoin must be monitored and adjusted as needed. Most neurologic problems are reversible.

Malignancy

Transplant patients have an increased incidence of *de novo* malignancies. The most commonly encountered malignancies, in decreasing order of frequency, are cancers of the skin and lips, lymphomas, carcinoma of the lung, Kaposi's sarcoma, and carcinoma of the uterus [14•]. In OLT patients, lymphomas account for almost 60% of *de novo* malignancies, 40% of which are PTLDs associated with Epstein-Barr virus infection, as discussed earlier. Lymphomas are more common in children, perhaps because they have more lymphoid tissue than adults and because they have a higher incidence of primary Epstein-Barr virus infection after OLT. The mean and median times to presentation of lymphoma post-transplant are 15 and 6 months, respectively. Treatments include reduction or cessation of immunosuppression, excision, antiviral agents, chemotherapy, radiation therapy, and interferon. Penn [14•] has reported a 33% complete remission rate in OLT patients treated for lymphoma.

■ SURVIVAL

Survival after OLT has improved dramatically during the last decade. One- to 4-year graft- and patient-survival rates reported by UNOS from 1987 to 1995 are shown in Table 117-9 (UNOS web site, July 1997). The 1-year survival rate for all OLT patients is greater than 80%. Improved survival is due to more effective immunosuppression, standardized operative techniques, improved organ preservation, better donor management, and training of new transplant teams.

Several factors affect patient survival after liver transplantation. These include type and stage of liver disease, retransplantation, patient immune response, and overall recipient health. Clearly, mortality and morbidity rates are higher in patients who are more severely ill, particularly those with long-standing chronic disease who acutely decompensate and require life support before OLT. Table 117-10 shows 1- and 5-year survival rates for patients transplanted from 1987 through 1994 based on primary diagnosis [5•]. The best 1- and 5-year survivals are achieved in patients with either cholestatic or metabolic liver disease; the worst outcome is in patients transplanted for malignant disease. The 1-year survival rates also are low in patients with fulminant liver failure. Table 117—11 shows the 1- and 3-year survival rates for the same years (1987–1994) based on UNOS status at the time of transplant. UNOS status 1 patients have a 20% lower survival at 1 year than do patients well enough to await transplant at home. Patients undergoing

Table 117-9. Graft and Patient Survival Rates, October 1987 to December 1995

	Survival Rates, %			
	1 Year	2 Year	3 Year	4 Year
Graft	71.2	66.6	63.3	60.6
Patient	80.6	76.9	74.1	71.8

Data from UNOS [5].

Table 117-10. Patient Survival Rates, October 1987 to December 1995

	Survival Rates, %	
Primary Diagnosis	1 Year	5 Year
Noncholestatic cirrhosis	80	66
Cholestatic liver disease	85	77
Biliary atresia	81	76
Fulminant failure	71	64
Metabolic disease	82	76
Malignancy	66	34

From UNOS [5].

Table 117-11. Survival Based on UNOS Status, October 1987 to December 1995

Waiting list status	1 Year	3 Year
1	70	64
2	81	73
3	90	82
4	90	82

Definition of status: 1) bound for intensive care unit, expected to live 7 days; 2) hospitalized in an acute care bed for at least 5 days; 3) requires continuous care; at home; 4) at home (no longer exists as a status).
From UNOS [5].

Table 117-12. Primary Versus Retransplant Survival Rates, October 1987 to December 1995

	Survival Rates, %	
	1 Year	5 Year
Primary transplant	83	71
Retransplant	58	48

From UNOS [5].

retransplantation have a greater than 20% reduction in 1-year survival rates compared with first-time transplant recipients (Table 117-12) [5•].

Five- and 10-year survival rates for patients who live through the first year following transplant are 85% to 92% and 63 to 80%, respectively [15•]. At least 60% of deaths that occur more than 1 year after transplant are caused by graft problems or complications of chronic immunosuppression. Causes of late death include recurrent primary disease, hepatitis or malignancy, delayed hepatic artery thrombosis, opportunistic infection, and *de novo* malignancy, especially lymphoma. The majority of the remaining late deaths are caused by cardiovascular events, such as myocardial infarction and cerebrovascular accident.

RETRANSPLANTATION

Retransplantation is necessary in 9% to 21% of OLT patients for either acute or chronic graft failure. Primary nonfunction, hepatic artery thrombosis, and acute rejection are the most frequent causes of acute graft failure. Chronic rejection, bile duct necrosis from preservation injury, and recurrent primary disease are the major causes of chronic graft failure.

The 1-year survival rate for patients undergoing elective retransplantation is approximately 80%, virtually the same as that in primary transplant recipients. However, only a 40% 1-year survival rate is achieved in patients requiring emergent retransplantation. Financial and ethical issues associated with retransplantation are becoming increasingly important.

QUALITY OF LIFE

Assessment of the quality of life after liver transplantation is important but subjective. Several questionnaires and tools, such as the Karnofsky Performance Status Scale, the Sickness Impact Profile, and the Index of Well-Being, have been used to assess changes in the quality of life after liver transplantation. Overall, 80% to 85% of patients have an improved quality of life by the end of the first year following transplant [16•]. This improvement is sustained through the fifth year following transplant and beyond with many patients returning to part- or full-time employment outside the home.

REFERENCES

Recently published papers of particular interest have been highlighted as follows:
• Of interest
•• Of outstanding interest

1.• Belle SH, Beringer KC, Murphy JB, *et al.*: The Pitt-UNOS Liver Transplant Registry: Clinical Transplantation 1992. Los Angeles, UCLA Tissue Typing Laboratory, 1992.

2.•• Wiesner RH: Current indications, contraindications, and timing for liver transplantation. In *Transplantation of the Liver.* Edited by Busuttil RW, Klintmalm GB. Philadelphia: WB Saunders, 1996:71–84.

3. Scott V, Miro A, Kang Y, *et al.*: Reversibility of the hepatopulmonary syndrome by orthotopic liver transplantation. *Transplant Proc* 1993, 25:1787–1788.

4. Bromley PN, Hilmi I, Tan KC, *et al.*: Orthotopic liver transplantation in patients over 60 years old. *Transplantation* 1994, 58:800–803.

5.• UNOS: The US Scientific Registry of Transplant Recipients and the Organ Procurement and Transplantation Network. Transplant data 1988–1995. US Department of Health and Human Services, Health Resources and Services Administration. 1996: 141, 143, 144.

6. Carey WD, Dumot JA, Pimentel RR, *et al.*: The prevalence of coronary artery disease in liver transplant candidates over age 50. *Transplantation* 1995, 59:859–864.

7.• Dickson ER, Grambsch PM, Fleming TR, *et al.*: Prognosis in primary biliary cirrhosis: a model for decision making. *Hepatology* 1989, 10:1–7.

8.• Gonwa TA, Morris CA, Goldstein RM, *et al.*: Long-term survival and renal function following liver transplantation in patients with and without hepatorenal syndrome: experience in 300 patients. *Transplantation* 1991, 51:428–435.

9. Starzl TE, *et al*: Refinements in the surgical technique of liver transplantation. *Semin Liver Dis* 1985, 5:349.

10.•• European FK506 Multicenter Liver Study Group: Randomized trial comparing tacrolimus (FK506) and cyclosporine in prevention of liver allograft rejection. *Lancet* 1994, 344:423–428.

11.•• The US Multicenter FK506 Liver Study Group: A comparison of tacrolimus (FK506) and cyclosporine for immunosuppression in liver transplantation. *N Engl J Med* 1994, 331:1110–1115.

12.• D'Alessandro AM, Ploeg RA, Knechtle SJ, *et al.*: Retransplantation of the liver—A seven year experience. *Transplantation* 1993, 55:1083–1087.

13.• Stein DP, Lederman RJ, Vogt D, *et al.*: Neurologic complications following liver transplantation. *Ann Neurol* 1992, 31:644–649.

14.• Penn I: Post transplantation de novo tumors in liver allograft recipients. *Liver Transplant Surg* 1996, 2:52–59.

15.• Asfar S, Metrakos P, Fryer J, *et al.*: An analysis of late deaths after liver transplantation. *Transplantation* 1996, 61:1377–1381.

16.• Levy MF, Jennings L, Abouljoud M, *et al.*: Quality of life at one, two, and five years after liver transplantation. *Transplantation* 1995, 59:515–518.

Gallbladder and Biliary Tract

Edited by Jacques Van Dam

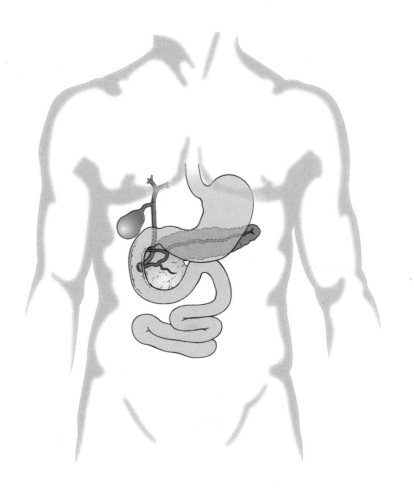

Contributors

Michael D. Apstein
David C. Brooks
William R. Brugge
Amitabh Chak
Francis P. Colizzo
Francis A. Farraye
Paul Fockens
Gerard Isenberg
Ira M. Jacobson
William V. Kastrinakis
Rabia Köksal
Glen A. Lehman
Simon K. Lo
John D. McKee

Stuart Sherman
Steven J. Shields
Adam Slivka
Roy Soetikno
Michael Sossenheimer
Assaad M. Soweid
Julie Spivack
Tony Tham
Jo Vandervoort
Dirk J. van Leeuwen
Irving Waxman
Richard C. K. Wong
Wisam F. Zakko

118 Anatomy and Developmental Anomalies
Jo Vandervoort, Roy Soetikno, and Tony Tham

EMBRYOLOGY OF THE BILIARY SYSTEM

Early in the fourth week of development, the liver, gallbladder, and biliary system arise as a ventral outgrowth from the caudal part of the foregut (see Chapter 87). This entodermal outgrowth or hepatic diverticulum subsequently divides into cephalic and caudal portions, the former giving rise to the liver and hepatic ducts, and the latter forming the gallbladder and cystic duct; the stalk of the hepatic diverticulum forms the common bile duct. By the seventh week of development, the initially solid structures have become vacuolized and their lumens established. The distal muscularis propria of the bile duct and pancreatic duct are independent from duodenal musculature [1••].

NORMAL ANATOMY OF THE BILIARY SYSTEM

Intrahepatic Bile Duct Anatomy

The liver is divided into two major portions: the right and left hepatic lobes and a dorsal (caudate) lobe (see Chapter 87). The separation between the right and left lobes (Cantlie's line) is an oblique plane that extends from the center of the gallbladder bed to the left side of the inferior vena cava. Within this plane lies the middle hepatic vein, an important landmark in radiologic and ultrasound investigations in identifying the two lobes [2••]. The right and left lobes of the liver are drained by the right and the left hepatic ducts, respectively, whereas the dorsal lobe (caudate lobe) is drained by one or several ducts joining both the right and left hepatic ducts. The intrahepatic ducts are tributaries of the corresponding hepatic ducts that form part of the major portal tracts and which penetrate the liver invaginating Glisson's capsule at the hilus. Thorough knowledge of hilar anatomy and the caudate lobe is important for surgical resection.

Extrahepatic Bile Duct Anatomy

The extrahepatic segments of the left and right hepatic ducts join to form the common hepatic duct. The common bile duct is the main biliary channel draining into the duodenum. The accessory biliary apparatus constitutes a reservoir for bile and is made up of the gallbladder and cystic duct. The confluence of the right and left hepatic ducts takes place to the right of the hilus of the liver anterior to the portal venous bifurcation and overlying the origin of the right branch of the portal vein (Fig. 118-1). The extrahepatic segment of the right duct is short but the left duct has a much longer extrahepatic course.

The main bile duct is divided into two segments; the segment proximal to the cystic duct insertion is called the common hepatic duct. The cystic duct joins the common hepatic duct to form the common bile duct. There is a considerable range of bile duct diameters; the upper limit of normal for the main bile duct diameter measured by ultrasonography is generally accepted as 4 to 5 mm. The common bile duct joins the duodenum anterior to the portal vein. It usually lies in a groove on the undersurface of the pancreas or may be completely surrounded by pancreatic tissue. The common bile duct approaches the second part of the duodenum obliquely from left to right and posterior to anterior. In its terminal course it lies against the medial wall of the duodenum, joined to it by connective tissue, for a distance of 8 to 22 mm. This anatomic orientation facilitates the safe performance of endoscopic sphincterotomy or operative sphincteroplasty. The terminal part of the common bile duct is accompanied by the terminal part of the duct of Wirsung. It runs adjacent to but separated from the bile duct by the transampullary septum to enter the duodenum at the papilla of Vater.

Gallbladder and Cystic Duct

The gallbladder is a reservoir for bile and is located on the inferior surface of the right lobe of the liver in the region of the junction between segments IV and V; it is covered by a layer of peritoneum. It varies in size and consists of a fundus, body, and neck. The tip of the fundus usually reaches the free edge of the liver and is adjacent to the cystic plate. The neck of the gallbladder creates an angle with the fundus. A large gallstone lodged in this part of the neck creates a Hartmann's pouch. The cystic duct arises from the neck or infundibulum of the gallbladder and extends to join the common hepatic duct, most often in its supraduodenal segment. Its lumen is usually approximately 1 to 3 mm and its length is variable. The mucosa of the cystic duct

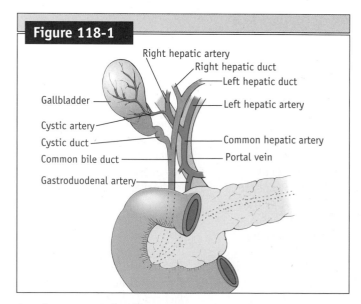

Figure 118-1

Right hepatic artery
Right hepatic duct
Left hepatic duct
Gallbladder
Left hepatic artery
Cystic artery
Cystic duct
Common hepatic artery
Common bile duct
Portal vein
Gastroduodenal artery

Anterior aspect of the biliary anatomy. The confluence of the hepatic bile ducts is situated anterior to the right branch of the portal vein. (*Adapted from* Smadja and Blumgart [2••].)

is arranged in spiral folds known as *Heister's valves*. Its wall is surrounded by a sphincteric structure called *Lütkens's sphincter*.

Anatomy of the Normal Sphincter of Oddi

The terminal parts of the common bile duct, pancreatic duct, common channel, and major duodenal papilla of Vater form the sphincter of Oddi segment (Fig. 118-2). The usual position of the papilla is in the second part of the duodenum, an average of 8 cm from the pylorus; however, this distance is variable. In 13% it may be located at or distal to the junction of the second and third parts of the duodenum; in 4% it may be found between 1.5 and 5 cm from the pylorus. Rarely it may be found in the stomach or pylorus. Although it is common to refer to the region beyond the common junction of the pancreatic duct and common bile ducts as the "ampulla of Vater," there is no such structure in humans.

The major part of the sphincter lies within the duodenal wall and enters the duodenum through a slit (choledochal window) in the duodenal muscle. The junction of the terminal common bile duct, pancreatic duct, and duodenum at the papilla assumes one of three configurations: 1) in approximately 70% of subjects the ducts open into a common channel that varies from 2 to 17 mm long and drains into the duodenum through a single orifice on the duodenal papilla of Vater; 2) in approximately 20% of subjects the common channel is almost nonexistent and the two ducts have a common opening on the papilla; 3) in 10% of subjects the common bile duct and pancreatic duct have separate openings on the tip of the papilla, lying adjacent to each other.

Before entering the duodenum, each duct becomes completely surrounded by circular muscle. The point at which the circular smooth muscle starts on each duct is identified radiologically as a notch. Distal to the notch, each lumen narrows as it passes through the duodenal wall. Throughout its course in the duodenal wall, the ducts are ensheathed by circularly oriented smooth muscle. Contrary to previous descriptions of three distinct sphincters (sphincter choledochus, sphincter pancreaticus, sphincter ampullae), it is now believed that the sphincter of Oddi consists of just one sphincter zone. The mucosa of the biliary system is lined by columnar epithelium and contains mucus-secreting glands. The mucosa is oriented into longitudinal folds like mucosal valvulae. These folds become maximal in the common channel.

▬ ABERRANT BILE DUCTS

Congenital variations or anomalies of the biliary system are common, with a reported prevalence of 18.5% [2••]. The most common biliary duct anomaly, an anomalous right hepatic duct that empties into the common hepatic duct or cystic duct, is seen in 4% to 5% of cholangiograms. It is important to recognize an aberrant right hepatic duct at cholangiography because of the potential risk of its injury during cholecystectomy (Fig. 118-3). The main variations of the hepatic duct confluence are shown in Figure 118-4. Several anomalies of drainage of the intrahepatic ducts into the neck of the gallbladder or cystic duct also have been reported and must be kept in mind during cholecystectomy to prevent ductal injury.

Anomalous ducts arising from the left lobe are rare and usually of no clinical significance. They do not drain into the common hepatic duct or cystic duct and, therefore, are not susceptible to injury during cholecystectomy. Anomalies of the accessory biliary apparatus with agenesis of the gallbladder, bilobar gallbladders with a single cystic duct but two fundi, and duplication of the gallbladder with two cystic ducts have been described. A double cystic duct may drain a unilocular gallbladder. Congenital diverticulum with a muscular wall also can be seen. The mode of union of the cystic duct with the common hepatic duct may be angular, parallel, or spiral. An angular union is the most frequent and is found in 75% of patients. The cystic duct may run parallel to the common hepatic duct in 20% of patients with connective tissue ensheathing both ducts. Finally, the cystic duct may go toward the common hepatic duct in a curled fashion, curving about it usually from the posterior aspect. Anomalies of location are uncommon but can lead to diagnostic dilemmas in patients with symptoms of pancreaticobiliary disease.

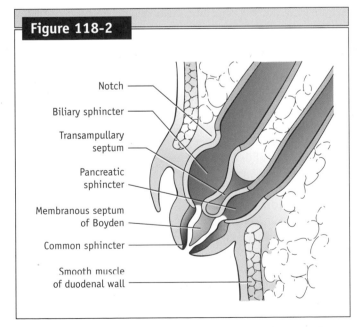

Figure 118-2

Notch
Biliary sphincter
Transampullary septum
Pancreatic sphincter
Membranous septum of Boyden
Common sphincter
Smooth muscle of duodenal wall

Normal anatomy of the sphincter of Oddi. (*Adapted from* Smadja and Blumgart [2••].)

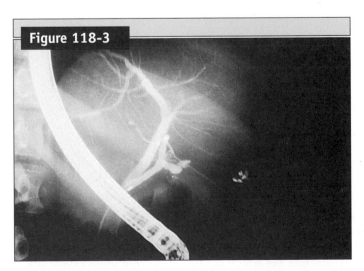

Figure 118-3

Aberrant right hepatic duct.

PANCREAS DIVISUM

Pancreas divisum is the most frequent congenital ductal anomaly of the pancreas, occurring in 3% to 7% of patients undergoing endoscopic retrograde cholangiopancreatography (ERCP) and in approximately 9% of autopsy studies [3]. The abnormality occurs when the dorsal pancreatic duct (duct of Santorini) and the ventral pancreatic duct drain into the duodenum through the major papilla and the dorsal pancreatic duct (duct of Wirsung) drains through the minor papilla. The relationship of pancreas divisum to pancreatitis is controversial. In patients with apparent idiopathic acute pancreatitis, there is a high prevalence of pancreas divisum reported in 12% to 50% of cases [4]. These patients usually develop symptoms during middle-aged years, and their pancreatitis

usually is mild but recurrent. Chronic relapsing pancreatitis also may occur and involve the ventral pancreas, dorsal pancreas, or both. In the young or middle-aged patient with recurrent pancreatitis without obvious cause, pancreas divisum must be considered and ERCP is recommended. No communication between the ventral and dorsal duct is demonstrated on injection of the major and minor papilla, respectively.

ANOMALOUS JUNCTION OF THE PANCREATICOBILIARY DUCTAL SYSTEM

Anomalous junction of the pancreaticobiliary system is defined as a union of the common bile duct and pancreatic duct outside the duodenum. The anomalous junction can occur as a long common channel, with the pancreatic duct inserting into the common bile duct. Alternatively, the common bile duct may insert into the pancreatic duct or via a more complex union. When an anomalous junction is present, pancreatic juice may reflux into the bile duct or bile can reflux into the pancreatic duct if a distal biliary obstruction is present. Such anomalous junctions may carry an increased risk of carcinoma.

CONGENITAL BILIARY CYSTS

In adult patients with persistent and unexplained symptoms, such as cholangitis, pancreatitis, jaundice, recurrent abdominal pain, nausea, and vomiting, a congenital anomaly of the pancreatic or bile duct must be considered and a diagnostic cholangiopancreatography performed. Although congenital pancreaticobiliary abnormalities are relatively uncommon, the increased prevalence of cholangitis, gallstones, and cholangiocarcinoma seen with the various types of biliary cystic disease and junctional anomalies, and the increased association of pancreatitis that occurs with pancreatic anomalies, make recognition of variant anatomy clinically important.

Cystic dilation of the biliary tree occurs in a variety of forms that involve isolated or combined dilation of the intra- and extrahepatic ducts. Congenital cystic anomalies are classified as choledochal cysts, cystic duct cysts, and gallbladder cysts. Because cystic duct cysts and gallbladder cysts are rare and are treated by cholecystectomy, the following discussion focuses on choledochal cystic disease (*ie*, choledochocele, choledochal cyst, Caroli's disease). Choledochal cysts are associated with significant morbidity and mortality. Understanding the etiology, classification, pathology, diagnosis, and management of choledochal cysts, in conjunction with proper use of endoscopic and surgical treatment modalities, are necessary to provide the optimal treatment of these patients.

Classification

The most commonly used classification of choledochal cyst disease is that of Todani [5•] (Fig. 118-5). Because the risks and causes of morbidity and mortality of choledochal cysts correlate with the type of cysts, an accurate classification is mandatory. Type I choledochal cyst is a diffuse cystic dilation of the common bile duct and hepatic duct (the hepatic duct bifurcation, intrahepatic ducts, and cystic duct are not involved); type II is a supraduodenal diverticulum with a relatively normal biliary tree; type III is also called *choledochocele* or *an isolated intraduodenal*

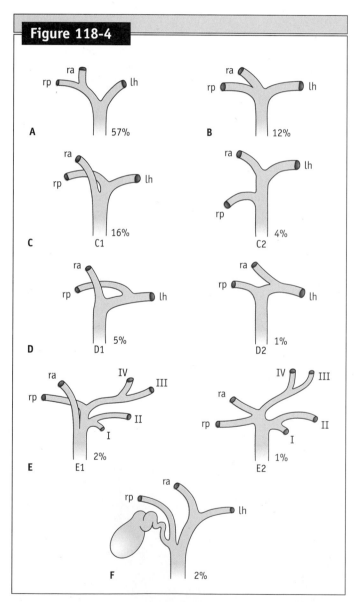

Figure 118-4

Main variations of the hepatic duct confluence. **A,** Typical anatomy of the confluence; **B,** triple confluence; **C,** ectopic drainage of a right sectoral duct into the common hepatic duct; **D,** ectopic drainage of a right sectoral duct into the left hepatic ductal system; **E,** absence of the hepatic duct confluence; **F,** absence of the right hepatic duct and ectopic drainage of the right posterior duct into the cystic duct. (*Adapted from* Smadja and Blumgart [2••].)

diverticulum; type IV is divided into two types—type IVa involves dilation of the intra- and extrahepatic ducts and type IVb is characterized by multiple extrahepatic cystic dilations and a choledochocele; type V, which is also called Caroli's disease, involves multiple dilations of the intrahepatic ducts without extrahepatic biliary abnormalities. Two types of Caroli's disease have been recognized. The most common form is accompanied by progressive hepatic fibrosis and cirrhosis whereas the less common form is not. Caroli's disease usually is confined to the left lobe, but it can involve both lobes together.

Etiology

The exact pathogenesis of choledochal cysts is unclear [6]. Theories that have been proposed include 1) a congenital anomalous pancreatobiliary junction, 2) abnormal canalization of the bile duct during embryogenesis, and 3) abnormalities of autonomic innervation of the extrahepatic bile duct. Additional theories specific for the type 3 choledochocele have been suggested, including that it is an acquired evagination of mucosa of the distal common bile duct into the duodenum resulting from an impacted stone, fibrosis, papillitis, or sphincter of Oddi dysfunction. None of these theories have gained widespread acceptance. There have been few reports of type 5 Caroli's disease occurring in twins, but, in general, choledochal cyst disease is not inherited [7].

Pathology

The size of the cyst varies from 1 cm in diameter to a cyst that can contain more than 5 L of bile. The wall of the cyst usually is fibrotic and can be a few millimeters to 1 cm in thickness. Incomplete columnar or cuboidal epithelial cells are typical except in type 3 choledochocele, which is lined by either biliary or duodenal epithelium. Chronic inflammation, intestinal metaplasia, and carcinoma may be present [8•,9]. Adenocarcinoma (cholangiocarcinoma) is most common, followed by squamous and undifferentiated types.

The fluid contained within the cysts may be sterile or may contain bacteria, typically gram-negative rods. Cystolithiasis has been associated with increased risk for concurrent cholangiocarcinoma. The liver may be fibrosed and cirrhotic.

Clinical Features

The classic presentation of choledochal cyst include a triad of abdominal pain, jaundice, and an abdominal mass; however, only up to one third of patients present with the triad. In an analysis of 740 cases, abdominal pain was present in slightly over half of patients, jaundice was present in approximately two thirds of patients, and a mass was found in over 50% of patients. There is a female to male ratio of 3 to 1. Typically there is a long delay before the diagnosis is made, although approximately 75% of patients are

Figure 118-5

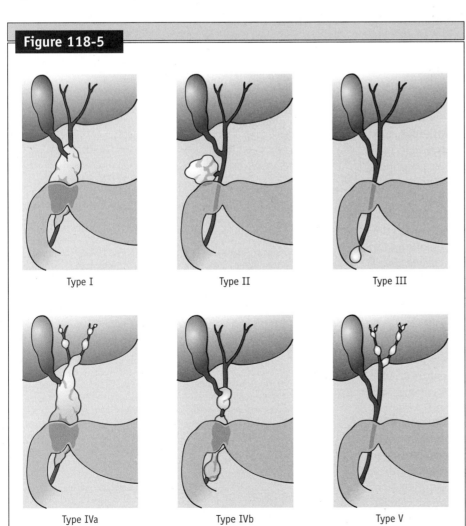

Type I   Type II   Type III

Type IVa   Type IVb   Type V

Biliary ductal cyst classification. Type I—the classic form of a choledochal cyst: saccular dilation of the common bile duct; type II—diverticulum originating from the common bile duct; type III—choledochocele; type IVa—cystic dilation of the intrahepatic biliary ducts: saccular dilation of the common bile duct; type IVb—multiple cystic dilations involving only the common bile duct; type V—Caroli's disease: cystic dilations of the intrahepatic bile ducts only. (*Adapted from* Todani *et al.* [5•]; with permission.)

diagnosed before adulthood. Recurrent cholangitis and abdominal pain are typical symptoms of patients with Caroli's disease.

Diagnosis

The diagnosis of choledochal cyst is made radiologically. Ultrasonography and computed tomography are useful initial studies, but many patients require further study with ERCP or percutaneous transhepatic cholangiography. ERCP allows precise definition of the anatomy of the pancreatic and biliary ductal systems and offers the possibility for tissue sampling or stenting when there is suspicion of malignancy [10] .

Complications

Biliary cystic disease may be complicated by jaundice, gallstones, cholecystitis, cholangitis, pancreatitis, or carcinoma of the biliary tree, gallbladder, and pancreas. Spontaneous cyst rupture is rare. Hepatic fibrosis, cirrhosis, and the complications of cirrhosis may occur after long-standing intermittent or partial biliary obstruction, and are mainly associated with a type V cyst (Caroli's disease).

The most common cancer associated with choledochal cyst is cholangiocarcinoma [8•,9]. The risk of cholangiocarcinoma varies according to the type of cyst and increases with age. The risk of developing cancer seems to be related to bile stasis and contact between bile and the epithelium. It also may be related to reflux of pancreatic juice into the biliary tree, which gives rise to chronic irritation and metaplasia. The incidence of cholangiocarcinoma has been reported to be up to 15%, but may be as low as 2.5% in type 3 choledochocele. Although cholangiocarcinoma has been reported in teenagers with choledochal cysts, it is most often found during the fourth decade of life. Survival after the diagnosis of cholangiocarcinoma is usually less than 1 year [1••]. Although excision of the cyst eliminates a potential source of cholangiocarcinoma, it does not exclude the possibility of cancer developing in the intrahepatic bile ducts. Therefore, long-term observation is indicated in all patients with choledochal cysts.

In infants and neonates, a choledochal cyst may present as bile peritonitis secondary to cyst rupture. The pathogenesis of spontaneous perforation of choledochal cysts is unknown, but underperfusion with acute inflammation of the dilated ductal wall and mural weakness caused by reflux of pancreatic juice are two possible factors. Cyst rupture due to trauma or during pregnancy also has been reported infrequently.

The association of pancreatitis with choledochal cysts, although infrequent, is well recognized. The pathophysiology of pancreatitis is related to the anomalous pancreaticobiliary junction with a long common channel. In such cases, obstruction of the pancreatic duct or the common channel by a stone or bile reflux through the dilated common channel can precipitate pancreatitis [11].

The course of Caroli's disease [12•] is dominated by recurrent episodes of bacterial cholangitis, the frequency of which varies widely from 2 to 20 episodes a year; the prognosis is poor in patients with frequent episodes of cholangitis. Most of these patients die 5 to 10 years after the onset of cholangitis, usually of an uncontrolled biliary bacterial infection. These recurrent episodes of cholangitis induce the formation of intrahepatic pigment stones. Cholangiocarcinoma can also develop in this condition.

Management

It generally is accepted that the ideal long-term management of choledochal cysts type 1, 2, and 4 is surgical, excising all cyst tissue and reconstructing the continuity between the liver and intestine using an intestinal limb by a Roux-en-Y hepaticojejunostomy [10,13,14,15]. This surgery minimizes the risk of cholangitis and presumably reduces the risk of carcinoma. Cholecystectomy also is performed. In patients who may require continuing postoperative surveillance of the biliary tree, such as those with incomplete resection, interposition of a short (15 cm) jejunal segment between the liver hilum and duodenum may allow subsequent endoscopy. Alternatively, in patients with associated dilation of the intrahepatic duct, partial hepatectomy may be appropriate, especially when the dilation involves a single lobe. The management of type 3 choledochal cyst usually involves endoscopic sphincterotomy to unroof the choledochocele. The long-term management of type 5 (Caroli's disease) is controversial, but usually involves supportive treatment for recurrent cholangitis and possibly surgical drainage if abscesses develop. Surgical therapy is most appropriate in unilobar disease (about 20% of cases are unilobar and usually involve the left lobe). In cases of unilobar disease, partial hepatectomy often is needed whereas orthotopic liver transplantation has been performed in cases with extensive bilateral liver involvement.

▅▅ REFERENCES

Recently published papers of particular interest have been highlighted as follows:
- •   Of interest
- •• Of outstanding interest

1.•• Rizzo RJ, Szucs RA, Turner MA: Congenital abnormalities of the pancreas and biliary tree in adults. *Radiographics* 1995, 15:49–68.

2.•• Smadja C, Blumgart LM: *Surgery of the Liver and Biliary Tract*, edn 2. Edited by Smadja C and Blumgart LM. Edinburgh: Churchill Livingstone; 1994:11–26.

3.   Sugawa C, Walt AJ, Nunez DC, Masuyama H: Pancreas divisum: is it a normal anatomic variant? *Am J Surg* 1987, 153:62–66.

4.   Bernard JP, Sahel J, Giovannini M, Sarles H: Pancreas divisum is a probable cause of acute pancreatitis: a report of 137 cases. *Pancreas* 1990, 3:248–254.

5.• Todani T, Watanabe Y, Narusue M, et al.: Congenital bile duct cysts: classification, operative procedures and review of 37 cases including cancer arising from choledochal cyst. *Am J Surg* 1977, 134:263–269.

6.   Flanigan DP: Biliary cysts. *Ann Surg* 1975, 182:635–643.

7.   Ribeiro A, Rajender KR, Bernstein D, et al.: Caroli's syndrome in twin sisters. *Am J Gastroenterol* 1996, 91:1024–1026.

8.• Ozawa K, Yamada T, Matumoto Y, Tobe R: Carcinoma arising in a choledochocele. *Cancer* 1980, 45:195–197.

9.   Todani T, Tabuchi K, Watanabe Y, Kobayashi T: Carcinoma arising in the wall of congenital bile duct cysts. *Cancer* 1979, 44:1134–1141.

10. Venu RP, Geenen JE, Hogan WJ, et al.: Role of endoscopic retrograde cholangiopancreatography in the diagnosis and treatment of choledochocele. *Gastroenterology* 1984, 87:1144–1149.

11. Greene FL, Brown JJ, Rubinstein P, Anderson MC: Choledochocele and recurrent pancreatitis: diagnosis and surgical management. *Am J Surg* 1985, 149:306–309.

12.• Tandon RK, Grewal H, Anand AC, Vashist S: Caroli's syndrome: a heterogeneous entity. *Am J Gastroenterol* 1990, 85:170–173.

13. Caudle SO, Dimler M: The current management of choledochal cysts. *Am Surg* 1986, 52:76–80.

14. Okada A, Nakamura T, Okumura K, et al.: Surgical treatment of congenital dilatation of bile duct (choledochal cyst) with technical considerations. *Surgery* 1987, 101:238–243.

15. Nagorney DM, Mc Ilrath DC, Adson MA: Choledochal cysts in adults: clinical management. *Surgery* 1984, 96:656–663.

119 Gallstones

Michael D. Apstein

Gallstone disease is very common in the United States, affecting 15% of the total population and 25% of women over 50 years of age. Of the million persons diagnosed annually with gallstones in the United States, half undergo biliary tract surgery. Despite the relative ease and popularity of laparoscopic cholecystectomy, major issues for clinicians remain: evaluation of patients for gallstones; determination of who should be treated and how; consideration of the role of endoscopic therapy; and recommendations for prevention of gallstones in persons at high risk, such as those undergoing rapid weight loss.

PATHOPHYSIOLOGY

Gallstones are composed primarily of either cholesterol or calcium bilirubinate salts (pigment). Typically, patients harbor one type or the other, not both. In the United States, 80% of gallstones are of the cholesterol variety. Identifying the type of gallstone has clinical importance because only cholesterol gallstones are amenable to dissolution or prevention with oral bile acid therapy.

Cholesterol Gallstones

The traditional hypothesis to explain cholesterol gallstone formation invokes three distinct pathophysiologic defects: supersaturation of bile with cholesterol, accelerated nucleation of cholesterol in the gallbladder, and gallbladder hypomotility [1••]. Persons who form cholesterol gallstones secrete excess cholesterol into bile, the primary excretory route for cholesterol. Recent studies suggest that a genetic defect responsible for the hypersecretion of cholesterol from the liver is the fundamental pathophysiologic abnormality in patients with cholesterol gallstones [2]. Hypersecretion of cholesterol into bile may trigger events in the gallbladder wall that accelerate cholesterol nucleation and inhibit gallbladder contractility [1••].

Cholesterol normally is solubilized effectively in bile by micelles and vesicles composed of bile salts and the phospholipid lecithin. Biliary cholesterol secretion is determined, in large measure, by biliary bile salt secretion. Relatively more cholesterol is secreted into bile at low bile salt secretion rates than at high ones. Thus, for example, during an overnight fast when the bile salt secretion rate is low, bile is more saturated with cholesterol than it is after a meal, when the secretion rate is high.

In persons with cholesterol gallstones, cholesterol nucleates in gallbladder bile five times more rapidly than normal. Accelerated nucleation may occur either because of an excess of pronucleating or a deficiency of antinucleating proteins. In addition, gelled gallbladder mucin hastens gallstone nucleation. Bile containing excess cholesterol stimulates gallbladder mucin synthesis and secretion. In animals, aspirin, which inhibits mucin production, can prevent gallstone formation despite the persistence of supersaturated bile. Cholesterol crystals enmeshed in mucin can agglomerate and grow into macroscopic gallstones in a poorly contracting gallbladder.

The speed at which cholesterol gallstones form varies with the patient's risk factors and underlying genetic predisposition for gallstone formation (see "Risk Factors"). In Pima Indians, the average time between the appearance of "lithogenic" bile and gallstones is 8 years. In patients whose gallstones have been dissolved with oral bile acids, new gallstones form at the rate of 10% per year. In contrast, patients with acute spinal cord injuries and obese patients ingesting a very low calorie diet form gallstones within months. For example, after ileal bypass surgery performed for obesity, gallstones can develop within 6 months, and by 2 to 4 years the prevalence of gallstones ranges from 20% to 60%.

Pigment Gallstones

There are two varieties of pigment gallstones, black and brown [3].

Black pigment gallstones. In Western populations black pigment gallstones form principally in the gallbladder. These gallstones are composed of bilirubin polymers and inorganic salts of calcium (carbonate and phosphate), the latter accounting for their radiopacity. Black pigment gallstones occur in the setting of overproduction and secretion of excess unconjugated bilirubin into bile, increased biliary concentration of ionized calcium, decreased biliary bile salt secretion, and poor gallbladder motility. Ionized calcium in bile bonds with unconjugated bilirubin, precipitates, and grows to form gallstones. Normally, bile salts solubilize unconjugated bilirubin and compete with it for binding with ionized calcium. Consequently, bile salt deficiency may promote pigment gallstone formation by making more unconjugated bilirubin and ionized calcium available for coprecipitation. Gallbladder hypomotility allows calcium bilirubinate precipitates to remain in the gallbladder and grow into macroscopic gallstones.

Brown pigment gallstones. Brown pigment gallstones usually form *de novo* in the bile ducts after cholecystectomy and occur in the setting of biliary tract infection. Bacterial deconjugation of conjugated bilirubin produces an excess of unconjugated bilirubin in bile. Bacterial phospholipase hydrolyzes biliary phospholipid producing fatty acids. Brown pigment gallstones are composed mainly of calcium bilirubinate and organic fatty acid (palmitate and stearate) salts of calcium; hence these gallstones are radiolucent.

EPIDEMIOLOGY

The prevalence of gallstones varies greatly throughout the world [4]. They are very common in certain populations, such as Native

American Indians of the Southwest United States, and rare in many Third World countries. In countries with high prevalence rates, the overall female-to-male ratio is approximately 2 to 1, reflecting a predominance of cholesterol gallstones. In countries with low prevalence rates, the gender ratio is 1 to 1, reflecting a predominance of pigment gallstones. The prevalence of cholesterol and pigment gallstone disease among the populations of Japan and China has changed markedly during the 20th century. Up until the end of World War II, both Japan and China had a low prevalence of gallstones, which were predominantly of the pigment variety. Over the past 40 years, the prevalence of cholesterol gallstones in this population has increased markedly and that of pigment gallstones has decreased.

Ultrasonography of large ambulatory populations has defined the true prevalence of gallstones in various populations. In Sirmione, Italy, for example, investigators screened nearly 2000 persons (70% of the population) and found that gallstone prevalence increased linearly in women and men, respectively, from 2.9% and 1.1% at the ages of 18 to 29 to 27% and 11% at the ages of 50 to 65. Importantly, 80% of persons with gallstones were unaware of their presence and had no history of biliary pain during the 5 years preceding the study [5].

Risk Factors for Gallstone Formation

Cholesterol gallstones form when environmental risk factors are added to genetic predisposition.

Cholesterol gallstones

The risk factors for formation of cholesterol gallstones are listed in Table 119-1.

Female gender. Endogenous estrogens increase biliary cholesterol secretion, offering a potential explanation for the increased risk of cholesterol gallstone formation in women between puberty and menopause. After menopause, women lose their increased risk for gallstone formation.

Parity. Pregnancy is an independent risk factor for cholesterol gallstones. Elevated estrogen and progesterone levels during pregnancy probably are responsible for increasing biliary cholesterol secretion and inhibiting gallbladder motor function, respectively.

Obesity. Obesity increases the risk of cholesterol gallstone formation and the development of symptomatic gallstones. Obese persons synthesize more cholesterol and secrete more of it into bile than do nonobese persons. Biliary cholesterol saturation reverts to normal after obese persons achieve ideal body weight.

Rapid weight loss. Obese persons undergoing rapid weight loss (approximately 1% to 2% of body weight, or 2 to 5 lb/wk) have an extraordinary (25% to 70%) chance of developing gallstones within 4 months. This phenomenon is explained by the observation that with weight loss, cholesterol is mobilized from adipose tissue and secreted into bile. Even less rapid weight loss has been associated with gallstone formation.

Native American heritage. A genetic predisposition may explain the very high prevalence of cholesterol gallstones among Pima Indians: 4% in 25- to 34-year-old men and 70% in men over 65 years of age. Pima Indian women have an even greater risk: 73% of 25- to 34-year-old women have gallstones.

Gallbladder stasis. Gallbladder stasis syndromes and poor gallbladder motility are associated with gallstone cholesterol formation in women during pregnancy, patients with somatostatinomas, patients receiving octreotide or total parenteral nutrition, and patients with spinal cord injury.

Medications. Fibric acid derivatives, such as clofibrate, that lower serum cholesterol by increasing biliary cholesterol secretion increase the risk of cholesterol gallstone formation.

Cholestyramine and other bile acid sequestrants lower serum cholesterol by binding bile acids in the intestine and causing bile acid malabsorption. These drugs do not increase the risk of gallstones because the liver compensates by increasing synthesis of bile salts to maintain the size of the bile salt pool.

Inhibitors of 3-hydroxy-3-methylglutaryl coenzyme A (HMG CoA) reductase, the rate-limiting enzyme of cholesterol synthesis (eg, lovastatin), decrease biliary cholesterol saturation and should protect against gallstone formation.

Estrogen therapy in men or women is associated with an increased risk of developing cholesterol gallstones secondary to up-regulation of the hepatic low-density lipoprotein receptor, increased hepatic uptake of cholesterol, and increased excretion of cholesterol into bile.

Serum lipids. The relations between serum and bile lipids are complex. Whereas plasma triglyceride concentration is positively correlated with gallstone prevalence (even within the normal range), high-density lipoprotein cholesterol levels are inversely correlated with gallstone prevalence.

Diet. Little reliable data are available concerning diet and cholesterol gallstone disease. Except for obesity and weight loss, dietary habits probably do not influence cholesterol gallstone formation.

Diabetes mellitus. Persons with diabetes potentially have several risk factors for cholesterol gallstone formation, including increased biliary cholesterol secretion (independent of obesity);

Table 119-1. Risk Factors for Cholesterol Gallstone Formation
Female gender
Parity
Obesity
Rapid weight loss
Native American heritage
Gallbladder stasis
Medications: fibric acid derivatives (clofibrate), estrogens, and octreotide
Elevated triglycerides, depressed high-density lipoprotein cholesterol

abnormal gallbladder motility, usually in diabetic patients with long-standing disease and autonomic neuropathy. Whether diabetes mellitus itself is an independent risk factor for cholesterol gallstone disease is controversial [5,6]. Most older epidemiologic studies of persons with diabetes that describe such a correlation fail to separate the effects of obesity and hypertriglyceridemia.

Pigment Gallstones

The risk factors for formation of pigment gallstones are given in Table 119-2 [4].

Chronic hemolysis. Inherited hemolytic anemias, sickle-cell disease, spherocytosis, thalassemia, chronic hemolysis associated with artificial heart valves, and malaria all dramatically increase the risk of pigment gallstone formation because of increased biliary excretion of bilirubin. A sonographic study of 226 nonrandom patients with sickle-cell disease showed the following: the overall prevalence of gallstones or biliary sludge was 33%; in both men and women, the prevalence increased from 12% in the 2- to 4-year-old age group to 43% in the 15- to 18-year-old age group; symptoms attributable to gallstones were rare [7].

Alcoholic cirrhosis. Patients with alcoholic cirrhosis or alcoholism have an increased prevalence of pigment gallstones that increases steadily with advancing age and severity of liver disease. The mechanism is not known.

Increasing age. Increasing age is a risk factor for pigment gallstone formation. Patients with pigment gallstones undergo cholecystectomy at a later age than do patients with cholesterol gallstones, suggesting that either pigment gallstones form later in life than do cholesterol gallstones or these persons remain asymptomatic for longer periods of time than those with cholesterol gallstones.

Ileal disease, resection, or bypass. Patients with ileal disease, resection, or bypass have a striking increased risk of gallstone formation that is directly proportional to the length of ileum involved or resected. Of patients with ileal Crohn's disease, 30% have gallstones. Heretofore it was believed that ileal disease led to cholesterol gallstone formation; however, more recent studies show that these patients are at risk for pigment gallstones.

Table 119-2. Risk Factors for Pigment Gallstone Formation

Chronic hemolysis
Alcoholic cirrhosis
Increasing age
Ileal disease, resection, or bypass
Biliary infection
Duodenal diverticula
Gallbladder stasis syndrome
Truncal vagotomy
Hyperparathyroidism
Primary biliary cirrhosis

Biliary infection. In Asia, brown pigment gallstones are found frequently in the intrahepatic bile ducts and are nearly always associated with bacterial infection (usually *Escherichia coli*) or parasitic infestation (*Clonorchis sinensis* or *Ascaris lumbricoides*). In patients in Western countries, intraductal gallstones that develop after cholecystectomy are associated with stasis and biliary tract infection; hence, they are almost invariably brown pigment gallstones, even in those patients whose original gallstones were cholesterol.

Duodenal diverticula. A strong association exists between diverticula near the ampulla of Vater and the presence of pigment gallstones in the gallbladder. An attractive working hypothesis is that decreased muscular tone and contractility of the sphincter of Oddi and the common bile duct caused by the presence of the diverticulum allows the biliary tract to become infected with bacteria. In addition, the diverticulum itself may harbor bacteria and be the source of biliary tract seeding.

Gallbladder stasis syndromes. Total parenteral nutrition (TPN) dramatically increases the likelihood of pigment and cholesterol gallstone formation secondary to decreased gallbladder motility. In a prospective study using ultrasonography, 43% of children on TPN for a mean time of 21 months developed gallstones, and all patients receiving TPN for more than 6 weeks developed biliary sludge [8].

The frequency of either pigment or cholesterol gallstone formation in patients receiving TPN depends on concurrent medical problems. Thus, for example, by 2 years of TPN, gallstones developed in 39% of patients with, and 25% of patients without ileal disease [8].

Other. Gallstone formation is associated with truncal vagotomy, hyperparathyroidism, and primary biliary cirrhosis. Vagotomy probably decreases gallbladder motility, and hyperparathyroidism increases biliary calcium levels. However, gallstone composition in these conditions is unknown at present.

▬ DIAGNOSIS

Because the patient's medical history and physical examination are neither sensitive nor specific for the diagnosis of gallstones, the clinician must rely on confirmational diagnostic tests. Ultrasonography is the initial diagnostic procedure of choice for patients in whom gallstones are suspected. It is easily performed and interpreted and does not involve patient preparation or irradiation.

In addition to demonstrating gallstones, ultrasonography can detect so-called "gallbladder sludge," which is indicated by multiple weak echoes without acoustic shadowing in the dependent part of the gallbladder (Fig. 119-1) [9]. Gallbladder sludge can form during prolonged fasting in debilitated hospitalized patients, during hyperalimentation of patients, in patients with extrahepatic biliary obstruction, and in women (40%) soon after pregnancy. Gallbladder sludge is composed of a mixture of mucin glycoproteins and microprecipitates of calcium bilirubinate, liquid crystals of bile lipids, and solid cholesterol monohydrate crystals. Mucin glycoproteins accumulate in the gallbladder during stasis and in response to lithogenic bile and can entrap microprecipitates of calcium bilirubinate and, less frequently, liquid crystals and solid cholesterol crystals.

The natural history of gallbladder sludge is unpredictable (Fig. 119-2). In many patients, gallbladder sludge may be innocuous and disappear soon after delivery or oral refeeding. In others, however, sludge may cause any of the symptoms or complications of gallstones: biliary pain, acute cholecystitis, or pancreatitis. There is no doubt that sludge can evolve into gallstones. It is likely that sludge represents an early but still reversible stage of gallstone formation [9].

CLINICAL SYNDROMES

Most patients with gallstones never develop symptoms and harbor so-called "silent stones." If gallstones or biliary sludge occlude the cystic duct transiently, biliary pain (misnamed *colic*) occurs. A more prolonged obstruction of the cystic duct can be followed by acute cholecystitis, an infection in the gallbladder. When left

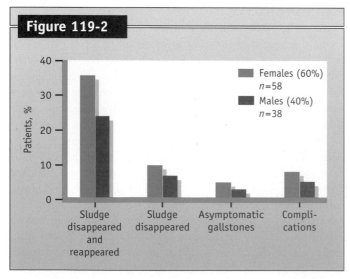

Figure 119-1

Gallbladder ultrasonography in a patient with biliary sludge. The *arrow* indicates the layering of the sludge dependently and the bile–sludge interface.

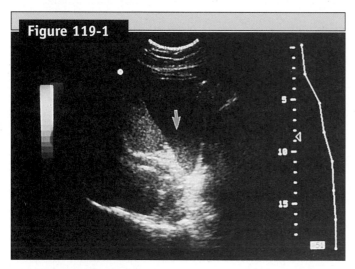

Figure 119-2

The natural history of biliary sludge. No patient under 40 years of age developed gallstones or complications. (*Adapted from* Lee *et al.* [33]; with permission.)

untreated, acute cholecystitis can progress to empyema, a pus-filled gallbladder, or gangrene of the gallbladder wall. Gallstones or sludge migrating from the gallbladder through the cystic duct into the common bile duct may cause biliary pain, jaundice, cholangitis, or pancreatitis. More rarely, gallstones erode through the gallbladder directly into the stomach or small intestine to cause obstruction, Bouveret's syndrome, or so-called "gallstone ileus," respectively. Finally, although rare, adenocarcinoma of the gallbladder is associated with long-standing gallstone disease.

Gallstones in Patients Who Are Asymptomatic

Multiple studies have demonstrated that most patients with gallstones never develop symptoms (Fig. 119-2) [10,11]. These "silent stones" are usually discovered incidentally on ultrasonography performed during pregnancy or for symptoms not associated with the biliary tract.

Two long-term prospective studies of asymptomatic patients with gallstones revealed similar results: patients have a 15% to 30% risk of developing symptoms over 10 to 20 years; most patients who develop symptoms usually do so within the first 5 years after the gallstones are discovered; and biliary pain, and not a complication of gallstones, is usually the first symptom [10,11] (Fig. 119-3).

Treatment of Patients Who Are Asymptomatic

Most asymptomatic patients with gallstones should be reassured and treated expectantly by watchful waiting because of the benign natural history of gallstones [10–12]. A decision analysis demonstrated that prophylactic cholecystectomy for men with asymptomatic gallstones resulted in a *loss* of 4 to 18 days of life [13]. Patients should be advised they are at risk for developing biliary pain over their predicted life span and that no lifestyle modifications, including diet, will modify that risk. If pain occurs, the patient must be reevaluated (see "Treatment of Patients with Biliary Pain").

The Role of Prophylactic Cholecystectomy

Prophylactic cholecystectomy is appropriate for several small categories of asymptomatic patients with gallstones [4] (Table 119-3).

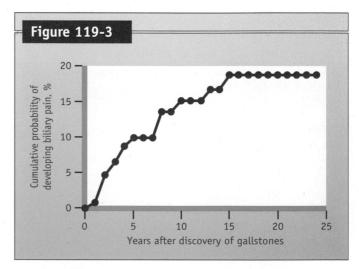

Figure 119-3

The natural history of gallstones in asymptomatic patients. (*Adapted from* Gracie and Ransohoff [11]; with permission.)

Occupation or lifestyle. Individuals working or vacationing for *extended* periods in remote parts of the world that lack rapid access to high-quality surgery should undergo cholecystectomy before embarking on their journey. Medical dissolution therapy would not be feasible in such circumstances because of time requirements and the risk of recurrence, as discussed later in this chapter.

Gallstones and gallbladder cancer. All patients with gallstones are at a slightly increased risk of developing gallbladder cancer. Even the very low risk of elective surgery in the average Western patient with gallstones, however, is much higher than are the patient's chances of developing gallbladder cancer. However, Native American women with gallstones and patients with a gallstone over 3.0 cm in diameter have a risk of developing gallbladder cancer that does outweigh the risk of surgery and, consequently, should undergo prophylactic cholecystectomy. Medical therapy to dissolve gallstones would not be appropriate in these patients because the gallstones themselves may not be the causative factor of the cancer.

Gallbladder cancer without gallstones. Four conditions require cholecystectomy even in the absence of gallstones because of the high risk of gallbladder cancer: calcification in the wall of the gallbladder (so-called "porcelain gallbladder") (Fig. 119-4), gallbladder polyps over 12 mm in diameter, anomalous pancreatico-biliary ductal junction, and carriers of *Salmonella typhosa*.

Diabetes and Prophylactic Cholecystectomy

In the past, prophylactic cholecystectomy for diabetic patients with asymptomatic gallstones was controversial. Anecdotal reports suggested that persons with diabetes were more prone to develop acute cholecystitis or other serious complications of gallstones without prior episodes of biliary pain. Also, diabetic patients with acute cholecystitis undergoing emergency cholecystectomy had an unacceptably high operative mortality (11% to 20%).

Taken together, these observations might support a role for prophylactic cholecystectomy in diabetic patients with asymptomatic gallstones. However, the natural history of gallstones in these patients is not known. Furthermore, two well-controlled retrospective studies of patients undergoing surgery for acute cholecystitis between 1960 and 1982 and a carefully performed decision analysis showed that diabetes was not an *independent* risk factor for operative mortality or serious postoperative complications [14], and that prophylactic cholecystectomy resulted

in 2 to 8 months of shortened life span in persons with diabetes in all age groups [15].

Thus, currently, prophylactic cholecystectomy for diabetic patients with asymptomatic gallstones cannot be recommended.

PREVENTION

Prevention is indicated in two groups of individuals at particularly high risk for the rapid formation of gallstones: patients receiving TPN and those undergoing rapid weight loss (see "Risk Factors"). The daily administration of intravenous cholecystokinin-octapeptide to patients receiving TPN prevents gallbladder stasis, gallbladder sludge, and gallstone formation [16•]. Oral administration of ursodiol, 8 to 10 mg/kg/d, to morbidly obese individuals undergoing rapid weight loss significantly reduces the formation of biliary sludge and gallstones [17] and is approved by the Food and Drug Administration (FDA) for this indication (Fig. 119-5).

TREATMENT OF SYMPTOMS
Biliary Pain

Biliary tract pain occurs when a gallstone or biliary sludge transiently obstructs the cystic or common bile duct. Typically, the pain, which is steady and *not colicky*, starts gradually, builds to a plateau, remains constant for several hours, and gradually resolves. Although most frequently localized to the right upper quadrant or epigastrium, biliary pain can occur in the left upper quadrant, subxiphoid region, or in the back. Radiation to the right shoulder or subscapular region is classic but not necessary for the diagnosis. Nausea and vomiting may accompany the pain. Despite anecdotal reports to the contrary, no evidence exists that ingestion of fatty or rich food, overeating, exercise, straining, or stress precipitates biliary pain.

Vague dyspeptic symptoms such as fatty food intolerance, postprandial bloating, indigestion, flatulence, and abdominal discomfort are no more common in patients with gallstones than they are in the general population. Therefore, these symptoms should not be attributed to gallstones and should not be expected to disappear or improve after cholecystectomy.

The results of a physical examination performed during an acute attack of biliary pain usually are normal. Occasionally,

Table 119-3. Conditions Prompting Prophylactic Cholecystectomy
Unusual occupation or lifestyle
Native American women
Large gallstones, over 3 cm
"Porcelain" gallbladder
Gallbladder polyps over 12 mm
Anomalous pancreatico-biliary ductal junction
Carrier of *Salmonella typhosa*

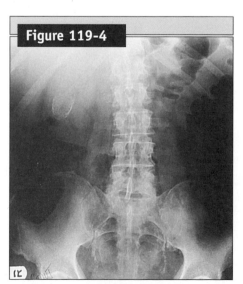

Figure 119-4

A "porcelain" gallbladder. Note the "eggshell" calcification in the gallbladder wall.

right upper quadrant tenderness may be present. Fever suggests progression to acute cholecystitis.

Laboratory studies, including a complete blood count and liver chemistry tests, should be obtained during an episode of suspected biliary pain. Elevated liver chemistry test results suggest transient obstruction of the common bile duct rather than of the cystic duct. Elevation of serum transaminase levels into the range indicative of hepatitis may be seen acutely with common bile duct obstruction. Typically, these elevations resolve within several days and are followed by an increase in the serum alkaline phosphatase level. Leukocytosis, especially with a "left shift," suggests the development of acute cholecystitis.

Ultrasonography, the initial diagnostic procedure of choice for patients with suspected biliary pain, has a 95% sensitivity and 98% specificity for gallbladder stones. It can also demonstrate common bile duct dilation and biliary sludge.

The natural history of patients with even one episode of biliary pain is less benign than that of asymptomatic patients with gallstones (Fig. 119-6). Half of these patients will experience recurrent pain over the subsequent 20 years. Additionally, acute cholecystitis and other complications (cholangitis and pancreatitis) occur at a linear rate of 1% annually [18].

Treatment Options for Patients with Biliary Tract Pain
Laparoscopic cholecystectomy is now the gold standard for treatment of patients with gallstones who have biliary tract pain. Over 95% of elective cholecystectomies use this approach [19]. Advantages of laparoscopic cholecystectomy include a smaller scar, a shortened hospital stay, and earlier return to normal activities [20]. The major disadvantage is a far higher rate of bile duct injury (0.8%) than occurs during traditional cholecystectomy [21,22••]. Nonetheless, the reduced overall morbidity explains its

acceptance into widespread clinical practice. A limited role still exists for medical dissolution with oral bile acids [12,23].

Although biliary physiology is profoundly altered after cholecystectomy, fat malabsorption does not occur and no special diet is indicated. Because the bile salt pool can no longer be sequestered by the gallbladder during an overnight fast, bile salt recirculation is continuous, thus eliminating low fasting bile salt secretion rates and high cholesterol saturation. As a result, cholesterol gallstones never re-form in the biliary ducts after cholecystectomy.

Medical dissolution therapy. Oral administration of the naturally occurring bile acid, ursodeoxycholic acid (ursodiol; Actigall, Novartis Pharmaceuticals Corp., East Hanover, NJ) decreases cholesterol secretion into bile. As a result, cholesterol molecules on the surface of a gallstone can be dissolved, gradually shrinking the gallstone [4,12].

Medical dissolution treatment with ursodiol completely dissolves small gallstones in up to 80% of highly selected patients. Its use is limited critically by the character and size of the gallstone and the severity of symptoms. It may be appropriate for those who are mildly symptomatic with small cholesterol (but not pigment or calcified) gallstones; those who are at high risk for surgery; those who refuse surgery; and those who have newly formed gallstones, such as those that occur after rapid weight loss or pregnancy. The major disadvantages of treatment with ursodiol are that gallstones dissolve slowly (1-mm shrinkage in radius per month) and will re-form in 50% of patients within 5 years of discontinuing therapy.

Before initiating ursodiol treatment, gallstone size, number, and calcium content must be evaluated with ultrasonography and abdominal flat plate radiography. Small noncalcified gallstones filling less than 50% of the gallbladder volume can be treated with a divided dose of ursodiol therapy, 8 mg/kg/d. Reassessment of gallstone size by ultrasonography after 6 months of therapy is the only follow-up required. Lack of dissolution at follow-up should prompt the physician to discontinue ursodiol therapy. Patients with repeated attacks of biliary

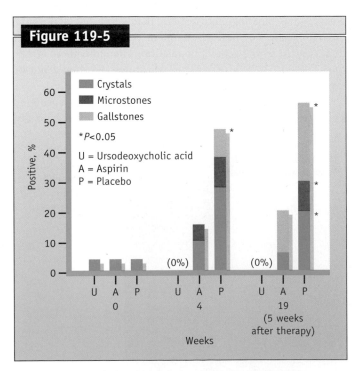

Figure 119-5

The effect of ursodiol and aspirin in preventing cholesterol gallstone formation during weight loss. (*Adapted from* Broomfield *et al.* [17].)

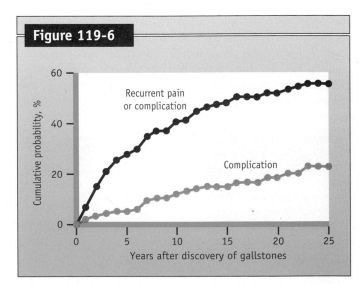

Figure 119-6

The natural history of gallstones in minimally symptomatic patients. (*Adapted from* Friedman *et al.* [18].)

pain during therapy require prompt surgery. Ursodiol should be continued for 3 months after complete gallstone dissolution has been confirmed by ultrasonography. Maintenance therapy with either low-dose ursodiol or dietary modifications to prevent recurrence are neither effective nor recommended.

Ursodiol, unlike its predecessor chenodiol, is remarkably free of side effects. However, patients should be advised that the drug is expensive ($1500 annually) and that gallstones re-form in 50% of patients over 5 years, requiring a second course of therapy for symptomatic recurrence.

After successful dissolution, patients should be reevaluated for recurrent gallstones only if symptoms of biliary tract disease recur. Surveillance ultrasonography for gallstone recurrence is not recommended.

Lithotripsy. Extracorporeal shock-wave lithotripsy is still investigational (FDA investigational new drug status required) and should be viewed only as adjuvant to ursodiol treatment to accelerate dissolution of cholesterol gallstones.

Treatment Recommendations for Patients With Biliary Tract Pain

Patients with one attack of biliary pain. After acute cholecystitis has been excluded, patients with suspected acute biliary tract pain should be treated with supportive care, narcotics, or intramuscular diclofenac (Voltaren; Novartis Pharmaceutical Corp., East Hanover, NJ), a potent nonsteroidal anti-inflammatory drug (NSAID) [24]. The management of nondiabetic patients after only one episode of biliary pain is controversial. In young healthy patients, as discussed previously in this chapter, cholecystectomy is reasonable. Similarly, a watch-and-wait approach to observe the frequency of attacks and confirm they are due to gallstones is also rational. Patients with small noncalcified gallstones, especially if they have developed during weight loss, recent pregnancy, or use of medications such as clofibrate (Novopharm USA Inc., Schaumberg IL), are ideal candidates for ursodiol therapy during the observation period.

Patients with more than one attack of biliary pain. Patients who have had more than one attack of biliary tract pain should be treated definitively to prevent repeated attacks, acute cholecystitis, cholangitis, and pancreatitis.

Otherwise healthy patients under age 55 years. Patients under 55 years of age who are otherwise in good health should have an elective cholecystectomy while their operative risk is small (<0.1%). Although the operative risk is real, half of patients with acute biliary tract pain will have attacks of pain over the next 20 years, and at least 20% will develop complications of their gallstones and need a cholecystectomy later in their lives when their operative risk is significantly higher [18]. Medical dissolution therapy has a very small role in these patients.

Patients with diabetes. Patients with diabetes should have an elective cholecystectomy after only one episode of biliary pain.

Patients of advanced age. Symptomatic patients of advanced age present the most difficult therapeutic dilemma because they are likely to have a concomitant medical problem that influences operative mortality and life expectancy. The clinician needs to balance the risks of waiting and possibly being forced to perform surgery under adverse conditions versus the chance that the patient will die of other causes before gallstones cause complications. For example, a man with his first attack of biliary pain at 65 years of age might be treated surgically if he were otherwise healthy and expected to live an additional 20 years. If the patient is a poor surgical risk, however, treatment for pain and dissolution therapy with ursodiol may be appropriate.

Patients who refuse surgery. Medical dissolution therapy with ursodiol can be attempted in patients with noncalcified gallbladder stones who refuse surgery.

▆▆▆ BILIARY COMPLICATIONS
Acute Cholecystitis

An acute inflammation of the gallbladder wall, acute cholecystitis, usually is due to transient obstruction of the cystic duct by gallstones. The best treatment for acute cholecystitis is early cholecystectomy. In patients who are poor surgical candidates, percutaneous cholecystostomy may be performed under local anesthesia. After recovery, if possible, a definitive biliary operation should be performed. The natural history of patients with acute cholecystitis who do not undergo cholecystectomy is poor. Half will have recurrent biliary colic or additional complications within 5 years. Bile acid therapy has no role in the management of acute cholecystitis.

Choledocholithiasis, or Common Bile Duct Gallstones

Of gallstones found in the common bile duct, 95% originate in and migrate from the gallbladder and only 5% form *de novo* in the duct. The prevalence of common bile duct gallstones increases exponentially from 8% to 15% in persons between 20 and 60 years of age to over 50% in those over 60 years of age.

The natural history of common bile duct gallstones is highly variable and unpredictable. At least 10% of patients will pass gallstones "silently" into the intestines via the common duct. Gallstones may remain in the common bile duct for years without causing symptoms. Patients with choledocholithiasis may present clinically with cholangitis, jaundice, acute pancreatitis, and biliary pain.

Cholangitis

Cholangitis is a potentially life-threatening bacterial infection of the bile and bile duct that occurs when the bile duct is obstructed by either a gallstone, stricture, or neoplasm.

Intermittent and Persistent Jaundice

Approximately 10% of patients with so-called "painless jaundice" have common bile duct gallstones. Medical history, physical examination, and routine laboratory tests can only suggest the diagnosis. Fluctuating levels, rather than a progressive increase, of serum alkaline phosphatase and bilirubin should raise the suspicion of a common bile duct stone. The serum bilirubin levels rarely exceed 10 to 15 mg/dL because common duct stones usually cause low-grade intermittent obstruction.

Abdominal ultrasonography and CT scan are unreliable in diagnosing choledocholithiasis. Only 15% of common bile duct stones are identified at ultrasonography, and even a normal-sized common bile duct does not exclude the presence of stones. Ductal dilation frequently does not occur because of the low-grade intermittent character of the obstruction. Similarly, an abdominal CT scan can detect the common duct stone directly in only half of all patients.

Endoscopic retrograde cholangiopancreatography (ERCP) is the diagnostic test of choice (Fig. 119-7). It allows the endoscopist to inspect the periampullary region of the duodenum, delineate the biliary and pancreatic ducts, and perform sphincterotomy with gallstone extraction (Fig. 119-8) or stent placement. Percutaneous transhepatic cholangiography should be reserved for failure or unavailability of ERCP.

Pancreatitis Caused by Gallstones

Gallstones migrating through the common bile duct into the duodenum can cause acute pancreatitis, which is indistinguishable clinically from any other cause. In contrast to pancreatitis from alcoholism, gallstone pancreatitis never results in chronic pancreatitis or pancreatic insufficiency even after recurrent attacks. Immediately after recovery from the acute attack, the patient should undergo a cholecystectomy because of the high likelihood of repeated attacks [4]. When cholecystectomy is delayed, 25% of patients with gallstone pancreatitis will have another attack of potentially fatal acute pancreatitis within 30 days, and 50% within 11 months. In contrast, only 2% to 7% of patients who have had a cholecystectomy and removal of common bile duct stones experience recurrent pancreatitis.

The role and timing of endoscopic sphincterotomy in patients who have recovered from acute gallstone pancreatitis remain controversial. Many experts opt to perform ERCP after cholecystectomy if signs or symptoms of choledocholithiasis persist [25,26]. Endoscopic sphincterotomy and removal of common bile duct stones, without choloecystectomy, is a reasonable alternative in patients who are at high surgical risk [27].

Up to 60% of patients with so-called "idiopathic pancreatitis" have biliary sludge–induced pancreatitis [28,29••,30••]. Biliary sludge causes pancreatitis, as do gallstones, as particulate matter or cholesterol crystals pass through the common bile duct. The diagnosis can be made by examining a sample of duodenal bile by microscopy for cholesterol or calcium bilirubinate crystals (Fig. 119-9*A* and *B*). Treatment with cholecystectomy, endoscopic sphincterotomy, or ursodiol reduces the rate of recurrent pancreatitis from 50% to 10% (Fig. 119-10) [29••,30••]. The duration and end point of treatment with ursodiol are difficult to determine.

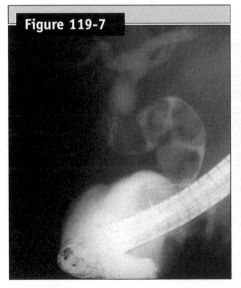

Figure 119-7

Multiple radiolucent gallstones in a dilated common bile duct as visualized by endoscopic photographs. (*Courtesy of* M.D. Apstein, MD.)

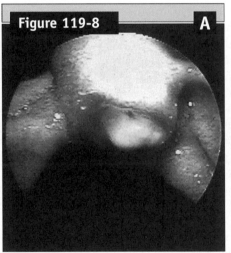

Figure 119-8 **A**

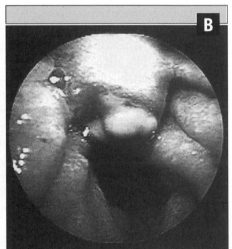

B

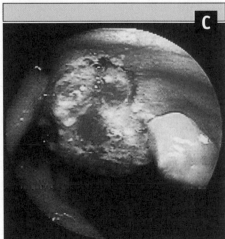

C

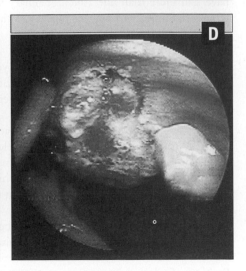

D

Endoscopic photographs of removal of common bile duct stone following an endoscopic sphincterotomy. See also **Color Plate**. (*Courtesy of* M.D. Apstein, MD)

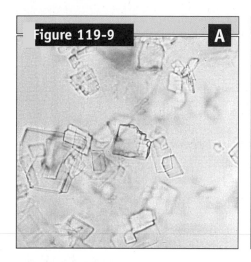

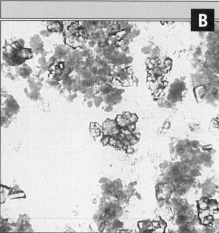

Cholesterol crystals (**A**) and calcium bilirubinate (**B**) from a sample of duodenal bile. (*From* Carey [34]; with permission.)

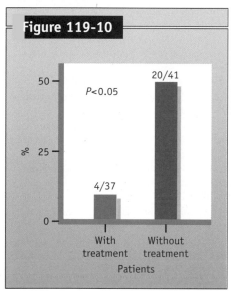

Recurrent pancreatitis in patients with biliary sludge. (*Data from* Ros *et al.* [29] and Lee *et al.* [30].)

Biliary Tract Pain Without Other Complications

The pain from uncomplicated choledocholithiasis is indistinguishable from biliary pain caused by gallbladder stones. Because biliary pain secondary to uncomplicated gallbladder stones rarely causes abnormal liver test results, elevation of serum bilirubin, alkaline phosphatase, or amylase in a patient with biliary pain should raise the suspicion of choledocholithiasis. ERCP is the diagnostic test of choice because of the low sensitivity of ultrasonography and CT scan. Cholescintigraphy has insufficient resolution to delineate the bile ducts adequately for diagnosis.

GALLSTONE ILEUS

Small bowel obstruction secondary to an impacted gallstone is called *gallstone ileus*. It usually results from a large gallstone that erodes through the gallbladder wall and into the small bowel. In the nondiseased small bowel, the gallstone usually becomes impacted at the ileocecal valve; however, in patients with small bowel disease or previous surgery, it can lodge at any site of narrowing. Clinically, gallstone ileus should be suspected in any elderly patient, especially women, with small bowel obstruction.

Although gallstone ileus often occurs in the setting of longstanding clinical gallbladder disease, 30% of patients give no antecedent clinical history of cholelithiasis and only half have right upper quadrant tenderness. Abdominal plain film radiography is critical in making the diagnosis, because air in the biliary tree is present in at least 60% of patients and a radiopaque gallstone may be seen outside the gallbladder.

The treatment of gallstone ileus is surgical removal of the impacted gallstone. Generally, the cholecystoduodenal fistula does not need repair because it rarely causes symptoms.

PROBLEMS AFTER CHOLECYSTECTOMY

Retained Common Duct Stones

Gallstones are overlooked and retained in the common bile duct after 1% to 8% of cholecystectomies and should be suspected in any patient with biliary symptoms or signs after cholecystectomy. Endoscopic sphincterotomy is the treatment of choice for retained common bile duct stones, with an overall mortality of approximately 1% [31]. Dissolution of retained common duct stones with T-tube infusion of cholesterol solvents, such as methyl tert-butyl ether, monooctanoin, or sodium cholate is neither safe nor effective. Surgical removal and exploration of the common bile duct should be considered the last resort.

Biliary Stricture

Bile duct injury and stricture formation after laparoscopic cholecystectomy occur far more commonly than after open cholecystectomy [32]. One third of the injuries become evident clinically within 30 days after surgery. The remainder usually occur within 2 years, and a symptom-free period of 25 years has been reported. Cholangitis appearing more than 5 years after cholecystectomy is most likely to be secondary to retained or newly formed gallstones rather than a biliary stricture. The diagnosis of biliary stricture is made by ERCP or percutaneous transhepatic cholangiography. An abdominal CT scan or ultrasonography may show dilated ducts but is rarely reliable in distinguishing a stricture from a retained gallstone. Surgical repair should be attempted as soon as the stricture is identified and the patient has recovered from acute cholangitis.

Postcholecystectomy Syndrome

Patients with any abdominal pain or discomfort after cholecystectomy are often given the diagnosis of "postcholecystectomy syndrome." This designation should be avoided because there are no known symptoms that predictably follow removal of the gallbladder. A systematic approach is needed to diagnose the specific cause for the discomfort in these patients, of which there are four major possibilities: biliary stricture; a retained common duct stone; the possibility that the symptoms after cholecystectomy are not related to gallstones but are similar to those that prompted the surgery; or true motor dysfunction of the sphincter of Oddi exists, which was present before the cholecystectomy but was mistaken for symptomatic gallstones.

▓▓ REFERENCES

Recently published papers of particular interest have been highlighted as follows:
- Of interest
- • Of outstanding interest

1.•• Apstein MD, Carey MC: Pathogenesis of cholesterol gallstones: a parsimonious hypothesis. *Eur J Clin Invest* 1996, 26:343–352.
This paper presents the current understanding of the pathophysiology of cholesterol gallstone formation.

2. Khanuja B, Cheah Y-C, Hunt M, *et al.*: Lith 1, a major gene affecting cholesterol gallstone formation among inbred strains of mice. *Proc Natl Acad Sci USA* 1995, 92:7729–7733.

3. Crowther RS, Soloway RD: Pigment gallstone pathogenesis: from man to molecules. *Sem Liver Dis* 1990, 10:171–180.

4. Apstein MD, Carey MC: Gallstones. In *Office Practice of Medicine*, edn 3. Edited by Branch WT. Philadelphia: WB Saunders Co; 1994:277–295.

5. Barbara L, Sama C, Labate AMM, *et al.*: A populations study on the prevalence of gallstone disease: the Sirmione study. *Hepatology* 1987, 7:913–917.

6. De Santis A, Attili AF, Corradini SG, *et al.*: Gallstones and diabetes: a case-control study in a free-living population sample. *Hepatology* 1997, 25:787–790.

7. Sarnaik S, Slovis TL, Corbett DP, *et al.*: Incidence of cholelithiasis in sickle cell anemia using the ultrasonic grey-scale technique. *J Pediatr* 1980, 96:1005–1008.

8. Quigley EMM, Marsh MN, Shaffer JL, *et al.*: Hepatobiliary complications of total parenteral nutrition. *Gastroenterology* 1993, 104:286–301.

9. Angelico M, De Santis A, Capocaccia L: Biliary sludge; a critical update. *J Clin Gastroenterol* 1990, 12.656–662.

10. Attili AF, De Santis A, Capri R, *et al.*: The natural history of gallstones: the GREPCO experience. *Hepatology* 1995, 21:656–660.

11. Gracie WA, Ransohoff DF: The natural history of silent gallstones: the innocent gallstone is not a myth. *N Engl J Med* 1982, 307:798–800.

12. Johnston DE, Kaplan MM: Pathogenesis and treatment of gallstones. *N Engl J Med* 1993, 328:412–421.

13. Ransohoff DF, Gracie WA: Treatment of gallstones. *Ann Intern Med* 1993, 119:606–619.

14. Ransohoff DF, Miller GL, Forsythe SB, *et al.*: Outcome of acute cholecystitis in patients with diabetes mellitus. *Ann Intern Med* 1987, 106:829–832.

15. Friedman LS, Roberts MS, Brett AS, *et al.*: Management of asymptomatic gallstones in the diabetic patient. A decision analysis. *Ann Intern Med* 1988, 109:931–939.

16.• Sitzmann JV, Pitt HA, Steinborn PA, *et al.*: Cholecystokinin prevents parenteral nutrition induced biliary sludge in humans. *Surg Gynecol Obstet* 1990, 170:25–31.
The authors report on the prevention of gallstones during administration of TPN.

17. Broomfield PH, Chopra R, Sheinbaum RC, *et al.*: Effects of ursodeoxycholic acid and aspirin on the formation of lithogenic bile and gallstones during loss of weight. *N Engl J Med* 1988, 319:1567–1572.

18. Friedman GD, Raviola CA, Fireman B: Prognosis of gallstones with mild or no symptoms: 25 years of follow-up in a health maintenance organization. *J Clin Epidemiol* 1989, 42:127–136.

19. The Southern Surgeons Club: A prospective analysis of 1518 laparoscopic cholecystectomies. *N Engl J Med* 1991, 324:1073–1078.

20. McMahon AJ, Russel IT, Baxter JN, *et al.*: Laparoscopic versus minilaparotomy cholecystectomy: a randomized controlled trial. *Lancet* 1994, 343:135–138.

21. Strasberg SM, Hertl M, Soper NJ: An analysis of the problem of biliary injury during laparoscopic cholecystectomy. *J Am Coll Surg* 1995, 180:101–125.

22.•• Barkun AN, Rezieg M, Mehta SN, *et al.*: Post-cholecystectomy biliary leaks in the laparoscopic era: risk factors, presentation, and management. *Gastrointest Endosc* 1997, 45:277–282.
In this report the authors discuss the management of bile leaks.

23. Strasberg SM, Clavien PA: Cholecystolithiasis: lithotherapy for the 1990s. *Hepatology* 1992, 16:820–893.

24. Akriviadis EA, Hatzigavriel M, Kapnias D: Treatment of biliary colic with diclofenac: a randomized, double-blind, placebo-controlled study. *Gastroenterology* 1997, 113:225–231.

25. Erickson RA, Carlson B: The role of endoscopic retrograde cholangiopancreatography in patients with laparoscopic cholecystectomies. *Gastroenterology* 1995, 109:252–263.

26. Strasberg SM, Soper NJ: Management of choledocholithiasis in the laparoscopic era. *Gastroenterology* 1995, 109:320–322.

27. Prat F, Malak NA, Pelletier G, *et al.*: Biliary symptoms and complications more than 8 years after endoscopic sphincterotomy for choledocholithiasis. *Gastroenterology* 1996, 110:894–899.

28. Steinberg WM: Acute pancreatitis: never leave a gallstone unturned. *N Engl J Med* 1992, 326:635–637.

29.•• Ros E, Navarro S, Bru C, *et al.*: Occult microlithiasis in "idiopathic" acute pancreatitis: prevention of relapses by cholecystectomy or ursodeoxycholic acid therapy. *Gastroenterology* 1991, 101:1701–1709.

30.•• Lee SP, Nicholls JF, Park HZ: Biliary sludge as a cause of acute pancreatitis. *N Engl J Med* 1992, 326:589–593.
This reference, along with reference 29, argues convincingly that biliary sludge can be important clinically.

31. Shields SJ, Carr-Locke D: Spincterotomy techniques and risks. *Gastrointest Endosc Clin North Am* 1996, 6:17–42.

32. Mehta SN, Pavone E, Barkum JS, *et al.*: A review of the management of post-cholecystectomy biliary leaks during the laparoscopic era. *Am J Gastroenterol* 1997, 92:1262–1267.

33. Lee SP, Maher K, Nicholls JF: Origin and fate of biliary sludge. *Gastroenterology* 1988, 94:170–176.

34. Carey MC: Bile salts and gallstones. In *AGA Undergraduate Teaching Project in Gastroenterology and Liver Disease*. American Gastroenterological Association, 1981.

120 Cholelithiasis and Cholecystitis

Francis P. Colizzo and Francis A. Farraye

It has been estimated that there are 20 to 25 million patients with gallstones in the United States, and over 1 million new cases are diagnosed yearly [1]. In 1991 there were 600,000 cholecystectomies, making cholecystectomy the most common operation after cesarean section (Fig. 120-1, see also *Color Plate*). Gallstones are the most costly digestive disease in the United States, with estimated costs of over $5 billion dollars annually in the United States.

EPIDEMIOLOGY AND NATURAL HISTORY OF CHOLELITHIASIS

Gallstones are three times more common in women than men and are more prevalent with increasing age. One in 5 women and 1 in 10 men above the age of 55 have gallstones (Fig. 120-2). Risk factors for the development of cholesterol gallstones include female gender, pregnancy and the use of oral contraceptives, race (*eg*, Hispanic, Native American), obesity, and rapid weight loss.

Cholesterol gallstones are the most common type of stone in the United States and the western world, accounting for approximately 80% of all stones; the remainder are pigment stones composed of bilirubin and calcium salts (pigment stones are discussed in greater detail later in this chapter). Approximately 10% of gallstones are calcified.

Almost 80% of patients with gallstones are asymptomatic. Approximately 10% of asymptomatic patients with stones develop symptoms within 5 years and 20% develop them within 20 years of the diagnosis [2,3]. Essentially, all patients will develop symptoms of biliary tract disease before they develop a complication (*ie*, cholecystitis, jaundice). Consequently, elective operation for asymptomatic and incidentally found gallstones is not indicated. Rare exceptions to this rule include patients with a porcelain gallbladder (Fig. 120-3), patients with gallbladder polyps larger than 1 cm, and, possibly, patients undergoing solid-organ transplantation.

Once symptoms of biliary colic develop, they are likely to continue. Cholecystectomy or an alternative treatment is recommended to prevent further attacks of biliary pain and associated complications. The most common complications are cholecystitis,

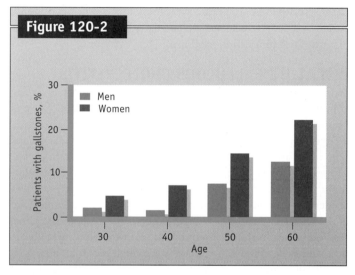

Figure 120-2

The prevalence of gallstone disease related to age and gender. (*From* Donovan [43].)

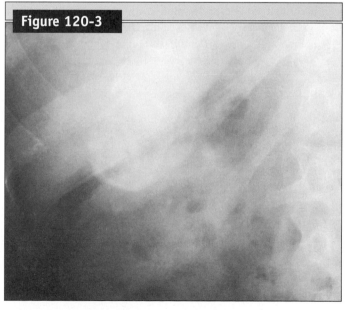

Figure 120-3

Plain radiograph of the abdomen demonstrating a porcelain gallbladder. (*Courtesy of* J. Braver, MD.)

Figure 120-1

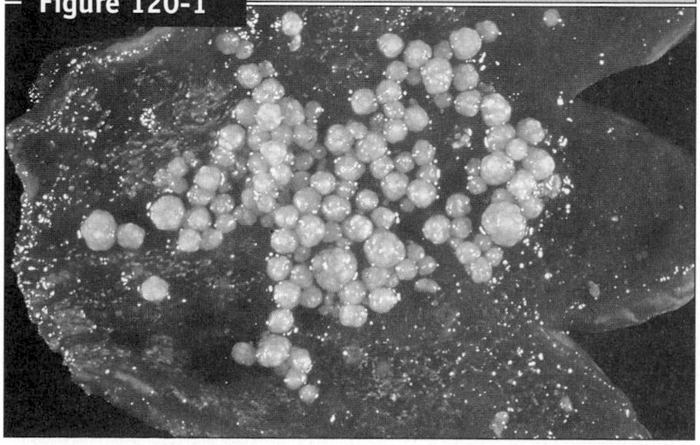

Chronic cholecystitis and cholelithiasis. (*Courtesy of* J. Guilizia, MD.) See also **Color Plate**.

choledocholithiasis, pancreatitis, and cholangitis. Most studies report a 1% to 2% complication rate per year in patients with symptomatic gallstones. Almost 25% of patients develop a complication 10 to 20 years after the onset of biliary pain.

CLINICAL MANIFESTATIONS OF CHOLELITHIASIS AND CHOLECYSTITIS

Biliary pain develops as a consequence of transient obstruction of the cystic duct by a stone. The term *biliary colic* is a misnomer, as patients classically describe episodic abdominal pain located in the epigastrium or in the right upper quadrant that lasts 1 to 5 hours, is associated with nausea and vomiting, and resolves spontaneously. The pain often awakens the patient at night and is not clearly postprandial. The pain increases in intensity, plateaus, and then resolves. It may radiate to the right subscapular area or chest. It can be misinterpreted by patients as cardiac pain when it seems to originate in or radiate to the chest. Nonspecific dyspeptic symptoms that are not commonly cured by cholecystectomy include fatty food intolerance with bloating, belching, and heartburn [4].

ACUTE CALCULOUS CHOLECYSTITIS

Acute cholecystitis (see Chapter 124) is the most common complication of cholelithiasis. Acute cholecystitis develops in as many as 10% of patients with symptomatic cholelithiasis, with a reported mortality rate approaching 5%. Cholecystitis begins with the same constellation of symptoms as biliary colic, but symptoms do not resolve and are associated with the development of fever and localized right upper quadrant pain and tenderness. Persistent obstruction of the cystic duct by a gallstone is the initiating factor in over 90% of patients with cholecystitis, resulting in gallbladder distention, inflammation of the gallbladder wall secondary to retained bile salts, bacterial infection, circulatory compromise, and if not treated, transmural gangrene (Fig. 120-4, see also *Color Plate*). A low-grade fever may be present. The physical examination reveals tenderness with guarding in the right upper quadrant. A palpable gallbladder can be seen in 30% of patients and is more common in patients without chronic cholelithiasis. Murphy's sign is right upper quadrant subcostal tenderness with worsening pain on inspiration (inspiratory

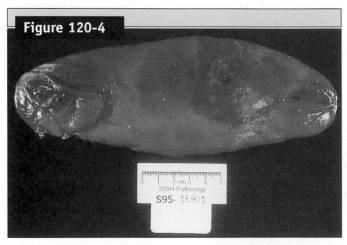

Figure 120-4

Gangrenous cholecystitis. (*Courtesy of* J. Guilizia, MD.) See also **Color Plate.**

arrest of the diaphragm). Elderly patients often may have a nonspecific clinical presentation that can lead to a delay in diagnosis.

Laboratory findings are not specific. The leukocyte count is usually elevated in the range of 11,000 to 15,0000 cells/mm^3, but it also may be normal. Minor elevations in the liver function tests can be seen in uncomplicated cholecystitis and do not necessarily imply the presence of a common bile duct stone, pancreatitis with common bile duct obstruction, hepatic abscess, or intrahepatic gallbladder. The differential diagnosis includes, but is not limited to, pancreatitis, cholangitis, acute hepatitis, hepatic abscess, pylenonephritis, peptic ulcer disease, and myocardial infarction.

Acalculous cholecystitis accounts for 10% of all cases of cholecystitis [5] and typically is seen in patients who are critically ill and hospitalized. Conditions that may predispose patients to the development of acalculous cholecystitis include complicated medical problems or multiple trauma requiring an intensive care unit (ICU) admission, postoperative state, posttransplantation, burns, or sepsis. In such settings, it is believed to be related to nonocclusive ischemia of the gallbladder associated with changes in biliary composition and abnormal gallbladder motility.

The lack of appreciation of the subtle signs of gallbladder inflammation in a critically ill, often intubated, patient can lead to a delay in diagnosis and, consequently, to increased morbidity and mortality. The diagnosis should be considered when the patient is deteriorating for unknown reasons. Abdominal imaging by ultrasound or computed tomography (CT) may demonstrate a thickened gallbladder wall, pericholecystic fluid, and tenderness on palpation. Depending on the clinical picture, the treatment is usually cholecystectomy or percutaneous cholecystostomy. Broad-spectrum antibiotics are indicated. The mortality is 10% if recognized early, but higher in patients with gangrenous cholecystitis and perforation.

Diagnosis

Radiologic imaging plays a vital role in the diagnosis and management of cholelithiasis and cholecystitis. Ultrasound and cholescintigraphy are the tests most used, with oral cholecystography being performed much less commonly than in years past.

The plain abdominal radiograph warrants mention as a historical note, as its clinical use for cholecystitis is limited. It may show calcified gallstones in 20% to 40% of patients (Fig. 120-5) [6], which is useful information in selecting candidates for oral dissolution therapy. It also may demonstrate a porcelain gallbladder and enable distinction between this and a large gallstone, which may be difficult to do by ultrasound [7]. Rarely, intestinal obstruction or air in the biliary tree from gallstone ileus or fistulization between the gallbladder and biliary tree or the gastrointestinal tract may be seen.

Oral cholecystography (OCG) was one of the first methods to become available for visualizing the gallbladder (Fig. 120-6). This imaging technique traditionally involved ingesting a lipid-soluble contrast agent after a high-fat meal to stimulate the enterohepatic circulation and improve absorption of the contrast agent for transport to the liver and concentration in the gallbladder [8]. Newer agents are less dependent on lipid solubilization and dietary fat intake, making a high-fat meal less important. Ingestion of the agent over a 2-day period reduces the likelihood of repeat examinations and a false-positive study [8].

Visualization of the gallbladder requires a patent cystic duct. Buoyancy is the most reliable predictor of cholesterol stones, although it is seen in only 35% of patients [8]. If the gallbladder cannot be seen, this suggests obstruction of the cystic duct; however, other causes, such as hepatic disease, recent pancreatitis, malabsorption, altered intestinal motility, noncompliance, insufficient dosage of contrast agent, and a poorly functioning gallbladder, need to be considered [8]. The test is generally well tolerated, although the side effects of the contrast agent include nephrotoxicity, dysuria, diarrhea, nausea, and vomiting [8].

The sensitivity and specificity of OCG for acute cholecystitis are reported to be 92% to 95% and 95% to 100%, respectively [7]. The addition of cholecystokinin to OCG has yielded no benefit. This test has been replaced by ultrasound and cholescintigraphy because of time and preparation requirements and technical limitations. It remains useful for confirmation after a nondiagnostic ultrasound in patients with a high clinical suspicion for cholelithiasis. It also can be used to identify candidates for extracorporeal shock-wave lithotripsy or dissolution therapy by assessing the size and composition of gallbladder stones and gallbladder function [7,8].

Ultrasonography has become the most commonly used imaging modality for the initial evaluation of suspected gallbladder disease, especially cholelithiasis (Fig. 120-7). Minimal patient preparation, ease of use, and rapid interpretation of results make this test highly useful. A detailed examination may be limited by the patient's body habitus, but in general, ultrasonography of the gallbladder is able to detect pericholecystic fluid, gallbladder wall thickening, biliary sludge, or cholelithiasis, with stone size ranging from 3 mm [7] to 20 mm [8]. It provides the additional advantage of being able to image the biliary tree and other organs within an area that can cause symptoms similar to those of cholecystitis. Detecting acute cholecystitis by ultrasound is 90% to 95% sensitive and 70% to 98% specific, although sensitivity is probably less for acalculous disease [7]. These values reflect the use of combining major and minor

criteria that have been defined to aid in the sonographic diagnosis of acute cholecystitis. Major criteria include gallstones or nonvisualization of the gallbladder (suggestive of a shrunken, diseased gallbladder) whereas minor criteria are wall thickening greater than 4 to 5 mm, pericholecystic fluid, a round shape, a gallbladder larger than 5 cm, or a positive sonographic Murphy's sign during examination [7]. Although biliary sludge may suggest microlithiasis and predispose to cholethiasis, at this time it cannot be listed as either a major or minor criterium. Its presence should be considered in conjunction with the patient's clinical presentation. The sonographic Murphy's sign generally is more sensitive than it is specific; the accuracy ranges from 68% to 87% [9], probably the result of operator variability.

Minor criteria are nonspecific, and any singular finding by itself is not considered diagnostic of cholecystitis. Gallbladder wall thickening, for example, can be seen with other underlying conditions, such as congestive heart failure, cirrhosis, nephrosis, or hypoalbuminemia [7]. When cholelithiasis is undetected in

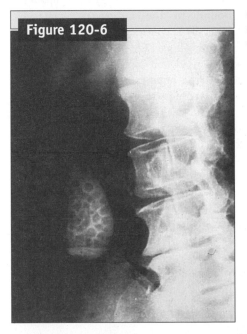

Figure 120-6

Oral cholecystogram of cholesterol gallstones. (*From* Donovan [43].)

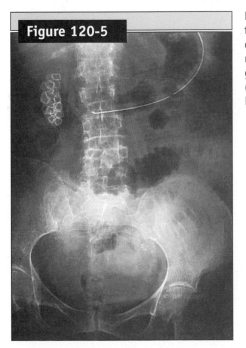

Figure 120-5

Plain radiograph of the abdomen demonstrating multiple calcified gallstones. (*Courtesy of* J. Braver, MD.)

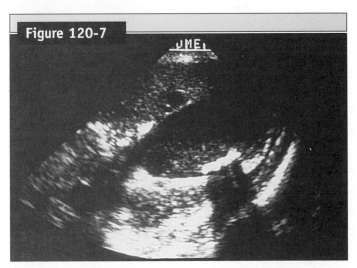

Figure 120-7

Ultrasound demonstrating gallstones and biliary sludge. (*From* Donovan [43].)

the setting of a thickened wall with right upper quadrant pain, closer examination may reveal the presence of stones in up to 50% of patients; the remaining patients will be equally distributed between those who have acalculous disease and those with another underlying condition [10]. A large dilated gallbladder is another nonspecific finding, but it may suggest the presence of a nonvisualized stone obstructing the cystic duct, a condition that could potentially lead to a perforation.

Biliary sludge by itself generally is not considered pathogenic and may be seen in patients who are fasting, critically ill, or receiving parenteral nutrition or ceftriaxone. It is, however, a precursor to stone formation and may represent stones too small to be detected by ultrasound. Some studies have suggested that sludge in the setting of right upper quadrant pain and a thickened gallbladder wall may represent cholecystitis [10,11]. Striations seen in a thickened wall are nonspecific, but when seen along with a clinical presentation of cholecystitis, they usually indicate a gangrenous gallbladder [12].

Cholescintigraphy involves the use of an organic compound, iminodiacetic acid, bound to the radioactive material, technetium-99m, and generally is considered most sensitive for detecting acute cholecystitis (Figs. 120-8 and 120-9). The names of the compounds used for biliary scintigraphy are derived from the nature of the organic ligands bound to the iminodiacetic acid, which confer slightly different hepatic excretion properties. The most commonly used agents are HIDA (hepato-iminodiacetic acid) and DISIDA (diisopropyl iminodiacetic acid), but occasionally PIPIDA (paraisopropyl iminodiacetic acid) also is used. DISIDA may have better excretion in the setting of hyperbilirubinemia [7]. Hepatocytes rapidly extract these agents following intravenous injection in a fasted patient. They are then excreted into the biliary system, allowing for visualization of the gallbladder, cystic duct, common bile duct, and a portion of the duodenum. The cholescintigraphic study may show one of several patterns that allow the determination of patency of the cystic and common bile ducts: complete gallbladder visualization, delayed gallbladder visualization, gallbladder nonvisualization, or the persistent hepatic phase [7].

The examination is normal if the biliary tract, gallbladder, and cystic duct are visualized within 60 minutes. Delayed visualization is reported if the gallbladder and cystic duct are not visualized until 1 to 4 hours later. Approximately 45% of patients with chronic cholecystitis will have such a result [7]. Other conditions resulting in delayed visualization include insufficient fasting, acute pancreatitis, chronic alcoholism, common bile duct obstruction, or hepatocellular dysfunction [13]. Nonvisualization of gallbladder and cystic duct results from obstruction of the cystic duct and is highly suggestive of acute cholecystitis. In all three of these settings, some contrast is usually noted in the duodenum. If contrast is not seen in either the gallbladder, cystic duct, or duodenum, or if duodenal appearance is delayed, this is termed *persistent hepatic phase*, and also suggests choledocholithiasis [7].

Modifications of the cholescintigraphic scans have been performed to enhance their diagnostic yield; cholecystokinin or morphine injections have been used to detect gallbladder dysfunction or to exclude acute cholecystitis, respectively. Morphine may be administered if there still is nonvisualization after 60 minutes. A dose of 0.04 mg/kg intravenously is used, which increases pressure in the sphincter of Oddi and common bile duct, facilitating entry into the gallbladder [14]. Images are then taken over the next 30 to 60 minutes, which reduces the need for delayed imaging up to 24 hours. This technique also may enhance the sensitivity of the test in patients likely to have a false-positive scan due to fasting, parenteral nutrition, or critical illness.

In the radiologic diagnosis of acute cholecystitis, CT has a very limited role, and perhaps is better used to diagnose complications. Ultrasound generally is more sensitive for detecting gallstones and is less expensive than CT [7]. Calcified stones may be seen on CT (Fig. 120-10). The sensitivities and specifics of the various imaging modalities are summarized in Table 120-1.

Figure 120-8

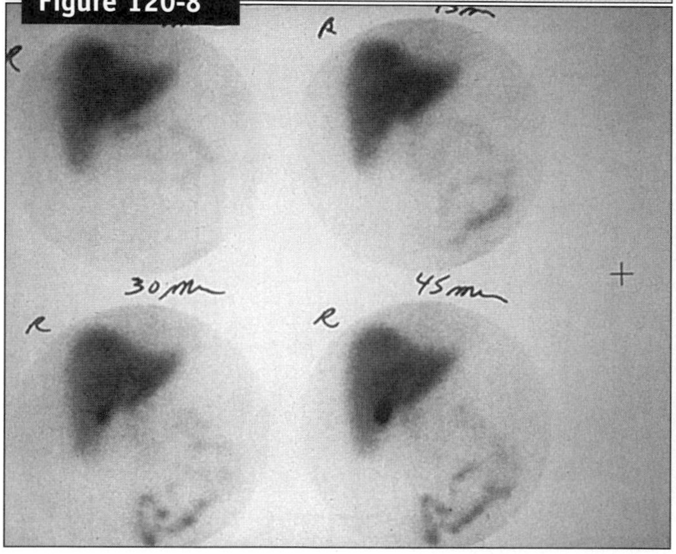

Normal hepato-iminodiacetic acid scan. (*Courtesy of* S. Nagel, MD.)

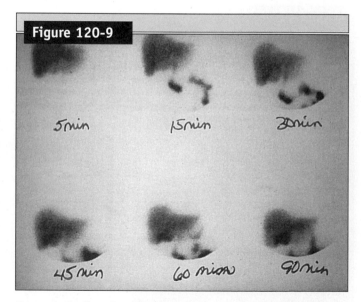

Figure 120-9

Hepato-iminodiacetic acid scan demonstrating nonfilling of the gallbladder at 45 minutes. (*Courtesy of* S. Nagel, MD.)

Complications

The most common complications of acute cholecystitis include gallbladder perforation, gallstone ileus, and emphysematous cholecystitis (Table 120-2). Mirizzi's syndrome is not really a complication of cholecystitis per se but may occur from cholelithiasis.

Rupture of the gallbladder wall has been reported to occur in up to 12% of cases of acute cholecystitis. A proposed mechanism [15] for rupture involves obstruction of the cystic duct, resulting in gallbladder distention from continued mucus secretion by the gallbladder mucosa. The overdistention results in compromised vascular flow leading to ischemia, necrosis, and perforation. The fundus of the gallbladder is most susceptible. The diagnosis can be difficult to make, as clinical findings are similar to those of uncomplicated cholecystitis, and some patients may note relief of pain after an acute rupture has occurred. The degree of perforation has been classified as acute, subacute, or chronic, resulting in bile peritonitis, abscess, or fistula, respectively [16]. Acute rupture may be more common in young people without chronic cholelithiasis who have an associated systemic disease (atherosclerosis, diabetes, carcinoma) or immunosuppression whereas fistulae are more likely in elderly patients with chronic cholecystitis or cholelithiasis [16].

The diagnosis is usually made intraoperatively or on postmortem examination. Ultrasound may demonstrate a pericholecystic fluid collection, edematous wall, or, simply, cholelithiasis, none of which are specific. Cholescintigraphy is better than ultrasound for the diagnosis, although both are relatively insensitive (sensitivities of 50% and 18%, respectively) [17]. The use of morphine with cholescintigraphy in this setting has not been studied well enough to define its place, although in theory it may confer some advantage. CT is believed to be superior for detecting perforation, and findings may include a wall defect, bulging gallbladder, or a "hole" resembling a perforated balloon [15]. Occasionally a hepatic abscess may be seen as a result of a well-localized perforation [18].

Once the diagnosis is made, therapy should be instituted with broad-spectrum antibiotics to cover enteric flora. Surgery remains the mainstay of treatment, and immediate surgical consultation is mandatory. Although there have been reports of percutaneous drainage for gallbladder perforations [19], this should be considered only as a temporizing measure and not a substitute for surgery in most cases. The mortality associated with perforation ranges from 0% to 23% in various reports [20].

Technically, gallstone ileus is a result of perforation with fistulization. Fistulae may occur between the gallbladder and any adjacent organs, or viscera. Biliary enteric fistulae are most common and are estimated to occur in about 1% of patients presenting with acute cholecystitis [21]. In order of decreasing frequency, they are cholecystoduodenal, cholecystocolonic, and cholecystoduodenocolonic [22]; fistulization is more common in the elderly [21,22]. Repetitive obstructive events result in inflammation of the gallbladder serosa, which forms adhesions with adjacent viscera. A final acute obstruction of the cystic duct by a stone causes a reaction in the wall reducing arterial, venous, and lymphatic supply, with reduced gallbladder wall absorption. The resulting distention further impairs vascular integrity, and the susceptible area becomes ischemic and gangrenous, allowing contents to penetrate the necrotic wall into the adjacent viscus [21]. Carcinoma of the gallbladder is more likely to be encountered in patients with biliary enteric fistula [21].

The clinical presentation of patients with biliary enteric fistula is similar to those with chronic cholecystitis and cholelithiasis. When intestinal obstruction by a gallstone is present, the obstructive symptoms are more dominant than the biliary symptoms. The obstructing stone is usually at least 2 to 2.5 cm in diameter [21]. Multiple stones may be seen in 3% to 40% of cases and are usually the cause for early recurrence [22].

Figure 120-10

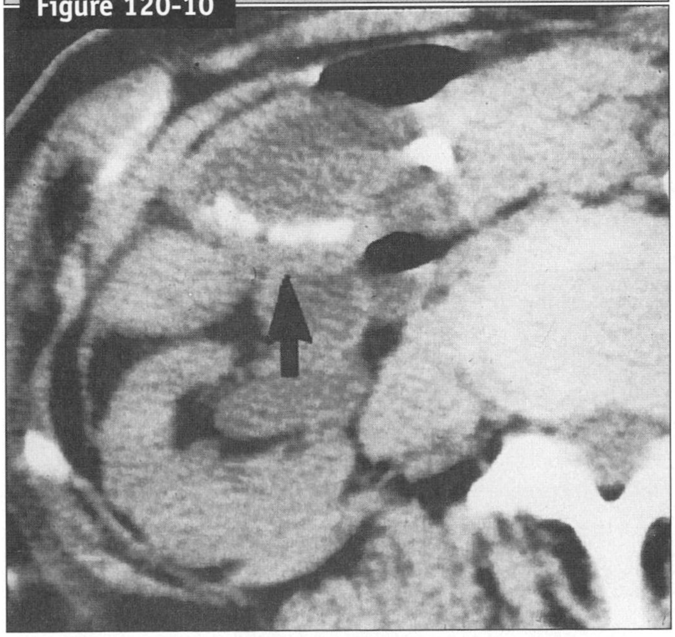

Calcified stones detected by CT scan. (*From* Thistle [44].)

Table 120-1. Comparison of Radiologic Tests for Acute Cholecystitis

Radiologic Test	Sensitivity, %	Specificity, %
Oral cholecystogram	92–95	95–100
Ultrasound (major criteria)	81–86	94–98
Ultrasound (major or minor)	90–95	70–98
Cholescintigraphy	95–97	90–97

Adapted from Marton and Doubilet [7].

Table 120-2. Complications of Cholecystitis

Complication	Incidence, %	Mortality, %
Perforation	12	0–23
Gallstone ileus	1	10–30
Mirizzi's syndrome	< 1	?
Emphysematous cholecystitis	< 1	?

The most common sites for impaction are the terminal ileum (50%–75%), proximal ileum and jejunum (20%–40%), and duodenum (10%) [22]. The colon is rarely involved, and when it is, there usually is a stenotic lesion in the sigmoid [22].

Less than 50% of patients are diagnosed preoperatively with biliary enteric fistula [21,22]. Plain radiograph of the abdomen may reveal pneumobilia, intestinal obstruction, an aberrantly located gallstone, or change in location of a gallstone [22]. Pneumobilia may be seen in up to 90% of cases [22]; however, it should be cautioned that this is a nonspecific finding and may be seen with perforated ulcer, post-sphincterotomy, biliary-intestinal anastomoses, or with a functioning biliary endoprosthesis. Ultrasound and contrast radiography also have been found to be useful in identifying fistula [22].

Surgery is the appropriate therapy for gallstone ileus to disimpact the offending stone via enterolithotomy and also to locate other stones in the bowel. Manual "lithotripsy" or "milking" a stone along an extensive distance of an impacted stone is to be avoided, as it may result in significant mucosal damage [22]. A single-stage procedure involving stone removal, fistula repair, and cholecystectomy is preferred for most patients who are clinically stable, whereas a two-stage procedure relieving bowel obstruction first is recommended for those who are debilitated and who are a higher surgical risk [22]. Mortality for this condition is reported to be 10% to 30%, a reflection of

the advanced age of the typical patient with or without concomitant disease [22].

Emphysematous cholecystitis is a rare variant of acute cholecystitis caused by gas-producing bacteria (Fig. 120-11). Elderly and diabetic patients appear to be most commonly affected when ischemia and necrosis occurs, allowing organisms such as *Clostridia* spp, enterococci, and gram-negative rods to proliferate [23]. Gallstones are not necessarily present. Although no controlled trials have compared the diagnostic value of CT with that of sonography, CT may be slightly better. Either may demonstrate the pathognomic findings of gas bubbles or linear air in the gallbladder wall [23]. Surgery and antibiotics are the appropriate therapies in this setting. Cholecystostomy has been used successfully in critically ill patients as a temporizing measure.

Mirizzi's syndrome occurs when the cystic duct is parallel to the common hepatic duct and a stone impacted in the cystic duct or neck of the gallbladder (Fig. 120-12) results in common hepatic duct obstruction and perhaps recurrent cholangitis [24]. Since the original description, the syndrome has been subdivided into type I, as described previously, and type II, where a cholecyst-choledochal fistula is present with a stone passing into the common bile duct. Mirizzi's syndrome is estimated to occur in less than 1% of patients presenting for cholecystectomy [25].

Patients usually present with obstructive jaundice and right upper quadrant pain. Ultrasound may show dilation of the biliary tree above the level of the gallbladder neck, presence of a stone impacted in the gallbladder neck, or an abrupt change in the width of the common bile duct below the level of the stone [24]. CT usually can suggest the absence of a malignancy but provides little information beyond ultrasound [24]. The diagnosis is usually confirmed at the time of retrograde cholangiography or surgery. Surgery is the proper therapy for Mirizzi's syndrome; however, the procedure done may vary depending on the type of obstruction present.

The presence of stones in the gallbladder increases the possibility of one escaping via the cystic duct and becoming impacted in the biliary tree. This can potentially result in infection of the biliary system, causing cholangitis (see Chapter 125).

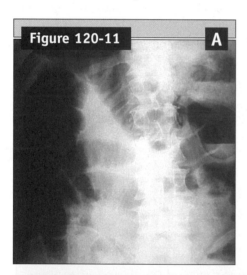

Figure 120-11   **A**

Emphysematous cholecystitis. (*From* Davis and Branch [45].)

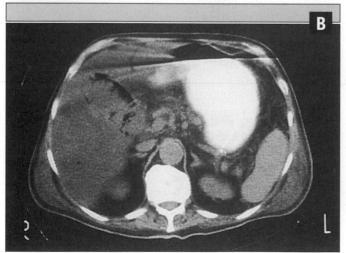

B

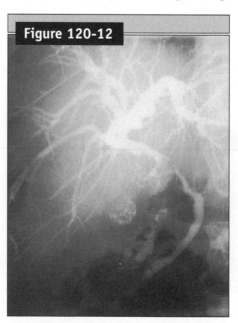

Figure 120-12

Mirizzi's syndrome. Endoscopic retrograde cholangiopancreatography demonstrating obstruction of the common bile duct by a stone-filled cystic duct. (*Courtesy of* D. Carr-Locke, MD.)

■ MANAGEMENT OF CHOLELITHIASIS AND CHOLECYSTITIS

In general, patients with asymptomatic gallstones may be managed expectantly. Those with an isolated episode of pain attributable to gallstones also may be observed. When symptoms become recurrent or progressive, cholecystectomy is the procedure of choice (see Chapter 121) [26,27]. Continued observation (realizing the recurrence rate over time) or nonoperative interventions may be used for those not willing to proceed with surgery or deemed to be at high surgical risk.

Patients with acute cholecystitis should be kept fasting and given intravenous fluid support. Nasogastric suction should be instituted if there is abdominal distention or persistent vomiting. In the setting of fever or elevated white blood cell count, appropriate antibiotic therapy should be initiated targeting gram-negative rods, streptococci, *Enterobacter*, enterococci, *Bacteroides*, and *Clostridial* spp (*eg*, cefoxitin, cefotaxime, ampicillin/sulbactam). Approximately 60% of patients will have resolution of an acute attack whereas those who fail to improve within 24 to 48 hours should receive urgent surgical intervention. Once the acute episode resolves, one of several surgical or nonsurgical options usually is recommended, as symptoms inevitably will recur.

Nonoperative therapies are most appropriate for patients with radiolucent stones and a patent cystic duct (Table 120-3). Smaller stones respond best to oral or contact dissolution therapies whereas larger (> 1 cm) and fewer stones respond best to shock-wave therapy. Such therapy is not definitive and can result in stone recurrence.

Altering the bile acid pool to dissolve gallstones has been clinically investigated for over 20 years (Fig. 120-13). Although chenodeoxycholic acid was originally investigated, current therapy uses ursodeoxycholic acid as it tends to have a safer side effect profile and better efficacy. Ursodeoxycholic acid primarily acts by reducing hepatic synthesis and secretion of cholesterol, thereby lowering the proportion of cholesterol in the gallbladder. This enables cholesterol from the gallstones to reenter into the cholesterol–bile salt–lecithin solution, eventually dissolving the stones. Thus, the best candidates for oral dissolution therapy are those with predominantly noncalcified cholesterol stones.

The usual dose of ursodeoxycholic acid is 8 to 10 mg/kg/d, which is generally well tolerated without hepatotoxicity, although up to 1% of patients may note mild diarrhea [28]. The dissolution rate is slow (about 1 mm per month) and its use is not recommended for stones greater than 20 mm in diameter [28]. Small stones (< 5 mm) have the greatest likelihood of complete dissolution (up to 90% success) [29]. Stones will dissolve completely in 30% to 60% of patients who meet optimal criteria, and symptoms may diminish before the stones are fully dissolved [30]. Adding chenodeoxycholic acid to ursodeoxycholic acid therapy, each in half of the usual doses, lessens the hepatotoxicity of the former, although the therapeutic advantage of this combined therapy is uncertain [28]. The 3-hydroxymethyl-glutaryl coenzyme A (HMG-CoA) inhibitors (*eg*, lovastatin, simvastatin) may prove useful in stone dissolution as well [29]. Ursodeoxycholic acid also can prevent stone formation in patients undergoing rapid weight loss [30]. The principal difficulty with this therapy is the high incidence of stone recurrence (in up to 50% of patients observed over long-term follow-up) [28,30]. If surgery is not a consideration, options include retreatment or a different nonoperative approach. Reports suggest that ursodeoxycholic acid continued at 300 mg/d may help to prevent stone recurrence [28].

The organic solvents methyl *tert*-butyl ether and *n*-propyl acetate can be used effectively to directly dissolve retained gallstones through a percutaneous cholecystostomy (Fig. 120-14). By instilling and draining the solvent with a pump system, cholesterol gallstones may dissolve into solution in as little as 24

Table 120-3. Summary of Nonoperative Therapies for Gallstones		
Therapy	**Stone Clearance, %**	**Mortality, %**
Oral Dissolution	30–90	0
Contact Dissolution	50–90	Insufficient Data
ESWL	70–90	<0.1

Adapted from Sauerbruch and Paumgartner [29].

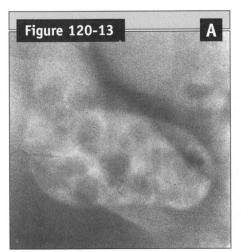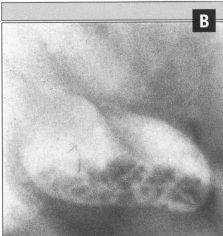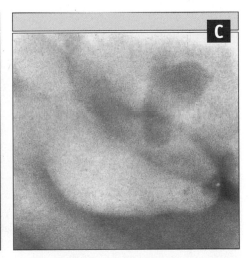

Figure 120-13   **A**   **B**   **C**

Oral dissolution of cholesterol gallstones using ursodiol as assessed by serial oral cholecystogram. (*From* Thistle [44].)

hours [30], but instillation for up to 4 days may be required [29]. Generally, the procedure is well tolerated, but patients may note biliary pain or nausea [30]. Spillage of solvent into the duodenum can cause mild sedation, although hemolysis or nephrotoxicity may result if solvent is absorbed into the systemic circulation [30]. Cholecystectomy may be required in up to 5% of patients due to leakage from gallbladder puncture. Endoscopic retrograde cannulation of the gallbladder has been accomplished but may be complicated by pancreatitis or cystic duct perforation [29]. Recurrence of gallstones after contact dissolution therapy may be as high as 29% at 1 year and 70% at 4 years [29,31]. The use of ursodeoxycholic acid after dissolution therapy for several months may diminish gallstone recurrence [29].

Extracorporeal shock-wave lithotripsy (ESWL) uses acoustic waves generated by electrohydraulic, piezoceramic, or electromagnetic methods to fragment gallstones [29]. Solitary stones up to 20 mm in diameter tend to respond best to ESWL methods. Approximately 90% of patients will have the debris

from a 30-mm stone cleared in about 18 months whereas stones of 20 mm will require 8 months to clear in 70% of patients [29]. Adjuvant therapy with ursodeoxycholic acid can double the 6-month success rate of ESWL [29]. A functioning gallbladder is necessary to mobilize the fragments into the duodenum [30]. Most of the adverse effects of ESWL result from passage of the fragments: pancreatitis (2%), cholestasis (1%), and cholecystitis (1%) [29]. Endoscopic therapy may be required in up to 5% of patients for fragments retained in the common duct [29].

Stone recurrence rates are probably lowest for ESWL among the nonoperative therapies. The percentage of patients without stones has varied according to the length of follow-up, initial size and number of stones, and whether adjuvant therapy with ursodeoxycholic acid has been used. "Stone-free" rates for patients with multiple stones or solitary stones larger than 20 mm have been quite low despite adjuvant therapy with ursodeoxycholic acid [32].

Although the incidence of carcinoma of the gallbladder in patients with gallstones is low, nonoperative therapies do not eliminate the risk of occurrence. Especially concerning findings include a porcelain gallbladder, which carries a 25% risk of carcinoma (Fig. 120-15, see also *Color Plate*), or gallbladder polyps larger than 1 cm and possibly larger stones [33]. In these situations, cholecystectomy should be given serious consideration.

There is little use for endoscopic management of cholelithiasis or cholecystitis aside from possible placement of a cystic duct catheter for contact dissolution, as discussed previously. Endoscopic therapy for choledocholithiasis is well documented and reviewed elsewhere in this book. On occasion, such as in an elderly patient with a gallbladder that contains many stones and obstructive jaundice from a common bile duct stone, sphincterotomy and stone removal may be done with the gallbladder left in situ. Methods for ablation of the gallbladder are still experimental.

Percutaneous drainage of the gallbladder allows for decompression of the gallbladder in cases of acute calculous or acalculous cholecystitis or of the biliary tree in choledocholithiasis if the cystic duct is patent. It may be performed by an interventional radiologist. This is generally not considered definitive therapy but a temporizing measure in critically ill patients or patients of

Figure 120-14

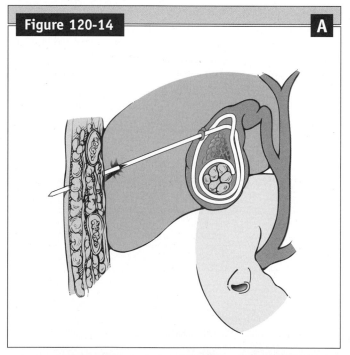

A

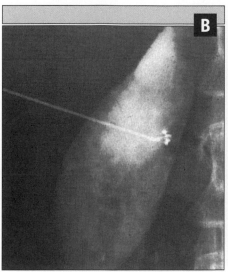

B

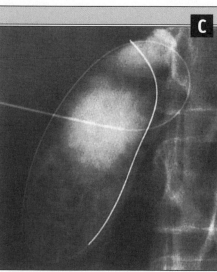

C

Percutaneous catheterization of the gallbladder for contact dissolution therapy.
A, Schematic of percutaneous transhepatic catheter placement on gallbladder.
B, Gallbladder localization confirmed by contrast injection under fluroscopy.
C, Guidewire placed through trocar prior to placement of pigtail catheter. Note gallstones in dependent portion of gallbladder in **B** and **C**. (*From* Thistle [44].)

high surgical risk. If symptoms fail to resolve within 24 hours, surgery may be necessary, as this may suggest necrosis or infarction of the gallbladder wall [34].

Aside from the risk of acute cholecystitis itself, cholecystostomy may be associated with intraperitoneal bile leak, bleeding, or visceral perforation. The added advantages of this procedure are allowance of antegrade cholangiography or instillation of a contact dissolution solvent. If the acute episode resolves and the patient is stable, a decision regarding observation versus elective cholecystectomy should be made. Study of patients undergoing cholecystostomy suggests when the original cause is acalculous disease, the catheter may be removed if cholecystography performed after 4 weeks shows contrast flowing into the common duct and duodenum. As long as the patient remains asymptomatic, cholecystectomy is not absolutely indicated [34]. For those who had calculous disease, cholecystectomy should be recommended, as the recurrence rate is 8% to 10% per year for the first 3 to 5 years after successful nonsurgical management [34].

The development of laparoscopic cholecystectomy has generally rendered nonoperative therapies less useful because of the ease and low morbidity and mortality associated with the surgery. It is now considered the procedure of choice among the surgical options for cholelithiasis and acute and chronic cholecystitis. Cholangiography and, sometimes, common duct exploration can be performed at the time of surgery as well, providing further diagnostic and therapeutic use. Unsuitable candidates for the laparoscopic procedure include patients who are medically unstable and those who have extensive adhesions or scarring around the gallbladder from chronic cholecystitis or prior abdominal surgery [30]. Extraction of large stones through the umbilical incision may be problematic, but complications such as bile duct injury, bleeding, ileus, bile leakage, or bowel injury occur in less than 5% of patients [29]. The conversion rate to open cholecystectomy is 5% in experienced hands, with a mortality rate of less than 1% [29]. The complication rate using laparoscopic techniques has been reported to be lower than that for open cholecystectomy [35]. Following laparoscopic cholecystectomy, patients experience

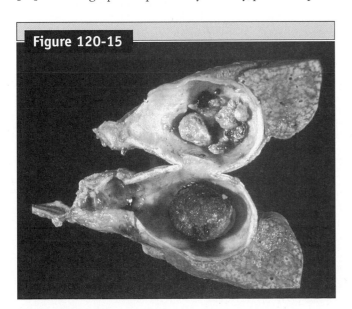

Figure 120-15

Porcelain gallbladder. (*Courtesy of* J. Guilizia, MD.)
See also **Color Plate.**

less pain, have shorter hospital stays, and return to their daily activities sooner as compared with open cholecystectomy [30]. Most patients will have complete relief of pain following cholecystectomy for calculous disease, but only half of patients with acalculous disease fall into this category [4]. As stated previously, nonpain dyspeptic symptoms are not usually cured by surgery [4].

Although cholecystectomy generally is not indicated for cholelithiasis detected incidentally, it has been recommended that patients found with incidental cholelithiasis at the time of laparotomy for nonbiliary indications undergo simultaneous cholecystectomy [33]. The rationale for this is that over 50% of patients, particularly those undergoing abdominal aortic surgery, will develop biliary symptoms attributable to cholelithiasis in 6 to 24 months [33]. Incidental cholecystectomy has not been demonstrated to add to the operative morbidity or mortality [33].

Cancer of the ascending colon has been reported to occur more commonly following cholecystectomy due to the higher levels of secondary bile acids exposed to the colon. This is currently a matter of debate, and no firm conclusions can currently be made without additional study.

Special Considerations

Pregnancy predisposes to cholelithiasis because of incomplete emptying of the gallbladder [36] and biliary cholesterol hypersaturation from the increased estrogen and progesterone [36]. Despite this, fewer than 1% of pregnant women develop biliary complications. When cholecystitis develops, the traditional approach has been to keep patients fasting and treat them with intravenous fluids, antibiotics, and, possibly, fetal monitoring, as cholecystectomy is believed to be too risky during pregnancy. The higher complication rate may have been due to the postponement of surgery in patients except those who were the most ill [36]. More recent evidence suggests that cholecystectomy may be feasible prior to delivery, although the data are taken from small groups in uncontrolled trials and do not allow generalized recommendations. Both open and laparoscopic cholecystectomy have been performed in the second trimester of pregnancy for both symptomatic cholelithiasis and acute cholecystitis, with no reported adverse effects on mother or fetus [37,38]. Cholecystostomy has also been used for acute cholecystitis in the third trimester [39]. Of the nonoperative methods, perhaps only ursodeoxycholic acid could be considered for symptomatic cholelithiasis; however, its effect may take too long for the patient to derive any benefit prior to delivery. Endoscopic retrograde cholangiography may be suitable in selected patients with choledocholithasis.

Of patients undergoing cholecystectomy, approximately 20% are found to have pigmented gallstones [40]. Pigmented gallstones are designated as either black or brown. Black stones typically are seen in hemolytic anemias, cirrhosis, alcoholism, pancreatitis, advanced age, or chronic parenteral nutrition, and usually are limited to the gallbladder. The majority of these black stones contain a higher proportion of calcium carbonate or calcium phosphate, which imparts a radiopaque property. Although hypercalcemia generally does not predispose to their formation, they also may be seen with primary hyperparathyroidism. The clinical manifestations of pigment stones are no different from those with cholesterol stones of the gallbladder.

Cholecystectomy usually is curative with recurrence or common duct stones seen in fewer than 5% of patients. Nonoperative therapies are not likely to be effective because of the stone composition. Infection usually is not associated with black stones [40].

Brown pigment stones are almost uniformly associated with bacterial infection of the bile, generally polymicrobial, although *Escherichia coli* is usually present [40]. Patients may have a juxtapapillary diverticulum. In contrast to the black stones, brown stones can be found throughout the biliary system and are almost never radiopaque. Surgical cholecystectomy with or without endoscopic papillotomy and stone retrieval is the best therapy, although stone recurrence is high [40].

Acalculous cholecystitis may be seen in patients with AIDS, although the exact incidence is not known. It usually manifests as right upper quadrant or epigastric pain with or without fever. Occasionally, jaundice is present. Elevation of the serum alkaline phosphatase is the most common biochemical abnormality. Ultrasound may show a dilated gallbladder with or without wall thickening, although this is nonspecific and may be normal. Cytomegalovirus, *Cryptosporidium*, and *Microsporidia* spp have been implicated most commonly. A detailed discussion of the hepatobiliary manifestations of AIDS is found elsewhere in this book (see Chapter 111).

From time to time, gastroenterologists may encounter patients with liver disease who have pigment or cholesterol gallstones. Therapeutic options may be complicated by the presence of a coagulopathy. Operative risk may be stratified according to the degree of hepatic compensation (Child's classification) as well as the urgency of the surgery. Based on these conditions, the operative mortality may range from 10% to over 80% [41]. The presence of jaundice may make it difficult to differentiate choledocholithiasis from underlying hepatocellular dysfunction. In the setting of cholecystitis, patients should be treated conservatively with intravenous fluids and antibiotics. Those who improve may be observed, but a worsening condition may require cholecystectomy. Cholecystostomy may be a safer alternative in this setting. New-onset jaundice or an increase in bilirubin from baseline may warrant endoscopic retrograde cholangiopancreatography and possible papillotomy following optimization of clotting parameters. Incidental cholecystectomy is not indicated for cirrhotic patients with asymptomatic cholelithiasis due to the low incidence of complications; however, close observation is warranted [42].

Xanthogranulomatous cholecystitis is a rare variant of chronic cholecystitis. Clinically, it is indistinguishable from calculous cholecystitis, and this diagnosis is made histologically. It tends to be more prone to the development of complications (*ie*, fistula, abscess). Eosinophilic cholecystitis is another rare diagnosis, also made histologically.

■ REFERENCES

1. National Institutes of Health: Consensus statement on gallstones and laparoscopic cholecystectomy. Am J Surg 1993, 165:390–396.
2. Friedman GD: Natural history of symptomatic and asymptomatic gallstones. *Am J Surg* 1993, 165:399–404.
3. Ransohoff DF, Gracie WA: Treatment of gallstones. *Ann Intern Med* 1993, 119:606–609.
4. Fenster LF, Lonborg R, Thirlby RC, *et al.*: What symptoms does cholecystectomy cure? *Am J Surg* 1995, 169:533–538.
5. Frazee RC, Nagorney DM, Mucha P: Acute acalculous cholecystitis. *Mayo Clin Proc* 1989, 64:163–167.
6. Rosenquist CJ: Radiology of the biliary tree. *Surg Clin North Am* 1981, 61:775–786.
7. Marton KI, Doubilet P: How to image the gallbladder in suspected cholecystitis. *Ann Intern Med* 1988, 109:722–729.
8. Maglinte DT, Tores WE, Laufer I: Oral cholecystography in contemporary gallstone imaging: a review. *Radiology* 1991, 178:49–58.
9. Bree RL: Further observations on the usefulness of the sonographic Murphy sign in the evaluation of suspected acute cholecystitis. *J Clin Ultrasound* 1995, 23:169–172.
10. Ekberg O, Weiber S: The clinical importance of a thickened, tender gallbladder without stones on ultrasonography. *Clin Radiol* 1991, 44:38–41.
11. Jennings WC, Drabek GA, Miller KA: Significance of sludge and thickened wall in ultrasound evaluation of the gallbladder. *Surg Gynecol Obstet* 1992, 174:394–398.
12. Teefey SA, Baron RL, Bigler SA: Sonography of the gallbladder: significance of striated (layered) thickening of the gallbladder wall. *AJR Am J Roentgenol* 1991, 156:945–947.
13. Kim CK, Juweid M, Woda A, *et al.*: Hepatobiliary scintigraphy: morphine-augmented versus delayed imaging in patients with suspected acute cholecystitis. *J Nucl Med* 1993, 34:506–509.
14. Krishnamurthy S, Krishnamurthy GT: Cholecystokinin and morphine pharmacological intervention during ^{99m}Tc-HIDA cholescintigraphy: a rational approach. *Semin Nucl Med* 1996, 26:16–24.
15. Kim PN, Lee KS, Kim IY, *et al.*: Gallbladder perforation: comparison of US findings with CT. *Abdom Imaging* 1994, 19:239–242.
16. Roslyn JJ, Thompson JE, Darvin H, *et al.*: Risk factors for gallbladder perforation. *Am J Gastroenterol* 1987, 82:636–640.
17. Swayne LC, Filippone A: Gallbladder perforation: correlation of cholescintigraphic and sonographic findings with the Niemeir classification. *J Nucl Med* 1990, 31:1915–1920.
18. Peer A, Witz E, Manor H, Strauss S: Intrahepatic abscess due to gallbladder perforation. *Abdom Imaging* 1995, 20:452–455.
19. van Sonnenberg E, D'Agostino HB, Casola G, *et al.*: Gallbladder perforation and bile leakage: percutaneous treatment. *Radiology* 1991, 178:687–689.
20. Ong CL, Wong TH, Rauff A: Acute gallbladder perforation: a dilemma in early diagnosis. *Gut* 1991, 32:956–968.
21. Glenn F, Reed C, Grafe WR: Biliary enteric fistula. *Surg Gynecol Obstet* 1981, 153:527–531.
22. Clavien P-A, Richon J, Burgan S, Rohner A: Gallstone ileus. *Br J Surg* 1990, 77:737–742.
23. Toscano RL, Taylor PH, Peters J, *et al.*: Mirizzi syndrome. *Am Surg* 1994, 60:889–891.
24. Csendes A, Diaz JC, Burdiles P, *et al.*: Mirizzi syndrome and cholecystobiliary fistula: a unifying classification. *Br J Surg* 1989, 76:1139–1143.
25. Andreu J, Pérez C, Cáceres J, *et al.*: Computed tomography as the method of choice in the diagnosis of emphysematous cholecystitis. *Gastrointest Radiol* 1987, 12:315–318.
26. Tait N, Little JM: The treatment of gallstones. *BMJ* 1995, 311:99–105.
27. Hussani SH: Clinical economics review: the management of gallstone disease. *Aliment Pharmacol Ther* 1996, 10:699–705.
28. Salen G, Tint GS, Shefer S: Treatment of cholesterol gallstones with litholytic bile acids. *Gastroenterol Clin North Am* 1991, 20:171–182.
29. Sauerbruch T, Paumgartner G: Gallbladder stones: Management. *Lancet* 1991, 338:1121–1124.
30. Johnston DE, Kaplan MM: Pathogenesis and treatment of gallstones. *N Engl J Med* 1993, 328:412–421.

31. Pauletzki J, Holl J, Sackmann M, *et al*.: Gallstone recurrence after direct contact dissolution with methyl *tert*-butyl ether. *Dig Dis Sci* 1995, 40:1775–1781.

32. Maher JW, Summers RW, Dean TR, *et al*.: Early results of combined electrohydraulic shockwave lithotripsy and oral litholytic therapy of gallbladder stones at the University of Iowa. *Surgery* 1990, 108:648–654.

33. Gibney EJ: Asymptomatic gallstones. *Br J Surg* 1990, 77:368–372.

34. Melin MM, Sarr MG, Bender CE, *et al*.: Percutaneous cholecystostomy: a valuable technique in high-risk patients with presumed acute cholecystitis. *Br J Surg* 1995, 82:1274–1277.

35. Jatzko GR, Lisborg PH, Pertl AM, *et al*.: Multivariate comparison of complications after laparoscopic cholecystectomy and open cholecystectomy. *Ann Surg* 1995, 221:381–386.

36. Davis A, Katz VL, Cox R: Gallbladder disease in pregnancy. *J Reprod Med* 1995, 40:759–762.

37. Swisher SG, Schmit PJ, Hunt KK, *et al*.: Biliary disease during pregnancy. *Am J Surg* 1994, 168:576–581.

38. Lanzafame RJ: Laparoscopic cholecystectomy during pregnancy. *Surgery* 1995, 118:627–633.

39. Allmendinger N, Hallisey MJ, Ohki SK, *et al*.: Percutaneous cholecystostomy treatment of acute cholecystitis in pregnancy. *Obstet Gynecol* 1995, 86:653–654.

40. Trotman BW: Pigment gallstone disease. *Gastroenterol Clin North Am* 1991, 20:111–126.

41. Gholson CF, Bacon BR: The liver in anesthesia and surgery. In *The Liver in Systemic Disease*. Edited by Rustgi VK, Van Thiel DH. New York: Raven Press; 1993:145–165.

42. Orozco H, Takahashi T, Mercado MA, *et al*.: Long-term evolution of asymptomatic cholelithiasis diagnosed during abdominal operations for variceal bleeding in patients with cirrhosis. *Am J Surg* 1994, 168:232–234.

43. Donovan JM: Pathogenesis of Gallstones. In *Gastroenterology and Hepatology: The Comprehensive Visual Reference*, vol. 6. Edited by LaRusso NF. Philadelphia: Current Medicine; 1996:7.4–7.20.

44. Thistle JL: Nonsurgical Treatment of Gallstones. In *Gastroenterology and Hepatology: The Comprehensive Visual Reference*, vol. 6. Edited by LaRusso NF. Philadelphia: Current Medicine; 1996:8.2–8.14.

45. Davis WZ, Branch MS: Biliary Tract Infections. In *Gastroenterology and Hepatology: The Comprehensive Visual Reference*, vol. 6. Edited by LaRusso NF. Philadelphia: Current Medicine; 1996:10.2–10.18.

121 Laparoscopic Cholecystectomy
William V. Kastrinakis and David C. Brooks

Cholecystectomy is the most common major surgical procedure in the United States today, with more than 500,000 such operations performed each year. Since its introduction in 1989, laparoscopic cholecystectomy has replaced the conventional open procedure and become the treatment of choice for patients with symptomatic gallstones. Approximately 90% of all cholecystectomies are now performed in this fashion. The widespread acceptance of laparoscopic cholecystectomy was fueled by a high degree of patient satisfaction resulting from decreased postoperative pain, less cosmetic disfigurement, markedly decreased hospital stay, and a rapid return to normal activity.

■ HISTORY OF GALLBLADDER SURGERY, LAPAROSCOPY, AND LAPAROSCOPIC CHOLECYSTECTOMY

The era of surgical management of gallstone disease followed the first human cholecystectomy performed by Carl Langenbuch in Berlin in 1882. Since then, surgical removal of the gallbladder has remained the gold standard for the treatment of symptomatic cholelithiasis. Other milestones in the treatment of gallstone disease included the first choledocholithotomy in 1890, through which Ludwig Courvoisier of Switzerland became the first person to remove a gallstone from the common bile duct. In 1924, Evert Graham and Warren Cole of the United States performed the first oral cholecystogram in humans, and in 1931,

Mirizzi described the technique and value of intraoperative cholangiography [1].

The term *laparoscopy* refers to the use of a laparoscopic telescope for examination of the abdominal cavity. Kelling first described laparoscopy in Germany in 1901, with reports of a cystoscope inserted into the abdominal cavity of a dog to examine the stomach. It was not until 1910, when the first laparoscope was built, that Jacobeus in Stockholm used laparoscopy in humans.

Laparoscopy has been used by gynecologists for many years to diagnose pelvic disease and for minor therapeutic procedures, such as tubal ligation. One of the limiting factors of this technology was visualization, as it was necessary to view the field directly through the instrument while simultaneously holding it. The evolution toward current video systems followed the development of the Hopkin's Rod-Lens system in 1966. Modern laparoscopy developed in 1986, when all members of the operating room team were able to view the abdominal cavity through the attachment of a charge-coupled device to the laparoscope.

The first laparoscopic cholecystectomy in humans was performed in Germany by Muhe in 1985. Most authors, however, give credit to Philip Mouret, a French gynecologist, who in 1987 changed the operative procedure to essentially that which is currently practiced. The technique was expanded in

France by Perissat in Bordeaux and Dubois in Paris. Laparoscopic cholecystectomy was first performed in the United States by McKernan and Saye in mid-1988, but was popularized by Reddick and Olsen, who subsequently performed hundreds of procedures with minimal morbidity. Laparoscopic cholecystectomy was subsequently introduced into the surgical community at an unprecedented rate of speed.

TECHNOLOGY REQUIREMENTS

Videolaparoscopy provides an indirect visualization of the peritoneal cavity in that the image is not viewed directly, but is electronically reconstructed on a video monitor. High-flow insufflation of carbon dioxide CO_2 is used to create the pneumoperitoneum needed for visualization of the abdominal cavity. Devices have been developed that elevate the abdominal wall by external retraction. This technique, referred to as *gasless laparoscopy*, can provide adequate visualization without the potential adverse local and systemic effects of pneumoperitoneum.

Imaging is achieved by attaching a charge-coupled device camera to a standard, rigid laparoscopic telescope and projecting the image onto a video monitor. A high-intensity light source is necessary to illuminate the peritoneal cavity through the laparoscope. Two-dimensional monocular imaging is the current industry standard. Three-dimensional imaging systems have been introduced because of limitations inherent in two-dimensional imaging, including diminished depth perception and monitor-induced variability of image resolution, color reconstruction, and lighting.

One of the controversies during the early development of laparoscopic cholecystectomy was whether the source of thermal energy used to facilitate dissection made a difference in outcome. Many of the pioneers of this procedure were advocates of laser laparoscopy because monopolar electrosurgery was thought to be dangerous and associated with a greater rate of thermal injury. Electrosurgery was shown to have significant advantages over laser surgery, including better hemostasis, less cost, and greater speed, and has thus become the standard source of thermal energy for dissection of the gallbladder during laparoscopic cholecystectomy [2].

Laparoscopic instrumentation has continued to evolve since the widespread introduction of laparoscopic cholecystectomy. Increased demand has resulted in a rapid increase in new technology and equipment availability. High-resolution video monitors afford greater clarity and definition as well as improved magnification of the operative field. Endoscopic clip appliers have been downsized to fit available trocars and are now routinely used. Basic instruments required for laparoscopic cholecystectomy include disposable or reusable access ports (trocar/cannula systems), grasping forceps, dissecting forceps, scissors, clip appliers, and extraction forceps for removing the gallbladder from the peritoneal cavity. Instruments that allow irrigation and aspiration of blood and bile are also necessary.

INITIAL REPORTS

Multiple series concerning the laparoscopic cholecystectomy experience in the United States have been published since the introduction of this technique. Redick and Olsen were the first to publish a comparison between laparoscopic and open cholecystectomy, showing advantages for the laparoscopic approach [3•]. Meyers organized a group of surgeons in the Southeastern United States, the Southern Surgeons Club, to publish the first large, multi-institutional series of laparoscopic cholecystectomies [4••]. This series demonstrated the low morbidity and mortality rates associated with laparoscopic cholecystectomy but revealed a higher bile duct injury rate than had been reported for standard open cholecystectomy.

The report of the National Institutes of Health Consensus Conference Development Panel on Gallstones and Laparoscopic Cholecystectomy published in 1993 concluded that laparoscopic cholecystectomy is a safe and effective treatment for most patients with symptomatic gallstones, and subsequently has become the treatment of choice for most of these patients. Furthermore, laparoscopic cholecystectomy provides distinct advantages over standard open cholecystectomy. It decreases pain and disability without increasing mortality and overall morbidity and can be performed at a treatment cost that is equal to, or slightly less than, that of open cholecystectomy [5].

DEMOGRAPHICS

Approximately 10% of the population of the United States has documented cholelithiasis. The prevalence of cholelithiasis has been associated with increasing age, female gender, obesity, diabetes, and rapid weight loss. The majority of candidates with symptomatic gallstones are candidates for laparoscopic cholecystectomy. Contraindications to performing laparoscopic cholecystectomy (Table 121-1) have changed as experience with this technique has grown. Many of the relative contraindications were previously considered as absolute contraindications; use of the laparoscopic approach in such patients is now dictated mostly by the surgeon's philosophy and expertise.

INDICATIONS

Cholecystectomy is indicated for the treatment of symptomatic gallstone disease. As laparoscopy has become the preferred approach for this procedure, an increase in the rate of cholecystectomies has been noted in several published series [6]. The growth in cholecystectomy rates is in part secondary to the liberalization of clinical thresholds for performing surgery. More patients with less severe gallstone-related disease have been

Table 121-1. Contraindications to Laparoscopic Cholecystectomy

Absolute	Relative
Inability to tolerate general anesthesia	Morbid obesity
Diffuse peritonitis	Previous upper abdominal surgery
Cholecystoenteric fistula	Cirrhosis, portal hypertension
Suspected gallbladder malignancy	Abdominal aortic, iliac aneurysm
Uncorrected coagulopathy	Suspected empyema or gangrenous cholecystitis
"Frozen" abdomen	Pregnancy
Other conditions requiring laparotomy	Severe obstructive lung disease
	Huge gallstones

attracted to undergo surgery because of the beneficial qualities of this approach. Likewise, as the skill level for this procedure among surgeons has evolved, so have the indications for surgery. Laparoscopic cholecystectomy can now be performed safely in many patients with acute inflammation of the gallbladder and may be appropriate for selected categories of asymptomatic patients. Occasionally, patients without gallstones, such as those with acute or chronic acalculous cholecystitis, biliary dyskinesia, HIV-associated biliary disease, or "crystal disease," will require removal of the gallbladder [7].

CHOLECYSTITIS: CHRONIC, ACUTE, AND GANGRENOUS

Chronic cholecystitis is characterized by recurrent episodes of nausea, vomiting, and colicky right upper quadrant or epigastric pain. The pain attack can last from 30 minutes to 24 hours, often follows meals, and can radiate to the scapula region. The discomfort of chronic cholecystitis is believed to represent biliary colic, not acute, inflammation. The treatment of chronic cholecystitis and cholelithiasis is cholecystectomy.

Acute calculous cholecystitis results from cystic duct obstruction by a stone impacted in Hartmann's pouch. Secondary bacterial invasion of the inflamed obstructed organ occurs in 50% of cases. The role of laparoscopic surgery in the management of acute cholecystitis remains controversial. Although acute cholecystitis was initially a contraindication to laparoscopic cholecystectomy, it now appears to be a safe and effective option in selected patients and should not preclude an initial laparoscopic approach by experienced surgeons.

Most of the controversy regarding laparoscopic cholecystectomy for acute cholecystitis centers around the higher risk of potential complications when acute edema and inflammation distort the biliary and vascular anatomy. Often, the gallbladder is found to be distended with a thick, inflamed wall. Decompression of the gallbladder with a large-gauge needle and syringe may facilitate application of the grasping forceps for retraction. Technical difficulties arise when the inflammation extends beyond the gallbladder to the porta hepatis. Edema and thickening of the tissues investing the cystic duct or the duct itself can obscure the anatomy, making blunt dissection techniques more difficult. If the anatomy is unclear, intraoperative cholangiography must be performed or the surgeon may need to convert from laparoscopic cholecystectomy to an open cholecystectomy.

Collective series have shown that conversion from laparoscopic cholecystectomy to open cholecystectomy occurs in approximately 5% of cases [8]. Conversion to an open cholecystectomy is usually due to inflammation, obscure anatomy, and, occasionally, intraoperative problems. In a review of 460 attempted cholecystectomies, Singer and McKeen [9] reported conversion rates to open cholecystectomy of 2.8% for chronic cholecystitis, 13.6% for acute cholecystitis, and 75% for gangrenous cholecystitis. The length of operation for laparoscopic compared with open cholecystectomy for acute cholecystitis was not significantly different. Laparoscopic cholecystectomy was found to be technically possible in the majority of patients with acute cholecystitis, and although the conversion rate is higher, if completed successfully, postoperative recovery is faster and the length of hospital stay is shorter than with the open method.

Conversely, the laparoscopic approach for gangrenous cholecystitis carries a much higher conversion rate, requires longer operative time, and shows no significant difference in length of stay when compared to the open procedure. Use of the laparoscopic approach when gangrenous cholecystitis is suspected should be questioned, and once diagnosed, warrants a low threshold for conversion to the open procedure [10].

Several reviews have evaluated different preoperative variables for identification of those patients with acute cholecystitis who require conversion to open cholecystectomy. The duration of symptoms prior to surgery repeatedly has shown predictive value for surgical outcome. Patients who undergo laparoscopic cholecystectomy within 72 hours of the onset of symptoms have lower rates of conversion to the open procedure. Delaying surgery for more than 72 hours is associated with significantly higher conversion rates, greater hospital costs, and a longer time of recovery following surgery [11]. Some authors advocate laparoscopic cholecystectomy for acute cholecystitis immediately after the diagnosis is made, as delaying surgery allows progression of the inflammatory process, thereby increasing the associated technical difficulty of the procedure [12]. Patients with symptoms lasting longer than 72 hours should be considered for initial medical management followed by interval cholecystectomy in 6 to 8 weeks after the acute attack.

BILIARY PANCREATITIS

As laparoscopic cholecystectomy has become the treatment of choice for uncomplicated cholelithiasis, it also has been applied to more complicated biliary tract disease, including biliary pancreatitis. Historically, cholecystectomy was delayed for 6 to 8 weeks following the diagnosis of acute gallstone pancreatitis; however, several studies have shown that cholecystectomy is best performed during the initial admission for biliary pancreatitis following clinical and chemical improvement. This strategy is meant to avoid the risk of recurrent pancreatitis, which may approach 50% to 75% within 30 days of the initial attack.

Preoperative endoscopic retrograde cholangiopancreatography (ERCP) has been used to confirm the presence of common bile duct stones and achieve stone removal; however, even with the best selection criteria, two thirds of patients undergoing preoperative ERCP will fail to demonstrate choledocholithiasis. Therefore, a selective approach for preoperative ERCP is generally recommended [13]. The majority of patients with mild biliary pancreatitis can be treated by laparoscopic cholecystectomy and intraoperative cholangiography, without preoperative ERCP, once symptoms have improved [14]. Patients with severe or unremitting biliary pancreatitis, concurrent cholangitis, or evidence of bile duct stones on abdominal ultrasound are managed best by early ERCP with sphincterotomy and stone extraction prior to removal of the gallbladder.

ASYMPTOMATIC PATIENTS

Prophylactic cholecystectomy may be advisable for selected asymptomatic patients. Children with gallstones almost always develop cholecystitis, and should be considered for cholecystectomy. Likewise, elective cholecystectomy is recommended for patients with sickle cell disease and gallstones, as diagnostic difficulties may arise during sickle cell crises.

Prophylactic cholecystectomy also may be advisable for patients at high risk for gallbladder cancer. Large gallstones and gallstones associated with calcification of the gallbladder appear to be markers for gallbladder carcinoma. The risk of gallbladder cancer is increased 10-fold in patients with gallstones greater than 3 cm in diameter; this corresponds to about 4% of patients with gallstones. The risk of gallbladder cancer also is dramatically elevated when plain radiography demonstrates calcification of the gallbladder wall or "porcelain gallbladder." In asymptomatic patients with these risk factors, laparoscopic cholecystectomy may prevent biliary malignancy and should be recommended. If gallbladder cancer is suspected on visual inspection during attempted laparoscopic cholecystectomy, either a definitive open procedure should be performed or the laparoscopic approach should be terminated and the patient referred for definitive therapy.

Adenomas of the gallbladder likely represent precursors of gallbladder carcinoma. Risk factors for carcinoma include size greater than 10 mm, age over 60, and the presence of a solitary lesion. Early laparoscopic cholecystectomy is indicated for polypoid lesions greater than 10 mm or for a polyp of any size associated with gallstones. Because the risk of advanced cancer increases with size, open cholecystectomy with partial liver resection are recommended once polyps reach 18 mm in size [15].

DIABETES

The management of gallstones in diabetic patients remains controversial. Earlier reports had suggested a higher prevalence of cholelithiasis in diabetics and a significantly higher perioperative morbidity and mortality in diabetics undergoing cholecystectomy for acute cholecystitis. The increased risk for these patients appears to be related to the higher incidence of comorbid medical problems rather than a direct result of the diabetes. Although the severity of acute cholecystitis is greater in diabetics when compared with the general population, there are no strong data supporting either routine screening of diabetics for gallstones or routine prophylactic cholecystectomy for asymptomatic gallstones.

TRANSPLANTATION

The potential for significant complications from gallstones in solid-organ transplant recipients is well known. Most of the morbidity from gallstone complications occurs in the early posttransplant period, with associated mortality approaching 40%. Growing evidence has suggested that the perioperative management of patients undergoing solid-organ transplantation should include evaluation for cholelithiasis and consideration of prophylactic cholecystectomy for asymptomatic gallstones. Laparoscopic cholecystectomy in transplant recipients has been associated with reduction in morbidity and mortality. Other advantages of this approach have included shorter hospitalization, rapid return to normal activity, and early resumption of oral immunosuppression [16].

SURGICAL TECHNIQUE

Laparoscopic cholecystectomy is generally performed under general anesthesia and controlled ventilation with the surgeon standing to the patient's left; the first assistant stands to the

patient's right to manipulate the gallbladder and provide exposure. The laparoscopic camera can be operated by the surgeon or designated camera operator. The operative setup for laparoscopic cholecystectomy is shown in Figure 121-1.

Pneumoperitoneum is first established by instilling CO_2 by either a closed or an open technique. In the open technique, a small supra or infraumbilical incision is made, and a 10-mm laparoscopic sheath is inserted under direct vision into the peritoneal cavity. In the closed technique, CO_2 is insufflated through a needle passed blindly into the abdominal cavity. Two secondary, 5-mm subcostal ports are then placed in the right upper quadrant under direct visualization. The last 10-mm port is placed under direct vision in the epigastrium. The position for insertion of the access ports is shown in Figure 121-2.

The assistant uses grasping forceps passed through the secondary ports to grab the fundus of the gallbladder and push the gallbladder in a cephalad direction over the liver edge, thereby exposing the gallbladder and porta hepatis. Dissecting forceps passed through the epigastric port are used by the surgeon to tease away any omentum or areolar tissue adherent to the gallbladder infundibulum. Electrocautery is used cautiously because of the proximity of the duodenum and transverse colon and the risk of thermal visceral injury. The peritoneum around the gallbladder neck is dissected and the structures of Calot's triangle (cystic artery, cystic duct, common bile duct) are identified. Once the junction between the infundibulum and origin of the cystic duct is identified, cholangiography is performed or the

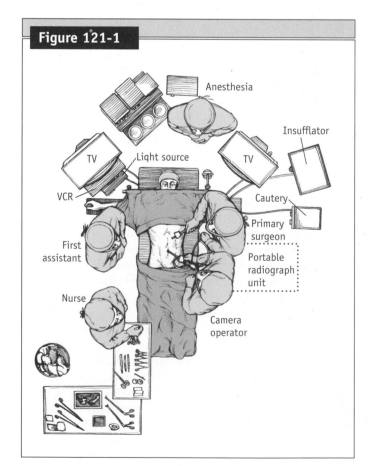

Figure 121-1

Typical organization of the operating room for laparoscopic biliary surgery. (*Adapted from* Fried *et al.* [35]; with permission.)

cystic duct is clipped and divided. The cystic artery is similarly identified, clipped, and divided. The neck of the gallbladder is then placed on traction in a superior direction and separation of the gallbladder from the liver bed is accomplished by dissection with electrocautery. After the cholecystectomy is completed, the gallbladder is removed from the abdominal cavity via the umbilical port. The abdominal cavity is then irrigated and the incisions are closed [17]. The majority of patients are discharged from the hospital the day of surgery or following overnight recovery and observation. Most patients will require a short-term oral analgesic following surgery. Patients can expect mild incisional discomfort and fatigue for 1 to 2 weeks postoperatively. No dietary or activity restrictions are necessary.

■ CONTROVERSIAL AREAS: CHOLANGIOGRAPHY

Choledocholithiasis has been identified in as many as 12% of patients undergoing routine intraoperative cholangiography during laparoscopic cholecystectomy [11,18]. Several authors have debated the question of when to perform laparoscopic cholangiography. The first description of intraoperative laparoscopic cholangiography was published by Spaw in 1991. Since then, refinements in technique and improvements in instrumentation have made intraoperative cholangiography routine in many medical centers. Opponents point out that routine cholangiography overlooks a certain percentage of common bile

duct stones, adds time and cost to the procedure, and may produce false-positive readings leading to a high incidence of unnecessary common bile duct explorations. When not routinely performed, the indications for selective intraoperative laparoscopic cholangiography remain controversial. Criteria have included a clinical history of passing a common bile duct stone, jaundice, elevated liver test results, pancreatitis, or ultrasound findings of choledocholithiasis or a dilated common bile duct.

Cholangiography provides a map of the entire biliary tree and aids in the dissection of the junction between the cystic and common bile ducts, a critical landmark that may be obscured when variations in normal ductal anatomy are found. Operative cholangiography generally involves one or two static cholangiograms (Fig. 121-3) performed after the injection of dilute, iodine-containing, water-soluble contrast medium into the common bile duct. Serious limitations of static cholangiography have included the failure to opacify the entire ductal system, difficulty in discriminating air bubbles within the biliary tree, and the absence of duodenal filling because of the high-pressure zone at the sphincter of Oddi. The introduction of digital fluoroscopic imaging to cholangiography has reportedly improved real-time visualization and decreased false-positive and false-negative results [19].

The routine use of intraoperative cholangiography during laparoscopic cholecystectomy is advocated and practiced in many medical centers; however, selective intraoperative cholangiography has been shown to be safe when the ductal anatomy is clearly defined and when there is no clinical, radiologic, or laboratory evidence of choledocholithiasis [21]. Symptomatic retained common duct stones are rare when cholangiography is performed for the appropriate indications [22].

The management of common bile duct stones identified during laparoscopic cholecystectomy is still evolving, but should depend on the clinical situation, the judgement of the surgeon, and the availability and expertise of a physician qualified to perform postoperative ERCP. Management options include laparoscopic common bile duct exploration (CBDE), conversion

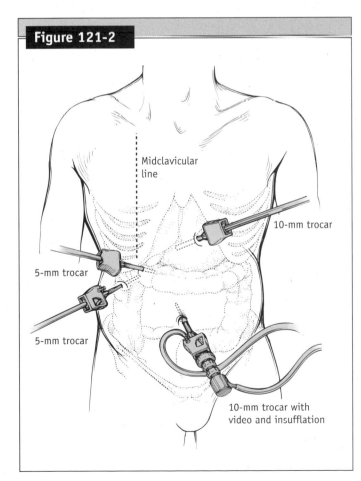

Typical laparoscopic cholecystectomy cannula insertion sites. (*Adapted from* Fried *et al.* [35]; with permission.)

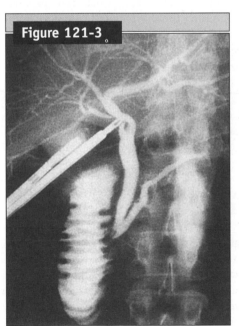

Radiograph obtained during intraoperative laparoscopic cholangiography. (*From* Clair and Brooks [20].)

to open cholecystectomy and open CBDE, or postoperative ERCP with or without papillotomy and stone extraction. Observation in anticipation of spontaneous passage may be appropriate for small solitary common duct stones.

Laparoscopic CBDE is performed through a transcystic duct approach or a laparoscopically placed choledochotomy. Instruments used in bile duct exploration include biliary balloon and basket catheters, tapered plastic dilators, and the (transcystic duct) choledochoscope [23]. Currently available flexible laparoscopic choledochoscopes can be threaded through the cystic duct after gentle dilation to approximately 2F. Following direct visualization of common bile duct stones, endoscopic baskets can be passed via either approach for stone retrieval. The limitations to transcystic CBDE include difficulties in examining the common hepatic duct and in extracting large stones (> 8 mm) through the cystic duct. Laparoscopic choledochotomy allows access to the proximal bile duct and removal of larger stones; however, this approach is technically more difficult and requires placement of a T-tube and drain. In experienced hands, laparoscopic CBDE should clear the bile duct of stones in greater than 90% of cases [24].

PREGNANCY

Complications of gallstones represent one of the most common indications for nonobstetric operations performed during pregnancy. The incidence of cholecystectomy is second only to appendectomy, performed in 0.05% and 0.1% of pregnancies, respectively [25]. Cholecystectomy for recurrent episodes of biliary colic should be postponed until the postpartum period, if possible. Pregnant patients with obstructive jaundice, peritonitis, or acute cholecystitis that is unresponsive to medical management should undergo immediate cholecystectomy, regardless of trimester.

Previously, published guidelines considered pregnancy to be a contraindication to laparoscopy. Recent data suggest that therapeutic laparoscopy during the first or second trimester of pregnancy can be performed safely. Surgery is safest during the second trimester, when uterine size does not preclude laparoscopy, as occurs during the third trimester, and when the risk of teratogenesis associated with surgery in the first trimester is no longer present. The rate of miscarriage is 5.6% in the second trimester, compared with 12% in the first trimester. Potential benefits of laparoscopic surgery to the pregnant patient include a decreased rate of premature delivery because of decreased uterine manipulation, decreased fetal depression secondary to decreased use of narcotics, a decreased rate of incisional hernias, and a quicker return of gastrointestinal activity [26].

PREOPERATIVE ENDOSCOPIC RETROGRADE CHOLANGIOPANCREATOGRAPHY

Preoperative ERCP is used selectively in most medical centers for patients suspected of having common bile duct stones. Although the reported success rates of ERCP for the removal of common bile duct stones approaches 95%, the predictive value of preoperative clinical parameters for choledocholithiasis is at best 50%. Therefore, routine use of preoperative ERCP may subject many patients to unnecessary examinations.

Preoperative ERCP should be considered for elderly patients with a clinical suspicion of choledocholithiasis or for those patients who are at high operative risk, as an increased operative time with cholangiography or duct exploration may be disadvantageous. The presence of multiple stones or a small cystic or common bile duct, which may preclude safe transcystic exploration, also are relative indications for preoperative ERCP if common bile duct stones are suspected.

COMPLICATIONS

Despite the advantages of laparoscopic cholecystectomy over the traditional open approach, there have been several reports of complications resulting from technical errors during the laparoscopic procedure. Complications may be secondary to either the laparoscopic technique or to removal of the gallbladder. Overall complication rates have been documented between 1.0% and 9.0% in most large series, with mortality rates of 0% to 1.0% [27].

Potential complications of the laparoscopic technique are related largely to trocar insertion and creation of pneumoperitoneum. Intestinal perforation or damage to major retroperitoneal vessels have been reported in 0.14% and 0.25% of cases, respectively, and are among the most lethal complications [28]. Bowel and vascular injuries most commonly occur during needle or trocar insertion, often in the setting of previous abdominal surgery, peritonitis, or bowel distention. Complications associated with creation of pneumoperitoneum include gas embolism, vagal reaction, ventricular arrhythmias, and hypercarbia with acidosis.

Meticulous hemostasis is essential in laparoscopic cholecystectomy. Hemorrhage may occur secondary to disruption of the cystic or hepatic artery during dissection of the structures of Calot's triangle. Hemorrhage during laparoscopic cholecystectomy often obscures visualization of the operative field and may result in conversion to an open procedure if the bleeding source cannot be readily identified or adequately controlled.

Bile duct injuries that occur during laparoscopic cholecystectomy can range from small bile collections of no clinical significance to major ductal disruption leading to irreversible liver damage and hepatic transplantation. The classic laparoscopic biliary injury occurs when the common bile duct or common hepatic duct is misinterpreted as the cystic duct during the initial dissection of Calot's triangle (Fig. 121-4).

Another common type of major biliary injury results when excessive or inappropriate use of electrocautery or laser leads to a biliary stricture. Patients with biliary strictures from thermal injury may present with progressive jaundice weeks to months following surgery, and these injuries are often difficult to reconstruct surgically.

Biliary injuries have generally been classified as main or accessory cystic duct leakage; bile duct leakage, stricture, or both; or major bile duct transection or excision. In a multi-institutional study, 81 bile duct injuries were reported from three referral centers. Among the described injuries, the incidence of cystic duct leakage was 19%, bile duct leakage, stricture, or both was 33%, and major bile duct transection or excision was 48% [29]. The risk of major bile duct disruption has generally been reported to be two to five times more likely with the laparoscopic method than with open cholecystectomy. A national survey of over 77,000 cases from 4292 hospitals broadly estimated the frequency of major operative complications of laparoscopic cholecystectomy and found the mean rate of bile duct injury to be 0.6% [30•]. This is comparable to published single and multi-institutional studies reporting bile duct injury rates of 0% to 2% during laparoscopic cholecystectomy compared with historical rates of 0% to 0.4% during open cholecystectomy.

The clinical manifestations and timing of presentation depend on the type of ductal injury. Patients with complete ductal disruption usually present within 10 days of surgery with anorexia, ileus, ascites, diffuse abdominal pain, and tenderness. Patients with complete bile duct obstruction but without bile extravasation usually present within the first 2 weeks of the laparoscopic procedure with progressive jaundice. Major bile duct strictures can be either early or late, and can vary in length and diameter. Biliary strictures have been grouped by the Bismuth classification according to their location and extent of injury. A level 1 stricture is greater than 2 cm from the hepatic bifurcation, level 2 is within 2 cm of the bifurcation, level 3 is at the bifurcation, and level 4 involves the right and left hepatic ducts [32]. If a biliary leak or obstruction is suspected, ERCP is the best method for delineating biliary anatomy. A treatment algorithm for biliary injury is shown in Figure 121-5. Early suspicion, recognition, and treatment of biliary injuries is critical in decreasing the risk for long-term morbidity and mortality.

Once recognized, postoperative bile leaks have been successfully treated with endoscopically placed long biliary endoprostheses that traverse the site of the leak. Recently, endoscopic placement of short transpapillary stents without sphincterotomy has been described to be equally effective by equalizing the bile duct and duodenal pressures, thereby facilitating leak closure [33]. Major injuries to the extrahepatic biliary tree are less amenable to endoscopic techniques. These injuries not only subject the patient to the immediate risks of a major biliary reconstruction, but also the life-long risk of recurrent stricture formation.

Cholangiography has been shown to increase the intraoperative detection of biliary tract injury by nearly twofold when completed and correctly interpreted. Although cholangiography may not prevent all biliary tract injuries, it may prevent the extension of a common duct injury and minimize the associated morbidity, as early identification and repair of bile duct injuries are advantageous over late identification and repair [29]. Cholangiography may be most helpful in avoiding injuries when abnormal anatomic variants are discovered during surgery.

Several studies have reported a correlation between the surgeon's experience with laparoscopic cholecystectomy and the risk of common bile duct injury. Although the experience of the surgeon appears to be an important factor, similar injuries have occurred during procedures by surgeons with considerable laparoscopic experience, suggesting that laparoscopic cholecystectomy

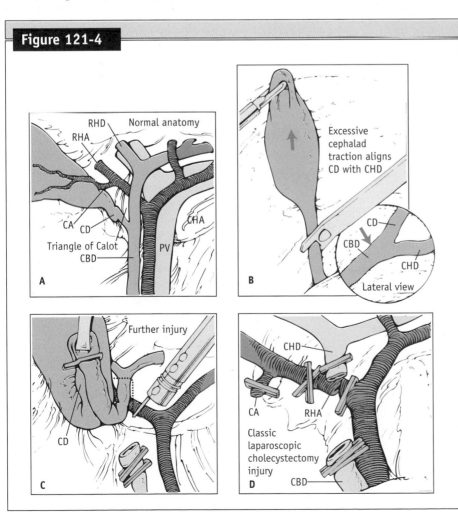

Figure 121-4

Mechanism of classic laparoscopic cholecystectomy common bile duct injury. **A**, Normal anatomy. **B**, Excessive cephalad traction aligns the cystic duct (CD) with the underlying common hepatic duct (CHD). **C**, Further injury. **D**, Classic laparoscopic cholecystectomy injury. The common bile duct (CBD) is mistaken for the CD. CA—cystic artery; CHA—common hepatic artery; PV—portal vein; RHA—right hepatic artery; RHD—right hepatic duct. (*Adapted from* Schirmer [27].)

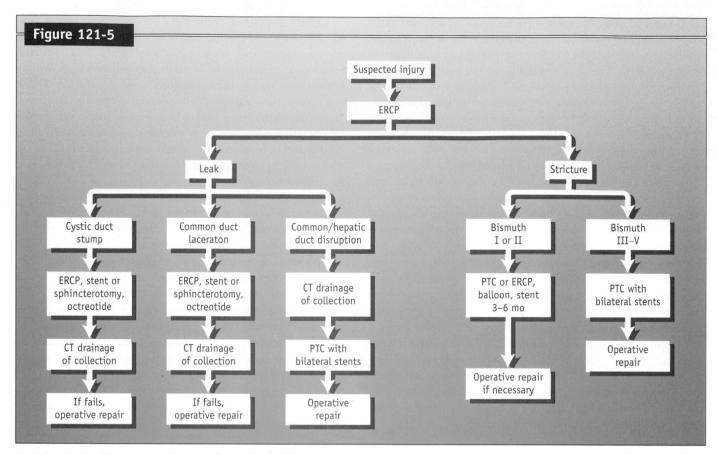

Figure 121-5

Algorithm for suspected common bile duct injury following laparoscopic cholecystectomy. CT—computed tomography; ERCP—endoscopic retrograde cholangiopancreatography; PTC—percutaneous transhepatic cholangiography. (*Adapted from* Branum and Pappas [31].)

Table 121-2. Factors Determining Conversion to Laparotomy in Patients Undergoing Laparoscopic Cholecystectomy

Inability to define anatomy
Hemorrhage
Inability to safely enter the peritoneal cavity
Common bile duct injury
Small-bowel or colon injury
Unexpected findings

---

may be associated with an inherently greater risk of bile duct injury than open cholecystectomy.

RESULTS

The rates of conversion to an open procedure range from 1.8% to 8.5% and have been noted to decrease with increasing operator experience [34]. Factors determining conversion to laparotomy in patients undergoing laparoscopic cholecystectomy are listed in Table 121-2.

The most common reason for conversion is inability to accurately define the anatomy. Fried *et al*. [35] have reported data that show significant predictors of conversion bhat include increasing age (especially 65 or older), acute cholecystitis, male gender, thickened gallbladder wall found by preoperative ultrasonography, and obesity. The mortality rate associated with laparoscopic cholecystectomy is comparable to that of the open approach, and is dependent on age and the presence of comorbid disease.

CURRENT STATUS

Laparoscopic cholecystectomy has become the standard operation for symptomatic gallstones. This procedure can be performed safely by surgeons with proper training and experience. The incidence of injuries to the bile duct is low, but slightly higher than with open cholecystectomy. Conversion to anopen cholecystectomy is required in approximately 5% of patients. The morbidity and mortality rates of laparoscopic cholecystectomy are low. Benefits to the patient are less postoperative discomfort and early return to normal activity. The multiple small incisions are cosmetically more appealing than the larger incision used during traditional cholecystectomy. Other clear advantages include the decreased length of hospital stay and the consequent reduction in hospital-related costs.

REFERENCES

Recently published papers of particular interest have been highlighted as follows:
•   Of interest
••   Of outstanding interest

1.   Glenn F, Grafe W: Historical events in biliary tract surgery. *Arch Surg* 1966, 93:848–852.

2.   Bordelon BM, Hobday KA, Hunter JG: Laser vs. electrosurgery in laparoscopic cholecystectomy: a prospective randomized trial. *Arch Surg* 1993, 128:233–236.

3.• Reddick EJ, Olsen DO: Laparoscopic laser cholecysterectomy: a comparison with minilap cholecystectomy. *Surg Endosc* 1989, 3:131–133.
This represents the first published comparison between laparoscopic cholecystectomy and open cholecystectomy showing advantages for the laparoscopic approach.

4.•• The Southern Surgeons Club: A prospective analysis of 1518 laparoscopic cholecystectomies. *N Engl J Med* 1991, 324:1073–1078.
This is the first large, multi-institutional series of laparoscopic cholecystectomies published in the United States in a widely read medical journal.

5. National Institutes of Health Consensus Conference: Gallstones and laparoscopic cholecystectomy. *JAMA* 1993, 269:1018–1024.

6. Escarce JJ, Chen W, Schwartz JS: Falling cholecystectomy thresholds since the introduction of laparoscopic cholecystectomy. *JAMA* 1995, 273:1581–1585.

7. Wind P, Chevallier JM, Jones D, *et al.*: Cholecystectomy for cholecystitis in patients with acquired immune deficiency syndrome. *Am J Surg* 1994, 168:244–246.

8. Larson GM, Vitale GC, Casey J, *et al.*: Multipractice analysis of laparoscopic cholecystectomy in 1,983 patients. *Am J Surg* 1992, 163:221–226.

9. Singer JA, McKeen RV: Laparoscopic cholecystectomy for acute or gangrenous cholecystitis. *Am Surg* 1994, 60:326–328.

10. Cox MR, Wilson TG, Luck AJ, *et al.*: Laparoscopic cholecystectomy for acute inflammation of the gallbladder. *Ann Surg* 1993, 218:630–634.

11. Koo KP, Thirlby RC: Laparoscopic cholecystectomy in acute cholecystitis: what is the optimal timing for operation? *Arch Surg* 1996, 131:540–545.

12. Rattner DW, Ferguson C, Warshaw AL: Factors associated with successful laparoscopic cholecystectomy for acute cholecystitis. *Ann Surg* 1993, 217:233–236.

13. Welbourn CR, Mehta D, Armstrong CP, *et al.*: Selective preoperative endoscopic retrograde cholangiography with sphincterotomy avoids bile duct exploration during laparoscopic cholecystectomy. *Gut* 1995, 37:576–579.

14. Soper NJ, Brunt M, Callery MP, *et al.*: Role of laparoscopic cholecystectomy in the management of acute gallstone pancreatitis. *Am J Surg* 1994, 167:42–51.

15. Schwesinger WH, Diehl AK: Changing indications for laparoscopic cholecystectomy: stones without symptoms and symptoms without stones. *Surg Clin North Am* 1996, 76:493–504.

16. Graham SM, Flowers JL, Schweitzer E, *et al.*: The utility of prophylactic laparoscopic cholecystectomy in transplant candidates. *Am J Surg* 1995, 169:44–49.

17. Brooks DC: Laparoscopic biliary surgery. In *Principles of Endosurgery*. Edited by Loughlin KR and Brooks DC. Cambridge, MA: Blackwell Science; 1996:176–190.

18. Duensing RA, Williams RA, Collins JC, Wilson SE: Managing choledocholithiasis in the laparoscopic era. *Am J Surg* 1995, 170:619–623.

19. Soper NJ, Brunt LM: The case for routine operative cholangiography during laparoscopic cholecystectomy. *Surg Clin North Am* 1994, 74:953–959.

20. Clair DG, Brooks DC: Laparoscopic cholangiography. In *Current Review of Laparoscopy*, edn. 2. Edited by Brooks DC. Philadelphia: Current Medicine; 1995:29.

21. Clair DG, Carr-Locke DL, Becker JM, Brooks DC: Routine cholangiography is not warranted during laparoscopic cholecystectomy. *Arch Surg* 1993, 128:551–555.

22. Clair DG, Brooks DC: Laparoscopic cholangiography: the case for a selective approach. *Surg Clin North Am* 1994, 74:961–966.

23. Hunter JG, Soper NJ: Laparoscopic management of bile duct stones. *Surg Clin North Am* 1992, 72:1077–1097.

24. Waters GS, Crist DW, Davoudi M, Gadacz TR: Management of choledocholithiasis encountered during laparoscopic cholecystectomy. *Am Surg* 1996, 62:256–258.

25. Curet MJ, Allen D, Josloff RK, *et al.*: Laparoscopy during pregnancy. *Arch Surg* 1996, 131: 546–551.

26. Lanzafame RJ: Laparoscopic cholecystectomy during pregnancy. *Surgery* 1995, 118:627–631.

27. Schirmer BD: Complications of laparoscopy. In *Current Review of Laparoscopy*. Edited by Brooks DC. Philadelphia: Current Medicine; 1995:61–75.

28. Crist DW, Gadacz TR: Complications of laparoscopic surgery. *Surg Clin North Am* 1993, 73:265–289.

29. Woods MS, Traverso LW, Kozarek RA, *et al.*: Characteristics of biliary tract complications during laparoscopic cholecystectomy: a multi-institutional study. *Am J Surg* 1994, 167:27–34.

30.• Deziel DJ, Millikan KW, Economou SG, *et al.*: Complications of laparoscopic cholecystectomy: a national survey of 4,292 hospitals and an analysis of 77,604 cases. *Am J Surg* 1993, 165:9–14.
This is a retrospective national survey of 77,604 laparoscopic cholecystectomies showing that this procedure is associated with reasonably low overall rates of morbidity and mortality, but with a significant rate of bile duct injury.

31. Branum GD, Pappas TN: Complications of laparoscopic cholecystectomy. In *Atlas of Laparoscopic Surgery*. Edited by Pappas TN, Schwartz LB, Eubanks S. Philadelphia: Current Medicine; 1996:9.2–9.11.

32. Blumgart LH, Kelley CJ, Benjamin IS: Benign bile duct stricture following cholecystectomy: critical factors in management. *Br J Surg* 1984, 71:836–843.

33. Bjorkman DJ, Carr-Locke DL, Lichtenstein DR, *et al.*: Post surgical bile leaks: endoscopic obliteration of the transpapillary pressure gradient is enough. *Am J Gastroenterol* 1995, 90:2128–2133.

34. Watters CR: Basic techniques of laparoscopic cholecystectomy. In *Atlas of Laparoscopic Surgery*. Edited by Pappas TN, Schwartz LB, Eubanks S. Philadelphia: Current Medicine; 1996:6.2–6.7.

35. Fried GM, Barkun JS, Sigman HH, *et al.*: Factors determining conversion to laparotomy in patients undergoing laparoscopic cholecystectomy. *Am J Surg* 1994, 167:35–41.

122 Endoscopic Management of Bile Duct Injuries

Irving Waxman and John D. McKee

Since Langenbuch performed the first cholecystectomy in 1882, various surgical injuries of the bile ducts have been recognized, including strictures with biliary obstruction, fistulas and leaks, and complete transection of the common bile duct. Complications arising from biliary obstruction include cholangitis and secondary biliary cirrhosis. Biliary fistulas or leaks can give rise to peritonitis and fluid collections or bilomas that may become secondarily infected. Bile duct injuries are more common in patients undergoing laparoscopic cholecystectomy than in patients who undergo open cholecystectomy [1–3,4•,5••,6,7].

Iatrogenic bile duct injury can result from several factors, including variant anatomy, obesity, fibrosis in the triangle of Calot, and intraoperative hemorrhage. Concomitant conditions, including cholecystitis, Mirizzi's syndrome, pancreatitis, and peptic ulcer disease, may increase the likelihood of bile duct injuries because of difficulty identifying anatomic structures. Routine intraoperative cholangiography may help to reduce the overall incidence of bile duct injuries, but this remains a source of controversy [8,9].

Although the same factors are evident during open and laparoscopic cholecystectomy, improved exposure and dissection probably account for decreased incidence of bile duct injuries in the former compared with the latter. The experience of the surgeon also plays an important role in the incidence of bile duct injuries during surgery. The Southern Surgeons Club described a learning curve for laparoscopic cholecystectomy, showing that the incidence of bile duct injuries in the first 13 patients was 2.2% compared with 0.1% for subsequent patients [5••]. Russell's

review of over 30,000 patients who underwent either laparoscopic cholecystectomy or open cholecystectomy showed that the incidence of major bile duct injuries during the shift from the open to laparoscopic technique went from 0.04% in 1989 to 0.24% in 1991, then decreasing to 0.11% in 1993 [10].

Bile duct injuries resulted from the following intraoperative errors: excessive dissection leading to a compromised blood supply or "skeletonization" of the biliary tree; inappropriate duct transection or ligation; trauma during dilation; thermal or mechanical trauma during dissection (Figs. 122-1*A* and *B*); and occlusion of the biliary tree during flush maneuvers [11].

In a study performed by Barkun *et al.* [12••] examining the clinical histories of 64 patients who developed postoperative bile leaks, 36% of the patients had intraoperative complications. This is in contrast to a complication rate of 0.6% in a control group of patients who did not develop postoperative leaks.

CLINICAL PRESENTATION AND TREATMENT OF BILE DUCT INJURIES

Classification of bile duct injuries has important implications regarding treatment and prognosis [13]. The classification of bile duct injuries adapted from Strasberg *et al.* [14] (Fig. 122-2) includes four major types of injuries: 1) type A—bile leak from minor duct or cystic duct still in continuity with the common bile duct; 2) type B—occlusion of part of the biliary tree with or without leak from the excluded segment (aberrant right hepatic ducts are particularly vulnerable); 3) type C—lateral injury to

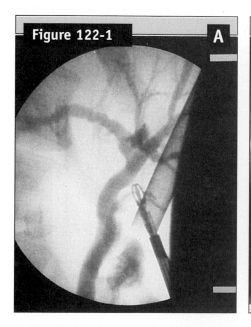
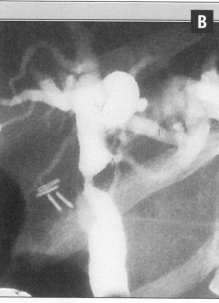

Figure 122-1

A, Intraoperative fluoroscopy showing instrument placement in relation to biliary tree. **B,** Postoperative bile duct stricture.

extrahepatic ducts; 4) type D—circumferential injury of the major bile ducts (bismuth class 1–5). Types A, C, and D are amenable to endoscopic treatment whereas type B is not.

Bile Leaks

The rates of postoperative bile leak in laparoscopic cholecystectomy patients range from 0.38% to 0.63% [15]. Cystic duct leaks, however, seem much more common than leaks involving the common bile duct, and in a series of 54 patients with bile duct injuries reported by Woods *et al.* [16], 17 patients (31%) had cystic duct leaks.

Approximately 50% of all bile leaks originate from the cystic duct stump (Fig. 122-3) [1]. Extrahepatic and gallbladder fossa leaks from the right intrahepatic ducts also occur, but are less common. The ducts of Luschka, which course through the gallbladder bed, are particularly vulnerable to injury during laparoscopic cholecystectomy (Fig. 122-4).

Elboim *et al.* [17] reported that bile leaks can be documented in 25% of patients who are evaluated by abdominal ultrasonography after cholecystectomy; however, the vast majority of postoperative bile leaks go unnoticed and are not clinically significant. Conversely, symptomatic bile leaks occur in less than 5% of all patients undergoing laparoscopic cholecystectomy [1–3, 5••, 6].

The clinical manifestations of bile leaks are best characterized as nonspecific. The spectrum of presentation ranges from minor complaints of vague abdominal or shoulder pain to sepsis with signs of peritonitis. Jaundice and biliary ascites may be present on physical examination; abdominal films may reveal an ileus; laboratory tests may show leukocystosis and abnormal liver test results. Computed tomography (CT) and ultrasonography often are able to show the presence of fluid collections. Scintigraphy effectively demonstrates bile leaks, but may be unnecessary, par-

ticularly if aspiration of the fluid collection is planned [18]. Hepato-iminodiacetic acid (HIDA) scan has an important role in confirming the diagnosis when other studies are inconclusive or when there is a need to assess whether the leak is active.

Initial treatment of patients with bile leaks is centered on optimizing their clinical status prior to intervention. Circulating blood volume and electrolyte imbalances are corrected and intravenous antibiotic therapy aimed at coverage of intra-abdominal infections is begun at the outset. Once the patient is stable, definitive therapy can be performed. Percutaneous aspiration is not considered definitive, as illustrated by Himal's report [19] on 11 minimally ill patients with bile leaks who underwent percutaneous aspiration of bile as their initial therapy. Only 2 of the 11 patients responded to this approach whereas the other 9 patients required emergent endoscopic retrograde cholangiopancreatography (ERCP).

Percutaneous transhepatic cholangiography offers both diagnostic and therapeutic potentials, but access to the biliary tree is

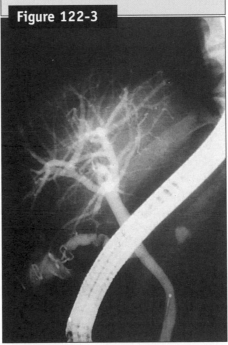

Figure 122-3

Cystic duct leak.

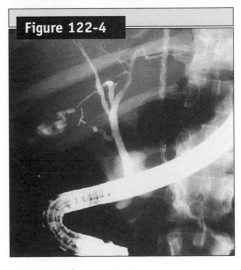

Figure 122-4

Duct of Luschka leak.

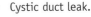

Figure 122-2

A–D, Bile duct injury classification.

B with leak

A

B

C

D

obtained with higher risks of bleeding, sepsis, and perforation compared with ERCP. Frequently the intrahepatic ducts are not dilated, making the procedure technically even more difficult. In addition to these concerns, the typical patient with a bile duct injury from laparoscopic cholecystectomy is relatively young (average age, 43 years old), and percutaneous drainage catheters are more cumbersome in comparison to the options with endoscopic therapy [20].

Although surgery offers diagnostic and therapeutic options in the acute setting, the morbidity and mortality of surgical intervention, reported to be around 31% and 8%, respectively, do not compare favorably with ERCP [4•,12••,21].

Endoscopic Diagnosis and Treatment of Bile Leaks

Endoscopic retrograde cholangiopancreatography offers both diagnostic and therapeutic potential in the management of bile leaks. The initial and diagnostic portion of ERCP can evaluate the biliary tract for obstruction caused by strictures, retained stones, and tumors, as well as determine the precise location of the leak. Biliary obstruction may be noted in up to 31% of patients presenting with postoperative bile leaks [11].

The treatment of a bile leak depends on the site of the leak and the underlying conditions noted at the time of ERCP. For instance, biliary obstruction secondary to gallstones may be seen if the surgeon did not obtain intraoperative cholangiography. Stone extraction followed by diversion of the flow of bile away from the bile leak can be achieved readily during ERCP.

Successful management of bile leaks hinges on removing the pressure gradient between the duodenum and the bile duct. Sphincterotomy, stent placement, or both are the mainstays of ERCP therapy for bile leaks. The need for sphincterotomy, the length of stents, and the optimal duration the stent should be maintained within the bile duct are controversial. Bjorkman *et al.* [22••] demonstrated that sphincterotomy, long stents, and short stents were equally effective in treatment of bile leaks, and Mergener *et al.* [23] reported 27 of 29 patients (93%) were successfully treated with endoscopic stenting alone, leading to complete resolution of leak and symptoms within a median of 29 days. Davids *et al.* [24••] reported endoscopic management of bile leaks in 54 patients; endoscopic treatment was successful in 43 of 48 patients (90%). Despite adequate treatment, five patients (10%) died of persistent sepsis. In this series, 27 patients had bile leaks after open cholecystectomy; 60% of the patients had distal bile duct obstruction.

Nasobiliary drain placement has been reported in lieu of stent placement. Its added benefit is that follow-up cholangiography can be obtained via the nasobiliary catheter, allowing for documentation that the leak has resolved prior to removal of the catheter [25]. Nasobiliary drain contrast studies, as well as removal of the drain, can be achieved without the need for further anesthesia or instrumentation.

After initial endoscopic therapy of a bile leak, repeat endoscopy often is required to remove intrabiliary stents. A general principle that is widely accepted is to leave a stent in place long enough to allow a leak to heal, but not so long that the stent will occlude and lead to cholangitis. The optimal period of stent placement, however, has not been determined. The authors generally remove stents from asymptomatic patients

between 1 to 3 months of the placement and do not routinely obtain follow-up cholangiography on retrieval of a stent in patients who demonstrated clinical recovery after stent placement. Patients who do not fair well after stent placement should be considered for ultrasound or CT imaging to exclude the possibility of additional fluid collections that should undergo percutaneous drainage if infection is suspected. HIDA scans in these cases provide valuable information when demonstrating persistent leaks. Scout films followed by repeat ERCP with appropriate intervention are indicated if technical failure due to stent migration or premature occlusion is suspected.

Bile Duct Strictures

Bile duct strictures represented 22% of all postoperative bile injuries reported by Gouma and Go [4•] in a series from the Netherlands that included over 11,000 cholecystectomies. Strictures resulting from open cholecystectomy have an incidence of approximately 0.1% [26]. The incidence of postlaparoscopic cholecystectomy bile duct strictures is generally accepted to be 5- to 10-fold greater than the incidence of strictures after the open procedure [1,5••] and may result from the use of laser, electrocautery, or from dissection with devascularization [27].

The clinical manifestations of bile duct strictures may be seen within days of the initial procedure or may present several months to years after the initial procedure [28]. Abdominal pain, jaundice, or fever during the postoperative period are cause for concern, and excessive biliary drainage in patients who have T tubes in place signifies a distal obstruction. Jaundice, fever, and abdominal tenderness also may result from biliary obstruction with cholangitis. Coexisting bile leaks may produce chemical peritonitis or result in bilomas that may become infected secondarily. Typically, elevations of the serum alkaline phosphatase and transaminase are noted as part of the laboratory serologic test profile. Bilirubin levels also are elevated, but the patient need not be clinically jaundiced.

Ultrasound and CT scans of the abdomen may show intrahepatic and, possibly, extrahepatic ductal dilation, depending on the site of the injury. Fluid collections secondary to bile leaks should be drained if indicated by the clinical circumstances and technically feasible. In general, large nonloculated fluid collections and collections where infection is suspected should be drained percutaneously. Most of the small fluid collections will resolve without intervention.

Magnetic resonance cholangiopancreatography is a novel technique employing heavily T_2-weighted images to demonstrate biliary anatomy. The technique is capable of demonstrating biliary pathology, such as strictures or stones, with a sensitivity of over 90% [29••,30–31]. The test is noninvasive, but it is purely diagnostic and is not widely available.

Traditional treatment of bile duct strictures has been surgical, involving hepaticojejunostomy, hepaticoduodenostomy, or end-to-end anastomoses. There is considerable morbidity of 20% to 30% associated with such biliary stricture repair [32–34]. Mortality of 5% is influenced largely by the presence of infection and underlying disease [32,35]. Patients with underlying cirrhosis are at particularly high risk and have a mortality rate of 30% [36].

Long-term follow-up of patients who undergo successful surgical bile duct repair reveals recurrent stricture formation in up to 30% of cases [34]. Thus, nonsurgical management has developed in the hands of the interventional radiologists and endoscopists. The minimally invasive endoscopic approach has gained favor because it typically is well tolerated and does not preclude additional surgical intervention should the need arise. The converse does not always hold true for surgery as the initial means of treatment in patients with bile duct strictures. Hepaticojejunostomy anastomoses are typically out of reach for even the most experienced endoscopists, with successful ERCP in patients with Roux-en-Y in only 33% of cases [37].

Endoscopic Treatment of Bile Duct Strictures

Reports of endoscopic treatment of bile duct strictures involving repeated balloon dilation and placement of stents within biliary strictures for a prolonged period describe success in 73% to 88% of patients (Figs. 122-5*A–D*, 122-6*A* and *B*) [38,39••,40••,41]. The hypothesis underlying such therapy is that a biliary stricture, once dilated, can, in effect, be held open by the biliary stents. Scar tissue and fibrosis fashion a scaffolding around the stents after repeated treatments and allow for removal of the stents on completion of therapy.

Endoscopic therapy was reported in 70 patients by Davids *et al.* [39••]. The technique involved use of metal-tip dilators of gradually increasing diameter and polyethylene balloons passed over guidewires into the biliary strictures for the purpose of dilating any tight strictures. Initially, one 7F to 10F stent was placed; this was followed by placement of two 10F stents within 6 weeks. Trimonthly, elective exchanges were performed to prevent cholangitis. Stents were successfully placed in 66 of the 70 patients (94%), with improvement of jaundice noted in all patients. Six of the 70 patients eventually required operation. Restricturing was noted in 17% of patients whose stents were removed. The mean follow-up was 42 months, with a range of 4 to 99 months.

Davids *et al.* [40••] also described a series of 101 patients who either had surgical or endoscopic therapy for their biliary strictures. Although the study was retrospective and nonrandomized, both groups of patients were similar with regard to the types and locations of strictures and underlying medical conditions. Although late complications were more common in the endoscopy group, at 50 months' follow-up approximately 83% of the patients who were endoscopically treated had a good result, as reflected by symptoms, laboratory parameters, and cholangiography, which was similar to the surgically treated group.

The use of expandable metal stents in the treatment of intractable bile duct strictures also has been described [42,43•],

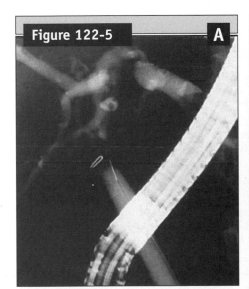
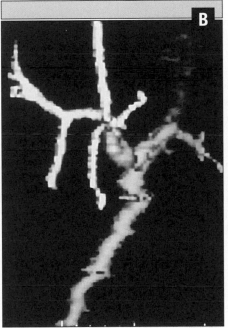
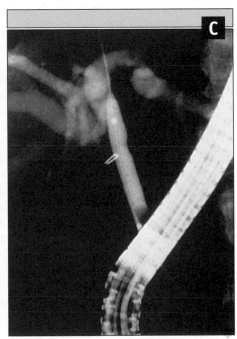
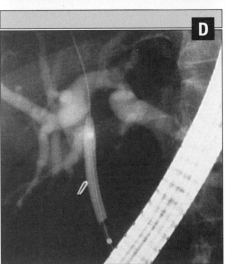

Figure 122-5

A, Common hepatic duct stricture from accidental clip placement. **B**, Computed tomography reconstruction revealing clip placement in relation to stricture. **C**, Endoscopic retrograde cholangiopancreatography (ERCP) with balloon dilation of stricture. **D**, ERCP dilation with disappearance of the balloon waist.

Figure 122-6

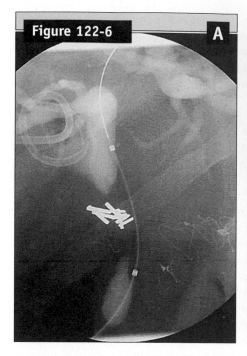
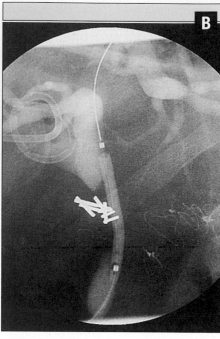

A, Endoscopic retrograde cholangiopancreatography (ERCP) demonstrating multiple clips placed on the common bile duct with significant stenosis. A dilating balloon placed over a guidewire is noted. **B**, ERCP dilation with disappearance of the waist.

but this approach is not commonly used at present. The uncovered metal stents, in general, are not retrievable, and tissue ingrowth occurs to give the stents a finite period of patency. Metal stents may render many surgical approaches impossible; therefore, widespread use for biliary strictures has not been observed.

The ideal endoscopic treatment of biliary strictures at present is unknown. The optimal dilation method, stent size, interval between sessions, and overall number of sessions also have yet to be determined. Despite this uncertainty, endoscopic techniques appear to compare favorably with surgery in selected patients.

▨ SUMMARY

The two principal postoperative bile duct injuries, bile leak and biliary stricture, typically can be managed successfully by endoscopic means. The minimally invasive nature of endoscopy and excellent safety profile of such therapy are well recognized. Additional data regarding long-term follow-up of patients treated by endoscopic means will help to define future practices.

▨ REFERENCES

Recently published papers of particular interest have been highlighted as follows:
- Of interest
- • Of outstanding interest

1. Deziel DJ, Millikan KW, Economou SG, *et al.*: Complications of laparoscopic cholecystectomy: A national survey of 4,292 hospitals and an analysis of 77,604 cases. *Am J Surg* 1993, 165:9–14.

2. Deveney KE: The early experience with laparoscopic cholecystectomy in Oregon. *Arch Surg* 1993, 128:627–632.

3. Cuschieri A, Dubois F, Mouiel J, *et al.*: The European experience with laparoscopic cholecystectomy. *Am J Surg* 1991, 161:385–387.

4.• Gouma DJ, Go PM: Bile duct injury during laparoscopic and conventional cholecystectomy. *J Am Coll Surg* 1994, 178:229–233.

5.•• The Southern Surgeons Club: A prospective analysis of 1518 laparoscopic cholecystectomies. *N Engl J Med* 1991, 324:1073–1078.

6. Albasini JL, Aledo VS, Dexter SP, *et al.*: Bile leakage following laparoscopic cholecystectomy. *Surg Endosc* 1995, 12:1274–1278.

7. Shea JA, Healey BS, Berlin JA, *et al.*: Mortality and complications associated with laparoscopic cholecystectomy: A meta analysis. *Ann Surg* 1996, 224:609–620.

8. Lorimer JW, Fairfull-Smith RJ: Intraoperative cholangiography is not essential to avoid duct injuries during laparoscopic cholecystecotomy. *Am J Surg* 1995, 169:344–347.

9. Panton ON, Nagy AG, Scudamore CH, Panton RJ: Laparoscopic cholecystectomy: A continuing plea for routine cholangiography. *Surg Laparosc Endosc* 1995, 5:43–49, 1995.

10. Russell JC, Walsh SJ, Mattie AS, Lynch JT: Bile duct injuries, 1983–1993: A statewide experience: Connecticut Laparoscopic Cholecystectomy Registry. *Arch Surg* 1996, 131:382–388.

11. Moosa AR, Easter DW, Van Sonnenberg E, *et al.*: Laparoscopic injuries to the bile duct: A cause for concern. *Ann Surg* 1992, 215:203–208.

12.•• Barkun AN, Rezieg M, Mehta S, *et al.*: Postcholecystectomy biliary leaks in the laparoscopic era: Risk factors, presentation, and management. *Gastrointest Endosc* 1997, 45:277–281.

13. Bergman J, van den Brink GR, Rauws EA, *et al.*: Treatment of bile duct lesions after laparoscopic cholecystectomy. *Gut* 1996, 38:141–147.

14. Strasberg SM, Hertl M, Soper NJ: An analysis of the problem of biliary injury during laparoscopic cholecystectomy. *J Am Coll Surg* 1995, 180:101–125.

15. Shea JA, Healey BS, Berlin JA, *et al.*: Mortality and complications associated with laparoscopic cholecystectomy: A meta analysis. *Ann Surg* 1996, 224:609–620.

16. Woods MS, Shellito JL, Santoscoy GS, *et al.*: Cystic duct leaks in laparoscopic cholecystectomy. *Am J Surg* 1994, 168:560–565.

17. Elboim CM, Goldman L, Hahn L, *et al.*: Significance of post-cholecystectomy subhepatic fluid collections. *Ann Surg* 1983, 198:137–141.

18. Trerotola SL, Savader SJ, Lund GB, *et al.*: Biliary tract complications following laparoscopic cholecystectomy: Imaging and intervention. *Radiology* 1992, 184:194–200.

19. Himal HS: The role of ERCP in laparoscopic cholecystectomy-related cystic duct stump leaks. *Surg Endosc* 1996, 10:653–655.

20. Kern KA: Medicolegal perspectives on laparoscopic bile duct injuries. *Surg Clin North Am* 1994, 74:979–983.

21. Brooks DC, Becker JM, Connors PL, Carr-Locke DL: Management of bile leaks following laparoscopic cholecystectomy. *Surg Endosc* 1993, 7:292–295.

22.•• Bjorkman DJ, Carr-Locke DL, Lichtenstien DR, *et al.*: Postsurgical bile leaks: Endoscopic obliteration of the transpapillary pressure gradient is enough. *Am J Gastroenterol* 1995, 90:2128–2133.

23. Mergener K, Jowell P, Branch M, *et al.*: The role of ERCP in the management of biliary leaks following laparoscopic cholecystectomy. *Gastrointest Endosc* 1996, 43:389.

24.•• Davids P, Rauws E, Coene P, *et al.*: Postoperative bile leakage: Endoscopic management. *Gut* 1992, 33:1118–1122.

25. Barthel J, Scheider D: Advantages of sphincterotomy and nasobiliary tube drainage in the treatment of cystic duct stump leak complicating laparoscopic cholecystectomy. *Am J Gastroenterol* 1995, 90:1322–1324.

26. Andren-Sandberg A, Alinder G, Bengmark S: Accidental lesions of the common bile duct at cholecystectomy: Pre-perioperative factors of importance. *Ann Surg* 1985, 201:452–455.

27. Davidoff AM, Pappas TN, Murray EA, *et al.*: Mechanisms of major biliary injury during cholecystectomy. *Ann Surg* 1992, 215:196–202.

28. Pitt HA, Miyamoto T, Parapatis SK, *et al.*: Factors influencing outcome in patients with postoperative biliary strictures. *Am J Surg* 1982, 144:14–21.

29.•• Ishizaki Y, Tatsuro W, Okada Y, Kobayashi T: Magnetic resonance cholangiography for evaluation of obstructive jaundice. *Am J Gastroenterol* 1994, 12:2072–2077.

30. Hall-Craggs MA, Allen CM, Owens CA, *et al.*: MR cholangiography: Clinical evaluation in 40 cases. *Radiology* 1993, 189:423–427.

31. Morimoto K, Shimoi M, Shirakawa T, *et al.*: Biliary obstruction: Evaluation with three-dimensional MR cholangiography. *Radiology* 1992, 183:578–580.

32. Pitt HA, Kaufman SL, Coleman J, *et al.*: Benign postoperative biliary strictures: Operate or dilate? *Ann Surg* 1989, 210:417–420.

33. Genest JF, Nanon E, Grundfest-Broniatowski S, *et al.*: Benign biliary strictures: An analytic review (1970–1984). *Surgery* 1986, 99:409–413.

34. Pelligrini CA, Thomas MJ, Way LW: Recurrent biliary stricture: Pattern of recurrence and outcome of surgical therapy. *Am J Surg* 1984, 147:409–413.

35. Saber K, El-Manialow M: Repair of bile duct injuries. *World J Surg* 1984, 8:82–89.

36. Blumgart LH, Kelley CJ, Benjamin IS: Benign bile duct stricture following cholecystectomy: Critical factors in management. *Br J Surg* 1984, 71:863–843.

37. Hintze RE, Veltzke W, Adler A, Abou-Rebyeh H: Endoscopic sphincterotomy using an S-shaped sphincterotome in patients with a Billroth II or Roux-en-Y gastrojejunostomy. *Endoscopy* 1997, 29:74–78.

38. Berkelhammer C, Kortan P, Haber G: Endoscopic biliary prostheses as treatment for benign postoperative bile duct strictures. *Gastrointest Endosc* 1989, 35:95–100.

39.•• Davids PH, Rauws AJ, Coene PP, *et al.*: Endoscopic stenting for postoperative biliary strictures. *Gastrointest Endosc* 1992, 38:12–18.

40.•• Davids PH, Andras KF, Rauws EA, *et al.*: Benign biliary strictures surgery or endoscopy? *Ann Surg* 1993, 217:237–243.

41. Geenen DJ, Geenen JE, Hogan WJ, *et al.*: Endoscopic therapy for benign bile duct strictures. *Gastrointest Endosc* 1989, 35:267–271.

42. Foerster EC, Hoepffner N, Domschke W: Bridging of benign choledochal stenoses by endoscopic retrograde implantation of mesh stents. *Endoscopy* 1991, 23:133–135.

43.• Rossi P, Salvatori FM, Bezzi M, *et al.*: Percutaneous management of benign biliary strictures with balloon dilation and self-expanding metallic stents. *Cardiovasc Intervent Radiol* 1990, 13:231–239.

123 Postcholecystectomy Syndrome

Steven J. Shields

Over 0.5 million cholecystectomies are performed annually in the United States [1,2], mostly with an excellent outcome. In approximately 20% to 40% of patients undergoing cholecystectomy, however, there is persistence or recurrence of symptoms [1,3], a condition referred to as *postcholecystectomy syndrome* (PCS). PCS encompasses numerous biliary, pancreatic, and other entities (Table 123-1); therefore, the term is nonspecific. In fact, the symptoms experienced by the patient postoperatively often do not differ from those prior to the cholecystectomy. Symptoms in most patients with PCS are mild to moderate, but in 10% to 25% of patients these symptoms are severe and debilitating [4,5].

PHYSIOLOGY AND PATHOPHYSIOLOGY

Upon removal of the gallbladder, the collection reservoir for hepatic bile no longer exists. As a result of this loss, the initial bolus secretion of bile, normally stimulated by a meal, does not take place. The concentration of bile salts in the upper gastrointestinal tract remains in physiologic range, however, and,

Table 123-1. Postulated Causes of Postcholecystectomy Syndrome

Biliary
Retained common bile duct stone, bile duct stricture, bile leak, cystic duct remnant, papillary stenosis, Sphincter of Oddi dyskinesia, ampullary neoplasm, periampullary diverticulum, choledochocele, incomplete cholecystectomy, neuroma, seroma, hematoma

Pancreatic
Pancreatitis, pancreas divisum, pancreatic pseudocyst, pancreatic neoplasm, annular pancreas

Nonpancreaticobiliary
Gastroesophageal reflux disease, peptic ulcer disease, postoperative adhesions, gastrointestinal motility disorders, irritable bowel syndrome, nonulcer dyspepsia, gastrointestinal malignancy, hepatitis, appendicitis, hernia (incisional, inguinal, internal), pyloric stenosis, retroperitoneal fibrosis, chronic mesenteric ischemia (intestinal angina)

Nongastrointestinal
Psychiatric disorders, neurologic disorders, coronary artery disease

therefore, digestion and absorption of food remains unimpaired [4]. Bile salts undergo a more rapid enterohepatic circulation [4]. The cholesterol concentration in bile is reduced and the percentage of deoxycholic acid is elevated due to the rapid recycling and longer exposure of bile to intestinal bacteria, respectively [4]. These physiologic changes occur in response to removal of the gallbladder and are not thought to be pathologic.

Cholecystectomy is associated with a significantly greater prevalence of bile reflux into the stomach [4,6], as well as an increased incidence of gastroesophageal reflux disease (GERD) and esophagitis [1,7,8], although there is no difference in the incidence of GERD in patients who undergo open or laparoscopic cholecystectomy [1]. Furthermore, although ambulatory 24-hour pH monitoring reveals a significant increase in acid reflux in both groups, esophageal manometry does not show abnormalities in lower esophageal sphincter (LES) pressure. It is postulated that, after cholecystectomy, increases in postprandial cholecystokinin (CCK) levels lead to increased transient LES relaxations and subsequent acid reflux [1,9]. Other studies have implicated a role of CCK in the cause of postcholecystectomy syndrome.

Postcholecystectomy syndrome may be associated with a long cystic duct remnant with resultant bile stasis, infection, stone formation or retention, and, possibly, neuroma [5], although the incidence of neuroma formation is similar in patients with and without PCS symptoms [5].

Papillary or sphincter of Oddi stenosis may occur as a primary event or as a consequence of repeated trauma from the passage of gallstones or biliary sludge (see Chapter 119). The resultant impediment to bile flow may herald the onset of obstructive biliary and pancreatic symptoms. After removal of the gallbladder, common bile duct diameter and pressure increase [10–13]. Whether these changes are physiologic and of no clinical consequence or pathologic and a cause of PCS has been the subject of debate [13]. Manometry can be used to detect abnormalities in biliary, pancreatic, and sphincter of Oddi pressure.

CLINICAL FEATURES

The majority of patients with PCS present with abdominal pain or discomfort, typically located in the right upper quadrant or epigastrium. Radiation of pain to the shoulder or back is not uncommon. The pain usually is postprandial, sharp, and often associated with nausea and vomiting. Episodes may last several hours and resolve spontaneously or with analgesics. Intervals of weeks or months may occur between acute episodes. Some patients describe a background of more constant daily discomfort but of a lesser degree than with the acute episodes. Fevers, chills, and jaundice suggest biliary tract obstruction as the underlying cause.

Other commonly described complaints include excessive belching, bloating, flatulence, heartburn, indigestion, and intolerance to certain foods. These symptoms have previously been labeled flatulent dyspepsia, are nonspecific, and may be seen with coexistent irritable bowel syndrome. Symptoms may begin any time from days to decades after cholecystectomy. Nonspecific dyspeptic symptoms existing prior to surgery are more likely to persist or recur after cholecystectomy as are

symptoms in patients without gallstones in the cholecystectomy specimen. It is axiomatic that the longer a patient has had symptoms preoperatively, the less likely it is that cholecystectomy will relieve their symptoms [3].

Postcholecystectomy syndrome may mimic angina pectoris [14]. In one report, a patient was correctly diagnosed with sphincter of Oddi spasms after being treated for angina pectoris for 15 years. Complete resolution of symptoms was achieved after endoscopic sphincterotomy.

Physical examination of patients with PCS is usually noncontributory. Often the only finding is nonspecific abdominal tenderness. The abdomen should be inspected carefully for unusual hernias. Rarely, a patient will have jaundice or scleral icterus on examination.

DIAGNOSIS
Laboratory Testing
Laboratory testing often reveals normal results in patients with PCS, especially if the serum is obtained between acute episodes. Transient fluctuations in liver tests, amylase, and lipase can be seen; therefore, serum analyses should be obtained during symptomatic episodes. A single set of normal laboratory values does not exclude biliary or pancreatic origin. Abnormal liver tests, amylase, and lipase are highly suggestive of a pancreaticobiliary origin.

Noninvasive Testing
Abdominal ultrasound is ordered frequently in patients suspected of having PCS. It can detect bile duct dilation, abnormal fluid collections (eg, biloma, abscess, hematoma), or liver disease. On occasion, a common bile duct stone can be identified. Abdominal ultrasound is limited in evaluating the pancreas because of the frequent interposition of bowel gas between the pancreas and the ultrasound transducer, a limitation that can be overcome by endoscopic ultrasonography. It is important to remember that a "negative" abdominal ultrasound does not eliminate the possibility of an underlying biliary or pancreatic abnormality.

Abdominal computed tomography (CT) scan is complementary to abdominal ultrasound. Advancements in technology with new spiral/helical CT scanners have improved the image resolution capabilities. Invasive radiologists can use the CT scan to guide therapeutic interventions, such as biopsy, aspiration, and drain placement.

Magnetic resonance cholangiopancreatography (MRCP) is an emerging tool for the evaluation of the hepatobiliary systems. It is a noninvasive imaging technique that does not require intravenous contrast. Preliminary studies have reported a high sensitivity and specificity for ductal pathology. It also has the advantage of imaging adjacent organs.

The dimethyl-iminodiacetic acid (HIDA) scan is a nuclear medicine imaging modality using a Tc-labeled iminodiacetate analogue. It is useful in the detection of postcholecystectomy bile leaks, which have become more common with the emergence of laparoscopic cholecystectomy. Quantitative HIDA, also referred to as *hepatobiliary scintigraphy*, has been a useful noninvasive test for patients suspected of having partial biliary obstruction, including sphincter of Oddi dysfunction (SOD) [12,15]. One limitation is the inability to differentiate a structural obstruction from a functional obstruction. False-negative results have been reported in patients with SOD with basal sphincter pressures as high as 40 mm Hg. A positive test result helps direct appropriate diagnostic and therapeutic interventions.

Ultrasound examination after a standard fatty meal has been used to help identify patients with SOD dysfunction. After ingestion of a fatty meal, CCK is released, which normally enhances bile flow. In SOD, bile flow is impeded paradoxically. As a result of which, bile duct pressure and diameter increase. Ultrasound detection of greater than a 2-mm increase in bile duct diameter after the fatty meal is considered positive.

Secretin ultrasound also has been used to diagnose patients with SOD. After the intravenous administration of secretin, pancreatic secretions are increased and there is an increase in the basal tone of the sphincter of Oddi. These changes result in an increase in the pancreatic duct diameter, which is more pronounced in patients with papillary stenosis and SOD. A major limitation of the test is the ability to image the pancreatic duct by ultrasound in a large percentage of patients [12].

The morphine-prostigmine provocation (NARDI) test failed in the noninvasive diagnosis of SOD. It was postulated that patients with SOD would have sphincter spasm following the administration of morphine and, with the prostigmine-induced biliary and pancreatic secretion, there would be a resultant onset of abdominal pain and a corresponding increase in the liver function tests, amylase, or lipase. The test has a low sensitivity and specificity, however, and no longer is recommended [16].

Invasive Testing

Since its introduction over two decades ago, endoscopic retrograde cholangiopancreatography (ERCP) has become the primary test for the evaluation of suspected PCS, especially in those individuals with signs and symptoms of biliary obstruction or pancreatitis [5,17]. ERCP not only offers the opportunity to accurately diagnose the cause, but also allows for therapeutic intervention. ERCP can identify and define postoperative strictures, retained common bile duct stones (Fig. 123-1), bile leaks (Fig. 123-2), anatomic variants (*eg*, pancreas divisum, choledochoceles), and tumors of the ampulla, bile duct, or pancreas (Fig. 123-3). Ampullary tumors can be difficult to diagnose but are suspected when there is a deformity of the ampullary region. Endoscopic biopsies before and after endoscopic sphincterotomy are suggested to confirm the diagnosis [18] (see Chapter 129). The possibility of papillary stenosis or SOD can be evaluated at the time of ERCP and is suggested when dilated biliary or pancreatic duct, delayed drainage of contrast, or difficult cannulation at the ampulla are present. Pain on contrast injection initially was considered to be suggestive of SOD [5] (see Chapter 127), but has since been shown to be a nonspecific finding [12]. A limited examination of the duodenum, stomach, and distal esophagus also can be accomplished at the time of ERCP. Potential causes of PCS, such as periampullary diverticula (Fig. 123-4, see also *Color Plate*), duodenal strictures, polyps, or ulcers (Fig. 123-5, see also *Color Plate*), gastric ulcers or tumors, and esophageal inflammation or ulceration, can be detected.

Endoscopic ultrasound (EUS) is a useful test in the evaluation of PCS and can reliably detect common bile duct stones (Fig. 123-6), ampullary and pancreatic neoplasms, chronic pancreatitis, and pancreatic pseudocysts [19–22]. EUS has a limited role in the diagnosis of sphincter of Oddi disorders. EUS is also technically demanding, limited by the available local expertise, and is being performed primarily at major academic centers (see Chapter 188).

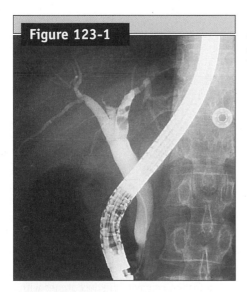

Figure 123-1

Retained common bile duct stone after cholecystectomy.

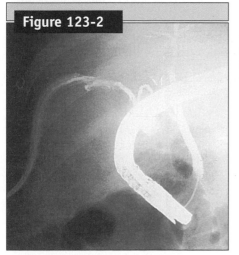

Figure 123-2

Postcholecystectomy bile leak. Note the contrast extravasation via the surgical drainage catheter.

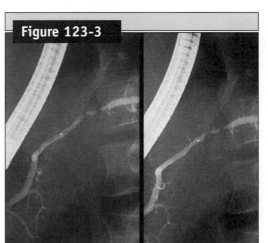

Figure 123-3

Pancreatic duct strictures documented at endoscopic retrograde cholangiopancreatography.

Sphincter of Oddi manometry (SOM) typically is performed via a side-viewing duodenoscope and a manometry catheter passed retrograde into the sphincter region. SOM allows determination of basal sphincter of Oddi pressure and amplitude, frequency, and direction of sphincter of Oddi contractions. In addition to assessment of the biliary sphincter, the manometry catheter can be directed into the pancreatic duct to assess the pancreatic sphincter [12].

During SOM, the finding of an elevated basal pressure greater than 40 mm Hg is thought to represent sphincter of Oddi stenosis [11,12,23]. Stenosis may be produced as a result of fibrosis of the sphincter segment by repeated episodes of localized inflammation, trauma during trans-sphincteric passage of gallstones or sludge, or from instrumentation during surgery. Localized smooth-muscle hypertrophy has also been postulated as a cause of sphincter of Oddi stenosis.

Other sphincteric manometric abnormalities have been described in patients with PCS with SOD. Patients with these findings have typically been classified as having sphincter of Oddi dyskinesia [23]. A sustained increase in the frequency of sphincter of Oddi contractions in excess of seven per minute is considered abnormal and is termed *tachyoddia*. Retrograde contractions in excess of 50% may represent an abnormally functioning sphincter that can retard biliary and pancreatic

flow. Intermittent elevations of basal sphincter pressure can be seen during manometry and may represent periods of sphincter spasm. The normal response of the sphincter of Oddi to CCK administration is a decrease in basal pressure and an inhibition of phasic contractions. In patients with sphincter of Oddi dyskinesia, a paradoxical response to CCK can be seen. Invasive testing in patients with PCS may require upper endoscopy, small-bowel enteroscopy, colonoscopy, or laparoscopy.

◼ TREATMENT

The goal of therapy in patients with PCS is aimed at alleviating their symptoms. To be effective, therapy should be directed toward the specific cause.

Retained common bile duct (CBD) stones after cholecystectomy are a frequent cause of PCS. Management typically involves endoscopic sphincterotomy with subsequent stone extraction by balloon or basket. Smaller stones occasionally can be removed without sphincterotomy by either initial balloon dilation of the sphincter (sphincteroplasty) or by simple extraction, sometimes using nitroglycerin to relax the sphincter without sphincterotomy or spincteroplasty. Large-diameter stones may require mechanical, laser, or electrohydraulic lithotripsy to fragment the stones.

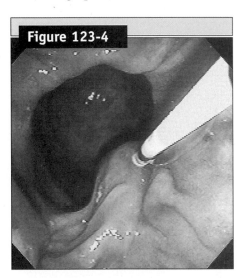

Figure 123-4

Large periampullary diverticulum as seen during endoscopic retrograde cholangiopancreatography. See also **Color Plate.**

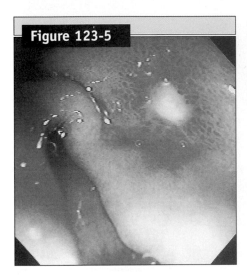

Figure 123-5

Acute ulcer in the duodenal bulb, a potential cause of postcholecystectomy syndrome. See also **Color Plate.**

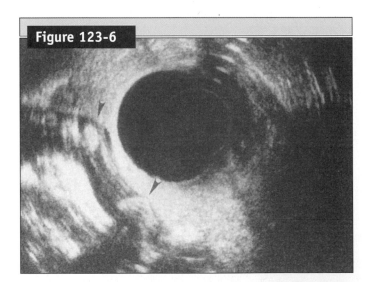

Figure 123-6

Endoscopic ultrasonography revealing common bile duct stones with acoustic shadowing. (*From* Sugiyama *et al.* [21]; with permission.)

Table 123-2. Treatment Options for SOD

Medical	Endoscopic	Surgical
Long-acting nitrates	Biliary sphincterotomy	Biliary sphincteroplasty
Calcium-channel blockers	Pancreatic sphincterotomy	Pancreatic sphincteroplasty
Anxiolytics	Botulinum toxin injection	
Analgesics	Balloon sphincteroplasty	
	Trans-sphincteric stenting	

Stricturing of the CBD after cholecystectomy can result from ischemic injury to the bile duct or from inadvertent clip placement during surgery. Successful management usually is accomplished by endoscopic stricture dilation with or without periods of bile duct stenting. Surgical intervention may be required for successful management for those patients unresponsive to endoscopic therapy or for those diagnosed with significant bile duct injury (*eg*, complete transection of the duct).

With the rapid expansion of laparoscopic cholecystectomy, there has been a corresponding increase in the frequency of postoperative bile leaks (see Chapter 122). Although some bile leaks may heal spontaneously, intervention is frequently necessary, especially when there is fever, cholangitis, or significant pain. Endoscopic management of bile leaks by biliary stenting, endoscopic sphincterotomy, a combination of sphincterotomy and stenting, and nasobiliary drainage have all proven successful [24,25].

Long cystic duct remnants have been linked to the development of postcholecystectomy syndrome [5]. Occasionally, patients have benefited from repeat surgery for removal of the cystic duct. If the cystic duct remnant is noted to contain sludge or stones, their endoscopic removal should be attempted.

Pancreas divisum, a congenital anomaly, is believed by many to cause recurrent attacks of pancreatitis. Diagnosis typically is made at the time of ERCP. Although controversial, studies have shown effective endoscopic management with minor papilla sphincterotomy [26]. Symptoms can recur if there is subsequent stenosis of the sphincterotomy site.

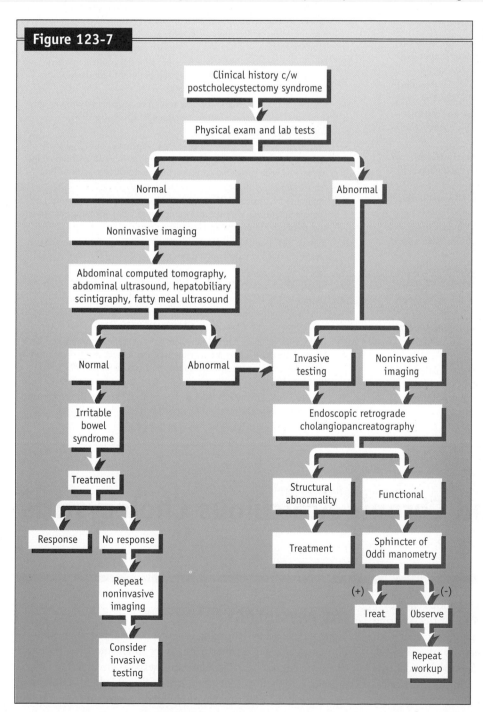

Figure 123-7

Algorithm for management of postcholecystectomy syndrome. FMUS—fatty meal ultrasound; HBS—hepatobiliary scintigraphy.

Several treatment options exist for those patients diagnosed as having SOD; these are listed in Table 123-2 and discussed in Chapter 127.

PROGNOSIS

Postcholecystectomy syndrome is a nonspecific term that encompasses many different disease entities (Table 123-1). Excellent prognosis is expected when the underlying disease is identified and treated; however, many patients suffering from this chronic pain syndrome do not have a specific disease identified despite exhaustive diagnostic evaluation (Fig. 123-7). These patients are likely to be frustrated with their medical care, seek multiple medical opinions, and consume a disproportional percentage of the health care resources.

REFERENCES

1. Rothwell JF, Lawlor P, Byrne PJ, et al.: Cholecystectomy-induced gastroesophageal reflux: is it reduced by the laparoscopic approach? Am J Gastroenterol 1997, 92:1351–1354.

2. Sawyers JL: Current status of conventional (open) cholecystectomy versus laparoscopic cholecystectomy. Ann Surg 1996, 223:1–3.

3. Ros E, Zambon D: Postcholecystectomy symptoms: a prospective study of gallstone patients before and two years after surgery. Gut 1987, 28:1500–1504.

4. Way LW, Sleisenger MH: Postoperative syndromes. In Gastrointestinal Disease. Edited by Sleisenger MH, Fordtran JS. Philadelphia: WB Saunders; 1993:1404–1409.

5. Lasson A: The postcholecystectomy syndrome: diagnosis and therapeutic strategy. Scand J Gastroenterol 1987, 22:897–902.

6. Abu Farsakh NA, Stietieh M, Abu Farsakh FA: The postcholecystectomy syndrome: a role for duodenogastric reflux. J Clin Gastroenterol 1996, 22:197–201.

7. Jazrawi S, Walsh TN, Byrne PJ, et al.: Cholecystectomy and oesophageal reflux: a prospective study. Br J Surg 1993, 80:50–53.

8. Bates T, Ebbs SR, Harrison M, et al.: Influence of cholecystectomy on symptoms. Br J Surg 1991, 78:964–967.

9. Clave P, Gonzalez A, Martin M, et al.: Endogenous cholecystokinin (CCK) enhances post-prandial gastroesophageal reflux in healthy volunteers. Gastroenterology 1996, 110:A649.

10. Rolny P, Geenen JE, Hogan WJ: Post-cholecystectomy patients with "objective signs" of partial bile outflow obstruction: clinical characteristics, sphincter of Oddi manometry findings, and results of therapy. Gastrointest Endosc 1993, 39:778–781.

11. Kalloo AN, Tietjen TG, Pasricha PJ: Does intrabiliary pressure predict basal sphincter of Oddi pressure: a study in patients with and without gallbladders. Gastrointest Endosc 1996, 44:696–699.

12. Funch-Jensen P: Defining sphincter of Oddi dysfunction. Gastrointest Endosc Clin North Am 1995, 6:107–115.

13. Lasson A, Fork FT, Tragardh B, Zedfeldt B: The postcholecystectomy syndrome: bile ducts as pain trigger zone. Scan J Gastroenterol 1988, 23:265–271.

14. Osawa H, Saito M, Fujii M, et al.: Postcholecystectomy syndrome mimicking angina pectoris detected by the morphine provocation test. Intern Med 1995, 34:51–53.

15. Coelho JCU, Weiderkehr JC: Motility of Oddi's sphincter: recent developments and clinical applications. Am J Surg 1996, 172:48–51.

16. Geenen JE, Hogan WJ, Dodds WJ, et al.: The efficacy of endoscopic sphincterotomy in post-cholecystectomy patients with sphincter of Oddi dysfunction. N Engl J Med 1989, 320:82–87.

17. Cooperman M, Ferrara JJ, Carey LC, et al.: Endoscopic retrograde cholangiopancreatography: its use in the evaluation of nonjaundiced patients with the postcholecystectomy syndrome. Arch Surg 1981, 116:606–609.

18. Ponchon T, Aucia N, Mitchell R, et al.: Biopsies of the ampullary region in patients suspected to have sphincter of Oddi dysfunction. Gastrointest Endosc 1995, 42:296–300.

19. Dancygier H, Nattermann C: The role of endoscopic ultrasonography in biliary tract disease, obstructive jaundice. Endoscopy 1994, 26:800–802.

20. Prat F, Amouyal G, Amouyal P, et al.: Prospective controlled study of endoscopic ultrasonography and endoscopic retrograde cholangiography in patients with suspected common bile duct lithiasis. Lancet 1996, 347:75–79.

21. Sugiyama M, Atomi Y: Endoscopic ultrasonography for diagnosing choledocholithiasis: a prospective comparative study with ultrasonography and computed tomography. Gastrointest Endosc 1997, 45:143–146.

22. Tenner SM, Banks PA, Wiersema MJ, Van Dam J: Evaluation of pancreatic disease by endoscopic ultrasonography. Am J Gastroenterol 1997, 92:18–26.

23. Hogan WJ, Geenen JE: Biliary dyskinesia. Endoscopy 1988, 20:179–183.

24. Bjorkman DJ, Carr-Locke DL, Lichtenstein DR, et al.: Postsurgical bile leaks: endoscopic obliteration of the transpapillary pressure gradient is enough. Am J Gastroenterol 1995, 90:2128–2133.

25. Barthel JS, Scheider DM: The advantages of sphincterotomy and nasobiliary tube drainage in the treatment of cystic duct stump leak complicating laparoscopic cholecystectomy. Am J Gastroenterol 1995, 90:1322–1324.

26. Lehman GA, Sherman S, Nisi R, Hawes RH: Pancreas divisum: results of minor papilla sphincterotomy. Gastrointest Endosc 1993, 39:1–8.

124 Acute and Chronic Acalculous Cholecystitis
William R. Brugge

Acalculous cholecystitis is less common than calculous cholecystitis and manifests as a large number of clinical entities, ranging from asymptomatic gallbladder inflammation unassociated with gallstones to life-threatening gallbladder necrosis in acutely ill patients. Its pathophysiology is not well understood, and diagnosis and treatment are based on extensive clinical experience. This chapter reviews acute and chronic acalculous cholecystitis.

PHYSIOLOGY

Normal gallbladder emptying is controlled via hormonal stimulation and cholinergic innervation. The small intestinal hormone cholecystokinin (CCK) is released in response to ingested fat and protein, and is a potent stimulator of gallbladder contraction. Approximately 50% to 80% of gallbladder contents are emptied in response to CCK or eating. Bile empties from the gallbladder through a patent cystic duct and a relaxed sphincter of Oddi.

Cholinergic innervation via the vagus nerve also contributes to normal gallbladder motility, particularly modulating the tone of the gallbladder in the fasting state. Normally, the gallbladder empties and fills several times a day and acts as a reservoir for bile; it preferentially fills by hepatic secretion of bile when the sphincter of Oddi is contracted. The gallbladder takes several hours to fill, although it may empty in 15 to 30 minutes.

■ PATHOPHYSIOLOGY

Three key features are involved in the pathophysiology of acute and chronic cholecystitis: 1) abnormal gallbladder emptying, 2) biliary sludge formation, and 3) infections of the gallbladder mucosa. At some point, at least in the development of necrosis, veno-occlusive ischemia plays a fundamental or adjunctive role.

Abnormal gallbladder emptying is an important factor in the development of both acute and chronic acalculous cholecystitis. Prolonged fasting, particularly in the acutely ill patient, results in stasis of gallbladder contents and often precedes or accompanies the appearance of biliary sludge. Gallbladder stasis also is common in patients receiving high doses of narcotics, anticholinergics, or octreotide. These agents inhibit normal gallbladder emptying by interfering with cholinergic and CCK-mediated gallbladder contraction. Similar effects are seen in patients with diabetic autonomic neuropathy. Obstruction of the biliary system can cause gallbladder stasis, which in turn can result in chronic inflammation of the gallbladder mucosa or wall.

Biliary sludge formation, a key step in the development of acalculous cholecystitis, is a result of both gallbladder stasis and inadequate solubility of cholesterol and bilirubin [1•]. Cholesterol crystals precipitate when relatively large amounts of cholesterol are secreted in bile in comparison with the amount of solubilizing bile salts available to keep them in solution. Obese patients who are on a highly restrictive diet commonly develop biliary cholesterol crystals as a result of gallbladder stasis and excess cholesterol secretion. The presence of cholesterol crystals and other biliary precipitants may cause gallbladder inflammation and further reduce gallbladder emptying.

Infections of the biliary system, either primary or secondary, also can result in gallbladder stasis, abnormal bile, and chole-cystitis. Sepsis often results in gallbladder stasis, and may contribute to bacterial seeding of bile. Infections localized to the biliary system, such as those that occur with clogged or obstructed biliary stents, also can lead to cholecystitis that may not be associated with gallstones. Primary infections of the gallbladder, which are especially common in immunocompromised patients, can lead to acute or chronic cholecystitis. In AIDS patients, cytomegalovirus, *Cryptosporidium*, and Microsporida organisms may cause mucosal infections of the gallbladder. An experimental treatment with interleukin-2 has been reported to cause acute acalculous cholecystitis in patients with AIDS [2].

■ CLINICAL FEATURES

Acalculous cholecystitis may be acute or chronic. Certain pathophysiologic derangements are common to both disease processes, but the clinical features and treatments differ.

Acute Acalculous Cholecystitis

Acute acalculous cholecystitis is commonly seen in very ill patients in intensive care units (ICUs) [3•]. The presentation varies, but most patients have multisystem failure such as that seen after major trauma, surgery, or an acute cardiovascular event [4]. In the comatose patient on a ventilator, abdominal tenderness may be difficult to detect, and the primary presentation may be unexplained fever, abdominal distention, loss of bowel sounds, leukocytosis, or abnormal liver function test results. Other patients may have focal right-upper-quadrant tenderness associated with a palpable mass or may complain of discomfort that is not easily localized. Sometimes gallbladder wall thickening is found incidentally in patients undergoing ultrasonography or computed tomography (CT) scanning for other reasons.

In a small percentage of patients, cholecystitis may be complicated by gangrene or suppuration that can lead to gallbladder perforation or a perihepatic abscess.

Several risk factors are associated with the development of acute acalculous cholecystitis (Table 124-1). Prolonged fasting is the most common, and often is the result of surgery, trauma, or an acute illness. Sepsis, transfusions, total parenteral nutrition (TPN), and chronic narcotic use also are risk factors. Up to 4% of high-risk patients may develop clinically evident acute acalculous cholecystitis, and many others will develop subclinical forms of the disease, such as a sludge-filled gallbladder.

Diagnosis

The diagnosis should be suspected in acutely ill patients with unexplained fever, abdominal tenderness, or even a sudden deterioration in clinical condition. Laboratory testing is usually nonspecific. Eighty-two percent of patients have an elevated leukocyte count and many have a leukocyte count of more than 20,000/mm^3 [3•]. Two thirds of patients have abnormal liver biochemical test results or increased serum amylase levels; however, despite having marked increases in bilirubin and amylase levels, patients may have no evidence of pancreatitis or bile duct obstruction [5].

Many radiographic tests are available for diagnosing acute acalculous cholecystitis, but ultrasonography is most commonly used, as it can be performed easily in an ICU setting (Fig. 124-1). Because laboratory test results and clinical features often are not diagnostic, acalculous cholecystitis is often diagnosed on the basis of ultrasound findings—sludge, hydrops, or gallbladder wall thickening—even though they may not necessarily indicate clinical cholecystitis nor the need for cholecystostomy [6]. An ultrasonographic Murphy's sign may improve the specificity of the ultrasound findings, as sludge or gallbladder wall thickening

Table 124-1. Risk Factors for Acute Acalculous Cholecystitis
Prolonged stay in the intensive care unit
Total parenteral nutrition with fasting
Chronic narcotic use
Sepsis
Gallbladder sludge

is seen in 25% of asymptomatic patients in ICUs. Similar non-specific findings also are seen on CT scanning (Fig. 124-2). Only air in the gallbladder wall, an unusual finding during CT scanning, is diagnostic of cholecystitis; so-called emphysematous cholecystitis is more common in patients with diabetes mellitus, and may be diagnosed by plain radiography of the abdomen.

Cholescintigraphy, which tests cystic duct patency, has been used to diagnose acute acalculous and calculous cholecystitis, but the gallbladder may not fill with radionuclide in 50% of acutely ill patients who do not show evidence of cholecystitis

[7]. Such poor filling probably reflects hyperviscous, sludge-containing bile within the cystic duct. Recently, morphine-augmented cholescintigraphy has been used to reduce the incidence of false-positive scans and improve overall accuracy for predicting cholecystitis [8]. Morphine causes the sphincter of Oddi to contract, thereby improving gallbladder filling.

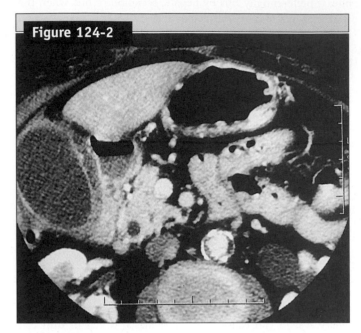

Figure 124-2

Abdominal computed tomography scan of acute acalculous cholecystitis. The distended gallbladder is filled with sludge and the wall is thickened.

Figure 124-1

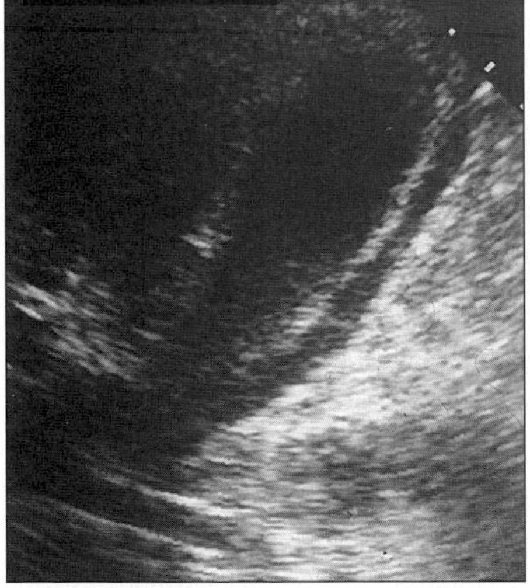

Transabdominal ultrasound image of acute acalculous cholecystitis. Note the thickening of the gallbladder wall with a hypoechoic layer suggesting inflammatory edema.

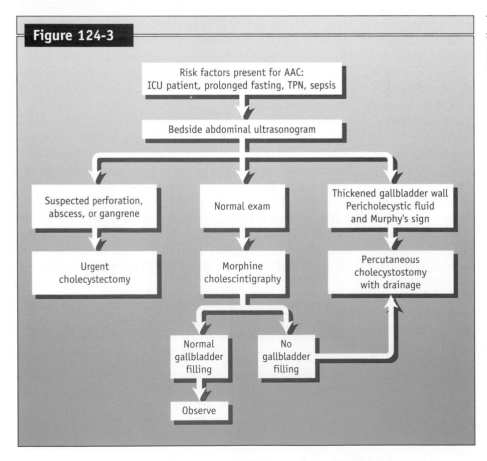

Figure 124-3

Treatment algorithm for patients with suspected acute acalculous cholecystitis (AAC). ICU—intensive care unit; TPN—total parenteral nutrition.

Risk factors present for AAC:
ICU patient, prolonged fasting, TPN, sepsis

Bedside abdominal ultrasonogram

Suspected perforation, abscess, or gangrene

Normal exam

Thickened gallbladder wall
Pericholecystic fluid
and Murphy's sign

Urgent cholecystectomy

Morphine cholescintigraphy

Percutaneous cholecystostomy with drainage

Normal gallbladder filling

No gallbladder filling

Observe

Treatment

The use of ultrasonography to pinpoint the location of the gallbladder and determine its shape, size, contents, and wall thickness also makes it possible to perform ultrasound-guided percutaneous cholecystostomy for acute acalculous cholecystitis in the ICU (Fig. 124-3). The clinical response to cholecystostomy may be dramatic and may determine whether unexplained fever or leukocytosis was the result of cholecystitis [9••]. A bedside approach to cholecystostomy that uses a transhepatic, single-stick trocar technique is often necessary in acutely ill patients [10]. An indwelling 7F to 10F pigtail catheter is used to drain the gallbladder over several days, and the bile can be sent to the laboratory for culture and Gram stain (Fig. 124-4). About 9% of patients treated with percutaneous cholecystostomy have complications, including bile peritonitis, bleeding, and vagal reactions [11•]. Percutaneous cholecystostomy with drainage is highly effective in acute acalculous cholecystitis, and recurrence after catheter removal is unusual [12].

An endoscopic approach to draining the gallbladder also has been described [13]. By means of retrograde cannulation of the bile duct (endoscopic retrograde cholangiopancreatography), a catheter can be placed through the cystic duct and into the gallbladder. The infected bile is drained through a nasobiliary catheter that can be removed easily after the cholecystitis has subsided. Although this technique is more invasive than cholecystostomy, it has the advantage of not requiring transperitoneal needle placement.

Laparoscopy also can be used to diagnose and treat acute acalculous cholecystitis. Reports indicate that only a small number of intubated and sedated patients have undergone diagnostic laparoscopy at the bedside [14], but this technique may be able to differentiate between a normal, an inflamed, and a gangrenous gallbladder [15]. Once cholecystitis has been diagnosed, a laparoscopic cholecystostomy or cholecystectomy can be performed [16]. Another therapeutic maneuver that should not

be forgotten is prophylaxis against the development of acalculous cholecystitis. To maintain a regular emptying schedule for the gallbladder, periodic intravenous administration of CCK has been suggested for patients who cannot take nutrition by mouth.

Pathology

Gross and microscopic examination of resected gallbladder specimens reveal acute inflammation with areas of necrosis and gangrene in more than 50% of patients with acute acalculous cholecystitis [3•]. Ischemic injury caused by vasculitis (especially with periarteritis nodosa) or by cholesterol emboli has been reported. In acute acalculous cholecystitis caused by cytomegalovirus, intranuclear inclusion bodies are seen in epithelial cells [17]; in acalculous cholecystitis caused by Microsporida or *Cryptosporidium*, these protozoa may be seen on or just below the mucosal surface of the gallbladder.

Chronic Acalculous Cholecystitis

The diagnosis of chronic acalculous cholecystitis is controversial in patients with chronic, biliary-like pain in the absence of gallstones (Table 124-2). Occasionally, the presentation also includes recurrent acute pancreatitis, presumably as a result of microlithiasis. A wide range of outpatient tests are used to detect abnormalities in bile and gallbladder function in these persons. Because laboratory test results and clinical features are usually nondiagnostic, chronic acalculous cholecystitis is often diagnosed on the basis of various radiographic procedures or bile analysis (Fig. 124-5).

Diagnosis

Few, if any, detectable structural abnormalities of the gallbladder are seen during ultrasound or CT scanning, but a thorough examination should be performed to exclude microlithiasis and sludge. Sludge in the gallbladder may be readily seen with ultrasonography (Fig. 124-6), and indicates the presence of cholesterol crystals and bilirubinate granules in bile, abnormalities suggestive of chronic cholecystitis. If the gallbladder appears normal on ultrasonography, the next diagnostic step is the use of cholescintigraphy to examine gallbladder motility.

Cholescintigraphy with CCK stimulation is an accepted clinical test of gallbladder emptying used in otherwise healthy outpatients with suspected acalculous cholecystitis. A large number of studies using a variety of doses, routes, and duration of a synthetic CCK octapeptide, (Kinevac; Bristol-Myers Squibb, Princeton, NJ) have documented abnormal gallbladder emptying [18•]. Following a low dose of CCK (0.01 µg/kg over a 3-minute period), an ejection fraction of less than 30%

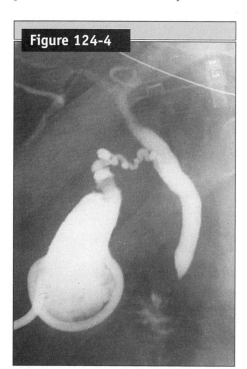

Figure 124-4

Cholecystostomy catheter in a gallbladder. Contrast has been injected, outlining the biliary tree and gallbladder.

Table 124-2. Clinical Features of Chronic Acalculous Cholecystitis
Intermittent upper abdominal pain
Gallbladder wall thickening
Gallbladder sludge
Gallbladder ejection fraction <30%
Abnormal bile analysis (crystals and granules)

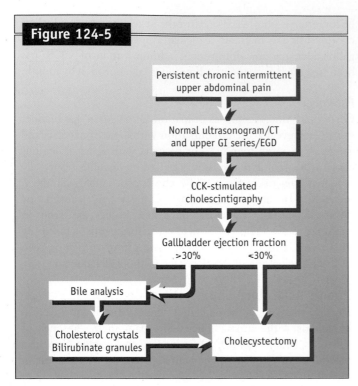

Figure 124-5

Algorithm for management of suspected chronic acalculous cholecystitis. EGD—esophagogastroduodenoscopy.

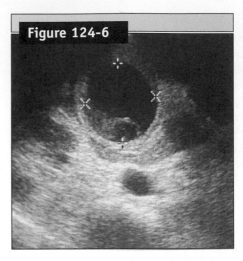

Figure 124-6

Transabdominal ultrasound of a gallbladder filled with sludge. The gallbladder wall has a normal appearance.

predicts that chronic cholecystitis is present and that pain will be relieved by cholecystectomy [19]. High doses of CCK should be avoided, as they may cause gallbladder spasm and actually inhibit gallbladder emptying. Patients with irritable bowel syndrome, or diabetes mellitus, or those who have had a vagotomy, may have abnormal gallbladder motility that interferes with the interpretation of stimulated cholescintigraphy. A large number of medications, including narcotics, calcium channel blockers, and anticholinergics, also may reduce gallbladder emptying and should be avoided during testing. Re-creation of the patient's pain during testing is of no use diagnostically, as CCK may cause painful contractions of the small intestine and colon.

Gallbladder bile stimulated by a CCK infusion can be collected with a duodenal catheter and examined microscopically under high power. So-called B bile is dark green and readily distinguishable from A bile (bile from the common bile duct or duodenum), and C bile (newly secreted hepatic bile). B bile from patients with chronic acalculous cholecystitis may reveal cholesterol crystals and bilirubinate granules [20]. The bile of immunocompromised patients may show evidence of *Cryptosporidium*, Microsporida, or other rare protozoa [21]. Most patients whose bile analysis is abnormal also will have a decrease in gallbladder emptying that is detectable with less invasive testing.

Treatment

Once the patients have been identified, the treatment of chronic acalculous cholecystitis is relatively simple. Laparoscopic cholecystectomy makes it possible to remove the gallbladder with relative ease and safety [22]. Although symptomatic improvement is seen in a majority of patients with abnormal gallbladder emptying, cholecystectomy may aggravate other causes of chronic abdominal pain, such as irritable bowel syndrome [23••].

A small percentage of patients with acalculous cholecystitis and normal gallbladder emptying respond to cholecystectomy. Endoscopic sphincterotomy probably has little value except for the small number of patients with microlithiasis and recurrent pancreatitis. No medical therapies are known to be effective for chronic acalculous cholecystitis.

Pathology

Resected gallbladder specimens from symptomatic patients with abnormal gallbladder emptying are usually histologically abnormal. Most patients have mild mucosal infiltration by lymphocytes and plasma cells; a smaller percentage have adenomyomatosis, cholesterosis, or prominent Rokitansky-Aschoff sinuses.

◼ REFERENCES

Recently published papers of particular interest have been highlighted as follows:
•   Of interest
••   Of outstanding interest

1.•   Janowitz P, Kratzer W, Zemmler T, *et al.*: Gallbladder sludge: spontaneous course and incidence of complications in patients without stones. *Hepatology* 1994, 20:291–294.
This is a retrospective study of the clinical course of patients with gallbladder sludge. The study determined that 71% of patients had resolution of their sludge and 13% had persistent gallstones.

2.   Powell FC, Spooner KM, Shawker TH, *et al.*: Symptomatic interleukin-2-induced cholecystopathy in patients with HIV infection. *AJR Am J Roentgenol* 1994, 163:117–121.

3.•   Schapiro MJ, Luchtefeld WB, Kurzweil S, *et al.*: Acute acalculous cholecystitis in the critically ill. *Am Surg* 1994, 60:335–339.
This is a study of 22 patients with acute acalculous cholecystitis and a description of the results of hepato-iminodiacetic acid (HIDA) scanning, ultrasonography, and computed axial tomography scans. Fifty-nine percent of the patients had gangrenous or a necrotic gallbladder.

4.   Sessions SC, Scoma RS, Sheikh FA, *et al.*: Acute acalculous cholecystitis following open heart surgery. *Am Surg* 1994, 59:74–77.

5.   Kurzweil SM, Shapiro MJ, Andrus CH, *et al.*: Hyperbilirubinemia without common bile duct abnormalities and hyperamylasemia without pancreatitis in patients with gallbladder disease. *Arch Surg* 1994, 129:829–833.

6.   Molenat F, Boussuges A, Valantin V, Sainty JM: Gallbladder abnormalities in medical ICU patients: an ultrasonographic study. *Intensive Care Med* 1996, 22:356–358.

7.   Fig LM, Wahl RL, Stewart RE, *et al.*: Morphine augmented hepatobiliary scintigraphy in the severely ill: caution is in order. *Radiography* 1990, 175:467–473.

8. Flancbaum L, Choban PS, Sinha R, Jonasson O: Morphine cholescintigraphy in the evaluation of hospitalized patients with suspected acute cholecystitis. *Ann Surg* 1994, 220:25–31.

9.•• Boland GW, Lee JM, Leung J, Mueller PR: Percutaneous cholecystostomy in critically ill patients: early response and final outcome in 82 patients. *AJR Am J Roentgenol* 1994, 163:339–342.
Eighty-two patients with sepsis underwent percutaneous cholecystostomy and the clinical course and sonographic abnormalities were determined and reported in this study. Fifty-nine percent of the patients had a response to percutaneous cholecystostomy.

10. Lo LD, Vogelzang RL, Braun MA, Nemcek AA Jr: Percutaneous cholecystostomy for the diagnosis and treatment of acute calculous and acalculous cholecystitis. *J Vasc Interv Radiol* 1995, 6:629–634.

11.• van Sonnenberg E, D'Agostino HB, Goodacre BW, *et al.*: Percutaneous gallbladder puncture and cholecystectomy: results, complications, and caveats for safety. *Radiology* 1992, 183:167–170.
One hundred twenty-seven patients underwent gallbladder puncture and cholecytsostomy. Complications occurred in 8.7%, and the 30-day mortality was 3%.

12. van Overhagen H, Meyers H, Tilanus HW, *et al.*: Percutaneous cholecystectomy for patients with acute cholecystitis and an increased surgical risk. *Cardiovasc Intervent Radiol* 1996, 19:72–76.

13. Johlin FC Jr, Neil GA: Drainage of the gallbladder in patients with acute acalculous cholecystitis by transpapillary endoscopic cholecystectomy. *Gastrointest Endosc* 1993, 39:645–651.

14. Almeida J, Sleeman D, Sosa JL, *et al.*: Acalculous cholecystitis: the use of diagnostic laparoscopy. *Journal of Laparoscopic Surgery* 1995, 5:227–231.

15. Brandt CP, Prelbe PP, Jacobs DG: Value of laparoscopy in trauma ICU patients with suspected acute acalculous cholecystitis. *Surg Endosc* 1994, 8:361–364.

16. Yang HK, Hodgson WJ: Laparoscopic cholecystectomy for acute acalculous cholecystitis. *Surg Endosc* 1996, 10:673–675.

17. Adolph MD, Bass SN, Lee SK, *et al.*: Cytomegaloviral acalculous cholecystitis in acquired immunodeficiency syndrome patients. *Am Surg* 1993, 59:679–684.

18.• Kloiber R, Molnar CP, Shaffer EA: Chronic biliary-type pain in the absence of gallstones: the value of cholecystokinin cholescintigraphy. *AJR Am J Roentgenol* 1992, 159:509–513.
This is a review of the radiographic and clinical aspects of chronic acalculous cholecystitis.

19. Sorenson MK, Fancher S, Lang NP, *et al.*: Abnormal gallbladder nuclear ejection fraction predicts success of cholecystectomy in patients with biliary dyskinesia. *Am J Surg* 1993, 166:672–674.

20. Brugge WR, Brand DL, Atkins HL, *et al.*: Biliary dyskinesia in chronic acalculous cholecystitis. *Dig Dis Sci* 1986, 31:461–467.

21. Wind P, Chevallier JM, Jones D, *et al.*: Cholecystectomy for cholecystitis in patients with acquired immune deficiency syndrome. *Am J Surg* 1994, 168:244–246.

22. Schwesinger WH, Diehl AK: Changing indications for laparoscopic cholecystectomy: stones without symptoms and symptoms without stones. *Surg Clin North Am* 1996, 76:493–504.

23.•• Reed DN, Fernancez M, Hicks RD: Kinevac-assisted cholescintigraphy as an accurate predictor of chronic acalculous gallbladder disease and the likelihood of symptom relief with cholecystectomy. *Am Surg* 1993, 59:273–277.
In this study, thirty patients with chronic abdominal pain and a negative ultrasound underwent CCK-stimulated cholescintigraphy. Ninety percent of the patients with an ejection fraction of less than 35% had symptomatic relief from a cholecystectomy.

125 Pyogenic Cholangitis
Rabia Köksal and Simon K. Lo

Cholangitis is an inflammatory condition of the bile duct caused by an infectious, ischemic, autoimmune, idiopathic, or drug-induced process. Virtually all cholangitic conditions may be complicated by acute pyogenic or suppurative cholangitis. Pyogenic cholangitis was first reported by Charcot in 1877 in patients with right upper quadrant abdominal pain, jaundice, and fever, now known as *Charcot's triad*. In 1959, Reynolds and Dargan [1] added hypotension and mental confusion to characterize a more severe form of the disease. Since death may result within hours of presentation, early recognition and immediate treatment of pyogenic cholangitis are essential [2•].

PATHOGENESIS

Three factors are involved in the development of cholangitis: the presence of bacteria within the bile duct, impedance of bile flow, and local multiplication of bacteria [2•,3•].

The human bile duct is a sterile environment under normal conditions [4]. The biliary tract is isolated from gastrointestinal pathogens by the sphincter of Oddi, which in the resting state is contracted. When stimulated to open, the flow of bile keeps it free from contamination. Once this barrier is disrupted, such as after sphincterotomy or with biliary-enteric reconstructive surgery, enteric organisms are recovered from the bile duct in the majority of cases. Many mechanisms of bacterial entry into the biliary tract have been proposed (Table 125-1) [2•,3•,5], but direct implantation by instrumentation and ascent via the duodenum are the best documented and, perhaps, most common

Table 125-1. Proposed Routes of Bacterial Entry into the Biliary Tract

Ascent via the duodenum

Direct implantation by instrumentation

Portal venous seeding

Extension from the gallbladder

Hepatic secretion

Lymphatic spread

Systemic circulation

[5–7]. Gallstone passage may dilate the sphincter and temporarily render it incompetent. Indwelling biliary stents and percutaneous biliary catheters violate the integrity of the sealed compartment and provide a continuous supply of microorganisms. Also, the instillation of contrast for cholangiography may introduce a sufficient quantity of bacteria to cause cholangitis.

Biliary defense mechanisms against local propagation and the systemic spread of bacteria include tight intercellular junctions, unidirectional bile flow, mucinous coating of bile duct epithelium, bacteriostatic bile salts, and the immunologic defenses of Kupffer's cells and secretory immunoglobulins [5,8]. Therefore, the mere presence of bactibilia usually does not induce clinical cholangitis, as evidenced by the rarity of cholangitis following sphincterotomy; however, bile duct obstruction can impair these defenses by allowing organisms to remain within the ductal system and by raising intraductal pressure, which secondarily reduces biliary secretions and disrupts the epithelial lining. The raised intraductal pressure may render this well-insulated system porous for bacterial spread into the systemic circulation, a phenomenon referred to as *cholangiovenous reflux* [9]. Finally, nutrient-rich bile fluid is a good culture medium to promote bacterial growth and multiplication.

With pyogenic cholangitis, prolonged infection and raised biliary pressure may result in histopathologic changes in the liver and biliary system; however, there is poor correlation between histopathologic alterations and clinical severity of the disease. Periductular neutrophilic infiltration, hepatic lobular microabscesses, fatty liver infiltration, focal necrosis, and portal thrombus are some of the more common findings [10•,11].

■ MICROBIOLOGY

Bile cultures are positive in 80% to 100% of patients with cholangitis; however, blood cultures are positive only in a minority of cases and usually are positive just for aerobes. Most microorganisms involved in acute pyogenic cholangitis are aerobes derived from the gut flora (Table 125-2) [2•, 3•,12•,13••,14–18]. *Escherichia coli* is involved in roughly half of cases, followed by *Klebsiella*. Thirty percent to 88% of cholangitis cases are caused by polymicrobial infection, which may include anaerobic organisms, most commonly, *Bacteroides*. Anaerobes tend to be isolated from patients with severed disease, especially the elderly, and in iatrogenic settings. *Pseudomonas* infection has been linked to rare outbreaks of biliary sepsis following endoscopic biliary instrumentation because of inadequate equipment disinfection [19,20]. *Serratia marcescens* also has been linked to

Table 125-2. Common Biliary Pathogens

Aerobes	Anaerobes
E. coli (35%–60%)	Bacteroides (2.5%)
Klebsiella (14%–40%)	Clostridium (1.5%)
Enterococcus (8%–16%)	Fungal Candida <4%
Proteus (4.5%–12%)	
Pseudomonas (5%–9%)	
Streptococcus 8%	
Enterobacter 8%	

post-endoscopic retrograde cholangiopancreatography (ERCP) infections [21]. Endoscopic equipment should be inspected if recurrent episodes of post-ERCP *Pseudomonas* infection have taken place. *Candida albicans* is the most common fungal cause of cholangitis, and present as an isolated biliary infection or as part of a systemic disease. It also may complicate or lead to pyogenic cholangitis. Predisposing conditions for fungal infection include systemic antibiotic treatment, malignancy, immunosuppression, and diabetes. Multiple irregular ductal masses or fungal balls seen on cholangiography or sonography are typical [22,23]. Actinomycosis may produce biliary fistulae and strictures (authors' personal observation).

■ CAUSE

Choledocholithiasis is the most common cause of acute pyogenic cholangitis in the western world, and accounts for 80% of such cases (Table 125-3) [15,24]. Factors that promote infection in choledocholithiasis are old age, prolonged illness, previous biliary surgery, immunosuppression, and bile duct obstruction [25]. The second most common cause of cholangitis is biliary stricture, usually a result of long-standing choledocholithiasis, chronic pancreatitis, papillary stenosis, malignancy, or bile duct injury.

A foreign body within the bile duct (*eg*, endoprostheses, surgical sutures, parasites, gallstones) may cause obstruction or serve as a nidus for the formation of gallstones. In the case of bile duct stents that traverse the biliary sphincter, bacterial colonization virtually is always present, but the risk of cholangitis is low until stent occlusion has taken place [26].

■ CLINICAL MANIFESTATIONS

The clinical presentation of cholangitis can vary substantially from vague abdominal symptoms or fever of unknown origin to a florid picture with Reynold's pentad and death. The mean age of patients is 50 to 60 years old. Both genders are equally affected.

Charcot's triad of right upper abdominal pain, fever and jaundice is present in 50% to 70% of patients, but certainly is not specific for cholangitis (Table 125-4). Fever is the most common presenting symptom and is seen in more than 90% of cases [2•,3•,15]. Chills or rigor, which suggests intermittent bacteremia, is experienced by two thirds of patients [2•]; jaundice is absent in one third of the cases. Abdominal pain often is present, but is usually mild and may not be localized to the right upper quadrant. Nonetheless, cholangitis occasionally presents with severe pain and should be considered in the differential diagnosis of an acute abdomen. Nausea and vomiting are nonspecific but common symptoms. Mental confusion and hypotension denote a particularly morbid form of the illness, and, fortunately, are seen in only a minority of the cases.

Physical findings of cholangitis are also variable. Abdominal tenderness, usually mild relative to the patient's complaint, is detected in two thirds of the cases. Disproportionately mild tenderness is an important clue to a bile duct process. Peritoneal signs are rare and should raise the suspicion of another diagnosis, such as perforated viscus, pancreatitis, or acute cholecystitis. A Murphy's sign (inspiratory arrest of the diaphragm) points to a gallbladder condition. Mirizzi's syndrome, causing concomitant cholecystitis and cholangitis or biliary obstruction, should be considered when Murphy's sign and significant jaundice coexist.

COMPLICATIONS

Cholangitis can spread rapidly to involve the portal and systemic circulations. If infection progresses to exhibit Reynold's pentad, morbidity and mortality will be very high (Table 125-5). Disseminated intravascular coagulopathy (DIC) and respiratory failure may develop in severe disease. Multifocal microabscesses or a large solitary liver abscess may be found, depending on the biliary anatomy and site of obstruction. Cholecystitis or pancreatitis may be complicated by cholangitis or caused by the same underlying process, further confusing and complicating diagnosis and management decisions. Residual strictures and secondary sclerosing cholangitis may result even after successful treatment of cholangitis. Severe biliary infection may lead to pyelophlebitis and portal vein thrombosis. Finally, recurrent, low-grade cholangitis may cause chronic epithelial inflammation and, ultimately, cholangiocarcinoma. Gigot and coworkers [27•] performed multivariate analysis to identify seven factors with independent significance of predicting mortality: (1) acute renal failure, (2) associated liver abscess, (3) high malignant biliary stricture, (4) liver cirrhosis, (5) radiologic evidence of cholangitis, (6) female gender, and (7) age over 50 years old.

LABORATORY FINDINGS

The most common laboratory finding is an elevated white cell count with a shift to the left. As in other infectious conditions, leukopenia and pancytopenia may be seen in patients who are severely ill and septic. Most patients have one or more abnormal liver tests. Depending on the duration and degree of underlying biliary obstruction, liver enzyme elevations can either reflect a cholestatic process or an acute hepatocellular condition. Cholangitis complicating a malignant biliary obstruction typically produces a cholestatic pattern. When biliary pressure suddenly increases, as with an acute gallstone impaction, the aminotransferases transiently dominate the liver profile.

Table 125-3. Causes of Pyogenic Cholangitis and Common Sites of Bile Duct Involvement

Etiology	Lesion location
Choledocholithiasis	Common ducts
Neoplastic biliary strictures	
Pancreatic cancer	Common bile duct
Cholangiocarcinoma	Any ducts
Metastatic cancer	Common hepatic duct
Papillary adenomatosis	Any ducts
Ampullary carcinoma	Papilla
Hepatocellular carcinoma	Intrahepatic ducts, main hepatic ducts
Gallbladder cancer	Common hepatic duct
Simple benign biliary strictures	
Congenital	Any ducts
Postoperative	Common hepatic duct, anastomosis
Ischemic	Surgery site
Chronic pancreatitis	Common bile duct
Papillary stenosis	Papilla
Multifocal benign strictures	
Primary sclerosing cholangitis	Any ducts
Hepatic arterial chemoinfusion	Common hepatic and intrahepatic ducts
AIDS cholangiopathy	Any ducts, papilla
Recurrent pyogenic cholangitis	Intrahepatic ducts, papilla
Foreign bodies	
Parasites	Any ducts
Surgical sutures	Common ducts
Stents	Common ducts
Sump syndrome	Distal common bile duct, common hepatic ducts
Nonobstructive biliary stasis	
Choledochal cyst	Any large ducts
Juxta-ampullary diverticulum	Duodenum
Mucin plugs	
Papillary adenomatosis, AIDS cholangiopathy, mucin-producing cancer	Any large ducts
Blood clots	
Transhepatic punctures, sphincterotomy, postoperative bleeding, hepatocellular carcinoma, cholangiocarcinoma, biliary stent, trauma	Any large ducts
Iatrogenic causes	
ERCP contamination	Any ducts
Clogged biliary stent	Any large duct
Transhepatic catheterization, TIPS, liver biopsy	Along the catheter tract

Table 125-4. Differential Diagnoses of Right Upper-Quadrant Pain, Fever, and Jaundice

Acute cholangitis

Viral hepatitis

Alcoholic hepatitis

Liver abscess

Severe nonbiliary abdominal infection

Complicated acute cholecystitis

Infected bile leak

Acute pancreatitis with bile duct obstruction

Cirrhosis with concomitant abdominal infection

Table 125-5. Common Complications of Pyogenic Cholangitis

Local	Systemic
Liver abscess (solitary or multiple)	Disseminated intravascular coagulopathy
Secondary sclerosing cholangitis/strictures	Acute renal failure
	Respiratory failure
Cholangiocarcinoma	Sepsis/septic shock
Portal vein thrombosis/ pylephlebitis	Mental obtundation
Cholecystitis	
Pancreatitis	

Irrespective of the serum enzyme pattern, hyperbilirubinemia is reported in 88% to 100% and alkaline phosphatase elevation is observed in 80% of the cases [3•]. Interestingly, the increase in bilirubin or alkaline phosphatase may lag behind the clinical symptoms by one or more days [2•,3•]. Although the vast majority of patients with cholangitis have some abnormalities in liver enzymes, normal results do not exclude the diagnosis [13]. Conversely, liver enzyme abnormalities are seen in many febrile conditions and are not specific for a biliary process.

Mild hyperamylasemia may occur in up to 40% of patients with cholangitis and does not necessarily imply concomitant acute pancreatitis. The tumor marker, CA19-9, has been found to be elevated in acute cholangitis and renormalize after successful therapy [28]. Prolongation of the prothrombin time is difficult to interpret, as it may be the result of biliary cirrhosis, depletion of fat-soluble vitamins due to long-standing biliary obstruction, or DIC from the cholangitis; normalization of this test within 24 to 48 hours following vitamin K administration implies biliary tract obstruction as its cause.

◼ IMAGING STUDIES

The diagnosis of cholangitis is generally made at the bedside. Because the only means to confirm the diagnosis is by discovering infected bile or obtaining cholangiographic evidence of the disease process, performing additional noninvasive studies often is of limited clinical value; however, ultrasound or computed tomography (CT) scan is important in patients with subtle complaints or equivocal findings, as it may occasionally identify a bile duct stone or an unrelated source of symptoms. Plain abdominal films are abnormal in 15% of patients and may show ileus, radio-opaque gallstones, biliary endoprostheses, or pneumobilia.

When cholangitis is supected, ultrasonography (US) usually is employed as the first imaging test to exclude cholecystitis and document cholelithiasis, choledocholithiasis, or bile duct dilation. Its accuracy in differentiating extrahepatic obstruction from intrahepatic cholestasis reaches 96%; however, US is highly operator dependent and is insensitive (<50%) in confirming choledocholithiasis [15,18,29]. Thus, it is a general practice to assume the presence of a bile duct stone when sonography reveals a dilated bile duct and gallstones inside the gallbladder. Recently, the sonographic finding of bile duct wall thickening has been suggested as a strong indicator of acute cholangitis. Lack of bile duct filling defect and ductal dilation does not exclude the diagnosis of cholangitis [30]. Despite its limitations in the evaluation of bile duct stones, ultrasonic imaging is a low-cost test that carries virtually no risk to the patients. Its portability and wide availability are particularly suitable to investigate a critically ill patient with possible cholangitis.

Computed tomography may be valuable in defining the level and cause of biliary obstruction, and is particularly useful when neoplasia is suspected. In one study, CT was shown to confirm the clinical diagnosis of acute cholangitis in 87% [31]. Overall, CT is only slightly more sensitive than US in diagnosing choledocholithiasis. Like US, an unremarkable CT examination does not rule out cholangitis or choledocholithiasis.

The role of nuclear scintigraphy is not well defined and is of limited clinical use in this setting. It is sometimes helpful in differentiating atypical acute cholecystitis from cholangitis; a nonvisualization of the duodenum in delayed scanning suggests a very-high-grade biliary obstruction. In febrile patients immediately following cholecystectomy, biliary scintigraphy is quite useful in diagnosing bile leaks [18]. Like most radionuclide studies, biliary scintigraphy produces inadequate anatomic details of the biliary tract and cannot be relied upon to diagnose choledocholithiasis or incomplete biliary obstruction.

Three relatively new imaging technologies are available on a limited basis for diagnosing biliary tract disorders. With special computer software, MR imaging and MR cholangiopancreatography (MRCP) is capable of producing detailed images of the gallbladder, bile, and pancreatic ducts. MRCP may replace ultrasound and diagnostic ERCP in the future. Using a similar approach with special computer software, CT cholangiography may achieve equivalent results.

Endoscopic US (EUS) is more invasive than MRCP and CT cholangiography and as safe as a diagnostic upper endoscopy. EUS combines the features of a flexible endoscope and an echoprobe at the tip of the scope. Thus, it is possible to scan the bile duct, gallbladder and pancreas and avoid the interference of bowel gas. Images of the bile duct can be obtained in great detail. Like MRCP, the surrounding structures are readily visualized with EUS. Its exact role in managing cholangitis is questionable at present.

Direct cholangiography is the diagnostic gold standard for cholangitis. It may be performed endoscopically (ERCP), percutaneously (transhepatic cholangiography [PTC]), or operatively (intraoperative cholangiography [IOC]). Besides identifying the anatomy of the bile ducts, cholangiography also allows retrieval of bile fluid, which consists of pus or contains microorganisms in virtually all cases of cholangitis. With each modality carrying the potential for significant iatrogenic complications, these tests should be performed only if there is a high index of suspicion of the diagnosis or when more likely sources of sepsis have been excluded. The risks of these diagnostic tests may be justifiable because of the possibility of providing therapy in the same setting as diagnosis. From a purely diagnostic standpoint, the choice of ERCP or PTC is a matter of anatomic considerations and availability of trained physicians; however, bleeding potential, patient discomfort, risk of leakage of infected bile, and a high rate of failure in nondilated bile duct favor the use of ERCP over PTC. IOC is generally not done in an acute setting because it is preferable to defer surgery unless the other options are not available or applicable.

◼ TREATMENT
Medical Management

Management of cholangitis begins with early recognition of the condition; therapy must be initiated once a presumptive diagnosis of cholangitis is made. Roughly 80% of patients respond to appropriate medical supportive treatment, with resolution of fever and pain; however, medical therapy is useful only in controlling the infection and stabilizing the patient [32,15]. The underlying pathology tends to persist and requires further cholangiographic investigations and definitive treatment.

Medical management consists of hydration with intravenous fluids, cessation of oral intake, and initiation of broad-spectrum antibiotics once blood cultures have been obtained. Patients who are seriously ill, very old, or frail should be monitored in an intensive care setting. Maintenance of euvolemia is of critical importance in ensuring adequate perfusion of vital organs. In the event that an emergency ERCP or surgery is needed, inadequate hydration predisposes to vascular collapse and other serious complications during the procedure. Mild to moderate coagulopathy occurs commonly in acute cholangitis and should be treated with vitamin K and perhaps fresh frozen plasma. If the prothrombin time does not respond to vitamin K administration, DIC or liver failure should be suspected.

The choice of antibiotics is dependent on their spectrum of antimicrobial activity and hepatobiliary penetration. In general, a single agent or combination of antibiotics with a broad spectrum of activities but particularly strong action against the enteric gram-negative rods should be used (Table 125-6) [7,13••,29,33]. Many antibiotics have been shown to be excreted in high concentrations into the biliary tract (Table 125-7). Unfortunately, cholangitis always is associated with biliary stasis which raises biliary ductal pressure and impairs biliary excretion of antibiotics [7,34,35]. This is the main reason why antibiotic therapy alone is often inadequate in treating this condition. Biliary penetrability is of less significance in patients who have already exhibited signs of septicemia; gentamicin, for instance, is as effective in controlling biliary sepsis as antibiotics with enhanced biliary penetration [36•]. The antibiotic regimen should be continued for 7 to 14 days, depending on the patient's response [29,33]; intravenous formulations can be switched to oral preparations once clinical resolution has been attained. Coverage for anaerobes and enterococcus also is important in patients who are severely ill, very

elderly, or with a prior history of biliary tract manipulation (Table 125-8) [13••,14].

Regardless of the severity at presentation, cholangitis demands close patient observation within the first 24 hours of management [14,18,29]. If available, a biliary interventional team should be on alert. Hypotension or toxic delirium calls for an emergency ERCP. Likewise, all nonresponders to initial medical management will need early endoscopic intervention. Failure of conservative measures is somewhat arbitrarily defined as fever, disabling pain, worsening leukocytosis, or rising liver enzymes for more than 24 to 36 hours [37]. Advanced age, comorbid illnesses, neoplastic biliary strictures, renal insufficiency, hypoalbuminemia, thrombocytopenia, or severe hyperbilirubinemia at the time of presentation are contributing factors to such failures [38,39].

Endoscopic Management

There had been numerous reports of successful endoscopic therapy of acute pyogenic cholangitis before the landmark study performed at Hong Kong University [32,38,40]. Investigators in that study randomly assigned patients with severe cholangitis

Table 125-6. Empiric Antibiotic Regimens Commonly Employed for Cholangitis

Ampicillin + aminoglycoside
Ureidopenicillin + aminoglycoside
Second-generation cephalosporin + aminoglycoside
Ciprofloxacin
Ciprofloxacin + ampicillin-sulbactam
Ciprofloxacin + ampicillin + metronidazole

Table 125-7. Biliary Secretion of Some Commonly Used Antibiotics

	Normal LT	Obstructed System	Obstruction relieved
Ampicillin	+++	None	NA
Mezlocillin	+++	None	NA
Cefoperazone	+++	None	+
Ceftazidime	+	None	+
Gentamicin	++	None	NA
Netilmicin	+	None	+
Imipenem	+	None	+
Ciprofloxacin	+++	++	+++
Metronidazole	+++	None	NA

LT = Liver tests; NA = not applicable; +++ = bile/serum>1; ++ = bile/serum~1; + = bile/serum<1

Table 125-8. In Vitro Susceptibilities to Commonly Used Antibiotics of Biliary Pathogens

	E. coli	Klebsiella	Enterococcus	Proteus	P. aeruginosa	Aerobic gram-negative bacteria
Ampicillin	-	-	++	-	-	-
Cefoperazone	++	+++	-	+++	-	-
Ceftazidime	+++	+++	-	+++	-	-
Netilmicin	++	+++	-	+++	++	++
Ciprofloxacin	+++	+++	++	+++	+++	+++

+++ = excellent activity (MIC90<2 mg/dL); ++ = good activity (MIC90 =2–8 mg/dL); + = fair activity (MIC90 =8–16 mg/dL); – = almost no activity (MIC90>16 mg/dL)

to receive emergency endoscopic or surgical drainage procedures. The morbidity and mortality rates were high in both groups because of the nature of this serious illness; however, only 10% of endoscopically treated patients died whereas the mortality rate was three times greater for the surgical treatment group. Additionally, morbidity was less in the endoscopic arm of the study. Today, ERCP is firmly established as the treatment of choice for cholangitis that has failed empiric medical therapy.

Endoscopic management begins with aggressive fluid resuscitation and good control of the airway. Patients should be sufficiently stabilized to undergo ERCP without serious concerns for their safety during the procedure. Extreme care must be exercised in patient sedation, as hypotension and respiratory failure may ensue precipitously, even with tiny doses of medications.

Endoscopic retrograde cholangiopancreatography may start with bile fluid collection for bacteriologic studies, accomplished with gentle aspiration of an empty cannula that has been inserted into the bile duct via the ampulla of Vater. Enteric contamination of the collected bile fluid is a genuine concern with regard to validity of its culture; however, clinical experience shows this to be a reliable way of sampling for Gram stain and culture. A diagnostic cholangiogram is performed to identify the cause of cholangitis. The ultimate goal is to establish patency of an obstructed bile duct, which can be achieved definitively by extracting a bile duct stone or temporarily by placing a biliary drainage catheter (Fig. 125-1). The advantages of a nasobiliary drainage include rapid placement, easy catheter removal, and continuous external access of the bile duct [32,37,41]. Following drain placement, biliary irrigation, bile fluid collection, cholangiographic imaging, and instillation of a biliary dissolution solvent can be done; however, a nasobiliary drain is a small-caliber catheter that may occlude, kink, or dislodge. Alternatively, a short and wider indwelling endoprosthesis can be placed and provides the security of a stable means of internal drainage [14]. Its disadvantages are the tendency to be clogged by thick pus because of the lack of access for irrigation and the requirement for a subsequent ERCP for stent removal. Whenever possible, eliminating the source of biliary obstruction is the most thorough form of therapy for cholangitis, but rapid decompression of the biliary tract with a nasobiliary catheter is the choice of treatment in patients who are moribund or have severe coagulopathy [29,32].

More than 80% of cholangitis is caused by gallstone retention within the bile duct, and definitive treatment usually involves the performance of endoscopic sphincterotomy to widen the biliary sphincter for stone extraction. In recent years, endoscopic sphincteroplasty carried out by balloon dilation has gained popularity in situations where bleeding or perforation is a serious concern [6]; however, balloon sphincteroplasty followed by stone extraction could be time consuming and should be avoided when treating acute suppurative cholangitis. Once a very difficult endoscopic procedure, sphincterotomy and stone extraction are considered routine by many community endoscopists. A greater than 95% rate of stone clearance is reported by most major biliary centers; however, this high rate of success may require precutting, mechanical lithotripsy, peroral choledochoscopy, endoscopic electrohydraulic lithotripsy (EHL), and extracorporeal shockwave lithotripsy (ESWL) [6]. As expected, the complication rate varies greatly according to the procedural difficulty and the endoscopist's clinical judgment and ERCP skill. The generally quoted morbidity and mortality rate is 7% to 10% and 0.1% to 0.5%, respectively, for therapeutic ERCP cases in a nonemergent setting, and performed by an experienced biliary endoscopist. The most common complication is pancreatitis, followed by bleeding, perforation, and aggravation of gallstone impaction [42]. Despite these considerations, endoscopy is still the safest procedure in treating retained bile duct stones.

Percutaneous Transhepatic Cholangiographic Drainage

Transhepatic access to the biliary tree is done under local anesthesia with a fine needle. Performed blindly or guided by ultrasound, multiple passes toward the liver hilum or a dilated duct are made until opacification of the biliary tract is achieved. The procedure is successful in identifying a dilated bile duct in greater than 90% of cases [2•,18,29]. The success rate falls to 60% when nondilated ducts are encountered. Because about 30% of the bile ducts that contain gallstones are nondilated, the use of percutaneous transhepatic cholangiographic (PTC)-mediated biliary drainage may be restricted. Major complications are catheter-related sepsis, which occurs frequently with prolonged drainage or additional catheter manipulations [43]. Bleeding occurs in 15% of the cases. Other potential complications are bile leak, biliary-vascular fistula, pneumothorax, and hemothorax [3•,15,18,44]. Patients with cirrhosis, coagulopathy, or ascites are particularly prone to adverse events. It is always of concern that PTC might lead to septic bile peritonitis when puncturing an infected bile duct under high pressure. Even if the duct has been drained safely, catheter-induced discomfort frequently is a complaint. The overall reported complication rate related to PTC-guided external biliary drainage is 30% to 80%, with a mortality rate of 5% to

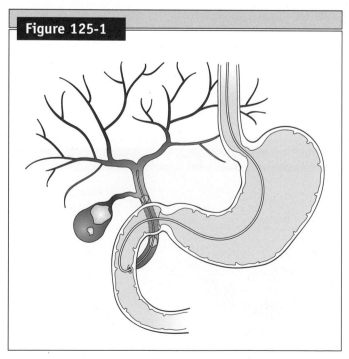

Figure 125-1

Schematic drawing of a nasobiliary drainage catheter.

17% [15,18]. Similar to endoscopic placement of biliary drains, this procedure provides only temporary relief. Definitive therapy is almost always needed.

Surgical Treatment

Long held as the treatment of choice for pyogenic cholangitis, urgent surgical exploration for ductal decompression is rarely done. Rather, bile duct exploration and biliary bypass procedures are reserved for definitive therapy of the underlying processes following the resolution of cholangitis. The major indication for an emergency operation is failure of biliary decompression by nonsurgical attempts. Surgical options are open choledochotomy, intraoperative choledochoscopy, surgical sphincteroplasty, T-tube placement, bile duct resection, or bypass. Whereas endoscopic therapy is superior to surgery in an acute setting, PTC-assisted external biliary drainage has not been carefully studied to compare its efficacy against surgery. Many institutions prefer a surgical approach once an endoscopic attempt has failed to bring about relief of cholangitis. Reported operative morbidity and mortality in emergency surgery for cholangitis is 7% to 40% and 17% to 60%, respectively [14,15,18,38]. If patients are able to undergo an elective operation, the operative mortality rate falls to only 2% to 3% [45].

▆▆ OTHER CONDITIONS PREDISPOSING TO CHOLANGITIS

The discussion so far has been focused on pyogenic cholangitis due to extrahepatic bile duct stone disease. Other causal factors exist and deserve to be considered separately. Although the general evaluation and therapeutic principles are applicable to both calculous and noncalculous conditions, there are some important distinguishing features that may influence management decisions.

Acquired Immunodeficiency Syndrome Cholangiopathy

Cholangiopathy generally takes place late in the course of illness and long after the patient has manifested the AIDS-defining complex (see Chapter 111). Cytomegalovirus, cryptosporidium, microsporidium, and *Mycobacterium avium* are the infections most commonly associated, although polymicrobial infection also has been described [10•]. Four morphologic forms of AIDS-related cholangiopathy have been described: (1) papillary stenosis, (2) sclerosing cholangitis, (3) long extrahepatic bile duct strictures, and (4) combined pathology of the bile duct and papilla. Pathologic examination of the biliary tract may reveal ductal dilatation, wall thickening, ulceration, edema, and nodular irregularities of its mucosal surface. The cholangiographic findings simulate, but are frequently distinguishable from, those of primary sclerosing cholangitis (PSC) (Fig. 125-2).

Approximately half of the patients with papillary stenosis may benefit from endoscopic sphincterotomy [46]. Biliary dilations and stenting can be performed for ductal obstruction. Recurrence of symptoms is common and repeated endoscopic therapy may be necessary. Because the prognosis of patients with AIDS-related cholangiopathy is poor because of significant underlying disease, endoscopic treatment should only be considered palliative.

Recurrent Pyogenic Cholangitis

Recurrent pyogenic cholangitis (RPC), also referred to as *oriental cholangiohepatitis* and *intrahepatic pigment stone disease*, is a syndrome characterized by bile duct strictures, intrahepatic duct stones, and recurrent low-grade biliary infections. The peculiar intrahepatic ductal appearance and numerous hepatic duct stones are pathognomonic of the disease in its classic form (Fig. 125-2). It is most prevalent in Southeast Asia and has been reported from India, Mexico, Central and South America, South Africa, and Italy [47–49].

Symptoms of recurrent pyogenic cholangitis may begin early in life, but the disease usually presents after the third or fourth

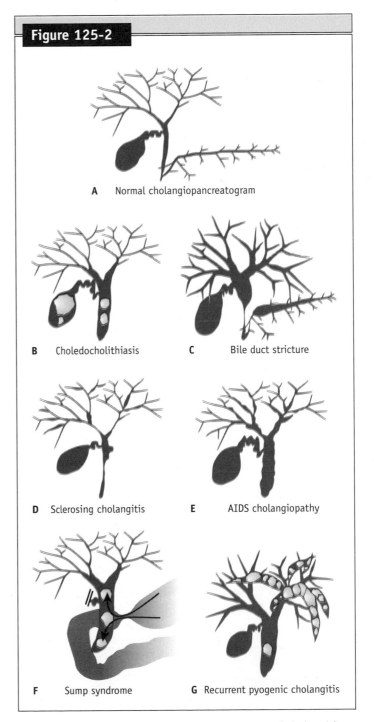

Figure 125-2

A   Normal cholangiopancreatogram

B   Choledocholithiasis

C   Bile duct stricture

D   Sclerosing cholangitis

E   AIDS cholangiopathy

F   Sump syndrome

G   Recurrent pyogenic cholangitis

Schematic cholangiograms of some common causes of cholangitis.

decade; it affects men and women equally. RPC may evolve because of chronic parasitic infestation of the bile duct leading to duct damage and strictures, bile stasis, and secondary bile duct stone formation (Fig. 125-3). *Clonorchis sinensis*, *Ascaris lumbricoides*, and *Fasciola hepaticas* may be recovered from the stool or bile fluid in 5% to 25% of patients. The same parasites or their fragments have been isolated in the core of brown pigment stones removed from these patients. A second potential cause for RPC is related to malnutrition, with frequent gastroenteritis and bacteremia. Poor protein intake also results in low production of glucaric acid, a beta-glucuronidase inhibitor, and increased susceptibility to infections of beta-glucuronidase-producing bacteria, such as *E. coli* [2•,3•,48–50].

Patients with RPC usually present with signs, symptoms and subtle laboratory findings of low-grade biliary obstruction or mild pyogenic cholangitis. Past history of fecal passage of worms is common. Physical findings are usually unremarkable, but many patients have undergone previous cholecystectomy because of clinical suspicion of gallbladder disease. Occasionally a patient may present with fever of unknown origin without biochemical or physical findings referable to the biliary tract. The gallbladder may be palpated in about one third of the patients [49].

Recurrent pyogenic cholangitis is suspected on the basis of clinical history and patient background. The diagnosis is best made on cholangiography; however, sonographic or CT findings of hepaticolithiasis and intrahepatic ductal dilation imply the diagnosis unless proven otherwise. Pooled data from the literature show a high incidence of concomitant common duct and intrahepatic duct stones [6]. Approximately 90% of the cases involve stones in the left hepatic system, which usually contains multiple high-grade stenoses located at the points of second-order ductal branching. The right hepatic system contains stones and strictures in only half of the cases. The major papilla may be hypertrophic and fibrotic, but usually is patent; sphincter of Oddi manometry suggests dysfunction of the biliary orifice in about half of these individuals [2•,3•,49,51]. In advanced and long-standing disease, the entire hepatic lobe becomes atrophic and is replaced by a huge number of small- to medium-sized brown pigment stones; however,

progression to cirrhosis is rare in this disease because it usually is localized to the left lobe of the liver [52].

The gallstones involved in RPC are constituted predominantly of calcium bilirubinate. They are typically brown, soft, and friable. As opposed to choledocholithiasis due to cholesterol or black pigment stones that originate from the gallbladder, these stones are formed de novo within the bile duct through bacterial conversion of bilirubin pigments. There often is biliary "mud" without discrete stones.

All patients suspected of RPC should undergo a CT scan of the liver, followed by cholangiography. CT provides a global picture of hepatic ductal involvement whereas cholangiography confirms the diagnosis and identifies locations of ductal strictures. Whereas cholangiographic details are comparable between the PTC and ERCP routes, ERCP is preferred because of the frequent finding of common duct stones. Because of the locations and high degree of ductal strictures, it may not be possible to opacify obstructed branches. As a result, the cholangiograms of these patients are frequently reported as normal or showing nonspecific abnormalities. A careful balloon occlusion cholangiographic study is usually needed to obtain the desired anatomic details.

Recurrent pyogenic cholangitis may be complicated by portal vein thrombosis, pancreatitis, gallbladder perforation, biliary-enteric fistula, and gram-negative sepsis [29,48,49,53]. Liver abscesses are particularly common, occurring in about 20% of the cases [48]. Cholangiocarcinoma has been observed in about 5% of RPC patients, prompting some authors to recommend careful evaluations for cholangiocarcinoma in patients who are older than 50 years of age [49,53]. Perhaps the most common and serious complications of RPC are iatrogenic. Endoscopic, transhepatic, or surgical biliary manipulations may introduce bacterial contaminants to the obstructed bile ducts and lead to cholangitis and abscess formation. Surgical mortality for RPC is 8%, mostly resulting from postoperative infection [6]. For this reason, careful planning and antibiotic prophylaxis prior to all invasive biliary procedures are mandatory.

The natural history of this disease is chronic progression. During the acute presentation of cholangitis, endoscopic biliary decompression should be carried out. Surgical resection of the liver segment that contains all the involved bile ducts constitutes definitive therapy; however, very-low lying or multisegmental disease cannot be cured by a simple lobectomy or segmentectomy. In such cases, surgical resection is best supplemented by percutaneous or endoscopic bile duct dilation and stone removal [48]. Information essential to this decision is obtained preoperatively by combining the findings on CT and ERCP. Cutaneous access of the bile duct for repetitive endoscopic treatment may be created in the form of an indwelling transhepatic catheter, a T-tube tract, or hepaticojejunostomy that connects to a subcutaneous or cutaneous stoma. Recent reports suggest that transhepatic choledochoscopic stricture and stone treatment is highly effective [6].

Biliary Strictures

Most benign biliary strictures are secondary to operative trauma. Other common causes include bile duct stones, extrinsic compression, ischemia, and primary sclerosing cholangitis. The most common neoplastic stricture in the distal bile duct is caused

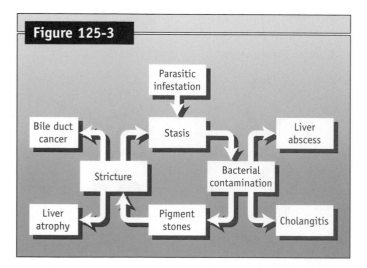

Figure 125-3

Pathogenesis and complications of recurrent pyogenic cholangitis.

by pancreatic cancer, whereas malignant hilar obstruction may result from metastasis or cancer of the gallbladder, bile duct, or the liver. Spontaneous occurrence of cholangitis complicating a biliary stricture is rare. Once the obstructed compartment has been contaminated, however, the incidence of cholangitis increases significantly. For instance, 21% of patients with malignant biliary obstruction undergoing ERCP develop septicemia [36•]. Therefore, it is recommended that prophylactic antibiotics be given prior to any endoscopic procedure of an obstructed bile duct.

Cholangitis in the setting of choledocholithiasis proximal to a biliary stricture poses a particularly challenging situation to the managing physicians. Following acute biliary decompression to relieve cholangitis, a biliary bypass procedure may be necessary to obtain an effective and lasting result. Stone fragmentation and extraction, followed by stricture stenting for 1 year, has resulted in very good and lasting responses. For recurrent strictures, surgical revisions should take into consideration future recurrences. When the surgeon transects the bile duct and constructs a long Roux-en-Y choledochojejunostomy, it becomes extremely difficult to study endoscopically.

Foreign Bodies

Foreign bodies, including surgical sutures, parasites, endoprostheses, and refluxed duodenal contents, may directly impede bile flow and become the nidus for gallstone formation within the bile duct. The sump syndrome is an interesting entity that involves entry of duodenal matter into the bile duct through the choledochoduodenal stoma. These materials then get impacted on the supra-ampullary portion of the bile duct or encourage the formation of bile duct stones, resulting in extensive choledocholithiasis, pancreatitis, and ascending cholangitis. The sump syndrome occurs in 0.14% to 1.3% of choledochoduodenostomy treated patients.

When dealing with cholangitis that is precipitated by foreign bodies, therapy must remove the foreign body and also treat the underlying pathology. In the case of the sump syndrome, a large endoscopic sphincterotomy to reduce retention of debris above the ampulla is generally therapeutic. Because endoscopic stenting of malignant biliary strictures has been accepted as a standard palliative modality, cholangitis due to stent clogging has become a regular occurrence. Failure to exchange an occluded indwelling stent invariably leads to cholangitis, even if antibiotics have been initiated. There is laboratory evidence that a bacterial colonized biofilm within a stent lumen promotes its occlusion and that prolonged usage of suppressive antibiotics may delay stent clogging and, hence, prevent cholangitis; however, this theoretical benefit has not been proven to be of significant clinical value.

■ ANTIBIOTIC PROPHYLAXIS AGAINST ENDOSCOPIC RETROGRADE CHOLANGIOPANCREATOGRAPHY–RELATED CHOLANGITIS

The incidence of cholangitis after ERCP is 2% to 8% [36•]. When performed for biliary strictures, ERCP may be followed by cholangitis in 8% to 25% of cases; therefore, it is logical to assume that the initiation of antibiotics before or during ERCP would prevent subsequent infection of the bile duct. It has been difficult, however, to prove the benefit of routine antibiotic

prophylaxis prior to ERCP in comparative trials [36•]. Even in high-risk cases, only one randomized, controlled study was able to show the benefit of antibiotic prophylaxis. Instead, immediate establishment of biliary drainage at the time of ERCP is a more important protective factor against postprocedural cholangitis. In addition, it is essential to maintain antibiotic treatment after a failed attempt to insert a biliary stent until adequate drainage of the obstruction is established. Other risk factors for post-ERCP cholangitis are a history of cholangitis, leukocytosis, contaminated instruments, dilation of biliary tract, and fever occurring less than 72 hours before the procedure [33].

Prophylactic antibiotics may be given parenterally in a single dose an hour prior to the invasive biliary procedure. The choice of antibiotics depends on local bacterial susceptibility. One may use the same antibiotics recommended for prophylaxis against infective endocarditis. Likewise, monotherapies of cefotaxime, piperacillin, cefonicid, ciprofloxacin, cefazolin, and cefuroxime have been studied in controlled trials. It is worthwhile to mention that ciprofloxacin is the only oral agent tested that is effective in prophylaxis against cholangitis.

■ REFERENCES

Recently published papers of particular interest have been highlighted as follows:
•   Of interest
••   Of outstanding interest

1.   Reynolds BM, Dargan EL: Acute obstructive cholangitis: a distinct clinical syndrome. *Ann Surg* 1959, 150:299–303.

2.• Sinanan MN: Acute cholangitis. *Infect Dis Clin North Am* 1992, 6:571–599.

3.• Hanau LH, Steigbigel NH: Cholangitis: pathogenesis, diagnosis and treatment. *Curr Clin Top Infect Dis* 1995, 15:153–178.

4.   Csendes A, Fernandez M, Uribe P: Bacteriology of the gallbladder bile in normal subjects. *Am J Surg* 1975, 129:629–631.

5.   Sung JY, Costerton JW, Shaffer EA: Defense system in the biliary tract against bacterial infection. *Dig Dis Sci* 1992, 37:689–696.

6.   Lo SK, Chen J: The role of ERCP in choledocholithiasis. *Abdom Imag* 1996, 21:120–132.

7.   Sung JJY, Lyon DJ, Suen R, *et al.*: Intravenous ciprofloxacin as treatment for patients with acute suppurative cholangitis: A randomized, controlled clinical trial. *J Antimicrob Chemother* 1995, 35:855–864.

8.   Sung JY, Shaffer EA, Olson ME, *et al.*: Bacterial invasion of the biliary by way of the portal-venous system. *Hepatology* 1991, 14:313–317.

9.   Raper SE, Barker ME, Jones AL, *et al.*: Anatomic correlates of bacterial cholangiovenous reflux. *Surgery* 1989, 105:352–359.

10.• Roberts SK, Ludwig J, Larusso NF: The pathobiology of biliary epithelia. *Gastroenterology* 1997, 112:269–279.

11. Shimada H, Nihmoto S, Matsuba A, *et al.*: Acute cholangitis: a histopathologic study. *J Clin Gastroenterol* 1988, 10:197–200.

12.• Brook I: Aerobic and anaerobic microbiology of biliary tract disease. *J Clin Microbiol* 1989, 27:2373–2375.

13.•• Leung JWC, Ling TKW, Chan RCY, *et al.*: Antibiotics, biliary sepsis and bile duct stones. *Gastrointest Endosc* 1994, 40:716–721.

14. Libby ED, Leung JW: Acute bacterial cholangitis. In *Consultations in Gastroenterology*. Edited by Snape WJ. Philadelphia: WB Saunders; 1996:877–881.

15. Shailesh LTC, Kadakia C: Biliary tract emergencies. *Medical Dis Clin North America* 1993, 77:1015–1036.

16. Shimada K, Noro T, Inamatsu T, *et al.*: Bacteriology of acute obstructive suppurative cholangitis of the aged. *J Clin Microbiol* 1981, 14:522–526.

17. Shimada K, Urayama K, Noro T, *et al.*: Biliary tract infection with anaerobes and the presence of free bile acids in bile. *Reviews of Infectious Diseases* 1984, 6:s147–s151.

18. Sievert W, Vakil NB: Emergencies of the biliary tract. *Gastroenterol Clin North Am* 1988, 17:245–264.

19. Allen JI, Allen MO, Olson MM, *et al.*: Pseudomonas infection of the biliary system resulting from use of a contaminated endoscope. *Gastroenterology* 1987, 92:759–763.

20. Classen DC, Jacobson JA, Burke JP, *et al.*: Serious pseudomonas infections associated with endoscopic retrograde cholangiopancreatography. *Am J Med* 1988, 84:590–596.

21. Gadiwala T, Andry M, Agrawal N, *et al.*: Consecutive *Serratia marcescens* infections following endoscopic retrograde cholangiopancreatography. *Gastrointest Endosc* 1988, 34:345–347.

22. Irani M, Truong LD: Candidiasis of the extrahepatic biliary tract. *Arch Pathol Lab Med* 1986, 110:1087–1090.

23. Uflacker R, Wholey MH, Amaral NM, *et al.*: Parasitic and mycotic causes of biliary obstruction. *Gastrointest Radiol* 1982, 7:173–179.

24. Grier JF, Cohen SW, Grafton WD, *et al.*: Acute suppurative cholangitis associated with choledochal sludge. *Am J Gastroenterol* 1994, 89:617–619.

25. Lygidakis NJ: Incidence of bile infection in patients with choledocholithiasis. *Am J Gastroenterol* 1982, 77:12–17.

26. Yu JL, Ljungh A: Infectiona associated with biliary drains. *Scand J Gastroenterol* 1996, 31, 625–630.

27.• Gigot JF, Leese T, Dereme T, *et al.*: Acute cholangitis: multivariate analysis of risk factors. *Ann Surg* 1989, 209:435–438.

28. Albert MB, Steinberg WM, Henry JP: Elevated serum levels of tumor marker CA19-9 in acute cholangitis. *Dig Dis Sci* 1988, 33:1223–1225.

29. Canto MIF, Diehl AM: Bacterial infections of the liver and biliary system. In *Gastrointestinal and Hepatic Infections*. Edited by Surawicz C and Owen RL. Philadelphia: WB Saunders; 1995:380–385.

30. Gaines P, Markham N, Leung J, *et al.*: The thick common bile duct in pyogenic cholangitis. *Clin Radiol* 1991, 44:175–177.

31. Balthazar EJ, Birnbaum BA, Naidich M: Acute cholangitis: CT evaluation. *J Comput Assist Tomogr* 1993, 17:283–289.

32. Leung JWC, Sung JJ, Chung SCS, *et al.*: Urgent endoscopic drainage for acute suppurative cholangitis. *Lancet* 1989, 1:1307–1309.

33. van del Hazel SJ, Speelman P, Tytgat GNJ, *et al.*: Role of antibiotics in the treatment and prevention of acute and recurrent cholangitis. *Clin Infect Dis* 1994, 19:279–286.

34. Dooley JS, Hamilton-Miller JMT, Brumfitt W, *et al.*: Antibiotics in the treatment of biliary infection. *Gut* 1984, 25:988–998.

35. Leung JW, Chan RC, Cheung SW, *et al.*: The effect of biliary obstruction on the biliary excretion of cefoperazone and ceftazidime. *J Antimicrob Chemother* 1990, 25:399–406.

36.• Lo SK: Failure of cefonicid prophylaxis for infectious complications related to endoscopic retrograde cholangiopancreatography [Editorial Response]. *Clin Infect Dis* 1996, 23:380–384.

37. Boender J, Nix JJ, deRidder AJ, *et al.*: Endoscopic sphincterotomy and biliary drainage in patients with cholangitis due to common bile duct stones. *Am J Gastroenterol* 1995, 90:233–238.

38.•• Lai ECS, Mok FPT, Tan ESY, *et al.*: Endoscopic biliary drainage for severe acute cholangitis. *N Engl J Med* 1992, 326:1582–1586.

39. O'Connor MJ, Schwartz ML, McQuarrie DG, *et al.*: Acute bacterial cholangitis. *Arch Surg* 1982, 117:437–441.

40. Barnett JL: Cholangitis and endoscopic drainage [Letter]. *Hepatology* 1992, 16:1302–1303.

41. Rohrmann CA Jr, Kimmey MB: Benign conditions of the bile ducts. In *Endoscopic Retrograde Cholangio-pancreatography*. Edited by Silvis SE, Rohrmann CA Jr, Ansel HJ. New York: Igaku-Shoin; 1995:195–200.

42. Freeman ML, Nelson DB, Sherman S, *et al.*: Complications of endoscopic biliary sphincterotomy. *N Engl J Med* 1996, 335:909–918.

43. Audisio RA, Bozzetti F, Severini A, *et al.*: The occurrence of cholangitis after percutaneous biliary drainage: evaluation of risk factors. *Surgery* 1988, 103:507–512.

44. Siegel JH, Rodriquez R, Cohen JA, *et al.*: Endoscopic management of cholangitis: clinical review of an alternative technique and report of a large series. *Am J Gastroenterol* 1994, 89:1142–1146.

45.• Lai ECS, Tam PC, Paterson IA, *et al.*: Emergency surgery for severe acute cholangitis: the high risk patients. *Ann Surg* 1990, 211:55–59.

46. Ducreux M, Buffet C, Lamy P, *et al.*: Diagnosis and prognosis of AIDS-related cholangitis. *AIDS* 1995, 9:875–880.

47. Khuroo MS, Dar MY, Yattoo GN, *et al.*: Serial cholangiographic appearances in recurrent pyogenic cholangitis. *Gastrointest Endosc* 1993, 39:674–679.

48. Stain SC, Incarbone R, Guthrie CR, *et al.*: Surgical treatment of recurrent pyogenic cholangitis. *Arch Surg* 1995, 130:527–533.

49. Scully RE, Mark EJ, McNeely WF, *et al.*: Case records of Massachusetts General Hospital. *N Engl J Med* 1990, 323:467–475.

50. Leung JWC, Chung SCS, Mok SD, *et al.*: Endoscopic removal of large common bile duct stones in recurrent pyogenic cholangitis. *Gastrointest Endosc* 1988, 34:238–241.

51. Khuroo MS, Zargar SA, Yattoo GN, *et al.*: Oddi's sphincter motor activity in patients with recurrent pyogenic cholangitis. *Hepatology* 1993, 17:53–58.

52. Kashi H, Lam FT, Giles GR: Recurrent pyogenic cholangiohepatitis. *Ann R Coll Surg Engl* 1989, 71:387–389.

53. Bonar S, Burrell M, West B, *et al.*: Recurrent cholangitis secondary to oriental cholangiohepatitis. *J Clin Gastroenterol* 1989, 11:464–468.

126 Endosonographic Evaluation of the Gallbladder and the Bile Duct

Assaad M. Soweid and Amitabh Chak

A variety of diagnostic tests are used to evaluate diseases of the gallbladder and the bile duct, including conventional transabdominal ultrasonography (US), computed tomography (CT), angiography, percutaneous transhepatic cholangiography (PTHC), endoscopic retrograde cholangiopancreatography (ERCP), and endoscopic US (EUS). Each has its advantages and disadvantages and may be indicated depending on the clinical situation.

Ultrasonography is a widely available, noninvasive test that offers the advantages of low cost, portability, and lack of exposure to radiation, all of which make it the preferred initial diagnostic test for patients suspected of having hepatic or biliary disorders; however, US imaging of deep anatomic structures, such as the distal bile duct and the head of the pancreas, is limited because of the marked attenuation of ultrasound waves by subcutaneous fat, bones, and intestinal gas. CT is also a popular screening test for biliary tract diseases. In most instances, however, it is unable to accurately detect biliary stones or localize and stage small biliary tumors. Cholangiography using PTHC or ERCP is considered the imaging "gold standard" for the biliary tree. Additionally, PTHC and ERCP offer therapeutic options, but they are technically difficult to perform and are invasive. Complications of PTHC and ERCP include bleeding, bile leak, infection, and pancreatitis.

EUS was developed in part as a method for obtaining high-resolution US images of the gastrointestinal (GI) tract and adjacent organs. EUS allows for intraluminal sonographic imaging of the biliary ductal system and the gallbladder. It can accurately diagnose stones and localize and stage even small tumors of the gallbladder and bile duct. EUS also can provide information concerning lesions that may not be immediately classified by other tests. The role of EUS in evaluating diseases of the gallbladder and the bile duct is rapidly evolving.

INSTRUMENTATION FOR ENDOSCOPIC ULTRASONOGRAPHY

Endosonographic systems include a probe (US transducer), an imaging device, a processor, and accessories (balloon, needles, pump). There are two basic types of commercially available ultrasound endoscopes—one with a mechanically rotating radial imaging transducer, the other with a curved or linear phased-array transducer. Both have standard endoscopic capabilities and oblique viewing optics, allowing advancement and positioning of the ultrasound transducer under direct endoscopic guidance. In the phased-array echoendoscope, the plane of scanning allows visualization of instruments and accessories introduced through the accessory channel, thus permitting needle aspiration of

imaged lesions. Mechanically rotating transducer echoendoscopes, which can image in the plane of the accessory channel and have EUS-guided biopsy capabilities, have also been developed. Most EUS applications have been defined with radial-type echoendoscopes.

Performance of EUS requires removal of a conventional endoscope and insertion of the echoendoscope; therefore, EUS is generally performed separately from endoscopy. Recently, catheter US probes have been introduced that can be inserted through the accessory port of standard endoscopes. These fine-caliber echoprobes, which can be inserted deep into the pancreaticobiliary system, have high operating frequencies, giving them enhanced resolution but limited depth of penetration. Images of the pancreatic or biliary duct walls and surrounding structures, such as the portal vein and hepatic artery, can be obtained with these probes.

TECHNIQUE OF ENDOSONOGRAPHIC EVALUATION OF THE BILIARY TRACT

Endosonographic examination of the biliary tree is performed by placing the tip of the echoendoscope into the descending duodenum. Scanning is performed through a water-filled balloon covering the US transducer, which is located at the tip of the echoendoscope and comes into contact with the duodenal wall. The water in the balloon displaces duodenal air, allowing good acoustic contact. Water also can be infused through the accessory channel as needed. During EUS imaging, the right lobe of the liver and pancreatic head serve as reference organs. The bile duct is identified as an anechoic tubular structure adjacent to the duodenal wall and ventral to the portal vein. At the start of the examination the transducer can be endoscopically positioned adjacent to the ampulla. From this position, the distal portion of the bile duct can be visualized. Slight manipulation of the scope tip at this position allows imaging of the distal common bile duct (CBD) as it courses through the pancreas into the ampulla. Upon withdrawal, the echoendoscope can be repositioned in the duodenal bulb apex in a *long position*, with the shaft bowed along the greater curve of the stomach, or in a *short-wedged position*, with the shaft along the lesser curve and the transducer held in place in the duodenal bulb with a water-inflated balloon. Most of the bile duct and portal vein can be seen in the longitudinal axis from this position (Fig. 126-1). By slowly withdrawing the instrument, the extrahepatic bile duct can be followed to the hilum of the liver (bifurcation of the right and left hepatic ducts). Thus, by using different positions the entire extrahepatic bile duct can be imaged. The gallbladder can easily be imaged by placing the transducer in the duodenal bulb or in the prepyloric region (Fig. 126-2). Vessels that can be routinely imaged by endosonographic scanning through the duodenal bulb and posterior gastric wall include the portal vein, hepatic artery, splenic artery and vein, celiac trunk, and the splenoportal confluence. Lymph nodes adjacent to the major blood vessels, such as the portal vein, mesenteric artery, aorta, inferior vena cava, and celiac trunk, also can be identified. Figure 126-3 presents the echoendoscopic positions in the duodenum and the stomach that are ideal for viewing the biliary system.

ROLE OF ENDOSONOGRAPHY IN THE EVALUATION OF OBSTRUCTIVE JAUNDICE

Endoscopic ultrasonography is highly accurate in demonstrating CBD dilation and in revealing the cause of obstruction in obstructive jaundice. In this regard, EUS is superior to US and CT; however, the noninvasiveness, low cost, and ease of performance of US make it the first choice. The accuracy of EUS is only challenged by ERCP, which additionally offers the capability of simultaneous therapy (stone extraction, stent placement, and so forth). EUS, ERCP, and CT were used to evaluate pancreaticobiliary disease in 60 patients who presented with obstructive jaundice [1•]. EUS provided significant information in 75% of cases, prompting a change in treatment in 32%. Compared with CT and ERCP, EUS proved to be more sensitive and specific (Table 126-1). EUS was reported to be 88% accurate in providing specific diagnosis in patients with obstructive jaundice. The sensitivity and specificity in the diagnosis of CBD stenosis were 93% and 91%, respectively, whereas the sensitivity and specificity in diagnosing tumor obstruction were 83% and 92%, respectively [2].

The accuracy of EUS compares favorably to ERCP for diagnosising the cause of obstruction in patients with obstructive jaundice or dilation of CBD; both tests are superior to CT and US. Accuracy is reported to be 29% to 95% for US, 20% to 66%

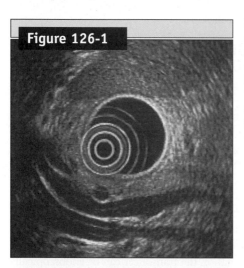

Figure 126-1

Endosonographic view of the bile duct and the portal vein in the longitudinal axis. The bile duct is closer to the central transducer.

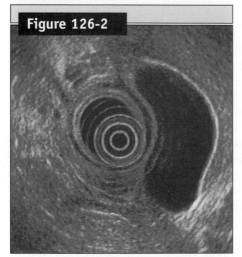

Figure 126-2

Endosonographic view of the gallbladder from the duodenal bulb.

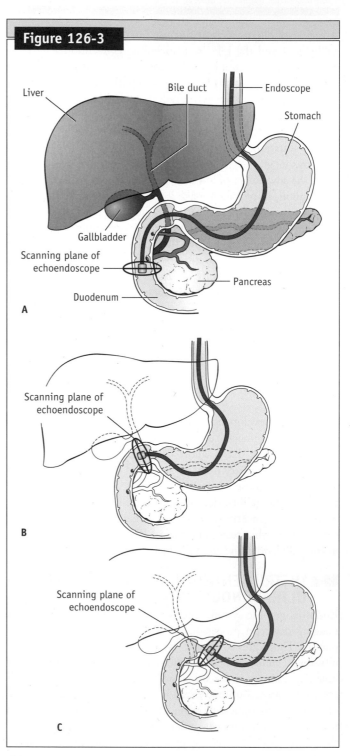

Figure 126-3

A

B

C

Schematic representation of echoendoscope in three different positions commonly used to image the gallbladder and bile duct.

for CT, 97% for ERCP, and 74% to 100% for EUS [3]. EUS is more sensitive than US and CT (100% vs 80% and 83%, respectively) in diagnosing biliary obstruction and in identifying the cause of obstruction (97% vs 49% and 66%, respectively). In addition, it is more effective in the assessment of the local or regional spread of tumor obstruction (75% vs 38% and 62%, respectively) [4].

Endoscopic ultrasonography should be considered in patients with obstructive jaundice if an initial noninvasive screening test, such as US or CT, is inconclusive. It can replace ERCP in cases when a patient is a surgical candidate, when no interventional procedures are necessary, or when ERCP fails. EUS cannot replace the therapeutic capability of ERCP. It should be considered a complementary test to ERCP and CT in patients with ampullary/pancreaticobiliary tumors, for which EUS provides more accurate local staging. The role of this powerful imaging technology is still evolving. The recent availability of phased-array and mechanically rotating transducer echoendoscopes, which have imaging planes that parallel the shaft of the endoscope and have larger accessory channels, may soon lead to the ability to access the pancreaticobiliary ductal system under EUS guidance in cases where ERCP fails.

■ CHOLEDOCHOLITHIASIS

A small but significant number of patients undergoing cholecystectomy will have CBD stones, even without symptoms, biliary dilation, or significant laboratory abnormalities. Choledocholithiasis may be a present in 3% to 35% of patients undergoing cholecystectomy for symptomatic gallstones, and may be a major source of morbidity in 10% to 20 % of patients. In addition, the widespread use of laparoscopic cholecystectomy with its technically more difficult access to the bile duct has renewed the search for noninvasive methods to detect stones preoperatively.

Up to 50% of subsequently discovered CBD stones may be missed on US. Failure may be secondary to the inability to identify the distal CBD because of adjacent duodenal air. CT is limited by its inability to detect noncalcified and smaller stones. The reported sensitivity of CT in detecting choledocholithiasis ranges from 50% to 90%. With helical CT, this sensitivity is unlikely to change because the cholesterol-predominant bile duct

stones will be isodense with the bile. MR imaging cholangiography offers encouraging results in the detection of choledocholithiasis, but further studies are needed to determine its sensitivity and specificity. Cholangiography by ERCP or PTHC is considered the gold standard for stone detection, but these modalities are invasive and are associated with significant complications. Also, technical aspects, such as air bubble introduction into the bile duct or density of contrast media used, hinder stone detection, limiting the sensitivity and specificity of this gold standard.

Endoscopic ultrasonography overcomes many technical difficulties of US because the transducer may be placed in close proximity to the biliary tree and interference from duodenal air is avoided. EUS can detect large (Figs. 126-4 and 126-5) and smaller stones (2–3 mm), even in nondilated ducts. It is less invasive than ERCP or PTHC, and the interpretation is not subject to artifacts introduced by air bubbles, as in cholangiography. The performance of EUS, however, does demand a high level of training and technical skill.

Many studies using radial-type EUS have demonstrated a high accuracy (up to 100%) in detecting bile duct stones [5] (Table 126-2). The diagnosis of bile duct stones using EUS versus ERCP was compared in a prospective, double-blind study in pre- and postcholecystectomy patients with suspected choledocholithiasis referred for ERCP [6•]. EUS was found to be equally accurate (94% overall accuracy) but much safer (complication rate 1.6% vs 12.6%) than ERCP. EUS followed by therapeutic ERCP (when indicated) was calculated to be less costly than ERCP. In addition, EUS provided further information or alternative diagnoses to bile duct stones in 21% of patients.

In another study, EUS was found to be as sensitive and specific as ERCP and superior to US in the detecting CBD stones. The sensitivity of EUS ranged from 88% to 97%, with a specificity of 97% to 100% [7•]. EUS was compared to direct cholangiography and surgical exploration in the evaluation of a total of 422 patients for CBD stones [8•]. Compared with surgery, EUS had a sensitivity of 94.9% and a specificity of 97.8%, with an accuracy of 95.9% in detecting choledocholithiasis. All CBD stones found by ERCP were seen by EUS. Concordance was obtained in 91.3% of cases.

In patients with known choledocholithiasis, ERCP is obviously the test of choice; however, even with careful selection,

Table 126-1. EUS Compared to ERCP in Evaluating Patients With Pancreaticobiliary Disease Presenting With Jaundice

		CT, %	CT + ERCP, %	ERCP, %	EUS, %
Detection of abnormality	Sensitivity	71	95	94	98
	Specificity	25	25	100	100
Differentiation between benign and malignant	Sensitivity	—	75	—	85
	Specificity	—	65	—	80
Prediction of specific diagnosis	Sensitivity	—	30	—	75
	Specificity	—	20	—	50

ERCP—endoscopic retrograde cholangiopancreatography; EUS—endoscopic ultrasonography.
From Snady [1].

about one half to three quarters of patients with suspected choledocholithiasis referred for ERCP do not have stones. EUS is less costly than ERCP and avoids the potential morbidity of pancreatitis. EUS may enable selective performance of therapeutic ERCP in the following patients:

Patients with a nondilated CBD on US who have abnormal liver tests prior to laparoscopic cholecystectomy

Patients with a relative contraindication to ERCP, such as contrast allergy or pregnancy

Patients with a history of post-ERCP pancreatitis

Patients with suspected CBD stones who had an unsuccessful ERCP

Low- or medium-risk patients (0%–20% risk of stones) with mildly elevated liver function tests, minimal or no biliary dilation, or remote history of jaundice or pancreatitis who have had a cholecystectomy

■ MALIGNANT LESIONS OF THE BILE DUCT

The most common malignancy of the extrahepatic bile duct is slow-growing cholangiocarcinoma that seldom produces distant metastases. Cancer of the extrahepatic bile duct is divided into distal and proximal for purposes of staging. The clinical presentation and management of distal cholangiocarcinoma is similar to carcinoma in the head of the pancreas. Proximal cholangiocarcinoma represents a more complicated problem from the standpoints of endoscopic and surgical management.

Ultrasonography and CT are useful for imaging advanced cancers of the biliary tree; however, they are of limited value in the identification of small biliary tumors, specifically those less than 2 to 3 cm. EUS can depict tumor masses involving the terminal end of the CBD more clearly than US or CT. In addition, EUS can detect small (<3 cm) bile duct tumors (Fig. 126-6) more often than other imaging modalities, such as CT, US, and angiography [9].

Cholangiography can identify ductal strictures in patients with biliary tumors, but the origin of the stricture can only be inferred from the radiographic appearance and clinical scenario. EUS can provide an accurate estimation of tumor size and also determine presence of vascular invasion and involvement of lymph nodes. Intraductal cytology may provide a diagnosis at ERCP in a minority of cases. EUS-guided fine-needle aspiration (FNA) appears to be a promising method for obtaining cytological material from tumors.

Angiography is sometimes used in assessing vascular infiltration, but is not accurate in detecting small bile duct cancers and determining invasion into adjacent organs, as these tumors are not very vascular. Intraductal ultrasonographic imaging with catheter-type echoprobes may be useful in the evaluation of tumor invasion into the adjacent portal vein and hepatic artery.

Characteristic EUS findings in distal bile duct cancer include intramural or transmural hypoechoic thickening of the bile duct with prestenotic dilation, but no evidence of penetration into

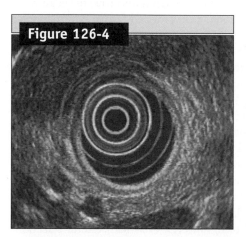

Endosonographic photograph of a typical bile duct stone (circular, hyperechoic particle with acoustic shadowing).

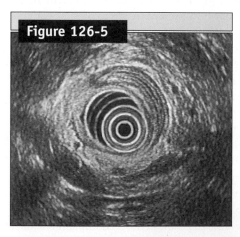

Another endosonographic view of a bile duct stone.

Table 126-2. Efficacy of EUS for Suspected Choledocholithiasis

Study, y	Patients, n	CBD stone frequency, %	Sensitivity, %	Specificity, %	Accuracy, %
Sakai, 1991	15	100	73	NA	NA
Edmundowicz, 1992	20	20	75	100	95
Denis, 1993	60	42	92	100	97
Amouyal, 1994	62	52	97	100	98
Canto, 1995	64	30	84	95	92
Palazzo, 1995	422	39	95	98	93
Total	643	38	86	99	95

CBD—common bile duct; EUS—endoscopic ultrasonography.
Data from Canto [5].

pancreatic tissue. When a tumor invades the pancreas, the distinction between biliary and pancreatic cancer on EUS is nearly impossible. Detection of small (<3 cm) biliary tumors with EUS is equal to ERCP (100%) and superior to other modalities (Table 126-3) [9,10•,11]. Accuracy of staging the depth of the tumor and presence of vascular invasion with EUS (T staging) is over 80% [10•,11]; however, EUS is not accurate in diagnosing lymph node metastases and distinguishing them from reactive adenopathy. The availability of EUS-guided FNA may improve the accuracy of EUS in staging local nodal disease.

Biliary tumors are staged according to the tumor-node-metastasis (TNM) system [12]. Endosonographically, the bile duct wall is comprised of three layers, roughly corresponding to mucosa, muscularis propria, and serosa. EUS staging of depth of tumor (T) is as follows:

T1—tumor is limited to the first two layers (mucosa/muscularis).

T1a—tumor limited to the first layer (mucosa).

T1b—tumor invasion into the second layer (muscularis).

T2—tumor involves all layers interrupting the outer margin of the bile duct, which is irregular because of invasion into the periductal connective tissue.

T3—tumor invades into adjacent structures, such as blood vessels, liver, pancreas, gallbladder, stomach, duodenum, or colon

Characteristics of malignant lymph nodes on EUS are round shape, well-demarcated border, relative hypoechogenicity, and enlarged size. Nodal staging of biliary tumors is as follows:

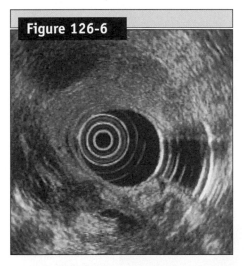

Figure 126-6

Endosonographic appearance of distal bile duct tumor. A hypoechoic 15-mm mass arising from the bile duct and invading the portal vein.

N0—no regional lymph node metastasis

N1—regional lymph node metastasis

N1a—metastasis along the CBD, cystic duct, or in the hilum of the liver

N1b—metastasis into the periduodenal and periportal regions or adjacent to the celiac trunk and mesenteric vessels.

M0/M1 refers to absence or presence of distant metastasis.

Because of its limited depth of penetration, EUS can only determine regional tumor status and is not reliable in assessing metastatic disease.

A major criticism of the TNM system of staging in biliary cancer is that T staging and resectability do not correlate well. Tumors infiltrating into the pancreas or duodenum are resectable whereas tumors invading the portal vein are not, yet they are both classified as T3 tumors. In addition, longitudinal spread, which also is important in assessing resectability (especially in Klatskin tumors), has not yet been included in the staging system.

Intraductal ultrasonography using catheter ultrasound probes eventually may be useful in the evaluation of bile duct lesions. Current models still have difficulty in traversing narrow bile duct strictures that limit their use. A preliminary report [13] has suggested that intraductal US may improve the accuracy of EUS staging of biliary ductal carcinomas.

Malignant tumors at the level of the bile duct bifurcation are generally defined as Klatskin tumors. Bifurcation of the bile duct can be imaged during EUS examination by following the CBD and common hepatic duct proximally to the hilum of the liver. For the more proximal branches of the intrahepatic bile duct, ultrasound penetration with EUS may not be sufficient to detect small tumors. Accurate staging of such tumors is important when surgery is a consideration.

Klatskin tumors can spread toward the distal bile duct or can spread proximally, and involve multiple branches of the intrahepatic biliary tree. When diagnosis is made using ERCP, there is always a risk of cholangitis from manipulating the bile duct and filling the proximal parts with contrast unsterile medium, especially if placement of a drain is unsuccessful. Unlike distal biliary cancers, Klatskin tumors do not have an increased incidence of lymph node metastasis with progression of tumor growth. Klatskin tumors are usually imaged during EUS as hypoechoic masses adjacent to a dilated hepatic duct. The mass is often surrounded by hyperechoic fibrotic tissue. Lymphomas, hepatomas, metastatic lymph nodes, fibrosis, purulent cholangitis, and even Mirizzi's syndrome should be considered in the

Table 126-3. Detection Route of CBD Carcinoma

Tumor size	Patients, n	EUS, %	ERCP, %	AG, %	CT, %	USG, %
≤ 20 mm	12	100	100	33	33	33
> 20 mm	9	100	100	89	67	56
Overall	21	100	100	57	48	43

AG—angiography; CBD—common bile duct; ERCP—endoscopic retrograde cholangiopancreatography; EUS—endoscopic ultrasonography; USG—ultrasonography. Data from Mukai [11].

differential diagnosis. The overall accuracy for EUS in patients with Klatskin tumors has been reported to be 85% for determining T-stage involvement and 53% for detecting nodal involvement [10•].

Intraductal ultrasonography using catheter-type echoprobes may eventually become the imaging method of choice when evaluating these subtle lesions. When the probe is able to traverse the lesion, this imaging technique is reported to have a 100% accuracy in assessing portal venous invasion [14], even in the case of proximal tumors.

▬ BENIGN LESIONS OF THE GALLBLADDER

Ultrasonography is very accurate in diagnosing cholelithiasis; however, it has limitations in evaluating other gallbladder diseases, such as gallbladder carcinomas and cholesterol polyps. During EUS, the gallbladder can be imaged from the duodenal bulb position and sometimes from the gastric antrum position. Endosonographically, the normal gallbladder wall is comprised of three layers: the first layer is slightly hyperechoic, the second layer is hypoechoic, and the third layer is hyperechoic. Comparison with histologic sections reveals that the first layer roughly corresponds to the mucosal layer, the second to the muscular layer, and the third to the serosal layer. Because it provides high-resolution images of the gallbladder wall, EUS is able to distinguish small lesions, such as adenomatous polyps and adenomyomatosis. As with US, the clinical significance of detecting these small lesions remains questionable.

Gallbladder stones occur in up to 10% of the general population that is over 50 years of age, but only 10% to 20% of these patients become symptomatic. US has a sensitivity of over 95% in detecting gallbladder stones, but because of the high prevalence of this disease in the general population, the number of symptomatic patients with normal US is still high.

The following criteria have been proposed for the diagnosis of cholelithiasis by EUS [15]:

Hyperechoic, mobile particles larger than 2 mm and with acoustic shadowing (Fig. 126-7)

Sludge, defined as mobile, low-amplitude echoes in lumen that layer in the most dependent part of the gallbladder without associated acoustic shadowing

Minilithiasis, defined as mobile, 1–2 mm hyperechoic signals without acoustic shadowing

Mobility is somewhat difficult to ascertain in a sedated patient who is undergoing endoscopy.

A few studies [5, 15] have been published involving selected patients suspected of having gallbladder stones who have normal US or in whom US is unsatisfactory because of body habitus. EUS is able to demonstrate cholelithiasis in obese patients who cannot be examined adequately by US. Because of the close proximity of the transducer to the gallbladder, EUS may be able to also identify sludge or microlithiasis more sensitively than US. Thus, EUS has a potential role in the following clinical situations when US is normal or inconclusive:

Idiopathic, acute pancreatitis

Obese subjects with suspected cholelithiasis

Patients with repeated episodes of colic

This condition is characterized by proliferation of the gallbladder epithelium with gland-like formation and outpouchings of mucosa into or through the thickened muscular layer (ie, Rokitansky-Aschoff sinuses). This process may be diffuse or localized. On EUS, the gallbladder wall is seen as two layers: a thick, low echoic inner layer, and a hyperechoic outer layer with small cystic echoes within the wall. On histologic comparison, muscle and perimuscular fibrosis match the hypoechoic layer, while the small cystic echoes correspond to the dilated Rokitansky-Aschoff sinuses. With EUS it also is possible to identify the polypoid type of gallbladder adenomyomatosis as protuberant lesions with small cystic echoes in the gallbladder wall [16].

On EUS the gallbladder wall appears thick and separated into three or more layers (especially in cases of severe cholecystitis) (Fig. 126-8). In cases with cholecystitis secondary to cholelithiasis, stone shadowing is seen in addition to the wall thickening. These findings may be imaged with better resolution by EUS than US; however there appears to be little clinical use for EUS in this setting.

Cholesterol polyps exhibit a typical sonographic appearance of multiple granular structures composed of hyperechoic foci. On occasion they may have the appearance of homogeneous hyperechoic masses and thus be wrongly diagnosed as neoplasms. Due to its higher resolution, EUS may be able to discern the characteristic granular appearance in these cases and be better able to characterize these benign lesions [16].

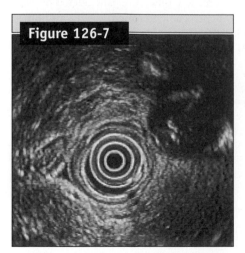

Figure 126-7

Endosonographic examination of the gallbladder showing multiple smaller stones.

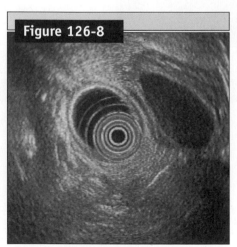

Figure 126-8

Endosonographic appearance of a markedly thickened gallbladder wall.

◼◼◼ MALIGNANT LESIONS OF THE GALLBLADDER

Endoscopic ultrasonography can demonstrate the polypoid type of gallbladder cancer as a papillary, irregular, hypoechoic mass. These carcinomas are not usually imaged by US. Tumor infiltration into the gallbladder wall is characterized by destruction of the three endosonographic layers. Gallbladder carcinoma may also present as a polypoid intraluminal mass of varying echo density and irregularity with progressive wall destruction and infiltration into the liver (depending on the stage). Involvement of the bile duct can be identified on EUS. This type of cancer is rare, and investigations on the accuracy of EUS in staging gallbladder cancer are limited; however, based on preliminary studies and its accuracy in staging other pancreaticobiliary cancers, it is reasonable to presume that EUS will be accurate in staging gallbladder cancers. The TNM method of classification is again used for staging gallbladder cancers, with T1 being a tumor limited to the mucosa of the gallbladder without penetration into the muscularis, T2 a tumor invading into the muscularis layer, and T3 tumor invasion into adjacent structures (duodenum, liver, major blood vessels). N0 and N1 refer to the absence or presence of regional lymph node involvement [17].

◼◼◼ CONCLUSION

Endoscopic ultrasonography is effective in diagnosing many benign and malignant lesions of the gallbladder and the bile duct. It is not as inexpensive or as technically easy to perform as conventional US and it lacks the therapeutic potential of ERCP; however, it is highly accurate in the diagnosis of choledocholithiasis, cholelithiasis, and in the diagnosis and staging of biliary tract and gallbladder carcinomas, including small tumors that may not be detected by the conventional diagnostic modalities. EUS may become the test of choice in screening patients with suspected choledocholithiasis instead of ERCP given its significantly lower rate of complications. The use of catheter US probes and EUS-guided fine-needle biopsy will undoubtedly increase the capability of EUS in the diagnosis of gallbladder and biliary tract diseases.

◼◼◼ REFERENCES

Recently published papers of particular interest have been highlighted as follows:
- • Of interest
- •• Of outstanding interest

1.• Snady H, Cooperman A, Siegel JH: Endoscopic ultrasonography compared with computed tomography and ERCP in patients with obstructive jaundice or small peripancreatic mass. *Gastrointest Endosc* 1992, 38:27–34.

2. Giovannini M, Seitz JF: Endoscopic ultrasonography with a linear-type echoendoscope in the evaluation of 94 patients with pancreatobiliary disease. *Endoscopy* 1994, 26:579–585.

3. Buscail L: Endoscopic ultrasonography in pancreatobiliary disease using radial instruments. *Gastrointest Endosc Clin North Am* 1995, 5:781–787.

4. Amouyal P, Palazzo L, Amouyal G, *et al.*: Endosonography: promising method for diagnosis of extrahepatic cholestasis. *Lancet* 1989, 2:1195–1198.

5. Canto M: Endoscopic ultrasonography and gallstone disease. *Gastrointest Endosc* 1996, 43:S37–S43.

6.• Canto MIF, Chak A, Stellato T, *et al.*: Endoscopic ultrasonography vs cholangiography for the diagnosis of choledocholithiasis in pre- and post-cholecystectomy patients. *Gastrointest Endosc* 1998, in press.

7.• Edmundowicz SA: Common bile duct stones. *Gastrointest Endosc Clin North Am* 1995, 5:817–824.

8.• Palazzo L, Girollet PP, Salmeron M, *et al.*: Value of endoscopic ultrasonography in the diagnosis of common bile duct stones: comparison with surgical exploration and ERCP. *Gastrointest Endosc* 1995, 42:225–231.

9. Yasuda K, Nakajima M, Kawai K: Diseases of the biliary tract and the papilla of Vater. In *Endoscopic Ultrasonography in Gastroenterology*. Edited by Kawai K. Tokyo/New York: Igaku Shoin Press; 1988:96–105.

10.• Tio TL, Cheng J, Wijers OB, *et al.*: Endosonographic TNM staging of extrahepatic bile duct cancer: comparison with pathological staging. *Gastroenterology* 1991, 100:1351–1361.

11. Mukai H, Yasuda K, Nakajima M: Tumors of the papilla and distal common bile duct: diagnosis and staging by endoscopic ultrasonography. *Gastrointest Endosc Clin North Am* 1995, 5:763–772.

12. Sobin LH, Hermanek P, Hutter RP: TNM classification of malignant tumors. *Cancer* 1988, 61:2310–2314.

13. Yasuda K: Ultrasonic probes for pancreaticobiliary strictures. *Gastrointest Endosc* 1996, 43:S35–S37.

14. Tamada K, Ido K, Ueno N, *et al.*: Assessment of portal vein invasion by bile duct cancer using intraductal ultrasonography. *Endoscopy* 1995, 27:573–578.

15. Amouyal G, Amouyal P: Endoscopic ultrasonography in gallbladder stones. *Gastrointest Endosc Clin North Am* 1995, 5:825–830.

16. Morita K, Nakazawa S, Kimoto E, *et al.*: Gallbladder diseases. In *Endoscopic Ultrasonography in Gastroenterology*. Edited by Kawai K. Tokyo/New York: Igaku Shoin Press; 1988:87–95.

17. Tio TL: The TNM staging system. *Gastrointest Endosc* 1996, 43:S19–S24.

127 Sphincter of Oddi Dysfunction

Stuart Sherman and Glen A. Lehman

Since its description by Rugero Oddi in 1887, the sphincter of Oddi (SO) has been the subject of study and controversy. Even its existence as a distinct anatomic or physiologic entity has been disputed. Hence, it is not surprising that the clinical syndrome of SO dysfunction and its therapy are controversial [1•]. This chapter reviews the anatomy and physiology of the SO, clinical presentations, and methods to diagnose and treat SO dysfunction.

DEFINITIONS

Sphincter of Oddi dysfunction refers to an abnormality of SO contractility. It is a benign, noncalculous obstruction to the flow of bile or pancreatic juice through the pancreaticobiliary junction (*ie*, the SO). SO dysfunction may manifest by pancreaticobiliary pain, pancreatitis, or deranged liver tests. SO dysfunction actually is made up of two entities. *SO dyskinesia* refers to a primary motor abnormality of the SO that may result in hypertonia or, less commonly, hypotonia of the sphincter. *SO stenosis*, in contrast, refers to a structural alteration of the sphincter, probably from an inflammatory process, with subsequent fibrosis. Because it often is impossible to distinguish patients with SO dyskinesia from those with SO stenosis, the term SO dysfunction has been used to encompass both groups of individuals. A variety of less accurate terms are listed in the medical literature to describe this entity, such as papillary stenosis, ampullary stenosis, biliary dyskinesia, and postcholecystectomy syndrome (even though SO dysfunction may occur with the gallbladder intact). In an attempt to deal with this overlap in etiology, and also to determine the appropriate use of SO manometry, a clinical classification system has been developed for patients

with suspected SO dysfunction [2•]—the Hogan-Geenen SO dysfunction classification system (Table 127-1).

ANATOMY, PHYSIOLOGY, AND PATHOPHYSIOLOGY

The SO is a complex of smooth muscles surrounding the terminal common bile duct, main (ventral) pancreatic duct of Wirsung, and the common channel (ampulla of Vater), when present (Fig. 127-1). It has both circular and "figure 8" components. The high-pressure zone generated by the sphincter varies from 4 to 10 mm in length. Its role appears to regulate bile and pancreatic exocrine juice flow and to prevent duodenum-to-duct reflux (*ie*, maintain sterile intraductal environment). The SO possesses basal pressure and phasic contractile activities; the former appears to be the predominant mechanism regulating flow of pancreaticobiliary secretions into the intestine. Although phasic SO contractions may aid in regulating bile and pancreatic juice flow, their primary role appears to be maintaining a sterile intraductal milieu. SO regulation is under both neural and hormonal control. Phasic wave activity of the SO is closely tied to the migrating motor complex (MMC) of the duodenum. Innervation of the bile duct does not appear to be essential, as SO function has been reported to be preserved following liver transplantation [3]. Cholecystokinin and secretin appear to be most important in causing SO relaxation, with contributions from nonadrenergic, noncholinergic neurons via vasoactive intestinal peptide (VIP) and nitric oxide [4].

Wedge specimens of the SO obtained at surgical sphincteroplasty from patients with SO dysfunction, show evidence of

---

Table 127-1. Hogan-Geenen Sphincter of Oddi Classification System Related to the Frequency of Abnormal Sphincter of Oddi Manometry and Pain Relief by Biliary Sphincterotomy

Patient group classifications	Approximate frequency of abnormal sphincter manometry	Probability of pain relief by sphincterotomy if manometry is		Manometry before sphincter ablation
		Abnormal	Normal	
Biliary I: Patients with biliary-type pain; abnormal aspartate aminotransferase or alkaline phosphatase >2 x the normal documented on two or more occasions; delayed drainage of ERCP contrast >45 min; and dilated common bile duct of >12 mm in diameter	75%–95%	90%–95%	90%–95%	Unnecessary
Biliary II: Patients with biliary-type pain but only one or two of the above criteria	55%–65%	85%	35%	Mandatory
Biliary III: Patients with only biliary-type pain and no other abnormalities	25%–55%	55%–65%	<10%	Mandatory

ERCP—endoscopic retrograde cholangiopancreatography.

inflammation, muscular hypertrophy, fibrosis, or adenomyosis within the papillary zone in approximately 60% of patients [5]; a motor disorder is suggested in the remaining 40% with normal histology. Infections with cytomegalovirus or *Cryptosporidium,* as may occur in patients with AIDS, or *Strongyloides* also have caused SO dysfunction.

How does SO dysfunction cause pain? Although unproven, it is theorized that abnormalities of the SO can give rise to pain by impeding the flow of bile and pancreatic juice, resulting in ductal hypertension, ischemia arising from spastic contractions, and "hypersensitivity" of the papilla.

EPIDEMIOLOGY

Sphincter of Oddi dysfunction may occur in children or adults, although most SO dysfunction occurs in middle-aged women. SO dysfunction most commonly occurs after cholecystectomy, but it may also arise with the gallbladder in situ. In a recent survey on functional gastrointestinal disorders, SO dysfunction appeared to have a relevant impact on quality of life and was highly associated with work absenteeism, disability, and healthcare use [6].

The frequency of manometrically documented SO dysfunction in patients prior to cholecystectomy has received limited study. Guelrud *et al.* [6a] performed SO manometry prior to cholecystectomy in 121 patients with symptomatic gallstones and normal common bile duct diameter. Basal SO pressure was elevated in 12% of patients and SO dysfunction was diagnosed in 4% and 40%, respectively, of individuals with a normal or elevated serum alkaline phosphatase level. Ruffolo *et al.* [7] performed

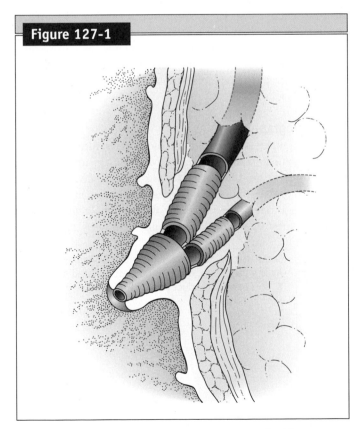

Figure 127-1

Schematic representation of the human sphincter of Oddi, demonstrating the circular smooth muscle that surrounds the distal common bile duct, pancreatic duct, and common channel.

scintigraphic gallbladder ejection fraction and endoscopic SO manometry in 81 patients with symptoms suggestive of biliary disease but normal endoscopic retrograde cholangiopancreatography (ERCP) and no gallbladder stones; 53% of patients had SO dysfunction and 49% had an abnormal gallbladder ejection fraction. SO dysfunction occurred with a similar frequency in patients with abnormal and normal ejection fractions.

Pain resembling preoperative biliary colic occurs in 10% to 20% of patients after cholecystectomy [8]. The frequency with which SO dysfunction is diagnosed in reported series varies considerably from 9% [9] to 68% [10]. Sherman *et al.* [11•] used SO manometry to evaluate 115 patients who had pancreaticobiliary pain without bile duct stones or tumors and found 51% showed abnormal basal SO pressure (>40 mm Hg). These patients were categorized further by the Hogan-Geenen SO dysfunction classification system (Table 127-1); abnormal SO manometry was found in 86%, 55%, and 28% of biliary type I, type II, and type III patients, respectively. These frequencies are similar to those reported by others for type I and type II [12,13•], whereas in type III patients, abnormal basal SO pressure is found in 12% to 55%. Dysfunction may occur in the pancreatic duct portion of the SO and cause recurrent pancreatitis. Manometrically documented SO dysfunction has been reported in 15% to 59% of patients with recurrent pancreatitis previously labeled as idiopathic [14•].

CLINICAL PRESENTATION

Abdominal pain is the most common presenting symptom of SO dysfunction, usually is epigastric or in the right upper quadrant, may be disabling, and lasts for 20 minutes to several hours. In some patients the pain is continuous with episodic exacerbations, may be precipitated by food or narcotics, and radiates to the back or shoulder, accompanied by nausea and vomiting. The pain may begin several years after a cholecystectomy and resemble the pain prompting the cholecystectomy. Alternatively, the pain may not be relieved by cholecystectomy. Jaundice, fever, or chills are rare. Physical examination is characterized by a paucity of abnormal findings. Most common is mild, nonspecific abdominal tenderness. Transient elevation of liver test results, typically during episodes of pain, are present in less than 50% of patients. The pain is not relieved by trial medications for acid-peptic disease or irritable bowel syndrome. Patients with SO dysfunction may also present with typical pancreatic pain and recurrent pancreatitis.

Clinical Evaluation

The diagnostic approach to suspected SO dysfunction may be influenced by the presence of key clinical features; however, the clinical manifestations of functional abnormalities of the SO may not always be easily distinguishable from those caused by organic ones (*eg,* common bile duct stones) or other functional non-pancreaticobiliary disorders (*eg,* irritable bowel syndrome).

General Initial Evaluation

Evaluation of patients with suspected SO dysfunction should be initiated with standard serum liver chemistries, serum amylase or lipase, or both, and abdominal ultrasonography, CT scans, or both. Serum enzyme studies should be drawn during bouts of pain, if possible. Mild elevations (< two times the upper limit of normal) are frequent in SO dysfunction whereas greater abnormalities are more suggestive of stones, tumors, and liver parenchymal disease. CT scans and abdominal ultrasound examinations usually are normal, but a dilated bile duct or pancreatic duct occasionally may be found, particularly in patients with type I SO dysfunction. Evaluation and treatment of more common upper gastrointestinal conditions, such as peptic ulcer disease and gastroesophageal reflux, should be performed simultaneously. In the absence of mass lesions, stones, or response to acid suppression therapeutic trials, the suspicion for sphincter disease is heightened. After initial evaluation, patients are commonly categorized according to the Hogan-Geenen SO dysfunction classification system (Table 127-1).

■ NONINVASIVE DIAGNOSTIC METHODS

Because SO manometry, which is considered by most authorities to be the gold standard for diagnosing SO dysfunction, is difficult to perform, invasive, not widely available, and associated with a relatively high complication rate, several noninvasive and provocative tests are used in an attempt to identify patients with SO dysfunction.

Morphine-Prostigmin Provocative Test (Nardi Test)

Morphine causes SO contraction. Neostigmine (Prostigmin; ICN Pharmaceuticals, Costa Mesa, CA) (1 mg subcutaneously) a potent cholinergic secretory stimulant, is added to morphine (10 mg subcutaneously) to make this challenge test. The morphine-prostigmin test, historically, had been used extensively to diagnose SO dysfunction. Reproduction of the patient's typical pain associated with a fourfold increase in aspartate aminotransferase, alanine aminotransferase, alkaline phosphatase, amylase, or lipase constitute a positive response. The usefulness of this test is limited by its low sensitivity and specificity in predicting the presence of SO dysfunction and its poor correlation with outcome after SO ablation. This test has been replaced by more sensitive tests.

Ultrasonographic Assessment of Extrahepatic Bile Duct and Main Pancreatic Duct Diameter After Secretory Stimulation

After a lipid-rich meal or cholecystokinin administration, the gallbladder contracts, hepatic bile flow increases, and the SO relaxes, resulting in bile entry into the duodenum. Similarly, after a lipid-rich meal or secretin administration, pancreatic exocrine juice flow is stimulated and the SO relaxes. If the SO is dysfunctional and causes obstruction to flow, the common bile duct or main pancreatic duct may dilate under secretory pressure; such dilation can be monitored by transcutaneous ultrasonography (Fig. 127-2). SO and terminal duct obstruction from other causes (stones, tumors, strictures, etc.) also may cause ductal dilation and must be excluded. Pain provocation should be noted if present. To date, limited studies comparing these noninvasive tests with SO manometry or outcome after sphincter ablation [15] show only modest correlation.

Quantitative Hepatobiliary Scintigraphy

Hepatobiliary scintigraphy assesses bile flow through the biliary tract. Impairment of bile flow from SO disease, tumors, stones, or parenchymal liver disease result in impaired radionuclide flow. The precise criteria to define a positive (abnormal) study remain controversial, but duodenal arrival time greater than 20 minutes and hilum to duodenum time greater than 10 minutes are most widely used [16]. Most studies are flawed by lack of correlation with SO manometry or outcome after SO ablation. Overall, it appears that patients with dilated bile ducts and high-grade obstruction are likely to have a positive scintigraphic study. Patients with lower-grade obstruction (Hogan-Geenen classification types II and III) generally have normal scintigraphy, even if done after cholecystokinin provocation.

Noninvasive testing for SO dysfunction has a relatively low or undefined sensitivity and specificity, and therefore is not recommended for general clinical use, except in situations where SO manometry is unsuccessful or unavailable.

■ INVASIVE DIAGNOSTIC METHODS

Because of their associated risks, invasive testing with ERCP and manometry should be reserved for patients with clinically significant or disabling symptoms. In general, invasive assessment of patients for SO dysfunction is not recommended unless definitive therapy (SO ablation) is planned if abnormal SO function is found.

Cholangiography

Cholangiography is essential to exclude stones, tumors, or other biliary obstructions that may cause symptoms identical to those of SO dysfunction. Once such lesions are excluded, ducts that are dilated or that drain slowly suggest obstruction at the level of the SO. A variety of methods to obtain a cholangiogram are available. Intravenous cholangiography has been replaced by

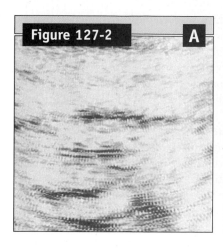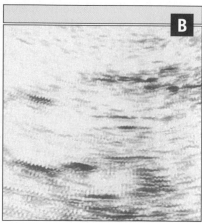

Figure 127-2   **A**   **B**

Secretin-stimulated pancreatic ultrasonography.
A, The pancreatic duct in the unstimulated state.
B, The pancreatic duct has dilated following administration of secretin.

more definitive methods. Helical computed tomographic cholangiography and MR cholangiography appear promising, but need further comparative analysis. Direct cholangiography can be accomplished by percutaneous or intraoperative methods, or more conventionally, at ERCP. Although some controversy exists, extrahepatic ducts that are greater than 12 mm in diameter (postcholecystectomy) when corrected for magnification are considered dilated. Drainage of contrast is influenced by drugs that affect the rate of bile flow and relaxation or contraction of the SO. Such drugs must be avoided to obtain accurate drainage times. Because the common bile duct angulates from anterior to posterior, the patient must be supine to assess gravitational drainage through the sphincter. Although definitive normal supine drainage times have not been well defined [17], a postcholecystectomy biliary tree that fails to empty all contrast media by 45 minutes is generally considered abnormal.

Endoscopic evaluation of the papilla and peripapillary area can yield important information that influences the diagnosis and treatment of patients with suspected SO dysfunction. Occasionally, ampullary cancer may simulate SO dysfunction. The endoscopist should do tissue sampling of the papilla, preferably after sphincterotomy, in suspicious cases [18•].

It is important to assess radiographic features of the pancreatic duct in patients with suspected SO dysfunction. Dilation of the pancreatic duct (>6 mm in the pancreatic head and >5 mm in the body) and delayed contrast drainage time (≥9 minutes in the prone position) may give indirect evidence for the presence of SO dysfunction.

Sphincter of Oddi Manometry

Sphincter of Oddi manometry is the only available method to measure SO motor activity directly. Although SO manometry can be performed intraoperatively and percutaneously, it is most commonly done in the ERCP setting. SO manometry is considered by most authorities to be the gold standard for evaluating patients for SO dysfunction [19]. The use of manometry to detect motility disorders of the SO is similar to its use in other parts of the gastrointestinal tract. Unlike techniques used to study other areas of the gut, SO manometry is more technically demanding and hazardous. Questions remain as to whether

these short-term observations (2–10 minute recordings per pull-through) reflect the "24-hour pathophysiology" of the SO.

Sphincter of Oddi Manometry Technique and Indications

Sphincter of Oddi manometry usually is performed at the time of ERCP. All drugs that relax (anticholinergics, nitrates, calcium channel blockers, glucagon) or stimulate (narcotics, cholinergic agents) the SO should be avoided for at least 8 to 12 hours prior to SO manometry and during the manometric session. Current data indicate that benzodiazepines do not affect the SO pressure, and therefore are acceptable sedation for SO manometry. Meperidine, at a dose of 1 mg/kg or less, does not affect the basal SO pressure, although it does affect the phasic wave characteristics [20]. Because the basal sphincter pressure generally is the only manometric criterion used to diagnose SO dysfunction and determine effectiveness of therapy, meperidine can be used to facilitate conscious sedation for manometry. If glucagon must be used to achieve cannulation, at least an 8- to 10-minute waiting period is required to restore the SO to its basal condition.

Sphincter of Oddi manometry requires selective cannulation of the bile duct, pancreatic duct, or both, often using special aspiration catheters [21]. The duct entered can be identified by gently aspirating on any port (Fig. 127-3; see also *Color Plate*). Yellow-colored fluid seen during endoscopy indicates entry into the bile duct; clear aspirate indicates that the pancreatic duct has been entered. A small amount of dilute contrast can be injected, but this may hinder accurate intraductal pressure measurements and offers no advantage over aspiration. One must be certain that the catheter is not impacted against the wall of the duct in order to ensure accurate pressure measurements. Once deep cannulation is achieved and the patient acceptably sedated, the catheter is withdrawn across the SO at 1- to 2-mm intervals by standard station pull-through technique. Ideally, both the pancreatic and bile ducts should be studied. Abnormal basal SO pressure may be confined to one side of the sphincter in 35%–65% of patients with abnormal manometry [22–24], and thus, one sphincter may be dysfunctional whereas the other may be normal. Raddawi *et al.* [22] reported that an abnormal basal SO was more likely to be confined to the pancreatic duct seg-

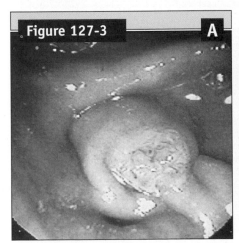
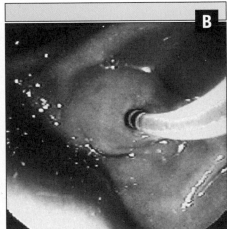
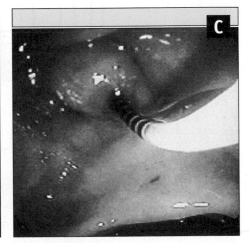

Figure 127-3

The duct entered during sphincter of Oddi manometry can be identified by aspirating the catheter (**A**). Yellow-colored fluid (**B**) signifies entry into the bile duct whereas clear fluid (**C**) indicates pancreatic duct entry. See also **Color Plate**.

ment in patients with pancreatitis and to the bile duct segment in patients with biliary-type pain and elevated liver test results.

Abnormalities of basal SO pressure ideally should be observed for at least 30 seconds in each lead and be seen on two or more separate pull-throughs. From a practical clinical standpoint, a single pull-through from each duct is sufficient if the readings are clearly normal or abnormal. Once the baseline study is done, agents to relax or stimulate the SO can be given and manometric and pain response monitored. The value of these provocative maneuvers for routine use needs further study before widespread application is recommended.

Criteria for interpretation of SO tracing are relatively standard, although there are some areas of disagreement. The basal sphincter pressure is usually defined as the baseline pressure between phasic waves (using the duodenal lumen pressure as the zero reference point) sustained for at least 30 seconds and observed in at least two leads (Fig. 127-4). The amplitude of phasic contraction waves is measured and the mean pressure determined. The number of phasic waves per minute and the duration of the phasic waves also is determined. Most authorities use only the basal SO pressure as an indicator of SO dysfunction; however, data from Kalloo et al. [25•] suggest that intrabiliary pressure, which is easier to measure than SO pressure, correlates with SO basal pressure. In this study, intrabiliary pressure was significantly higher in patients with SO dysfunction than in those with normal SO pressure (20 vs 10 mm Hg; P<0.01). These results await confirmation but support the theory that increased intrabiliary pressure is a cause of pain in SO dysfunction.

The study establishing normal values for intraductal pressure, basal SO pressure, and phasic wave parameters on SO manometry was reported by Guelrud et al. [26••] (Table 127-2); 50 asymptomatic control patients were evaluated, 10 of whom had repeat studies. Thirty-five mm Hg or 40 mm Hg is used as the upper limits of normal for mean basal SO pressure.

Several studies have indicated that pancreatitis is the most common major complication after SO manometry [21]. Using standard perfused catheters, pancreatitis rates as high as 31% have been reported, especially following manometric evaluation of the pancreatic duct in patients with chronic pancreatitis. In one study, Rolny et al. [27•] reported an 11% incidence of pancreatitis following pancreatic duct manometry that rose to 26% in patients with chronic pancreatitis undergoing SO manometry. A variety of methods to decrease the incidence of postmanometry pancreatitis have been proposed and in a prospective randomized study, Sherman et al. [21] found that the aspirating catheter, allowing for aspiration of the perfused fluid from end and side holes while accurately recording pressure from the two remaining sideports, reduced the frequency of pancreatic duct manometry–induced pancreatitis from 31% to 4%. The reduction in pancreatitis with use of this catheter and the very low incidence of pancreatitis after bile duct manometry lend support to the notion that increased pancreatic duct hydrostatic pressure is a major cause of this complication.

Sphincter of Oddi manometry is recommended in patients with idiopathic pancreatitis or unexplained disabling pancreaticobiliary pain with or without hepatic enzyme abnormalities. An attempt can be made to study both sphincters, but clinical decisions can be made if the first sphincter evaluated is found to be abnormal. If an adequate study is not available, an ERCP usually is performed immediately after SO manometry to exclude other potential causes for the patient's symptoms. Indications for the use of SO manometry have also been developed according to the Hogan-Geenen SO dysfunction classification system (Table 127-1). In type I patients there is a general consensus that a structural disorder of the SO (eg, SO stenosis) exists. Although SO manometry may be useful in documenting SO dysfunction, it is not essential before endoscopic or surgical SO ablation. Such patients uniformly benefit from

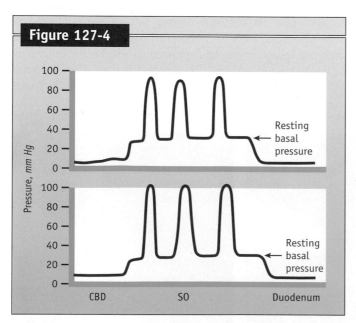

Figure 127-4

Schematic representation of a sphincter of Oddi (SO) manometry recording. Note that the basal sphincter pressure is the baseline pressure between phasic waves (using the duodenal pressure as the zero reference point). CBD—common bile duct.

Table 127-2. Suggested Standard for Abnormal Values for Endoscopic Sphincter of Oddi Manometry Obtained From 50 Volunteers Without Abdominal Symptoms*

Basal sphincter pressure†	>35 mm Hg
Basal ductal pressure	>13 mm Hg
Phasic contractions	
Amplitude	>220 mm Hg
Duration	>8 s
Frequency	>10 min

*Values were obtained by adding 3 standard deviations to the mean (mean obtained by averaging the results on 2–3 station pull-throughs); data combine pancreatic and biliary studies.

†Basal pressures determined by (1) reading the peak basal pressure (ie, highest single lead as obtained using a 3 Lumen catheter), (2) obtaining the mean of these peak pressures from multiple station pull-throughs.

Adapted from Guelrud et al. [26••]. with permission.

SO ablation regardless of the SO manometry results. Type II patients demonstrate SO motor dysfunction in 55% to 65% of cases. In this group, SO manometry is mandatory, as the results of the study predict outcome from SO ablation. Type III patients have pancreaticobiliary pain without objective evidence of SO outflow obstruction, and SO manometry is mandatory to confirm the presence of SO dysfunction. Although not well studied, it appears that the results of SO manometry may predict outcome from SO ablation in these patients.

Stent Trial as Diagnostic Test

Placement of a pancreatic or biliary stent on a trial basis in an attempt to achieve pain relief and predict the response to more definitive therapy (*ie*, SO ablation) has received only limited application. Pancreatic stent trials, especially in patients with normal pancreatic ducts, are strongly discouraged because serious ductal and parenchymal injury may occur if stents are left in place for more than several days [28]. Goff [29] reported a biliary stent trial in 21 type II and III SO dysfunction patients with normal biliary manometry. Stents, 7F, were left in place for at least 2 months if symptoms resolved, and removed sooner if they were judged ineffective. Relief of pain with the stent was predictive of long-term pain relief after biliary sphincterotomy; however, 38% of the patients developed pancreatitis (14% were graded severe) following stent placement. Because of this high rate of complications, biliary stent trials are strongly discouraged.

▮ THERAPY FOR SPHINCTER OF ODDI DYSFUNCTION

The therapy of SO dysfunction is evolving. Historically, most emphasis has been placed on definitive intervention (*ie*, surgical sphincteroplasty or endoscopic sphincterotomy). This appears appropriate for patients with high-grade obstruction (type I, as per Hogan and Geenen criteria). In patients with lesser degrees of obstruction, the clinician must carefully weigh the risks and benefits before recommending invasive therapy. Most reports indicate that patients with SO dysfunction have a complication rate from endoscopic sphincterotomy of at least twice that of patients with ductal stones [30].

Medical Therapy

Medical therapy for documented or suspected SO dysfunction has received only limited study. Because the SO is a smooth muscle structure, it is reasonable to assume that drugs that relax smooth muscle might be effective treatment for SO dysfunction. Sublingual nifedipine and nitrates have been shown to reduce the basal SO pressures in asymptomatic volunteers and symptomatic patients with SO dysfunction [1•]. Khuroo *et al.* [31•] evaluated the clinical benefit of nifedipine in a placebo-controlled crossover trial, and found 21 of 28 patients (75%) with manometrically documented SO dysfunction had a reduction in pain scores, emergency room visits, and use of oral analgesics during short-term follow-up. In a similar study, Sand *et al.* [32•] found that 9 of 12 patients (75%) with suspected type II SO dysfunction improved with nifedipine. Although medical therapy may be an attractive initial approach in patients with SO dysfunction, several drawbacks exist [1•]. First, medication side-effects may be seen in up to one third of patients. Second,

smooth muscle relaxants are unlikely to be of any benefit in patients with the structural form of SO dysfunction (*ie*, SO stenosis), and the response is incomplete in patients with a primary motor abnormality of the SO (*ie*, SO dyskinesia). Finally, long-term outcome from medical therapy has not been reported. Nevertheless, because of the "relative safety" of medical therapy and the benign, although painful, character of SO dysfunction, this approach should be considered in all type III and less severely symptomatic type II patients with SO dysfunction before considering more aggressive SO ablation therapy. Guelrud *et al.* [33] have demonstrated that transcutaneous electrical nerve stimulation (TENS) lowers the basal SO pressure in patients with SO dysfunction by a mean of 38% (but, unfortunately, generally not into the normal range). This stimulation was associated with an increase in serum VIP levels.

Surgical Therapy

Surgery was the traditional therapy of SO dysfunction. The surgical approach, most commonly, is a transduodenal biliary sphincteroplasty with a transampullary septoplasty (pancreatic septoplasty). Sixty percent to 70% of patients were reported to have benefited from this therapy during a 1- to 10-year follow-up [34,35•]. Patients with an elevated basal SO pressure determined by intraoperative SO manometry were more likely to improve from surgical sphincter ablation than those with a normal basal pressure [35•]. Some reports have suggested that patients with biliary-type pain have a better outcome than patients with idiopathic pancreatitis whereas others suggested no difference [34,35•]; however, most studies found that symptom improvement following surgical SO ablation alone was relatively uncommon in patients with established chronic pancreatitis [35•].

The surgical approach for SO dysfunction has largely been replaced by endoscopic therapy. Patient tolerance, cost of care, morbidity, mortality, and cosmetic results are some of the factors that favor an initial endoscopic approach. At present, surgical therapy is reserved for patients with restenosis following endoscopic sphincterotomy and for when endoscopic evaluation and therapy is not available or technically feasible.

Endoscopic Therapy

Endoscopic sphincterotomy is the current standard therapy for patients with SO dysfunction. Most data on endoscopic sphincterotomy relate to biliary SO ablation alone. Clinical improvement following therapy has been reported to occur in 55%–95% of patients (Table 127-1). These variable outcomes are reflective of the different criteria used to document SO dysfunction, the degree of obstruction (type I biliary patients appear to have a better outcome than types II and III), the methods of data collection (retrospective vs prospective), and the techniques used to determine benefit. Using SO manometry, Rolny *et al.* [36] studied 17 type I postcholecystectomy biliary patients, 65% of whom had abnormal SO manometry. During a mean follow-up interval of 2.3 years, all patients benefited from biliary sphincterotomy. The results of this study suggested that since type I biliary patients invariably benefit from biliary sphincterotomy, SO manometry in this patient group is not only unnecessary, but also may be misleading. The results of this study, however, await independent validation.

Table 127-3. Change in the Mean Pain Score and Hospitalization Requirement*

Therapy	Follow-up, y	Mean pain score		Days/months in hospital, n		Patients improved, %
		Pre-Rx	Post-Rx	Pre-Rx	Post-Rx	
ES (n=19)	3.3	9.2	3.9†	0.85	0.23†	68§
S-ES (n=17)	2.2	9.4	7.2	0.87	0.89	24
SSp ± Ccx (n=16)	3.4	9.4	3.3†	0.94	0.27‡	69§

RX—treatment.

*Using a 0 (none) to 10 (most severe) linear pain scale and number of hospital days per month required for pain in patients with manometrically documented sphincter of Oddi dysfunction randomized to endoscopic sphincterotomy (ES), sham sphincterotomy (S-ES), and surgical sphincteroplasty with or without cholecystectomy (SSp±CCx).

†P < 0.04.

‡P = 0.002.

§P = 0.009; ES and SSp±CCx vs S-ES.

Adapted from Sherman et al. [38]; with permission.

Table 127-4. Clinical Benefit Correlated With Sphincter of Oddi Dysfunction Type

SO dysfunction type*	Patients improved, n/total patients, n		
	ES	S-ES	SSp±CCx
II	5/6 (83%)†	1/7 (14%)	8/10 (80%)†
III	8/13 (62%)	3/10 (30%)	3/6 (50%)

ES—endoscopic sphincterotomy; S-ES—sham sphincterotomy; SSP±CCx—surgical sphincteroplasty with or without cholecystectomy.

*Sphincter of Oddi (SO) dysfunction type based on Hogan-Geenen SO dysfunction Classification System.

†P < 0.02; ES and SSp±CCx vs S-ES.

Adapted from Sherman et al. [38]; with permission.

Although most of the studies reporting efficacy of endoscopic therapy in SO dysfunction have been retrospective, two notable randomized trials have been reported. In a landmark study by Geenen *et al.* [37••], 47 patients with postcholecystectomy type II biliary were randomized to biliary sphincterotomy or sham sphincterotomy; SO manometry was performed in all patients but not used as a criterion for randomization. During a 4-year follow-up, 95% of patients with an elevated basal SO benefited from sphincterotomy. In contrast, only 30% to 40% of patients with an elevated sphincter pressure treated by sham sphincterotomy or with a normal SO pressure treated by endoscopic sphincterotomy or sham sphincterotomy benefited from this therapy. The two important findings of this study were that SO manometry predicted the outcome from endoscopic sphincterotomy and that endoscopic sphincterotomy offered long-term benefit in type II biliary patients with SO dysfunction.

Sherman *et al.* [38] reported their preliminary results of a randomized study comparing endoscopic sphincterotomy, surgical biliary sphincteroplasty with pancreatic septoplasty (with or without cholecystectomy) to sham sphincterotomy for type II and III biliary patients with manometrically documented SO dysfunction; the results are shown in Tables 127-3 and 127-4. During a 3-year follow-up period, 69% of patients undergoing endoscopic or surgical SO ablation improved compared with 24% in the sham sphincterotomy group (P=0.009). There was a trend for type II patients to benefit more frequently from SO ablation than type III patients (13 of 16 [81%] vs 11 of 19 [58%]; P=0.14). Evidence is now accumulating that the addition of a pancreatic sphincterotomy to an endoscopic biliary sphincterotomy in such patients may further improve outcome. Long-term outcome studies are awaited.

Balloon Dilation and Stenting

Balloon dilation of strictures in the gastrointestinal tract has become commonplace. In an attempt to be less invasive and preserve SO function, adaptation of this technique to treat SO dysfunction has been described. Unfortunately, because of the unacceptably high complication rates, primarily pancreatitis, this technology has little role in the management of SO dysfunction [39]. Similarly, although biliary stenting might offer short-term symptom benefit in patients with SO dysfunction and predict outcome from sphincter ablation, it too has unacceptably high complication rates and cannot be advocated in this setting [29].

Botulinum Toxin Injection

Botulinum toxin (Botox; Allergan, Irvine, CA), a potent inhibitor of acetylcholine release from nerve endings, has been successfully applied to smooth muscle disorders of the gastrointestinal tract, such as achalasia. In a preliminary clinical trial, Botox injection into the SO resulted in a 50% reduction in the basal sphincter pressure and improved bile flow [40]. This reduction in pressure may be accompanied by symptom improvement in some patients. Although further study is warranted, Botox may serve as a therapeutic trial for patients with SO dysfunction, with responders undergoing permanent SO ablation.

SPHINCTER OF ODDI DYSFUNCTION IN RECURRENT PANCREATITIS

Sphincter of Oddi dysfunction has been documented manometrically in 15% to 59% of patients with recurrent pancreatitis, previously labeled as idiopathic [14•]. Biliary sphincterotomy alone has been reported to prevent further pancreatitis episodes in more than 50% of such patients. From a scientific, but not practical viewpoint, care must be taken to separate out subtle biliary pancreatitis [41•] that also will similarly respond to biliary sphincterotomy. The value of ERCP, SO manometry, and SO ablation therapy was studied in 51 patients with idiopathic pancreatitis [19], 24 (47.1%) of whom had an elevated basal SO pressure. Twenty patients were treated by biliary sphincterotomy and 10 had surgical sphincteroplasty with septoplasty. Fifteen of 18 patients (83%) with an elevated basal SO pressure had long-term benefit from SO ablation therapy (including 10 of 11 treated by biliary sphincterotomy) in contrast to only 4 of 12 (33.3%) with a normal basal SO pressure (including 4 of 9 treated by biliary sphincterotomy). However, Guelrud *et al.* [42] found that severance of the pancreatic sphincter was necessary to resolve the pancreatitis (Table 127-5). In this series, 69 patients with idiopathic pancreatitis due to SO dysfunction underwent treatment by standard biliary sphincterotomy, 24 patients had biliary sphincterotomy with pancreatic sphincter balloon dilation, 13 patients had biliary sphincterotomy followed by pancreatic sphincterotomy in separate sessions, and 14 patients had combined pancreatic and biliary sphincterotomy in the same session; 81% of patients undergoing pancreatic and biliary sphincterotomy had resolution of their pancreatitis compared with 28% of patients undergoing biliary sphincterotomy alone. These data are consistent with the theory that many such patients who benefit from biliary sphincterotomy alone have subtle gallstone pancreatitis. The results of Guelrud *et al.* [42] also support the anatomic findings of separate biliary and pancreatic sphincters and the manometry findings of residual pancreatic sphincter hypertension in more than 50% of persistently symptomatic patients who undergo biliary sphincterotomy alone. Currently, the best method to treat residual pancreatic sphincter stenosis (after biliary sphincterotomy) awaits further study. Patients with idiopathic pancreatitis who fail to respond to biliary sphincterotomy alone should have their pancreatic sphincter reevaluated and be considered for sphincter ablation if residual high pressure is found.

Table 127-5. Response to Sphincter Therapy in Pancreatic Sphincter Dysfunction and Recurrent Pancreatitis

Treatment	Number of patients improved/ Total number of patients, %
Biliary sphincterotomy alone	5/18 (28%)
Biliary sphincterotomy followed by pancreatic sphincter balloon dilation	13/24 (54%)
Biliary sphincterotomy plus pancreatic sphincterotomy at later session	10/13 (77%)*
Biliary sphincterotomy and pancreatic sphincterotomy at same session	12/14 (86%)*

* P < 0.005 vs biliary sphincterotomy alone.
Adapted from Guelrud et al. [42].

FAILURE TO ACHIEVE SYMPTOMATIC IMPROVEMENT AFTER BILIARY SPHINCTEROTOMY

There are several potential explanations as to why patients may fail to achieve symptom relief after biliary sphincterotomy is performed for well-documented SO dysfunction (Table 127-6). First, the biliary sphincterotomy may have been inadequate or restenosis may have occurred. Although the biliary sphincter commonly is not totally ablated [43•], Manoukian *et al.* [44] indicate that clinically significant biliary restenosis occurs relatively infrequently. If no "cutting space" remains in such a patient, balloon dilation to 8 to 10 mm may suffice, but long-term outcome from such therapy is unknown [39].

Second, the importance of pancreatic sphincter ablation is increasingly being recognized, as noted in the data preliminarily reported by Guelrud *et al.* [42]. Soffer and Johlin [45] reported that 25 of 26 patients (mostly type II) who failed to respond to biliary sphincterotomy had elevated pancreatic sphincter pressure. Endoscopic pancreatic sphincterotomy was performed with overall symptomatic improvement in two thirds of patients.

Third, patients may fail to respond to sphincterotomy because they have chronic pancreatitis; such patients may or may not have abnormal pancreatograms. Intraductal pancreatic juice aspiration and analysis for volume, amylase, and bicarbonate concentration after secretin stimulation may help make this diagnosis. Endoscopic ultrasound may show parenchymal and ductular changes, suggesting chronic pancreatitis in some of these patients [46].

Fourth, some patients may be having pain from altered gut motility of the stomach, small bowel, or colon (irritable bowel or pseudo-obstruction variants). There is increasing evidence that upper gastrointestinal motility disorders may masquerade as pancreatobiliary-type pain [47•]. This area needs more study to determine the frequency, significance, and possible coexistence of these motor disorders along with SO dysfunction.

SUMMARY

In summary, SO dysfunction and the manometric techniques used to assist in this diagnosis are evolving. Successful endoscopic SO manometry requires good ERCP skills and careful attention to detail. If SO dysfunction is suspected in a patient with type III or mild to moderate pain level type II, medical therapy should be attempted first. If medical therapy fails, ERCP and manometric evaluation are recommended. The role of less invasive studies

Table 127-6. Causes for Failure to Achieve Symptom Relief After Biliary Sphincterotomy in Sphincter of Oddi Dysfunction

Residual or recurrent biliary sphincter dysfunction
Pancreatic sphincter (major papilla) dysfunction
Chronic pancreatitis—subtle, pancreatogram normal
Other obstructive pancreaticobiliary pathology (stones, strictures, tumor, pancreas divisum)
Nonpancreatobiliary disease, especially gut motor disorders or irritable bowel syndrome

remains uncertain because of their undefined sensitivity and specificity. SO ablation is generally warranted in symptomatic type I patients and in type II and III patients with abnormal manometry with a symptom relief rate of 55% to 95%. Initial nonresponders require thorough pancreatic sphincter and pancreatic parenchymal evaluation. Patients with SO dysfunction have relatively high complication rates after diagnostic or therapeutic ERCP. Thorough review of the risk-to-benefit ratio is mandatory for each patient.

ACKNOWLEDGMENT

The authors are grateful to Tina Jackson for the technical preparation of this document.

REFERENCES

Recently published papers of particular interest have been highlighted as follows:
• Of interest
•• Of outstanding interest

1.• Kalloo AN, Pasricha PJ: Therapy of sphincter of Oddi dysfunction. *Gastrointest Endosc Clin North Am* 1996, 6:117–125.
Current therapies of sphincter of Oddi dysfunction are reviewed in this paper.

2.• Hogan W, Sherman S, Pasricha P, Carr-Locke DL: Position paper on sphincter of Oddi manometry. *Gastrointest Endosc* 1997, 45:342–348.
This position paper on sphincter of Oddi manometry was developed by the biliary motility subspecialty group of the American Motility Society. The use and methodology of sphincter of Oddi manometry are detailed. Issues regarding training in sphincter of Oddi manometry and its impact on patient care are reviewed.

3. Richards RD, Yeaton P, Shaffer HA, *et al.*: Human sphincter of Oddi motility and cholecystokinin response following liver transplantation. *Dig Dis Sci* 1993, 38:462–468.

4. Becker JM, Parodi JM: Basic control mechanisms of sphincter of Oddi motor function. *Gastrointest Endosc Clin North Am* 1993, 3:41–66.

5. Anderson TM, Pitt HA, Longmire WP: Experience with sphincteroplasty and sphincterotomy in pancreatobiliary surgery. *Ann Surg* 1985, 201:399–406.

6. Drossman DA, Zhiming L, Andruzzi E, *et al.*: US Householder Survey of functional gastrointestinal disorders: prevalence, sociodemography, and health impact. *Dig Dis Sci* 1993, 38:1569–1580.

6a. Guelrud M, Mendoza S, Mujica V, Uzcategui: Sphincter of Oddi (SO) motor function in patients with symptomatic gallstones. *Gastroenterology* 1993, 104:A361.

7. Ruffolo TA, Sherman S, Lehman GA, Hawes RH: Gallbladder ejection fraction and its relationship to sphincter of Oddi dysfunction. *Dig Dis Sci* 1994, 39:289–292.

8. Black NA, Thompson E, Sanderson CFB, ECHSS Group: Symptoms and health status before and six weeks after open cholecystectomy: a European cohort study. *Gut* 1994, 35:1301–1305.

9. Neoptolemos JA, Bailey IS, Carr-Locke D: Sphincter of Oddi dysfunction: results of endoscopic sphincterotomy. *Br J Surg* 1988, 75:454–459.

10. Roberts-Thomson IC, Toouli J: Is endoscopic sphincterotomy for disabling biliary-type pain after cholecystectomy effective? *Gastrointest Endosc* 1985, 31:370–373.

11.• Sherman S, Troiano FP, Hawes RH, *et al.*: Frequency of abnormal sphincter of Oddi manometry compared with the clinical suspicion of sphincter of Oddi dysfunction. *Am J Gastroenterol* 1991, 86:586–590.
This study examines the frequency of abnormal sphincter of Oddi manometry based on a sphincter of Oddi dysfunction classification system. For patients with type I, II, or III sphincter of Oddi dysfunction, the frequency of an abnormal manometry was approximately 89%, 57%, and 32%, respectively.

12. Meshinpoor H, Mollot M: Sphincter of Oddi dysfunction and unexplained abdominal pain: clinical and manometric study. *Dig Dis Sci* 1992, 37:257–261.

13.• Botoman VA, Kozarek RA, Novel LA, *et al.*: Long term outcome after endoscopic sphincterotomy in patients with biliary colic and suspected sphincter of Oddi dysfunction. *Gastrointest Endosc* 1994, 40:165–170.
In this study, seventy-three highly selected patients (35 type II, 38 type III) with biliary type pain underwent sphincter of Oddi manometry. The frequency of sphincter of Oddi dysfunction (60% vs 55%), improvement after endoscopic sphincterotomy at a mean follow-up of 3 years (68% vs 56%), and the postprocedure pancreatitis rates (16% vs 15%) were similar for the two groups.

14.• Lehman GA, Sherman S: Sphincter of Oddi dysfunction. *Int J Pancreatol* 1997, 20:11–25.
Pathogenesis, diagnosis, and therapy of sphincter of Oddi dysfunction are reviewed.

15. Warshaw AL, Simeone J, Schapiro RH, *et al.*: Objective evaluation of ampullary stenosis with ultrasonography and pancreatic stimulation. *Am J Surg* 1985, 149:65–72.

16. Sostre S, Kalloo AN, Spiegler EJ, *et al.*: A noninvasive test of sphincter of Oddi dysfunction in postcholecystectomy patients: the scintigraphic score. *J Nucl Med* 1992, 33:1216–1222.

17. Elta GH, Barnett JL, Ellis JH, *et al.*: Delayed biliary drainage is common in asymptomatic post-cholecystectomy volunteers. *Gastrointest Endosc* 1992, 38:435–439.

18.• Ponchon T, Aucia N, Mitchell R, *et al.*: Biopsies of the ampullary region in patients suspected to have sphincter of Oddi dysfunction. *Gastrointest Endosc* 1995, 42:452–456.
In this study, 69 patients with presumed sphincter of Oddi dysfunction (18 type I, 51 type II) were treated with endoscopic sphincterotomy. Three patients (4.3%) were found to have an ampullary adenocarcinoma on biopsies of the intra-ampullary region done an average of 7 weeks after the sphincterotomy. The authors advocated biopsying all patients suspected of having sphincter of Oddi dysfunction and treated by endoscopic sphincterotomy.

19. Lans JL, Parikh NP, Geenen JE: Application of sphincter of Oddi manometry in routine clinical investigations. *Endoscopy* 1991, 23:139–143.

20. Sherman S, Gottlieb K, Uzer MF, *et al.*: Effects of meperidine on the pancreatic and biliary sphincter. *Gastrointest Endosc* 1996, 44:239–242.

21. Sherman S, Troiano FP, Hawes RH, Lehman GA: Sphincter of Oddi manometry: decreased risk of clinical pancreatitis with the use of a modified aspirating catheter. *Gastrointest Endosc* 1990, 36:462–466.

22. Raddawi H, Geenen J, Hogan W, *et al.*: Pressure measurements from biliary and pancreatic segments of sphincter of Oddi: comparison between patients with functional abdominal pain, biliary, or pancreatic disease. *Dig Dis Sci* 1991, 36:71–74.

23. Rolny P, Ärlebäck A, Funch-Jensen P, *et al.*: Clinical significance of manometric assessment of both pancreatic duct and bile duct sphincter in the same patient. *Scand J Gastroenterol* 1989, 24:751–754.

24. Silverman WB, Ruffolo TA, Sherman S, *et al.*: Correlation of basal sphincter pressures measured from both the bile duct and pancreatic duct in patients with suspected sphincter of Oddi dysfunction. *Gastrointest Endosc* 1992, 38:440–443.

25.• Kalloo AN, Tietjen TG, Pasricha PJ: Does intrabiliary pressure predict basal sphincter of Oddi pressure: study in patients with and without gallbladders. *Gastrointest Endosc* 1996, 44:696–699.
The intrabiliary pressure is an easier parameter to record at manometry than the basal sphincter pressure. The results of this study suggest that intrabiliary pressure correlates with the sphincter of Oddi basal pressure. This study needs to be confirmed at other centers.

26.•• Guelrud M, Mendoza S, Rossiter G, Villegas MI: Sphincter of Oddi manometry in healthy volunteers. *Dig Dis Sci* 1990, 35:38–46.
This is the best study in establishing normal values for intraductal pressure, basal sphincter pressure, and phasic wave parameters. The study population was 50 asymptomatic patients.

27.• Rolny P, Anderberg B, Ihse I, *et al.*: Pancreatitis after sphincter of Oddi manometry. *Gut* 1990, 31:821–824.

28. Kozarek RA: Pancreatic stents can induce ductal changes consistent with chronic pancreatitis. *Gastrointest Endosc* 1990, 36:93–95.

29. Goff JS: Common bile duct sphincter of Oddi stenting in patients with suspected sphincter of Oddi dysfunction. *Am J Gastroenterol* 1995, 90:586–589.

30. Sherman S, Ruffolo TA, Hawes RH, Lehman GA: Complications of endoscopic sphincterotomy. *Gastroenterology* 1991, 101:1068–1075.

31.• Khuroo MS, Zargar SA, Yattoo GN: Efficacy of nifedipine therapy in patients with sphincter of Oddi dysfunction: a prospective, double-blind, randomized, placebo-controlled, crossover trial. *Br J Clin Pharmacol* 1992, 33:477–485.
The clinical benefit of nifedipine was studied in this placebo-controlled crossover trial. Twenty-one of 28 patients (75%) with manometrically documented sphincter of Oddi dysfunction had a reduction in pain scores, emergency room visits, and use of oral analgesics during short-term follow-up.

32.• Sand J, Nordback I, Koskinen M, *et al.*: Nifedipine for suspected type II sphincter of Oddi dyskinesia. *Am J Gastroenterol* 1993, 88:530–535.

33. Guelrud M, Rossiter A, Souney P, *et al.*: The effect of transcutaneous nerve stimulation on sphincter of Oddi pressure in patients with biliary dyskinesia. *Am J Gastroenterol* 1991, 86:581–585.

34. Moody FG, Vecchio R, Calabuig R, Runkel N: Transduodenal sphincteroplasty with transampullary septectomy for stenosing papillitis. *Am J Surgery* 1991, 161:213–218.

35.• Sherman S, Hawes RH, Madura J, Lehman GA: Comparison of intraoperative and endoscopic manometry of the sphincter of Oddi. *Surg Gynecol Obstet* 1992, 175:410–418.

36. Rolny P, Geenen JE, Hogan WJ: Post-cholecystectomy patients with "objective signs" of partial bile outflow obstruction: clinical characteristics, sphincter of Oddi manometry findings, and results of therapy. *Gastrointest Endosc* 1993, 39:778–781.

37.•• Geenen JE, Hogan WJ, Dodds WJ, *et al.*: The efficacy of endoscopic sphincterotomy after cholecystectomy in patients with suspected sphincter of Oddi dysfunction. *N Engl J Med* 1989, 320:82–87.
This landmark study showed that sphincter of Oddi manometry predicted the outcome from endoscopic sphincterotomy and that endoscopic sphincterotomy offered long-term benefit in type II biliary patients with manometrically documented sphincter of Oddi dysfunction.

38. Sherman S, Lehman GA, Jamidar P, *et al.*: Efficacy of endoscopic sphincterotomy and surgical sphincteroplasty for patients with sphincter of Oddi dysfunction (SOD): Randomized, controlled study. *Gastrointest Endosc* 1994, 40:A125.

39. Kozarek RA: Balloon dilation of the sphincter of Oddi. *Endoscopy* 1988, 20:207–210.

40. Pasricha PJ, Miskovsky EP, Kalloo AN: Intrasphincter injection of botulinum toxin for suspected sphincter of Oddi dysfunction. *Gut* 1994, 35:1319–1321.

41.• Ros E, Navarro S, Bru C, *et al.*: Occult microlithiasis in idiopathic acute pancreatitis: prevention of relapses by cholecystectomy or ursodeoxycholic acid therapy. *Gastroenterology* 1991, 101:1701–1709.

42. Guelrud M, Plaz J, Mendoza S, *et al.*: Endoscopic treatment in type II pancreatic sphincter dysfunction. *Gastrointest Endosc* 1995, 41:A398.

43.• Heinerman PM, Graf AH, Boeckl O: Does endoscopic sphincterotomy destroy the function of Oddi's sphincter? *Arch Surg* 1994, 129:876–880.

44. Manoukian AV, Schmalz MJ, Geenen JE, *et al.*: The incidence of post-sphincterotomy stenosis in group II patients with sphincter of Oddi dysfunction. *Gastrointest Endosc* 1993, 39:496–498.

45. Soffer EE, Johlin FC: Intestinal dysmotility in patients with sphincter of Oddi dysfunction: a reason for failed response to sphincterotomy. *Dig Dis Sci* 1994, 39:1942–1946.

46. Wiersema MJ, Hawes RH, Lehman GA, *et al.*: Prospective evaluation of endoscopic ultrasonography and endoscopic retrograde cholangiopancreatography in patients with chronic abdominal pain of suspected pancreatic origin. *Endoscopy* 1993, 25:555–564.

47.• Koussayer T, Ducker TE, Clench MH, Mathias JR: Ampulla of Vater/duodenal wall spasm diagnosed by antroduodenal manometry. *Dig Dis Sci* 1995, 40:1710–1719.

128 Primary Sclerosing Cholangitis
Wisam F. Zakko

Primary sclerosing cholangitis (PSC) is a chronic cholestatic liver disease of unknown cause characterized by inflammation, destruction of the intrahepatic and extrahepatic bile ducts, and fibrosis. The disease is progressive, leading to cirrhosis, portal hypertension, and liver failure. Although a rare cause of liver disease, PSC is the fourth leading indication for liver transplantation in the United States. The disease typically occurs in patients with inflammatory bowel disease (IBD) but may be seen alone or in association with other disorders.

◼ CLASSIFICATION AND ASSOCIATED DISORDERS

Sclerosing cholangitis may be either primary or secondary to a variety of disorders, including surgical trauma, bile duct stones,

ischemia, and toxic agents. In 70% to 80% of patients with PSC, an associated disorder exists (Table 128-1).

Inflammatory bowel disease, most commonly ulcerative colitis, is the disorder most frequently associated with PSC, occurring in approximately 75% of patients (Table 128-2) [1]. When IBD is associated with PSC, early onset of colitis and more extensive disease tend to occur; however, most of these patients are mildly symptomatic at presentation [2••,3]. Although the course of PSC does not parallel that of colitis, its presence seems to be a risk factor for increased mortality, dysplasia, colorectal cancer [4,5], and pouchitis when an ileal pouch–anal anastomosis is performed [6]. Smoking cigarettes appears to protect against development of PSC in patients with ulcerative colitis [7].

An abnormal pancreatogram occurs in a varying number of patients with PSC (0%–77%) [8]. It is not clear whether these radiographic changes are nonspecific secondary effects of cholestasis or whether the same pathologic process involves the pancreatic ducts. Other disorders are rarely associated with PSC (Table 128-2).

EPIDEMIOLOGY

The prevalence of PSC in the United States is unknown. It occurs in 2.3% to 6% of patients with ulcerative colitis, for an estimated incidence of 2 to 7 per 100,000 population. This is probably an underestimate because *most but not all* patients with PSC have ulcerative colitis. The median age at diagnosis is 39 years; however, PSC can affect persons of any age. Of patients with PSC, 60% to 70% are male [9•].

PATHOGENESIS

The cause of PSC is unknown. Portal bacteremia, increased hepatic copper levels, viral infections of the biliary tract, and toxic bile acid metabolites have all been suggested as possible pathogenic mechanisms, albeit without supporting evidence.

Immune and genetic factors appear more likely to be involved in the pathogenesis of PSC based on the high frequency of auto-antibodies; association with other autoimmune diseases; and association with HLA-B8, DR3, DR2, and DR4. Furthermore, an aberrant expression of major histocompatibility class II HLA molecules in biliary epithelial cells occurs, suggesting that bile duct epithelial cells act as autoantigens to host lymphocytes.

PATHOLOGY

Primary sclerosing cholangitis may involve the intrahepatic or extrahepatic bile ducts, or both. In less than 5% of cases, PSC involves only the small intrahepatic ducts. When affected, the large ducts appear as thickened cords with marked intraluminal narrowing. Layers of fibrous tissue and chronic inflammation surround the ductal walls.

As in other cholangiopathies of the small ducts, involvement of the intrahepatic bile ducts can be divided into four stages. In stage I, the disease is confined primarily to the portal tract, with enlargement of the portal area and an increase in inflammatory cells and collagen. Infiltration of the bile ducts with lymphocytes and ductular proliferation may be noted (Fig. 128-1, see also **Color Plate**) [10]. In stage II, the lesion involves the periportal area where tongues of ductular profiles surrounded by collagen, inflammatory cells, and edema extend into the parenchyma. Ductopenia is a prominent feature of this stage. Stage III marks the onset of septal fibrosis, the periportal reaction leading to formation of fibrous bands bridging one portal tract to the other. Stage IV is that of biliary cirrhosis with loss of normal architecture, the formation of portal-central septa, and nodular regeneration.

In less than 40% of cases a characteristic lesion called *fibrous obliterative cholangitis* is seen. The presence of concentric periductal fibrosis that progressively obliterates medium-sized ducts in the portal space characterizes this lesion (Figs. 128-2 and 128-3, see also **Color Plate**) [10]. This obliteration leads to progressive atrophy and in some cases complete disappearance of the duct, leaving only fibrous scar remnants [11].

Table 128-1. Classification of Sclerosing Cholangitis	
Primary sclerosing cholangitis	**Secondary sclerosing cholangitis**
Associated with other diseases	Choledocholithiasis
No associated disease	Surgical trauma
	Cholangiocarcinoma
	Ischemia (liver allograft rejection, vascular trauma during surgery)
	Infection (AIDS cholangiopathy)
	Chronic pancreatitis
	Toxic agents:
	Injection of hepatic echino-coccal cysts with formalde-hyde or hypertonic saline
	Intra-arterial infusion of floxuridine

Table 128-2. Disorders Associated With Primary Sclerosing Cholangitis	
Common disorders	**Rare disorders**
Inflammatory bowel disease:	Autoimmune hemolytic anemia
Ulcerative colitis (65–70%)	Celiac disease
Crohn's disease (5–10%)	Diabetes mellitus
Pancreatitis	Riedel's thyroiditis
	Retroperitoneal fibrosis
	Rheumatoid arthritis
	Sarcoidosis
	Sjögren's syndrome

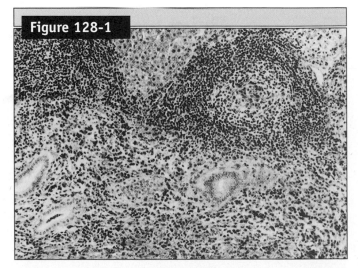

Figure 128-1

Intense inflammatory reaction surrounding a bile duct. The bile duct epithelium is infiltrated with lymphocytes. This patient had pruritus, elevated alkaline phosphatase, and a cholangiogram typical of PSC (hematoxylin and eosin stain; original magnification × 200). See also **Color Plate**. (*From* Gitlin and Strauss [10]; with permission.)

■ CLINICAL FEATURES

In primary sclerosing cholangitis, patients may present with right upper quadrant abdominal pain, pruritus, fatigue, and weight loss, or with symptoms related to complications such as cholangitis, cirrhosis, or cholangiocarcinoma. At presentation, however, up to 44% of patients are asymptomatic. These patients are diagnosed only because of abnormal test results of a screening liver biochemistry profile (Table 128-3) [9•,12].

Chronic cholestasis. Pruritus is most likely caused by the accumulation of endogenous opiates and stimulation of neurogenic opioid receptors and not by retention of bile acids and their sequestration in the skin, as previously thought. Itching is worse at night and in warm weather, and it is exacerbated by eating fatty meals. Pruritus can be debilitating and can lead to severe excoriations.

Steatorrhea and fat malabsorption occur late in the course of PSC and are due to decreased secretion of conjugated bile acids into the lumen of the small intestine. Low levels of vitamins A, D, and E have been demonstrated in a significant number of patients [13]. Metabolic bone disease and compression fractures occur more frequently than previously thought and are due to osteoporosis rather than osteomalacia [14]. Because of colonic bacterial synthesis of vitamin K, clinical vitamin K deficiency rarely occurs. It is seen in advanced disease and in patients treated with cholestyramine.

Cholangitis. Severe acute cholangitis is rare in the absence of previous biliary surgery or interventional endoscopic procedures. Fluctuating symptoms of low-grade fever, mild abdominal pain, and jaundice occur in up to 15% of patients with PSC who have not had previous surgery. These symptoms are probably caused by microlithiasis, leading to transient biliary obstruction in a strictured area.

End-stage liver disease and periostomal varices. Primary sclerosing cholangitis is progressive and ultimately leads to cirrhosis. End-stage liver disease occurs in 30% of patients with PSC after a follow-up period longer than 7 years. These patients may present with variceal bleeding, ascites, and encephalopathy. Patients with PSC and ulcerative colitis who undergo total colectomy and ileostomy may develop stomal or peristomal varices, leading to bleeding that is often difficult to control (Fig. 128-4, see also **Color Plate**).

Cholangiocarcinoma. Cholangiocarcinoma complicates PSC in up to 30% of cases, as shown at autopsy or on examination of the explanted liver [15]. Symptoms suspicious for malignant transformation include progressive weight loss, worsening jaundice, abdominal pain, sudden onset of bacterial cholangitis, and superficial thrombophlebitis [16]. Risk factors for cholangiocarcinoma

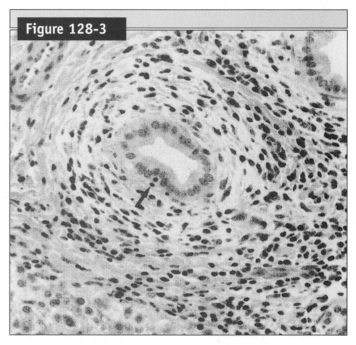

Figure 128-3

"Onion skin" lesion. The bile duct is surrounded by concentric fibrosis. Note two lymphocytes in the epithelium of the bile duct (*arrow*) (hematoxylin and eosin stain; original magnification × 200). See also **Color Plate**. (*From* Gitlin and Strauss [10]; with permission.)

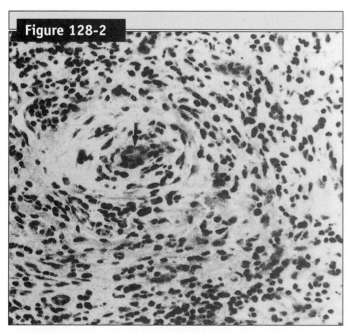

Figure 128-2

Concentric fibrosis surrounding a bile duct with an intense inflammatory reaction. The bile duct contains lymphocytes (*arrow*) (hematoxylin and eosin stain; original magnification × 200). See also **Color Plate**. (*From* Gitlin and Strauss [10]; with permission.)

Table 128-3. Symptoms of Primary Sclerosing Cholangitis at Presentation

Symptom	Patients, %
Asymptomatic	44
Abdominal pain	37
Pruritus	30
Jaundice	30
Fever	17
Ascites	4
Variceal hemorrhage	4

From Broom et al. [9]; with permission.

are older age, presence of liver cirrhosis, and long-standing ulcerative colitis. The tumor is most commonly located at the hepatic bifurcation and can be multicentric in origin. Prognosis is poor, with patients rarely surviving beyond 2 years from the time of diagnosis.

DIAGNOSIS

The diagnosis of PSC can be made in any patient with a cholestatic liver chemistry profile and typical cholangiogram or liver histology and in whom all other secondary causes of sclerosing cholangitis have been excluded.

Laboratory Findings

Alkaline phosphatase levels are commonly elevated, averaging fourfold normal, but may be normal in 8% of patients with PSC. The level does not correlate with the histologic severity of disease. Transaminase levels are mildly to moderately elevated in most patients. Bilirubin levels fluctuate and are usually normal on presentation [9•].

The test for perinuclear antineutrophil cytoplasm antibodies (pANCAs) is 65% sensitive and 72% specific in diagnosing PSC. Using a higher dilution of serum increases the specificity but decreases the sensitivity of the test. The presence of pANCAs is correlated with involvement of the extrahepatic and intrahepatic biliary tree but not with histologic severity. pANCAs are also seen in patients with autoimmune hepatitis type 1; however, it is not seen in other forms of chronic liver disease or large duct obstruction (Table 128-4) [17]. Antinuclear antibodies and anti–smooth muscle antibodies are seen in low titer in one third of cases. Serum IgM levels are mildly elevated in about half the cases, and generalized hyper-gammaglobulinemia occurs in one third of patients.

Imaging Studies

Endoscopic retrograde choleangiopancreatography. Imaging the biliary tree is essential to make the diagnosis of PSC and is usually accomplished endoscopically. Endoscopic retrograde cholangiopancreatography (ERCP) is performed to make the

initial diagnosis, to provide therapy for known symptomatic dominant strictures, and to exclude the presence of cholangio-carcinoma in patients who are deteriorating. Cholangiographic features of PSC include the presence of multiple strictures alternating with normal or slightly dilated ducts, giving the ducts a beaded appearance (Fig. 128-5). Other findings include diverticulum-like outpouchings, which are thought to be characteristic, and mural irregularities, particularly in the common bile duct. Changes are diffuse, usually involving both the intrahepatic and extrahepatic ducts. The extrahepatic ducts are involved in most patients; however, in 20% to 30% of cases the involvement of the extrahepatic ducts is either absent or, more commonly, is confined to a short segment at the hilum of the liver near the hepatic bifurcation. One caveat is that under-filling of the ducts can give the radiographic appearance of strictures, falsely suggesting PSC.

Magnetic resonance cholangiopancreatography. Magnetic resonance cholangiopancreatography (MRCP) is an evolving imaging tool for evaluation of the biliary system and the pancreatic duct. MRCP is noninvasive and requires neither intravenously nor orally administered contrast material. This technique has been used successfully to detect common bile duct stones and dilated hepatic and pancreatic ducts caused by neoplasms. Recently, MRCP has been reported to be useful in diagnosing PSC and cholangiocarcinoma (Fig. 128-6) [18]. Presently, because of its low spatial resolution, discrete irregu-larities of the peripheral bile ducts and subtle ectasia of the common bile duct can be missed (Fig. 128-7) [18,19].

Ultrasonography and CT scan. Ultrasonography and CT scan are rarely diagnostic of PSC, and these techniques are more often used when cholangiocarcinoma is suspected. Features suggestive of PSC include mural thickening of the extrahepatic ducts, segmental dilation, intrahepatic stones, and gallbladder

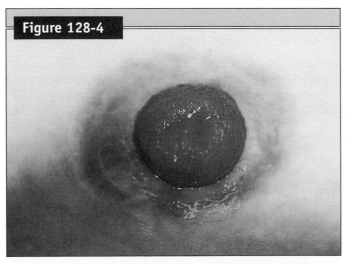

Figure 128-4

Peristomal blue halo due to portal hypertension and varices in a patient with Crohn's disease, primary sclerosing cholangitis, and recurrent stomal bleeding. See also **Color Plate.**

Table 128-4. pANCA in PSC and Other Liver Disease		
Liver disease	**pANCA at 1:5, %**	**pANCA at 1:50, %**
PSC with ulcerative colitis	70	54
PSC with Crohn's disease	67	50
PSC only	29	14
All PSC	65	49
Autoimmune hepatitis	49	11
Primary biliary cirrhosis	6	3
Alcoholic cirrhosis	0	–
Large duct obstruction	0	–
Hemochromatosis	0	–
Cryptogenic cirrhosis	0	–
Control group	0	–

pANCA—Perinuclear antineutrophil cytoplasm antibody; PSC—primary sclerosing cholangitis.
Modified from Bansi, Chapman, and Fleming [16].

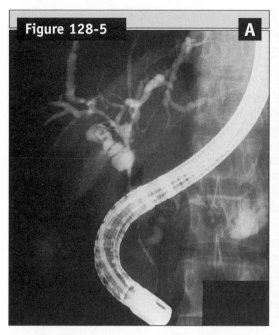

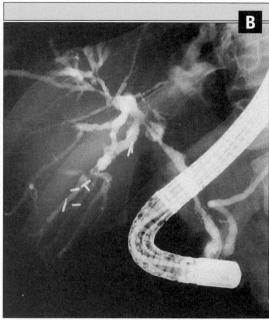

Figure 128-5

Endoscopic retrograde cholangiopancreatography in sclerosing cholangitis. **A,** Changes in the intrahepatic and extrahepatic biliary tree. The cystic duct is particularly dilated proximal to a distal bile duct stricture. **B,** Mural irregularities in the common bile duct, stricture in the common hepatic duct and typical changes in the intrahepatic ducts. (*Courtesy of* D. Carr-Locke, MD.)

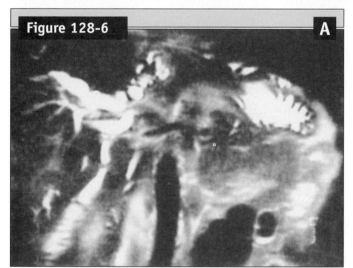

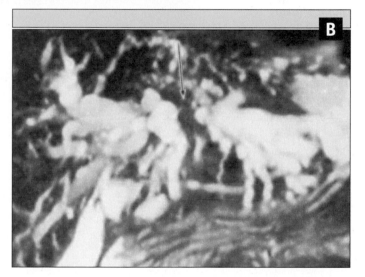

Figure 128-6

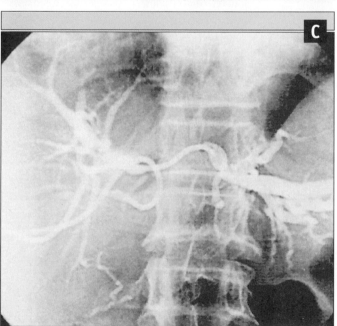

MRI cholangiopancreatography (MRCP) in a man 62 years of age with hilar cholangiocarcinoma. **A,** Coronal source image of MRCP shows severe dilation of the right intrahepatic bile ducts caused by hilar obstruction. **B,** Maximum intensity projection image of MRCP demonstrates hilar obstruction (*arrow*) and dilated intrahepatic bile ducts in both lobes. **C,** Percutaneous transhepatic cholangiogram in the same patient shows the typical appearance of hilar obstruction with separation and dilation of intrahepatic ducts in both lobes. (*From* Choi *et al.* [18]; with permission.)

wall thickening. Cross-sectional imaging also can help confirm the presence of advanced disease by demonstrating heterogeneity of the liver and signs of portal hypertension.

Liver Biopsy

Although liver biopsy is almost always abnormal in PSC, it has a limited role. Liver biopsy is diagnostic in less than 40% of cases and only when fibrous obliterative cholangitis is seen. In most cases the biopsy is nonspecific, showing only portal and periportal inflammation, and may be interpreted as chronic hepatitis. Liver biopsy, however, is useful to stage the disease (see previous section on "Pathology"), and it is the only diagnostic tool in patients with small duct PSC. Sampling variability has been noted with percutaneous liver biopsies [20].

Diagnosis of Cholangiocarcinoma in Patients with Primary Sclerosing Cholangitis

Diagnostic tools include tumor markers, imaging, and cytology. The diagnosis is notoriously difficult to make in patients with PSC, despite the use of all three modalities.

Tumor Markers

CA19-9 in values over 100 μ/mL was found to be 89% sensitive and 86% specific for diagnosing cholangiocarcinoma in patients

with PSC [21]. A more recent study showed that a combination of serum carcinoembryonic antigen (CEA) and serum CA19-9 (using the formula CA19-9 + [CEA x 40]) has a sensitivity of 66% and specificity of 100% (Table 128-5) [22].

Imaging and Cytology

Cholangiocarcinoma occurs most commonly at the bifurcation of the common bile ducts, followed in frequency by the middle and distal bile ducts. Cholangiographic findings suggestive of malignant change include the presence of a severe stricture with marked ductal dilation (Fig. 128-8), progression in a stricture compared with a baseline cholangiogram, and the presence of an intraductal polypoid mass over 1 cm in diameter.

Brushings and biopsies of suspicious strictures may be obtained during ERCP and provide 100% specificity and 30% to 70% sensitivity in detecting cholangiocarcinoma. Delivering the brush within the sheath to the laboratory improves yield.

Thickening of the extrahepatic bile duct of more than 6 mm detected by CT scan or ultrasonography is highly suspicious of cholangiocarcinoma. These modalities allow guided needle biopsies and also can detect a mass or the presence of metastases.

Endoscopic ultrasonography (EUS) features of cholangiocarcinoma include markedly dilated ducts and a hypoechoic

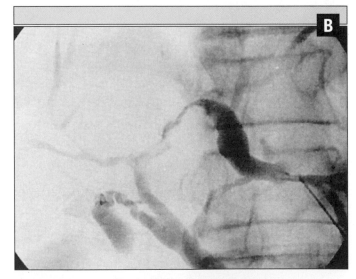

Figure 128-7

The low spatial resolution and limitation of MRI cholangiopancreatography in detailed evaluation of the tumor extent in a patient with hilar cholangiocarcinoma. **A,** Coronal source image of MRCP shows mild dilation of the intrahepatic bile ducts in the lateral segment of the left lobe. Slight irregularity (*arrows*) is suspected in the central portion of the left intrahepatic bile duct. **B,** Percutaneous intrahepatic cholangiogram shows diffuse irregularity involving central portion of both intrahepatic ducts and common hepatic duct. (*From* Choi *et al.* [18]; with permission.)

Table 128-5. Tumor Marker Index in the Diagnosis of Cholangiocarcinoma

CA19-9 + (CEA x 40)	PSC with cholangiocarcinoma (*n* = 15)	PSC without cholangiocarcinoma (*n* = 22)
<400	10	0
>400	5	22

PSC—primary sclerosing cholangitis.
Modified from Ramage et al. [20].

mass surrounded by a hyperechoic fibrotic tissue. EUS is useful to stage tumors, to detect encasement of vessels by color flow Doppler imaging, and to sample tissues by fine-needle aspiration. More recently, intraductal probes have been used for early detection of these tumors [23].

■ TREATMENT
Drug Therapy
No specific therapy apart from liver transplantation has been shown to be beneficial for patients with PSC. Because PSC is rare, most of the studies available are open-label or small controlled trials, with only a few being large controlled randomized trials (Table 128-6). Bile acid therapy and immunosuppressant, antifibrotic, and cupruretic agents have been studied. The most widely used agent is ursodeoxycholic acid. Because no specific treatment exists that has proved to be effective, patients with PSC should be enrolled in treatment trials whenever possible.

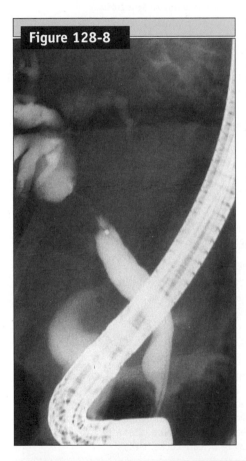

Figure 128-8

Endoscopic retrograde cholangiopancreatography (ERCP) showing proximal bile duct cancer with intrahepatic duct dilation, note the ERCP catheter at the distal extent of the stricture. (*Courtesy* of D. Carr-Locke, MD.)

Ursodeoxycholic acid. In open-label and small controlled trials, ursodeoxycholic acid (Ursodiol; Novartis Pharmaceuticals Co., East Hanover, NJ) has been shown to be effective in improving symptoms, liver biochemical test results, and histologic stage. In a recent randomized placebo-controlled double-blind study of 105 patients with PSC, ursodiol, 13 to 15 mg/kg/d, was beneficial in improving serum alkaline phosphatase, aspartate aminotransferase, bilirubin, and albumin levels. The treatment was not found to increase the relief of symptoms; increase the time to treatment failure, defined as death; lessen the need for liver transplantation; or slow the histologic progression of disease or the progression to cirrhosis [24•,25•]. Despite the lack of evidence supporting its efficacy, most physicians use ursodiol to treat patients with PSC because it is safe, well-tolerated, and improves biochemical tests results and pruritus.

Colchicine. Because of its antifibrotic properties and effectiveness in treating primary biliary cirrhosis, colchicine was evaluated in a double-blind study in 84 patients with PSC and was found not to be better than placebo with regard to survival, symptoms, biochemistry profile test results, and histologic stage [26].

Penicillamine. Because of its immunosuppressive and cupruretic properties, penicillamine was evaluated in a randomized double-blind trial. The drug showed a high incidence of side effects without benefiting symptoms, liver biochemical tests, histologic stage, or survival [27].

Tacrolimus. Tacrolimus (FK506) was studied in a preliminary open-label trial involving 10 patients with PSC with 1-year follow-up. A reduction of serum bilirubin, alkaline phosphatase, alanine aminotransferase, and aspartate aminotransferase levels was noted without adverse effects on renal function [28]. Evaluating FK506 in a large randomized study will further define its role in treatment.

Cyclosporine. In a double-blind study of 35 patients with PSC, cyclosporine improved alkaline phosphatase levels but did not improve symptoms, prevent histologic progression, or prevent the complications of cirrhosis [29].

Methotrexate. In an open-label trial of 21 patients with PSC, improvement in symptoms, liver biochemistry profile test results, and histologic stage were noted in patients without advanced disease. In a small randomized study, however, methotrexate

Table 128-6. Summary of Therapeutic Trials in Primary Sclerosing Cholangitis

Results	Large randomized trials	Small randomized trials	Open-label studies
No benefit	Penicillamine Colchicine	Colchicine and corticosteriods	Methotrexate and ursodeoxycholic acid (ursodiol)
Biochemical improvement	Ursodiol	Methotrexate Cyclosporine	Tacrolimus (FK506) Corticosteriods Ursodiol
Symptomatic improvement			Methotrexate Ursodiol
Prevention of disease progression			

improved serum alkaline phosphatase levels but had no effects on the levels of serum bilirubin, aminotransferase, or albumin or on the need for liver transplantation. However, half of the patients already had cirrhosis, which may have limited the effectiveness of the drug [30]. A more recent pilot study compared methotrexate in combination with ursodiol and ursodiol alone, finding no benefit for symptoms or liver test results from adding methotrexate. Moreover, significant toxicity occurred [31].

Corticosteroids. The concern over the progression of osteoporosis may have prevented a controlled evaluation of corticosteroids in patients with PSC. In one report, 10 patients treated with prednisone showed improvement in results of liver biochemistry profiles [32]. Combined treatment with corticosteroids and colchicine was not shown to benefit progression of the disease or biochemical parameters [33].

Management of Chronic Cholestasis

Cholestyramine usually reduces pruritus within 2 to 4 days; cholestipol hydrochloride is an alternative if cholestyramine is not tolerated. The mechanism of action of bile acid resins in reducing pruritus is unknown and presumably is due to binding and biliary excretion of an unidentified pruritogenic agent.

If pruritus is not responsive to bile acid binding resins, other therapies are ursodiol, rifampin, activated charcoal, flagyl, and opiate and serotinin antagonists (Table 128-7). Antihistamines, ultraviolet light, and phenobarbitol are ineffective in pruritus associated with cholestasis.

Bone disease is prevented by ensuring an adequate intake of calcium supplements, ample exposure to sunlight, and vitamin D supplementation, if needed, and by avoiding prolonged immobilization. Other fat-soluble vitamins also should be monitored and deficiencies supplemented. Clinically significant steatorrhea is treated with a low-fat diet or the use of medium chain triglycerides.

Endoscopic Intervention

Endoscopic interventions include balloon dilation of dominant strictures with or without stent placement (Figs. 128-9 and 128-10), stone extraction with or without sphincterotomy, and nasobiliary lavage with corticosteroid solutions.

Although endoscopic intervention for PSC has not been evaluated in a randomized way, one study involving 85 patients with PSC used endoscopic intervention in the form of biliary dilation, stent placement, or stone extraction and showed improved symptoms, test results of biochemistry profiles, and

Table 128-7. Antipruritic Agents for Management of Primary Sclerosing Cholangitis

Agent	Administration
Cholestyramine	4–8 g orally 2 to 3 times daily. Response seen in 2 to 4 days. Main side effect is constipation. Malabsorption of fat-soluble vitamins may be aggravated.
Ursodiol	300 mg orally 2 to 3 times daily.
Rifampin	150 mg, 2 to 3 times daily for 7 to 14 days. Treatment can be repeated as needed. Long-term treatment with 150 mg, 1 to 2 times daily, may be used for severe pruritus unresponsive to other modalities. Side effects are hepatotoxicity and pseudomembranous colitis.
Flagyl	250 mg, 3 times daily for 7 days [30].
Ondansetron	Effective when tested in intravenous form. Oral ondansetron for refractory pruritus was without benefit in a recent report [31].
Naloxone	Effective when tested in intravenous form. Oral opioid antagonists are potential antipruritic agents.
Activated charcoal	6 g daily.
Plasmapheresis	Expensive, with only a transient response.

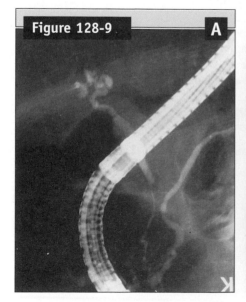
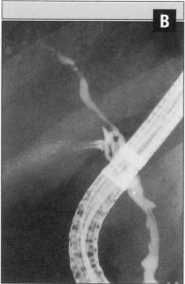

Figure 128-9   **A**   **B**

Endoscopic retrograde cholangiopancreatography in a patient with sclerosing cholangitis undergoing long-term endoprosthesis therapy. **A**, Cholangiogram in 1990 showing long distal common bile duct stricture. **B**, Repeat study five years later after stent removal. (*Courtesy of* D. Carr-Locke, MD.)

less often, cholangiographic appearance. One of these three parameters was shown to improve in 70% of patients, with a complication rate of 15% [36].

Endoscopic balloon dilation with or without stent placement is clearly indicated for patients with symptomatic dominant strictures causing jaundice, in cases of acute obstruction with cholangitis, and in patients with recurrent cholangitis. It is less obvious whether these measures should be applied to asymptomatic or mildly symptomatic patients with dominant high-grade strictures. Endoscopic intervention is not effective in diffuse disease and when multiple intrahepatic strictures are present. It is associated with an increased risk of sepsis because adequate biliary decompression may not be achieved. Likewise, endoscopic interventions are not recommended for patients with advanced liver disease, except for the presence of acute cholangitis, because these patients are unlikely to benefit and there is an increased risk of complications that may preclude or delay liver transplantation [37].

Placement of metallic stents is not advisable because it may increase technical difficulty with liver transplantation and also because of poor results in one retrospective study [38]. Anecdotal reports from Amsterdam [39] of benefit from nasobiliary bile duct perfusion with corticosteroids in patients with PSC were offset by the results of a small controlled study showing lack of benefit and a risk of inducing cholangitis [40].

Surgical Intervention

Resection and biliary reconstruction. Earlier reports on resection of an extrahepatic biliary stricture with choledochoenterostomy with or without long-term transhepatic stenting, showed an increased survival in patients without cirrhosis when compared with survival in a prognostic model from the Mayo Clinic

[41,42]. The surgery, however, may be complicated by recurrent cholangitis and scarring in the porta hepatis, increasing the technical difficulty of future transplantation. It was later demonstrated that patients who underwent biliary reconstructive surgery have longer operative time, increased blood transfusion requirements, and decreased survival after liver transplantation [43•,44]. Furthermore, these reports showed no survival benefit of biliary reconstruction when compared with a prognostic model. Biliary reconstruction therefore is not recommended at present.

Liver transplantation. Orthotopic liver transplantation (OLT) is the treatment of choice for patients with advanced liver disease and is the only effective treatment for PSC. Transplantation provides a definite survival benefit in patients with PSC when compared with all other modalities and with prognostic models. The 5-year survival rate after OLT is over 80%.

Orthotopic liver transplantation is recommended for patients with decompensated cirrhosis, a history of spontaneous bacterial peritonitis, progressive encephalopathy, recurrent variceal bleeding, and intractable ascites. Patients with PSC who have intractable pruritus, progressive bone disease, and recurrent bleeding from periostomal varices are also candidates for OLT.

Transplantation seems to obviate the risk of developing cholangiocarcinoma. In one report, cholangiocarcinoma occurred in 8 of 23 patients on medical therapy versus none of 23 patients after transplantation [44]. The high incidence of biliary malignancy in these patients and the poor outcome with cholangiocarcinoma argue for early transplantation in patients with PSC. A multicenter study group–modified Mayo Clinic Index has been used as a prognostic model to predict biliary malignancy and to time liver transplantation. This model, which uses the age of the patient, total serum bilirubin levels, size of the enlarged spleen, and

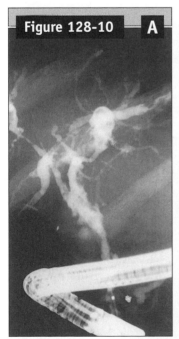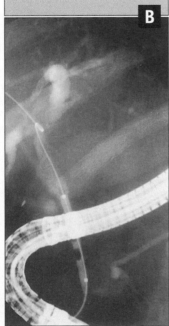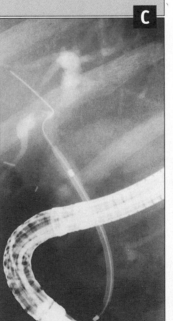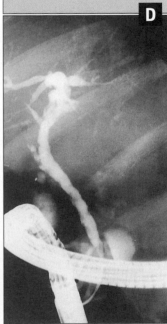

Figure 128-10

Endoscopic retrograde cholangiopancreatography (ERCP) in a patient with sclerosing cholangitis showing effects of balloon dilation with short-term endoprosthesis therapy. **A**, Initial ERCP appearance demonstrating widespread changes of sclerosing cholangitis with distal common bile duct stricture. **B**, Balloon dilation to a 4 mm diameter. **C**, Insertion of a 10F diameter stent. **D**, Cholangiographic appearance 2 months later after stent removal, cytology was negative for malignancy. (*Courtesy of* D. Carr-Locke, MD.)

histologic stage, demonstrated a risk of biliary malignancy with a score over 4.4, and therefore, it was suggested to consider transplantation at scores over 4 [45]. Because of the risk of malignancy, it is suggested that patients with dominant strictures and histologic evidence of cirrhosis be considered for OLT [37].

There are other important issues with regards to liver transplantation in patients with PSC. First, after transplantation, intrahepatic and nonanastomotic extrahepatic strictures are more common in patients with PSC compared with other liver diseases. The strictures may occur secondary to recurrence of the disease, infection, ischemia, or rejection [46,47]. Second, evidence exits that intensive immunosuppression may increase the risk of colonic carcinoma in patients who undergo OLT [43•]. Therefore, these patients should undergo frequent colonoscopic screening postoperatively, and the gastroenterologist should have a low threshold in recommending proctocolectomy preoperatively.

Algorithm for Management of Primary Sclerosing Cholangitis

In the appropriate setting the diagnosis of PSC can be made when the typical findings are demonstrated during ERCP; a

normal cholangiogram, however, may be seen in patients with "small duct PSC". In patients with a dominant stricture, cholangiocarcinoma should be ruled out by obtaining brushings and biopsies. Symptomatic benign strictures may be treated with balloon dilation and stenting. In patients with a dominant stricture and liver cirrhosis, liver transplantation should be considered. Patients with PSC should be enrolled in a treatment protocol whenever possible (Fig. 128-11).

Treatment of Cholangiocarcinoma Complicating Primary Sclerosing Cholangitis

Surgical resection. Surgical resection with negative biopsy results for lesion margins provides the only hope for cure. Results of surgery, however, are disappointing.

Distal lesions are usually amenable to pancreaticoduodenectomy, with a 5-year survival rate near 30%. The prognosis of hilar lesions, however, is poor. These tumors are rarely resectable, and even when a local resection is performed the 5-year survival rate is less than 5%. More recently, hepatic lobectomy in addition to bile duct resection has been performed for hilar lesions and has resulted in a 5-year survival rate near

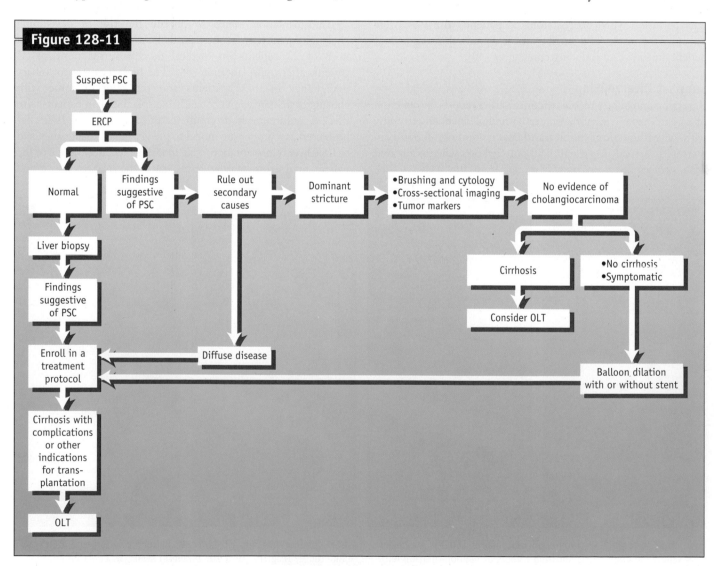

Figure 128-11

Algorithm for the management of primary sclerosing cholangitis. ERCP—endoscopic retrograde cholangiopancreatography; OLT—orthotopic liver transplantation.

30% [48]. Liver transplantation in these patients has been disappointing as well, and recurrence is the rule. Because the 5-year survival rate after OLT is less than 20%, transplantation is not recommended for cholangiocarcinoma.

Bile duct stenting and surgical bypass. Because most of these lesions are not resectable, patients with cholangiocarcinoma are usually managed with bile duct stenting or a surgical bypass procedure. Endoscopic or transhepatic stenting has a lower complication rate than and similar initial success to surgery

(Fig. 128-12); however, it carries a higher risk for recurrent jaundice and duodenal obstruction.

Distal lesions are more suitable for endoscopic stenting when compared with hilar lesions, and stenting results in significant palliation of symptoms with minimal morbidity. Hilar lesions are more difficult to approach endoscopically and may require bilateral stents. When endoscopic approaches fail, biliary drainage with metallic stent placement can be accomplished transhepatically by an interventional radiologist. This approach is particularly useful for hilar lesions and may be the preferred method in these cases.

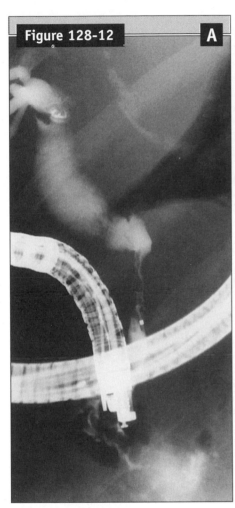
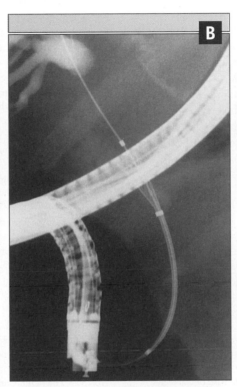
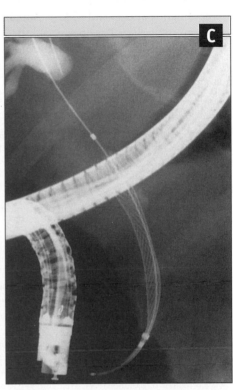
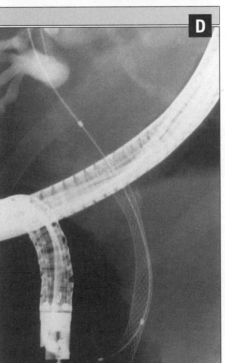
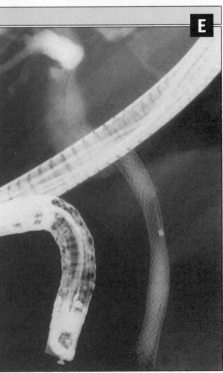
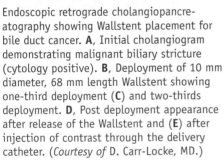

Endoscopic retrograde cholangiopancreatography showing Wallstent placement for bile duct cancer. **A**, Initial cholangiogram demonstrating malignant biliary stricture (cytology positive). **B**, Deployment of 10 mm diameter, 68 mm length Wallstent showing one-third deployment (**C**) and two-thirds deployment. **D**, Post deployment appearance after release of the Wallstent and (**E**) after injection of contrast through the delivery catheter. (*Courtesy of* D. Carr-Locke, MD.)

Oncologic treatment. External beam radiation and brachytherapy with or without chemotherapy have been used as adjuvant therapies after surgical resection and as palliation for nonresectable lesions. Most of the studies, however, fail to show a survival benefit from radiation therapy or chemotherapy.

■ PROGNOSIS

Primary sclerosing cholangitis is a progressive disease that ultimately leads to liver failure, resulting in death or liver transplantation. Prognosis varies depending on the presence or absence of symptoms. The 10-year survival rate is 93% in asymptomatic patients and 47% in patients with symptoms.

Prognostic indices have been published by the Mayo Clinic, King's College Hospital, and a multicenter study group, which further refined the original Mayo Clinic Index. These models help define risk groups and may be useful in identifying potential candidates for liver transplantation [49]. The most widely used is the modified Mayo Clinic Index, which stratifies patients with PSC into low-, moderate-, and high-risk groups. The 5-year survival probabilities for these risk groups are 0.91, 0.55, and 0.18, respectively.

■ REFERENCES

Recently published papers of particular interest have been highlighted as follows:
* Of interest
** Of outstanding interest

1. Broome U, Glaumann H, Hellers G, et al.: Liver disease in ulcerative colitis: an epidemiological and follow-up study in the county of Stockholm. *Gut* 1994, 35:84–89.

2.** Lee Y-M, Kaplan M: Primary sclerosing cholangitis. *N Engl J Med* 1995, 332:924–933.

3. Lundqvist K, Broome U: Differences in colonic disease activity in patients with ulcerative colitis with and without primary sclerosing cholangitis: a case control study. *Dis Colon Rectum* 1997, 40:451–456.

4. Loftus EV Jr, Sandborn WJ, Tremaine WJ, et al.: Risk of colorectal neoplasia in patients with primary sclerosing cholangitis. *Gastroenterology* 1996, 110:331–338.

5. Broome U, Lofberg R, Veress B: Primary sclerosing cholangitis and ulcerative colitis: evidence for increased neoplastic potential. *Hepatology* 1995, 22:1404–1408.

6. Penna C, Dozois R, Tremaine W, et al.: Pouchitis after ileal pouch-anal anastomosis for ulcerative colitis occurs with increased frequency in patients with associated primary sclerosing cholangitis. *Gut* 1996, 38:234–239.

7. Loftus-EV Jr, Sandborn WJ, Tremaine WJ, et al.: Primary sclerosing cholangitis is associated with nonsmoking: a case control study. *Gastroenterology* 1996, 110:1496–1502.

8. Lillemore KD, Pitt HA, Cameron JL: Primary sclerosing cholangitis. *Surg Clin North Am* 1990, 70:1382–1402.

9.* Broom U, Olsson R, Loof L, et al.: Natural history and prognostic factors in 305 Swedish patients with primary sclerosing cholangitis. *Gut* 1996, 38:610–615.

10. Gitlin, Strauss, eds: *Atlas of Clinical Hepatology.*Philadelphia: W.B. Saunders Co.; 1995.

11. Desmet VJ: Histopathology of cholestasis. *Verh Dtsch Ges Pathol* 1995, 79:233–240.

12. Okolicsanyi L, Fabris L, Viaggi S, et al.: Primary sclerosing cholangitis: clinical presentation, natural history and prognostic variables: an Italian multicenter study. The Italian PSC Study Group. *Eur J Gastroenterol Hepatology* 1996, 8:685–691.

13. Jorgensen RA, Lindor KD, Sartin JS, et al.: Serum lipids and fat soluble vitamin levels in PSC. *J Clin Gastroenterol* 1995, 20:215–219.

14. Therneau T, Jorgensen R, Dickson ER, et al.: Prevalence and progression of bone disease in primary sclerosing cholangitis. *Gastroenterology* 1997, 112:A1213.

15. Knechtle SJ, D'Alessandro AM, Harms BA, et al.: Relationships between sclerosing cholangitis, inflammatory bowel disease, and cancer in patients undergoing liver transplantation. *Surgery* 1995, 118:615–619.

16. Martins EB; Fleming KA, Garrido MC, et al.: Superficial thrombophlebitis, dysplasia and cholangiocarcinoma in primary sclerosing cholangitis. *Gastroenterology* 1994, 107:537–542.

17. Bansi D, Chapman R, Fleming K: Antineutrophil cytoplasmic antibodies in chronic liver diseases: prevalence, titre, specificity and IgG subclass. *J Hepatology* 1996, 24:581–586.

18. Choi BI, Kim TK, Han JK: MRI of clonorchiasis and cholangiocarcinoma. *JMRI* 1998, 8:359–366.

19. Feldman DR, Kay CL, Cotton PB, et al.: MR Cholangiography (MRC) in primary sclerosing cholangitis. *Gastroenterology* 1997, 112:A1263.

20. Olsson R, Hagerstrand I, Broome U, et al.: Sampling variability of percutaneous liver biopsy in primary sclerosing cholangitis. *J Clin Pathol* 1995, 48:933–935.

21. Nichols JC, Gores GJ, LaRusso NF, et al.: Diagnostic role of serum CA19-9 for cholangiocarcinoma in patients with primary sclerosing cholangitis. *Mayo Clin Proc* 1993, 68:874–879.

22. Ramage JK, Donaghy A, Farrant JM, et al.: Serum tumor markers for the diagnosis of cholangiocarcinoma in primary sclerosing cholangitis. *Gastroenterology* 1995, 108:865–869.

23. Tio TL: Proximal duct tumors in GI endoscopy. *Clin North Am* 1995, 5:773–780.

24.* Lindor K: Ursodiol for primary sclerosing cholangitis. *N Engl J Med* 1997, 336:691–695.

25.* Kaplan M: Toward better treatment of primary sclerosing cholangitis. *New Engl J Med* 1997, 336:719–721.

26. Olson R, Broome U, Danielsson A, et al.: Colchicine treatment of primary sclerosing cholangitis. *Gastroenterology* 1995, 108:1199–1203.

27. LaRusso NF, Wiesner RH, Ludwig J, et al.: Prospective trial of penicillamine in primary sclerosing cholangitis. *Gastroenterology* 1988, 95:1036–1042.

28. Van Thiel DH, Carroll P, Abu-Elmaged K, et al.: Tacrolimus (FK 506), a treatment for primary sclerosing cholangitis: results of an open label preliminary trial. *Am J Gastroenterol* 1995, 90:455–459.

29. Wiesner RH, Steiner B, LaRusso NF: A controlled trial evaluating cyclosporine in the treatment of primary sclerosing cholangitis. *Hepatology* 1991, 14:63A.

30. Knox TA, Kaplan MM: A double blind trial of oral pulse methotrexate therapy in the treatment of primary sclerosing cholangitis. *Gastroenterology* 1994, 106:494–499.

31. Lindor KD, Jorgensen RA, Anderson ML, et al.: Ursodeoxcholic acid and methotrexate for primary sclerosing cholangitis: a pilot study. *Am J Gastroenterol* 1996, 91:511–515.

32. Burgert SL, Brown BP, Kirkpatrick RB, et al.: Possible corticosteroid response in early primary sclerosing cholangitis. *Gastroenterology* 1984, 86:1307.

33. Lindor KD, LaRusso NF, Wiesner RH: Prednisone and colchicine are not of benefit after two years in patients with primary sclerosing cholangitis. *Hepatology* 1989, 10:638.

34. Berg C, Gollan J: *Pharmacotherapy of Hepatobiliary Disease in Gastrointestinal Pharmacotherapy.* Philadelphia: WB Saunders Co.; 1994.

35. Donohue JWO, Haigh C, Williams R: Ondansetron in the treatment of pruritus of cholestasis: a randomized controlled trial. *Gastroenterology* 1997, 112:A1349.

36. Lee JG, Schutz SM, England RE, et al.: Endoscopic therapy of sclerosing cholangitis. *Hepatology* 1995, 21:661–667.

37. Eckhauser F, Colleti L, Knol J: The changing role of surgery for sclerosing cholangitis. *Dig Dis* 1996, 14:180–191.

38. Huibregtse KA, Kugler C, Lammer J, *et al.*: Benign biliary obstruction: is the treatment with Wallstent advisable? *Radiology* 1996, 200:437–441.

39. Grijim R, Huibregtse KA, Barteksman J, *et al.*: Therapeutic investigations in PSC. *Dig Dis Sci* 1986, 31:792–798.

40. Allison MC, Burroughs AK, Noone P, *et al.*: Biliary lavage with corticosteroids in primary sclerosing cholangitis. A clinical cholangiographic and bacteriological study. *J Hepatology* 1986, 3:118–122.

41. Pitt HA, Thompson HH, Tompkins RK, *et al.*: Primary sclerosing cholangitis: results of an aggressive surgical approach. *Ann Surg* 1982, 2196:259.

42. Cameron JL, Pitt HA, Zinner M, *et al.*: Resection of hepatic duct bifurcation and transhepatic stenting for sclerosing cholangitis. *Ann Surg* 1988, 207:614–622.

43.• Narumi S, Roberts JP, Edmond JC, *et al.*: Liver transplantation for primary sclerosing cholangitis. *Hepatology* 1995, 22:451–457.

44. Fargas O, Malassagne B, Sebagh M, *et al.*: Primary sclerosing cholangitis: liver transplantation or biliary surgery. *Surgery* 1995, 117:146–155.

45. Nashan B, Schlitt HJ, Tusch G, *et al.*: Biliary malignancies in primary sclerosing cholangitis: timing for liver transplantation. *Hepatology* 1996, 23:1105–1111.

46. Sheng R, Zajko AB, Campbell WL, *et al.*: Biliary strictures in hepatic transplants: prevalence and types in patients with primary sclerosing cholangitis vs those with other liver diseases. *AMJ Am J Roentgenol* 1993, 161:297–300.

47. Campbell WL, Sheng R, Zajko AB, *et al.*: Intrahepatic biliary strictures after liver transplantation. *Radiology* 1994, 191:735.

48. Baer HU, Stain SC, Dennison AR, *et al.*: Improvements in survival by aggressive resections of hilar cholangiocarcinoma. *Ann Surg* 1993, 217:20.

49. Dickson ER, Murtaugh PA, Wiesner RH, *et al.*: Primary sclerosing cholangitis; refinement and validation of survival models. *Gastroenterology* 1992, 103:1893–1901.

129 Benign and Malignant Ampullary Tumors
Gerard Isenberg and Richard C. K. Wong

Ampullary tumors are uncommon, with approximately 3000 cases being reported every year in the United States. Perry reported the first description of an ampullary tumor in 1893. In 1899, Halsted performed the first local excision of a neoplastic lesion of the ampulla of Vater using a transduodenal approach in a woman with jaundice. Unfortunately, the patient died 7 months later of local recurrence. In 1935, Whipple pioneered the field of radical resection by introducing pancreaticoduodenectomy for recurrence of carcinoma after a local excision. Whereas Whipple's operation was plagued by a high mortality rate of 15% to 25%, the current rate is 5% to 15% [1••].

ETIOLOGY AND PATHOGENESIS

Adenoma and carcinoma of the ampulla of Vater are frequently associated. As in the case of colon cancer, an adenoma-to-carcinoma sequence of development has been shown [2–4]. Carcinogens in bile or pancreatic secretions also may play a role in ampullary tumor development [5]; however, no convincing association has been found with gallstones (present in 35% to 50% of cases). Liver flukes are thought to have a predisposing influence to neoplasia in Asia; however, the high rate of infection in this area may make this association incidental.

PATHOLOGY

Ampullary tumors are small, rarely more than 2 to 3 cm in diameter, typically soft, polypoid, and rarely metastasize. Benign tumors represent the minority and include villous adenomas (the most common), leiomyomas, lipomas, hemangiomas, lymphangiomas, carcinoids, and neurogenic tumors. Although the exact incidence of malignant transformation of adenomas is unknown, 25% to 85% have been reported to harbor either carcinoma in situ or invasive carcinoma (Fig. 129-1, see also **Color Plate**). Tumor size is not predictive of malignan-

cy, except in adenomas over 4 cm in diameter; 30% to 35% of all cancers have an associated adenomatous component [5–9].

Malignant tumors are invariably adenocarcinomas. Most arise from the mucosa of the ampulla of Vater; the remaining arise from the pancreas (Fig. 129-2, see also **Color Plate**) or the pancreatic duct epithelium, epithelium of the terminal portion of the common bile duct, or duodenal mucosa. The distinction is made by review of surgical histologic sections.

The classification and staging of ampullary carcinoma are shown in Table 129-1. Survival rates of treated patients correlate well with staging. The 5-year survival rates can be as high as 100% for stage I to as low as 0% for stage IV lesions. The epithelium of origin also appears to influence survival; one study

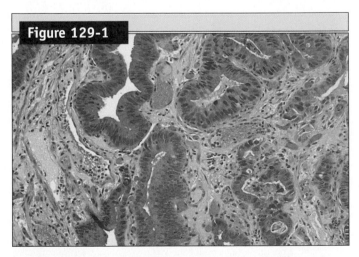

Figure 129-1

Primary malignant ampullary tumor (hematoxylin and eosin stain, original magnification × 400). Invasive adenocarcinoma (*right*) arising in an adenomatous ampullary polyp (*left*). See also **Color Plate**. (*Courtesy of* J. Willis, MD.)

has shown that tumors of pancreatic duct origin have a worse prognosis than do others [10].

Because of their small size, ampullary carcinomas rarely metastasize. They infiltrate locally, sometimes spreading to the lymph nodes of the porta hepatis or to the liver. The extent of lymph node involvement appears to be the most critical prognostic indicator; however, the presence of lymph node metastases does not preclude the possibility of cure by radical surgery. Patients with lymph node metastases have been reported as having 20-year survival rates of 20%, contrary to findings in pancreatic cancer [11–13].

EPIDEMIOLOGY

Ampullary adenomas of the papilla of Vater are rare premalignant lesions with occurrence rates of 0.04% to 0.12% at autopsy. Malignant tumors of the ampullary region constitute 0.063%

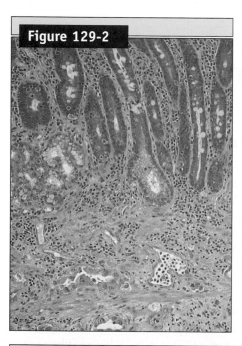

Figure 129-2

Invasion of ampulla by pancreatic carcinoma (hematoxylin and eosin stain, original magnification × 250). Invasive pancreatic adenocarcinoma (*base*) infiltrating into normal ampullary mucosa (*top*). See also **Color Plate.** (*Courtesy of* J. Willis, MD.)

to 0.21% of all cancers of the digestive tract; however, they account for 10.2% to 36% of all surgically operable pancreaticoduodenal tumors [9].

Tumors of the ampulla occur at all ages but more often between 50 and 70 years. The male-to-female ratio is about 1.5 to 1. Adenomas of the papilla and the adjacent duodenum have been reported in half or more of patients with familial adenomatous polyposis. Malignancy of the duodenum, particularly involving the ampulla, represents one of the most common causes of mortality in patients with familial adenomatous polyposis, and therefore, upper endoscopy surveillance is performed at periodic intervals in these patients [14].

CLINICAL FEATURES

Table 129-2 depicts the clinical features associated with ampullary tumors. Initially, patients present with jaundice, which may fluctuate owing to the cyclic necrosis of the tumor with corresponding relief of biliary obstruction. The duration of symptoms before diagnosis is approximately 30 days for jaundice; for abdominal pain, nausea, and anorexia, the diagnosis is made approximately 2 to 4 months later. Aspartate aminotransferase, alanine aminotransferase, alkaline phosphatase, and bilirubin levels are abnormal in 60% to 85% of patients.

The classic "silver stool sign of Thomas," caused by the mixture of acholic stools owing to biliary obstruction and blood issuing from the tumor, is rare. Of cancers of the ampulla, 25% to 35% are associated with a palpably enlarged gallbladder (Courvoisier's sign).

The differential diagnosis of ampullary lesions includes cholelithiasis, choledocholithiasis, pancreatic neoplasms, and cholangiocarcinoma. Indeed, many patients initially are misdiagnosed as having gallstone disease and undergo cholecystectomy.

DIAGNOSIS AND STAGING

Findings on upper gastrointestinal barium examination in patients with ampullary tumors are abnormal 50% to 80% of the

Table 129-1. The Primary Tumor, Regional Nodes, Metastasis (TNM) System of Classification and Staging Ampullary Carcinoma

T	Indicates the primary tumor	N	Indicates the regional lymph nodes	M	Indicates distant metastasis	Stage grouping			
TX	Primary tumor cannot be assessed	NX	Regional lymph nodes cannot be assessed	MX	Presence of distant metastasis cannot be assessed	Stage 0	Tis	N0	M0
T0	No evidence of primary tumor	N0	No regional lymph node metastasis	MO	No distant metastasis	Stage I	T1	N0	M0
Tis	Carcinoma in situ	N1	Regional lymph node metastasis	M1	Distant metastasis	Stage II	T2 or 3	N0	M0
T1	Tumor limited to ampulla of Vater					Stage III	T1, T2, or T3	N1	M0
T2	Tumor invades duodenal wall					Stage IV	T4	Any N	M0
T3	Tumor invades 2 cm or less into the pancreas						Any T	Any N	M1
T4	Tumor invades more than 2 cm into the pancreas, into other adjacent organs, or both								

time, but a high false-negative rate exists. Occasionally, villous tumors produce a "soap bubble" appearance when multiple lucent rounded areas are interspersed in a fine reticular pattern, with barium lying within the interstices of the tumor fronds.

Transabdominal ultrasonography followed by abdominal CT scan are useful in initial screening but lack specificity for identifying ampullary lesions because of their small size. Findings on ultrasonography or CT scan that may suggest an ampullary lesion include bile ducts dilated to the level of the duodenum without intraductal filling defects and with the absence of a mass at the head of the pancreas.

Endoscopy is the most accurate diagnostic test for detecting ampullary lesions, particularly when using a side-viewing instrument (Fig. 129-3*A* to *C*, see also **Color Plate**). Although endoscopy also provides the opportunity for a biopsy, specimens often are not taken deeply enough from tissue to be diagnostic. The overall rate of false-negative biopsy results in ampullary malignancies is 17% to 40%. In particular, small intra-ampullary carcinomas can be difficult to diagnose, and a tumor sphincterotomy can be used to improve diagnostic yield. A forceps biopsy can be taken at the same time as the tumor sphincterotomy is performed. It has been suggested, however, that higher specimen yields and less complications may occur (*ie*, bleeding) when the biopsy is delayed for 1 to 2 weeks [15].

In a recent study using a monoclonal anti-p53 antibody test, on review of surgical resection specimens it was found that ampullary tumors with false-negative biopsy results for malignancy but positive for p53 contained carcinoma [16•]. Larger studies are needed to confirm these findings.

Endoscopic ultrasonography has been shown to be accurate in the preoperative staging of ampullary neoplasms (Fig. 129-

Table 129-2. Symptoms and Signs of Ampullary Tumors

Symptoms and signs	Patients, %
Jaundice	60–85
Abdominal pain	40–60
Weight loss	20–50
Nausea and vomiting	20–30
Melena	10–20
Anemia	30–40
Courvoisier's sign	25–35
Hepatomegaly	20–30
Silver stool sign of Thomas	< 5

Figure 129-3

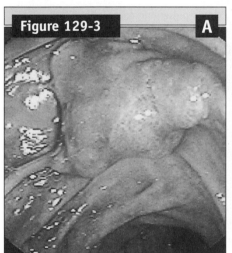
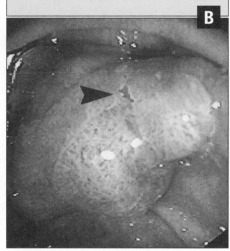
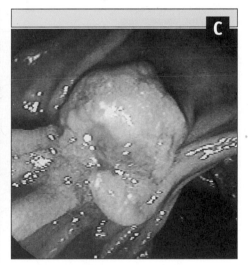

A, Ampulla of Vater: tubulovillous adenoma. **B**, *Arrowhead* indicates ampullary orifice. **C**, Ampulla of Vater: poorly differentiated adenocarcinoma. See also **Color Plate**.

Figure 129-4

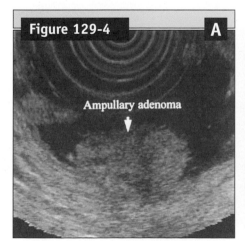
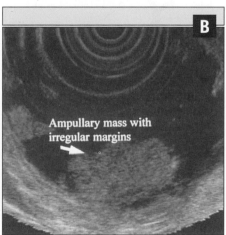

Endoscopic ultrasound images using a mechanical sector scanning echoendoscope. **A**, Ampullary adenoma. **B**, An ampullary mass with irregular margins.

4*A* and *B*). Endoscopic ultrasonography may facilitate the decision to perform local or radical resection by accurately defining the depth of invasion and presence of lymph node metastases.

■ TREATMENT

Despite the introduction of alternative modes of therapy, surgical resection still remains the gold standard of treatment [17]. Benign tumors, if confirmed by frozen sections, often are treated curatively by local transduodenal resection (Fig. 129-5). The difficulty lies in accurately determining the presence of malignancy on frozen sections, and occasionally, malignant tumors are found outside the biopsy margins. If the test results on the marginal sections specimens are positive for carcinoma, the local resection can be converted to a radical resection intraoperatively, usually by a pylorus-sparing pancreaticoduodenectomy (Fig. 129-6).

The long-term efficacy of more recent endoscopically based treatment modalities, including snare resection (Fig. 129-7), laser photoablation, and photodynamic therapy, is not yet known. Endoscopic treatment is usually reserved for high-risk surgical patients [18•]. The immediate risks of endoscopic therapy include bleeding, biliary obstruction, acute pancreatitis, perforation, and an existing carcinoma not being diagnosed. Long-term

Figure 129-5

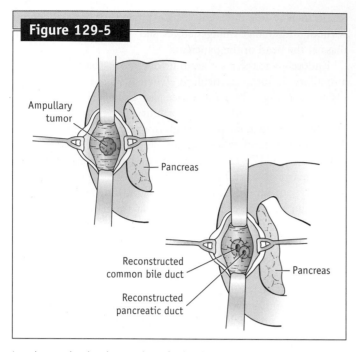

Local transduodenal resection of a benign ampullary tumor with reconstruction of the common bile duct and pancreatic duct.

Figure 129-6

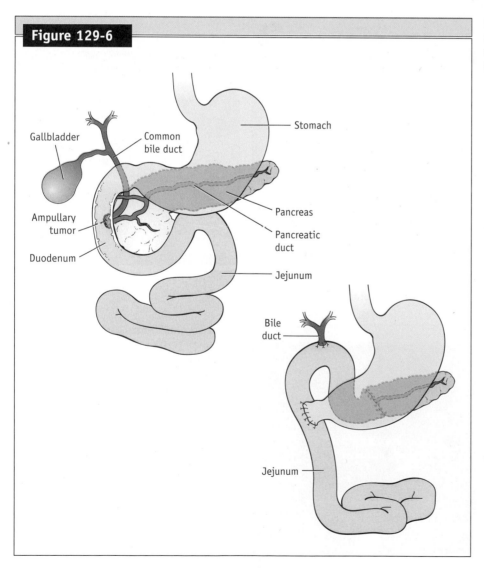

Pylorus-preserving pancreaticoduodenectomy; resection of a malignant ampullary tumor with anatomy before and after the procedure.

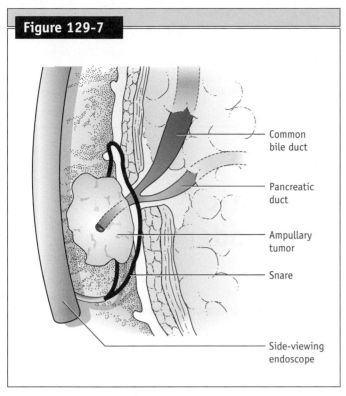

Figure 129-7

Common bile duct

Pancreatic duct

Ampullary tumor

Snare

Side-viewing endoscope

Endoscopic snare papillectomy.

risks include local stenosis of the pancreatic and biliary ductal orifices secondary to scarring and tumor recurrence. Regular endoscopic surveillance is therefore essential in all patients treated by endoscopically based modalities.

Whipple's pancreaticoduodenectomy has an operative mortality rate of 5% to 15%, with a morbidity rate of 20% to 30%. Complications include delayed gastric emptying, pancreaticojejunostomy leak or fistula, gastrojejunal anastomotic leakage, wound infection, sepsis, hemorrhage, and metabolic disorders (ie, diabetes mellitus and pancreatic exocrine insufficiency). In most series, the resectability rate is 90% to 100%. Adjuvant chemoradiation is poorly tolerated and without survival benefit.

PROGNOSIS

Ampullary carcinoma is the most curable of all cancers of the upper gastrointestinal tract. Untreated patients with adenocarcinoma of the ampulla of Vater die within months as a result of cholestasis. The overall 5-year survival rate after treatment is 10% to 40%. Generally, for stages I and II disease, the 5-year survival rate is 75% to 80%; for stages III and IV disease, it is 0% to 25%, a marked decrease.

FOLLOW-UP AND SURVEILLANCE

Benign ampullary tumors have been reported to progress to adenocarcinoma after local resection, and therefore, when local resection is performed, repeat endoscopic surveillance every 6 to 12 months is warranted. A prospective controlled multicenter study is needed to assess the optimal surveillance period.

Patients with familial adenomatous polyposis should have routine surveillance endoscopies (with both forward- and side-viewing instruments) every 1 to 2 years owing to the predilection for adenomatous change in the ampulla of Vater (reported in up to 50% of patients with familial adenomatous polyposis).

No recommendation can be made regarding the use of colonoscopy in assessing for polyps of the colon in patients with ampullary tumors. It is not known whether patients with ampullary tumors are at increased risk for these polyps; however, many patients undergo colonoscopy to determine the cause of anemia or guaiac-positive stools during their diagnostic evaluation.

REFERENCES

Recently published papers of particular interest have been highlighted as follows:
• Of interest
•• Of outstanding interest

1.•• Michelassi F, Erroi F, Dawson PJ, et al.: Experience with 647 consecutive tumors of the duodenum, ampulla, head of the pancreas, and distal common bile duct. *Ann Surg* 1989, 210:544–554.
A large retrospective study analyzing data collected from 1946 to 1987 which demonstrated that the 5-year survival rate was dependent on intent of operation (palliative vs resection for cure), histologic type, and site of tumor.

2. Perzin KH, Bridge MF: Adenomas of the small intestine: a clinicopathologic review of 51 cases and a study of their relationship to carcinoma. *Cancer* 1981, 48:799–819.

3. Gouma DJ, Obertop H, Vismans J, et al.: Progression of benign epithelial ampullary tumor to adenocarcinoma. *Surgery* 1987, 101:501–504.

4. Sellner F: Investigations on the significance of the adenoma-carcinoma sequence in the small bowel. *Cancer* 1990, 66:702–715.

5. Ryan DP, Schapiro RH, Warshaw AL: Villous tumors of the duodenum. *Ann Surg* 1986, 203:301–306.

6. Komorowski RA, Cohen EB: Villous tumors of the duodenum: a clinicopathologic study. *Cancer* 1981, 47:1377–1386.

7. Rosenberg J, Welch JP, Pyrtek LJ, et al.: Benign villous adenomas of the ampulla of Vater. *Cancer* 1986, 58:1563–1568.

8. Hayes DH, Bolton JS, Willis GW, et al.: Carcinoma of the ampulla of Vater. *Ann Surg* 1987, 206:572–577.

9. Yamaguchi K, Enjoji M: Carcinoma of the ampulla of Vater *Cancer* 1987, 59:506–515.

10. Mori K, Ikei S, Yamane T, et al.: Pathologic factors influencing survival of carcinoma of the ampulla of Vater. *Eur J Surg Oncol* 1990, 16:183–188.

11. Roder JD, Schneider PM, Stein HJ, et al.: Number of lymph node metastases is significantly associated with survival in patients with radically resected carcinoma of the ampulla of Vater. *Br J Surg* 1995, 82:1693–1696.

12. Klempnauer J, Ridder GJ, Pichlmayr R: Prognostic factors after resection of ampullary carcinoma: multivariate survival analysis in comparison with ductal cancer of the pancreatic head. *Br J Surg* 1995, 82:1686–1691.

13. Allema JH, Reinders ME, van Gulik TM, et al.: Results of pancreaticoduodenectomy for ampullary carcinoma and analysis of prognostic factors for survival. *Surgery* 1995, 117:247–253.

14. Sivak MV, Jagelman DC: Upper gastrointestinal endoscopy in polyposis syndromes: familial polyposis coli and Gardner's syndrome. *Gastrointest Endosc* 1984, 30:102–104.

15. Ponchon T, Berger F, Chavaillon A, et al.: Contribution of endoscopy to diagnosis and treatment of tumors of the ampulla of Vater. *Cancer* 1989, 64:161–167.

16.• Younes M, Riley S, Genta RM, et al.: p53 protein accumulation in tumors of the ampulla of Vater. *Cancer* 1995, 76:1150–1154.
Using a monoclonal anti-p53 antibody, sections of normal ampullas, adenomas, carcinomas, and initial biopsy specimens of tumors that had no morphologic evidence of carcinoma were stained immunohistologically: Test results for 16 of 17 carcinomas were positive for p53, and test results for 7 of 9 biopsy specimens initially determined to be either normal or adenomatous were positive for p53 (all 9 were subsequently diagnosed as carcinoma). Currently experimental, this technique offers potential for further refinement in accurate diagnosis.

17. Rivera JA, Rattner DW, Fernandez-del Castillo C, *et al.*: Surgical approaches to benign and malignant tumors of the ampulla of Vater. *Surg Oncol Clin North Am* 1996, 5:689–711.

18.• Binmoeller KF, Boaventura S, Ramsperger H, *et al.*: Endoscopic snare excision of benign adenomas of the papilla of Vater. *Gastrointest Endosc* 1993, 39:127–131.
The first study to evaluate this nonsurgical treatment modality in a large series of patients. This technique was limited by the high number of recurrences (6/25 patients) in a median follow-up of 37 months. However, in high-risk surgical patients, this procedure may have its place in treatment of these lesions.

130 Tumors of the Extrahepatic Biliary Tract and Gallbladder

Dirk J. van Leeuwen and Paul Fockens

Tumors of the biliary tract and gallbladder present specific diagnostic and therapeutic challenges. Most are malignant and require a multidisciplinary approach with input from a gastroenterologist, radiologist, surgeon, and pathologist. Imaging studies often fail to differentiate the more common malignant tumor from the rarer benign condition. Symptomatic biliary tract tumors are rarely curable; however, treatment may provide prolonged palliation of symptoms. Unfortunately, management decisions for the treatment of cholangiocarcinoma and gallbladder carcinoma are complicated by a lack of randomized clinical trials to support the choice of therapy.

FUNCTIONAL AND ANATOMIC ASPECTS

The presentation of biliary tract tumors may be varied and is partially determined by the location of the tumor. Depending on the level of obstruction of the biliary system (Fig. 130-1),

Figure 130-1

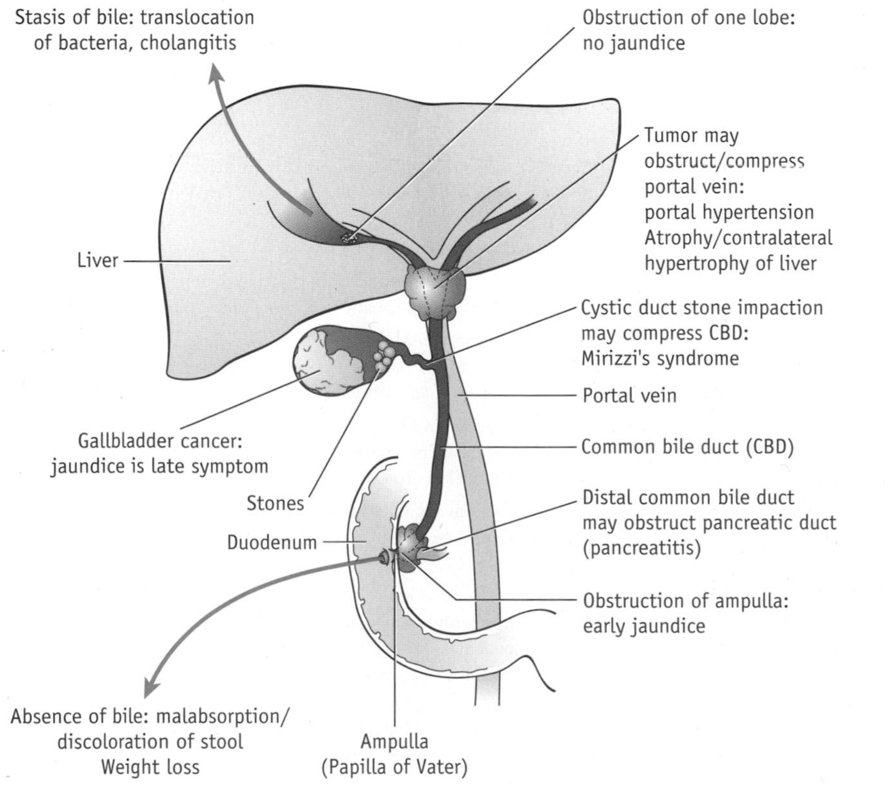

Stasis of bile: translocation of bacteria, cholangitis

Obstruction of one lobe: no jaundice

Tumor may obstruct/compress portal vein: portal hypertension Atrophy/contralateral hypertrophy of liver

Liver

Cystic duct stone impaction may compress CBD: Mirizzi's syndrome

Portal vein

Common bile duct (CBD)

Gallbladder cancer: jaundice is late symptom

Stones

Distal common bile duct may obstruct pancreatic duct (pancreatitis)

Duodenum

Obstruction of ampulla: early jaundice

Absence of bile: malabsorption/ discoloration of stool Weight loss

Ampulla (Papilla of Vater)

Major pathophysiologic events related to bile duct obstruction.

such tumors may lead to jaundice as a presenting symptom. In the case of gallbladder carcinoma, however, the disease may be fairly advanced before jaundice occurs as a consequence of common bile duct obstruction.

Obstruction of the biliary system usually is accompanied by an increase in serum levels of alkaline phosphatase and γ-glutamyl transpeptidase and followed by an increase in serum bilirubin concentration. Both benign and malignant obstruction may cause weight loss, which at least is partially due to fat malabsorption caused by diminished bile excretion. Tumors that arise from the papilla of Vater or the distal common bile duct may show symptoms at an early stage of disease in contrast to intrahepatic biliary tumors that may be at a much more advanced stage before causing symptoms of obstruction; one unobstructed liver lobe often provides sufficient excretion of bilirubin to prevent jaundice.

Long-standing obstruction may cause biliary cirrhosis and portal hypertension. The proximal part of the extrahepatic biliary system is located adjacent to the portal vein. Tumors in this location may therefore compromise the portal vein and in more extensive cases the hepatic artery; they may also result in portal hypertension due to portal vein obstruction, liver atrophy, and compensatory hypertrophy of the contralateral lobe. Surgery in patients with long-standing obstruction therefore may be accompanied by major blood loss because of portal hypertension. Varices may develop subsequently in a surgical anastomosis or stoma and cause significant bleeding. Variants of biliary anatomy require recognition to avoid surgical accidents.

EPIDEMIOLOGY

Cholangiocarcinoma

The prevalence of cholangiocarcinoma of the extrahepatic biliary system in the United States is 0.5 to 1.0 per 100,000 persons. The peak incidence occurs in the seventh decade of life, and there is a small male predominance. Predisposing factors include congenital anomalies and various conditions associated with chronic inflammation. Cholangiocarcinoma is not directly associated with gallstone disease.

A number of congenital conditions (*eg*, choledochal cysts) are often grouped together under the name of fibropolycystic disease of the liver and are developmental disorders of the biliary ductal plate. Congenital hepatic fibrosis, (multiple) hamartomas (von Meyenberg's complexes), and polycystic liver disease are only very rarely associated with the development of cancer. However, the risk is increased in the case of choledocal cyst and Caroli's disease (biliary ductectasia). Malignancies associated with such anomalies may not present until early adulthood. In recent years, a long common channel has been recognized as a predisposing factor for the development of biliary tract malignancy [1,2].

In some cases these tumors are directly associated with infestation by parasites such as *Clonorchis sinensis* in China and *Opisthorchis viverrini* in Thailand. Oriental hepatolithiasis [3,4] is a condition frequently encountered in Japan, Thailand, and Hong Kong in which the biliary system is filled with a soft or friable brown-to-black–colored pigment. Years of recurrent episodes of cholangitis and abscesses may be followed by the development of cholangiocarcinoma. All these conditions are less common in the West, except in places with a significant Asian immigrant population. The biliary malignancies encountered with such predisposing conditions are mainly intrahepatic as are the peripheral cholangiocarcinomas associated with the use of Thorotrast, a radiocontrast agent that is no longer in use. The serum α-fetoprotein levels in patients with these types of tumors are usually normal, although the carcinoembryonic antigen level may be elevated.

Other diseases associated with carcinoma of the biliary system include primary sclerosing cholangitis and ulcerative colitis. These two diseases, which are often found together, are also independently associated with an increased risk of cholangiocarcinoma.

Gallbladder Carcinoma

Adenocarcinoma of the gallbladder ranks as the fourth most common malignant tumor of the gastrointestinal tract in the West, after colorectal, stomach, and pancreatic tumors. The incidence in the United States is about 1 per 100,000 men and 2 per 100,000 women. In some parts of the world the prevalence is much higher, and in Israel, Chile, and Mexico the male-to-female ratio may be as high as 2 to 3:1, with a peak incidence in the seventh decade of life. Native American women (with an incidence of 21.1 per 100,000), women in Japan, and Northern Europeans are at especially high risk. Gallstones are the main predisposing factor, although the cancer risk is not high enough to warrant prophylactic cholecystectomy. Other associations include any predisposing factors for gallstone formation and gallbladder calcification (so-called porcelain gallbladder). Recently, an association between Mirizzi syndrome and gallbladder carcinoma has been reported [5].

PATHOLOGY

A variety of tumors may arise from the biliary system [6,7] (Table 130-1). Rare tumors are not discussed in any detail herein. If biliary tract obstruction results, the changes in liver biopsy specimens typically are those indicative of large bile duct

Table 130-1. Tumors of the Gallbladder and Extrahepatic Biliary System

Cell of origin	Benign	Malignant
Epithelial	Adenoma Cystadenoma Papillomatosis	Adenocarcinoma (various types) Squamous cell Adenosquamous cell Oat cell Others
Nonepithelial	Granular cell tumor Soft tissue tumors	Rhabdomyosarcoma
Miscellaneous (including pseudotumors)	Benign inflammatory tumor Neuroma (including postsurgical) Reactive lymphoid hyperplasia	

Abbreviated and modified according to Albores-Saavredra and Henson [6] and Anthony [7].

obstruction with features such as periductal fibrosis, periportal edema, and inflammation. Malignant spread may not be present in random liver biopsy specimens, explaining the limited use of performing a blind liver biopsy to assess whether extrahepatic bile duct obstruction is caused by malignant or benign disease.

Childhood Tumors

Rhabdomyosarcoma is the most common soft-tissue tumor in children and accounts for 10% to 15% of all soft-tissue tumors in children, including 0.8% involving the biliary system. Peak incidence occurs between 4 and 5 years of age. Current imaging techniques allow the recognition of tumor growing into the biliary system and therefore differentiation from choledochal cysts. Although the prognosis is usually poor, combination therapy consisting of surgery, chemotherapy, and radiotherapy has improved outcome. Benign inflammatory tumor of the common bile duct is rare but has an excellent prognosis.

Benign Tumors

Bile duct adenomas are found in approximately 0.5% to 1% of resected gallbladders. Bile duct cystadenoma invariably is a multilocular condition in contrast to developmental cysts, which are usually solitary. Biliary papillomatosis may involve the intrahepatic and extrahepatic biliary system and the gallbladder. This progressive condition has a fatal outcome due to cholangitis, hemobilia, or malignancy. Other rare benign tumors include granular cell tumors found primarily in black women, neuromas (both *de novo* and after surgery), and mesenchymal tumors such as lipomas and fibromas.

Malignant Tumors

Cholangiocarcinoma and gallbladder carcinoma are found incidentally at cholecystectomy or in the evaluation of jaundice more frequently than any other tumors with the exception of ampullary lesions. Obstruction may be due to intrinsic tumor growth in the biliary system or extrinsic compression by tumor,

metastasis, or enlarged lymph nodes. Enlarged periductal or perihilar lymph nodes may be caused by either benign inflammatory reaction or malignant disease. Perihilar varices also may cause compression, mimicking cholangiocarcinoma.

Primary biliary tract malignancies are nearly always cholangiocarcinomas. When present at the liver hilum (bifurcation), they are referred to as *Klatskin tumors* [8,9]. Approximately 70% are mucin-producing sclerosing tumors. The more distal tumors are more likely to be papillary tumors. Ampullary carcinomas often begin as villous adenomas, a premalignant condition. Other unusual tumors are diagnosed by review of the resected surgical specimen or at autopsy (Fig. 130-2) and include carcinoid, neuroma, metastatic carcinoma (*eg*, kidney, breast, malignant melanoma), and non-Hodgkin's lymphoma. Gallbladder cancer and hepatocellular carcinoma may invade the biliary system and pose diagnostic challenges.

Biliary Tract Strictures

Diagnosis of biliary strictures using cytologic or fine-needle aspirate samples obtained during endoscopic retrograde cholangiopancreatography (ERCP) or percutaneous transhepatic cholangiography (PTC) remains problematic. Cholangiocarcinomas often have strong desmoplastic features with abundant fibrosis and a limited number of cells that can be identified as malignant. Stents used to treat biliary tract obstruction may cause reactive changes in the bile duct wall and induce mucosal changes that may mimic in situ malignancy, thus adding to the difficulty of interpretation of brush cytology and fine-needle aspiration biopsy (Fig. 130-3). The yield of brush cytology or fine-needle aspirate obtained via intraluminal techniques is higher when the tumor is located within the biliary system than when it is an extrinsic tumor compressing the biliary system.

Gallbladder Carcinoma

Chronic inflammation and dysplasia are associated with the development of malignancies, though this may take a decade or more

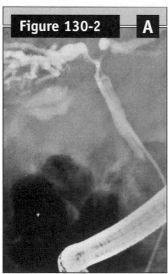
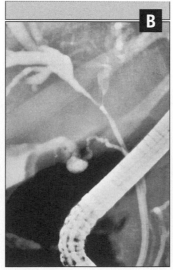
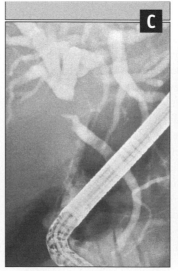
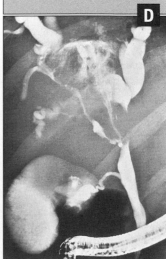

Figure 130-2

Cholangiocarcinoma at the liver hilum and some imitators. **A**, A Klatskin tumor (Type II) with tight strictures. **B**, After resection this tumor at the hilum appeared to be benign fibrosing disease (?PSC). **C**, Invading gallbladder carcinoma. Note some displacement of the common bile duct. **D**, A peculiar stricturizing process. Pathologic examination revealed non-Hodgkin's lymphoma restricted to the liver hilum. (*From* van Leeuwen *et al.* [9]; with permission of the editor and publishers of *Seminars in Liver Disease*, Thieme Publishers.)

[10]. Most malignancies of the gallbladder are adenocarcinomas; 60% are found in the fundus, 30% in the body, and 10% in the neck of the gallbladder. Gallbladder carcinoma is most often found incidentally in the resected cholecystectomy specimen.

■ CLINICAL PRESENTATION

Medical History

The medical history of patients with extrahepatic cholangiocarcinoma or gallbladder carcinoma is often unrevealing and may be limited to general malaise, mild fever, and weight loss without localized symptoms. On rare occasions, a sensation of fullness or presence of a mass may be experienced by the patient. In certain patients, laboratory evidence of cholestasis (*eg*, a high serum alkaline phosphatase and γ-glutamyl transpeptidase level) may point toward a biliary tract problem. In patients with biliary tract obstruction, jaundice may be the presenting sign. Distal common bile duct obstruction may manifest by acute pancreatitis and steatorrhea. Fever, cholangitis, or abscess may be associated with tumor. Fever is occasionally caused by lymphoma.

Physical Examination

The physical findings of jaundice, cachexia, a distended palpable gallbladder (Courvoisier's sign), or a right upper quadrant mass should be sought. Usually, however, they are absent. Palpable metastatic lymph nodes are rarely encountered.

Laboratory Studies

Liver test results indicating cholestasis (*eg*, elevated alkaline phosphatase and γ-glutamyl transpeptidase) may precede elevation of serum bilirubin. Tumor markers, such α-fetoprotein in hepatocellular carcinoma and carcinoembryonic antigen in metastatic colon cancer, may be useful once imaging studies have detected a lesion in the liver. Cholangiocarcinoma, specifically in association with primary sclerosing cholangitis, may be reflected in persistently high levels of CA19-9.

Imaging Studies

Cross-sectional noninvasive imaging techniques such as Doppler ultrasonography, CT scan, and magnetic resonance cholangiopancreatography (MRCP) have dramatically changed the clinical approach to patients with biliary tract tumors [9,11–14]. Modern imaging techniques can assess the biliary system and precisely determine the proximal and distal extent of the disease. They are very safe compared with invasive imaging techniques. Whereas cross-sectional imaging infrequently allows a specific diagnosis of cholangiocarcinoma, biliary

Figure 130-3

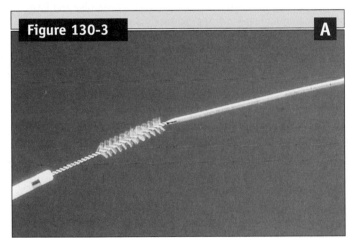
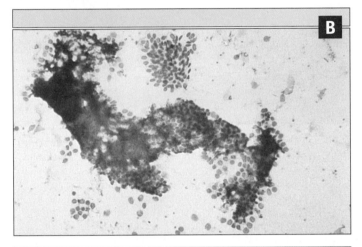
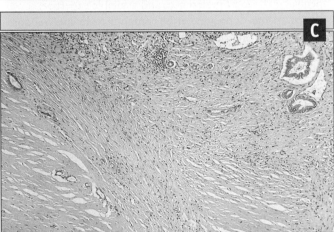
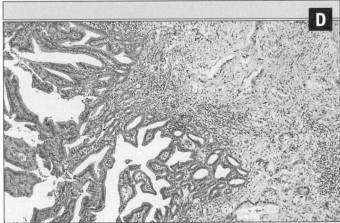

Pathology of cholangiocarcinoma and endoscopic cytology. **A**, The brush is protected from contamination by a covering catheter. At the level of the stricture the brush can be passed through the stricture and retracted into the catheter to allow removal and processing of brushed material. **B**, A group of malignant cells (cholangiocarcinoma). **C**, An extensive desmoplastic reaction (*lower 75% of the field*) may obscure malignant cells (*top*) or cytologic aspirates of both lobes.
D, A cholangiocarcinoma protruding into the lumen: The yield of brush cytology will increase in this situation (hematoxylin and eosin stain, original magnification X 16). (*Courtesy of* A. Bosma, MD.)

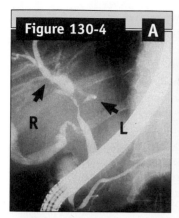
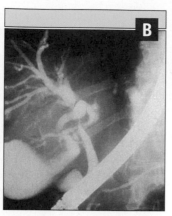
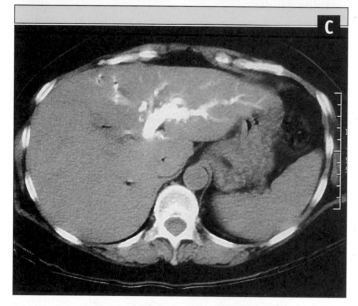

Complementary images from endoscopic retrograde cholangiopancreatography (ERCP) and computed tomography (CT) scan of a woman 64 years of age with persistent itching and test results showing a mildly cholestatic liver. After initial negative results on ultrasonography, a second study suggested mild intrahepatic biliary dilation. **A** and **B** ERCP shows a hilar stricture. Note the initially limited filling of the left system (*arrow*) and of a branch of the right biliary system (*arrow*). An endoprosthesis was inserted into the right system, with abundant drainage. **C**, A few hours later, a CT scan showed contrast in a dilated left system, (not appreciated on fluoroscopy) whereas adequate drainage of the right system is reflected by the absence of a visible biliary system. Surgical exploration confirmed a small extrahepatic cholangiocarcinoma. Also note that the CT scan does not show a tumor, which is very characteristic for this tumor type.

dilation caused by the obstructing tumor often is easily identified. Cross-sectional imaging techniques also are limited in their ability to differentiate benign and malignant disease. Tumor and fibrosis cannot be differentiated with certainty, although in the appropriate clinical setting (*eg*, a patient with long-standing ulcerative colitis who becomes jaundiced and loses weight) strictures should be considered malignant until it is proved otherwise. Intrahepatic lesions secondary to the obstructive process may be abscesses or metastases; the latter are rarely seen in small cholangiocarcinomas. Enlarged lymph nodes in the hilar area can be metastases or reactive lymph nodes. Gallstones may be the cause of biliary obstruction, or sludge and stone formation may be secondary to a benign or malignant stricture.

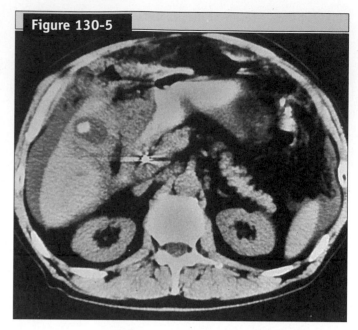

CT scan showing complications of PTC. Endoscopic retrograde cholangiopancreatography (ERCP) was attempted on a man 42 years of age with obstructive jaundice. Cannulation failed, and he was referred for PTC. As can be seen on this CT scan, PTC was complicated by intrahepatic hematoma and subcapsular and intra-abdominal biliary leakage. Approximately 6 weeks later, the puncture site revealed metastatic carcinoma, illustrating the risk of tumor seeding in the abdomen and in scars during percutaneous interventions.

One should be particularly aware of this possibility in the elderly. Cross-sectional images need to be carefully compared with findings obtained by direct cholangiography (Fig. 130-4).

Direct Cholangiography

When a proximal bile duct obstruction is suspected clinically and because of the results of noninvasive studies, direct cholangiography should be considered [15,16•]. Both ERCP and PTC allow tissue sampling and drainage. The selection of procedure depends on the local preferences and available expertise.

Percutaneous drainage may be complicated by intra-abdominal leakage of bile that may lead to infection and peritonitis. Even more important, spillage of malignant cells may occur. Unlike the intestine, the intra-abdominal cavity is an excellent growth medium for malignant cells. Therefore, the risks of percutaneous invasive procedures must be balanced with the potential for cure or prolonged palliation. The true risk for seeding of tumor cells is difficult to assess. We have observed patients who, within weeks after PTC, developed skin metastases at the puncture site where a drain exited the biliary system (Fig. 130-5). Another reflection of the risk is the high positive yield of malignant cells in bile when surgical resection is undertaken. Reports are now increasing of gallbladder carcinoma metastasizing to surgical scars after laparoscopic cholecystectomy, reemphasizing the risk of percutaneous manipulation [17].

The risks of percutaneous drainage procedures have decreased in recent years with the development of thin self-expandable metallic stents. Introduction of these stents causes only minimal duct trauma compared with less sophisticated systems and therefore allows drainage in a one-stage procedure. Ultrasonography also helps greatly to diminish the number of attempts to access the biliary system. A major advantage of PTC is that in emergency cases, such as a patient with cholangitis who does not respond to resuscitation and antibiotics, external percutaneous drainage can be relatively easily performed. In contrast, endoscopic drainage usually requires more advanced therapeutic skills. The greatest advantage of having ERCP performed by an experienced endoscopist is the diminished risk of abdominal contamination. Also an internal drain is much more patient friendly. Change of occluded drains is more easily done with external drains.

OBSTRUCTIVE JAUNDICE IN SUSPECTED MALIGNANT PROXIMAL BILE DUCT OBSTRUCTION

Certain considerations assist the clinician in making adequate management decisions for patients with suspected malignant bile duct obstruction.

Medical history and physical examination. A detailed medical history and physical examination are essential in arriving at a correct diagnosis; a history of (complicated) biliary tract surgery, ulcerative colitis, primary sclerosing cholangitis, or malignancy elsewhere is particularly helpful. Occasionally, fever unassociated with the typical features of cholangitis and nonresponsiveness to broad spectrum antibiotics may point toward a diagnosis of lymphoma.

Symptoms. Potentially life-threatening symptoms may be more acutely attributable to biliary tract obstruction and resultant cholangitis, rather than to the tumor itself. In these circumstances, patient survival may be determined as much by the feasibility of obtaining effective biliary drainage as by achieving control of tumor growth. Biliary interventional procedures may provide relief of symptoms or, if drainage is incomplete, may lead to clinically overt cholangitis and significantly worsen the patient's condition.

Imaging. Imaging tests often may be very effective in assessing the level of obstruction but usually fail in differentiating malignant from benign conditions.

Surgical Versus Nonsurgical Approaches to Proximal Bile Duct Obstruction

Surgery is the only treatment modality that provides the potential for cure of malignant biliary tract obstruction [15,16•,18, 19,20•,21•]. In cases selected for surgical resection, cure may be achieved in only 10% of patients with a malignancy of the proximal biliary tract; cure is very rarely achieved in cases of cholangiocarcinoma. Even if a cure cannot be achieved, patients may benefit from a palliative surgical procedure if it provides prolonged relief from biliary tract obstruction.

Adjuvant radiotherapy, chemotherapy, or both, may further prolong bile duct patency. The major advantage of successful surgical drainage is that patients may not require any additional intervention, such as changes of internally or externally clogged drains, for an extended period of time. Also, permanently

inserted external drains may cause the patient mechanical and other discomforts that can significantly reduce the quality of palliation. Surgical drainage depends on the feasibility of establishing adequate bilio-enteric anastomoses. The role of imaging therefore is to identify opportunities for drainage. It is with this in mind that various classifications [22,23•] of proximal bile duct obstruction should be used such as the one according to Bismuth and Corlette [22] (Fig. 130-6). A drainage procedure also may include partial surgical resection of the liver, currently feasible with acceptable morbidity and mortality.

Adequate biliary drainage usually can be achieved in types I and II lesions by any of the currently available techniques. Surgical resection can be done in anticipation that types I and II lesions progress toward type III. Once obstruction is of type III, surgical, percutaneous, and endoscopic drainage becomes very difficult, because an increasing number of bile ducts require separate drainage. Subhilar stenosis can be caused by a 2- to 3-cm long cholangiocarcinoma, a tumor of such limited size usually can be resected; alternatively, such a small lesion can be part of a large, invading gallbladder carcinoma, reemphasizing the role of adequate imaging before surgery. Drainage of one part of the biliary system may provide excellent palliation.

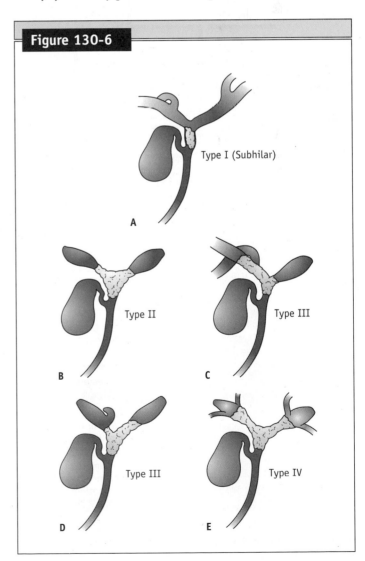

Figure 130-6

Type I (Subhilar)

A

Type II

B

Type III

C

Type III

D

Type IV

E

Classification of hilar lesions according to Bismuth and Corlette [22].

◼◼ A PATIENT-TAILORED MANAGEMENT PLAN

The design of a management plan must take into account the previously mentioned considerations. The algorithm provided in Figure 130-7 summarizes the surgical and nonsurgical options for proximal biliary tract obstruction. Ideally, a multidisciplinary team should review each case. Unfortunately, such a team often is dismayed when the actual level and extent of pathology are recognized after initiation of invasive procedures.

The initial strategy is determined by combining clinical data and noninvasive imaging to identify the extent of pathology and the suitability of the patient for surgical therapy. Vascular involvement, now assessed using Doppler ultrasonography, usually precludes surgery. In a limited number of patients, surgery will be undertaken without any invasive imaging. In cases of doubt and in patients for whom surgical therapy is not an option, direct cholangiography confirms and more precisely assesses the extent of disease; helps obtain a pathologic diagnosis, in some cases; and is used to establish biliary drainage, all in

the same session. The more apparent the surgical risks, the more emphasis is put on nonsurgical drainage for long-term palliation [24] (Fig. 130-8). Nonsurgical drainage can be done with various types of prostheses. Increasingly, metallic self-expandable stents are being used (Fig. 130-9). It must be emphasized that manipulation of the biliary system, particularly in the case of proximal biliary tract obstruction, is potentially risky and should be performed only by an experienced radiologist or therapeutic endoscopist. If drainage cannot be obtained, a patient with jaundice may become septic within hours. Optimal (re)hydration and intravenous antibiotic prophylaxis are important in helping to prevent infectious complications.

The difficulties in obtaining pathologic confirmation of the malignant nature of a stricture have been discussed. They are further exemplified by our own critical review of the pathologic findings in 86 patients in whom a presumptive preoperative diagnosis was made of cholangiocarcinoma at the bifurcation. Experienced surgeons believed even peroperatively that malignancy was obvious in a number of these cases. Postoperatively, 13.6% were found to have benign inflammatory changes mimicking a Klatskin tumor [11] (Fig. 130-1). Others have described similar cases before our more extensive report. The finding of benign disease offers the opportunity for alternative therapeutic options, including liver transplantation; transplantation should be considered for extensive benign stricturing with liver failure as well as for symptomatic primary sclerosing cholangitis. Liver transplantation for malignant disease is investigational and has a poor outcome. Patients with extrahepatic metastases should not be considered for such therapy [21•, 25•].

Major surgical intervention is not a desirable option in patients with comorbid cardiac, pulmonary, or renal disease; however, a patient with severe cholangitis, septicemia, and multiple organ failure may quickly recover after nonsurgical drainage. Thus, candidacy for surgery may require reassessment after biliary drainage has been established.

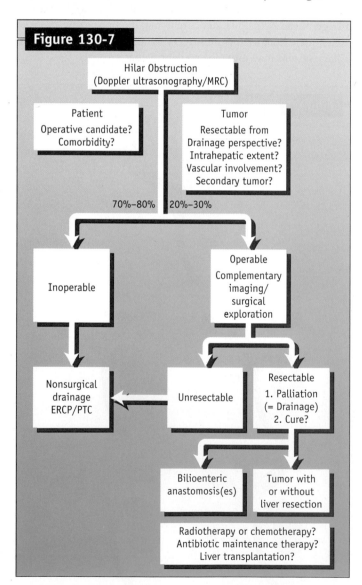

Figure 130-7

Algorithm for diagnosis and treatment of patients with obstruction of the bifurcation of the hepatic ducts. ERCP—endoscopic retrograde cholangiopancreatography; PTC—percutaneous transhepatic cholangiography.

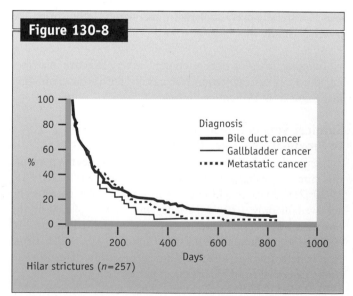

Figure 130-8

Survival of a large group of patients with biliary obstruction from a variety of causes and treated with endoprostheses placed at the bifurcation of the hepatic ducts. (*From* Coene [24]; with permission from the author.)

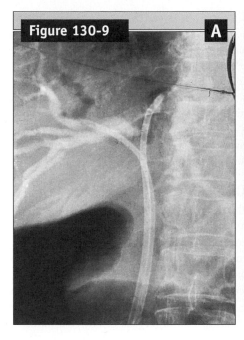 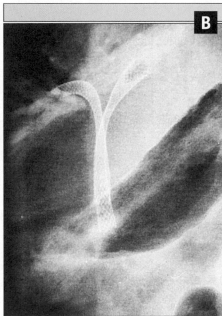

Figure 130-9

A, Two conventional endoprostheses (right and left systems) placed in the patient shown in Figure 130-1, a woman 78 years of age who quickly recovered from severe cholangitis after placement of these stents. She was subsequently deemed a candidate for surgery and underwent resection of the bifurcation of the hepatic ducts with two hepaticojejunostomies. She lived for another 2 years without recurrence of cholangitis or jaundice, then rapidly deteriorated and had extensive spread of malignancy within and outside of the liver. **B**, Two self-expandable metal stents for drainage of a hilar malignancy.

Role of Laparoscopy

Laparoscopy has gained renewed interest in staging malignancies and diagnosing peritoneal metastases that may defy detection using current imaging technology. However, noninvasive imaging techniques may identify patients with proximal biliary malignancies in whom surgery is a preferred approach. These patients typically have less extensive disease and therefore are less likely to have peritoneal metastases. In this respect, proximal cholangiocarcinoma probably differs from pancreatic cancer, in which laparoscopy is likely to be of greater benefit in identifying patients who may benefit from radical pancreaticoduodenectomy (Whipple's operation).

Specific Surgical Treatment

In properly selected patients, surgical resection may be attempted. Although there is a very limited chance for cure it may result in reestablishment of biliary drainage for a prolonged period. Resectability usually refers to the feasibility of resection of the bifurcation and may imply partial resection of the liver followed by multiple hepaticojejunostomies to reestablish biliary drainage. Peroperative intubation can be performed, or "access" loops can be created to allow subsequent external manipulations of the biliary system, including intraluminal radiotherapy. However, these access loops are not always useful and occasionally allow new problems to develop such as stomal varices in patients with tumor-associated portal vein obstruction.

In some cases a firm diagnosis of malignancy may not be established even at laparotomy. In well-selected cases, explorative laparotomy may be indicated to establish a diagnosis and explore surgical options.

Radiotherapy

Clinical trials have failed to establish a role for radiotherapy. Nonetheless, in some medical centers radiotherapy in combination with 5-FU (5-fluorouracil) is an important part of the management of hilar cholangiocarcinoma (Fig. 130-10). Some patients with nonradical resection of malignant tumors compli-

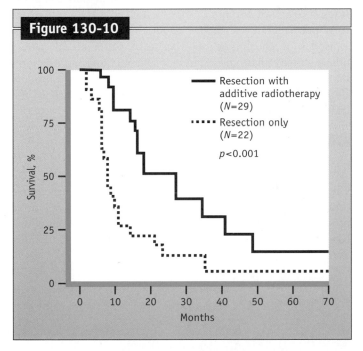

Figure 130-10

Survival outcome of resection of the bifurcation of the hepatic ducts for hilar cholangiocarcinoma (Klatskin tumor) with and without postoperative radiotherapy. Note that this was *not* a randomized trial but compared two treatment protocols. The differences in survival may indicate the potential benefit of radiotherapy, because careful comparison of clinical data showed that the group that did not receive radiotherapy had less severe disease compared with patients who received adjuvant radiotherapy. Not only is survival prolonged but recurrent biliary obstruction is delayed. (*From* Verbeek *et al* [29].)

cated by lymph node metastasis and neuroinvasive growth have survived more than 5 years after a combination of surgical therapy with radiotherapy. Some patients who underwent subsequent radiotherapy in the hilar area after surgery, later on autopsy had no local tumor recurrence, but were found to have multiple intra-abdominal metastases elsewhere. This is only rarely seen in patients who are managed without surgery. This observation reemphasizes the risk of intra-abdominal metastasis during surgery when tumor spread cannot be avoided. Although some investigators advocate surgery in combination with radiotherapy and chemotherapy, others doubt its benefit [23•]. Radiotherapy can be given externally alone or in combination with brachytherapy, allowing a relatively high dose to control local tumor load or recurrence while avoiding the complications of more extensive abdominal irradiation. Theoretically, the combination of 5-FU, a radiosensitizing agent, with radiotherapy should enhance the efficacy of radiotherapy; this has become the treatment of choice at many institutions.

Antibiotics

Cholangitis is a major problem in patients with hilar cholangiocarcinoma [26,27]. Antibiotics may be given as a single prophylactic dose to prevent cholangitis when manipulating the biliary system, as therapy for 5 to 7 days in doses to treat acute cholangitis, or as maintenance therapy. The patient with one or more biliary stents occasionally may become febrile. Because stent exchange may fail or be associated with new complications, a course of antibiotics may be used in certain patients to treat persistent fevers before attempting invasive procedures. Episodes of cholangitis may occur in patients with patent biliary-enteric anastomoses; in most patients, antibiotic maintenance therapy decreases the severity of this problem. Randomized clinical trials of such treatments are lacking and difficult to perform in this category of patients.

◼ DISTAL COMMON BILE DUCT OBSTRUCTION CAUSED BY CHOLANGIOCARCINOMA

Cholangiocarcinoma of the distal common bile duct may mimic cancer of the pancreatic head. Endoscopic drainage, the initial procedure of choice and often the definitive palliative procedure, usually can be achieved. Tumors of the pancreatic head are easily

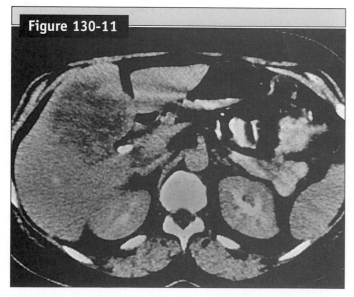

Figure 130-11

Computed tomography scan showing an intrahepatic mass, which was determined to be carcinoma of the gallbladder. Unfortunately, symptomatic gallbladder carcinoma usually has a poor outcome.

identified at ERCP; however, it can be difficult, even in the resected specimen, to differentiate between a cholangiocarcinoma invading the pancreas and a pancreatic carcinoma invading the common bile duct. Possible distal cholangiocarcinoma should be approached as pancreatic head malignancy, and a radical pancreatoduodenectomy is the treatment of choice for this condition in the appropriate patient. The 5-year survival rate of approximately 20% in most series of studies is slightly better than is that of pancreatic carcinoma. Ampullary tumors tend to present earlier and have a 5-year survival rate of 30% to 50%.

◼ GALLBLADDER CANCER

Gallbladder cancer has a 5-year survival rate of 4% and a 1-year survival rate of approximately 12%. In patients in whom cancer was found incidentally at cholecystectomy for benign disease, the 5-year survival rate still was only 15%. Despite attempts to improve the outcome with surgery and adjuvant therapies, results have remained poor. Surgery is the only therapy with the potential for a cure in properly selected patients; however, the debate over how aggressive the surgery should be continues.

Diagnosis

Unfortunately, symptomatic gallbladder cancer nearly always indicates advanced and incurable disease (Fig. 130-11). Symptoms include pain, jaundice, and weight loss, along with nonspecific complaints such as nausea. Pain can become a predominant complaint in advanced cases, more so than in cholangiocarcinoma.

Gallbladder cancer still is commonly diagnosed incidentally. A patient undergoing cholecystectomy for what is believed to be chronic cholecystitis with significant inflammation and gallstones may have widespread carcinoma. Inflammatory changes may mimic malignancy clinically. At the other extreme, a patient may undergo laparoscopic cholecystectomy for mild symptomatic gallstone disease with a resultant unexpected finding of carcinoma in situ or nonpenetrating gallbladder carcinoma, which may be identified during surgery or only by examination of the resected specimen. Metastatic tumors (eg, breast cancer and malignant melanoma) or other rare primary malignancies may be found occasionally.

Treatment

Although a variety of therapies are under investigation, no data are available from prospective randomized clinical trials that optimally guide management of patients with gallbladder carcinoma. Guidelines are based on small studies combined with common sense. The staging for gallbladder carcinoma is summarized in Table 130-2.

Table 130-2. Simplified Staging of Gallbladder Carcinoma

Stage	Criteria
I	Gallbladder wall involvement only
II	Perimuscular tissue involvement
III	Nodal involvement, with liver invasion of <2 cm
IV	Extensive local disease or metastatic disease

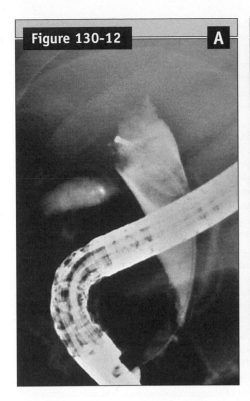
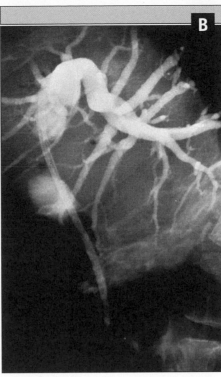

Figure 130-12

A

B

Endoprosthesis for gallbladder carcinoma. **A**, Endoscopic cholangiographic appearance of mid–common bile duct involvement by carcinoma. **B**, Endoprosthesis positioned within the left biliary system. The patient survived for several years, requiring infrequent stent exchanges for symptomatic biliary obstruction.

Guidelines for Treatment of Gallbladder Carcinoma

Nonsurgical palliation. Three types of patients should undergo nonsurgical palliation: 1) those with extensive disease, including a large tumor mass, ascites, or distant metastasis; 2) those in whom extensive malignancy is diagnosed after pathologic examination of the resected specimen and in whom many cuts through tumor were made and tumor spread in the abdominal cavity is likely to have occurred; and 3) those with significant comorbid diseases who are poor surgical candidates. Age is not a contraindication for consideration of surgical therapy.

Radical surgical treatment. Three types of patients are candidates for radical surgical treatment: 1) those who have limited disease (stage II and early stage III), preferably diagnosed or assumed before surgery, who have had detailed preoperative imaging studies to assess the feasibility of radical resection; 2) those with stage I disease who do not need more extensive surgery, as opposed to patients with advanced stage III or stage IV disease who cannot be cured by extensive surgery; and 3) those in whom the gallbladder has been opened immediately after removal, a suspicious lesion seen, and a frozen specimen examined, revealing gallbladder cancer. If discovered during laparoscopic surgery, conversion to open cholecystectomy should be considered and a more extensive procedure should be done.

Biliary endoprosthesis. Gallbladder carcinoma usually is amenable to endoscopic biliary drainage, unless extensive hilar invasion has occurred. Endoscopic drainage may provide excellent palliation for obstruction and its complications (Fig. 130-12). If endoscopic drainage fails, however, percutaneous drainage still may be beneficial.

Other therapies. Chemotherapy and radiotherapy, alone or in combination, are used to treat patients with gallbladder carcinoma but have uncertain benefit. Radiotherapy is unlikely to be useful in the case of a very large mass, because the necessary dosages would lead to significant morbidity. If extensive tumor spread has occurred during surgery, radiotherapy alone is less likely to benefit the patient because total abdominal radiation would be required and would add to morbidity.

■ REFERENCES

Recently published papers of particular interest have been highlighted as follows:
• Of interest
•• Of outstanding interest

1.• Bloustein PA: Association of carcinoma with congenital cystic conditions of the liver and bile ducts. *Am J Gastroent* 1997, 67:40–46
According to the author, choledochal cyst and biliary ductectasia are members of the family of polyfibrocystic disease which should be approached as a high risk premalignant condition.

2. Chijiiwa K, Tanaka M: Surgical strategy for patients with anomalous pancreaticobiliary ductal junction without choledochal cyst. *Int Surg* 1995, 80:215–217.

3. Nakanuma Y, Yamaguchi K, Ohta G, Terada T: The Japanese Hepatolithiasis Study Group. Pathologic features of heptolithiasis in Japan. *Hum Pathol* 1988, 19:1181–1186.

4. Chou ST, Chan CW: Mucin-producing cholangiocarcinoma: an autopsy study in Hong Kong. *Pathology* 1976, 8:321–328.

5. Redaelli CA, Buchler MW, Schilling MK, *et al.*: High Coincidence of Mirizzi syndrome and gallbladder carcinoma. *Surgery* 1997, 121:58–63.

6. Albores-Saavedra J, Henson DE, eds: *Atlas of Tumor Pathology.* Washington, DC: Armed Forces Institute of Pathology; 1986.

7. Anthony PP: Tumors of the hepatobiliary system. In *Diagnostic Histopathology of Tumors.* Edited by Fletcher CDM. Edinburgh: Churchill Livingstone; 1995:275–320.

8. Klatskin G: Adenocarcinoma of the hepatic duct at its bifurcation within the porta hepatis. *Am J Med* 1965, 38:241–256.

9. van Leeuwen DJ, Huibregtse K, Tytgat GNJ: Carcinoma of the hepatic confluence 25 years after Klatskin's description: diagnosis and endoscopic management. *Sem Liver Dis* 1990, 10:102–114.

10. Roa I, Araya JC, Villaseca M, *et al.*: Preneoplastic lesions and gallbladder cancer: an estimate of the period required for progression. *Gastroenterology* 1996, 111:232–236.

11. Verbeek PCM, van Leeuwen DJ, De Wit L Th, *et al.*: Benign hepatic confluence obstruction mimicking hilar malignancy. *Surgery* 1992, 112:866–871.

12. Hann LE, Getrajdman GI, Brown KT, *et al.*: Hepatic lobar atrophy: association with ipsilateral portal vein obstruction. *AJR Am J Roentgenol* 1996, 167:1017–1021.

13. Hann LE, Greatrex KV, Bach AM, *et al.*: Cholangiocarcinoma at the hepatic hilus: sonographic findings. *AJR Am J Roentgenol* 1997, 168:985–989.

14. Bach AM, Hann LE, Brown KT, *et al.*: Portal vein evaluation with US: comparison to angiography combined with CT arterial portography. *Radiology* 1996, 201:149–154.

15. Silverman W, Slivka A: New technique for bilateral metal mesh stent insertion to treat hilar cholangiocarcinoma. *Gastrointest Endosc* 1996, 43:61–63.

16.• Schima W, Prokesch R, Osterreicher C, *et al.*: Biliary Wallstent endoprosthesis in malignant hilar obstruction: long-term results with regard to the type of obstruction. *Clin Radiol* 1997, 52:213–219.
Extensive experiences with percutaneous and endoscopic drainage techniques are provided here. The authors report that self-expandable stents are increasingly taking over for long-term palliation of hilar obstruction.

17. Fong Y, Brennan MF, Turnball A, *et al.*: Gallbladder cancer discovered during laparoscopic surgery: potential for iatrogenic tumor dissemination. *Arch Surg* 1993, 128:1054–1056.

18. Cameron JL, Pitt HA, Zinner MJ, *et al.*: Management of proximal cholangiocarcinomas by surgical resection and radiotherapy. *Am J Surg* 1992, 159:91–98.

19. Bismuth H. Nakoche R, Diamond T: Management strategies in resection of cholangiocarcinoma. *Ann Surg* 1992, 215:311–338.

20.• Kuvshinott BW, Fong Y, Blumgart LH. Proximal bile duct tumors. *Surg Oncol Clin North Am* 1996, 6:317–336.
This is an article from one of the leading surgical centers reporting its experience with cholangiocarcinoma.

21.• Klempnauer J, Ridder GJ, Werner M, *et al.*: What constitutes longterm survival after surgery for hilar cholangiocarcinoma? *Cancer* 1997, 79:26–34.
This is an article from one of the leading surgical centers reporting its experience with cholangiocarcinoma, including results of liver transplantation.

22. Bismuth H, Corlette MB: Intrahepatic cholangio-enteric anastomosis in carcinoma of the hilus of the liver. *Surg Gynecol Obstet* 1975, 140:170–178.

23.• Nakeeb A, Pitt HA, Sohn TA, *et al.*: Cholangiocarcinoma. A spectrum of intrahepatic, perihilar, and distal tumors. *Ann Surg* 1996, 224:463–475.
This article provides a classification of obstruction of the biliary system with related treatment perspectives.

24. Coene PPLO: Endoscopic biliary stenting: mechanisms and possible solutions of the clogging phenomenon [PhD thesis]. Amsterdam: University of Amsterdam; 1990

25.• Washburn WK, Lewis WD, Jenkins RL: Aggressive surgical resection for cholangiocarcinoma. *Arch Surg* 1995, 130:270–276.
This is a report from a center that included liver transplantation in its aggressive surgical therapies. The authors conclude that unlike its usefulness in the treatment of benign disease, transplantation remains a doubtful alternative for treatment of malignant disease.

26. van den Hazel SJ, Speelman P, Tytgat GNJ, *et al.*: Acute and recurrent cholangitis. The role of antibiotics in the treatment and prevention. *Clin Infect Dis* 1994, 19:279–286.

27. van den Hazel SJ, Speelman P, Tytgat GNJ, van Leeuwen DJ: Successful treatment of recurrent cholangitis with antibiotic maintenance therapy. *Eur J Clin Microbiol Infect Dis* 1994, 13:662–665.

28. Verbeek PCM, van Leeuwen DJ, van der Heyde MN, Gonzalez DG: Does additive radiotherapy after hilar resection improve survival of cholangiocarcinoma? *Ann Chirug* 1991, 45:350–354.

131 Endoscopic Management of Biliary Obstruction

Julie Spivack and Ira M. Jacobson

Malignant obstruction of the extrahepatic biliary tract is a common consequence of carcinoma of the pancreas, ampulla, bile duct, or gallbladder, but it also may result from metastatic spread of nonpancreaticobiliary tumors or lymphoma (Table 131-1). Appropriate management relies on accurate staging of the primary lesion and determination of resectability in surgically fit candidates. Unfortunately, fewer than 20% of patients have resectable disease at the time of presentation. Since the introduction of endoscopic retrograde cholangiopancreatography (ERCP) in 1970, endoscopic sphincterotomy (ES) in 1974, and transpapillary stenting in 1979, ERCP has been essential to diagnose and treat malignant biliary obstruction. The endoscopic management of malignant biliary obstruction is reviewed and compared with other modalities, such as surgery and percutaneous transhepatic cholangiography.

ANATOMY OF THE EXTRAHEPATIC BILIARY TREE

The right and left hepatic ducts emerge from the transverse fissure of the liver where they join to form the common hepatic duct (CHD). The cystic duct, which arises from the gallbladder, converges with the CHD to form the common bile duct (CBD). The CBD then passes posterior to the first portion of the duodenum and traverses behind or within the head of the pancreas before it tangentially enters the second portion of the duodenum and opens into the major papilla (Fig. 131-1). The CBD and main pancreatic duct may join outside the duodenum or form a common channel as they course through the duodenal wall or even enter the papilla separately. (Fig. 131-2).

The extrahepatic biliary tract typically is divided into three anatomic areas: the upper third, comprising the confluence of the left and right hepatic ducts plus the CHD; the middle third, comprising the CBD between the cystic duct and the upper border of the duodenum; and the lower third, between the upper border of the pancreas and the ampulla of Vater [1]. Malignant obstruction of the biliary tree may occur at any level from the hilum of the liver to the major papilla.

PATHOPHYSIOLOGY

Malignant obstruction of the biliary tree results in cholestasis and reduced excretion of bile into the small intestine. When luminal bile acid levels fall below the critical micellar concentration, steatorrhea and fat-soluble vitamin deficiencies may result, with ensuing malnutrition, weight loss, and coagulopathy. Pruritus may relate to retained bile acids, whereas jaundice and acholic stools result from impaired biliary excretion of bilirubin. Impaired cholesterol excretion leads to the formation of xanthelasma, xanthomas, and alterations in the erythrocyte membrane, leading to target cell and spur cell formation. Prolonged biliary obstruction may cause hepatic failure. The adverse physiologic sequelae of biliary obstruction warrant strong consideration of biliary drainage in patients with malignant obstruction even in the absence of infection or pruritus.

CLINICAL FEATURES

Unfortunately, the early clinical features of pancreaticobiliary cncers are very subtle and often nonspecific. These include anorexia, nausea, weight loss, epigastric or back pain, and depression. In addition, painless jaundice is a characteristic hallmark of malignant biliary obstruction. In contrast, acute illness with the abrupt onset of jaundice, fever or abdominal pain in a patient who has otherwise been well suggests choledocholithiasis, especially in a patient with demonstrable gallbladder stones or a history of cholecystectomy. However, there are no absolute distinguishing signs between benign and malignant obstruction. Occasionally, patients with CBD stones may present with painless jaundice and patients with malignant obstruction may present with an acute illness, including infection.

Other than jaundice, physical findings may include a palpable abdominal mass, a palpable, nontender gallbladder, (Courvosier's sign), or hepatomegaly. Uncommonly, ascites from peritoneal carcinomatosis may be present.

In some cases, jaundice may be wrongly attributed to choledocholithiasis or pancreatitis, and thus, the clinician must maintain a high index of suspicion to avoid missing a poten-

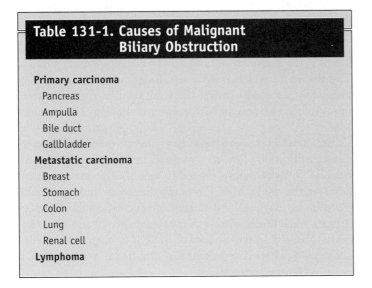

Table 131-1. Causes of Malignant Biliary Obstruction

Primary carcinoma
  Pancreas
  Ampulla
  Bile duct
  Gallbladder
Metastatic carcinoma
  Breast
  Stomach
  Colon
  Lung
  Renal cell
Lymphoma

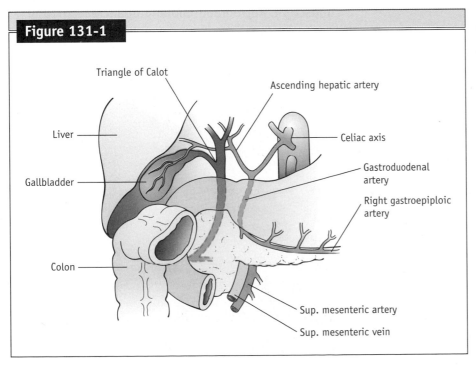

Figure 131-1

Relationship of the gallbladder and extrahepatic biliary tract to the liver, duodenum, colon, and pancreas. (*From Yamada et al.* [24].)

Triangle of Calot
Ascending hepatic artery
Liver
Celiac axis
Gallbladder
Gastroduodenal artery
Right gastroepiploic artery
Colon
Sup. mesenteric artery
Sup. mesenteric vein

tially resectable tumor. Warning signs of malignancy in the patient with obstructive jaundice include age over 40 years, unexplained loss of more than 10% of body weight, unexplained lumbar pain, new onset of dyspepsia, new onset of diabetes mellitus without family history or other predisposing factors, idopathic pancreatitis, or unexplained steatorrhea. A trap is occasionally sprung on the unwary clinician by the patient who presents with obstructive jaundice, gallbladder stones, and a distal biliary stricture without a pancreatic mass on computed tomography (CT) scan. It may be tempting to attribute this picture to an inflammatory stricture or "papillary stenosis" and monitor the patient. All too often, it becomes clear later that the patient has cancer of the pancreas.

Approximately 80% to 90% of patients with cancer of the head of the pancreas present with jaundice, as opposed to only 6% of patients with cancer in the pancreatic body or tail. Patients with ampullary cancers and cholangiocarcinomas almost always present with jaundice, whereas this is a late complication of cancer of the gallbladder.

■ DIAGNOSIS

Ultrasonography

Real-time ultrasonography is an excellent modality for the initial evaluation of persons with jaundice. In patients with intact gallbladders, biliary ductal dilation is defined as an extrahepatic duct over 7 mm wide or intrahepatic ducts over 5 mm wide. Sonography is as accurate as CT scan in detecting the presence of bile duct obstruction, though it may reveal less information about the underlying cause. Sonography reveals bile duct stones in 25% to 50% of patients in whom they are present. If the obstruction is distal in a patient with suspected malignancy, pancreatic cancer is most likely, whereas if it is hilar, cholangiocarcinoma or metastatic disease to the porta

hepatis is probable. Although an inexpensive and noninvasive tool for initial investigation, ultrasonography is highly dependent on the skill of the ultrasonographer. It is further limited in patients who are obese, in those with previous upper abdominal operations, and in patients requiring evaluation of the retroperitoneum.

Computed Tomography Scan

When malignant biliary obstruction is suspected, the diagnostic test of choice is an abdominal CT scan using both oral and intravenous contrast agents. An oral contrast agent must be given immediately before the scan to delineate the duodenum. Thin sections (5-mm collimation) through the extrahepatic biliary tree and pancreas and acquisition of images during the dynamic phase of iodinated contrast enhancement are important. The use of helical CT scans allows for excellent identification of the adjacent vasculature and has greatly decreased the need for angiography.

Magnetic Resonance Imaging

Magnetic resonance (MR) imaging has been used to a limited extent in the diagnosis and staging of pancreaticobiliary tumors. The degree to which it adds to current noninvasive imaging techniques, especially helical CT scan, requires further evaluation. A major advance in MR imaging technology has been the advent of magnetic resonance cholangiopancreatography (MRCP), which has the capacity to provide excellent noninvasive identification of the pancreatic and bile ducts (Fig. 131-3). Because it lacks biopsy capability and therapeutic potential, however, the role of MRCP is purely diagnostic and its ultimate place in the diagnosis and staging of pancreaticobiliary tumors remains to be determined. The preponderance of attention thus far has focused on the capacity of MRCP to diagnose choledocholithiasis, where if negative it may obviate the need for ERCP prior to cholecystectomy.

Endoscopic Retrograde Cholangiopancreatography

The sensitivity of CT scans is diminished for lesions less than 1 to 2 cm and for lesions in the periampullary region. Thus, when malignant biliary obstruction is suspected but cannot be

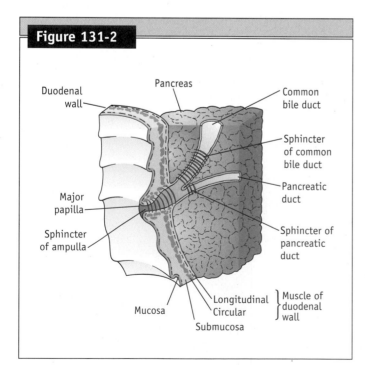

Figure 131-2

Duodenal wall · Pancreas · Common bile duct · Sphincter of common bile duct · Pancreatic duct · Sphincter of pancreatic duct · Major papilla · Sphincter of ampulla · Mucosa · Longitudinal · Circular · Submucosa · Muscle of duodenal wall

Muscular apparatus at the terminal end of the common bile duct. (*From* Yamada *et al.* [24].)

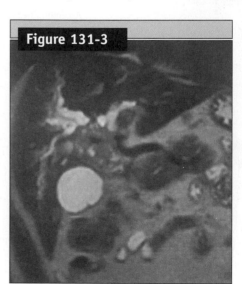

Figure 131-3

Magnetic resonance cholangiopancreatogram (MRCP) revealing obstruction of right and left hepatic ducts by a hilar mass. (*Courtesy of* L. Schwartz, MD.)

confirmed by ultrasonography and CT scan, ERCP is the next step. Characteristic signs of malignancy seen on ERCP include an abrupt termination of any part of the biliary tree or pancreatic duct with proximal dilation; a shelf defect; an irregular stricture; and narrowing of both the distal CBD and the pancreatic duct, the so-called double duct sign (Figs. 131-4, 131-5, and 131-6). ERCP is most sensitive for lesions in the extrahepatic biliary tree and offers the added advantage of potentially providing a tissue biopsy specimen for diagnosis with wire-guided brush cytology or forceps biopsy. The ability to identify and sample small intraductal lesions may be enhanced by the use of a "mother-baby" scope system in which a slim choledochoscope is passed through the biopsy channel of the larger scope and into the bile duct. Overall, specificity of pathologic diagnosis with endoscopic tissue sampling techniques approaches 100%; however, sensitivity ranges from 15% to 70%. Hence the positive predictive value is excellent; however, the negative predictive value is poor and malignancy cannot be excluded based on a negative result. Despite the imperfect sensitivity, ERCP is not considered complete in a patient with a potentially malignant stricture unless, at the least, cytologic samplings have been obtained from the stricture before stent placement.

A recent prospective study from Europe compared the sensitivity of ultrasonography, CT scan, and ERCP in the diagnosis of extrahepatic and intrahepatic malignant obstruction. ERCP was found to be superior in patients with extrahepatic disease (57%, 80%, and 83% sensitivity, respectively), and ultrasonography to be superior in detecting intrahepatic lesions (100%, 77%, and 60%, respectively) [2]. Although the superiority of sonography over CT scan in the latter setting may be questioned, it is difficult to dispute the conclusion of the study that these three methods of imaging often complement one another; all may be necessary to evaluate patients with jaundice who have a suspected malignancy. Of course, ERCP does not provide accurate staging of disease or determination of resectability.

Endoscopic Ultrasonography

The newest diagnostic tool available is endoscopic ultrasonography (EUS). EUS is a minimally invasive technique using a high-frequency transducer placed directly in the gastric and duodenal lumen adjacent to the pancreas, biliary tree, and gallbladder to provide high-resolution sonographic images of these structures. EUS can detect lesions smaller than 2 cm, as well as lymph node and vascular involvement by tumor. The latest lin-

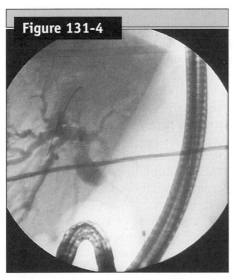

Figure 131-4

Proximal dilation of the biliary tree with cut-off caused by a cholangiocarcinoma.

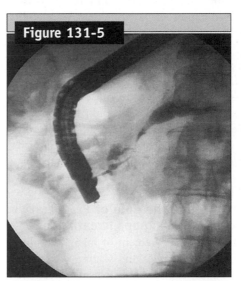

Figure 131-5

Malignant stricture of the pancreatic duct secondary to carcinoma of the pancreatic head.

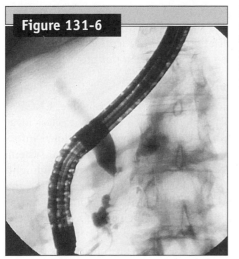

Figure 131-6

Malignant stricture of the bile duct in a patient with carcinoma of the head of the pancreas.

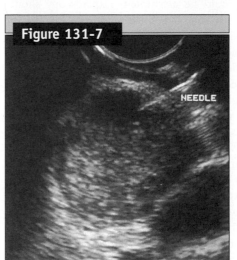

Figure 131-7

Needle aspirate of a pancreatic mass under linear array endoscopic ultrasound guidance. The cytologic specimen revealed adenocarcinoma.

ear array EUS scopes also allow the endoscopist to obtain fine-needle aspiration of suspicious lesions (Fig. 131-7). Recent studies suggest that EUS is superior to conventional sonography, CT scan, and angiography in assessing resectability [3]. In expert hands, radial and linear array scopes offer equal accuracy in staging; however, the capacity to obtain a tissue specimen for biopsy to determine the diagnosis with linear array scopes may make them preferable for this purpose [4•]. Experience with EUS is becoming more widespread.

Endoscopic Retrograde Cholangiopancreatography Versus Endoscopic Ultrasonography

In some clinical situations in which ERCP was traditionally performed, it now is questioned if EUS should precede or even replace it. This seems an appropriate question when the CT scan suggests a mass in the body or tail of the pancreas. Previously, pancreatography was undertaken to determine whether the ductal anatomy was suspicious for neoplasia. EUS offers the advantages of better definition of the mass, information about local invasion, and the capacity to obtain a tissue specimen for biopsy, all at lower risk. Even for lesions in the pancreatic head, for which ERCP offers the capacity to obtain cytologic or biopsy samples, EUS offers a superior yield of tissue specimen to determine the diagnosis and more information for staging and determination of potential for resectability. Thus, for lesions in the pancreatic head considered potentially resectable, EUS can precede ERCP, and the latter may not be required at all when preoperative biliary drainage is not considered necessary (see the discussion later in this chapter). When biliary drainage is planned or when the cause of the biliary obstruction is unclear, however, ERCP should be performed first. EUS should be employed later if the results of cytologic sampling by ERCP are negative or if critical staging information is still considered necessary.

▮ TREATMENT
Resectable Malignancy and the Role of Preoperative Endoscopic Retrograde Cholangiopancreatography

Several options exist for the management of malignant biliary obstruction. When initial assessment and staging suggest that the tumor is resectable and the patient is medically fit, curative surgical resection should be attempted. Laparoscopy should precede laparotomy to rule out small peritoneal or hepatic metastases that would prevent cure, thus avoiding unnecessary surgery. Laparascopic ultrasound is receiving increasing attention as a means of detecting vascular invasion or occult metastasis. Initial laparoscopy is not necessary in patients who have evidence of duodenal obstruction and who will require surgical bypass regardless of whether the tumor can be resected.

Controversy persists regarding the utility of preoperative ERCP. Diagnostic ERCP is indicated if the cause of jaundice is obscure. After opacification of the biliary tree in such cases, it is essential to provide drainage by placement of an intraductal stent to prevent postprocedural cholangitis. Although a nasobiliary tube provides adequate temporary drainage for this purpose, a 10F or an 11.5F endoprosthesis is preferred even when surgery is planned because it cannot be pulled out inadvertently and is far better tolerated by the patient.

When the diagnosis is clear based on ultrasonography and CT scan, the question arises whether preoperative biliary drainage reduces surgical morbidity and mortality. Proponents argue that the potential benefits of preoperative decompression include faster recovery of liver function, correction of coagulopathy, improved nutritional status, and improved renal function. Opponents state that cannulation of the biliary tree only succeeds in introducing infection, which in turn, leads to an increase in postoperative septic complications. Additionally, the reversal of metabolic derangements seen with biliary decompression takes weeks to occur, leading to the argument that it is unlikely to benefit the patient without incurring an undue delay in surgery. Three randomized prospective studies from the 1980s failed to demonstrate any reduction in morbidity or mortality with preoperative biliary drainage [5•]; however, these studies used percutaneous transhepatic stenting, and therefore, it is unclear if endoscopically placed stents would offer an advantage owing to the lower complication rate associated with this approach. Anecdotally, some hepatobiliary surgeons note that preoperative biliary stenting triggers an inflammatory response in the bile duct, leading to a thickened wall and adherence to local structures that make surgical dissection more tedious.

Unresectable Malignancy

The role of ERCP in the treatment of malignant obstructive jaundice is greatest in the large number of patients who, unfortunately, are found to have unresectable disease. Palliation of jaundice relieves pruritus and also may improve nausea, anorexia, and abdominal discomfort [6]. Nevertheless, not every person with incurable disease requires palliation. Patients who are asymptomatic or patients who have a preterminal stage of disease are unlikely to attain any meaningful benefit from decompression of the biliary tree. In those patients who are symptomatic, it is essential to document that the symptoms derive from biliary obstruction and not from diffuse hepatic parenchymal infiltration by tumor or metastases.

Palliation of biliary obstruction may be achieved endoscopically, percutaneously, or surgically. Because each of these methods achieves biliary decompression in over 90% of patients with distal bile duct strictures, choice of technique depends on local expertise, the patients' symptoms and performance status, disease bulk, and level of obstruction. The nonoperative techniques have diminished rates of success (70% to 75%) and a concomitant increase in complication rates in patients with hilar lesions; however, surgery is also more difficult in this group.

Endoscopic Stent Placement

When therapeutic endoscopic expertise is available, ERCP is preferable to the transhepatic approach because it is less invasive, has fewer complications, and provides additional information about the major papilla and pancreatic ductal system. The patient scheduled for ERCP is fasted after midnight. Before the procedure, coagulopathy, if severe, is corrected and prophylactic intravenous antibiotics with good biliary penetration are given. Third-generation penicillins or a quinolone is suitable; use of aminoglycosides is avoided in patients who are significantly jaundiced from malignant biliary obstruction because of enhanced susceptibility to nephrotoxicity. After intravenous conscious sedation, a therapeutic side-viewing endoscope with a channel capable of accommodating at least a 10F stent is passed into the second portion of the duodenum, and the major papilla is identified. Decisions regarding the need for pancreatography should be individualized. When the cause of obstruction is ambiguous or when cytologic brushings from the pancreas are desired, attempts should be made to cannulate the pancreatic duct before the bile duct. If the diagnosis is known before ERCP, pancreatography is not necessary. A catheter is then passed through the papillary orifice into the CBD, and contrast is injected under fluoroscopy to delineate the exact length and location of the obstruction, which is necessary to select the appropriate length of endoprosthesis to be inserted. Selection of stent diameter and type are discussed subsequently.

After biliary cannulation is accomplished, a guidewire is passed through the catheter and advanced across the strictured segment. Although no randomized studies exist that evaluate the role of ES before stent placement, some experts advocate making a small incision to facilitate stent insertion and avoid recannulation of an intact papilla if future ERCP is necessitated by stent occlusion. Moreover, a recent study strongly suggests that ES reduces the risk of postprocedural pancreatitis in patients with proximal biliary strictures. It is theorized that proximal lesions serve as a fulcrum, leading to medial deflection of the stent and compression of the pancreatic orifice [7]. Presently, we individualize our approach, preferring to perform ES when cannulation of the ampulla or traversal of the stricture has been difficult, in case ERCP may be necessary again. We also generally perform ES in patients with proximal biliary lesions, which are often scirrhous and may offer considerable resistance to stent passage. Presently, no prospective randomized trials exist that evaluate the merits of ES before stent placement.

In preparation for stent placement, the guidewire should be placed well beyond the stricture into an intrahepatic duct to minimize the risk of it being pulled out inadvertently during subsequent maneuvers (Fig. 131-8). A stiff 6F polyethylene inner catheter is then passed over the guidewire beyond the stricture, and the stent is inserted over the catheter. Important

technical considerations include the need to keep the tip of the endoscope close to the papilla, and for the assistant to maintain tension on the inner catheter and guidewire as the endoscopist pushes the stent in the patient. The length of the stent should be selected to ensure that its proximal end will be located at least 1 to 2 cm above the proximal aspect of the stricture (Fig. 131-9).

Once the stent is correctly positioned, the inner catheter and guidewire can be withdrawn and drainage observed. Failure to observe immediate spontaneous bile flow at this point or, at the very least, bile flow when suction is applied via the endoscope, should raise concern over whether the stent is in proper position (Fig. 131-10, see also **Color Plate**).

Self-expandable metallic stents such as the Wallstent have a preassembled delivery system. Once in correct position, the stent expands. Full expansion may take up to 24 hours. Radiopaque markers delineate the proximal and distal ends of the stent. Deployment is initiated with the end of the stent positioned well above the stricture, because the stent shortens during deployment (Figs. 131-11 and 131-12). For distal strictures, such as those associated with pancreatic cancer, the stent should be pulled back during deployment so that its distal end protrudes about 1 cm beyond the papilla (Fig. 131-13,

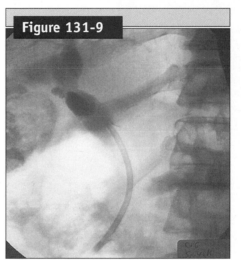

Figure 131-9

A patient with distal bile duct stricture and marked proximal biliary dilatation from a pancreatic head tumor. A guidewire has been placed well into the intrahepatic biliary tree, providing a secure anchor in preparation for stent placement.

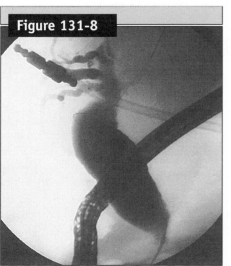

Figure 131-8

Guidewire in place in preparation for stent placement.

Figure 131-10

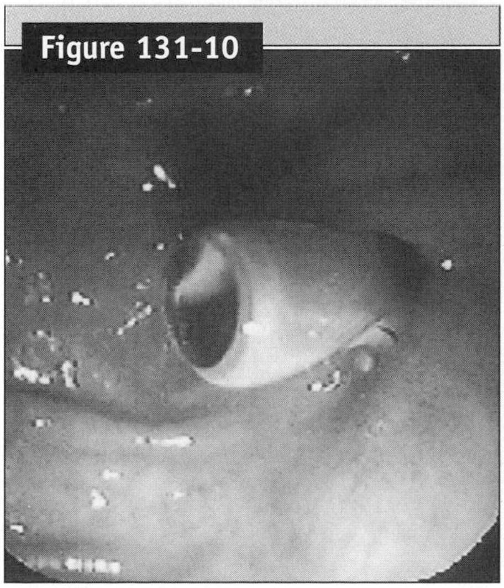

Bile draining from the distal end of a polyethylene stent immediately after stent placement. See also **Color Plate**.

see also **Color Plate**). For proximal biliary strictures, the metal stent may be left entirely within the bile duct above the papilla.

Metal stents become embedded in the bile duct wall and cannot be removed. When the stent is fully deployed but the position is suboptimal, another metal stent can be placed inside the first one, extending beyond it in either direction. Epithelialization of the stent eliminates the complication of future migration that may be seen with plastic stents; however, the open strut configuration of metal stents may permit tumor ingrowth and subsequent stent occlusion (see the discussion later in this chapter).

After stent placement, patients usually are hospitalized overnight. However, some patients may be discharged the same day. We continue administration of intravenous or oral antibiotics after the procedure to prevent cholangitis until adequate biliary drainage is documented by improvement in liver function test results.

Technical success is achieved in at least 85% of patients. Endoscopic failures most often are due to the inability to access the papilla secondary to duodenal obstruction by tumor; unusual anatomy, as seen in patients with diverticuli; previous Billroth II or Roux-en-Y anastomosis; inability to traverse the stricture with a guidewire; or inability to obtain a deep cannulation in the case of proximal lesions. Occasionally, the papilla cannot be cannulated; however, with the use of needle-knife sphincterotomy, successful overall cannulation rates exceed 95%. In the case of endoscopic failure, percutaneous drainage may be necessary or a combined percutaneous-endoscopic approach may be undertaken.

Cholangitis and pancreatitis are the most common immediate complications after endoprosthesis insertion. When performed, the small ES rarely results in significant bleeding or retroperitoneal perforation. Complication rates vary up to 36%; however, major procedural morbidity is less than 10% (Table 131-2) [8–11]. The 30-day mortality rate ranges from 6% to 20%, with a median survival of only 6 months owing mostly to the advanced nature of the underlying malignancy [8–10]. A recent meta-analysis of series published between 1981 and 1990 reports that late complications from endoscopic stent placement vary from 13% to 45% and may include stent occlusion with recurrent jaundice and cholangitis, stent migration, duodenal perforation, stent fracture, and cholecystitis [10]. Late development of duodenal obstruction by tumor occurs in 5% to 14% of patients who initially received nonsurgical palliation [8,10].

Stent Migration

The published rate of stent migration is 5% [12]. Distal stent migration may result in damage to the duodenal wall, with subsequent hemorrhage and perforation. The major problems with proximal migration are loss of adequate biliary drainage and resultant cholangitis. These problems can be managed by placing a second stent alongside the first or extracting the original stent with a balloon, basket, snare, or guidewire-assisted stent extractor.

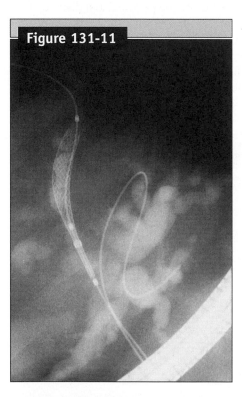

Figure 131-11

Partial deployment of a metal stent within a malignant stricture. Note the radiopaque markers on either end of the stent to assist in positioning prior to deployment. (*Courtesy of* M. Sossenheimer, MD.)

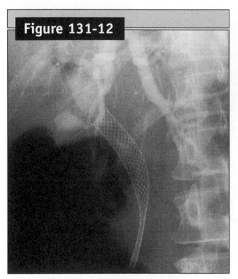

Figure 131-12

Metal stent fully deployed within a malignant stricture. (*Courtesy of* M. Sossenheimer, MD.)

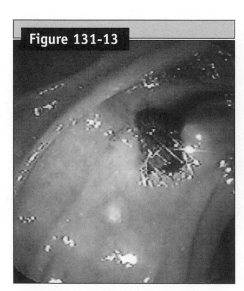

Figure 131-13

Wallstent with distal tip protruding out of the papilla. See also **Color Plate**.

Table 131-2. Complications of Biliary Stent Placement

Mechanism	Clinical manifestation	Incidence, %
Placement-related	Failed placement	15–20
	Hemorrhage	4
	Perforation	5
Obstruction-related	Jaundice	8*
	Cholangitis	8*
	Pancreatitis	3
	Liver abscess	2
Migration-related	Perforation	0–8
	Cholangitis and jaundice	8
Stent fracture	Cholangitis	Rare

*Early incidence, approaches 100% at average of 5 months.
Modified from Smilanich and Hafner [11].

Stent Occlusion and Stent Diameter

The most common late complication of endoprosthesis placement is stent occlusion, which may occur days to years after deployment. Because many patients will die from their underlying malignancy before occlusion occurs, stent exchange may never be necessary and is required in only 20% to 30% of patients. The pathogenesis of plastic stent occlusion is related to the formation of a bacterial biofilm and subsequent deposition of sludge containing products of bacterial metabolism such as calcium bilirubinate. Pharmacologic means of preventing stent occlusion are not consistently effective.

Various characteristics of endoprostheses may contribute to occlusion, including stent shape, position, diameter, length, design, and material. Inner stent diameter has been shown to be a critical factor in determining stent patency; 11.5F stents have twice the flow rate of 10F stents, which in turn, have 170% the flow rate of 8F stents, translating into mean patencies of 67 and 144 days for 7F and 10F stents, respectively [13]. The greater flow seen in stents larger than 10F, however, does not correlate with a clinically significant difference in outcome [14••].

The potential for cholangitis and sepsis when stents occlude has led some authorities to favor scheduled stent exchanges. The optimal timing of such exchanges, however, is unclear. Given the low occlusion rates with 10F to 11.5F stents of 4.2% and 10.8% at 3 and 6 months, respectively, Frakes and coworkers [15] recommended a 6-month interval between stent replacements to minimize cost and patient inconvenience. Alternatively, one may choose to follow patients closely and change the stent at the first sign of occlusive symptoms (eg, low-grade fever, malaise, pruritus, and jaundice). Patients must be advised to contact their physician promptly should any of these symptoms appear. Patients not ill enough to require immediate hospitalization should be given oral antibiotic therapy (eg, with a quinolone like ciprofloxacin) after any febrile episode until stent exchange has been accomplished.

Endoscopic management of occluded stents is simple and is associated with resolution of obstructive symptoms. Typically, endoscopy is performed to the duodenum, the stent is grasped with a minisnare or basket and extracted through the endoscopic channel, and a new one is placed across the stricture using standard technique. Because the tumor may have enlarged in the interim, careful measurement of the stricture length should be made before selecting the size of the replacement stent. Devices are available that, after placement of a guidewire through the old stent, permit its removal over the wire without loss of access to the biliary tree.

Metallic Versus Plastic Stents

The problem of plastic stent occlusion led to the development of large-diameter self-expandable metallic stents. FDA-approved metallic stents available for use in the United States include, the Gianturco-Rosch Z Stent and the Wallstent. These stents are delivered in a compressed and sheathed form such that removal of the sheath results in spontaneous expansion without the need for balloon dilation. The Gianturco Z stent is delivered in a 12F system and expands to 25F and 30 mm in length. The Wallstent is a stainless steel mesh deployed from an 8F system. It expands to 30F when it is fully opened and is available in 42- and 68-mm lengths.

The US Wallstent Study Group performed the largest randomized multicenter trial comparing the Wallstent to 10F plastic endobiliary prostheses [16••]. The trial randomized 182 patients with biliary strictures such that 94 received Wallstents and 88 received plastic stents; placement was successful in 97% and 95%, respectively. Early complication rates included 3% stent occlusion with plastic stents (none with Wallstents) and 7% mortality in each group owing to underlying disease. Late complications included stent occlusion in 5% of Wallstents and an additional 25% of plastic stents. Tumor ingrowth or overgrowth was seen in 10% of Wallstents and was not observed with plastic stents, resulting in an overall complication rate of 16% for Wallstents and 31% for plastic stents. This advantage was observed regardless of stricture site and was even more pronounced in patients who had a previously occluded plastic stent. The probability of a plastic stent occlusion was determined to be 2.8 times greater than for Wallstents. No difference in patient survival based on life table analysis was seen. The study concluded that there are significant clinical and economic advantages to Wallstent placement, despite higher initial cost, owing to the reduced need for subsequent interventions. A second prospective study from Europe confirmed these results [17•].

Occlusion caused by tumor ingrowth is by far the most common complication of metal stents. Other reported complications include duodenal ulceration and hemobilia related to erosion of the stent into a blood vessel adjacent to the bile duct.

As stated earlier, plastic stents can easily be removed and replaced; however, occluded metallic stents cannot be extracted owing to epithelialization of the stent. Recannalization of the stent lumen may be achieved by placement of a second metallic or plastic endoprosthesis within the existing lumen. Development of covered, closed framework, and removable stents is underway and may lead to a further advantage for metallic stents [18].

PERCUTANEOUS TRANSHEPATIC BILIARY DRAINAGE

The percutaneous transhepatic biliary drainage (PTBD) approach was introduced in the 1970s. The procedure requires hospitalization and is routinely performed with ultrasonography or CT guidance after administration of prophylactic antibiotics, intravenous sedation, and local anesthesia. Once the biliary tree is accessed, a guidewire is passed through the obstruction over which a drainage catheter is then placed. Success of external drainage approaches 100%; however, whenever possible, drainage should be internalized to avoid losing large volumes of bile and resulting severe dehydration, electrolyte disturbances, and malabsorption. Patients also prefer internal drainage for cosmetic reasons. Internalization can be achieved by placing a plastic or self-expanding metallic endoprosthesis across the stricture and through the papilla so that bile flows into the duodenum. External drainage may be maintained for a day or two and then clamped to ensure successful internal drainage before extracting the external catheter. An option with plastic stents is to place an external-internal drain in which one end is in the duodenum and the other end protrudes, remains capped, and is taped to the skin. This approach is advantageous because it provides ready access for exchange in the event of future stent occlusion. Complication rates vary and include bleeding, cholangitis, bile leakage, and pneumothorax. All patients should receive prophylactic antibiotics before and after the procedure.

In one prospective trial, 70 patients were randomized to undergo endoscopic or percutaneous placement of a plastic endoprosthesis [19••]. Relief of jaundice (81% vs 61%), complication rates (19% vs 67%), and procedure-related mortality (13% *vs* 36%) were significantly better in patients treated endoscopically. Higher mortality in the transhepatic technique was due to bleeding and bile leakage that were consequences of hepatic puncture. Nonrandomized trials have yielded similar results. Therefore, endoscopic stenting is preferable to the percutaneous approach and should be the nonoperative palliative procedure of choice, except perhaps in proximal hilar lesions. Percutaneous biliary drainage should be reserved for endoscopic failures or in centers where ERCP expertise is not available.

In cases of endoscopic failure, a combined percutaneous-endoscopic procedure may be considered. After percutaneous transhepatic cholangiography by the interventional radiologist, a guidewire is advanced through the papilla and then pulled into the endoscope using a polypectomy snare, creating a pulley system over which a stent is placed endoscopically.

HILAR STRICTURES

When the right and left hepatic ducts do not communicate with each other, a single stent will not provide drainage of the entire liver. No consensus exists about the need to place stents into each lobe of the liver in this situation. Drainage of one lobe is usually sufficient to result in resolution of jaundice; however, cholangitis in the undrained lobe remains a concern. Cholangiography itself may increase the risk of cholangitis, and dense opacification of the intrahepatic biliary tree should be avoided, particularly if there is any question about the capacity to provide drainage later.

The advantages of metal over polyethylene stents may be particularly pronounced with hilar strictures [20•]. Two factors to which this may relate include 1) the capacity for bile to flow through the meshwork along the side of metal stents, as opposed to the occlusion of side branches by plastic stents; and 2) the lower likelihood of tumor ingrowth by relatively scirrhous proximal cholangiocarcinomas. Relatively high success rates have been reported with percutaneously or endoscopically placed Wallstents, even in patients with high hilar strictures (Bismuth types II and III) [21•].

SURGICAL BILIARY BYPASS

The overall success rates of surgical palliation of obstructive jaundice are comparable to those of endoscopic and percutaneous methods. Results of prospective randomized trials indicate that nonoperative palliation results in a shorter initial hospitalization and lower procedure-related morbidity and mortality (Table 131-3) [10]. These benefits, however, are counterbalanced by a higher incidence of late complications in the group treated endoscopically, primarily owing to stent occlusion that results in jaundice and cholangitis requiring repeat ERCP, hospitalization, or both. The most recent study in England confirms these results with procedure-related

Table 131-3. Percutaneous Versus Endoscopic Stent Placement Versus Surgical Bypass in Malignant Biliary Obstruction

	Percutaneous stent (*n*=490)	Endoscopic stent (*n*=689)	Surgical bypass (*n*=1807)
30-day mortality, %	6–33	0–20	0–31
Hospital stay, *d*	13–18	3–26	9–30
Success rate, %	76–100	82–100	75–100
Early complications*, %	4–67	8–34	6–56
Late complications, %	7–38	13–45	5–47

*First 30 days.

Modified from Watanapa and Williamson [10].

mortality rates of 3% versus 14% and major complication rates of 11% versus 29% in endoscopically versus surgically managed patients, respectively [22••]. No difference in median survival between the two groups was seen (21 vs 26 weeks). These data suggest that whereas surgical palliation of jaundice is preferable in patients with concomitant duodenal obstruction, endoscopic therapy is favorable in patients without gastric outlet obstruction at initial presentation and in those who are unfit for surgery. Another European study demonstrated that endoscopic endoprosthesis is the best option for patients expected to survive for less than 6 months and surgical biliary bypass for those with an expected survival of more than 6 months [23]. This conclusion necessitates the development of prognostic criteria to predict survival: the Cox proportional-hazards survival analysis found advanced age, male sex, liver metastases, and large diameters of tumors to be poor prognostic factors.

THE FUTURE

The studies listed previously compare polyethylene endoprostheses with surgical bypass. The future widespread use of metallic stents, with their improved patency, may decrease the incidence of late occlusive complications of endoscopic stenting, and the balance would then further favor endoscopic over surgical palliation of jaundice. Conversely, if sufficient expertise develops in the evolving technique of laparoscopic biliary-enteric anastomosis, initial mortality, morbidity, and length of hospitalization should all decrease in patients treated surgically, and the pendulum could swing back to favor this method. A final procedure awaiting further evaluation is endoscopic "double bypass," which would allow the endoscopist to insert a stent in both the duodenum and the biliary tree, obviating the need for surgical intervention in incurable patients with duodenal obstruction who are at high operative risk (Fig.131-14).

REFERENCES

Recently published papers of particular interest have been highlighted as follows:
- Of interest
- •• Of outstanding interest

1. Lindner HH: Embryology and anatomy of the biliary tree. In *Surgery of the Gallbladder and Bile Ducts*. Edited by Way LW, Pellegrini CA. Philadelphia: WB Saunders Co.; 1987.

2. Pasanen PA, Partanen KP, Pikkarainen PH, *et al.*: A comparison of ultrasound, computed tomography and endoscopic retrograde cholangiopancreatography in the differential diagnosis of benign and malignant jaundice and cholestasis. *Eur J Surg* 1993, 159:23–29.

3. Rösch T, Braig C, Gain T, *et al.*: Staging of pancreatic and ampullary carcinoma by endoscopic ultrasonography: comparison with conventional sonography, computed tomography, and angiography. *Gastroenterology* 1992, 102:188–189.

4.• Gress F, Savides T, Cummings O, *et al.*: Radial scanning and linear array endosonography for staging pancreatic cancer: a prospective randomized comparison. *Gastrointest Endosc* 1997, 45:138–144.
This carefully performed randomized trial demonstrates that linear array EUS is as accurate as radial scanning EUS for staging pancreatic cancer, and offers the additional benefit of fine needle aspiration for cytologic sampling.

5.• McPherson GAD, Benjamin IS, Hodgson HJF, *et al.*: Preoperative percutaneous transhepatic biliary drainage: results of a controlled trial. *Br J Surg* 1984, 71:371–375.
This is one of several trials which cumulatively failed to show a benefit for preoperative percutaneous biliary drainage in patients with malignant biliary obstruction.

6. Ballinger AB, McHugh M, Catnach SM, *et al.*: Symptom relief and quality of life after stenting for malignant bile duct obstruction. *Gut* 1994, 35:467–470.

7. Tarnawsky PR, Cunningham JT, Hawes R, *et al.*: Transpapillary stenting of proximal biliary strictures: does biliary sphincterotomy reduce the risk of postprocedure pancreatitis? *Gastrointest Endosc* 1997, 45:46–51.

8. Huibregtse K, Katon RM, Coene PP, Tytgat GNJ: Endoscopic palliative treatment in pancreatic cancer. *Gastrointest Endosc* 1986, 32:334–338.

9. Lillemoe KD, Pitt HA: Palliation of pancreatic carcinoma. *Cancer* 1996, 78:605–614.

10. Watanapa P, Williamson RCN: Surgical palliation for pancreatic cancer: developments during the past two decades. *Br J Surg* 1992, 79:8–20.

Figure 131-14

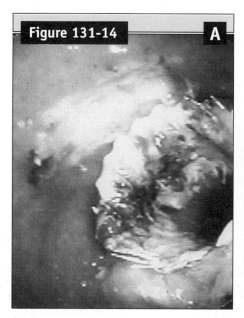 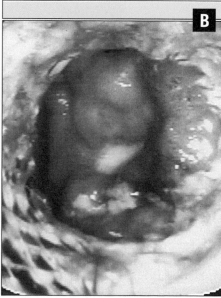

A patient with cancer of the head of the pancreas, managed with biliary stents, presenting with late duodenal obstruction. A metal stent has been placed across the obstruction. Several weeks later the proximal end, in the bulb (**A**) and the distal end, well beyond the ampulla (**B**) are patent and the patient is able to eat well.

11. Smilanich RP, Hafner GH: Complications of biliary stents in obstructive pancreatic malignancies. *Dig Dis Sci* 1994, 39:2645–2649.

12. Johanson JF, Schmaltz MJ, Geenen JE: Incidence and risk factors for biliary and pancreatic stent migration. *Gastrointest Endosc* 1992, 38:341–346.

13. Pedersen FM: Endoscopic management of malignant biliary obstruction. Is stent size of 10 French gauge better than 7 French gauge? *Scand J Gastroenterol* 1993, 28:185–89.

14.•• Sherman S, Lehman G, Earle D, *et al.*: Multicenter randomized trial of 10 French versus 11.5 French plastic stents for malignant bile duct obstruction. *Gastrointest Endosc* 1995, 41:415.

This clinical trial involving leading endoscopists demonstrated that, for practical purposes, bigger is not necessarily better. Patients who have 10F stents placed are served about as well (and sometimes more easily and with more readily available equipment, such as scopes with 3.7-3.8 mm channels) as patients with 11.5F stents.

15. Frakes JT, Johanson JF, Stake JJ: Optimal timing for stent replacement in malignant biliary obstruction. *Gastrointest Endosc* 1993, 39:164–167.

16.•• Carr-Locke DL, Ball TJ, Connors PJ, *et al.*: Multicenter randomized trial of Wallstent biliary endoprosthesis versus plastic stents. *Gastrointest Endosc* 1993, 39:310.

This major US study demonstrated the advantages of metal stents over plastic stents.

17.• Davids PHP, Groen AK, Rauws EAJ, *et al.*: Randomized trial of self-expanding metal stents versus polyethylene stents for distal malignant biliary obstruction. *Lancet* 1992, 340:1488–1492.

This trial from a world-class group also demonstrates the benefits of metal stents.

18. Thurner SA, Drammer J, Thurner MM, *et al.*: Covered self-expanding transhepatic biliary stents: a clinical pilot study. *Cardiovasc Intervent Radiol* 1996, 19:310–314.

19.•• Speer AG, Cotton PB, Russell RCG, *et al.*: Randomized trial of endoscopic versus percutaneous stent insertion in malignant obstructive jaundice. *Lancet* 1987, 2:57–62.

This oft-quoted study helped to establish endoscopic stent placement as the preferred means of providing nonsurgical biliary drainage in unresectable patients.

20.• Wagner HJ, Knyrim K, Yakil N, Klove KN: Plastic endoprostheses versus metal stents in the palliative treatment of malignant hilar biliary obstruction: a prospective and randomized trial. *Endoscopy* 1993, 25:213–218.

These authors report that metal stents may offer particular advantages in patients with malignant hilar strictures.

21.• Peters RA, Williams SG, Lombard M, *et al.*: The management of high-grade hilar strictures by endoscopic insertion of self-expanding metal endoprostheses. *Endoscopy* 1997, 29:10–16.

This is another study showing that the benefits of metal stents extend to patients with proximal biliary strictures.

22.•• Smith AC, Dowsett JF, Russell RCG, *et al.*: Randomised trial of endoscopic stenting versus surgical bypass in malignant low bile duct obstruction. *Lancet* 1994, 344:1655–1660.

This is an important trial demonstrating that the results of endoscopic stenting compare favorably with those of surgical biliary drainage.

23. Van den Bosch RP, Van der Schelling GP, Klinkenbijl JHG, *et al.*: Guidelines for the application of surgery and endoprostheses in the palliation of obstructive jaundice in advanced cancer of the pancreas. *Ann Surg* 1994, 219:18–24.

24. Yamada T, Alpers DH, Owyan C, *et al.*: Textbook of Gastroenterology, edn 3. Philadelphia: Lippincott-Raven, 1998.

132 Endoscopic Management of Biliary Disorders After Liver Transplantation

Michael Sossenheimer and Adam Slivka

Biliary tract complications occur in 13% to 34% of patients receiving liver transplantation and are an important cause of postoperative morbidity [1–4,5••,6–8,9•]. The range of biliary complications after transplantation is broad and can be classified according to their time of onset: Early complications are those occurring within 30 days after surgery, and late complications are those occurring after 30 days (Table 132-1) [4,9•]. As more experience in the management of biliary complications after transplantation is gained, optimal management algorithms can be constructed by a multidisciplinary team of experienced surgeons, hepatologists, therapeutic endoscopists, and interventional radiologists. Although one third of all biliary complications after transplantation eventually require additional surgical intervention [2,3,7,10–12], recent experience suggests that a nonoperative approach using endoscopic or percutaneous techniques may be palliative and allow definitive surgical repair to be performed months after transplantation, when the patient is fit for repeat surgical intervention [9•,13•]; furthermore, these techniques may be definitive in

certain patients. The following are reviewed: aspects of the vascular and biliary anatomy of the liver; the harvesting and transplantation operations; pathophysiology and clinical presentations of biliary complications after transplantation; and diagnostic studies used to optimally manage patients after transplantation; and outcome of nonoperative interventions in the treatment of these complications, with an emphasis on endoscopic management. A basic understanding of hepatic and biliary anatomy, the transplant operations, and pathologic and histologic manifestations of biliary complications is critical to the successful recognition, evaluation, and treatment of biliary complications after liver transplantation.

ANATOMY

The transplanted liver and extrahepatic bile ducts are highly dependent on the integrity of both the hepatic artery and portal vein. Vascular complications during harvesting and transplantation attributed to anatomic variations or technical errors may result in ischemic biliary strictures and graft failure.

Hepatic Artery

A single common hepatic artery is found in 50% to 67% of all patients, typically arising from the celiac axis and branching into a right hepatic and a left hepatic artery. Anatomic anomalies of hepatic arterial supply are frequent, the most common (25%) being an aberrant common hepatic artery arising from the superior mesenteric artery [14]. The left hepatic artery may originate from the left gastric artery in 14% to 25% of cases, and the right hepatic artery may originate from the superior mesenteric artery in 10% of cases. Rarely, anomalies of the right and left hepatic arteries may occur simultaneously, or the common hepatic artery may be absent. Each of these aberrant vessels may be the only hepatic arterial blood supply. Other rare vascular anomalies have also been reported. Thus, great care must be taken during the harvesting operation to identify the arterial supply of the graft and to recognize any anomalies.

Portal Vein

The splenic and superior mesenteric veins unite to form the portal vein, which is joined by the superior pancreaticoduodenal vein and left gastric vein. Before entering the liver, the main portal vein, carrying blood from the small and large bowel, spleen, pancreas, and gallbladder divides into the right and left portal veins. The right portal vein receives blood from the cystic vein, and the left portal vein is joined by the umbilical and paraumbilical veins. In addition, the left portal vein receives blood from branches of the caudate and quadrate lobes of the liver before entering the hepatic parenchyma. Unlike the hepatic arteries, anomalies of the portal vein are quite rare. In the most commonly described anomaly, the anterior segment of the right lobe of the liver is drained by a branch from the proximal left portal vein.

Extrahepatic Bile Ducts

The common hepatic duct arises from the confluence of the left and right hepatic ducts and is joined by the cystic duct to form the common bile duct. The union of the cystic duct to the common hepatic duct varies, and its recognition is important during the dissection. Other anatomic anomalies of the extrahepatic biliary tree are rare. Reports of accessory bile ducts draining the gallbladder and cystic duct drainage into the right hepatic duct have been described (Fig. 132-1). The right and left hepatic ducts may join close to the intraduodenal segment of the biliary tree, with the right hepatic duct receiving bile from the cystic duct. In such cases, the common hepatic duct may be absent.

Operative Techniques

The successful outcome of liver transplantation is dependent on organ procurement, recipient hepatectomy, and subsequent grafting. A detailed review of the operative techniques is beyond the scope of this chapter; however, a general understanding of these techniques is critical because technical variations may directly affect the subsequent development of postoperative biliary complications.

Organ Harvesting

The organ harvesting and subsequent preparation (the so-called back table procedure) establish the anatomy of the donor organ and contribute to overall ischemic time. When arterial anomalies are encountered, arterial reconstruction may be performed, allowing for a single anastomotic site with the recipient's artery.

Recipient Hepatectomy and Grafting

Care must be taken during the recipient hepatectomy and grafting to avoid trauma to the vascular and biliary trees, guarantee optimal "fit" of the anastomosis, and establish optimal flow in the vascular and biliary trees. Because the graft and its extrahepetic and intrahepatic biliary epithelia are highly dependent on the integrity of the hepatic artery, arterial reconstruction is the crucial step for graft function, and hepatic artery thrombosis is a dreaded technical complication [13•,14,15]. Anastomosis of the portal veins is usually performed in an end-to-end fashion. Portal vein thrombosis may call for a thromboendovenectomy, or when the portal vein is unusable, a portal venous conduit constructed from

Table 132-1. Biliary Complications After Liver Transplantation	
Early complications (within 30 d)	**Late complications (after 30 d)**
Anastomotic leak	Anastomotic obstruction/stricture
Hepatic artery thrombosis	Hepatic artery thrombosis
Extrinsic obstruction	Hemobilia
Hemobilia	Biliary fistula
Biliary stones and casts	Biliary stones and casts
Diffuse bile duct dilation/SOD	Diffuse bile duct dilation/SOD
	Ischemic-type biliary injury
	Cystic duct remnant mucocele
	T-tube leak

SOD—Sphincter of Oddi dysfunction.
Adapted from Van Thiel et al. [4] and Sossenheimer, M. et al. [9•].

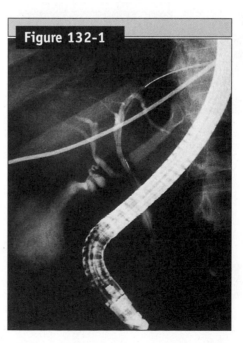

Figure 132-1

Cystic duct arising from the right hepatic duct.

donor iliac vein may be anastomosed to the recipient superior mesenteric vein. Excessive length of the anastomosed portal vein must be avoided to prevent kinking, folding, and obstruction to flow [14]. Successful vena cava reconstruction requires maximal preservation of the right and left hepatic veins during organ harvesting, perfect intimal adaptation during the grafting operation, and avoidance of excessive vena cava length.

Biliary Reconstruction

After earlier innovations in the surgical management of the donor-recipient biliary anastomosis, a choledochocholedochostomy (67% to 75% of transplants) and choledochojejunostomy Roux-en-Y anastomosis (25% to 33% of transplants) are now favored [1–4,9•,10,13•,15–17,18•,19]. A choledochocholedochostomy is used in a minority of children (10%) but is the preferred anastomosis in adults because it saves operative time, may provide T-tube access, avoids disruption of intestinal continuity, preserves endoscopic access to the biliary tree, and avoids intestinal complications from a choledochojejunostomy Roux-en-Y anastomosis [1–3,9•,10,13•,16,17,18•,19]. Furthermore, sphincter of Oddi integrity is preserved, thereby preventing biliary reflux of intestinal contents and cholangitis from a poorly draining Roux-en-Y limb. Typically, a choledochocholedochostomy is constructed over a short T-tube limb or an internal stent is used to buttress the duct-to-duct anastomosis [14]. As with vascular anastomoses, excessive length of the bile ducts must be avoided. The donor cystic duct, if not resected, must be allowed to drain freely into the common bile duct to prevent cystocele or mucocele formation [14].

A choledochojejunostomy Roux-en-Y anastomosis becomes necessary when bile ducts are inadequate to construct a choledochocholedochostomy, or if the native bile duct is diseased, absent, or inadequate for biliary drainage (*eg*, patients with sclerosing cholangitis, biliary atresia, or cholangiocarcinoma, or those with very large biliary collateral veins from portal vein thrombosis or Budd-Chiari syndrome). Adults undergoing repeat transplantation and surgical reconstruction

after transplantation and children require a choledochojejunostomy Roux-en-Y anastomosis [1,2,4,9•,13•,16]. The choledochus is anastomosed to a 20- to 40-cm jejunal limb, using a temporary internal plastic stent to guarantee postoperative anastomotic patency.

◼ ETIOLOGY

Biliary tract complications after liver transplantation are dependent on many factors, for example, the type of biliary reconstruction, possible harvesting injuries, cold ischemic time, technical skill of the surgeon, and vascular anastomotic integrity [1,2,4,5••,8,9•,13•,15,16]. It is convenient to categorize postoperative biliary complications as obstructions or leaks. Obstructive complications may be due to ischemic and anastomotic strictures, sludge, stones, bile cast syndrome, T-tube migration or obstruction, retained surgical stents, sphincter of Oddi dysfunction, cystoceles, mucoceles, and pancreatitis. Bile leaks may result from ischemic injury with dehiscence or necrosis of the biliary anastomosis after T-tube removal or as a result of rejection.

A recent survey of major transplant centers assessed the frequency of biliary complications as diagnosed by endoscopic retrograde cholangiopancreatography (ERCP) or percutaneous transhepatic cholangiography (PTC) [9•]. Major biliary complications after liver transplantation included stones, strictures, leaks, and sphincter stenoses. Strictures accounted for most complications (28% to 46%), followed by leaks (17% to 31%), sphincter stenoses (11% to 30%), and stones (15% to 21%) (Table 132-2). Furthermore, diffuse dilation of the recipient common bile duct presents a frequent obstructive complication in up to 20% of all biliary tract complications after liver transplantation in which a choledochocholedochostomy anastomosis has been performed.

Two thirds of all biliary complications are classified as early and tend to be related to technical problems associated more with a choledochojejunostomy than with a duct-to-duct anastomosis (Table 132-3). This corresponds to a time when patients are most unstable and on maximal immunosuppressive therapy. The morbidity and mortality of repeat operative intervention during this time period are extraordinarily high [3]. Complications after duct-to-duct anastomosis may be seen with a more even distribution in time.

Table 132-2. Frequency of Major Biliary Complications as Diagnosed by Endoscopic Retrograde Cholangiopancreatography or Percutaneous Transhepatic Cholangiography*		
	ERCP	PTC
Leak	17	31
Stricture	28	46
Stones	21	15
Sphincter stenosis	11	30

* Numbers represent mean percentage of total cases evaluated by each modality

ERCP—endoscopic retrograde cholangiopancreatography; PTC—percutaneous transhepatic cholangiography.

Adapted from Sossenheimer M. et al. [9•].

Table 132-3. Predisposing Factors for Biliary Complications
Reduced-sized grafts
Hepatic artery thrombosis
Hepatic artery stenosis
Portal vein thrombosis
Harvesting injuries
Ischemia and reperfusion injuries
Cold ischemic time of the harvested graft
Recurrent biliary tract disease
Recurrent viral infection
Acute and chronic rejection
Reflux cholangitis caused by choledochojejunostomy Roux-en-Y

Harvesting injuries during organ procurement, preservation-reperfusion injuries, and allograft ischemia are other important causes of biliary complications, leading to nonanastomotic strictures of the intrahepatic and extrahepatic biliary trees; biliary epithelial sloughing; or sludge, casts, or stone formation [5••,20,21•,22,23]. Formation of biliary sludge and casts have been related to inadequate flushing of the procured organ during reperfusion.

Ischemic biliary complications typically occur 1 to 4 months after transplantation. They are associated with hepatic artery thrombosis, chronic ductopenic rejection, transplantation in the setting of ABO-incompatible blood group donors, and prolonged allograft ischemia before transplantation [5••,20,21•,22–25]. Ischemia and reperfusion injuries correlate with the duration of cold ischemic time. Allograft preservation for 11, 13, and 15 hours has been shown to be associated with a 10%, 22%, and 38% probability of ischemic biliary complications [22]. Ischemic preservation-reperfusion injuries remain a major indication for repeat transplantation because diffuse intrahepatic biliary strictures cannot be managed surgically, endoscopically (ERCP), or radiologically (PTC).

PATHOPHYSIOLOGY

Although only one third of the hepatic blood supply normally is provided by the hepatic artery, its thrombosis is a dreaded complication after transplantation because the donor bile duct blood supply is dependent solely on the reconstructed hepatic artery. Hepatic artery thrombosis after liver transplantation occurs in 4% to 10% of adults and up to 26% of children; furthermore, 86% of patients with hepatic artery thrombosis have resultant biliary tract complications [1,4,20,26,27]. Loss of vascular integrity of the donor bile duct may result in stricturization and necrosis anywhere in the donor biliary tree and should be suspected if bile duct strictures, leaks, intrahepatic abscesses, or cholangitis occur [2,5••,9•,13•,25–27]. The strictures seen after hepatic artery thrombosis are most often multiple and diffuse. Technical difficulties (*eg*, harvesting injuries), preservation-reperfusion injuries, rejection, hypotension, hypercoagulable state, transplantation in the setting of ABO-incompatible blood group donors, and prolonged allograft ischemia may all cause hepatic artery thrombosis; however, in up to 60% of cases the cause of hepatic artery thrombosis remains unknown.

The pathogenesis of preservation and reperfusion injuries has been discussed in great detail elsewhere [21•]. Harvesting injuries can be avoided by refraining from excessive dissection of periductal tissues, excessive cleaning of donor and recipient bile ducts, and thorough adequate sizing of the donor common bile duct to ensure satisfactory blood supply, thereby minimizing devascularization of the extrahepatic bile ducts [15]. Use of fine monofilament suture material is preferred over braided absorbable sutures or electrocautery to reduce inflammatory responses and tissue necrosis [13•,28]. Inadequate flushing of the biliary tree of the graft may contribute further to biliary sludge and cast formation [5••].

Ischemia and reperfusion injuries correlate with the duration of cold ischemic time. Procured livers preserved in University of Wisconsin solution for less than 11.5 hours showed fewer biliary complications (< 10%), whereas grafts preserved for more than 13 or 15 hours showed an increase in biliary complications of 22% and 38%, respectively [22]. In the absence of hepatic artery thrombosis or stenosis, development of multiple or late intrahepatic strictures is suggestive of ischemic preservation-reperfusion injuries.

Transplantation in the setting of ABO-incompatible blood group donors causes ABO blood group antigen expression on cells of bile ducts, sinusoids, arteries, and veins, where they may act as potential sites of immunologic injury. Biliary complications are found more frequently in transplantation with ABO-incompatible donors than with ABO-matched donors (82% vs 6%) [18•,24]. Hepatic artery thrombosis is also found with increased frequency in patients who receive transplanted organs having an ABO-incompatible donor [18•].

Diffuse dilation of the recipient bile duct is a common complication seen with choledochocholedochostomy reconstructions, accounting for about 20% of all biliary tract complications after liver transplantation [4,16,17,18•]. The recipient native bile duct is dilated progressively from the sphincter zone to the site of the choledochocholedochostomy (Fig. 132-2). Donor duct involvement may also be seen (Fig. 132-3). Diffuse bile duct dilation after liver transplantation may be equivalent to sphincter of Oddi dysfunction in the nontransplant population; however, the entity continues to be poorly defined [29,30]. There is some evidence it is due to denervation of the native bile duct during the grafting operation, yet normal sphincter of Oddi function has been demonstrated after transplantation [10,17,31,32]. ERCP with manometry should be considered to confirm sphincter of Oddi dysfunction and to differentiate it from distal biliary obstruction caused by stones, strictures, choledochocele, and tumors.

PATHOLOGY

Because liver histology is an important component of the diagnosis and treatment of biliary complications after transplantation, knowledge of basic histologic features of bile duct injuries caused by harvesting injuries, vascular occlusion, rejection, infection, and primary biliary recurrent diseases is crucial. Because it is often difficult to identify the exact mechanism of injury in a poorly functioning allograft and histologic patterns of injury are often similar, liver biopsies must be interpreted with the clinical presentation in mind [33].

Harvesting Injury

Harvesting injuries, a result of nonimmunologic damage to the liver, are difficult to distinguish from large duct obstruction or rejection. All show portal tract expansion, edema, and peripheral bile duct proliferation. Two injury patterns with varying severity are typically seen: intracellular edema and necrosis. Whereas well-functioning grafts may show only minimal edema with small clusters of necrosis, more severe cases may show confluent necrosis with centrilobular or periportal distribution [33].

Hepatic Artery Thrombosis

Manifestations of hepatic artery thrombosis range from occult allograft dysfunction to major bile duct necrosis, abscess formation, graft infarction, and graft loss. The histologic evaluation mirrors this varying degree of injury and ranges from normal biopsy tissue to confluent or complete coagulative necrosis [33].

Rejection

Rejection represents the host immune response against the allograft. Rejection has been classified as acute or chronic, as hyperacute, humoral, cellular, or arteriopathic. Synonyms such as cellular rejection, nonductopenic rejection, rejection without duct loss, and reversible rejection have been used in the past but recently have been challenged at the Third Banff Conference on Allograft Pathology [34•]. The Banff consensus document proposes a definition of hepatic allograft rejection as inflammation of the allograft elicited by a genetic disparity between donor and recipient, primarily affecting interlobular bile ducts and vascular endothelium, including portal veins, hepatic venules, and occasionally the hepatic artery and its branches. Biologic rejection and clinically relevant rejection need to be distinguished because histopathologic evidence of acute rejection does not necessarily warrant treatment. To complete a diagnosis of acute rejection, as per the Banff consensus document, two of the following three histologic findings need to be present: 1) mixed but predominantly mononuclear portal inflammation, 2) bile duct inflammation and damage, and 3) subendothelial inflammation of portal veins or hepatic venules [34•]. An international grading system for acute liver allograft rejection as a measure of the severity of the necro-inflammatory process has been proposed [34•].

■ DIAGNOSIS

Biliary complications after transplantation should always be suspected in patients who manifest liver dysfunction, jaundice, fever, ascites, abdominal pain, or ileus, or in whom ultrasonography demonstrates biliary dilation. In addition, biliary abnormalities may be noted in asymptomatic patients who present for T-tube cholangiography before T-tube removal. Symptoms may occur early or late after transplantation and may be insidious, as seen in chronic rejection. If one of the signs or symptoms listed previously develops in the patient after transplantation, immediate and aggressive steps must be taken to establish the cause. Integrity of the vascular supply, biliary tract abnormalities, and abdominal fluid collections are demonstrated by conventional ultrasonography and color flow Doppler imaging [4,9•,18•]. Hepatic artery thrombosis may be confirmed on angiography. Suspected biliary tract complications may require T-tube, ERCP, or PTC. Liver biopsy plays an important part in diagnosing complications after transplantation, providing valuable information about rejection, harvesting injury, recurrent viral infection, and ischemia, or suggesting extrahepatic obstruction [33,34•].

In addition, computed tomography (CT), Magnetic resonance (MR), or hydroxyiminodiacetic acid (HIDA) imaging may be helpful to delineate other complications, such as abscess formation, biloma, and leaks. Endoscopic evaluation and biopsies may be warranted to exclude disorders, such as posttransplant lymphoproliferative disorder or cytomegalovirus infection. The development of peritonitis after T-tube removal suggests an intra-abdominal bile leak. These leaks occur more frequently in patients after transplantation, and it has been suggested that this is due to the failure of formation of a mature cutaneous tract as a result of immunosuppression. Leaks can be diagnosed by HIDA scan or ERCP. ERCP may be favored because therapy can be implemented simultaneously. Biliary strictures and stones may be diagnosed at routine T-tube cholangiography or suggested by a cholestatic liver injury pattern after T-tube clamping, or in evaluation of unexplained fever, jaundice, or abdominal pain.

■ TREATMENT

The management of biliary complications after liver transplantation is best approached by a multidisciplinary team of surgeons, hepatologists, therapeutic endoscopists, and interventional radiologists. Although further surgical intervention after transplantation may be necessary in 30% to 50% of patients with biliary complications, endoscopic and radiologic interventions are being increasingly used as diagnostic and therapeutic modalities [2,7,8,9•,10–12,13•,18•,35–46].

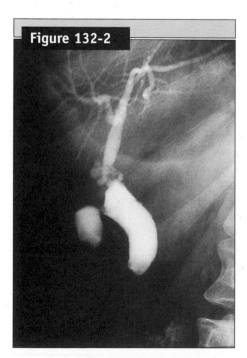

Figure 132-2

Sphincter dysfunction with dilation of the native bile duct after liver transplantation.

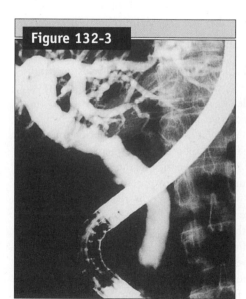

Figure 132-3

Sphincter dysfunction with diffuse dilation of both the donor and recipient biliary trees after liver transplantation.

Successful endoscopic treatment of biliary complications after liver transplantation was reported by Stratta [2] and O'Connor [40] using sphincterotomy for papillary stenosis; stent placement for bile leak; anastomotic stricture balloon dilation; and sphincterotomy for sludge, stones, and cast removal. Wolfsen [10] reported a 85% successful therapeutic outcome of patients treated endoscopically with biliary complications after liver transplantation. Sphincterotomy for bile leaks, removal of sludge or debris, and diffuse ductal dilation, as well as balloon dilation of anastomotic strictures were the reported therapeutic interventions. Ostroff and coworkers [36] described successful endoscopic management of patients after liver transplantation with bile leakage after T-tube removal with nasobiliary catheter drainage. Rask-Madsen and coworkers [41] have reported their experience of diagnostic and therapeutic endoscopy in patients with choledochocholedochostomy anastomosis and resultant biliary leaks or strictures. Cholangiography was successful in 94%, with subsequent successful sphincterotomy in 100%. Balloon stricture dilation was successful in 33% of cases. Morbidity and mortality rates were 6% and 3%, respectively. More recent reports have further stressed the emergence of endoscopic techniques in patients after transplantation as a viable therapeutic modality, making endoscopy the method of choice for acquiring cholangiography in patients with choledochocholedochostomy anastomoses. Bernstein and coworkers [42] reported a therapeutic endoscopic success rate of 76% (using sphincterotomy, nasobiliary drains, stents, balloon dilation, and stone extraction), whereas Burton and coworkers [43] noted 100% successful endoscopic treatment of biliary complications (ie, choledocholithiasis and bile leaks) after liver transplantation.

Recently, Sherman and coworkers [12,44] assessed the efficacy and safety of endoscopic management of biliary tract complications with a prospective evaluation of 50 patients with biliary complications after transplantation. Suspected bile leaks were correctly identified by ERCP in 89% of cases and successfully treated in all cases (using nasobiliary tube and stent placement). Furthermore, patients were successfully treated for stones, sludge,

and anastomotic or intrahepatic strictures. Overall, ERCP identified biliary tract complications in 84% of the patients in this series and was therapeutic in 97% of attempted procedures. A second study by the same investigators reported successful therapeutic endoscopic outcome of bile leaks and peritonitis as a result of T-tube removal or migration in 94.4% (using nasobiliary tube drainage, sphincterotomy and stent placement, or stent placement alone) [12]. Sherman concluded that endoscopic management of biliary fistulas complicating liver transplantation and other hepatobiliary operations is safe and obviates the need for surgery. Osorio and coworkers [11] retrospectively evaluated the endoscopic and radiologic management of bile leaks after liver transplantation (leakage occurred at the T-tube insertion site or the choledochocholedochostomy anastomosis). Successful ERCP with nasobiliary drainage catheter placement was used in 77% of cases, and PTC was employed in 23% because endoscopy was unsuccessful or unavailable. No complications were reported with ERCP, whereas 12% of patients treated with PTC experienced complications, such as bleeding, hemobilia, and infection.

Results of a recent questionnaire of major transplant centers in the United States reporting on the management experience of over 6000 patients who received liver transplantations revealed that biliary complications occurred in 16% [9•]. About 40% of biliary complications were treated with endoscopic therapy (ERCP) and 41% with radiologic intervention (PTC). ERCP was therapeutic in 72% of cases and PTC in 62%. Of patients with biliary complications, 32% required additional surgery.

The published experience for endoscopic management of biliary complications after liver transplantation is summarized in Tables 132-4, 132-5, and 132-6. Additional unpublished experience with the endoscopic management of biliary leaks and strictures after transplantation is included in Tables 132-4 and 132-5. Biliary stents, nasobiliary decompression tubes, endoscopic sphincterotomy, and balloon dilation are part of the endoscopic armamentarium used to treat such complications, and reports of successful outcomes continue to grow in number. Sphincterotomy

Table 132-4. Endoscopic Therapy of Leaks After Liver Transplantation (T-tube, Anastomotic)

Study	Year	n	Therapy	Success rate, %	Comments
Ostroff	1990	12	NBD	100	Leak closure at x=6.5 d
Reveille	1991	7	Stent	86	1 failed stent placement
Wolfsen	1992	8	ES	75	Closure within 72 h
Sherman	1993	18	NBD:13, stent:3 stent+ES:3	94	Closure at x=6.3 d
Osorio	1993	17	NBD	82	3 failures (anastomotic leak, suture line disruption)
Burton	1993	4	—	100	—
Rask-Madsen	1994	10	ES:1, stent:2, stent+ES:5	80	1 patient treated conservatively 1 patient treated surgically 1 patient with cholangitis after ERCP
Bourgeois	1995	3	ES, NBD	100	—
Catalano	1995	2	Stent	100	—
UPMC	1995	25	Stent:19, ES:4 ES+stent:2	100	unpublished
Total		106		91.7	

ES—sphincterotomy; NBD—nasobiliary drain; UPMC—University of Pittsburgh Medical Center.

Table 132-5. Endoscopic Therapy of Strictures After Transplantation

Study	Year	n	Therapy	Success, %	Comments
Stratta	1989	3	Dilation	33	—
O'Connor	1991	1	ES, passage dilation	0	Requires biliary reconstruction
Wolfsen	1992	3	Balloon:2 Balloon+stent:1	66	1 patient with diffuse strictures required liver transplantation
Rask-Madsen	1994	6	Dilation, stent	25	3 patients with multiple and intrahepatic strictures associated with failure
Theilmann	1994	6	ES, dilation, stent	66	Multiple strictures and intrahepatic strictures associated with failure
Bourgeois	1995	11	Dilation, stent	91	Early stricture, Rx 3 months, late stricture, Rx 1 year
Catalano	1995	5	Dilation, stent	60	—
UPMC	1995	23	Dilation, stent, ES	91	Intrahepatic stricture required retransplantation (unpublished)
Total		58		54	

ES—sphincterotomy; UPMC—University of Pittsburgh Medical Center.

Table 132-6. Endoscopic Therapy of Stones After Transplantation

Study	Year	n	Therapy	Success, %	Comments
Stratta	1989	2	ES, Sludge extraction	50	—
O'Connor	1991	7	ES, Sludge extraction	57	Failed in 3 with gallbladder conduit
Wolfsen	1992	4	ES, Sludge extraction	100	3 patients required second ERCP
Burton	1993	6	ES, Sludge extraction	100	—
Catalano	1995	1	ES, Sludge extraction	100	—
Total		20		81.4	

ES—sphincterotomy; ERCP—endoscopic retrograde cholangiopancreatography.

is the mainstay of therapy for papillary stenosis; diffuse ductal dilatation; and removal of sludge, stones, and casts.

In the treatment of bile leaks, the goal of therapy is to equilibrate biliary pressure with that of the duodenum. This goal can be accomplished with biliary stents, nasobiliary drainage catheters, or papillotomy. The most common scenario is a leak from the T-tube tract after T-tube removal (Fig. 132-4*A* and *B*). Although conservative observational management has been successfully applied for these T-tube leaks [38,47], we prefer a proactive approach that uses short stents to relieve pain quickly and reduces the infectious complications of bile peritonitis. The leaks usually seal within days and the stents can be removed at elective endoscopy 3 to 4 weeks later. Alternative treatment includes nasobiliary drains and sphincterotomy. Symptomatic bilomas causing peritonitis should be drained percutaneously because of the high incidence of superinfection in patients with immunosuppression.

Biliary strictures may be treated with balloon dilation and biliary stenting (Fig. 132-5) [5••]. Repeat dilation and stenting may be required. For anastomotic leaks associated with strictures, internal stenting is preferred and bridging of the stricture appears to be most effective. Endoscopic treatment of high-

grade biliary strictures appears less definitive than does therapy for leaks but may play an important role in stabilizing patients before surgical reconstruction. Multiple strictures from hepatic artery thrombosis require repeat transplantation.

Diffuse dilation of the biliary tree may be related to ampullary dysfunction after transplantation; however, the syndrome remains poorly characterized. When a patient has progressive biliary dilation and cholestasis that are corrected with draining the T-tube externally and cholangiography fails to reveal distal strictures or stones, an empiric endoscopic sphincterotomy appears reasonable. When a T-tube is not in place, or the diagnosis is in question, sphincter of Oddi manometry should be considered. Establishing a diagnosis of sphincter dysfunction justifies an endoscopic sphincterotomy that may obviate the need for surgical conversion of the choledochocholedochostomy reconstruction to choledochojejunostomy Roux-en-Y, currently the standard approach for sphincter dysfunction in some transplant centers [1,4,17,30]. One report suggests that this condition is transient, describing effective endoscopic therapy with temporary biliary stenting [30].

The overall cited complication rate for ERCP is 4% to 6%, with most complications being pancreatitis, bleeding after

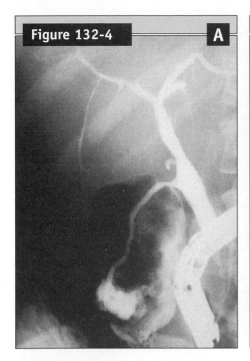

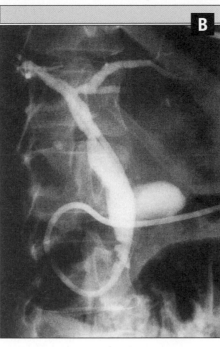

A, Bile leak demonstrated at endoscopic retrograde cholangiopancreatography from a T-tube tract. **B**, This leak was successfully treated with a nasobiliary drain.

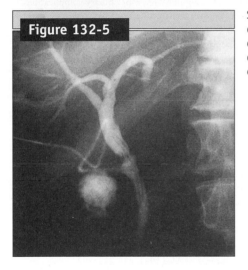

Stricture at duct-to-duct anastomosis demonstrated during T-tube cholangiography.

biliary reconstructions. ERCP identifies biliary tract complications in more than 84% of cases and provides therapeutic intervention in up to 97% of attempted procedures. Definitive therapy for biliary leaks or biliary fistulas can be expected in 90% of cases, and thus ERCP should be considered the treatment of choice for these lesions. Endoscopic treatment of biliary strictures is more problematic, with definitive therapy provided in only half of all cases.

Endoscopic management of biliary complications after liver transplantation is safe and should be explored before additional surgery because it may obviate the need for it. Long-term follow-up data for endoscopic therapy are lacking, warranting prospective studies comparing endoscopic to surgical management.

CONCLUSIONS

A basic understanding of hepatic and biliary anatomy, the transplantation operations, and pathologic and histologic manifestations of biliary complications is critical to the successful recognition, evaluation, and treatment of biliary disorders after liver transplantation. Biliary complications in patients after transplantation should be considered if liver dysfunction, fever, ascites, abdominal pain, ileus, or biliary dilation occur. Color flow Doppler imaging, liver biopsy, and direct cholangiography (ERCP or PTC) should be obtained promptly. Extensive experience in patients who are not immunocompromised and growing experience in liver transplant patients have shown that endoscopic therapy may provide definitive treatment for many biliary complications and avoid further surgical intervention. In addition, definitive surgery may be delayed and performed at a time when patients are fit, by using endoscopic techniques. Therefore, many centers are moving toward endoscopic management of biliary tract complications after orthotopic liver transplantation, reserving surgical biliary reconstruction for endoscopic failures. Randomized prospective trials are needed to assess the most cost-effective approach for managing these patients.

papillotomy, and retroperitoneal perforation. Most endoscopic complications are mild and can be managed conservatively. Recent prospective studies have demonstrated that complications of ERCP and sphincterotomy vary widely depending on the indications for the procedure [48,49]. Prospective data for ERCP complications after liver transplantation are scarce and incomplete [50]. Reported complications of PTC (up to 12%) include bleeding, hemobilia, and infection. The endoscopic 30-day all-cause mortality rate of 1% to 2% compares favorably with the reported surgical mortality for repeat transplantation (as high as 32%). This significant increase in mortality associated with early surgical interventions after transplantation justifies the use of endoscopic and radiologic therapies as alternatives to surgery [3]. Surgical reconstruction should be reserved for endoscopic or radiologic failures. ERCP is preferred for all patients with duct-to-duct anastomoses, reserving PTC for patients with a Roux-en-Y reconstruction.

Overall, cholangiography can be obtained safely and successfully in over 98% of patients with choledochocholedochostomy-

■■■ REFERENCES

Recently published papers of particular interest have been highlighted as follows:
* Of interest
** Of outstanding interest

1. Lerut J, Gordon RD, Iwatsuki S, *et al.*: Biliary tract complications in human orthotopic liver transplantation. *Transplantation* 1987, 43:47–51.

2. Stratta RJ, Wood P, Langnas AN, *et al.*: Diagnosis and treatment of biliary tract complications after orthotopic liver transplantation. *Surgery* 1989, 106:675–684.

3. Lebeau G, Yanaga K, Marsh JW, *et al.*: Analysis of surgical complications after 397 hepatic transplantations. *Surg Gynecol Obstet* 1990, 170:317–322.

4. Van Thiel DH, Fagiuoli S, Wright Hl, *et al.*: Biliary complications of liver transplantation. *Gastrointest Endosc* 1993, 39:455–460.

5.•• Donovan J: Nonsurgical management of biliary tract disease after liver transplantation. *Gastroenterol Clin North Am* 1993, 22:317–336.

This is a detailed review of nonsurgical management options of biliary complications in liver transplantation categorized by the type of biliary complication.

6. Kuo PC, Lewis WD, Stokes K, *et al.*: A comparison of operation, endoscopic retrograde cholangiopancreatography, and percutaneous transhepatic cholangiography in biliary complications after hepatic transplantation. *J Am Coll Surg* 1994, 179:177–181.

7. Delgado M, de Dios JF, Mino G, *et al.*: Role of endoscopic retrograde cholangiopancreatography in liver transplantation. *Revista Espanola de Enfermedades Digestivas* 1993, 84:319–325.

8. Theilmann L, Küppers B, Kadmon M, *et al.*: Biliary tract strictures after orthotopic liver transplantation: diagnosis and management. *Endoscopy* 1994, 26:517–522.

9.• Sossenheimer M, Slivka A, Carr-Locke DL: Management of extrahepatic biliary disease after orthotopic liver transplantation. *Endoscopy* 1996, 25:565–571.

This US survey of transplant centers, summarizes the current use of ERCP and PTC in diagnosis and treatment of biliary complications after liver transplantation.

10. Wolfsen HC, Porayko MK, Hughes RH, *et al.*: Role of endoscopic retrograde cholangiopancreatography after orthotopic liver transplantation. *Am J Gastroenterol* 1992, 87:955–960.

11. Osorio RW, Freise CE, Stock PG, *et al.*: Nonoperative management of biliary leaks after orthotopic liver transplantation. *Transplantation* 1993, 55:1074–1077.

12. Sherman S, Shaked A, Cryer HM, *et al.*: Endoscopic management of biliary fistulas complicating liver transplantation and other hepatobiliary operations. *Ann Surg* 1993, 218:167–175.

13.• Gholson CF, Zibari G, McDonald JC: Endoscopic diagnosis and management of biliary complications following orthotopic liver transplantation. *Dig Dis Sci* 1996, 41:1045–1053.

This is a well written, recent review of biliary complications related to liver transplantation and endoscopic management options.

14. Emre S: The donor operation. In *Transplantation of the Liver*. Edited by Busuttil RW. Philadelphia: WB Saunders; 1996:392–404.

15. Starzl TE, Demitris AJ, Van Thiel D: Liver transplantation. *N Engl J Med* 1989, 321:1014–1022.

16. Porayko MK, Kondo M, Steers JL: Liver transplantation: late complications of the biliary tract and their management. *Sem Liver Dis* 1995, 15:139–155.

17. Steiber AC, Ambrosino G, Kahn D, *et al.*: An unusual complication of choledochocholedochostomy in orthotopic liver transplantation. *Transplant Proc* 1988, 20:619–621.

18.• Vallera RA, Cotton PB, Clavien PA: Biliary reconstruction for liver transplantation and management of biliary complications: overview and survey of current practices in the United States. *Liver Transplant Surg* 1995, 1:143–152.

This paper provides an overview of surgical practices and a US survey of management strategies of biliary complications in liver transplantation.

19. Friend PJ: Overview: biliary reconstruction after liver transplantation. *Liver Transplant Surg* 1995, 1:153–155.

20. Sanchez-Urdazpal L, Gores GJ, Ward EM, *et al.*: Clinical outcome of ischemic-type biliary complications after liver transplantation. *Transpant Proc* 1993, 25:1107–1109.

21• Clavien PA, Harvey PR, Strasberg SM: Preservation and reperfusion injuries in liver allografts. *Transplantation* 1992, 53:957–978.

This paper represents an extensive physiologic and pathophysiologic review of preservation and reperfusion injuries in liver transplantation and synthesis of current studies.

22. Sanchez-Urdazpal L, Gores GJ, Ward EM, *et al.*: Ischemic-type biliary complications after orthotopic liver transplantation. *Hepatology* 1992, 16:49–53.

23. Li S, Stratta RJ, Langnas AN, *et al.*: Diffuse biliary tract injury after orthotopic liver transplantation. *Am J Surg* 1992, 164:536–540.

24. Sanchez-Urdazpal L, Batts KP, Gores GJ, *et al.*: Increased bile duct complications in liver transplantation across the ABO barrier. *Ann Surg* 1993, 218:152.

25. Mor E, Schwartz ME, Sheiner PA, *et al.*: Prolonged preservation in University of Wisconsin solution associated with hepatic artery thrombosis after orthotopic liver transplantation. *Transplantation* 1993, 56:1399–1402.

26. Northover J, Terblanche J: Bile duct blood supply: its importance in human liver transplantation. *Transplantation* 1978, 26:67–69.

27. Zajko AB, Campbell WL, Logsdon GA, *et al.*: Biliary complications in liver allografts after hepatic artery occlusion: a 6-1/2-year study. *Transplant Proc* 1988, 20:607–609.

28. Klein AS, Savader S, Burdick JF, *et al.*: Reduction of morbidity and mortality from biliary complications after liver transplantation. *Hepatology* 1991, 14:818–823.

29. Douzdjian V, Abecassis MM, Johlin FC: Sphincter of Oddi dysfunction following liver transplantation. Screening by bedside manometry and definitive manometric evaluation. *Dig Dis Sci* 1994, 39:253–256.

30. Clavien PA, Camargo CA, Baille J, *et al.*: Sphincter of Oddi dysfunction after liver transplantation [letter]. *Dig Dis Sci* 1995, 40:73–75.

31. Yeaton P, Weber F, Pambianco D, *et al.*: Sphincter of Oddi manometry via T-tube tract following orthotopic liver transplantation [abstract]. *Gastroenterology* 1992, 102:A331.

32. Richards RD, Yeaton P, Shaffer HA Jr, *et al.*: Human sphincter of Oddi motility and cholecystokinin response following liver transplantation. *Dig Dis Sci* 1993, 38:462–468.

33. Hertzler GL, Millikan WJ: The surgical pathologist's role in liver transplantation. *Arch Pathol Lab Med* 1991, 115:273–282.

34.• Banff schema for grading liver allograft rejection: an international consensus document. *Hepatology* 1997, 25:658–663.

This international consensus conference report establishes a unified reporting system, classification, and grading of liver allograft rejection to overcome obstacles created by multiple currently existing schemes.

35. Ward EM, Kiely MJ, Maus TP, *et al.*: Hilar biliary strictures after liver transplantation: cholangiography and percutaneous treatment. *Radiology* 1990, 177:259–263.

36. Ostroff JW, Roberts JP, Gordon RL, *et al.*: The management of T-tube leaks in orthotopic liver transplant recipients with endoscopically placed nasobiliary catheters. *Transplantation* 1990, 49:922–924.

37. Donovan JP, Sorrell MF, Stratta RJ, *et al.*: Endoscopic placement of expandable prosthesis as therapy for biliary strictures following liver transplantation [abstract]. *Hepatology* 1991, 14:60A.

38. Katkow WN, Dienstag JL, Rubin RH, *et al.*: Conservative management of bile leaks following T-tube removal in liver transplant patients [abstract]. *Hepatology* 1991, 14:51A.

39. Reveille RM, Ghin GSL, Goff JS, *et al.*: Bile leaks after T-tube removal following orthotopic liver transplantation: successful management by endoscopic stent placement [abstract]. *Hepatology* 1991, 14:56A.

40. O'Connor HJ, Vickers CR, Buckels JAC, *et al.*: Role of ERCP after orthotopic liver transplantation. *Gut* 1991, 32:419–423.

41. Rask-Madsen C, Svendsen LB, Bondesen S, *et al.*: Diagnosis and therapeutic ERCP after liver transplantation. *Transplant Proc* 1994, 26:1796.

42. Bernstein GP, Roberts JP, Ascher NL, *et al.*: The role of ERCP after orthotopic liver transplantation [abstract]. *Hepatology* 1992, 16:273A.

43. Burton FR, Li SCY, Solomon H, *et al.*: Incidence and endoscopic management of early biliary lithiasis complicating orthotopic liver transplantation. Am J *Gastroenterol* 1993, 88:182A.

44. Sherman S, Jamidar P, Shaked A, *et al.*: Endoscopic diagnosis and therapy of biliary tract complications [btc] after orthotopic liver transplantation [OLT] [abstract]. *Am J Gastroenterol* 1993, 88:240A.

45. Catalano MF, Van Dam J, Sivak MV Jr: Endoscopic retrograde cholangiopancreatography in the orthotopic liver transplant patient. *Endoscopy* 1995, 27:584–588.

46. Ward EM Wiesner RH, Hughes RW, *et al.*: Persistent bile leak after liver transplantation: biloma drainage and endoscopic retrograde cholangiopancreatographic sphincterotomy. *Radiology* 1991, 179:719–720.

47. Jabbour N, Karavias D, Felekouras E, *et al.*: Bile leak following T-tube removal in patients having had an orthotopic liver transplant [abstract]. *Hepatology* 1993, 18:1114.

48. Freeman ML, Nelson DB, Sherman S, *et al.*: Complications of endoscopic biliary sphincterotomy. *N Engl J Med* 1996, 335:909–918.

49. Cotton PB, Geenen JE, Sherman S, *et al.*: Endoscopic sphincterotomy for stones by experts is safe; even in younger patients with normal ducts. *Ann Surg* 1998, 227:201–204.

50. Bourgeois N, Deviere J, Yeaton P, *et al.*: Diagnostic and therapeutic endoscopic retrograde cholangiography after liver transplantation. *Gastrointest Endosc* 1995, 42:527–534.

7 Pancreas

Edited by C. S. Pitchumoni

Contributors

Nanakram Agarwal
Simmy Bank
Russell D. Brown
Charles F. Frey
Vivek V. Gumaste
Richard A. Kozarek
Eric J. Kraut
Irvin M. Modlin

Jean Perrault
C.S. Pitchumoni
Howard A. Reber
Stefan W. Schmid
Karen E. Todd
L. W. Traverso
Jorge E. Valenzuela
Rama P. Venu

133 Pancreatic Anatomy and Physiology
Jorge E. Valenzuela

▧ ANATOMY

The pancreas, a gland resembling a bunch of grapes, lies across the abdomen in the retroperitoneum at the approximate level of the second lumbar vertebral body. It is 12 to 15 cm long and weighs 70 to 100 g. The head and uncinate process are encircled by the duodenum; the tail extends to the hilum of the spleen. The common bile duct approaches the intestine from behind the pancreas and, as it descends, traverses the head of the pancreas to enter the duodenum, together with the pancreatic duct at the main papilla.

Blood Vessels

Arterial blood supply is provided by branches of the celiac artery, the pancreaticoduodenal arcades, and the superior mesenteric and splenic arteries. The superior mesenteric artery crosses the pancreas posteriorly at the angle between the head and the body of the gland; the splenic artery runs posteriorly in the upper border of the gland. These two main arteries and their branches appear to provide enough blood to make the pancreas relatively resistant to splanchnic ischemia, although in certain conditions, such as prolonged extracorporeal circulation, pancreatitis may be triggered by ischemia [1]. The splenic and superior mesenteric veins merge posteriorly to the head of the pancreas to form the portal vein (Fig. 133-1). Inflammatory and neoplastic processes involving the pancreas may cause thrombosis in these vessels and produce splenomegaly, hypersplenism, and varicosities of the gastric fundus.

Embryologically, the pancreas develops from two separate buds, one dorsal and one ventral, both of which contain axial ducts. During intrauterine development the dorsal bud enlarges to the left and constitutes the main portion of the gland; the ventral bud rotates behind the duodenum to fuse with the dorsal portion. The respective ducts also fuse. The ventral duct joins with the dorsal duct at the junction of the head and body of the pancreas. It becomes the main duct of Wirsung by draining most of the gland; the more proximal part of the dorsal duct empties into the intestine through the minor papilla. A wide assortment of anomalies or anatomic variations may result from this complicated process of fusion. Among the most common is failure of the ducts to fuse, which causes pancreas divisum. This condition occurs in about 5% of the population (Fig. 133-2). In some persons pancreas divisum causes obstruction at the minor papilla and possibly obstructive pancreatitis.

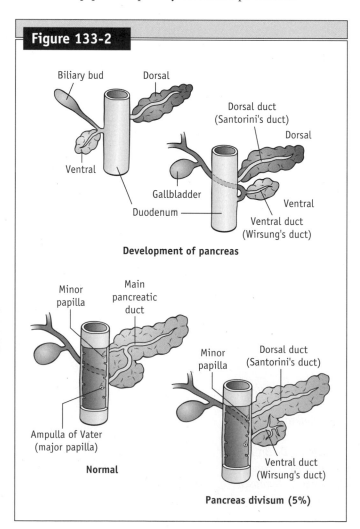

Figure 133-2

Development of pancreas

Normal

Pancreas divisum (5%)

Development of pancreas and pancreas divisum.

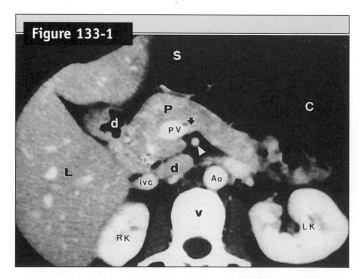

Figure 133-1

Transverse CT of the pancreas (P) showing its relationship with the stomach (S), colon (C), duodenum (d), liver (L), right kidney (RK), left kidney (LK), aorta (Ao), portal vein (PV), inferior vena cava (ivc), common bile duct (*open arrow*), superior mesenteric artery (*arrowhead*), and superior mesenteric vein (*black arrow*). V—vertebra. (*Courtesy of* M. Fernandez, MD.)

Nerves

The pancreas is innervated by sympathetic, parasympathetic, sensory afferent, peptidergic, and enteropancreatic nerves, which contribute to the regulation of exocrine function. Preganglionic parasympathetic fibers originate in the dorsal motor nucleus and descend along the vagus nerve to synapse at the intrapancreatic ganglion. Neurotransmission at the ganglion is mediated by acetylcholine via nicotinic receptors. Postganglionic fibers exert their effects by releasing mainly acetylcholine, although other neuropeptides also serve as neurotransmitters.

The sympathetic pathways originate from preganglionic fibers of the sympathetic chain, from level C8 to level L3. Splanchnic nerves reach the paravertebral and celiac ganglia, where they synapse with postsynaptic α and β fibers. In the sympathetic pathways the main preganglionic neurotransmitter is acetylcholine, whereas norepinephrine is a postganglionic neurotransmitter. As with other neural pathways, effects mediated by receptors may be antagonized by certain substances, (eg, muscarinic receptors by atropine, nicotinic receptors by hexamethonium, α-adrenergic receptors by phentolamine, and β-adrenergic receptors by propranolol). Afferent fibers originating in the pancreas travel within splanchnic nerves to the spinal cord and play a role in regulation of pancreatic blood flow, also contributing to regulation of endocrine and exocrine pancreatic functions.

◼ HISTOLOGY

The exocrine portion of the pancreas, occupying most of the gland, consists of lobules and acini separated by connective tissue, which carries small vessels and terminal nerves. The endocrine portion of the pancreas constitutes about 5% to 10% of the gland and is scattered throughout the gland. It is represented mainly by the islets of Langerhans, with α cells that secrete glucagon, β cells that secrete insulin, D cells that release somatostatin, and F cells that contain pancreatic polypeptide (PP). Some of the blood vessels that reach the acini have previously irrigated the islets, making them a true portal system. Therefore, this blood contains high levels of gastrointestinal peptides, that, by affecting exocrine secretion, play an important role in the control of exocrine function.

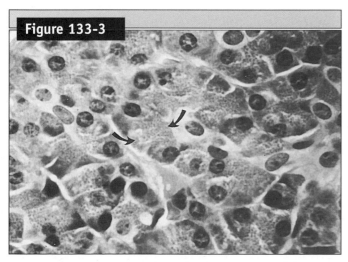

Figure 133-3

Pancreatic acinar cell (between *arrows*) with typical zymogen granules. (*Courtesy of* A. Ibarra, MD.)

The acini are composed of cells with a characteristic pyramid-like shape. The digestive enzymes are stored toward the apical portion of the cell as zymogen granules and are easily observed by light microscopy (Fig. 133-3). In the center of the acini, the ducts are lined with the flatter centroacinar or ductular cells.

The acinar cell is a highly polarized, regulated, secretory cell. Synthesis of proteins occurs toward the base of the cell at the endoplasmic reticulum, according to the encoding instructions contained in the DNA. The message is transmitted by the RNA to the ribosomes, where amino acids are aggregated and the protein molecule is synthesized. Proenzymes contain a terminal amino acid, the signal peptide, which is cleaved after transport through the microsomal membranes and the rough endoplasmic reticulum. The remaining protein undergoes conformational changes and then is transported to the trans-Golgi network, where lysosomal and secretory enzymes are sorted [2]. Lysosomal enzymes receive a molecule of ribose in position 6, which is then phosphorylated and is recognized by specific receptors at the Golgi complex. Lysosomal enzymes are separated and stored in the lysosomes, where acidic pH facilitates dissociation from receptors. Alteration of this smooth, well-coordinated trafficking and sorting of enzymes, with the almost-complete inhibition of exocytosis of enzymes by the acinar cell, is common in the early stages of acute experimental pancreatitis. By understanding the intrinsic mechanisms of this phenomenon, one may be able to comprehend the triggering processes that eventually limit or prevent the development of pancreatitis.

◼ CELLULAR PHYSIOLOGY

As shown in Figure 133-4, the acinar cell may be stimulated by agonists that reach the basolateral membrane through blood vessels, nerve terminals, or paracrine pathways. Interaction with specific plasma membrane receptors triggers the cascade of events that eventually leads to discharge of secretory proteins. In general, it is believed that each agonist activates the cell mainly through a common second messenger. One intracellular pathway is related to an increase in cellular cyclic AMP (cAMP). Coupled to

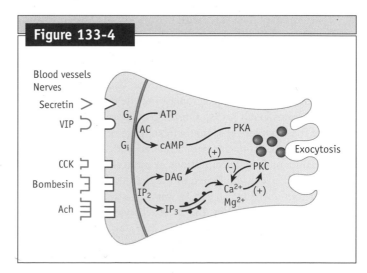

Figure 133-4

Diagram of the pancreatic acinar cell, the membrane receptors for agonists, and intracellular events related to secretion of enzymes. AC—adenyl cyclase; PKA—protein kinase A; PKC—protein kinase C; VIP—vasoactive intestinal polypeptide.

membrane receptors are low-molecular weight guanine nucleotide-binding G proteins, with G_s stimulating and G_i inhibiting the formation of cAMP. Another family of G proteins, G_p, activates phospholipase C and is associated with hydrolysis of inositol 4,5-diphosphate (IP_2), resulting in the generation of inositol 1,4,5-triphosphate (IP_3), which in turn increases cytoplasmic Ca^{2+}, mainly by release from intracellular stores. Intracellular magnesium regulates mobilization of Ca^{2+}. Hydrolysis also leads to the formation of diacylglycerol (DAG), which stimulates the affinity of protein kinase C for Ca^{2+} [3]. Protein kinase C (PKC) sustains formation of DAG and decreases intracytosolic Ca^{2+}. Protein kinase C plays a crucial role in signal transmission, exocytosis, cell growth, and gene expression [4••]. Evidence indicates that in addition to transmitting external signals, G proteins may participate in the control of transport between intracellular compartments and exocytosis. In addition, studies on the effect of secretin on acinar cell response have shown that secretagogues, such as secretin, may stimulate secretion by activating more than one exclusive pathway.

PANCREATIC JUICE

The human pancreas secretes approximately 1500 mL/24 h of a clear, slightly alkaline (pH 7 to 8) fluid, with a high concentration of ions. The ions consist mainly of bicarbonate, with lesser amounts of chloride, sodium, potassium, calcium, magnesium, and proteins. At slow rates of secretion (eg, during the interdigestive state), pancreatic juice is derived mainly from the acinar cells, and its electrolyte composition is similar to that of plasma. After a meal, secretin is released, and the centroacinar and ductular cells actively secrete water and bicarbonate. This process is mediated by two main mechanisms:

1) Activation of cAMP-regulated chloride channels (the cystic fibrosis transmembrane conductance regulator [CFTR]) and Cl^- and HCO_3^- exchanges in the luminal membrane in duct cells results in an electrogenic active secretion of HCO_3^- while Cl^- returns to the cytoplasm.

2) At the same time, proton pumps inserted in the basolateral membrane lead to active H^+ ion secretion. This H^+ ion may then react with plasma HCO_3^-, generating CO_2, which diffuses into the duct cells. Thus, secretion of HCO_3^- originates in the bloodstream and is associated with a downward CO_2 gradient from blood to pancreatic juice. Carbonic anhydrase II, present in high concentrations in the cytoplasm of the ductular cells, generates H_2CO_3 [5•]. On the basolateral membrane of the ductular cells, another exchange of Na^+ and H^+ provides CO_2 to the cytoplasm and Na^+, K^+-ATPase maintains low concentrations of intracellular Na^+. K^+ and Na^+ reach the lumen of the ducts by the paracellular route, which also carries water passively and maintains osmolality (Fig. 133-5). Exchange of HCO_3^- and Cl^- is mediated by cytoplasmic carbonic anhydrase as the juice flows to the intestine, and this exchange is inversely correlated with the secretion rate.
Concentration of chloride in the juice varies inversely with the rate of water and HCO_3^- secretion, so that the sum of the concentrations of HCO_3^- and Cl^- remains constant at any rate of secretion.

Proteins

Most pancreatic juice proteins are hydrolases. Pancreatic juice also contains small amounts of lysosomal enzymes, glycoproteins, trypsin inhibitor, lithostatin, lactoferrin, and plasma proteins, along with tiny amounts of antigens such as CA 19-9, α-fetoprotein, carcinoembryogenic antigen, and certain gastrointestinal peptides like somatostatin and insulin. Depending on the substrate, hydrolases can be categorized as proteases, amylases, or lipases (Table 133-1).

Proteases constitute about 10% of the pancreatic juice proteins and are secreted mainly as proenzymes. Trypsinogen is activated in the lumen of the duodenum by the hydrolytic action of enterokinase, resulting in trypsin and a small peptide fragment. Trypsinogen-activated peptide is usually degraded; however, it may be detected in the peritoneal fluid, urine, or blood in persons with acute pancreatitis and may indicate the severity of the disease. Active trypsin, in turn, activates the remaining proenzymes.

Enzymes have been assumed to secrete at fixed ratios, according to a concept that implies parallel secretion of enzymes. However, current evidence shows that protein secretion may occur in a nonparallel pattern, supporting the concept of a complex system of regulation and a nonhomogenous source of enzymes.

REGULATION OF PANCREATIC SECRETION

Pancreatic secretion is regulated through an interplay involving many complex neural and hormonal pathways [6••]. Between meals, while a person is at rest, there is a modest flow of pancreatic secretion, about 10% of that observed postprandially. This basal, or interdigestive, secretion is not steady; it fluctuates in volume and in HCO_3^- and protein concentration, relative to the phases of the migrating motor complex (MMC). Maximal concentrations of bicarbonate and protein in this situation are observed toward the end of phase 2 of the MMC, which corresponds with gastrointestinal peristalsis. The cyclic pattern of secretion seems to be

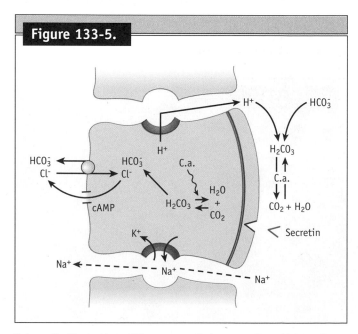

Figure 133-5.

Schematic illustration of the pancreatic ion secretion. (*Adapted from* Raeder [5•].)

regulated mainly by cholinergic neural input involving M_1 receptors. Ingestion of a meal elicits a strong pancreatic secretory response. Interdigestive cyclic secretion does not seem to be suppressed by ingestion of a meal but rather is superimposed on the MMC. According to this concept, the response following a meal may vary, depending on the phase of the MMC during which the food is ingested; a more prompt response is seen late in phase 1 or phase 2. Postprandial pancreatic secretion is triggered by mechanisms originating in different levels of the body and is thereby divided into cephalic, gastric, and intestinal phases. This division is rather artificial, as the mechanisms interact and complement each other. Also, although the net final response is an increase in the flow and in bicarbonate and protein secretion, each phase has stimulatory and inhibitory components. The interplay of these mechanisms produces a well-coordinated, proportional, and time-limited response to the meals.

Cephalic Phase

Anticipation, smell, sight, chewing, taste, and deglutition of a meal stimulate pancreatic secretion through mechanisms mediated mainly by the vagus nerve [7]. Secretion during the cephalic phase is relatively low in volume and bicarbonate but rather high in proteins, accounting for about 25% of the postprandial response. Owing to observations that atropine abolishes cephalic enzyme secretion, it is generally accepted that this effect is mediated by muscarinic receptors. However, because atropine does not clearly affect the volume and bicarbonate secretion of this phase, secretion of these components may be mediated by another transmitter—possibly vasoactive intestinal polypeptide (VIP). Vagal stimulation of enzymes is probably mediated by cholinergic receptors at the acinar cell, but recent evidence suggests that preganglionic fibers synapse at intrapancreatic ganglia, where the neurotransmitter is acetylcholine. Postganglionic fibers affect acinar cells through cholinergic and peptidergic receptors, the latter responding to cholecystokinin (CCK), gastrin-releasing peptide, and VIP. Because stimulation of the cephalic phase also releases PP, a known inhibitor of pancreatic secretion, the secretory response of the cephalic phase represents the net result of the interplay between stimulatory and inhibitory impulses.

Gastric Phase

Arrival of food in the stomach stimulates pancreatic secretion by two mechanisms: 1) gastric distention and activation of vagovagal and gastropancreatic reflexes; 2) stimulation by protein digestion products of gastric chymoreceptors with release by the antrum of certain peptides such as gastrin, and suppression of others, such as somatostatin. Overall, this phase represents a modest contribution to the postprandial response of about 10%.

Intestinal Phase

This phase is the most important component of the pancreatic postprandial secretory response, representing approximately 75% of the total response. Individual nutrients appear to induce different enzymatic responses: carbohydrates have little effect, amino acids an intermediate effect, and lipids a maximal effect. These effects may be important when planning the feeding of a patient recovering from acute pancreatitis. As with previous phases, stimulatory and inhibitory regulatory mechanisms exist, some of them mediated by nerves and others by release of gastrointestinal peptides into the circulation. Distention of the duodenum and administration of hyperosmolar solutions, as occurs after a meal, stimulates secretion of enzymes mainly by a cholinergic mechanism. In contrast, enteropancreatic inhibitory reflexes release peptides that inhibit cholinergic transmission, including that of PP, peptide YY, neuropeptide Y, neurotensin, enkephalin, calcitonin gene-related peptide, and pancreastatin. The exact modulatory input of the reflexes releasing these peptides in the intestinal phase of pancreatic secretion is unknown [8].

The hormonal control of pancreatic secretion was firmly established at the beginning of this century in the classic studies by Bayliss and Starling, in which acidification of the duodenum was found to increase the flow of pancreatic juice [9]. Lowering the pH of the duodenal mucosa to a concentration below 4.5 releases secretin, a potent stimulant of water and HCO_3^- secretion and a weak stimulant of protein secretion. The presence of fatty acids in the duodenum also releases secretin. These same conditions also release VIP, which has similar but weaker effects on pancreatic secretion.

When fatty acids, peptides, amino acids, and calcium come into contact with the duodenal mucosa, CCK is released, which stimulates pancreatic enzyme secretion. CCK receptors have been detected in human acinar cells [10], where CCK_B receptors are predominantly expressed. The physiologic effects of CCK on the in situ human pancreas appear to be more complex. Based on observations in several species, CCK has been proposed as a mediator of afferent nerves that activate central mechanisms and other efferent fibers that stimulate enzyme secretion. These mechanisms could be the main pathways by which CCK stimu-

Table 133-1. Enzymes Secreted in Pancreatic Juice

Enzymes	Substrate	Site of action	Products
Amylase	Amylase	1–4 links between hexoses	Oligosaccharides
	Amylopectin		Dextrins
Peptidases	—	—	—
Endopeptidases (trypsin, chymotrypsin, elastase)	Proteins	Internal peptides	Smaller peptides
Exopeptidases	Proteins	C-terminal bonds	Terminal amino acids
Lipase	Triglycerides	Ester bonds 1 and 3	Diglycerides, monoglycerides, fatty acids
Phospholipase	Fatty acids	Ester bond 2	Lysolecithin

lates pancreatic secretion. Other studies in humans point toward the interaction between CCK and the cholinergic system [11]. Earlier observations showed that pancreatic enzyme and bicarbonate secretion occurring after a meal is significantly suppressed by vagotomy [12] and that atropine inhibits the stimulatory effect of a meal on the pancreas without affecting circulatory CCK levels [13]. From all these observations, it may be concluded that cholinergic impulses play a modulatory role in the pancreatic secretory response to CCK and secretin.

In addition, release of CCK by the intestinal mucosa appears to be mediated by a releasing factor that is digested by trypsin under resting conditions. After a meal, the amount of substrate that reaches the duodenum competes for the hydrolytic tryptic activity that would free CCK-releasing factor [14] (Fig. 133-6). Indirect evidence for this regulatory mechanism in humans is provided by studies in which the administration of trypsin and chymotrypsin into the intestine decreased CCK release. This feedback mechanism is the basis for therapies designed to alleviate pain in patients with chronic pancreatitis who have decreased trypsin output and increased plasma levels of CCK [15••].

Another autoregulatory mechanism is also involved in elevated plasma CCK. It has been observed that elevated plasma CCK elicits somatostatin release, which in turn inhibits release of CCK-releasing peptide [14]. A similar mechanism involving the participation of an intermediate-releasing peptide appears to mediate the release of secretin by the duodenal mucosa [16].

As food moves through the intestine, inhibitory mechanisms of pancreatic secretion become increasingly evident. First, hyperglycemia and hyperaminoacidemia decrease pancreatic secretion, an effect that may be mediated by increased release of somatostatin. Second, the presence of fats in the terminal ileum inhibit pancreatic secretion, probably by a hormonal mechanism releasing enteroglucagon and neuropeptide Y.

ENDOCRINE AND EXOCRINE INTERACTION

The islet-acinar portal system exposes acinar cells to high concentrations of gastrointestinal peptides, such as insulin, glucagon, PP, somatostatin, and pancreastatin (of which chromogranin A is the precursor), which originate in the islet cells and have well-known effects on acinar cells. Glucagon, somatostatin, and PP are

inhibitors of enzyme secretion, whereas insulin potentiates CCK and secretin effects [17]. Furthermore, some differences exist in the staining of the acinar cells surrounding the islets; more intense staining occurs on the acinar cells near the islets than on those more distal. This so-called halo phenomenon may represent some functional differences among acinar cells, determined by the influence of peptides released by the islets. Such differences between acinar cells are difficult to demonstrate.

REFERENCES

Recently published papers of particular interest have been highlighted as follows:
•   Of interest
••   Of outstanding interest

1.   Lefor AT, Vuocolo P, Parker FB Jr, Sillin LF: Pancreatic complications following cardiopulmonary bypass: factors influencing mortality. *Arch Surg* 1992, 127:382–387.

2.   Gaisano HY, Sheu L, Grondin G, *et al.*: The vesicle-associated membrane protein family of protein in rat pancreatic and parotid acinar cells. *Gastroenterology* 1996, 111:1661–1669.

3.   Williams JA, Blevins GT Jr: Cholecystokinin and regulation of pancreatic acinar cell function. *Physiol Rev* 1993, 73:701–723.

4.•• Bruzzone R: The molecular basis of enzyme secretion. *Gastroenterology* 1990, 99:1157–1176.
This article provides an excellent review of the molecular events that take place during enzyme secretion.

5.• Raeder G Morten: The origin of and subcellular mechanisms causing pancreatic bicarbonate secretion. *Gastroenterology* 1992, 103:1674–1684.
This article provides a comprehensive review of the mechanisms and regulation of bicarbonate secretion.

6.•• Adler G, Nelson KD, Katschinski M, Beglinger C: Neurohormonal control of human pancreatic exocrine secretion. *Pancreas* 1995, 10:1–13.
This article covers the different mechanisms that participate in the control of pancreatic secretion.

7.   Katschinski M, Dahmen G, Reinshagen M, *et al.*: Cephalic stimulation of gastrointestinal secretory and motor responses in humans. *Gastroenterology* 1992, 103:383–391.

8.   Bradish RJ, Kuvshinoff BW, MacFadden DW: Somatostatin inhibits cholecystokinin-induced pancreatic protein secretion via cholinergic pathways. *Pancreas* 1995, 10:401–406.

9.   Bayliss WM, Starling EH: Mechanisms of pancreatic secretion. *J Physiol* 1902, 28:325–353.

10. Tang Ch, Biemond I, Lamers BHW: Cholecystokinin receptors in human pancreas and gallbladder muscle: a comparative study. *Gastroenterology* 1996, 111:1621–1626.

11. Thimister PW, Hopman WP, Sloots CE, *et al.*: Role of intraduodenal proteases in plasma cholecystokinin and pancreaticobiliary responses to protein and amino acids. *Gastroenterology* 1996, 110:567–575.

12. Malagelada JR, Go VLW, Summerskill WHJ: Altered pancreatic and biliary function after vagotomy and pyloroplasty. *Gastroenterology* 1974, 66:22–27.

13. Soudah HC, Lu Y, Hasler WL, Owyang C: Cholecystokinin at physiological levels evokes pancreatic enzyme secretion via a cholinergic pathway. *Am J Physiol* 1992, 263:G102–G107.

14. Li Y, Hao Y, Owyang C: Evidence for autoregulation of cholecystokinin secretion during diversion of bile pancreatic juice in rats. *Gastroenterology* 1995, 109:231–238.

15.•• Slaff J, Jacobson D, Tillman CR, *et al.*: Protease-specific suppression of pancreatic exocrine secretion. *Gastroenterology* 1984, 87:44–52.
This notable article is the only study of its kind in human subjects.

16. Li P, Chang TM, Chey WY: Neuronal regulation of the release and action of secretin-releasing peptide and secretin. *Am J Physiol* 1995, 269:305–312.

17. Lee KY, Krusch D, Zhou L, *et al.*: Effect of endogenous insulin on pancreatic exocrine secretion in perfused dog pancreas. *Pancreas* 1995, 11:190–195.

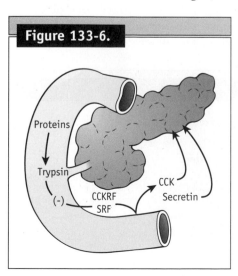

Figure 133-6. Feedback regulation of peptide release on stimulation of pancreatic secretion. CCKRF—cholecystokinin-releasing factor; SRF—secretin-releasing factor.

134 Acute Pancreatitis

Simmy Bank

Acute pancreatitis varies from clinically mild to fulminating disease and has been recorded as a cause of sudden death. Advances made in establishing biochemical and clinical criteria for the severity and prognosis of an attack have markedly influenced our therapeutic approach. Early administration of improved antibiotics, the role of cytokine inhibitors, and the judicious use of endoscopic or surgical techniques to establish the etiology and treat the complications of the disease have reduced the mortality rate from acute pancreatitis to about 5% to 10% for the acute attack. However, our inability to reduce this mortality rate further, despite the increased understanding of the pathophysiology, is one of the more disappointing aspects of the disease.

ANATOMY

There are four critical anatomic areas relative to acute pancreatitis. The first is the gland's, or pancreas' relation to surrounding vital vascular structures, in particular the splenic and portal veins and splenic and pancreaticoduodenal arteries. These can be compressed, thrombosed, or eroded by an enlarged pancreas, an abscess, or a cyst.

The second is the close relationship of the pancreas to the duodenal loop and the greater curvature of the stomach and splenic flexure also are important. These features make these organs vulnerable to obstruction, compression, and erosion as well as pressure on the celiac axis and its connections that transmit pain fibers from the gland.

A third area of anatomic importance is the intimate relationship between the common bile duct and pancreatic duct. These ducts traverse the head of the pancreas as they enter the duodenum, either as a "common channel" (in approximately 70% of people) or through separate openings. This anatomic feature is important in gallstone pancreatitis and, more practically, the ability to cannulate the ducts at endoscopic retrograde cholangiopancreatography (ERCP). The ampulla is also richly innervated and may be a trigger zone for nervous impulses to the rest of the gland.

The fourth area of anatomic importance is the relationship of the ductal-acinar and islets of Langerhans. The peripheral ducts are divided into primary, secondary, and tertiary radicals. The tertiary radicals drain the acini and, embryologically, probably give rise to the islets. The islets of Langerhans are concentrated in the body and tail of the pancreas, so that disease or necrosis in this area has a greater tendency to result in transient hyperglycemia. The head of the gland contains a higher concentration of the hormone *pancreatic polypeptide*, which is under the influence of cholinergic impulses and may play a role in the genesis of acute pancreatitis.

Anatomic Abnormalities

There are two developmental abnormalities significant to acute pancreatitis. The first is *pancreas divisum*, an important cause of recurrent acute attacks. About 6% of pancreases at autopsy show that the dorsal duct (Santorini) rather than the major duct (Wirsung) is the dominant drainage site for pancreatic secretion. In these patients, the major duct may end blindly in the head of the pancreas, communicate inadequately with the dorsal duct, or drain equally with it (see Fig. 133-2 in Chapter 133). The accessory papilla, which drains the duct of Santorini, may be inadequate to sustain pancreatic flow and therefore lead to partial obstruction and retrograde pancreatitis [1].

The second developmental abnormality significant to acute pancreatitis is *annular pancreas*, in which a ring of pancreatic tissue surrounds the second portion of the duodenum, possibly causing it to become obstructed, especially in childhood. The pancreatic ducts supplying the annular pancreas may drain insufficiently, causing recurrent attacks of acute pancreatitis [2]. Other abnormalities of pancreatic ductal anatomy have been implicated as causes of hereditary forms of pancreatitis, but these are more speculative, especially in the light of a recently described gene deletion in hereditary forms of pancreatitis (trypsinogen [TCBR complex] genes) and even the rarer association of pancreatitis and pancreatic cysts with von Hippel-Landau disease (cerebellar arteriovenous malformations).

PHYSIOLOGY

Pancreatic physiology is intimately connected to acute pancreatitis [3]. The two main hormonal pancreatic stimuli, secretin for volume and bicarbonate and cholecystokinin (CCK) for enzymes, may be implicated in attacks of pancreatitis. For example, the sudden surge of pancreatic volume flow after a large meal, caused by secretin release against an impacted stone in the ampulla, may be a major cause of acute gallstone pancreatitis. Alcohol given orally or intravenously, either by vagal or local release of CCK from the duodenum, may cause ampullary spasm or excessive enzyme secretion, thereby causing acute pancreatitis against a closed ampulla or by producing protein plugs of enzymes in centroacinar or larger ducts. CCK hyperstimulation usually causes an edematous type of pancreatitis in experimental animals. In the acini themselves, conversion of trypsinogen (and possibly a specific mesotrypsinogen) to trypsin is considered to be the initiating mechanism in acute pancreatitis, resulting in intra-acinar enzyme release. Fusion of digestive enzymes with lysosomal enzymes (*eg*, cathepsin B) at a critical pH level may result in the release of lipases, esterases, phospholipases, and so forth, which lead to progressive parenchymal and vascular necrosis. Other etiologic factors (*eg*, toxins) may prevent the release of enzymes from the acini (exostosis) into the centroacinar ducts, resulting in autoactivation of intracellular enzymes.

ETIOLOGY
Alcohol and Gallstones

Alcohol and gallstones account for about 90% of all cases of acute pancreatitis worldwide. The predominance of one cause over the other depends on socioeconomic, ethnic, and cultural differences. For example, gallstones are extremely common among Navajo Native Americans; people with a sedentary lifestyle; and those who are obese or have metabolic illnesses, such as hyperlipidemias, hypercholesterolemia, diabetes, and hypothyroidism. Alcohol-induced pancreatitis is more common in young and middle-aged people in whom an idiosyncratic sensitivity to alcohol may exist at levels of alcohol consumption exceeding 80 g/d (ie, 5 fl oz or "shots" of hard liquor or three quarters of a bottle of wine per day). Other predisposing factors may be the level of alcohol dehydrogenase activity in the gastric mucosa and the liver.

Medications

There is hardly a drug that has not been incriminated anecdotally in the cause of acute pancreatitis [4]. However, drugs for which a direct association can be elucidated are azathioprine (Imuran); chemotherapeutic agents; sulfonamides, including azulfidine; drugs used in the treatment of acquired immunodeficiency syndrome (AIDS), such as didanosine and zalcitabine; valproic acid; tetracycline; estrogens in hyperlipidemic patients; and more controversially, diuretics. The mechanism of pancreatitis for many of these medications is obscure. Some, such as didanosine and tetracycline, appear to sensitize the patient to the effects of alcohol. Occupational exposure to organophosphorus compounds is a rare cause for acute pancreatitis.

Cancer of the Pancreas

Cancer of the pancreas is a rare cause of acute pancreatitis. However, the increase in prevalence of pancreatic cancer, especially with the increasing longevity of populations in developed countries, has made this an important cause to consider in patients initially considered to have *idiopathic pancreatitis*. In fact, cancer of the pancreas is probably the most important entity to rule out once gallstones have been entirely excluded in patients initially believed to have the idiopathic form of the disease [5•].

Endoscopic Retrograde Cholangiopancreatography

Endoscopic retrograde cholangiopancreatography has become an extremely common diagnostic and therapeutic technique in clinical practice. The incidence of post-ERCP hyperamylasemia is approximately 50%; mild pancreatitis occurs in 7% to 10% of patients and severe attacks in 1% to 3%, with a mortality rate near 0.01% in those receiving optimum care. Many techniques are being attempted to reduce the incidence of ERCP pancreatitis, including the use of pre-ERCP medications, such as gabexate and cytokines. Octreotide (Sandostatin) has not been found to reduce the incidence of post-ERCP pancreatitis.

Idiopathic Pancreatitis

Idiopathic pancreatitis is the designation applied to patients who have an attack of pancreatitis for which no cause can be found. The initial investigation usually does not include an ERCP [6]. The author usually recommends gallbladder ultrasonography at 3- to 6-month intervals for 2 to 3 years to entirely exclude a gallstone etiology. The question of gallbladder sludge on sonography is currently a gray area. However, with careful follow-up and extensive evaluation of recurrent attacks, including ERCP, episodes initially appearing to be "idiopathic" usually are not caused by gallstones. The difficulty is in determining how many sonograms and duodenal aspirates are warranted after one attack to exclude a gallstone etiology and whether ERCP or even laparoscopic cholecystectomy is indicated after recurrent severe attacks.

Other Causes

Hyperlipidemia (trigylcerides >600 mg), hypercalcemia, and uremia should be excluded in seeking a cause for pancreatitis. Occult duodenal disease that may obstruct the flow of pancreatic juice, such as Crohn's disease and villous tumors of the ampulla, are excluded by endoscopy. After these possible causes have been excluded, other anatomic abnormalities, such as pancreas divisum, and viral or other infectious etiologies should be investigated. The diagnosis of pancreas divisum is nearly always made at ERCP, after recurrent attacks. The diagnosis occasionally is made by ultrasonography following an intravenous dose of secretin that shows that the duct remains dilated, thereby impeding the flow of pancreatic juice. Pancreatitis is common after organ transplantation. This may be due to the therapy that is used to prevent or treat rejection, and it seems to be particularly common after bone marrow transplantation in patients who suffer graft-versus-host disease. *Traumatic pancreatitis* is usually obvious and follows blunt or open trauma. *Ascaris lumbricoides* is a common cause of pancreatitis in the Far East, as are scorpion bites in Trinidad.

MECHANISMS
Duct Obstruction

Duct obstruction may be caused by obstruction of a common channel between the bile duct and the pancreatic duct or obstruction of the pancreatic duct itself. Increased pressure in the pancreatic ductal system or neurohormonal stimulation from the ampulla may affect pancreatic secretion or cause vascular constriction or other as yet undetermined factors that may initiate the attack. Examples of duct obstruction are gallstone impaction, pancreas divisum, ascariasis, ampullary stenosis, carcinoma of the pancreas, and a single stone in the pancreatic duct.

Direct Toxic Effect on Acinar Cells

Direct toxic effect on acinar cells cause fusion between zymogen granules and lysosomes. This mechanism might be incriminated in such diverse causes as acute alcoholism, drugs, scorpion venom, viral etiologies, and heroin or cocaine toxicity.

Neurohormonal Mechanisms

Cholecystokinin overstimulation by alcohol and other peptides, hypercalcemia, and perhaps sympathetic overstimulation or an estrogen effect after menopause have been suggested as possible mechanisms in the induction of acute pancreatitis.

Vascular Insufficiency

Vascular insufficiency, such as in pancreatic ischemia caused by hypotension or that induced by swelling of the gland itself, may be an important factor in the progression to hemorrhagic pancreatitis. A role for oxygen-free radical release or nitric oxide generation in vascular injury is highly speculative.

Although not all of the above mechanisms are immediately apparent, they do form a cohesive pathophysiologic schema that might cause pancreatic acinar cell disruption with release of enzymes and lysosomes, thereby giving rise to pancreatic autodigestion and necrosis.

Enzyme-Cytokine Cascade

After activation of trypsinogen to trypsin and the release of elastases, esterases, and phospholipases, the inflammatory and necrotic processes cause an influx of neutrophils. The neutrophils become activated and release a number of cytokines, particularly tumor necrosis factor-α (TNF-α), interleukins (IL-6, IL-8), and platelet activating factors. In addition, vasoconstrictive peptides, such as kallikrein and bradykinin, may lead to vascular compromise and necrosis. The inflammatory process may give rise to further obstruction of the pancreatic duct, liquefaction of necrosis, and cyst formation. In severe pancreatitis, increased intestinal permeability associated with ileus and the translocation of intestinal (particularly colonic) bacteria to the necrotic area is extremely common. By the fifth day after the onset of the attack, contamination by *Esherichia coli*, *Streptococcus faecalis*, and other bacteria results in infected necrotic tissue and subsequent abscess formation. The release of unspecified cytokines, endotoxins, and enzymes into the bloodstream give rise to extra-abdominal organ involvement of the type usually seen in patients with multiple organ system failure (MOSF), that is, cardiac, renal, pulmonary, hepatologic, neurologic, and hematologic effects that form the basis of the clinical criteria of severity (Bank's signs).

▮ PATHOLOGY

The pathology of changes from acute pancreatitis includes the following:

- *Cellular changes only*, as manifested by high serum enzymes after an attack (*eg*, gallstones) but normal CT scan or sonogram. Such attacks are usually mild and subside after several days.
- *Edematous pancreatitis* with only slight enlargement of the pancreas on CT scan or sonogram; histologically, the gland may show edema and a mild acute cellular reaction. These attacks are usually mild but may occasionally become severe.
- *Necrotic and hemorrhagic pancreatitis*, as evidenced by areas of poor uptake of contrast media on contrast-enhanced CT scan (Fig. 134-1). Examples are Cullen's signs, a grayish discoloration of altered blood around the umbilicus; Grey Turner's signs, a gray discoloration of altered blood in the flanks; and a brown peritoneal aspirate. This form of pancreatitis usually is accompanied by cellular infiltration and followed by infection. Attacks are nearly always severe or fulminating. Necrosis may be so severe that it eliminates enzyme production with only slight, if any, elevation of enzymes.

- *Infected necrosis*, as evidenced by extensive CT scan changes, either intrapancreatic or extrapancreatic, and eventual abscess formation. A marked inflammatory reaction is present with neutrophils. These attacks are always severe.

▮ OUTCOME

The outcome of the acute attack depends in part on the etiology and in part on the severity of the attack. For example, in alcohol-induced pancreatitis the first attack probably occurs because of long-standing alcohol abuse that has caused silent histologic damage [7]. If the attack occurs in an already compromised gland, it may be followed by diabetes and steatorrhea. Abnormal pancreatic function on secretion testing and abnormal duct morphology on ERCP will be evident. There is an increasing body of opinion that even alcohol-induced pancreatitis may occur on a "virgin" gland and that the chronicity may be due to repetitive attacks of alcohol-induced pancreatitis (see Chapter 137, *Chronic Pancreatitis*).

With most causes (eg, gallstones) once the attack subsides, the pancreas returns to a normal histology and functional capacity. Although there may be temporary endocrine and histologic changes that last up to 6 months, it is rare to get abnormal pancreatic function or abnormal duct morphology. Alternatively, after a fulminating or severe attack with necrosis or with multiple acute attacks, the necrosis may be replaced by cell atrophy, fibrous tissue, stricture of the main or branched ducts, and parenchymal fibrosis, all of which ultimately lead to abnormal morphology on ERCP. So-called *small duct disease*, with no ductal change on ERCP but recurrent episodes of pain, may be the most difficult type of acute attack to diagnose and treat. Most acute attacks of pancreatitis unrelated to alcohol rarely result in exocrine or endocrine insufficiency after the attack has subsided and in subsequent years.

▮ CLINICAL FEATURES

The dominant symptom of acute pancreatitis is abdominal pain that is usually excruciatingly severe and appears as an acute abdominal emergency [4,8••]. Occasionally, the pain may be less

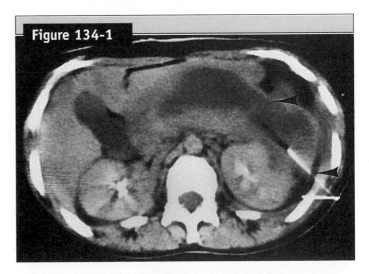

Figure 134-1

Computed tomography scan of abdomen shows virtually no uptake of intravenous contrast by pancreas compared liver and kidneys, indicating severe necrosis (*arrow*). Fine-needle aspiration for bacteria (*arrow*) is being performed.

severe and localized to the right or left upper quadrant or the back. In rare cases, the pain may be insignificant, with the main finding being fever or an abdominal mass. Vomiting, constipation, and diarrhea may occur but rarely are prominent. The attack may occur after a heavy meal or an alcoholic binge. It is typically persistent and constant, which distinguishes it from peptic ulcer or a gallstone attack. The severity of the pain tends to exceed the findings on examination; guarding and rigidity on palpation are slight unless there is diffuse peritonitis. Acute pancreatitis and acute mesenteric ischemia are the two diseases in which severe pain may be associated with a relative paucity of abdominal signs. Every patient with moderate or severe abdominal pain should have a serum amylase determination. The finding of hyperamylasemia in a patient with abdominal pain becomes the pivotal starting point for three questions regarding patient management:

1. Is the hyperamylasemia due to pancreatitis, another abdominal emergency, or concomitant coincidental disease?
2. If pancreatitis is present, how severe is the attack?
3. What is the etiology of the pancreatitis, and does it need urgent correction?

Differential Diagnosis of Hyperamylasemia and Abdominal Pain

There are approximately three dozen causes of raised serum amylase, most of which may be associated with abdominal pain [9] (Table 134-1). However, the main diagnostic problems occur in patients presenting with an acute abdominal catastrophe. This is because the same degree of hyperamylasemia may be seen in patients with perforated viscous, intestinal obstruction or strangulation, ruptured aortic aneurysm, ectopic pregnancy, strangulated ovarian cyst, and other problems. A plain film of the abdomen should be the first diagnostic test; it may show air under the diaphragm, intestinal obstruction, or an abdominal aneurysm. Pelvic examination may confirm an ectopic pregnancy. However, if any doubt as to the diagnosis exists (diagnostic difficulty exists in some 5%–30% of patients) an immediate CT scan of the abdomen should be obtained. Severe pancreatitis that may be confused with other abdominal catastrophes will always require a CT

scan. Alternatively, a CT scan may help confirm one of the other conditions requiring urgent operation. Although a CT scan may be normal in approximately 20% of patients with pancreatitis, such attacks are usually mild and amenable to more leisurely evaluation. In these less severe cases, other causes of hyperamylasemia should be considered, including abdominal pain occurring in patients with incidental macroamylasemia, acute or chronic renal disease in which amylase is not excreted, or one of the hematologic conditions or tumors that secrete salivary-type amylase [10].

Assessment of Severity

About 30% of patients with a severe attack of pancreatitis will show obvious signs of a catastrophic illness as evidenced by hypotension; tachycardia; acidosis; abdominal ileus; evidence of hemorrhagic pancreatitis, such as Grey Turner's signs or Cullen's signs; and evidence of a central loop of distended bowel over the pancreas or colon cutoff sign, caused by a gas-filled colon up to the splenic flexure and probably due to exudative obstruction of the colon. The remaining 70% of patients with pancreatitis will require consideration of the current criteria used to assess disease severity. The most commonly used criteria are

- *Ranson's early objective signs* (1974) [11••], which are assessed on admission and at 48 hours (Table 134-2)
- *Bank's clinical criteria* (1983) [12], or signs of multiple organ system failure (MOSF) (Table 134-3)
- the *Apache II physiologic score* [8••], which is available in most intensive care units (ICUs) but is not practical outside the ICU setting.

Three or more Ranson's signs, one Bank's sign, and more than eight Apache signs indicate severe disease [13]. Estimates of severity may be enhanced by the extent of the disease on CT scan (graded from A through E) [14]. The most important characteristic is the extent of necrosis, that is, non-uptake of contrast on a contrast-enhanced CT scan (Fig. 134-1). Necrosis of more than 30% of the gland signifies a severe attack. However, a CT scan should not be done only to assess severity because the contrast may impair the pancreatic and renal microcirculation [15•]. Contrast scanning should be reserved for those patients who do not

Table 134-1. Causes of Hyperamylasemia

Acute Abdominal Emergencies

Penetrating peptic ulcer

Acute cholecystitis with hyperamylasemia

Intestinal obstruction with strangulation

Intestinal infarction

Ruptured aortic aneurysm or dissection

Ruptured ectopic pregnancy

Acute salpingitis

Torsion of ovarian cyst or carcinoma

Abdominal trauma with hematoma formation

Perforated diverticulitis

Postgastrectomy afferent loop obstruction

Crohn's disease

Physiologic

Pregnancy

? Genetic S hyperamylasemia

Protein-Bound Hyperamylasemia

Inborn macroamylasemia attached to albumin or globulin (macroamylase)

IgA-bound: celiac disease, lymphoma, IPSID

IgG-bound: chronic infections, liver disease

Immune-complex-bound: AIDS, collagen disease, Sjögren's syndrome

Decreased Excretion of Amylase

Acute and chronic renal failure

Tumor-Associated Amylase

Cancer of the ovary

Cancer of the lung

Lymphoma

Hematologic malignancy

Other tumors

Miscellaneous

Salivary gland disease, *eg*, mumps, tumors

Diabetic ketosis

Postictal

Post-ERCP

improve after 72 hours and those who are suspected of having complications. There have been many refinements to these criteria (notably from Imre in Glasgow [13], and Agarwal and Pitchumoni in New York [16]) as well as development of newer biochemical and radiologic refinements to improve prognostic accuracy at an earlier stage of the disease. Most of these prognostic criteria have a specificity of 75% to 80%. Elevation of quantitative C reactive protein levels and interleukin-6 elevation within 5 hours may prove to be early indicators of severe disease. Treatment in an ICU, when once deemed a severe attack, becomes mandatory. This meticulous approach and supportive therapy in the ICU has been solely responsible for reducing the mortality of the acute attacks from approximately 15% to 5% [13]. Comorbid conditions, such as obesity, cardiac, renal and pulmonary insufficiency, and other diseases, increase the mortality rate and are independent indicators of a severe attack.

Early Assessment of Etiology

Early consideration of the etiology of the attack has taken on renewed importance since the suggestion that early endoscopic stone removal from a common channel may ameliorate or prevent further deterioration in a patient with gallstone pancreatitis. To date, two studies [17,18] have shown such a benefit, whereas one has not demonstrated a significant decrease in morbidity or mortality [19••]. However, there are two definitive indications for early ERCP. One is the presence of cholangitis, as evidenced by chills, fever, raised bilirubin greater than 4 mg/dL, abnormal liver tests (especially alkaline phosphatase), and a bile duct greater than 8 mm on sonography. The other indication is if the severity of the illness worsens, as evidenced by increasing Ranson's, Bank's, or Apache signs. In either of these cases an urgent ERCP and stone removal should be carried out. Other etiologic factors are less evident and do not demand such urgent therapy: alcohol is often denied; hyperlipemia may be induced by an attack; hypercalcemia may be

masked by the low serum calcium consequent to the attack; and drugs that may induce pancreatitis might not be recalled immediately. A careful history and evaluation of the etiology of the attack are required. Once the attack has subsided or recurrent acute attacks occur, these causes need to be reevaluated. If no etiology is apparent, diagnostic ERCP and possibly sphincter manometry should be considered, especially for recurrent attacks or recurrent pain. The pancreatic duct morphology should be evaluated for pancreas divisum, the sphincter of Oddi should be evaluated for dysfunction, and the pancreas should be evaluated for neoplasia.

▉ COMPLICATIONS

Early mortality results almost solely from extra-abdominal organ failure and usually occurs in the first 2 to 7 days. Delayed mortality is due to intra-abdominal complications, which occur most frequently in patients with severe attacks. The major delayed complications (7 days to 21 days), all of which require extreme vigilance while treatment for the acute attack is in progress, are as follows.

- *Infected necrosis or abscess*—A high fever and white blood cell count, continuing severe signs, CT scan that shows necrosis or an extrapancreatic collection, and a thin needle aspirate that is positive for bacteria will confirm infected necrosis or abscess formation (Fig. 134-1) [20].
- *Noninfected continued massive necrosis*—A high fever and white blood cell count; a CT scan that shows more than 30% necrosis; and continued Ranson's, Bank's, or Apache II signs with a fine-needle aspirate that is negative for bacteria suggest continued massive necrosis of the pancreas. In these situations, a needle aspiration may need to be repeated [8••].
- *Gastrointestinal or intra-abdominal hemorrhage*—Hematemesis, melena, sudden hypotension, decrease in hemoglobin or hematocrit, and subcutaneous ecchymosis in the flanks are indications that an incidental or pancreatitis-associated hemorrhage is occurring [21].

Table 134-2. Ranson's Signs

		Alcohol and other	Gallstone
Ranson's early objective signs (1974)			
0 h	Age	>55 y	>70 y
	Leukocyte count	>16,000 mm	>18,000 mm
	Blood sugar	>200 mg/100 mL	>220 mg/100mL
	LDH	>350 U/L	>250 U/L
	AST	>250 U/L	>250 U/L
48 h	HCT	<10%	<10%
	BUN	>5 mg/100 mL	2mg/100 mL
	Ca²⁺	<8 mg/100 mL	<8 mg/100 mL
	P₀	<60 mm Hg	—
	Base deficit	>4 mEq/L	>5 mEq/L
	Fluid sequestration	>6000 mL	>4000 mL

Interpretation: < 3–5 signs indicates mild disease; 3–5 signs indicate moderate disease; > 5 signs indicates fulminating disease.

AST—aspartate aminotransferase; BUN—blood urea nitrogen; LDH—lactate dehydrogenase; greater than—increase; less than—decrease.

Table 134-3. Bank's Criteria

	Bank's clinical criteria (1983)
Cardiac	Shock, tachycardia >130, arrhythmia, EcG changes
Pulmonary	Dyspnea, rales, P₀ <60, adult respiratory distress syndrome
Renal	Urine output <50 mL/h, rising BUN or serum creatinine level
Metabolic	Low or falling Ca²⁺, pH, serum albumin decrease
Hematologic	Falling HCT, diffuse intravascular coagulation (low platelets, split products)
Neurologic	Irritability, confusion, localizing signs
Hemorrhagic disease	On physical (Grey Turner, Cullen) signs or peritoneal tap
Tense distention	Severe ileus, fluid ++

Interpretation:One or more abnormalities in any of the previously mentioned categories indicate severe disease (the greater the number of extra-abdominal organs involved, the worse the prognosis).

• *Cyst formation, ascites, and massive pleural effusion*—High amylase-containing fluid collections may manifest in abdominal distention or mass, recurrent pain; a CT scan or sonogram showing a cyst (Fig. 134-2), ascites, or pleural fluid. An ERCP at 3 to 6 weeks may show communication with the ductal system or non-communication between the ductal system, cyst, ascites, or pleural effusion (Fig. 134-3) [22].

Some of these complications can be so protracted and need so much attention that ICU or in-hospital therapy may be required for 6 or 12 months.

Transient minor complications include the following:

• Acute diabetes, as evidenced by glycosuria and hyperosmolar nonketotic coma
• Peripheral fat necrosis, which occurs 1 or 2 weeks after the attack and manifests with subcutaneous erythematous nodules, fever, eosinophilia, and arthralgia; biopsy of skin lesions shows fat necrosis, and radiographs of the bones may show intramedullary defects, reflecting intramedullary fat necrosis
• Retinal changes, as evidenced by visual difficulties, macular or retinal hemorrhagic exudates, and hemorrhages (Puertscher's retinopathy) [23].

▆ SPECIAL TESTS
Serologic Tests Other than Serum Amylase
In the majority of patients, there is little evidence that determination of serum esterase, phospholipase A_2, fractionation of the serum amylase into salivary (S) and pancreatic (P) isoenzymes, or the amylase-creatinine excretion ratio narrows the diagnosis or differential diagnosis of acute pancreatitis. The total serum amylase level remains the most useful and readily available test [24]. Tests for "benign" macroamylasemia or fractionation of the

amylase into its S and P components are warranted when the diagnosis of acute pancreatitis is uncertain and the serum amylase level is moderately elevated.

Although serum lipase elevation is not as widely used as serum amylase, this test is considered by some as more specific for pancreatic injury than amylase levels [25]. In the past, methodologic problems have been cited as the reason for the unpopularity of lipase determination [9]. However, with the advent of newer technologies, most of the shortcomings of the previous methods have been overcome. Modern techniques and the use of appropriate diagnosis levels (more than three times normal) may make serum lipase elevation a more useful test than the serum amylase.

A number of potential advantages exist for using serum lipase levels instead of serum amylase levels. Serum lipase levels tend to remain elevated longer than do serum amylase levels and therefore may be useful in patients who present late in their course. By the fourth day of hospital admission, 90% of patients maintain increased lipase levels, whereas only 60% have elevated amylase levels.

Another advantage of estimating serum lipase is that the ratio of serum lipase to amylase (L/A ratio) may shed some light on the etiology of the pancreatitis. Although studies have produced conflicting results regarding the precise diagnostic level, a high L/A ratio (>3) is highly indicative of acute alcoholic pancreatitis, whereas a low L/A ratio is more suggestive of gallstone pancreatitis.

Serum lipase levels, like serum amylase levels, may be elevated in patients with non-pancreatic abdominal disorders, such as ruptured aortic aneurysm, cholelithiasis, choledocholithiasis, small bowel obstruction, and nephrolithiasis. The elevation seen in these conditions, however, is usually less than three times normal, so that a serum lipase level more than three times normal differentiates between abdominal pain of pancreatic from non-pancreatic origin. However, it should be stressed that the accuracy of the lipase test should be verified for individual laboratories.

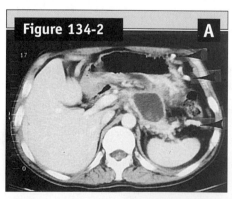
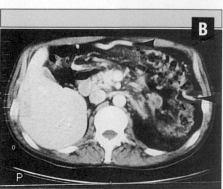

A, Computed tomography (CT) scan of pancreatic cyst with thick wall. *Arrows* indicate contrast material in dilated blood vessels due to vascular compression from the long-standing cyst. **B,** Large vein near anterior abdominal wall. These vessels precluded endoscopic or radiologic drainage and necessitated open surgery.

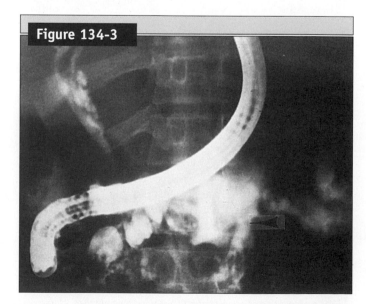

ERCP in a patient with pancreatic ascites persisting 2 months after an acute attack and showing dilated pancreatic duct with extravasation of contrast into the peritoneal cavity (*arrow*).

Computed Tomography Scan

Computed tomography scanning without contrast is not a sensitive test to detect pancreatic necrosis but can be used to evaluate pancreatic size and mass, extent of associated inflammation, and complications, such as pseudocyst formation. CT scanning should *not* be done routinely because of the danger of contrast-induced prolongation of the attack or renal impairment [15•]. It should be reserved for cases in which there is doubt about the diagnosis early in its course; to detect complications such as necrosis, abscess, and cyst; and in patients with non-resolution of the attack in whom a fine-needle aspiration or radiologic drainage of the cyst or abscess is required. In patients with severe disease requiring repeated surgery, CT scan may have to be performed frequently. After an attack has subsided and no diagnosis has been made, a CT scan is important for evaluation of persistent pain or to exclude carcinoma of the pancreas.

Endoscopic Retrograde Cholangiopancreatography

There are a number of scenarios in which ERCP is indicated, *ie* when cholangitis is suspected or when the pancreatitis changes from mild to severe and an impacted stone in the common duct is suspected [26]. There are now two studies showing improved morbidity and mortality if urgent stone removal is performed, although there is at least one controlled study showing no benefit from such urgent sphincterotomy [19••]. If a cyst develops later in the course of the disease, ERCP may be required to determine whether the cyst communicates with the ductal system. In traumatic pancreatitis, ERCP may be indicated to evaluate duct fracture or disruption [27]. Another indication is for unresolving pancreatic ascites or pleural effusion to elucidate the site of the leak.

Idiopathic pancreatitis, possibly because of the passage of a single stone, is often a "once only" disease. ERCP should be performed only after a second attack to exclude possible causes, including ampullary disease (stenosis or tumor); unsuspected gallstones (biliary drainage or manometry may be done at this time); carcinoma or pancreas divisum; and diffuse duct abnormalities, as in chronic pancreatitis, cystic fibrosis, and so forth.

▰ TREATMENT

There are two definitive treatment periods in acute pancreatitis: early treatment of the acute attack and late treatment of complications (Fig. 134-4).

Early Treatment

It is implicit that the 20% of attacks that are severe be managed in an ICU to treat or *anticipate* extra-abdominal organ system failure requiring intervention for cardiac, pulmonary, renal, hepatologic, or neurologic complications and to treat ileus (Table 134-4). It is important to both perform nasogastric suction, nasal oxygen, careful measurements of intake and output, frequent determination of serum electrolytes, and evaluation of metabolic function and treat each abnormality promptly. In addition, blood replacement, dextran supplementation, and parenteral nutrition should be instituted if hemorrhagic pancreatitis is evident or a prolonged course of treatment is expected. Determination of the need for Swan-Ganz catheter placement and endotracheal intubation must be individualized.

The role of antibiotic therapy is still uncertain, but it now appears that such treatment is warranted. Studies from Ulm (Germany) using needle aspiration of the pancreas have shown bacterial colonization of necrotic areas, often beginning after the fifth day of disease. In these studies, the administration of antibiotics before this time (ie, at the onset of attack)—especially with those antibiotics that penetrate the pancreas and necrotic tissue, such as imipenem and ciprofloxacin, has decreased morbidity, and perhaps mortality, rates. It may be expedient to start one of these antibiotics early in the attack to prevent overt infection of necrosis or cyst [28•]. More specific therapy, such as peritoneal dialysis, antitrypsins (*eg*, aprotinin or gabexate), and the universal inhibitor of secretion, octreotide, are used in specific centers but have not yet gained wide acceptance [29]. Multicenter trials in England and the United States are being conducted using cytokines and their inhibitors. One of these inhibitors, a platelet-activating factor inhibitor (lexipafant), has shown some benefit in reducing morbidity and mortality. With these measures, most patients will show progressive improvement in 1 to 2 weeks. Oral feeding may be reinstituted, and the patient can be weaned off critical care attention despite some residual CT scan findings. The remaining 70% to 80% of patients with a mild attack usually require no more than intravenous fluid and electrolyte replacement and discontinuation of oral feedings for 3 to 7 days while considering the extent of investigations required to establish etiology.

Late Treatment
Continuing Necrosis

If fine-needle aspiration or surgery has failed to show bacterial contamination despite a "septic course," ICU monitoring, antibiotic therapy, and total parenteral nutrition (TPN) should be continued and CT scans should be repeated to evaluate progress (Fig. 134-5). In some centers, if signs of organ failure develop, surgery is performed to remove the necrotic tissue. This procedure is known as a *necrosectomy*. However, there seems to be little difference in mortality rates (approximately 30%) between medically and surgically treated groups. The physician should explain to the patient and his or her family that in-hospital therapy (with possible recurrent surgery) may be required for months or even 1 year.

Infected Necrosis or Abscess

The diagnosis of infection in and around the pancreas virtually mandates extensive surgical debridement and removal of all necrotic and infected material (see Chapter 135, *Surgical Treatment of Acute Pancreatitis*). This may have to be done repeatedly, using multiple drainage tubes and retroperitoneal irrigation, leaving the abdomen open, and taking cultures for change in organisms or fungal overgrowth. Erosion of an abscess with multiple fistulas into the duodenum, stomach, and colon is common and prolongs hospitalization. This usually is treated with long-term antibiotic therapy, TPN, or repeated surgeries. Erosion into blood vessels may cause catastrophic bleeding. Survival rates are improved if necrosis is not extensive and there are fewer biochemical and clinical criteria for severe pancreatitis. Some patients with infected necrosis will survive when treated with the newer antibiotics even if they are not surgical candidates or refuse surgery.

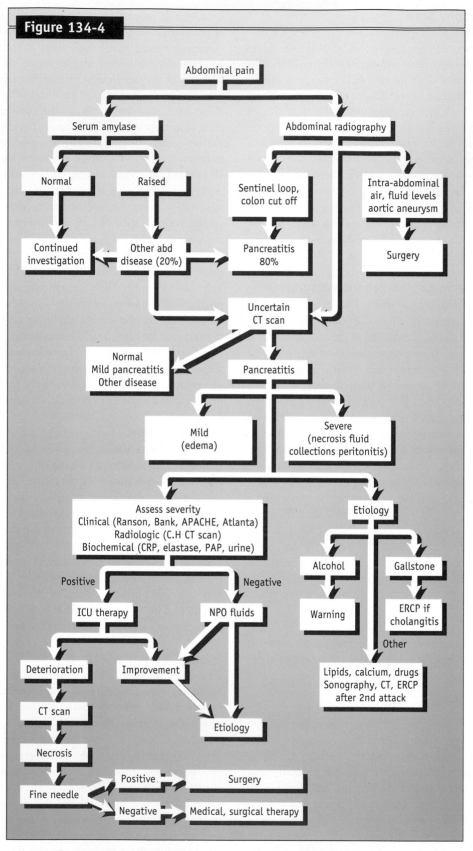

Algorithm for diagnosis and investigation in acute pancreatitis.

Gastrointestinal Hemorrhage

Gastrointestinal hemorrhage in acute pancreatitis is often due to coincidental causes, such as acute stress ulceration due to the disease or as a result of an aspirin- or nonsteroidal anti-inflammatory drug–induced ulcer, a preexisting duodenal or gastric ulcer, or gastric varices. Upper tract endoscopy to diagnose and control the bleeding is the first consideration. However, there are four causes of bleeding directly related to the pancreatitis. One cause is compression or thrombosis of the splenic (or portal) vein resulting in varices from the short gastric fundic veins, which may require sclerosis or surgical ligation. Erosion of a large artery by an abscess,

causing gastric, duodenal, or colonic bleeding, usually is diagnosed and treated by angiography and embolization of bleeding vessels. Other causes of bleeding directly related to the pancreatitis are weakening of a blood vessel adjacent to a cyst, resulting in hemorrhage into the cyst, and communication between an eroded vessel or an aneurysm and the pancreatic duct, leading to bleeding from the ampulla, a condition known as *hemosuccus pancreaticus*. These last two causes require angiography and embolization or Pitressin infusion and perhaps surgical tamponade. Whatever the cause, bleeding in the setting of acute pancreatitis, especially in a severe attack, is a formidable complication with a high mortality.

Pancreatic Cyst, Ascites, and Pleural Effusion

About 40% to 60% of cysts will subside spontaneously and may be observed for 3 to 4 weeks. If the cyst enlarges and pain persists, [31], drainage should be considered. Although a common practice is to wait 4 to 6 weeks for a mature cyst wall to form before beginning therapy to facilitate surgical anastomosis, this is a hazardous approach and should be regarded as obsolete. Complications arising from the cyst are frequent within 3 to 4 weeks. TPN may be required, and octreotide (Sandostatin) in doses ranging from 100 to 200 µg three times per day may be helpful in reducing the flow of pancreatic juice into the cyst [29]. Failure of the cyst to resolve in 3 to 4 weeks should lead to consideration of endoscopic transpapillary or transgastric drainage, internal radiologic drainage, or cyst-gastrostomy [27]. Lengthy observations of cysts that form after acute pancreatitis allow the dangers of infection, rupture, ascites, pleural effusion, and aneurysm formation of blood vessels in and around the cyst with hemorrhage. Pancreatic ascites and pleural

Table 134-4. Benefits of Treatment Options		
Definite benefits	**Possible benefit**	**Experimental benefit**
ICU therapy	Dextran 60	0-Radical scavengers
Surgery	Peritoneal lavage	(allopurinol, dismutase,
for complications	for 7 days	and catalase)
Angiography	Antibiotics,	Interleukins 10, 11,
for bleeding	antifungals	TNF-α antibody
	Octreotide	Calcium channel blockers
	Gabexate	
	ERCP and	
	stone removal	
	Platelet factor	
	inhibitor	
	(Lexipifant)	

Figure 134-5

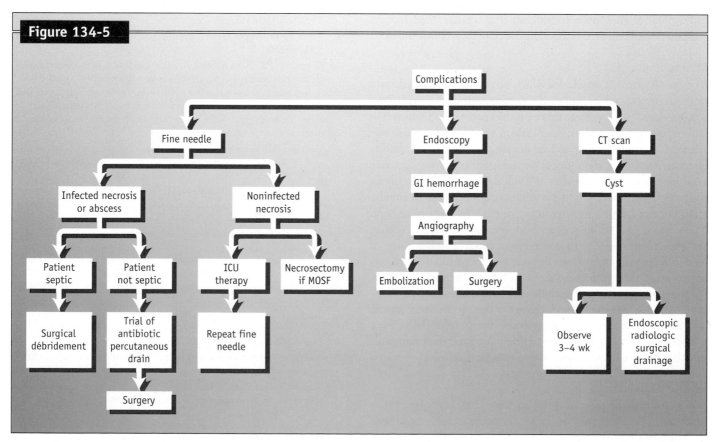

Algorithm for investigation and treatment of complications.

effusion may improve after internal stenting at ERCP; if surgery is contemplated, an ERCP is essential to localize the site of the leak so that resection distal to the leak is prevented (Fig. 134-3).

Transient Diabetes

Diabetic coma is extremely uncommon, therefore insulin should be used only with caution because the diabetes may resolve as pancreatic inflammation subsides. A conservative approach is suggested that allows hyperglycemia rather than trying to achieve euglycemia and prompt hypoglycemia.

Treatment of Etiology

During the Attack

During the attack, alcohol and pancreatitis-producing drugs must be stopped. Hyperlipemia may be temporary, but if it is severe (eg, >1000 mg/dL) it may require plasmapheresis. Hypercalcemia requires correction. Cholangitis, an impacted stone in the common channel, or deterioration of the pancreas usually necessitates ERCP with sphincterotomy and stone removal or, in the elderly and patients with significant comorbid disease, merely placing a biliary stent to facilitate drainage [30].

After the Attack Has Subsided

After the attack has subsided, treatment should continue as during the attack. If gallstones are present, cholecystectomy should be performed while the patient is still in the hospital. For patients with severe comorbid disease, an endoscopic sphincterotomy *without* cholecystectomy is a option to allow the stones to pass. About 30% of patients with an in situ gallbladder will have a subsequent attack of gallstones or cholecystitis [30]. Alcohol should be forbidden. If there has been foreign travel, a 3-day course of mebendazole may be recommended.

Recurrent Attacks

In cases of recurrent attacks for which no etiology is found despite extensive investigation, some authors recommend an empiric trial of high-dose (8 tablets three times per day) pancreatin (Viokasc) to reduce pancreatic secretion; vitamins A, C, and E and methionine-selenium as antioxidants; and in desperate situations, octreotide injections and even translumbar or transgastric endoscopic celiac axis block. Suspected sphincter of Oddi stenosis or spasm requires endoscopic manometry, and some endoscopists resort to empiric biliary or pancreatic sphincterotomy or trials of stent placement. These endoscopic techniques are best reserved for research centers and expert endoscopists. In nonsevere attacks, the judicious use of narcotics such as oxycodone (Percocet) or meperidine (Demerol) during attacks might prevent recurrent hospital admissions.

Newer diagnostic tests include endoscopic ultrasound to diagnose common bile duct stones or cancer during the acute attack, and magnetic resonance cholangiopancreatography (MRCP), a noninvasive method of demonstrating pancreatic duct morphology that may be useful in evaluating recurrent attacks.

■ PROGNOSIS

Eighty percent of patients with an acute attack of pancreatitis (excluding recurrent pain or attacks in patients with established chronic pancreatitis) have a relatively mild episode that subsides in 7 to 10 days, and only about 1% to 3% of these patients will progress to more severe involvement or develop a complication. Twenty percent of patients with an acute attack will have an attack that may be categorized as severe by one of the criteria for the grading of severity. Of these patients, 2% to 3% will die within 72 hours of multiple organ failure. In some of these patients, their death may be prolonged by peritoneal dialysis. Thirty to 50% of the remaining patients with a severe attack will die after a more protracted course from one of the devastating complications of the disease. The overall mortality has declined at Long Island Jewish Medical Center, from 13.5% between 1978 and 1982 to 8% between 1986 and 1990, since stratification of severity by Ranson's or Bank's signs became generally employed, thus allowing more directed and selective therapy. A more dramatic decline in mortality rates has been demonstrated in some Scottish and German series, and our own current mortality is 5%. Despite this, one of the major disappointments of treating this disease has been the inability to reduce the mortality below the 5% to 10% level despite better understanding of its pathophysiology, etiology, and therapy.

■ REFERENCES

Recently published papers of particular interest have been highlighted as follows:
- • Of interest
- •• Of outstanding interest

1. Warshaw AL, Simeone JF, Schapiro RH, Flavin-Warshaw B: Evaluation and treatment of the dominant dorsal duct syndrome (pancreas divisum redefined). *Am J Surg* 1990, 159:59–66.
2. England RE, Newcomer MK, Leung JW, Cotton PB: Case report: annular pancreas divisum causing pancreatitis—a report of two cases and review of the literature. *Br J Radiol* 1995, 68:325–328.
3. Steer ML: How and where does acute pancreatitis begin? *Arch Surg* 1992, 127:1350–1353.
4. Steinberg W, Tenner S: Acute pancreatitis. *N Engl J Med* 1995, 330:1198–1210.
5.• Greenberg RE, Bank S, Stark B: Adenocarcinoma of the pancreas producing pancreatitis and pancreatic abscess. *Pancreas* 1990, 5:108–113.
Although cancer of the pancreas is a relatively rare cause of acute severe pancreatitis, this article presents three such cases and highlights the difficulty in diagnosing the underlying carcinoma during the protracted course of the pancreatitis in these patients.
6. Ballinger AB, Barnes E, Alstead EM, Fairclough PP, et al.: Is intervention necessary after a first episode of acute idiopathic pancreatitis? *Gut* 1996, 38:293–295.
7. Amman RW, Heitz PU, Kloppel G: Course of alcoholic chronic pancreatitis: a prospective clinicomorphological study. *Gastroenterol* 1996, 111:224–231.
8.•• Banks P: Practice guidelines in acute pancreatitis. *Am J Gastroenterol* 1997, 92:377–386
This recent review details a step-by-step approach to the diagnosis and management of acute pancreatitis and its complications. It is a valuable addition to state-of-the-art references and should be kept in a readily accessible place when seeing patients with pancreatitis.
9. Bank S, Burns GP: Diagnosis of acute abdomen associated with hyperamylasemia. In *Disorders of the Pancreas*. Edited by Bank S, Burns GP. New York: McGraw-Hill; 1992:52–63.
10. Sachdeva C, Bank S, Greenberg R, et al.: Fluctuations in serum amylase in patients with macroamylasemia. *Am J Gastroenterol* 1995, 90:800–803.
11.•• Ranson JHC, Rifkind KM, Roses DF, et al.: Prognosic signs and the role of operative management in acute pancreatitis. *Surg Gynacol Obstet* 1974, 139:69–81.
This is Ransom's classic article on the early prognostic signs of acute pancreatitis that initiated the concept of trying to classify patients into severe or mild disease. Ransom's 11 early prognostic signs are found in Table 134-2.

12. Bank S, Wise L, Gersten M: Risk factors in acute pancreatitis. *Am J Gastroenterol* 1983, 78:637–640.

13. Lam S, Bank S: Risk factors for morbidity and mortality in pancreatitis. *Dig Dis* 1996, 14:83–95.

14. Balthazar EJ, Robinson DL, Megibow AJ, Ranson JH: Acute pancreatitis: value of CT in establishing prognosis. *Radiology* 1990, 174:331–336.

15.• McNemamin DA, Gates LK Jr: A prospective analysis of the effect of contrast-enhanced CT on the outcome of acute pancreatitis. *Am J Gastroenterol* 1996, 91:1384–1387.

Although there is considerable controversy whether early use of contrast-enhanced CT is detrimental in acute severe pancreatitis, this study shows that patients who underwent CT scan in the first 48 hours had a hospital stay of 11 days compared with 7 days in those who underwent a CT scan later. Mortality was not changed. Intravenous contrast produced a higher mortality from pancreatitis in experimental animals.

16. Agarwal N, Pitchumoni CS: Assessment of severity in acute pancreatitis. *Am J Gastroenterol* 1991, 86:1385–1391.

17. Fan ST, Lai ECS, Mok FPT, *et al*: Early treatment of acute pancreatitis by endoscopic papillotomy. *N Engl J Med* 1993, 328:228–232.

18. Neoptolemos JP: Endoscopic sphincterotomy in acute gallstone pancreatitis. *Br J Surg* 1993, 80:547–549.

19.•• Fölsh U, Nitshe R, Ludtke R, *et al.*, and the German Study Group on Acute Biliary Pancreatitis: early ERCP and papillotomy compared with conservative treatment for acute biliary pancreatitis. *N Engl J Med* 1997, 336:237–242.

This prospective study in patients without obvious biliary obstruction investigated the role of urgent ERCP and stone removal in 126 patients compared with 112 who had medical ICU therapy. The study failed to show a beneficial effect of the endoscopic therapy and was thus at variance with two other studies showing improved mortality and morbidity by the emergent ERCP approach.

20. Gerzof SG, Banks PA, Robbins AH, *et al.*: Diagnosis of pancreatic infection by CT guided aspiration: an update. *Pancreas* 1988, 3:590–595.

21. Ho HS, Frey CF: Gastrointestinal and pancreatic complications associated with severe pancreatitis. *Arch Surg* 1996, 130:817–923.

22. Bank S, Siegel D, Stark B: Pancreatic cysts: a new dimension. *Am J Gastroenterol* 1994, 89:1766–1767.

23. Semlacher AU, Chan-Yan C: Acute pancreatitis presenting with visual disturbance. *Am J Gastroenterol* 1993, 88:756–759.

24. Sternby B, O'Brien JF, Zinsmeister AR, DiMagno EP: What is the best biochemical test to diagnose acute pancreatitis: a prospective clinical study. *Mayo Clin Proc* 1996, 71:1138–1144.

25. Gumaste VV: Diagnostic tests for acute pancreatitis. *Gastroenterologist* 1994, 2:119–130.

26. Santucci L, Natalini G, Sarpi L, *et al.*: Selective endoscopic retrograde cholangiography and preoperative bile duct stone removal in patients scheduled for laparoscopic cholecystectomy: a prospective study. *Am J Gastrtoenterol* 1996, 91:1326–1330.

27. Kozarek RA, Ball TJ, Patterson DJ, *et al.*: Endoscopic transpapillary therapy for disrupted pancreatic duct and peripancreatic fluid collections. *Gastroenterol* 1991, 100:1362–1370.

28.• Sainio V, Kempainen E, Puolakkainen P, *et al.*: Early antibiotic treatment in acute necrotizing pancreatitis. *Lancet* 1995, 346:663–666.

These authors found that the use of prophylactic cefuroxime decreased not only urinary infections and bloodstream infections but also reduced pancreatic infection. It appears to confirm an Italian study of antibiotic benefit using impenum.

29. Pezzilli R, Gullo L, DiStefano M, *et al.*: Treatment of pancreatic ascites with somatostatin. *Pancreas* 1993, 8:120–122.

30. Uomo G, Manes G, Laccetti M, *et al.*: Endoscopic sphincterotomy and recurrence of acute pancreatitis in gallstone patients considered unfit for surgery. *Pancreas* 1997, 14:28–31.

31. Maringhini A, *et al.*: Ascites, pleural and pericardial effusions in acute pancreatitis: a prospective study of incidence, natural history and prognostic role. *Dig Dis Sci* 1996, 91:1384.

135 Surgical Intervention in Acute Pancreatitis
Nanakram Agarwal

HISTORY

In 1889, Reginald Fitz provided the first accurate description of acute pancreatitis and initiated the controversies surrounding the role of surgery in its management [1]. Regarding surgical management, Fitz observed "an operation...in the early stages of this disease, is extremely hazardous." In 1903, however, he stated "in cases of acute pancreatitis...laparotomy in an increasing number of cases has proven the most satisfactory method of treatment, and like most abdominal operations for the relief of acute symptoms, is the most helpful the earlier in the course of the disease it is performed." Nearly a century later, confusion regarding the timing and role of surgical intervention in acute pancreatitis persists [2•].

NATURAL COURSE

Figure 135-1 illustrates the outcome probabilities after acute pancreatitis. In most patients (70% to 80%), acute pancreatitis is mild, with only minimal to moderate abdominal pain that usually resolves within a few days of fasting and intravenous fluid therapy. However, in nearly 20% to 30% of cases it can be extremely severe and associated with multiple organ failure, significant morbidity, and mortality.

MANAGEMENT

The most important step in the management of patients with acute pancreatitis is the differentiation between the mild and severe forms of the disease. This discrimination is achieved based on assessment of various prognostic signs, Acute Physiology and Chronic Health Evaluation (APACHE) II scores, serum C-reactive protein level and contrast-enhanced computed tomography (CT) findings [3,4••] (Chapter 134).

Mild pancreatitis has an excellent prognosis, with minimal morbidity and no mortality. All patients with severe pancreatitis should be monitored and treated in an intensive care unit. The pancreas is extremely susceptible to ischemia in shock, and hypoperfusion is a critical factor in the progression of disease. Close monitoring of intravascular volume and adequate replacement of fluid

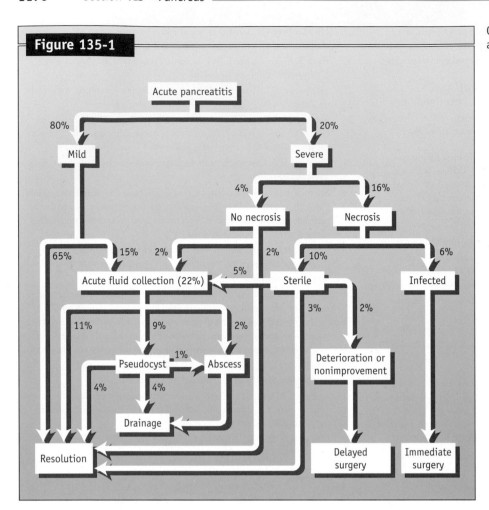

Figure 135-1

are critical to a successful outcome. Prophylactic use of antibiotics, especially imipenem-cilastatin or quinolones, has been shown to significantly reduce the subsequent development of infection and should be part of standard care. Other strategies that need further validation include peritoneal lavage, selective decontamination of the gut, isovolemic hemodilution, and octreotide therapy.

■ INDICATIONS FOR SURGICAL INTERVENTION

Acute pancreatitis infrequently necessitates surgical intervention, but current indications for surgery can be divided into three main categories: 1) diagnostic (when diagnosis is uncertain), 2) management of complications, and 3) management of etiology (Table 135-1).

In clinical practice, the diagnosis of acute pancreatitis is hinged on the clinical picture and elevated serum amylase levels. The greatest disadvantage of serum amylase assay is its overall low specificity. Besides pancreatitis, conditions that increase total serum amylase levels include many disorders of the biliary tract, the liver, the intestines, and the genitourinary tract. In such cases, CT should be performed early to exclude other catastrophic intra-abdominal conditions, such as perforated viscus, intestinal obstruction, dissecting or leaking aortic aneurysms, or tubo-ovarian pathology. Pancreatic enlargement, particularly when associated with features of peripancreatic inflammation, is pathognomonic of acute pancreatitis; abdominal paracentesis or peritoneal lavage may clarify the diagnosis further. Nonetheless,

there may remain a few instances when it is necessary to distinguish acute pancreatitis from a surgically correctable disorder—especially when a patient is critically ill or in shock. In such circumstances diagnostic laparotomy does not exacerbate the attack of acute pancreatitis, and without prompt operative intervention intra-abdominal catastrophes that may mimic acute pancreatitis usually are lethal.

When acute pancreatitis is found at laparotomy, abdominal exploration should be completed with careful attention to the gallbladder, duodenum, and pancreas. The lesser sac should be opened by dividing the gastro-colic ligament to inspect the pancreas. Needless manipulation of the pancreas and duodenum should be avoided. The gallbladder and common bile duct are palpated for cholelithiasis.

If cholelithiasis is present and acute pancreatitis is mild, definite biliary surgery is recommended. Cholecystectomy with a cystic duct cholangiogram is performed. If common duct stones are found, full exploration of the common duct, including choledoscopy and transduodenal sphinteroplasty, can be performed safely. If pancreatitis is severe, biliary surgery is limited to cholecystostomy, removal of all palpable gallstones, and performance of cholangiography. Simple insertion of a T-tube may be indicated in the presence of a dilated common bile duct. More extensive surgery, specifically transduodenal sphinteroplasty, is hazardous at this time.

If there is no evidence of cholelithiasis and only mild acute pancreatitis, the abdomen is closed without placement of lavage

Table 135-1. Indications for Surgical Intervention

Diagnostic
  Uncertain diagnosis
    Acute abdomen
    Shock
    Sepsis
  Management of complications
    Sterile necrosis: deteriorating condition
    Infected pancreatic necrosis
    Pseudocyst
    Pancreatic abscess
    Pancreatic ascites
    Pancreatic fistula
    Massive hemorrhage
    Bowel necrosis
  Management of etiology
    Biliary pancreatitis

catheters. Drainage of pancreas has been found to provide no benefit while increasing the incidence of subsequent infection. If pancreatitis is severe, a Tenckhoff catheter may be inserted for peritoneal lavage.

STERILE PANCREATIC NECROSIS

Approximately 20% of patients with acute pancreatitis develop pancreatic or peripancreatic necrosis, or both. Contrast-enhanced computed tomography (CECT) is the best test for early detection of pancreatic necrosis. The degree of pancreatic necrosis as estimated on CT (<30%, 30% to 50%, > 50% of the pancreas) correlates well with morbidity and mortality. Few patients with severe acute pancreatitis and no pancreatic necrosis on initial CT scanning subsequently develop necrosis. The phenomenon of late necrosis is seen only in patients who demonstrate peripancreatic changes or fluid collections on initial CT examination. A repeat CT scan, therefore, should be done in all patients with these findings [5].

Sterile necrosis precedes infected necrosis, with infection following in approximately 40% of cases. Management of patients with sterile pancreatic necrosis is primarily medical. In the largest series reported [6], a retrospective analysis of 172 subjects in Germany with sterile pancreatic necrosis managed between 1982 and 1993, 107 subjects had necrosectomy with continuous postoperative closed lavage, and 65 were treated nonsurgically. Although not statistically significant, the mortality rate of 13.1% in the surgically treated subjects was twice that of nonsurgically treated subjects (6.2%). The surgical group had statistically significant longer median (44.5 vs 20 days, $P<0.001$) hospital and intensive care unit stays (16.5 vs 7 days, $P<0.001$). Overall, more complications were observed in the surgical group: 27% of subjects developed secondary abscesses, 26% fistula, and 42% sepsis syndrome. In the nonsurgical group, only one subject (2%) had abscesses and five (8%) sepsis syndrome. However, the two groups were not comparable; the surgically treated subjects were sicker, as evidenced by higher Ranson's

and APACHE II scores and greater C-reactive protein levels on admission. Furthermore, whereas 94% of the nonsurgically treated subjects responded to intensive care therapy, local and systemic complications persisted or increased in 77% of surgical subjects. These authors now recommend that most patients with sterile pancreatic necrosis should be managed conservatively, with surgery reserved for patients who do not respond to intensive therapy.

Bradley [7] also concluded that the presence or extent of sterile pancreatic necrosis is not an absolute indication for surgical intervention, even when organ failure is present. A retrospective review by Bradley [7] demonstrated that the mortality for 287 subjects with severe sterile necrotizing pancreatitis who were managed nonsurgically was approximately 10%. The author concluded that delayed surgical débridement after 5 to 6 weeks is indicated very rarely in patients who have persistent symptoms of abdominal pain, nausea, vomiting, or recurrent pancreatitis.

In contrast, Rattner et al. [8] advocate early débridement of symptomatic necrotic tissue irrespective of the results of pancreatic cultures. They think that surgeons should operate on the basis of symptoms and clinical picture even in the absence of proven infection. In their retrospective review of 73 subjects who underwent surgery for necrotizing pancreatitis, mortality rates for sterile and infected necrosis were not significantly different, and a 10% false-negative rate was observed for needle aspiration. However, the overall mortality rate of 25% observed in this study is much greater than that reported for sterile necrosis treated conservatively, and recurrent infected collections occurred in 39% of subjects who had sterile necrosis initially.

In summary, the past decade has seen the development of a new strategy in the management of sterile pancreatic necrosis. Patients with sterile necrosis involving less than 50% of the gland and who are stable or improving are best managed conservatively. Controversy exists, however, for patients with more extensive necrosis or those with persisting and worsening organ complications. There is increasing consensus that even these patients should be managed medically as long as possible and that surgery should be delayed for at least 3 to 5 weeks, enabling the possibility of spontaneous recovery. In the first week, surgery is more likely to result in incomplete débridement of necrotic tissue because of incomplete demarcation, whereas there is far more complete demarcation of necrotic tissue by the third week, increasing the possibility of performing débridement safely (Fig. 135-2). Finally, late surgery is indicated in the few patients who do not recover completely, that is, those with lingering respiratory insufficiency requiring ventilatory support or refractory pain resulting in inability to eat, weight loss, intermittent hyperamylasemia, and recurrent hospitalization [9].

INFECTED PANCREATIC NECROSIS

Infected pancreatic necrosis is seen in only 5% to 10% of patients with acute pancreatitis. It is the most serious complication resulting from acute pancreatitis, accounting for more than 80% of deaths associated with the disease. Infection is time dependent and is related to the extent of necrosis; more widespread necrosis leads to earlier development of infection. Although infection may occur as early as the first day, it is seen

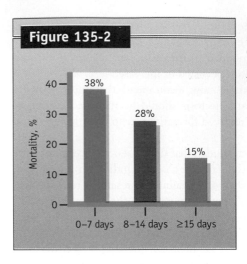

Figure 135-2

Relationship between the timing of an operation and mortality in necrotizing pancreatitis. From Bradley [2].

within 1 week of the onset of abdominal pain in approximately 25% of patients. Infection peaks to 51.4% between the second or third week and then decreases to 32.5% after the fourth week. The extent of necrosis, as assessed by CT, also correlates significantly with the development of infection. Necrosis appears to be a prerequisite for infection because patients with non-necrotizing pancreatitis usually do not develop pancreatic or peripancreatic infection.

The precise mechanism by which infection of necrotic areas occurs appears to be related to bacterial translocation, reticuloendothelial dysfunction, and other transient immunologic disturbances.

Pancreatic infections are most commonly caused by gram-negative enteric bacteria. With the use of broad-spectrum antibiotics, there has been a change in the bacterial flora causing these infections: resistant bacteria are now the most frequently isolated pathogens (*ie*, *Enterococcus fecalis* in 48%, *Pseudomonas aeruginosa* in 36%, *Escherichia coli* in 20%, and *Klebsiella pneumonia* in 16%). Furthermore, fungal isolates are also much more frequent, with *Candida albicans* found in 16% and non-*Candida* yeast species found in another 16% [10,11].

Without surgical drainage, infected pancreatic necrosis usually is lethal. Delaying surgery in the presence of infected necrosis increases mortality, in contrast to non-infected necrosis, in which surgical intervention is associated with increased incidences of complications and mortality. Differentiating sterile from infected necrosis is therefore crucial, although difficult. Clinically, both types of necrosis may present with similar findings, such as fever, leukocytosis, abdominal tenderness, ileus, and organ dysfunction. There is no consistently reliable clinical or biochemical test that indicates the presence of infection. Percutaneous needle aspiration under ultrasonographic or CT guidance of pancreatic and extrapancreatic necrotic area or fluid collections for bacteriology is the test of choice for diagnosing pancreatic infections. A false-negative rate of 10% has been reported [8], and repeated CT-guided aspirations at weekly intervals is the safest and most reliable method for distinguishing infected pancreatic necrosis from sterile pancreatic necrosis [4••].

Surgical Techniques

The optimal form of surgical intervention for infected pancreatic necrosis is controversial. Surgical management can be divided into three distinct methods: conventional, necrosectomy with continuous local lavage, and open management.

Conventional

The conventional technique advocated by Warshaw [9], uses a midline abdominal incision to allow unrestricted exploration of the entire abdomen. The necrotic pancreatic tissue is accessed through the transverse mesocolon and as much devitalized tissue as possible is débrided, largely by means of finger dissection. Then the cavity is filled and packed with a combination of Penrose and suction drains, which are brought out through separate incisions. The abdominal incision is closed primarily. Drains are removed sequentially, starting after 1 week.

Necrosectomy with Local Lavage

Surgical débridement-necrosectomy supplemented by intraoperative and postoperative closed continuous local lavage of the lesser sac, as proposed by Beger *et al.* [12], has gained popularity in recent years. The abdomen is opened through upper midline or bilateral subcostal incision; the gastrocolic and duodenocolic ligaments are divided, the duodenum is kocherized, and the right and left colon are mobilized. Débridement or necrosectomy, either digitally or by the careful use of instruments, is performed to remove all demarcated devitalized tissue while preserving vital pancreatic tissue. After surgical débridement, meticulous hemostasis with transfixing stitches is mandatory. Extensive intraoperative lavage with 4 to 6 L of normal saline follows. The success of postoperative closed lavage depends on the number and size of the drainage tubes, and two or more large (28F to 34F) double-lumen silicon rubber tubes are inserted to lie in the pancreatic region and retroperitoneal spaces. The gastrolic and duodenocolic ligaments are sutured to create a closed compartment for lavage. Continuous local postoperative lavage results in evacuation of vasoactive and toxic substances, bacteria, local active enzymes, and necrotic tissue. Postoperative lavage is done using a slightly hypertonic fluid at a rate of 1 L every hour in the first day. Subsequently, the quantity is reduced rapidly depending on the clinical course and appearance of the outflow fluid. Lavage is stopped when there are no more signs of acute pancreatitis, as confirmed by amylase level in the draining fluid and absence of necrotic tissue. Finally, drainage tubes are removed successively.

Open Management

The "open management" or "open drainage" approach, proposed by Bradley [2•], involves blunt débridement of infected necrosis, placement of laparotomy packs over nonadherent gauze to protect adjacent intestinal surfaces, partial abdominal closure, and scheduled reexploration every 2 days for redébridement and packing changes. Variations include using a mesh, which is sutured to fascial edges with continuous nonabsorbable sutures to contain the abdominal viscera and prevent evisceration and daily débridement. The basic principle of this technique is scheduled reexploration, which is undertaken irrespective of the patient's general condition and stopped only when there is formation of retroperitoneal granulation tissue and no evidence of infected necrotic debris. Secondary closure of the abdominal wound is accomplished over lavage catheters placed in the area of the débridement.

COMPARISON OF THE SURGICAL METHODS

Results of the three surgical strategies were reviewed by D'Edigio and Schain [13] (Table 135-2). Mortality after conventional treatment (42%) was significantly greater than that seen after necrosectomy followed by lavage (18%) or open management (21%); there were no significant differences between necrosectomy followed by lavage or open management. Approximately one third of patients treated by the conventional method or necrosectomy followed by lavage require reexploration for persistent intra-abdominal infection or ongoing necrosis. However, decisions regarding surgery and its timing are difficult, and delay in surgery contributes to the high mortality. With both the conventional method or necrosectomy followed by lavage, there should be a very low threshold for reexploration. The open management techniques avoids the issue of reexploration but carries a higher risk of complications, such as colonic necrosis or fistula (13%), small bowel fistula (14%), and postoperative hemorrhage (16%).

PANCREATIC RESECTION

Total to near-total pancreatectomy, first suggested by Watts [14], is needlessly radical and associated with significant morbidity and mortality (33%–100%). Besides major complications of hemorrhage and continued sepsis, viable pancreatic tissue is removed, resulting in serious exocrine and endocrine deficiency states, such as brittle diabetes, steatorrhea, polyneuropathy, and so on in the survivors.

OTHER OPTIONS

Although surgical intervention is mandatory for infected pancreatic necrosis, there are recent case reports [15] of subjects with infected pancreatic necrosis in whom surgery was not performed because of unstable medical condition or subject's refusal. Following antibiotic therapy, all subjects survived [15]. It appears that with the availability of antibiotics that are capable of achieving a high concentration in the diseased pancreas and infected necrotic tissue, some patients can be managed nonsurgically.

Percutaneous drainage of infected pancreatic necrosis under CT or ultrasound guidance is not recommended: failure results from the small size of the catheters and the thick consistency of

the necrotic debris. As reported by Rattner *et al.* [8], all subjects on whom percutaneous drainage was the initial therapeutic procedure required subsequent surgical débridement and drainage for recurrent sepsis. Percutaneously placed large-bore tubes may have a temporizing effect, allowing time to stabilize a critically ill patient.

ACUTE PANCREATIC FLUID COLLECTIONS

Acute fluid collections are seen in approximately 40% of patients with acute pancreatitis, and they can be intrapancreatic or extrapancreatic. Spontaneous resolution occurs in over 50% of cases. In the remainder, these collections evolve into pseudocysts, or abscess. CT is the best diagnostic test for evaluating acute fluid collections; it determines their number, location, size, extent, and anatomic relationship to other structures.

No specific treatment is indicated unless these collections get infected, a situation usually confirmed by CT-guided fine needle aspiration. Percutaneous drainage under CT or sonographic guidance is the treatment of choice if the fluid collection is infected, causing pain, of increasing size, or if it involves contiguous organs or structures. Such drainage procedures are contraindicated if there is coexisting pancreatic necrosis, recent or active bleeding into the fluid collection, or a pseudoaneurysm within the collection.

PANCREATIC PSEUDOCYSTS

More than 50% of pseudocysts resolve spontaneously. Indications for drainage are size (> 6 cm), pain, enlargement of cyst, and complications (infection, hemorrhage, rupture, and obstructions). Treatment options, including percutaneous, endoscopic, or surgical drainage, are discussed in Chapter 141.

PANCREATIC ABSCESS

A pancreatic abscess is a loculated walled-off collection of pus resulting from liquification of necrotic areas or secondary infection of an acute pseudocyst. They may or may not communicate with the major pancreatic duct. Abscesses occur at a relatively late stage, most commonly in the third to fifth week after the onset of acute pancreatitis. CT scanning is the test of choice for diagnosis. Acute pancreatic fluid collections tend to be poorly walled off and can track into the retroperitoneum, the peritoneal cavity, the mediastinum, the pleura, or the soft tissues. A pancreatic abscess is a low-density fluid collection in a defined cavity that contains gas bubbles. On occasion, however, gas bubbles may be absent and the margins not clear. Diagnosis of pancreatic abscess is confirmed by percutaneous aspiration, after which percutaneous drainage is the treatment of choice. This procedure is successful in approximately 60% to 90% of cases. Surgical drainage is done when percutaneous drainage is not curative. Prognosis for pancreatic abscess is extremely good, with few incidences of mortality.

PANCREATIC ASCITES

Pancreatic ascites is most commonly secondary to a leakage from a pseudocyst (70%) or a pancreatic duct (10% to 20%). It rarely develops after duct disruption following trauma, lymphatic blockage, or portal hypertension. Pancreatic ascites is characterized by straw-colored or blood-tinged ascitic fluid with high amylase levels (usually > 1000 U/dL; range, 205 to 97,000 U) and protein (usually > 2.5 g/dL; range, 2.1 to 5.7 g). Endoscopic retrograde cholangiopancreatography (ERCP) is the procedure

Table 135-2. Comparison of Surgical Techniques for Infected Pancreatic Necrosis

—	Conventional, %	Necrosectomy with lavage, %	Open management, %
Mortality	42	18	21
Complications			
Small bowel	5	4	14
Colonic	8	2	13
Hemorrhage	14	8	16
Pancreatic fistula	16	17	17
Reoperations	36	33	100

From D'Egidio and Schein [13].

of choice to demonstrate the site of leakage. Medical management consists of total parenteral nutrition and octreotide and should not be continued for more than 2 to 3 weeks. Definitive surgical treatment, which entails either resection of the body and tail of the pancreas or internal drainage, results in 100% survival rates, low morbidity rates, and no recurrence of ascites.

■ PANCREATIC FISTULA

Most pancreatic fistula result from external drainage of a pseudocyst or abscess. They eventually close spontaneously. Octreotide is helpful in decreasing the output of the fistula and expediting closure. Surgical intervention may be indicated if the fistula persists.

■ MASSIVE HEMORRHAGE

Upper gastrointestinal bleeding is common in acute pancreatitis and usually results from stress ulcers, peptic ulcer disease, hemorrhagic gastroduodenitis, or Mallory-Weiss tears. Massive hemorrhage occurs in approximately 2% of patients, most commonly into the gastrointestinal tract, less commonly into the abdominal cavity, and rarely into the pancreatic duct ("hemosuccus pancreaticus"). Erosion of a major pancreatic or peripancreatic vessel leads to free rupture or formation of a pseudoaneurysm that subsequently ruptures. The splenic artery is the most commonly involved vessel, followed by the pancreaticoduodenal and gastroduodenal arteries; the left gastric, hepatic, and small intrapancreatic arteries are implicated infrequently. Pseudoaneurysm formation should be suspected with repeated episodes of gastrointestinal bleeding, an enlarging pulsatile abdominal mass, an abdominal bruit, and in patients with increasing abdominal pain. Bolus dynamic CT scan is the most useful initial diagnostic test to detect hemorrhage (attenuation > 30 Hounsfield units) and pseudoaneurysms. Angiography is the procedure of choice for both identifying the source of bleeding and therapy by embolization.

Surgical intervention is indicated in patients who are hemodynamically unstable or when embolization is technically not possible or fails to stop the bleeding. However, angiography should be attempted preoperatively. Identification of the site and the source of bleeding facilitates surgical control of bleeding and eliminates unnecessary harmful dissection. Surgical options consist of 1) proximal and distal ligation of the bleeding vessels with drainage of a pseudocyst or necrotic tissue or 2) distal pancreatectomy if bleeding arises from the body or tail of the pancreas.

■ BOWEL NECROSIS

Colonic, duodenal, or gastric necrosis, in order of frequency, are secondary to either infarction from thrombosis of blood vessels involved in an extrapancreatic necrotizing process or as a complication of external drainage. In pancreatic necrosis, diagnosis is difficult and prognosis is poor. Colonic necrosis necessitates resection and creation of an ileostomy or colostomy and mucus fistula. Duodenal and gastric necrosis are managed best by external drainage.

■ BILIARY PANCREATITIS

All patients with acute pancreatitis, even those with alcoholic pancreatitis, should have ultrasonography of the gallbladder to determine whether gallstones are present. If gallstones are detected, biliary surgery should be performed during the index admission. Deferring such surgery carries a 32% to 48% risk of recurrent pancreatitis. Kelly and Wagner [16] demonstrated in a prospective randomized study that in subjects with mild pancreatitis (*ie*, three or fewer Ranson's signs) the timing of surgery, either early (within 48 hours of admission) or delayed until resolution of the pancreatitis, has little effect on the outcome. However, in subjects with more than three signs, early surgery is associated with significantly increased rates of complications (83% early vs 18% delayed) and mortality (47.8% early vs 11.8% delayed).

Patients who have cholangitis or progressive jaundice should undergo ERCP and biliary decompression with sphincterotomy. ERCP in absence of biliary obstruction or cholangitis is controversial. Recently Folsch *et al.* [17•] have shown that early ERCP and papillotomy was not beneficial in patients with acute biliary pancreatitis without obstructive jaundice. Patients with biliary pancreatitis who fail to improve with conservative management also should undergo ERCP. When stones are found in the common bile duct, they should be extracted endoscopically. Preoperative ERCP in patients undergoing laparotomy for complications such as infected necrosis or abscess also avoids the need for and risks of exploring the common bile duct. Because endoscopic sphincterotomy has a complication rate of approximately 10% and a 1% mortality rate [18], routine preoperative ERCP is not recommended. Even in patients who might benefit from this procedure, the preferred approach depends on the availability and expertise of the endoscopist and the surgeon.

Peritoneal Lavage

Peritoneal lavage in acute pancreatitis is performed to assess its severity or for therapy. McMahon *et al.* [19] have shown that the volume and color of peritoneal fluid are indicators of the severity of pancreatitis. Severe acute pancreatitis is indicated by the presence of 20 mL of free intraperitoneal fluid irrespective of its color; free fluid of a dark color (prune juice); and lavage fluid darker than a pale straw color obtained after peritoneal lavage with 1 L normal saline.

The major advantages of peritoneal lavage are early assessment of severity and diagnosis of other etiologies of acute abdomen in approximately 2% of patients. However, there is an approximate 1% risk of inadvertent visceral puncture.

It may be expected that removal of enzyme-rich "broth" and toxins (*eg*, histamine, trypsin, kinin, prostaglandins, myocardial depressant factor) from the peritoneal cavity would reduce their systemic absorption and improve disease outcome. Although peritoneal lavage improved survival in experimental studies, its therapeutic value in humans has been controversial. Controlled clinical trials or peritoneal lavage done for 2 to 4 days demonstrate dramatic improvement in cardiovascular and respiratory function with subsequent reduction of early deaths but no statistically significant differences in the overall hospital mortality rate or the incidence of major complications. Almost all death in lavage patients is due to pancreatic sepsis, suggesting that lavage only delays early mortality.

Ranson and Berman [20] have proposed longer periods of peritoneal lavage. They compared short periods (2 days) of peritoneal lavage in 15 subjects with long periods (7 days) of peritoneal lavage in 14 subjects with severe acute pancreatitis (three or more positive prognostic signs). Longer periods of lavage reduced the frequency of both pancreatic sepsis (21% vs 40%) and death from sepsis (0% vs 20%) but not overall mortality (14% vs 20%). Differences were more pronounced in the 17 subjects with five or more positive prognostic signs in whom longer lavage was associated with a reduction in pancreatic sepsis (30% vs 57%), septic deaths (0% vs 43%) and overall mortality (20% vs 43%). However, to demonstrate a statistically significant difference in subjects with five or more prognostic signs, the authorities had to include all their previously reported subjects (prospective and retrospective) treated with short–term peritoneal lavage and also those managed nonoperatively and without peritoneal lavage. This study demonstrated important trends in favor of long peritoneal lavage for reducing early systemic and septic complications but has no proven efficacy in improving overall survival.

■ REFERENCES

Recently published papers of particular interest have been highlighted as follows:
•   Of interest
•• Of outstanding interest

1. Leach SD, Gorelick FS, Modlin IM: Acute pancreatitis at its centenary. The contribution of Reginald Fitz. *Ann Surg* 1990, 212:109–113.
2.• Bradley EL III: Surgical indications and techniques in necrotizing pancreatitis. In *Acute Pancreatitis: Diagnosis and Therapy* . Edited by Bradley EL III. New York: Raven; 1994:105–117.
3. Agarwal N, Pitchumoni CS: Assessment of severity in acute pancreatitis. *Am J Gastroenterol* 1991, 86:1385–1391.
4•• Banks PA: Practice guidelines in acute pancreatitis. *Am J Gastroenterol* 1997, 92:377–386.
5. Balthazar EJ, Freeny PC Van Sonnenberg E: Imaging and intervention in acute pancreatitis. *Radiology* 1994, 193:297–306.
6 Rau B, Pralle U, Uhl W, *et al.*: Management of sterile necrosis in instances of severe acute pancreatitis. *J Am Coll Surg* 1995, 181:279–288.
7. Bradley EL III: Débridement is rarely necessary in patients with sterile pancreatic necrosis. *Pancreas* 1996, 13:220–223.
8. Rattner DW, Legemate DA, Mueller PR, Warshaw AL: Early surgical débridement of pancreatic necrosis is beneficial irrespective of infection. *Am J Surg* 1992, 163:105–110.
9. Warshaw AL: What to do about sterile pancreatic necrosis? *Pancreas* 1996, 13:223–225.
10. Stephan RN, Bradley EL III: Pancreatic infections. *Gastroenterologist* 1996, 4:163–168.
11. Savino JA, LaPunzna C, Agarwal N, *et al.*: Open versus closed treatment of necrotizing pancreatitis. *Shock* 1996, 6 (suppl):65–70.
12. Beger HG, Uhl W, Buchler M: Pancreatic necrosis. Deliberation on débridement. In *Difficult Decisions in Gastroenterology*, edn 2. Edited by Barkin J, Rogers AI. St. Louis: Mosby Year Book; 1996:113–119.
13. D'Egidio A, Schein M: Surgical strategies in the treatment of pancreatic necrosis and infection. *Br J Surg* 1991, 78:133–137.
14. Watts GT: The total pancreatectomy for fulminant pancreatitis. *Lancet* 1963, 384:24–31.
15. Dubner H, Steinberg W, Hill M, *et al.*: Infected pancreatic necrosis and pancreatic fluid collections: serendipitous response to antibiotics and medical therapy in three patients. *Pancreas* 1996, 12:298–302.
16. Kelly TR, Wagner DS: Gallstone pancreatitis: a prospective randomized trial of the timing of surgery. *Surgery* 1988, 104:600–605.
17.• Folsch UR, Nitscher, Ludther, *et al.*: Early ERCP and papillotomy compared with conservative treatment for acute biliary pancreatitis. *N Engl J Med* 1997, 336:237–242.
18. Freeman M, Nelson D, Sherman S, *et al.*: Complications of endoscopic biliary sphincterotomy. *N Engl J Med* 1996, 335:909–918.
19. McMahon MJ, Playforth MJ, Pickford R: A comparison study of methods for the prediction of severity of attacks of acute pancreatitis. *Br J Surg* 1980, 67:22–25.
20. Ranson J, Berman R: Long peritoneal lavage decreases pancreatic sepsis in acute pancreatitis. *Ann Surg* 1990, 211:708–718.

136 Pancreatic Fistulas and Ascites
Richard A. Kozarek and L.W. Traverso

Pancreatic fistulas may be internal or external and result from acute or chronic pancreatitis; trauma, including pseudocyst drainage, pancreatic surgery, and percutaneous biopsy; or neoplasm. Treatment options include minimizing pancreatic secretion (by eliminating oral intake or by providing hyperalimentation, pancreatic enzymes, or octreotide), attempts at serosal apposition (by thoracentesis or paracentesis), and performing percutaneous tube manipulation or surgery. The success of these therapies depends, in part, on the presence or absence of concomitant pseudocysts, ongoing ductal obstruction, or a disconnected duct syndrome. Recently, transpapillary pancreatic duct stents or drains have been used to treat refractory ductal leaks. Such stents may cause direct fistula occlusion or lower the duodenal-pancreatic pressure gradient.

■ PATHOPHYSIOLOGY

Pancreatic fistulas are the consequence of pancreatic autodigestion or necrosis that results in a persistent pancreatic duct disruption. Traditionally, such fistulas have been considered either internal or external based on the presence or absence of a cutaneous communication (Table 136-1) [1,2•,3•,4].

Internal fistulas usually result from active inflammation, which is often associated with downstream duct hypertension caused by an inflammatory stricture [5–8]. Less commonly, this ductal obstruction is neoplastic. Ductal obstruction may be associated with a ruptured duct and the release of pancreatic juice and enzymes into pancreatic and peripancreatic tissue [9]. Clinical symptoms depend on the site of ductal decompression. An anteriorly ruptured pancreatic duct may cause a direct communication with contiguous bowel, resulting in a pancreaticoenteric fistula [10]. Alternatively, free rupture into the peritoneal space causes pancreatic ascites, which may be associated with a pseudocyst [5]. Rupture into the retroperitoneal space allows pancreatic juice to track through the aortic or esophageal hiatus and may be associated with a mediastinal pseudocyst or bronchopleural fistula [7,8]. Usually, however, intrathoracic dissection of pancreatic juices tracks into one or both pleural cavities with resultant chronic pleural effusions. In patients with preexisting lung disease, such as tuberculosis or bronchiectasis, the risk of pancreaticopleural communication from an internal fistula appears to increase significantly [2•].

External fistulas communicate with the skin. They are usually iatrogenic and are caused by percutaneous biopsy, drainage of a pancreatic fluid collection, or surgery such as pancreatic resection or decompression [5]. The most common predisposing event appears to be percutaneous pseudocyst drainage in conjunction with downstream pancreatic duct obstruction. External fistulas also may result from attempts to drain pancreatic necrosis. A postoperative incidence of up to 20% for external fistulas has been reported in patients who undergo extensive pancreatic resection [3•,4,5]. Conditions that have been associated with internal and external pancreatic fistulas are summarized in Table 136-2.

Table 136-1. Pancreatic Fistula Classification

Internal
  Intra-abdominal
    Pseudocyst
    Pancreatic ascites
    Pancreatico-gut communication
  Intrathoracic
    Pseudocyst
    Pancreatic pleural effusion
    Pancreaticobronchial communication
External
  Abdominal
  Thoracic

Table 136-2. Etiology of Pancreatic Fistula

Internal
  Pancreatitis
    Acute (necrosis)
    Chronic
  Trauma
    Surgery
    Blunt injury
    Spontaneous or percutaneous pseudocyst drainage
  Neoplasm
  Miscellaneous
    (eg, duplication cyst)
External
  Trauma
    Surgery
    Percutaneous biopsy or drainage of pancreatic fluid collections
    Penetrating injury

■■ DIAGNOSIS

The clinical signs and symptoms of internal pancreatic fistulas depend on both the rate of leakage and whether dissection of pancreatic juice is above or below the diaphragm. Lipsett and Cameron reviewed 50 subjects with internal pancreatic fistulas who were treated at Johns Hopkins over a 30-year period. Nine subjects presented with pleural effusions that contained high levels of amylase, and 34 subjects presented with pancreatic ascites [1]; seven subjects had both. Subjects with pancreaticopleural fistulas had varying degrees of cough, chest pain, or shortness of breath, whereas those presenting with pancreatic ascites had abdominal distention. Discomfort and weight loss, despite increased abdominal girth, also were common. Approximately half of the subjects had a history of pancreatitis.

Diagnosis of an internal pancreatic fistula is contingent on demonstrating the pancreatic duct connection to the chest or abdominal cavities or finding pancreatic juice (ie, high levels of amylase) in ascitic or pleural fluid, or both (Table 136-3) [1,4,5]. Often, serum amylase also is elevated, possibly because of enzyme diffusion across the peritoneal or pleural surface. The ascitic fluid albumin concentration usually is greater than 3 g/dL, helping to distinguish pancreatic from cirrhotic ascites.

Plain radiographs of the abdomen are marginally useful. They may show the nonspecific changes of ascites (ground-glass appearance, loss of the psoas margin) or pleural effusions, which can be primarily left-sided and sometimes massive. Calcifications of chronic pancreatitis may be present. Ultrasound or abdominal CT scans also may be nonspecific and usually fail to demonstrate the site of ductal leakage. However, abnormalities are noted in up to 80% of patients and include ductal dilation, pseudocyst, pancreatic calcifications, ascites, and pleural effusions (Fig. 136-1A) [4]. Endoscopic retrograde cholangiopancreatography (ERCP) should be undertaken in all patients with suspected or proved internal fistulas; it is essential in directing their subsequent management (Fig. 136-1B–D) [6,9]. Pancreatography not only defines the site of ductal disruption, it also may demonstrate anatomic factors that would

---

Table 136-3. Diagnosis of Pancreatic Fistula

Internal
  Laboratory tests
    High amylase ascites/pleural effusion
  Imaging
    Plain films
      Ground-glass appearance
      Loss of psoas shadows
      Pleural effusions
    Computed tomography/ultrasound
      Pancreatic duct dilation, ± calculi
      ± Pseudocyst
      ± Effusion/ascites
  Endoscopic retrograde cholangiopancreatography
    Ductal disruption/obstruction/pseudocyst
External
  High amylase fluid
  Percutaneous tube study
  ERCP

preclude a response to conservative therapy, such as obstructing strictures or stones or a duct that has been completely disconnected, leaving the pancreatic parenchyma in two separate pieces (disconnected duct syndrome) (Fig. 136-2) [6,9].

In contrast to pancreatic pleural effusions or ascites, pancreaticoenteric fistulas are often a natural consequence of spontaneous pseudocyst decompression. They also can occur secondary to a percutaneously placed tube that has eroded into a contiguous loop of bowel. This type of fistula may be asymptomatic and is diagnosed at a follow-up evaluation of the tube [10]. This type of fistula usually resolves after the catheter is removed and replaced with a tube of smaller diameter or one made of more compliant material. An exception to resolution occurs when tracts or catheters communicate directly with the colon to produce a superinfection.

External pancreatic fistulas usually are easier to diagnose than internal fistulas [5]. They are often recognized perioperatively after pancreatic surgery as ongoing drainage, and may present as a leakage of clear fluid following penetrating abdominal trauma. Another common presentation is persistently high fluid production following percutaneous drainage of a pseudocyst (Fig. 136-3). The secretions from external fistulas have a high amylase concentration. However, fistula fluid production varies, depending on the site of disruption (tail, body, or head of the pancreas; major duct or side branch) and the presence or absence of downstream ductal obstruction [11••]. If the fistula tract becomes superinfected, as occurs in up to one third of these patients, fever, tachycardia, progressive abdominal pain, and ileus are common clinical features [1].

TREATMENT

The choice of therapy for pancreatic fistulas is contingent on the clinical status of the patient and on whether the fistula is internal or external. Treatment also depends on both the site of ductal disruption and the presence or absence of downstream ductal obstruction or the disconnected duct syndrome [6]. Pancreaticoenteric communications that have undergone fistulization into the small bowel or stomach often require no intervention and may be one mechanism for "spontaneous" pseudocyst resolution [10]. If fistula formation is the consequence of percutaneous tube erosion into a contiguous loop of bowel, the fistula often resolves following catheter repositioning, replacement with one of a smaller size, or removal.

Historically, the medical treatment for most types of pancreatic fistulas has included attempts to inhibit pancreatic secretions. This often has been accomplished by feeding the patient clear

Figure 136-1

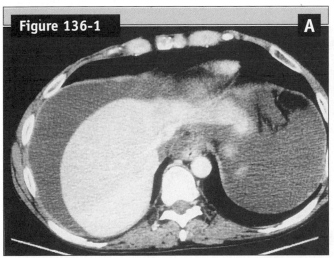
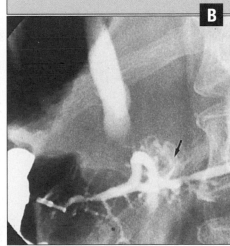
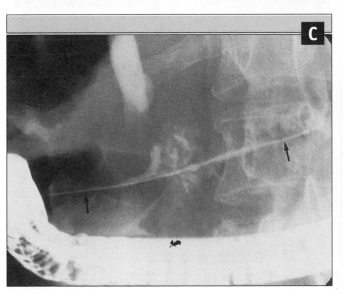
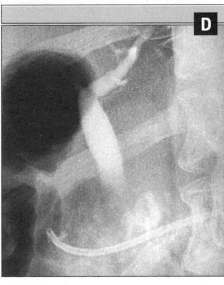

A, Abdominal CT scan demonstrating intraperitoneal fluid in a patient with pancreatic ascites. **B**, Pancreatogram demonstrating leak site (*arrow*) in patient with pancreas divisum, chronic alcoholic pancreatitis, and high amylase ascites. **C**, Note guidewire (*arrows*) placed across leak site. **D**, Transpapillary endoprosthesis inserted through duct of Santorini and across leak site. The latter plus single large volume paracentesis resulted in resolution of pancreatic ascites.

liquids only or by not allowing the patient to have anything orally and initiating total parenteral nutrition (TPN) (Table 136-4) [1,2•,3•,4]. Some authorities have attempted to achieve serosal apposition through multiple paracenteses or thoracenteses. Long-term chest tube placement also has been advocated. Additional attempts to minimize pancreatic secretion have included the use of acetazolamide or other diuretics; atropine; high doses of pancreatic enzymes in conjunction with a low-fat diet [1,2•,3•,4,12]; and more recently, somatostatin analogs (octreotide) at doses ranging between 50 and 300 µg given subcutaneously every 8 hours [13–15,16••,17]. Other, less conventional treatments of internal fistulas have been advocated, including low-dose irradiation and fluid re-infusion by means of a peritoneojugular shunt [4]. Surgical treatment, usually reserved for situations in which medical therapy has failed, has included either duct decompression in conjunction with Roux-en-Y cyst-jejunostomy or localized resection of the pancreatic head or tail.

Because the more conventional approaches to healing pancreatic fistulas often fail, an attempt has been made to use transpapillary endoprostheses to achieve fistula closure, precluding the need for surgery [6–10]. Transpapillary stents also have been used in acutely ill patients in an attempt to allow elective surgery to be performed in a controlled situation [18]. Sometimes these stents are effective by bypassing a downstream stricture or stone, at other times, they also may "plug" a ductal disruption. They also may bypass the sphincter of Oddi, thereby converting the pancreatic duct to a low-pressure system and accelerating closure, much the same way that stents placed across the papilla repair cystic duct leakage [5,6]. Stents alone appear to be of little use in complete ductal transection if the pancreas becomes disconnected as a result of acute trauma or pseudocyst [19].

Internal Fistula

Approximately half of patients with internal fistulas respond to repeated paracenteses or thoracenteses in conjunction with hyperalimentation and bowel rest [20•]. In the Hopkins series, for instance, 21 of 42 subjects responded to such conservative therapy, and approximately 70% (15 of 21) were discharged within 2 weeks of admission [1]. Of the five deaths recorded in the medically managed group, all occurred in subjects who had been managed conservatively for more than 3 weeks, suggesting that surgery should be considered as an option in those whose fistulas do not close after 2 to 3 weeks of therapy. Uchigama and colleagues reviewed 37 cases of pancreatic ascites reported in the Japanese literature [21]: 12 subjects healed with conservative measures alone, 18 subjects required surgery, and seven high-risk subjects were treated solely with external drainage.

Octreotide has been used in most recent series to treat pancreatic fistulas. Octreotide is a somatostatin analog, and it appears to accelerate fistula healing and possibly improve the percentage of patients responding to medical management [13–15,16••,17]. For example, Parekh and Segal reported 23 subjects with high amylase ascites or pleural effusions, 10 of

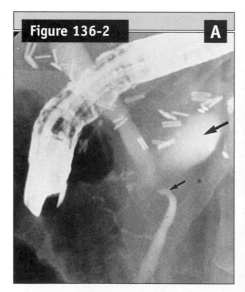
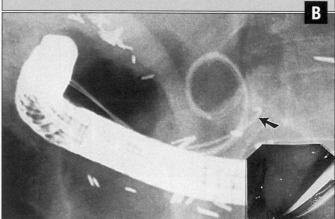
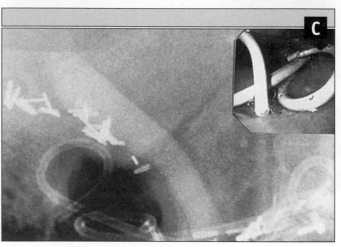

Figure 136-2

A, Small *arrow* indicates site of duct obstruction; large *arrow* indicates a pseudocyst (filled by transduodenal puncture) in a patient with disconnected duct syndrome. **B-C,** *Arrow* depicts insertion of guidewires across fistula through duodenal wall followed by insertion of two pigtail stents. Note surgical clips, contrast in bile duct. The pseudocyst resolved in 4 weeks, but long-term clinical success is uncertain.

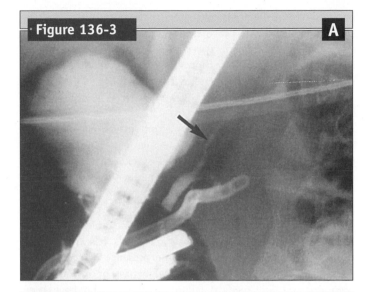

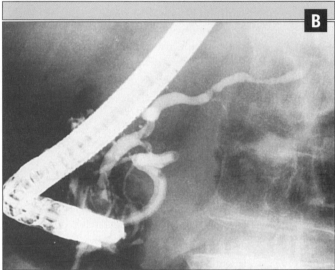

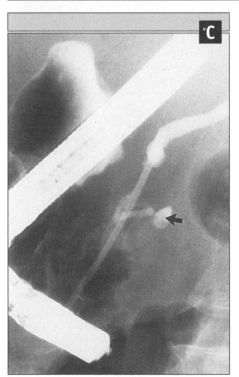

A, ERCP demonstrating tight stricture (*arrow*) in patient with residual pancreatic fistula following pseudocyst drainage. Note percutaneous drain. **B**, Percutaneous tube study demonstrating body and tail of pancreas in same patient. **C**, *Arrow* delineates small residual pseudocyst in patient whose external fistula closed 24 hours after transpapillary stent placement. Note that the external drain has been removed.

whom improved with medical therapy alone at a mean of 30 days [2•]. Five additional subjects (three with ascites, two with effusion) subsequently responded to octreotide. This study also suggested that ductal anatomy was the major correlate of successful therapy: nine of 11 subjects with mild to moderate chronic pancreatitis as judged by ERCP responded to conservative therapy, octreotide, or both, in contrast to only one of 10 with advanced changes of chronic pancreatitis.

Historically, surgical therapy has been limited to patients who failed several weeks of conservative treatment [1,4]. Lipsett and Cameron performed pancreatic resection or decompression in 24 of 50 subjects with internal fistulas, resulting in a single surgical failure and an 8.3% mortality rate (two deaths) [1]. These authors believed that both type and timing of surgery should be dictated by preoperative ERCP. Others have reported recurrence rates as high as 50% if surgery is undertaken without delineation of the ductal anatomy by either ERCP or operative pancreatography. Mortality rates for medical or surgical management of internal fistulas have been in the range of 15% to 25%. Moreover, approximately 15% of patients with internal fistulas develop recurrent fistulas, whether treated medically or surgically.

Because of the significant morbidity and mortality in patients with internal fistulas treated by the modalities noted previously, it appeared reasonable to attempt transpapillary stent or drain insertion in patients with pancreatic ascites or effusions (see Fig. 136-1) [18]. For example, four subjects with pancreatic ascites and an additional two subjects with high amylase effusions were stented [20•]. All of the subjects underwent

Table 136-4. Therapy of Pancreatic Fistula

Internal
  Medical
    High-dose pancreatic enzymes
    NPO
    Hyperalimentation
    Octreotide
    ? Diuretics
  Mechanical
    Percutaneous drainage of any concomitant pseudocyst
    Remove or downsize drain (pancreaticoenteric fistula)
    Transpapillary stent
  Surgical
    Resection
    Decompression
External
  Medical
    High-dose pancreatic enzymes
    NPO
    Hyperalimentation
    Octreotide
    ? Diuretics
  Mechanical
    Percutaneous drainage of any concomitant pseudocyst
    Remove or downsize drain (pancreaticoenteric fistula)
    Transpapillary stent
  Surgical
    Resection
    Decompression

subsequent percutaneous drainage of pleural effusions and ascites and two concomitant pseudocyst drainage under ultrasound control. The subjects were fed a low-fat diet within 12 hours of prosthesis placement, and all were discharged within 7 days, having had their fluid collections resolved without complications. Prostheses were removed after a mean of 4 weeks. Neither ascites nor effusion has recurred at a mean follow-up of 30 months. Further experience suggests that endoscopic therapy for internal pancreaticoenteric fistulas also may be effective. As such, we reported eight subjects with pancreaticoduodenal (five subjects) or pancreaticocolonic fistulas (three subjects) [10]. Three (38%) healed simply by removing or downsizing a percutaneous drainage catheter. An additional three closed their leak after transpapillary endoprosthesis placement. Two of the eight subjects (25%) required pancreatic resection [10].

External Fistula

It is often best to try to prevent the development of external pancreatic fistulas rather than attempt treatment after they have formed. Because pancreatic resection or decompression is the most common etiology of external fistulas in many institutions, some surgeons have adopted measures to minimize persistent perioperative leak. These measures range from local therapy in the operative field, such as fibrin glue [22] and modified pancreaticojejunal anastomosis [23], to use of medications pre- and postoperatively to decrease pancreatic secretion. Büchler *et al.*, for example, randomized 246 subjects undergoing pancreatic resection to receive either octreotide 100 μg or placebo subcutaneously three times daily for 7 days perioperatively [24••]. Complications occurred in more than half of the subjects receiving placebo and less than one third of those receiving octreotide, the latter set of complications being mainly a consequence of decreased anastomotic leak in subjects at significant risk.

External fistula therapy depends on the etiology and the output of the fistula as well as the presence or absence of bacterial superinfection. Martin and colleagues treated 27 subjects with external fistulas and nine subjects with internal fistulas using hyperalimentation and maintaining subjects NPO [1]. Eighty-three percent of the subjects (30 of 36) ultimately required surgery. There was an overall operative success rate of 83% and a single (3%) postoperative death. Saari and colleagues reported the results in 19 subjects with external fistulas, 14 of whom had either necrotizing or chronic pancreatitis [15]. All subjects were treated with hyperalimentation and received constant infusion of octreotide. Sixty-eight percent (13 of 19) of the subjects in this series had fistula closure after a median treatment of 7 days (range 2–14 days). Only one of six subjects with an obstructed pancreatic duct responded to medical management, whereas all subjects without bacterial contamination of their tract responded medically. High-dose pancreatic enzyme supplementation also may accelerate the healing of external pancreatic fistulas in some situations. For example, Garcia-Pugés and colleagues reported five subjects with external pancreatic fistulas who had reduction of fistula flow and trypsin output after starting enzymes and fistula closure within 1 to 12 days [12].

Finally, transpapillary stents have been used in nine patients with refractory pancreaticocutaneous fistulas (Fig. 136-2) [5]. Of the nine patients, eight experienced fistula closure: five patients within 48 hours and three patients within 7 days of stent placement. One prosthesis migrated into the duodenum and required replacement. A second stent occluded, causing an iatrogenic pseudocyst infection. This was successfully treated with antibiotics and prosthesis exchange.

▰▰ CONCLUSION

Pancreatic fistulas imply a ductal disruption whether they result from acute or chronic pancreatitis, obstructing neoplasm, trauma, or surgery. Whether this disruption responds to medical treatment or requires surgery depends on a number of interdependent factors, including the etiology, the size and site (main duct versus side branch) of the ductal disruption, and the presence of an ongoing downstream obstruction and concomitant bacterial infection. Response to therapy also depends on whether the fistula is external or internal and the presence of a persistent pseudocyst [25]. Historically, surgical bypass or resection has been reserved for "medical failures," patients who have been treated variably with high-dose pancreatic enzymes, TPN, or octreotide in combination with percutaneous drainage procedures. The use of transpapillary endoprostheses has proved successful in selected patients and deserves additional study.

▰▰ REFERENCES

Recently published papers of particular interest have been highlighted as follows:
- •   Of interest
- •• Of outstanding interest

1. Lipsett PA, Cameron JL: Internal pancreatic fistulas. *Am J Surg* 1992, 163:216–220.

2.• Parekh D, Segal I: Pancreatic ascites and effusion. Risk factors for failure of conservative therapy and the role of octreotide. *Arch Surg* 1992, 127:707–712.
A good clinical study from Johannesburg, South Africa that attempts to identify possible risk factors for failure of conservative medical therapy in 23 subjects with pancreatic ascites and effusion. The study recommends conservative medical therapy for mild to moderate effusions.

3.• Martin FM, Rossi RL, Munson JL, *et al.*: Management of pancreatic fistulas. *Arch Surg* 1989, 124:571–573.
This study from the Lahey Clinic, Massachusetts, reviews the authors' experience in the management of 35 subjects with pancreatic fistulas. Subject selection is noted to be important in the decision to resect or drain and is based in part on imaging the pancreatic duct and fistula.

4. Eckhauser F, Raper SE, Knol JA, Mulholland MW: Surgical management of pancreatic ascites, and pancreaticopleural fistulas. *Pancreas* 1991, 6(suppl):66–75.

5. Kozarek RA, Ball TJ, Patterson DJ, *et al.*: Endoscopic treatment of pancreaticocutaneous fistulas. *J Gastrointest Surg* 1997, 1:357–361.

6. Kozarek RA, Traverso LW: Endotherapy for chronic pancreatitis. *Int J Pancreatol* 1996, 19:93–102.

7. Burgess NA, Moore HE, Williams JO, Lewis MH: A review of pancreaticopleural fistula in pancreatitis and its management. *HPB Surgery* 1992, 5:79–86.

8. Rockey DC, Cello JP: Pancreaticopleural fistula. Report of 7 patients and review of the literature. *Medicine* 1990, 69:332–344.

9. Kozarek RA: Endoscopic drainage of pancreatic pseudocysts. In: *Advanced Therapeutic Endoscopy*, vol 2. Edited by Barkins JS, O'Phalen C. New York: Raven Press, 1994:401–402.

10. Wolfsen HC, Kozarek RA, Ball TJ, *et al.*: Pancreaticoenteric fistula. *J Clin Gastroenterol* 1992, 4:117–121.

11.•• Szentes MJ, Traverso LW, Kozarek RA, Freeny PC: Invasive treatment of pancreatic fluid collections with surgical and nonsurgical methods. *Am J Surg* 1991, 161:600–605.
This paper is based on the 14-year experiences of the authors' group at Virginia Mason Medical Center. The paper compares the operative and nonoperative management of symptomatic pancreatic fluid collections and identifies subgroups of patients who may benefit from nonsurgical drainage.

12. Garcia-Pugés AM, Navarro S, Fernandez-Cruz L, *et al.*: Oral pancreatic enzymes accelerate closure of external pancreatic fistulas. *Br J Surg* 1988, 75:824–825.

13. Secchi A, DiCarlo V, Martinenghi S, *et al.*: Octreotide administration in the treatment of pancreatic fistulae after pancreas transplantation. *Transplant Int* 1992, 5:201–204.

14. Lansden FT, Adams DB, Anderson MC: Treatment of external pancreatic fistulas with somatostatin. *Am Surg* 1989, 55:695–698.

15. Saari A, Schroder T, Kivilaasko LE, *et al.*: Treatment of pancreatic fistulas with somatostatin and total parenteral nutrition. *Scand J Gastroenterol* 1989,24:859–862.

16.•• Torres AJ, Landa JI, Moreno-Azcoita M, *et al.*: Somatostatin in the management of gastrointestinal fistulas. *Arch Surg* 1992, 127:97–100.
A multicenter, controlled, randomized prospective trial evaluating the effectiveness of TPN versus TPN plus somatostatin in the conservative management of postoperative gastrointestinal fistulas.

17. Ohta T, Nagakawa T, Mori K, *et al.*: Effect of SMS 201-995 on exocrine pancreatic secretion in a patient with external pancreatic fistula. *Int J Pancreatol* 1992, 11:185–189.

18. Kozarek RA, Ball TJ, Patterson DJ, *et al.*: Endoscopic transpapillary therapy for disrupted pancreatic duct and peripancreatic fluid collections. *Gastroenterology* 1991, 100:1362–1370.

19. Devière J, Bueso H, Baise M, *et al.*: Complete disruption of the main pancreatic duct: endoscopic management. *Gastrointest Endosc* 1995, 42:445–451.

20.• Kozarek RA, Jiranek GC, Traverso LW: Endoscopic treatment of pancreatic ascites. *Am J Surg* 1994, 168:223–228.
This paper indicates the benefits of transpapillary pancreatic duct endoprothesis based on the authors' experience in the management of four patients with pancreatic ascites.

21. Uchigama T, Yamamoto T, Mizuta F., Suzuki T: Pancreatic ascites—A collected review of 37 cases in Japan. *Hepatogastroenterology* 1989, 36:244–248.

22. Kram HB, Clark SR, Ocampo IIP, *et al.*: Fibrin glue sealing of pancreatic injuries, resections, and anastomoses. *Am J Surg* 1991, 161:479–481.

23. Maki IIS, Kolts RL, Kuehner ME: Prevention of pancreatic fistula by modified pancreaticojejunal anastomosis. *Am J Surg* 1990, 160:533–534.

24.•• Büchler M, Friess M, Klempa I, *et al.*: Role of octreotide in the prevention of postoperative complications following pancreatic resection. *Am J Surg* 1992, 163:125–131.
This excellent publication from the Ulm Group of investigators suggests that perioperative administration of octreotide reduces the occurrence of complications following pancreatic resection, including pancreatic fistula.

25. Kozarek RA, Traverso LW: Endoscopic treatment of chronic pancreatitis—An alternative to surgery? *Dig Surg* 1996, 13:90–100.

137 Chronic Pancreatitis
C. S. Pitchumoni

Chronic pancreatitis is characterized clinically by recurrent or persistent abdominal pain, although the disease may also present without pain. Steatorrhea, diabetes, or both, may occur in late stages of the disease, heralding pancreatic insufficiency. Morphologically, chronic pancreatitis is characterized by irregular sclerosis, with destruction and permanent loss of exocrine parenchyma that may be focal, segmental, or diffuse. These changes may be associated with varying degrees of stricture and dilation of the duct system; protein plugs or calculi may be seen inside the ducts. A distinct morphologic form of chronic pancreatitis is obstructive pancreatitis, secondary to obstruction of the duct by tumors or scars.

In affluent nations, alcoholism is generally considered the leading cause of chronic pancreatitis, whereas in many developing nations nonalcoholic calculous pancreatitis of undetermined etiology (*ie*, tropical, nutritional, or Afro-Asian pancreatitis) is more common [1••]. Table 137-1 summarizes the important data on various types of chronic pancreatitis.

EPIDEMIOLOGY

Because alcohol is the most important cause of chronic pancreatitis, the epidemiology of the disease parallels the prevalence of alcohol abuse in the community. Along with the increase in alcohol consumption in Western nations, a parallel rise in the incidence of chronic pancreatitis has been observed. In the United States, nearly 75% of chronic pancreatitis cases are caused by chronic alcoholism. Hospitalization rates are higher for black men than for white men with chronic pancreatitis (20.7/100,000 vs 5.7/100,000), respectively, and for black men than for black women (20.7/100,000 vs 14.6/100,000, respectively) (Fig. 137-1). Pima Indians have the lowest predisposition to the disease. The relatively low hospitalization rates for Native Americans with chronic pancreatitis are surprising, given the high prevalence of gallstones and alcoholism among this group.

Overall, chronic pancreatitis occurs less frequently than acute pancreatitis; the ratio is 1:1.5 to 1:17, depending on the population group studied. The relatively low incidence of chronic pancreatitis is explained in part by the fact that diagnostic criteria for the disease often are not clear; alcoholics who present with typical signs and symptoms of acute pancreatitis (*eg*, elevated amylase levels) and whose symptoms usually resolve in a few days are usually categorized as having acute pancreatitis, even though they may actually have chronic pancreatitis.

PATHOLOGY

Most observations on the pathology of chronic pancreatitis are based solely on information gathered from surgery (usually many years after onset) or autopsy (involving very late stage disease) of the pancreas performed on patients with alcoholic pancreatitis. Sequential changes from early to late stages of pancreatitis have not been well studied, mostly because pancreatic biopsies are not performed routinely. In surgery, the pancreas may appear enlarged, but at autopsy the gland is often atrophic and may adhere to adjacent structures. The gland feels nodular and gritty in areas of calculi and cystic over areas of dilated ducts and pseudocysts [2•].

Microscopic features of the pancreas vary according to the stage of the disease. Involvement of the gland is patchy and focal [2•]. The earliest changes are atrophy of the acinar cells and a decrease in or disappearance of the zymogen granules within them. In a diseased pancreas, some areas appear almost normal or show only minimal changes, whereas in other areas all exocrine cells may be replaced by loose areolar tissue or dense collagen (Fig. 137-2).

The ductal system shows an increase in ductules, the result of dedifferentiation of acinar cells. Long strictures or short-segment strictures and proximal dilations may be seen in the main pancreatic duct. Squamous and goblet cell metaplasia are notable in the ductal epithelium. Intraductal calculi are usually seen in late cases. In alcoholic pancreatitis, these stones appear infrequently (about 30%) and are small, speckled, and ill defined, in contrast to tropical pancreatitis where they are more frequent (about 90%), large, dense, and knobby. Typically, the larger stones are near the head, probably because they migrate from small ductules toward the head where they get lodged and grow. Stones in the pancreas may become smaller or even disappear with progression of disease. Disappearance of pancreatic calculi ("vanishing pancreatic calcifications") is *not* considered a sign of malignancy, as indicated in some previous reports.

The nerves appear hypertrophied and prominent and may demonstrate accumulation of inflammatory cells in the perineural regions [3] (Fig. 137-3). The islet cells show atrophy in some areas but may appear well preserved in others. Immunohistochemical studies have shown that many of these islets are newly formed from the ductular epithelium (nesidioblastosis).

PATHOGENESIS

The pathogenesis of chronic pancreatitis is not well understood. The following are proposed hypotheses pertaining to alcohol-induced chronic pancreatitis, the type most frequently found and best studied [4••].

Table 137-1. Chronic Pancreatitis: Types, Clinical Features, and Pathogenesis

Types	Clinical features	Pathogenesis

Alcoholic	Common in Western Hemisphere
	Mean age of onset 30–35 y
	Alcoholism for >15 y, >80 g/d
	Painful episodes followed by calculi (9 y), later steatorrhea (13 y), diabetes (20 y)
		I. Unfavorable secretory changes
		  Viscous pancreatic juice—protein plugs
		  Pancreatic stone protein (lithostathine)
		  deficiency—calculi
		II. Early acinar cell injury

Tropical	Prevalent in Afro-Asian countries Affects poor children and young adults Episodes of abdominal pain Early onset of diabetes and calculi High incidence of pancreatic cancer	Nonalcoholic No proven etiologic factor, probably malnutrition
Hereditary	Caucasians Abdominal pain in childhood Calculi later in life Pancreatic cancer at a young age	Autosomal dominant

Idiopathic	Two types:
	  1) Early onset
	    Painful
	    Calculi, steatorrhea, diabetes
	    2–3 decades later
	  2) Late onset (senile)
	    Painless
	    Pancreatic calculi are incidental
		Idiopathic

Obstructive	Calculi rare, markedly dilated ducts Relieved by surgery	Posttraumatic ductal stricture Periampullary tumors Pancreas divisum
Miscellaneous	Hyperlipidemia Hyperparathyroidism Celiac disease Billroth II gastrectomy α_1-antitrypsin deficiency Autoimmune Hemochromatosis	Not known Not known Lack of stimulus to pancreas Lack of stimulus to pancreas Not known Iron deposition

Small Duct Hypothesis (Unfavorable Secretory Changes, Protein Plug Theory)

Sarles and coworkers hypothesized that the pathophysiologic events begin with protein plug formation and subsequent calcification with calcium carbonate crystals, resulting in the formation of intraductal stones [5••]. Obstruction caused by protein plugs and calculi leads to atrophy of acinar cells and periductular fibrous tissue formation. Sequential changes in the composition of pancreatic juice in chronic alcoholics appear to promote protein plug formation. The viscosity of pancreatic juice increases as a result of increased enzymatic as well as nonenzymatic (eg, lactoferrin) proteins. Inherited or acquired deficiency of lithostathine, a special protein secreted by the acinar cells and formerly known as pancreatic stone protein, is the primary factor in the pathogenesis of chronic calculous pancreatitis. Large amounts of lithostathine are present in the pancreatic juice of healthy individuals and prevent calcium carbonate crystallization. Deficiency of lithostathine promotes crystal formation of calcium carbonate, with resultant formation of calculi. Hereditary and nutritional factors, and possibly alcoholism, may be involved in decreased lithostathine secretion. Opposing views exist concerning the role of lithostathine in the pathogenesis of chronic pancreatitis. Some observers have been unable to associate low lithostathine levels with chronic pancreatitis, whereas others have demonstrated increased lithostathine levels in acute and chronic pancreatitis.

Other proteins, such as enzymatic proteins and an iron-containing protein, lactoferrin, may also play a role in lithogenesis. The protein plug hypothesis has been challenged by many pathologists and clinicians, who note that calculus formation is not a feature of early chronic pancreatitis and that all patients with alcoholic pancreatitis do not necessarily develop calculi.

Big Duct Hypothesis

Opie's "common channel" theory (1901) proposed that impaction of a gallstone in the distal common bile duct would cause reflux of bile into the pancreatic duct if there were a common biliopancreatic channel proximal to the obstruction. Refluxed bile was suspected of activating of pancreatic enzymes, causing autodigestion of the pancreas. The extrapolation of Opie's theory to the pathogenesis of alcoholic pancreatitis presumes that alcohol induces obstruction at the papilla by spasm of sphincter of Oddi or duodenitis but proof of this is lacking. The current belief is that the "big duct" theory may have a role only in biliary pancreatitis.

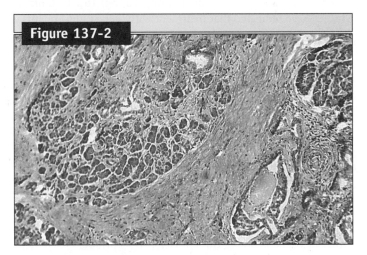

Figure 137-2

The section shows scattered acinar tissue separated by extensive fibrosis. The ductal epithelium shows metaplasia. Intraductular protein precipitate and calculi also can be seen.

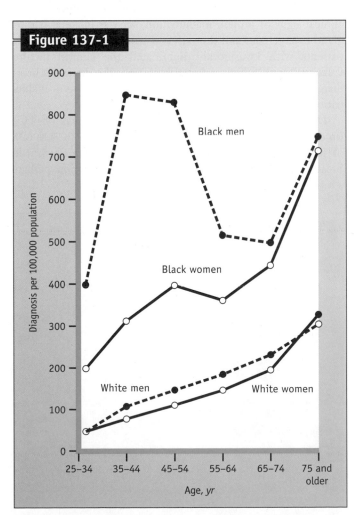

Figure 137-1

Rate of hospital discharges with the diagnosis of pancreatic disorders in the United States. (*From* Go [1••].)

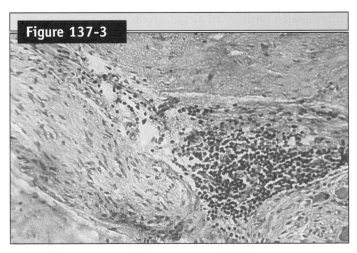

Figure 137-3

Two giant nerves, close to each other, capped by an area of accumulation of inflammatory cells.

Early Acinar Cell Injury

The crux of this hypothesis is that acinar cells are injured first, secretory changes follow morphologic alterations, and fibrosis, ductular abnormalities, and stone formation develop as late sequelae [4••].

Toxic Metabolite Hypothesis

The pathogenesis of chronic pancreatitis, according to this theory, is somewhat similar to that for alcoholic liver disease, in that the acinar cell injury results from a direct cytotoxic effect of alcohol. Ethanol is, to some extent, metabolized in the pancreas by alcohol dehydrogenase (ADH). Chronic alcohol consumption induces intrapancreatic lipid deposition, fibrosis, and atrophy by direct toxic and metabolic effects, possibly through acetaldehyde. Pancreatic biopsies in alcoholic patients without pancreatitis have shown that the acinar cells are often injured very early, before clinical pancreatitis appeared.

Free Radical Injury

Patients with chronic pancreatitis have a significantly lower dietary intake of antioxidants, such as vitamins (A, C, β-carotene, E) and trace elements (Zn, Cu, Se) [6]. Preliminary studies have indicated that treatment with dietary antioxidants is beneficial to patients with chronic pancreatitis. It is postulated that acetaldehyde oxidation by xanthine oxidase releases free radicals that cause blockade of the intracellular pathway ("pancreastasis"), fusion of lysosomal and zymogen components, and membrane lipid oxidation. These events, believed to occur in both acute and chronic pancreatitis, lead to mast cell degranulation, platelet activation, and inflammatory responses with zymogen activation. The free radical injury hypothesis is supported by recent epidemiological studies noting a high incidence of alcoholic pancreatitis in smokers [7]. Cigarette smoking induces free radicals and alcoholism depletes antioxidant vitamins and trace elements involved in scavenging free radicals.

The initial injury by free radicals may be accentuated by other factors enhancing the severity of the episode. Free radicals produce chemotactic factors for neutrophils, macrophages, and platelets. Excessive stimulation of neutrophils releases lysosomal enzymes from the acinar cells.

Increased Fragility of Organelles

The increased fragility of organelles containing lysosomal enzymes, leading to premature activation of zymogens, is believed to initiate acinar cell injury. Trypsinogen, the most important zymogen, can be activated to trypsin, which in turn could initiate a cascade of activation of other zymogens.

One or more of the above mechanisms may initiate acinar cell injury and induce acute pancreatitis in an alcoholic patient. Alcoholic chronic pancreatitis may indeed be only a late manifestation of recurrent acute pancreatitis (necrosis - fibrosis sequence) [8].

It is not clear why all alcoholics do not develop chronic pancreatitis. The role of nutrition in the pathogenesis of alcoholic pancreatitis is debatable. A previous observation from Europe that a diet high in fat and protein predisposes the individual to chronic pancreatitis is not supported by data from the United States and Australia. A weak correlation has been observed between HLA-B13 and alcoholic chronic pancreatitis.

▇ OTHER FORMS OF CHRONIC PANCREATITIS

Tropical Calculous Pancreatitis

A nonalcoholic form of chronic pancreatitis, tropical calculous pancreatitis (TCP), occurs mostly in children and young adults in many developing nations. The multiplicity of terms used to describe this disease entity indicates uncertainty about its etiology but emphasizes a strong association with malnutrition (nutritional pancreatitis), predominant occurrence in children (juvenile tropical pancreatitis), a high prevalence of diabetes and calculi formation (fibrocalcific pancreatic diabetes), and the occurrence of the disease in the tropical and Afro-Asian countries (tropical, Afro-Asian pancreatitis), and sparsity of inflammatory cells (tropical calculous pancreatopathy) in surgical biopsies of the pancreas [9].

The cardinal clinical manifestations of TCP are recurrent abdominal pain in childhood, followed by onset of diabetes mellitus a few years later [9•]. Prevalence of pancreatic calculi in TCP is nearly 90%, which is much higher than that found in patients with alcoholic pancreatitis (30%). Pancreatic calculi varying in size and shape are demonstrable throughout the markedly dilated main duct, in some cases forming a ductogram and in the dilated ductules mimicking a pancreatogram (Fig. 137-4).

Early reports on TCP identified patients only in late stages of the disease when extreme emaciation, and other obvious clinical signs of protein malnutrition, such as bilateral parotid gland enlargement and the skin and hair changes that occur in patients with kwashiorkor dominated the clinical picture. Currently, with a high index of suspicion, the disease is being diagnosed very early, even when such advanced signs of malnutrition are nearly absent.

Diabetes is almost an inevitable consequence of TCP (in contrast to alcoholic pancreatitis in which only 30% to 60% of patients develop diabetes) and is characteristically brittle. Steatorrhea is a surprisingly rare clinical manifestation, perhaps a reflection of very low dietary fat intake.

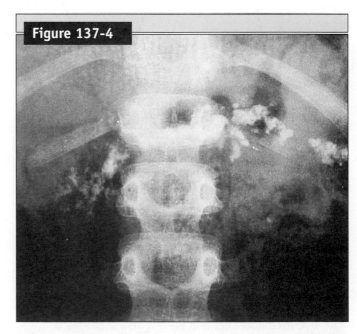

Figure 137-4

Intraductal calculi in the main pancreatic duct in a patient with TCP.

The etiologic factors for TCP are not known, but, based on the fact that the disease mostly affects the poor populations of Third World Nations, malnutrition is strongly suspected. High-carbohydrate/low-protein diets, typical of those of developing nations, have been shown to induce malnutrition, cause acinar cell injury, and produce pancreatic fibrosis. However, no correlation exists between the prevalence of TCP and kwashiorkor-marasmus syndromes (protein-energy malnutrition) in different geographic areas, casting doubts on malnutrition being the sole factor in the etiology. Other factors considered frequently, but not confirmed, include consumption of cassava root (manioc, manihot, esculenta), which besides being associated with a high-carbohydrate/low-protein diet, is known to contain cyanogens. Hypothetically, cyanogens induce free radicals and deplete micronutrients many of which such as zinc and selenium necessary for the integrity of acinar cells.

Hereditary Pancreatitis

Hereditary pancreatitis is discussed in detail in Chapter 143. Onset in childhood, presence of pancreatic calculi (40% to 60%), occurrence of the disease in successive generations, autosomal dominant inheritance, and increased incidence of pancreatic cancer are some important features.

Idiopathic Chronic Pancreatitis

The prevalence of idiopathic pancreatitis is variable and may represent 10% (South Africa) to 40% (Europe) of all cases of chronic pancreatitis. Idiopathic pancreatitis has two subsets [10••]. The juvenile form is characterized by male preponderance, age of onset before 25 years, and a long history of recurrent attacks of abdominal pain. The hallmarks of chronic pancrea-titis such as calculi formation, pancreatic insufficiency, and diabetes develop 25 to 28 years after the onset of the disease. Prognosis is poor.

There is also a late-onset idiopathic calculous pancreatitis (senile pancreatitis), which may occur after the age of 60. This type of pancreatitis, which is often painless, is diagnosed by the fortuitous discovery of pancreatic calculi in a routine abdominal radiograph or during evaluation of a patient with steatorrhea of uncertain etiology. Routine autopsies have shown a prevalence of pancreatic calculi in about 4% of individuals above 70 years of age. The pathogenesis of asymptomatic calculi in the elderly is attributed to ductal changes as a result of aging.

Rare Forms of Chronic Pancreatitis

Minimal-change chronic pancreatitis is a form of idiopathic chronic pancreatitis in which the macroscopic and radiologic changes are minimal, although pain is a chief clinical feature. The histology of the pancreas predominantly shows chronic inflammatory cells.

Obstructive pancreatitis results from a blockage of flow in the large pancreatic ducts as a result of a scar or tumor. Although earlier, pancreatic calculi were reported to be rare, they are not always absent. This form of chronic pancreatitis may be reversible, or at least the progression can be arrested if obstruction is promptly relieved by surgery. There is enormous dilation of the ductal system proximal to the occlusion of one of the major ducts by tumor or scars, diffuse atrophy, and fibrosis of the exocrine parenchyma (Fig. 137-5).

Acute pancreatitis is the usual complication of hypertriglyceridemia and is seen when serum triglyceride levels are elevated above 1000 mg/dL. Although rare, chronic pancreatitis has been reported as a result of hyperlipidemia. The mechanism of pancreatic injury resulting in hyperlipidemic acute or chronic pancreatitis is not clear.

Hypercalcemic states including hyperparathyroidism have been suspected to cause acute as well as chronic pancreatitis. Hypercalcemia is a potent stimulus to pancreatic secretion. Chronic hypercalcemia is reported to be responsible for pancreatic injury by increasing pancreatic calcium secretion and permeability of calcium. The incidence of chronic pancreatitis in individuals with hyperparathyroidism is infrequent.

Pancreas divisum, a congenital anomaly in which the ventral and dorsal buds of the embryonic pancreas fail to unite properly, is a debatable cause of chronic pancreatitis. Isolated case reports exist describing localized chronic pancreatitis of the ventral pancreas.

Groove pancreatitis is a rare and special form of segmental chronic pancreatitis involving the "groove" among pancreatic head, duodenum, and common bile duct. The disease is often preceded by peptic ulcer, gastric resections, or biliary tract diseases. Abdominal pain, vomiting due to duodenal stenosis, obstructive jaundice, and weight loss are the common presenting symptoms; these symptoms may mimic pancreatic carcinoma.

Other etiologic associations of chronic pancreatitis include α_1-antitrypsin deficiency, celiac disease, sclerosing cholangitis Sjögren's syndrome, autoimmune disturbances, Crohn's disease, Waldenström's macroglobulinemia, previous abdominal radiotherapy, hemachromatosis, systemic lupus erythematosus, abdominal trauma, and congenital ductal abnormalities. Chronic pancreatitis may also occur after partial gastrectomy and Billroth II anastomosis.

▆▆ CLINICAL FEATURES
Pain

Recurrent abdominal pain, the dominant symptom in nearly 85% of patients with chronic pancreatitis, is the most common reason for patients to seek medical attention. The pain can be

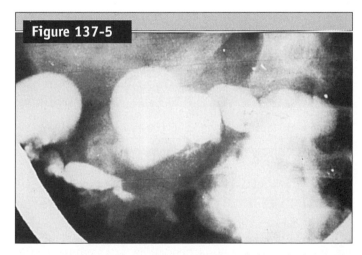

Figure 137-5

Obstructive pancreatitis. Prestenotic dilation of the main duct. Note the giant dilation of the pancreatic duct, which is two to three times the size of the scope.

quite debilitating and intractable, causing disruption of lifestyle and often leading to functional incapacity, drug and alcohol addiction, a poor quality of life, and even suicidal tendencies.

The patient typically presents with steady, boring, and agonizing pain in the epigastrium or sometimes in the left upper quadrant with radiation directly to the back between the T12 and L2 vertebrae or to the left shoulder. Patients sit up and lean forward in the so-called pancreatic position or lie in the knee-chest position on their side. The severity of pain varies greatly among patients; it may even vary in the same individual during different episodes. Postprandial pain may occur, associated with nausea and persistent vomiting. Vomiting does not relieve the pain, in contrast to that of gastritis or pyloric obstruction. Although pain is often precipitated by bouts of drinking, exacerbation of pain may occur even during abstinence from alcohol and with no other identifiable cause. The duration of pain-free intervals is unpredictable and may last from weeks to months, making it difficult to assess the value of different types of pain therapy. The pain may decrease, remain stable, or worsen with advancing disease. Ammann and associates [11] from Switzerland state that about 50% of patients with alcoholic pancreatitis obtain lasting pain relief spontaneously with a long duration of disease, onset of pancreatic dysfunction, and/or abstinence from alcohol. However, in the experience of many others, pain relief resulting from the "burning out" of the exocrine pancreas occurs infrequently and is unpredictable. Development of calculi, pancreatic insufficiency, and pain relief usually does not occur until after 18 years of disease.

The pathogenesis of pancreatic pain appears to be multifactorial, which explains why pain relief does not always occur with medical, endoscopic or surgical treatment (Table 137-2).

Intraductal/interstitial hypertension. Outflow obstructions resulting from strictures lead to prestenotic dilatation and increased ductal pressure, especially when such an anatomic abnormality is associated with fairly well-preserved pancreatic function. Pancreatic secretory activity and intraductal pressure decrease during fasting, which relieves the pain. Many surgical decompression procedures such as lateral pancreaticojejunostomy (eg, Puestow procedure) may help in immediate pain relief but are associated with a fall in ductal pressures.

Table 137-2. Mechanisms of Pain in Chronic Pancreatitis

Pancreatic causes	Extrapancreatic causes
Increased intraductal pressure (stones, strictures)	Pseudocysts
Increased interstitial pressure	Stenosis of common bile duct/duodenum/colon
Pancreatic ischemia	
Acute inflammation of the pancreas	
Perineural inflammation, lack of nerve sheath	

A poor correlation exists, however, between ductal abnormalities and degree of pain and exocrine function. In many alcoholics with pancreatitis, endoscopic retrograde cholangiopancreatography (ERCP) findings show normal ducts even though the patient may still have severe pancreatic pain. By using a special technique, pancreatic tissue pressure was often noted to be increased in chronic pancreatitis. Tissue pressure changes occur independent of changes in the main pancreatic duct. After surgical drainage of the pancreas the tissue pressure drops, coinciding with pain relief.

Conceivably, a high interstitial pressure could cause pancreatic ischemia as a result of increased vascular resistance and reduced blood flow; ischemia may be another cause of pancreatic pain.

Neuronal changes. The absence of the normal perineurium exposes the pancreatic nerves to activated enzymes, plasma components, and bioactive materials released from inflammatory cells (Fig. 137-3). The many weaknesses of the neuronal theory of pain constitute its failure to explain why individuals with end-stage chronic pancreatitis have pain despite cessation of pancreatic function or after surgical procedures, which reduce intraductal pressure but do not alter the neuronal pathology.

Ongoing pancreatic injury. Surgical specimens of pancreatic tissue from patients with chronic pancreatitis show that fat necrosis and pseudocysts are common in the early and advanced stages of the disease [8]. The disease itself, rather than its end result, is a possible factor for pain. During the progressive scarring of the pancreas, nerves, ducts, islets, and vessels become irregularly entrapped in fibrotic tissue. Recurrent tissue necrosis causes pain in the early stages of the disease, while the persistent pain experienced in advanced chronic pancreatitis is a result of incomplete obstruction of ducts.

Malabsorption

Steatorrhea and azotorrhea occur when pancreatic enzymes are insufficient to maintain normal digestion. In the natural history of chronic pancreatitis, steatorrhea occurs usually only after 10 years of the onset of the disease. Steatorrhea does not occur until enzyme secretion is reduced to less than 10% of normal [12]. Lipolytic activity decreases much faster than tryptic activity, which explains why steatorrhea occurs sooner and is more severe than azotorrhea. Bicarbonate secretion also decreases in patients with severe chronic pancreatitis, in turn lowering the pH of the duodenum. Lipase is a fragile enzyme that is inactivated by an intraluminal pH of less than 4 and by proteolytic digestion. Stools may be bulky and formed, as opposed to the watery diarrhea seen in malabsorptive disorders secondary to small intestinal causes. Passage of oil droplets in the stool is often reported in chronic pancreatitis. Lower weight and higher fat (>20 g/24 h) typify fecal content of patients with pancreatic insufficiency, compared with those with steatorrhea from other causes.

A few patients with chronic pancreatitis do not develop overt steatorrhea despite far-advanced exocrine pancreatic insufficiency; one explanation is that non-pancreatic lipases such as lingual lipase may be involved in the digestion of 20% to 50% of dietary fat.

Pancreatic Diabetes

Although glucose intolerance is common early in the course of chronic pancreatitis, clinical diabetes occurs relatively late in the disease. The prevalence of pancreatic diabetes depends on duration of the disease, genetic predisposition to diabetes and other factors. Nearly 30% of patients develop diabetes after 10 years of having chronic pancreatitis. Pancreatic diabetes may complicate known pancreatitis or be the presenting symptom as in patients with painless pancreatitis. The diabetic syndrome secondary to pancreatic disease is an example of acquired β- and α-cell insufficiency associated with insulin resistance [13].

Pancreatic diabetes is usually mild and ketoacidosis is rare (Table 137-3). The risk and characteristics of retinopathy in patients with pancreatic diabetes are similar to those of patients with non–insulin-dependent diabetes melitis. Neuropathy is common, probably because of the additive effect of alcohol abuse and malnutrition. The most dramatic manifestation is the frequent and profound hypoglycemic episodes which may be fatal if not managed promptly. Such episodes are common because of the lack of the usual protective response of glucagon.

Complications

Pancreatic complications. Pancreatic complications such as pseudocysts, abscesses, and pancreatic ascites are discussed in other chapters.

Stenosis of the common bile duct. Obstructive jaundice in chronic pancreatitis, as a result of common bile duct stenosis, is another frequent complication. The distal common bile duct that traverses the head of the pancreas is most often involved in common bile duct stenosis. This is seen in acute exacerbations of chronic pancreatitis, as a result of fibrosis of the region or by compression from a pseudocyst. Clinical manifestations are similar to those of pancreatic carcinoma and include chronic pain, jaundice, and persistent elevation of serum alkaline phosphatase levels. Ultrasonography, percutaneous transhepatic cholangiography, and ERCP delineate the stricture and proximal dilation of the common bile duct and intrahepatic biliary radicles (Fig. 137-6). It is prudent to adopt conservative treatment for 2 to 3 weeks because in some cases obstruction due to edema may be reversible. Use of appropriate antibiotic therapy and decompression of the biliary tract by choledochoenterostomy averts complications such as acute cholangitis and secondary biliary cirrhosis.

Peptic ulcer disease. A decrease in pancreatic bicarbonate secretion is the postulated cause for the observed increase in peptic ulcer disease. The role of *Helicobacter pylori* in this regard is not clear.

Stenosis of the duodenum or colon. Fibrosis of the head of the pancreas may involve the adjacent gastric antrum or the duodenum, causing epigastric pain, postprandial fullness, nausea, and vomiting. Diagnosis is established by an upper gastrointestinal series (Fig. 137-7) and by esophagogastroduodenoscopy. Surgical treatment may be needed to relieve obstruction.

The anatomic relationship of the pancreas to the transverse colon allows the inflammatory exudate to seep down through the transverse mesocolon and cause colonic necrosis and stricture formation near the splenic flexure.

Gastrointestinal bleeding. Thrombosis of the splenic vein, splenic artery aneurysm, and pseudoaneurysm are complications of chronic pancreatitis. The splenic and portal veins may also be compressed by a pseudocyst or occluded by fibrosis from adjacent inflammation. A segmental form of portal hypertension develops,

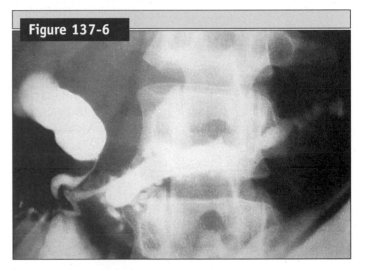

Figure 137-6

ERCP shows fibrotic CBD obstruction and narrowing of the pancreatic duct in the head region.

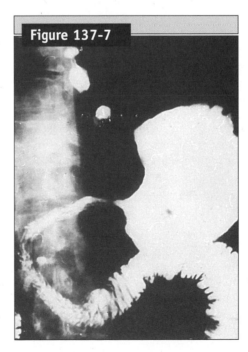

Figure 137-7

Upper GI series shows smooth extrinsic compression of the antrum in the greater curvature region, indicating either enlargement of the head of the pancreas or a pseudocyst.

Table 137-3. Pancreatic Diabetes

Late manifestation of chronic alcoholic, idiopathic pancreatitis
Earlier and more frequent in tropical pancreatitis
Ketoacidosis is rare
Brittle diabetes and hypoglycemic reactions are common
Retinopathy and neuropathy not uncommon
Judicious insulin therapy
Liberal-calorie, low-fat diet

characterized by gastric and esophageal varices, and life-threatening variceal bleeding may occur. Splenectomy is curative. Hemorrhage from a vascular lesion into the pancreas is diagnosed by endoscopy. Exclusion of other causes of bleeding and visualization of blood arising from the ampulla suggests pancreatic bleeding. Retroperitoneal or intraperitoneal bleeding is diagnosed by a computed tomography (CT) scan of the abdomen and is localized by celiac or superior mesenteric angiography, which also permits a transcathether embolectomy. Surgical treatment may be required if bleeding does not stop with the aforementioned procedure.

Pleural effusions. Unilateral or bilateral effusions, rich in amylase, are most often the result of a leaking pseudocyst or pleuropancreatic fistula, both of which can be demonstrated by ERCP.

Extrapancreatic malignancies. Men with chronic pancreatitis have a higher than normal incidence of cancer of the tongue, larynx, bronchus, colon, rectum, liver, skin, lip, bladder, and stomach; women with the disease have a higher incidence than normal of breast, bone, and liver cancers [14]. Cigarette smoking may be the etiologic factor for some but not all of these cancers.

Pancreatic cancer. A recent multinational cooperative study has shown that any form of chronic pancreatitis—alcoholic, hereditary, or idiopathic—is associated with a high incidence of cancer of the pancreas [15••]. In a separate study [9•], the risk for pancreatic cancer in tropical pancreatitis was also much higher than that in the general population. The role of tumor markers, including CA 19-9, in the follow-up of patients with chronic pancreatitis is not clear.

■■■ DIAGNOSIS

Chronic pancreatitis should be considered in all patients with unexplained abdominal pain. Very few patients present with the classic triad of pancreatic calculi, diabetes mellitus, and steatorrhea. The diagnosis is usually based on a typical history of abdominal pain in a patient with a long-standing history of alcoholism. Even in the absence of steatorrhea, weight loss may be a feature because the postprandial pain forces many patients to reduce their food intake. Steatorrhea and diabetes mellitus, being late features, help only to document associated exocrine and endocrine deficiency. Jaundice resulting from extrahepatic bile duct obstruction or edema of the head of the pancreas in an acute exacerbation may occasionally be a feature on initial presentation. A small number of patients with atypical abdominal pain and absence of alcoholism may pose a diagnostic challenge.

Physical examination findings in patients with alcoholic pancreatitis are nonspecific and include epigastric tenderness, occasional associated hepatomegaly, and signs of chronic alcoholism. A number of tests are available (Table 137-4), which are briefly discussed here, but in clinical practice the most useful ones are plain abdominal radiography, sonogram or CT scan of the abdomen, and ERCP [16].

Serum Pancreatic Enzyme/Hormone Levels

In early stages of chronic pancreatitis and during acute exacerbations, serum amylase and lipase values are elevated, but these tests are of no value between acute exacerbations. Low levels of pancreatic isoamylase are found in patients with severe exocrine insufficiency. In evaluating patients with atypical abdominal pain one should remember that the prevalence of macroamylasemia in the general population is about 5%. This high–molecular-weight amylase, bound to serum proteins, is not cleared in the urine. A persistent elevation of the enzyme in the serum may exist, although the increase is only about two- to threefold. The temptation to make a diagnosis of chronic pancreatitis solely based on mild elevations of serum amylase is not justifiable.

It remains controversial whether the serum lipase-amylase ratio differentiates acute episodes of alcoholic pancreatitis from those of nonalcoholic pancreatitis [17]. Patients with alcoholic pancreatitis have significantly lower serum amylase levels and significantly higher lipase-amylase ratios than those with nonalcoholic pancreatitis. It appears that the higher the lipase-amylase ratio, the greater the specificity of alcohol as causing the acute episode of pancreatitis. Low serum levels of pancreatic polypeptides noted in advanced chronic pancreatitis have no diagnostic value.

Radiologic Studies

Plain film of the abdomen including a chest film is the first radiologic study in all patients with initial or subsequent episodes of suspected chronic pancreatitis, to detect pancreatic calculi and to exclude other intra-abdominal causes of pain. Calcification may also occur in the walls of the pseudocysts and cystadenomas. Demonstration of pancreatic calculi, although unusual in the early stages of chronic pancreatitis, is highly specific for the diagnosis of the disease.

Ultrasound and computed tomography of the abdomen. The two diagnostic modalities serve to assess the many morphologic

---

Table 137-4. Tests for Chronic Pancreatitis

Imaging studies
  Plain film of abdomen
  Ultrasound of abdomen
  CT scan
  Endoscopic retrograde cholangiopancreatography
  Endoscopic ultrasound
  MRI/MRCP
Serum studies
  Enzymes: amylase, lipase, trypsin-like immunoreactivity
  Isoamylase levels
  Pancreatic polypeptide levels
  Aminoacid consumption test
Pancreatic function studies
  Tubeless tests
    Bentiromide test
    Pancreatolauryl test
    Vitamin B_{12} absorption test (Schilling IV)
    Fecal chymotrypsin
    Stool fat
  Tube tests
    Secretin; CCK, cerulein stimulation tests
    Lundh test

CCK—cholecystokinin; MRCP—magnetic resonance cholangiopancreatogram; MRI—magnetic resonance imaging.

abnormalities of the pancreas: its size, presence or absence of cysts, irregularities and size of ducts, parenchymal heterogeneity, presence or absence of calculi, extrapancreatic complications such as common bile duct obstruction and dilation, and other contiguous organ involvement [18].

Despite its low cost, easy availability, and lack of radiation, ultrasound has limited usefulness in obese patients and in those with increased bowel gas. Changes in gland size often are not diagnostic of chronic pancreatitis when the gland is enlarged or atrophic. Many prefer computed tomography to ultrasound because of its increased sensitivity (nearly 20% more) and because it is not an operator-dependent technique (Fig. 137-8). No data exist to demonstrate that magnetic resonance imaging is superior to computed tomography.

Endoscopic retrograde cholangiopancreatography (ERCP).

This is the new gold standard for chronic pancreatitis diagnosis. ERCP findings are highly sensitive (70% to 90%) and specific (90% to 100%) (see Chapter 142). Pancreatogram findings in chronic pancreatitis may be classified as showing normal, equivocal, mild, moderate, and severe alterations. Normal or equivocal duct changes are said to occur when only one or two side branches are affected. In mild ductular abnormalities, three or more side branches are altered but the main duct is normal. In moderate changes, the main duct also is irregular. With severe alterations, in addition, large cavities, duct obstruction, intraductular filling defects, and mild dilatation or irregularity of the main pancreatic duct are notable (Fig. 137-9). The limitations of ERCP include its high cost, risk of inducing acute pancreatitis (2% to 3%) and even death (0.1% to 0.2%). Ductal changes may be absent or minimal in many patients with mild alcoholic pancreatitis and in early idiopathic pancreatitis in which such findings may be delayed. It is also difficult to differentiate pancreatic cancer from chronic pancreatitis, based solely on the ductal morphology. However, ERCP offers valuable information on ductal morphology, which is needed before endoscopic or various surgical intervention techniques are decided on and to diagnose extrahepatic biliary obstruction.

Other imaging techniques. Endoscopic ultrasound appears to complement other radiologic studies in improving the accuracy of diagnosis for chronic pancreatitis. This technique identifies parenchymal changes, including cystic abnormalities and hyperechoic foci in the gland; presence of stones or protein plugs in the ducts; and small pseudocysts. Magnetic resonance cholangiopancreatogram appears to be an excellent tool in the evaluation of patients with chronic pancreatitis.

The sonographic secretin test involves ultrasound of the pancreas after secretin stimulation. Patients with chronic pancreatitis demonstrate a longer-lasting dilation of the main pancreatic duct than do control subjects. Currently, there is no clinical value for this test.

Pancreatic Exocrine Function Tests

These tests are traditionally classified as either tubeless tests (indirect tests of pancreatic insufficiency) or tube tests (tests involving duodenal drainage).

Tubeless Tests

The *bentiromide (NBT-PABA) test* depends on intraduodenal hydrolysis by chymotrypsin of a synthetic peptide (bentiromide) bound to *p*-aminobenzoic acid (PABA). The liberated PABA is absorbed, conjugated in the liver, and excreted in the urine. The concentration of conjugated PABA excreted in the urine measures pancreatic secretion of chymotrypsin. The test has marked limitations. Because the pancreas possesses an ample reserve, the test result is positive only in those with marked exocrine insufficiency. In patients with diseases of malabsorption and with liver or kidney disorders, a false-positive test result occurs. Many medications such as sulfonamides, sulfonylureas,

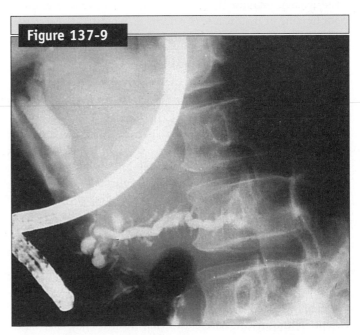

CT scan of the abdomen, showing multiple small calculi distributed throughout the pancreas.

ERCP in chronic pancreatitis. The main pancreatic duct shows strictures and dilations. Many side branches are dilated.

laxatives, diuretics, and pancreatic enzymes, and some foods such as prunes and cranberries, interfere with the test result. False-positive test results may also occur in patients with intestinal bacterial overgrowth syndromes of the gut because some bacteria cleave to NBT-PABA peptide. However, it is a simple test for follow-up in patients with chronic pancreatitis and to determine the need for oral enzyme therapy.

In the *pancreolauryl test* the digestion of di-dodeoic ester of fluorescein by pancreatic lipase is tested after oral administration of the agent. Fluorescein-dilaurate is given with a standard breakfast. The water-soluble molecule is absorbed by the intestine, conjugated by the liver, and excreted in the urine. The conjugate can also be measured in the serum. The test has a low sensitivity in the diagnosis of early chronic pancreatitis and is not available in the United States.

The *fecal chymotrypsin test* has a low sensitivity in the diagnosis of mild or moderate chronic pancreatitis. However, estimation of chymotrypsin in random stool samples is simple and is helpful in follow-up studies of established cases of chronic pancreatitis to assess the progress of the disease. False-positive results are obtained in other malabsorptive diseases, after partial gastrectomy celiac disease, in Crohn's disease, and in cirrhosis.

In the amino-acid consumption test, patients with chronic pancreatitis demonstrate less of a decrement in plasma amino acid concentration than healthy individuals following intravenous administration of secretin and CCK, or cerulein. The decrease in amino acid measures amino acid incorporation into newly synthesized pancreatic enzymes. The test is not sensitive enough to diagnose chronic pancreatitis or even exocrine pancreatic insufficiency.

The *Schilling test*, when used to diagnose chronic pancreatitis, is based on the observation that dietary vitamin B_{12} is bound first to the R-binding protein of saliva, which is then cleaved by pancreatic enzymes at a duodenal pH of 7 or higher, allowing intrinsic factor to bind to the B_{12} molecule. In severe pancreatic insufficiency, vitamin B_{12} absorption is defective as a result of poor binding of B_{12} because of a decrease in bicarbonate secretion and pancreatic enzymes. Although clinically evident, B_{12} deficiency is rare in patients with chronic pancreatitis. The Schilling test result may be abnormal unless bicarbonate supplementation is added. In the dual-labeled Schilling test, (57CO) cobalamin bound to intrinsic factor and (58CO) cobalamin bound to the R protein are simultaneously given and the elimination of both is measured in the urine. In pancreatic insufficiency cobalamin bound to the R protein is poorly absorbed. This test is not clinically useful and complicated to perform, and its validity has not been confirmed.

The principle of the *triolein breath test* is that in pancreatic insufficiency the functional deficiency is in neutral fat hydrolysis and not in fatty acid malabsorption. After ingestion of labeled triolein and a standard breakfast, elimination of (^{14}C) carbon dioxide in the breath is tested. In patients with intestinal malabsorption absorption of both is impaired. In patients with pancreatic insufficiency, triolein not hydrolyzed by lipase reaches the colon, where it is digested by bacteria, liberating (^{14}C) CO_2. This test is not useful except in those with severe exocrine insufficiency, and false-positive results may occur in patients with other causes of malabsorption, hepatic failure, and diabetes mellitus.

The *72-hour stool fat estimation test* does not diagnose chronic pancreatitis, but evaluates steatorrhea and pancreatic insufficiency. The highest fecal excretion of fat is seen in pancreatic insufficiency, with values commonly exceeding 20 g/24 h.

Tube Tests

The *secretin-cholecystokinin test* used to be considered the gold standard but now has become increasingly unpopular and currently is available in only a few specialized medical centers. The test is time consuming and difficult to perform because a special double-lumen tube must be passed, with fluoroscopic guidance, into the second part of the duodenum. After a dose of secretin alone, or with cholecystokinin or cerulein, the volume of pancreatic secretion aspirated and the concentrations of bicarbonate and enzyme concentrations are determined in the duodenal aspirate. As a functional test, the secretin-cholecystokinin test is the most sensitive test for detection of mild to moderate chronic pancreatitis. When properly performed, it correlates well with the histology of the pancreas established by pancreatic wedge biopsy—the real gold standard, available only at surgery. The doses recommended are intravenous 0.6 to 1.0 U /kg/h of secretin and 75 ng/kg/h of cerulein or 40 to 50 ng/kg/h of cholecystokinin for 60 minutes. The bicarbonate concentration gives the best discriminatory value. The test is not to be performed during an acute episode of chronic pancreatitis.

Endoscopic retrograde cholangiopancreatography has replaced the secretin-CCK test as the most reliable and easily available test to diagnose chronic pancreatitis, although interpretation of subtle changes in side branches is often difficult and subjective. The secretin-CCK test is complementary to ERCP in the diagnosis of early chronic pancreatitis. Furthermore, the advantage of secretin-CCK test is that it has no side effects and no risks for patients or investigators. Pure pancreatic juice collected at ERCP can be analyzed for volume, bicarbonate, and enzymes, but it is invasive, expensive, and associated with the risks of ERCP.

The *Lundh test* (an indirect pancreatic stimulation test) is not commonly used in the United States. In this test, a meal containing fat (6%), protein (5%), and carbohydrate (15%) is given to stimulate the pancreas, and tryptic activity is measured in the duodenal aspirate. Pure pancreatic juice collected at ERCP can be analyzed for volume, bicarbonate, and enzymes, but it is invasive, expensive, and associated with the risks of ERCP. Estimations of lactoferrin, pancreatic stone protein, or tumor markers in pure pancreatic juice obtained at ERCP have no value in the diagnosis of chronic pancreatitis. An algorithmic approach to the diagnosis of chronic pancreatitis is given in Figure 137-10.

■ TREATMENT

Continued use of alcohol, narcotic dependence, personality problems, aggressive behavior, and manipulative tendencies (to gain narcotics) are common traits in many patients with chronic pancreatitis. Pain may be the only clinical feature in some patients, whereas in others diabetes and steatorrhea may be complications requiring prompt additional care. Many patients visit several hospital emergency rooms to satisfy their need for narcotics.

All of these features emphasize the need for a multidisciplinary team approach. Participation of an internist as the "gatekeeper" to coordinate care, and a gastroenterologist, psychiatrist, experienced pancreatic surgeon, social worker, and diabetologist as consultants, should be included in this approach. The management of an acute exacerbation of chronic pancreatitis is the same as that of acute pancreatitis. Long-term management and care plans for the most important symptoms or complications are discussed in the following sections [19].

Pain Management

The options available to manage pain are shown in Table 137-5. Before initiating therapy, treatable complications such as pseudocysts, bile duct obstructions, and peptic ulcer disease should be ruled out.

The importance of abstinence from alcohol cannot be overemphasized. Pain relief is usually greater and deterioration of pancreatic function slower in patients who abstain from drinking alcohol. The help of a psychiatrist and/or an Alcoholics Anonymous group is often necessary. The clinical stage of the disease influences the effect of alcohol on pain. In the early stage of the disease with well-preserved pancreatic function, secretagogues, such as alcohol, exaggerate pain; whereas in the advanced stages, alcohol may have very little stimulatory effect on the pancreas, as it is almost totally fibrotic by that time.

For pain relief, the first step is to try nonopioid analgesics such as acetaminophen, salicylates, and nonsteroidal anti-inflammatory drugs, with or without antidepressants. Most patients however, need opioid analgesics for symptomatic relief; initial doses should be low and administered infrequently. Drugs of choice include Darvocet U100 or small doses of codeine derivatives with acetaminophen.

Small, frequent low-fat meals are recommended to minimize pancreatic stimulation. Diet should be nutritious, adequate in calories to achieve and maintain usual body weight, high in protein (24% of calories), moderate in carbohydrates (40%), and low in fat (30%). In patients with severe pain, hospitalization, total cessation of oral intake of food, and short-term use of partial parenteral nutrition or total parenteral nutrition may be needed. Supplementation with vitamins having antioxidant properties reduces recurrence of pain.

The role of oral enzyme therapy in the treatment of pain is controversial. Advocates of enzyme therapy base their opinions on the following:

Intraductal pressure is influenced by the secretory status of the exocrine tissue and obstruction to pancreatic outflow. A protease-dependent, negative-feedback mechanism contributes to the physiologic regulation of pancreatic secretion. Based on these concepts, it is speculated that extremely low levels of intraduodenal proteases in chronic pancreatitis stimulate pancreatic enzyme secretion and increase intraductular pressure

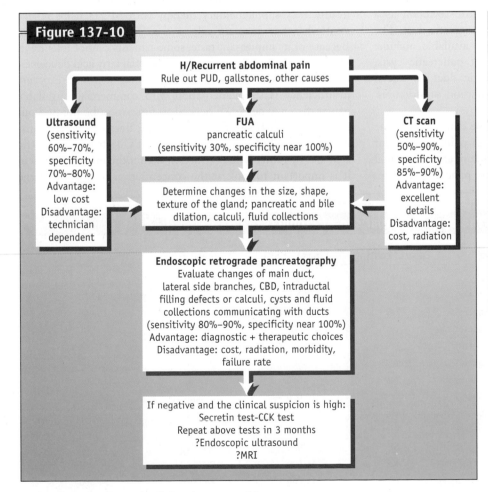

Figure 137-10

H/Recurrent abdominal pain
Rule out PUD, gallstones, other causes

Ultrasound
(sensitivity 60%–70%, specificity 70%–80%)
Advantage: low cost
Disadvantage: technician dependent

FUA
pancreatic calculi
(sensitivity 30%, specificity near 100%)

CT scan
(sensitivity 50%–90%, specificity 85%–90%)
Advantage: excellent details
Disadvantage: cost, radiation

Determine changes in the size, shape, texture of the gland; pancreatic and bile dilation, calculi, fluid collections

Endoscopic retrograde pancreatography
Evaluate changes of main duct, lateral side branches, CBD, intraductal filling defects or calculi, cysts and fluid collections communicating with ducts (sensitivity 80%–90%, specificity near 100%)
Advantage: diagnostic + therapeutic choices
Disadvantage: cost, radiation, morbidity, failure rate

If negative and the clinical suspicion is high:
Secretin test-CCK test
Repeat above tests in 3 months
?Endoscopic ultrasound
?MRI

Approach to the diagnosis of chronic pancreatitis.

Table 137-5. Management of Pain in Chronic Pancreatitis

Medical
  Abstinence from alcohol
  Low-fat diet
  Nonopioid analgesics
  ? High-dose pancreatic enzymes
    (in small duct disease)
  ? Parenteral nutrition
  ? Octreotide injections (investigational)
Endoscopic therapy
  Sphincterotomy, stone extraction
  Septotomy
  Stent placement (short-term)
  Direct chemical dissolution of stones
Surgical therapy
Neurolytic therapy celiac ganglion blockade
Extracorporeal shock wave lithotripsy ?

proximal to strictures. The converse is that adequate amounts of proteases should decrease pancreatic secretion and intraductal pressure. In order to effect feedback inhibition of pancreatic secretion and offer pain relief, it is important to administer large doses of a commercially available nonenteric coated pancreatic enzyme preparation with a high concentration of proteases. However, the best clinical response is seen in a small group of female patients with idiopathic pancreatitis and normal fecal fat excretion. Enzyme therapy is of little value in patients with large duct disease. However, in view of its simplicity and lack of adverse reactions, enzyme therapy may be tried in all patients for 2 to 3 months before attempting other alternatives.

Other modes of medical therapy include the following. Octreotide acetate is a synthetic analogue of somatostatin. When given subcutaneously, it is rapidly absorbed and inhibits pancreatic enzyme release while also suppressing insulin and glucagon secretion. Recent studies have shown conflicting results [20]. If pain relief is achieved, it is often transient and continuous treatment is expensive and impractical.

Dissolution of pancreatic calculi with orally administered citrate and depot secretin therapy to "wash out" the sticky protein-rich secretions and protein plugs in the pancreatic duct are interesting approaches that need further study.

Endoscopic Therapy

The underlying principle of all endoscopic therapies is that the sole or the most important mechanism of pain in chronic pancreatitis is impaired outflow of pancreatic secretion as a result of strictures or calculi in the main pancreatic duct. The forms of endoscopic procedures currently available include: 1) sphincterotomy, 2) internal drainage of pancreatic cysts, 3) extraction of stones from the pancreatic duct, 4) ductal ablation by glues, 5) guidewire-catheter dilation of strictures, and 6) placement of pancreatic stents.

Currently, endoscopic intervention can be considered in the following situations: 1) biliary strictures, 2) pain or recurrent pancreatitis associated with a dominant stricture at the proximal end (head), 3) recurrent pancreatitis with pancreas divisum,

4) pancreatic cysts, 5) pancreatic stones, and 6) sphincter of Oddi dysfunction. The optimistic belief is that these methods may achieve the same results as surgical drainage but without its operative morbidity (20% to 40%) or mortality (2% to 5%). These interventional techniques are all relatively new, and are discussed in detail in Chapter 142.

Neurolytic Therapy

Afferent fibers from the pancreas traverse the celiac plexus along with afferent and efferent sympathetic fibers and some parasympathetic nerves. Celiac plexus block using alcohol or phenol as a neurolytic agent is not only technically difficult, but resultant pain relief is often transient, sometimes lasting only for a few days. Complications include hypotension, epidural or intraperitoneal hematomas, and sexual dysfunction. Neurolytic block is thus considered a therapy of last resort. Surgical management is discussed in Chapter 138.

Management of Pancreatic Insufficiency

A low-fat diet (30 g/d) and frequent small meals, prohibiting alcohol altogether, should be recommended. Substitution of dietary fat with medium-chain triglycerides (MCTs), which are fatty acids 8 to 10 carbon atoms long, may be indicated temporarily to provide calories and promote weight gain in severely malnourished patients. MCTs are better absorbed than the usual dietary fats even in the presence of very small amounts of lipase and in the absence of bile salts. In patients with exocrine insufficiency supplementary therapy with MCTs helps relieve steatorrhea and increase calorie absorption and weight gain. Because of its unpleasant taste, some patients cannot tolerate it. Use of MCTs exclusively may cause essential fatty acid deficiency.

The definitive therapy for the management of exocrine insufficiency is supplementation with commercially available pancreatic enzymes [21]. Several factors are to be pointed out on the scientific basis of enzyme therapy. Because orally administered lipase (but not protease) is mostly destroyed by gastric acid and by proteolytic destruction within the intestinal lumen, it is important to look at the concentration of lipase and the

Table 137-6. Pancreatic Enzyme Therapy: A Comparison of Products

Enzyme preparation	Tablet/capsule	Enteric coating	Lipase (USP)	Protease (USP)	Amylase (USP)
Cotazym (Organon)	Capsules (powder)	No	8000	30,000	30,000
Cotazym-S	Capsules (microsphere)	Yes	5000	20,000	20,000
Creon 5 (Solvay)	Capsules (microsphere)	Yes	5000	18,750	16,600
Creon 10	Capsules (microsphere)	Yes	10,000	37,500	32,200
Creon 20	Capsules (microsphere)	Yes	20,000	75,000	64,400
Pancrease (McNeil)	Capsules (microsphere)	Yes	4500	25,000	20,000
Pancrease MT 4	Capsules (microsphere)	Yes	4000	12,000	12,000
Pancrease MT 10	Capsules (microsphere)	Yes	10,000	30,000	30,000
Pancrease MT 16	Capsules (microsphere)	Yes	16,000	48,000	48,000
Pancrease MT 20	Capsules (microsphere)	Yes	20,000	44,000	56,000
Viokase (Robins)	Tablets	No	8000	30,000	30,000
	Powder (1/4 spoon)	No	16,800	70,000	70,000
Zymase (Organon)	Capsules (spheres)	Yes	12,000	24,000	24,000

form of the enzyme preparation (tablet vs acid-resistant enteric-coated tablets or capsules) (Tables 137-6 and 137-7). It is necessary to administer up to 5- to 10-fold more lipase than that normally required in the duodenum. To deliver such high concentrations one has to take a large number of tablets, up to eight with each meal, which, because of the high cost and other factors, may decrease patient compliance.

Enteric-coated tablets or capsules have a tendency to be retained in the stomach during digestion of a meal and delivered into the duodenum only in the subsequent interdigestive state—an asynchrony that makes the enzymes less effective. However, the lipase released subsequently may shift fat digestion and absorption to the distal small intestine.

Layer and Holtmann [21] recommend enteric-coated microspheres (in contrast to the nonenteric-coated preparation that is preferred in pain management), stating that they are more effective, less expensive, and better tolerated. Choosing an enzyme preparation from the many different preparations in the form of tablets, capsules, powders, and enteric-coated and acid-resistant capsules is difficult. To diminish severe steatorrhea (>20 g/24 h of fecal fat) to a lower, more acceptable range (<15 g/24 h of fecal fat) it is usually necessary to administer at least 25,000 to 40,000 U of lipase/meal. A common mistake is not in the choice of the preparation but in the dosage, which is often too small. Weight gain and improvement in stool consistency are the markers of satisfactory enzyme therapy. When the response is poor, one has to check the compliance of the patient taking such large quantities of enzymes or to exclude other associated causes of malabsorption, including bacterial overgrowth or *Giardia lamblia* infestation. The addition of an H_2-receptor antagonist or proton-pump inhibitor (to decrease gastric acidity and prevent destruction of enzymes), and bicarbonate (to achieve a suitable pH for the enzymes to act), is needed in some patients. Fat-soluble vitamin deficiency is a rare problem. Supplementation of vitamins A and D is to be given if symptoms of night blindness, bone pain, or a high bone alkaline phosphatase is noted. In those with excessive bruising or a bleeding tendency vitamin K supplementation is required. There is insufficient evidence to prohibit a high-fiber diet; some studies, however, have indicated that in patients with severe exocrine insufficiency such a diet may inhibit pancreatic lipase.

Table 137-7. Pancreatic Enzyme Therapy

Interaction
 A high-fiber diet may inhibit enzymes

Contraindication
 Allergy to pork protein

Side effects
 Hyperuricosuria (high doses in CF)
 Impairment of folate absorption
 Impairment of iron absorption
 ? Colonic stricture (high doses)

For steatorrhea
 Enteric-coated capsules

For pain
 High-dose nonenteric-coated tablets

Management of Pancreatic Diabetes

Hypoglycemia is a common cause of death in individuals with diabetes secondary to chronic pancreatitis. Patients must be educated to recognize its early symptoms and to initiate prompt self-management. Abstinence from alcohol use should be emphasized. Problems with steatorrhea, malabsorption of carbohydrate and proteins, and associated liver disease should be considered when prescribing a diet for these patients. The diet for persons with pancreatic diabetes should help to effect weight gain and not weight loss. In those with malabsorption, calories should be increased by at least 50%, by increasing the protein and carbohydrate to compensate for the erratic absorption. Food intake should be divided into six meals per day instead of the traditional three meals.

Oral hypoglycemic agents are of value in the early stages of pancreatic diabetes. In administering insulin therapy, caution must be used in its dosage, timing of injections, frequency, and type of insulin used. It is important to err on the side of under-insulinization rather than to aim for normoglycemia. The insulin requirement varies because of the insulin resistance seen in many patients. The incidence of diabetes and worsening of preexisting diabetes increases after pancreatic resection.

■ PROGNOSIS

The typical patient with alcoholic pancreatitis returns to the emergency room more and more frequently with pain, which becomes constant and requires round-the-clock doses of a narcotic analgesic. In course, the patient starts losing weight, develops steatorrhea, demonstrates evidence of nutritional deficiency, and ultimately develops brittle diabetes.

Patients who continue to drink alcohol have a lower survival rate than those who discontinue or decrease alcohol intake. Pancreatic calculi may increase in density, number, and size with increasing duration of disease. The development of pancreatic calculi is closely related to the onset of steatorrhea. In a subgroup of patients with alcoholic chronic pancreatitis, individuals do not progress to advanced chronic pancreatitis and are considered to have chronic nonprogressive pancreatitis.

The concomitant presence of alcoholic liver disease and alcoholic pancreatitis is much more common than previously reported. Significant liver disease may be seen in up to 40% of patients with chronic pancreatitis. The adverse prognostic factors in chronic pancreatitis include continued alcoholism, cigarette smoking, insulin-dependent diabetes mellitus–associated liver disease, and advancing age.

■ REFERENCES

Recently published papers of particular interest have been highlighted as follows:
- • Of interest
- •• Of outstanding interest

1.•• Go VLW, Everhart JE: Pancreatitis in digestive diseases in the United States: epidemiology and impact. US Department of Health and Human Services. Public Health Service. National Institute of Diabetes and Digestive and Kidney Diseases. May 1994; 693–712.
This is an outstanding paper on the epidemiologic aspects of acute and chronic pancreatitis in the United States. The varying prevalence of the disease in different ethnic groups points to genetic, environmental, and nutritional factors in the etiology of alcoholic pancreatitis.

2.• Kloppel G, Maillet B: Pathology of acute and chronic pancreatitis. *Pancreas* 1993, 8:659–670.

In this paper, Kloppel challenges the Marseille concept of alcoholic pancreatitis being chronic from its onset. In the necrosis-fibrosis sequence, chronic alcoholic pancreatitis is the result of recurrent attacks of acute pancreatitis.

3.   Buchler M, Weihe E, Friess H, *et al.*: Changes in peptidergic innervation in chronic pancreatitis. *Pancreas* 1992, 7:183–192.

4.•• Pitchumoni CS, Bordalo O: Evaluation of hypotheses on pathogenesis of alcoholic pancreatitis. *Am J Gastroenterol* 1996, 91:637–647.

This is an updated review on the pathogenesis of alcoholic pancreatitis.

5.•• Sarles H, Bernard JP: Lithostathine and pancreatic lithogenesis. *View Points on Digestive Diseases* 1991, 23:6–12.

In this article, Sarles and coworkers, who pioneered the concept of stone protein, nicely summarize the complex biochemical details of pancreatic stone protein or lithostathine.

6.   Braganza JB: The pancreas. In *Recent Advances in Gastroenterology*. Edited by Pounder RE. Edinburgh: Churchill Livingstone. 1986; 251–280.

7.   Cavallini G, Talamini G, Vaona P, *et al.*: Effect of alcohol and smoking on pancreatic lithogenesis in the course of chronic pancreatitis. *Pancreas* 1994, 9:42–46.

8.   Kloppel G, Maillet B: The morphological basis for the evolution of acute pancreatitis into chronic pancreatitis. *Virch Arch A Pathol Anat Histopathol* 1992, 420:1–4.

9.• Pitchumoni CS: Juvenile Tropical Pancreatitis in Pediatric Gastrointestinal Disease. Edited by Walker WA, Durie PR, Hamilton JR, *et al.* St Louis: CV Mosby; 1996:1502–1510.

This article provides a comprehensive review of the data on tropical pancreatitis, studied in many Afro-Asian countries.

10.•• Layer P, Yamamoto H, Kalthoff L, *et al.*: The different courses of early-and-late-onset idiopathic and alcoholic pancreatitis. *Gastroenterology* 1994, 107:1481–1487.

This elegant study distinguishes for the first time the two types of idiopathic pancreatitis and describes their natural history.

11.   Ammann RW: Natural history of chronic (progressive) pancreatitis. A life experience In *Chronic Pancreatitis*. Edited by Beger HG, Buchler M, Ditschuneit H, Malfertheiner P. Berlin Heidelberg: Springer-Verlag; 1990:47–62.

12.   DiMagno EP: Laboratory assessment of pancreatic impairment. In *Bockus Gastroenterology*. Edited by Haubrich WS, Schaffer F, Berk JE. Philadelphia: WB Saunders; 1995:2835–2850.

13.   Cavallini G, Vaona B, Bovo P, *et al.*: Diabetes in chronic alcoholic pancreatitis: role of residual β cell function and insulin resistance. *Dig Dis Sci* 1993, 38:497–501.

14.   Rocca G, Gaia E, Juliano M: Increased incidence of cancer in chronic pancreatitis. *J Clin Gastroenterol* 1987, 9:175–179.

15.•• Lowenfels AB, Maisonneuve P, Cavallini G, *et al.*: Pancreatitis and the risk of pancreatic cancer. *N Engl J Med* 1993, 38:1433–1437.

This international cooperative study clearly documents that all forms of chronic pancreatitis are associated with a high incidence of pancreatic cancer.

16.   Bank S, Chow KW: Diagnostic tests in Chronic Pancreatitis. *The Gastroenterologist* 1994, 2:224–232.

17.   Gumaste VK, Dave PB, Weissman D, *et al.*: Lipase/Amylase ratio: a new index that distinguishes episodes of alcoholic from non-alcoholic acute pancreatitis. *Gastroenterology* 1991, 101:1361–1366.

18.   Freeny PC: Imaging of Chronic Pancreatitis: a synopsis in chronic pancreatitis. *Edited by Beger HG, Buchler M, Ditschuneit H, Malfertheiner P. Berlin: Springer-Verlag* 1990;330–341.

19.   Toskes PP: Medical management of chronic pancreatitis. *Scand J Gastroenterol* 1995, (suppl)208:74–80.

20.   Malfertheiner P, Mayer D, Buchler M, *et al.*: Treatment of pain in chronic pancreatitis by inhibition of pancreatic secretion with Octreotide. *Gut* 1995, 36:450–454.

21.   Layer P, Holtmann G: Pancreatic enzymes in chronic pancreatitis. *Int J Pancreatol* 1994, 15:1–11.

138 Surgical Management of Chronic Pancreatitis

Eric J. Kraut and Charles F. Frey

Surgical indications for chronic pancreatitis are intractable epigastric back pain, local complications, and suspicion of cancer.

■ PAIN
Surgical Indications

Not all patients with chronic pancreatitis have significant or persistent pain. Many patients with only mild pain often have spontaneous pain relief over the course of a decade ("pancreas burnout") [1••]. Nevertheless, pain remains the most common reason for operative intervention in patients with chronic pancreatitis. Surgical intervention is indicated for pain relief in chronic pancreatitis when pain interferes substantially with the patient's quality of life or the patient requires frequent use of narcotics for pain relief.

In patients with a dilated pancreatic duct (>3 mm), and in some patients with narrower ducts [2], it is believed that the pain may be caused by ductal hypertension (normal pressure 8–12 cm H_2O) stimulating the stretch fibers in the duct wall. Neural or perineural inflammation may initiate or contribute to pancreatic pain [1••]. Although patients may have more than one cause of pain, fibrosis and inflammation are the underlying pathophysiologic disturbances; a duct may be obstructed by calcium carbonate calculi or by single or multiple fibrotic strictures. The effects of abstinence from alcohol on pain are unpredictable [2], although abstinence does seem to slow but not prevent the progression of exocrine and endocrine insufficiency. The pain is managed medically until it is intractable or the patient is at risk of developing narcotic dependence. Medical measures used in the treatment of chronic pancreatitis include a low-fat diet and oral pancreatic enzyme therapy with trypsin and chymotrypsin to inhibit the cholecystokinin-releasing factor (see Chapter 137). Pharmacologic suppression of pancreatic secretions using somatostatin also has been used with variable success to diminish the pain of chronic pancreatitis.

Morphologic findings that are indicative of potential benefit from surgical intervention are an inflammatory mass in the head of the pancreas, a pseudocyst, diffuse alterations of the pancreatic ductal system, and extensive pancreatic calcifications. Nealon has reported that decompression of the major ductal systems may slow the progressive loss of pancreatic endocrine and exocrine function characteristic of chronic pancreatitis, although it does not reverse the damage that has already been done [3••]. If Nealon's work is confirmed, amelioration of exocrine and endocrine insufficiency could be an important indication for operation in chronic pancreatitis even in the absence of pain.

Surgical Procedures for Pain

Surgical procedures for pain relief include splanchnic nerve ablation, duct decompression, and pancreatic resection. There is no one best operation for pain relief for all patients with chronic pancreatitis. The surgeon must address the structural abnormalities, the site and severity of disease, and the degree of remaining pancreatic endocrine and exocrine function as well as the patient's emotional and physical health. A nutritional assessment should be done. Patients who have lost more than 20% of their ideal body weight [4] may require preoperative parenteral nutrition. To compare the results of various therapeutic modalities in the care of patients with chronic pancreatitis, it is necessary to use reproducible objective assessments of the severity of pain and quality of life pre- and postoperatively. We use a pain scale of 0 (no pain) to 10 (worst pain imaginable). Narcotic intake is categorized as minimal (Vicodin or equivalent required once or twice a month), moderate (Vicodin weekly to daily), and major (Demerol or equivalent weekly to daily). The patient's quality of life also is assessed [5]. This assessment attempts to quantify to what degree the patient's pain interferes with activities of daily living.

Splanchnic Nerve Ablation

Pain relief has been reported after splanchnicectomy using either a thoracotomic or thoracoscopic approach [6]. Midepigastric and left-sided pain is treated with left splanchnic nerve resection, and right-sided pain is treated with right splanchnic nerve resection. Studies have not been large enough and follow-up has not been long enough to propose splanchnicectomy as a routine treatment.

Drainage Procedures

The rationale for duct decompression is based on evidence showing high pressure in the pancreatic ducts of patients with chronic pancreatitis [7••]. Normal duct pressure averages 8 to 12 cm of water; in patients with chronic pancreatitis this pressure averages 33 cm of water. Visceral pain is thought to be initiated when the obstructed duct dilates. Duct decompression is an effective treatment and at least 80% of patients initially report complete or significant relief of pain. Controversy exists over how large the main pancreatic duct should be before successful

duct decompression can be expected. Some surgeons believe that pain relief is less likely to result when the duct is smaller than 3 to 5 mm in diameter [8], although we have found it possible to decompress ducts as small as 2.5 to 3 mm with comparable pain relief to that experienced by patients who have had a large duct decompressed [8]. The most commonly performed operation for pain relief is longitudinal pancreaticojejunostomy (LPJ). LPJ may fail to control pain if the duct is not opened to the tail or the duodenum [9] (Fig. 138-1) and when disease is not limited to the main pancreatic duct. LPJ does not address disease in the head of the pancreas and uncinate process, areas drained by the duct of Santorini and the duct of the uncinate process along with their tributary ducts (Fig. 138-2). This may explain why, in some patients, initial reports of pain relief are not sustained over 3 to 5 years [7,10].

Resection Procedures

In the 1960s and 1970s, the most common operation for chronic pancreatitis was an 80% to 95% distal pancreatectomy, which left the remaining 15% to 20% of the proximal pancreas intact. Such distal pancreatectomy resulted in a high incidence of endocrine and exocrine insufficiency; the incidence of diabetes mellitus was found to increase from 28% preoperatively to 72% postoperatively [11••]. Pancreaticoduodenectomy was less frequently employed because it was associated with high mortality rates [7]. Currently performed procedures, including local resection of the head of the pancreas combined with LPJ (Figs. 138-3 and 138-6) and duodenum-preserving local resection (DPLR) of the head of the pancreas resect only 5% to 35% of the gland. Both operations have a lower incidence of endocrine and exocrine insufficiency while providing adequate pain relief [12,13••]. Local resection of the head of the pancreas combined with LPJ (LR-LPJ) was designed to treat the patient with chronic pancreatic pain who has a combination of the following conditions: a multiple-strictured main pancreatic duct; a markedly enlarged fibrotic pancreatic head and uncinate process

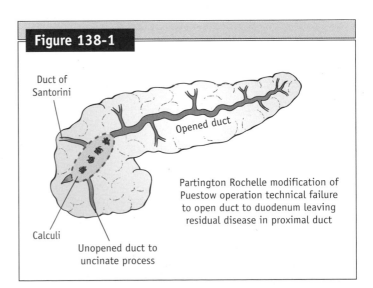

Figure 138-1

Duct of Santorini

Opened duct

Partington Rochelle modification of Puestow operation technical failure to open duct to duodenum leaving residual disease in proximal duct

Calculi

Unopened duct to uncinate process

In the Partington Rochelle operation the main pancreatic duct is opened longitudinally from the tail of the pancreas to the duodenum. Failure to open the duct to the duodenum leaves residual disease in the proximal duct and does not accomplish the operation as it was concieved.

with calculi; and small pseudocysts along the ducts of Santorini and Wirsung, the uncinate duct and their tributary ducts, and a dilated duct in the body and tail of the pancreas (Fig. 138-4, see also **Color Plate**). Total pancreatectomy rarely is used as the initial procedure in the management of pain in patients with chronic pancreatitis because pancreatic endocrine and exocrine insufficiency are inevitable consequences of this procedure and the pain relief it offers is not much better than that of other procedures [14].

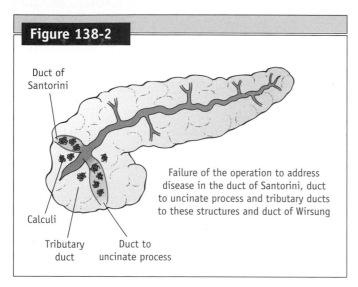

Figure 138-2

Duct of Santorini

Calculi

Tributary duct

Duct to uncinate process

Failure of the operation to address disease in the duct of Santorini, duct to uncinate process and tributary ducts to these structures and duct of Wirsung

Failure of the Partington Rochelle modification of the Puestow operation to address disease in the duct of Santorini, duct to uncinate, tributary ducts to these structures, and duct of Wirsung.

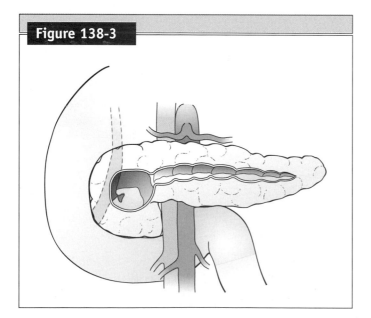

Figure 138-3

The main pancreatic duct is opened longitudinally in the body and the tail; the head of the pancreas is cored out. A margin of at least 4-mm is maintained medially between the coring-out process and the superior mesenteric and portal veins. A cuff of at least 3 to 4mm of pancreas is retained along the medial aspect of the duodenum. The depth of the coring-out process is gauged with the surgeon's hand behind the Kocherized duodenum and the head of the pancreas. If the position of the common bile duct is not readily discernible its position can be ascertained by intubating it with a Bakes dilator.

Whole organ or islet autotransplantation has been used in small populations of patients with chronic pancreatitis. It has been demonstrated that total or near-total pancreatectomy combined with autologous islet transplantation may prevent long-term diabetes in more than 33% of patients [15••]. Islets are freed from acinar tissue using collagenase. They are washed and placed in sterile syringes. The mean time required for this process is 105 ± 7 minutes. The pancreatic islets are returned to the patient by injecting them into the portal venous system or beneath the kidney capsule in cases of portal vein thrombosis. Eighty percent of the patients with islet autotransplantation in Sutherland's report had pain relief from this procedure [15••]. The main predictor of insulin independence was the number of islets transplanted. In patients who received more than 300,000 islets, 74% were insulin independent in 2 years. Autotransplantation can only be used in a small percentage (probably < 5%) of subjects with chronic pancreatitis. Candidates for islet autotransplantation may be those with small ducts (< 2.5 mm) who are non-diabetic and whose gland is not too fibrotic because the number of recoverable islet cells correlates with the degree of fibrosis [15••]. Segmental pancreatic autotransplantation also has been performed in 13 subjects with 11 successful grafts [16••].

Results

Operative Mortality

Table 138-1, which is based on collective series of retrospective and prospective studies reported since 1986, lists the operative and late mortality rates of a variety of operations to relieve the pain associated with chronic pancreatitis [9,10,16••,17,18••, 19,20]. The lowest operative mortality rate is associated with preservation of the duodenum; the highest rate is associated with pancreatectomy. The operative mortality of pancreaticojejunostomy has decreased from 10% to 20% in the 1970s and 1980s to as low as 1.1% in the late 1980s early 1990s [21]. The most common complication following pancreaticoduodenectomy is delayed gastric emptying; the most serious complication is an anastomic leak at the pancreaticojejunostomy site. The incidence of leak at the pancreaticojejunostomy site is dependent on the type of anastomosis performed—duct-to-mucosa (6%)

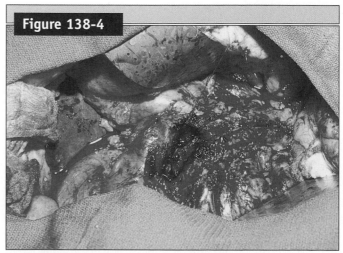

Figure 138-4

Local resection of the head of the pancreas with longitudinal pancreaticojejunostomy. See also **Color Plate**.

[22] or stuffing or invaginational (12%–18%) [23,••,24] —and the degree of fibrosis in the gland (ie, the more fibrosis the lower the incidence of leak) [23••].

Late Mortality

Most late deaths after operations for management of pain or complications of chronic pancreatitis are due to the effects of continued alcoholism and chronic pancreatitis. The incidence of late death is considerably higher in the alcoholic than in the nonalcoholic patient. In the United States, less than 60% of alcoholic patients survive 10 years after a 80% to 95% distal pancreatectomy or a longitudinal pancreaticojejunostomy. Table 138-2 lists the causes of late deaths for chronic pancreatitis [9,10,16••,17,18••,19,20]. Forty-nine percent of late deaths are due to the effects of alcoholism. Complications of diabetes account for another 10% of deaths. The incidence and cause of late deaths are unrelated to the type of procedure performed [25]. Long-term survival rates have been better in some of the series from Europe than in series from the United States [26••], perhaps because of the different patient populations. In European cultures, the percentage of patients with alcoholic pancreatitis who drink because of social custom exceeds the percentage of those who binge drink, whereas in the United States, addicted binge drinkers predominate (Gullo and Ammann, Personal communication).

Pain Relief

Longitudinal pancreaticojejunostomy provides initial relief in 80% of patients, but Bradley [27••] and the Lahey Clinic group [28••] found that pain recurred in 30% at 5 years. Long-term pain relief is 80% with proximal and distal resections if the most diseased portion of the gland is removed [12]. An 80% to 95% distal pancreatectomy provides long-term pain relief in 75% to 80% of subjects at 6.7-year follow-up; a less than 80% distal pancreatectomy is associated with an 85% rate of pain relief at 5.8-year follow-up [11••]; 50% to 60% distal pancreatectomy results in pain relief in 80% of the subjects [29••] if there is no evidence of disease in the head of the pancreas based on computed tomography (CT) scan, endoscopic retrograde cholangiopancreatography (ERCP), and assessment at operation.

Table 138-1. Operative Mortality, Late Mortality, Pain Relief, and Average Length of Follow-up After Surgical Procedures for Chronic Pancreatitis

Procedures*	Operative mortality, (%)	Late mortality, (%)	Pain relief, %	Average length of follow-up, y
LPJ	12/425 (2.8)	67/413 (16.2)	81	6.5
TP	10/163 (6.1)	67/153 (43.8)	73	5.8
TP-AIT	1/43 (2.3)	6/43 (4.0)	81	5.0
DP	4/187 (2.1)	15/183 (8.2)	85	5.5
PD	6/555 (1.1)	73/443 (16.5)	82	4.0
DPLR	5/582 (0.9)	38/537 (7.1)	88	4.4
LR-LPJ	0/75 (0)	5/75 (6.7)	88	3.2

*LPJ—longitudinal pancreaticojejunostomy; TP—total pancreatectomy; TP-AIT—total or near total pancreatectomy with islet cell transplantation; DP—less than 80% distal pancreatectomy; PD—pancreaticoduodenectomy; DPLR—duodenum-preserving local resection of the head of the pancreas; LR-LPJ—local resection of the head of the pancreas combined with longitudinal pancreaticojejunostomy.

Data from references 9,10,16••,17,18••,19,20.

Table 138-2. Etiology of Late Death After Procedures for Chronic Pancreatitis

Procedures*	n	Alcohol-related causes, (%)	Diabetes complications, (%)	Pancreatic cancer, (%)	Other cancers, (%)	Unrelated causes, (%)
LPJ	67	25 (37.4)	7 (10.4)	7 (10.4)	11 (16.4)	17 (25.4)
TP	26	1 (3.8)	5 (19)	0	16 (64)	4 (16)
DP	15	3 (20)	1 (6.7)	2 (13.3)	2 (13.3)	7 (46.7)
PD	77	38 (32)	8 (11)	0	11 (15.1)	20 (16.9)
DPLR	15	13 (86.6)	1 (6.7)	0	1 (6.7)	0
LR-LPJ	5	3 (60)	0	0	0	2 (40)
Total	205	98 (40)	22 (8.9)	9 (3.7)	26 (10.6)	50 (20)

*LPJ—longitudinal pancreaticojejunostomy; TP—total pancreatectomy; DP—less than 80% distal pancreatectomy; PD—pancreaticoduodenectomy; DPLR—duodenum-preserving local resection of the head of the pancreas; LR-LPJ—local resection of the head of the pancreas combined with longitudinal pancreaticojejunostomy.

Data from references 9,10,16••,17,18••,19,20.

If there is disease in the head, tail, and body of the pancreas, the newer operations (*ie*, LR-LPJ and DPLR of the head of the pancreas) are indicated. These operations give similar results at mean follow-up of 3.2 and 4.4 years and have lower operative mortality rate than other procedures for chronic pancreatitis (Table 138-1). Izbicki prospectively compared duodenum-preserving pancreatic head resection and LR-LPJ and found no difference in either the safety of operation or its efficacy in pain relief [13••].

Endocrine and Exocrine Function

All pancreatic resection procedures diminish the endocrine and exocrine functions of the gland (Table 138-3) [16••,18••]. Eighty to 95% distal resection is followed by a 72% incidence of diabetes mellitus, whereas a less than 80% distal pancreatectomy results in a 45% incidence of diabetes.

Pancreaticoduodenectomy is associated with 53% incidence of diabetes within 4.2 years [21,22,23••,24]. In part, the loss of endocrine and exocrine function following operation is attributable to progressive sclerosis of the gland and continuing disease, not the operation. Even patients who undergo longitudinal pancreaticojejunostomy and from whom no pancreatic tissue has been removed and patients with chronic pancreatitis with mild pain who avoid operation will be seen to develop endocrine and exocrine insufficiency the longer they are followed [3,16••].

▄▄ LOCAL COMPLICATIONS OF CHRONIC PANCREATITIS

Local complications of chronic pancreatitis include disruption of the pancreatic ductal system, obstruction of the biliary or gastrointestinal tract, and vascular damage.

Disruption of the Pancreatic Ductal System

Disruption of the pancreatic ductal system occurs in 20% to 50% of patients operated on for chronic pancreatitis and can result in pancreatic and peripancreatic fluid collections. If these fluid collections persist, they will develop a wall and qualify as pseudocysts, pancreatic fistula, or pancreatic ascites.

Persistent collections of fluid become enclosed by a fibrous wall in 6 to 8 weeks, thus forming a pseudocyst. Not all pseudocysts require operative management. Regardless of their size, pseudocysts that are asymptomatic and not compressing vital structures do not require operative intervention. Pain, infection, hemorrhage, enlargement, rupture, and common bile duct or duodenal obstruction are indications for operation.

Pseudocysts are the most common complication of chronic pancreatitis, developing in the head (37.8%), body (14.6%), tail (37.5%), and multiple sites (10.2%) of the pancreas [30]. A key to successful operative management of pseudocysts is to define the structural pathology in the main pancreatic ducts of Wirsung, Santorini, and the uncinate process. When there are multiple sites of obstruction, the entire pancreatic ductal system must be decompressed by longitudinal pancreaticojejunostomy to prevent pain or recurrent pseudocyst formation.

In chronic pancreatitis, pancreatic fistulas can occur between the disrupted duct and the chest, the gastrointestinal tract, or the free peritoneal cavity if the fluid is not contained as a pseudocyst (Fig. 138-5).

Pancreatic ascites also can occur when a pseudocyst or retention cyst ruptures and pancreatic juice leaks into the peritoneal cavity. Pancreatic ascites often resolves spontaneously (45% of the cases resolve in 2 weeks). If the pancreatic ascites persists for more than 3 weeks, the mortality and treatment failure are higher with nonoperative management, including fasting and parenteral alimentation, than with operative management [31]. If there is a single point of obstruction in the main pancreatic duct proximal to the ductal disruption, a Roux-en-Y pancreaticojejunostomy to the fistula will drain the fistula or ascites. If there are multiple sites of obstruction, a Roux-en-Y longitudinal pancreaticojejunostomy will be necessary.

Obstruction of the Biliary or Gastrointestinal Tract

Obstruction of the biliary or pancreatic ductal system may be caused by fibrosis of the pancreatic parenchyma or a pseudocyst. Fibrosis or pseudocyst also can obstruct the duodenum, resulting in gastrointestinal obstruction; or it can obstruct the common bile duct, producing jaundice, and thrombose the portal or splenic vein, causing portal vein hypertension and gastric variceal hemorrhage.

Table 138-3. Endocrine and Exocrine Function Before and After Surgical Intervention in Chronic Pancreatitis

Procedures*	Diabetes		Steatorrhea		Average length
	Preoperative, %	Postoperative, %	Preoperative, %	Postoperative, %	Follow-up, *y*
LPJ	19	35	25	35	6.5
> 80% DP	4	72	29	74	5.5
< 80% DP	22	45	27	70	5.5
PD	20	51	46	73	4.3
DPLR	19	35	55	70	2.7
LR-LPJ	20	29	24	41	3.2

*LPJ—longitudinal pancreaticojejunostomy; PD—pancreaticoduodenectomy; DPLR—duodenum-preserving local resection of the head of the pancreas; LR-LPJ—local resection of the head of the pancreas combined with longitudinal pancreaticojejunostomy.
From Adloff et al. [17], with permission.

Biliary stricture is the most common complication of chronic pancreatitis other than pseudocyst. ERCP examinations of the biliary tract will show narrowing or distortion of the duct in 50% to 60% of patients, but these anatomic abnormalities are biochemically and clinically significant in only 6% of patients. Indications for operation on patients with biliary stricture in chronic pancreatitis include proximal dilation of the intrahepatic biliary tree, persistence of serum alkaline phosphatase levels of three to four times the upper limit of normal for 4 to 6 weeks, or jaundice for a similar period. Surgery is performed to prevent recurrent attacks of cholangitis (a 9.5% incidence) and biliary cirrhosis (a 5.2% incidence). Surgical options include choledochojejunostomy if the patient is having no pancreatic pain and either LR-LPJ or DPLR in patients experiencing pancreatic pain. The operative mortality of LR-LPJ or DPLR is 1.5%. If the duodenum is obstructed, gastrojejunostomy is required. When both biliary and duodenal obstruction are present, pancreaticoduodenectomy may be necessary.

Vascular Complications

Pseudoaneurysm, thrombosis, and rupture of peripancreatic vessels may occur in as many as 17% of patients with chronic pancreatitis [32]. Pseudoaneurysms of the pancreatic and peripancreatic vessels are more often a complication of a pseudocyst (occurring in 5% of patients with pseudocysts) than the sclero-

sis accompanying chronic pancreatitis. Pseudoaneurysms most commonly involve the splenic artery and, in decreasing order of frequency, the gastroduodenal, pancreaticoduodenal, gastric, and hepatic arteries. If a pseudoaneurysm is identified by angiography in either the bleeding or asymptomatic patient, an effort should be made to embolize the involved artery at the time of the procedure. The site of active bleeding from pseudoaneurysms and feeding vessels is difficult to identify and control during surgery because of the intense inflammatory reaction in pseudocysts in and around the pancreas.

Splenic vein thrombosis occurs most commonly in association with pseudocysts of the body or tail of the pancreas and almost invariably occurs when there is a pseudoaneurysm of the splenic artery. Splenic vein thrombosis may be associated with left-sided portal hypertension severe enough to cause gastric varices; however, bleeding gastric varices are seen in only 10% to 20% of such patients. Splenectomy is curative. Preoperative embolization of the splenic artery will prevent unnecessary blood loss at splenectomy. Portal vein thrombosis is less common than splenic vein thrombosis but also may be responsible for portal hypertension and bleeding esophageal varices.

■ SUSPICION OF CANCER

Malignancy may masquerade as benign disease in patients believed to have alcoholic or idiopathic chronic pancreatitis. Chronic pancreatitis is a known risk factor for cancer of the pancreas [33••,34••]. Between 1.8% and 3% of patients with chronic pancreatitis develop cancer after 10 years, and 4% develop cancer after 20 years [2,33••]. The incidence of cancer in chronic pancreatitis is 26.3 times that of a country-specific group without cancer adjusted for age and sex. Cancer risk is

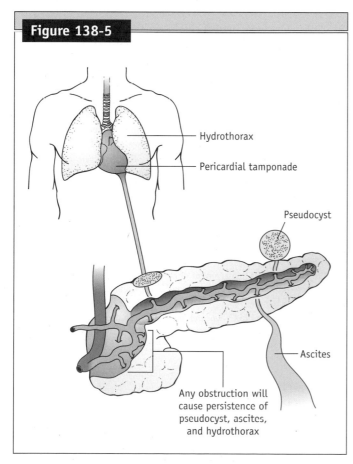

Figure 138-5

Obstruction of the main pancreatic duct may cause persistent communication of the pancreatic duct to the peritoneal cavity or the chest leading to pancreatic ascites, pericardial tamponade, or hydrothorax.

Labels in figure: Hydrothorax; Pericardial tamponade; Pseudocyst; Ascites; Any obstruction will cause persistence of pseudocyst, ascites, and hydrothorax

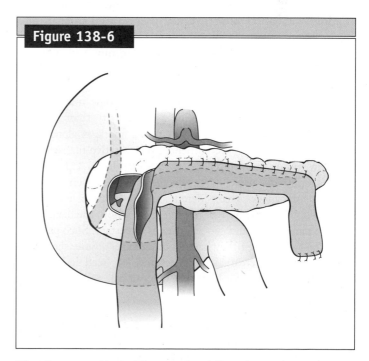

Figure 138-6

After the pancreatic duct is opened and the pancreas is cored out, a Roux-en-Y limb is sutured to the main pancreatic duct and the cored-out head of the pancreas in two layers: an inner layer of continuous 000 PDS (polydioxanone) and an outer layer of interrupted 000 silk.

believed to be due to chronic inflammation and appears to be independent of the type of chronic pancreatitis (ie, alcoholic, idiopathic, tropical) [33••]. Conversely, cancer of the pancreas may induce obstructive pancreatitis, pseudocysts, and acute pancreatitis by obstructing the major pancreatic duct. These latter conditions may divert the clinician's attention from the underlying cancer. Even when the diagnosis of cancer is considered preoperatively, in 10% to 20% of patients it may be difficult to distinguish between chronic pancreatitis and cancer.

Clues in the history, laboratory, and radiologic findings favor one diagnosis over the other. A history of alcohol abuse does not exclude cancer, but the absence of alcohol abuse in a patient who appears to have a new onset of chronic pancreatitis should raise concern of cancer. A progressive rise of total serum bilirubin to 15 to 20 mg/dL or greater is very suggestive of cancer. Patients with common bile duct obstruction secondary to chronic pancreatitis rarely have a total serum bilirubin level greater than 10.9 mg/dL (average of 3.9 mg/dL). Elevated bilirubin levels in patients with chronic pancreatitis often fluctuate as the pancreatitis waxes and wanes. In chronic pancreatitis, this elevated bilirubin level normally subsides 1 week after the inflammation has resolved.

The CA 19-9 serum marker is often helpful in differentiating chronic pancreatitis from cancer of the pancreas. In a patient without bile duct obstruction or liver disease, progressive elevation of the CA 19-9 is characteristic of pancreatic cancer.

Radiologic features characteristic of pancreatic cancer are 1) ERCP-documented "double duct" sign, which is due to obstruction of both biliary and pancreatic ducts; 2) smooth or shoulder tapering of the intrapancreatic portion of the common bile duct with dilation of the intrahepatic biliary ducts; and 3) a solid pancreatic mass on CT or a cystic lesion with striations, lobulation, or an irregular wall or solid components. A pancreatic mass on CT that appears as a less vascularized region after intravenous contrast has been administered is characteristic of pancreatic cancer.

In patients with chronic pancreatitis or a high suspicion for pancreatic cancer, the combined use of radiologic imaging and serum tumor markers yields a higher sensitivity than imaging alone and a higher specificity than tumor markers alone [35]. Therefore, we routinely recommend a preoperative management of serum tumor markers (CEA, CA 19-9) and a CT scan in patients with high suspicion for pancreatic cancer. Even when the diagnosis of cancer is considered and appropriate assessment performed, there may be 10% of patients in whom the distinction between pancreatitis and cancer remains uncertain. Such patients should be treated as if they had cancer, and resections should be performed (ie, pancreaticoduodenectomy for head lesions and distal pancreatectomy for body and tail lesions).

CYSTIC TUMORS

The distinction between pseudocysts and pancreatic cystic tumors may be as difficult as that between chronic pancreatitis and pancreatic cancer. The presence of serrations within the cyst on CT scan, nodularity, or lobulations is pathognomonic for tumor. Aspiration of the cyst fluid should be performed and its CEA, CA 125, and tissue polypeptide antigen levels determined; cytology should be done. The CA 19-9 is not particularly helpful

in the diagnosis of cystic tumors [36–38]. High viscosity and mucoid staining of cyst fluid are diagnostic of cystic tumor. In patients with the preoperative diagnosis of pancreatic pseudocyst, we recommend preoperative evaluation of tumor markers and either a radiologically guided needle aspiration for cytologic studies or an intraoperative biopsy of the cyst wall with frozen section to look for an epithelial lining. This lining is inconsistent with the diagnosis of pseudocyst and establishes the diagnosis of cystic tumor. In the case of cystic tumor, a resection of the pancreas is performed instead of the internal drainage that is usually done for a pseudocyst.

REFERENCES

Recently published papers of particular interest have been highlighted as follows:
•   Of interest
••   Of outstanding interest

1.•• Bockman DE, Buchler M, Malfertheiner P, Beger HG: Analysis of nerves in pancreatitis. *Gastroenterology* 1988, 94:459–469.

2. Lankisch PG, Löhr-Happe A, Otto J, Creutzfeldt W: Natural course in chronic pancreatitis. Pain, exocrine and endocrine pancreatic insufficiency and prognosis of the disease. *Digestion* 1993, 54:148–155.

3.•• Nealon WH, Thompson JC: Progressive loss of pancreatic function in chronic pancreatitis is delayed by main pancreatic duct decompression: a longitudinal prospective analysis of the modified Puestow procedure. *Ann Surg* 1993, 217:458–466.

4. Sabiston DC: The small intestine. In *Textbook of Surgery*, edn 14. Philadelphia: WB Saunders; 1991:851.

5. Medical Outcomes Trust: SF-36TM Health Survey, Standard US Version 1.0. The Medical Outcome Trust 1992:5.

6. Maher JW, Johlin FC, Pearson D: Thoracoscopic splanchnicectomy for chronic pancreatitis pain. *Surgery* 1996, 120:603–609.

7.•• Frey CF, Amikura K: Local resection of the head of the pancreas combined with longitudinal pancreaticojejunostomy in the management of patients with chronic pancreatitis. *Ann Surg* 1994, 220:492–507.

8. Keith RG, Saibil FG, Sheppard RH: Treatment of chronic alcoholic pancreatitis by pancreatic resection. *Am J Surg* 1989, 157:156–162.

9. Markowitz JS, Rattner DW, Warshaw AL: Failure of symptomatic relief after pancreaticojejunal decompression for chronic pancreatitis: strategies for salvage. *Arch Surg* 1994, 129:374–379, disc 379–380.

10. Büchler MW, Friess H, Müller MW, *et al.*: Randomized trial of duodenum-preserving pancreatic head resection versus pylorus-preserving Whipple in chronic pancreatitis. *Am J Surg* 1995, 169:65–69, disc 69–70.

11. Frey CF, Child CG, Fry W: Pancreatectomy for chronic pancreatitis. *Ann Surg* 1976, 184:403–413.

12. Frey CF: Current management of chronic pancreatitis. In *Advances in Surgery*, vol 28. Edited by Cameron JL. St. Louis: Mosby; 1994:299–328.

13.•• Izbicki JR, Bloechle C, Knoefel WR, *et al.*: Comparison of the two techniques of duodenum-preserving resection of the head of the pancreas in chronic pancreatitis. *Dig Surg* 1994, 11:331–337.

14. Fleming WR, Williamson RC: Role of total pancreatectomy in the treatment of patients with end-stage chronic pancreatitis. *Br J Surg* 1995, 82:1409–1412.

15.•• Wahoff DC, Papalois B E, Najarian JS, *et al.*: Autologous islet transplantation to prevent diabetes after pancreatic resection. *Ann Surg* 1995, 222:562–575; discussion 575–579.

16.•• Rossi RL, Soeldner JS, Braasch JW, *et al.*: Long-term results of pancreatic resection and segmental pancreatic autotranplantation for chronic pancreatitis. *Am J Surg* 1990, 159:51–57.

17. Adloff M, Schloegel M, Arnaud JP, Ollier JC: Role of pancreaticojejunostomy in the treatment of chronic pancreatitis: a study of 105 operated patients. *Chirurgie* 1991, 117:251–256.

18.•• Izbicki JR, Bloechle C, Knoefel WT, *et al.*: Duodenum-preserving
resection of the head of the pancreas in chronic pancreatitis: a prospective, randomized trial. *Ann Surg* 1995, 221:350–358.

19. Büchler MW, Friess H, Bittner R, *et al.*: Duodenum-preserving pancreatic head resection: long-term results. *J Gastrointestinal Surg* 1997, 1:13–19.

20. Frey CF, Ho HS: Chronic pancreatitis: surgical treatment and procedures. In *Practical Gastroenterology*. Edited by Berk JE. Philadelphia:
WB Saunders; 1996:40–62.

21. Howard JM, Zhang Z: Pancreaticoduodenectomy (Whipple resection)
in the treatment of chronic pancreatitis. *World J Surg* 1990, 14:77–82.

22. Fernandez del Castillo C, Raftner DW, Warshaw AL: Standards for
pancreatic resection in the 1990s. *Arch Surg* 1995, 130:295–300.

23.•• Yeo CJ, Cameron JL, Maher Mm, *et al.*: A prospective randomized
trial of pancreaticogastrostomy versus pancreaticojejunostomy after
pancreaticoduodenectomy. *Ann Surg* 1995, 222:580–592.

24. Barens SA, Lillemoe KD, Kaufman HS, *et al.*:
Pancreaticoduodenectomy for benign disease. *Am J Surg* 1996,
171:131–134; disc 134–135.

25. Frey CF: The surgical treatment of chronic pancreatitis. In *The
Pancreas: Biology, Pathobiology and Disease*, edn 2. Edited by Go VLW,
DiMagno EP, Gardner JD,*et al*. New York: Raven; 1993:707–740.

26.•• Beger HG, Büchler M: Duodenum-preserving resection of the head of
the pancreas in chronic pancreatitis with inflammatory mass in the
head. *World J Surg* 1990, 14:83–87.

27.•• Bradley EL III: Long-term results of pancreatojejunostomy in patients
with chronic pancreatitis. *Am J Surg* 1987, 153:207–213.

28.•• Taylor RH, Bagley FH, Braasch JW, Warren KW: Ductal drainage or
resection for chronic pancreatitis. *Am J Surg* 1981, 141:28–33.

29.•• Sawyer R, Frey CF: Is there still a role for distal pancreatectomy in
surgery for chronic pancreatitis. *Am J Surg* 1994, 168:6–9.

30. Walt AJ, Bouwman DL, Weaver DW, Sachs RJ: The impact of technology on the management of pancreatic pseudocyst. *Arch Surg* 1990,
125:759–763.

31. Cameron JL, Kieffer RS, Anderson WJ, Zuidema GD: Internal pancreatic fistulas, pancreatic ascites and pleural effusions. *Ann Surg* 1976,
184:587–593.

32. Woods MS, Traverso LW, Kozarek RA,*et al.*: Successful treatment of
bleeding pseudoaneurysms of chronic pancreatitis. *Pancreas* 1995,
10:22–30.

33.•• Lowenfels AB, Maisonneuve P, Cavallini G, *et al.*: Pancreatitis and the
risk of pancreatic cancer. *New Engl J Med* 1993, 328:1433–1437.

34.••Ekbom A, McLaughlin JK, Karlsson BM, *et al.*: Pancreatitis and pancreatic cancer: a population-based study. *J Nati Cancer Inst* 1994,
86:625–627.

35. Pasanen PA, Eskelinen M, Partanen K, *et al.*: A prospective study of
the value of imaging, serum markers and their combination in the
diagnosis of pancreatic carcinoma in symptomatic patients. *Anticancer
Res* 1992, 12:2309–2314.

36. Lewandrowski KB, Southern JF, Pins MR, *et al.*: Cyst fluid analysis in
the differential diagnosis of pancreatic cysts: a comparison of pseudocysts, serous cystadenomas, mucinous cystic neoplasms, and mucinous
cystadenocarcinoma. *Ann Surg* 1993, 217:41 –47.

37. Yang JM. Southern JF, Warshaw AL, Lewandrowski KB: Proliferation
tissue polypeptide antigen distinguishes malignant mucinous cystade-
nocarcinomas from benign cystic tumors and pseudocysts. *Am J Surg*
1996, 126–129; disc 129–130.

38. Centeno BA, Lewandrowski KB,Warshaw AL, *et al.*: Cyst fluid
cytologic analysis in the differential diagnosis of pancreatic cystic
lesions. *Am J Clin Pathol* 1994, 101:483–487.

139 Adenocarcinoma of the Pancreas
Karen E. Todd and Howard A. Reber

Adenocarcinoma of the pancreas causes approximately 28,000 deaths per year in the United States [1] and is second only to colorectal cancer as a cause of death from gastrointestinal neoplasms. The peak incidence of pancreatic carcinoma is in the seventh decade of life, and there is a slight male-to-female predominance [2]. The incidence of the disease in the United States is approximately 30% to 40% higher among blacks than whites [3]. Pancreatic cancer is an aggressive lesion with an extremely poor prognosis. Surgical resection offers the only hope of cure, but the median survival rate is 10%. Nevertheless, significant advances have occurred in both the diagnosis and treatment of this disease in the last decade.

ANATOMY

The pancreas is a retroperitoneal organ that weighs approxi-mately 100 g in adults. It is divided arbitrarily into the head, neck, body, and tail. The main pancreatic duct (Wirsung) and the accessory duct (Santorini) drain the pancreatic exocrine secretions into the duodenum.

The head of the pancreas lies to the right of the superior mesenteric vein and is closely related to the duodenum. The distal 3 to 4 cm of the common bile duct passes through this part of the pancreas. Together, the bile duct and main pancreatic duct terminate at the papilla of Vater. This explains why cancers in the head of the pancreas usually obstruct both ducts, producing jaundice and possibly malabsorption from pancreatic insufficiency. The neck of the pancreas overlies the superior mesenteric and portal veins. If these vessels become involved by the cancer, the tumor is usually considered to be unresectable. The body and tail of the pancreas extend from the left of the superior mesenteric vein to the hilum of the spleen. The anterior surface of the gland lies behind the posterior wall of the stomach. The rich arterial supply of the pancreas is provided by numerous anastomoses formed by the celiac and the superior mesenteric arteries. Venous drainage is through the hepatic portal system.

PHYSIOLOGY

The exocrine pancreas is composed of acinar cells, which synthesize and store digestive enzymes, and the cells that line the ducts and secrete water and bicarbonate. The endocrine pancreas is comprised of the islets of Langerhans, which produce insulin, glucagon, somatostatin, and pancreatic polypeptide [4]. Most pancreatic adenocarcinomas originate from the ductal cells, although all of the other cell types may be the source of neoplasms. Because only about 10% of the pancreatic parenchyma are necessary to provide sufficient digestive enzymes and insulin for normal exocrine and endocrine function, a Whipple resection done for cancer in the head of the gland would not be expected to cause pancreatic insufficiency; the remaining body and tail of the pancreas are adequate for pancreatic enzyme production. Nevertheless, some patients experience fat malabsorption and benefit from enzyme replacement. This is probably due to poor mixing of the food with the pancreatic enzymes, which is caused by altered anatomy (described later). Diabetes does not occur if the remaining pancreas is normal.

EPIDEMIOLOGY

Various factors have been studied as possible risk factors for pancreatic cancer. The carcinogen most strongly linked to the disease is cigarette smoke. United States military veterans who were heavy smokers had a nearly doubled risk compared with nonsmokers [3]. Both the length of smoking history and the number of cigarettes smoked appear to be important [5•].

A study demonstrated that a history of chronic pancreatitis, regardless of the etiology, significantly increased the risk of developing pancreatic cancer (odds ratio of 3.42) [6]. However, the association between chronic pancreatitis and pancreatic cancer remains unclear because many patients develop chronic pancreatitis secondary to duct obstruction from pancreatic cancer. Thus, it may be impossible to determine which came first.

Although diabetes has been reported as a risk factor for pancreatic cancer, one group followed subjects with diabetes for up to 24 years and [7] found no increased risk. A history of recent onset of diabetes often precedes the diagnosis of the neoplasm, but this does not imply that the diabetes caused the cancer to develop.

Protein and fat have been shown to be promoters of pancreatic carcinogenesis in experimental animals [2]. In Japan, two clinical studies have shown a correlation between meat consumption and the development of pancreatic cancer [3]. Several studies examined the role of coffee consumption in the development of pancreatic cancer, but it remains unclear whether this is a risk factor [8,9].

PATHOLOGY

Most pancreatic cancers originate from the exocrine pancreas, and 80% are adenocarcinomas. Adenocarcinomas usually are of ductal origin, and 60% are located in the head of the gland [2]. The remainder occur in the body and tail (18%–26%), or are diffusely situated throughout the gland (10%–19%).

The staging system most commonly used for this neoplasm is the American Joint Committee for Cancer (AJCC) TNM system shown in Table 139-1. Because pancreatic cancer has usually spread to lymph nodes by the time the diagnosis is made, most patients have at least stage III disease. Stage IV disease (distant metastases) is unresectable.

MOLECULAR BIOLOGY

Recent studies have begun to characterize the genetic abnormalities associated with pancreatic cancer. The most common one identified so far is in the oncogene K-*ras*, where a point mutation in codon 12 has been found in as many as 90% of patients with the disease [10]. The tumor suppressor gene *P53* has been found to be abnormal in about 50% of patients with pancreatic cancer. Because some data suggest that the genetic abnormalities predate the development of the cancer, this raises the possibility of earlier diagnosis by genetic screening of pancreatic secretions or stool samples. This is an area of active investigation.

CLINICAL FEATURES

Patients with adenocarcinoma of the head of the pancreas usually present with obstructive jaundice, abdominal pain, and some degree of weight loss. Frequently, the pain is due to the distention of the bile ducts and gall bladder, which occurs when the bile duct is obstructed by the cancer. Back pain is a more ominous symptom that, when persistent and severe, often signifies tumor invasion of the retroperitoneal nerves, which is incurable. *Painless* jaundice is an uncommon symptom. Because most tumors in the head of the pancreas produce jaundice, they are usually diagnosed at an earlier stage than cancers in the body or tail of the gland. The latter produce more vague symptoms, such as back pain and weight loss or even depression, which may mask the pancreas as the source of the problem. Tumors of the body and tail are often advanced by the time the diagnosis is made.

In advanced cases of pancreatic cancer, physical examination may reveal hepatomegaly from liver metastases, a palpable abdominal mass, or ascites, which often reflects peritoneal seeding by tumor. A distended palpable gall bladder (Courvoisier's sign) is present about half the time when cancer obstructs the bile duct [11]. Abnormal laboratory values include elevated serum total bilirubin, which is usually greater with malignant than benign obstruction (15 mg/dL vs 5 mg/dL), increased serum conjugated bilirubin concentrations, and elevated serum levels of alkaline phosphatase.

Table 139-1. American Joint Committee on Cancer (AJCC) Staging of Carcinoma of the Pancreas

TNM Classification	Characteristics
T1	Limited to the pancreas
T2	Direct extension to duodenum, bile duct, or peripancreatic tissues
T3	Direct extension to stomach, spleen, colon, adjacent large vessels
N0	Regional lymph nodes not involved
N1	Regional lymph nodes involved
M0	No distant metastasis
M1	Distant metastasis present

TNM Staging System	Characteristics
Stage I	T1–2, N0, M0
Stage II	T3, N0, M0
Stage III	T1–3, N1, M0
Stage IV	T1–3, N0–1, M1

DIAGNOSIS AND STAGING

All patients with a suspected pancreatic cancer should undergo an abdominal CT scan, which is the best single study for both diagnosis and staging. The current state of the art is the helical (spiral) CT, which provides information about the nature and site of the lesion, its ressectability (eg, hepatic metastases, vascular invasion), and details of the vascular anatomy (Fig. 139-1). Indeed, it may be the only test required. If the patient has presented with classic signs and symptoms of pancreatic cancer and the CT shows a mass in the head of the pancreas with extra- and intrahepatic dilation but lacking evidence of metastatic disease, laparotomy may be undertaken without further diagnostic studies.

Endoscopic retrograde cholangiopancreatography (ERCP) has both diagnostic and therapeutic applications. It may be the first study performed because the clinician may be focused on the biliary obstruction due to the jaundice. Malignant obstruction of both the bile and pancreatic ducts in the head of the pancreas is manifested as the "double-duct sign," which is almost a pathognomonic sign of pancreatic cancer (Fig. 139-2). Direct brushing of the pancreatic duct can be done to obtain material for cytologic study. ERCP should be followed by a helical CT scan to further characterize and determine the resectability of the lesion. If the CT scan was done first, ERCP is indicated when a tumor was not seen or in other circumstances when the CT findings were atypical for cancer. ERCP may reveal findings that suggest pancreatic cancer even when the CT scan does not show a tumor. However, if both the CT scan and ERCP are normal, the diagnosis of pancreatic cancer is extremely unlikely.

The routine placement of a bile duct stent for preoperative decompression in patients with obstructive jaundice is not indicated. There is no evidence that preoperative stent placement has decreased the morbidity or mortality rates os subsequent surgery. Exceptions include circumstances in which operation must be delayed for several weeks or more, or when cholangitis is present or likely to develop. When a stent is inserted, effort should be made to use one that is at least 10F in size; smaller stents are more likely to obstruct. In patients with bile duct obstruction who are not operative candidates, stents are an effective form of palliation (described later). It should be stressed that metal (Wallstent) stents should *never* be placed in patients who are candidates for resection. The inflammatory response and the potential for tumor ingrowth into the interstices of the stent may complicate or prevent the resection.

Endoscopic ultrasound is a valuable technique to detect small tumors that may not be evident on CT; assess vascular involvement by the tumor; and when required, guide fine needle aspiration for cytologic diagnosis. Nevertheless, endoscopic ultrasound is not indicated in every patient, and it should be used selectively. Helical CT appears to provide equivalent information about vascular involvement and tumor resectability. Most experienced pancreatic surgeons do not require preoperative confirmation of the diagnosis, therefore fine needle aspiration should not be done routinely.

Fine needle aspiration guided by endoscopic ultrasound, CT, or transcutaneous ultrasound is most valuable in patients who are not candidates for operation and in whom tissue proof of the diagnosis is required to guide further therapy. For example, in a patient with a tumor in the body of the pancreas who has no symptoms for which surgical palliation is required, fine needle aspiration could confirm the diagnosis, and chemotherapy or radiation, or both, could be given. In a patient with obstructive jaundice and a mass in the head of the pancreas who may not be a candidate for resection because of coexisting medical problems, fine needle aspiration would be useful to confirm the diagnosis. Then a stent could be placed for palliation, avoiding surgery. It is important to stress that a negative fine needle aspiration never excludes the possibility of malignancy. Complications of fine needle aspiration include hemorrhage, pancreatitis, pancreatic fistula, and seeding of the needle tract with cancer cells, all of which are uncommon.

Laparoscopy should not be used prior to laparotomy in patients with pancreatic cancer who appear to have resectable lesions, as

Figure 139-1

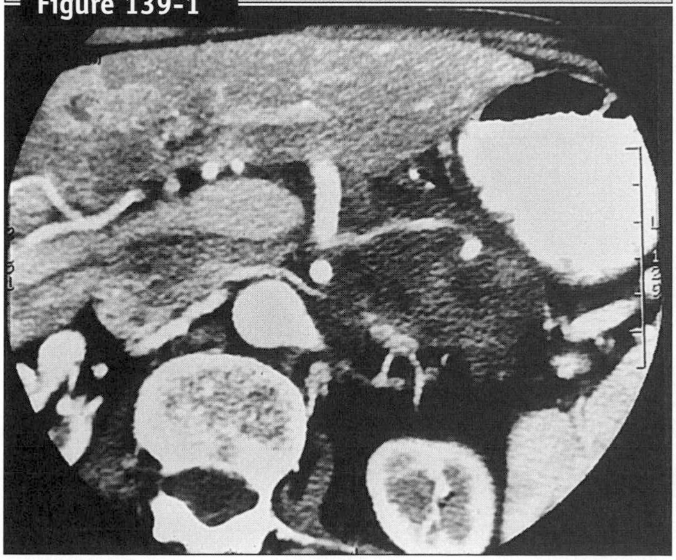

Pancreatic phase of a helical CT scan. There is a large tumor in the body and tail of the pancreas which invades the splenic artery and therefore is not resectable. (Courtesy of D. Lu, MD.)

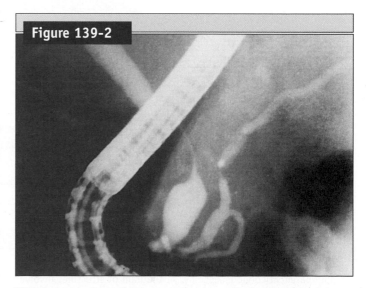

Figure 139-2

ERCP from a patient with pancreatic cancer. Both the bile and pancreatic ducts are obstructed which gives the characteristic "double duct sign."

judged by helical CT scan. In that situation, 75% to 80% of tumors will be amenable to resection. Half of the remaining 20% to 25% will be found to have unresectable lesions because of unsuspected vascular involvement that would not have been apparent with laparoscopy. Thus, in only 10% to 12% of patients would laparoscopic examination have avoided laparotomy by the detection of small liver or peritoneal metastases. This is too small a number to justify the added time, risk, and expense of the procedure. Laparoscopy is useful when there appears to be a high likelihood of unresectability that could not be confirmed preoperatively (*eg*, when what appears on CT to be metastatic lesions is not confirmed by fine needle aspiration). Laparoscopy also may become more useful as a therapeutic tool as surgeons gain experience with laparoscopic biliary and gastric bypass procedures for palliation.

◼ TREATMENT

Preoperative Management

Most patients with pancreatic cancer come to the surgeon in reasonable nutritional and metabolic shape for operation. This is probably because the diagnosis is made more rapidly and their condition has not deteriorated to the degree once common. Nevertheless, a complete preoperative assessment should be done to optimize their cardiac, pulmonary, and general medical condition for a major operation. When it is necessary to delay surgery more than a few weeks and the patient is jaundiced, a biliary stent should be placed endoscopically.

Operative Management

The Whipple pancreaticoduodenectomy (Fig. 139-3) is the standard operation for adenocarcinoma of the head of the pancreas. It consists of a partial gastrectomy (antrectomy), cholecystectomy, and resection of the distal common bile duct, the head of the pancreas, the duodenum, the proximal jejunum and the regional lymph nodes. Reconstruction of gastrointestinal continuity requires a pancreaticojejunostomy, an hepaticojejunostomy, and a gastrojejunostomy. In the hands of experienced pancreatic surgeons around the world the operative mortality rate of this operation is about 2% to 3%. There are numerous series of more than 100 consecutive subjects with no deaths [12•, 13].

Because of the association of the standard Whipple resection with excessive morbidity (excessive weight loss, diarrhea, dumping syndrome), many surgeons adopted a modification in which the stomach, the pylorus, and several centimeters of the duodenum are preserved (pylorus-preserving Whipple resection) (Fig.139-4). Although this procedure maintains gastric reservoir function and postoperative gastric emptying is closer to normal, patients probably do not fare any better nutritionally when the stomach is preserved. The pylorus-preserving Whipple resection does not appear to compromise the chance for cure of the cancer.

To improve the cure rates for pancreatic cancer, Japanese surgeons have advocated a more radical operation [14]. It consists of the standard Whipple resection with removal of more retroperitoneal soft tissue and lymph nodes and, if they appear to be involved by tumor, resection of segments of the superior mesenteric and portal veins. Western surgeons generally have been skeptical of this more aggressive approach.

Determination of Resectability

Pancreatic resection is done if it appears that all gross tumor can be removed and a cure is possible. Hepatic or peritoneal metastases, evidence of tumor in the lymph nodes, or soft tissue outside the usual limits of the resection indicate unresectability. In the absence

Figure 139-3

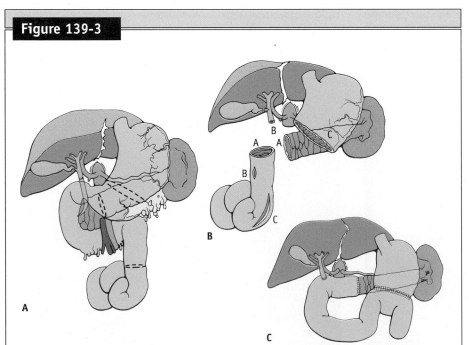

Figure 139-4

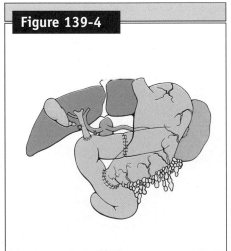

Pylorus-preserving pancreaticoduodenectomy.

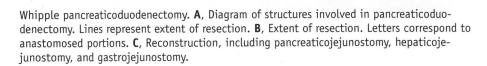

Whipple pancreaticoduodenectomy. **A**, Diagram of structures involved in pancreaticoduodenectomy. Lines represent extent of resection. **B**, Extent of resection. Letters correspond to anastomosed portions. **C**, Reconstruction, including pancreaticojejunostomy, hepaticojejunostomy, and gastrojejunostomy.

of such findings, tumors usually are resectable if they have not invaded the nearby major blood vessels, including the celiac and hepatic arteries, the superior mesenteric artery and vein, the portal vein, and the vena cava. Although small pancreatic tumors (< 2 cm diameter) are more likely to be resectable than larger ones, patients should not be denied a chance for resection because their tumor is "too big." Regardless of tumor size, if the CT scan shows no evidence of unresectability, the abdominal exploration should be done.

Experienced pancreatic surgeons do not require histologic evidence of cancer before undertaking a resection, and efforts to establish the diagnosis preoperatively do not simplify the operation. On the contrary, such procedures are uncomfortable for the patient, may be associated with complications, and represent an additional expense. Finally, a negative diagnosis does exclude cancer. In a patient with signs and symptoms that suggest pancreatic cancer, with CT and ERCP evidence for the disease, and with typical operative findings, there is only about a 5% chance that the diagnosis of cancer will be wrong. Then the underlying problem will prove to be chronic pancreatitis, for which a Whipple resection also may be appropriate.

Palliation

Patients with pancreatic cancer may require palliation from obstructive jaundice, gastric outlet obstruction, or pain.

Jaundice

In patients who are not operative candidates, endoscopic placement of biliary stents provides effective relief of biliary obstruction with minimal risk. However, plastic stents (at least 10F) require placement every 3 to 4 months because biliary sludge eventually obstructs the stent lumen and patients may develop recurrent jaundice and cholangitis. Metal Wallstents have a larger diameter and are less likely to become obstructed.

Biliary obstruction also can be relieved surgically. Cholecystojejunostomy and choledochojejunostomy are safe and effective procedures. They are the procedures of choice if an operation is to be performed [11] (Figs. 139-5 and 139-6). Jaundice is relieved in about 90% of patients, but it may persist in patients with liver damage from long-standing obstruction [11].

Gastric Outlet Obstruction

Up to one third of patients develop gastric outlet obstruction during the course of their disease. Gastrojejunostomy (Fig. 139-7) is effective palliation for this and often is done prophylactically when patients undergo a biliary bypass. Neither the morbidity nor the mortality rates are increased by the addition of the gastric bypass procedure. Occasionally, gastrojejunostomy fails to relieve the vomiting symptoms that mistakenly led to the diagnosis of gastric outlet obstruction. In such patients, the problem may be a gastric motility disturbance. Surgical treatment for this is unsatisfactory, but patients may get some relief from prokinetic agents.

Pain

Many patients with pancreatic cancer develop severe, persistent abdominal and back pain. This is due to the invasion of the retroperitoneal neural plexuses by the tumor. Celiac plexus block, given either at the time of operation or later, percutaneously, often helps. Narcotic analgesics remain the mainstay of treatment, and they are used most effectively by specialists in pain management, who should be involved in the care of these patients.

Radiation Therapy and Chemotherapy

Neither radiation therapy given alone nor single agent chemotherapy are effective. A combination of 5-fluorouracil and external beam radiation therapy has been shown to increase survival in patients who have undergone pancreatic resection for pancreatic cancer compared with those who had resection alone (2-year survival rates, 43% vs 18%; median survival rates, 18 months vs 10 months) [15]. Anecdotal reports of the effectiveness of certain multiple drug regimens remain to be confirmed in prospective and randomized studies.

▉ RESULTS

Operative mortality rates for the Whipple resection are now 2% to 3% in major centers that are experienced in the management of these patients. There is evidence that care is delivered with lower morbidity and mortality rates, and at less cost, in institutions where at least 20 pancreatic resections are performed yearly.

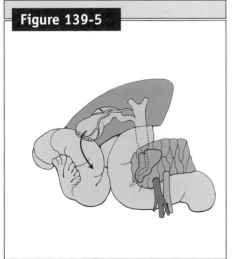

Figure 139-5

Cholecystojejunostomy.

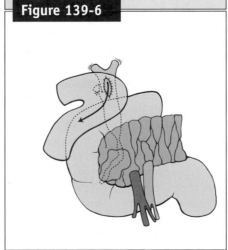

Figure 139-6

Choledochojejunostomy.

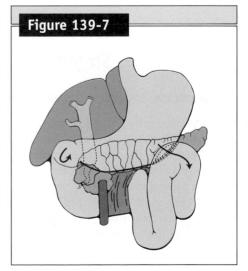

Figure 139-7

Gastrojejunostomy.

The median survival after pancreatic resection is 18 to 20 months, with an overall 5-year survival rate of 10%. Up to 50% of patients alive at 5 years still die from recurrent cancer. However, if the tumor is removed with clear surgical margins and no lymph node metastases are found, the 5-year survival rate is as high as 25% [16••].

The prognosis after resection depends on a number of factors, including the presence of lymph node metastases, the degree of differentiation of the tumor, and the tumor size. In one series, the median survival was 55.8 months in node-negative subjects versus 11 months in "node-positive" subjects [17]. In another series, subjects with well-differentiated tumors had an actuarial 5-year survival rate of about 50%; those with poorly differentiated cancer had a survival rate of about 10% [18]. In general, patients with small (< 2 cm) tumors fare better than those with larger ones.

▮▮▮ REFERENCES

Recently published papers of particular interest have been highlighted as follows:
* Of interest
•• Of outstanding interest

1. Gold EB: Epidemiology of and risk factors for pancreatic cancer. *Surg Clin North Am* 1995, 75:819–843.

2. Wanebo HJ, Vezeridis MP: Pancreatic carcinoma in perspective: a continuing challenge. *Cancer* 1996, 78:580–591.

3. Ahlgren JD: Epidemiology and risk factors in pancreatic cancer. *Semin Oncol* 1996, 23(2):241–250.

4. Bockman DE: Anatomy of the pancreas. In *The pancreas: Biology, pathobiology, and disease*, 2nd edn. Edited by Go VLW, DiMagno EP, Gardner JD, *et al.* New York: Raven, 1993:1–8.

5.• Ji B, Chow W, Dai O, *et al.*: Cigarette smoking and alcohol consumption and the risk of pancreatic cancer: A case-control study in Shanghai, China. *Cancer Causes and Control* 1995, 6:369–376.
This case-control study from China showed that the number of cigarettes smoked per day, and the duration of smoking increase the risk of developing pancreatic cancer.

6. Bansal P, Sonnenberg A: Pancreatitis is a risk factor for pancreatic cancer. *Gastroenterology* 1995, 109:247–251.

7. Chow W, Gridley G, Nyren O, *et al.*:Risk of pancreatic cancer following diabetes mellitus: a nationwide cohort study in Sweden. *J Natl Cancer Inst* 1995, 87:930–931.

8. Gullo L, Pezzilli R, Moraelli-Labate A, and the Italian Pancreatic Cancer Study Group: Coffee and cancer of the pancreas: An Italian multicenter study. *Pancreas* 1995, 11:223–229.

9. Nishi M, Ohba S, Hirata K, Miyake H: Dose-response relationship between coffee and the risk of pancreatic cancer. *Jpn J Clin Oncol* 1996, 26:42–48.

10. Sarkorafas G, Lazaria A, Tsiotou A, *et a.*:Oncogenes in cancer of the pancreas. *Eur J Surg Oncol* 1995, 21:251–253.

11. Ashley SW, Reber HA: Surgical management of exocrine pancreatic cancer. In *The pancreas: Biology, Pathobiology, and Disease*, 2nd edn. Edited by Go VLW, DiMagno EP, Gardner JD, *et al.*: New York: Raven, 1993:913–929.

12.• Trede M, Schwall G, Saeger H: Survival after pancreaticoduodenectomy: 118 consecutive reaction without an operative mortality. *Ann Surg* 1990, 211:477–458.
From November of 1985 to 1989, 118 consecutive pancreaticoduodenectomies were performed without an operative mortality. This study is important in emphasizing that the Whipple procedure can be performed safely by experienced pancreatic surgeons.

13. Cameron JL, Pitt HA, Yeo CJ, *et al.*: One hundred and forty-five consecutive pancreaticoduodenectomies without mortality. *Ann Surg* 1993, 217(5):430–438.

14. Takahashi S, Ogata Y, Tsuzuki T: Combined resection of the pancreas and portal vein for pancreatic cancer. *Br J Surg* 1994, 81:1190–1193.

15. Kalser M, Ellenberg S, Levin B, *et al.*: Pancreatic cancer: adjuvant combined radiation and chemotherapy following potentially curative resection. *Proc Am Soc Clin Oncol* 1983, 2:122.

16.•• Yeo CJ, Cameron JL, Lillemoe KD, *et al.*: Pancreaticoduodenectomy for cancer of the head of the pancreas. 201 patients. *Ann Surg* 1995, 221 (6):721–733.
This retrospective review is the largest single-institution experience reported to date. This group concluded that survival of patients with pancreatic cancer is improving. Aspects of tumor biology are the strongest predictors of outcome.

17. Cameron JL, Crist DW, Sitzmann JV, *et al.*: Factors influencing survival after pancreaticoduodenectomy for pancreatic cancer. *Am J Surg* 1991, 161:120–125.

140 Endocrine Neoplasms of the Pancreas

Stefan W. Schmid and Irvin M. Modlin

The endocrine cells of the pancreas are located mainly in the pancreatic islets, although a few isolated endocrine cells may be scattered in the exocrine pancreas. Neoplasms of the pancreas may be of exocrine or endocrine origin, although the latter are comparatively rare. Nevertheless, endocrine pancreatic tumors represent the majority of neuroendocrine neoplasms of the gastrointestinal tract [1••]. Overall, endocrine pancreatic tumors, also known as islet cell tumors, are rare neoplasms with an annual incidence of 0.1 to 0.4/100,000. They are identified generically as a component of the group of neuroendocrine neoplasms, as it is believed that they originate from neuroectodermal cells that possess the potential to differentiate into various endocrine tumors. These tumors have been labeled as APUDomas because they arise from cells that are capable of amine precursor uptake and decarboxylation, resulting in synthesis of amines or peptides. In general, most (70% to 80%) endocrine pancreatic tumors are relatively benign, slow-growing neoplasms and are therefore often found incidentally at autopsy (1% to 3%) [2]. The release of the amines and peptides from the tumors leads to the development of specific clinical symptoms and syndromes that characterize the type of endocrine pancreatic tumor.

ISLET ARCHITECTURE

Interspersed in the connective tissue of the exocrine pancreas are clusters of endocrine cells called the islets of Langerhans, which in the adult pancreas, represent 1% to 2% of the total mass of the gland (about 1 g) [3]. Islet size and diameter may vary from a few cells of less than 40 μm to 5000 cells of 400 μm. The small islets (<160 μm) represent 75% of the number of islets but only 15% of the volume, whereas the large islets (>250 μm) account for 15% of the number and 60% of the volume. Various peptide hormones, including insulin, glucagon, somatostatin, vasoactive intestinal peptide (VIP), and pancreatic polypeptide (PP), are secreted by the islets. The four major islet endocrine cell types are, in order of abundance: the insulin-producing B cells, the glucagon-producing A cells, the somatostatin-producing D cells, and the PP-producing cells. Other, less-abundant cell types release VIP, substance P, serotonin, and gastrin (only during the perinatal period). A regulatory unit of endocrine cells with direct neural input and local paracrine modulation is evident. The distribution within the islet cells shows a core of B cells surrounded by a mantle of non–B cells. The regional distribution of the islet cells is different: the tail, body, and anterior portion of the head are rich in B and A cells and poor in PP cells, whereas the posterior part of the head is poor in A cells and rich in PP cells.

Each islet cell group is surrounded by a thin capsule consisting of fibroblasts, but this capsule is often absent between the islets and the exocrine tissue itself. Islets are disproportionately vascularized and, although constituting only 1% to 2% of the pancreatic mass, they are supplied by 10% to 20% of the total pancreatic blood flow.

Each group of cells has a direct arteriolar blood flow, and the capillaries are fenestrated, providing a high permeability. A closely applied venous drainage system provides a configuration similar to the local portal venous drainage scheme of the pituitary gland. The nerves follow the blood vessels and terminate within the pericapillary space closely apposed to the endocrine cells.

PHYSIOLOGY

Endocrine pancreatic function is very complex, and hormone secretion is regulated by multiple independent signals, which, in many instances, are still poorly understood. Known regulators include levels of blood glucose, amino acids, and other nutrients; paracrine and systemic hormones (gastrointestinal hormones); as well as the autonomic nervous system. At a local level, islet cells can modulate other islet cells by junctional interactions, paracrine interactions, and blood-borne feedback loops (intra-islet portal system). In this respect, insulin can inhibit the A and D cells, somatostatin inhibits the A and B cells, and glucagon can stimulate the B and D cells. Autonomic neural regulation is via the vagus nerve and the adrenergic system, the postganglionic fibers of which originate in the celiac ganglion. The sensory innervation of the pancreas is provided by fibers arising from the nodose ganglia and spinal ganglia and conveyed by the vagus and splanchnic nerves. Nerve fibers that terminate in the islets and intrapancreatic ganglia contain many different neuropeptides, and, indeed, nerve terminals may store chemical messengers similar to those found in endocrine cells. These include substance P, VIP, somatostatin, cholecystokinin, serotonin, gastrin-releasing peptide, galanin, neuropeptide Y, neurotensin, calcitonin, gene-related peptides, and enkephalin-like peptides, which are all capable of neural or endocrine activity.

HISTOPATHOLOGY AND IMMUNOPATHOLOGY

Tumor nodules with a diameter of less than 5 mm, known as microadenomas, usually behave in a benign fashion, often without any hormonal syndrome. Tumors greater than 5 mm are known as macrotumors; these may be associated with hormonal syndromes, thus representing the group of functioning tumors. The functioning tumors have been broadly characterized according to their secreted hormone and the resultant development of a definable syndrome. Consequently, nonsecreting tumors have been designated simplistically as nonfunctioning tumors, although this reflects only the current lack of knowledge of the secretory product or its demonstrable metabolic effect.

The usual histologic patterns of malignancies (nuclear pleomorphism, mitotic activity, infiltration into the surrounding tissue) are often unreliable in diagnosis of endocrine pancreatic tumors [4•]. The clearest evidence of malignancy is provided by local or capsular extension to adjacent organs or demonstration of vascular invasion and metastases. Because metastases may only become apparent many months or even years after the removal of the primary tumor, a prolonged clinical follow-up is required to establish the precise nature of a tumor.

Endocrine pancreatic tumors are evenly distributed throughout the pancreas with the exception of gastrinomas, pancreatic polypeptide tumors, somatostatinomas, and nonfunctioning endocrine pancreatic neoplasms, which are located mainly in the head of the pancreas. Although macroscopically most tumors appear well demarcated, they often fail to exhibit a well-defined capsule; they are usually white-gray to pinkish-brown and of a firm consistency. Their size generally ranges from 1 to 5 cm in diameter. Tumor size, however, is not correlated with severity of clinical hormonal symptoms.

Microscopically the tumors usually reveal uniform cuboidal cells, with eosinophilic cytoplasm and centrally located round-to-oval nuclei. The histologic picture shows a trabecular, ribbon-like, or gyriform pattern, sometimes combined with glandular or acinar elements, and a solid medullary pattern. Both patterns may be present within the same neoplasm. The histologic architecture usually is not indicative of a specific tumor type or hormonal product; two exceptions are glandular structures that contain psammoma bodies and are often observed in somatostatinomas of the ampullary region, and the amyloid deposits (islet amyloid polypeptide) in insulinomas.

The hormonal product of functioning tumors can usually be detected by immunocytochemistry, but the staining intensity is not associated with the severity of clinical symptoms. Many tumors exhibit staining for multiple hormones, and metastases may produce hormones not found in the primary tumor. For example, 50% of gastrinomas are multihormonal, containing PP, glucagon, and insulin, in addition to gastrin. Appropriate fixation is necessary to identify the relevant peptides in the tumor, as tissue preserved in formalin is often inappropriate for diagnostic immunohistochemistry of endocrine pancreatic tumors. In such fixation, peptide antigenicity may be destroyed and peptides may either be extracted during processing or denatured by hot paraffin.

CLASSIFICATION

Endocrine pancreatic tumors are classified according to the hormone responsible for the clinical syndrome (*eg*, insulin = insulinoma, gastrin = gastrinoma). The exact diagnosis requires specific immunocytochemistry and extraction and assay of the hormonal content in the tumor. To confirm the neuroendocrine origin of the tumor, neuron-specific enolase, chromogranin, or neurofilament content should be determined. The clinical and biochemical features of endocrine pancreatic tumors are summarized in Table 140-1.

INSULINOMA

Insulinomas represent 70% to 80% of symptomatic endocrine pancreatic tumors and are found in all age groups, with a peak from the third to the fifth decade. The tumors are usually solitary and evenly distributed throughout the pancreas, although in ±1%

they are ectopic (stomach, duodenum, Meckel's diverticulum, bile duct, ovary, omentum). Insulinomas are usually (±90%) benign and only occasionally (10%) multicentric, in which case they are often associated with the multiple endocrine neoplasia type 1 (MEN1) syndrome. About 30% of all insulinomas are part of the MEN1 syndrome.

Most tumors have a diameter less than 2 cm, but malignant tumors are usually greater than 3 cm; metastases are evident in about one third at the time of initial diagnosis. Permanent cure rates with surgery approach 90%, but metastases can occur several years after apparent surgical cure.

Clinical Features

Patients usually present with symptoms caused by hypoglycemia or attributable to the consequent catecholamine responses, including weakness, sweating, tremulousness, tachycardia, hunger, fatigue, headache, dizziness, visual difficulties, disorientation, seizures, and unconsciousness. Because the hypoglycemic episodes occur sporadically with symptom-free intervals over

Table 140-1. Clinical and Biochemical Features of Endocrine Pancreatic Neoplasms

Endocrine tumor	Frequency, %	Clinical presentation	Malignancy, %	Biochemical abnormalities and diagnostic testing
Insulinoma	60–70	Weakness, sweating, tremulousness, tachycardia, fatigue, headache, dizziness, disorientation, seizures, and unconsciousness	< 10	Glucose levels decrease Insulin levels increase, C-peptide levels increase, proinsulin levels increase Fasting provocation test
Gastrinoma	15–20	Recurrent peptic ulcer disease (hemorrhage, perforation), diarrhea	50–60	Gastrin levels increase, basal acid output decreases Secretin provocation test
Nonfunctioning tumors/PPoma	10–15	Obstructive jaundice, pancreatitis, duodenal obstruction, epigastric pain, weight loss, dyspepsia, fatigue	70	PP levels increase Atropine inhibition test
VIPoma	>4	Watery diarrhea, flushing, hypotension, abdominal pain	80	VIP levels increase, K^+ levels decrease, Cl^- levels decrease
Glucagonoma	>4	Migrating skin rash, glossitis, stomatitis, angular cheilitis, diabetes, weight loss, diarrhea	80	Glucagon levels increase, amino acids decrease Arginine provocation test
Somatostatinoma	<5	Weight loss, cholelithiasis, diarrhea	50	Somatostatin levels increase Pentagastrin provocation test Glucose tolerance test
Carcinoid	<2	Flushing, sweating, diarrhea, borborygmi, wheezing, edema, lacrimation	94	5-HT increases, PP levels increase, SP levels increase, urine 5-HIAA increases Pentagastrin provocation test
ACTHoma	>1	Cushing's syndrome	> 90	ACTH increases, urinary cortisol levels increase Dexamethasone test
GRFoma	>1	Acromegaly	30	GRF levels increase
PTH-like-oma	>1	Hypercalcemia, bone pain	> 90	Ca^{2+} levels increase, PTH-like factor levels increase, PTH levels greatly decrease
Neurotensinoma	>1	Hypotension, tachycardia, malabsorption	> 80	Neurotensin increases
Mixed endocrine-exocrine tumor	—	Obstructive symptoms/any of the aforementioned	—	—

*Percentage of pancreatic carcinoids of 6100 reviewed gut carcinoids.

ACTH—adrenocorticotropic hormone; GRF—growth hormone release factor; PP—pancreatic polypeptide; PTH—parathyrin; SP—substance P.

weeks or months, the diagnosis may be difficult in the initial stage of the disease. In addition, the ephemeral or otherwise odd nature of the symptoms is often erroneously ascribed to neurotic or dysfunctional behavior.

Diagnosis

Diagnostic biochemical parameters include hypoglycemia and elevation of insulin, proinsulin, and C-peptide plasma levels. Given the relatively wide normal variations, fasting plasma levels of insulin may not always be increased in patients with insulinoma. However, with the use of prolonged fasting (up to 72 hours) hypoglycemia can almost always be provoked (glucose <2.2 mmol/L or 40 mg/dL). Relief of symptoms following food ingestion is also diagnostic.

■ GASTRINOMA (ZOLLINGER-ELLISON SYNDROME)

About 80% of gastrinomas are found centered around the pancreatic head and duodenum, the so-called gastrinoma triangle, although rarely other sites (stomach, jejunum, biliary tract, and liver, kidney, heart) have been documented. The mean age of patients with gastrinomas is 45 to 50 years of age, and children are rarely affected. The majority of gastrinomas (60% to 70%) are sporadic, 20% to 30% are metastatic, and the remainder (10% to 20%) exhibit a MEN1 background. The tumor size in the pancreas is usually greater than 2 cm and in the duodenum less than 1 cm—often very tiny. At diagnosis pancreatic gastrinomas are often metastatic, with up to 60% having spread to regional lymph nodes. Only a small percentage of these patients(15% to 30 %), however, develop life-shortening liver metastases. Duodenal gastrinomas seem to have a lower incidence of malignancy, but metastases may be evident even when the primary neoplasm is evident only microscopically. MEN1-associated gastrinomas often exhibit a duodenal component and are multicentric.

Clinical Features

Under the influence of hypergastrinemia, gastric acid secretion is increased. Patients with gastrinomas clinically present with symptoms of peptic ulcer disease often not responsive to the usual therapy or with recurrent peptic ulcers after surgery. Complications, such as hemorrhage and perforation, are common. Suspicion of gastrinoma should be aroused if ulcers are in unusual locations (second part of duodenum or jejunum) or are multiple. However, duodenal ulcers associated with gastrinoma are mostly singular and in the usual location (ie, duodenal bulb). Occasionally, acid inactivation of pancreatic lipase leads to unexplained diarrhea due to steatorrhea. Gastrinomas are diagnosed based on an elevated fasting serum gastrin level and an increased basal acid output. The diagnosis may be confirmed by intravenous injection of secretin, which results in a paradoxical increase of serum gastrin concentration.

■ GLUCAGONOMA

Glucagonomas represent less than 1% of all endocrine tumors of the enteropancreatic system. They are slightly more prevalent in female than in male patients and occur in all adult age groups, with a peak between the fifth and seventh decades. Glucagonomas are usually solitary, malignant (80%) and located in the pancreas tail (50%). Clinically active tumors are usually larger, having a diameter of greater than 5 cm. Metastatic spread affects predominantly the liver and adjacent lymph nodes, and less frequently the vertebra, ovary, peritoneum, and adrenals.

Clinical Features

Migrating skin rash and mild diabetes are the predominant signs in the glucagonoma syndrome (approximately 90%). The rash, a necrolytic migratory erythema, exhibits a 7- to 14-day sequence of erythema, blister, secondary breakdown, infection, healing, and hyperpigmentation. Mucosal lesions (eg, glossitis, stomatitis, angular cheilitis) are associated with the cutaneous rash in about 70% of patients. Diabetes usually precedes skin rash (and diagnosis) by years. Further clinical features are weight loss due to the hypercatabolic effect of glucagon, venous thrombosis with pulmonary embolism, diarrhea, and various psychiatric and neurologic disturbances. Blood investigations reveal anemia, hypoaminoacidemia, hypoalbuminemia, and hypocholesterolemia as the most common disorders.

Diagnosis

Basal plasma glucagon concentrations are elevated in almost all patients with glucagonomas. Many other conditions (eg, diabetic ketoacidosis, acute pancreatitis, and chronic renal failure) are associated with hyperglucagonemia, but only in cirrhosis of the liver do the plasma glucagon levels exceed the upper level by the threefold, as is common in glucagonomas. An arginine provocation test may be helpful in diagnosis. The tumors are usually more than 3 cm and can be imaged by somatostatin receptor scintigraphy, celiac angiography, CT scanning, and endoscopic sonography.

■ SOMATOSTATINOMA

Less than 5% of endocrine pancreatic tumors belong to the group of somatostatinomas. As somatostatin cells are frequently evident in endocrine pancreatic tumors, the definition of somatostatinoma requires some restriction. These neoplasms are usually large (>3 −5 cm) at the time of diagnosis, are usually malignant, and are found mostly in the pancreatic head or the periampullary region of the duodenum. The latter group of somatostatinomas are often associated with von Recklinghausen's disease and pheochromocytoma.

Clinical Features

A symptom complex of diarrhea with steatorrhea, weight loss, an abnormal glucose tolerance test result, cholecystomegaly, and cholelithiasis (probably due to bile stasis because of gallbladder atony) may be evident. Additional nonspecific symptoms include bloating, epigastric fullness, and dyspepsia. These are the result of cholelithiasis or of the influence of somatostatin on intestinal function (inhibition of gastric emptying, delayed intestinal nutrient absorption, reduction of splanchnic blood flow, inhibition of gastric acid secretion). The prolonged inhibition of pancreatic enzyme secretion, gallbladder emptying, and intestinal absorption leads to steatorrhea.

Diagnosis

Plasma somatostatin levels are usually massively elevated, but if this is not the case, a provocation test with tolbutamide or calcium plus pentagastrin can be given. Endoscopic ultrasound may be useful in localization because the tumors are usually in the pancreatic head or periampullary region.

VASOACTIVE INTESTINAL POLYPEPTIDE TUMORS

In adults, vasoactive intestinal polypeptide tumors (VIPomas), which include Verner-Morrison, pancreatic cholera, and watery diarrhea, hypokalemia, hypochlorhydria (WDHA) syndrome, are usually found in the pancreas, but other rare sites of VIP production include VIP-producing pheochromocytomas and intestinal carcinoids. In the majority (80%) VIPomas exhibit a malignant pattern of behavior with distant metastases mainly located in the liver, lung, or bone. The tumors occur in all age groups with a peak of frequency in the fourth decade and a male-female ratio of 1:3. Usually VIPomas are isolated, but up to 6% are associated with MEN1. The tumor size is generally large with a mean diameter of 4 cm to 5 cm.

Clinical Features

Vasoactive intestinal peptide is a humoral mediator of intestinal secretion; diarrhea is thus induced by malabsorption or secretion of water and electrolytes in the jejunum and ileum, or both. The classic syndrome consists of profuse watery diarrhea, hypokalemia, and achlorhydria, which is occasionally associated with vasomotor symptoms such as flushing and hypotension (20%). Half of the patients involved experience a chronic secretory diarrhea that is continuous; in the other half it is intermittent. The volume of stools may range from 1 to 8 L/day but can exceed 10 L/day; stools often resemble water with rice grains and are usually afecal. Because the delay between onset of symptoms and diagnosis may be up to 32 months, most patients have weight loss and dehydration as a result of the chronic diarrhea. Other clinical signs and symptoms include vomiting, abdominal pain, and flushes; the electrolyte disturbances (hypokalemia, hypercalcemia, hypomagnesemia) may result in paresia, muscle weakness, cardiac arrhythmias, and tetany.

Diagnosis

Diagnosis is based on evidence of an elevated plasma VIP level in up to 90% of the patients and the presence of a concomitant secretory diarrhea. The tumor size is usually large (>3 cm in 78% of cases) and may be easily demonstrated by noninvasive imaging methods such as somatostatin receptor scintography, sonography, CT scan, or magnetic resonance imaging.

GROWTH HORMONE–RELEASING FACTOR TUMORS

Growth hormone–releasing factor tumors (GRFomas) are extremely rare subtypes of endocrine pancreatic tumors. Defined as extracerebral tumors, they synthesize and release GRF, resulting in acromegaly and growth hormone hypersecretion. GRFomas occur in age groups from 15 to 60 years of age (average 40 years), with a male-female ratio of 1:3. The preferential location is the pancreatic tail, and approximately 30% of these tumors are malignant. GRFomas are associated in 40% with other endocrine disorders such as MEN1, hyperparathyroidism, Zollinger-Ellison syndrome, hypoglycemia, Cushing's syndrome,

and pheochromocytoma. Multiple tumors are observed mainly in association with MEN1. Usually, the pancreatic tumor is detected before the diagnosis of acromegaly is made.

Clinical Features

These patients present with acromegaly. Imaging of the sella turcica by CT scan or magnetic resonance imaging shows a normal sella in nearly 50%; however, in 40% to 45% a hypophyseal mass resembling a true adenoma is evident. Whether this is a true adenoma or represents hyperplasia of the somatotrophs remains controversial. In the remaining few percent, the sella is enlarged without evidence of a hypophyseal mass.

Diagnosis

Plasma concentrations of immunoreactive growth hormone are elevated in all patients, and diagnosis is based on documentation of high levels of plasma GRF by radioimmunoassay. Hyperprolactinemia is also observed in approximately 70% of cases. Imaging methods and treatment are indicated, as they are in patients with other endocrine pancreatic tumors.

PANCREATIC POLYPEPTIDE TUMORS

Pure pancreatic polypeptide tumors (PPomas) are extremely rare; no specific clinical syndrome has been identified, even in association with extremely high plasma levels. PP is often produced in nonfunctioning neoplasms (>50%) or in mixed functioning tumors together with other peptides. Rarely, increased PP levels may derive from colonic PP cells in various diarrheal conditions. As PPomas fail to cause any clinical symptoms, they are often included within the group of nonfunctioning tumors.

CARCINOIDS

Overall, carcinoids are the most common endocrine gut tumor, usually located in the small bowel and appendix. The latter type of tumor is usually discovered by chance, whereas the former type is often found during abdominal laparotomy for intestinal obstruction or bleeding. Less than 1% of gut carcinoids are located in the pancreas and are often discovered incidentally, having usually metastasized (hepatic and mesenteric) by the time of diagnosis. The humoral secretions (serotonin, bradykinins, tachykinins, substance P, and substance K/neurokinin A) are generally inactivated in the liver. Therefore, the presence of the syndrome is usually evidence of significant hepatic metastatic spread or extension into the retroperitoneal tissues, with consequent systemic venous drainage of tumor-derived humoral factors.

Clinical Features

The nonspecific symptomatology, which includes flushing, sweating, diarrhea, borborygmi, wheezing, edema, and lacrimation may be initially difficult to identify until recognized as a constellation of related symptoms. The characteristic carcinoid facial flush may be induced by small amounts of alcohol, coffee, or cheese.

Diagnosis

Classic biochemical identification of carcinoid tumors involves quantitation of 24-hour urinary excretion of 5-hydroxyindolacetic acid, which exhibits a sensitivity of 73%. Further plasma examinations show an elevation of 5-HT, PP, and SP levels. In patients with negative or equivocal biochemical evaluation, provocative testing with pentagastrin may substantiate the diagnosis. The most effective localization study is somatostatin receptor scintigraphy.

■ NONFUNCTIONING TUMORS

Nonfunctioning endocrine pancreatic tumors (N/F) are usually found incidentally during intra-abdominal surgery or autopsy. Patients with N/F fail to present any clinical symptoms, owing to hormone overproduction. Therefore, tumors with detectable increases of plasma hormone levels (*eg*, PPomas) but not associated with distinct hormonal manifestations are included in the nonfunctioning group. However, this definition is controversial, as some authors require no hormonal symptoms, no elevated peptide plasma levels, and no positive immunocytochemistry as the criteria for an N/F. The proportion of N/F among endocrine pancreatic tumors ranges from 15% to 30%. In some circumstances, a tumor initially considered nonfunctioning may later be considered a functioning tumor (*eg*, gastrinoma).

The absence of hormonal syndromes may make N/Fs difficult to distinguish from exocrine malignancies. The reasons for the nonfunctioning pattern are numerous: 1) elevated plasma peptide levels (PP, hCG-α, and hCG-β subunits, neurotensin, islet amyloid polypeptide, and chromogranins) do not produce any specific clinical symptoms; 2) peptide levels may be too low to produce hormonal symptoms; 3) inactive molecular precursor forms may be present; 4) there may be downregulation of peripheral receptors or simultaneous production of an inhibitory peptide (somatostatin); 5) synthesis of a peptide without release may occur. Overall, immunocytochemistry reveals the same pattern as seen in functioning endocrine pancreatic tumors.

Nonfunctioning endocrine pancreatic neoplasms are relatively benign but often exhibit a far more malignant pattern than their functional counterparts. N/Fs are usually unifocal and originate in the pancreatic head, where they behave in a malignant fashion, with metastatic spread of 60% to 90% at diagnosis. The tumor size is usually greater than 5 cm, as diagnosis is made late because of an absence of clinical hormonal symptoms. N/Fs often secrete PP (50%) and are sometimes, therefore, designated as PPomas. In MEN1, multiple tumors always occur, either synchronously or metachronously.

Clinical Features

These lesions do not exhibit specific clinical features and are usually found incidentally at surgery in patients who initially present with symptoms caused by the tumor location (obstructive jaundice, pancreatitis, or duodenal obstruction), regarded as pancreatic adenocarcinoma. Other nonspecific symptoms evident in these patients include epigastric pain, weight loss, steatorrhea, upper gastrointestinal bleeding, dyspepsia, and fatigue.

■ MULTIPLE ENDOCRINE NEOPLASIA TYPE 1

Multiple endocrine neoplasia type 1 is a simultaneous or successive, benign or malignant cellular proliferation of at least two endocrine glands—mainly the parathyroid gland, pancreatic islets, pituitary glands, and adrenal glands. Neoplastic pancreatic

tumors develop in about 30% of clinical studies and are shown in up to 100% of autopsy studies. The syndrome often is familial (up to 60%) and may be inherited as an autosomal-dominant trait caused by a defect on chromosome 11.

The differentiation between sporadic and multiple endocrine adenomatosis is important, as sporadic cases frequently have pancreatic tumors and liver metastases. Patients with MEN1 have multiple endocrine glands, each expressing primary tumors. It may be difficult therefore to determine which of the multiple tumors is producing a particular syndrome. Diagnosis and management of endocrine pancreatic tumors in association with MEN1 is more difficult because the islet cell tumors are usually multiple, disseminated throughout the pancreas, and small. The pathologic picture of pancreatic lesions in MEN1 is diffuse microadenomatosis, in combination with one or more macrotumors. Clinically nonfunctioning PPomas are most frequently found, followed by glucagonomas and insulinomas.

Clinical Features

Given the discrepancy of the incidence in clinical and autopsy studies, which report endocrine pancreatic tumors in about 30% and 100%, respectively, many neoplasms are probably nonfunctioning. Hyperfunctional syndromes are generally gastrinomas (>50%) and insulinomas (20%), followed by VIPomas, glucagonomas, and GRFomas. The malignancy rates of endocrine pancreatic tumors in MEN1 were initially regarded as lower than in sporadic cases, but more recent studies suggest a similar risk. Somatostatinomas do not develop in MEN1, although they are evident in neurofibromatosis, which has a different genomic origin.

Diagnosis and Localization

The history of the diagnostic saga of an individual with an endocrine pancreatic tumor is fraught with misadventure. It is characterized initially by failure to identify the affected person, followed by misdiagnosis caused by lack of a specific recognizable syndrome or inability to identify the appropriate diagnostic marker. As a consequence, endocrine pancreatic tumors may be detected in as few as 25% of patients preoperatively. Insulinomas, because of their typical clinical pattern, are diagnosed more easily, although in some instances of exotic psychiatric behavior the diagnosis may be delayed. For the most part the other tumors are often not recognized at all or diagnosed late in the course of the disease [5••]. In particular, the clinical features, including diarrhea, dyspepsia, skin rash, weight loss, flushing, or a pancreatic mass, are often overlooked as reflections of more banal disease such as diabetes, inflammatory bowel disease, peptic ulcer disease, or functional disorders. The diagnostic algorithm of endocrine pancreatic tumors is given in Figure 140-1.

Clinical Presentation

Although the specific symptom complex is classic, it may often not be clear-cut in individual patients. Thus, there may initially be a delay in identifying the relationship between obvious or less obvious symptoms with a particular endocrine lesion. Clear examples of this exist in patients with insulinoma, in whom the often-vague early symptoms of hypoglycemia are misinterpreted (functional), as are the secondary manifestations of the catecholamine response (thyroid malfunction). Such individuals may be considered neurotic, anxiety-prone, hyperthyroid, or even delusionary. Sometimes the symptoms may be initiated by fasting. Similarly, the vague symptom of dyspepsia or even recalcitrant peptic ulcer disease may not be initially identified as gastrinoma. The identification of diarrhea in such individuals, particularly if not taking antacids, should lead to a suspicion of gastrinoma. An almost classic example of diagnostic confusion is the carcinoid tumor, the protean manifestations of which (flushing, sweating, diarrhea, asthma) often result in a vast series of unsuccessful investigations before correct diagnosis is finally established.

Biochemistry

Once a symptom complex has been identified as consistent with a particular endocrine pancreatic tumor, the initial requirement is biochemical confirmation of its presence. The general or non-specific plasma markers of endocrine pancreatic tumors include plasma PP and chromogranin. In general, chromogranin appears to be the best tumor marker for endocrine pancreatic tumors [6]. However, it is not specific for endocrine pancreatic tumors, as it is also elevated in carcinoid and other neuroendocrine tumors. PP is a useful nonspecific gut neuroendocrine tumor marker that is predominantly produced by the PP cells of pancreatic islets. Although up to 75% of endocrine pancreatic tumors exhibit increased levels, serum PP can be produced also by carcinoid tumors as well as by certain inflammatory diseases, and it is elevated in patients with impaired renal function. Food ingestion provokes an increase in serum PP. Non–tumor-related increases in plasma PP levels can be diminished by atropine, whereas tumor

PP secretion is autonomous in vagal cholinergic regulation. A less common nonspecific plasma marker is calcitonin, which, although usually a marker for thyroid C-cell tumors, may also be produced by endocrine pancreatic tumors, particularly in patients presenting with secretory diarrhea. Occasionally, human chorionic gonadotropin (hCG-α or hCG-β) levels may be elevated. In patients who are suspected of having the MEN1 syndrome, biochemical screening using a meal test increases the sensitivity of lesion identification. After fasting, a standard carbohydrate, fat, and protein meal is administered and blood sampled at 10-minute intervals for 2 hours. The extensive use of biochemical screening programs in MEN1 kindreds has enabled the biochemical diagnosis of endocrine pancreatic tumors to be made an average of 3.5 years before it is radiologically detectable.

If a classic symptom complex is identified, the specific peptide or amine should be measured. For practical purposes, the specific neuroendocrine markers are insulin and C-peptide, gastrin, VIP, substance P, serotonin, glucagon, and somatostatin. False-negative results should be avoided by meticulously following the instructions for specimen collection and storage. To ensure correct biochemical analysis of peptide markers, the blood sample should be taken in the morning after an overnight fast. Individual peptides have varying stability in blood samples: gastrin and PP are particularly stable, whereas VIP and somatostatin are rapidly degraded. Samples for analysis of such labile peptides should be taken in prechilled heparin tubes, immediately cooled in ice, cold centrifuged within 45 minutes, and then frozen until analysis. The use of aprotinin or other enzyme inhibitors to prevent degradation is recommended.

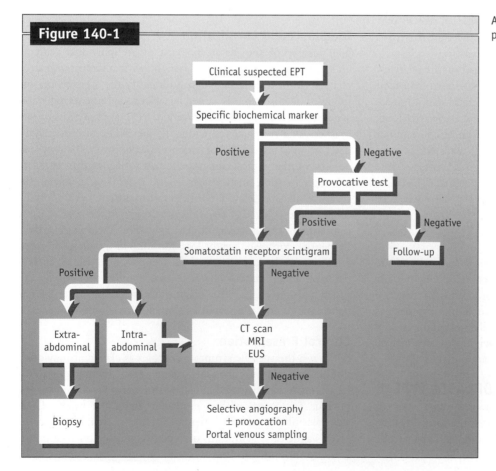

Figure 140-1

Algorithm for diagnosis of endocrine pancreatic tumors.

False-positive results are uncommon, but when they do occur, this usually reflects a different reason for elevation of the substance in the plasma. Thus, in gastrinoma patients, elevated gastrin levels may reflect nonfasting, gastric distension, achlorhydria, or the use of an acid-inhibiting agent. In suspected insulinoma patients, it is necessary to consider the factitious use of insulin or the possibility of an insulin-like peptide secreted by a non-neuroendocrine tumor (*eg*, mesothelioma, small cell lung carcinoma, retroperitoneal sarcoma). Patients believed to have glucagonomas may have elevated glucagon levels caused by unrecognized catabolic states. In patients with the WDHA syndrome, surreptitious use of laxatives or medullary carcinoma of the thyroid should be considered, even though elevated VIP levels are highly specific.

Elevated serum or plasma levels of peptides or amines need to be interpreted with caution in patients with evidence of renal disease. The use of a provocative study is usually unnecessary, except in rare cases of paroxysmal symptoms and repeated equivocal biochemic test results. Marginally elevated plasma levels of peptides may require the application of provocative agents, to demonstrate significant plasma increments consistent with the diagnosis of the neoplasm. The pentagastrin test [7] is useful for carcinoids in the presence of marginally elevated urinary 5-hydroxyindolacetic acid or equivocally elevated plasma amine (substance P, serotonin) levels. The secretin provocation test [8] for gastrinomas has been widely used, but the calcium provocation study is now held in less regard. Arginine infusion for glucagonoma is probably of minimal value.

In the interest of both time- and cost-effectiveness, the initial strategy should be to measure the presumed plasma agent of interest under the correct conditions. If results are equivocal, the test should be repeated and chromogranin level measured. If the latter is elevated and the agent of interest is still equivocal, then a provocation test should be given. If the provocation study results are positive or the agent of interest alone was initially positive, topographic localization, preferably by somatostatin receptor scintigraphy, should be undertaken. Patients with equivocal biochemic test results, negative nonspecific markers and negative somatostatin receptor scintigraphy should probably not be further investigated but followed up regularly (Fig. 140-1).

Imaging

Somatostatin Receptor Scintigraphy

In order to develop an appropriate management strategy, the precise location of the primary tumor and its metastases, whether overt or covert, is of critical relevance. The most significant and important advance has been the development of somatostatin receptor scintigraphy, which uses indium-111–labeled octreotide in individuals with the putative diagnosis of endocrine pancreatic tumors. This compound preferentially identifies such tumors since these lesions express large numbers of somatostatin receptors (SST_R), particularly subtype 2 (SST_R2) for which octreotide has a high affinity (Fig. 140-2A). By use of a gamma camera, uptake is estimated at 4 hours, and further studies may be undertaken at 24 and 48 hours (rarely necessary), by which time renal and hepatic background activity has significantly dissipated. The associated use of single positron emission computed tomography imaging provides further enhancement of the sensitivity of this study and precise identification of covert and often unsuspected lesions. The fact that the entire body can be imaged at one time is of considerable advantage, as it enables the detection of covert lesions that might otherwise be either undetectable (outside of evaluated area) or require multiple different imaging studies for identification. Somatostatin receptor scintigraphy is actually more sensitive than any other imaging method for the identification of primary gastrinomas, and its sensitivity alone is equal to that of all other conventional methods combined [9•]. A certain percentage of neuroendocrine tumors fail to exhibit SST_R2 in quantities sufficient to enable visualization by somatostatin receptor scintigraphy. This is particularly evident for insulinomas because up to 40% of such lesions do not express SST_R2 and are thus cannot be visualized. However, an undetectable primary insulinoma tumor may often generate hepatic and extrahepatic secondary tumors that are identifiable by somatostatin receptor scintigraphy (Fig. 140-2B). This may reflect the increased level

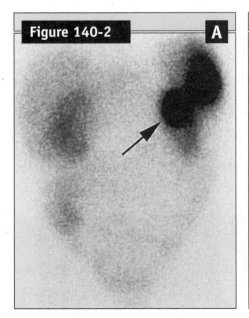 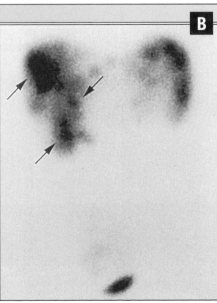

Figure 140-2   **A**   **B**

Somatostatin receptor scintigram of (*A*) a glucagonoma in the pancreatic tail (*arrow*) and (*B*) diffuse liver metastases (*arrows*).

of SST_R2 expression on tumor neovascularization. In the identification of extrahepatic tumors, the sensitivity of somatostatin receptor scintigraphy alone is equal to that of conventional imaging methods combined. The combination of the use of conventional imaging methods in addition to somatostatin receptor scintigraphy results in the identification of more than 95% of hepatic metastases.

Endoscopic Ultrasonography

The experienced use of endoscopic ultrasonography seems to be particularly useful in the diagnosis of endocrine pancreatic tumors, especially in the identification of small tumors in the pancreatic head and the localization of duodenal microgastrinomas (usually <1 cm). Endoscopic ultrasonography has the highest sensitivity (80% to 85%) and specificity (95%) in the detection of endocrine pancreatic tumors, compared with ultrasound, CT scan, or magnetic resonance imaging. The procedure is performed by passing an endoscope through the stomach and duodenum or using an endoscopic ultrasonograph probe passed through a conventional endoscope. A balloon is inflated with saline solution and a 5- to 10-MHz transducer is used to scan the pancreas and duodenal wall (Fig. 140-3) [10•].

Abdominal Ultrasonography

This examination exhibits a low sensitivity (20% to 30%) for primary endocrine pancreatic tumors. Small tumors are not well visualized by this method, which has little to recommend it.

Computed Tomography Scan

Approximately 50% of primary and metastatic tumors can be detected with this method, but the sensitivity for small tumors (<2 cm) can be as low as 35% [11]. The use of dynamic CT with pancreatic protocol is more effective, with sensitivity ranging from 75% to 80%.

Magnetic Resonance Imaging

This technique has a relatively low sensitivity for the detection of endocrine pancreatic tumors (eg, only 25% for gastrinomas)

(Fig. 140-4) [11]. Short inversion recovery magnetic resonance imaging appears to exhibit a significant advantage in detecting hepatic metastatic disease, with a sensitivity of 83% [12].

Selective and Provocative Angiography

With this method, a sensitivity of about 70% for extrahepatic lesions and 86% for hepatic gastrinomas is accompanied by a specificity of greater than 97% for both lesions [11]. Combined with the administration of secretagogues (Ca^{2+} or secretin), a greater proportion of tumors can be localized, with a 90% positive predictability rate. For this procedure, secretin in gastrinoma patients or calcium in insulinoma patients is selectively injected into specific mesenteric arteries, while serial blood samples from the hepatic and peripheral veins are assayed for gastrin levels [13]. A rapid rise of the specific hormone (gastrin or insulin) in the hepatic vein indicates that the injected artery probably supplies the lesion. Selective angiography can provide a reasonable degree of localization (regionalization) of gastrinomas and insulinomas with respect to their site in the pancreas or the liver.

Portal Venous Sampling

In this technique, a catheter is passed percutaneously through the liver into the portal vein and its branches, and multiple blood samples are collected for hormone assay. The closer the catheter is placed to the tumor, the higher the hormone concentration. The sensitivity of portal venous sampling is 70% to 90%, with a specificity ranging from 30% to 90% [11,14]. However, this highly invasive method is time consuming, expensive, and technically difficult; it is associated also with a high rate of complications. In addition, in most cases this procedure does not specifically localize the tumor but rather provides only evidence of a region of interest. This procedure is rarely recommended and indicated only in special, doubtful cases.

Intraoperative Ultrasonography

This method is performed by the operating surgeon and an ultrasonographer. Endocrine pancreatic tumors appear as sonolucent masses on an ultrasound scan. Intraoperative ultrasonography images pancreatic insulinomas and gastrinomas in

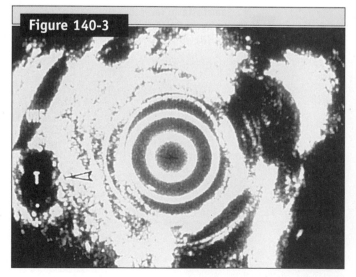

Figure 140-3

Endoscopic ultrasonogram of a gastrinoma (T) in the pancreatic head. (*From* Ruszniewski *et al.* [24]; with permission.)

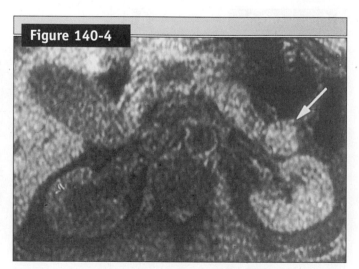

Figure 140-4

Magnetic resonance image of a glucagonoma in the pancreatic tail (*arrow*).

approximately 90% and is particularly useful in that it may often detect tumors that are not palpable. The ultrasonographic detection of endocrine pancreatic tumors is supported by the uniform echo-dense background of the pancreas [15].

▊ TREATMENT

The pattern of endocrine pancreatic tumors, with their generally slow growth, should be taken into account before extensive therapy is undertaken; treatment may have side effects that are worse than the untreated state, thereby decreasing the quality of life. In general, it is wise to adopt the adage that the treatment should not be more aggressive than the disease [16•]. The therapeutic algorithms of endocrine pancreatic tumors are shown in Figures 140-5 and 140-6.

Surgery

If the diagnosis has been biochemically established and metastases have been excluded, then surgery should be aimed at tumor removal and cure of the endocrine syndrome. Even in malignant endocrine pancreatic tumors, when a curative resection is not possible a debulking procedure (cytoreductive surgery) should always be considered, if the general health of the patient warrants intervention. The advantages of cytoreductive surgery include:

1) reduction of the hormone-producing cell mass, which decreases hormone levels and improves the related syndrome; 2) facilitation of the medical management of symptoms; 3) decreased tumor mass for optimization of cytotoxic dosage; and 4) induction of a clinical remission by a palliative surgical resection, as the tumor growth beyond the capsule of the pancreas is often slow and removal of a large lesion relieves mass effect. Thus, regional lymph node or liver metastases are not necessarily contraindications to surgery but need to be evaluated in the context of each individual patient. Nevertheless, although an aggressive surgical approach is still the best chance for cure, relatively few patients fulfill the criteria for surgical intervention.

The type of resection depends on the localization and the extent of the neoplasm. In principle, the surgeon has two options available to remove an endocrine pancreatic tumors—enucleation or resection. Enucleation is indicated in small, benign tumors, mainly insulinomas or occasionally gastrinomas. Resection should be considered for all other classes of endocrine pancreatic tumors, as the higher malignancy rate favors a resective procedure. A Whipple procedure or a partial or total pancreatectomy may be undertaken, depending on tumor location. If the neoplasm is not resectable and biliary obstruction is present, a biliary bypass procedure should be performed.

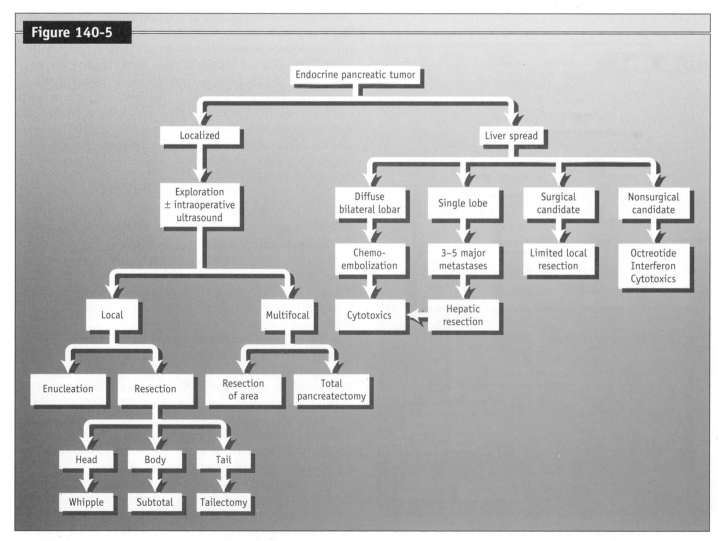

Figure 140-5

Algorithm for the therapy of endocrine pancreatic neoplasms.

Particularly important at surgery is the establishment of tumor multicentricity, lymph node involvement, and hepatic metastasis. Multiple sites should therefore be sampled. Intraoperative sonography is an especially useful method of tumor localization. Once a complete tumor map of the area has been established, the operative procedure should be undertaken. After mobilizing the pancreas, an experienced surgeon can palpate the tumor in most cases and remove the neoplasm, either by enucleation or partial resection of the pancreas. Intraoperative ultrasonography should be performed to confirm tumor removal.

For sporadic gastrinomas, an aggressive surgical approach is justified because a complete cure is attainable in some patients. Surgery for the MEN1 syndrome, however, is particularly controversial, as most MEN1 gastrinomas are multicentric, microscopic, and not only disseminated but also associated with other endocrine neoplasia. Current opinion regarding the management of gastrinomas includes: 1) enucleation/resection if a clear gradient in portal venous gastrin levels is detected; 2) resection if a tumor can be imaged, in order to prevent local and metastatic spread; and 3) resection if tumor is associated with an insulinoma [17]. The other types of islet cell tumors in MEN1 are often large but may be resected, despite the development of recurrent disease, because MEN1 appears to involve most of the islet cell mass at some time.

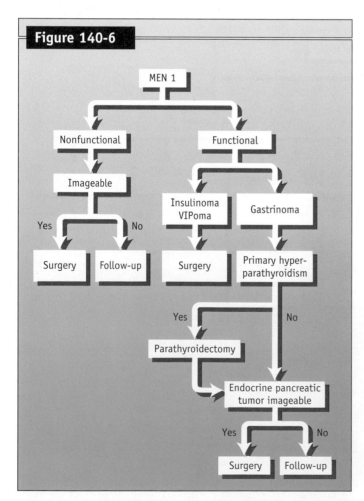

Figure 140-6

Algorithm for the therapy of endocrine pancreatic lesions in the multiple endocrine neoplasia type 1 (MEN1) syndrome.

The therapeutic procedure for insulinomas is less a matter of controversy. Even in metastatic disease an aggressive surgical approach can improve the quality and duration of life. Untreated patients rarely survive 12 months, whereas in advanced disease complete resection of metastatic insulinoma results in a long-term survival in almost 50% of individuals with biochemical remission. The localization of the functional tumor, especially in patients with MEN1, however, is often difficult, even with transhepatic venous sampling and endoscopic and intraoperative ultrasound.

Besides the problems of abdominal surgery (pulmonary complications, infection, ileus), specific postoperative complications after removal of an endocrine pancreatic tumor include pancreatic fistula, abscess, pancreatitis, pseudocysts, and duodenal leak. The overall morbidity rates may be as high as 15% to 30% [16•]. The routine perioperative and postoperative administration of octreotide to inhibit pancreatic secretion has been proposed because it reduces complications after pancreatic surgery.

Somatostatin Analogues, Interferons

If complete surgical removal is not possible because of extensive liver metastases, wide local invasion, or rapid growth, the use of long-acting somatostatin analogues are indicated. Somatostatin and its analogues have a dual action: they not only suppress the release of gastroenteropancreatic amines or peptides from neoplastic cells but also inhibit their action on target tissues [18]. Thus, octreotide reduces the plasma glucagon levels in patients with glucagonomas and improves the skin lesions and metabolic condition. The same is true in those with VIPomas, in whom a reduction of VIP levels is often associated with a dramatic improvement in the volume of diarrhea. In patients with metastatic disease, octreotide, at dosages of 450 to 600 µg/day, reduces or even halts diarrhea but larger doses may be required. Unfortunately, patients may become resistant to octreotide after long-term therapy owing to increases in tumor bulk or the development of tachyphylaxis.

Overall, almost all clinical symptoms in patients with endocrine pancreatic tumors can be pharmacologically controlled. Although adequate data on survival are still incomplete, it appears that the quality of life is improved by somatostatin analogues. In addition, octreotide may have an antiproliferative effect on the tumor itself. The mechanism of this growth inhibitory effect reflects a direct inhibition of tumor growth and the effects on associated concomitant growth factors such as insulin-like growth factor 1 and transforming growth factor–α.

Mild adverse effects of octreotide occur in about 30% of patients and are generally transient. These include diarrhea, abdominal discomfort, nausea, vomiting, and flatulence. Because of decreased gallbladder motility, the incidence of cholelithiasis may be increased in up to 30% to 50% of patients after long-term administration. In addition, a worsening of the tendency to develop hypoglycemia in patients with metastatic insulinoma is described, as somatostatin and its analogues also suppress glucagon and growth hormone secretion.

Interferon is regarded as a biologic modifier that decreases the tumor peptides and also has an antitumor effect. Overall, the results indicate a mean biochemical response rate of about 40% and a reduction in tumor size of about 10% [19]. The adverse reactions of interferon, which may be severe, include fatigue, weight loss, anemia, and autoimmune reactions (thyrotoxicosis, hypothyroidism, thyroiditis, vasculitis).

Arterial Embolization

Endocrine pancreatic tumors generally metastasize to lymph nodes, to the liver, and, less frequently, to the bones. Consequences of liver metastases include disruption of hepatic physiologic capacity, a large painful liver, and a substantial release of active peptides or amines into the systemic circulation, with a consequent unpleasant amplification of clinical symptoms. If an operative procedure is too risky and cytostatic therapy has failed, local treatment of liver metastases should be considered, to improve the quality of life.

One possibility includes the blockade of blood flow to liver metastases, as they are often hypervascular and derive most of their blood supply from the hepatic artery (Fig. 140-7). Transcutaneous sequential selective hepatic arterial embolization is a most effective strategy and may result in long-lasting remissions [20]. An additional step is the administration of local chemotherapeutic agents through an arterial catheter (chemoembolization). A side effect of this method, caused by liver or tumor necrosis, or both, is a postembolization syndrome characterized by right upper quadrant pain associated with nausea, vomiting, and high fever. Severe complications may occur, including acute hepatic failure, infection with abscess and septicemia, cholecystitis (probably of ischemic origin), and massive release of peptides (symptomatic paroxysm) during this procedure (a consequence of tumor necrosis). The latter problem can be obviated by the pre-embolic administration of octreotide.

Chemotherapy

Systemic chemotherapy in metastatic endocrine pancreatic tumors is usually a second choice for several reasons: unpredictable response rates, toxic side effects, and the temporary and often short-lasting response. Because cure cannot be achieved by chemotherapy, quality of life is a most important issue; inhibition of symptoms with octreotide is in most instances preferable.

The recommendations for well-differentiated endocrine carcinomas consist of a number of combinations, which usually include streptozotocin, doxorubicin, 5-fluoro-uracil, cisplatin, and etoposide [21]. The response rate in insulinomas or carcinoids

may be as high as 60%, but this rate is unpredictable and often associated with debilitating side effects.

Symptomatic Drugs

The management of endocrine pancreatic tumors has been dramatically altered by the introduction of octreotide. This long-lasting somatostatin analogue dramatically decreases all endocrine symptoms and is relatively free of side effects. Its routine use has considerably increased the quality of life in almost all patients. Except for gastrinomas, in which proton pump inhibitors are more effective, octreotide is the symptomatic therapy of choice.

Diazoxide is an effective inhibitor of insulin secretion from normal and neoplastic β-cells and is therefore useful in preventing fasting hypoglycemia in patients with insulinoma. The dose of diazoxide has to be determined individually, on the basis of tolerance and effectiveness, and may vary from 50 to 600 mg daily. Its side effects may be severe and include hirsutism and renal and cardiac failure.

The management of patients with gastrinomas has changed dramatically with the availability of the proton pump inhibitors. Formerly, total gastrectomy was a usual therapeutic option; currently, this procedure is almore obsolete.

Emergent correction of dehydration and abnormal serum electrolyte value is often necessary, particularly in VIPomas and glucagonomas. Parenteral nutrition may be introduced as a perioperative procedure or in patients with prolonged periods refractory to surgical and medical treatment.

▉ PROGNOSIS AND FOLLOW-UP MANAGEMENT

Most patients with abdominal endocrine tumors, even if associated with metastases, have a longer survival than do similar patients with nonendocrine tumors. As mentioned earlier, endocrine pancreatic tumors usually metastasize to the liver or local lymph nodes. Recurrence of the tumor is usually at a local site in the retroperitoneum and lymph nodes, but late hepatic metastases may also occur. The clinical diagnosis is best made by the identification of recurrent symptoms; before such manifestations, however, measurement of the relevant peptide or amine in the plasma may be an earlier indication of tumor regrowth. Topographic localization is best obtained using somatostatin receptor scintigraphy, which may in itself become the earliest test for identification of lesion recurrence. The results of magnetic resonance imaging or CT scan may be difficult to interpret due to the interference of previous surgery with image reconstruction and interpretation.

Reliable data on survival rates are available for insulinomas and gastrinomas, which represent the majority of endocrine pancreatic tumors. Surgical cure of benign insulinomas is attainable in more than 90% of cases. Survival rates for sporadic, localized gastrinomas are lower, having a short-term cure of 60% to 85%, decreasing to 30% to 40% in the long term as a result of recurrent disease. Patients with metastatic gastrinoma show a 5-year survival rate of 20% [22].

Each patient needs a personalized follow-up, which includes history, physical examination, biochemical testing, and imaging studies. Measurement of plasma PP or amines, or both, is

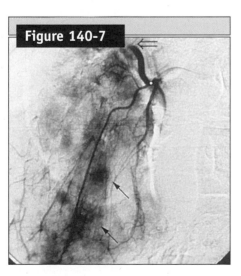

Figure 140-7

Angiogram of multiple liver metastases (*arrows*) along a branch of the right hepatic artery. Following embolization (*open arrow*) most of the peripheral branches are occluded.

suggested every 3 months for the first 12 months, and then every 6 months. Urine 5-hydroxyindolacetic acid levels and chest radiography are indicated every 6 months. Octreoscan, abdominal CT scan or short inversion recovery magnetic resonance imaging, and panendoscopy once a year are recommended [23].

ACKNOWLEDGMENT

The authors would like to thank Dr. Eugene Cornelius from the Yale New Haven Hospital, Diagnostic Radiology (nuclear medicine), for providing the radiologic pictures.

REFERENCES

Recently published papers of particular interest have been highlighted as follows:
• Of interest
•• Of outstanding interest

1.•• Modlin IM, Tang LH: Approaches to the diagnosis of gut neuroendocrine tumors: the last word (today). *Gastroenterology* 1997, 112:583–590.
This is a very useful and logical overview of management strategies for identifying endocrine pancreatic tumors.

2. Kimura W, Kuroda A, Morioka Y: Clinical pathology of endocrine tumors of the pancreas. Analysis of autopsy cases. *Dig Dis Sci* 1991, 36:933–942.

3. Bonner-Weir S: Anatomy of the islet of Langerhans. In *The Endocrine Pancreas*. Edited by Samols E. New York: Raven Press; 1991:15–27.

4.• Klöppel G, Schröder S, Heitz PU: Histopathology and immunopathology of pancreatic endocrine tumors. In *Endocrine Tumors of the Pancreas*. Edited by Mignon M. Basel: Karger; 1995:99–120.
This is a concise outline of pathological function enabling identification of lesions.

5.•• Mignon M, Jensen RT: Endocrine tumors of the pancreas. In *Recent Advances in Research and Management*. Edited by Modlin IM. Basel: Karger; 1995.
This is a comprehensive overview of all aspects of endocrine pancreatic tumors in significant detail both for lesions and management strategies.

6. Eriksson B, Arnberg H, Lindgren PG, et al.: Neuroendocrine pancreatic tumours: clinical presentation, biochemical and histopathological findings in 84 patients. *J Intern Med* 1990, 228:103–113.

7. Ahlman H, Dahlstrom A, Gronstad K, et al.: The pentagastrin test in the diagnosis of the carcinoid syndrome: blockage of gastrointestinal symptoms by ketanserin. *Ann Surg* 1985, 201:81–86.

8. Frucht H, Howard JM, Slaff JI, et al: Secretin and calcium provacative tests in the Zollinger-Ellison syndrome: a prospective study. *Ann Intern Med* 1989, 111:713–722.

9.• Gibril F, Reynolds JC, Doppman JL, et al.: Somatostatin receptor scintigraphy: its sensitivity compared with that of other imaging methods in detecting primary and metastatic gastrinomas. A prospective study. *Ann Intern Med* 1996, 125:26–34.
This is a current assessment of utility of somatostatin receptor scintigraphy in diagnosis of management.

10.• Rosch T, Lightdale CJ, Botet JF, et al.: Localization of pancreatic endocrine tumors by endoscopic ultrasonography. *N Engl J Med* 1992, 326:1721–1726.
This paper provides an outline of applications and advantages of endoscopic ultrasonography.

11. Orbuch M, Doppman JL, Strader DB, et al.: Imaging for pancreatic endocrine tumor localization: recent advances. In *Endocrine Tumors of the Pancreas*. Edited by Mignon M. Basel: Karger; 1995:268–281.

12. Pisegna JR, Doppman JL, Norton JA, et al.: Prospective comparative study of ability of MR imaging and other imaging modalities to localize tumors in patients with Zollinger-Ellison syndrome. *Dig Dis Sci* 1993, 38:1318–1328.

13. Doppman JL, Miller DL, Chang R, et al.: Insulinomas: localization with selective intraarterial injection of calcium. *Radiology* 1991, 178:237–241.

14. Miller DL, Doppman JL, Metz DC, et al.: Zollinger-Ellison syndrome: technique, results, and complications of portal venous sampling. *Radiology* 1992, 182:235–241.

15. Norton JA: Surgical treatment of islet cell tumors with special emphasis on operative ultrasound. In *Endocrine Tumors of the Pancreas*. Edited by Mignon M. Basel: Karger; 1995:309–332.

16.• Norton JA: Neuroendocrine tumors of the pancreas and duodenum. *Curr Probl Surg* 1994, 31:77–156.
This is a detailed overview with special reference to diagnosis and treatment of endocrine pancreatic tumors.

17. Mignon M, Cadiot G, Rigaud D, et al.: Management of islet cell tumors in patients with multiple endocrine neoplasia type 1. In *Endocrine Tumors of the Pancreas*. Edited by Mignon M. Basel: Karger; 1995:342–359.

18. Scarpignato C: Octreotide, the synthetic long-acting SST analogue: pharmacological profile. In *Octreotide: From Basic Science to Clinical Medicine*. Edited by Scarpignato C. Basel: Karger; 1996:54–72.

19. Oberg K: Interferon-α versus somatostatin or the combination of both in gastro-enteropancreatic tumours. *Digestion* 1996, 57:81–83.

20. Arcenas AG, Ajani JA, Carrasco CH, et al.: Vascular occlusive therapy of pancreatic endocrine tumors metastatic to the liver. In *Endocrine Tumors of the Pancreas*. Edited by Mignon M. Basel: Karger; 1995:439–450.

21. Moertel CG, Lefkopoulo M, Lipsitz S, et al.: Streptozocin-doxorubicin, streptozocin-fluorouracil or chlorozotocin in the treatment of advanced islet-cell carcinoma. *N Engl J Med* 1992, 326:519–523.

22. Norton JA, Doppman JL, Jensen RT: Curative resection in Zollinger-Ellison syndrome. Results of a 10-year prospective study. *Ann Surg* 1992, 215:8–18.

23. Modlin IM: Islet cell neoplasia. In *Follow-up of Cancer*. Edited by Fischer DS. Philadelphia: Lippincott-Raven; 1996:108–109.

24. Ruszniewski P, Amouyal P, Amouyal G, et al.: Endocrine tumors of the pancreatic area: localization by endoscopic ultrasonography. In *Endocrine Tumors of the Pancreas*. Edited by Mignon M. Basel: Karger; 1995:258–267.

141 Pancreatic Pseudocyst

Vivek V. Gumaste and C.S. Pitchumoni

As defined by the Atlanta International Symposium, a pseudocyst of the pancreas is a collection of pancreatic juice enclosed by a nonepithelialized wall that arises as a consequence of acute pancreatitis, pancreatic trauma, or chronic pancreatitis [1]. Pseudocyst formation is a well-documented complication of pancreatitis. In developing countries, gallstones are the leading cause for chronic pancreatitis. The only population-based study of pancreatitis in the United States is from Rochester, Minnesota. The study shows a steadily increasing incidence of pancreatitis to 17 per 100,000 per year, which is comparable with the rates quoted from Europe [2]. Earlier studies, based on upper gastrointestinal series, reported an extremely low incidence (1%–3%) of pseudocyst formation with pancreatitis [3••]. CT scanning and ultrasound, which are more accurate than barium studies, demonstrate that 10% to 15% of patients will develop pseudocysts.

PATHOGENESIS

The pathogenesis of pseudocyst formation is not clear. Several theories have been proposed. In acute pancreatitis (*eg,* secondary to biliary tract diseases) cysts may develop as a result of accumulation of enzyme-rich fluid, blood, and products of tissue digestion in the lesser sac. In early stages, the cyst is not well demarcated, and it takes nearly 4 to 6 weeks for an inflammatory capsule to develop. In chronic alcoholic pancreatitis, pseudocysts may occur without an identifiable episode of acute pancreatitis and have a mature capsule at the time of diagnosis. The pathogenesis in chronic alcoholic pancreatitis is related to ductular obstruction and increased intraductal pressure, which occur as a result of protein plugs, calculi, or stricture formation. Leakage of enzymes may occur into the pseudocyst. Some authors believe that chronic pseudocysts develop from retention cysts secondary to ductal hypertension [3••]. The fluid of pseudocysts is relatively clear because it does not contain blood products and tissue debris.

PATHOLOGY

Macroscopic Features

Pseudocysts can be single or multiple. Single, unilocular cysts are seen in nearly 90% of cases. Multiple pseudocysts are more commonly seen with acute alcoholic pancreatitis. Some pseudocysts are as large as 30 cm, but most are usually 4 to 8 cm (Fig. 141-1). Small pseudocysts lie within the pancreas. Nearly one third of pseudocysts are located in the head and two thirds in the body or tail of the gland. The lesser sac is also a common location. Extension into the transverse mesocolon may occur because of the close anatomic relationship between it and the pancreas. Additional sites include the anterior and posterior pararenal spaces, the mediastinum, and the retroperitoneum. Posterior pseudocysts are rare and may extend inferiorly into the pelvic area and groin; in rare cases they have been reported to occur in the liver or spleen. Pseudocysts may or may not have a grossly demonstrable communication with the pancreatic ductal system (Fig. 141-2) [4].

In chronic pancreatitis, pseudocysts are more common in glands with focal fibrosis and few calcifications than in those with advanced fibrosis and numerous calcifications [5]. Pseudocysts are more likely to be smooth and rounded, with a fibrous

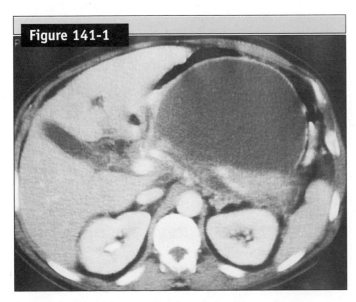

Figure 141-1

Computed tomography scan showing pancreatic pseudocyst.

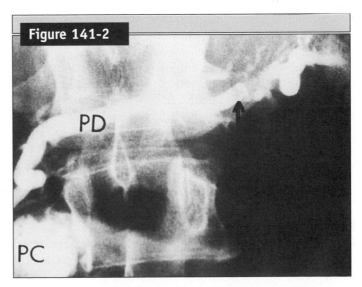

Figure 141-2

An endoscopic retrograde cholangiopancreatography showing communication between the main pancreatic duct and pseudocyst. (*From* Toskes and Forsmark [4]; with permission.)

granulation tissue capsule separating the cysts from other structures. The capsule is highlighted on contrast-enhanced CT scan.

The fluid in the pseudocyst is watery, but it may be xanthochromic or brown in color because of blood or necrotic tissue. The electrolyte content of the fluid is similar to that of plasma. Its amylase, lipase, and trypsin contents tend to be higher and the albumin and protein concentrations lower than those of the serum [6]. There is evidence to indicate that the fluid in the cyst can exchange with the plasma, perhaps accounting for the decrease in amylase values noted in aged pseudocysts. The same mechanism may be responsible for the reabsorption of small pseudocysts.

Microscopic Features

The characteristic feature of a pseudocyst is its lack of an epithelial lining; instead, its wall is composed of granulation and fibrous tissue. In an acute pseudocyst, four zones usually can be distinguished in the wall: zone 1 is the narrow inner zone containing hemosiderin pigment and loose connective tissue; zone 2 is made up of inflammatory and capillary-rich fibrous tissue; and zone 3 is composed of cell-poor hyalinized connective tissue that merges with the outer zone, zone 4, consisting of capillary-rich fibrous stroma [6].

■ CLINICAL PRESENTATION

Development of a pseudocyst should be suspected when

1. an episode of acute pancreatitis fails to resolve
2. a patient has persistently raised serum amylase levels
3. a patient has persistent abdominal pain
4. an epigastric mass is present

Other forms of presentation may be related to pseudocyst complications, including infection, rupture, and hemorrhage. Infection is the most common complication, occurring in roughly 10% of patients. It is characterized by fever and abdominal pain.

Sudden rupture into the peritoneum produces severe peritonitis necessitating emergency surgery and is often fatal. Spontaneous drainage and amelioration of symptoms results when a pseudocyst ruptures into the gastrointestinal tract. This may be accompanied by vomiting or bloody diarrhea, especially when the colon is involved. Hematemesis or melena may occur. A slow leak into the peritoneum produces pancreatic ascites.

Hemorrhage results from erosion of the small vessels lining the cyst wall or from erosion of major blood vessels, such as the splenic artery. Intracystic bleeding leads to a rapid enlargement of the cyst, producing pain and shock. Sometimes bleeding into the pancreatic duct occurs, a condition referred to as "hemosuccus pancreaticus" [3••]. This complication is associated with a very high mortality. Angioembolization is extremely effective in controlling the hemorrhage. Table 141-1 lists some of the rare presentations of a pseudocyst.

■ LABORATORY FINDINGS

Laboratory investigations are of limited value in the diagnosis of a pseudocyst. A persistently elevated serum amylase level may be present in up to 76% of patients with pseudocysts, and in some patients the serum may demonstrate "old amylase" when it is tested electrophoretically [3••]. An increased serum bilirubin level is found when the pseudocyst produces biliary obstruction.

■ IMAGING STUDIES
Plain Radiographs

Frequently, a plain radiograph of the abdomen is not helpful in diagnosing pseudocysts. Occasionally, abdominal radiographs may demonstrate displacement of the gastric bubble or calcification in the cyst wall. A chest radiograph may show elevation of the diaphragm, pleural effusion, or rarely a mediastinal mass.

Ultrasound and Computed Tomography Scanning

Ultrasound has a sensitivity of only 75% to 90% in detecting pseudocysts [3••]. CT scanning is a much more accurate and precise modality to delineate pseudocysts, with a sensitivity of 90% to 100%. Even pseudocysts smaller than 1 cm can be

Table 141-1. Complications of a Pancreatic Pseudocyst

Local
  Infection
  Hemorrhage
  Rupture
    Pancreatic ascites
    Shock
    Peritonitis
Involving adjacent organs
  Gastrointestinal tract
    Esophagus
      Secondary achalasia
      Mechanical dysphagia
    Stomach
      Gastric outlet obstruction
      Fistula
      Intramural gastric mass
    Duodenal
      Obstruction
      Fistula
    Colonic
      Fistula
      Colonic stenosis
      Obstruction
      Rectal bleeding
    Liver
      Common bile duct obstruction
    Spleen
      Splenic vein thrombosis
      Splenic rupture
  Genitourinary tract
    Pelvis
      Stricture
      Fistula
    Ureter
      Obstruction
  Chest
    Pleural effusion
    Mediastinal extension
  Vascular
    Arterial
      Erosion of gastroduodenal artery
      Erosion of splenic artery
    Venous
      Splenic vein thrombosis
      Portal vein thrombosis
  Skin
    Subcutaneous fat necrosis

detected by this technique [7]. A CT scan is also more effective than sonography in detecting the secondary complications of a pseudocyst, such as infection; hemorrhage; and involvement of adjacent structures, such as the spleen, the liver, blood vessels, the urinary tract, and the kidneys. Gas bubbles seen on a CT scan may indicate an infection. Normally, the density of fluid in an uncomplicated pseudocyst ranges from 0 to 25 Hounsfield units (HU). A significant increase in the density of the fluid collection (50–100 HU) is suggestive of hemorrhage into the pseudocyst [8]. Finally, CT scanning is an important adjunct in the therapy of pseudocysts.

In summary, CT scanning is useful for the precise definition and localization of a pseudocyst, whereas an ultrasound examination, because of its convenience and less cost, is an ideal method for follow-up of patients managed conservatively.

Endoscopic Retrograde Cholangiopancreatography

Endoscopic retrograde cholangiopancreatography (ERCP) is not a routine method for diagnosing a pseudocyst. ERCP may be useful in patients who require surgery to delineate the ductal anatomy and help devise optimal therapy. Often ERCP findings alter the operative plan, resulting in an improved outcome. However, there is a danger of introducing infection, and surgery should be planned within 24 hours of performing the ERCP. ERCP also may be used as a therapeutic modality when draining pseudocysts through the transpapillary approach. This method will be discussed later in this chapter. Another role that ERCP may play is in deciding which patients will benefit from percutaneous drainage. If there is an obstruction between the communication and the papilla, the chances for the success of percutaneous drainage are minimal. ERCP is not routinely indicated in patients undergoing percutaneous drainage. It should be reserved for those patients who fail percutaneous therapy.

Endoscopic Ultrasound

Small cysts are usually imaged well with endoscopic ultrasound [9]. Large cysts that extend into peripancreatic areas cannot be seen in their entirety. Endoscopic ultrasound accurately defines the proximity of the cyst to the gut lumen; is the only technique able to determine whether a large blood vessel is present close to the puncture site, which greatly reduces the chance of post-procedure hemorrhage; and can determine whether septae are present in the pseudocyst, which may be an indicator of post-procedure infection [10]. This information may prove especially helpful in selecting patients who can be managed successfully by endoscopic therapy.

Once a pseudocyst is diagnosed, it must be determined whether the pseudocyst can be treated conservatively, in the hope of spontaneous resolution, or whether immediate intervention is necessary to prevent complications. If intervention is necessary, it must be determined whether surgical, percutaneous, or endoscopic drainage is the best approach.

▬ SPONTANEOUS RESOLUTION

To choose the correct approach to the management of a pseudocyst, it is necessary to be aware of its natural history. Spontaneous resolution of pseudocysts has been reported in 7% to 85% of subjects [3••]. This wide range can be attributed to

many factors that influence healing of pseudocysts, including size, chronicity, wall thickness, multiplicity, and etiology. Overall, 40% of pseudocysts will resolve spontaneously [3••].

Timing

Most pseudocysts that are likely to heal do so within 6 weeks, but resolution may be seen after 24 weeks or even 28 months [3••]. Cysts that persist for 8 to 10 weeks are unlikely to resolve spontaneously.

Size

Size is an important determinant of spontaneous resolution. Cysts less than 4 to 6 cm will usually resolve by themselves. As the size of the cyst increases, so does the need for intervention (Table 141-2) [11••]. However, some large pseudocysts (> 6 cm) may undergo spontaneous resolution. In one study, 3 of 11 pseudocysts larger than 10 cm resolved spontaneously [11••].

Chronicity

Chronicity affects healing adversely. Most series that comprise a large number of subjects with chronic pancreatitis report a low incidence of spontaneous healing. In one study the rate of spontaneous resolution in subjects with chronic pancreatitis was 9%, compared with 20% for the group with acute pancreatitis [12]. Pancreatic calcification also is a poor prognostic indicator.

Multiplicity

The presence of multiple pseudocysts augurs badly. Patients with more than one cyst eventually require surgical intervention for cure.

Change in Size

If serial ultrasound examinations demonstrate an increase in size or show no change, the chance of resolution is small. Conversely, a decrease in size is a good sign. In a series of 24 subjects with pseudocysts undergoing spontaneous resolution, a decrease in the size of the cyst was seen on the second or third ultrasound examination [3••].

Etiology

Etiology also may have some bearing on the outcome. In one study, subjects with pseudocysts related to alcohol abuse had a more favorable outcome [13]. No pseudocysts associated with postoperative or biliary pancreatitis resolved spontaneously in

Table 141-2. Size and Outcome of Pancreatic Pseudocysts

Size, cm	Operated, %	Not operated, %
0–2	33	67
2–4	37	63
4–6	45	55
6–8	63	37
8–10	64	36
> 10	73	27

From [11••]; with permission.

this study. Traumatic pseudocysts may have a high percentage of spontaneous resolution.

Communication With Pancreatic Duct

The opinion that the presence of a communication with the pancreatic duct might enhance spontaneous resolution is controversial.

CONSERVATIVE MANAGEMENT

Initial studies showed that conservative treatment in the hope of spontaneous resolution was not without risk. A complication rate ranging from 0% to 41% has been noted during the waiting period, most within 13.5 ± 6 weeks. The overall mortality rate for conservative therapy ranges from 0% to 12%. However, with improved medical care, the incidence of complications and mortality has decreased considerably. In a study of 75 subjects with pseudocysts, nearly 50% resolved spontaneously [11••]. Although two thirds of cysts larger than 6 cm remained symptomatic and required surgery, diameter was not an absolute predictor of the need for interventional therapy. Three of 11 cysts larger than 10 cm resolved spontaneously. Indications for operation in the remaining 39 subjects were continuous pain, cyst enlargement, infection, hemorrhage, cyst rupture, common bile duct obstruction, and gastric outlet obstruction. During the follow-up period (1–9 years) in 36 conservatively treated subjects, only one pseudocyst-related complication occurred, and there was no mortality [11••]. Therefore, most physicians opt for a conservative approach for asymptomatic small pseudocysts or even larger asymptomatic pseudocysts that show signs of regression [14].

SURGICAL INTERVENTION

Surgical procedures for pancreatic pseudocysts include excision, external drainage, and internal drainage, the latter of which can take the form of a cystogastrostomy, a cystoduodenostomy, or a cystojejunostomy.

Complication rates for these operations range from 10% to 65%, with a mean of 35%. Early complications include pneumonia, intra-abdominal sepsis, postoperative bleeding, and pancreatitis; late complications include the onset of diabetes, chronic pancreatic fistula, and chronic pancreatic insufficiency. Fistulas are more common with external drainage.

The mortality for all surgical procedures ranges from 0% to 21%, with a mean of 8.5% [3••]. However, the mortality varies depending on the type of procedure performed. Earlier studies with internal drainage reported mortality rates in excess of 5%;

however, mortality rates in more recent studies have dropped significantly (0%–4%). External drainage is associated with a higher mortality rate (10%) because of the poor condition of the subjects in whom it is employed [15]. External drainage is reserved for patients in whom the cyst is infected or the cyst wall is not sufficiently thick to allow proper anastomosis. Resection carries a mortality rate of 8% [15].

Recurrence is another problem that can result from surgical procedures. Recurrence is seen in about 8% but it can be as high as 17%. Excision is associated with a very low recurrence rate but is feasible only for pseudocysts in the tail of the gland.

Low mortality and complication rates make internal drainage the surgical procedure of choice. However, internal drainage cannot be performed in high-risk patients. Furthermore, it cannot be attempted until the cyst wall is mature and usually is not performed in cases of infected cysts.

PERCUTANEOUS DRAINAGE

Ever since Hancke and Pedersen successfully performed percutaneous drainage of a pseudocyst, in 1976, this method has become increasingly popular [16]. Percutaneous drainage is usually done by the retroperitoneal or transperitoneal approach. A transgastric approach [3••] has several advantages: communication with the stomach means that any leakage will empty into the stomach and be drained, thereby preventing recurrence, and the chances of a patient developing a pancreaticocutaneous fistula are minimized. A transduodenal approach or a transhepatic route rarely has been used. Percutaneous pancreatic cystogastrostomy is a modification of this technique in which, with the aid of endoscopy and ultrasound imaging, one end of a pigtail catheter is placed in the stomach and the other end in the cyst.

Needle aspiration is useful to detect infection in a pseudocyst. However, when used as a therapy for pseudocysts, it carries a high rate of recurrence (63%) with a failure rate of 54% (Table 141-3). No complications or mortality have been noted in this procedure.

Continuous catheter drainage (Fig. 141-3) has demonstrated more impressive results than needle aspiration (Table 141-3) [3••].

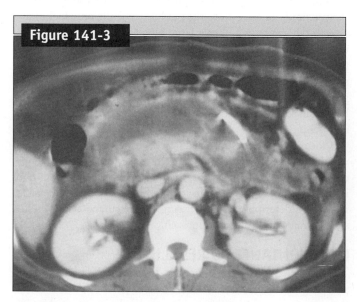

Figure 141-3

Computed tomography scan showing pseudocyst with a percutaneous drainage catheter in place.

Table 141-3. Results of Percutaneous Drainage for Pancreatic Pseudocysts With and Without an Indwelling Catheter

	Without, %	With, %
Complications	0	18
Recurrence	63	7
Failure	54	16
Mortality	0	0

Adapted from [17]; with permission.

The recurrence rate decreases to about 7%. The complication rate is about 18%, the most serious complication being secondary infection of a noninfected pseudocyst, which occurs in about 10% of patients. Other complications include catheter occlusion or displacement, cellulitis at the site of entry, and accidental puncture of the spleen. Fistula to the stomach, the jejunum, or the cecum also complicates this procedure. The mortality rate in most studies is negligible.

ENDOSCOPIC DRAINAGE

Endoscopic drainage of a pseudocyst is another alternative [17,18]. Cysts that communicate with the pancreatic duct can be drained through a transpapillary approach (Fig. 141-4) [19]. Pseudocysts that impinge on the stomach or the duodenum can be drained by making a fistulous communication between the cyst and the gastrointestinal lumen (Fig. 141-5). Before cysto-gastrostomy or cystoduodenostomy is performed, adherence between the cyst and the intestinal wall must be ensured by CT scanning. This is a prerequisite for performing this technique.

Success with endoscopic drainage ranges from 61% to 88%. Recurrence rates are approximately 6% to 12%, with a complication rate of 0% to 16%. No mortality directly related to this procedure has been reported.

Experience with endoscopic drainage is increasing. Creemer and coworkers [17] successfully performed endoscopic cysto-toenterostomy in 27 of 33 subjects, a success rate of 81%. Benign complications occurred in three subjects, and there was no mortality. Four subjects suffered relapse, and in two of them the relapse was managed successfully by repeat endoscopic cystoduodenostomy or cystogastrostomy. Complications of endoscopic drainage include bleeding, perforation, fever, and apnea. Stent-related complications, such as stent clogging, stent migration, and kinking also can occur. There have been no reports of procedure-related mortality.

ROLE OF SOMATOSTATIN

Somatostatin has a profound inhibitory effect on pancreatic exocrine secretion, a property utilized in the treatment of pseudo-cysts. Gullo and Barbara [20] used somatostatin (octreotide 100 μg three times daily for two weeks) as the primary therapy in seven subjects with pseudocysts, and four of the subjects demonstrated reduced pseudocysts. A definite decrease in the intensity of the pain was more significant. Octreotide also has been used in conjunction with percutaneous catheter drainage of pseudocysts, resulting in a shortened drainage time. The role of somatostatin in the management of pseudocysts is not clear. Prospective controlled trials are necessary to prove its efficacy.

INDICATIONS FOR INTERVENTION

Infected pseudocysts need to be drained immediately. Sterile pseudocysts smaller than 4 cm have such a high rate of spontaneous resolution that careful observation is all that is required. Pseudocysts in acute pancreatitis or those that occur immediately

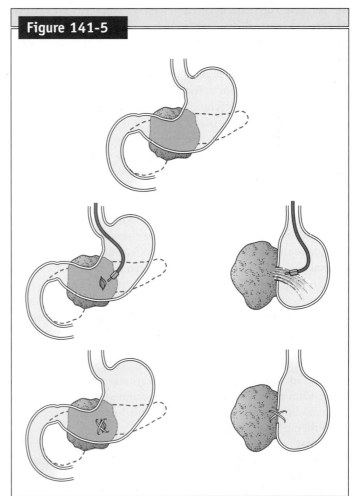

Figure 141-5

Schematic representation of endoscopic cyst-gastrostomy (coronal and saggital view). (*From* Lawson and Baillie [10]; with permission.)

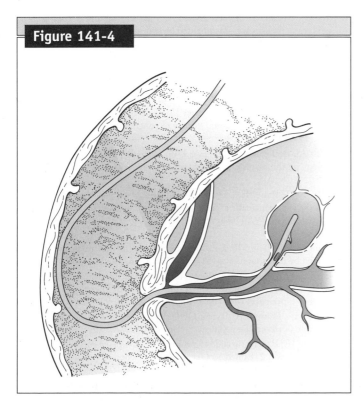

Figure 141-4

Transpapillary drainage of pancreatic pseudocyst using an endoscopically placed nasopancreatic tube. (*From* Geenen [19]; with permission.)

after an acute episode also may resolve spontaneously, even if larger than 4 cm. In such situations, serial CT scans for several weeks are recommended to monitor the size of the pseudocyst and to assess the potential of healing before considering intervention, especially in an asymptomatic patient. Only if the cyst is enlarging rapidly or the patient's symptoms worsen is intervention recommended. If the cyst is regressing, a conservative approach is adopted.

Pseudocysts in chronic pancreatitis are less likely to heal spontaneously, and drainage is warranted in symptomatic patients. However, observation alone may suffice in those with very small chronic pseudocysts.

CONCLUSION

An ideal therapeutic technique should have a high success rate with few complications and a low mortality, and it should also be universally applicable and inexpensive. None of the available methods fulfills these criteria.

When evaluating treatment outcomes, percutaneous drainage must be compared with the combined results of all surgical procedures rather than with internal drainage alone. Unlike the percutaneous technique, surgical internal drainage is not an option for all patients with pseudocysts. Internal drainage is limited to approximately 60% of patients undergoing surgical intervention. Furthermore, because cyst wall maturity is essential for surgical internal drainage, it is feasible only after 6 weeks. The mortality rate for all types of surgery is high compared with the mortality rate of percutaneous drainage; however, recent studies show a decrease in mortality for surgical patients [3••].

Increasing experience with percutaneous drainage has convinced us that the technique has few contraindications, an almost nonexistent mortality, and a low complication rate. Studies do not appear to select only low-risk patients. Such drainage can be performed in all patients, including those at high risk. Maturity of the cyst wall is not a prerequisite, as it is for surgical internal drainage, making percutaneous drainage a procedure available at any time without the stipulated 6-week delay for wall maturity. Performed under local anesthesia, percutaneous drainage is less expensive than a major operation. Most patients with noninfected pseudocysts are observed in the hospital for only 1 day after the procedure before discharge (van Sonnenberg E, Personal communication). These factors contribute to making percutaneous continuous catheter drainage the procedure of choice, provided adequately trained personnel are available. Needle aspiration alone is associated with a very high recurrence rate, so that continuous catheter drainage is the procedure of choice. Somatostatin may establish itself as an adjunct to continuous catheter drainage in the future. One note of caution must be sounded: cystic neoplasm masquerading as pseudocyst must be ruled out before percutaneous therapy is employed [21•].

Surgery may be reserved for those patients for whom percutaneous drainage does not work or is contraindicated; when associated conditions are present that favor a surgical option; or in patients in whom the diagnosis is uncertain, for example, in patients with suspected cystadenomas. Many pseudocysts require both surgery and percutaneous therapy, and close cooperation between the gastroenterologist, the surgeon,

and the radiologist is necessary for the proper management of these cases.

REFERENCES

Recently published papers of particular interest have been highlighted as follows:
- • Of interest
- •• Of outstanding interest

1. Bradley EL: The necessity for a clinical classification of acute pancreatitis: The Atlanta System. In *Acute Pancreatitis*. Edited by Bradley EL. New York: Raven; 1994:27–32.

2. Go VW, Everhart JE: *Pancreatitis in Digestive Diseases in the United States*. National Institutes of Health; May 1994. NIH Publication no. 94-1447:693–712.

3.•• Gumaste VV, Pitchumoni CS: Pancreatic pseudocysts. *Gastroenterologist* 1996, 4:33–43.
This is a good review article with 88 references and detailed tables that compare the different modalities.

4. Toskes P, Forsmark CE: Chronic pancreatitis. Sandoz Nutrition Corporation, 1993. Pamphlet.

5. Kloppel G, Maillet B: Pseudocysts in chronic pancreatitis: a morphological analysis of 57 resection specimens and 9 autopsy pancreata. *Pancreas* 1991, 6:266–274.

6. Pour PM, Thompson JS, Baxter BT, Murayama K: Pathology of pancreatic pseudocysts. In *Acute Pancreatitis*. Edited by Bradley EL. New York: Raven; 1994:181–189.

7. Thoeni RF, Blankenberg F: Pancreatic imaging. *Radiol Clin North Am* 1993, 31:1085–1113.

8. Balthazar E: Contrast-enhanced computed tomography in severe acute pancreatitis. In *Acute Pancreatitis*. Edited by Bradley EL. New York: Raven; 1994:57–68.

9. Hawes HR, Zaidi S: Endoscopic ultrasonography of the pancreas. *Gastrointest Clin North Am* 1995, 5:61–80.

10. Lawson MJ, Baillie JB: Endoscopic therapy for pancreatic pseudocysts. *Gastrointest Clin North Am* 1995, 5:181–193.

11.•• Yeo CJ, Bastides JA, Lynch-Nyhan A, et al.: The natural history of pancreatic pseudocysts documented by computed tomography. *Surg Gynecol Obstet* 1990, 170:411–447.
This study reinforces the role of expectant therapy and emphasizes the decreasing mortality rates with surgical techniques.

12. Bourliere M, Sarles H: Pancreatic cysts and pseudocysts associated with acute and chronic pancreatitis. *Dig Dis Sci* 1989, 34:343–348.

13. Nguyen BT, Thompson JS, Edney JA, et al.: Influence of the etiology of pancreatitis on the natural history of pancreatic pseudocysts. *Am J Surg* 1991, 162:527–531.

14. Walt AJ, Bouwman DL, Weaver DW, Sachs RJ: The impact of technology on the management of pancreatic pseudocyst. *Arch Surg* 1990, 125:759–763.

15. Maule WF, Reber HA: Diagnosis and management of pancreatic pseudocysts, pancreatic ascites and pancreatic fistulas. In *The Pancreas*. Edited by Go VW, Dimagno EP, Gardner JD, et al. New York: Raven; 1993:741–750.

16. Hancke S, Pedersen JF: Percutaneous puncture of pancreatic cysts guided by ultrasound. *Surg Gynecol Obstet* 1976, 142:551–552.

17. Cremer M, Deviere J, Engelholm L: Endoscopic management of cysts and pseudocysts in chronic pancreatitis: long-term follow-up after 7 years of experience. *Gastrointest Endosc* 1989, 35:1–9.

18. Smits ME, Rauws EAJ, Tytgat GNJ, et al.: Efficacy of endoscopic drainage of pancreatic pseudocyst. *Gastrointest Endosc* 1995, 42:202–207.

19. Geenen JE: Pancreatic endoscopy. In *Techniques in Therapeutic Endoscopy*, edn 2. Edited by Geenen JE, Fleischer DE, Waye JD. New York: Gower; 1992:9–11.

20. Gullo L, Barbara L: Treatment of pancreatic pseudocyst with octreotide. *Lancet* 1991, 338:540–541.

21.• Warshaw AL: Pancreatic cysts and pseudocysts. New rules for a new game. *Br J Surg* 1989, 76:533–534.
This is an excellent editorial.

142 Endoscopic Retrograde Cholangiopancreatography in Pancreatic Disorders

Rama P. Venu and Russell D. Brown

Endoscopic retrograde cholangiopancreatography (ERCP) has become an integral part of the diagnostic approach and management of pancreatic disorders. ERCP plays a pivotal role in the diagnosis of pancreatic disorders, such as pancreas divisum, pancreatic cancer, and chronic pancreatitis. Malignant cells also can be acquired in patients with suspected pancreatic ductal adenocarcinoma by introducing a cytology brush into the main pancreatic duct followed by brushing. In patients with recurrent pancreatitis related to sphincter of Oddi motor dysfunction (SOD), sphincter of Oddi manometry (SOM) can be performed at the time of ERCP. Besides these diagnostic applications, ERCP has emerged in recent years as a valuable technique for therapeutic intervention in a number of disorders, including acute gallstone pancreatitis, pancreas divisum, pseudocyst of the pancreas, and chronic pancreatitis.

▄▄ PROCEDURE

Patient Preparation

Prior to performing ERCP, informed consent must be obtained. The procedure, its benefits, its potential complications, and therapeutic alternatives are discussed in detail, preferably using one or more audiovisual aids, which are available through the American Society of Gastrointestinal Endoscopy or the American College of Gastroenterology. The patient should not eat or drink for at least 8 hours prior to the procedure. Although coagulation studies, such as prothrombin time, partial thromboplastin time, or bleeding time, are not ordered routinely, they are indicated in patients suspected to have coagulopathy or liver disease and for those who are taking anticoagulants or nonsteroidal anti-inflammatory drugs. Prophylactic antibiotics generally are not indicated *except* in patients with history of sepsis; suspected bile duct or pancreatic duct obstruction; pseudocyst of the pancreas; and certain other medical conditions, such as a prosthetic heart valve, a history of endocarditis, a systemic pulmonary shunt, or a synthetic vascular graft within the last year. Commonly used antibiotics include third-generation cephalosporins, ciprofloxacin, or the combination of ampicillin and aminoglycoside. The majority of ERCPs are done under conscious sedation using meperidine, midazolam, diazepam, or a combination thereof. About 4% of patients may require general anesthesia, including those with mental retardation, unstable cardiovascular status, a previous failed attempt with conscious sedation, and tolerance to medications secondary to substance abuse or narcotic use for pain.

Technical Aspects

The patient lies in the recumbent prone position with the head turned to the right side, facing the endoscopist. Sedatives are administered through an intravenous line already in place, preferably in the left hand. Oropharyngeal anesthesia using gargle or cetacaine spray is helpful to suppress the gag reflex. A lateral viewing duodenoscope (10–11.5 mm in outer diameter) is introduced gently into the mouth and guided into the stomach. The endoscope is then advanced into the descending duodenum. The technique of traversing the pylorus and stationing the endoscope close to the papilla has been described previously [1]. For successful duct cannulation, the endoscope should follow the lesser curvature of the stomach or the "short position." The depth of insertion of the endoscope in this position is usually between 65 and 70 cm from the incisor teeth. The papilla should be visualized *en face* to allow identification of the papillary orifice. A preliminary radiograph of the entire abdomen should be taken prior to contrast instillation to identify previously administered barium or calcification in and around the pancreas. A 3F to 5F catheter filled with contrast material is introduced into the papillary orifice. By gently injecting contrast material under close fluoroscopic monitoring, a cholangiogram and a pancreatogram are obtained. As a rule, selective cannulation of the bile duct is obtained by directing the catheter cephalad at the 11 to 1 o'clock position of the papillary orifice, and selective cannulation of the pancreatic duct is achieved by directing the catheter at the 1 to 3 o'clock position. Because disease of the pancreatic head can cause structural changes in the common bile duct, a satisfactory cholangiogram is essential for optimal evaluation of pancreatic disorders.

During contrast instillation, especially into the pancreatic duct, close fluoroscopic monitoring is necessary to prevent over injection leading to acinar filling or "acinarization." This can cause abdominal pain during the procedure and significantly increase the chance of post-ERCP pancreatitis. Spot radiographs also should be obtained during the early phase of contrast injection into the pancreatic duct and bile duct. This is especially helpful to evaluate the intramural segments of these ducts, which may be involved in ampullary neoplasia or a choledochocele. Radiographs taken in the upright position are also helpful to evaluate the terminal ends of the bile duct and pancreatic duct. Radiographs taken in the supine position are useful to study the duct in the tail of the pancreas because, being the most dependent portion of the pancreatic duct, contrast fills this segment selectively by gravity. Delayed films taken at 15 and 45 minutes can provide useful information about ductal drainage; contrast retained in the pancreatic duct 10 to 15 minutes after injection is indicative of delayed drainage.

ENDOSCOPIC EVALUATION

Endoscopic inspection of the major duodenal papilla, minor papilla, and peripapillary duodenum is a vital part of ERCP. The major duodenal papilla is located in the posteromedial wall of the descending duodenum. It is a nipple-like structure about 5 to 7 mm in diameter, covered with smooth pinkish mucous membrane. The papillary orifice is located at its summit, and the surrounding mucosa is often reticulated. Small finger-like structures may be seen at the margins of the papillary orifice. In approximately 85% of subjects, a single papillary orifice provides the exodus for both the pancreatic duct and the bile duct, whereas in 10% to 15% of subjects there are separate openings for each of these ducts [2]; in such cases, the pancreatic duct aperture is always beneath the biliary orifice.

The papilla may be involved in a variety of pathologic conditions. Acute inflammation of the papilla, or papillitis, is characterized by an enlarged, erythematous and edematous papilla. Acute pancreatitis and an impacted gallstone at the ampulla are commonly associated with papillitis. Chronic inflammation of the papilla may lead to papillary stenosis, resulting in a papilla that may appear small and fibrotic. Chronic pancreatitis occasionally is associated with papillary stenosis. An unusually large papilla protruding into the duodenal lumen, often referred to as a "bulging papilla," may be seen in a choledochocele, impacted stone, or ampullary neoplasm [3••].

The papillary orifice is commonly recognized by its golden yellow drainage of bile. A clear watery secretion at the papillary orifice indicates the pancreatic ductal opening. In chronic pancreatitis, whitish precipitates may be seen and pus may escape through the orifice in infected pseudocysts that communicate with the pancreatic duct. Seepage of blood through the papillary orifice occasionally is seen in patients with chronic pancreatitis and hemosuccus pancreaticus. A papillary orifice appearing widely patent and with clear mucus at the orifice is pathognomonic for mucinous ductal ectasia of the pancreas.

Peripapillary Region

The most common abnormality of the peripapillary region is duodenal diverticula. The incidence of diverticula increases with age and is about 20% in patients older than 70 years. Diverticulae are almost always asymptomatic. However, an increased incidence of bile duct stones and pancreatitis have been reported by some in association with peripapillary diverticula [4]. Duodenal nodularity, friability, and luminal narrowing can be seen proximal to the papilla in carcinoma of the pancreas that invades the duodenal wall; forceps biopsy of this area during ERCP can establish a tissue diagnosis. Similarly, a smooth bulge on the duodenum proximal to the papilla may be seen with large pseudocysts or cystic neoplasms of the head of the pancreas. Duodenal duplication cysts also may produce a bulge in the duodenal wall and present clinically with acute pancreatitis [5]. The papilla is often contained in the cyst. Patients with annular pancreas might have a concentric narrowing of the peripapillary duodenal lumen.

Minor Papilla

The minor duodenal papilla is smaller than the major papilla, measuring 2 to 3 mm in diameter. It is usually located 1 to 2 cm proximal and medial to the major papilla. The duct of Santorini, derived from the duct of the dorsal pancreatic analge, opens at the summit of the minor papilla. However, the orifice of this duct is patent in only 15% to 50% of patients. In patients born with pancreas divisum, the minor papilla provides the orifice for the duct of the dorsal pancreas.

The minor papilla may be prominent in some patients with chronic pancreatitis, especially when there is a dominant stricture involving the terminal end of the main pancreatic duct. In this situation, the duct of Santorini, which opens at the minor papilla, offers an alternate path of drainage. In some patients with pancreas divisum and pancreatitis the minor papilla may be large and the terminus of the dorsal duct dilated, causing a bulge in the minor papilla. Some investigators have coined the term *Santorinicele* to describe this abnormality [6••].

RADIOGRAPHIC EVALUATION

Following endoscopic inspection, contrast material is injected into the pancreatic duct. The entire ductal system should be delineated for proper interpretation but monitored carefully during injection to avoid acinarization.

Normal Anatomy

From the papilla, where the pancreatic duct terminates, the main duct courses upward and to the left, crossing the spine at the L2 vertebral level (Fig. 142-1). The main duct tapers toward the tail, where usually it ends in a bifurcation. The pancreatic duct is widest at the head, measuring up to 5 mm in diameter. It has a mean diameter of 3.8 mm in the body and about 1 to 2 mm at the tail [7]. The main duct and the side branches may be wider in older people. The length of the main pancreatic duct is highly variable, from 45 to 250 mm. There are at least two unpaired lateral branches terminating in the main duct: the duct of Santorini, directed superiorly from the main duct and terminating at the minor papilla, and the duct directed inferiorly from the main duct and draining the uncinate process. Other side branches terminate at the main pancreatic duct. There are

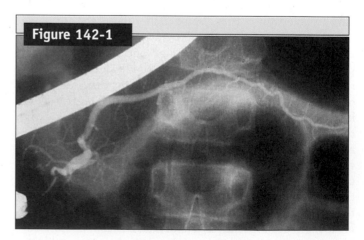

Figure 142-1

Normal pancreatogram. The main pancreatic duct is widest at the head, tapers towards the tail, and ends in a bifurcation. Note the lateral branches, more numerous in the head.

about 20 to 30 side branches seen in the body of the gland. These lateral branches, which are more numerous at the head, taper toward the periphery.

Abnormal Pancreatic Duct

Pancreatography demonstrates characteristic findings in a number of entities, such as pancreas divisum, annular pancreas, papillary stenosis, choledochocele, chronic pancreatitis, pancreatic ductal adenocarcinoma, pseudocyst of the pancreas, and mucinous ductal ectasia. Similarly, ductal disruption and fistulae also produce characteristic pancreatographic features, which are discussed later.

■ TISSUE SAMPLING

Beside demonstrating characteristic radiographic findings, ERCP provides a unique opportunity for exfoliative cytology. There are number of different techniques currently available for cytology, including pancreatic juice aspiration, and brushing ductal strictures.

Pancreatic juice cytology has been acquired by aspirating duodenal samples with a Dreiling tube after administration of intravenous secretin to stimulate pancreatic secretion. Cannulating catheters have been advanced into the duct during ERCP to aspirate pancreatic juice directly from the pancreatic duct for cytologic analysis. The yield of malignant cells using this technique has been reported to be 50% to 84% [8••]; however, experience with pancreatic juice cytology is limited in this country.

Brush cytology is a more widely used technique for acquisition of malignant cells. For this procedure, a pancreatogram is obtained to delineate the location and morphology of the stricture. A guidewire is then advanced beyond the stricture. A cytology sheath is passed over the guidewire, and the guidewire is exchanged with a cytology brush. The cytology brush has a flexible tip to facilitate negotiations through strictured areas. The brush segment is stationed across the stricture under fluoroscopic guidance (Fig. 142-2). Brushing is done with multiple to-and-fro movements. The brush is withdrawn into the sheath, and the whole assembly is removed. The brush is then smeared onto a slide, and the slide is fixed and examined. Endopancreatic brush cytology generally gives a positive yield for malignant cells in more than 50% of cases [8••], with a specificity of almost 100% and only minimal complications.

Studies have shown that the yield of positive cytology depends on the location of the malignancy [9]. Cancer located at the ampulla, genu, and tail regions of the main pancreatic duct gives a low yield compared with that of the head and body. In patients with cancer involving the head of the pancreas, concurrent brushing of the common bile duct stricture can enhance the overall diagnostic yield [9]. When there is strong clinical suspicion for malignancy, alternate methods of tissue acquisition, such as endoscopic ultrasonography, computed tomography (CT)-directed fine needle aspiration cytology, or even laparotomy should be considered if endopancreatic brush cytology is negative.

■ SPHINCTER OF ODDI MANOMETRY

The terminal ends of the bile and pancreatic ducts are entwined by smooth muscle fibers constituting the sphincter of Oddi, the physiologic role of which is to regulate the flow of bile and pancreatic secretions. The sphincter is a dynamic structure maintaining a basal tone with superimposed phasic contractions at a frequency of 3 to 5 per minute. These phasic waves normally are propagated in an antegrade direction and seem to be peristaltic. High basal pressure ($\geq$ 40 mm Hg), rapid phasic contractions, and retrograde propagation of phasic waves either alone or in combination can impede biliary and pancreatic flow, an occurrence designated as sphincter of Oddi dysfunction. Some investigators believe that sphincter of Oddi dysfunction can lead to recurrent pancreatitis, presumably by impeding the flow of pancreatic juice and thereby producing pancreatic ductal hypertension [10•].

During the past decade, significant technical developments have allowed assessment of the motility characteristics of the sphincter of Oddi in health and disease. To perform SOM, a minimally compliant, constantly perfused manometry catheter is introduced into the pancreatic duct during ERCP. The catheter is stationed within the sphincter zone, recording the basal pressure and other pressure phenomena. Studies have demonstrated a high basal pressure ($\geq$ 40 mm Hg) of the pancreatic sphincter in a cohort of subjects with idiopathic recurrent pancreatitis, some of whom had biliary sphincter pressures within the normal range. Endoscopic sphincterotomy of the biliary sphincter, the pancreatic sphincter, or both, has been shown to prevent further episodes of pancreatitis in these patients [10•]. Although useful in selected patients, pancreatic SOM is limited by a relatively high incidence of post-procedure pancreatitis, approaching 25% in some studies. A decrease in the incidence of pancreatitis has been reported by using the middle manometry port for continuous aspiration of fluid from the pancreatic duct during the procedure, perhaps avoiding pancreatic ductal hypertension [11].

■ THERAPEUTIC PROCEDURES

Commonly employed therapeutic interventions in pancreatic disorders include endoscopic sphincterotomy (ES) of the pancreatic sphincter, minor papillotomy, dilation of ductal strictures,

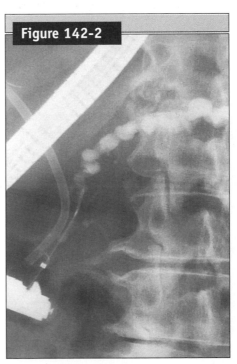

Figure 142-2

Endopancreatic brush cytology. The brush is stationed at the stricture in the head of the pancreas. A stent placed across the bile duct stricture to establish biliary drainage also is seen.

extraction of pancreatic calculi, placement of endoprotheses (stents), and drainage of pseudocysts. ES of the pancreatic sphincter through the major duodenal papilla often is required to enlarge the pancreatic ductal orifice and allow passage of accessory devices, such as dilators, Dormia wire baskets, balloons, and endoprostheses. As an initial step for pancreatic ES, a pancreatogram is obtained. A sphincterotome similar to the one used for biliary sphincterotomy is introduced into the pancreatic duct, and its position is verified by fluoroscopy. The sphincterotome is slowly withdrawn until 50% of the cutting wire is visible outside the papillary orifice. The sphincterotome is partially opened and incremental incisions are made with the wire directed to the 1 to 3 o'clock position. A 7 to 10 mm incision is sufficient in most instances. Dilation of strictures is commonly done with dilating catheters that are passed over guidewires advanced beyond the stricture. Hydrostatic balloons (4–6 mm) also can be used for dilating strictures. Extraction of stones usually is done using Dormia wire baskets (Fig. 142-3). The basket is advanced beyond the stone, and the wires are opened. The stone is trapped inside the basket with to-and-fro movements, and the basket with the entrapped stone is pulled out. Stent placement is another technique used to facilitate drainage. Stents with outer diameters of 5F, 7F, and 8.5F are advanced directly over the guidewire with a pusher tube. A guide catheter (7F) is passed over the guidewire first before larger stents (10F, 11.5F) are placed across the stricture.

COMPLICATIONS

Endoscopic retrograde cholangiopancreatography is associated with a number of complications. Among these complications, drug reactions; cardiorespiratory problems, including hypoxemia and arrhythmias; and injury to the esophagus, stomach, or duodenum are similar to those seen with esophagogastroduodenoscopy. Untoward side effects of drugs may be seen in at least 6% of patients; these include hypersensitivity reactions, phlebitis at the site of injection, and respiratory depression. Complications specific to ERCP include acute pancreatitis, cholangitis, pancreatic sepsis, sphincterotomy bleeding and instrumental injury to the bile and pancreatic ducts [12].

Although hyperamylasemia is seen in up to 70% of patients following ERCP, acute pancreatitis occurs in only 1% to 7.4% of

patients. The exact mechanism of pancreatitis is not known, but contributing factors include repeated attempts at cannulation, trauma to the ampulla, increased injection pressure and volume of injectate, and the underlying condition of the pancreas.

Infection is the most serious complication of diagnositc ERCP. Although bacteremia has been reported in up to 14% of patients, cholangitis occurs in only 0.81% of patients [12]. Ductal obstruction related to stricture or calculi as well as pseudocyst of the pancreas may predispose patients to infection. Pancreatic abscess has been reported in 0.3% of patients. Mortality consequent to ERCP is seen between 0.1% to 0.2% of patients. Ascending cholangitis and pancreatitis with sepsis constitute the major causes of death.

INDICATIONS AND DIAGNOSTIC FEATURES

Endoscopic retrograde cholangiopancreatography is indicated in acute pancreatitis, chronic pancreatitis, pancreatic cancer, cystic neoplasm, mucinous ductal ectasia, and other conditions (Table 142-1).

Acute Pancreatitis

Alcohol and gallstones are responsible for approximately 80% to 85% of acute pancreatitis in the United States, Europe, and most developed countries. In the remaining 15% to 20%, acute pancreatitis is caused by a variety of uncommon mechanisms. Pancreas divisum, choledochocele, sphincter of Oddi dysfunction, papillary tumors, pancreatic ductal adenocarcinoma, and ascariasis are some of the abnormalities identified in these patients [13••]. In addition, studies have reported finding microlithiasis or cholesterol crystals and calcium bilirubinate precipitate in up to 60% of patients with acute pancreatitis of unknown etiology [14••]. Pancreatic trauma resulting in ductal disruption also can cause acute pancreatitis, or rarely, pancreatic ascites rich in amylase.

Endoscopic retrograde cholangiopancreatography plays an important role in the evaluation of patients with acute pancreatitis when an etiology is not evident after routine history and physical examination and conventional studies, such as ultrasonography of the gallbladder [13••]. The major entities causing acute pancreatitis and their diagnostic features follow.

Pancreas Divisum

Pancreas divisum is the most common congenital variant of the pancreas, reported in approximately 6% of the population. In pancreas divisum, besides parenchymal malfusion, the dorsal and ventral embryologic ducts fail to fuse and form one main duct. As a result, the larger dorsal duct opens into the duodenum via the minor papilla and the smaller ventral duct opens into the duodenum through the major papilla along with the bile duct.

When contrast is instilled into the major papilla, a short pancreatic duct with immediate arborization is demonstrated; the bile duct also can be delineated with contrast injected through the major papillary orifice (Fig. 142-4). Early spot films are important to delineate the ventral pancreas because overfilling of the ventral pancreatic acini can occur quickly, masking the ductal anatomy and making the diagnosis difficult (Fig. 142-5).

When pancreas divisum is suspected on the basis of such findings, it is imperative to identify the minor papilla and delineate

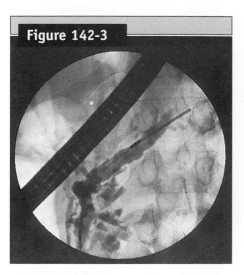

Figure 142-3

Basket extraction of stone. A Dormia basket with entrapped stone is seen in the main pancreatic duct. The main pancreatic duct and the lateral branches are markedly dilated indicating chronic pancreatitis.

Table 142-1. Diagnostic Indications of Endoscopic Retrograde Cholangiopancreatography

Pancreatitis
   Idiopathic recurrent pancreatitis
   Chronic pancreatitis (undiagnosed)
Fistulae
   Unexplained ascites*
   Unexplained pleural effusion*
Tumors
   Obstructive jaundice
   Suspicious mass lesion by other imaging studies
Preoperative evaluation
   Chronic pancreatitis
   Pseudocyst
Miscellaneous
   Unexplained weight loss*
   Steatorrhea*
   Brush cytology
   Pancreatic juice cytology
   Sphincter of Oddi manometry

With clinical and laboratory findings suggesting pancreatic disease.

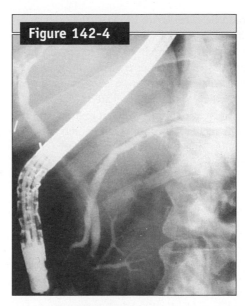

Figure 142-4

Pancreas divisum. The ventral pancreatic duct and the common bile duct terminate at the major papilla. The dorsal duct crossing the common bile duct is seen terminating at the minor papilla cephalad to the ventral duct.

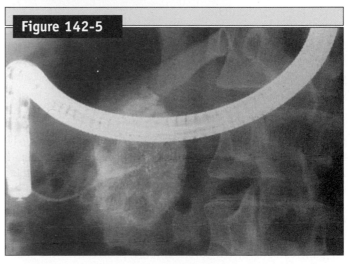

Figure 142-5

Acinarization or overfilling of the ventral pancreas during endoscopic retrograde cholangiopancreatography; the glandular structure of the pancreas is filled, causing a generalized radiodensity.

the dorsal pancreatic duct, thus confirming the diagnosis. Additionally, structural abnormalities involving the dorsal duct, such as stricture, ectasia, or calculi can be detected, which may account for the clinical presentation.

Intravenous administration of secretin (1 U/kg) is helpful to identify the minor papillary orifice. The orifice becomes dilated and clearly visible within minutes after secretin injection as bicarbonate-rich pancreatic juice pours out from it [15]. Using a tapered-tip cannula (3F), contrast can be injected into the duct and radiographs obtained. The anatomy of the dorsal duct is similar to that of a normal main pancreatic duct. In a subgroup of patients, the dorsal pancreatic duct communicates with the ventral duct through a tiny branch. This entity is usually referred to as communicating or incomplete pancreas divisum.

Choledochocele

Choledochocele is characterized by cystic dilation involving the terminal end of the common bile duct (Fig. 142-6). The pancreatic duct often terminates within this cystic structure. Endoscopically, the papilla may appear enlarged and bulging with the papillary orifice usually eccentric in location. The bile duct may be normal or dilated. Upright radiographs are helpful to demonstrate a choledochocele as contrast material fills the dependent cystic structure by gravity.

Sphincter of Oddi Dysfunction

Sphincter of Oddi dysfunction is a rare cause of acute pancreatitis. Routine ERCP may be entirely normal in sphincter of Oddi dysfunction. Occasionally, the bile duct, the pancreatic duct, or both may be dilated and drainage of contrast delayed from one or both ducts. In such a situation, ampullary carcinoma or

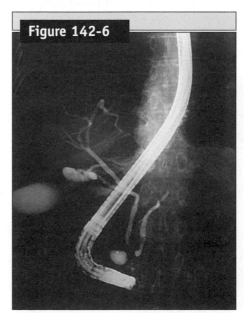

Figure 142-6

Endoscopic retrograde cholangiopancreatography in a patient who presented with acute recurrent pancreatitis. The cystic structure at the terminal end of the bile duct represents a choledochocele. The incompletely filled pancreatic duct is also visible.

papillary stenosis should be considered. SOM is the gold standard for establishing the diagnosis of sphincter of Oddi dysfunction. Basal sphincter of Oddi pressure ≥ 40 mm Hg is the most common abnormality reported in patients with sphincter dysfunction. Although such elevated pressure usually is present in both the pancreatic and biliary sphincters, elevated basal pressure may be limited to the pancreatic sphincter in approximately 15% of patients. Therefore, pancreatic sphincter manometry should be performed along with biliary sphincter manometry in the subset of patients with recurrent pancreatitis.

Posttraumatic Pancreatitis

Endoscopic retrograde cholangiopancreatography is helpful in patients who suffer abdominal pain after blunt abdominal trauma and who are believed to have pancreatitis. Pancreatography often can demonstrate extravasation of contrast material at the site of a ductal disruption [16]. In selected patients, wire-guided endoprosthesis placement across the disrupted duct maybe helpful to bridge the disruption.

Ductal Adenocarcinoma

Ductal adenocarcinoma of the pancreas rarely can present with obstructive pancreatitis. The diagnostic features of pancreatic cancer are discussed later.

Neoplasms of the Papilla

Neoplasms of the papilla, especially villous adenoma, may cause recurrent pancreatitis. The papilla is often enlarged and nodular but smooth (Fig. 142-7, see also **Color Plate**). The diagnosis is established by biopsy.

Chronic Pancreatitis

Chronic pancreatitis is associated with characteristic findings on pancreatography. In severe chronic pancreatitis, the main pancreatic duct often demonstrates alternating areas of stricture and dilation, an appearance referred to as a "chain-of-lakes." Pseudocysts communicating with the main pancreatic duct and intraductal calculi also may be seen in chronic pancreatitis.

Based on pancreatographic findings, chronic pancreatitis is classified into equivocal, mild, moderate and severe. In *equivocal* chronic pancreatitis, fewer than three side branches show irregularity or

ectasia, and the main duct is normal [17••]. In *mild* chronic pancreatitis, more than three side branches are involved, and the main pancreatic duct is normal. In *moderate* pancreatitis, the main duct is dilated along with changes in the side branches. In *severe* cases, there are strictures, dilation, calculi, and pseudocysts in addition to the earlier findings (Fig. 142-8). Pseudocysts appear as contrast-filled cavities that are adjacent to and communicate with the main duct. Calculi appear as filling defects in the duct (Fig. 142-9).

It may be difficult to differentiate chronic pancreatitis from carcinoma of the pancreas because both these entities demonstrate stricture and dilation. However, pancreatic duct strictures longer than 10 mm along with associated findings discussed later are supportive of a diagnosis of carcinoma.

Pancreatic Ductal Adenocarcinoma

Ductal adenocarcinoma accounts for 80% of pancreatic neoplasms. As they arise from the ductal epithelium, most cause a stricturing of the main pancreatic duct (Fig. 142-10). The distal duct leading up to the stricture is usually normal in caliber, whereas the duct proximal to the stenosis is dilated. A long irregular stricture is a less common finding in carcinoma of the pancreas. Absence of side branches at the location of the neoplasm is another characteristic finding of malignant pancreatic lesions. In

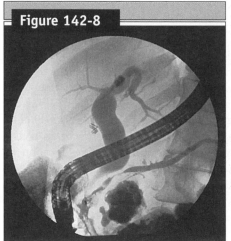

Figure 142-8

Pancreatogram in a patient with chronic alcoholic pancreatitis showing a stricture involving the common bile duct and pancreatic duct. A pseudocyst filled with contrast also is present beneath the pancreatic duct at the uncinate process.

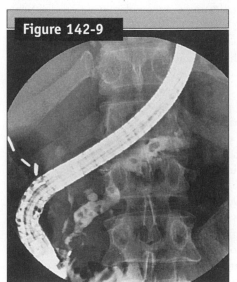

Figure 142-9

Pancreatogram in a patient with chronic pancreatitis showing multiple calculi in the main pancreatic duct.

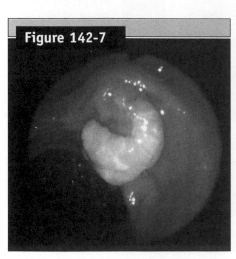

Figure 142-7

Endoscopic image demonstrating a villous adenoma involving the papilla from a patient who presented with recurrent pancreatitis. See also **Color Plate**.

rare cases, tumor necrosis may give the lesion a cavitary appearance similar to that of a pseudocyst. In carcinoma arising in the head of the pancreas, the intrapancreatic segment of the common bile duct may be involved and compressed by tumor, typically producing a stricture (Fig. 142-11). The presence of adjacent strictures of the common bile duct and the pancreatic duct causes the characteristic radiographic finding of a "double duct sign," where the ducts proximal to each stricture are dilated. Although this finding is typical for carcinoma of the head of the pancreas, it is not pathognomic and may be seen in chronic pancreatitis.

Overall, ERCP carries ≥ 90% sensitivity and specificity for the diagnosis of pancreatic ductal adenocarcinoma. Nevertheless, it may miss malignancies in the so-called "blind areas" in the tail, the uncinate process, and the area of pancreatic head drained by the duct of Santorini. Demonstration of the accessory duct through the minor papilla may be helpful in the last instance.

Mucinous Ductal Ectasia

Mucinous ductal ectasia is another neoplastic condition characterized by a dilated main pancreatic duct that usually contains multiple filling defects caused by mucin plugs (Fig. 142-12). Endoscopic inspection often shows a patulous papillary orifice with mucin extruding into the duodenal lumen (Fig. 142-13, see also **Color Plate**) [18]. Cytologic studies of the mucus can show neoplastic cells, in which case pancreatectomy may be appropriate.

Cystic Tumors of the Pancreas

Cystic tumors of the pancreas, such as serous cystadenoma, mucinous cystadenoma, and cystadenocarcinoma, generally do not produce any ductal changes on pancreatography. Rare findings in these

Figure 142-10

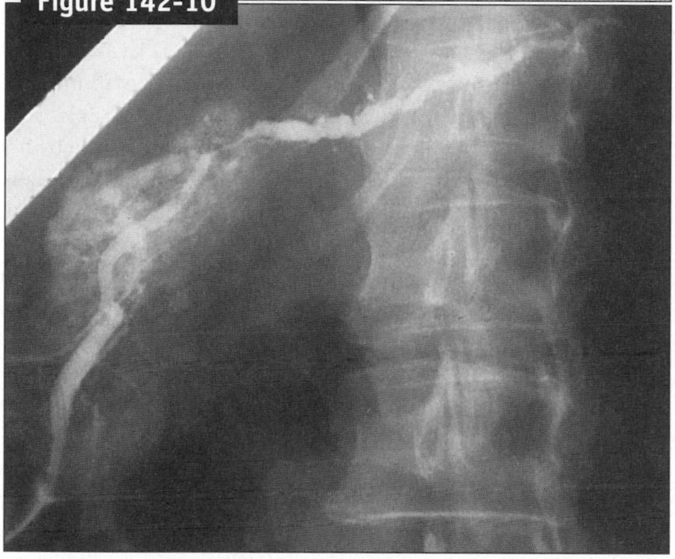

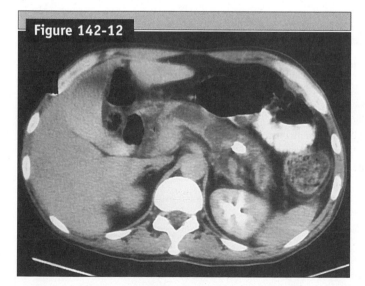

Pancreatic cancer at the body demonstrating a short irregular stricture. Contrast also has extravasated into the neoplasm.

Figure 142-11

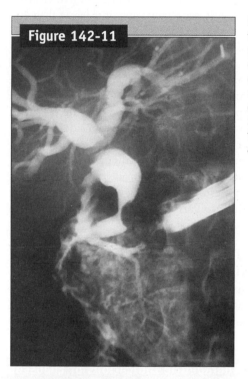

Carcinoma of the head of the pancreas with complete obstruction of the main pancreatic duct. The common bile duct is also involved, causing a stricture.

Figure 142-12

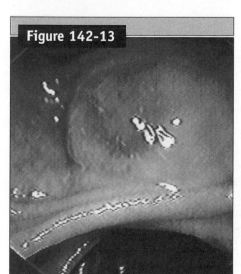

Computed tomography scan of the abdomen in a patient with mucinous ductal ectasia showing dilated pancreatic duct containing inhomogenous densities representing mucus plugs. (*Courtesy of* J. Baillie, MD.)

Figure 142-13

Endoscopic view demonstrating a mucus plug at the papillary orifice in a patient with mucinous ductal ectasia. Note the papilla is enlarged from mucus filling up the ampulla. See also **Color Plate**. (*Courtesy of* J. Baillie, MD.)

cystic neoplasms include a smooth narrowing of the duct resulting from extrinsic compression and absence of lateral branches.

Miscellaneous

Endoscopic retrograde cholangiopancreatography often is indicated when other imaging studies, such as ultrasonography or CT scan of the abdomen, are suspicious for pancreatic tumor or chronic pancreatitis. This is especially true when the patient has symptoms or laboratory studies suggestive of a pancreatic disorder. Patients suspected of having a pancreatic fistula either to the peritoneal or pleural cavity also benefit from ERCP. In these situations contrast instilled into the pancreatic duct during pancreatography may be seen to extravasate from the duct either into the peritoneal or pleural cavity during fluoroscopy. On spot radiographs, this extravasation can be identified as a collection of contrast material in close proximity to the pancreatic duct. Another indication for ERCP is the evaluation of patients with a nonresolving pseudocyst, especially when it is larger than 4 to 6 cm and associated with symptoms. A "road map" of the anatomy of the pancreatic duct is helpful in planning appropriate surgical or endoscopic therapy. In this situation, ERCP should be performed just prior to therapy and in consultation with the surgical team to limit the risk of infection due to injection of contrast. Similarly, pancreatography can demonstrate the site of ductal disruption in pancreatic trauma when considering possible therapeutic intervention.

Hemosuccus pancreaticus is an uncommon cause of gastrointestinal bleeding that should be considered in patients with obscure upper gastrointestinal hemorrhage. In such cases, blood escaping through the papillary orifice may be identified with the side-viewing duodenoscope.

▬ THERAPEUTIC PROCEDURES AND INDICATIONS

Besides its diagnostic role, ERCP offers therapeutic possibilities in acute pancreatitis, chronic pancreatitis, pancreatic fistulae, pseudocysts, and pancreatic cancer (Table 142-2).

Acute Pancreatitis

Acute pancreatitis is a common clinical manifestation of gallstone disease. Migration of gallstones from the gallbladder to the ampulla of Vater has been documented in patients with acute biliary pancreatitis by recovering stones from the feces of such patients as well as by direct observation of stones at the ampulla during early ERCP and surgery [19]. Pancreatic duct hypertension caused by stone-induced ampullary obstruction plays a major role in the pathogenesis of acute gallstone pancreatitis. Thus, early ERCP and stone extraction by endoscopic sphincterotomy seems an attractive approach in the management of patients with biliary pancreatitis.

Three randomized studies have evaluated the role of early (24–72 hours) ERCP and ES in the treatment of acute gallstone pancreatitis. Although, in an early study, ERCP with biliary decompression and stone removal reduced morbidity in a subgroup of subjects with severe pancreatitis [20••], a beneficial effect was not observed in a more recent study that excluded patients with ongoing biliary obstruction [21•]. Evidence that early endoscopic intervention and biliary drainage will improve the morbidity associated with biliary obstruction and sepsis seen in conjunction with biliary pancreatitis was demonstrated in a large study from Hong Kong [22•]. On the basis of these data, ERCP and ES can be recommended when biliary obstruction, sepsis, or both complicate gallstone pancreatitis and may still be considered in patients who are clinically deteriorating with severe pancreatitis even when biliary obstruction is not obvious.

Pancreas Divisum

It is estimated that 95% of subjects with pancreas divisum remain asymptomatic, and whether pancreas divisum is responsible for the clinical findings in the 5% who develop symptoms is controversial. However, histologic findings of significant fibrosis at the orifice of the minor papilla, pancreatitis limited to the dorsal pancreas, a narrow minor papillary orifice, dilation of the dorsal duct, and delayed pancreatic ductal drainage support a causal relationship. Additionally, enlarging the orifice of the

Table 142-2. Therapeutic Indications of Endoscopic Retrograde Cholangiopancreatography

Diagnoses	Potential Therapy
Acute pancreatitis	
Acute biliary pancreatitis	Sphincterotomy and stone extraction
Pancreas divisum	Minor papillotomy
Choledochocele	Unroofing via needle knife or standard sphincterotomy
Papillary tumors	Endoscopic resection/papillectomy
SOD	Sphincterotomy
Chronic pancreatitis	
Intractable pain	Pancreatic sphincterotomy, dilation of strictures, stone extraction,
Relapsing pancreatitis	stent placement
Pseudocyst of the pancreas	Cyst gastrostomy/duodenostomy or transpapillary drainage
Pancreatic cancer	
Bile duct obstruction with jaundice	Endoprosthesis across the bile duct stricture
Pancreatic duct obstruction with pain	Endoprosthesis across the pancreatic duct stricture

SOD—sphincter of Oddi motor dysfunction.

dorsal pancreatic duct by ES or surgical sphincteroplasty can lead to improvement in clinical symptoms in selected patients.

The major clinical presentations of pancreas divisum include abdominal pain, acute recurrent pancreatitis, and chronic pancreatitis. A functional impedance to pancreatic flow at the relatively narrow minor papillary orifice is considered to be the pathophysiologic basis of these clinical disorders [23]. The underlying principle behind endoscopic therapy for pancreas divisum consists of enhancing drainage of the dorsal duct through the minor papilla by enlarging the papillary orifice. This can be accomplished by dilation, stent placement, or minor papillotomy. Dilation using catheters or hydrostatic balloons rarely is performed because therapeutic effects, if any, are transient. Both stent placement and papillotomy of the minor papilla have been performed successfully in patients with pancreas divisum presenting with abdominal pain, acute recurrent pancreatitis, and chronic pancreatitis.

Identification of the minor papilla is the first step before undertaking endoscopic interventions. A meticulous search for its orifice is the next step. Intravenous administration of secretin (1 U/kg body weight) can facilitate localization of the papillary orifice. Copious flow of clear pancreatic juice indicates the location of the papillary orifice, which becomes dilated following secretin injection. A tapered-tip catheter (3F) is then introduced into the papillary orifice and contrast is instilled into the duct slowly under fluoroscopic monitoring. The pancreatogram is carefully studied for ductal dilation, strictures, or calculi. A hydrophilic guidewire (0.018 in) is introduced into the dorsal duct through the catheter. Once advanced well inside the duct, this wire is exchanged for a standard guidewire and the catheter is removed (Fig. 142-14*A*, see also **Color Plate**). A 3F or 5F (3 cm) stent is pushed over the wire and stationed across the papilla (Fig. 142-14*B*, see also **Color Plate**). Using a needle knifc sphincterotome, a 3 to 5 mm incision is made in a cephalad direction to enlarge the aperture (Fig. 142-14*C* and *D*, see also **Color Plate**). Unlike ES of the major papilla, minor papillotomy is less precise due to the absence of distinct anatomic landmarks. The stent serves as a splint for a safe incision. Following papillotomy, the stent may migrate spontaneously into the duodenum in the next few days or can be removed within the next few weeks. Placement of a 5F to 7F stent alone without papillotomy also has been performed to widen the orifice of the dorsal duct. However, stents must be replaced periodically, and long-term stent placement carries the risk of stent-induced pancreatic ductal damage [24•]. Papillotomy of the minor papilla also can be done using a tapered-tip sphincterotome. This technique is easier in patients with chronic pancreatitis and pancreas divisum, especially when the minor papilla is prominent. In patients with a bulging minor papilla or Santorinicele, an unroofing procedure can be done using a needle knife without a stent.

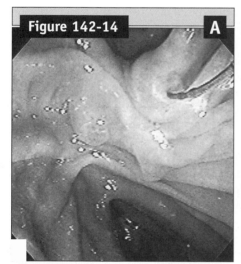
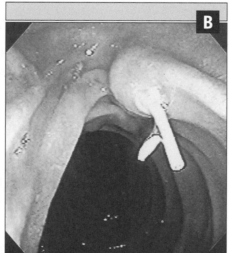
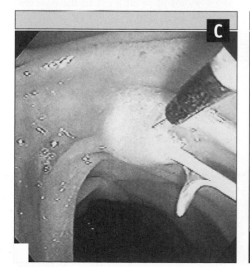
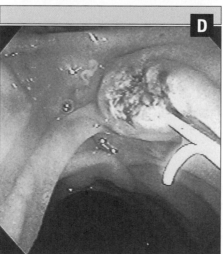

Figure 142-14

Technique of minor papillotomy. **A**, Note the guidewire introduced through the minor papilla. **B**, Endoscopic view showing the stent at the minor papilla placed in the dorsal duct. **C**, The needle is placed just above the stent. **D**, An incision is made in the cephalad direction. See also **Color Plate**.

In a randomized study, endoprothesis therapy has been reported to prevent recurrent episodes of pancreatitis in 90% of patients with idiopathic recurrent pancreatitis compared with 11% of controls. The stent was left in place for 12 months with replacement every 3 to 4 months. Long-term benefit was noted for a mean period of 24 months after removing the stent [25•]. Papillotomy of the minor papilla over a short stent in patients with recurrent pancreatitis was noted to be beneficial in preventing recurrent episodes of pancreatitis in 74% of patients undergoing such therapy [26•]. However, when performed in patients with pancreas divisum and abdominal pain without documented pancreatitis, papillotomy was only marginally beneficial.

The immediate complications of these endoscopic techniques include pancreatitis, bleeding, sepsis, and intestinal perforation. Long-term complications include papillary stenosis of the minor papilla, stent-induced pancreatic duct stricture, and recurrence of pancreatitis. Although endoscopic therapy offers an attractive, minimally invasive treatment for the various clinical disorders associated with pancreas divisum, careful patient selection and adherence to proper technique are of utmost importance. Patients with acute recurrent pancreatitis remain the best candidates for therapy; the presence of a Santorinicele might indicate a favorable outcome. Endoscopic therapy also may be useful in pancreas divisum with chronic pancreatitis. It is probably not helpful in patients presenting with pain alone. Given the expertise required and the relative rarity of such patients, these procedures are best undertaken in specialized centers.

Choledochocele

Intermittent obstruction with retrograde flow of bile into the pancreatic duct might play a role in the pathogenesis of pancreatitis associated with choledochocele. Unroofing the choledochocele by use of a sphincterotome relieves such obstruction by establishing drainage and has been shown to be highly successful in preventing recurrent pancreatitis.

Sphincter of Oddi Dysfunction

Sphincter of Oddi dysfunction causing recurrent pancreatitis can be managed by ES of the sphincter choledochus, the sphincter pancreaticus, or both.

Tumors of the Papilla

Tumors of the papilla that lead to recurrent pancreatitis can be treated by endoscopic or surgical excision.

Chronic Pancreatitis

Patients suffering from chronic pancreatitis often present with disabling abdominal pain. The pathogenesis of such pain is poorly understood. High pressure in the pancreatic duct, often referred to as ductal hypertension, is considered to be a major cause of severe abdominal pain but probably does not explain the chronic persistent pain found in many of these patients. A variety of structural abnormalities, such as dominant strictures, calculi, periductal fibrosis, and papillary stenosis can create an impedance to pancreatic drainage and lead to elevated pressure.

Endoscopic therapy is aimed at correcting such abnormalities and reestablishing drainage and seems best suited in patients with intermittent pain, relapsing pancreatitis, or both. Pancreatic sphincterotomy, dilation of strictures, extraction of stones, and placement of stents constitute the commonly employed techniques during endoscopic therapy. For these procedures, a satisfactory pancreatogram is obtained first. The morphology of the pancreatic duct is analyzed for the number and location of strictures and calculi. Communicating pseudocysts also should be identified. A pancreatic sphincterotomy is performed, and strictures are dilated using a dilating catheter or hydrostatic balloon. These accessories are usually advanced over a standard guidewire (0.035 in) already positioned in the duct. Calculi from the pancreatic duct are extracted using a Dormia wire basket. Following stricture dilations and stone extraction, an endoprothesis (5F to 11.5F and 7–10 cm long) is left in the duct to facilitate drainage (Fig. 142-15). The stent is replaced every 3 to 4 months for up to 12 months to prevent recurrence of strictures.

In two studies, endoscopic therapy was performed in 84 patients with chronic pancreatitis, and stent insertion was successful in 80% [27,28]. Clinical improvement followed in 74% to 82% of patients. Early complications, such as acute pancreatitis, bleeding, sepsis, or intestinal perforation, were observed in almost 20% of patients. Late complications, including stent clogging, stent migration, stent-induced duodenal ulcer and recurrence of pseudocyst were seen in about 50% of patients. Stent-induced damage to the pancreatic duct is a potential problem when stents are left in place for prolonged intervals; however, this complication is relatively uncommon in chronic pancreatitis.

In summary, endoscopic therapy for chronic pancreatitis offers a viable alternative to operative intervention. Endoscopic treatment is associated with low and acceptable morbidity and mortality rates. However, careful selection of patients is the key to the success. These procedures are best undertaken in specialized centers.

Common bile duct stricture complicating chronic pancreatitis and causing bile duct obstruction also can be managed by stent placement. However, recurrence of obstruction is the rule following removal of such stents.

Pseudocysts

Pseudocysts of the pancreas are fluid collections that typically lack a lining epithelium and are found in or adjacent to the pancreas.

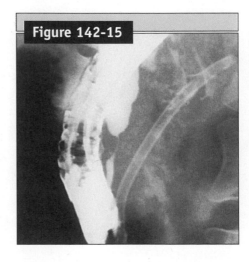

Figure 142-15

Radiograph showing a stent placed in the pancreatic duct after extraction of stones. The common bile duct is strictured. Note the calcification suggestive of chronic pancreatitis.

They are caused by acute pancreatitis, chronic pancreatitis, and traumatic damage to the pancreatic duct. Pseudocysts are seen in 10% to 15% of patients with chronic pancreatitis. The natural history of pancreatic pseudocyst is variable and poorly understood. Spontaneous resolution of pseudocysts occurs more commonly in those associated with acute pancreatitis. Based on several reports, about 50% of pseudocysts resulting from acute pancreatitis and 7% of those seen in chronic pancreatitis can be expected to reabsorb spontaneously [29].

Indications for Drainage

Size, underlying pancreatic pathology, duration of the pseudocyst, and the presence of symptoms are major factors determining the need for drainage. Upper abdominal pain that is usually worse after meals, vomiting related to duodenal compression, jaundice related to bile duct compression, and exacerations of pancreatitis from pancreatic duct compression are among the common signs and symptoms of pseudocysts. Pseudocysts that are 4 to 6 cm, symptomatic, and unresolved after 6 weeks of observation in patients with chronic pancreatitis should be drained. Enlarging pseudocysts should also undergo drainage. Patients left untreated are at risk for complications such as bleeding, rupture, or infection of the cyst.

Endoscopic Retrograde Cholangiopancreatography in Pseudocyst

Once a decision for drainage is made, an ERCP can provide valuable information in selecting appropriate therapy.

Communicating cysts. Approximately 60% of pseudocysts communicate with the main pancreatic duct. These can often be drained through the transpapillary route. Presence of communication indicates a high risk of recurrence when such pseudocysts are drained percutaneously.

Morphology of main pancreatic duct. A "road map" of the ductal morphology often will influence endoscopic or surgical therapy; in one surgical series, 50% of surgical approaches were influenced by the ERCP findings [30]. Endoscopic therapy also may be altered based on the morphology of the pancreatic duct. Patients with strictures of the pancreatic duct or calculi may benefit from dilation and stone removal during ERCP in addition to pseudocyst drainage; patients selected for surgery who demonstrate obstructed pancreatic ducts often require pancreatic resection in addition to drainage.

Table 142-3. Criteria for Successful Drainage of Pseudocyst

Visible bulge (by endoscopy)

Mature wall (by CT scan)

Close apposition to stomach or duodenum
   (by CT or endoscopic ultrasonography)

? Absence of vascular structure at the interface
   (by endoscopic ultrasonography)

Communication with main duct (for transpapillary drain)

Endoscopic Drainage

Three different techniques are used for endoscopic pseudocyst drainage: cystgastrostomy, cystduodenostomy, and transpapillary drainage. To accomplish successful drainage and avoid complications, experience, proper technique, and careful patient selection are essential. For cystgastrostomy and cystduodenostomy there must be a visible bulge of the cyst on the stomach or duodenal wall (Table 142-3), and the pseudocyst should be located no more than 10 mm from the gastric or duodenal wall; this can be assessed by CT scan or endoscopic ultrasonography (Fig. 142-16). Endoscopic ultrasonography with Doppler also may be helpful to avoid any vascular structure at the interface of the cyst and gastric or duodenal wall, which could cause severe bleeding during incision. Although some endoscopists routinely perform endoscopic ultrasonography and Doppler studies to identify vascular structures, the practice is not universal and the need for this additional step has not been firmly established by controlled studies.

Transpapillary Drainage

Transpapillary drainage is the most common endoscopic technique employed. It is indicated and indeed only possible when the pseudocyst communicates with the main pancreatic duct. During ERCP the pancreatic duct is selectively cannulated and injected with contrast material (Fig. 142-17). The morphology of the duct, including ductal strictures, and the site of communication between cyst and duct are identified. A hydrophilic guidewire is then introduced through the duct and advanced into the cyst cavity. After advancing the catheter into the cyst cavity over the hydrophilic wire, it is exchanged for a regular guidewire (0.035 in). Using the wire as the lead, a 7F, 10F, or 11.5F straight Amsterdam-type stent is placed in the cyst, with the other end of the stent lying freely in the duodenal lumen. If there is a stricture present in the main pancreatic duct, it first must be dilated using a Soehendra-type dilator or hydrostatic balloon.

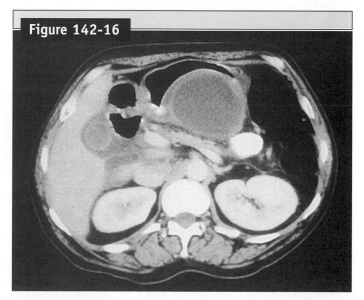

Figure 142-16

Computed tomography scan of the abdomen showing pseudocyst of the pancreas fulfilling the following criteria for endoscopic drainage: size (6.5 cm), position adjacent to stomach, and fibrous wall indicating a mature cyst.

Cystgastrostomy and Cystduodenostomy

For cystgastrostomy and cystduodenostomy, the site of maximum bulge on the stomach or duodenal wall is identified during endoscopy. This spot is next punctured using a needle knife and electrocautery (Fig. 142-18*A*, see also **Color Plate**). Once the cyst is entered, a gush of fluid into the stomach or duodenum is observed. After removing the needle, the cyst fluid should be aspirated for analysis to exclude a cystic neoplasm. The catheter is advanced deep into the pseudocyst lumen under fluoroscopic guidance, and contrast is instilled into the cyst cavity. Next, a guidewire is introduced through the sheath and coiled gently inside the cyst. If the puncture site is small, it should be dilated using a hydrostatic balloon prior to attempts at stent placement (Fig. 142-18*B*, see also **Color Plate**). Using the guidewire as a lead, one or multiple straight or pigtail stents can be placed bridging the cyst lumen and the stomach or duodenum (Fig. 142-18*C*, see also **Color Plate**).

Although an endoprothesis is preferred for draining the pseudocyst by many endoscopists, a nasocystic tube with intermittent flushing sometimes is employed. However, some of the problems associated with this technique include nasal and oropharyngeal irritation, accidental removal, kinking, and blockage of the tube. Following the drainage procedure, the size of the cyst is assessed by CT scan or ultrasonography in

4 to 6 weeks. When the cyst is completely resolved, the stents are removed.

Endoscopic drainage has been shown to be successful in 80% to 90% of patients [31•]. However, complications are reported in about 20% of patients with endoscopic pseudocyst drainage [32••]. Bleeding is the most serious complication and can be life-threatening. Sepsis, intestinal perforation, and pancreatitis also may occur. Inadvertent puncture of the gallbladder is another rare complication. Recurrence of pseudocyst is seen in up to 23% of patients [31•]. Based on some reports, bleeding and recurrence are more common with cystogastrostomy compared with the other techniques.

Although endoscopic drainage is seemingly more attractive and cost-effective and less invasive than the traditional surgical approaches, questions regarding optimal patient selection and clinical outcomes among various techniques remain unanswered. Moreover, there are no randomized studies available comparing endoscopic drainage with surgical therapy.

Pancreatic Cancer

Endoscopic therapy can be beneficial to patients with unresectable pancreatic cancer who have abdominal pain or obstructive jaundice. Common bile duct obstruction, resulting from direct extension of carcinoma of the head of the pancreas, is responsible for jaundice and pruritus. Placing an endoprosthesis across the bile duct stricture during ERCP establishes biliary drainage and effective palliation with relief of jaundice and pruritus in 90% of patients treated. A major limitation of polyethylene stents is plugging, which may be overcome with expandable stents made of wire mesh.

Abdominal pain, another common presenting symptom in pancreatic cancer, may be related to pancreatic ductal stricture with resultant pancreatic ductal hypertension. Placing an endoprosthesis across such stricture has been reported to improve abdominal pain in small groups of patients with intermittent or post-prandial pain related to pancreatic duct obstruction. However, more experience is needed before this treatment modality can be recommended widely.

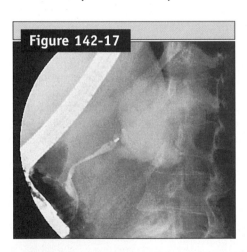

Figure 142-17

Pancreatogram demonstrating a communicating pseudocyst. This cyst was treated by transpapillary drainage.

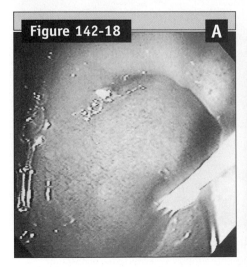
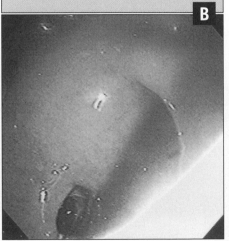
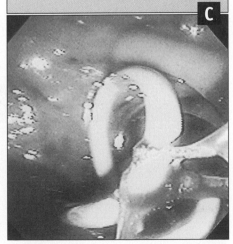

Figure 142-18   **A**   **B**   **C**

Technique of cystoduodenostomy. **A**, The cyst is bulging into the lumen and punctured through the duodenal wall. **B**, The puncture site is being dilated with a hydrostatic balloon. **C**, Endoscopic view showing two pigtail stents placed across the puncture site into the cyst cavity. See also **Color Plate**.

■ REFERENCES

Recently published papers of particular interest have been highlighted as follows:
- Of interest
- •• Of outstanding interest

1. Cotton PB, William CB: Using a lateral viewing gastroduodenoscope. In *Practical Gastrointestinal Endoscopy*. Oxford: Blackwell Scientific; 1980:30–32.

2. Venu RP, Geenen JE: Diagnosis and treatment of diseases of the papilla. In *Clinics in Gastroenterology*. Edited by Classen M. London: WB Saunders; 1986:439–456.

3.•• Venu RP, Geenen JE, Hogan WJ, *et al.*: Role of endoscopic retrograde cholangiopancreatography: in the diagnosis and treatment of choledochocele. *Gastroenterology* 1985, 87:1144–1149.

4. Shemesh E, Fredman E, Czesniak A, *et al.*: The association of biliary and pancreatic abnormalities with periampullary duodenal diverticuli. *Arch Surg* 1987, 122:1055–1057.

5. Johanson JF, Geenen JE, Hogan WJ: Endoscopic therapy of a duodenal duplication cyst. *Gastrointest Endosc* 1992, 38:60–64.

6.•• Eisen G, Schutz S, Metzler D, *et al.*: Santorinicele: new evidence for obstruction in pancreas divisum. *Gastrointest Endosc* 1994, 40:73–76.

7. Cotton PB: The normal pancreatogram. *Endoscopy* 1974, 6:65–70.

8.•• Venu RP, Brown RD, McGuire DE: Exfoliative cytology for pancreatic cancer: a review. *Int Gastroenterol* 1998, 9:133–138.

9. McGuire DE, Venu RP, Brown RD, *et al.*: Brush cytology for pancreatic carcinoma: an analysis of factors influencing results. *Gastrointest Endosc* 1996, 44:300–304.

10.• Raddawi HM, Geenen JE, Hogan WJ, *et al.*: Pressure measurements from biliary and pancreatic segments of sphincter of Oddi. *Dig Dis Sci* 1991, 36:71–74.

11. Sherman S, Troiano F, Hawes R, *et al.*: Pancreatitis following bile duct sphincter of Oddi manometry: utility of the aspirating catheter. *Gastrointest Endosc* 1992, 38:347–350.

12. Bilbao MK, Dottoer CT, Lee TG, Katon RM: Complications of endoscopic retrograde cholangiopancreatography (ERCP). *Gastroenterology* 1976, 70:314.

13.•• Venu RP, Geenen JE, Hogan WJ, *et al.*: Idiopathic recurrent pancreatitis: an approach to diagnosis and treatment. *Dig Dis Sci* 1989, 34:55–60.

14.•• Lee SP, Nicholls JF, Park HZ: Biliary sludge as a cause of acute pancreatitis. *N Engl J Med* 1992, 326:589–593.

15. O'Connor KW, Lehman GA: An improved technique for accessory papilla cannulation in pancreas divisum. *Gastrointest Endosc* 1985, 31:13–17.

16. Barkins JS, Ferstenberg RM, Panullo W, *et al.*: Endoscopic retrograde cholangiopancreatography in pancreatic trauma. *Gastrointest Endosc* 1988, 34:102–105.

17.•• Axon ATR, Classen M, Cotton PB, *et al.*: Pancreatography in chronic pancreatitis. *Gut* 1984, 25:1107.

18. Lichtenstein DR, Ferrari AP, Carr-Locke DL, *et al.*: Intraductal mucin secreting neoplasms of the pancreas. *Am J Gastroenterol* 1993, 88:1535.

19. Acosta JM, Ledesma CL: Gallstone migration as a cause of acute pancreatitis. *N Engl J Med* 1974, 290:484–487.

20.•• Neoptolemos JP, Carr-Locke DL, London NJ, *et al.*: Controlled trials of urgent endoscopic retrograde cholangiopancreatography and endoscopic sphincterotomy versus conservative treatment for acute pancreatitis due to gallstones. *Lancet* 1988, 2:979–983.

21.• Folsch UR, Nitsche R, Ludtke R, *et al.*, and the German Study Group on Acute Biliary Pancreatitis: Early ERCP and papillotomy compared with conservative treatment for acute biliary pancreatitis. *N Engl J Med* 1997, 336:237–242.

22.• Fan ST, Lai ECS, Mok FPT, *et al.*: Early treatment of acute biliary pancreatitis by endoscopic papillotomy. *N Engl J Med* 1993, 328:228–232.

23. Cotton PB: Congenital anomaly of pancreas divisum as a cause of obstructive pain and pancreatitis. *Gut* 1980, 21:105–114.

24.• Kozarek RA: Pancreatic stent can induce ductal changes consistent with chronic pancreatitis. *Gastrointest Endosc* 1990, 36:93–95.

25.• Lans JI, Geenen JE, Johanson JF: Endoscopic therapy in patients with pancreas divisum and acute pancreatitis: a prospective randomized, controlled clinical trial. *Gastrointest Endosc* 1992, 38:430–434.

26.• Lehman GA, Sherman S, Nisi R, *et al.*: Pancreas divisum: results of minor papilla sphincterotomy. *Gastrointest Endosc* 1993, 39:1–8.

27. Smits ME, Badiga M, Rauws EAJ, *et al.*: Long-term results of pancreatic stents in chronic pancreatitis. *Gastrointest Endosc* 1995, 42:461–466.

28. Ponchon T, Bory RM, Hedelius F, *et al.*: Endoscopic stenting for pain relief in chronic pancreatitis: results of a standardized protocol. *Gastrointest Endosc* 1995, 42:452–456.

29. Grace PA, Williamson RCN: Modern management of pancreatic pseudocysts. *Br J Surg* 1993, 80:573–581.

30. Laxon LC, Fromkes JJ, Cooperman M: Endoscopic retrograde cholangiopancreatography in the management of pancreatic pseudocysts. *Am J Surg* 1985, 50:683.

31.• Binomoeller KF, Siefert H, Walter A, Sohendra N: Transpapillary transmural drainage of pancreatic pseudocysts. *Gastrointest Endosc* 1995, 42:219–224.

32.•• Smits ME, Rauws EAJ, Tytgat GNJ, Huibregtse K: The efficacy of endoscopic treatment of pancreatic pseudocysts. *Gastrointest Endosc* 1995, 42:202–207.

143 Hereditary Pancreatitis
Jean Perrault

The first family with hereditary pancreatitis was described by Comfort and Steinberg in 1952 [1•]. The authors presented four definite and two probable cases, the disease spectrum, included pancreatic calcifications, steatorrhea, diabetes, and an autosomal dominant inheritance was suggested. Since then, more than 100 families worldwide have been added to the literature [2••]. The clinical picture is indistinguishable from that of acute pancreatitis, but it is recognizable by an onset in early age, usually in the first decade of life; equal sex distribution; similar disease in other family members; and frequently, progression to chronic pancreatitis. The transmission of hereditary pancreatitis is autosomal dominant, with 80% penetration [3] and variable expressivity in age of onset. Identical twins have been affected [4]. A hereditary pancreatitis gene locus on chromosome 7 shared by at least five separate families [5,6] has been identified.

The term *hereditary pancreatitis* is preferred to familial pancreatitis because other conditions causing pancreatitis may affect many members of a single family, such as hyperlipidemia, hyperparathyroidism, or even alcoholism.

ETIOLOGY AND PATHOGENESIS

With the gradual addition of families with hereditary pancreatitis over the years, many phenotypes have been described. Many patients in the initial families had an aminoaciduria (lysine, cystine, and occasionally arginine) possibly related to a defect in renal tubular reabsorption [7,8]. Subsequent families did not show this defect or had different types of aminoaciduria that were more generalized [9] or selective (hyperglycinuria) [10]. Other family members exhibited aminoaciduria but no pancreatitis [11]. Four family members were described with hyperparathyroidism and pancreatitis [12], all of whom had increased urinary lysine and cystine concentrations. Only two of the four family memebers who went to surgery had parathyroid pathology, and it is not clear if the pancreatitis resolved after normocalcemic control. Another family was described with apolipoprotein C-II deficiency that led to marked hypertriglyceridemia (values >1000 mg/dL), and five of seven family members had pancreatitis [13]. The cause of pancreatitis in that family is not clear, although we do know that patients with severe hypertriglyceridemia or abnormal catabolism of chylomicron remnants may have secondary pancreatitis, which resolves once the serum lipid profile is controlled. In other families, anatomic abnormalities of the sphincter of Oddi or the pancreatic duct have been observed, suggesting that genetic abnormalities might be expressed in structural and anatomic defects [14,15]. However, many patients have normal endoscopic retrograde pancreatography in the first stages of the disease, whereas patients with nonhereditary pancreatitis may show similar anatomic abnormalities after longstanding disease. Another family with a possible decrease in antioxidant protection has been reported [16]; decreased levels of glutathione peroxidase were found in the red blood cells of affected and unaffected members, but only the affected family members had decreased levels of selenium and vitamin E. Further studies are required, however, because in the same report, patients with nonhereditary pancreatitis also had decreased levels of glutathione peroxidase and selenium.

Patients with hereditary pancreatitis have been known to develop stones, often quite large ones, in the ducts. Usually these are recognized by calcifications seen on abdominal plain radiographs. In a large, three-generation family, human leukocyte antigen types were determined without identifying any clear relationship to the occurrence of pancreatitis [17]. In a separate study, there did not appear to be a clear relationship between human leukocyte antigens and the formation of stones in different types of pancreatitis [18]. Sarles and colleagues suggest that hereditary pancreatitis might present in two forms: 1) *calcific lithiasis*, in which the stones are deeply calcified and the concentration of lithostatin (pancreatic stone protein) is low in the pancreatic fluid, and 2) *protein lithiasis*, which appears as

radiolucent stones with normal lithostatin [19,20]. Protein lithiasis is more common than calcific lithiasis and more difficult to identify [20]. However, a study from Japan seems to exclude any genetic alteration of the lithostatin gene in hereditary pancreatitis [21]. Gene analysis in two families with hereditary pancreatitis did not disclose any rearrangement or gross deletion of the gene in affected members, and the immunoreactive lithostatin level in acinar cells of one patient who underwent surgery was normal. The time of appearance of the stones, often years after the first attack of pancreatitis, led Comfort and Steinberg to conclude that the stones are the result of the pancreatitis rather than the cause [1•]. Further studies will help clarify this apparent phenotypic presentation.

With the variety of phenotypes, the ability to identify a gene for hereditary pancreatitis would improve our diagnostic capabilities, provide deeper insight into the molecular pathogenesis of the disorder, enable genetic counseling, and make possible the development of new therapeutic strategies. The phenomenal advances in molecular genetics along with the rapidly expanding human genome project have set the stage for remarkable findings of two groups of researchers. Each group was able to retrace a large number of family members in two different families [22••,23]. The two groups then identified almost exactly the same site as the most likely locus for the hereditary pancreatitis gene [5,6].

Whitcomb and colleagues, seeking to identify the site of the disease-carrying mutation, concentrated their efforts on a narrow strip where the five-gene trypsinogen locus is located among the T-cell receptor β chain gene (TRCB) locus on chromosome 7q35 [24••]. They identified a single mutation of arginine to histidine at position 117 of the cationic trypsinogen gene, which rendered this altered trypsinogen molecule resistant to trypsin-like proteases, thereby preventing the inactivation of activated trypsin in the pancreas through self-protective mechanisms. Small amounts of trypsinogen normally are activated to trypsin but are rendered harmless by at least two separate protective mechanisms [25]. If trypsin overwhelms the system, or resists inactivation, then it may lead to autodigestion of the pancreas and eventually pancreatitis. To date, four different families from the United States, and one from Italy, have shown this same anomaly [24••]. More recently, a second cationic trypsinogen gene mutation has been identified in two unrelated families [26].

CLINICAL FEATURES

There are no distinguishing clinical features between patients who present with an acute episode of hereditary pancreatitis and patients with any other type of acute pancreatitis. Typically, they present with epigastric pain, at times severe and radiating to the back, that is somewhat relieved by the fetal or knee–chest position. The pain often is accompanied by vomiting. The onset is often at an early age—as early as 2 years of age—although the symptoms usually present in the second decade of life [3,11,27,28]. Both sexes are affected equally. Hereditary pancreatitis is one of the most common causes of recurrent pancreatitis in children (Tudor RB, Personal communication).

The presentation of hereditary pancreatitis is not necessarily the same for all members of a family; some may even have painless pancreatitis and the diagnosis is made by the identification of pancreatic calcifications or because of other complications from the disease [29]. However, hemorrhagic pancreatitis is rare in hereditary pancreatitis. Acute symptoms usually last from 2 days to 2 weeks, with an occasional patient who remains symptomatic for weeks. In some families, the disease can skip two or more generations [22••], making it important to request as much information about as many members of the family as possible. There are no distinguishing features on physical examination to help differentiate hereditary pancreatitis from other types of pancreatitis, although minor developmental anomalies have been described, such as internal strabismus and nystagmus [27]. Patients with hereditary pancreatitis typically will have two to four recurrences a year, although recurrences may be more frequent. The severity and frequency of the attacks seem to be reduced in young adulthood [3,7,29].

The presentation and complications of 42 young patients with hereditary pancreatitis seen at our institution were compared with 28 young patients who had idiopathic relapsing pancreatitis [30]. Included in this comparison were 42 members of one of the most extensive genealogies, studied by LeBodic and colleagues [22••], who compiled data on 249 members of a family covering eight generations (Table 143-1). In general, patients with hereditary pancreatitis presented at a younger age and had a more severe disease (Table 143-1).

COMPLICATIONS

Patients with hereditary pancreatitis, as can be predicted by the relapsing nature of the disease, are at particular risk of developing complications (Table 143-2). Some of these complications, such as ascites or effusions [31,32], portal hypertension, or pseudocyst formation, may accompany an acute episode; the portal hypertension is usually the result of splenic or portal vein

thrombosis that follows pancreatic inflammation [3,7,9,33]. Another vital structure, the common bile duct, also may be affected, resulting in obstructive jaundice. Diabetes, steatorrhea, or pancreatic lithiasis may develop [3,7,9]. LeBodic and colleagues [22••] encountered similar complications as we did in our group of patients [30] but at a higher rate. The higher rates of complications may be attributed to that study's older population. The development of carcinoma was not observed in either study, although it is one of the most severe complications that result from this condition [34–36,37•]. The cancers themselves are the usual types of ductal adenocarcinoma, with the same grim prognosis; the onset is often at an early age, with a progressive rise in cancer risk, reaching 40% by age 70 years [37•]. An interesting observation from the International Hereditary Pancreatitis Study Group suggests that pancreatic carcinoma is associated with a paternal inheritance pattern [37•].

The development of pancreatic lithiasis is not uncommon [3,7,9] and has the potential of precipitating numerous attacks or prolonging individual episodes. Stones are found more often in the ducts than in the parenchyma [15], thus increasing the risk for ductal obstruction [3,9,35,38].

LABORATORY EVALUATION

Until recently, only a positive family history could help distinguish hereditary pancreatitis from other types of pancreatic inflammation. Now it should be possible to identify at least some cases of hereditary pancreatitis that share the anomaly on chromosome 7. Tests such as amylase and lipase usually are used to diagnose an acute event.

A plain radiograph of the abdomen may reveal calcified stones or help in following the development, enlargement, or even disappearance of stones. An ultrasound of the abdomen is

Table 143-1. Comparison of Clinical Features in Hereditary Pancreatitis as Compared to Idiopathic Pancreatitis in Young Age

| | Type of pancreatitis | | |
| | Hereditary | | |
Symptoms	Group 1 %, (n = 35)	Group 2, %, (n = 25)	Idiopathic, %, (n = 35)
At presentation			
n	42	42	28
Mean age, y	7	6.6	12
Abdominal pain	100	100	100
Vomiting	62	—	39
Back pain	40	—	43
Complications			
Follow-up, y	18	*	17
Steatorrhea	10	55.7	5
Diabetes	3	40†	5
Pseudocysts	17	11	4
Surgical intervention	55	50	14
Cancer	0	0	0

*Not specified, but "were followed-up regularly" [22].
†Diabetes after age 30.

Table 143-2. Complications of Hereditary Pancreatitis

Acute
  Ascites, effusions
  Pseudocyst
  Extrahepatic portal hypertension
  Obstructive jaundice
Chronic
  Diabetes mellitus
  Steatorrhea
  Lithiasis
  Extrahepatic portal hypertension
Carcinoma

important during an acute event to support the diagnosis of pancreatitis by demonstrating edematous enlargement of the gland; pseudocysts and ductal dilatation can be followed serially [39]. Doppler scanning helps in the assessment of the patency of the vascular structures surrounding the pancreas, especially the splenic vein. Computed tomography (CT) reinforces the findings seen at ultrasound (Figure 143-1) and may help in following the course of the disease (Figure 143-2). Endoscopic retrograde pancreatography is used more often for therapy than diagnosis: biliary and pancreatic stone extraction (Figure 143-3), or before surgery to delineate the pancreatic duct [27]. Endoscopic ultrasound, with guided fine needle biopsies, has the potential to improve on the diagnosis of carcinoma, although the differentiation of neoplastic masses from inflammatory masses may continue to be difficult.

DIFFERENTIAL DIAGNOSIS

As noted earlier, an episode of pancreatitis with a positive family history for pancreatitis is strongly indicative of a hereditary type of disease. Unfortunately, pancreatitis often is overlooked in children. Because pancreatic attacks start in childhood, it can take years before the diagnosis is made unless one of the parents has already been affected or is aware of the family history. Without a history of inheritance, the pancreatitis is indistinguishable from any other type. The physician must ask about trauma to the epigastrium or any recent accident. Many viruses can target the pancreas, such as the mumps agent, Rubella, measles, and coxsackie virus. Ascaris worms also can insinuate themselves into the bile and pancreatic ducts, causing inflammatory changes.

Congenital lesions of the duodenum (diverticulum), the bile duct (choledochocysts), the pancreas (pancreas divisum, ductal polyp), or other genetic diseases (cystic fibrosis), also may cause pancreatitis. More common causes of acute pancreatitis, especially in adults, include alcohol, gallstones, and various medications. Certain conditions associated with pancreatitis and a propensity for a familial occurrence include hereditary hyperparathyroidism [8,40] and the syndrome of hypocalciuria and hypercalcemia [41,42]. A few cases have been described of parenchymal fibrosis or chronic fibrosing pancreatitis [43]. Hyperlipidemia with triglyceride levels greater than 1000 mg/dL also may be accompanied by pancreatitis [13].

TREATMENT

The identification of the chromosome, and now the gene, that is responsible for hereditary pancreatitis is bringing us closer to a more specific therapy, but until then we continue to treat the patient symptomatically, watching for potential complications and trying to reduce recurrences with maintenance therapy.

Medical Therapy

Acute Episodes

The approach to treatment of an acute episode of hereditary pancreatitis is essentially the same as for any attack of acute pancreatitis: nothing by mouth; administration of intravenous fluids; correction of hyperglycemia, hypocalcemia, or other electrolyte disorders; and control of pain. We usually advocate injectable ketorolac (0.5 mg/kg in children, 30 mg in adults) or meperidine (2 mg/kg in children, 50–100 mg in adults) every 6 hours to control pain. If vomiting is causing distress, nasogastric aspiration may be used, although *not* on a routine basis. Once vomiting and pain have subsided oral fluids are offered, but fluids are limited to carbohydrates without proteins or fat to limit the stimulation of the exocrine pancreas for the first 24 to 48 hours. Nutrition in a more prolonged episode may be achieved by a chemically defined diet given through a jejunostomy feeding tube; the more distal the infusion, the less likely the stimulation of the pancreas.

In the event of severe or prolonged pain, octreotide (Somatostatin) at a dose of 25 to 50 µg four times per day may be used [44]. Octreotide also has been successful in controlling a pleural effusion from a pancreaticopleural fistula [45]. Long-term use can lead to sludge formation in the gallbladder if not gallstone formation [46]. In some patients with prolonged pain, evaluation for the possibility of a pancreatic duct stone obstructing the pancreatic duct may be rewarded with the identification of a progressively dilating pancreatic duct. An endoscopic removal of the stones may lead to resolution of symptoms.

Interest has resurfaced for a trypsin inhibitor, gabexate mesylate, which has been used to prevent symptomatic pancreatitis following endoscopic retrograde pancreatography. Because the pathophysiology for hereditary pancreatitis is most likely a mutant trypsinogen resistant to autoinactivation, interest in gabexate mesylate is probably well-founded. However, while the drug is useful in prophylaxis, its potential effectiveness as a treatment is debatable: it is impossible to predict when an attack will develop, and by the time pancreatitis has started, use of the drug is probably too late. So, although it is effective for prophylaxis, it is not useful in acute disease.

Recurrent Episodes or Chronic Pain

Many patients with hereditary pancreatitis will have more than just one or two episodes of pancreatitis per year or will have chronic pain. In these patients, disability may be great, not only because of incapacity but also because of the possibility of analgesic or narcotic abuse. The first therapeutic approach is to use diet manipulation in an attempt to reduce pancreatic stimulation; avoidance of alcohol and medications known to complicate pancreatitis is mandatory. The addition of pancreatic enzyme supplementation, such as pancreatin, may decrease pancreatic secretion and reduce pain [47]. Because intraduodenal perfusion

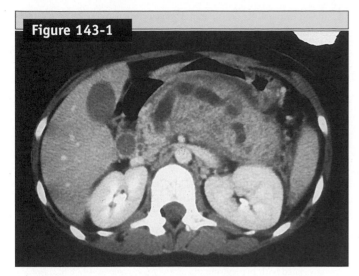

Contrast-enhanced computed tomography scan showing marked enlargement and inhomogeneous enhancement of the pancreas, marked dilation of the pancreatic duct, and inflammatory thickening of the peripancreatic fascia near the tail of the pancreas. All the changes are indicative of pancreatitis. (*Courtesy of* R. MacCarty, MD.)

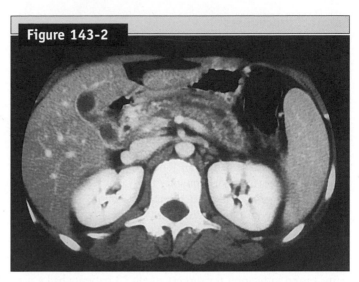

Contrast-enhanced computed tomography scan done 8 weeks after scan in Figure 143-1. The scan shows resolution of the pancreatitis with a normal size gland but with some residual dilation of the pancreatic duct. (*Courtesy of* R. MacCarty, MD.)

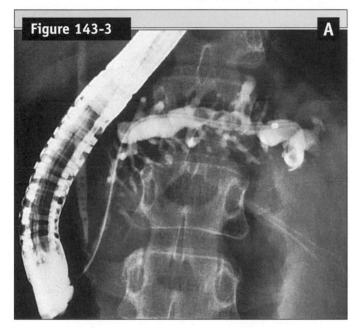

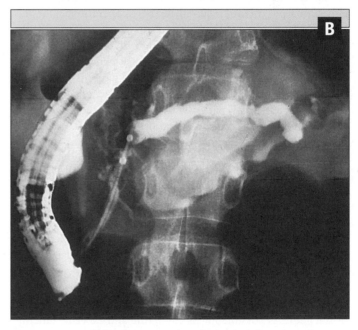

A, Retrograde pancreatogram showing a dilated pancreatic duct containing several lucent stones. A balloon catheter has been passed into the distal pancreatic duct for stone extraction.

B, Pancreatogram following extraction shows that the stones have been removed. There is residual dilation of the pancreatic duct. (*Courtesy of* R. MacCarty, MD.)

of extracts has maximum effect, nonencapsulated preparations usually are prescribed. In many instances, however, the effect is moderate at best, and antioxidants may be added to the regimen. Patients with chronic pancreatitis usually have a low intake of one or more antioxidants. Accordingly, a group taking a "cocktail" of selenium (600 μg), beta carotene (9000 IU), vitamin C (0.54 g), and vitamin E (270 IU) with 2 g of methionine per day was studied and compared with a placebo-controlled group in a 20-week crossover trial [48]. Six of 20 patients had an attack while using the placebo, but none had any symptoms during active treatment. Because low antioxidants levels have been noted in hereditary pancreatitis [16], this approach

requires further study. A celiac block is reserved for patients with intractable pain.

Endoscopic Procedures

Patients with a dilated and stone-obstructed pancreatic duct are ideal candidates for a therapeutic endoscopic procedure. Our experience with stent placement in the pancreatic duct in hereditary pancreatitis has not yet been positive. Complications occur, such as infections and sepsis, which are relieved by removing the stent and use of parenteral antibiotics. Sphincteroplasty and basket extraction of stone material and debris from the pancreatic duct have been performed successfully. Lithotripsy also has been suggested [49].

Surgical Procedures

Indications for surgery are straightforward: chronic pain; mechanical complications, such as obstructive jaundice, pseudocyst, ascites, and perhaps intestinal obstruction; and differentiating between pancreatitis and carcinoma in the case of an indeterminate mass [50]. The goals of surgery are to relieve intractable pain and remedy local complications while preserving as much of the exocrine and endocrine function of the pancreas as possible [51]. Of the many procedures that have been advocated, lateral pancreaticojejunostomy (modified Puestow procedure) is performed frequently [52]; if it fails, or if a more severely damaged gland is encountered, a duodenal-preserving resection of the head of the pancreas combined with longitudinal pancreaticojejunostomy of the body and the tail of the pancreas has been advocated [53].

In 22 adults with hereditary pancreatitis treated surgically, pain was an indication for surgery in all; 13 patients had a pancreaticojejunostomy (three of whom had concomitant distal pancreatectomy, four had a cholecystectomy with sphincteroplasty, and one each had an enteric drainage of a pseudocyst or drainage of a pancreatic abscess)[50]. Eighteen patients obtained marked improvement to complete relief of symptoms, although five patients required further reoperation; none died and only three patients had some form of complication (intraabdominal abscess, wound infection, and urinary tract infection) [50]. In 25 children with hereditary pancreatitis, surgery was undertaken to relieve pain in 55% of patients and to treat complications in 45%. A longitudinal pancreaticojejunostomy was performed in 21 patients, whereas the others underwent cyst decompression, transduodenal pancreatic duct sphincteroplasty, pancreatic resection, or a splenorenal shunt for portal hypertension. Seventy-seven percent of the patients reported good to excellent results after 15 years of follow-up. There was no mortality following the procedure. Surgical complications occurred in 16% of the patients and included pneumonia, pulmonary edema, and wound or intraperitoneal infection.

Generally, we advocate medical therapy for patients with hereditary pancreatitis with close follow-up. When pain is intractable or when the pancreatic duct remains persistently dilated or reveals stony material, then surgery is an attractive alternative. The intent of surgery should be to preserve as much of the gland as possible for its endocrine and exocrine function. When all else fails, total pancreatectomy with pancreas or islet cell transplantation may be considered (see Chapter 117, Liver Transplantation).

■■ REFERENCES

Recently published papers of particular interest have been highlighted as follows:
- Of interest
- • Of outstanding interest

1.• Comfort MW, Steinberg AG: Pedigree of a family with hereditary chronic relapsing pancreatitis. *Gastroenterol* 1952, 21:54–63.
This is the first publication to refer to hereditary pancreatitis.

2.•• Perrault J: Hereditary pancreatitis. *Gastroenterol Clin North Am* 1994, 23:743–752.
This is a review on the subject, with a complete bibliography.

3. Sibert JR: Hereditary pancreatitis in England and Wales. *J Med Genet* 1978, 15:189–201.

4. Freud E, Barak R, Ziv N, *et al.*: Familial chronic recurrent pancreatitis in identical twins: case report and review of the literature. *Arch Surg* 1992, 127:1125–1128.

5. LeBodic L, Bignon JD, Raguénès O, *et al.*: The hereditary pancreatitis gene maps to long arm of chromosome 7. *Hum Mol Genet* 1996, 5:549–554.

6. Whitcomb DC, Preston RA, Aston CE, *et al.*: A gene for hereditary pancreatitis maps to chromosome 7q35. *Gastroenterol* 1996, 110:1975–1980.

7. Gross JB: Hereditary pancreatitis. In *The Exocrine Pancreas: Biology, Pathobiology, and Diseases.* Edited by Go VLW. New York: Raven Press; 1986:829–839.

8. Gross JB, Ulrich JA, Jones JD: Urinary excretion of amino acids in a kindred with hereditary pancreatitis and aminoaciduria. *Gastroenterol* 1964, 47:41–48.

9. Sato T, Saitoh Y: Familial chronic pancreatitis associated with pancreatic lithiasis. *Am J Surg* 1974, 127:511–517.

10. Bergstrom K, Hellstrom K, Kallner M, *et al.*: Familial pancreatitis associated with hyperglycinuria. *Scand J Gastroenterol* 1973, 8:217–223.

11. Gross JB, Ulrich JA, Maher FT: Further observations on the hereditary form of pancreatitis. In *Ciba Foundation Symposium on the Exocrine Pancreas: Normal and Abnormal Functions.* Edited by de Reuck AVS, Cameron MP. Boston: Little, Brown & Co., 1961, 278–305.

12. Carey MC, Fitzgerald O: Hyperparathyroidism associated with chronic pancreatitis in a family. *Gut* 1968, 9:700–703.

13. Cox DW, Breckenridge WC, Little JA: Inheritance of apolipoprotein C-II deficiency with hypertriglyceridemia and pancreatitis. *N Engl J Med* 1978, 299:1421–1424.

14. Robechek PJ: Hereditary chronic relapsing pancreatitis: a clue to pancreatitis in general. *Am J Surg* 1967, 113:822–825.

15. Hardy M, Cornet E, Dupon H, *et al.*: Chronic pancreatitis associated with familial dilatation of the pancreatic ducts: 6 operated cases. *Bibl Gastroenterol* 1965, 7:189–216.

16. Nordback I, Saarenpaa-Heikklla O, Koskimies S: Screening a family for hereditary chronic pancreatitis. *Panminerva Med* 1990, 32:19–24.

17. Forbes A, Schwarz G, Mirakian R, *et al.*: HLA antigens in chronic pancreatitis. *Tissue Antigens* 1987, 30:176–183.

18. Mathew P, Wyllie R, Van Lente F, *et al.*: Antioxidants in hereditary pancreatitis. *Am J Gastroenterol* 1996, 91:1558–1562.

19. Sarles H, Camarena J, Bernard JP, *et al.*: Lithiase próteique et lithiase calcique héréditaires: deux formes différentes de pancréatite héréditaire. *Bull Acad Natle Méd* 1993, 177:565–574.

20. Sarles H, Camarena J, Bernard JP, *et al.*: Two forms of hereditary chronic pancreatitis. *Pancreas* 1996, 12:138–141.

21. Suzuki T, Matozakt T, Matsuda K: Analysis of pancreatic stone protein gene of HEPE. *Japanese J Gastroenterol* 1992, 89:63–68.

22.•• LeBodic L, Schnee M, Georgelin T, *et al.*: An exceptional genealogy for hereditary chronic pancreatitis. *Dig Dis Sci* 1996, 41:1504–1510.
In this report the authors study 249 family members from one family, born between 1800 and 1993.

23. It takes a family [editorial]. *Nature Genetics* 1996, 14:117–118..

24.•• Whitcomb DC, Gorry MC, Preston RA, *et al.*: Hereditary pancreatitis is caused by a mutation in the cationic trypsinogen gene. *Nature Genetics* 1996, 14:141–145.

25. Rinderknecht H, Adham NF, Renner IG, Carmack C: A possible self-destruct mechanism preventing pancreatic autodigestion. *Int J Pancreatol* 1988, 3:33–34.

26. Gabbaizadeh D, Gates L, Ulrich CD, *et al.*: Clinical features of hereditary pancreatitis in a family with a new genotype. *Gastroenterol* 1997, 112:A442.

27. Crane JM, Amoury RA, Hellerstein S: Hereditary pancreatitis: report of a kindred. *J Pediatr Surg* 1973, 8:893–900.

28. Vantini I, Piubello W, Ederle A, *et al.*: Hereditary pancreatitis: morphological pictures (ERCP) in the youngest member of a family. *Acta Hepatogastroenterol* 1979, 26:253–256.

29. Riccardi VM, Shih VE, Holmes LB, *et al*.: Hereditary pancreatitis: nonspecificity of aminoaciduria and diagnosis of occult disease. *Arch Intern Med* 1975, 135:822–825.

30. Konzen KM, Perrault JP, Moir C, Zinsmeister AR: Long-term follow-up of young patients with chronic hereditary or idiopathic pancreatitis. *Mayo Clin Proc* 1993, 68:449–453.

31. Nash FW: Familial calcific pancreatitis: an acute episode with massive pleural effusion. *Proc R Soc Med* 1971, 64:17–18.

32. Rao SSC, Riley SA, Foster PN, *et al*.: Hereditary pancreatitis presenting with ascites. *Postgrad Med J* 1986, 62:873–875.

33. McElroy R, Christiansen PA: Hereditary pancreatitis in a kinship associated with portal vein thrombosis. *Am J Med* 1972, 52:228–241.

34. Mlan TA, Zuberi SJ: Familial pancreatitis with lithiasis. *JPMA* 1980, 30:275–278.

35. Logan A Jr, Schlicke CP, Manning GB: Familial pancreatitis. *Am J Surg* 1968, 115:112–117.

36. Bartholomew LG, Gross JB, Comfort MW: Carcinoma of the pancreas associated with chronic relapsing pancreatitis. *Gastroenterol* 1958, 35:473–477.

37.• Lowenfels A, Maisonneuve P, DiMagno EP, *et al*.: Hereditary pancreatitis and the risk of pancreatic cancer. *J Natl Cancer Inst* 1997, 89:442–446.
This is a multicenter study comparing the expected frequency of pancreatic cancer with hereditary pancreatitis in 10 countries.

38. Perrault J, Gross JB, King JE: Endoscopic retrograde cholangiopancreatography in familial pancreatitis. *Gastroenterol* 1976, 71:138–141.

39. Telander RL, Charbonneau WL, Haymond MW: Intraoperative ultrasonography of the pancreas in children. *J Pediatr Surg* 1986, 21:262–266.

40. Jackson CE: Hereditary hyperparathyroidism associated with recurrent pancreatitis. *Ann Intern Med* 1958, 49:829–836.

41. Davis M, Klimiuk PS, Adams PH, *et al*.: Familial hypocalciuric hypercalcemia and acute pancreatitis. *Br Med J* 1981, 282:1023–1025.

42. Heath H: Familial benign (hypocalciuric) hypercalcemia. *Endocrinol Metab Clin North Am* 1989, 18:723–740.

43. Williams TE Jr, Sherman NJ, Clatworthy HW Jr: Chronic fibrosing pancreatitis in childhood: a cause of recurrent abdominal pain. *Pediatrics* 1967, 40:1019–1023.

44. Müller MK, Beglinger C: Effects of somatostatin on the exocrine pancreas. *Scand J Gastroenterol* 1991, 26:129–136.

45. Guez T, Baetz A, Sicard D, *et al*.: Intérêt de la somatostatine dans le traitement d'une fistule pancréatico-pleurale. *Gastroenterol Clin Biol* 1990, 14:286–295.

46. Fisher RS, Rock E, Levin G, Malmud L: Effects of somatostatin on gallbladder emptying. *Gastroenterol* 1987, 92:885–890.

47. Isaksson G, Ihse I: Pain reduction by an oral pancreatic enzyme preparation in chronic pancreatitis. *Dig Dis Sci* 1983, 28:97–102.

48. Uden S, Bilton D, Nathan L, *et al*.: Antioxidant therapy for recurrent pancreatitis: placebo-controlled trial. *Aliment Pharmacol Ther* 1990, 4:357–371.

49. Pitchumoni CS, Mohan AT: Pancreatic stones. *Gastroenterol Clin North Am* 1990, 19:873–893.

50. Miller AR, Nagorney DM, Sarr MG: The surgical spectrum of hereditary pancreatitis in adults. *Ann Surg* 1992, 215:39–43.

51. Rumenapf G, Kamm M, Rupprecht H, Scheele J: Surgical management of hereditary pancreatitis: report of a case and presentation of a new family. *Pancreas* 1994, 9:398–399.

52. Crombleholme TM, deLorimier AA, Way LW, *et al*.: The modified Puestow procedure for chronic relapsing pancreatitis in children. *J Pediatr Surg* 1990, 25:749–754.

53. Frey CF, Smith GJ: Description and rationale of a new operation for chronic pancreatitis. *Pancreas* 1987, 2:701–707.

Pediatric Gastroenterology

8

Edited by Fredric Daum

Contributors

Harvey W. Aiges
Estella M. Alonso
R. Peter Altman
Stephen M. Borowitz
William J. Byrne
Anupama Chawla
Mitchell B. Cohen
Richard B. Colletti
Arnold G. Coran
Stanley E. Fisher
Joseph F. Fitzgerald
Donald E. George
Mark S. Glassman
Eric Hassall
James E. Heubi
Jay A. Hochman
Jeffrey S. Hyams
Esther Jacobowitz
 Israel
Ellen Kahn
Kenneth Kenigsberg
William J. Klish
Neil D. Kutin
Eric L. Lazar
Carlos H. Lifschitz

Kathleen M. Loomes
Eric S. Maller
James F. Markowitz
Karan E. McBride
Marvin S. Medow
Adam G. Mezoff
Parvathi Mohan
Andrew E. Mulberg
Maria M. Oliva-Hemker
David A. Piccoli
Roy Proujansky
Philip Rosenthal
Thomas M. Rossi
José M. Saavedra
Sarah Jane
 Schwarzenberg
Linda Shalon
Harvey L. Sharp
Edwin Simpser
Robert H. Squires, Jr
Francis P. Sunaryo
Vasundhara Tolia
William R. Treem
Jon A. Vanderhoof

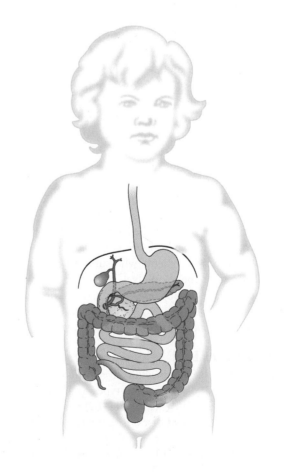

144 Esophageal Atresia and Tracheoesophageal Fistula

Arnold G. Coran

This chapter focuses on three main variants of esophageal atresia (EA) and tracheoesophageal fistula (TEF): EA with distal TEF, pure EA without TEF, and TEF without EA. The very rare variant laryngotracheoesophageal cleft is not discussed.

■ EMBRYOLOGY

The trachea and esophagus appear as a ventral diverticulum of the foregut at 22 to 23 days of gestation [1]. As the diverticulum elongates, masses of endodermal cells form ridges of tissue that ultimately divide the foregut into tracheal and esophageal channels. This process begins at the carina and extends cephalad. By the 26th day of gestation, the esophagus and trachea have become completely separated to the level of the larynx. By the 6th week of gestation, the circular muscular coat of the esophagus has appeared, and the vagus nerves appear shortly thereafter. Blood vessels from the aorta are present by the 7th week, and the longitudinal muscle of the esophagus is seen in the 9th week of gestation. The lining of the esophagus is initially ciliated, but by the 20th week of gestation it is replaced by stratified squamous epithelium. It is probably at about the 4th week of gestation, when the trachea and esophagus are being separated by the ingrowth of ectodermal ridges, that an interruption in this process occurs and results in a TEF.

The process by which EA develops is less clear. One theory suggests that the elongation of the trachea in a caudal direction is so rapid that when there is a fistula producing fixation of the esophagus to the trachea, the dorsal wall of the esophagus is drawn forward and downward to be incorporated into the trachea. Atresia of the esophagus results because of the presence of the fistula. This does not explain how isolated EA occurs, however. A vascular deficiency has been postulated as the cause.

Clinical data suggest there is some genetic cause for the transmission of the abnormality. Deletions or duplications of a number of chromosome loci have been described in single cases of EA [2•]. A number of patients who survived repair of their EA have children with the anomaly. Cases of siblings with EA have been reported, including one family with three affected children. A recent series reported an incidence of 9% of both twins with EA in 102 patients with the anomaly.

■ CLASSIFICATION

The incidence of EA is one in 4000 live births. Figure 144-1 illustrates the three most common types of EA and TEF. Proximal EA with distal TEF (Fig. 144-1*A*) is most common, accounting for 85% to 90% of cases. Isolated EA (Fig. 144-1*B*), the second most common form of this entity, occurs in about 5% to 7% of affected infants. TEF without EA (Fig. 144-1*C*) is

the least common, accounting for between 2% and 6% of cases. Rare forms of these anomalies include EA with proximal TEF and EA with both proximal and distal TEF.

■ ESOPHAGEAL ATRESIA WITH DISTAL TRACHEOESOPHAGEAL FISTULA

Newborn infants with proximal atresia with distal TEF develop significant respiratory difficulty immediately after birth. The EA impedes the swallowing of saliva, resulting in the accumulation of fluid in the proximal esophageal pouch and putting the infant at risk for airway obstruction, atelectasis, and aspiration pneumonia. The distal TEF produces the most serious physiologic disturbance. Because most newborns have free gastroesophageal reflux, acidic gastric juice can reflux into the tracheobronchial tree, causing chemical pneumonitis. Saliva is far better tolerated by the lungs than is gastric juice. In addition, passage of air from the trachea into the distal TEF promotes intestinal and abdominal distention, causing elevation of the diaphragm—the major respiratory muscle—which may seriously impair the neonate's ventilatory capacity. The larger the distal TEF, the greater is the intestinal distention and subsequent respiratory compromise. If an associated distal congenital obstruction of the intestine, such as duodenal atresia or imperforate anus (eg, the vertebral, anal, cardiac, tracheal, esophageal, renal, and limb [VACTERL] syndrome) is present, distention of the proximal intestine is even greater and the respiratory compromise even more severe.

Associated Anomalies

The overall incidence of congenital defects associated with EA is between 50% and 70% [2•] (Table 144-1). The most common associated anomalies are cardiac (30%; patent ductus arteriosus, ventricular septal defect, and atrial septal defect being most common) and gastrointestinal (12%; especially imperforate anus, duodenal atresia, annular pancreas, and pyloric stenosis). Every newborn with imperforate anus should be evaluated for EA, and vice versa. Infants with VACTERL anomalies are increasing in incidence (25% to 30% of all cases of EA).

Diagnosis and Clinical Findings

Polyhydramnios is seen in EA with distal TEF but is more common in pure EA without distal fistula. Infants with EA tend to drool soon after birth and accumulate an excessive amount of secretions in their posterior pharynx, resulting in early onset of choking, coughing, and cyanosis.

The simplest way to rule out EA is to pass a nasogastric tube very carefully and gently through the mouth or nose into the

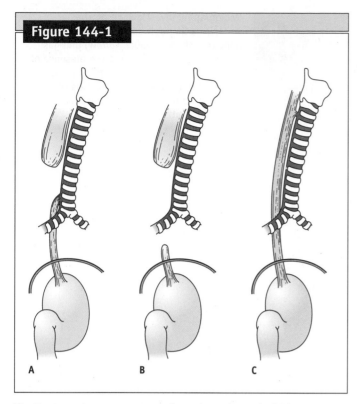

Figure 144-1

The three most common types of esophageal atresia (EA).
A, Proximal atresia and distal tracheoesophageal fistula (TEF).
B, Esophageal atresia without fistula. **C**, Tracheoesophageal fistula without esophageal atresia.

Table 144-1. Incidence of Associated Anomalies	
Type	**Incidence, %**
Cardiovascular	35
Gastrointestinal	15
Neurologic	5
Genitourinary	5
Skeletal	2
VACTERL	25
Overall Incidence	50–70

VACTERL—vertebral, anal, cardiac, tracheal, esophageal, renal, and limb syndrome.

stomach. If the tube meets with obstruction, a plane radiograph in the frontal and lateral projections (Fig. 144-2*A*) is taken to document atresia. Contrast studies can then be performed to confirm the diagnosis. Thin barium (0.5 to 1.0 mL) infused through the tube into the upper pouch outlines an upper esophageal pouch with a blind ending (Fig. 144-2*B*). Thin barium is preferred over Hypaque because it is less irritating to the lungs if aspirated. This type of contrast study, along with preoperative bronchoscopy and esophagoscopy, is helpful in ruling out a proximal fistula. If air is present in the gastrointestinal tract on the abdominal portion of the film, a distal fistula is present. A gasless abdomen confirms the diagnosis of EA without TEF (Fig. 144-3).

Preoperative Treatment

Pneumonitis resulting from both aspiration of pharyngeal contents and reflux of gastric juice into the tracheobronchial tree must be treated vigorously before surgery. Further aspiration and reflux are prevented by elevating the infant, and any pneumonitis is treated by placing a sump catheter into the upper pouch. A gastrostomy can be performed if necessary, but in most cases gastrostomy is not done. The infant also is placed on broad-spectrum antibiotic coverage.

Operative Treatment

The goal of surgery is to correct the anomaly completely with one operation. The procedure includes division of the TEF and primary repair of the EA. Modern survival data reflect the birth weight of the infant and the presence or absence of major cardiac anomalies [3•].

Postoperative Complications

There are three types of complications related to the esophageal anastomosis: leak, stricture, and recurrent fistula. The incidence of leaks ranges from 5% to 10%, depending on the type of anastomosis and the degree of tension at the anastomosis. Virtually all leaks managed with parenteral nutrition (NPO) close spontaneously within 1 to 3 weeks. One exception is an anastomotic disruption. The rate of stricture—defined as narrowing requiring at least two dilatations—is between 10% and 15%. Most strictures respond to periodic dilatations every 3 to 6 weeks over a period of 3 to 6 months. Those that do not respond to this conservative approach usually are associated with severe gastroesophageal reflux. The frequency of recurrent TEF ranges from 5% to 10%. Most recurrent fistulas are the result of leak, recognized or unrecognized, and do not close spontaneously. Occasionally, a very small recurrent TEF closes spontaneously within 3 to 4 weeks. If the recurrent TEF is still present after 4 weeks, however, surgery usually is required. Recurrent fistulas are difficult to repair and are associated with a further recurrence of 20%. It is critical that tissue such as pleura, muscle, or pericardium be placed between the esophageal and tracheal suture lines during the repair [4].

Two other significant postoperative complications are gastroesophageal reflux (GER) and tracheomalacia. The incidence of GER observed in various series ranges from 20% to 40% and is probably secondary to extensive mobilization of the distal esophagus. It often can be treated with simple medical maneuvers, including upright thickened feedings, prokinetic agents, and H$_2$-blockers. Between 30% and 50% of infants, however, continue to have significant reflux, leading to a recurrent anastomotic stricture that is resistant to dilatation. In this group of infants, fundoplication is often necessary. However, the Nissen fundoplication, which involves a 360° wrap, may obstruct the esophagus (no matter how loosely it is made) because of the esophageal dysmotility present in these children [5]. We prefer, therefore, to use an anterior, 230° to 270° fundoplication (Thal), which is not obstructing [6,7].

Severe tracheomalacia has been reported as a complication not of the repair but of the EA itself. Symptomatic tracheomalacia has been reported in up to 25% of patients with EA and TEF. The diagnosis of tracheomalacia is best made at bronchoscopy, where the typical finding is the "fishmouthing" or

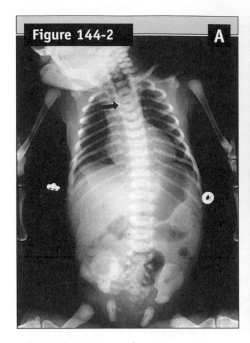
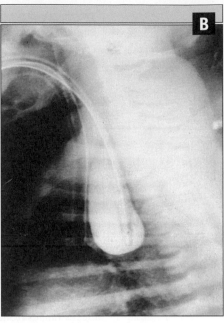

Radiographic investigation of atresia.
A, Plain radiograph demonstrates a blind upper esophageal pouch (*arrow*) and gas in the abdomen, indicating the presence of a proximal EA (esophageal atresia) and a distal TEF (tracheoesophageal fistula). **B,** The blind upper pouch is outlined by 0.5 to 1 mL of thin barium.

collapsing of the trachea during inspiration at the level of the aortic arch. This diagnostic finding is subtle and requires an experienced endoscopist. Most infants with tracheomalacia improve with time; however, a small percentage develop chronic severe respiratory difficulty, which can result in respiratory arrest and death. Aortopexy, a procedure in which the transverse aorta is sutured to the undersurface of the sternum, has been successful in treating most of these patients by suspending the trachea open. Pediatric surgeons reserve aortopexy for those infants who cannot be extubated or who have suffered a well-documented respiratory arrest. More recently, intratracheal stents have been used for severe tracheomalacia.

Results

The vast majority of children born with EA and TEF can look forward to survival with a normal quality of life. The overall survival rate ranges between 90% and 95%. For those in the good-risk categories, survival is close to 100%.

Changing referral patterns in most parts of the Western world have led to an increased proportion of neonates with severe associated congenital anomalies or significant prematurity undergoing treatment at referral institutions. In spite of the increasing number of severely affected infants being treated, operative mortality has continued to decline in recent years. Continued advances in the perioperative intensive care management of high-risk neonates account for much of this decrease in operative mortality.

ISOLATED ESOPHAGEAL ATRESIA

Neonates with isolated EA represent 5% to 7% of patients with the anomaly and present with a clinical picture similar to that seen in infants with EA and distal TEF [8–13]. The main differences are that infants with EA only have less severe pneumonitis and do not have abdominal distention because there is no TEF. Diagnosis is usually made early in the neonatal period, as with EA and distal TEF, because of excessive drooling and the discovery that a nasogastric tube cannot be inserted into the stomach.

Diagnosis

The diagnosis of isolated EA is suggested when the previously described clinical signs and symptoms are associated with a gasless abdomen on an abdominal radiograph (Fig. 144-3). The diagnosis is confirmed with a contrast study of the upper blind pouch, which also rules out a proximal TEF. The frequency and distribution of associated anomalies are the same as seen in the more common form of EA and distal TEF.

Treatment

Suction of the upper pouch must be initiated immediately to prevent aspiration. Operative gastrostomy (not a percutaneous gastrostomy) is mandatory (as opposed to EA and distal TEF) and can be carried out during the first 24 to 48 hours of life. Gastrostomy can be problematic because the stomach is always small and is easily confused with the transverse colon. In addition, gastrostomy placement can be technically difficult because of the small size of the stomach. Once the gastrostomy is in place, feedings are begun to provide nutritional support and to allow enlargement of the stomach so that it can be used for the later definitive repair.

During the first 3 to 6 weeks, while gastrostomy feedings are proceeding, the upper pouch (and sometimes the lower one) is stretched once or twice daily to elongate the esophageal segments. Most surgeons believe the lower segment cannot be adequately stretched and thus do not bother with stretching the lower pouch. The upper pouch is usually stretched with a mercury bougie. This technique results in 2 to 4 cm of additional length. Some surgeons believe that the stretching is irrelevant and that the esophagus grows faster than the thoracic cavity, resulting in a reduction in the gap between the two esophageal ends. Stretching of the upper pouch is done for 8 to 12 weeks.

Once it is deemed that maximal length has been achieved with stretching, the anastomosis is usually done, but it is under significant tension despite the use of myotomies. Other options for accomplishing a difficult anastomosis are to take an anterior flap from the upper pouch [14] or use a Collis gastroplasty

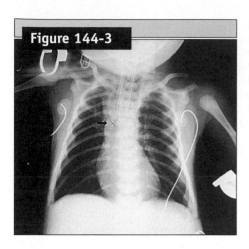

Gasless abdomen confirms the diagnosis of isolated esophageal atresia. The arrow points to the blind upper pouch.

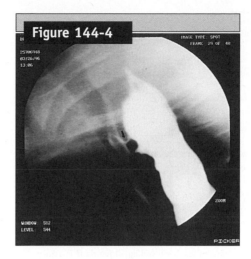

Isolated tracheoesophageal fistula (*arrow*). No esophageal atresia is present.

[15]. It is far better to preserve the esophagus and tolerate an anastomotic leak, stricture, or both than to resort to esophageal replacement. If the anastomosis is impossible (*ie*, presence of a gap >4 cm between the two esophageal segments after all of the maneuvers described have been done), two options are available. The first, more traditional, approach is to perform a cervical esophagostomy (preferably on the left side to make esophageal replacement at a later date easier) and then to perform an esophageal replacement with colon or stomach at 6 months to 1 year of age. More recently, some centers have elected to try an esophageal replacement (usually with a gastric transposition) at the time of the initial thoracotomy.

Postoperative Care

All patients have significant GER if a primary esophagoesophagostomy has been done because of the significant mobilization of the distal esophageal segment. GER can result in pulmonary aspiration and anastomotic stricture and can also compromise nutrition.

If a cervical esophagostomy has been done, local skin irritation can be a significant problem. It can best be managed with a collecting device or placement of A and D ointment around the stoma. If an esophageal placement has been done at the time of initial thoracotomy (and especially if a gastric transposition has been used), there is no gastrostomy, and feedings initially have to be administered through an oro- or nasogastric tube or through a feeding jejunostomy.

Complications

Esophageal anastomotic leaks are managed conservatively, as described in the section on EA and distal TEF. Strictures are likewise managed as described in the previous section except in these cases they are probably universally aggravated by GER.

Results

The results of esophagoesophagostomy are not as good as those seen in EA with distal TEF because of the higher incidence of leak, stricture, and GER. Mortality is essentially the same and is related to the associated severe cardiac anomalies.

◼ ISOLATED TRACHEOESOPHAGEAL FISTULA

Isolated TEF accounts for 2% to 6% of all cases [16]. The clinical findings in this group of infants are quite different from those in other forms of this anomaly in which EA is present. Patients usually present in the first few months of life, rather than in the newborn period, with a history of choking and coughing with feeding. These findings often are disregarded initially as being due to GER or formula intolerance. A high index of suspicion is necessary to make the diagnosis. Continual contamination of the tracheobronchial tree often results in chronic pneumonia with failure to thrive.

Diagnosis

Isolated TEF usually can be diagnosed with a barium esophagogram using thin barium (Fig. 144-4). Visualization of the fistula is aided by passing a Foley catheter into the distal esophagus and inflating the balloon to create distal obstruction. Before making a radiologic diagnosis, it is very important to exclude the possibility of aspiration of barium into the tracheobronchial tree.

If the diagnosis cannot be made radiologically, then simultaneous bronchoscopy and esophagoscopy under general anesthesia are required. If double endoscopy does not reveal the fistula, dilute methylene blue can be injected into the bronchoscope or endotracheal tube and visualized dripping out of the fistula via esophagoscopy.

Treatment

All of these fistulas are located at the junction of the cervical and thoracic trachea and join the esophagus a little more cephalad, thus forming an "N" rather than the classic "H." The results of fistula repair are excellent. Postoperative care is routine. Antibiotics are discontinued after 24 hours, and feedings are restarted after 48 hours.

Results and Complications

The results are excellent, with normal swallowing and freedom from pneumonia in almost all cases. Recurrent fistulas are extremely rare, much rarer than in cases of EA with distal TEF. If the operation is done through a left cervical incision, injury to the thoracic duct can occur, manifested either as a lymph leak in the neck with a persistent lymphocele or as lymphatic obstruction from ligation of the duct with the development of chylothorax.

REFERENCES

Recently published papers of particular interest have been highlighted as follows:

• Of interest
•• Of outstanding interest

1. Skandalakis JE, Gray SW: *Embryology for Surgeons*, edn 2. Baltimore: Williams & Wilkins; 1994.

2.• Spitz L: Esophageal atresia: past, present, and future. *J Ped Surg* 1996, 31:19–25.
This is an updated review of the experience at the Hospital for Sick Children, Great Ormond Street, London. The article also provides an extensive history of this anomaly.

3.• Spitz L, Kiely EM, Morecroft JA, Drake DP: Esophageal atresia: at-risk groups for the 1990's. *J Ped Surg* 1994, 29:723–725.
This article describes the new risk groups for survival.

4. Wheatley MJ, Coran AG: Pericardial flap interposition for the definitive management of recurrent tracheoesophageal fistula. *J Ped Surg* 1992, 27:1122–1126.

5. Wheatley MJ, Coran AG, Wesley JR: The efficacy of the Nissen fundoplication in the management of gastroesophageal reflux following esophageal atresia repair. *J Ped Surg* 1993, 28:53–55.

6. Kazerooni N, VanCamp JM, Hirschl RB, *et al.:* Fundoplication in 160 children less than 2 years of age. *J Ped Surg* 1994, 29:677–681.

7. Bliss D, Hirschl RB, Oldham KT, *et al.:* Efficacy of the anterior gastric fundoplication in the treatment of gastroesophageal reflux in infants and children. *J Ped Surg* 1994, 29:1071–1075.

8. Ein SH, Shandling D: Pure esophageal atresia: a 50-year review. *J Ped Surg* 1994, 29:1208–1211.

9. Spitz L, Kiely EM, Drake DP, Pierro A: Long-gap esophageal atresia. *Ped Surg Int* 1996, 11:462–465.

10. Lindahl H, Rintala R: Long-term complications in cases of isolated esophageal atresia treated with esophageal anastomosis. *J Ped Surg* 1995, 30:1222–1223.

11. Rescorla FJ, West KW, Sherer LR, Grosfeld JL: The complex nature of type A (long-gap) esophageal atresia. *Surgery* 1994, 116:658–664.

12. Coran AG: Long-gap esophageal atresia: how long is long? *Ann Thorac Surg* 1994, 57:528–529.

13. Boyle EM, Irwin ED, Foker JE: Primary repair of ultra-long-gap esophageal atresia: results without a lengthening procedure. *Ann Thorac Surg* 1994, 57:576–579.

14. Brown AK, Glugh MH, Nicholls SG, Tam PKH: Anterior flap repair of esophageal atresia: a 16-year evaluation. *Ped Surg Int* 1995, 10:525–528.

15. Evans M: Application of Collis gastroplasty to the management of esophageal atresia. *J Ped Surg* 1995, 30:1232–1235.

16. Crabb ED, Kiely EM, Drake DP, Spitz L: Management of isolated congenital tracheo-esophageal fistula. *Eur J Ped Surg* 1996, 6:67–69.

145 Gastroesophageal Reflux in Infants and Children

Vasundhara Tolia

Transient backflow of gastric contents into the esophagus is called gastroesophageal reflux (GER). It is a normal physiologic event in children of all ages and is usually of little clinical significance. GER is common in infancy and is manifested by spitting following feedings and during burping. However, when reflux occurs excessively often, or in large volumes, and the patient experiences discomfort with subsequent irritability and poor feeding, GER is of greater concern to the family and the physician. This chapter reviews the pathophysiology, spectrum of clinical presentation, differential diagnosis, diagnostic evaluation, and management of GER in infancy and childhood.

ANATOMY AND PHYSIOLOGY OF THE GASTROESOPHAGEAL JUNCTION

The intrinsic and extrinsic factors that constitute the natural barrier mechanisms to reflux in children are essentially the same as those in adults [1,2]. Crying and other infant behaviors that increase intra-abdominal pressure do not overwhelm the antireflux barrier because of the intra-abdominal position of the distal esophagus.

Physiologic reflux that occurs in the postprandial state is normally cleared by secondary peristalsis, gravity, and salivation.

PATHOPHYSIOLOGY

Symptomatic GER in children is caused primarily by transient lower esophageal sphincter (LES) relaxation, which occurs asynchronously with swallowing, resulting in equalization of pressures in the stomach and esophagus. This equalization creates a common cavity across the hollow viscera, thereby facilitating GER. Increased intragastric pressure that overwhelms the LES may occur as a result of delayed gastric emptying, leading to persistent gastric distention. Finally, diminished LES pressure can also cause GER. The presence of a hiatal hernia may weaken the antireflux barrier [3], as can a number of medications, hormones, and dietary constituents, which can decrease the LES pressure. Recent studies have also demonstrated that psychological stress may influence the LES pressure and esophageal peristalsis [4]. Most episodes of GER are cleared as previously described. However, the degree of reflux, the volume and nature of the refluxate, the duration of acid exposure within the esophagus, and the ability of the esophagus to clear its contents determine the extent and degree of mucosal injury from the refluxate. The mechanism of GER in healthy, thriving infants who regurgitate postprandially is different. Reflux most commonly occurs synchronously with swallowing; however, the LES relaxation persists for a longer period of time than in infants who do not have GER [5]. Low basal LES pressures are seen only in the presence of severe esophagitis or neurologic disorders. Coordination and maturation of both esophageal motility and LES pressure is important during maturation of the upper gastrointestinal tract, as observed by studies in preterm [6] and term infants [7]. This maturation is related more to postnatal age than to weight or other factors.

EPIDEMIOLOGY

During the past two decades, GER has been diagnosed more frequently in infants and children because of an increased awareness of the condition and also because of the more sophisticated diagnostic techniques that have been developed for identifying and quantifying the disorder. Estimates of the prevalence of GER in normal infants in the first 6 months of life as reflected by regurgitation range from 18% to 50%. Physiologic GER occurs less often in healthy breast-fed newborns than in formula-fed babies. There are no data regarding sex or ethnicity variations. Furthermore, the prevalence of pathologic GER in infancy has yet to be defined accurately because there are no standardized criteria for defining, diagnosing, or quantifying reflux in this age group. The prevalence of nonregurgitant reflux also remains uncertain. Spontaneous improvement with ultimate resolution of GER eventually occurs towards the end of the first year. The natural history of GER as diagnosed with esophageal pH monitoring on formula feeding was retrospectively reviewed in 456 infants at Children's Hospital of Michigan to evaluate their management and outcome. All these infants were <1 year of age at presentation with one or more of these symptoms: regurgitation, choking, irritability, failure to thrive, acute life threatening episodes, feeding difficulties, and/or hematemesis. Pathologic GER was detected in 243 infants. A prokinetic agent, cisapride or metoclopramide was used in 228 infants. Additional acid suppression was necessary in 57 of these patients. The mean time of resolution from the time of diagnosis was 6.91 months in 158 infants, 38 infants had ongoing but controlled symptoms on treatment, 2 required surgery and the rest were lost to follow-up. Of the 213 infants with normal esophageal pH monitoring, 174 had resolution of symptoms in a mean period of 1.93 months. Recently, the prevalence of the frequency of regurgitation and its resolution in 948 normal, term infants <13 months of age was also reported [8]. This prospective study included a white, nonhispanic population from suburban pediatric practices in Illinois. The parents completed a GER questionnaire. It was noted that the symptoms of spitting peaked at 4 months in 67% of infants and was resolved by 7 months in a majority of infants. It should be noted that the reported treatments included a formula change in 8.1%, thickening of feedings in 2.2%, termination of nursing in 1.1% and medication in 0.2% of patients. None of these infants were referred to subspecialists. A study of GER in normal children older than 3 years suggests that they require chronic medical therapy and that they have a less favorable prognosis than do otherwise normal infants with GER [9]. Nonregurgitant reflux may be a significant etiologic factor in conditions such as recurrent sinusitis and otitis media as well as in laryngotracheobronchial diseases.

A variety of conditions predispose children to pathologic GER (Table 145-1). Neurologically impaired children are at increased risk for severe GER, esophagitis, and Barrett's esoph-

agus. Many of these children also have autonomic neuropathy, which leads to prolonged esophagogastric transit and delayed gastric emptying [10].

CLINICAL MANIFESTATIONS

The spectrum of clinical manifestations of GER in children of all ages is diverse (Table 145-2). GER has a different course and prognosis depending on the child's age, the clinical presentation, and the presence of complications [11].

Effortless regurgitation is the hallmark of GER in an otherwise healthy infant. Reflux may cause projectile vomiting, but the baby does not appear to be in distress and often smiles immediately afterward, in contrast to babies of the same age whose vomiting is caused by pyloric stenosis. The emesis seen in pyloric stenosis is not only projectile but also effortful.

During the first several months of life, most infants vomit or spit up small amounts of formula or breast milk shortly after feedings. This spitting up is associated with burping, crying, or a Valsalva movement. Air swallowing may exaggerate the spitting. GER in early infancy initially must be regarded as physiologic, unless the baby exhibits irritability, difficulty with feedings, or both. The introduction of solid feedings and the assumption of a more upright posture after about 6 months of age may result in a decreased frequency of regurgitation. Reflux may be precipitated or exacerbated by intercurrent illnesses and may persist for days after the acute insult. However, infants with physiologic reflux continue to thrive, and extensive evaluation and aggressive pharmacologic intervention should not be instituted once the association is appreciated.

Pathologic manifestations of GER can be broadly classified as regurgitant or nonregurgitant. Is the baby spitting up or vomiting, or is the refluxate flowing only partially retrograde up the esophagus and then back into the stomach? In babies, postprandial regurgitation or vomiting becomes more problematic between 4 and 8 weeks of age as the volume of feedings is increased. With more persistent and chronic GER, the infant becomes irritable and often inconsolable. Feeding may be fraught with fussing and refusal to feed. GER may also cause what appears to be a neuropsychiatric disturbance, with arching, stiffening, and torticollis (ie, Sandifer syndrome). Sleep may be interrupted, and the baby appears uncomfortable. Such symptoms suggest esophagitis. Failure to thrive, bleeding, or anemia from chronic blood loss may ensue. On occasion, an infant may present with symptoms of colic

Table 145-1. Conditions Predisposing to Pathologic Gastroesophageal Reflux
Tracheoesophageal fistula (post repair)
Neurologic impairment
Chronic respiratory conditions
Asthma
Cystic fibrosis
Bronchopulmonary dysplasia
Hiatal hernia
Orthopedic abnormalities, *eg,* kyphoscoliosis

without significant regurgitation. In older children, esophagitis is almost always manifested by odynophagia. Dysphagia is also commonly associated with esophagitis without stricture, probably from dysmotility. Heartburn, chest pain, pyrosis, water brash, and hematemesis also may be present, as in adults.

The spectrum of nonregurgitant manifestations of GER is diverse (Table 145-2). GER may contribute significantly to hoarseness, stridor, wheezing, recurrent pneumonia, and apparent life-threatening events (ALTE). Considerable controversy surrounds the association between GER and respiratory diseases, especially ALTE. Up to 75% of affected infants with such life-threatening events may have pathologic GER. Reflux is more likely to be the cause of such an event if it occurs when the infant is awake or within 2 hours of a feeding. It is crucial to note that the presence of vomiting is a poor indicator of pathologic reflux. A better indicator is quantification of the mean duration of reflux episodes during sleep. In reflux-induced respiratory symptoms, the mean duration of reflux episodes usually is more than 4 minutes.

GER also aggravates the symptoms of diseases such as cystic fibrosis, asthma, bronchopulmonary dysplasia (BPD), and trachoesophageal fistula after repair.

◼ DIFFERENTIAL DIAGNOSIS

A wide range of conditions must be considered in the differential diagnosis of GER (Table 145-3). Regurgitant manifestations of GER must be differentiated from gastric outlet obstruction, acid-peptic disease, food allergy or intolerance, malrotation, cyclic vomiting, and central nervous system lesions. Infants with intractable vomiting should also be evaluated for immunologic, neurologic, metabolic, and renal disor-

Table 145-2. Spectrum of Pediatric Manifestations of Gastroesophageal Reflux

Physiologic	Pathologic
Regurgitation only	Esophagogastric symptoms and signs
	Persistent irritability
	Feeding problems (failure to thrive)
	Arching, torticollis (Sandifer syndrome)
	Rumination with destruction of dental enamel and caries
	Odynophagia
	Dysphagia
	Water brash
	Salivation/spitting
	Hematemesis/melena
	Protein-losing enteropathy
	ENT
	Stridor, hoarseness, recurrent sinusitis, recurrent otitis media
	Pulmonary
	Aspiration, apnea/ALTE, chronic cough, refractory asthma
	Others
	Halitosis, hypertrophic osteoarthropathy

ALTE—apparent life-threatening events; ENT—ear, nose, throat.

Table 145-3. Differential Diagnosis of Gastroesophageal Reflux Symptoms

Gastrointestinal Manifestations	Pulmonary manifestations	Otolaryngologic manifestations	Neurobehavioral manifestations	Other manifestations
Spitting/vomiting	Chronic cough, wheezing, life-threatening events	Stridor, recurrent otitis media	Tics	Metabolic diseases
Achalasia	Reactive airway disease	Sandifer syndrome	Chromosomal disease
Pyloric stenosis	Apnea	Laryngomalacia		Sepsis (eg, urinary tract infection)
Malrotation	Foreign-body aspiration	Laryngeal webs	Seizures	
Dysmotility		Laryngeal stenosis	Toxins, medications	
Acid-peptic disorders		Infections	Congenital malformations of central nervous system	
Gastritis		Vascular rings		
Allergic gastroenteropathy			Neoplasms and other space-occupying lesions	
Disaccharide intolerance				
Psychogenic cause				
Bulimia				
Abdominal pain				
Acid peptic disease				
Gallbladder disease				
Colic				
Gastritis				
Hematemesis				
Acid peptic disease				
Mallory-Weiss tears				
Gastritis				
Esophageal varices				

ders and sepsis. With severe respiratory symptoms, vascular ring and foreign body aspiration should be considered.

DIAGNOSTIC EVALUATION OF PEDIATRIC GER

The diagnosis in infancy usually is suggested by the history and careful observation of the infant during and after a feeding. Having the caretaker feed the baby in the office is often revealing. One can observe whether the episode is effortless, whether the baby is irritable, and how the caretaker and the baby interact. A general physical examination is important to exclude other causes of vomiting, and stool should be checked for occult blood.

No single diagnostic test has emerged as the best way to evaluate the child with possible GER. Tests are best performed in a stepwise fashion as shown in Figure 145-1. Individualized planning of the order of investigations must be based on the individual patient's symptoms.

Esophageal pH Monitoring

Twenty-four-hour intraesophageal pH monitoring is usually the procedure of choice for the evaluation of GER in infants and is well tolerated. However, this test does have limitations. For instance, pH monitoring does not detect reflux for as long as 2 hours following the feeding of regular formula, which buffers gastric acid [12]. The advantages of pH monitoring are that it allows for evaluation in association with feedings, variations in position, and sleep–wake status, and for possible documentation of a temporal association between reflux episodes and symptoms or signs of respiratory distress. This latter correlation is best achieved by using half-strength apple juice (pH <4.0) to facilitate the observation of all reflux episodes; otherwise, neutral reflux episodes

would be missed. Normal values for differentiating between physiologic and pathologic GER for different age groups are available. Esophageal clearance also can be determined by measuring the number of episodes of reflux that are longer than 5 minutes in duration and by determining the duration of the longest episode. A wide variety of methods, guidelines, and feedings have been used in different studies. A reflux index is defined as the percentage of time the esophageal pH is less than 4.0 for the total duration of the test. Two of the more commonly used criteria for diagnosing pathologic GER include a reflux index of >5% of the duration of the test with formula feeding, or a Euler and Byrne score of $x + 4y \geq 50$ (where x = total number of reflux episodes, and y = number of episodes lasting >5 minutes). Guidelines for pH monitoring in children have been published [13].

Radiologic and Radionuclide Tracer Studies

The barium study and gastroesophageal scintigraphy are the tests most commonly chosen from the different radiologic modalities available for evaluating patients with GER.

Barium Esophagram

The purpose of a barium esophagram is to exclude structural abnormalities that may present as or be associated with GER-type symptoms and to enable assessment of esophageal motility and swallowing. However, the esophagram should not be considered a means of determining whether a child has or does not have gastroesophageal reflux. False-positive and false-negative results are common, and there is no clear distinction between normal and abnormal amounts of barium refluxate. There are also no studies correlating the level to which barium refluxes in the esophagus with the severity of symptoms, results

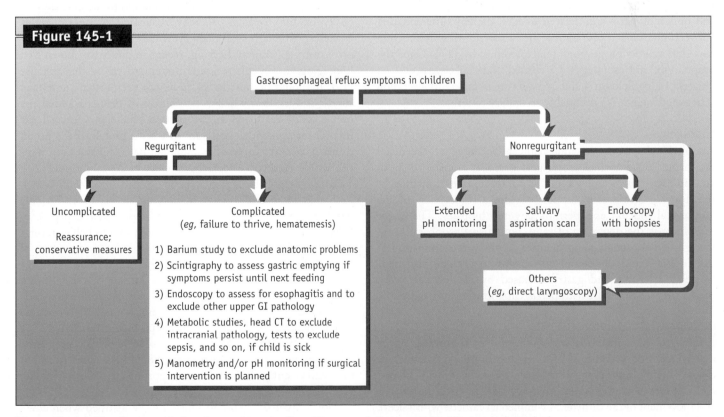

Figure 145-1

Diagnostic algorithm for suspected gastroesophageal reflux. CT—computed tomography; GI—gastrointestinal.

of pH monitoring, or the response to treatment [14•]. Detection of the presence of GER radiographically is of no help in determining whether the GER is primary or secondary unless the radiologist ensures evaluation of the gastric outlet and the position of the ligament of Treitz. As an example, it is well known that babies with pyloric stenosis and gastric outlet obstruction may also have significant gastroesophageal reflux. This reflux may not remit after a successful pyloromyotomy. The process of "spitting" by a baby at the time of a barium esophagram is usually interpreted by the radiologist as severe reflux. This interpretation should be discouraged, because it may be misleading and in itself result in further unnecessary studies, medical interventions, or both.

Gastroesophageal Scintigraphy

The normal scintigraphic range of values to differentiate physiologic from pathologic GER has not been established for different pediatric age groups. The presence or absence of GER as shown by scintigraphy does not correlate with pathologic GER as diagnosed by extended pH monitoring, even when the two studies are performed simultaneously [12]. Alternatively, scintigraphy may be helpful in evaluating gastric emptying, non-acidic reflux, and pulmonary aspiration. Calculation of gastric emptying at 1 hour is adequate with the usual infant formula, and routine delayed images are not recommended [15•]. By obtaining scintigraphic images of the lungs 4 to 6 hours later, one may also detect whether the infant has aspirated as a result of gastroesophageal reflux [16].

Radionuclide Salivagram

The salivagram test is performed by placing a small amount of technetium Tc 99m sulfur colloid on the tip of the infant's tongue and obtaining early and delayed images, thereby differentiating between pulmonary aspiration related to swallowing dysfunction and that caused by gastroesophageal reflux by [17]. Once the oropharynx and esophagus are cleared of radioactivity, delayed images of lung fields at 4 and 24 hours are obtained. If aspiration is detected later, it is presumably secondary to reflux.

Endoscopy

An obviously abnormal endoscopic appearance of the distal esophagus, or abnormal esophageal mucosal biopsies, or both are indicative of pathologic GER. Endoscopic examination of the upper gastrointestinal tract provides a direct view of the esophageal mucosa and permits targeted biopsies. The major advantage is the detection of mild, nonerosive esophagitis and low-grade endoscopic abnormalities. Moreover, examination of the stomach and duodenum also helps to exclude acid-peptic–related lesions and gastritis caused by *Helicobacter pylori*, which may also present with persistent vomiting in children.

Esophageal Manometry

Esophageal manometry is seldom helpful in the evaluation or management of pediatric GER. The test is poorly tolerated by awake infants, and even when they are sedated with chloral hydrate, infants and children invariably awaken with the passage and movement of the catheter. A commercial catheter with a sleeve within a sleeve is not routinely available for pediatric patients.

MANAGEMENT

Most infants with GER do not require medical intervention. Advice with regard to feeding techniques and attention to the infant's position after feedings and during sleep usually are adequate (Fig. 145-2). Several studies have demonstrated a decrease in GER when the infant is in a prone position so that the GE junction is on the same plane as the stomach air bubble. In this position the burp is more likely to be dry than wet. Although the prone sleeping position may diminish GER, this position has been suggested as a possible factor in sudden infant death syndrome (SIDS) [18] and probably should be avoided in the first 6 months of life, when SIDS usually occurs. The prone position also is not easy to maintain once the infant becomes more mobile.

Other factors that might lead to the exacerbation of GER must also be considered. Passive smoke inhalation should be avoided, and treatment with theophylline, caffeine and β-adrenergic-agonists, which may decrease lower esophageal sphincter pressure, should be used judiciously. Mechanical effects of chest physiotherapy may also induce GER through forced expiration and cough maneuvers, so such therapy is best performed during the fasting state after antacid treatment.

Dietary Therapy

Overfeeding should be avoided. A careful history is required to determine whether the frequency of feedings or the volume of feeding is excessive. An extremely wet diaper may be indicative of excessive liquid intake. Improper feeding practices are particularly common with first children and after a child has had significant diarrhea. In the latter situation, mothers fearful of dehydration often force-feed excessive volumes of liquid.

Thickening the feedings with cereal (from 1 teaspoon to 1 tablespoon per ounce of formula) is believed to increase the viscosity of the feedings, thereby reducing regurgitant reflux episodes. Although such maneuvers may decrease the frequency of overt spitting and crying, recent studies have shown that nonregurgitant occult reflux is not improved by this practice [19]. It should be noted that, although the protein content of cereals is very low, when 1 tablespoon of cereal is added per ounce of 24-cal formula, the protein intake may exceed the infant's recommended daily allowance for protein if the infant drinks 1 quart or more of formula per day. This does not happen with 1 teaspoon of cereal per ounce of 20-cal formula [20]. Various dietary manipulations are listed in Table 145-4. Although the use of a whey-hydrolysate or soy-based formula has been shown to promote gastric emptying, the degree of GER was not significantly different from that in babies receiving standard cow's milk–based formula [21•]. Modification of formula by replacing long chain with medium chain triglycerides has shown no improvement in the rate of GER during the first two postprandial hours [22]. In older children, avoidance of liquid or solid intake for several hours before bedtime may be helpful if GER is a nocturnal problem. Restricting fatty foods at dinnertime may alleviate problems of delayed gastric emptying, but severe fat restriction should be avoided so as not to inadvertently fall short of appropriate caloric intake. Avoidance of caffeine may be helpful.

Use of hypoallergenic formulas can be justified when cow's milk protein allergy presents as GER. GER may be associated

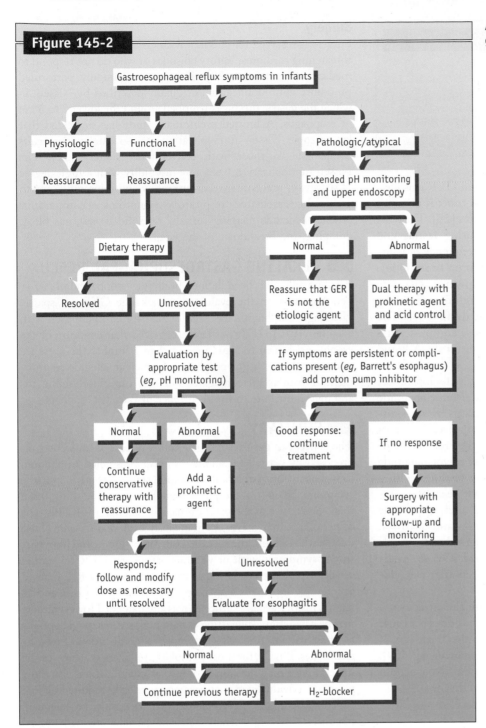

Figure 145-2

Algorithm for management of gastroesopageal reflux (GER) in infants.

with cow's milk protein allergy in up to 42% of infants under 1 year of age. There is a characteristic pattern of pH monitoring tracing that helps to distinguish between those infants who have GER with cow's milk protein allergy and those who have GER without it. In infants with cow's milk protein allergy, a constant, progressive, and persistent fall in esophageal pH to less than 4.0 is evident in the postprandial period, and persists until the next feeding, when the pH rises steeply [23•].

■ PHARMACOTHERAPY OF GER
Prokinetic Agents
Judicious use of medications is appropriate when nonmedical measures have failed. Prokinetic agents enhance the transit of

nutrients through the gastrointestinal tract. Unfortunately, there are few studies evaluating the use of these medications in children [24]. Currently, cisapride is the most commonly used prokinetic agent in children with GER. Cisapride is a far safer medication than metoclopramide, because the latter crosses the blood–brain barrier and may cause neurologic symptoms. Drugs that inhibit the hepatic cytochrome P450 system (eg, macrolide antibiotics and some antifungal agents) should not be used simultaneously with cisapride, because cardiac arrhythmias have been reported in children when they are used concomitantly with cisapride [25]. The primary practitioner and the patient's guardian should be advised of this potential problem. Although cisapride has been shown to

Table 145-4. Dietary Measures	
Nonspecific	**Specific**
Avoid overfeeding	Thicken formula
Give small, frequent feedings	Use formula with faster gastric emptying (whey hydroysate)
	Use hypoallergenic formula

lower the frequency and duration of prolonged GER episodes, as well as the total esophageal acid exposure time, it does not appear to modify the number of reflux episodes [26]. The beneficial effects of cisapride are consistent during fasting and sleep periods. Cisapride also decreases the frequency of vomiting in patients, including those with chronic bronchopulmonary diseases associated with GER. However, cisapride does not appear to improve the clearance of refluxate from the distal esophagus in patients with neurologic dysfunction. The recommended dosage is 0.2 to 0.3 mg/kg/dose administered 3 to 4 times each day 15 to 30 minutes before meals. A liquid preparation is available.

Despite the possible adverse side effects of metoclopramide, it is currently a second-line drug for GER. Metoclopramide may improve GER in preterm babies and infants by accelerating gastric emptying. Weight gain has been improved in infants older than 3 months of age with GER when they receive metoclopramide [27]. The recommended dosage of metoclopramide is 0.1 mg/kg orally 15 to 30 minutes before feedings, with a maximum daily dose of 0.5 mg/kg/d. Adverse reactions commonly associated with higher dosages of metoclopramide include drowsiness, restlessness, dry mouth, and diarrhea. Extrapyramidal side effects cause the most alarm but are usually reversible when the medication is stopped. Gynecomastia with galactorrhea has been reported in children after metoclopramide usage [28].

Although domperidone has the advantage that it does not readily enter the central nervous system and thus does not cause extrapyramidal side effects, its usefulness in the treatment of GER in pediatric patients has not been convincing [29]. Bethanechol is not commonly used in the pediatric population because of its limited spectrum of action and efficacy.

Acid Control

Gastric antacids and H_2-receptor blockers are used in infants and children with dyspepsia. Gastric antacids must be used frequently throughout the day to effect relief, and the timing of the doses is difficult because the baby's feeding and sleep patterns are unpredictable. Therefore, it is common for the primary practitioner to use ranitidine twice or three times per day in such situations. The recommended dosage, extrapolated from dosages used in adults, is 4 to 6 mg/kg/d in two or three divided doses. Liquid preparations of cimetidine (5 to 10 mg/kg/dose qid) and famotidine (0.6 mg/kg/d in two divided doses) are also available.

Omeprazole and lansoprazole are seldom used unless the patient has documented esophagitis (see Chapter 146).

Surgery

Surgery is reserved for children with GER who experience life-threatening cardiorespiratory episodes or who do not respond to medical management [30]. The most commonly performed procedure is fundoplication, originally described by Nissen, in which the gastric fundus is wrapped around the lower 2 to 3 cm of esophagus. A limited preliminary study has suggested that laparoscopic Nissen fundoplication is also safe, with results comparable to those with conventional surgery [31]. The Nissen fundoplication has a low morbidity with a high degree of success in preventing recurrent reflux and improving growth and reflux-associated respiratory symptoms. Postoperative problems include gagging (usually on solid foods), gas bloat, dumping, and breakdown of the wrap.

■ ALKALINE GASTROESOPHAGEAL REFLUX

Alkaline reflux has been defined by an intraesophageal pH >7.0. Pediatric data on the evaluation of alkaline GER are sparse. Histologic esophagitis has been demonstrated in children with alkaline GER [32]. It has been suggested that exposure of the esophageal lumen to a pH greater than 7 implies the presence of duodenal juice in the esophagus. In such an alkaline environment, trypsin and deconjugated bile salts can cause esophagitis and may contribute to the occurrence of Barrett's esophagus.

■ SUMMARY

The concept of gastroesophageal reflux disease as an iceberg, as proposed by Castell for adults, can also be applied to children [33]. The majority of infants with mild spitting or other sporadic symptoms belong to the physiologic group, and nothing more than reassurance of the parent is usually required [34]. This type of reflux usually resolves spontaneously by 1 year of age. Those infants who fall into the so-called functional group and have persistent symptoms with or without pathologic GER by studies usually experience resolution of their problems by 1 to 2 years of age. Simple explanation of the pathophysiology of GER and its natural history usually suffice to reassure parents. However, there may be a benefit in suggesting certain nonpharmacologic options for these patients, including appropriate modification of feeding techniques. Finally, for those pathologic refluxers at the tip of the iceberg, who may develop a variety of complications, carefully planned individualized management is usually required. These patients should be closely monitored to ensure an adequate response to medical therapy. Realistic expectations with regard to duration of therapy must be discussed with the family, especially for children with documented nocturnal reflux [35].

■ REFERENCES

Recently published papers of particular interest have been highlighted as follows:
• Of interest
•• Of outstanding interest

1. Glassman M, George D, Grill B: Gastroesophageal reflux in children. *Gastroenterol Clin North Am* 1995, 24:71–98.
2. Tovar JA, Arana J, Tapia I: Effects of sedation on motor function of the refluxing esophagus. *Pediatr Surg Int* 1990, 5:418–421.
3. Mittal RK, Balaban DH: The esophagogastric junction. *N Engl J Med* 1997, 336:924–932.

4. Mittal RK, Stewart WR, Ramahi M, *et al.*: The effect of psychological stress on the esophagogastric junction pressure and swallow-induced relaxation. *Gastroenterology* 1994, 106:1477–1484.

5. Mahoney MJ, Migliavacca M, Spitz K, Milla PJ: Motor disorders of the oesophagus in gastro-esophageal reflux. *Arch Dis Child* 1988, 63:1333–1338.

6. Newell SJ: The lower esophageal sphincter in the preterm infant. In *Disorders of Gastrointestinal Motility in Childhood.* Edited by Milla PJ. Chichester, UK: Wiley; 1988:39–50.

7. Boix-Oshoa J, Canals J: Maturation of the lower esophageal sphincter. *J Pediatr Surg* 1976, 11:749–756.

8. Nelson SP, Chen EH, Syntar GM, *et al.*: Prevalence of symptoms of gastroesophageal reflux during infancy. *Arch Pediatr Adolesc Med* 1997, 151:569–572.

9. Treem WR, Davis PM, Hyams JS: Gastroesophageal reflux in the older child: presentation, response to treatment and long-term follow-up. *Clin Pediatr* 1991, 30:435–440.

10. Cunningham K, Riddell P, Maddern R, *et al.*: Relationships between autonomic nerve dysfunction, gastric emptying, and esophageal transit in gastroesophageal reflux. *Gastroenterology* 1990, 98:A34–A40.

11. Sondheimer JM: Gastroesophageal reflux in children: clinical presentation and diagnostic evaluation. *Gastrointest Endosc Clin North Am* 1994, 4:55–74.

12. Tolia V, Kuhns L, Kauffman RE: Comparison of simultaneous 2-hour scintigraphy and pH monitoring in infants with gastroesophageal reflux. *Am J Gastroenterol* 1993, 88:661–664.

13. Colletti RB, Christie DL, Orenstein SR: Indications for pediatric esophageal pH monitoring. *J Pediatr Gastroenterol Nutr* 1995, 21:253–262.

14.• Johnston BT, Troshinski MB, Castell JA, Castell DO: Comparison of barium radiology with esophageal pH monitoring in the diagnosis of gastroesophageal reflux disease. *Am J Gastroenterol* 1996, 91:1185–1189.

15.• Tolia V, Kuhns L, Kauffman RE: Comparisons of gastric emptying of formulas at 1 and 2 hours following a feeding. *Pediatr Radiol* 1993, 23:26–28.

16. Boonyapara S, Alderson PA, Garfinkel DJ, *et al.*: Detection of pulmonary aspiration in infants and children with respiratory distress. Concise communication. *J Nucl Med* 1980, 21:314–318.

17. Heyman S, Respondek M: Detection of pulmonary aspiration in children by radionuclide "Salivagram." *J Nucl Med* 1989, 30:697–699.

18. Michell EA: Sleeping position of infants and the sudden infant death syndrome. *Acta Paediatr* 1993, 389–395.

19. Orenstein SR, Magill HL, Brooks P: Thickening of infant feedings for therapy of gastroesophageal reflux. *J Pediatr* 1987, 110:181–186.

20. Pennington JAT: Infant, junior and toddler foods. In *Food Values of Portions Commonly Used*, edn 15. Edited by Pennington JAT. New York: Harper and Row; 1989:121–122.

21.• Tolia V, Lin CH, Kuhns LR: Gastric emptying using three different formulas in infants with gastroesophageal reflux. *J Pediatr Gastroenterol Nutr* 1992, 15:297–301.

22. Sutphen JL, Dillard VL: Medium chain triglyceride in the therapy of gastroesophageal reflux. *J Pediatr Gastroenterol Nutr* 1992, 14:38–40.

23.• Cavataio F, Iacono G, Montatto G, et al: Gastroesophageal reflux associated with cow's milk allergy in infants: which diagnostic examinations are useful? *Am J Gastroenterol* 1996, 91:1215–1220.

24. Grill BB, Flores AE: Pharmacotherapy. In *Pediatric Gastrointestinal Motility Disorders*. Edited by Hyman PE, Di Lorenzo C. New York: Academy Professional Information Services; 1994:377–386.

25. Lewin MB, Bryant RM, Fenrich AL, *et al.*: Cisapride induced long QT internal. *J Pediatr* 1996, 128:279–281.

26. Cuchiara S: Cisapride therapy for gastrointestinal disease. *J Pediatr Gastroenterol Nutr* 1996, 22:259–269.

27. Tolia V, Calhoun J, Kuhns L, *et al*: Randomized, prospective double-blind trial of metclopramide and placebo for gastroesophageal reflux in infants. *J Pediatr* 1989, 115:141–145.

28. Madani S, Tolia V: Gynecomastia and galactorrhea with metoclopramide. *J Clin Gastroenterol* 1997, 24:79–81.

29. Bines JE, Quinlan JE, Treves S, *et al.*: Efficacy of domperidome in infants and children with gastroesophageal reflux. *J Pediatr Gastroenterol Nutr* 1992, 14:400–405.

30. Fonkalsrud E, Ament M: Gastroesophageal reflux in childhood. *Curr Probl Surg* 1996, 1:3–70.

31. Lloyd DM, Robertson GSM, Johnstone JMS: Laparoscopic Nissen fundoplication in children. *Surg Endosc* 1995, 9:781–785.

32. Malthaner RA, Newman, KD, Parry R, *et al.*: Alkaline gastroesophageal reflux in infants and children. *J Pediatr Surg* 1991, 26:986–991.

33. Castell DO: Introduction of pathophysiology of gastroesophageal reflux. In *Gastroesophageal Reflux Disease: Pathogenesis, Diagnosis, Therapy.* Edited by Castell DO, Wu WC, Ott DJ. Mount Kisco, NY: Future Publishing Co; 1985:3–9.

34. Vandenplas Y, Beili D, Benhamow PH, *et al.*: Current concepts and issues in the management of regurgitation in infants: a reappraisal. *Acta Pediatr* 1996, 85:531–534.

35. Tolia V: Evaluation and management of pediatric gastroesophageal reflux. *Family Practice Recertification* 1997, 19:35-58.

146 Esophagitis and Barrett's Esophagus in Children

Eric Hassall

ESOPHAGITIS

Gastroesophageal (GE) reflux is responsible for most cases of esophagitis in children. This chapter focuses on the special features of reflux esophagitis as they pertain to children. The section on esophagitis in adults (see Section 1) discusses entities other than reflux esophagitis [1].

Reflux Esophagitis

Pathophysiology

The specific mechanisms that lead to reflux esophagitis in children are similar to those in adults, *ie*, transient lower esophageal sphincter relaxations (TLESR), hypotonic lower esophageal sphincter (LES), poor esophageal clearance, hiatal hernia, and delayed gastric emptying [2].

Predisposing Conditions

Certain underlying disorders predispose children to pathologic GE reflux. These include neurologic impairment, repaired esophageal atresia, chronic lung disease (especially cystic fibrosis), and hiatal hernia (Table 146-1).

The term *neurologic impairment* refers to mental retardation or cerebral palsy (CP) of any cause, alone or as a feature of various syndromes. Disorders that cause neurologic impairment usually are congenital or genetic, or arise from perinatal asphyxia, head injury, or cerebral hypoxia. Whatever the etiology, children with neurologic impairment often have many factors predisposing to severe GE reflux, *eg*, esophageal dysmotility, poor esophageal acid clearance, gastroduodenal dysmotility, LES dysfunction, and hiatal hernia. They also may have kyphoscoliosis, muscle spasticity, and seizures, and may be nursed or fed in the recumbent position for prolonged periods. In addition, mental retardation, CP, or both conditions result in verbal or motor responses to esophageal symptoms or pain that are subtle, nonspecific, or absent. These factors contribute to the relative silence of GE reflux in this group, so that complications often have already developed before GE reflux is diagnosed.

Repaired esophageal atresia is another cause of GE reflux. Children with esophageal atresia have a congenitally abnormal (*ie*, dysmotile) esophagus. Although at birth surgical anastomosis establishes continuity of the esophagus, of necessity the esophagus is often shortened, and a hiatal hernia brought up. As a result, there are many factors that predispose these children to severe GE reflux [3].

Because of several pathogenetic mechanisms, including chronic cough, negative intrathoracic pressure, raised intra-abdominal pressure, LES dysfunction, and hiatal hernia, children with cystic fibrosis or other chronic lung diseases have a marked predilection for developing pathologic GE reflux [4]. Conversely, severe GE reflux may cause acute or chronic pulmonary disease or exacerbate existing disease [5•,6].

Hiatal hernia has long been ignored as a major factor predisposing to pathologic reflux in children. Although hiatal hernia often accompanies the disorders discussed earlier, on its own and in otherwise healthy children without underlying disease, it is a primary cause of pathologic GE reflux [7•].

Clinical Presentation

Older children (approximately 5 years or older) usually manifest GE reflux and esophagitis similarly to adults. Infants, in whom nonregurgitant GE reflux is much more common than is vomiting due to reflux, present with such symptoms and signs as failure to thrive, nonspecific "irritability" that often is worse postprandially, and anemia from chronic blood loss. Neurobehavioral symptoms or torticollis also may occur. In all of these circumstances, esophagitis is almost always present. Whereas recurrent vomiting may be a presenting symptom at all ages in children, frank hematemesis is less common. As in adults, children may present with peptic stricture. Silent or late presentation with complications of reflux is more common in

---

Table 146-1. Conditions Predisposing to Severe Gastroesophageal Reflux in Children

Neurologic impairment
  Intrauterine infection/hypoxemia
  Syndromes (Cornelia de Lange, Down, many others)
  Microcephaly
  Leukodystrophy/other progressive neurologic disorders
  Cerebral palsy/mental retardation of any cause
  Perinatal asphyxia
  Postmeningitis, postencephalitis
  Cerebral trauma/hypoxemia
Repaired esophageal atresia/tracheoesophageal fistula
Chronic lung disease
  Cystic fibrosis
  Bronchopulmonary dysplasia
  Asthma
Hiatal hernia
Miscellaneous
  Esophageal dysmotility
  Esophageal surgery, *eg*, resection of stricture

neurologically impaired children, in children with cystic fibrosis, and in children with nocturnal reflux [4,8].

Chest pain alone is an uncommon presentation of reflux esophagitis in children, and, unlike in adults, the differential diagnosis of reflux esophagitis in children hardly ever includes chest pain of cardiac origin. It does include other causes of esophagitis, *eg*, motility disorders of the esophagus, gastritis, peptic ulcer disease, and non-ulcer dyspepsia. Chest pain of musculoskeletal origin usually is differentiated by history and physical examination.

Diagnostic Studies

Upper gastrointestinal series. As in adults, barium esophagram testing is insensitive and nonspecific for diagnosing esophagitis. However, an upper GI series is essential to exclude intestinal malrotation or other anatomic abnormalities that can cause partial obstruction and recurrent vomiting, or GE reflux; it may reveal a hiatal hernia or esophageal stricture. Although it is important as a "road map," the presence or absence of contrast reflux on such a study usually is not helpful—reflux into the distal half of the esophagus may merely reflect physiologic reflux occurring at the time of the study, and even reflux occurring more proximally may merely reflect the child's anxiety. Conversely, absence of reflux on a barium study does not exclude pathologic reflux. Reflux to the level of the clavicles on fluoroscopy may be a clue that pathologic reflux is present, but it does not establish the diagnosis. Reflux with aspiration of contrast is significant. A small bowel study is seldom necessary in the evaluation of GE reflux, and malrotation or nonrotation of the small bowel usually can be determined by examination of contrast passage to the ligament of Treitz.

Upper gastrointestinal endoscopy with biopsies. As in adults, upper GI endoscopy usually is the definitive study to determine the presence of esophagitis or Barrett's esophagus (BE). Careful documentation of the locations of the lower esophageal sphincter (LES), diaphragmatic pinchcock and Z-line is important. Endoscopes with a biopsy channel smaller than 2.8 mm in diameter usually yield biopsies that are small, difficult to orient and mount properly, and that often have crush artifact, making meaningful interpretation difficult or impossible. Sedation or anesthesia should be adequate to allow safe passage of an endoscope of such a size that at least a 2.8-mm biopsy channel is present. Issues specific to the performance of safe, accurate GI endoscopy in children are addressed in other sources [9] and in Chapter 188. Biopsies should always be taken from the body of the esophagus, and from the gastric cardia, *ie*, at and immediately below the Z-line. Even in the presence of a normal endoscopy, the presence of carditis on biopsy may indicate the presence of reflux [10]; the differential diagnosis of carditis includes *Helicobacter pylori* in adults [11] and in children (Hassall and Dimmick, Unpublished data). Biopsies from the Z-line region also may reveal specialized intestinal metaplasia [10].

Erosive esophagitis occurs in children with severe, chronic GE reflux, especially in association with the predisposing conditions mentioned previously (see Table 146-1). Erosive esophagitis is uncommon in children younger than 4 to 6 months of age. In children, as in adults, histologic evidence of esophagitis usually is considerably more prevalent than is macroscopic erosive esophagitis, but there are several pitfalls in the use of esophageal body histology alone to diagnose and quantify reflux esophagitis [12]. For example, biopsies taken within 2 cm of the Z-line may show abnormalities even in asymptomatic healthy subjects, probably resulting from physiologic reflux; even in erosive esophagitis, biopsies may show severe, few, or no histologic changes, because esophagitis often is a patchy lesion. The changes produced by crush artifact from grasp biopsies, mounting techniques, and variations of interpretation by pathologists using differently weighted histologic criteria lead to findings that are not easily interpretable, and often are not even reproducible in the same patient.

As in adults, peptic strictures in children usually occur in the LES region. However, when they are associated with BE, they tend to occur in the mid- or proximal esophagus, often in the region of the proximally located Z-line [13•].

Treatment of Reflux Esophagitis

In nonerosive (*ie*, histologic only) reflux esophagitis, so-called "endoscopy-negative" esophagitis symptoms usually respond to "low-level" measures such as lifestyle changes and prokinetic drugs or H_2-receptor antagonists. Cessation of pharmacotherapy after a trial of treatment is important to determine whether esophagitis is transient, or whether it is chronic and relapsing, requiring long-term therapy. Erosive esophagitis usually is chronic and relapsing, with the risk of stricture formation, and usually requires "big league" therapy, *ie*, antireflux surgery or long-term proton pump inhibitor (PPI) use.

Recent studies have shown that healing of erosive esophagitis and maintenance of remission can be accomplished in children, as in adults, with PPI [14,15,16•]. Thus, effective and safe medical therapy in the form of long-term use of omeprazole is now a viable alternative to antireflux surgery for children. Although antireflux surgery may be the treatment of choice for documented GE reflux disease in selected patients, children often have undergone antireflux surgery without clearly documented indications. The perioperative morbidity, the failure rate of antireflux surgery, and even mortality are high in certain high-risk groups—ironically, in those children most at risk for severe reflux: those with neurologic impairment, repaired esophageal atresia, and chronic lung disease [7•].

Many factors must be considered in the choice of long-term therapy with PPIs or antireflux surgery [7•]. Cost is one of them. The high initial costs of antireflux surgery can be justified when there are no other ongoing costs for morbidity, further investigations, need for repeat operations, or the cost of repeated hospitalizations, in addition to the psychosocial costs of absences from school and family. These costs must be weighed against the substantial costs of using PPIs for long periods. A recent study in the United States [17] showed that even when antireflux surgery was performed laparoscopically, the costs of medical therapy were equal to those of surgery at 10 years postoperatively; thus, much hinges on maintenance of the long-term antireflux effect of surgery, *ie*, its long-term success. Most pediatric studies only offer data regarding short-term follow-up [7•]. A sobering study by Luostarinen *et al.* [18] found that antireflux surgery failed in at least 30% of adults followed for 20 years, and these adults did not have the same high-risk factors as do many children with GE reflux.

Children who should be considered for long-term or lifetime PPI therapy include those who have failed antireflux surgery or those who have a major risk factor for surgical failure, morbidity, or mortality.

Informed judgment as to appropriate therapy for a given child requires more data. For example, it is not known what degree or specific nature of neurologic impairment or chronic lung disease constitutes high risk for surgical failure; whether failed antireflux surgery places a child at risk for further surgical failure; whether upper GI motility studies might be predictive of surgical success or failure; and whether fundoplications in even low-risk children remain functional with time or inevitably require revision.

It is notable that although antireflux surgery has been performed in children for 30 years, an "ideal" operative approach for all has not been determined. Whereas the morbidity and failure rates of antireflux surgery are apparent in carefully performed studies reviewed in detail elsewhere [7•], some pediatric surgical reports provide a misleadingly favorable impression of outcomes [19,20].

Antireflux surgery should be reserved for children with complicated GE reflux disease who would otherwise require lifetime therapy and who have the greatest chance for operative success; those who are neurologically normal with no previous esophageal surgery for esophageal atresia; and those with normal esophageal motility. At present, for high-risk children, perhaps surgery should be reserved for documented failures of optimized medical treatment.

Many neurologically impaired children require gastrostomy tubes for feeding; in some such children, pathologic reflux develops after G-tube placement. This may occur, in part, because with a G-tube, the child begins to receive adequate volumes of nutrition and GE reflux is unmasked, and in part because G-tube placement may cause reflux by mechanical means, *eg*, change of the angle of His. Despite these potential mechanisms, only some children develop pathologic reflux. We do not advocate routine antireflux measures in children who have G-tube placement.

▇▇ BARRETT'S ESOPHAGUS

There are important differences between BE in children and in adults [13•]. It is much less prevalent in children than in adults, and in childhood BE there is a high prevalence of serious, underlying coexisting disorders [8]. An understanding of these issues may be helpful to the adult gastroenterologist who "inherits" adolescent or young adult patients with BE.

Definition

Because BE has neoplastic potential, the diagnosis calls for surveillance in childhood and beyond, and often has implications with respect to longevity, life insurance, and medical insurance. Accurate diagnosis is, therefore, important.

There is increasing agreement that the diagnosis of BE should be made only when specialized columnar epithelium is present in the tubular esophagus, *ie*, epithelium containing goblet cells that stain positive with Alcian blue pH 2.5. This

mucosa is preneoplastic, and surveillance endoscopy is indicated [13•]. In contrast, neither fundic nor cardiac mucosa has been shown to carry a risk of neoplastic progression. In many reports of BE in children, the diagnosis has been based solely on the presence of a "prominent" Z-line at endoscopy, or on the presence of only fundic or cardiac columnar epithelium in one, or perhaps two, biopsies reportedly taken from the tubular esophagus [8,13•]. In most pediatric reports, the locations of biopsy sites relative to the endoscopic landmarks of Z-line, top of gastric folds, and diaphragmatic pinchcock have not been documented. One may conclude from this, as well as from evidence presented elsewhere [13•], that the fundic or cardiac mucosa–containing biopsies have come from hiatal hernias or normal cardia, and that the diagnosis of BE often has been made erroneously in children.

Prevalence

The true prevalence of BE in children is unknown. However, its prevalence may be estimated from experiences at two children's hospitals. In unpublished data from British Columbia Children's Hospital in Vancouver, British Columbia, from 1985 to 1996, only seven children, for a prevalence of 0.02% of all pediatric upper GI endoscopies, were newly diagnosed as having BE (*ie*, with specialized metaplasia) during that period. The children's ages were 8 to 17 years, with a mean of 14 years. In that unit, it is routine at endoscopy to document esophagogastric landmarks and to take biopsies from the Z-line region and tubular esophagus, making it unlikely that BE would be missed. A study at the Boston Children's Hospital found only seven children with BE from 1982 through 1986, for a prevalence of 0.6% of all pediatric upper GI endoscopies [21]. The patient's ages ranged from 13 to 27 years, with a mean of 20 years, and all seven patients had severe neurologic diseases.

One major reason for the rarity of BE in children, as opposed to adults, is that it is an acquired disorder that results from prolonged exposure to severe GE reflux. The true prevalence of BE in childhood depends in part on the definition of "child," and also on the group under study.

Comorbidities

In children with BE, coexisting underlying systemic disorders (*ie*, comorbidities) have been reported in four categories—neurologic impairment, chronic lung disease (primarily cystic fibrosis), esophageal atresia, and malignancies treated with chemotherapy. In addition, there is a group of children with BE who are otherwise healthy, *ie*, without a significant underlying systemic disorder; they almost always have hiatal hernias.

Neurologic Impairment
The association between major underlying or systemic disorders in BE was first reported in adults [22]. Snyder and Goldman [21] subsequently drew attention to the presence of comorbidities in children and young adults with BE.

By far the most prevalent comorbidities are those in which significant neurologic impairment is present [8]. Factors that predispose children with neurologic impairment to severe GE reflux, discussed earlier in this chapter, also compound the often silent and late presentation of BE. Late presentation of BE is a problem at all ages, perhaps because Barrett's epithelium exhibits decreased esophageal pain sensitivity.

Chronic Lung Disease

Another major comorbidity with BE is chronic lung disease, specifically cystic fibrosis (CF). Reflux is silent in most CF patients. In some cases, GI symptoms are truly absent, whereas in others, symptoms may be ignored because of the plethora of other problems. Some children with CF consider upper GI symptoms such as heartburn, chest pain, and occasional vomiting to be part of CF, and, therefore, may not report them. This delays diagnosis, resulting in a presentation that includes complications of GE reflux.

Barrett's esophagus in association with cystic fibrosis was first described in detail in two children with CF in 1993 [4]. Given the high prevalence of pathologic reflux in CF patients, it is surprising that there had been no earlier description. The probable explanation for this is that, because of reluctance to perform endoscopy and multiple esophageal biopsies in these patients, clinicians have missed BE in children and young adults with CF. The presence of GE reflux is important in CF, because it is a major cause of added morbidity for these children. For example, children with CF and GE reflux present earlier, and spend 10 times more time in the hospital, than do CF patients without reflux [8]. However, effective antireflux treatment may lead to a dramatic improvement in pulmonary and gastrointestinal symptoms and to improved quality of life. BE carries its own morbidity and implications, but in CF its additional importance is that it is a marker for particularly severe reflux, which may exacerbate the nutritional and pulmonary problems of CF patients.

Esophageal Atresia

Patients with esophageal atresia are at high risk for complications of severe GE reflux and, therefore, are candidates for the development of BE. However, because of their surgically altered anatomy, the diagnosis of BE in these patients should be made only if landmarks are carefully documented and specialized mucosa is present. Thus far none of the patients with esophageal atresia reported in the literature have had specialized Barrett's epithelium [8]. Of the many patients with repaired esophageal atresia followed at our institution, only two have BE.

Chemotherapy for Malignancies

Barrett's esophagus has been reported in patients who received chemotherapy for leukemia, but the specialized mucosa with goblet cells was present in only a few adult cases. The putative mechanism is chemotherapy-induced severe mucositis, which, in a milieu of ongoing reflux caused by chemotherapy-induced chronic emesis, heals in the distal tubular esophagus by columnar metaplasia [23]. However, Peters *et al.* [24] found no increased prevalence of BE in patients treated with chemotherapy for testicular cancer or breast cancer. In addition, three children reported to have columnar metaplasia following chemotherapy did not have goblet cell metaplasia [25]. A prospective study of a large cohort of patients is needed to test the hypothesis that chemotherapy poses a substantially increased risk for the development of BE.

It is estimated that some 60% to 70% of children with BE have a significant comorbidity [8]. Those without a significant comorbidity are otherwise healthy children, usually with hiatal hernias or, perhaps, transient lower esophageal sphincter relaxations (TLESRs). In our experience, hiatal hernia is present in almost all children with BE, whether or not a comorbidity is present. In adults with BE, the main comorbidities reported are neurologic impairment, scleroderma, and Heller myotomy for achalasia, all conditions recognized to predispose to GE reflux and poor acid clearance. Other than neurologic impairment, these conditions were reported in small numbers, and appear to constitute a tiny fraction of cases of BE in adults [8].

Conclusions and Implications

Barrett's esophagus is much less prevalent in children than in adults. Children with BE have a high prevalence of serious underlying disorders. Associated comorbidities usually are congenital, genetic, or arise from perinatal asphyxia. These conditions may result in BE by causing severe, chronic GE reflux, which often is silent.

Adenocarcinoma occurs in children with BE [26], though rarely, and endoscopic surveillance is indicated [27]. Given the marked heterogeneity of associated comorbidities and the wide variation in longevity among affected children, surveillance should be on a case-by-case basis. Recognizing that certain children may have severe but silent reflux, endoscopy with biopsies is warranted in children at high risk.

Treatment

The treatment of erosive esophagitis in Barrett's mucosa is the same as that for erosive esophagitis, as discussed earlier in this chapter, *ie*, antireflux surgery or PPIs. Ulcers in Barrett's mucosa often require higher doses of PPIs and a longer duration of such therapy for healing, compared with peptic "squamous esophagitis" [16•]. The ideal treatment goal in BE is elimination of the risk of adenocarcinoma, which requires eradication of the Barrett's mucosa.

To date, there has not been a well-documented case of complete regression of BE after medical or surgical therapy [27]. Unfortunately, partial regression does not eliminate the risk of cancer.

Various therapies aimed at ablation of Barrett's mucosa are currently in trials in adults. These include ablation by a variety of techniques: laser, heater-probe, and photodynamic therapy. A combination of antireflux and ablative therapies is likely to be the future treatment for children with BE, but as yet, there is no defined role for these modalities in the absence of dysplasia.

▮ REFERENCES

Recently published papers of particular interest have been highlighted as follows:
*   Of interest
**   Of outstanding interest

1. Lewin KS, Riddell RH, Weinstein WM: Inflammatory disorders of the esophagus. In: *Gastrointestinal Pathology and Its Clinical Implications.* New York: Igaku-Shoin; 1992:401–439.

2. Orenstein SR: Gastroesophageal reflux. In: *Pediatric Gastrointestinal Disease: Pathophysiology, Diagnosis and Management.* Edited by Wyllie R, Hyams JS. Philadelphia: WB Saunders; 1993:337–369.

3. Langer JC: Neonatal surgery and the acute abdomen. In *Gastroenterology and Hepatology: The Comprehensive Visual Reference*, vol 4: *Pediatric GI Problems*. Edited by Hyman PE. Philadelphia: Current Medicine, 1997:3.1–3.21.

4. Hassall E, Israel DM, Davidson AGF, Wong LTK: Barrett's esophagus in children with cystic fibrosis: not a coincidental association. *Am J Gastroenterol* 1993, 88:1934–1938.

5.• Sontag S: Pulmonary complications of gastroesophageal reflux. In *The Esophagus*. Edited by Castell DO. Boston: Little, Brown and Co; 1995:555–570.
This report provides a review of the complex interrelationship between GE reflux and pulmonary disease, and a critical analysis of the reports of therapeutic interventions.

6. Orenstein SR, Orenstein DM: Gastroesophageal reflux and respiratory disease in children. *J Pediatr* 1988, 112:847–858.

7.• Hassall E: Wrap session: is the Nissen slipping? *Am J Gastroenterol* 1995, 90:1212–1220.
This article provides a critical review of the results of antireflux surgery in children and identification of risk factors for failure of surgery. The potential role of PPI therapy is discussed as an alternative to surgery in some children.

8. Hassall E: Co-morbidities in childhood Barrett's esophagus. *J Pediatr Gastroenterol Nutr* 1997, 25:255–260.

9. Hassall E: NASPGN Position Paper: requirements for training to ensure competence of endoscopists performing invasive procedures in children. *J Pediatr Gastroenterol Nutr* 1997, 24:345–347.

10. Riddell RH: The biopsy diagnosis of gastroesophageal reflux disease, "carditis", and Barrett's esophagus, and sequelae to therapy. *Am J Surg Pathol* 1996, 20:531–550.

11. Genta RM, Huberman RM, Graham DY: The gastric cardia in *Helicobacter pylori* infection. *Hum Pathol* 1994, 25:915–919.

12. Hassall E: Macroscopic vs microscopic diagnosis of esophagitis: erosions or eosinophils? *J Pediatr Gastroenterol Nutr* 1996, 22:321–325.

13.• Hassall E: Barrett's esophagus: new definitions and approaches in children. *J Pediatr Gastroenterol Nutr* 1993, 16:345–364.
This article offers a review of several aspects of Barrett's esophagus, including history, definition, morphology, and pathogenesis. The reports of BE in children are critically examined and proposals made for stringent diagnostic criteria, and an approach to treatment and surveillance.

14. Gunasekaran TS, Hassall E: Efficacy and safety of omeprazole for severe gastroesophageal reflux in children. *J Pediatr* 1993, 123:148–154.

15. Hassall E, Israel DM, Shepherd R, *et al.*: Omeprazole for chronic erosive esophagitis in children: a multicenter study of dose requirements for healing [abstract]. *Gastroenterology* 1997, 112:143.

16.• Israel DM, Hassall E: Omeprazole and other proton pump inhibitors: pharmacology, efficacy and safety, with special reference to use in children. *J Pediatric Gastroenterol Nutr*, in press.
This article provides a detailed review of omeprazole use, including recent pediatric efficacy, safety and dosing data, and methods of administration in children. Some data regarding lansoprazole and pantoprazole are mentioned, although there are few or no pediatric use data with these agents as yet.

17. Heudebert G, Marks R, Wilcox C, Centor R: Cost-effectiveness of omeprazole vs fundoplication in the long-term treatment of reflux esophagitis. *Gastroenterology* 1997, 112:1078–1086.

18. Luostarinen M, Isolauri J, Laitinen J, *et al.*: Fate of Nissen fundoplication after 20 years. *Gut* 1993, 34:1015–1020.

19. Fonkalsrud EW, Ashcraft KW, Coran AG, *et al.*: The surgical management of gastroesophageal reflux in children: a combined hospital study of 7467 patients. *Pediatrics* 1998, 101:419–422.

20. Hassall E: Antireflux surgery in children: time for a harder look. *Pediatrics* 1998, 101:467–468.

21. Snyder JD, Goldman H: Barrett's esophagus in children and young adults: frequent association with mental retardation. *Dig Dis Sci* 1990, 10:1185–1189.

22. Roberts IM, Curtis RL, Madara JL: Gastroesophageal reflux and Barrett's esophagus in developmentally disabled patients. *Am J Gastroenterol* 1986, 81:519–523.

23. Spechler SJ: Barrett esophagus: a sequela of chemotherapy. *Ann Intern Med* 1991, 114:243–244.

24. Peters FRM, Sleijfer DT, van Imhoff GW, Kleibeuker JH: Is chemotherapy associated with development of Barrett's esophagus? *Dig Dis Sci* 1993, 38:923–926.

25. Dahms BB, Greco MA, Strandjord SE, Rothstein FC: Barrett's esophagus in three children after antileukemia chemotherapy. *Cancer* 1987, 60:2896–2900.

26. Hassall E, Dimmick JE, Magee JF: Adenocarcinoma in childhood Barrett's esophagus. *Am J Gastroenterol* 1993, 88:282–288.

27. Hassall E: Columnar-lined esophagus in children. *Gastroenterol Clin North Am* 1997, 26:533–548.

147 Achalasia and Esophageal Motility Disorders

Mark S. Glassman and Marvin S. Medow

The esophagus propels food from the mouth to the stomach by a process called peristalsis, which results from the complex interactions of skeletal and smooth muscle, and the enteric and central nervous systems (see Chapter 6). Sphincters at the proximal and distal ends of the esophagus are zones of high pressure that allow the luminal contents to progress in an aboral direction while preventing retrograde movement. Primary peristaltic contractions are initiated by a swallow and are associated with pharyngeal muscle contraction and relaxation of the upper esophageal sphincter (UES), whereas secondary peristaltic waves result from distention of the esophagus by food and are not accompanied by pressure changes in the pharynx or UES. The term *tertiary peristalsis* refers to spontaneous contractions of the esophagus that are not peristaltic or physiologic [1,2]. Details on the anatomy and physiology of the esophagus are presented in Chapter 6.

DIAGNOSIS OF ESOPHAGEAL MOTILITY DISORDERS

Motor function of the proximal esophagus can be altered in patients with diseases that affect striated muscle, such as poliomyelitis, botulism, multiple sclerosis, and inflammatory myopathies. Such proximal esophageal motor dysfunctions are poorly defined and are associated with pharyngeal dyscoordination, cricopharyngeal achalasia or hypertension, and delayed relaxation of the UES in response to swallow. Symptoms associated with UES dysfunction can include choking, coughing with meals, poor eating, and aspiration pneumonia. Radiographic or laryngoscopic evidence of oropharyngeal dysfunction confirms the diagnosis of UES dysfunction. Manometry may be useful in defining the pathophysiology of UES dysfunction, but it has not yet been validated in children.

In children, primary esophageal motility abnormalities of the lower esophagus are classified using the same manometric, radiographic, and endoscopic criteria applied to adult patients [3,4]. Most motility disorders are classified as follows:

Achalasia: a hypertonic lower esophageal sphincter (LES) fails to relax with swallowing. Peristalsis is absent, and the esophageal contractions are of low amplitude (Fig. 147-1). Endoscopic examination reveals a quiet esophagus with normal mucosa and a LES zone that transiently resists passage of the endoscope.

Diffuse esophageal spasm (DES): esophageal contractions are spontaneous, simultaneous, or nonperistaltic, with contraction waves of variable intensity and duration (Fig. 147-2).

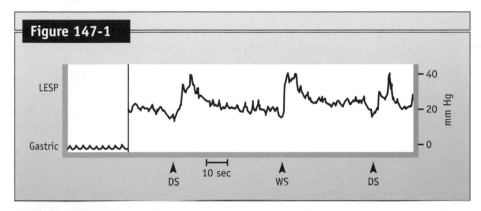

Figure 147-1

Incomplete LES relaxation after both wet (WS) and dry swallows (DS) in a patient with achalasia. Note that mean LES pressure (LESP) (23 mm Hg) falls within the normal range. (*From* Castell *et al.* [2], with permission.)

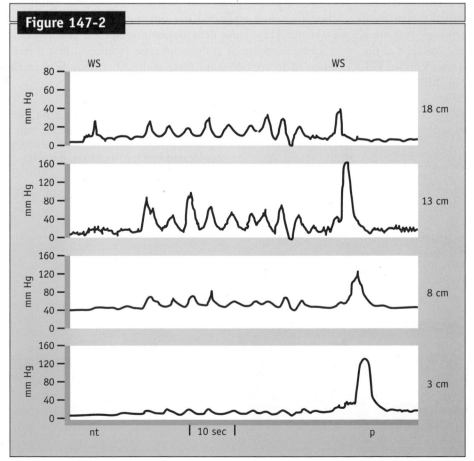

Figure 147-2

Classic repetitive contractions in a patient with diffuse esophageal spasm. In this case, the nontransmitted (nt) wet swallow (WS) resulted in pooling of fluid in the body of the esophagus and subsequent repetitive, simultaneous contractions. This is terminated by a peristaltic contraction (p) after a wet swallow. (*From* Castell *et al.* [2], with permission.)

Nutcracker esophagus: peristaltic pressures are elevated in both intensity (>180 mm Hg) and duration (>6 minutes) (Fig. 147-3).

Hypertensive LES: pressure in the esophageal body exceeds 45 mm Hg, but there is complete relaxation of the LES to gastric baseline.

Hypotensive LES: pressures in the esophageal body are <10 mm Hg.

Aperistalsis: there are no contractions in the esophageal body after a swallow [2].

Glassman *et al.* evaluated the manometric data from 83 children presenting with noncardiac chest pain and found that 21 children (25%) had abnormal esophageal motility [5]. Diffuse esophageal spasm was diagnosed in seven, achalasia in four, hypotensive LES in three, aperistalsis in three, and nutcracker esophagus or hypertensive esophagus in two each. These findings are similar to those reported in studies of adult patients [6,7].

ESOPHAGEAL DYSFUNCTION AND CHEST PAIN

Disruption of the muscular or neurologic control of esophageal function, known as dysmotility, can result in symptoms that include chest pain, dysphagia, or regurgitation. Chest pain is a common complaint during adolescence, affecting as many as 15% of inner-city youths [8]. However, the role of esophageal dysmotility as a cause of this symptom is poorly understood. Studies of children presenting to the emergency department with complaints of chest pain report a high frequency of idiopathic or functional pain. The value of these studies is limited, however, by their failure to exclude a gastrointestinal cause of the pain. In 1988, Berezin *et al.* reported that in 16 of the 27 children (62%) referred for gastroenterologic evaluation of chest pain, the pain had an esophageal cause, and in 5 of the 16 (30%) esophageal motor abnormalities were identified [9]. The age at presentation, duration of symptoms before referral,

and site of pain did not distinguish between children with or without an esophageal cause of pain [10].

To further characterize the spectrum of esophageal disorders that can cause chest pain in the pediatric population, Glassman and associates reviewed their experience in 83 children presenting with chest pain or dysphagia [5]. Fifty-seven percent had normal esophageal histology and motility, 18% had esophagitis, 18% had esophageal dysfunction, and 8% had both esophageal inflammation and dysmotility. Age, gender, and symptoms of chest pain, dysphagia, and vomiting did not distinguish between children with normal esophageal physiology and histology and those with primary esophageal disorders. However, children with esophageal dysfunction tended to have a longer duration of symptoms before diagnosis.

Among the children identified as having esophageal dysfunction, diffuse esophageal spasm (DES) was the most common disorder, affecting 33% of the children with esophageal dysmotility. Achalasia, hypotensive LES pressure, aperistalsis, nutcracker esophagus, and hypertensive LES were the other causes of esophageal motor disorders. The overall prevalence and the distribution of esophageal disorders were similar to that in the numerous reports surveying the causes of chest pain in adult patients. However, the relative frequency of motor disorders that cause chest pain differs from the prevalence in adult patients [5] (Fig. 147-4).

Until recently, the relationship between gastroesophageal reflux and esophageal motor dysfunction was poorly understood. Ganatra *et al.* reported that in three of eight children undergoing evaluation of chest pain, intraesophageal perfusion of 0.1 N hydrochloric acid produced esophageal spasm and chest pain that replicated the symptoms that had prompted evaluation [11]. These data suggest that in these children DES is a manifestation of gastroesophageal reflux and that therapy intended to control esophageal acidification may prevent the chest pain associated with this motor disorder.

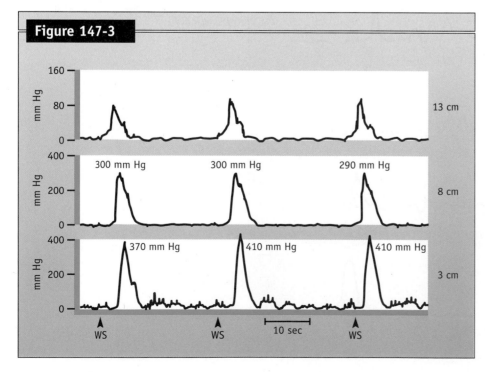

Figure 147-3

Baseline motility tracing from a patient with a nutcracker esophagus demonstrating high-amplitude peristaltic contractions. Recording sites located at 13, 8, and 3 cm above the LES. WS—wet swallow.

The effect of inflammatory lesions on the manometric characteristics of the esophagus remains controversial. Cucciara reported that children with severe esophagitis had esophageal manometric abnormalities characterized by frequent tertiary contractions, double-peaked peristaltic waves, and decreased peristaltic amplitude. These abnormalities improved after successful treatment of the inflammatory process [12]. In contrast, Berezin *et al.* found no difference in the esophageal manometry of children with and without esophagitis [13]; results of their study indicate that LES pressure and the amplitude, duration, and conduction velocity of esophageal contraction are independent of the occurrence and degree of esophageal inflammation. Additionally, manometric abnormalities in patients with both esophagitis and esophageal dysmotility persist, despite healing of inflammatory lesions. It appears that esophagitis and esophageal motor dysfunction may be independent disorders.

SECONDARY MOTOR DISORDERS

Esophageal motility disorders can result from disease processes limited to the musculature and the enteric nervous system of the esophagus (primary esophageal disease) or may be part of a more generalized disorder (secondary esophageal disease). Diseases that affect the central nervous system, such as cerebral palsy, are associated with swallowing dysfunction. Myotonia or muscular dystrophy can disrupt the normal peristaltic patterns within the esophageal body. Inflammatory myopathies associated with connective tissue disorders such as scleroderma, dermatomyositis, polymyositis, systemic lupus erythematosus, and CREST (calcinosis, Raynaud's, esophageal dysmotility, sclerodactyly, telangiectasia) syndrome can disrupt normal esophageal motili-

ty. Endocrinopathies such as hypothyroidism and diabetes mellitus, various medications, metabolic disorders such as hypothyroidism and hyperparathyroidism, and idiopathic intestinal pseudo-obstruction or neuronal intestinal dysplasia may alter normal esophageal motility as well. In a study of esophageal manometry in children with scleroderma, Flick *et al.* found abnormalities of esophageal motor function in five of seven children [14], including low-amplitude esophageal contractions, tertiary waves, and decreased LES pressure. These data were similar to those in published reports of esophageal dysfunction in children with intestinal pseudo-obstruction. Staiano *et al.* found that in children with Hirschsprung's disease, abnormalities of esophageal motility persisted after successful correction of the colonic pathology (Fig. 147-5) [15]. These data suggest that Hirschsprung's disease may be the colonic manifestation of a more generalized intestinal motility disorder.

TREATMENT

Experience in treating children with proximal esophageal disorders is limited. The nature of the lesion(s) responsible for the dysfunction of the esophageal skeletal muscle is unknown, but appears to be developmental. Treatment by dilation or myotomy in this population has been complicated by postoperative aspiration and should be avoided if possible. Symptoms of esophageal dysfunction in these children actually improve spontaneously over time, and in many instances without treatment. Therefore, conservative management using enteral nutritional support appears preferential to more aggressive intervention. More invasive dilation or surgical treatment should be reserved for patients who fail to improve over a prolonged period.

The distribution of esophageal manometric abnormalities in 21 children and 255 adults. LES—lower esophageal sphincter.

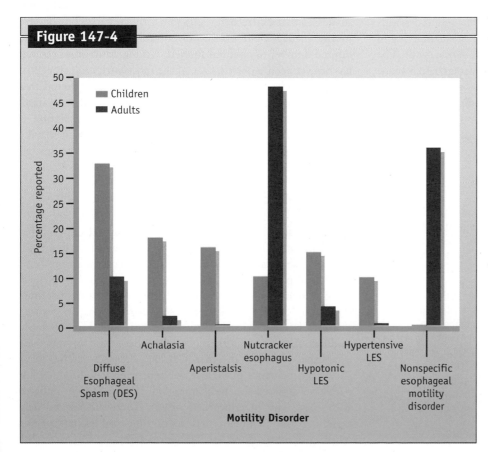

Figure 147-4

In general, the results of therapy for children with motility disorders of the esophagus have been disappointing. Glassman *et al.* reported that 73% of 21 children with primary esophageal dysmotility remained symptomatic despite disease-specific treatment [5]. In comparison, 80% of the children with esophagitis improved after therapy with H_2-receptor antagonists. Esophageal dilation, and the use of H_2-receptor antagonists (ranitidine) and Ca^{2+} channel blockers are effective in the majority of children with achalasia, whereas esophageal dilation, ranitidine, and prokinetic agents control the symptoms of other motility disorders [5].

ACHALASIA AND HYPERTENSIVE LOWER ESOPHAGEAL SPHINCTER

Balloon dilation of the hypertensive LES has been effectively used for the treatment of achalasia in children for almost 40 years. Boyle *et al.* [16], and Berquist *et al.* [3] reported success rates of approximately 80% using pneumatic dilation, results comparable to those reported in the treatment of adult patients. Complications of this procedure, including perforation, pleural effusion, and fever, occur in less than 4% of children. Repeat dilations for recurrent symptoms are required frequently to achieve successful resolution of this condition.

Experience with pharmacologic treatment of achalasia in children is limited. Isosorbide dinitrate effectively lowers LES pressure, but causes postural hypotension and often must be discontinued. Calcium channel blocking agents to lower LES pressure in children are as effective in the younger patient as in the adult and have fewer side effects when used for short periods (2 weeks) [17]. Clinical trials in which botulinum toxin is injected directly into the LES of patients with achalasia have shown successful results [18]. Botulinum toxin reduced symptom scores, LES pressure and enhanced esophageal emptying in adults with achalasia by acting as an anticholinergic agent. The duration of response following this therapy averaged 1.25 years. Characteristics such as the duration of illness prior to therapy, previous response to injection therapy, and radiographic characteristics of the esophagus were not predictive of an individual's response to this treatment modality; younger patients with lower LES pressures were less likely to respond.

There are few studies reporting the results of therapy in children with hypertensive LES. Based on the similar manometric characteristics of both achalasia and hypertensive LES, which indicate smooth muscle hyperactivity, the therapeutic approach to treatment of a patient with hypertensive LES initially should parallel that of achalasia.

Surgical myotomy of the LES has been successful in relieving the symptoms of achalasia in approximately 80% of children. However, postoperative morbidity is quite high, and the development of gastroesophageal reflux approaches 50% in children reevaluated over a span of 10 years. These children may suffer significant complications of reflux, resulting in the formation of peptic strictures. Studies have shown that the success and complication rate of myotomy in children is not affected by previous attempts at LES dilatation [3]. Thus, a rational approach to the child with achalasia includes initial treatment with calcium channel blockade followed by balloon dilation if long-term drug therapy is unsuccessful or is associated with unacceptable side effects. Surgical myotomy is a last resort.

DIFFUSE ESOPHAGEAL SPASM

There is no defined approach to the treatment of a child with DES. Milov *et al.* reported that of five children treated with DES using sublingual nitrates, three became asymptomatic while on therapy. However, the medication had to be discontinued because of the development of severe postural hypotension in all five patients [19]. Glassman *et al.* used calcium channel blockade in five children with DES and had success in only one patient [5]. Ganatra *et al.* described the relationship between intraesophageal acidification and the development of DES and suggested that H_2-receptor antagonist therapy may be effective in the management of this disorder [11]. However, in the limited number of children studied, symptomatic improvement has not yet been reported. One of the most intriguing aspects of DES in children was reported by Milov *et al.*, who found that symptoms resolved without specific therapy after 2 years in all five of their patients [19]. The reason for this resolution is unknown, but it suggests that DES in this population may be a transient phenomenon, which should, therefore, be treated conservatively.

NONSPECIFIC ESOPHAGEAL MOTOR DISORDERS

Although advances in manometric analysis have permitted the delineation of several types of esophageal dysfunction, including achalasia and diffuse esophageal spasm, a significant number of patients with swallowing difficulties and esophageal motor abnormalities do not fall into any clearly defined diagnostic category. The term *nonspecific esophageal motility disorders* has been used to describe esophageal manometric findings that are abnormal, but not diagnostic for any one established motility disorder [20,21]. Previous studies have shown an incidence of NEMD of approximately 40% in adult patients evaluated for dysphagia, and 25% to 50% in patients with chest pain of noncardiac origin. There are limited data regarding the treatment and natural history of nonspecific esophageal motor disorders in children [22].

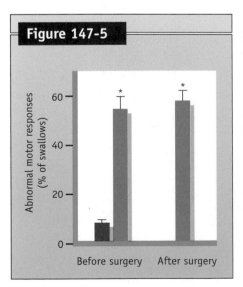

Figure 147-5

Manometric findings in six children 3 months after operative treatment of Hirschsprung's disease (*green bars*). Findings in the control children (*gray bar*) are included for comparison. Asterisk indicates *P* < 0.001 compared with control children. (*From* Staiano et al [15]; with permission.)

■ SUMMARY

Although the experience in children is not as extensive as that in adults, it appears that a significant percentage of children with vomiting, chest pain, and dysphagia have an esophageal cause for their complaints. As many as 25% of these children have an esophageal motor disorder characterized as diffuse esophageal spasm, achalasia, or a nonspecific motor disorder. Almost 75% of these children remain symptomatic despite treatment of the underlying dysmotility with calcium channel blockade, sublingual nitrates, or H_2-receptor antagonists. In contrast, balloon dilation or myotomy are successful in treating children with achalasia. The prevalence of esophageal pathology and the spectrum of esophageal disorders causing chest pain in children is comparable to the experience in the adult population. The response to specific therapeutic interventions in children and adults is similar as well. Of note, however, is the tendency for proximal esophageal motor disorders and diffuse esophageal spasm to resolve spontaneously over prolonged time intervals (approximately 2 years) in children.

■ REFERENCES

1. Herbst J: Achalasia and other motor disorders. In *Pediatric Gastrointestinal Disease: Pathophysiology, Diagnosis, Management.* Edited by Wyllie R, Hyams JS. Philadelphia: WB Saunders, 1993:391–401.

2. Castell DO, Richter JE, Dalton CB: *Esophageal Motility Testing.* New York: Elsevier, 1987.

3. Berquist WE, Byrne WJ, Ament ME, *et al*: Achalasia: diagnosis, management and clinical course in 16 children. *Pediatrics* 1983, 71:798–805.

4. Weinstock LB, Clouse RE: Esophageal physiology: normal and abnormal motor function. *Am J Gastroenterol* 1987, 81:399–405.

5. Glassman MS, Medow MS, Berezin S, Newman LJ: Spectrum of esophageal disorders in children with chest pain. *Dig Dis Sci* 1992, 37:663–666.

6. McCallum RW: The spectrum of esophageal motility disorders. *Hosp Pract* 1987, 22:71–83.

7. Richter JE, Bradley LA, Castell DO: Esophageal chest pain: current controversies in pathogenesis, diagnosis and therapy. *Ann Intern Med* 1989, 110:66–78.

8. Brunswick AP, Bovie JM, Tanca C: Who sees the doctor? A study of urban black adolescents. *Soc Sci Med* 1979, 13A:45–46.

9. Berezin S, Medow MS, Glassman MS, Newman LJ: Chest pain of gastrointestinal origin. *Arch Dis Child* 1988, 63:1457–1460.

10. Berezin S, Medow MS, Glassman M, Newman LJ: Use of intraesophageal acid perfusion test in provoking nonspecific chest pain in children. *J Pediatr* 1989, 115:709–712.

11. Ganatra JV, Medow MS, Berezin S, *et al*: Esophageal dysmotility elicited by acid perfusion in children with esophagitis. *Am J Gastroenterol* 1995, 90:1080–1083.

12. Cucciara S, Staiano A, DiLorenzo C: Esophageal motor abnormalities in children with reflux and peptic esophagitis. *J Pediatr* 1986, 108:907–910.

13. Berezin S, Halata MS, Newman LJ, *et al*: Esophageal manometry in children with esophagitis. *Am J Gastroenterol* 1993, 88:680–682.

14. Flick JA, Boyle JT, Tuchman DN, *et al*: Esophageal motor abnormalities in children and adolescents with scleroderma and mixed connective tissue disease. *Pediatrics* 1988, 82:107–111.

15. Staiano AS, Corazziari E, Andreotti MR, Clouse RE: Esophageal motility in children with Hirschsprung's disease. *Am J Dis Child* 1990, 145:310–313.

16. Boyle JT, Cohen S, Watkins JB: Successful treatment of achalasia in childhood by pneumatic dilation. *J Pediatr* 1981, 99:35–40.

17. Maksimak M, Perlmutter DH, Winter HS: The use of nifedipine for the treatment of achalasia in children. *J Pediatr Gastroenterol Nutr* 1986, 5:883–886.

18. Bhutani MS: Gastrointestinal uses of botulinum toxin. *Am J Gastroenterol* 1997, 92:929–933.

19. Milov DE, Cynamon HA, Andres JM: Chest pain and dysphagia in adolescents caused by diffuse esophageal spasm. *J Pediatr Gastroenterol Nutr* 1989, 9:450–453.

20. Richter JE, Wu WC, Johns DN, *et al*: Esophageal manometry in 95 healthy adult volunteers: variability of pressures with age and frequency of "abnormal" contractions. *Dig Dis Sci* 1987, 32:583–592.

21. Achem SR, Crittenden J, Kolts B, Burton LS: Long-term clinical and manometric follow-up of patients with non-specific esophageal motor disorders. *Am J Gastroenterol* 1992, 87:825–830.

22. Katz PO, Dalton CB, Richter JE, *et al*: Esophageal testing of patients with noncardiac chest pain or dysphagia. *Ann Intern Med* 106:593–597, 1987.

148 Caustic and Foreign Body Ingestion
Donald E. George

Children, especially very young children, enjoy putting things in their mouths. During early development, the mouth is used as a tool for exploring the environment. Such behaviors are part of the normal developmental process and are not necessarily indicative of mental deficiency or other pathology. The tendency of children to put things in their mouths, coupled with the development of mobility and curiosity, makes them particularly vulnerable to injury of the gastrointestinal tract from ingestion of various agents, especially foreign bodies or corrosive substances. The pathophysiology of corrosive exposures is detailed in Chapter 11. The tools and techniques available to manage foreign bodies are reviewed by Kim and Benjamin. This chapter focuses on the clinical issues involved in the care of young patients who have ingested corrosive or foreign bodies.

■ CAUSTIC INGESTION

Accidental ingestion of caustic agents is seen predominantly in children. Indeed, the bulk of cases occurs in toddlers, although there is another peak in young adults related to suicide gestures. Studies from Denmark indicate that ingestions leading to esophageal burns are 10 times more common in children than in adults and that 94% of these children are under 5 years of age [1,2]. Surprisingly, the incidence of caustic ingestions has not decreased since the Poison Prevention Packaging Act of 1970 was enacted. In 1990, more than 16,000 caustic ingestions (11,000 of alkali) were reported to the Association of Poison Control Centers (APCC), of which 66% were in children under 6 years of age [3]. In 1995, the APCC reported more than 26,000 exposures to corrosives, 11,400 of which involved alkali products. Again, the majority were in children less than 6 years of age [4]. Deaths related to caustic ingestion are more common in adults intent on suicide than in children who accidentally ingest caustic substances. The products most frequently ingested are personal care products, household bleaches, automatic dishwasher products, swimming pool products, and bathroom and oven cleaners (Table 148-1). Household bleaches have a low concentration of sodium hypochlorite and pose little risk [5]. However, swimming pool products have a much higher concentration of alkali and are capable of causing severe tissue damage. Cosmetic products, especially hair relaxers, are often ingested and produce mucosal injury. Fortunately, this injury is rarely severe [6,7].

Lye is the most feared ingestant because of the ability of strong alkali to cause liquefaction necrosis and deep tissue injury [8]. Crystalline forms are less likely to cause esophageal burns because they cause such severe mouth pain that they are often spit out before they can be swallowed. However, liquid products are odorless, do not always cause immediate pain, and, therefore, are more completely swallowed. They often have a pleasant color that can attract children. Acids have a bitter taste and often are spit out quickly. If they are swallowed, they generally produce a more superficial lesion with less risk of perforation. Rapid coagulation with eschar formation limits the depth of injury. Because of the relative resistance of the squamous epithelium to acid, and the effect of gravity, liquids quickly pass into the dependent portions of the stomach, which may be severely injured; reflex pylorospasm increases damage to the antrum and pylorus by prolonging contact times [8,9].

Clinical Features

Symptoms usually develop immediately after ingestion. The child is often frightened and presents with coughing, spitting, or drooling. In many cases the bottle for the ingested material is found nearby. Often the corrosive has been decanted by an adult before the child gets to it from its original protective container to another, more attractive one, such as a soda bottle or milk bottle. Mouth pain and odynophagia are frequently noted. Stridor or vomiting is of particular concern, because these symptoms signal severe tissue damage. Burns are present on the lips and in the oropharynx in most children who have ingested alkali, but only in about one third of patients who have ingested acid. Signs and symptoms of ingestions are listed in Table 148-2.

The more severe the symptoms and signs, the more likely it is that there are esophageal burns. The presence of oral burns often is used mistakenly as the sole indication that esophageal burns are present [10]. Esophageal burns may be noted in the absence of oropharyngeal burns, however, and esophageal strictures may develop in patients who had no burns of the oropharynx [11]. Although several studies have documented the relation between the number of initial symptoms and signs and the presence and severity of esophageal burns, no single symptom or group of symptoms has been found to be predictive of the presence or depth of esophageal burns [12,13•]. Therefore, all symptomatic patients require evaluation. Suggested algorithms are provided in Figures 148-1 and 148-2.

Evaluation and treatment of children who have experienced caustic ingestion most often are based on the experience and expertise of the care provider. Development of guidelines and algorithms is hampered by the lack of controlled studies with large series of patients. Most recommendations are based on expert opinion.

Chest radiographs and, rarely, airway films may be useful in patients with respiratory symptoms. Aspiration pneumonia may be detected, and widening of the mediastinum or an air–fluid level in the mediastinum indicates perforation of the esophagus. If the child has abdominal pain, or if there are signs of peritonitis, abdominal radiographs should be obtained to look for free air. Although they are very important for follow-up and for detection of late complications, most providers think radiographic studies using barium or water-soluble contrast have little value in the ini-

---

Table 148-1. Common Caustic Agents

Chemical	Products
Alkali	
Sodium hydroxide (lye)	Drain openers
	Oven cleaners
	Clinitest tablets
	Hair relaxers
	Epoxy activators
	Tile cleaners
Potassium hydroxide	Disk batteries
Acid	
Sulfuric acid	Drain openers
Hydrochloric acid	Toilet bowl cleaners
Sodium bisulfate	Toilet bowl cleaners
Detergents	
Sodium phosphates	Dishwashing products
and sodium carbonates	Laundry detergents
Miscellaneous	
Sodium hypochlorite,	Bleach,
hydrogen peroxide	swimming pool products

Table 148-2. Symptoms of Caustic Ingestion

Symptoms	Signs
	Oropharyngeal burn
Dysphagia	Drooling
Odynophagia	Abdominal tenderness
Respiratory distress	Vomiting
Chest pain	Hoarseness
Nausea	Wheezing, rales
Abdominal pain	Stridor
Vomiting	Respiratory distress

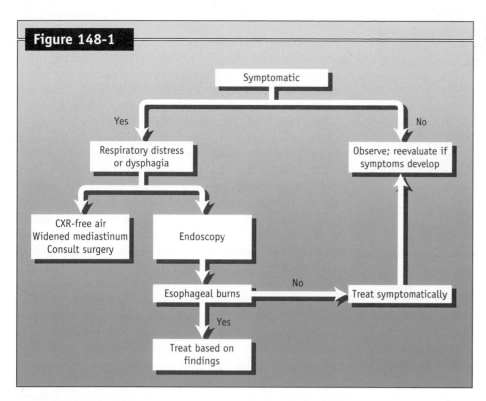

Figure 148-1

Management of ingestion of a caustic agent. CXR—chest radiograph.

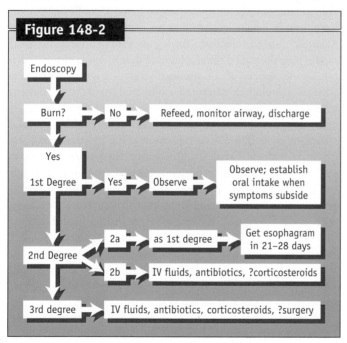

Figure 148-2

Management of esophageal burns. IV—intravenous.

tial evaluation of a child with suspected ingestion of a caustic substance. Those who favor imaging studies argue that a well-performed upper gastrointestinal series with careful fluoroscopic guidance provides evidence of ulceration, perforation, or necrosis in the esophagus, stomach, or duodenum. Opponents argue that endoscopy is ultimately necessary no matter what the results of the upper gastrointestinal series. In addition, drinking barium is unpleasant for a child with dysphagia and potentially increases the risk of aspiration.

Endoscopy is the most reliable way to evaluate the upper gastrointestinal tract. The decision for flexible versus rigid endoscopy is made based on the experience and expertise of the physician caring for the patient. However, flexible endoscopy with an appropriate-sized instrument is considered the procedure of choice. The stomach and duodenum, as well as the esophagus, may be examined, with only a small risk of perforation or tissue damage if gentle technique is used.

Burns of the esophagus are classified by depth of injury. First-degree burns involve only the mucosa, which appears hyperemic and edematous. Second-degree burns result in damage to the mucosa and submucosa. Exudate, erosions, and ulcers are present. Third-degree burns indicate injury to the deeper tissue layers with deep ulcerations and necrosis. Third-degree burns limit the extent of endoscopic evaluation and probably increase the risk of the procedure.

Recently a modified classification of esophageal burns has been developed [14•] (Table 148-3) that differentiates injuries with shallow ulcerations (IIa) from those that are deep and circumferential (IIb). Furthermore, it differentiates grade III injuries based on extent of necrosis. This classification has been shown to be predictive of complications.

In the past, when only rigid instruments were available, common practice dictated that endoscopy should be discontinued at the level of first burn. It is now clear that with flexible instruments it is safe to evaluate the upper gastrointestinal tract more thoroughly. Endoscopy may be continued beyond mild to moderate burns [8]. The first burn encountered may not give complete information about the degree and depth of damage, and a large percentage of patients with esophageal injury also have gastric injury [15]. As soon as a third-degree burn is seen, however, the instrument should not be advanced any further.

Endoscopy of children, especially very young children, must always be done in a controlled environment. Whether intravenous sedation or general anesthesia is used depends not only on the comfort and experience of the endoscopist but also on

Table 148-3. Endoscopic Classification of Esophageal Burns

Grade	Description
I	Mucosal hyperemia and edema Occasional desquamation
IIa	Superficial erosion or ulceration White membranes
IIb	As in IIa with deep or circumferential ulceration
IIIa	Multiple ulcerations with areas of necrosis
IIIb	Extensive necrosis

From Zargar et al. [14].

that of the endoscopy assistants and support staff. The age of the child and his or her ability to cooperate must be considered. Although examination under intravenous sedation can be done safely and accurately, if there is a concern about the airway, or if the patient's cooperation cannot be ensured, general anesthesia should be used. Endoscopy should not be done in a stridorous child without first obtaining airway control.

Whether all patients with a caustic ingestion require endoscopy is controversial [8,11,13,16]. At issue is how the information obtained will alter treatment or outcome. Use of medication such as corticosteroids and antibiotics is controversial, especially for lower grade injuries. Very early endoscopy (ie, <6 hours after ingestion) may underestimate the degree of damage, because the maximum change may not be visible for 24 to 48 hours. Although it is known that the maximum damage may not be visible for 48 hours, endoscopy is usually done 12 to 24 hours after ingestion.

The child with signs or symptoms of caustic injury (Table 148-2) is admitted for observation and further evaluation and treatment. Stridor and respiratory distress are particularly ominous signs, and children showing those signs should be admitted to an intensive care area.

Children who are severely symptomatic or who have grade IIb or III esophageal burns should be stabilized and considered for transport to a tertiary children's center. Both the acute management and the chronic care and rehabilitation of these patients require an integrated multidisciplinary team of providers, including gastroenterologists; otolaryngologist, general, and thoracic surgeons; speech therapists; and feeding specialists who are particularly familiar with children.

Treatment

The asymptomatic child requires no treatment, but he or she may be observed for 4 to 6 hours and given liquids to drink. Reassessment is mandatory if symptoms develop. The child may be discharged to home with a follow-up appointment in 48 hours. Endoscopic evaluation usually is unnecessary. The primary care provider should be alerted because of the remote possibility that symptoms may develop 6 to 8 weeks later. It is exceedingly rare for strictures to develop in a child without antecedent symptoms.

The symptomatic child should be admitted and given appropriate resuscitation and intravenous fluids. Vomiting should not be induced, because regurgitation of caustic material may further damage the esophagus. Neutralizing agents have not been shown to be effective, and they add the potential risk of thermal injury. Charcoal is not effective in neutralizing acid or alkali and can hinder endoscopic evaluations. Special care must be taken to avoid aspiration during and after stabilization.

Blind passage of a nasogastric tube should be avoided so as not to aggravate injury or cause perforation. Gagging during passage of a tube can induce vomiting and potentiate the risk of aspiration. A tube, string, or stent may be placed at the time of endoscopy to provide access for feeding or to maintain patency and provide a guide for future dilations should severe stenosis develop.

There are no generally accepted guidelines for the routine use of antibiotics. They are not indicated in patients with oropharyngeal burns only or first-degree esophageal burns. Broad-spectrum antibiotics are freely used in patients with severe (grade IIb or higher) esophageal burns or evidence of aspiration. Certainly, patients in whom perforation may have occurred should receive antibiotic coverage. In addition, patients with signs of infection (eg, fever, pneumonia) should be treated. Ampicillin alone or in combination with gentamycin, erythromycin, or third-generation cephalosporins may be used.

The use of corticosteroids has long been debated and remains highly controversial [8,9,16,17,18••,19•]. Although animal studies indicate there may be benefit, studies in humans have been inconclusive. Differences in the corticosteroids used, dosages, patient selection, timing of intervention, and study design have precluded development of a clear consensus as to their efficacy. A review of 13 studies found that 41% of untreated patients developed strictures, compared to 19% of patients treated with corticosteroids and antibiotics [17]. This review compared patients from studies with different designs and, therefore, is open to criticism because of the lack of controls and extensive statistical analysis. One consistent feature was that no patient with first-degree burns developed strictures. In a controlled study of 131 children, 60 of whom had serious burns, Anderson and coworkers [18••] found that strictures developed with equal frequency in corticosteriod treated (11 of 29) and untreated (10 of 30) patients. Fewer treated patients required esophageal replacement, but this trend was not significant. A recent study has suggested that dexamethasone (1 mg/kg/d) is more effective than prednisolone (2 mg/kg/d) in preventing complications, but this awaits confirmation [19•].

Advocates of the use of corticosteroids argue that they must be started early to be beneficial. Opponents argue that they are potentially risky and increase morbidity because they may induce infection. Corticosteroid treatment is not indicated for patients with mild (grade I or IIa) injury. Furthermore, because of the increased risk of sepsis, corticosteroids are not indicated in the patient who has perforation or extensive (grade IIIb) necrosis. The dosage, duration, and use of corticosteroids for moderate injury will continue to be debated until consensus can be reached by a well-designed multicenter trial.

Esophageal motor function is altered by caustic ingestion, placing patients at increased risk for gastroesophageal reflux both acutely and chronically. Treatment with an H_2-blocker or a proton pump inhibitor may be indicated, therefore, both acutely and for a prolonged period [20–22].

Children with first-degree burns require little specific therapy. Depending on the presence of oropharyngeal burns, oral intake usually can be reestablished within 24 to 48 hours. Follow-up is important, but there are no recommendations for routine radiographic studies or repeat endoscopy. Decisions as to the need for further studies are made on a case-by-case basis, based on symptoms. Children with grade IIa burns at 24 hours should be closely monitored, because it is known that early endoscopy may underestimate the severity of injury. Corticosteroids and antibiotics are not necessary. Feedings should be started as soon as the child is pain free and can tolerate his or her secretions. Follow-up with an upper gastrointestinal series is advised.

The management of extensive second-degree (grade IIb) and third-degree burns requires an aggressive multidisciplinary approach. Special attention is paid to nutritional support and tube feeding via gastrostomy or percutaneous endoscopic gastrostomy (PEG). The use of a string or stent for early treatment depends on the expertise of the surgeon. A string or endoscopically placed narrow-bore nasogastric tube provides a guide for future dilations. Early placement of an esophageal stent has not been extensively studied in children but may be useful [23].

Complications

Early complications within the first 24 to 72 hours after injury include fever, pneumonia, and perforation [24] (Table 148-4). The most common late complication is formation of an esophageal stricture, which may occur as soon as 21 days after ingestion or may present much later in the course. Caustic strictures are fragile, and dilation is done with caution. If a string is in place, retrograde dilation with the Tucker dilator is probably safest. Dilation with balloons, Eder-Pustow or Savary-Gillard dilators, or bougies is also acceptable. Most strictures require frequent dilation, and even with dilation some patients require esophageal replacement.

Patients who have caustic esophageal burns are at much greater subsequent risk for squamous cell carcinoma (as much as 1000 times greater) than the general population. This complication typically develops more than 30 or 40 years after ingestion, which emphasizes the need for lifelong follow-up and surveillance [8,9].

Caustic ingestion remains a severe, catastrophic, and preventable problem. Treatment is largely ineffective, and efforts must be made at prevention. Legislative mandates, not only to improve package safety but also to limit access to injurious material, such as those that have been instituted in other countries, are necessary. Education is also important. Caustics

Table 148-4. Complications of Caustic Ingestion	
Early (< 48 h)	**Late**
Mediastinitis	Tracheoesophageal fistula
Sepsis	Pseudodiverticula
Gastrointestinal bleeding	Esophageal stricture
Perforation	Gastric outlet obstruction
	Hiatal hernia
	Squamous cell cancer (> 30 y later)

should not be transferred to alternative nonprotective vessels. Children should be taught "If you can't touch it, don't taste it."

■ FOREIGN BODIES

Ingestion of foreign bodies is common in children. The APCC reported 75,021 instances in 1995, 53,972 of which were in children under 6 years of age [4]. The peak incidence of foreign body ingestion is between the ages of 6 months and 3 years, the ages during which children place objects in their mouths as a means of exploring the environment. The actual incidence of foreign body ingestion is higher, because the majority of episodes go unreported [25•]. This makes recommendations for a universal standard of care based on hospital-acquired data difficult to develop.

Fortunately, the majority of foreign bodies that reach the gastrointestinal tract pass without difficulty and require no intervention (Fig. 148-3). However, serious complications can occur. Because the true incidence of the problem is uncertain, it is difficult to estimate the associated morbidity and mortality. It is estimated that 10% of patients receive some intervention, and approximately 1500 deaths resulting from foreign body ingestion occur annually. Guidelines for management have been published [26].

Anatomy

Foreign bodies become lodged at areas of physiologic or pathologic narrowing. Pointed objects may become trapped in the hypopharynx at the vallecula or in the pyriform sinuses. The esophagus has four areas of narrowing: 1) the cricopharyngeus and upper esophageal sphincter; 2) the area compressed by the aortic arch; 3) the area compressed by the left mainstem bronchus; and 4) the lower esophageal sphincter. Once an object clears the esophagus it usually passes through the remainder of the gastrointestinal tract without difficulty. However, the pylorus, ileocecal valve, and anus are potential sites of obstruction. Congenital or acquired strictures may also be sites of impaction.

Clinical Features

In contrast to emergency room–based data, which indicate that most foreign body ingestion occurs at night, office-based data suggest the peak time of ingestion is between noon and 6 PM [27]. Although several studies have identified contributory social, developmental, or psychiatric factors in such ingestions, these factors are more common in adolescents and adults. The majority of children who ingest foreign bodies are normal and from functional environments and are in the care of their parents. Commonly swallowed objects are listed in Table 148-5.

Most patients or their parents are able to give a clear history of foreign body ingestion. Older children and adults often are able to point to the location of discomfort. However, in toddlers or mentally impaired older children or adults, the ingestion may go unrecognized. In addition, the onset of symptoms such as choking, refusal to eat, wheezing, or regurgitation may be remote from the time of ingestion.

Esophageal foreign bodies most often are associated with odynophagia, dysphagia, or regurgitation (Table 148-6). Because the tracheal cartilage of young children, especially those less than 3 years of age, is more compliant and is easily compressed, respiratory symptoms often predominate. A young child may present with wheezing or symptoms of upper respiratory infection when a foreign body has been ingested but nobody witnessed the event [28]. Occasionally the only symptom of an ingestion is refusal to take textured feedings.

Gastric foreign bodies most often are asymptomatic. Occasionally there is sporadic vomiting when the object obstructs the pylorus. There may be early satiety and weight loss. Once an object has passed the pylorus, onset of symptoms usually indicates perforation or obstruction.

Radiography

Radiography identifies most but not all foreign bodies [29]. It also identifies free air in the mediastinum, abdomen, or subcutaneous tissue. Biplane films of the neck, chest, and abdomen are obtained in most instances. Special attention is paid to the airway to assess tracheal compression. A flat object, such as a coin, is oriented in the frontal plane if it is lodged in the esophagus but in the sagittal plane if it is in the trachea.

Contrast examinations are not routinely performed. If symptoms are confusing or the diagnosis is not clear, a cautiously performed study may be helpful. Careful attention must be paid to avoid aspiration.

Many foreign bodies are radiolucent, and objects such as some fish bones, wood, plastic, or glass may not be seen by radiographs. Therefore, endoscopy is indicated in the patient with persistent symptoms even if the radiograph is unrevealing.

Treatment

Foreign body ingestion that causes severe respiratory symptoms is a medical emergency. In children older than 6 years of age, the Heimlich maneuver is useful, but in infants and young children the abdominal thrust of this maneuver may be dangerous, carrying the risk of rib fracture and injury to the abdominal organs. Instead, four blows to the back between the shoulder blades are recommended.

Once a foreign body ingestion has been diagnosed, the physician must decide if an intervention is necessary and, if so,

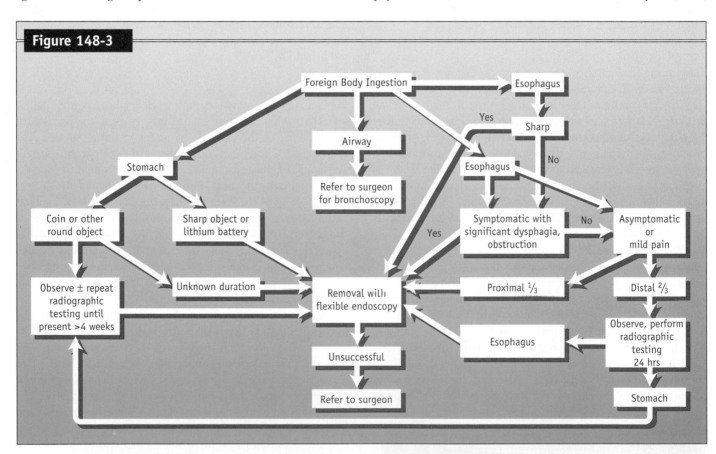

Figure 148-3

Management of foreign body ingestion.

Table 148-5. Commonly Swallowed Objects		
Coins	Toothpicks	Seashells
Safety pins	Disk batteries	Crayons
Straight pins	Tacks	Bones (fish, chicken)
Marbles	Screws	Bottletops

Table 148-6. Symptoms of a Foreign Body in the Esophagus	
Odynophagia	Cough
Dysphagia	Pulmonary aspiration
Sialorrhea	Choking
Feeding difficulty	Stridor

with what degree of urgency. The decision to remove a foreign body is based on the size, shape, and type of foreign body; its location; and the age and condition of the patient [26]. The techniques available also play a role. Objects that usually require removal are listed in Table 148-7. The timing of intervention is based on the perceived risks of aspiration or perforation. For example, urgent intervention is required for sharp objects or disk batteries lodged in the esophagus. If the object causes obstruction severe enough to prevent swallowing of secretions (sialorrhea), urgent removal is necessary. Children who show no evidence of high-grade obstruction and who are not in distress do not require emergency intervention, because spontaneous passage may occur [28]. Blunt, rounded objects, such as coins, located in the mid- or distal esophagus will pass spontaneously; therefore a 12- to 24-hour period of observation is recommended. Objects impacted at the cricopharyngeus or in the upper third of the esophagus are unlikely to pass and should be removed, especially if the child is symptomatic. Because it is known that complications such as mucosal erosion and perforation occur with prolonged impaction, no object should remain in the esophagus for more than 24 hours even if the child is asymptomatic [30].

Once a coin is in the stomach the family can be reassured. Stools should be examined, and if the coin has not passed, a repeat radiograph should be obtained. If the coin remains in the stomach for 4 weeks it should be removed. Dimes (17 mm) or pennies (18 mm) are rarely retained in the stomach, but quarters (24 mm) may be too large to pass the pylorus of the young child.

Disk or button batteries deserve special mention [31••]. They contain potassium hydroxide, and unsealed batteries may deliver caustic material directly to the mucosa. Button batteries impacted at any level of the esophagus should be removed emergently. Once they have entered the stomach they usually pass without difficulty. If the battery has not passed within 48 hours, a repeat abdominal film should be obtained. If the battery is still in the stomach it should be removed. Use of cathartics to hasten transit has not been studied systematically but appears unnecessary.

Sharp or elongated objects impacted in the esophagus should be removed. Once they enter the stomach they usually pass without problem. In adults it is suggested that objects longer than 7 cm be removed. The figure is proportionately shorter for children. General guidelines for removal are objects longer than 6 cm in older children and objects longer than 3 to 4 cm in infants and toddlers. Most smaller sharp objects pass spontaneously without problem. In situations in which the blunt end of the object is larger (eg, screws, tacks, nails), the object usually is propelled through the gut with the blunt end forward, reducing the risk of damage. Toothpicks and wires have a high risk of perforation, and removal is recommended.

Food bolus impaction is not common but is well reported in children. In contrast to impaction with coins and toys, food impaction happens more often in older children and adolescents than in infants and toddlers. Sausages and hot dogs are the most common offenders. As with adults, there is a high incidence of underlying esophageal disease, stricture, or dysmotility in these patients. If the obstruction is high grade, as evidenced by sialorrhea and chest pain, removal must be done urgently. If the patient is comfortable, a 12- to 24-hour observation period may be indicated [32]. Use of effervescent agents or papain (meat tenderizer) can cause perforation and is to be discouraged. Bougienage without visualization of the esophagus distal to the impaction is risky because of the high incidence of underlying pathology such as stricture. Once the food bolus passes, an esophagram or upper endoscopy should be done to evaluate for dysmotility or organic lesions, respectively.

Several techniques for removal are available, and the choice depends on the expertise of the clinician [33,34] (Table 148-8). The fluoroscopically controlled Foley catheter technique is safe and effective for blunt objects such as coins located in the hypopharynx or proximal one third of the esophagus [35,36]. The child is positioned prone and in Trendelenburg position. A deflated Foley catheter is passed beyond the foreign body, inflated, and removed, dragging the foreign body before it. It is especially effective in young children and when the impaction is less than 72 hours old. An attempt with this technique does not hamper subsequent attempts at endoscopic therapy.

Should endoscopy be required, flexible endoscopy is preferred over rigid endoscopy in most cases. It allows examination of the esophagus, stomach, and duodenum. Equipment is available to allow the retrieval of most ingested objects, including those in the stomach. Rigid esophagoscopy and direct laryngoscopy are preferred for sharp objects impacted in the hypopharynx and may be preferable for removal of objects such as razor blades from the esophagus.

Regardless of the technique used, maintenance of the airway is the prime consideration. As noted previously, the decision to use general anesthesia or conscious sedation depends on the age and cooperation of the patient, the experience of the endoscopist and support staff, and the nature of the object to be removed.

Table 148-7. Foreign Bodies That Require Removal

Coin proximally located in esophagus causing respiratory symptoms

Button battery in esophagus

Coin in distal esophagus > 24 h

Coin in stomach > 4 wk

Disk batteries in stomach > 2 d

Objects longer than 6 cm

Objects > 2.5 cm in diameter

Sharp, jagged, or irregular objects in esophagus

Razor blades

Table 148-8. Techniques for Removal of a Foreign Body

Technique	Object
Flexible endoscopy	Most commonly used
Rigid endoscopy	Certain sharp objects
Foley catheter	Round, recently ingested, proximally located objects
Bougienage	Coins and distally located objects

Sedation of children requires special training and monitoring. In children who have clinical evidence of respiratory distress or airway compression, general anesthesia with airway control is preferable. If the object is particularly long or sharp, or an overtube is necessary in a small child, the procedure is facilitated by general anesthesia and airway control. However, in most situations adequate patient cooperation and safety can be maintained using sedation alone.

Complications

Complications increase with the length of time a foreign body stays in the esophagus and most often occur in children in whom ingestion of the object has not been recognized [27,30]. Early complications include perforation and respiratory distress. Mucosal ulceration around the object is often seen but rarely causes a chronic problem [37]. Stricture formation after foreign body impaction has been described but is uncommon [38]. Blunt objects that are free but are retained in the stomach rarely cause problems. Foreign bodies retained in the esophagus for long periods of time have been known to cause perforation, with tracheoesophageal and even aorto-esophageal fistula [39].

As with corrosive exposure, prevention is most important. Toddlers need a protected environment as they explore. Modification of the design of toys and other products for use by children is an important part of this safety process. Parental education and avoidance of objects and foods that produce the greatest risk will further reduce injury.

■ REFERENCES

Recently published papers of particular interest have been highlighted as follows:
• Of interest
•• Of outstanding interest

1. Christesen HB: Caustic ingestion in adults. Epidemiology and prevention. *J Toxicol Clin Toxicol* 1994, 32:557–568.

2. Christesen HB: Epidemiology of caustic ingestion in children. *Acta Paediatr* 1994, 83:212–215.

3. Litovitz TL, Bailey KM, Schmitz BF, *et al.*: 1990 Annual report of the American Association of Poison Control Centers National Data Collection System. *Am J Emerg Med* 1991, 9:461–509.

4. Litovitz TL, Felberg L, White S, *et al.*: 1995 Annual report of the American Association of Poison Control Centers Toxic Exposure Surveillance System. *Am J Emerg Med* 1996, 14:487–537.

5. Harley EH, MD Collins: Liquid household bleach ingestion: a retrospective review. *Laryngoscope* 1997, 107:122–125.

6. Stenson K, Bruber B: Ingestion of caustic cosmetic products. *Otolaryngol Head Neck Surg* 1993, 109:821–825.

7. Forsen JW, Muntz HR: Hair relaxer ingestion: a new trend. *Ann Otol Rhinol Laryngol* 1993, 102:781–784.

8. Byrne WJ: Foreign bodies, bezoars, and caustic ingestion. *Gastrointest Endosc Clin North Am* 1994, 4:99–119.

9. Gryboski JD: Traumatic injury of the esophagus. In *Pediatric Gastrointestinal Disease*, edn 2. Edited by Walker WA, Durie PR, *et al.* St. Louis: Mosby; 1996.

10. Gaudreault P, Parent M, McGuigan MA, *et al.*: Predictability of esophageal injury from signs and symptoms: a study of caustic ingestion in 378 children. *Pediatrics* 1983, 71:767–770.

11. Previtera C, Giusti F, Guglielmi M: Predictive value of visible lesions (cheeks, lips, oropharynx) in suspected caustic ingestion: may endoscopy be omitted in completely negative pediatric patients? *Pediatric Emergency Care* 1990, 7:126–127.

12. Gorman RL, Khin-Maung-Gyi MT, Klein-Schwartz W, *et al.*: Initial symptoms as predictors of esophageal injury in alkaline corrosive ingestion. *Am J Emerg Med* 1992, 10:189–194.

13.• Christesen HB: Prediction of complications following unintentional caustic ingestion in children. Is endoscopy always necessary. *Acta Paediatr* 1995, 84:1177–1182.
In this paper the authors report that signs and symptoms do not always predict esophageal burn.

14.• Zargar SA, Kochhar R, Mehta S, *et al.*: The role of fiberoptic endoscopy in the management of corrosive ingestion and modified endoscopic classification of burns. *Gastrointest Endosc* 1991, 37:165–169.
This article provides a detailed and useful classification system that is predictive of complications.

15. Zargar SA, Kochhar R, Nagi B, *et al.*: Ingestion of strong corrosive alkalis: spectrum of injury to upper gastrointestinal tract and natural history. *Am J Gastroenterol* 1992, 87:337–341.

16. Oakes DD: Reconsidering the diagnosis and treatment of patients following ingestion of lye [editorial]. *J Clin Gastroenterol* 1995, 21:85–86.

17. Howell JM, Dalsey WC, Hartsell FW, *et al.*: Steroids for the treatment of corrosive esophageal injury: a statistical analysis of past studies. *Am J Emerg Med* 1992, 10:421–425.

18.•• Anderson KD, Rouse TM, Randolph JG, *et al.*: A controlled trial of corticosteroids in children with corrosive injury of the esophagus. *N Engl J Med* 1990, 323:637–640.
In this well controlled study of 131 children, no statistically significant benefit was seen.

19.• Bautista A, Varela R, Villanueva A, *et al.*: Effects of prednisolone and dexamethasone in children with alkali burns of the oesophagus. *Eur J Pediatr Surg* 1996 6:198–203.
In this report, data are presented that patients treated with dexamethasone have fewer complications than those given prednisolone or no treatment.

20. Cadranel S, DiLorenzo C, Rodesch P, *et al.*: Caustic ingestion and esophageal function. *J Pediatr Gastroenterol Nutr* 1990, 10:164–168.

21. Dantas RO, Mamede RC: Esophageal motility in patients with esophageal caustic injury. *Am J Gastroenterol* 1996, 91:1157–1161.

22. Bautista A, Varela R, Villanueva A, *et al.*: Motor function of the esophagus after caustic burn. *Eur J Pediatr Surg* 1996, 6:204–207.

23. Berkovits RN, Bos CE, Wijburg FA, *et al.*: Caustic injury of the oesophagus: sixteen years experience and introduction of a new model oesophageal stent. *J Laryngol Otol* 1996, 110:1141–1145.

24. Nuutinen M, Uhari M, Karvala T, *et al.*: Consequences of caustic ingestion in children. *Acta Paediatr* 1994, 83:1200–1205.

25.• Conners GP, Chamberlain JM, Weiner PR: Pediatric coin ingestion: a home based survey. *Am J Emerg Med* 1995, 13:638–640.
Questionnaire data suggest that most coin ingestions go unreported and cause no problems.

26. Guideline for the management of ingested foreign bodies: American Society of Gastrointestinal Endoscopy. *Gastrointest Endosc* 1995, 42:622–625.

27. Paul RI, Christoffel KK, Binns HJ, *et al.*: Foreign body ingestions in children: risk of complication varies with site of initial health care contact. *Pediatrics* 1993, 91:121–127.

28. Conners GP, Chamberlain JM, Ochrinlager DW: Symptoms and spontaneous passage of esophageal coins. *Arch Pediatr Adolesc Med* 1995, 149:36–39.

29. Macpherson RI, Hill JG, Othersen HB, *et al.*: Esophageal foreign bodies in children: diagnosis, treatment and complications. *AJR Am J Roentgenol* 1996, 166:919–924.

30. Reilly J, Thompson J, MacArthur C, *et al.*: Pediatric aerodigestive foreign body injuries are complications related to timelines of diagnosis. *Laryngoscope* 1997, 107:17–20.

31.•• Litovitz T, Schmitz BF: Ingestion of cylindrical and button batteries: An analysis of 2,382 cases. *Pediatrics* 1992, 89:747–757.
This paper represents an exhaustive study of a large number of cases. Conservative management is suggested.

32. Conners GP, Chamberlain JM, Oscksenschlager DW: Conservative management of pediatric distal esophageal coins. *J Emerg Med* 1996, 14:723–726.

33. Dokler ML, Bradshaw J, Mollitti DL, *et al.*: Selective management of pediatric esophageal foreign bodies. *Am Surg* 1995, 61:132–134.

34. Emslander HC, Bonadio W, Klatzo M: Efficiency of esophageal bougienage by emergency physicians in pediatric coin ingestion. *Am Emerg Med* 1996, 6:726–729.

35. Harned RK, Strain JD, Hay TC, *et al.*: Esophageal foreign bodies: safety and efficiency of Foley catheter extraction of coins. *AJR Am J Roentgenol* 1997, 168:443–446.

36. Schunk JE, Harrison AM, Corneli HM, Nixon GW: Fluoroscopic Foley catheter removal of esophageal foreign bodies in children: experience with 415 episodes. *Pediatrics* 1994, 94:709–714.

37. Bonadio WA, Emslander H, Milner D, *et al.*: Esophageal mucosal changes in children with acutely ingested coins in the esophagus. *Pediatr Emerg Care* 1994, 10:333–334.

38. Doolin EJ: Esophageal stricture: an uncommon complication of foreign bodies. *Ann Otol Rhinol Laryngol* 1993, 102:863–866.

39. Tucker JG, Kim HH, Lucas GW: Esophageal perforation caused by coin ingestion. *South Med J* 1994, 87:269:208–272.

149 Developmental Abnormalities of the Stomach

Stephen M. Borowitz

▮▮▮ DEVELOPMENT OF THE STOMACH

The primitive gastrointestinal tract is typically divided into the foregut, midgut, and hindgut. During the 5th week of gestation, the foregut dilates in a fusiform fashion to give rise to the primitive stomach. During the following 2 weeks, the primitive stomach makes a 90° clockwise rotation around its longitudinal axis, resulting in the left side facing anteriorly and the right side facing posteriorly. As a result, the left vagus nerve innervates the anterior gastric wall and the right vagus nerve innervates the posterior gastric wall. Because the stomach is attached to the posterior and anterior walls of the embryo by the dorsal and ventral mesogastrium, this rotation results in the formation of the omental bursa. During this time, there is differential growth of the anterior and posterior walls of the primitive stomach, which gives rise to the greater and lesser curvatures. The abdominal esophagus gradually elongates, and by the 4th month of gestation it has bent nearly 90° to enter the stomach through a funnel-shaped expansion [1] (Fig. 149-1).

Microscopic rugae and the circular muscular layer first can be identified in the fetal stomach during the 8th week of gestation. The longitudinal layer of muscle appears between weeks 8 and 10, and the oblique layer develops between weeks 12 and 14. The pyloric ring is well developed between the 4th and 5th months of gestation. Although we have a good understanding of the neuromuscular development of the stomach, little is known about fetal gastric motility.

Glandular pits first appear along the lesser curvature at approximately 6 weeks of gestation, and by week 10 they are present throughout the body of the stomach and the pyloric channel. Parietal cells are first recognizable at 11 weeks, and chief cells appear during the 12th week of gestation. Pepsin can first be identified in the gastric mucosa during the last half of the 6th month, but neither pepsin nor hydrochloric acid appears in the stomach contents until near term. Although stomach contents are nearly neutral at birth, gastric acid increases rapidly within several hours. (This increase occurs in the absence of food.)

▮▮▮ CONGENITAL MICROGASTRIA
Anatomy and Pathophysiology

Congenital microgastria is characterized by a small tubular stomach, megaesophagus, and incomplete gastric rotation [2]. Although the cause of congenital microgastria is uncertain, it is usually thought to result from a failure of the stomach to become differentiated from the primitive foregut [3]. In most reported cases, the stomach is an incompletely formed tube lined with normal gastric mucosa [4,5]. The total cell mass of the stomach is significantly reduced, which may lead to decreased production of gastric acid and intrinsic factor [4,5].

Clinical Features
Symptoms

Congenital microgastria is an extremely rare anomaly, with fewer than 30 cases reported in the medical literature. This disorder has rarely been observed in isolation. Asplenia has been observed in approximately two thirds of the reported cases [4,5], and a variety of other anomalies also have been described, including malrotation, situs inversus, asplenia, micrognathia, radial and ulnar hypoplasia, and hypoplastic nails [2,4,5].

Most affected infants present with severe feeding intolerance beginning at birth [2,4,5]. As a consequence of severe gastroesophageal reflux, these infants usually experience persistent vomiting and growth failure. Recurrent episodes of aspiration and pneumonia may develop as a result of a dilated esophagus and incompetent lower esophageal sphincter. Some infants suffer from chronic diarrhea as a result of very rapid gastric emptying or dumping syndrome [6].

Diagnosis

The diagnosis of microgastria is established radiographically. On upper gastrointestinal (GI) series, a small, fusiform stomach is identified in the midline without any apparent curvature or rotation. The fundus, body, and antrum generally cannot be distinguished [3]. Typically, the distal esophagus is very dilated (megaesophagus), and the lower esophageal sphincter is incompetent, resulting in very prominent gastroesophageal reflux [4,5].

Treatment

Most infants with congenital microgastria have been managed with either prolonged parenteral nutrition or some form of continuous gastrostomy or jejunostomy feedings. More recently, some authors have reported good results following the creation of an artificial food reservoir termed a Hunt-Lawrence pouch [4].

CONGENITAL GASTRIC OUTLET OBSTRUCTION

Anatomy and Pathophysiology

Atresia of the stomach with extensive obliteration of the lumen is an extraordinarily rare anomaly.

More often, atresia or stenosis of the stomach results when a membranous diaphragm (pyloric membrane, or an antral web 1 cm proximal to the pylorus) obstructs the lumen [7]. Typically, the obstructing membrane is composed of mucosa with or without submucosa and is located within several centimeters of the pyloroduodenal junction [8]. Very thin membranes may perforate spontaneously from the pressure of gastric contents and leave an annular stenosis or narrowing [8].

The reason for development of these membranes remains uncertain. It had been suggested that they were the result of incomplete recanalization of the embryonic foregut [9], but more recent studies have shown that, unlike the development of the esophagus and small intestine, epithelial perforation does not occur during gastric development. It has, therefore, been suggested that these membranous diaphragms develop as a result of excessive endodermal proliferation [10].

In older infants and adults, rather than being congenital, a membrane may be acquired from the alternate healing and expansion of gastric ulcers [11].

Clinical Features

Symptoms

Congenital gastric outlet obstruction is an extremely rare disorder and is far less common than atresia or stenosis in other portions of the intestinal tract [6,8]. Approximately 30% of affected infants have other anomalies, but no consistent pattern of malformations has been identified [7]. Epidermolysis bullosa has been associated with congenital gastric outlet obstruction (Fig. 149-2) [12]. There are several reports of familial gastric outlet obstruction that appears to be inherited as an autosomal recessive trait [12,13].

The presence of a congenital gastric obstruction may be suggested by a history of maternal polyhydramnios [7]. Infants with congenital gastric outlet obstruction present with persistent, nonbilious vomiting that begins with the first feeding. They may develop progressive distention of the upper abdomen as a result of gastric distention. Rarely, gastric perforation develops [6]. Infants with incomplete gastric outlet obstruction may experience episodic symptoms of obstruction as a result of inflammation and edema around the central orifice of the membrane [6].

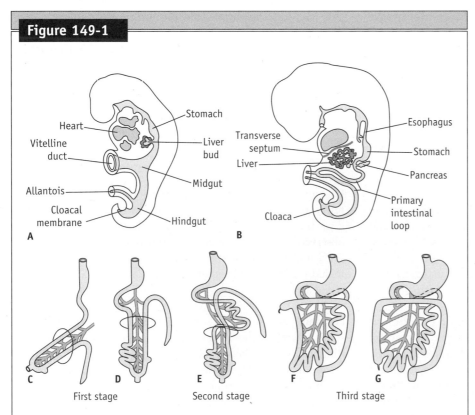

Figure 149-1

Normal embryological development of the stomach and intestines. **A**, At 25 days' gestation, the stomach appears as a fusiform dilation of the foregut. **B**, At 32 days' gestation, the beginnings of the greater and lesser curvatures of the stomach can be identified. **C**, At 6 weeks' gestation, there is little or no rotation of either the stomach or intestine. **D**, At 8 weeks' gestation, the stomach has begun to rotate clockwise along its longitudinal axis while the intestine has begun to rotate counterclockwise. **E**, At 9 weeks' gestation, the stomach has nearly completed its rotation and the pylorus has begun to develop. **F**, At 11 weeks' gestation, the stomach and intestine have nearly completed their rotations, and the greater and lesser curvatures of the stomach are well established. **G**, At 12 weeks' gestation, the stomach and intestine are completely rotated, and the abdominal esophagus is beginning to elongate to enter the stomach through a funnel-shaped extension.

Heart, Stomach, Vitelline duct, Liver bud, Allantois, Cloacal membrane, Midgut, Hindgut

Transverse septum, Liver, Esophagus, Stomach, Pancreas, Primary intestinal loop, Cloaca

A   B   C   D   E   F   G

First stage   Second stage   Third stage

Diagnosis and Therapy

Plain films of the abdomen demonstrate an air- and fluid-filled stomach, with no air in the duodenum or more distal portions of the gastrointestinal tract (*ie*, single bubble). The onset of vomiting immediately after birth distinguishes congenital gastric outlet obstruction from hypertrophic pyloric stenosis, which rarely develops before the second week of life. A slender radiolucent line running perpendicular to the long axis of the gastric antrum may be seen on an upper GI series; however, gastrointestinal endoscopy should be used to corroborate the diagnosis [7].

Once the obstruction has been identified, prompt surgical intervention is warranted. The actual surgical procedure employed depends on the specific abnormality; however, essentially, the surgery consists of excision of the obstructing membrane or atretic segment, combined with pyloroplasty, gastroduodenostomy, or gastrojejunostomy [3].

More recently, there have been reports of endoscopic balloon dilation or transection of the membrane [14–16].

■ CONGENITAL DIVERTICULUM OF THE STOMACH

Anatomy and Pathophysiology

Most congenital diverticula of the stomach are true diverticula involving all layers of the stomach wall, but mucosal herniation may occur through congenitally aplastic areas of the muscularis. Most congenital gastric diverticula arise along the posterior wall of the stomach, approximately 2 cm below the junction of the esophagus and stomach and 3 cm from the lesser curvature [17] (Fig. 149-3). Most gastric diverticula are less than 4 cm in length. Occasionally it is difficult to distinguish larger diverticula from communicating duplications [6].

In most cases, the etiology of a gastric diverticulum is obscure. A localized region of muscle weakness along the posterior wall of the stomach has never been identified. In most cases, the gastric diverticulum is an isolated finding without any other abnormalities either inside or outside of the gastrointestinal tract.

Clinical Features

Symptoms

The absolute prevalence of gastric diverticula is difficult to ascertain, because they often go undetected or are found incidentally during gastrointestinal radiographic or endoscopic procedures, during abdominal surgery, or at autopsy. Diverticula are less common in the stomach than elsewhere in the gastrointestinal tract and account for approximately 3% of gastrointestinal diverticula [6]. Only a very small minority of gastric diverticula are identified during childhood or young adulthood. Most often, they are detected during the fifth decade of life [17].

Between 66% and 85% of gastric diverticula are not associated with symptoms [6]. When symptoms are present, the patient may experience epigastric or lower chest pain, with or without vomiting or indigestion.

Diagnosis and Therapy

The diagnosis of a gastric diverticulum is usually made radiographically. The diverticulum appears as a smoothly rounded, sharply defined, mobile pouch that often contains an air bubble above the barium contrast medium. Emptying is usually but not always delayed [6]. Endoscopically, the diverticulum appears as a round hole with sharply defined edges. Active contractions of the diverticular mouth may be seen. There usually is no local alteration in the pattern of rugae.

The diverticulum must be distinguished from hypertrophied gastric folds or some form of ulceration. Although ulcers are often found within diverticula, there does not appear to be any association between gastric diverticula and other forms of gastric disease.

■ GASTRODUODENAL DUPLICATIONS

Anatomy and Pathophysiology

Gastric duplications are closed, spherical or tubular cystic structures that are typically lined with gastric epithelium. The cyst is contiguous with the gastric wall and is surrounded by smooth muscle [18]. Most often, gastric duplications develop along the greater curvature of the stomach [18,19]. They may be associated with enterogenous cysts in the posterior mediastinum, the esophagus, or the duodenum [18,19]. The cysts are usually less than 12 cm in diameter, and in most cases they do not communicate with the remainder of the intestinal tract [18]. When a communication is identified, it may enter directly into the stomach (Fig. 149-4) as well as into the duodenum or into a Meckel's diverticulum [6,18,19].

Figure 149-2

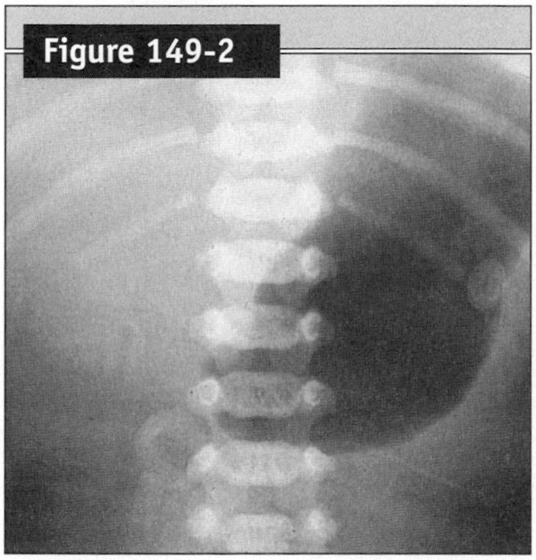

Abdominal radiograph taken of a six year old child with epidermolysis bullosa demonstrating gastric outlet obstruction.

Figure 149-3

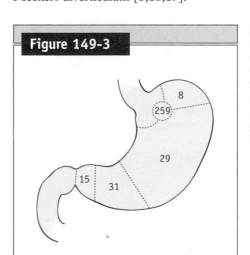

Location of 342 diverticula of the stomach, 76% of which were located along the posterior wall of the upper portion of the stomach. (*From* Palmer [34].)

Clinical Features

Symptoms

Gastroduodenal duplications are rare lesions, accounting for less than 10% of all gastrointestinal duplications [6]. Fifty percent of children with gastric duplications have additional congenital anomalies. Most commonly there is a cyst of the esophagus or duodenum; however, vertebral anomalies and ectopic pancreas also have been observed [18,19]. Several reports have emphasized the association between gastric duplications and pulmonary sequestration [20,21].

Gastric duplications typically are diagnosed during childhood, with more than half diagnosed during the first year of life. Vomiting is the most common complaint and is present in approximately 60% of cases. The vomiting usually results from partial or complete obstruction of the gastric antrum. In nearly two thirds of cases there is a palpable abdominal mass. Other common complaints include chronic or recurrent abdominal pain, weight loss, and growth failure. Hematemesis, melena, or both are seen in approximately 30% of affected children. Rarely, a large duplication cyst may perforate secondary to ulceration caused by stasis of gastric enzymes and hydrochloric acid within the cyst [22]. Large noncommunicating duplications may compress the adjacent stomach and lead to gastritis or peptic ulceration. When there is coexisting gastric and pancreatic duplication, pancreatitis or erosion into a contiguous viscus may occur [23].

Diagnosis and Therapy

In most cases, the diagnosis of a gastric duplication is suspected when an extrinsic defect is identified along the greater curvature of the stomach during an upper GI series. If the cyst is more distal, it may distort the pylorus or duodenal channel and delay gastric emptying. An abdominal ultrasound or CT scan may aid in defining the anatomy.

In most cases, the treatment of choice is excision of the cyst, either by dissection from a common wall or by excision of the cyst within a margin of normal stomach with primary closure [18]. In 10% of patients the cyst perforates into the peritoneal space or fistulizes into adjacent structures. Overall mortality is less than 3% [18].

■ GASTRIC VOLVULUS

Anatomy and Pathophysiology

Gastric volvulus occurs when there is laxity or absence of the normal stomach attachments provided by the gastrophrenic or gastrocolic ligaments (Fig. 149-5). Distention of the stomach with gas or fluid, or displacement by other organs, may serve as precipitating factors [24]. The volvulus can be either organoaxial, along the stomach's long axis (Fig. 149-6), or mesenteroaxial, around a line that is perpendicular to the line joining the cardia and pylorus (Fig. 149-7). Mesenteroaxial volvulus appears to be the most common form of gastric volvulus [25]. Mixed forms of volvulus also occur.

Clinical Features

Symptoms

Gastric volvulus is a rare disorder, with fewer than 100 cases having been reported in the medical literature [25,26]. It is predominantly a disorder of childhood, with most cases reported being in children younger than 5 years of age [25]. Typically, there is an abrupt onset of severe epigastric pain, which is soon followed by gastric distention and nonproductive retching. In infants, this condition may be manifest as recurrent attacks of screaming or inconsolable crying [3]. Seventy percent of affected children demonstrate Borchardt's classic triad of acute painful

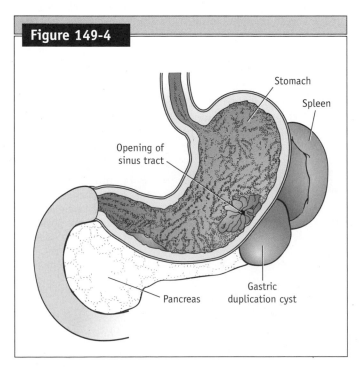

Figure 149-4

Gastric duplication cyst originating along the greater curvature of the stomach with a communication directly into the stomach.

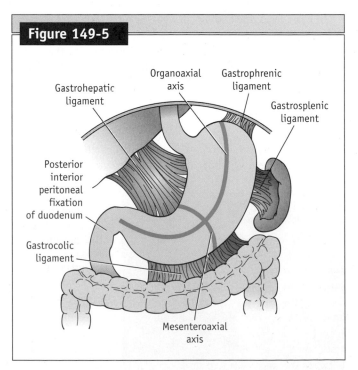

Figure 149-5

Normal ligamentous attachments of the stomach include the gastrophrenic, gastrosplenic, gastrocolic, and gastrohepatic ligaments. The stomach is anchored inferiorly to the descending portion of the duodenum.

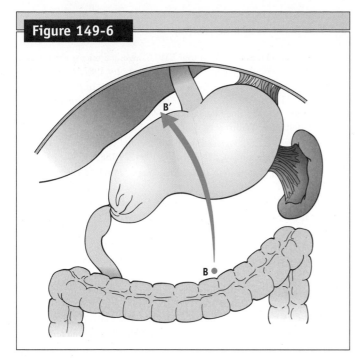

Diagram of an organoaxial gastric volvulus. Due to laxity or absence of the gastrocolic ligament, the stomach rotates along its long (horizontal) axis.

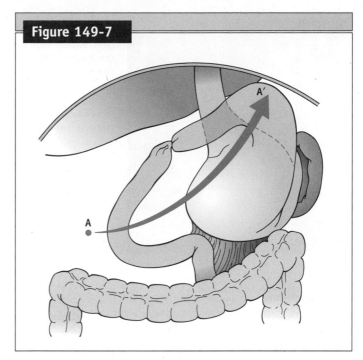

Diagram of a mesenteroaxial gastric volvulus. Due to laxity or absence of the gastrocolic or gastrohepatic ligaments, or both, the stomach rotates along its short (vertical) axis.

distention of the stomach, inability to pass a nasogastric tube, and nonproductive retching. Other symptoms can include chest pain, dysphagia, dyspnea, dyspepsia, and borborygmi [25].

Diagnosis and Therapy
The diagnosis of acute gastric volvulus usually is suggested by plain abdominal radiographs. There is massive dilation of the stomach, with paucity of gas throughout the remainder of the stomach. The presence of the volvulus usually is confirmed with an upper GI series. With a mesoaxial volvulus, the entire stomach may appear to be inverted, whereas with an organoaxial volvulus there may be conical narrowing of the gastric antrum and pyloric obstruction [3,25].

Acute gastric volvulus is a true surgical emergency. Nonoperative mortality approaches 80% [25]. After the stomach is decompressed with a nasogastric tube or an emergent gastrostomy, it is fixed by either a permanent gastrostomy or gastropexy to prevent any future recurrences [27].

▆ HETEROTOPIC PANCREATIC TISSUE IN THE STOMACH
Anatomy and Pathophysiology
Heterotopic pancreatic tissue in the stomach is often termed a *pancreatic rest*. Pancreatic rests are most often found incidentally during gastrointestinal radiographic or endoscopic procedures, during surgery, or at autopsy. Although pancreatic tissue has been identified throughout the stomach, it most commonly is identified in the gastric antrum [28] (Fig. 149-8). Pancreatic rests range from less than 1 mm to 5 cm in diameter, with most between 0.6 and 3 cm in diameter [29]. The majority of identified lesions are limited to the submucosa and only rarely extend into the muscularis. Larger lesions are characteristically smooth round masses that occasionally demonstrate central umbilication

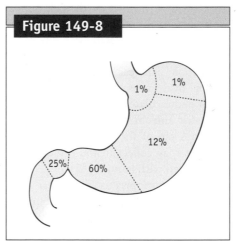

Intragastric distribution of pancreatic heterotopic tissue in 174 patients. 85% of cases were located within the pylorus or antrum. (*From* Palmer [35].)

[29]; the umbilication represents the aborted pancreatic duct. Histologically, the lesions resemble normal pancreatic tissue with identifiable acini, ducts, and islet cells.

The mechanism by which pancreatic tissue ends up in the stomach remains uncertain. Histologic investigations have suggested two potential etiologies [30]: either fetal pancreatic tissue migrates from the dorsal pancreatic bud into the distal stomach, or there is defective differentiation of fetal gastric tissue into pancreatic tissue.

Clinical Features
Symptoms
Pancreatic rests are the most common congenital defect involving the stomach; as many as 2% of the population may have ectopic pancreatic tissue within the stomach [29,31,32]. In most cases, no symptoms can be attributed to pancreatic rests [29]. Some patients, however, appear to experience intermittent nausea and

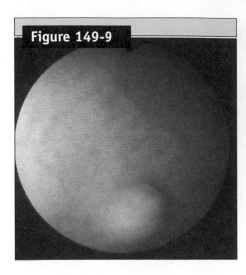

Figure 149-9

Endoscopic view of heterotopic pancreatic tissue in the gastric antrum. The lesion is limited to the submucosa and has the characteristic smooth, round appearance.

epigastric pain [31–33]. Large lesions in the gastric antrum may result in intermittent obstruction, and, even more rarely, overlying ulceration may result in hemorrhage. There have been isolated reports of gastrointestinal obstruction, recurrent vomiting with growth failure, hemorrhage, and intussusception associated with pancreatic heterotopia [33].

Diagnosis and Therapy

In most cases, pancreatic rests are identified incidentally during an upper GI series, gastrointestinal endoscopy, or abdominal surgery. They do not appear to be associated with any other congenital abnormalities.

Radiographically, the ectopic pancreas usually appears as a small, smooth, round, or oval mass with a broad base. Occasionally, it may appear pedunculated. Most commonly, the mass is identified in the gastric antrum along the posterior wall of the stomach within 3 to 6 cm of the pylorus. In approximately half of cases, contrast may collect in the center of the mass, representing the duct filled with barium [31].

Endoscopically, pancreatic heterotopias usually appear as an irregularly surfaced yellowish mass, often with a central umbilication representing the orifice of a duct [31] (Fig. 149-9).

The mass is generally broad-based and appears to project into the lumen of the stomach. On some occasions, the ductular orifice may be sufficiently large to be confused with a diverticulum.

In most cases, pancreatic rests are incidental findings, and no specific intervention is warranted once the diagnosis is established. In the small group of patients with symptoms attributable to pancreatic heterotopia, endoscopic or surgical resection of the ectopic pancreatic tissue is usually curative.

■ REFERENCES

1. Langman J: Special embryology. In *Medical Embryology*. Baltimore: Williams & Wilkins; 1975:282–290.

2. Hoehner JC, Kimura K, Soper RT: Congenital microgastria. *J Pediatr Surg* 1994, 29:1591–1593.

3. Dodge JA: The stomach. In *Pediatric Gastroenterology and Hepatology*, edn 3. Edited by Gracey M, Burke V. Oxford: Blackwell Scientific Publications; 1993:77–110.

4. Velasco AL, Holcomb GW, Templeton JM, Ziegler MM: Management of congenital microgastria. *J Pediatr Surg* 1990, 25:192–197.

5. Aintablian NH, Slim MS, Antour BW: Congenital microgastria. Case report and review of the literature. *Pediatr Surg Int* 1987, 2:307–310.

6. Shandalakis JE, Gray SW, Ricketts R: The stomach. In *Embryology for Surgeons: The Embryological Basis for the Treatment of Congenital Anomalies*, edn 2. Edited by Skandalakis JE, Gray SW, Rickets RR, *et al.* Baltimore: Williams & Wilkins; 1994:150–183.

7. Lugo-Vicente H: Congenital (prepyloric) antral membrane: prenatal diagnosis and treatment. *J Pediatr Surg* 1994, 29:1589–1590.

8. Conway N: Pyloric antral mucosal diaphragm. *Br Med J* 1965, 1:970–971.

9. Mitchell KG, McGowan A, Smith DC, *et al.*: Pyloric diaphragm, antral web, congenital antral membrane—a surgical rarity? *Br J Surg* 1979, 66:572–574.

10. Bell MJ, Ternberg JL, McAlister W, *et al.*: Antral diaphragm—a cause of gastric outlet obstruction in infants and children. *J Pediatr* 1977, 90:196–202.

11. Spitz L, Zail SS: Serum gastrin levels in congenital hypertrophic pyloric stenosis. *J Pediatr Surg* 1976, 11:33–35.

12. Malhem RE, Salem G, Mishalany H, *et al.*: Pyloroduodenal atresia: a report of three families with several similarly affected children. *Pediatr Radiology* 1975, 3:1–5.

13. Olson L, Grotte G: Congenital pyloric atresia: report of a familial occurrence. *J Pediatr Surg* 1976, 11:181–184.

14. Bill MJ, Ternberg JL, Keating JP, *et al.*: Prepyloric gastric antral web: a puzzling epidemic. *J Pediatr Surg* 1978, 13:307–313.

15. Tunell WP, Smith EI: Antral web in infancy. *J Pediatr Surg* 1980, 15:152–155.

16. Brandt, Boley, Daum: *Dig Dis* 1978, 23:

17. Palmer ED: Gastric diverticula. *Surg Obstet Gynecol* 1951, 92:417–428.

18. Wieczorek RL, Seidman I, Ransom JH, *et al.*: Congenital duplication of the stomach: case report and review of the English literature. *Am J Gastroenterol* 1984, 79:597–602.

19. Bartels RJ: Duplication of the stomach: case report and review of the literature. *Ann Surg* 1976, 33:747–748.

20. Braffman B, Keller R, Gendal ES, Finkel SI: Subdiaphragmatic bronchogenic cyst with gastric communication. *Gastrointestinal Radiol* 1988, 13:309–311.

21. Stanley P, Vachon L, Gilsanz V: Pulmonary sequestration with congenital gastroesophageal communication: report of two cases. *Pediatr Radiol* 1985, 15:343–345.

22. Sieunarine K, Manmohansingh E: Gastric duplication cysts presenting as an acute abdomen in a child. *J Pediatr Surg* 1988, 24:1152.

23. Rosenlund ML, Schnaufer L: Gastric duplications presenting as cyclical abdominal pain. *Clin Pediatr* 1978, 17:747–748.

24. Cameron AEP, Howard ER: Gastric volvulus in childhood. *J Pediatr Surg* 1987, 22:944–947.

25. Miller DL, Pasquale MD, Seneca RP, Hodin E: Gastric volvulus in the pediatric population. *Arch Surg* 1991, 126:1146–1149.

26. Senocak ME, Buyukpamukcu N, Hicsonmez A: Chronic gastric volvulus in children—a ten year experience. *Z Kinderchir* 1990, 45:159–163.

27. Idowu J, Aitken DR, Georgeson KE: Gastric volvulus in the newborn. *Arch Surg* 1980, 115:1046–1049.

28. Palmer ED: Benign intramural tumors of the stomach: a review with special reference to gross pathology. *Medicine* 1951, 30:81–96.

29. Lai ECS, Tompkins RK: Heterotopic pancreas: review of a 26 year experience. *Am J Surg* 1986, 151:697–700.

30. Yamagiwa H, Onishi N, Nishii M: Heterotopic pancreas of the stomach: histogenesis and immunohistochemistry. *Acta Pathologica Japonica* 1992, 42:249–254.

31. Thoeni RF, Gedgaudas RK: Ectopic pancreas: usual and unusual features. *Gastrointest Radiol* 1980, 5:37–42.

32. Dolan RV, ReMine WH, Docerty MB: The fate of heterotopic pancreatic tissue: a study of 212 cases. *Arch Surg* 1974, 109:762–765.

33. Mollitt DL, Golladay S: Symptomatic gastroduodenal pancreatic rest in children. *J Pediatr Surg* 1984, 19:449–450.

34. Palmer ED: Gastric diverticula. *Surg Obstet Gynecol* 1951, 43:32–433.

35. Palmer ED: Benign intramural tumors of the stomach: a review with special reference to gross pathology. *Medicine* 1951, 30:81–86.

150 Neonatal Intestinal Obstruction
Kenneth Kenigsberg

Obstruction of the intestine in the newborn is a serious condition. Error or delay in diagnosis or treatment may lead to death, whereas timely management usually is curative.

The signs of intestinal obstruction are distention and vomiting. Presentation depends on three factors: 1) the level of the blockage; 2) the fetal age at which the blockage develops; and 3) the cause of the blockage.

■ DUODENAL OBSTRUCTION

Anatomy
Early in the development of the fetus, the duodenum is a solid rod of cells. Then tubulation occurs and a passage from stomach to small bowel is formed. If this tubulation is incomplete, the pathway from stomach to small bowel is completely blocked, a condition called *atresia* or significantly narrowed, a condition called *stenosis* [1]. Incomplete tubulation is the usual cause of duodenal obstruction. In one third of cases, the obstruction is caused by a ring of pancreas that completely encircles the duodenum. This ring is called the *annular pancreas* [2].

Pathophysiology
Obstruction of the duodenum caused by atresia, stenosis, or annular pancreas usually occurs distal to the ampulla of Vater. Therefore, the regurgitation or vomitus is bile stained. In a small number of duodenal obstructions, the block is proximal to the ampulla and the vomitus is clear [2]. The part of the gastrointestinal (GI) tract that is distended is the bowel proximal to the blockage—the first part of the duodenum and the stomach. Occasionally, distention of the stomach is so great that it makes the upper abdominal wall protrude (Fig. 150-1). Because the blockage occurs early in fetal development and is high in the GI tract, the fetus can swallow and absorb very little of the amniotic fluid. Therefore, there is increased fluid in the amniotic sac, a condition called *hydramnios*, which often can be seen prenatally by sonography. Approximately one fourth of all duodenal obstructions occur in children with Down syndrome [3].

Diagnosis
Diagnosis can be made by prenatal sonography or by a plain radiograph of the abdomen, which shows a double bubble created by the air-filled distended stomach and duodenum (Fig. 150-2).

Treatment
Duodenal obstruction does not constitute an emergency. The baby should be hydrated, the stomach should be decompressed, and other systems should be evaluated for congenital anomalies. The most serious concomitant anomaly is cardiac disease. The definitive repair of duodenal obstruction consists of bypassing the duodenal obstruction (atresia, stenosis, or annular pancreas) via a shunt between the proximal distended duodenum and the collapsed distal bowel as close to the obstruction as possible.

Prognosis
The shunt around the duodenal blockage, a duodenoduodenostomy, corrects the GI pathophysiology, and these children thrive [1,2].

■ JEJUNOILEAL ATRESIA

Anatomy
Blockage of the small intestine can occur anywhere between the ligament of Treitz and the ileocecal valve. Small bowel atresia is not caused by failure of tubulation, as is the case in duodenal atresia. Rather, it is due to an in utero vascular accident such as thrombosis, which leads to sterile necrosis and atresia or stenosis of the involved bowel. The atresia often is associated with volvulus, intussusception, or herniation of some part of the bowel [4].

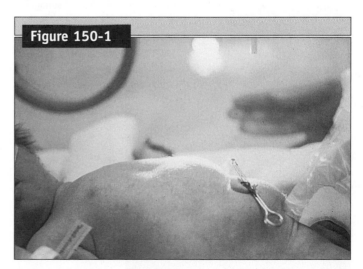

Figure 150-1

Distention of upper abdomen indicates duodenal atresia.

A vascular accident may be caused by maternal cocaine ingestion [5]. The atresia may be high or low, single or multiple, with necrosis of nearly all of the small bowel or only a small portion.

Pathophysiology

If the obstruction is high in the jejunum, the fetus swallows little of the amniotic fluid, and, consequently, the mother has hydramnios. If the obstruction is in the distal ileum, on the other hand, there may be no hydramnios. Again, the level of the obstruction determines the area of bowel distention. A high jejunal obstruction may cause considerable distention of the duodenum with collapse of the rest of the small bowel.

Diagnosis

Prenatal sonography usually shows dilated proximal bowel and hydramnios (Fig. 150-3). At birth, the presenting signs of jejunoileal atresia are bilious vomiting and abdominal distention.

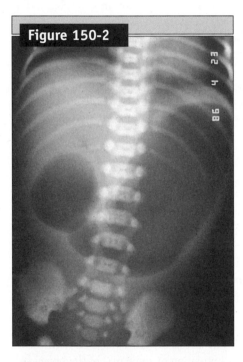

Figure 150-2

Radiograph shows "double bubble" characteristic of duodenal atresia.

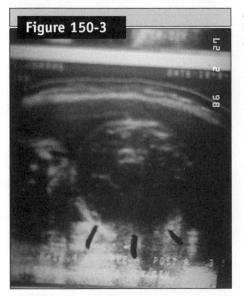

Figure 150-3

Antenatal sonogram shows jejunoileal atresia.

Bilious vomiting tends to occur earlier in high obstructions, whereas abdominal distention is predominant with lower obstructions. Nasogastric aspiration obtains more than 25 mL of bilious material, and a plain film of the abdomen shows multiple abdominal distended loops of bowel and an airless distal abdomen (Fig. 150-4). No further studies are necessary to make the diagnosis.

Treatment

The goal of therapy is to restore bowel continuity and sufficient mucosal surface to allow normal digestion. As is the case with obstruction of the duodenum, small bowel atresia is not an emergency. Other systems should be evaluated, and intravenous fluids should be started. The goal of surgery is to restore bowel continuity with an end-to-end anastomosis. This procedure often requires bowel tapering to overcome the disparity between the distended bowel proximal to the obstruction and the collapsed bowel distal to the obstruction. The entire length of small bowel must be examined to exclude other sites of obstruction.

Prognosis

The outcome is excellent in infants with sufficient length of small bowel. Occasionally there is such extensive loss of bowel that a short-gut syndrome results, but this condition is much more common after midgut volvulus (See Chapter 164).

■ MALROTATION AND MIDGUT VOLVULUS

Anatomy

At the 6th week of fetal development, the intestine, which is growing more rapidly than the coelom, is squeezed into the umbilical cord. By week 10, the abdominal cavity has grown sufficiently to contain the intestine. As the intestine returns to the abdomen, its coils are laid down and anchored by the base of the mesentery in a specific pattern that prevents kinking or twisting [6].

Pathophysiology

Ordinarily, the small bowel mesentery becomes fixed along the longest axis in the abdomen, from the left upper quadrant to the

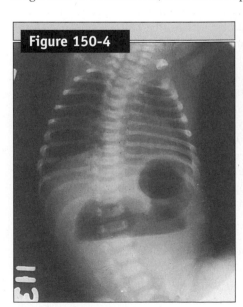

Figure 150-4

Flat film radiograph shows high small bowel atresia with multiple fluid levels and a distal airless abdomen.

right lower quadrant. With this arrangement, the small bowel falls into gentle folds along the greatest diameter in the abdomen. If the returning bowel does not follow the prescribed course, the mesentery base may be very narrow, and the bowel suspended from it may be prone to twisting.

In addition, the cecum, eager to cement itself in the right lower quadrant, sends out adhesive strands (Ladd's bands) that may cross and obstruct the duodenum when the bowel is malrotated. The cecum misses the right lower quadrant and therefore embraces the duodenum.

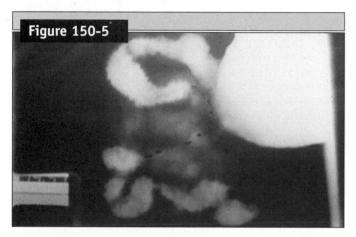

Figure 150-5

Upper GI radiograph shows malrotation. The fourth portion of the duodenum does not cross the spine from right to left.

Diagnosis

The main symptom of malrotation is bilious vomiting, which indicates obstruction of the upper small bowel by Ladd's bands, volvulus of the intestine, or both. If rectal bleeding also is present, it indicates that the bowel is undergoing volvulus, vascular obstruction, and ischemia. Definitive diagnosis is made by an upper gastrointestinal series that shows the fourth portion of the duodenum on the right side of the spine [7] (Fig. 150-5).

Treatment

In contrast to atresia of the duodenum and small bowel, malrotation with midgut volvulus is an acute emergency. Vascular obstruction, as indicated by rectal bleeding, may result within hours in necrosis of all or most of the midgut. Diagnosis of malrotation calls for prompt exploration. The need for operation is particularly urgent in the presence of the "traffic light sign:" green (bile) above and red (blood) below. The Ladd procedure is performed, correcting malrotation by untwisting the bowel and dividing all obstructing bands [7] (Figs. 150-6 through 150-9, see also *Color Plate*).

Prognosis

If volvulus with extensive loss of bowel has not occurred in utero, and if postnatal treatment is accomplished before there is torsion and loss of bowel, the prognosis is excellent. The gastrointestinal tract functions normally, and the life span is not shortened. Unfortunately, however, malrotation and midgut volvulus

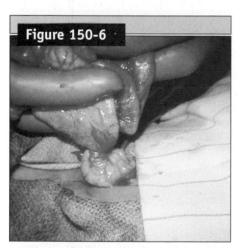

Figure 150-6

Malrotation. Volvulus of the midgut and a small mesenteric base are seen. See also **Color Plate**.

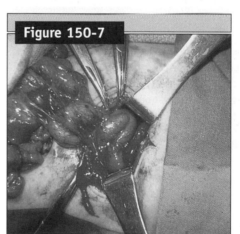

Figure 150-7

Malrotation. Ladd's bands are seen crossing the duodenum. See also **Color Plate**.

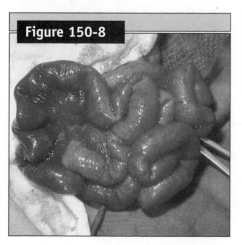

Figure 150-8

Malrotation and volvulus. Venous engorgement is seen; the bowel is viable. See also **Color Plate**.

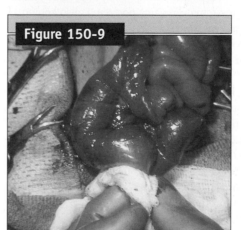

Figure 150-9

Volvulus with gangrene. (Only a few hours passed between the condition pictured in Fig. 150-8 and that shown in Fig. 150-9.) See also **Color Plate**.

remains the leading cause of mortality in neonatal intestinal obstruction, usually because of delayed diagnosis and treatment. If extensive loss of bowel occurs either before or after birth, the infant becomes a gastrointestinal cripple dependent on parenteral nutrition [8]. Such nonenteral nutrition ultimately results in liver failure. Methods are available for expediting bowel adaptation [9], and transplantation of liver, small bowel, or both has prolonged survival (see Chapter 164). Children with liver transplantation may have normal life spans; intestinal transplantation is too recent to evaluate.

OTHER CONDITIONS ASSOCIATED WITH INTESTINAL OBSTRUCTION

Two other conditions associated with intestinal obstruction are discussed elsewhere in this text. For more information about meconium ileus, see Chapter 170. For a discussion of Hirschsprung's disease, see Chapter 172.

REFERENCES

1. Moore SW, deJongh G, Bouic P, et al.: Immune deficiency in familial duodenal atresia. *J Pediatr Surg* 1996, 31:1733–1735.
2. Spigland N, Yazbeck S: Complications associated with surgical treatment of congenital intrinsic duodenal obstruction. *J Pediatr Surg* 1990, 25:1127–1130.
3. Coppens B, Vos A: Duodenal atresia. *Pediatr Surg Int* 1992, 7:435–437.
4. Ashcraft KW, Holder TM: *Pediatric Surgery*, edn 2. Philadelphia: WB Saunders; 1993:308.
5. Spinazzola R, Kenigsberg K, Usmani S, Harper R: Neonatal gastrointestinal complications of maternal cocaine abuse. *N Y State J Med* 1992, 92:22–23.
6. Torres AM, Ziegler MM: Malrotation of the intestine. *World J Surg* 1993, 17:326–331.
7. Lin JN, Lou CC, Wang KL: Intestinal malrotation and midgut volvulus: a 15-year review. *J Formos Med Assoc (Taiwan)* 1995, 94:178–181.
8. Galea MH, Holliday H: Short bowel syndrome: a collective review. *J Pediatr Surg* 1992, 27:592–596.
9. Georgeson K, Halpin D: Sequential intestinal lengthening procedures for refractory short bowel syndrome. *J Pediatr Surg* 1994, 29:316–321.

151 Vomiting
Francis P. Sunaryo

Vomiting is a common symptom in children, caused by a wide range of such diverse conditions as physiologic regurgitation of infancy to increased intracranial pressure. The diagnostic challenges are to decide when it is necessary to investigate, to determine what diagnostic tests should be performed and in what sequence, and to avoid unnecessary studies.

NEUROANATOMY

The act of vomiting is coordinated by a center in the medulla that is probably composed of a number of areas, including the parvicellular reticular formation, the solitary tract nucleus, and the medullary visceral-somatic motor nuclei. The afferent input to the medullary vomiting center comes from abdominal splanchnic and vagus nerves, vestibular receptors, the cerebral cortex, and the area postrema. The area postrema, also known as the chemoreceptor trigger zone (CTZ), is a vascular structure on the floor of the fourth ventricle. The location of the CTZ is important because it contains neuroreceptors that can monitor both the blood and the cerebrospinal fluid. Dopamine (D_2), serotonin (5-HT_3), histamine (H_1), and muscarinic receptors are found in abundance in the CTZ and in the gastrointestinal tract; they are of particular interest because they are the basis for antiemetic pharmacotherapy. The efferent motor output is derived from cranial nerves V, VII, and IX, which cause the prodromes of vomiting (*ie*, salivation, licking, and chewing); from somatomotor nuclei, which lead to complex contractions of the diaphragm and abdominal and gastercostal muscles; and from vagus and sympathetic nuclei in the medulla, which result in gastrointestinal motility changes [1,2].

PATHOPHYSIOLOGY

Vomiting is the forceful expulsion of gastric contents through the mouth. It usually is preceded by nausea and retching. *Retching*, which may occur without vomiting, is a series of spasmodic contractions of the muscles of the diaphragm and the abdominal wall. The sequential motor activities of vomiting start with proximal stomach relaxation and contraction of the antrum and pylorus. The cardia is pulled into the chest cavity through the crural hiatus by contraction of the longitudinal striated muscles of the upper esophagus. This temporary hiatal hernia eliminates the antireflux barrier produced by abdominal pressure on the lower esophageal sphincter. The gastric contents are pushed into the esophagus. At this point the diaphragm ascends rapidly, producing positive intrathoracic pressure, followed by upper esophageal relaxation and expulsion of the vomitus [1,3].

Regurgitation, or spitting up, in contrast to vomiting, is an effortless return of gastric contents to the mouth. Regurgitation is a frequent symptom of, but is not synonymous with, gastroesophageal reflux in infants. It usually is not associated with nausea or retching.

DIAGNOSTIC APPROACH

The diverse list of causes for vomiting (Tables 151-1, 151-2, and 151-3) emphasizes the need for an orderly approach to the differential diagnosis. The history and physical examination usually determine what, if any, laboratory studies are necessary. Routine laboratory or radiologic studies are unwarranted in straightforward cases such as acute viral gastroenteritis or in the infant with recurrent regurgitation who is feeding normally and gaining weight.

Table 151-1. Causes of Vomiting in the Newborn

Gastroesophageal reflux
Congenital obstructive gastrointestinal anomalies
   Atresias, stenosis, webs
   Malrotation, with or without volvulus
   Meconium ileus or plug
   Hirschsprung's disease
   Enteric duplications
Acquired gastrointestinal disorders
   Necrotizing enterocolitis
   Milk allergy
   Lactobezoar
Infections
   Sepsis
   Meningitis
   Urinary tract infection
Neurologic
   Subdural hematoma
   Hydrocephalus
Renal
   Obstructive uropathy
   Renal insufficiency
Metabolic (Table 151-5)

Table 151-3. Causes of Vomiting in Childhood and Adolescence

Obstructive gastrointestinal disorders
   Malrotation, with or without volvulus
   Intussusception
   Esophageal stricture (peptic or caustic)
   Foreign bodies, bezoar
   Adhesions
   Incarcerated hernia
   Intestinal pseudoobstruction
   Superior mesentery artery syndrome
Infectious or inflammatory gastrointestinal disorders
   Gastroenteritis
   Appendicitis
   Peptic ulcer
   Pancreatitis
   Gastroduodenal Crohn's disease
Neurologic
   Brain tumor
   Intracranial bleeding
   Migraine
   Ventriculoperitoneal shunt dysfunction
Abdominal trauma (accidental or nonaccidental)
   Duodenal hematoma
   Pancreatitis
Metabolic
   Diabetic ketoacidosis
   Reye's syndrome
   Adrenal insufficiency
Cyclic vomiting syndrome
Renal
Toxins or drugs
Miscellaneous
   Pregnancy
   Bulimia

Table 151-2. Causes of Vomiting in Infancy

Gastroesophageal reflux
Congenital obstructive gastrointestinal anomalies
   Malrotation, with or without volvulus
   Stenosis or webs
   Hirschsprung's disease
   Enteric duplications
Acquired gastrointestinal disorders
   Pyloric stenosis
   Intussusception
   Incarcerated hernia
   Milk or food allergy
   Foreign bodies
   Celiac disease
   Intestinal pseudoobstruction
Infections
   Gastroenteritis
   Urinary tract infection
   Sepsis or meningitis
   Pertussis
Metabolic (Table 151-5)
Rumination
Neurologic
   Brain tumor
   Intracranial bleeding
   Hydrocephalus, ventriculoperitoneal shunt dysfunction
Renal
Toxins or drugs

■ HISTORY

The history considers the age of the child, the contents of the vomitus, the effort and force of vomiting, the timing of the vomiting, associated symptoms, and any additional medical history.

Various conditions are seen exclusively in newborns, infants or older children, and adolescents (Tables 151-1, 151-2, and 151-3).

The contents of the vomitus give clues to the cause of the vomiting. Bilious vomiting suggests obstruction distal to the ampulla of Vater. In the newborn, bilious vomiting is indicative of intestinal obstruction until proven otherwise and requires emergency evaluation (see Chapter 150). Bilious vomiting in the neonate also may be a sign of sepsis or central nervous system infection. Bloody vomitus in the newborn may be caused by maternal blood swallowed during delivery. In breast-fed babies, swallowed blood from cracked nipples is a possible cause of hematemesis.

Because parents often do not distinguish between vomiting and regurgitation, the clinician must differentiate between the two. Effortful, projectile vomiting in an infant younger than 3 months of age typically is associated with gastric outlet obstruction (hypertrophic pyloric stenosis). Effortless vomiting is seen with gastroesophageal reflux. In the older child with effortful vomiting, the possibility of pyloric stricture caused by corrosive ingestion, chronic granulomatous disease, or gastroduodenal Crohn's disease should be considered (Fig. 151-1).

Vomiting of undigested food many hours after its ingestion suggests delayed gastric emptying. Vomiting on awakening, particularly if it is associated with headache, is suggestive of an intracranial lesion. Early morning vomiting also may be seen in children with sinusitis who gag from a postnasal drip. In the adolescent female, pregnancy also may be manifested by early morning vomiting.

Diarrhea accompanying vomiting may suggest infectious gastroenteritis or food poisoning. Epigastric pain with vomiting is suggestive of acid peptic disease, cholecystitis, or pancreatitis. Jaundice is seen in infants with urinary tract infection, hepatitis, or malformations of the biliary tract.

The additional medical history to be considered includes preexisting illnesses, prescribed medications, drug abuse, trauma, and previous abdominal surgery. In newborns with vomiting, maternal drug use, infection, and hydramnios also are important.

■ PHYSICAL EXAMINATION

Assessment of the child's general appearance helps to decide the necessity and urgency of evaluation and treatment of vomiting. Hydration and circulatory status are determined by blood pressure, pulse, respiratory rate, capillary refill, and skin color and turgor. Plotting the infant's weight and height on a growth

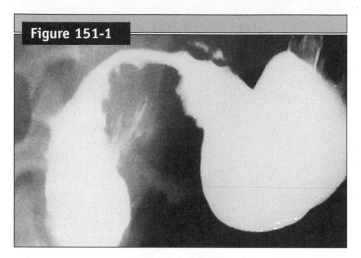

Figure 151-1

Gastroduodenal Crohn's disease. Antral and duodenal narrowing, mucosal irregularities, and deep linear ulceration are seen in a 12-year-old girl with recurrent epigastric pain, vomiting, and weight loss.

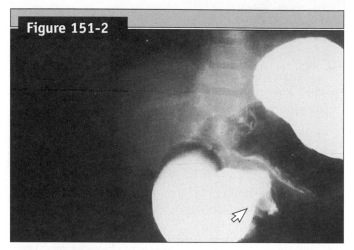

Figure 151-2

Duodenal web (*arrow*) in a 6-month-old infant born with duodenal atresia. The web was not recognized during the initial surgery. Bilious vomiting recurred after surgery.

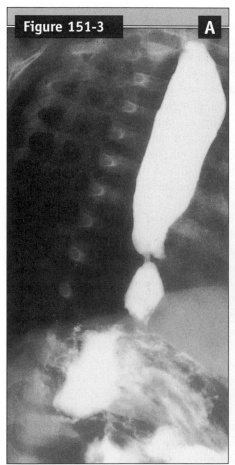

Figure 151-3 **A**

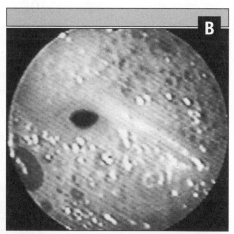

B

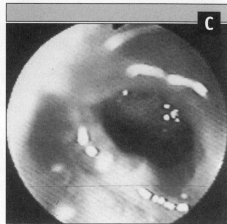

C

A, Esophageal stricture in a 10-month-old infant with AIDS and a history of poor feeding and recurrent vomiting. A small diverticulum is noted just proximal to the stricture. **B**, Endoscopic view of the stricture before dilation. **C**, Endoscopic view after dilation of the stricture.

chart may reveal failure to thrive. Localized abdominal tenderness, distention, organomegaly, masses, and scars from previous surgical procedures help to refine the differential diagnosis. Burn marks, ecchymoses, or linear contusions suggest possible abdominal trauma resulting from child abuse. A neurologic examination should include assessment of the child's mental status, as well as a funduscopy. A tense fontanel suggests meningitis, subdural hematoma, tumor, or pseudotumor cerebri. Observing the caretaker feed the child may reveal improper feeding techniques such as bottle propping or failure to burp the baby adequately, a swallowing disorder, or disturbances in the maternal–infant relationship.

LABORATORY STUDIES

The need for any initial laboratory studies or more definitive tests is determined by the data from the history and physical examination. Depending on the age of the child and the clinical presentation, only one or two specific diagnostic studies may be necessary, for example, ultrasound of the upper abdomen for suspected hypertrophic pyloric stenosis or a barium enema in the child with a possible intussusception. Vomiting without specific urinary tract symptoms may be the only symptom of a urinary tract infection. A urinalysis and urine culture are usually appropriate screening tests. Plain radiographs of the abdomen are important in evaluating children with bilious vomiting and suspected obstruction. An upper gastrointestinal series is particularly useful for revealing whether there are structural abnormalities of the esophagus, stomach, or proximal small bowel (Fig. 151-2). In children with suspected acid peptic disease or suspected anatomic abnormalities, endoscopy of the upper gastrointestinal tract may be helpful (Fig. 151-3). Therapeutic endoscopy also can be used. Recurrent unexplained episodes of metabolic acidosis should prompt evaluation for a metabolic disorder (Table 151-4). In the child with vomiting that is ill defined, initial evaluation should include a complete blood count, serum electrolytes, and blood urea nitrogen, as well as a urinalysis and culture.

CAUSES OF VOMITING ACCORDING TO AGE GROUPS

The clinical approach to vomiting in children is determined to some extent by the age of the child. Therefore, it is convenient to organize the many different causes of vomiting into three age periods: 1) newborn, 2) infancy, and 3) childhood and adolescence. Although there is considerable overlap in some cases, most entities tend to fall into specific age groupings.

Newborn

Physiologic gastroesophageal reflux is common in neonates and young infants. Effortless regurgitation usually is the presenting symptom, although occasionally forceful vomiting is seen. The baby grows normally and has a normal physical examination. Evaluation generally is not indicated.

Congenital obstructive gastrointestinal anomalies should be of concern in newborns who present with persistent vomiting shortly after the initiation of feeding, particularly if the vomiting is bilious [4•,5•] (see Chapters 144, 150, and 172).

Infection, including sepsis, meningitis, or urinary tract infection, is a serious cause of vomiting in the newborn.

Necrotizing enterocolitis (NEC) is seen primarily in premature infants, although approximately 10% of affected neonates are born at term. The classic triad of symptoms includes abdominal distention, bilious vomiting, and bloody stools (see Chapter 168).

Inborn errors of metabolism such as the urea cycle disorders and organic acidemias usually present in the newborn period with recurrent or persistent vomiting. The vomiting is usually associated with lethargy, seizures, failure to thrive, and coma [6].

Congenital adrenal hyperplasia, particularly of the salt-losing variety, should be suspected in the infant with persistent vomiting who is failing to thrive. In girls, the genitalia are usually ambiguous, whereas in boys the genitalia may appear normal. The clinical manifestations are often confused with those of pyloric stenosis: decreased serum sodium and chloride concentrations with an elevated serum potassium level are common. Elevated serum 17-hydroxyprogesterone is diagnostic for 21-hydroxylase deficiency, which accounts for 95% of patients with congenital adrenal hyperplasia [7•].

Miscellaneous conditions such as inspissated milk or lactobezoar (Fig. 151-4) are occasionally seen in premature infants

Table 151-4. Laboratory Tests for Suspected Metabolic Disorders

Initial tests
  Electrolytes, bicarbonate, glucose, pH
  AST, ALT, bilirubin
  Ammonia
  Lactate, pyruvate
  Urine ketones and reducing substances
More specific tests
  Serum total and free carnitine
  Blood and urine for amino acids
  Urine organic acids

ALT—alanine aminotransferase; AST—asparte aminotransferase.

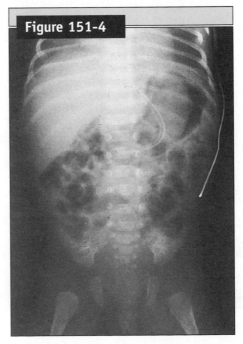

Figure 151-4

Lactobezoar. A well-formed intraluminal cast surrounded by air.

Table 151-5. Some Important Metabolic Disorders Associated With Vomiting

Urea cycle defects
  Ornithine transcarbamylase
    deficiency
  Carbamyl phosphate synthetase
    deficiency
  Citrullinemia
  Argininosuccinic aciduria
  Hyperargininemia

Organic acidemias
  Methylmalonic acidemia
  Propionic acidemia

Metabolic carbohydrate disorders
  Galactosemia

Hereditary fructose intolerance
  Diabetic ketoacidosis

Fatty acid oxidation defects
  Medium-chain acyl-CoA
    dehydrogenase deficiency
Congenital adrenal hyperplasia
  21-hydroxylase deficiency

Figure 151-5

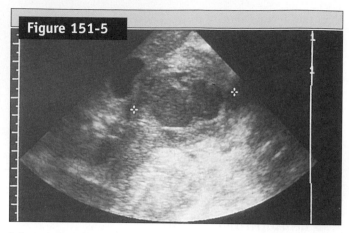

Infected pancreatic pseudocyst of the head of the pancreas in a 20-month-old boy with suspected child abuse.

Figure 151-6

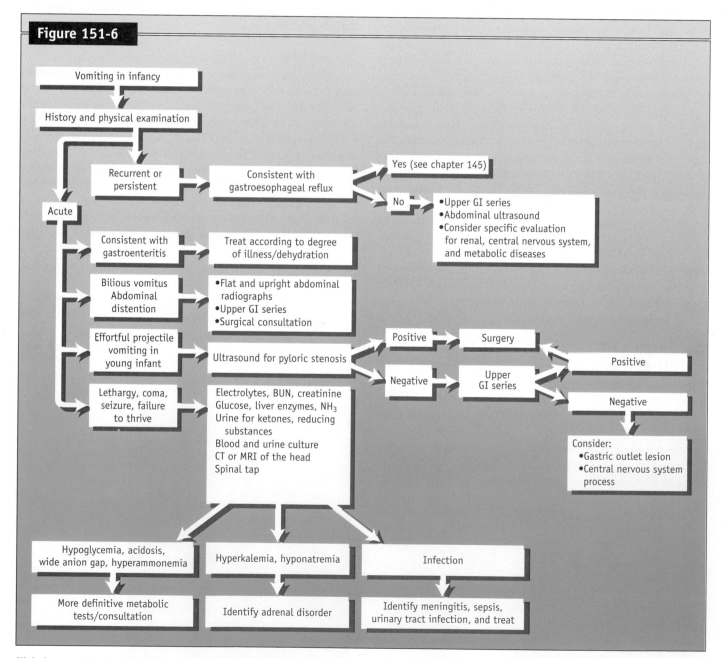

Clinical approach to the infant with vomiting. BUN—blood urea nitrogen; CT—computed tomography; GI—gastrointestinal; MRI—magnetic resonance imaging.

and present with abdominal distention and vomiting. Factors that may contribute to lactobezoar formation include respiratory distress, birth asphyxia, delayed gastric emptying, continuous feeding, and high caloric–density formula [8]. Treatment consists of withholding feedings for 24 to 48 hours.

Infancy

Gastroesophageal reflux and food allergy are common causes of vomiting in infants (see Chapters 145 and 169)

Obstructive gastrointestinal lesions (*eg*, hypertrophic pyloric stenosis, malrotation, volvulus, intussusception, and incarcerated hernia) are discussed individually in other chapters (see Chapters 154 and 162). Malrotation must be considered promptly in newborns, older infants, and children with bilious vomiting, because volvulus around the superior mesenteric artery may result in bowel ischemia and infarction.

Infection is the likely cause of vomiting in an infant who previously was well. Such infections include acute gastroenteritis, sepsis, meningitis, urinary tract infection, and pertussis.

Rumination often is seen in infants with reflux, or it may be voluntary and self-induced. Regurgitated food may be mouthed and reswallowed. The material that is mouthed, if not spit out, often causes destruction of the dental enamel and caries. Rumination may be a response to pain [9,10•], a result of gastroesophageal reflux in an otherwise normal infant, or seen in infants with a disturbed parent–child relationship [11].

Neurologic causes of vomiting include mass lesions, as well as meningitis and encephalitis. Occlusion of a ventriculoperitoneal shunt in children with hydrocephalus may produce vomiting. Vomiting may occur initially in the absence of increased intracranial pressure in patients with tumor involving the vomiting center in the medulla. Other neurologic causes of vomiting include migraine and familial dysautonomia [12].

Many metabolic disorders (Table 151-5) manifest themselves in the newborn during catabolic stress (*eg*, fasting and intercurrent illness).

Childhood and Adolescence

Infectious diseases continue to be the most common cause of vomiting in childhood, although peptic ulcer disease, pancreatitis, and inflammatory bowel disease also should be considered. Blunt trauma to the abdomen may cause pancreatitis or a duodenal hematoma (Fig. 151-5). Reye's syndrome has been reported in Kawasaki disease, one of the few conditions in which salicylates are still used therapeutically in children [13]. In adolescents, pregnancy and drug abuse should be considered.

Cyclic vomiting is characterized by recurrent and intense bouts of vomiting with intervals of normal health in between episodes. The problem commonly starts in preschool- or early school-aged children. Episodes tend to be similar in time of onset and duration. Vomiting often occurs during the night or on arising in the morning, or both. The duration of vomiting ranges from several hours to 5 to 7 days, with 12 to 48 hours being most common [14•]. Attacks often are precipitated by emotional stress, nonnoxious excitement, minor infections, and physical exhaustion. Migraine headaches occur in up to 38% of patients [15]. Treatment should be institut-

Table 151-6. Antiemetics and Recommended Dosages

Drug (brand name*)	Mechanisms	Indication and remarks	Route and dosages
Dimenhydrinate (Dramamine)	H₁ antagonist, anticholinergic	Motion sickness, **not for children < 2 y**	PO, IM, IV 5 mg/kg/24 h ÷ q 6 h
Prochlorperazine (Compazine)	D₂ and H₁ antagonists at CTZ	Chemotherapy, cyclic vomiting. Side effects: hypotension, drowsiness, extrapyramidal	PO, PR 0.4 mg/kg/24 h ÷ q 6–8 h **Do not use IV in children**
Metoclopramide (Reglan)	D₂ antagonist at CTZ and enteric nervous system	Gastroesophageal, chemotherapy, gastroparesis. Side effect: extrapyramidal	PO, IV 0.1 mg/kg qid
Ondansetron (Zofran)	5-HT₃ Antagonist at enteric nervous system and CTZ	Chemotherapy, postoperation, cyclic vomiting. Side effects: headache, bronchospasm, tachycardia	PO: < 4 y: 2 mg q 4 h 4–11 y: 4 mg q 4 h > 12 y: 8 mg q 4 h IV: 0.15–0.45 mg/kg, 30 min before, 4 and 8 h after emetogenic drug
Granisetron (Kytril)	Similar to ondansetron	Chemotherapy	IV: 10–20 µg/kg, 30 min before emetogenic drug as a single dose
Lorazepam (Ativan)	Anxiolytic, GABA inhibition at limbic system	In conjunction with other antiemetic in chemotherapy. Side effects: respiratory depression, dizziness	IV: 0.04–0.08 mg/kg q 6 h

Manufacturer information is as follows: Dramanine: Upjohn Co., Kalamazoo, MI; Compazine: SmithKline Beecham Pharmaceuticals, Philadelphia, PA; Reglan: A.H. Robins Company, Richmond, VA; Zofran: Galaxo Wellcome Oncology/HIV, Research Triangle Park, NC; Kytril: SmithKline Beecham Pharmaceuticals; Ativan: Wyeth-Ayerst Laboratories, Philadelphia, PA.

CTZ—chemoreceptor trigger zone; GABA—gamma-aminobutyric acid; IM—intramuscularly; IV—intravenously; PO—per oral.

Data from Leslie et al. [19•], Ettinger [20•], and Barone [21].

ed as early as possible after the onset of symptoms in an attempt to interrupt the attack. Ondansetron, a serotonin antagonist, given intravenously is more effective than chlorpromazine, droperidol, trimethobenzamide, or metoclopramide [14•]. Propranolol, cyproheptadine, pizotifen, and erythromycin have been used prophylactically with some efficacy [16,17].

Bulimia nervosa is characterized by recurrent episodes of binge eating associated with recurrent inappropriate behavior to avoid weight gain, such as self-induced vomiting, laxative or diuretic abuse, fasting, or excessive exercise. Most patients are white adolescent and college-age females from middle to upper socioeconomic class families. Parotid and submandibular swelling, dental enamel defects and caries, scars on the knuckles, and widely fluctuating body weight and intermittent edema provide clues to the diagnosis [18••] (see Chapter 190).

■ THERAPY

Therapy is directed toward the specific cause of vomiting (Fig. 151-6). The dosages, mechanisms, and side effects of the most commonly used antiemetics are noted in Table 151-6 [19•,20•,21]. The use of prokinetic agents in children with GER or other gastrointestinal motility disorders is discussed in Chapters 145 and 147.

■ REFERENCES

Recently published papers of particular interest have been highlighted as follows:
• Of interest
•• Of outstanding interest

1. Grundy D, Reid K: The physiology of nausea and vomiting. In *Physiology of the Gastrointestinal Tract.* Edited by Johnson LR. New York: Raven Press; 1994:879–901.

2. McCallum RW, Kendall BJ: Diagnostic decisions in chronic nausea and vomiting. *Contemp Int Med* 1993, 5:60–68.

3. Orenstein SR: Vomiting and regurgitation. In *Practical Strategies in Pediatric Diagnosis and Therapy.* Edited by Kliegman RM. Philadelphia: WB Saunders; 1996:301–331.

4.• Hechtman DH, Stylianos S: Surgical conditions in the newborn. *Pediatr Ann* 1994, 23:231–239.
This article discusses the evaluation of neonates with surgical conditions, including obstructive gastrointestinal anomalies. Rapid identification of the conditions that require prompt surgical treatment is emphasized.

5.• Reyna TM, Reyna PA: Gastroduodenal disorders associated with emesis in infants. *Semin Pediatr Surg* 1995; 4:190–197.
This is a review of the common surgical conditions in infancy that present with vomiting.

6. Korson M: Metabolic etiologies of cyclic or recurrent vomiting. *J Pediatr Gastroenterol Nutr* 1995, 21: S15–S19.

7.• Miller WL: Genetics, diagnosis, and management of 21-hydroxylase deficiency. *J Clin Endocrinol Metab* 1994, 78:241–246.
This is a review of the most common form of congenital adrenal hyperplasia with emphasis on the newer molecular genetic findings and clinical management.

8. Erenberg A, Shaw RD, Yousefzadeh D: Lactobezoar in the low-birth-weight infant. *Pediatrics* 1979, 63:642–646.

9. Herbst J, Friedland GW, Zboralske FF: Hiatal hernia and rumination in infants and children. *J Pediatr* 1971, 78:261–265.

10.• Orenstein SR: Gastroesophageal reflux. In *Current Problems in Pediatrics.* Edited by Stockman J, Winter R. St. Louis: Mosby-Year Book, 1991:193–241.
This is an excellent review of the pathophysiology, clinical manifestations, diagnostic evaluation, and therapy of gastroesophageal reflux in children.

11. Fleisher DR: Functional vomiting disorders in infancy: innocent vomiting, nervous vomiting, and infant rumination syndrome. *J Pediatr* 1994, 125:S84–S94.

12. Johns DW: Disorders of the central and autonomic nervous systems as a cause for emesis in infants. *Semin Pediatr Surg* 1995, 4:166–175.

13. Takahashi M, Mason W, Thomas D, Sinatra F: Reye syndrome following Kawasaki syndrome confirmed by liver histopathology. In *Kawasaki Disease.* Proceedings of the Fifth International Kawasaki Disease Symposium, Fukuoka, Japan, May 22–25, 1995. Edited by Kato H. Amsterdam: Elsevier Press; 1995:436–444.

14.• Fleisher DR, Matar M: The cyclic vomiting syndrome: a report of 71 cases and literature review. *J Pediatr Gastroenterol Nutr* 1993, 17:361–369.
In this report, the authors describe their personal observations of 71 patients with this uncommon disorder.

15. Symon DNK, Russell G: The relationship between cyclic vomiting syndrome and abdominal migraine. *J Pediatr Gastroenterol Nutr* 1995, 21:S42–S43.

16. Forbes D, Withers G: Prophylactic therapy in cyclic vomiting syndrome. *J Pediatr Gastroenterol Nutr* 1995, 21:S57–S59.

17. Vanderhoof JA, Young R, Kaufman SS: Treatment of cyclic vomiting in childhood with erythromycin. *J Pediatr Gastroenterol Nutr* 1993, 17:387–391.

18.•• Kreipe RE: Eating disorders among children and adolescents. *Pediatr Rev* 1995, 16:370–379.
This is a comprehensive review of the epidemiology, pathogenesis, clinical aspects, and management of eating disorders.

19.• Leslie RA, Shah Y, Thejomayen M, Murphy KM: The neuropharmacology of emesis: the role of receptors in neuromodulation of nausea and vomiting. *Can J Physiol Pharmacol* 1990, 68:279–288.
This is a review of the neuromodulation of nausea and vomiting.

20.• Ettinger DS: Preventing chemotherapy-induced nausea and vomiting: an update and a review of emesis. *Semin Oncol* 1995, 22(Suppl 10):6–18.
This is a good review of chemotherapy-induced vomiting and guidelines for selecting antiemetics.

21. Barone MA: Drug doses. In *The Harriet Lane Handbook.* St. Louis: Mosby; 1996:475–665.

152 Chronic Abdominal Pain

Jeffrey S. Hyams

Chronic abdominal pain and recurrent abdominal pain are common gastrointestinal complaints. Studies suggest that about 10% to 15% of school-age children [1–3] and 15% to 25% of adolescents [4•] have recurrent abdominal pain. The definition of *recurrent abdominal pain* that originated with Apley and Naish [1] and is often used in both practice-based and community-based studies requires three episodes of abdominal pain severe enough to limit activity and occurring over a period longer than 3 months, with symptom-free intervals between episodes of pain. There are no generally accepted criteria for minimum duration of pain or its severity for a diagnosis of *chronic abdominal pain*. In this chapter, chronic abdominal pain is defined as discomfort that has existed for 1 month or longer.

The term *recurrent abdominal pain* is often used interchangeably with terms such as *functional abdominal pain, psychogenic abdominal pain*, and *nonorganic abdominal pain*. These terms are often used in a pejorative sense, and labeling recurrent abdominal pain as primarily a psychosomatic disorder has done a great disservice to many children. Recurrent abdominal pain represents a heterogeneous group of disorders. Although some of these disorders may have a psychogenic component, most of them do not. The term *functional abdominal pain* should be reserved to describe the pain of a distinct subgroup of children with recurrent abdominal pain who have a clearly defined constellation of findings, as described later. This chapter provides a framework within which to approach the child or adolescent with chronic or recurrent abdominal pain.

CLASSIFICATION

Patients with chronic or recurrent abdominal pain are divided into three categories. The first classification includes those children in whom a distinct cause for the pain can be identified and for whom there is an objective test that substantiates the diagnosis. Examples of such causes include inflammatory bowel disease, ulcer disease, pancreatitis, and ureteropelvic junction obstruction. The second includes those children whose symptoms show a distinct clinical pattern but in whom the pattern is nonspecific. No specific tests for diagnosis exist, and evaluation is directed toward excluding other disorders with a similar presentation. Examples include the irritable bowel syndrome and functional dyspepsia. The third group includes those patients whose symptoms are not suggestive of a specific disease and in whom no cause can be identified. In these patients somatization is sometimes a diagnostic consideration.

Historically, patients in the first group have been labeled as having *organic* disease and those in the second group as having *functional* disease. Because the basic pathophysiologic mechanisms involved in the pathogenesis of functional disorders are unknown, these disorders are classified as *nonorganic*.

CAUSES

The list of disorders associated with chronic or recurrent abdominal pain in children and adolescents is extensive (Table 152-1).

Irritable Bowel Syndrome

A recent community-based study of a suburban adolescent population in the United States suggested that 14% of high school students and 6% of middle school students had abdominal pain and defecatory symptoms consistent with a diagnosis of irritable bowel syndrome [4•]. The frequency of abdominal pain and irritable bowel–type symptoms was similar in girls and boys.

The clinical spectrum of irritable bowel syndrome in children is similar to that in adults. There are pediatric subjects with diarrhea predominance, constipation predominance, and a variable defecatory pattern. Although lower abdominal, cramping pain is the most common complaint, younger children sometimes have difficulty localizing their discomfort. Autonomic symptoms such as light-headedness, pallor, and diaphoresis are common.

The diagnosis of IBS in children is based on a suggestive history and a normal physical examination. Similar symptoms may be seen in other disorders such as lactose intolerance, inflammatory bowel disease, allergy, and giardiasis. The extent

Table 152-1. Causes of Recurrent or Chronic Abdominal Pain in Children and Adolescents

Gastrointestinal	Genitourinary
Gastroesophageal reflux	Urinary tract infection
Peptic disease	Hydronephrosis
Functional dyspepsia	Ureteropelvic junction obstruction
Carbohydrate intolerance	
Irritable bowel syndrome	Nephrolithiasis
Constipation	Gynecologic
Aerophagia	Endometriosis
Inflammatory bowel disease	Pelvic inflammatory disease
Celiac disease	Ovarian cyst or tumor
Allergic bowel disease	Dysmenorrhea
Parasitic infestation (*eg*, giardiasis, ascariasis)	Imperforate hymen
	Vaginal atresia
Pancreatitis	Other
Biliary colic (*eg*, cholelithiasis, choledochal cyst)	Abdominal migraine
	Porphyria
Intestinal obstruction (*eg*, malrotation, intussusception)	Angioneurotic edema
	Neurally mediated hypotension
	Familial Mediterranean fever
Meckel's diverticulum (with diverticulitis or intussusception)	Somatization
	Abdominal muscle tear
Intestinal duplication	Tumor

to which the clinician should pursue these other diagnoses depends on the specifics of each case. The symptoms of weight loss, rectal bleeding, nocturnal awakening, or fever should prompt an aggressive evaluation. Chronic absenteeism from school is a common stimulus for the performance of "tests" when the patient's family has difficulty accepting a clinical diagnosis of IBS.

The same general principles that guide treatment in adults can be applied to children. They include a thorough explanation of the presumed pathophysiology of symptoms, reassurance that there are no more severe underlying disorders, recommendations for modification of the patient's diet, with particular reference to increasing dietary fiber intake, and occasionally, the use of medications. Anticholinergic medications such as dicyclomine or low-dose tricyclic antidepressants may be helpful, but they may also lead to further constipation and worsening symptoms. Patients and families are told that there is no cure for irritable bowel syndrome but that palliative treatment is available. Psychological intervention, particularly biofeedback, can be effective in recalcitrant cases. Anxiolytics are of little benefit.

Dyspepsia

Although most children with dyspeptic symptoms complain of upper abdominal pain, some just describe an "ill feeling" in the epigastrium with a sense of nausea and bloating. Early satiety and anorexia are also common. There are many potential causes of dyspepsia in children (Table 152-2). Most children with dyspepsia do not have frank ulcer disease. In the strictest sense, a diagnosis of functional dyspepsia can be established only after a thorough biochemical, ultrasonographic, and endoscopic search has excluded the possibility of organic disease. In most cases, however, it is hard to justify this aggressive approach. Unfortunately, it may be very difficult when using only the initial clinical history to distinguish between pediatric patients with functional dyspepsia and those with biopsy-proven upper gastrointestinal inflammation.

Upper gastrointestinal endoscopy is warranted in the presence of persistent vomiting, hematemesis, weight loss, or significant school absenteeism. This procedure quickly establishes whether peptic ulcer or inflammation (including *Helicobacter pylori*-induced), allergic gastroenteropathy, or gastroduodenal Crohn's disease is present. In the absence of the symptoms listed, an empiric trial of H_2-receptor antagonist therapy is worthwhile.

Table 152-2. Causes of Dyspepsia in Children and Adolescents

Gastroesophageal reflux

Peptic esophagitis

Allergic bowel disease

Gastritis (peptic, allergic, *Helicobacter pylori*-induced)

Duodenitis

Medications (*eg*, nonsteroidal anti-inflammatory drugs)

Functional dyspepsia

Gastroduodenal Crohn's disease

Cholelithiasis

This therapy is offered for 6 weeks and then discontinued. Failure to respond to therapy or prompt recurrence of symptoms is an indication for endoscopy.

Carbohydrate Intolerance

Although most attention to carbohydrate malabsorption has focused on lactose, malabsorption of a variety of dietary carbohydrates (*eg*, fructose, starch, sorbitol) may result in a similar clinical picture. Lactase deficiency is classified as either primary or secondary. Primary lactase deficiency occurs when the intestinal morphology is normal and the decreased amount of lactase present in the intestinal epithelium is the result of a congenital condition (very rare) or as the result of a process by which normal aging is associated with diminished lactase activity. This deficiency is not seen in the White population before 5 years of age nor in the Black or Hispanic populations before 3 years of age. Secondary lactase deficiency can occur when the intestinal epithelium has suffered an injury resulting in diminished lactase activity.

Causes of secondary lactase deficiency in children include viral enteritis, *Giardia lamblia* infestation, allergic bowel disease, and celiac disease. Although either primary or secondary lactase deficiency may result in lactose malabsorption, not all children with lactase deficiency develop clinical symptoms following ingestion of a lactose load. Factors that influence whether symptoms develop include the severity of the lactase deficiency, the amount of lactose ingested, whether other foods are ingested concomitantly, the rate of gastric emptying, the fermentative activity of the colonic flora, and interindividual variability in response to colonic distention. Sorbitol and fructose intolerance may mimic lactose intolerance [5•].

Breath hydrogen testing is the most accurate and least invasive method of detecting lactose malabsorption (see Chapter 157). Treatment of lactose intolerance includes either decreasing or eliminating dietary lactose or using exogenous lactase enzyme supplements to aid in digestion. If milk products are severely restricted, calcium supplements should be considered.

Aerophagia

The classic history for aerophagia is that of a child who is well in the morning when awakening, but over the course of the day develops abdominal distention, may note abdominal pain, and often has marked belching and flatulence. Abdominal distention may be severe enough to decrease the appetite. Other conditions such as malabsorption and intestinal obstruction are commonly considered first in the evaluation of these children [6,7]. Aerophagia must be differentiated from carbohydrate malabsorption.

The diagnosis of aerophagia should be considered after a detailed history has been obtained. An abdominal radiograph reveals massive amounts of gas *without* the presence of air–fluid levels. Depending on the severity of the symptoms, as well as accompanying findings such as weight loss, the clinician determines how extensive an evaluation is required. The differential diagnosis of marked abdominal distention in the younger child includes Hirschsprung's disease, ascites, tumor, celiac disease, giardiasis, carbohydrate malabsorption, and massive organomegaly. Physical examination readily rules out several of these entities. The child with aerophagia has a tympanitic, distended abdomen without tenderness. Treatment usually consists of making the patient and family aware of the cause of the symptoms. In selected cases psychological evaluation and biofeedback may be of value [8].

Abdominal Migraine

Abdominal migraine is a periodic syndrome of acute-onset abdominal pain (epigastric or periumbilical) with accompanying symptoms that may include nausea, vomiting, pallor, diarrhea, irritability, and somnolence [9]. When these symptoms are accompanied by a history of migraine headaches, the diagnosis is straightforward. Rarely, there is no history of headaches and the diagnosis becomes presumptive. The affected individual usually has a stereotypical clinical presentation, is asymptomatic between attacks, and has a family history of migraine headaches. Lethargy commonly signals the end of an attack, and after a period of sleep the person is fine. When this constellation of findings occurs along with an abnormal electroencephalogram, and improvement is seen with anticonvulsant therapy, a diagnosis of abdominal epilepsy is made. The cyclic vomiting syndrome also observed in children may be part of the clinical expression of abdominal migraine. In cyclic vomiting syndrome, children have repeated, stereotypical bouts of vomiting lasting 12 to 24 hours (see Chapter 151).

Several modalities have been used in the treatment of abdominal migraine [10]. Most of them are directed toward prophylaxis, because therapy for established attacks is usually not helpful. Cyproheptadine and propranolol are two of the more common medications used; more refractory cases may prompt consideration of amitriptyline or carbamazepine.

Neurally Mediated Hypotension

Neurally mediated hypotension, also known as neurocardiogenic syncope, vasovagal reflex, and autonomic dysfunction, is a recently recognized cause of recurrent abdominal pain in adolescents [11,12]. Although it is classically associated with recurrent light-headedness and syncope, nausea and abdominal pain occur in some affected individuals. Symptoms may be precipitated by physical exertion, a warm environment, prolonged upright posture, or stress. A purplish discoloration of the hands and feet may be seen. The diagnosis is suggested by an abnormal response to a tilt-table test. Treatment may include increased ingestion of salt and fluid to expand the intravascular volume or mineralocorticoids or β-blockers.

Idiopathic Abdominal Pain

There is a group of patients in whom no organic disease is demonstrable and who have no recognizable constellation or association of symptoms that would fall into the category of a functional disorder. The abdominal pain does not appear to relate temporally to eating, defecation, or exercise. It may be recurrent or continuous and usually affects daily functioning. In children it is often continuous. The children state that it hurts all the time, from the moment of awakening until the time of sleep. These patients are often considered to have underlying psychological disturbances, and a diagnosis of somatoform disorder can be made in selected patients [13••]. The literature on the relationship between recurrent abdominal pain in children and psychopathology is prolific and occasionally conflicting [14,15]. Some studies have demonstrated that children with recurrent abdominal pain have an increased frequency of depression and anxiety compared with healthy children [14]. Mothers of children with recurrent abdominal pain have been shown to have higher measures of anxiety and depression than mothers of healthy children [15]. Organic pathology, functional bowel disease, and psychological disturbances may coexist in the same patient, however.

▊▊▊ GENERAL APPROACH

Without a reasonable diagnostic evaluation, the clinician cannot conclude with certainty that a child with chronic or recurrent abdominal pain does not have organic disease. Nonetheless, with no accompanying features suggestive of more serious disease, it may be appropriate to refrain from laboratory investigations early in the evaluation of such a patient. The history and physical examination are of paramount importance and usually point the clinician in the correct diagnostic direction (Table 152-3). Screening tests that may be helpful include a complete blood cell count, platelet count, erythrocyte sedimentation rate, urinalysis, and breath hydrogen test for lactose malabsorption. Specific disorders are described elsewhere in this text.

▊▊▊ REFERENCES

Recently published papers of particular interest have been highlighted as follows:
* •   Of interest
* ••   Of outstanding interest

1.   Apley J, Naish N: Recurrent abdominal pain: a field survey of 1,000 school children. *Arch Dis Child* 1958, 33:165–170.

2.   Alfven G: The covariation of common psychosomatic symptoms among children from socio-economically differing residential areas. An epidemiological study. *Acta Paediatr* 1993, 82:484–487.

3.   Linna SL, Miilanen I, Keistinen H, *et al.*: Prevalence of psychosomatic symptoms in children. *Psychother Psychosom* 1991, 56:85–87.

4.• Hyams JS, Burke G, Davis PM, *et al.*: Abdominal pain and irritable bowel syndrome in adolescents: a community-based study. *J Pediatr* 1996, 129:220–226.

Table 152-3. Characteristics of Chronic Recurrent Abdominal Pain

Organic
  Localized with or without radiation
  May awaken patient
  Accompanied by tenesmus
  Associated with systemic symptoms
  Associated with headaches
  Associated with vomiting
Functional
  Often migratory
  Does not awaken patient (except in patient with carbohydrate intolerance who has a carbohydrate snack shortly before bedtime)
  Relieved by flatus or defecation
  Associated with dietary intolerance

5.• Rumessen JJ: Fructose and related food carbohydrates. Sources, intake, absorption, and clinical implications. *Scand J Gastroenterol* 1992, 27:819–828.

6. Rosenbach Y, Zahavi I, Nitzan M, Dinari G: Pathologic childhood aerophagy: an under-diagnosed entity. *Eur J Pediatr* 1988, 147:422–423.

7. Gauderer MW, Halpin TC Jr, Izant RJ Jr: Pathologic childhood aerophagia: a recognizable clinical entity. *J Pediatr Surg* 1981, 16:301–305.

8. Bassotti G, Whitehead WE: Biofeedback as a treatment approach to gastrointestinal disorders. *Am J Gastroenterol* 1994, 89:158–163.

9. Fenichel GM: Headache. In *Clinical Pediatric Neurology. A Signs and Symptoms Approach*, edn 3. Edited by Fenichel GM. Philadelphia: WB Saunders; 1997:77–90.

10. Igarashi M, May WN, Golden GS: Pharmacologic treatment of childhood migraine. *J Pediatr* 1992, 120:653–657.

11. Rowe PC, Bou-Holaigah I, Kan JS, Calkins H: Is neurally mediated hypotension an unrecognized cause of chronic fatigue? *Lancet* 1995, 345:623–624.

12. Bou-Holaigah I, Rowe PC, Kan J, Calkins H: The relationship between neurally mediated hypotension and the chronic fatigue syndrome. *JAMA* 1995, 274:961–967.

13.•• Campo JV, Fritsch SL. Somatization in children and adolescents. *J Am Acad Child Adolesc Psychiatry* 1994, 33:1223–1235.

14. Garber J, Zeman J, Walker LS: Recurrent abdominal pain in children: psychiatric diagnoses and parental psychopathology. *J Am Acad Child Adolesc Psychiatry* 1990, 29:648–656.

15. Walker LS, Greene JW: Children with recurrent abdominal pain and their parents: more somatic complaints, anxiety, and depression than other patient families? *J Pediatr Psychol* 1989, 14:231–243.

153 Gastritis and Peptic Ulcer Disease in Children

Eric Hassall

GASTRITIS

The terms *gastropathy* and *gastritis* are both used to refer to the presence of macroscopic or histologic abnormalities of the gastric mucosa. However, in gastropathies, although histologic abnormalities may be present, inflammation is not a prominent feature; in gastritis, as the suffix "-*itis*" implies, inflammatory cells are a major feature, sometimes with atrophy resulting from chronic inflammation.

Gastritis is not a clinical diagnosis, nor is it a radiologic diagnosis. Most often it is a purely histologic diagnosis, made by targeted or random endoscopic biopsies [1••,2•,3]. Gastritis in children remains under-recognized and poorly characterized because of the flawed tendency to rely on macroscopic appearances at endoscopy and a reluctance to take multiple gastric biopsies (from several zones of the stomach).

Anatomy and Physiology

There are no anatomic differences between the upper gastrointestinal tracts of children and adults other than size. After early infancy, the physiology of acid secretion in children is the same as that in adults [4]. In the newborn human, gastric contents of pH <4 can be shown almost immediately after birth. The highest acid concentrations occur within 7 to 10 days, diminishing to adult levels in 60 to 90 days.

Etiology, Pathology, and Clinical Features

It is useful to classify gastritis in children by endoscopic and histologic appearance as erosive and hemorrhagic; nonerosive, nonspecific; or specific and distinctive [1••](Table 153-1). The gastritides in each of these categories are then specified by cause (Table 153-2).

Erosive and Hemorrhagic Gastropathies

Erosive and hemorrhagic gastropathies are diagnosed endoscopically. Inflammatory cell infiltrates are only a minor part of the injury pattern. The changes are primarily epithelial in the

Table 153-1. Classification of Gastritis Based on Endoscopic and Histologic Appearances

Type	Primary diagnosis by
Erosive and hemorrhagic gastropathy	Endoscopy
Nonerosive, nonspecific gastritis* (*ie*, chronic gastritis)	Histology
Specific (distinctive) gastritis†	Histology (endoscopy distinctive in some)

* *Pattern of inflammation is not diagnostic of a disorder or group of disorders.*

† *Distinctive histologic features that are diagnostic of or compatible with a narrower group of disorders; findings commonly have prognostic or other therapeutic implications.*

From Lewin KJ et al. [1••]; with permission.

case of erosions, and vascular in subepithelial hemorrhages. Most of the conditions discussed in this section are, therefore, gastropathies rather than gastritides.

"Stress" Gastropathy

"Stress" gastropathy occurs in the seriously ill child and is related to physiologic (not psychologic) stresses—such as shock, acidosis, sepsis, burns, or head injury—that result in mucosal ischemia. Early lesions predominate in the fundus and proximal body and spread to the antrum, producing a diffuse erosive and hemorrhagic appearance.

Prolapse Gastropathy

Forceful retching or vomiting (most often resulting from viral infections in children) produces typical subepithelial hemorrhages or petechiae in the fundus and proximal body, caused by knuckling of the proximal stomach into the distal esophagus—hence the term *prolapse gastropathy*. Mallory-Weiss tears of the cardia also may occur. Although the gastropathy and tears tend to resolve quickly, significant blood loss may occur.

Gastropathy Secondary to NSAIDs and Aspirin

Early erosions and hemorrhages occur in the gastric body and antrum and are of little clinical significance; the ulcers associated with nonsteroidal anti-inflammatory drugs (NSAIDs) are usually gastric and occasionally duodenal, and it is these lesions that may perforate or bleed [5]. Not infrequently, infants and young children treated with even small doses of aspirin for a febrile illness present with hematemesis and significant blood loss; in this circumstance, the characteristic finding is one or more ulcers on the incisura.

Table 153-2. Gastritides in Children

Erosive and hemorrhagic gastropathy
  Stress gastropathy
  Traumatic or prolapse gastropathy
  Aspirin or NSAIDs gastropathy
  Portal hypertensive gastropathy
  Henoch-Schönlein gastropathy
  Caustic injury
  Bile reflux gastropathy
Nonerosive, nonspecific gastritis
  Helicobacter pylori
  Postoperative stomach
  Pernicious anemia
Specific/distinctive gastritis
  Crohn's disease
  Chronic granulomatous disease
  Eosinophilic gastropathy
  Ménétriers' disease
  Chronic varioliform gastritis
  Graft-versus-host disease
  Cytomegalovirus
  Very rare specific gastritides in children are infectious, such as tuberculosis, syphilis, actinomycosis, phlegmonous and emphysematous gastritis, herpes, candida, histoplasmosis, mucormycosis, aspergillosis, cryptosporidiosis, anisakiasis, schistosomiasis, amebiasis, toxoplasmosis, and sarcoidosis.

Portal Hypertensive Gastropathy

In children with portal hypertension, congestive gastropathy often is present [6], with typical "mosaic lesions" and hemorrhages in the fundus and body.

Caustic Injury

In contrast to injuries to the esophagus, which usually are caused primarily by alkali ingestion, antral gastric injury is typical of ingested acid. Lesions range from erosions to ulcers to gangrene. Iron poisoning also may result in gastric mucosal necrosis. Caustic injuries may extend into the submucosa, and gastric antral stricture may occur as a late complication [7].

Henoch-Schönlein Gastropathy

Even when the clinical diagnosis is uncertain or when severe upper gastrointestinal symptoms are present, endoscopy may show a hemorrhagic and erosive picture suggestive of Henoch-Schönlein gastropathy [8]. The underlying vasculitis is not apparent in mucosal biopsies.

Other

Other, much less common erosive and hemorrhagic gastropathies in children are related to alcohol ingestion, ischemia, duodenogastric reflux, radiation, and chronic varioliform (also known as chronic erosive) gastritis (see "Chronic Varioliform Gastritis" later in this chapter).

Nonerosive, Nonspecific Gastritis or Chronic Active Gastritis

Chronic active gastritis of the antrum (formerly called "type B gastritis") is associated with peptic ulcer disease, whereas that of the body (formerly called "type A gastritis") is associated with pernicious anemia. Both types may be associated with the development of adenocarcinoma in adults, but that is an extremely rare occurrence in children. Nonerosive, nonspecific or chronic active antral gastritis is by far the most common gastritis in children; in nonerosive gastritis there usually is a poor correlation between endoscopic appearance and histologic findings, *ie*, it usually is a purely histologic diagnosis.

Helicobacter pylori Gastritis

In children, *Helicobacter pylori* is the most common cause of chronic active gastritis. Typically, this is solely an antral gastritis, although occasionally the gastric body may be involved. *H. pylori* gastritis without an associated ulcer is accompanied by a striking diffuse and confluent nodularity of the antrum in about 50% of cases. In children, when *H. pylori* antral gastritis is associated with duodenal ulcer, the nodularity is always present [9]; this finding recently has been reported in adults as well. Antral biopsies in children typically show chronic active superficial or panmucosal gastritis, often with hyperplastic lymphoid aggregates [9]. Because the antral mucosa appears endoscopically normal in about half the cases of primary *H. pylori* gastritis in children, tissue biopsy should always be done, regardless of endoscopic appearance. Biopsies also are necessary to determine the presence of *H. pylori* when there is nodularity. Nodularity may remain for months or longer after eradication of *H. pylori*.

The significance of primary *H. pylori* gastritis alone (*ie*, without duodenal ulcer) is unclear. In some cases it may be an incidental finding at endoscopy performed for another indication; at present, routine eradication of the organism under these circumstances is not indicated in children [10]. More data are required in this area. In *H. pylori*–associated ulcer disease, however, treatment is definitely recommended (see "Peptic Ulcer Disease" later in this chapter). Biopsies from the gastric cardia may show carditis due to *H. pylori* or gastroesophageal reflux in adults [11,12] and in children (E. Hassall, J Dimmick, unpublished data). In cases of possible or suspected *H. pylori* disease, biopsies should be taken from the antrum, body, and cardia, as *H. pylori* may cause different types of gastritis with different implications [13].

Lymphocytic Gastritis
Lymphocytic gastritis may be seen in childhood celiac disease [14,15]. It is characterized by a marked infiltration of the surface and pit epithelium of the antrum with T lymphocytes. In contrast, the lymphocytic gastritis of *H. pylori* is largely in the lamina propria, with intraepithelial lymphocyte counts of 4 per 100 epithelial cells, compared with 5 per 100 epithelial cells in healthy controls [14,15]. A lymphocytic gastritis also occurs in association with cytomegalovirus-induced Ménétrier's disease, as described later in this chapter.

The Postoperative Stomach
After partial gastrectomy, and, to a lesser degree, pyloroplasty, histologic changes occur in the gastric remnant or intact stomach that may be grouped under the term *reactive gastropathy* [1••].

Pernicious Anemia in Children With Portal Hypertension
Childhood or juvenile pernicious anemia (PA) is a rare condition in which achlorhydria occurs without gastric atrophy. Although uncommon, the classic form of PA also occurs in children.

Specific or Distinctive Types of Gastritis
The designation "specific or distinctive" indicates that histologic (and often endoscopic) features are present that markedly narrow the differential diagnosis, or are pathognomonic.

Crohn's Disease
Macroscopic or histologic abnormalities, or both, are present in the esophagus, stomach, or duodenum in up to 80% of children with Crohn's disease. In many of these children, however, the changes are nonspecific and occur also in ulcerative colitis. If only histologic features specific to Crohn's disease are included, such as giant cells and noncaseating granulomas, that figure becomes 20% to 33% [16,17]; if focal deep gastritis is included, the figure rises to around 50% to 60% [2•]. Upper gastrointestinal tract disease is present in over 20% of adults with Crohn's disease [18]. These figures may depend in large part on the number and location of biopsy specimens taken at endoscopy and whether serial sections of those specimens are carefully examined. The presence of noncaseating granuloma is diagnostic in the appropriate clinical context, but differentiation from other granulomatous gastritides, such as idiopathic granulomatous gastritis, chronic granulomatous disease (CGD) (discussed later in this chapter), foreign

body granulomas, tumor-associated granulomas, sarcoidosis, Whipple disease, and vasculitis-associated and unclassifiable granulomas [2•], is important. In our experience, Crohn's disease is by far the most common cause, followed distantly by chronic granulomatous disease. There usually is antral involvement. Even in children without upper gastrointestinal tract symptoms, upper tract endoscopy may be useful to help differentiate between Crohn's disease and ulcerative colitis. When growth or pubertal delay occurs, poor caloric intake and early satiety may be caused by upper gastrointestinal Crohn's disease [16].

Chronic Granulomatous Disease
Chronic granulomatous disease (CGD) is a rare X-linked immune deficiency disorder of boys. Gastric involvement is common and usually manifests as symptoms of delayed gastric emptying with a narrowed, poorly mobile antrum on contrast radiography. At endoscopy, the antral mucosa is often pale, lustreless, and swollen. Mild chronic inflammation and granulomas are often present on biopsy, but the diagnostic feature is the presence of vacuolated histiocytes laden with brown-pigmented material [19].

Eosinophilic Gastropathy
Eosinophilic gastropathy, also known as eosinophilic gastroenteropathy, also may involve the small bowel (and, less often, the colon); it usually presents with upper gastrointestinal tract symptoms, growth failure, iron deficiency anemia, and hypoalbuminemia [20]. The serum IgE is elevated, and peripheral eosinophilia is variably present. All layers of the gastric wall may be involved, but there may be selective predominance of eosinophilic infiltrates in the mucosa, muscle layers, or subserosa. Therefore, diagnosis by endoscopy is not always possible. Endoscopic features are nonspecific and include swollen folds or scattered nodules of swollen mucosa. The nodules seen in eosinophilic gastropathy are quite unlike the nodularity seen in *H. pylori* gastritis in that they are scattered, few in number, and not of uniform size; in *H. pylori*, small nodules of uniform size cover the antral mucosa diffusely, as a continuous carpet. The endoscopic findings can be striking, and are usually more impressive in the antrum. Targeted biopsies from lesions at endoscopy often reveal eosinophilic infiltrates; even in the absence of florid lesions, random biopsies are often diagnostic. Thus, the diagnosis in this disorder is made by microscopy alone or together with endoscopic findings.

Allergic Gastropathy
Allergic gastropathy may be considered to be a variant of eosinophilic gastropathy in which a specific allergen is identified, withdrawal of which results in resolution of the condition. The usual offending agent is cow's or soy milk protein, the mainstay of an infant diet. Milk protein–induced colitis also is common in these babies. Reintroduction of cow's or soy milk is almost always possible by 18 to 24 months of age. Eosinophils are present in gastric tissue obtained by mucosal biopsy [21].

Ménétrier's Disease
The typical childhood presentation of Ménétrier's disease includes upper gastrointestinal symptoms accompanied by edema following a viral illness. In the past, many children under-

went full-thickness gastric biopsy at laparotomy or even partial gastric resection, but with the development of endoscopy and biopsy techniques, surgery for diagnosis or treatment is virtually never necessary. The childhood form of the disease has been linked to cytomegalovirus (CMV) infection [22], and the natural history is one of self-resolution in weeks or months. In contrast, the adult disease is usually chronic, and partial gastrectomy has been required in some cases to alleviate persistent abdominal symptoms, hypoproteinemia, and blood loss [1••,2•].

Chronic Varioliform Gastritis
Chronic varioliform gastritis, also known as chronic erosive gastritis, appears to be more prevalent in Europe than in the United States and affects primarily older men. Nevertheless, it does occur in children. It presents with symptoms and signs similar to those of other acid peptic disorders, including gastrointestinal blood loss [23]. The clinical and histologic findings overlap with those of collagenous gastritis in children [24].

Graft-Versus-Host Disease
Graft rejection after bone marrow transplantation is manifested by changes in the gastrointestinal tract and the liver. Graft-versus-host disease (GVHD) appears to involve the stomach much less often than it involves the small and large bowel. Endoscopy may be normal, or show erythema, swelling, or erosions (although these may be due to CMV); necrosis of gland cells and apoptosis are the histologic characteristics of GVHD.

Cytomegalovirus
Cytomegalovirus infection of the stomach occurs very rarely in immunocompetent children or adults [1••,2•]. In children, it causes Ménétrier's disease and also causes gastritis following solid organ or bone marrow transplantation and immune suppression. CMV infection is so common in immune-suppressed patients that it is difficult to know in a given patient whether an area of gastritis is actually caused by the virus, or is simply a lesion resulting from physiologic stress, GVHD, or chemotherapy that happens to be colonized by the virus. It is considered to be caused by the virus if the pattern of injury is unique and not otherwise explainable.

Other
Less common specific causes of gastritis in children are noted in Table 153-2 and are discussed elsewhere.

◼ PEPTIC ULCER DISEASE
Primary Peptic Ulcer Disease
In children with chronic peptic ulcer disease, duodenal ulcers are far more prevalent than are gastric ulcers. When NSAID-related ulcers are excluded, duodenal ulcers are 20 to 30 times more common than gastric ulcers.

Helicobacter pylori
Infection with *H. pylori* may cause primary gastritis alone (see "Gastritis"), or primary gastritis in association with peptic ulcer. Such ulcers in children are almost always duodenal. Most but not all duodenal ulcer disease in children is *H. pylori*-related (Table 153-3) [25,26].

H. pylori-negative duodenal ulcer is an important entity in children; about 15% to 20% of children with duodenal ulcers have no serologic or histologic evidence of *H. pylori* [27]. Whereas children with *H. pylori*-associated duodenal ulcers have a nodular antrum and impressive histologic gastritis, those who are *H. pylori*-negative by histology and serology have no nodularity and virtual absence of histologic gastritis [27]. Children with *H. pylori*-negative duodenal ulcers do not appear to have greater acid secretion than do *H. pylori*-positive subjects, and at this time are regarded as having "idiopathic" duodenal ulcers. Genetic factors probably play a major role.

Hypersecretory conditions. Zollinger-Ellison syndrome and antral G-cell hyperplasia or hyperfunction are very rare in children [28,29]. Systemic mastocytosis, a disease in which mast cells accumulate in skin, bone marrow, liver, spleen, and gastrointestinal tract, is associated with acid hypersecretion, as is hyperparathyroidism. Hypergastrinemia with ulcer disease occurs in chronic renal failure, but whether in increased prevalence is unclear.

Secondary Peptic Ulcer Disease
Secondary peptic ulcer disease usually occurs in association with an identifiable ulcerogenic agent or circumstance. The ulcers are more often acute and are more prevalent in the stomach than in the duodenum.

Ulcers Caused by Physiologic Stress
In addition to stress gastropathy, shock, sepsis, acidosis, and hypoxemia may cause ulceration, more commonly in the stomach than in the duodenum, and sometimes in both. Gastric ulcers usually are located in the antrum or at the junction of the body and antrum. Curling's ulcer occurs after extensive burns and is more common in the stomach; Cushing's ulcer occurs with head injury, encephalopathy, or surgery, and occurs in the duodenum or stomach. Stress-related ulcers often bleed or perforate. These serious complications occur less often than they did in the past, probably because of improvements in postoperative and intensive care.

Table 153-3. Causes of Peptic Ulcer Disease in Children

Primary peptic ulcers	Secondary peptic ulcers
Helicobacter pylori-associated	Physiologic stress
	Shock, sepsis, hypoxemia
Non-*H. pylori*/idiopathic	Curling's ulcer
	Cushing's ulcer
Hypersecretory states	
Zollinger-Ellison syndrome	Drugs
G-cell hyperplasia/	Aspirin/NSAIDs
hyperfunction	Potassium chloride
Systemic mastocytosis	Iron
Chronic renal failure	Caustic agents
	Other diseases
	Sickle cell disease

Ulcers Caused by Drugs

The major offenders causing drug-related ulcers are aspirin and other NSAIDs. In children, steroids have not been shown to be an independent cause of ulcer disease. Other agents that occasionally cause ulceration are those that cause caustic injury (see "Gastritis") and potassium chloride, the latter in areas of stasis, eg, the antrum in delayed gastric emptying.

Ulcers Associated With Other Diseases

Sickle cell disease has been associated with an increased prevalence of duodenal ulcer [30]. Sickle cell disease has also been associated with splenic infarction and, small bowel ischemia.

▊▊ DUODENITIS

Like gastritis, duodenitis is neither a clinical nor a radiologic diagnosis. It may be a purely endoscopic or histologic diagnosis, but usually it is both.

Nonspecific duodenitis confined to the duodenal bulb. Multiple duodenal erosions and duodenitis occur as part of the spectrum of duodenal ulcer disease. They also may occur as a result of physiologic stress or NSAID ingestion, usually with, and occasionally without, their gastric counterparts.

Duodenitis in continuity with disorders of the rest of the small bowel. Nonspecific lesions may be postinfectious, or associated with celiac sprue or immunodeficiency states (eg, AIDS). Specific lesions are those of Crohn's disease, giardiasis, CMV, and graft-versus-host disease.

Clinical Presentation

Peptic disorders account for less than 5% of children presenting with abdominal pain, and are far less prevalent in pediatrics than in a practice of adult gastroenterology.

Symptoms of gastritis, peptic ulcer, and duodenitis may be similar, and in school-age children, they may be similar to those in adults. Being awakened from sleep by epigastric pain is a typical symptom of peptic ulcer disease in children. Most peptic ulcers occur in children between 7 and 16 years of age (mean 11 years) [9,27,32]. Younger children may not be able to localize the pain to the epigastrium, and may present with anorexia and irritability, especially with meals. Gastrointestinal bleeding may occur with long-standing antecedent epigastric pain or other symptoms, but painless bleeding may be the only manifestation of ulcer disease; in the experience at our hospital, about 30% to 40% of children with duodenal ulcers have this "silent" presentation. On physical examination, epigastric tenderness is an unreliable sign of gastritis or ulcer disease. Perforation and penetration are less common complications in children than in adults.

Diagnosis

As in adults, the symptoms of gastritis or peptic ulcer can be mimicked by esophagitis, nonulcer dyspepsia, gallbladder or liver disease, pneumonia, pancreatitis, or giardiasis. Pain that is truly localized to the epigastrium is relatively uncommon in children, and always requires investigation, as does upper gastrointestinal bleeding, with or without pain.

As in adults, the definitive diagnosis is made with gastroscopy, which can confirm or exclude the presence of ulcers and effect hemostasis in cases of active bleeding. The performance of endoscopy in children is a highly specialized undertaking, the *least* problematic aspect of which is actual passage of an appropriate-sized endoscope and the taking of biopsy specimens or performance of endoscopic hemostasis. Many other cognitive and practical pediatric skills are important to ensure the appropriate, safe, and humane performance of endoscopy in children [31].

The causes of ulcer disease and gastritis often can be differentiated by endoscopic examination and by biopsies of appropriate areas of the stomach. Diagnosis of a specific type of gastritis, or determination of the cause of peptic ulcer, obviously has important implications for treatment, as clearly illustrated by the very different treatment approaches to H. pylori–associated and non–H. pylori ulcer disease. When an H. pylori–negative ulcer is diagnosed, a fasting plasma gastrin level should be obtained to exclude one of the G-cell disorders or Zollinger-Ellison syndrome, and biopsy specimens should be carefully examined for signs of Crohn's disease.

A positive urea breath test does not indicate that ulcer disease is present; it indicates only that H. pylori is present in the stomach. Conversely, a negative urea breath test does not exclude ulcer disease. Once H. pylori–associated disease has been definitively diagnosed by endoscopy and biopsy, the urea breath test may be useful to establish that H. pylori has been eradicated, once the test is approved for children.

In children, upper gastrointestinal series are highly unreliable for the diagnosis of peptic diseases, with false-positives (eg, duodenal spasm or irritability) being as problematic as false-negatives. Even when an ulcer crater is shown, barium studies cannot distinguish between H. pylori–associated and non–H. pylori ulcers. Although marked antral nodularity occasionally is detected on barium studies, it usually is present whether or not H. pylori has been eradicated.

Barium studies are indicated mainly to evaluate complaints of early satiety or recurrent vomiting, to exclude intestinal malrotation, gastric outlet obstruction, or duodenal deformity.

Treatment

Treatment of Specific Disorders

The treatment of specific disorders in children is similar to that in adults. The difference in treatment results from the issues specific to children—the management of fluid and electrolyte balance in resuscitation; dosage, palatability and appropriate form (tablets/capsules/liquid) of medications; and the potential adverse effects of medications.

"Stress" gastritis is treated by managing the underlying hypoxemia, acidosis, sepsis, and with acid suppression and antacids. Traumatic gastritis is treated supportively and with attention to the underlying cause of forceful vomiting. Peptic disease caused by aspirin or NSAIDs may respond to dose reduction or switching of medication; treatment with prostaglandin- (misoprostol) or acid-suppressing agents alleviates symptoms and may prevent ulceration. Portal hypertensive gastropathy usually is asymptomatic but may be a source of bleeding; it responds when the underlying portal hypertension is treated. Caustic injuries are managed with acid suppression and supportive treatment. Whereas allergic gastropathy may respond to withdrawal of identified antigens, eosinophilic gastropathy often requires steroid therapy.

Currently, the major debate is how best to treat the most prevalent peptic disease—duodenal ulcer associated with *H. pylori* gastritis. Although eradication of *H. pylori* with antibiotics heals the ulcer, an ideal regimen for children has not yet been established.

Compliance is a problem in children with some regimens, but a 2-week course of MOC (metronidazole, omeprazole, and clarithromycin) has been highly efficacious [32]. Unless *H. pylori* gastritis is present, duodenal ulcers should not be treated with antibiotics. Those cases of true *H. pylori*–negative duodenal ulcer should be treated with 6 weeks of acid suppression. Peptic ulcer disease is not yet an approved indication for proton pump inhibitors in children. Currently, we perform follow-up endoscopy to determine ulcer healing and eradication of *H. pylori*. Serologic tests do not allow definitive diagnosis of *H. pylori*: a positive test indicates only that *H. pylori* may be present or has been present in the past. A positive serologic test does not determine whether an ulcer is present; a negative test does not rule out the presence of an *H. pylori*–negative ulcer. Following treatment, titers fall slowly. Antibody titers with appropriate cut-offs for children have not been established. Symptoms also are a poor guide to ulcer healing or cure, because a high percentage of children initially present with painless bleeding. For these reasons, endoscopic and histologic proof of ulcer healing and *H. pylori* eradication is important in children. At a future date, once urea breath tests (UBT) are approved for use in children, it may be justifiable to use the UBT to document eradication of *H. pylori* in children presenting with uncomplicated ulcer disease. Because ulcer disease is uncommon in children and because it has a high morbidity, definitive diagnosis and proof of successful treatment is warranted [33].

Routine eradication of *H. pylori* is not currently indicated in the presence of gastritis without an ulcer, because there is no good evidence that it is a cause of nonulcer dyspepsia. At present there is no indication to eradicate *H. pylori* in children with the intent of preventing cancer later in life.

Recently, the Canadian Consensus Conference on *H. pylori* disease published guidelines for an approach to diagnosis and treatment of *H. pylori* disease. These guidelines include recommendations for children that are different from those for adults [33].

Endoscopic therapy for children follows the same guidelines as in adults.

There is no evidence that restrictive diets are helpful other than in eosinophilic or allergic gastropathy, or when a patient reports symptoms from a particular food.

Acid-reducing operations such as vagotomy or antrectomy have a high morbidity and failure rate in children [29]. With the highly effective acid-suppressing medications that have become available in the last several years [34], these operations have become virtually obsolete in children. Current indications for surgery in peptic diseases are perforation of the stomach or duodenum; active bleeding that cannot be controlled by medical therapy or endoscopic hemostasis; gastric outlet or duodenal obstruction caused by scarring from peptic disease; or failure of medical therapy in hypersecretory syndromes.

REFERENCES

Recently published papers of particular interest have been highlighted as follows:
• Of interest
•• Of outstanding interest

1.•• Lewin KJ, Riddell RH, Weinstein WM: In *Gastrointestinal Pathology and its Clinical Implications. Part 4: Stomach and Proximal Duodenum*, vol 1. New York: Igaku-Shoin; 1992:493–587.
This standard text highlights the essential endoscopist-pathologist dialogue, with outstanding endoscopic and histologic photos accompanying the text, which directly pertain to clinical problems. The clinical classification of gastritis set forth by these authors was used as a basis for the pediatric approach described in this chapter.

2.• Jevon G, Dimmick JE, Hassall E: Pediatric gastritis. *Perspect Pediatr Pathol* 1997, 20:35–76.
This article provides a classification of gastritis in children, by etiology and pathogenesis. It deals with the necessity for endoscopist-pathologist communication, and comprehensively discusses the gastritides and gastropathies of childhood.

3. Carpenter HA, Talley NJ: Gastroscopy is incomplete without biopsy: clinical relevance of distinguishing gastropathy from gastritis. *Gastroenterology* 1995, 108:917–924.

4. Hyman PE, Clarke D, Everett SL, *et al.*: Gastric secretory function in preterm infants. *J Pediatr* 1985, 106:467–470.

5. Mulberg AE, Linz C, Bem E, *et al.*: Identification of nonsteroidal antiinflammatory drug-induced gastroduodenal injury in children with juvenile rheumatoid arthritis. *J Pediatr* 1993, 122:647–649.

6. Hyams JS, Treem WR: Portal hypertensive gastropathy in children. *J Pediatr Gastroenterol Nutr* 1993, 17:13–18.

7. Byrne WJ: Foreign bodies and caustic ingestions. *Gastrointest Endosc Clin North Am* 1994:99–119.

8. Tomomasa T, Hsu JY, Itoh K, Kuroume T: Endoscopic findings in pediatric patients with Henoch-Schönlein purpura and gastrointestinal symptoms. *J Pediatr Gastroenterol Nutr* 1987, 6:725–729.

9. Hassall E, Dimmick JE: Unique features of *H. pylori* disease in children. *Dig Dis Sci* 1991, 36:417–423.

10. Gormally SM, Prakesh N, Durnin MT, *et al.*: Association of symptoms with *Helicobacter pylori* infection in children. *J Pediatr* 1995, 126:753–756.

11. Genta RM, Huberman RM, Graham DY: The gastric cardia in *Heliobacter pylori* infection. *Hum Pathol* 1994, 25:915–919.

12. Riddell RH: The biopsy diagnosis of gastroesophageal reflux disease, "carditis", and Barrett's esophagus, and sequelae of therapy. *Am J Surg Pathol* 1996, 20:S31–S50.

13. Rubin CE: Are there three types of *H. pylori* gastritis? *Gastroenterology* 1997, 112:2108–2110.

14. De Giacomo C, Gianatti A, Negrini R, *et al.*: Lymphocytic gastritis: a positive relationship with celiac disease. *J Pediatr* 1994, 124:57–62.

15. Jevon GP, Dimmick JE, Dohil R, Hassall E: The spectrum of gastritis in celiac disease in childhood. *Ped Pathol Dev Med* 1998, in press.

16. Ruuska T, Vaajalahti P, Aräjarvi P, Mäki M: Prospective evaluation of upper gastrointestinal mucosal lesions in children with ulcerative colitis and Crohn's disease. *J Pediatr Gastroenterol Nutr* 1994, 19:181–186.

17. Lenaerts C, Roy CC, Vaillancourt M, *et al.*: High incidence of upper gastrointestinal tract involvement in children with Crohn's disease. *Pediatrics* 1989, 83:777–781.

18. Freeman HJ: Upper gastrointestinal tract Crohn's disease. *Can J Gastroenterol* 1990, 4:26–32.

19. Chin TW, Stiehm ER, Falloon J, Gallin JI: Corticosteroids in treatment of obstructive lesions of chronic granulomatous disease. *J Pediatr* 1987, 111:349–352.

20. Whitington PF, Whitington GL: Eosinophilic gastroenteropathy in childhood. *J Pediatr Gastroenterol Nutr* 1988, 7:379–386.

21. Goldman H, Proujansky R: Allergic proctitis and gastroenteritis in children. Clinical and mucosal biopsy features in 53 cases. *Am J Surg Pathol* 1986, 10:75–86.

22. Sferra TJ, Pawel BR, Qualman SJ, Li BU: Ménétrier disease of childhood: role of cytomegalovirus and transforming growth factor alpha. *J Pediatr* 1996, 128:213–219.

23. Couper R, Lasky B, Drumm B, *et al.*: Chronic varioliform gastritis in childhood. *J Pediatr* 1989, 115:441–444.

24. Colletti RB, Cameron DJS, Hassall E, *et al*: Collagenous gastritis: an international puzzle. *J Pediatr Gastroenterol Nutr* 1998, 26:540.

25. Graham DY, Go MF: Helicobacter pylori: current status. *Gastroenterology* 1993, 105:279–282.

26. Drumm B: Helicobacter pylori in the pediatric patient. *Gastroenterol Clin North Am* 1993, 22:169–182.

27. Hassall E, Hiruki T, Dimmick JE: True Helicobacter pylori-negative duodenal ulcer disease in children. *Gastroenterology* 1993, 104:96.

28. De Giacomo C, Fiocca R, Villani L, *et al.*: Omeprazole treatment of severe peptic disease associated with antral G cell hyperfunction and hyperpepsinogenemia I in an infant. *J Pediatr* 1990, 117:989–993.

29. Hyman PE, Hassall E: Marked basal gastric acid hypersecretion and peptic ulcer disease: medical management with combination H$_2$-histamine receptor antagonist and anticholinergic. *J Pediatr Gastroenterol Nutr* 1988, 7:57–63.

30. Rao S, Royal JE, Conrad JE, *et al.*: Duodenal ulcer in sickle cell anemia. *J Pediatr Gastroenterol Nutr* 1990, 10:117–120.

31.• Hassall E: NASPGN Position Paper: requirements for training to ensure competence of endoscopists performing invasive procedures in children. *J Pediatr Gastroenterol Nutr* 1997, 24:345–347.

This paper discusses the cognitive skills required and the minimum training requirements for attaining competence in performing endoscopic procedures in children.

32. Dohil R, Israel DM, Hassall E: Effective two-week antibiotic therapy for *H. pylori* disease in children. *Am J Gastroenterol* 1997, 92:244–247.

33.•• Hunt R, Thomson ABR, Consensus Conference Participants: Canadian Helicobacter pylori Consensus Conference. *Can J Gastroenterol* 1998, 12:31–41.

This is the first national consensus document to include guidelines for an approach to suspected peptic ulcer disease and to *H. pylori* disease in children.

34. Israel DM, Hassall E: Omeprazole and other proton pump inhibitors: pharmacology, efficacy, and safety, with special reference to use in children. *J Pediatr Gastroenterol Nutr*, in press.

154 Infantile Hypertrophic Pyloric Stenosis
Neil D. Kutin

Pyloric stenosis is the most common condition requiring abdominal surgery in infancy. Earlier literature referred to this condition as *congenital* or *idiopathic hypertrophic pyloric stenosis*. It is now called *hypertrophic pyloric stenosis* or *infantile hypertrophic pyloric stenosis* (IHPS). The development of successful surgical treatment in the early 1900s by Fredet and Ramstedt [1] made possible the survival of infants throughout the world, and modern pediatric anesthetic techniques have virtually eliminated mortality from surgical management. Recent advances in ultrasonography have resulted in earlier diagnoses, leading to fewer fluid- and nutritionally depleted infants and briefer hospitalizations.

ANATOMY

The pylorus is the anatomic area that joins the stomach to the duodenum (Fig. 154-1). The elongated distal part of this region is called the *pyloric canal*. The circular muscle layer of the stomach is thickest in the pyloric region, resulting in an actual ring of muscle, the *pyloric sphincter*, which can close the pylorus. Hypertrophy of the normal circular muscle of the pyloric canal produces a reduction in the size of the lumen. In time, the affected region increases in length as well as thickness, which results in a gastric outlet obstruction by a "tumor" large enough to be felt or diagnosed by appropriate imaging techniques.

EPIDEMIOLOGY

The reported incidence of IHPS ranges from 1.7 per 1000 [2] to 6.2 per 1000 [3] live births. It is more prevalent in whites than in blacks or Asians [4]. There is also a consistent gender differential, with a male preponderance ranging from 2.5:1 to 5.5:1 [4]. Several large series have shown that 40% of patients needing surgery for IHPS are firstborn males [5]. IHPS is often associated with congenital anomalies, including orthopedic, urologic, cardiac, and other gastrointestinal conditions [2]. There is a higher rate of IHPS in the children of women who have had

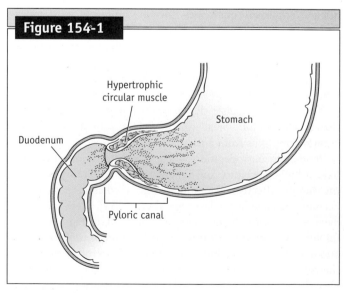

Figure 154-1

Anatomy of the pylorus.

surgery for IHPS than in children of men who were operated on for this condition (20% vs 5%) [6], and there are reports of twin and triplet females with IHPS, supporting the familial tendency [7].

ETIOLOGY

The cause of IHPS remains unknown. Any explanation must take into consideration genetic factors, age of presentation, and the results of histologic and hormonal studies.

Although some clinicians classify it as a congenital disorder, the condition is rarely present at birth. An ultrasound study reported from Northern Ireland in 1989 showed that muscle hypertrophy developed after birth in nine babies with IHPS confirmed at surgery [8••]. A relationship between IHPS and erythromycin estolate, when taken by the neonate, was reported in 1976 [9], but this association has not received further mention.

Anatomic studies of biopsy specimens obtained during pyloromyotomy demonstrate abnormalities of the myenteric plexus of the affected muscle. However, review suggests that these abnormalities are the result rather than the cause of the hypertrophy [10•].

A canine model of IHPS described in 1970 suggested a causal association between gastrin and IHPS [11]. Further work, however, has demonstrated that gastrin does not cross the human placenta [10•].

Recently, immunohistochemical analyses of biopsy specimens obtained during pyloromyotomy have been performed to evaluate substances active in the relaxation of smooth muscle. One study showed a loss of peptide-containing nerve fibers in the muscle, but not in the myenteric plexus [12]. There is evidence that ganglionic expression of vasointestinal peptide (VIP) in IHPS muscle is increased [13]. Of greatest interest is a report that levels of nitric oxide synthase (NOS) are selectively diminished in the circular muscle of IHPS material obtained at biopsy [14••].

PATHOPHYSIOLOGY

The pathophysiologic sequence begins with failure of the pyloric sphincter to relax. This failure may be the result of some predisposition to spasm as a result of a VIP- or NOS-mediated neuromuscular abnormality, as mentioned earlier. The response to the spasm is muscular hypertrophy, which narrows the pyloric canal. Once emesis becomes frequent, there is no further progression of the muscle hypertrophy. At the time the infant presents with IHPS, there is general uniformity in the size of the pyloric "tumor." Measurement of the DNA concentration in biopsy specimens has shown that the amount of hypertrophy is not related either to the infant's age or to the duration of symptoms [15]. The muscle thickening progresses to the point that it causes luminal obstruction on both mucosal and submucosal levels. This obstruction causes the infant to become symptomatic.

CLINICAL FEATURES

Infantile hypertrophic pyloric stenosis usually is suspected in an infant at the age of 2 weeks to 3 months because of worsening episodes of emesis. The emesis may have been occurring since birth, but it becomes more frequent and forceful as time goes on. The emesis is nonbilious, is not related to the infant's

position, and often is projectile in nature. Many infants are hungry soon after vomiting. Weight loss usually is present.

The differential diagnosis includes gastrointestinal and other causes (Table 154-1). Incorrect diagnoses of esophagogastric reflux, poor feeding technique, or formula intolerance have been made in an infant subsequently diagnosed with IHPS. IHPS has been seen in infants with hiatal hernias [16]. Increased intracranial pressure from congenital and acquired conditions also can cause projectile emesis, which may lead to an incorrect diagnosis of IHPS. Finally, infants with salt-losing adrenogenital syndrome, metabolic problems, or sepsis may persistently vomit and fail to thrive.

IHPS can cause hematemesis. Studies have shown the site of the bleeding in IHPS to be the esophageal mucosa, caused by acid reflux resulting from gastric outlet obstruction [17].

Physical examination of the infant suspected of having IHPS does not require sedation. The examination should begin in the inguinal area because an incarcerated inguinal hernia may present with severe vomiting.

The pyloric muscle is a hard moveable "olive" measuring about 2 cm by 1.5 cm in the upper abdomen near and usually to the right of the midline (Fig. 154-2). The stomach should be emptied with an 8- or 10F feeding tube before any attempt is made to palpate the pylorus. Decompression makes it easier to feel an abnormal pylorus, and the volume of gastric fluid aspirated can also aid in diagnosis. A volume of 60 mL or greater in an infant who has not been fed for several hours suggests gastric outlet obstruction.

The "tumor" can be successfully palpated about 80% of the time. When the history is suggestive of IHPS, an imaging study (ultrasonographic or upper gastrointestinal [UGI] series) is indicated if the pylorus is not palpable.

Laboratory values obtained should include a complete blood count (CBC), serum electrolytes, and urinalysis. There may be mild abnormalities in the level of hemoglobin, but severe anemia is rare. It is not unusual to see a mild to moderate elevation of the neutrophil count.

Vomiting secondary to gastric outlet obstruction results in the loss of hydrochloric acid, which causes a depletion of serum chloride and hypokalemic metabolic alkalosis. Severe electrolyte and acid–base disturbances have become less frequent with

---

Table 154-1. Differential Diagnosis of Projectile Emesis

Gastrointestinal
  Esophagogastric reflux
  Antral web
  Gastric duplication
  Nonrotation or malrotation
  Improper feeding techniques
  Formula intolerance
Other
  Increased intracranial pressure
  Salt-losing adrenogenital syndrome
  Metabolic disorders
  Sepsis

earlier detection. In a 1989 study of 216 infants, more than 50% of infants with IHPS presented with abnormal serum electrolyte values [18]. More recently, 85% and 90% of infants with IHPS had normal serum electrolyte levels [19••,20].

The urinalysis is usually normal in affected infants. Because the kidneys are still immature, even mild elevations of the specific gravity may indicate dehydration. Dehydration leads to increased production of aldosterone, which leads to increased renal excretion of potassium. Depletion of chloride also leads to an exchange of hydrogen and of potassium for sodium in the distal tubule. This paradoxic aciduria in the face of alkalosis is an indication of gastric outlet obstruction.

Jaundice is present in 2% of infants with IHPS. It may be caused by a decrease in hepatic glucuronyl transferase activity that results in an elevated unconjugated hyperbilirubinemia. It clears quickly after surgery [21].

▰ DIAGNOSIS

In the typical case of IHPS in which there is an easily palpable pyloric mass, no further diagnostic tests are needed. However, in the infant with an atypical presentation, or when the physical diagnosis is negative but the history is suspicious, an imaging test is indicated. In the past, the preferred study was a UGI barium study of the stomach and duodenum (UGI series) (Fig. 154-3). The UGI series gives a picture of the inner anatomy of the pyloric canal. Abnormal length of the canal, narrowing of the lumen, and delayed gastric emptying all are typical of IHPS. The UGI series also can detect esophagogastric reflux, hiatal hernia, errors of intestinal rotation, and other gastrointestinal abnormalities.

The preferred imaging test now is ultrasonography, which shows the thickness of the pyloric muscle. There are strict sonographic criteria for the diagnosis of IHPS (Fig. 154-4). The

pyloric muscle must be thicker than 5 mm and longer than 2.1 cm [22]. Some recent studies have claimed 100% accuracy with ultrasonographic diagnosis [23]. It is recommended that ultrasonography be reserved for the nonpalpable or atypical variety of IHPS [23].

The premature infant who is being evaluated for IHPS presents a special diagnostic problem. Because ultrasonography criteria may not be met in the premature infant, a UGI series may be needed in addition to ultrasonography. Premature infants who require transpyloric enteral feeds may be at particular risk for IHPS [24].

In 1994, a group from Brussels reported their experience with the endoscopic diagnosis of IHPS [25•]. Their criteria for endoscopic diagnosis included a cauliflower-like narrowing of the lumen, the inability to pass a 7.8-mm endoscope, and gastric stasis. Accuracy was 97% in their series of 63 infants.

▰ TREATMENT

Even in the least depleted infants there is some degree of dehydration, and fluid replacement is needed. In the infant with moderate to severe dehydration, a bolus of normal saline 20 mL/kg begins the correction. It may take several days to correct imbalances in infants with severe metabolic alkalosis. The infant's renal immaturity must be taken into consideration when determining the plan for restoration of normal electrolyte values.

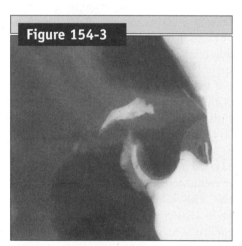

Figure 154-3

Infantile hypertrophic pyloric stenosis diagnosed by upper gastrointestinal series.

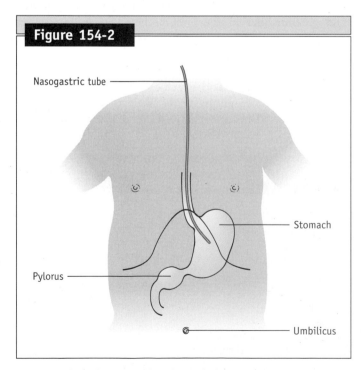

Figure 154-2

Nasogastric tube

Stomach

Pylorus

Umbilicus

Location of the hypertrophic pylorus during typical physical examination.

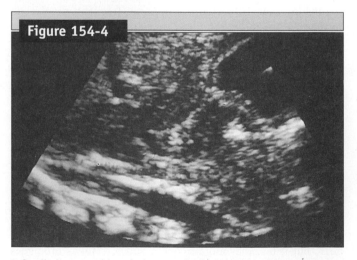

Figure 154-4

Infantile hypertrophic pyloric stenosis diagnosed by ultrasonography.

For the past 80 years the treatment for IHPS has been operative pyloromyotomy. This procedure almost always requires general anesthesia, but in the typical infant with IHPS and no associated cardiovascular anomalies, the anesthetic risk is minimal.

The most common operative complication is wound infection, which occurs in 3% of patients [19•]. Infection often appears after discharge from the hospital and is almost always managed successfully with topical antibiotic ointments on an outpatient basis. Next in frequency is perforation of the mucosa at the duodenal end of the canal [19•], but this complication has been shown recently to have markedly decreased.

Recently there have been some modifications in the surgical procedure. Surgery has been performed through an umbilical skin fold incision that leaves almost no visible scar [26]. Several groups have demonstrated that laparoscopic pyloromyotomy is possible [27]. However, the standard treatment is still open pyloromyotomy, a successful operation that takes less than 30 minutes.

Most of the experience with nonoperative management of IHPS has been reported by European groups [28•] and includes the use of intravenous atropine [29, 30].

Because of refinements in instrumentation, there is renewed interest in the role of balloon dilatation for IHPS (Fig. 154-5, see also **Color Plate**). Balloon dilatation has been especially helpful postoperatively, performed via the pediatric endoscope with or without fluoroscopic control [31••]. Successful endoscopic dilatation has been reported in a girl who developed IHPS following repair of a giant omphalocele [32].

PROGNOSIS

Most infants who undergo pyloromyotomy for IHPS have excellent results, resuming full feeding within a day or two of surgery. However, some infants continue to have emesis in the early postoperative period. This problem does not correlate with the postoperative feeding schedule, which varies widely among institutions. Marked weight loss, severe alkalosis, and hematemesis are associated with feeding difficulty after surgery. Most patients stop vomiting when the volume, strength, or interval of postoperative feedings is changed.

There are, however, infants with persistent postoperative emesis that does not respond to feeding manipulations. In these cases concern as to whether there is an incomplete division of the pyloric muscle or a recurrence of the stenosis is warranted.

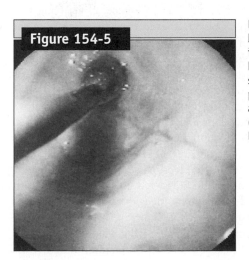

Figure 154-5

Endoscopic view of balloon dilation of infantile hypertrophic pyloric stenosis after failed pyloromyotomy. See also **Color Plate**. (*Courtesy of* V. Khoshoo, MD.)

Imaging studies are not helpful in these patients because it takes 2 to 12 weeks for the muscle hypertrophy to resolve after pyloromyotomy [33]. In these rare cases of refractory emesis following pyloromyotomy, there may be a role for atropine or endoscopic balloon dilatation.

REFERENCES

Recently published papers of particular interest have been highlighted as follows:
•   Of interest
•• Of outstanding interest

1. Ravitch MM: The story of pyloric stenosis. *Surgery* 1960, 48:1117–1143.
2. Applegate MS, Druschel CM: The epidemiology of infantile hypertrophic pyloric stenosis in New York State. *Arch Pediatr Adolesc Med* 1995, 149:1123–1129.
3. Jedd MB, Melton LJ, Griffen MR, *et al.*: Factors associated with infantile hypertrophic pyloric stenosis. *Am J Dis Child* 1988, 142:334–337.
4. Mitchell LE, Risch N: The genetics of infantile hypertrophic pyloric stenosis. *Am J Dis Child* 1993, 147:1203–1211.
5. Scharli A, Sieber WK, Kieswetter WB: Hypertrophic pyloric stenosis at the Children's Hospital of Pittsburgh from 1912 to 1967. *J Pediatr Surg* 1969, 4:108–114.
6. Carter CO, Evans KA: Inheritance of congenital pyloric stenosis. *J Med Genetics* 1969, 6:233–254.
7. Hicks LM, Morgan A, Anderson MR: Pyloric stenosis—a report of triplet females and notes on its inheritance. *J Pediatr Surg* 1981, 16:739–740.
8.•• Rollins MD, Shields MD, Quinn RJM, Wooldridge MAW: Pyloric stenosis: congenital or acquired? *Arch Dis Child* 1989, 64:138–139.
This paper confirmed the congenital nature of pyloric stenosis.
9. SanFilippo JA: Infantile hypertrophic pyloric stenosis related to ingestion of erythromycin estolate: a report of five cases. *J Pediatr Surg* 1976, 11:177–180.
10.• Spicer RD: Infantile hypertrophic pyloric stenosis: a review. *Br J Surg* 1982, 69:128–135.
This article presents an excellent review of the topic of infantile hypertrophic pyloric stenosis, with special emphasis on the etiology as well as clinical management in the early 1980s.
11. Dodge JA: Production of duodenal ulcers and hypertrophic pyloric stenosis by administration of pentagastrin to pregnant and newborn dogs. *Nature* 1970, 225:284–285.
12. Wattchow DA, Cass DT, Furness JB, *et al.*: Abnormalities of peptide-containing nerve fibers in infantile hypertrophic pyloric stenosis. *Gastroenterology* 1987, 92:443–448.
13. Abel RM: The ontogeny of the peptide innervation of the human pylorus, with special reference to understanding the aetiology and pathogenesis of infantile hypertrophic pyloric stenosis. *J Pediatr Surg* 1996, 31:490–497.
14.•• Vanderwinden JM, Mailleux P, Schiffmann SN, *et al.*: Nitric oxide synthase activity in infantile hypertrophic pyloric stenosis. *N Engl J Med* 1992, 327:511–515.
This experimental study has been cited frequently since its publication. The authors report a very promising avenue of research that might explain the cause of IHPS and may eventually alter its treatment.
15. Ukabiala O, Lister J: The extent of muscle hypertrophy in infantile hypertrophic pyloric stenosis does not depend on age and duration of symptoms. *J Pediatr Surg* 1987, 22:200–202.
16. Iijima T, Okamatsu T, Matsumura M, Yatsuzuka M: Hypertrophic pyloric stenosis associated with hiatal hernia. *J Pediatr Surg* 1996, 31:277–279.
17. Takeuchi S, Tamate S, Nakahira M, Kadowaki H: Esophagitis in infants with hypertrophic pyloric stenosis: a source of hematemesis. *J Pediatr Surg* 1993, 28:59–62.
18. Breaux CW, Hood JS, Georgeson KE: The significance of alkalosis and hypochloremia in hypertrophic pyloric stenosis. *J Pediatr Surg* 1989, 24:1250–1252.

19.• Poon TSC, Zhang AL, Cartmill T, Cass DT: Changing patterns of diagnosis and treatment of infantile hypertrophic pyloric stenosis: a clinical audit of 303 patients. *J Pediatr Surg* 1996, 31:1611–1615.
This group reports a clinical series typical of what is currently expected for the management of patients with infantile hypertrophic pyloric stenosis.

20.   Chen EA, Luks FI, Gilchrist BF, *et al*.: Pyloric stenosis in the age of ultrasonography: fading skills, better patients? *J Pediatr Surg* 1996, 31:829–830.

21.   Wooley MM, Felsher BF, Asch MJ, *et al*.: Jaundice, hypertrophic pyloric stenosis, and hepatic glucuronyl transferase. *J Pediatr Surg* 1974, 9:359–363.

22.   Blumhagen JD, Maclin L, Krauter D, *et al*.: Sonographic diagnosis of hypertrophic pyloric stenosis. *AJR Am J Roentgenol* 1988, 150:1367–1370.

23.   Godbole P, Sprigg A, Dickson JAS, Lin PC: Ultrasound compared with clinical examination in infantile hypertrophic pyloric stenosis. *Arch Dis Child* 1996, 75:335–337.

24.   Cosman BC, Sudekum AE, Oakes DD, deVries PA: Pyloric stenosis in a premature infant. *J Pediatr Surg* 1992, 27:1534–1536.

25.• De Backer A, Bove T, Vandenplas Y, *et al*.: Contribution of endoscopy to early diagnosis of hypertrophic pyloric stenosis. *J Pediatr Gastroenterol Nutr* 1994, 18:78–81.
These authors present a convincing argument for the role of endoscopy in the diagnosis of IHPS.

26.   Fitzgerald PG, Lau GYP, Langer JC, Cameron GS: Umbilical fold incision for pyloromyotomy. *J Pediatr Surg* 1990, 25:1117–1118.

27.   Greason KL, Thompson WR, Downey EC, Lo Sasso B: Laparoscopic pyloromyotomy for infantile hypertrophic pyloric stenosis: report of 11 cases. *J Pediatr Surg* 1995, 30:1571–1574.

28.• Rasmussen L, Hansen LP, Pedersen SA: Infantile pyloric stenosis: the changing trend in treatment in a Danish county. *J Pediatr Surg* 1987, 22:953–955.
The contrast between medical and surgical treatment for IHPS is well summarized in this historical review.

29.   Rudolph CD: Medical treatment of idiopathic hypertrophic pyloric stenosis: should we marinate or slice the "olive"? *J Pediatr Gastroenterol Nutr* 1996, 23:399–401.

30.   Nagita A, Yamaguchi J, Amemoto K, *et al*.: Management and ultrasonographic appearance of infantile hypertrophic pyloric stenosis with intravenous atropine sulfate. *J Pediatr Gastroenterol Nutr* 1996, 23:172–177.

31.•• Khoshoo V, Noel RA, LaGarde D, *et al*.: Endoscopic balloon dilatation of failed pyloromyotomy in young infants. *J Pediatr Gastroenterol Nutr* 1996, 23:447–451.
These authors suggest a role for the endoscopic management of infants with failed pyloromyotomy for IHPS.

32.   Ogawa Y, Higashimoto Y, Nishijima E, *et al*.: Successful endoscopic balloon dilatation for hypertrophic pyloric stenosis. *J Pediatr Surg* 1996, 31:1712–1714.

33.   Okorie NM, Dickson JAS, Carver RA, Steiner GM: What happens to the pylorus after pyloromyotomy? *Arch Dis Child* 1988, 63:1339–1340.

155 Upper Gastrointestinal Bleeding In Children
Adam G. Mezoff

Gastrointestinal bleeding is a relatively common problem in children. Approximately 1% of all inpatient admissions to a pediatric hospital and 10% of new referrals to pediatric gastroenterologists are for hematemesis or hematochezia [1••]. Additionally, many children with gastrointestinal bleeding are treated by their primary care physicians without hospitalization or referral. In most cases, bleeding in children stops spontaneously or is easily controlled. Its cause is usually easily determined.

PHYSIOLOGY AND PATHOPHYSIOLOGY

Pathophysiologic events that lead to a disruption in the integrity of the upper gastrointestinal mucosa and consequently cause bleeding are similar in children and adults.

The newborn stomach begins to produce hydrochloric acid soon after birth. By 6 hours of age, acid secretion in term infants is equal to basal acid output in an older control population [2]. The intragastric pH drops from 5.3 immediately after birth to 4.0 at 8 hours. The initially more alkaline gastric pH is attributed primarily to the pH of swallowed amniotic fluid. Gastric acid secretion decreases from day 10 to day 30, but by 3 to 4 months of age maximal secretion of acid approximates that in the adult [3,4]. Maximal pepsin secretion parallels maximal acid output during infancy. Pepsin output is proportional to hydrogen secretion during the first 4 months of life [5,6•].

INITIAL EVALUATION OF ACUTE GASTRO-INTESTINAL BLEEDING IN CHILDREN

The initial diagnostic evaluation of gastrointestinal bleeding focuses on four main issues: 1) ensuring that the child is indeed passing blood and not some other substance; 2) verifying that the blood is the child's blood; 3) evaluating the severity of the bleed; and 4) identifying the cause or source of bleeding.

Many foods mimic vomited blood, especially those with either natural or artificial red coloring (Table 155-1). Melena may be confused with dark-colored or black stools seen with iron supplementation, bismuth, or dark chocolate. It is, therefore, important to test stools or emesis appropriately to ensure that the color is correctly attributed to blood.

Once it has been established that blood has been passed, it is important to verify that the blood passed is that of the child. This is a primary concern in breast-fed infants, in whom vomited maternal blood from the mother's cracked nipples may be mistaken for neonatal blood. The Apt test, based on the conversion of oxyhemoglobin to hematin when blood is mixed with alkali (Table 155-2), can be used to differentiate infant from maternal hemoglobin. Fetal hemoglobin is resistant to denaturation, unlike maternal blood, and does not change color when this test is performed.

Gastrointestinal bleeding in children occasionally is fabricated (Munchausen syndrome by proxy; see Chapter 183). The blood found in these cases often is that of the parent reporting the problem. Therefore, blood typing and forensic testing may be important. The possibility of factitious bleeding should be considered in any child in whom the source of repeated upper gastrointestinal bleeding cannot be determined.

It is imperative to determine the hemodynamic consequences of the blood loss. In children, as in adults, the most reliable signs of significant blood volume loss are an increased pulse rate, signs of decreased perfusion (eg, capillary refill), and, eventually, a decrease in blood pressure. Alterations in vital signs can be correlated with the approximate blood volume lost (Table 155-3).

ETIOLOGY

The etiology of upper gastrointestinal bleeding in infants and children can be established in more than 90% of cases. Specific clinical conditions may be associated with distinct causes. Children with immune compromise often have gastrointestinal bleeding from infection. Viral agents such as cytomegalovirus or herpes simplex and fungi such as *Candida* may result in esophagitis, and, consequently, hematemesis. Chemotherapeutic agents can induce immune suppression, and, in addition, produce mucositis with upper gastrointestinal bleeding. Patients with severe burns (Curling's ulcers) or head trauma (Cushing's ulcers) also may develop peptic ulceration and bleeding. Patients in the pediatric intensive care unit with life-threatening illness are prone to bleeding from stress ulcers or gastritis. The causes of upper gastrointestinal bleeding are best categorized on the basis of age (Table 155-4).

Table 155-1. Foods That May Mimic Gastrointestinal Bleeding

Hematemesis	Melena
Red food coloring (ie, cereals)	Bismuth-containing substances
Beets	Blueberries
Red Jell-O	Cranberries
Red Kool-Aid	Dark chocolate
Fruit Juices	Grape juice
Catsup	Iron supplements
Tomato juice or skin	Spinach

Table 155-2. The Apt Test to Differentiate Fetal From Adult Hemoglobin

Mix one part of bloody stool or emesis with five parts water

Centrifuge at 2000 RPMs for 2 minutes

Mix the supernatant with 1 mL of 0.1 N sodium hydroxide

Adult hemoglobin turns the mixture brown, and fetal hemoglobin, more resistant to denaturation, remains pink

Neonates and Infants

Severe gastritis or localized ulcer disease associated with stress (eg, difficult delivery, respiratory distress, or necrotizing enterocolitis) can cause severe bleeding in the neonate. Massive bleeding often requires multiple transfusions of red blood cells, as well as platelets, which rapidly become depleted. If endoscopy is performed and a pulsating clot without active bleeding is noted, no attempt should be made to wash off the clot because of the possibility of uncontrollable bleeding. Once the bleeding has stopped, in conjunction with the above measures and acid suppression, these newborns usually have no further upper gastrointestinal hemorrhage. One of the most common causes of apparent upper gastrointestinal bleeding in the newborn period is swallowed maternal blood. This occurs in breast-fed infants when blood from the mother's cracked nipples is ingested by the infant and induces emesis. The Apt test (Table 155-3) can be used to differentiate maternal from fetal hemoglobin. Children with reflux esophagitis may present initially with

Table 155-3. Hemodynamic Significance of Vital Signs in Children

Vital Signs	Approximate loss of blood volume
Tachycardia without orthostasis	5%–10%
Tachycardia with orthostasis	> 10%
Tachycardia with hypotension	30%
Nonpalpable pulse	40%

Table 155-4. Age-Dependent Causes of Bleeding in the Upper Gastrointestinal Tract

Neonates and Infants (0–12 months)
  Swallowed maternal blood
  Newborn hemorrhagic gastritis:
    (eg, after stressful delivery, with respiratory distress)
  Coagulopathy
  Epistaxis
  Esophagitis
  Esophageal varices
  Gastritis
  Gastric or duodenal ulcer
  Mallory-Weiss tear
  Gastric duodenal duplication
Children (>12 mo)
  Epistaxis
  Tonsillitis or sinusitis
  Peptic esophagitis
  Esophageal ulcer
  Esophageal varices
  Mallory-Weiss tear
  Gastric or duodenal ulcers
Miscellaneous
  Hemobilia
  Munchausen's syndrome by proxy
  Henoch Schönlein purpura
  Hemophilia
  Mucositis from chemotherapy

hematemesis, even at this age. Esophageal varices with portal hypertension also can be seen in children by 6 months of age.

Children Older Than 12 Months

Epistaxis, hemorrhagic tonsillitis, and sinusitis occur quite commonly in children older than 12 months and can present with hematemesis. Peptic ulcers become more common as children get older, and may be painless. Forty percent or more of children with duodenal ulcers have a positive parental history of *Helicobacter pylori*–positive duodenal ulcer disease. The incidence of duodenal ulcers is three times higher in boys than it is in girls [7]. Gastric ulcers in children tend to be secondary, often related to medications such as salicylates or other nonsteroidal anti-inflammatory drugs or antimetabolites used for chemotherapy. The incidence of gastrointestinal bleeding from corticosteroids is unknown in children.

Helicobacter pylori is a leading cause of secondary gastritis and gastric ulcer disease in the older pediatric patient [8]. Anecdotal experience suggests that in the Asian population, children with hemorrhage from acid-peptic disease usually are *H. pylori*–positive by biopsy or urease slant but often are negative by *H. pylori* serology (Daum, unpublished data). Many different forms of esophagitis may be present with upper gastrointestinal bleeding at this age, including reflux esophagitis, infectious esophagitis, and mucositis caused by chemotherapy (Fig. 155-1, see also **Color Plate**). Mallory-Weiss tears, seen in children as young as

16 weeks of age, often are esophagogastric and may be best seen by a "J" maneuver of the endoscope. In most pediatric patients with bleeding from a Mallory-Weiss tear, the bleeding resolves spontaneously (Fig. 155-2, see also **Color Plate**).

◼ DIAGNOSTIC EVALUATION

A neonatal history of umbilical vein catheterization, omphalitis, or intra-abdominal sepsis has been associated with cavernous transformation of the portal vein, leading to later extrahepatic portal hypertension and esophageal varices (Fig. 155-3, see also **Color Plate**). The initial episode of bleeding occurs months to years after the inciting event.

Excessive bleeding from minor injuries or surgery may be an important clue that there is an underlying bleeding diathesis. An individual or family history of ulcers, telangiectasia, or liver disease, as well as a careful history of medication ingestion, are important considerations. The acute onset of intermittent, severe, colicky abdominal pain with dark blood mixed with mucus per rectum ("currant jelly stools") should alert the physician to the possibility of intussusception (see Chapter 162).

Physical examination and diagnostic evaluation, including nasogastric lavage and laboratory, endoscopic, and imaging studies, are used as in adults. Lavage amounts are different for children. We use approximately 10 mL/kg per lavage of normal saline (maximum amount, 10 to 12 oz) and repeat the lavage until clear.

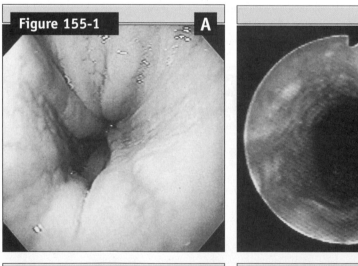
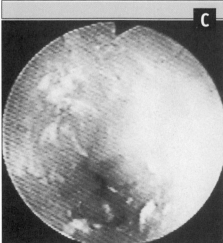
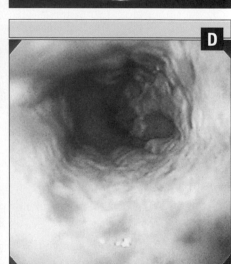

Figure 155-1

Causes of upper gastrointestinal bleeding in children. **A**, Peptic esophagitis. **B**, Viral esophagitis. **C**, Candida esophagitis. **D**, Mucositis from chemotherapy. See also **Color Plate**.

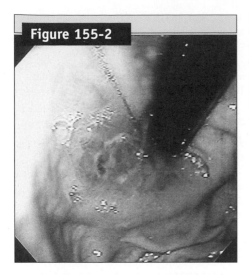

Mallory-Weiss tear in the cardia of a pediatric patient with retching and upper GI bleeding. See also **Color Plate**.

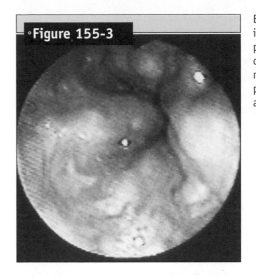

Esophageal varices in a 3-year-old patient with cavernous transformation of the portal vein. See also **Color Plate**.

TREATMENT

As in adults, stabilization of the patient and replacement of volume deficits are critical. Intravenous H_2 antagonists usually are the treatment of choice, at least until endoscopy has been accomplished. An initial dose of ranitidine at 1 mg/kg to a maximum of 50 mg every 6 to 8 hours usually is effective. Gastric pH is monitored every 2 to 4 hours, and if this dose of ranitidine does not maintain gastric pH above 5, bolus ranitidine is modified to a continuous drip, with an initial dose of 150 mg/1.73 m^2 every 24 hours. Antacids may be added at 0.5 mL/kg as needed to achieve a gastric pH higher than 5 once endoscopy has been accomplished. Other H_2 antagonists such as famotidine (40 mg/1.73 m^2 every 24 hours) or cimetidine (900 mg/1.73 m^2 every 24 hours) also may be used. Proton-pump inhibitors also are used in the treatment of upper gastrointestinal bleeding in children, with doses extrapolated from those used in adults.

Therapeutic Endoscopy

Three primary modalities exist for the endoscopic treatment of active, nonvariceal upper gastrointestinal bleeding: injection, thermo-electrocoagulation, and laser therapy [6•,9]. There is little published information on the safety and efficacy of these procedures in children, however. Extreme caution should be used in newborns, in whom bleeding usually stops spontaneously with pharmacologic therapy, red blood cell transfusions, and replacement of platelets.

Thermo-electrocoagulation typically is accomplished using the heater probe, or bipolar electrical current (Bicap Circon-ACMI, Stamford, CT). Bipolar electrocoagulation is accomplished using a 5-, 7-, or 10F probe. The 10F probe requires a therapeutic channel of 3.2 mm or larger, and therefore may be difficult to use for young or small children. Bicap therapy of gastroduodenal lesions in children is safe and efficacious when settings of 10 to 20 W and 2-second pulses are used. There is little information on the use of the argon or neodymium:yttrium-aluminum-garnet (Nd:YAG) laser in children. Therapeutic endoscopic treatments for variceal bleeding are discussed in Chapters 34 and 187.

Vasoactive Agents

Treatment of exsanguinating upper gastrointestinal hemorrhage may require an intravenous agent such as vasopressin or octreotide (*ie*, somatostatin analog). These agents produce peripheral vasoconstriction and decrease splanchnic blood flow, with a resulting decrease in portal vein pressure. Although there is little definitive evidence that these agents are effective in controlling nonvariceal lesions in children, patients with continued hemorrhage in whom a bleeding source cannot be localized may benefit. Vasopressin is given as a bolus of 0.3 U/kg (maximum 20 U) diluted in 2 mL/kg of 5% dextrose in water, and then followed by a continuous infusion of 0.2 to 0.4 U /1.73 m^2/min (the maximum adult dose is 1.5 U/min). The infusion is maintained at the rate required to control the bleeding for at least 12 hours, and then gradually tapered over the next 24 to 36 hours.

Somatostatin (octreotide) reduces gastric blood flow and inhibits gastric acid and gastrin production. Its use has been advocated for upper gastrointestinal bleeding in adults, but there is little published information on its use in pediatric patients.

Sengstaken-Blakemore or Linton Tubes

Sengstaken-Blakemore or Linton tubes, used to tamponade bleeding esophageal varices, are rarely employed in pediatric patients but are available in pediatric as well as adult sizes.

PROGNOSIS

In children, death from severe upper gastrointestinal bleeding usually is associated with the presence of a severe coagulation disorder, a systemic life-threatening disease, or both. In the patient with a hematocrit level higher than 20% and minimal transfusion requirements in whom the source of bleeding can be identified, bleeding usually is well-tolerated and the prognosis is excellent.

REFERENCES

Recently published papers of particular interest have been highlighted as follows:
- •   Of interest
- ••   Of outstanding interest

1.•• Mezoff AG, Preud'Homme DL: How serious is that GI bleed? *Contemp Pediatr* 1994, 11:60–92.

2. Euler AR, Byrne WJ, Cousins LM, *et al.*: Increased serum gastrin concentrations and gastric acid hyposecretion in the immediate newborn. *Gastroenterol* 1977, 72:1271–1273.

3. Agunod M, Yamaguchi N, Lopez R, *et al.*: Correlative study of hydrochloric acid, pepsin, and intrinsic factor secretion in newborns and infants. *Am J Dig Dis* 1969, 14:400–414.

4. Euler AR, Byrne WJ, Meis TJ, *et al.*: Basal and pentagastrin stimulated acid secretion in newborn human infants. *Pediatr Res* 1979, 13:36–37.

5. Deren JS: Development of structure and function in the fetal and newborn stomach. *Am J Clin Nutr* 1971, 34:144–159.

6.• Wyllie R, Kay M: Therapeutic intervention for nonvariceal gastrointestinal hemorrhage. *J Pediatr Gastroenterol Nutr* 1996, 22:123–133.

7. Mezoff AG, Balistreri WF: Peptic ulcer disease in children. *Pediatr Rev* 1995, 16:257–265.

8. Preud'Homme DL, Mezoff AG: Helicobacter pylori: a pathogen for all ages. *Contemp Pediatr* 1996, 13:27–49.

9. Fox V: Upper gastrointestinal endoscopy. In *Pediatric Gastrointestinal Disease*. Edited by Walker J. Philadelphia: Decker; 1996:1522–1523.

10. Goenka AS, Dasilva MS, Cleghorn GJ, *et al.*: Therapeutic upper gastrointestinal endoscopy in children: an audit of 443 procedures and literature review. *J Gastroenterol Hepatol* 1993, 8:44–51.

11. Yavorski RT, Wong RK, Maydonovitch C, *et al.*: Analysis of 3,294 cases of upper gastrointestinal bleeding in military medical facilities. *Am J Gastroenterol* 1995, 90:568–573.

12. Katz PO, Salas L: Less frequent causes of upper gastrointestinal bleeding. *Gastroenterol Clin North Am* 1993, 22:875–889.

13. Goyal A, Treem WR, Hyams JS: Severe upper gastrointestinal bleeding in healthy full-term neonates. *Am J Gastroenterol* 1994, 89:613–616.

14. Wilcox CM, Alexander LN, Cotsonis G: A prospective characterization of upper gastrointestinal hemorrhage presenting with hematochezia. *Am J Gastroenterol* 1997, 92: 231–235.

156 Evaluation of Fat Malabsorption and Maldigestion: Steatorrhea

Stanley E. Fisher

Steatorrhea is described by the child's parent or caregiver as loose, bulky or greasy, foul-smelling (rancid) stools. They may refer to it as diarrhea. Free oil may be seen in the diaper or toilet, particularly when the problem involves intraluminal fat maldigestion (*eg*, pancreatic insufficiency). Accompanying findings may be weight loss or poor weight gain, often with poor linear growth. A pediatric growth chart is an essential tool for identifying the failure to thrive that accompanies malabsorption as a result of caloric deficiency and loss of other essential nutrients, including the fat-soluble vitamins: A, D, E, and K. Other findings may be edema, abdominal distention, vomiting, increased or decreased appetite, jaundice, and a myriad of laboratory abnormalities, depending on the nature of the fat malabsorption or maldigestion and its underlying cause.

Excess excretion of fat, *ie*, steatorrhea, can result from a defect at any step in the normal process of fat absorption. For the purpose of discussing the differential diagnosis of steatorrhea in children, disorders accompanied by fat malabsorption or maldigestion are divided into five categories (Table 156-1).

As a rule, steatorrhea does not present as an isolated finding; rather, it is usually part of a constellation of signs and symptoms specific to a disease state. Isolated steatorrhea without malabsorption or maldigestion of other major nutrients (carbohydrate, protein, or both) is uncommon. Some disorders in which steatorrhea predominates without loss of other major dietary elements are indicated by *asterisks* in Table 156-1. The rare disorders of congenital absence of lipase or colipase may present in infancy. These disorders are characterized by particularly profuse steatorrhea.

FAILURE OF INTRALUMINAL DIGESTION

When fat does not undergo intraluminal digestion, neutral fats (primarily triglycerides) remain intact and pass to the colon in excessive amounts. In the colon, the fat ferments, resulting in loose stools with steatorrhea. The most common cause of failure of intraluminal fat digestion is exocrine pancreatic insufficiency. In infancy and childhood, this is most commonly due to cystic fibrosis (CF) (see Chapter 172), which affects all pancreatic enzymes and secretions. Other pediatric disorders associated with pancreatic insufficiency and steatorrhea are the Shwachman-Diamond syndrome, characterized by cyclic neutropenia, pancreatic insufficiency, and skeletal abnormalities; chronic familial pancreatitis, an autosomal dominant disorder with symptoms that are mild in the first decade; isolated enzyme deficiencies, including lipase and colipase deficiency; Johanson-Blizzard syndrome, characterized by pancreatic insufficiency, deafness, microcephaly, midline scalp defects, psychomotor retardation, hypothyroidism, dwarfism, absent permanent teeth, and aplasia of the alae nasae; sideroblastosis with pancreatic insufficiency; congenital rubella; and idiopathic pancreatic insufficiency. Gastrinomas may be associated with steatorrhea, because acid hypersecretion effectively creates pancreatic insufficiency by inhibiting pancreatic lipase and colipase activity. Gastrinomas are rare in childhood, however.

Pancreatic insufficiency of any cause results in maldigestion of fats, proteins, and complex carbohydrates. To compensate for these global losses, infants and children often have increased, even voracious, appetites. Even in the face of pancreatic insufficiency, however, symptoms of steatorrhea may not surface in the very young infant because of the compensatory action of gastric and breast milk lipases.

Inspection of the stools may reveal free oil, the presence of which is highly suggestive of pancreatic insufficiency. The results of stool fat smear for neutral fat and fatty acids and the steatocrit [1] usually are abnormal [2••]. Sometimes there are reducing substances in the stool (if the child is ingesting starch or long chain glucose polymers, which may require pancreatic amylase for digestion), but more often the pH is low (<5.0) from starch maldigestion. Stool chymotrypsin should be absent, but the feces have color and stool α_1-antitrypsin (a measure of protein loss) is normal. Serum folate usually is normal, as is the D-xylose absorption test. The 72-hour fecal fat excretion is abnormal, and a secretin-cholecystokinin test is definitive in non–CF cases; the sweat test and genotyping are definitive in CF.

◼ FAILURE OF FAT MICELLIZATION

Fat digestion and absorption requires bile salts in addition to secretion of the pancreatic enzymes lipase and colipase. A critical micellar concentration of conjugated bile salts is required for intraluminal digestion, penetration of the unstirred layer, and release of fats for uptake into the enterocytes. Depletion of the bile salt pool or biliary obstruction can, therefore, impair fat digestion. Depletion may result from small bowel bacterial overgrowth (intestinal stasis), ileal resection, or inflammatory diseases of the terminal ileum. Biliary obstruction can result from various hepatobiliary disorders, all manifested by cholestasis. Cholestasis in the neonate or young infant is most often the result of biliary atresia or intrahepatic paucity of the interlobular bile ducts. In both infants and older children, biliary obstruction occasionally is caused by congenital anomalies (eg, choledochal cyst) or stones.

CF, α_1-antitrypsin deficiency, and rare defects in bile salt metabolism also may cause cholestasis in the newborn or infant.

Steatorrhea is not a common presenting complaint in infants or children with cholestasis, but it may contribute to failure to thrive (see Chapter 182). Conjugated hyperbilirubinemia is the heralding sign of cholestasis. In infants it most often becomes evident within the first 4 weeks of life. In infants, the stool is acholic (gray to very pale yellow) when there is complete failure of bile excretion, as seen in biliary atresia. Pale yellow stools alone are not a definitive sign of cholestasis, because they can also result from back diffusion of bilirubin into the intestine, especially when there is a high serum bilirubin. However, if the stools are truly green or brown, it is virtually certain that the infant does not have biliary atresia or complete biliary obstruction.

In addition to abnormal stool color, the fat smear or steatocrit results may be positive, and the serum cholesterol and aminotransferase levels are elevated in most forms of cholestasis. Liver biopsy is the definitive diagnostic procedure in evaluating cholestasis of infancy. Whenever a newborn or young infant has a direct-reacting bilirubin level in excess of 2.0 mg/dL, referral to a pediatric gastroenterologist and evaluation for conjugated hyperbilirubinemia are recommended (see Chapter 173).

◼ FAILURE OF ENTEROCYTE UPTAKE

Once long chain fatty acids are released from triglycerides, they, along with monoglycerides, phospholipids, and cholesterol, must be taken up by the enterocytes. The major normal limiting factor for mucosal uptake of lipids is the small intestinal surface area of the enterocytes. The villi per se increase the surface area for absorption, which is magnified by the brush border on normal mature enterocytes. Hence, any illness that

Table 156-1. Disorders Accompanied by Steatorrhea

Failure of intraluminal digestion	Failure of fat micellization	Failure of enterocyte uptake	Failure of enterocyte processing*	Failure of post-enterocyte transport
Pancreatic insufficiency	Depletion of bile salt pool*	Short bowel syndrome	Anderson's disease (chylomicra retention disease)	Intestinal lymphangiectasia
Cystic fibrosis	Intestinal bacterial overgrowth (intestinal stasis syndrome)	Gluten-sensitive enteropathy	Abetalipoproteinemia	
Schwachman-Diamond syndrome		Dietary protein sensitivity (eg, cow's milk or soy)	Hypobetalipoproteinemia	
Familial pancreatic insufficiency	Ileal dysfunction	Tropical sprue		
Johanson-Blizzard syndrome	Ileal surgery	Immunodeficiency		
Sideroblastosis with pancreatic insufficiency	Inflammatory disease (eg, Crohn's disease)	Giardiasis		
Congenital rubella with pancreatic insufficiency	Cholestasis syndromes*	Crohn's disease		
Idiopathic	Biliary atresia			
Isolated lipase and colipase deficiency*	Intrahepatic paucity of the interlobular bile ducts			
Gastrinoma (Zollinger-Ellison)	Congenital anomalies (eg, choledocal cyst)			
	Cholelithiasis			
	α_1-Antitrypsin deficiency			
	Defects in bile salt metabolism			

Isolated steatorrhea without significant protein or carbohydrate loss.

results in loss of villous architecture or enterocyte brush border integrity may cause steatorrhea as well as malabsorption of many other nutrients. Likewise, surgical loss of intestinal length (short bowel syndrome) may compromise the effective surface area available for fat absorption. Diarrhea with loss of water and electrolytes is common.

A classic example of mucosal injury that may present with steatorrhea in childhood is gluten-sensitive enteropathy [3]. Gluten-sensitive enteropathy, like any cause of mucosal damage, reduces surface area and disaccharidase levels, leading to malabsorption of sugar, protein, and fat. In gluten-sensitive enteropathy and other malabsorption syndromes with diminished absorptive surface area, stool screening is positive for fat (smear or steatocrit); stool-reducing substances are positive; and stool pH is low. The serum folate level may be low, and the D-xylose absorption test results are usually abnormal. In contrast to pancreatic insufficiency, mucosal injury is likely to cause the child to have a decreased appetite. Failure to thrive is almost the rule in long-standing cases, and abdominal distention is common; in some cases, however, short stature (poor linear growth) may be the only presenting complaint. In the most severe cases of any diminished mucosal surface disorder, chronic diarrhea predominates. When protein loss or blood loss accompanies the mucosal injury, as may occur in sensitivity to dietary protein (eg, cow's milk or soy protein), the patient may present with edema, hematochezia, or anemia, and the stool α_1-antitrypsin usually is positive. Children with immunodeficiency syndromes, including human immunodeficiency virus (HIV), may develop opportunistic infections that impair mucosal absorption, leading to chronic diarrhea and, occasionally, steatorrhea. Regardless of the underlying cause of mucosal injury, documentation of excessive fat excretion must be viewed as merely one manifestation of an underlying disorder that requires more definitive tests.

▰ FAILURE OF ENTEROCYTE PROCESSING

In the enterocyte, long chain fatty acids are reesterified and, along with other lipids, transported into the lymph via chylomicrons. Congenital disorders of enterocyte processing of fat include Anderson's disease (chylomicron retention disease), abetalipoproteinemia, and hypobetalipoproteinemia. All three of these disorders present with steatorrhea and failure to thrive in infancy. There is severe anemia in the two abnormalities of β-lipoprotein, and acanthocytes are common on the blood smear. In contrast, Anderson's disease does not present with anemia or acanthocytosis. Cholesterol is low in all three disorders, but it is least affected in hypobetalipoproteinemia and most severe (<50 mg/dL) in abetalipoproteinemia.

▰ FAILURE OF POST-ENTEROCYTE TRANSPORT

The most common disorder of post-enterocyte transport is intestinal lymphangiectasia [2••]. It can be either congenital or secondary to many different disorders, such as cardiovascular anomalies or congestive heart failure, tumors of the mesenteric lymphatic system, inflammatory diseases (eg, Crohn's disease), intestinal malrotation, and thoracic duct obstruction from surgery or tumor. Lymphangiectasia, presenting with steatorrhea, edema, hypogammaglobulinemia, and lymphopenia (from protein and lymphocyte loss), is not uncommon in childhood. When the problem is congenital, it usually presents in infancy, may be associated with hemihypertrophy, and sometimes involves the lung.

In lymphangiectasia, the stool fat smear or steatocrit and α_1-antitrypsin are positive, the latter indicating protein-losing enteropathy. Stool-reducing substances are absent, and the D-xylose absorption test is normal. Blood cholesterol, albumin, immunoglobulins, and absolute lymphocyte count may all be low. Lymphocytes may be present in the stool. Small bowel biopsy is useful in making the definitive diagnosis (see Chapter 161).

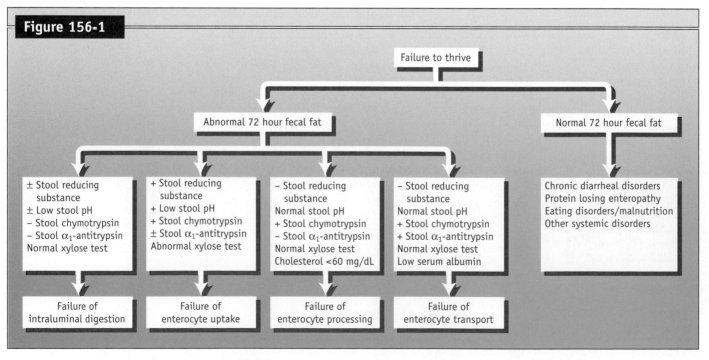

Figure 156-1

Guide to diagnostic priorities in suspected steatorrhea.

Table 156-2. Tests for Steatorrhea

Screening	Additional screening tests (indirect indicators of steatorrhea or malabsorption)	Other specific or definitive tests
Fat smear	Serum cholesterol	Sweat test and genotyping for cystic fibrosis
Steatocrit	Serum β-carotene	Lipoprotein electrophoresis
Functional	Serum vitamin E	Intestinal biopsy
^{13}C-triolein breath test (not generally available)	Serum calcium, phosphorus, and alkaline phosphatase	Liver biopsy
Fat loading (oral tolerance) tests	Serum folate	Secretin-cholecystokinin test
Definitive	Serum gastrin	Serum and urine bile acid analysis
72-hour fecal fat collection	Serum aminotransferases and bilirubin	Breath hydrogen test
	Serum immunoreactive trypsinogen	
	Quantitative serum immunoglobulins	
	Prothrombin time	
	Stool pH and reducing substances	
	Stool chymotrypsin	
	Stool α_1-antitrypsin	
	Antiendomysial and antigliadin antibodies	

GUIDE TO DIAGNOSTIC PRIORITIES IN SUSPECTED STEATORRHEA

Figure 156-1 provides a schematic guide for evaluating a child with suspected steatorrhea. This algorithm is only a rough guide, because there is overlap in the clinical and laboratory findings among the many causes of fat malabsorption. For example, cow's milk protein sensitivity can have the same appearance as gluten-sensitive enteropathy, or it can present as a protein-losing enteropathy, mimicking disorders of post-enterocyte transport.

Although there are many screening and definitive tests that may be useful in the evaluation of steatorrhea (Table 156-2), the approach in Figure 156-1 uses a core of commonly available and frequently used tests to assist in the differential diagnosis. It must be emphasized, however, that tests for malabsorption, like any laboratory investigation, require proper execution and interpretation. As a rule, when the stool is being examined for abnormal substances (eg, fat or reducing substances), the child must have been ingesting an adequate amount of the substance. Table sugar (sucrose), for example, is not a reducing sugar, and examination of the stool from a patient ingesting primarily sucrose requires acid hydrolysis before testing for reducing substances is performed. Serum folate levels or β-carotene may be falsely low if the diet is deficient in foods containing those substances.

The 72-hour fecal fat collection, upon which the diagnosis of steatorrhea often hinges, is accurate only if the child has ingested an adequate amount of fat for 48 hours before and during the entire collection. A rule of thumb for intake is 60 g of regular dietary fat per square meter of body surface area per day. The test should be done with normal dietary fat because specialized formulas with medium chain triglycerides can bypass the intraluminal digestion and micellization phases. (As a point of reference, a quart of whole milk contains 40 g of fat.) The dietary fat intake must be accurately recorded, and the stool collection must not be interrupted by lost specimens or contamination by urine. Although these guidelines are relatively easy to follow with older children, infants may require hospitalization and stool collection by experienced hospital personnel.

The D-xylose absorption test, a common test for malabsorption due to loss of mucosal surface area, depends in part on the rate of gastric emptying. After the child has ingested the appropriate amount of xylose (1g/kg; 50 g maximum), blood xylose levels should be obtained at 0.5, 1, and 2 hours. Urinary xylose collection usually is not performed in children.

SUMMARY

Steatorrhea may be a presenting sign of malabsorption syndrome in childhood. Like many serious pediatric problems, fat malabsorption is usually associated with poor growth and poor weight gain, ie, failure to thrive. With a careful history, evaluation of a pediatric growth chart, and a fat smear (or steatocrit), steatorrhea is not likely to be overlooked. A 72-hour fecal fat collection and judicious use of a few additional laboratory tests help to set the focus of the evaluation for steatorrhea and its many causes.

REFERENCES AND RECOMMENDED READING

Recently published papers of particular interest have been highlighted as follows:
- • Of interest
- •• Of outstanding interest

1. Tran M, Forget P, Van den Neucker A, et al.: The acid steatocrit: a much improved method. J Pediatr Gastroenterol Nutr 1994, 19:299–303.

2.•• Vanderhoof JA: Diarrheal disease in infants and children. In Pediatric GI Problems. Edited by Hyman PE. Philadelphia: Current Medicine; 1997:6.1–6.17.

3. Trancone R, Greco L, Auricchio S: Gluten-sensitive enteropathy. Pediatr Clin North Am 1996, 43:355–373.

4.• Branski D, Lerner A, Lebenthal E: Chronic diarrhea and malabsorption. Pediatr Clin North Am 1996, 43:307–331.

5.• Talusan-Soriano K, Lake AM: Malabsorption in childhood. Pediatr Rev 1996, 17:135–142.

157 Carbohydrate Malabsorption

José M. Saavedra

Carbohydrates constitute 40% to 60% of the average energy intake in humans. They are not simply a source of energy, however, but an important determinant of intestinal function through several physiologic mechanisms, most of which depend on a balance between their digestion and absorption and the luminal effects of the unabsorbed portions that are subjected to fermentation by the intestinal flora. This balance can significantly affect mucosal growth, as well as the absorption of water, nutrients, and minerals. The extent and rate of carbohydrate absorption have varying effects on insulin secretion and the regulation of other mediators such as thyroid and growth hormones [1–3]. Excessive delivery of sugars to the distal bowel can have significant and deleterious effects (*eg*, diarrhea and acidosis).

DIETARY CARBOHYDRATE

Dietary carbohydrate may be ingested in the form of starches (long complex chains of monosaccharides), oligosaccharides (polymers or shorter chains of monosaccharides), disaccharides (lactose, sucrose, and maltose), and monosaccharides (glucose, galactose, and fructose). A few major dietary nonstarch polysaccharides are resistant to human enzymatic digestion. These are principally plant cell-wall components, including cellulose and noncellulose polysaccharides such as pectin and hemicellulose, which are usually categorized as dietary fibers. Finally, modern diets contain a significant amount of nondigestible sugars, including stachyose, raffinose, and sugar alcohols such as sorbitol and mannitol, found in fruits, juices, soft drinks, and prepared foods.

PHYSIOLOGY

Figure 157-1 illustrates the general pathways of digestion of dietary carbohydrates by luminal and brushborder saccharidases [4–6]. Following mucosal digestion, the resulting monosaccharides—glucose and galactose—are actively transported into the enterocyte by a sodium–glucose cotransporter system. Fructose

Figure 157-1

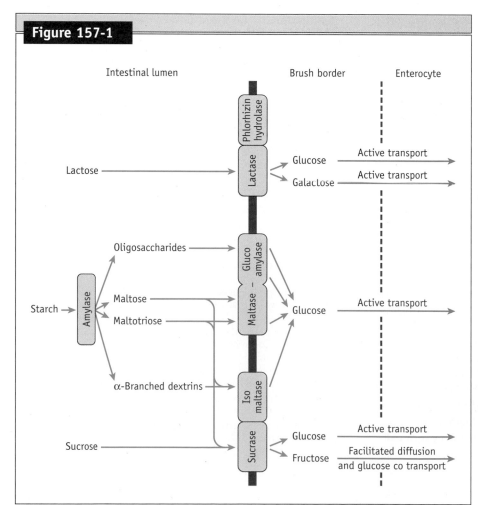

Major pathways for digestion and absorption of dietary carbohydrates. Following ingestion, salivary and pancreatic amylase initiate the hydrolysis of starches into smaller oligosaccharide chains, maltose, maltotriose, and α-limit dextrins (the branching portions of complex starch polymers). These sugars are further hydrolyzed by distinct glycosidases found in three glycosylated protein complexes that are anchored in the intestinal brush border membrane with hydrolytic sites facing the intestinal lumen. These are glucoamylase–maltase, sucrase–isomaltase, and lactase–phlorhizin hydrolase. Lactose is hydrolyzed to glucose and galactose by lactase, and sucrose is hydrolyzed to glucose and fructose by sucrase. Maltose is hydrolyzed to two glucose molecules by maltase activity. The sucrase–isomaltase complex is responsible for 80% of maltase activity, all sucrase activity, most isomaltase activity, and some α-limit dextrinase activity. The glucoamylase–maltase complex hydrolyzes all glucoamylose, most α-limit dextrins, 20% of maltose, and a small percentage of isomaltose. It is an important alternate pathway for starch digestion when there is reduced or absent pancreatic amylase activity. The lactase–phlorhizin hydrolase complex is responsible for hydrolyzing lactose to glucose and galactose.

is thought to be absorbed by two separate mechanisms [7]. One of them is a low-capacity facilitated transport and the other a high-capacity, glucose-dependent cotransport system.

In general, brush border glucoamylase and sucrase activities proceed at a faster rate than the final absorption of the component monosaccharides of glucose polymers and sucrose. Conversely, the hydrolysis of lactose to glucose and galactose proceeds at a rate below the maximum rates of absorption of the individual monosaccharides. Thus, lactase activity is the rate-limiting step in the digestion and absorption of lactose. Additionally, lactase activity usually is greater at the tip of the microvillus, whereas the activity of other glycosidases is greater in the body of the microvillus and in less mature enterocytes. Consequently, injuries to small bowel mucosa typically result in a greater impact on lactase activity as compared to that of other glycosidases.

On reaching the colon, nonabsorbed sugars are fermented by colonic bacteria. In healthy people, a small amount of carbohydrates and varying amounts of fermentable dietary fiber are metabolized by bacteria to short-chain fatty acids (SCFAs; acetate, lactate, propionate, and butyrate), gas (hydrogen, methane, CO_2) and other larger molecules [8,9]. The SCFAs resulting from fermentation have well-described trophic effects in the distal small bowel and colonic mucosa [10]. Butyrate in particular is the most important energy source of the colonocyte. Additionally, SCFAs can be absorbed and used as a source of energy. This colonic absorption of organic acids may represent a significant salvage pathway of energy that has escaped small bowel absorption and, thus, may be of benefit particularly to normal neonates and preterm infants, who have relatively low lactase levels [11].

PATHOPHYSIOLOGY

The pathophysiologic events that result from carbohydrate malabsorption are, in essence, an exaggeration of the normal balance among digestion, absorption, and fermentation (Fig. 157-2). Sugars that are not digested and are not absorbed in the proximal bowel exert an osmotic effect in the jejunum, increasing the secretion of water and sodium into the lumen and accelerating transit of small bowel contents [12,13]. Absorption of nutrients, particularly of protein, magnesium, calcium, and phosphate, also may be affected adversely [14]. The greater the amount of unabsorbed sugar presented to the distal bowel, the greater is the water loss, gas production, and degree of diarrhea.

The increased concentration of acids lowers the pH of the stool, reduces water absorption, and, at least in animal studies, causes mucosal injury [15]. When the rate of production and absorption of organic acids from the colon overwhelms the capacity of these acids to be used as a source of energy, their accumulation in the bloodstream may lead to metabolic acidosis, particularly in small infants [16] or in individuals with severe short bowel syndrome or gastrojejunal bypass. Bacterial flora capable of producing D-lactate can more easily lead to (D-lactate) acidosis, because this acid cannot be metabolized by human cells.

The increase in luminal gas leads to related symptoms. The production of hydrogen gas in the distal bowel, which readily diffuses to the portal circulation and eventually is exhaled from the lungs, provides the basis for the breath hydrogen test, which is used to diagnose carbohydrate malabsorption (discussed later in this chapter).

These pathophysiologic events result in increased looseness of stools or watery, acidic stools, which may contain some of the unabsorbed sugars; abdominal pain associated with the

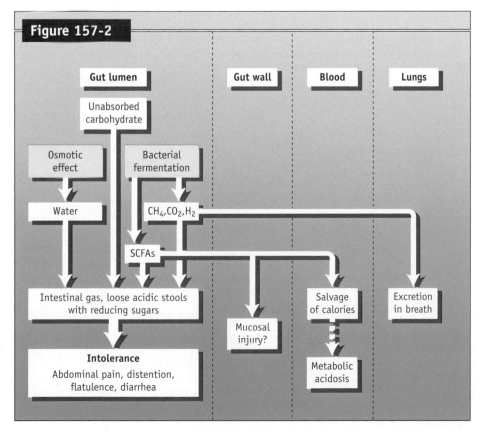

Figure 157-2

The pathophysiologic mechanisms in carbohydrate malabsorption are depicted. SCFAs—short-chain fatty acids.

increased amount of intraluminal fluid and gas; abdominal distention or bloating; and flatulence. When caused by malabsorption, this constellation of signs and symptoms is called *carbohydrate intolerance.*

These symptoms can present in a wide range of ways, from very mild abdominal discomfort to severe watery diarrhea and metabolic acidosis, depending on a number of factors (Fig. 157-3). Thus, not all malabsorption is accompanied by signs of carbohydrate intolerance, nor are the symptoms of intolerance diagnostic of malabsorption of a particular sugar.

■ ETIOLOGY AND CLINICAL PRESENTATION

Table 157-1 lists the most common conditions associated with carbohydrate malabsorption. Developmentally associated low levels of disaccharidases may be present in premature infants and newborns (Fig. 157-4).

Congenital Deficiencies

Congenital causes of carbohydrate malabsorption are uncommon. Congenital lactase deficiency is an extremely rare condition in which lactase activity is decreased or absent at birth, a deficiency that persists throughout life. It is managed by excluding lactose from the diet. Other congenital forms of malabsorption include glucose–galactose malabsorption, which results from the lack of a normal sodium–glucose cotransporter in the brush border [5]. In affected individuals, the only carbohydrate that can be tolerated is fructose. Sucrase–isomaltase deficiency usually becomes evident with the introduction of sucrose, sucrose-containing formula, or fruit into the diet during infancy. Sucrase–isomaltase deficiency is the most common of the congenital disaccharidase deficiencies, and is seen among Greenland and Canadian Eskimos and Canadian Indians, with an incidence as high as 10% [6].

Fructose Malabsorption

Fructose is absorbed more slowly than is glucose. Free fructose in monosaccharide form is present in significant quantities only in honey and a few fruits (dates, figs, apples, grapes, and berries), so it contributes only a small proportion of fructose to the average carbohydrate intake. Most fructose intake in modern diets is from added sources; it was not until the introduction of high-fructose syrup as an additive sweetener to prepared foods and beverages that fructose absorption became an area of clinical interest. Fructose is significantly sweeter than sucrose (table sugar) and is sweetest when cool, dilute, and slightly acidic, a property that makes it attractive for soft-drink manufacturers. Because of this, fructose intake in the United States has increased 10-fold in the last 15 years. The general population is heterogeneous with respect to its capacity for fructose absorption. Up to 70% of adults in some series have been shown to malabsorb a dose of 50 g of fructose, and some individuals can become symptomatic with doses of less than 25 g of fructose, the amount in 12 oz of a standard carbonated soft drink. When that individual threshold dose is exceeded, the signs and symptoms of carbohydrate intolerance ensue [17]. The presence of a cotransport mechanism of glucose and fructose explains the observation that malabsorption of fructose is reversed when it is ingested with an equivalent amount of glucose. In children, excessive consumption of fruit juices has been associated with intermittent loose stools, chronic nonspecific diarrhea, and recurrent abdominal pain. In adults, fructose malabsorption has been associated with the irritable bowel syndrome. From a nutritional point of view, excessive consumption of fruit juice by children has been associated with both increased caloric intake and overweight status, as well as with failure to thrive in toddlers [7,17].

Figure 157-3

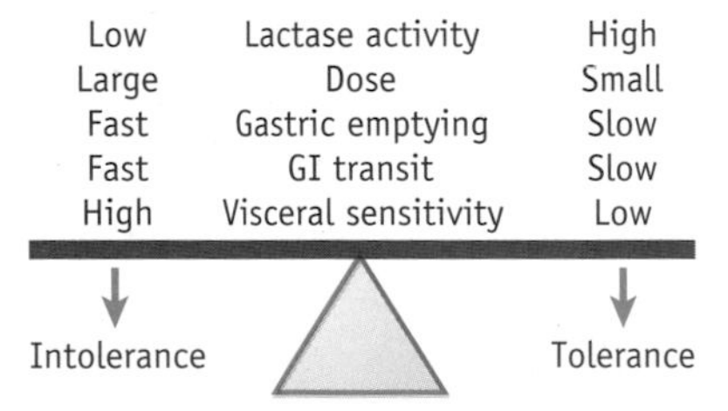

Low	Lactase activity	High
Large	Dose	Small
Fast	Gastric emptying	Slow
Fast	GI transit	Slow
High	Visceral sensitivity	Low

Intolerance   Tolerance

Factors determining intolerance in lactose-malabsorbing individuals. The development of clinical signs of intolerance varies from person to person, depending on multiple factors. Total lactase activity may be decreased permanently because of a normal autogenetic decline in activity, permanent loss of intestinal surface (*eg*, as a result of surgery) or transient loss, as in an acute viral gastroenteritis. Decreasing the quantity ingested or slowing gastric emptying of a sugar (as when taken with a meal) may allow for better tolerance, even though the degree of malabsorption remains the same.

Table 157-1. Conditions Associated With Carbohydrate Malabsorption

| | Presentation more common in: | | |
	Children	Adults	Can present in both
Primary			
Congenital lactase deficiency	x		
Glucose-galactose malabsorption	x		
Sucrase-isomaltase deficiency	x		
Fructose malabsorption			x
Sorbitol malabsorption			x
Ontogenetic			
Lactase deficiency of the premature infant	x		
Lactase nonpersistence (adult onset)		x	
Pancreatic amylase deficiency in infancy	x		
Secondary			
Acute gastroenteritis	x		
Small bowel bacterial overgrowth			x
Giardia lamblia infestation			x
Protein-sensitive (allergic) enteropathy	x		
Short bowel syndrome			x
Radiation enteritis			x
Crohn's disease			x

Except for specific enzyme deficiencies, as in the primary causes mentioned, and normally declining lactase levels, most secondary causes mentioned above affect absorption of multiple types of sugars, particularly those due to diffuse intestinal injury or decreased absorptive surface.

Sorbitol Malabsorption

Sorbitol is a naturally occurring sugar. A polyalcohol sugar, sorbitol is not absorbed by the gut. It is found in many plants, particularly fruits and juices of the Rosaceae family, including apples, cherries, plums, and pears; the sorbitol content is particularly high in pears. Thus, sorbitol is commonly ingested together with fructose, and, as with fructose, most sorbitol in standard modern diets comes from that added to commercial food, particularly candy, chewing gum, and sugar-free products. Sorbitol exacerbates the fermentation and potentiates the symptoms associated with fructose malabsorption. When taken together with fructose, sorbitol probably inhibits fructose transport [17].

Lactose Malabsorption

Lactase activity in humans, as in all mammals, is characterized by a genetically predetermined postweaning (ontogenetic) decline. Thus, the majority of the world's adult population has lactose malabsorption. Mammalian evolution "designed" lactose-containing milk as a food to be consumed primarily by newborns and the young, and did not include among its determining factors the development of dairying, which leads even adult humans to consume milk as a staple food. In the absence of the development of dairying in several cultures, primary or ontogenetic lactose "malabsorption," a normal phenomenon, would not be considered a pathologic condition [18].

Lactose malabsorption resulting from ontogenetic lactase nonpersistence is the most common form of carbohydrate malabsorption in adults [19]. This age-associated decline of lactase activity is compatible with a "hardwired" transcriptional control of lactase expression, and is a recessive phenotypic characteristic [6]. Lactase is a noninducible enzyme, so the degree of intake of lactose or dairy products does not alter its ontogenetic decline. This decline is influenced by ethnicity (Table 157-2), and can occur as early as 2 to 4 years of age in Thais, or as late as 15 years of age in Finns.

Malabsorption is not always accompanied by signs of intolerance. It is clear, however, that many people with lactose malabsorption can consume nutritionally significant amounts of milk or milk products with minimal or no signs of intolerance.

Secondary Carbohydrate Malabsorption

Any condition that causes injury to the intestinal mucosa and thus decreases the functional absorptive surface of the brush border may lead to carbohydrate malabsorption. The degree of injury determines the presence of signs and symptoms of intolerance. Table 157-1 lists the most common secondary causes of lactose malabsorption. Acute gastroenteritis from rotavirus infection in infants and children is the most common cause of transient carbohydrate intolerance.

Decreased absorption of lactose and other carbohydrates has been well described in multiple conditions [19,20], including inflammatory bowel disease, intestinal injury from chemotherapy or radiation, or extensive small bowel resection. Intestinal giardiasis can present with signs of carbohydrate malabsorption, which typically resolves following antiparasitic treatment. Contamination of the small bowel by bacteria, as occurs in intestinal dysmotility syndromes, diabetes mellitus, and immunodeficiency states, can lead to disaccharide deficiency and symptoms of malabsorption. Bacterial proteases and glycosidases appear to degrade brush border enzymes, and products of bacterial metabolism may interfere with glucose transport. Sugar malabsorption also is described in cow's milk– and soy protein–sensitive enteropathy, as well as in celiac disease. Lactase deficiency also appears to be common in children with the human immunodeficiency virus (HIV).

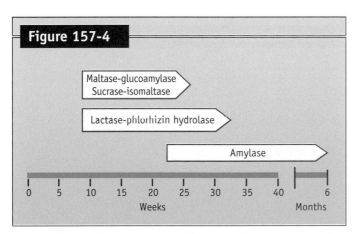

Figure 157-4

Embryologic development of intestinal saccharidases. Intestinal sucrase–isomaltase and maltase activity increases slowly from 10 to 26 weeks gestation and reaches 70% of that seen in term infants by 34 weeks gestation. Lactase activity is detected at about 12 weeks but develops slowly, reaching 70% of term infant activity by 35 to 38 weeks gestation. Glucose transport proteins are evident by the 11th week. Of all the saccharidases, lactase is the only one that undergoes a well-defined ontogenetic decline in activity with age, as in most mammals post-weaning.

Location	Individuals with malabsorption, %
Table 157-2. Prevalence of Lactose Malabsorption in Selected Healthy Adult Populations	
North America	
Native American (Arizona)	95
Black	70–75
White	5–10
Eskimo (Canada)	73–100
Mexico	74
Peru	80
Brazil	45–95
Denmark	3
Finland	8–17
Italy	39–100
Africa	
Bantu	100
Yoruba	83
Fulani	60
Israeli Jews	45–85
India	50–100
China	76–100
Thailand	100
Japan	75–100

Recurrent abdominal pain in children with the irritable bowel syndrome has been associated with lactose malabsorption in 5% to 95% of afflicted persons [19].

■ DIAGNOSIS

The clinical history may be helpful in identifying a malabsorptive problem and a specific offending sugar. Identifying intakes of large doses of lactose-, fructose-, and sorbitol-containing foods is helpful. Although the dietary history can be suggestive, it is never conclusive. Symptoms (mostly due to intestinal fermentation) may occur many hours after ingestion of the potential culprit, making the recognition of an association with symptoms quite difficult. The presence of any underlying primary or secondary gastrointestinal pathology that causes mucosal injury or motility abnormalities increases the risk of malabsorption.

Demonstration of decreased levels of mucosal disaccharidase in the small bowel by small bowel biopsy is the only means of measuring enzyme activity directly and is recommended when congenital carbohydrate malabsorption is suspected.

Oral glucose tolerance tests, which rely on an increase in blood glucose following the administration of a specific sugar, provide no information as to which component of the sugar is malabsorbed. Multiple blood sampling is required, and results are affected by alterations in intestinal motility or glucose metabolism. False-positive and false-negative results can occur in up to 30% of children [21].

Parameters that measure the effects of unabsorbed carbohydrates usually are more practical and more directly associated with the pathophysiologic mechanisms that lead to carbohydrate intolerance than are glucose tolerance tests. These indirect methods for detecting carbohydrate malabsorption are shown in Table 157-3.

Stool Tests

The detection of reducing sugars in stool provides a measure of how much carbohydrate is escaping absorption and fermentation. This is a useful bedside test for infants and children, particularly those with watery diarrhea, whose feedings of formula or food contain reducing sugars. The presence of more than 0.5% concentration of sugar in the stool may be an indication to modify the formula the child is receiving, particularly if there is moderate to severe dehydration associated with diarrhea. A stool pH <5.5 typically is associated with a high production of SCFAs from fermentation.

Breath Hydrogen Tests

Breath hydrogen testing has become the gold standard for the diagnosis of carbohydrate malabsorption [20,21]. Breath hydrogen testing is sensitive, noninvasive, and inexpensive, and can be performed easily in patients of all ages. Hydrogen is produced exclusively by intestinal bacterial fermentation, absorbed into the portal circulation, and excreted in the breath. The test is performed after an overnight fast on samples of expired air obtained before and at 30-minute intervals for a minimum of 3 hours after the administration of the test sugar in aqueous solution. The most commonly used testing dose is 2 g/kg (to a maximum of 50 g) given in a 20% solution. There are multiple methods for sample collection that use syringes or small collection bags. A gas chromatograph apparatus is used to analyze breath hydrogen samples. Under normal circumstances, with adequate digestion and absorption of the test sugar, there should be no significant rise in breath hydrogen measurements. A rise of 20 or more parts per million above the baseline is a positive test, usually indicating carbohydrate malabsorption. A hydrogen rise in the first 120 minutes following ingestion of sugar adequately identifies individuals with biopsy-proven lactase deficiency.

Breath hydrogen tests most commonly are used to diagnose lactose malabsorption. However, any sugar substrate can be tested, including fructose. Glucose breath hydrogen tests may be useful for evaluating the possibility of small bowel bacterial overgrowth. A high baseline fasting concentration with an early

---

Table 157-3. Indirect Methods for Detection of Carbohydrate Malabsorption

Test	Technique	Interpretation
Carbohydrates in feces	Place small amount of liquid stool in test tube	Negative ≤ 0.25%
	Dilute with twice its volume of water	Borderline 0.25%–0.5%
	Place 15 drops of the resulting suspension in a second test tube and add a Clinitest tablet	Positive ≥ 0.5%
	Compare the resulting color with the chart provided for testing of urine Note: sucrose and some glucose polymers are not reducing sugars and require 1N HCl instead of water, followed by brief boiling, to be hydrolyzed and tested as reducing sugars	
Fecal pH	Dip Nitrazine paper into liquid part of stool	Positive ≤ 5.5
	Compare resulting color of paper with chart provided	
Breath hydrogen	Patient fasts overnight	Negative < 10 ppm rise above baseline
	Obtain fasting sample of expired air	
	Administer oral load of test sugar, usually 1–2 g/kg to a maximum of 50 g/kg as 20% solution	Borderline 10–20 ppm
	Measure breath hydrogen concentration in expired air at 30 minutes, then hourly for 4 hours	Positive > 20 ppm

ppm—parts per million.

Table 157-4. Average Sucrose, Glucose, and Fructose Content of Selected Foods (g/100 g Edible Portion)

Fruit	Fructose	Glucose	Sucrose	Sorbitol
Apple	6.2	2.7	1.2	0.5
Pear	6.4	2.3	0.0	2.0
White grape	7.5	7.1	0.0	0.0
Orange	2.4	2.4	4.7	0.0

The absorptive capacity of fructose is dose dependent, unless administered with glucose, in which case its absorption is enhanced. Foods, fruits, or juices containing equivalent amounts of glucose and fructose (eg, orange and white grape juices) are better tolerated than those in which fructose content is three times that of glucose (eg, apple and pear juices).

rise in the first 30 minutes following sugar ingestion may indicate bacterial overgrowth.

False-positive tests may occur as a result of diets that are high in fiber or other complex fermentable sugars ingested hours before the test. For that reason, a standardized meal of protein (meat) and easily fermentable carbohydrate (rice) the night before the morning of the test is recommended. False-negative tests can result from the existence of non–hydrogen-producing flora, a relatively rare occurrence, or the use of antibiotics in the days preceding the test.

The developmental lack of lactase in premature infants typically is managed using formulas that contain glucose polymers, specifically designed for this population. In many normal newborns, the development of loose, watery, slightly acidic stools is not unexpected. These infants usually continue to thrive, and formula changes are rarely necessary, unless there is concurrent gastrointestinal disease. Glucose–galactose malabsorption presenting at birth, and sucrase–isomaltase deficiency, which usually presents when children are first introduced to juice or fruit at 4 to 6 months of age, is managed by avoiding the offending sugars.

If a potential dietary culprit such as consumption of large amounts of fructose or sorbitol is identified, simple measures such as decreasing the daily intake of juice, high fructose drinks, or sorbitol-containing foods, or the amount ingested at one time, may be all that is needed. Simultaneous ingestion of glucose and fructose, such as that found in white grape juice, can enhance fructose absorption (Table 157-4). Dilution of juices or substitution with white grape juice has been reported to improve chronic nonspecific diarrhea in children [17]. If there is clinical evidence of malabsorption of lactose in infants and children following acute gastroenteritis with moderate to severe dehydration, it can be managed easily with a variety of non–lactose-containing infant formulas. In most instances, adequate lactase levels return in a few days or weeks, and the malabsorption resolves. For this reason, change to a non–lactose-containing formula is indicated only in cases of severe or prolonged diarrhea, accompanied by dehydration or acidosis. In older children who are already receiving other weaning foods, simple restriction of dairy products and juices and drinks with high fructose content is all that is necessary. Breast-fed children who develop acute gastroenteritis appear to tolerate a decrease in lactase activity with less severe symptoms and rarely require significant intervention beyond maintaining adequate hydration with oral electrolyte solutions.

The more common problem of adult-onset lactose deficiency can be managed in a number of ways. A therapeutic trial of lactose restriction may not be helpful, and in cases of marked intolerance, even the small amounts of lactose contained in prepared foods or that found as filler in medication tablets may cause symptoms. In these situations, a specific diagnosis by breath hydrogen testing is indicated, to avoid unnecessary restrictions. Elimination of dairy products from the diet may compromise nutritional status, particularly in areas such as North America, where dairy products represent up to 75% of calcium and 20% of vitamin D intake.

Once the diagnosis of lactose intolerance is made, additional strategies are available. Consumption of whole cow's milk, with its relatively high fat content, tends to delay gastric emptying, and, if taken with meals, may reduce symptoms of intolerance by reducing the rates at which lactose is presented to the small bowel and unabsorbed carbohydrate reaches the colon. Fermented milk products such as cheese or yogurt can significantly reduce the symptoms of lactose intolerance. When yogurts with active live cultures (most commonly *Lactobacillus bulgaricus* and *Streptococcus thermophilus*) are ingested, the bacteria in the product express lactase activity in vivo, enhancing digestion of the lactose in the intestinal lumen [22,23]. Additionally, yogurts may improve intolerance by modifying the kinetics of delivery of unabsorbed sugar to the distal bowel.

More recently, milks that have been prehydrolyzed with commercially prepared lactase as well as oral preparations of lactase (eg, Lactaid and Lactrase) have become available. The lactase in most of these products is of fungal origin (*Kluyveromyces lactis* and *Aspergillus oryzae*). The enzyme, dispensed in the form of drops or tablets, can be added to milk, which is incubated for 12 to 24 hours and then can be ingested. Alternatively, tablets or drops of lactase may be taken by mouth just before ingestion of dairy products.

In patients with significant bacterial overgrowth, the use of oral antibiotics including metronidazole or nonabsorbable antibiotics such as neomycin or aminoglycosides, can reduce the enteric bacterial population, decrease fermentation, and thereby reduce malabsorption symptoms.

■ REFERENCES

1. Schneeman BO: Carbohydrates: significance for energy balance and gastrointestinal function. *J Nutr* 1994, 124(suppl 9):1747S–1753S.

2. Kien CL, Heitlinger LA, Li BU, *et al.*: Digestion, absorption, and fermentation of carbohydrates. *Semin Perinatol* 1989, 13:78–87.

3. Azizi F: Effect of dietary composition on fasting-induced changes in serum thyroid hormones and thyrotropin. *Metabolism* 1978, 27:935–942.

4. Southgate DAT: Digestion and metabolism of sugars. *Am J Clin Nutr* 1995, 62(suppl):2035–2115.

5. Levin RJ: Digestion and absorption of carbohydrates—from molecules and membranes to humans. *Am J Clin Nutr* 1994, 59(suppl):690S–698S.

6. Semenza G, Auricchio S: Small-intestinal disaccharidases. In *The Metabolic Basis of Inherited Disease*, edn 6. Edited by Scriver CR, Stanbury JB, Wyngaarden JB, Fredrickson DS. New York: McGraw-Hill; 1989:2975–2997.

7. Riby JE, Fujisawart, Kretchmer N: Fructose absorption. *Am J Clin Nutr* 1993, 59(suppl):7485–7535.

8. Bond JH, Currier BE, Buchwald H, Levitt MD: Colonic conservation of malabsorbed carbohydrate. *Gastroenterology* 1980, 78:444–447.

9. Bond JH, Levitt MD: Quantitative measurement of lactose absorption. *Gastroenterology* 1976, 70:1058–1062.

10. Reilly KH, Rombeau JL: Metabolism and potential clinical applications of short-chain fatty acids. *Clin Nutr* 1993, 12:97–105.

11. Kien CL: Digestion, absorption and fermentation of carbohydrates in the newborn. *Clinics in Perinatology* 1996, 23:211–228.

12. Bond JH, Levitt MD: Investigation of small bowel transit time in man utilizing pulmonary hydrogen (H$_2$) measurements. *J Lab Clin Med* 1975, 85:546–555.

13. Launiala K: The effect of unabsorbed sucrose or mannitol-induced accelerated transition absorption on the human small intestine. *Scand J Gastroenterol* 1969, 4:25–32.

14. Debongnie JC, Newcomer AD, McGill DB, Phillips SF: Absorption of nutrients in lactase deficiency. *Dig Dis Sci* 1979, 24:225–231.

15. Saunders DR, Sillery J: Effect of lactate and H$^+$ on structure and function of rat intestine. *Dig Dis Sci* 1982, 27:33–41.

16. Lifshitz G, Diaz-Bensussen S, Martinez-Garza V, *et al.*: Influence of disaccharides on the development of systemic acidosis in the premature infant. *Pediatr Res* 1971, 5:213–225.

17. Perman JA: Digestion and absorption of fruit juice carbohydrates. *J Am Coll Nutr* 1996, 15:125–175.

18. Saavedra J, Perman JA: Lactose malabsorption and intolerance. In *Encyclopedia of Human Biology*, vol 5. Edited by Dulbecco R. San Diego and London: Academic Press; 1997:215–225.

19. Saavedra JM, Perman JA: Current concepts in lactose malabsorption and intolerance. *Annu Rev Nutr* 1989, 9:475–502.

20. Montes RG, Perman JA: Disorder of carbohydrate absorption in clinical practice. *MMJ* 1990, 39:383–388.

21. Newcomer AD, McGill DB, Thomas PJ, Hoffman AF: Prospective comparison of indirect methods of detecting lactase deficiency. *N Engl J Med* 1975, 293:1232–1236.

22. Kolars JC, Levitt MD, Aoujim M, Savaiano DA: Yogurt—an autodigesting source of lactose. *N Engl J Med* 1984, 310:1–3.

23. Shermak MA, Saavedra JM, Jackson TL, *et al.*: Effect of yogurt on symptoms of kinetics of hydrogen production in lactose-malabsorbing children. *Am J Clin Nutr* 1995, 62:1003–1006.

158 Acute Diarrhea: Nonbloody and Bloody

Jay A. Hochman and Mitchell B. Cohen

Diarrhea is a nearly universal human experience. Most episodes are self-limited and mild; however, acute diarrhea remains a major cause of morbidity and mortality, particularly in the pediatric population. As many as 200,000 children per year are hospitalized in the United States for management of diarrheal illnesses [1••]. Childhood mortality due to diarrhea and dehydration in the United States is estimated at 500 deaths per year [2•,3] (Fig. 158-1). By improving the approach to the pediatric patient with diarrhea, most of these pediatric deaths can be averted [2•].

PHYSIOLOGY

Developmental regulation of disaccharidases and receptors and age-related changes in diet, microflora, and behavior coordinate the response of the host to an infectious or noninfectious insult. The physiologic changes with age can be either deleterious or protective. For example, the host response to *Clostridium difficile* is age-dependent. Infants are often colonized (40% to 70%) with this organism but rarely develop antibiotic-associated colitis. Therefore, even toxin-producing strains of *C. difficile* are considered a normal part of the bacterial microflora in children up to 1 to 2 years of age [4]. In contrast, the infant's intestine may be more responsive to STa, the heat-stable toxin elaborated by enterotoxigenic *E. coli*, than that of an older child due to increased expression of the STa receptor guanylate cyclase C and decreased degradation of STa [5] in the infant.

Many other physiologic factors, including motility, mucus production, gastric secretions, intestinal surface area, and, probably most importantly, cellular and humoral immunity, undergo age-related developmental changes and influence the host's response to diseases that cause acute diarrhea.

PATHOPHYSIOLOGY

The pathophysiology of acute diarrheal diseases in children is differentiated from that seen in the adult by several factors. These include the following: the immature immune system; a larger surface area-to-volume ratio; and dependence on a caretaker for fluid administration and health supervision.

Pediatric patients more often develop systemic infections from bacterial enteric pathogens, dehydration from fluid losses, and metabolic derangements (*eg*, electrolyte abnormalities, hypoglycemia, and acidosis) than do adults. Systemic spread of the offending microbe is particularly increased in infants. For example, osteomyelitis, bacteremia, and meningitis more commonly develop following enteric salmonella infection in newborns without underlying immunodeficiency. Associated malnutrition is an additional risk factor that promotes complications of diarrheal disease in childhood [6].

Age-related variation in susceptibility to enteric infections is explained by differences in infectious exposures and previous antigen challenge. Young children are at increased risk of acquiring microbial pathogens due to poor hygiene and close proximity with other children. Inadequate handwashing, sharing toys, and attendance at day care centers allow for fecal–oral transmission of pathogens. Furthermore, cellular and humoral immunity have not been fully developed in these children because they have had no previous exposure to specific microbes.

Infants in the first months of life who have acute diarrhea must be evaluated cautiously because of the increased likelihood that they may have congenital deficiencies and congenital structural lesions. Profound diarrhea in the immediate perinatal period is expected with the most severe defects (*eg*, congenital microvillus inclusion disease, congenital chloride diarrhea); however, other abnormalities, such as sucrase-isomaltase deficiency, Hirschsprung's disease, or intestinal duplication, can present with acute diarrhea beyond the neonatal period. Bloody diarrhea in the infant may represent a life-threatening infection or an acute abdominal catastrophe; nonbloody diarrhea may lead to hypovolemic shock, postenteritis enteropathy, or the diagnosis of a congenital defect.

■ CLINICAL FEATURES
Diagnostic Overview
The approach to the pediatric patient with acute diarrhea, whether nonbloody or bloody, begins with a thorough history and physical examination. As in the adult patient with diarrhea, important information to elicit includes stool volume, abdominal pain, tenesmus, the presence of bloody stools, the duration of symptoms, likelihood of exposure to infectious agents, diet, family history, recent medication use, past medical history, travel, and the presence of systemic symptomatology (*eg*, fever or weight

loss). However, the age of the patient is another important factor because the most common diagnoses differ from age group to age group (Tables 158-1 and 158-2). Certain diagnoses, such as allergic colitis, Hirschsprung's disease, and rotavirus-induced diarrhea, are seen almost exclusively in infants.

A careful physical examination is needed to focus the management and evaluation of the patient with diarrhea. The first task is to assess the patient's circulatory status, because the correction of volume depletion is more important than establishing the specific cause of the diarrhea. Physical examination may reveal important clues that help to determine the cause of the diarrhea, including an abdominal mass, perianal disease, signs of anemia, fever, edema, lymphadenopathy, skin lesions (*eg*, purpura), hepatosplenomegaly, and fecal impaction. Inspection of a stool specimen also may be helpful. The presence of blood, pus, or fat droplets in the stool may alter the diagnostic work-up.

Important Infectious Etiologies of Acute Diarrhea
Although children may be exposed to the same variety of enteropathogens that infect adults, the relative frequency, clinical symptoms, and sequelae caused by infectious agents differ vastly between these two populations. In all age groups, viral pathogens are isolated in acute diarrheal disease more often than are bacterial or parasitic pathogens; however, in a large percentage of diarrheal illness, no pathogen is identified [7] (Fig. 158-2).

Viral Pathogens
Rotavirus
In 1973, Bishop and colleagues identified rotavirus by electron microscopy of duodenal epithelial cells [8]. This infectious agent causes more pediatric diarrheal illness than any other single agent, both in the United States and worldwide [9].

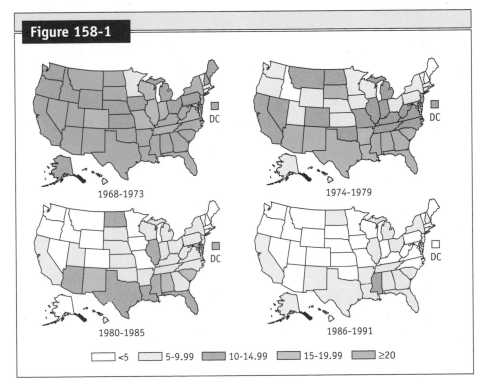

Figure 158-1

1968-1973   1974-1979

1980-1985   1986-1991

☐ <5   ☐ 5-9.99   ☐ 10-14.99   ☐ 15-19.99   ☐ ≥20

Mortality from diarrhea (per 100,000 live births) from 1968 through 1991 in the United States. DC indicates District of Columbia. (*Adapted from* Kilgore *et al.* [3]; with permission.)

Table 158-1. Acute Diarrhea: Differential Diagnosis by Age*

Newborn (0–1 mo)	Infancy (1–12 mo)	Childhood (1–12 y)	Adolescence and adulthood (>12 y)
*Allergic colitis	Antibiotic-induced diarrhea	*Antibiotic-induced diarrhea	*Food poisoning
Congenital disaccharidase deficiency (eg, sucrase-isomaltase deficiency)	*Allergic colitis	Fecal impaction (overflow)	*Infection (particularly Norwalk virus, all bacterial infections)
Congenital transport defect (eg, congenital chloride diarrhea)	Congenital disaccharidase deficiency (eg, sucrase-isomaltase deficiency)	*Food poisoning	Inflammatory bowel disease
Hirschsprung's colitis	*Gastroenteritis (particularly rotavirus, adenovirus, caliciviruses, and salmonella)	*Gastroenteritis (particularly rotavirus, Norwalk virus, astroviruses, all bacterial enteropathogens, giardia)	
*Gastroenteritis (particularly adenovirus, and salmonella)	Hirschsprung's colitis	Henoch-Schönlein purpura	
Necrotizing enterocolitis	Inflammatory bowel disease	Inflammatory bowel disease	
Parenteral infections (eg, urinary tract infections)	Intussusception	Intussusception	
	Munchausen syndrome by proxy	Munchausen syndrome by proxy	
		*Toddler's diarrhea	

Many diseases that are considered frequently as causes of chronic diarrhea are listed because many present in an acute fashion. More common diseases are denoted by an asterisk.

Table 158-2. Differential Diagnosis of Acute Diarrhea

Causes of bloody diarrhea	Causes of nonbloody diarrhea
Infectious Agents*	Infectious Agents
Aeromonas spp	Adenovirus
Campylobacter spp	Astrovirus
C. difficile	Bacteroides fragilis
Echerichia histolytica	Balantidium coli
Echerichia coli 0157:H7	Brachyspira aalborgii (intestinal spirochetosis)
Plesiomonas spp	Calicivirus
Shigella spp	Cryptosporidium spp
Yersinia spp	Cyclospora spp
Cytomegalovirus	Cytomegalovirus
Noninfectious Agents	Food poisoning
Allergic colitis	Giardia spp
Henoch-Schönlein purpura	Isospora beli
Hirschsprung's colitis	Listeria spp
Inflammatory bowel disease	Norwalk virus
Intussusception	Nonintestinal infection (eg, urinary tract infection)
Ischemic colitis	Rotavirus
Munchausen syndrome by proxy	Strongloides spp
Necrotizing enterocolitis	Noninfectious Agents
	Antibiotic-induced diarrhea
	Appendicitis
	Congenital transport defect
	Fecal impaction
	Heavy metal poisoning
	Medications
	Munchausen syndrome by proxy
	Partial obstruction
	Stevens-Johnson syndrome
	Toddler's diarrhea
	Toxic shock syndrome

Infectious agents that cause bloody diarrhea may also cause nonbloody diarrhea. This table does not list rare entities that can cause diarrhea.

Figure 158-2

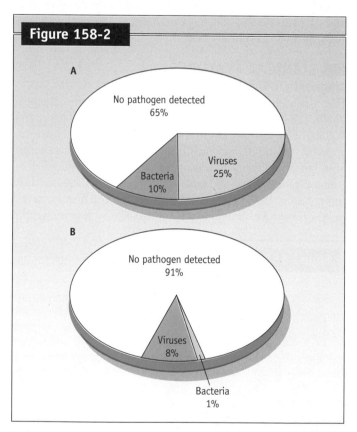

Isolation of enteropathogens from pediatric outpatients less than 2 years old with diarrheal illnesses (**A**) and in a control population of asymptomatic children (**B**). No ova or parasites were detected in any patient. (*Adapted from* Kotloff *et al.* [11]; with permission.)

Children between 6 and 24 months of age are most commonly affected. Adults with rotavirus infection typically are asymptomatic or demonstrate only mild symptoms, perhaps due to rotavirus antibody acquired early in life [10].

After a 48- to 72-hour incubation period following exposure, most affected subjects experience the sudden onset of vomiting with watery diarrhea, often with fever. The diarrhea, which usually is nonbloody, persists for 2 to 8 days. The volume of stool loss is usually 30 to 100 mL/kg/d but has been as high as 160 mL/kg/d and can result in dehydration and shock.

In addition to causing direct cytolytic damage to the villi, rotavirus may cause diarrhea by elaborating an enterotoxin. This enterotoxin is a nonstructural glycoprotein (NSP4) that potentiates chloride secretion by a calcium-dependent signaling pathway [11]. The effect of NSP4 is age dependent and dose related when tested in mice. In addition, the diarrhea induced by rotavirus may be the result of malabsorption subsequent to villous damage and secondary disaccharidase deficiencies (*eg*, lactase deficiency) along with crypt hyperplasia, which cannot be adequately compensated in the infant. The destructive effects of rotavirus on the intestinal villi (Fig. 158-3) may result in persistent diarrhea caused by a postenteritis enteropathy. Therefore, nutritional therapy for this type of damage may require prolonged enteral drip feedings with or without parenteral nutrition until the villi recover. Diagnosis of rotavirus typically is accomplished by using enzyme-linked immunosorbent assays (ELISAs) that detect rotaviral agents.

The mainstay of therapy has been effective supportive care with rehydration and nutritional support as needed. Vaccine development is being actively pursued, and clinical trials are under investigation. It is likely that a multivalent, live attenuated rotavirus vaccine will be considered for licensing in the United States in the near future.

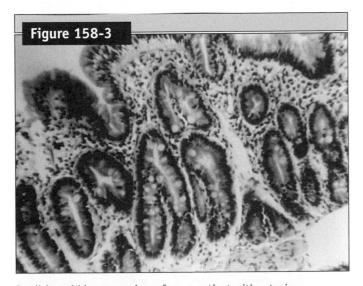

Figure 158-3

Small-bowel biopsy specimen from a patient with rotavirus enteritis. Most viruses result in injury to the proximal small intestine. The lesion is not unlike many other small-bowel disorders with partial flattening of the villi, increase in inflammatory cells, and loss of polarity of the surface epithelium. The lesion is often quite patchy and variable, as are many other small intestinal lesions. Combined secretory and osmotic diarrhea occurs in these patients, in whom the disorder is typically transient.

Other Viral Pathogens

Enteric adenoviruses (serotypes Ad40 and Ad41) are thought to be the second most common cause of viral gastroenteritis among children [12]. After contact through the fecal–oral route, children, usually less than 2 years of age, may develop vomiting and diarrhea. The diarrhea may persist as long as 14 days, whereas the vomiting is often mild and shorter in duration. Detection techniques to rapidly identify enteric adenovirus infection are not widely available. Treatment is supportive and consists of adequate hydration therapy.

Norwalk virus often causes gastroenteritis in older children and adults. Unlike adenoviruses, this virus is often acquired through exposure to a common source rather than via person-to-person contact. Vomiting is a more prominent symptom in most cases along with nausea, and cramping abdominal pain. Norwalk-induced illness is typically brief in duration (12 to 48 hours) and uncommonly results in significant dehydration.

Many other viral pathogens result in acute gastroenteritis. Caliciviruses have been documented in diarrheal illnesses in children from 3 months to 6 years, particularly in daycare centers. Astroviruses affect children in the 1- to 3-year age group, causing vomiting, diarrhea, fever, and abdominal pain. Other enteropathogens include coronavirus, pestivirus, and torovirus.

Cytomegalovirus (CMV) can also result in acute diarrhea. In the immunocompromised host, CMV causes a multitude of diseases, including a colitis with diarrhea. In immune competent children, CMV has been associated with a hypertrophic gastropathy, a form of Ménétrier's disease, which is acute and self-limited [13]. This infection often presents with diarrhea and results in a protein-losing enteropathy.

Bacterial Pathogens
Salmonella

Salmonella enterocolitis usually results from ingestion of contaminated poultry, meats, or dairy products. Because it requires a relatively large inoculum, person-to-person transmission is rare. Nevertheless, large outbreaks continue to occur [14], and an estimated 1 to 2 million infections per year are attributable to this enteropathogen . Infants represent the group at greatest risk. Infection with *Salmonella* species not only causes acute gastroenteritis (bloody and nonbloody) but also can result in bacteremia, focal nonintestinal infections, and enteric fever (*eg*, typhoid fever). *Salmonella* organisms invade epithelial cells in the ileum and colon, causing inflammatory diarrhea. These organisms may then reach the systemic circulation, causing numerous sequelae, including septicemia, meningitis, osteomyelitis, and pneumonia.

An additional problem following infection with *Salmonella* species in children is prolonged excretion of the organism. Although the median time of excretion is 7 weeks in children less than 5 years of age, 26% continue to excrete the bacterium for more than a year [7]; this may be tenfold higher than in adult patients. This propensity for a carrier state has led to the recommendation that antibiotics be avoided in patients with mild, uncomplicated disease because they have not been shown to decrease the excretion period. Antimicrobial therapy is recommended for patients of any age who are severely ill or at increased risk for sequelae (Table 158-3). The latter category includes all children less than 3 months of age, immunocompromised children, patients with sickle cell anemia, and individuals with surgically implanted medical devices. Some experts recommend parenteral antibiotics in all children younger than 6 to 18 months of age.

Escherichia coli 0157:H7

Escherichia coli bacteria that cause diarrheal illnesses have been divided, based on their serotyping or pathogenic mechanisms, into five major groups: enteropathogenic (EPEC), enterotoxigenic (ETEC), enteroinvasive (EIEC), enterohemorrhagic (EHEC), and entero-adherent (EAEC) or entero-aggregative (EAggEC). The spectrum of illnesses caused by these organisms includes severe infantile diarrhea in developing countries (ETEC), traveler's diarrhea (ETEC), dysentery-like illness (EIEC), and hemorrhagic colitis (EHEC). EHEC infections, including *E. coli* O157:H7, are particularly important because they are so common and because they may have significant sequelae.

E. coli O157:H7 may be the pathogen most often isolated from children with grossly bloody infectious diarrheal illnesses. This organism, which is also the most common cause of the hemolytic uremic syndrome (HUS), occurs more often among children than among adults [15,16] (Fig. 158-4). Undercooked hamburger meat is the most frequent source; however, other foods contaminated with bovine feces, including apple cider and raw milk, have been shown to be vehicles for outbreaks. In addition, 10% to 20% of cases occur through person-to-person spread because the inoculum needed to result in clinical disease is low.

Gastrointestinal symptoms associated with *E. coli* O157:H7 range from mild, watery diarrhea to hemorrhagic colitis. With hemorrhagic colitis, the diarrhea does not typically become bloody until the second or third day of the illness. Vomiting occurs in about half of patients; high fever is uncommon. Fecal shedding averages about 17 days but can persist for more than 30 days [17]. Approximately 10% of pediatric patients develop HUS, characterized by a microangiopathic hemolytic anemia, thrombocytopenia, and acute renal failure.

HUS is a significant public health concern because the mortality rate is approximately 10% and some patients develop severe long-term renal morbidity. Measures to control transmission of this organism focus on adequate cooking of hamburger meat as well as ensuring identification of *E. coli* O157:H7 in symptomatic patients. Guidelines for cooking hamburger issued by the U. S. Food and Drug Administration require that hamburgers reach an internal temperature high enough to kill the organism (160°). They should be cooked until the interior is no longer pink and the juices are clear. Identification of the organism may rely on a specific request to check for it because some laboratories do not routinely culture for this pathogen. Although no specific treatment, including antimicrobial agents, has proved helpful in preventing HUS , early identification of *E. coli* O157:H7 is important to prevent secondary transmission and to permit surveillance reporting.

Campylobacter

Infection with *Campylobacter* organisms is frequent in children less than 1 year old and in young adults. Like the diarrhea seen with other bacterial pathogens, the diarrhea caused by *Campylobacter* species is quite variable, ranging from watery stools to frank dysentery. Infection is acquired via the fecal–oral route or from contaminated food products, particularly chicken and raw milk. Associated symptoms often include fever and abdominal pain and may mimic appendicitis. Complications include Reiter's syndrome and Guillain-Barré syndrome [18]. A long period of excretion is typical, but it may be decreased with antibiotic treatment. Antibiotic therapy may be helpful if given early in the illness but usually does not shorten the course of illness when given more than 3 to 4 days after the onset of diarrhea.

Table 158-3. Antimicrobial Selection in Infectious Diarrhea

Organism	Drug Choices
Aeromonas spp	Ampicillin, trimethoprim-sulfamethoxazole, or a quinolone
Campylobacter spp	Erythromycin
Clostridium difficile	Metronidazole or vancomycin
Cryptosporidium spp	Paromomycin or azithromycin (unproven)
Cyclospora spp	Trimethoprim-sulfamethoxazole
Entamoeba histolytica	Metronidazole followed by iodoquinol or paromomycin
Enterotoxigenic *Escherichia coli* (traveler's diarrhea)	Trimethoprim-sulfamethoxazole, or a quinoline
Giardia lamblia	Furazolidone or metronidazole
Plesiomonas spp	Ampicillin, trimethoprim-sulfamethoxazole, or a quinolone
Salmonella spp	Ampicillin, amoxicillin, trimethoprim-sulfamethoxazole, or a quinolone
Shigella spp	Ampicillin, trimethoprim-sulfamethoxazole, or a quinolone
Vibrio cholerae	Tetracycline, trimethoprim-sulfamethoxazole, or a quinolone

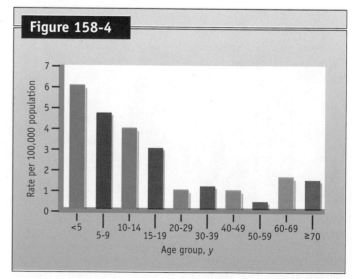

Figure 158-4

Age-specific attack rates of infection with *E.coli* 0157:H7 in the state of Washington in 1987. (*Adapted from* Ostroff *et al.* [16]; with permission.)

Shigella

Diarrhea caused by infection with *Shigella* species may be mild and watery; however, the classic picture is one of fever, malaise, abdominal cramping, and watery diarrhea followed by scant stools containing blood and mucus (bacillary dysentery). *Shigella* infection often is complicated by seizures. These seizures were formerly attributed to a neurotoxic effect of the Shiga toxin, but they are now considered a subgroup of simple febrile seizures caused by the fever rather than by the bacterium. Shigella has been identified often in daycare settings [7]. A very low inoculum (about 10 organisms) is sufficient to allow transmission via the fecal–oral route. Identification of *Shigella* organisms in stool specimens may be hampered in the initial phase following infection due to its low inoculum.

By the time a definitive diagnosis is established, many patients have improved clinically. Patients who remain symptomatic at the time of a positive stool culture usually warrant a course of antibiotic therapy (Table 158-3). Except for the severely ill patient, empiric antimicrobial therapy while awaiting the results of stool culture is not indicated. Furthermore, in epidemic situations, use of antibiotics promotes the development of bacterial resistance. Proper handwashing technique is just as effective in limiting the spread of the infection.

Clostridium difficile

Despite widespread use of antibiotics in children, the incidence of *Clostridium difficile*–associated colitis in children is less common than in adults. Antibiotic-associated diarrhea unrelated to *C. difficile* is common, whereas symptomatic infection associated with *C. difficile* is uncommon in children. Infection with this organism may result in symptoms ranging from asymptomatic carriage to life-threatening pseudomembranous colitis. In contrast to adults, in whom asymptomatic carriage is rare, asymptomatic carriage occurs in half of the newborn infants in special care nurseries. In most patients there is a history of antibiotic administration, but the disease has been noted without any antibiotic exposure. In severe disease, pseudomembranes may be present throughout the colon. The colitis from *C. difficile* causes edema of the bowel wall and thickening of the haustral markings that can be seen by computed tomography or with an abdominal radiograph. A characteristic histologic lesion, the summit lesion, is considered pathognomic. When severe disease is present, close clinical monitoring is essential. Evidence of deterioration includes ileus, as manifested by a rapid decrease in stool output, mental status changes, profuse hemorrhage, and toxic megacolon [4].

Treatment for *C. difficile* infection must be individualized. Mild disease may require no more than discontinuation of antibiotics. With more severe symptoms, treatment with metronidazole or vancomycin in addition to discontinuation of the antimicrobial therapy is indicated. In the most severe form of infection, colectomy may be life saving. Another difficult management problem is therapy for recurrent disease, which occurs in 10% to 20% of patients [4]. Treatment in this situation may necessitate a second course or pulsed courses of metronidazole or vancomycin. An alternative therapy for multiple relapses is the use of probiotic therapy with nonpathogenic yeast *Saccharomyces boulardii* [19] or *Lactobacillus GG* in addition to antimicrobials.

Other Bacterial Pathogens

Many other bacterial infections result in acute diarrhea, nonbloody and bloody. *Aeromonas hydrophilia* and the closely related *Plesiomonas shigelloides* both cause diarrhea in children. Disease caused by *Aeromonas* species is most often seen in children less than 2 years of age. Clinical presentations include mild watery diarrhea, bloody diarrhea, and persistent diarrhea. Similarly, *Plesiomonas* species have been associated with a variable presentation. However, this organism most often causes small-volume diarrheal stools with associated abdominal pain [20].

Yersinia enterocolitica typically affects children less than 5 years of age. The presentation is most often watery or mucoid diarrhea, with about 10% of cases having gross blood. Abdominal pain, headache, fever, arthritis, and pharyngitis often accompany the enteritis. Particularly in older patients, infection with *Yersinia* species may cause mesenteric adenitis, which can be confused with appendicitis, or ileitis, which can be confused with Crohn's disease. Most cases are self-limited. This infection is much more common in Canada and northern Europe than in the United States.

Many bacteria, including *Clostridium perfringens*, *Bacillus cereus*, *Vibrio parahaemolyticus*, and *Staphylococcus aureus* can cause food poisoning, which often presents as diarrhea along with abdominal cramps, vomiting, or fever. These infectious agents are discussed in detail elsewhere (see Chapter 62). Other agents that may cause bacterial gastroenteritis in children include enterotoxigenic *Bacteroides fragilis*, *Listeria monocytogenes* [21], and *Brachyspira aalborgi*, or intestinal spirochetosis.

Parasitic Pathogens

Giardia lamblia is the most common intestinal parasite in the United States. Giardiasis is particularly important in pediatrics because *G. lamblia* more often results in symptomatic illness in children than in adults, is readily spread in daycare centers [22], and can adversely affect growth [7]. *G. lamblia* infection is acquired via contaminated food and water (eg, well water) in addition to person-to-person transmission. Acute infection is characterized by the sudden onset of watery, foul-smelling diarrhea, often associated with flatus and belching. Acute symptoms typically last 3 to 4 days but may evolve to a chronic infection. Most individuals infected with *G. lamblia* are thought be asymptomatic carriers; however, infected children are more likely to be symptomatic than are infected adults.

Diagnosis of giardiasis has traditionally relied on the microscopic examination of stool specimens. Obtaining stool specimens on alternate days has been recommended to improve the diagnostic yield. Duodenal fluid and small intestinal biopsies may also be examined for *Giardia* organisms (Fig. 158-5*A* and *B*) [23]. More recently, ELISA methods have become available to detect *Giardia* antigens in the stool. After establishing the diagnosis, appropriate antiparasitic therapy should be prescribed (Table 158-3).

Although it is uncommonly encountered in the United States, *Entamoeba histolytica* is an important worldwide pathogen with a high rate of morbidity and mortality in infancy and childhood [24]. Like *Giardia*, *E. histolytica* is spread via cysts in contaminated food and water and by person-to-person transmission. There is a high frequency of asymptomatic carriers (80% to 90%), but infection can result in severe disease.

Infection with *E. histolytica*, *ie*, amebiasis, should be considered in the differential diagnosis of acute and chronic colitis, particularly with a history of foreign travel. Acute amebiasis produces symptoms indistinguishable from bacterial dysentery; in its most severe form, this infection may cause colonic dilation and toxemia. Chronic colitis resulting from amebiasis may mimic inflammatory bowel disease. Amebic liver abscess is an infrequent but well-known complication of *E. histolytica* infection and can occur days or years after intestinal infection. As with *Giardia* infection, diagnosis of amebiasis relies on fecal microscopic examination. Alternatively, amebiasis infection can be established by obtaining serology for IgG antibodies, which is positive in more than 70% of patients with amebic colitis and nearly all patients with liver involvement.

Cryptosporidium is another parasitic enteropathogen of increased importance in both immunocompetent and immunosuppressed individuals. *Cryptosporidium* infection is acquired via exposure to farm animals and person-to-person spread. Contamination of water supplies, presumably from the excrement of farm animals, has been implicated in large outbreaks in several locations, including one in Milwaukee in which about 370,000 people were infected [25]. In immunocompetent hosts, the symptoms of watery diarrhea, nausea, vomiting, and flu-like symptoms are self-limited. In contrast, in immunodeficient individuals, *Cryptosporidium*-induced diarrhea can be prolonged and severe (3–6 L/d), with spread of the organism to the biliary tract and the lungs. Definitive therapy for *Crytosporidium* infection has not been determined. Anecdotal reports indicate that several drugs, including paromomycin and azithromycin, have some promise (Table 158-3).

Cyclospora cayetanensis, like *Cryptosporidium*, are acid-fast organisms that may cause a prolonged diarrheal illness. *Cyclospora*, which can be treated with trimethoprim-sulfamethoxazole, has been implicated in recent epidemics of diarrhea following the ingestion of contaminated fruit. Additional parasites, including *Strongyloides stercoralis*, *Isospora belli*, and *Balantidium coli*, may present with acute diarrhea. A full discussion of these parasitic infections is beyond the scope of this chapter.

Important Noninfectious Causes of Acute Diarrhea

Awareness of noninfectious causes (Table 158-2) of acute diarrhea, nonbloody or bloody, is essential because these illnesses cause significant morbidity and mortality. Examples of potentially life-threatening disorders that may mimic gastroenteritis include intussusception, necrotizing enterocolitis, acute appendicitis, and Hirschsprung's disease. All of these problems may be difficult to recognize without a high index of suspicion and a careful physical examination. Recognition of nonsurgical, noninfectious causes of acute diarrhea, including allergic colitis, fecal impaction, sucrase-isomaltase deficiency, and Munchausen syndrome by proxy, also is necessary to provide appropriate therapy. These noninfectious disorders are more fully discussed in other chapters of this text (see Chapters 70, 157, and 183).

▬ EVALUATION

In the United States, the incidence of diarrhea in children younger than 3 years has been estimated to be 1.3 to 2.3 episodes per child per year; rates in children attending daycare centers are higher [1••]. Nine percent of hospital admissions in children younger than 5 years of age (220,000 children) are due to acute diarrhea [1••]. Therefore, even though acute diarrhea most often is self limited, caution still must be exercised in the evaluation of pediatric patients because of the frequency of dehydration and other complications.

Uncomplicated acute gastroenteritis requires a careful assessment of the patient's clinical status; usually a stool culture and laboratory evaluation are not necessary. In most of these cases, laboratory results do not alter management decisions and obtaining these tests is not cost effective. However, evaluation for infectious etiologies of acute diarrhea is warranted under the following circumstances: bloody diarrhea; severely ill patient; immunocompromised patient; age less than 3 months; hospitalized patient; community outbreak; and traveler's diarrhea.

A stool culture is diagnostic for bacterial enteropathogens. Communication with the laboratory helps to ensure the use of appropriate selective media for certain pathogens; *eg*, *E. coli* O157:H7, *Yersinia* species, and *V. cholerae*. A *C. difficile* toxin assay should be considered in all patients who developed their diarrhea within the hospital and in all patients who have had antibiotic

Figure 158-5

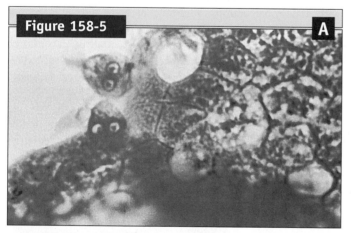

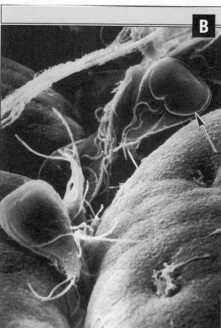

A, Duodenal biopsy demonstrating *Giardia lamblia* trophozoites attached to the epithelium. **B**, Scanning electron microscopy reveals the organism in a crevice over the intestinal epithelium (*arrow*). (*A*, Courtesy of D. Heyneman, MD. *B*, Courtesy of R. Owen, MD. *From* Soave [23]; with permission.)

exposure within the preceding 30 days. If these studies are unrevealing and the symptoms persist, additional evaluation, including sigmoidoscopy or colonoscopy, should be considered. Because the sensitivity of stool samples depends on the difficulty of culturing the organism and the precision of the laboratory, many infectious agents are diagnosed by endoscopy.

If the diarrhea persists and remains unexplained, noninfectious diseases should be considered in the differential diagnosis (Table 158-2) (see Chapter 183). Munchausen syndrome (child-initiated) or Munchausen syndrome by proxy (caretaker-initiated) resulting in diarrhea is seen in pediatrics and should be considered in the differential diagnosis (Table 158-2). Several tests can assist in detecting laxative use. These tests include alkalinization of the stool to detect phenolphthalein; measurement of magnesium, sulfate, or phosphate in fecal fluid; and measurement of senna in urine. Addition of water to the stool can be detected by measurement of stool osmolality.

■ TREATMENT
Rehydration and Refeeding
No matter what has caused the diarrhea, the first goal of therapy is to ensure adequate hydration. In mild to moderate dehydration (<10%), this can be accomplished with oral rehydration solutions (ORS) [26] (Table 158-4). These solutions provide glucose and electrolytes in concentrations that take advantage of the glucose–sodium cotransport mechanism. ORS is clinically as effective as intravenous therapy, and is also less invasive, less expensive, and more practical; it can be administered at home. The ideal ORS has 2% to 2.5% glucose and a sodium concentration ranging from 30 mEq/L to 90 mEq/L as well as additional electrolytes (eg, potassium, bicarbonate, and chloride). Although taste is a limiting factor for some adults and older children, infants with dehydrating diarrhea usually are able to consume ORS in sufficient quantities.

In adolescents, as with many therapies, poor compliance with ORS necessitates consideration of other means of rehydration. One option is the use of "sports drinks"; however, these beverages are not optimal replacements for diarrheal losses because they contain excessive glucose and too little sodium.

After ensuring adequate hydration, the next consideration in the pediatric patient is addressing the nutritional status. Particularly in infants, any insult to the gastrointestinal tract may lead to a persistent diarrhea because of a postenteritis syndrome. Therefore, to hasten recovery, prompt resumption of a normal, age-appropriate diet is necessary. This approach increases intestinal disaccharidases and pancreatic secretion, and stimulates mucosal cell growth and proliferation. Early refeeding also minimizes interruption of breast-feeding.

The debate about which foods are best for refeeding continues. In breast-fed infants, nursing should be resumed early. In formula-fed infants, debate regarding the use of diluted and lactose-free formulas is ongoing. No clinical benefit has been demonstrated from the incremental reintroduction of diluted formulas [1••]. Similarly, despite the transient lactase deficiency that may develop, the benefit of a lactose-free formula in most cases is uncertain. For these reasons, the American Academy of Pediatrics recommends an unrestricted age-appropriate diet, including full-strength milk, in children with mild, self-limited diarrhea [1••]. However, when the diarrhea is severe, when the patient is very young (<3 months of age), or when careful follow-up observation cannot be ensured, a lactose-free formula is recommended for 3 to 5 days, until disaccharidase activity returns to normal. In older children, complex carbohydrates (eg, rice, wheat, potatoes, bread, and cereals), lean meats, yogurt, fruits, and vegetables are recommended. Fatty foods and foods high in simple sugars (including juices and soft drinks) are discouraged [1••].

Antimicrobial Therapy
Antimicrobial agents and other drugs have limited usefulness in the management of acute diarrhea. Because viral agents are the predominant cause of acute diarrhea, antimicrobial therapy is not indicated. Furthermore, by the time a bacterial or parasitic enteropathogen is identified, treatment may no longer be necessary. Antimicrobial therapy is usually indicated when a susceptible enteropathogen is identified in a symptomatic patient (Table 158-3).

Table 158-4. Commercially Available Oral Rehydration Solutions

Solution	Carbohydrate (g/dL)	Sodium (mEq/L)	Potassium (mEq/L)	Chloride (mEq/L)	Base (mEq/L)
Pedialyte (Ross Laboratories, Columbus, OH)	2.5 (dextrose)	45	20	35	30 (citrate)
Rehydralyte (Ross)	2.5 (dextrose)	75	20	65	30 (citrate)
Infalyte (Mead Johnson, Evansville, IN)	3.0 (rice syrup solids)	50	25	45	30 (citrate)
Ceralyte* (Cera Products, Columbia, MD)	4.0 (rice syrup solids)	90	20	80	30 (citrate)
Kao Lectroyte (Pharmacia-Upjohn, Kalamazoo, MI)	3.0 (dextrose)	50	20	40	30 (citrate)
WHO Solution*, †	2.0 (glucose)	90	20	80	30 (bicarbonate)

*Must be reconstituted with water.

†Available in the United States from Jianas Bros. Packaging, Kansas City, MO. Many generic oral rehydration solutions with similar electrolyte composition are also available.

Therapy with Antidiarrheal Compounds

A variety of medications have been used to treat diarrhea. Their mechanisms of action include the alteration of intestinal motility, the alteration of secretions, the adsorption of toxins, and the alteration of intestinal microflora.

In general, these agents are not recommended for children with gastroenteritis [1••]. The opiate analogs, including loperamide and diphenoxylate, may exacerbate a toxigenic illness as well as promote additional adverse effects; ileus and death have been reported as complications. Similarly, anticholinergic agents can have unacceptable side effects in children, especially considering their unproved efficacy in ameliorating diarrhea. The beneficial effects of bismuth subsalicylate, likewise, are modest; potential toxicity exists due to overadministration. Adsorbents such as attapulgite have no proven value in decreasing diarrhea fluid losses or duration, although they may alter the appearance of the stool. Lactobacillus-containing compounds have not been tested adequately to be recommended for widespread use; there are no known toxic effects, however.

■ PROGNOSIS AND PERSISTENT DIARRHEA

The vast majority of infants and children recover uneventfully from acute diarrhea, both nonbloody and bloody. Persistent diarrhea (longer than 2 weeks) is another source of morbidity with increased frequency in pediatric patients. The causes of persistent diarrhea include the following: enteropathogens with a propensity for prolonged episodes of diarrhea; postenteritis enteropathy; noninfectious diarrhea; and toddler's diarrhea.

Certain infectious agents, including Giardia, *Clostridium difficile*, Salmonella, Aeromonas, Cryptosporidium, and Yersinia, are recognized as causing diarrhea that may last several weeks. Postenteritis enteropathy following an acute insult may occur. Many noninfectious disorders can cause prolonged diarrhea (Table 158-2). In the infant, allergic colitis should be considered strongly, whereas in the older child inflammatory bowel disease must be considered; in all ages, the possibility of Munchausen syndrome by proxy has to be considered when evaluating unexplained persistent diarrhea. Finally, the young child is particularly susceptible to diarrheal symptoms often related to dietary factors. In children with chronic, nonspecific diarrhea of infancy, also referred to as *toddler's diarrhea* or *sloppy stool syndrome* an acute episode of diarrhea is often perceived as an inciting event. In fact, a combination of causes may explain this condition, including excessive fluid intake, malabsorption of carbohydrates in fruit juices, restriction of dietary fat, and abnormal intestinal motility. Children with this condition often respond to dietary manipulation, including eliminating excessive fruit juices, increasing dietary fiber intake, and increasing fat consumption; in the absence of treatment, this condition resolves spontaneously at the time of toilet training.

Although much progress has been made in treating both acute and persistent diarrhea, the prevention of acute diarrhea through vaccine development and improved hygiene remains the best hope for reducing the morbidity and mortality caused by diarrhea. Currently, candidate vaccines for rotavirus, enterotoxigenic *E. coli*, *V. cholerae*, and Shigella are being evaluated. Even when vaccines do become available, however, they are likely not to be 100% effective. Therefore, therapies such as oral rehydration and nutritional therapy will still be important in minimizing the impact of acute diarrhea on children.

■ REFERENCES

Recently published papers of particular interest have been highlighted as follows:
•   Of interest
••   Of outstanding interest

1.•• Committee on Quality Improvement, Subcommittee on Acute Gastroenteritis, American Academy of Pediatrics: Practice parameter: the management of acute gastroenteritis in young children. *Pediatrics* 1996, 97:24–435.
This practice parameter formulates recommendations for health care providers about the management of acute diarrhea for children. This article discusses the scientific data regarding the complications and management of acute diarrheal illnesses. An expert consensus opinion is given regarding oral rehydration solutions, refeeding after rehydration, and the use of antidiarrheal agents.

2.• Ho MS, Glass RI, Pinsky PF, *et al*.: Diarrheal deaths in American children: are they preventable? *JAMA* 1988, 260:3281–3285.
This retrospective review of United States mortality data for 1973 through 1983 identified an average of 500 children, aged 1 month to 4 years, each year with diarrhea reported as the cause of death. Risk factors for children included age less than 1 year, black race, living in the South, and the winter season. Maternal risk factors included black race, young age, unmarried status, low level of education, and little prenatal care.

3. Kilgore PE, Holman RC, Clarke MJ, Glass RI: Trends of diarrheal disease—associated mortality in US children, 1968 through 1991. *JAMA* 1995, 274:1143–1148.

4. Kelly CP, Pothoulakis C, LaMont JT: *Clostridium difficile* colitis. *N Engl J Med* 1994, 330:57–262.

5. Sherman PM, Lichtman SN: Pediatric considerations relevant to enteric infections. In *Infections of the Gastrointestinal Tract*. Edited by Blaser MJ, Smith PD, Ravdin JI, *et al*. New York: Raven Press; 1995:143–152.

6.• Gracey M: Diarrhea and malnutrition: a challenge for pediatricians. *J Pediatr Gastroenterol Nutr* 1996, 22:6–16.
The influence of nutrition on the morbidity and mortality of acute infectious diarrheal diseases in childhood is discussed in this article. The impact of the most common enteric pathogens is described. In addition, the approach to the pediatric patient with an acute infectious diarrhea is outlined.

7. Laney DW Jr., Cohen MB: Approach to the pediatric patient with diarrhea. *Gastroenterol Clin North Am* 1993, 22:499–516.

8. Bishop RF, Davidson GP, Holmes IH, *et al*.: Virus particles in epithelial cells of duodenal mucosa from children with acute non-bacterial gastroenteritis. *Lancet* 1973, 2:1281–1283.

9. Blacklow NR, Greenberg HB: Viral gastroenteritis. *N Engl J Med* 1991, 325:252–264.

10. Ho MS, Glass RI, Pinsky PF, *et al*.: Rotavirus as a cause of diarrheal morbidity and mortality in the United States. *J Infect Dis* 1988, 158:1112–1116.

11. Ball JM, Tian P, Zeng CQY, *et al*.: Age-dependent diarrhea induced by a rotaviral nonstructural glycoprotein. *Science* 1996, 272:101–103.

12. Kotloff KL, Losonsky GA, Morris JG Jr., *et al*.: Enteric adenovirus infection and childhood diarrhea: an epidemiologic study in three clinical settings. *Pediatrics* 1989, 84:219–225.

13. Hochman JA, Witte D, Cohen MB: Diagnosis of pediatric Ménétrier's disease with *in situ* hybridization. *J Clin Microbiol* 1996, 34:2588–2589.

14. Hennessy TW, Hedberg CW, Slutsker L, *et al*.: A national outbreak of *Salmonella enteritidis* infections from ice cream. *N Engl J Med* 1996, 334:1281–1286.

15. Boyce TG, Swerdlow DL, Griffin PM: *Escherichia coli* O157:H7 and the hemolytic-uremic syndrome. *N Engl J Med* 1995, 330:364–367.

16. Ostroff SM, Kobayshi JM, Lewis JH: Infections with *Escherichia coli* O157:H7 in Washington state: the first year of statewide disease surveillance. *JAMA* 1989, 262:355.

17. Belongia EA, Osterholm MT, Soler JT, *et al.*: Transmission of *Escherichia coli* O157:H7 infection in Minnesota child daycare facilities. *JAMA* 1993, 269:883–888.

18. Rees JH, Soudain SE, Gregson NA, Hughes RAC: *Campylobacter jejuni* infection and Guillain-Barré syndrome. *N Engl J Med* 1995, 333:1374–1379.

19. Buts J-P, Corthier G, Delmee M: *Saccharomyces boulardii* for *Clostridium difficile* -associated enteropathies in infants. *J Pediatr Gastroenterol Nutr* 1993, 16:419–425.

20. Kain KC, Kelly MT: Clinical features, epidemiology, and treatment of Plesiomonas shigelloides diarrhea. *J Clin Microbiol* 1989, 27:998–1001.

21. Dalton CB, Austin CC, Sobel J, *et al.*: An outbreak of gastroenteritis and fever due to *Listeria monocytogenes* in milk. *N Engl J Med* 1997, 336:100–105.

22. Sealy DP, Schuman SH: Endemic giardiasis and day care. *Pediatrics* 1983, 72:154–158.

23. Soave R: Parasitic enteritis. In *Atlas of Infectious Diseases*, vol 7: *Intra-abdominal Infections, Hepatitis, and gastroenteritis*. Edited by Farber B. Philadelphia: Current Medicine;1996:6.3.

24. Merritt RJ, Coughlin E, Thomas DW, *et al.*: Spectrum of amebiasis in children. *Am J Dis Child* 1982, 136:785–789.

25. Sherman PM, Petric M, Cohen MB: Infectious gastroenterocolitides in children. An update on emerging pathogens. *Pediatr Clin North Am* 1996, 43:391–407.

26. Cohen MB, Mezoff AG, Laney W, *et al.*: Use of a single solution for oral rehydration and maintenance therapy of infants with diarrhea and mild to moderate dehydration. *Pediatrics* 1995, 95:639–645.

159 Chronic Diarrhea in Children
Carlos H. Lifschitz

Chronic diarrheal disorders, which for the purposes of this chapter are defined as lasting more than 2 weeks, are relatively common in children and usually are not caused by serious illnesses. Causes vary depending on the age of the child. In most instances, diarrhea is malabsorptive rather than secretory. Most secretory diarrhea is infectious. Before embarking on a series of complicated tests, the physician should consider the most common causes of a change in stool pattern: excessive intake of formula or other fluid (*eg*, water, fruit juice, high-carbohydrate beverages); chronic nonspecific diarrhea of the toddler; irritable bowel syndrome; and encopresis (overflow diarrhea).

■ ETIOLOGY, PATHOGENESIS, AND TREATMENT

Diagnosis, evaluation, and treatment of chronic diarrhea in children are illustrated in Table 159-1 and Figure 159-1.

Children Aged 1 to 6 Months

Acquired carbohydrate malabsorption. During the first few months of life, most infants receive lactose as the only carbohydrate in their diets, in the form of either breast milk or formula. Most lactose-free formulas contain glucose polymers; very few formulas have a mixture of glucose polymers and sucrose.

Following acute gastroenteritis, transient lactose intolerance, which resolves in 10 to 15 days, occurs in approximately 10% of well nourished infants [1]. More prolonged lactose intolerance is not common in well nourished, otherwise healthy infants and may be secondary to a relatively severe gastroenteritis (*eg*, rotavirus or adenovirus) [2] or changes in the intestinal mucosa caused by protein hypersensitivity [3]. Prolonged lactose intolerance can complicate acute gastroenteritis in malnourished infants [4•].

Glucose polymers are digested by glucoamylase and maltase, enzymes resistant to damage of the intestinal mucosa [5•]. However, in cases of severe damage to the integrity of the intestinal villi, malabsorption of glucose polymers also can occur [6].

Diarrhea follows the ingestion of formula or other carbohydrate-containing foods and improves when hydration is maintained with intravenous fluids or oral rehydration solution.

Following intake of the suspect carbohydrate, explosive diarrhea ensues and stools become watery and acidic, with a pH less than 5.5 and the presence of reducing substances.

The breath hydrogen test is difficult to interpret in infants [7], and false-negative results occur during episodes of acute diarrhea [8]. If carbohydrate malabsorption is suspected, a breath hydrogen test should be repeated after the child has recovered from the diarrheal episode.

Diarrhea caused by acquired carbohydrate malabsorption usually does not call for bowel rest. A formula containing glucose polymers should be substituted for one containing lactose. If the infant is intolerant to glucose polymer formulas, the possibility of protein hypersensitivity should be considered, and a formula with hydrolyzed protein should be tried. Alternatively, formula may be administered via a constant intragastric infusion. If the infant is unable to tolerate formula by constant infusion, parenteral nutrition should be initiated.

The duration of lactose intolerance in chronic diarrhea is difficult to predict. It can last from 10 days to several weeks or months [4,9••]. Gradual reintroduction of lactose and monitoring of stools are the best way to determine tolerance or sensitivity [10]. Feeding lactose to a lactose-intolerant child with chronic diarrhea can have adverse effects on nutritional recovery [4].

Congenital carbohydrate malabsorption. *Congenital sucrase–isomaltase deficiency* is the most common cause of the congenital disaccharide deficiencies. It is caused by complete or almost complete lack of sucrase activity, a decrease of maltase activity to about one third of normal, and a marked reduction in isomaltase activity [11]. When diarrhea with evidence of carbohydrate malabsorption follows the introduction of cereals to the diet, congenital deficiency of sucrase–isomaltase must be considered.

Diagnosis can be made by a breath hydrogen test using a sucrose challenge. Confirmation requires a small bowel biopsy with assay for disaccharidases. The small bowel histology is normal by routine microscopy.

Congenital sucrase–isomaltase deficiency requires elimination of complex starches and sucrose from the diet until the child is

---

Table 159-1. Differential Diagnosis of Chronic Diarrhea According to Age Groups

Children 0–6 mo
  Carbohydrate malabsorption
    Acquired
    Congenital
  Protein hypersensitivity
  Excessive intake of formula, water, or fruit juice
  Postenteritis syndrome and intractable diarrhea
  Infections
  Cystic fibrosis and other causes of fat malabsorption
  Immunodeficiency
  Lymphangiectasia
  Neuroblastoma
  Congenital chloridorrhea
  Intestinal villus inclusion disease
  Congenital defective jejunal Na+/H+ exchange

Children 7–23 mo
  Chronic nonspecific diarrhea ("toddler's diarrhea")
      (usually ≥ 11 mo)
  Small bowel bacterial overgrowth
  Celiac disease
  Immunodeficiency
  Munchausen's syndrome by proxy
  Graft versus host enteropathy
  Autoimmune enteropathy
  Carbohydrate malabsorption
  Protein hypersensitivity
  Excessive intake of fruit juice or high-carbohydrate drinks
  Postenteritis syndrome
  Cystic fibrosis
  Infections
  Fat malabsorption
  Neuroblastoma

Children ≥ 24 mo
  Irritable bowel syndrome
  Adult-type hypolactasia
  Encopresis
  Inflammatory bowel disease
  Excessive intake of laxatives
  Excessive intake of fruit juice or high-carbohydrate drinks
  Infections
  Small bowel bacterial overgrowth
  Celiac disease
  Munchausen's syndrome by proxy
  Graft versus host enteropathy
  Carbohydrate malabsorption

---

older, when colonic fermentation of malabsorbed carbohydrate may result in increased gas and short-chain fatty acid formation, but little if any diarrhea [12].

Glucose–galactose malabsorption is a rare congenital disease that results from a specific defect in the intestinal glucose and galactose sodium cotransporter. The discovery of the cDNA probe for the cotransporter in chromosome 22 has permitted the identification of the molecular basis of this transport defect [13]. Infants present with profuse diarrhea of the malabsorptive type (with presence of carbohydrate in stools) soon after the first feeding. Initially the fecal pH is not less than 5.5 because the fecal flora has not developed yet; thus, there is no colonic fermentation of malabsorbed carbohydrate. Diarrhea rapidly resolves when the infant is kept NPO and receives intravenous fluids only. Glucose–galactose malabsorption is suspected when diarrhea occurs soon after the first feeding of breastmilk or any kind of formula and if diarrhea resolves if feedings are discontinued, yet recurs once feedings are begun again. Small bowel biopsy demonstrates normal histology, and disaccharides are also normal.

The only effective treatment is the use of fructose as the carbohydrate source. It can be added to an infant formula that does not contain any carbohydrate (*eg*, RCF, Ross Carbohydrate-Free, Ross Laboratories, Columbus, OH). In the second or third year of life, as the colonic capacity to ferment carbohydrates improves, children can ingest limited amounts of a greater variety of carbohydrates. This results in formation of gas, but generally there is no significant diarrhea.

Congenital lactase deficiency is an extremely rare condition characterized by diarrhea with acidic stools and the presence of carbohydrate following the ingestion of lactose-containing milk. Symptoms resolve when the infant is fed lactose-free milk.

Protein hypersensitivity. Diarrhea caused by hypersensitivity to dietary protein occurs primarily in the first month of life, and secondarily in the first 6 months of life, or at any time after an episode of severe gastroenteritis [14••,15]. There may be carbohydrate malabsorption (enteritis) caused by small bowel involvement, as demonstrated by carbohydrates in the stool (positive reducing substances) and fecal pH less than 5.5, or diarrhea may be accompanied by mucus, blood, or both, suggesting colitis or proctitis [16,17]. If there is no enteritis or colitis, stools are looser and more frequent than normal, but excessive water loss is uncommon.

Protein hypersensitivity may occur in infants who are exclusively breast-fed because protein ingested by the mother can be excreted in breast milk and act as an allergen to the infant [16]. Intrauterine passage of antigens from the mother to the infant can result in symptoms immediately after birth when the infant ingests the antigen to which he is sensitized via breastmilk or formula.

Because there is no test diagnostic of dietary protein hypersensitivity [14••], diagnosis may be difficult. The most specific way to diagnose protein hypersensitivity is to elicit symptoms by challenge with the suspect antigen. A negative skin test to the antigen in itself does not rule out hypersensitivity; it must be confirmed by a double-blind oral challenge with the suspect antigen. Measurement of serum IgE and radioallergosorbent tests

(RAST) are of little help, particularly in infants under 6 months of age, because many infants without evidence of allergies have elevated titers to milk proteins. Response to an allergen challenge may not always be consistent. A child who previously has experienced milk protein–induced diarrhea or colitis may develop eczema or vomiting in response to a subsequent challenge.

The diagnosis of protein hypersensitivity is supported by the appearance of Charcot-Leyden crystals in the stool. A tissue biopsy from the small bowel or rectum showing a mucosa infiltrated by chronic inflammatory cells and eosinophils supports the diagnosis [14••,15–17].

Elimination of the noxious dietary protein is the only effective treatment of diarrhea caused by protein hypersensitivity.

Substitution of a soy-based formula for a formula containing casein may resolve the problem in some children. However, soy protein often acts as a sensitizing protein and, therefore, produces the same symptoms [18]. In many cases, a formula containing hydrolyzed protein must be used. In the United States, there are four such formulas for infants: Nutramigen (Mead Johnson, Evansville, IN) has partially hydrolyzed protein and glucose polymers; Alimentum (Ross Laboratories, Columbus, OH) and Pregestimil (Mead Johnson, Evansville, IN) contain medium-chain triglycerides; and, for cases in which symptoms persist despite the use of one of these formulas, a product that contains peptides, such as Neocate (SHS North America, Gaithersburg, MD), can be used. There are also formulas appropriate for children older than 1 year of age.

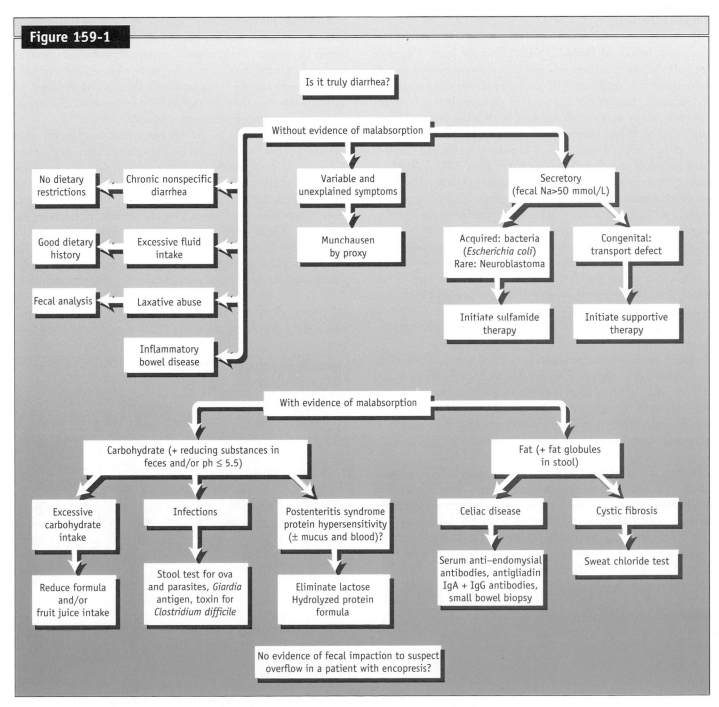

Figure 159-1

Algorithm for the evaluation and management of common causes of childhood chronic diarrhea.

Infants who are breast fed and present with chronic diarrhea caused by protein hypersensitivity may continue to breast-feed at times if the mother avoids cow's milk and soy protein in her diet. However, even if the mother does choose to eliminate these possible allergens from her diet, 40% of babies who appear allergic to milk protein continue to have symptoms and signs of protein hypersensitivity. In such instances, it is recommended that breast feeding be discontinued. Diarrhea may not resolve immediately following withdrawal of the noxious protein, and it may be necessary to administer formula as a constant infusion to overcome carbohydrate malabsorption. Total intravenous nutrition, or a combination of intravenous glucose and an enteral formula with partially hydrolyzed protein containing a reduced amount of carbohydrate, may be needed until the intestinal mucosa is repaired.

Excessive intake of formula, water, or fruit juice. Excessive formula intake can overwhelm the carbohydrate-digesting capacity of the small bowel or the water absorption capacity of the small and large bowel and result in diarrhea. It is not unusual to see children walking all day long with a bottle or a "sippy-cup" of juice. When questioned, parents may acknowledge juice intakes by the child as high as 2 L a day. Infants and children have difficulty absorbing volumes larger than 200 mL/kg/d; an excess results in diarrhea. Diarrhea, abdominal pain, or both can occur at much lower volumes with fruit juices, particularly those, such as apple juice, in which carbohydrates are mixed in a proportion that impairs absorption [19,20].

A high index of suspicion helps make the diagnosis. Such suspicion may be aroused, for example, if the caretaker offers juice to the child during the visit to soothe or entertain him or her. Stools may contain carbohydrate and have an acidic pH, but stool tests also may be normal. Sometimes parents continue to offer the child excessive amounts of fluids to prevent dehydration after an episode of acute diarrhea.

Fluid intake should be reduced to allow a milk intake of up to 1 L per day in the child aged 1 1/2 to 2 years and up to 500 mL in older children. Total fluid intake should be no more than 200 mL/kg/d during the first 2 years of life. Parents of infants who have diarrhea caused by excessive formula intake need to be educated regarding appropriate feeding practices.

Postenteritis syndrome and intractable diarrhea. Persistence of diarrhea following an episode of acute gastroenteritis is called *postenteritis syndrome*. This syndrome is characterized by carbohydrate malabsorption and, at times, protein hypersensitivity [21,22]. Typically, a previously healthy infant, formula- or (less commonly) breast-fed, develops acute gastroenteritis, and instead of improving over the following 3 to 7 days, the infant continues to suffer from loose, watery, explosive stools, with evidence of carbohydrate malabsorption [21]. Usually, oral hydration and small amounts of diluted formula are tolerated somewhat, but because the infant is unable to ingest an appropriate amount of calories, weight loss occurs.

Intractable diarrhea or idiopathic prolonged diarrhea, also known as acquired monosaccharide intolerance [23], is a syndrome in which the patient has persistent malabsorptive diarrhea with severe villous atrophy and acquired disaccharidase

deficiency with complete intolerance to all oral and enteral nutrition (Fig. 159-2) [24•]. It is possible that this is the extreme of postenteritis syndrome. In developed countries, intractable diarrhea is more common among formula-fed than breast-fed infants, and occurs predominantly in the first 3 months of life. In the developing world, this syndrome still is seen in large numbers of infants after weaning (6 to 18 months of age) [23]. Intractable diarrhea rarely is seen in developed countries, probably as a consequence of one or more of the following therapeutic modalities for acute gastroenteritis: oral rehydration; elimination of the "bowel rest" (prolonged fasting) formerly recommended for treatment of acute diarrhea; elimination of lactose in cases of persistent diarrhea; and the use of protein hydrolysates when clinically indicated.

There are no specific tests for the diagnosis of postenteritis syndrome or intractable diarrhea. A history of acute diarrhea with partial recovery and relapse is suggestive. Carbohydrate intolerance and an inability to provide the infant with sufficient calories to gain weight are often associated with the diarrhea. A biopsy of the small intestine from the patient who has postenteritis reveals villus atrophy with variable degrees of inflammation

Early identification of the problem and substitution of a formula that can be tolerated is the only effective approach in the treatment of postenteritis syndrome. When diarrhea becomes chronic and does not respond to carbohydrate substitution, temporary dilution of the formula, or small, frequent feedings, protein hypersensitivity should be considered. Elimination of sensitizing dietary proteins (*eg*, casein and soy) is necessary to prevent further inflammation of the small bowel mucosa and consequent villus damage. Total intravenous nutrition and complete bowel rest may be necessary in cases of intractable diarrhea.

Infections. A wide variety of extraintestinal and intestinal infections and systemic disorders (*eg*, cystic fibrosis) can cause

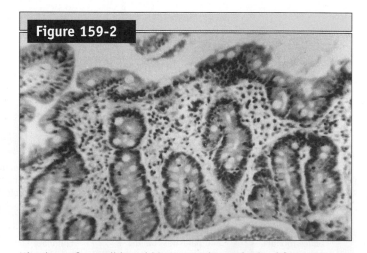

Figure 159-2

Histology of a small bowel biopsy specimen obtained from an infant with chronic diarrhea. There is blunting of the villi and increased inflammatory cells. The lesion may be patchy, as in protein-sensitive enteropathy and in celiac disease during gluten challenge. There is no good correlation between degree of small bowel mucosal injury and duration of the disease process. Patients with this kind of biopsy may require intravenous nutrition for a period of 2 weeks until repair occurs. (*Courtesy of* Robert Kruger, MD.) (*From* Vanderhoof JA [24]; with permission.)

chronic diarrhea in infants and children. Urinary tract infections, pneumonia, sepsis, and various bacterial and parasitic intestinal infections are the most common causes. Viral infection usually does not produce chronic diarrhea, but may be the cause of the initial illness, which may lead to postenteritis syndrome or predispose to protein hypersensitivity enteropathy or even intractable diarrhea.

Congenital immunodeficiency states. Congenital immunodeficiency usually does not become symptomatic until children are older than 6 months of age, particularly if they are breast fed, because maternal immunoglobulins protect them during the first few months of life. Therefore, this problem is discussed with others that may affect children older than 6 months.

Acquired immunodeficiency syndrome (AIDS). Perinatal transmission of human immunodeficiency virus (HIV) infection can present as failure to thrive with or without diarrhea (see Chapter 184). Diffuse lymphadenopathy, oral candidiasis resistant to therapy, and hepatosplenomegaly are common. Recurrent diarrhea or intractable diarrhea with malabsorption is common and difficult to manage. Organisms known to produce disease of the gastrointestinal tract are similar to those affecting adult patients with AIDS. Children diagnosed in the first few months of life have a worse outcome than those who present later in life. Children with AIDS suffering from chronic diarrhea may benefit from nutritional supplements delivered by nasogastric tube as a constant infusion. Formulas that are lactose-free and contain hydrolyzed protein and medium-chain triglycerides may be better tolerated.

Lymphangiectasia. Intestinal lymphangiectasia impairs lymphatic flow from the intestine (Fig. 159-3; also see Chapter 53). It can be caused by a congenital malformation or may be secondary to cardiovascular anomalies or operations (*eg*, the Fontan procedure), infection, inflammatory bowel disease, or drugs. Primary intestinal lymphangiectasia is associated with hypoalbuminemia, hypogammaglobulinemia, hypolipidemia, and lymphopenia. Diarrhea and edema are commonly found.

Neuroblastoma. Neuroblastoma occasionally is associated with secretory diarrhea, the result of catecholamines produced by the tumor. Seventy-seven percent of neuroblastomas occur in children under 5 years of age, and 90% occur in children under the age of 7 years. The peak age of occurrence is 1 to 3 years. Increased amounts of urine homovanillic acid and urine vanillylmandelic acid are found in 75% of patients.

Other disorders. Other disorders that may result in chronic diarrhea include *congenital chloridorrhea*, *intestinal villus inclusion disease*, and *congenital defective jejunal Na+/H+ exchange* [25].

Children 7 to 23 Months of Age

Chronic nonspecific diarrhea. The exact cause of chronic nonspecific diarrhea ("toddler's diarrhea") is not known, but it may result from an inability of the colon to adequately reabsorb fluid. Typically, the patient is a healthy child, 11 to 24 months of age, whose only problem is the presence of watery, runny

stools [26••]. If no dietary restrictions are imposed in an attempt to control the diarrhea, the child continues to gain weight normally. Unfortunately, many times parents or physicians discontinue milk, milk products, and other foods in an attempt to stop the diarrhea so that eventually the child experiences failure to thrive or actual weight loss. In many cases, excessive fluid intake can be identified as the cause, as discussed later. Sleep is not interrupted, and dehydration does not occur. However, at times parents or physicians may encourage the child to take more fluids in an attempt to prevent dehydration, which worsens the symptoms, creating a vicious circle, or overhydration diarrhea.

The diagnosis is suspected by a combination of the following factors. The child, 11 to 24 months of age, looks healthy (unless dietary restrictions result in failure to thrive) and has stools that may contain mucus but no blood. There is no abdominal pain, or abdominal pain is relieved by defecation, and there may have been dietary "transgressions" (*eg*, ingestion of an excessively low-fat diet, or excessive milk, water, juices, or fruit) [27]. The feces contain less than 40 mEq/L of sodium. There is no evidence of carbohydrate malabsorption (negative test for reducing substances). The stool pH is less than 5.5. There are no parasites and no bacteria, and tests for *Giardia lamblia* antigen and *Clostridium difficile* toxin are negative.

If dietary transgressions can be identified, correction can improve or resolve the problem completely [26••]. However, prolonged dietary restrictions should be avoided. Fiber supplementation can give bulk to the stools. Parental education is very important.

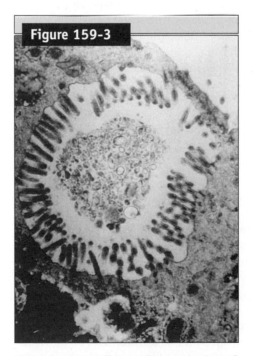

Figure 159-3

Histology of a small bowel biopsy specimen from an infant with intestinal lymphangiectasia. The photograph shows a widely dilated lacteal. Clinical features include steatorrhea and lymphocytopenia as loss of lymphocytes occurs through the gut. Dietary therapy includes the use of formulas containing medium-chain triglycerides that can be absorbed without transportation through the lymphatics (Portagen, Mead Johnson, Evansville, IN); however, products containing high carbohydrate and low-fat formula, as in some elemental diets, may be even more efficacious. (*From* Vanderhoof JA [24]; with permission.)

Small bowel bacterial overgrowth. The causes of small bowel bacterial overgrowth in children are the same as those in adults. Bacterial overgrowth also may occur after infection with *G. lamblia* or prolonged diarrhea, as a component of a postenteritis syndrome [28], or in association with cystic fibrosis and previous abdominal surgery for intestinal atresia, intestinal pseudo-obstruction, and tropical enteropathy [29].

Symptoms are excessive burping, abdominal distention, pain, excessive passage of gas, or diarrhea, which may be malabsorptive, secretory, or a combination of both.

The diagnosis is mainly clinical. The breath hydrogen test can be helpful if the baseline is elevated or if a peak is obtained at 10 or 20 minutes after ingestion of lactulose (0.5 g/kg). Later peaks can be explained by colonic fermentation, because transit time, particularly in young children, is short compared to that in adults.

Children may respond to metronidazole (30 mg/kg/d divided into 3 doses a day, for 7 to 10 days). A combination of trimethoprim and sulfamethoxazole (8 mg/kg of trimethoprim divided into 3 doses a day, for 7 to 10 days) also can be used.

Celiac Disease. (see Chapter 160)

Immunodeficiency. Congenital immunodeficiency can present in the first few months of life but may be delayed until after 6 months of age in infants who are breast fed and thereby receiving immunoglobulins from their mother. The following are the most common immunodeficiencies associated with chronic diarrhea:

X-linked agammaglobulinemia. This disorder typically presents in males during infancy with severe respiratory infection or meningitis and diarrhea that may or may not be associated with pathogens or bacterial overgrowth.

Secretory IgA deficiency: Diarrhea and malabsorption are associated with *Giardia* infection.

Severe combined immunodeficiency. The infant presents with severe infections, chronic diarrhea, malabsorption, and failure to thrive. Persistent diarrhea and oral thrush are common presentations. Diarrhea may become bloody or mucopurulent.

Munchausen syndrome by proxy. (see Chapter 183)

Graft-versus-host enteropathy. Following bone marrow transplantation, graft-versus-host disease can affect the intestine, causing protein-losing enteropathy [30]. Fecal excretion of α_1-antitrypsin is elevated. Usually this problem improves with corticosteroid therapy.

Autoimmune enteropathy. Autoimmune enteropathy is a rare entity in which infants have chronic diarrhea with severe villous atrophy and increased lymphocytic infiltrate in the lamina propria. Autoantibodies against enterocytes can be detected in the blood. Treatment with tacrolimus has shown some promise.

Children Aged 24 Months and Older

Irritable bowel syndrome. Irritable bowel syndrome in children is similar to that in the adult. Children can have alternating episodes of diarrhea and constipation, or abdominal pain, or both. Many preadolescent and adolescent patients use these symptoms as an excuse to miss school or to pay frequent visits to the nurse's office at school. Characteristically, constipation and abdominal pain occur during the day, with improvement on weekends and during vacations. Episodes of diarrhea alternate with episodes of constipation, particularly under stressful situations. Some parents who are separated or divorced report diarrhea when the child returns from visiting the other parent and may use this against the other parent for the purpose of restricting visitation rights.

Adult-type hypolactasia. Genetically determined hypolactasia can become symptomatic at 10 or 11 years of age, causing chronic diarrhea, abdominal pain, or both. Incidence is higher in non-Caucasians. Diagnosis is by elimination of lactose and is confirmed by a lactose breath hydrogen test.

Encopresis. (see Chapter 171)

Inflammatory bowel disease. (see Chapter 163)

Excessive intake of laxatives. In children, excessive use of laxatives can be seen in Munchausen syndrome by proxy and in anorexia nervosa. Male anorexia nervosa is rare. Laxatives to consider include diphenolic laxatives (phenolphthalein), anthraquinones (senna, cascara, rhubarb aloe, frangula, and dantheron); and osmotic laxatives such as sodium sulfate, sodium phosphate, magnesium sulfate, and magnesium citrate and ricinoleic acid.

This work is a publication of the USDA/ARS Children's Nutrition Research Center, Department of Pediatrics, Baylor College of Medicine, Houston, TX. This project has been funded in part with federal funds from the US Department of Agriculture, Agricultural Research Service under Cooperative Agreement number 58-6250-1-003. The contents of this publication do not necessarily reflect the views or policies of the US Department of Agriculture, nor does mention of trade names, commercial products, or organizations imply endorsement by the US government.

▩ REFERENCES

Recently published papers of particular interest have been highlighted as follows:
- • Of interest
- •• Of outstanding interest.

1. Sack DA, Rhoads M, Molla A, *et al.*: Carbohydrate malabsorption in infants with rotavirus diarrhea. *Am J Clin Nutr* 1982, 36:1112–1118.

2. Davidson GP, Goodwin D, Robb TA: Incidence and duration of lactose malabsorption in children hospitalized with acute enteritis: study in a well-nourished urban population. *J Pediatr* 1984, 105:587–590.

3. Iyngkaran N, Robinson MH, Sumithron E: Cow's milk protein sensitive enteropathy: an important factor in prolonging diarrhoea in acute infective enteritis in early infancy. *Arch Dis Child* 1978, 53:150–153.

4.• Penny ME, Paredes P, Brown KH: Clinical and nutritional consequences of lactose feeding during persistent post-enteritis diarrhea. *Pediatrics* 1989, 84:835–844.

5.• Lebenthal E, Lee PC: Glucoamylase and disaccharidase activities in normal subjects and in patients with mucosal injury of the small intestine. *J Pediatr* 1980, 97:389–393.

6. Lifschitz CH, Irving CS, Gopalakrishna GS, *et al.*: Carbohydrate malabsorption in infants with diarrhea studied with the breath hydrogen test. *J Pediatr* 1982, 102:371–375.

7. Perman JA: Breath analysis. In *Pediatric Gastrointestinal Disease: Pathophysiology, Diagnosis, Management*, vol 2. Edited by Walker WA, Durie PR, Hamilton JR, *et al*. Philadelphia: BC Decker; 1991:1354–1362.

8. Solomons NW, Garcia R, Schneider R, *et al*.: H₂ breath test during diarrhea. *Acta Paediatr Scand* 1979, 68:171–172.

9.•• Brown KH: Dietary management of acute diarrheal disease: contemporary scientific issues. *J Nutr* 1994, 124:1455S–1460S.

10. Lifschitz CH, Bautista A, Gopalakrishna GS, *et al*.: Absorption and tolerance of lactose in infants recovering from severe diarrhea. *J Pediatr Gastroenterol Nutr* 1985, 4:942–948.

11. Auricchio S: Genetically determined disaccharidase deficiencies. In *Pediatric Gastrointestinal Disease: Pathophysiology, Diagnosis, Management*, vol 1. Edited by Walker WA, Durie PR, Hamilton JR, *et al*. Philadelphia: BC Decker; 1991:647–667.

12. Argenzio RA, Moon HW, Kenny LJ, Whipp SC: Colonic compensation in transmissible gastroenteritis of swine. *Gastroenterology* 1984, 86:1501–1509.

13. Hediger MA, Coady MJ, Ikeda TS, Wright EM: Expression cloning and cDNA sequencing of the Na+/glucose co-transporter. *Nature* 1987, 330:379–381.

14.•• Sampson HA: Food allergy. *JAMA* 1997, 278:1888–1894.

15. Businco L, Benincori N, Cantani A, *et al*.: Chronic diarrhea due to cow's milk allergy. A 4 to 10 year follow-up study. *Ann Allergy* 1985, 55:844–847.

16. Lake AM, Whitington PF, Hamilton SR: Dietary protein-induced colitis in breast-fed infants. *J Pediatr* 1982, 101:906–910.

17. Goldman H, Proujanski R: Allergic proctitis and gastroenteritis in children: clinical and mucosal biopsy features in 53 cases. *Am J Surg Pathol* 1986, 10:75–86.

18. Ament ME, Rubin CE: Soy protein—another cause of the flat intestinal lesion. *Gastroenterology* 1972, 62:227–234.

19. Greene HL, Ghishan FK: Excessive fluid intake as a cause for chronic diarrhea in young children. *J Pediatr* 1983, 102:836–840.

20. Smith MM, Davis M, Chasalow FI, Lifshitz F: Carbohydrate absorption from fruit juice in young children. *Pediatrics* 1995, 95:340–344.

21. Rossi TM, Lebenthal E: Pathogenic mechanisms of protracted diarrhea. *Adv Pediatr* 1983, 30:595–633.

22. Walker-Smith JA: Cow's milk intolerance as a cause of post-enteritis diarrhoea. *J Pediatr Gastroenterol Nutr* 1982, 1:163–173.

23. Nichols VN, Fraley JK, Evans KD, Nichols BL: Acquired monosaccharide intolerance in infants. *J Pediatr Gastroenterol Nutr* 1989; 8:51–57.

24.• Vanderhoof JA: Diarrheal disease in infants and children. In *Gastroenterology and Hepatology: The Comprehensive Visual Reference*, vol 4. *Pediatric GI Problems*. Edited by Hyman PE. Philadelphia: Current Medicine; 1997:6.1–6.17.

25. Desjeux J-F: Congenital transport defects. In *Pediatric Gastrointestinal Disease*. Edited by Walker WA, Durie PR, Hamilton JR, *et al*. 1991, Philadelphia: BC Decker; 1991:668–688.

26.•• Kneepkens CM, Hoekstra JH: Chronic nonspecific diarrhea of childhood: pathophysiology and management. *Pediatr Clin North Am* 1996, 43:375–390.

27. Hoekstra JH: Fructose breath hydrogen tests in infants with chronic non-specific diarrhoea. *Eur J Pediatr* 1995, 154:362–364.

28. Forstner G, Sherman P, Lichtman S: Bacterial overgrowth. In *Pediatric Gastrointestinal Disease: Pathophysiology, Diagnosis, Management*, vol 1. Edited by Walker WA, Durie PR, Hamilton JR, *et al*. Philadelphia: BC Decker; 1991:689–700.

29. Perman JA, Modler S, Barr RG, Rosenthal P: Fasting breath hydrogen concentration: normal values and clinical applications. *Gastroenterology* 1984, 87:1358–1363.

30.• Tutschka PJ: Early complications of bone marrow transplantation in children and adults. *Bone Marrow Transplant* 1989;4(Suppl):22–26.

160 Celiac Disease
Thomas M. Rossi

Childhood celiac disease, also known as gluten-sensitive enteropathy, is characterized by malabsorption and disturbed growth in association with a specific histologic lesion of the small intestine. It was not until 1950 that the relationship between grain consumption and idiopathic steatorrhea was recognized. Dicke observed that the gastrointestinal symptoms of many affected children improved during World War II, when wheat and rye flour were unobtainable in Holland. Their symptoms worsened when wheat flour again became available after the war. Dicke and his associates are credited with identifying gluten, the water-insoluble protein fraction in wheat, as the toxic dietary substance responsible for this disease.

Celiac disease is a potentially debilitating illness for affected infants and young children and, in the past, was associated with substantial morbidity and mortality. Malnutrition and its complications continue to be associated with celiac disease, although it now is rarely fatal.

EPIDEMIOLOGY

Epidemiologic studies report regional differences in the incidence of celiac disease [1•]. Most clinicians believe that clinically overt celiac disease is uncommon in the United States, a theory supported by one study that documented 1.29 cases per 10,000 live births in the Western New York area [2], an incidence much lower than that of 1 or more per 1000 reported in most European centers.

In some countries, most notably Great Britain and Ireland, there has been a decline in the incidence of celiac disease. A delay in age at presentation, however, rather than an actual decline in the incidence of the disease may be the true explanation [3]. Most new cases are discovered in older children with minor symptoms. Explanations offered for this change have focused on trends in infant feeding practices. A resurgence in breast-feeding and the introduction of cow's milk and gluten to the diet at a later age correlate with the delay in onset of celiac symptoms. This delay may occur because breast-fed children are less likely to have gastroenteritis with its resultant mucosal atrophy and propensity for greater antigen absorption.

PATHOPHYSIOLOGY

The molecular mechanisms that account for the pathogenesis of celiac disease are still not known. The sera of patients with celiac disease contain antibodies that bind to a variety of tissues, including human umbilicus and fetal lung. Human placenta recently has been found to express embryonic celiac antigens (ECA), which bind to IgA in the sera of patients with celiac disease but not to the IgA or IgG in the sera of healthy patients or those with inflammatory bowel disease or other immunologic conditions [4].

People with celiac disease have a variety of antibodies directed at normal tissue antigens, even fetal antigens. Celiac disease may be genetically encoded from birth, and gliadin may alter the signal transduction pathway. The toxic antigen contained in gliadin is the major substance involved in turning on the signal transduction pathway, causing the immune system to mistakenly recognize normal tissue antigens as foreign.

The fact that antigliadin antibodies (AGA) are present in many conditions, and even in healthy individuals, suggests that these antibodies probably are not involved directly in the pathogenesis of celiac disease. Antireticulin antibodies (ARA), endomysium antibodies (EMA), and ECA, in contrast, are confined, for the most part, to those persons with active celiac disease and may have a role in the process that leads to intestinal atrophy. EMA, which are produced in the intestine, rise early in response to a gliadin challenge, and therefore appear in the earliest phases of celiac disease. Gliadin, either of itself or acting through AGA, may alter connective tissue antigens so that they are recognized as foreign and, in turn, turn on the production of ARA, EMA, and ECA. Gliadin may make self-antigens, normally hidden from the immune system, available for immunologic recognition, thus allowing recognition of cryptic epitopes [6]. These antibodies, particularly EMA, may attack components of the extracellular matrix of the mucosa such as collagen, reticulin, and muscle, unmasking cryptic reticulin endomysial epitopes. The antibodies may induce or disrupt the anchoring mechanism of fibroblasts and villous structural elements. Gliadin also may be involved as the stimulus for cell-mediated immunologic events, including proliferation of mononuclear cells and production of cytokines such as tumor necrosis factor, thereby perpetuating the immune response and tissue injury.

CLINICAL FEATURES

Because celiac disease results from the injurious effects of dietary gluten on the small intestinal mucosa, abdominal symptoms and malabsorptive stigmata are its classic features (Table 160-1). Celiac disease usually presents in infancy or early childhood. The period between the introduction of gluten and the onset of symptoms is quite variable. Some infants are exquisitely sensitive to gluten and present with violent vomiting and diarrhea soon after the introduction of cereals into the diet. Such symptoms may be easily confused with those of infectious gastroenteritis. In other children, there may be a delay of 6 months or even years

before the onset of symptoms. Celiac disease sometimes is even diagnosed for the first time in adulthood because symptoms have been ignored or misinterpreted as being normal.

Early Presentation

In general, symptoms seem to correlate with age at presentation, and age at presentation, in turn, relates to the age when gluten is introduced into the diet (see Table 160-1). The earlier in life gluten is introduced, the shorter is the time before symptoms appear. Gastrointestinal symptoms predominate in young infants, whereas short stature is more frequently seen in children over 5 years of age with late-onset celiac disease. Symptoms typically develop between 9 and 18 months of age and within weeks to months following gluten ingestion. The classical presentation includes the progressive development of frequent, loose, foul-smelling bowel movements, anorexia, apathy, and irritability. Failure to thrive and malnutrition ensue. The abdomen gradually becomes distended, and there is loss of subcutaneous fat as well as hypotonia with muscle wasting, especially of the buttocks and proximal limbs (Fig. 160-1). Stools may sometimes be bulky, suggestive of constipation. Constipation is reported in approximately 10% of cases. Young infants are more prone to developing celiac crisis, characterized by profuse watery diarrhea, with or without vomiting and dehydration. Malabsorption of calcium, magnesium, iron, and the fat-soluble vitamins A, D, E, and K, as well as enteric protein loss, may result in rickets, osseous fractures, tetany, anemia, bleeding, and pitting edema.

Late Presentation

An insidious onset is common in older children, with iron deficiency anemia, short stature, and delayed puberty. Older children may present solely with growth disturbances associated with subtle changes in the stool pattern, anorexia, abdominal distention, and microcytic or macrocytic anemia. Constipation is common in the older child. Most of the children reported with

Table 160-1. Clinical Features of Celiac Disease

Early Presentation (< 2 y)

Diarrhea	Constipation
Weight loss	Malnutrition
Vomiting	Growth failure
Anorexia	Pallor
Abdominal distention	Delayed development
Irritability	Bruising
Apathy	Rickets

Late presentation (> 5 y)

Lactose intolerance	Clubbing
Abdominal pain	Short stature
Anorexia	Anemia
Growth failure	Osteopenia
Pubertal delay	Bruising
Diarrhea	Dental enamel hypoplasia
Arthritis/arthralgia	

isolated growth failure have a markedly delayed bone age, and some show a blunted growth response to hormonal stimulation that is reversible following therapy with a gluten-free diet.

Atypical Presentation and Associated Features

Celiac disease can be associated with a number of systemic symptoms and signs as well as with other conditions. Arthralgia, arthritis, isolated megaloblastic anemia, pericarditis, menstrual disturbances, and infertility have been reported. Mood and mental changes, recurrent aphthous ulcers, anorexia, glossitis, hypoplasia of dental enamel, and abdominal pain secondary to transient intussusception also have been reported.

Celiac disease has been associated with several other conditions. A high proportion of adults with dermatitis herpetiformis have intestinal mucosal pathology similar to that seen in celiac disease. The enteropathy and skin lesions may respond to gluten restriction. Dermatitis herpetiformis is not commonly seen in children (see Fig. 54-7 in Chapter 54). The association of celiac disease with juvenile diabetes mellitus is now well established. HLA-B8 and DR3 antigens are shared by patients with celiac disease and those with diabetes. Other clinical entities that have been associated with celiac disease include IgA deficiency, cystic fibrosis, alpha$_1$-antitrypsin deficiency, Down's syndrome, and inflammatory bowel disease [7].

Intestinal malignancy is the most dreaded complication of celiac disease. The exact incidence of malignancy among patients with celiac disease is unknown, but one study in 1989 indicated that malignancy develops in as many as 14% of patients. Carcinoma of the esophagus and pharynx as well as intestinal lymphomas occur at a rate higher than expected. There still are reservations about the association between celiac disease and various cancers, and it is recommended that the association be presented to patients only as a hypothesis [8].

■ DIAGNOSIS

Antigliadin Antibodies

Circulating antigliadin antibodies (AGA) are antibodies to the cereal protein gliadin, which presumably is absorbed intact

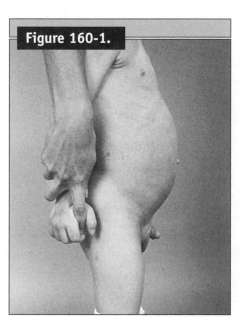

Figure 160-1. Physical appearance of a child with celiac disease. There is a protuberant abdomen, and loss of subcutaneous tissue is manifested by prominent ribs and thin extremities.

across the intestinal mucosa. Specificity and sensitivity range between 65% and 100% and 52% and 100%, respectively, for IgA antibodies, and 50% to 100% and 82% to 100%, respectively, for IgG antibodies. IgG antibodies, unfortunately, are found in healthy control subjects as well as in control subjects with other diseases, such as Crohn's disease and liver disease. Furthermore, IgG-AGAs increase with age in healthy controls, making the presence of those antibodies even less specific for the purpose of diagnosing celiac disease in older persons [9•]. IgA-AGA, in contrast, although more specific for celiac disease, are not found in all persons with celiac disease.

Antireticulin Antibodies

The specificity of IgG–antireticulin antibodies (ARA) for celiac disease is controversial. The range of specificity is between 59% and 100%, and sensitivity is between 30% and 95%, indicating a specificity and sensitivity similar to that of IgA-AGA. ARA also have been reported in patients with Crohn's disease and other conditions [10•].

Endomysial Antibodies

The endomysial antibodies (EMA) are sensitive and specific markers of celiac disease. These are primarily IgA antibodies directed against the intermyofibril substance of monkey esophagus smooth muscle. Unlike ARA, EMA have been demonstrated to be species-specific, reacting by direct immunofluorescence only with the endomysium in the gastrointestinal tract of primates. The sensitivity and specificity of the EMA approaches 100%. Some false-positive results have been reported, including those in an individual with cow's-milk protein allergy and in another with *Giardia lamblia* infection. False-negative results are less common than false-positive results but have been reported [11•,12]. Absence of EMA may be more frequent in patients younger than 2 years of age with celiac disease. Because the EMA tests for IgA antibody, one must always consider IgA deficiency, which occurs in approximately 2% of the healthy population as well as 3% of celiac patients, as a possible explanation for a false-negative result. Serum immunoglobulins should be evaluated for IgA deficiency at the same time a celiac panel is requested. In a study in Israel that compared EMA, AgA, and ARA in a group of celiac patients, the specificity of EMA was 98% and the sensitivity was 97%. EMA appears to be the most reliable serologic marker for the diagnosis of celiac disease. The positive predictive values of EMA and ARA were comparable (97% and 100%, respectively). However, EMA had the highest negative predictive value (98%). Additionally, EMA were found to be more diet sensitive. After 3 months of gluten withdrawal, more children had a negative EMA than had a negative AGA or ARA. EMA titers also appear to rise more quickly in response to gluten challenge [13]. Of all the markers, EMA is currently the best serologic test for diagnosing celiac disease and the most useful in tracking compliance with a gluten-free diet.

Oral Tolerance Tests

Oral absorption of the pentose sugar D-xylose is one of the more widely available screening tests for testing intestinal absorptive function. D-xylose undergoes active transport through the small intestinal brush border region of mature epithelial cells of the duodenum and proximal jejunum. It is given in a standard oral dose of 5 g for children weighing less than 30 kg, and a 1-hour serum sample is assayed for the concentration of the sugar. Values below 20 mg/dL indicate malabsorption secondary to villus atrophy. However, the test may be abnormal in conditions associated with mucosal atrophy other than celiac disease, and false-negative and false-positive test results are possible.

Other oral tolerance tests that measure intestinal permeability and are based on the differential intestinal absorption of two nonmetabolizable sugars recently have emerged as screening tests. A monosaccharide that requires diffusion for absorption, such as mannose or rhamnose, is given in solution with a poorly absorbable disaccharide, such as lactulose or cellobiose. With mucosal atrophy, monosaccharide absorption is decreased because of a reduction in intestinal surface area, whereas absorption of the larger molecule is increased or normal, perhaps secondary to widening of tight junctions. These sugar permeability tests have the same nonspecificity for celiac disease as do many other nonimmunologic screening tests. Because of the problems still associated with these screening tests, the small intestinal biopsy remains the single most reliable test for establishing the diagnosis of celiac disease.

■ DIAGNOSTIC CRITERIA

The European Society for Pediatric Gastroenterology and Nutrition (ESPGAN) recently revised the criteria for the diagnosis of celiac disease [14]. Previous criteria set forth in 1969 required at least three small intestinal biopsies. The salient histologic features of celiac disease were required to be present at the time of initial suspicion of the enteropathy. The histologic findings were expected to resolve following a period of gluten elimination and to reappear during a gluten challenge. The success of newer diagnostic markers—AGA, ARA, and EMA—since that time in serving as indicators of active disease has prompted a revision of these criteria. Current requirements include a characteristic histologic appearance of the mucosa at the time of presentation, with resolution of the symptoms following gluten

elimination. The presence of the previously mentioned circulating antibodies at time of diagnosis and disappearance following gluten withdrawal supports the diagnosis, especially in those who are asymptomatic. In certain circumstances, one may choose to perform a gluten challenge. This challenge is especially useful in patients in whom there is a diagnostic dilemma. In children younger than 2 years of age one may not be able to distinguish histologically between milk protein intolerance and celiac disease. Patients who have been empirically started on a gluten-free diet before referral and who have negative antibody studies also should be challenged with gluten. The challenge may last for more than 1 year before intestinal biopsy if symptoms do not develop. Serial determinations of serum antibodies may be helpful.

Small Intestinal Biopsy

The gluten-induced enteropathy that affects the small intestinal mucosa and leads to the symptoms of malabsorption with associated abnormalities is characterized by a number of histologic features. The main histologic findings (Fig. 160-2) include an absence of villi, crypt hyperplasia, and infiltration of the lamina propria with chronic inflammatory cells. The total thickness of the mucosa is normal or only slightly reduced, because hypertrophy of the crypts compensates for the absence or shortening of the villi. The mucosa is, therefore, in a hyperkinetic state, with the increased rate of cell proliferation by the crypts compensating for damage to the surface enterocytes. The hyperkinetic state has been established in a number of studies investigating the incorporation rate of tritiated thymidine into the in vitro–maintained mucosa of celiac patients. The cell cycle time is more than halved when compared with control mucosa, and the mitotic duration is increased. The crypt cell production rate is greatly increased, from the normal rate of 25 cells per crypt per hour to 155 cells per hour.

A small percentage of patients have partial villus atrophy with shortened villi in association with crypt hyperplasia and infiltration of the lamina propria with inflammatory cells (Table 160-2).

The enterocytes are reduced in height and become cuboidal, and intraepithelial lymphocytes are interspersed between the enterocytes. These lymphocytes originate in the lamina propria

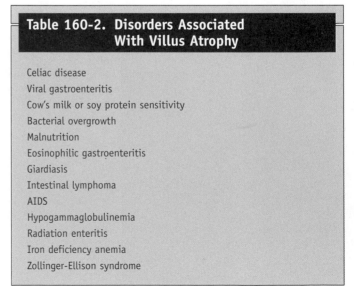

Figure 160-2.

Severe crypt hyperplasia and villus atrophy of the duodenum consistent with celiac disease. Note the absence of villi, elongated crypts, and increased cellularity of the lamina propria.

Table 160-2. Disorders Associated With Villus Atrophy
Celiac disease
Viral gastroenteritis
Cow's milk or soy protein sensitivity
Bacterial overgrowth
Malnutrition
Eosinophilic gastroenteritis
Giardiasis
Intestinal lymphoma
AIDS
Hypogammaglobulinemia
Radiation enteritis
Iron deficiency anemia
Zollinger-Ellison syndrome

and enter the space between the enterocytes through a break in the basal lamina of the epithelium. The ratio of lymphocytes to epithelial cells is increased in celiac disease, although the total number of lymphocytes per unit length of intestine may not be increased. The normal range of intraepithelial lymphocytes is 6 to 40 for every 100 epithelial cells. Most untreated celiac patients have lymphocyte counts higher than 40.

A reduction in mucosal enzymes (disaccharidases, peptidases, alkaline phosphatase, adenosine triphosphatase, and esterase) has been described. The reduction in brush border enzymes may be shown by either histochemistry or biochemical analysis [11•].

The histologic changes just described are not pathognomonic for celiac disease. Conditions other than celiac disease may be associated with a flat or otherwise abnormal mucosa. In children, these include gastroenteritis, cow's-milk protein intolerance, soy protein intolerance, protein-calorie malnutrition, intractable diarrhea of infancy, heavy infestation with *G. lamblia*, immunodeficiency states, severe iron deficiency anemia, tropical sprue, bacterial overgrowth syndrome, intestinal lymphoma, and Zollinger-Ellison syndrome.

■ MANAGEMENT

The specific therapy for celiac disease is a gluten-free diet, which excludes wheat, barley, oats, and rye. There is controversy regarding the toxicity of oats, which do not contain gliadin but rather contain avenin, which may or may not be injurious to the mucosa of patients with celiac disease. Some studies indicate that oats are well tolerated and produce no mucosal adverse affects. These studies, however, limited trial periods to only 6 to 12 months [15].

Further controversy surrounds the length of time for which it is necessary to restrict gluten intake. A gluten-restricted diet usually is prescribed for life, justified by the assumption that gluten elimination can prevent future development of malignancies. Agreement with this theory, however, is not universal. The histologic lesions of some patients with celiac disease who continue with a gluten-containing diet for many years actually improve, indicating that tolerance to gluten can occur in celiac disease. Further studies are necessary to clarify these issues before an alternative to lifelong gluten restriction can be offered definitively to patients with celiac disease[16].

In most instances, strict adherence to a gluten-free diet leads to improvement in clinical symptoms within a few days; full remission, however, may take weeks or months. The most dramatic improvements occur in the number and character of the stools, which usually improve within days to weeks. Irritability and anorexia also reverse in an equally short period of time. Weight gain accompanies the child's improved behavior and appetite. Improvement in height velocity usually follows the observed weight gain after several months. Abdominal distention, however, may require months of treatment to subside. The appearance of the mucosa improves to normal, usually within 1 year, but may take longer for complete recovery.

Symptoms continue or recur in 7% to 30% of treated celiac disease patients, suggesting either deliberate or inadvertent gluten ingestion. This can be assessed by a careful dietary history (Table 160-3). Monitoring the IgA, AGA, ARA, and EMA also can provide information regarding dietary intake of gluten, because levels nearly disappear by 1 to 3 months and, similarly, rise following gluten challenge. Transient disaccharidase deficiency, particularly lactase deficiency, secondary to mucosal atrophy must be considered in patients who continue to be symptomatic. In this setting, one must consider an accompanying milk, soy, or other dietary protein sensitivity, which can perpetuate the mucosal injury accompanying celiac disease. Occasionally, prolonged mucosal injury is associated with intestinal lymphoma. Also, some nonresponders are found to have a layer of dense collagen located directly below the surface epithelial cells. It is not known whether this "collagenous sprue" is a distinct pathologic entity or whether it simply represents long-standing disease. The presence of exocrine pancreatic insufficiency is yet another cause of persistence of symptoms after a gluten-free diet has been instituted. The association of exocrine pancreatic insufficiency with celiac disease probably represents either impaired secretion of cholecystokinin-pancreozymin from the injured mucosa or malnutrition and hypoproteinemia. Pancreatic enzyme supplementation may be helpful in both transient and permanent pancreatic insufficiency states [17].

Some patients with nonresponsive celiac disease continue their progressive decline in nutritional status. In these patients, treatment with elemental diets or total parenteral nutrition should be considered. In severe, unremitting cases, a variety of pharmacologic therapies can be considered, including corticosteroids, cyclosporine, and azathioprine. Pentagastrin has been found to accelerate the recovery of the jejunal mucosa when given to patients with severe celiac disease in the initial period of treatment. The success of immunosuppressive agents underscores the immunologic nature of this disorder [18••].

■ REFERENCES

Recently published papers of particular interest have been highlighted as follows:
•   Of interest
••   Of outstanding interest.

1.• Greco L, Maki M, Di Donato F, Visakorpi JK: Dynamic nutrition research. In *Common Food Tolerances 1: Epidemiology of Coeliac Disease.* vol 2. Edited by Auricchio S, Visakorpi JK. Basel: Karger; 1992:25–44.
This chapter traces the epidemiology of celiac disease in Europe and the Mediterranean area and provides a summary report on the multicenter study performed by the European Society of Pediatric Gastroenterology and Nutrition.

2. Rossi TM, Albini CH, Kumar V, *et al.*: Incidence of celiac disease identified by the presence of serum endomysial antibodies in children with chronic diarrhea, short stature, or insulin-dependent diabetes mellitus. *J Pediatr* 1993, 123:262–264.

3. Visakorpi JK, Maki M: Changing clinical features of coeliac disease [Review]. *Acta Paediatrica* 1994, 83(suppl 395):10–13.

4. Zhou JZ, Rossi TM, Lee K, *et al.*: Embryonic celiac antigens(ECA). *J Pediatr Gastroenterol Nutr* 1996, 23:342–374.

Table 160-3. Continuation of Symptoms

Erroneous diagnosis

Gluten ingestion (voluntary or inadvertent)

Lactase deficiency

Cow's milk, soy, "food" sensitivity

Intestinal lymphoma

Collagenous sprue

Pancreatic insufficiency

5. Picarelli A, Majuri L, Frate A, *et al.*: Production of antiendomysial antibodies after in-vitro gliadin challenge of small intestine biopsy samples from patients with coeliac disease. *Lancet* 1996, 348:1065–1067.

6. Rossi TM, Tjota A: Serological diagnosis of celiac disease. *J Pediatr Gastroenterol Nutr* 1998, 26:205–210.

7. Aurrichio S, Greco L, Troncone R: Gluten sensitive enteropathy in childhood. *Pediatr Clin North Am* 1988, 35:157.

8. Holmes GKT, Prior P, Lane MR, *et al.*: Malignancy in coeliac disease—effect of gluten free diet. *Gut* 1989, 30:333–338.

9.• Kumar V, Jain N, Lerner A, *et al.*: Comparative studies of different gliadin preparations in detecting antigliadin antibodies. *J Pediatr Gastroenterol Nutr* 1986, 5:730.
This important article provides perspective on the usefulness of antigliadin antibodies.

10.• Lerner A, Kumar V, Iancu TC, *et al.*: Immunological diagnosis of childhood coeliac disease: comparison between antigliadin, antireticulin and antiendomysial antibodies. *Clin Exp Immunol* 1994, 95:75–82.
This paper provides an important comparison of the three most common immune markers for celiac disease.

11.• Rossi TM, Kumar V, Lerner A, *et al.*: Relationship of endomysial antibodies to jejunal mucosal pathology: specificity towards both symptomatic and asymptomatic celiacs. *J Pediatr Gastroenterol Nutr* 1988, 7:858–863.
This paper documents the use of antiendomysial antibodies in asymptomatic family members and in enteropathies other than celiac disease.

12. Chan KN, Phillips AD, Mirakian R, *et al.*: Endomysial antibody screening in children. *J Pediatr Gastroenterol Nutr* 1994, 18:316–332.

13. Kumar V, Lerner A, Valeski JE: Endomysial antibodies in the diagnosis of celiac disease and the effect of gluten on antibody titers. *Immunol Invest* 1989, 18:533-544.

14. Walker-Smith JA, Guanalini S, Schmitz J, *et al.*: Revised criteria for diagnosis of coeliac disease. *Arch Dis Child* 1990, 65:909–911.

15. Kumar PJ, Farthing MGJ: Oats and celiac disease [Editorial]. *N Engl J Med* 1995, 333:1033–1037.

16. Seldon W. Prognosis in early adult life of coeliac children treated with a gluten-free diet. *Br Med J* 1969, 2:401–404.

17. Weizman Z, Hamilton JR, Kopelman LTR, *et al.*: Treatment failure in celiac disease due to co-existent exocrine pancreatic insufficiency. *Pediatrics* 1987, 80:924–926.

18.•• O'Mahony S, Howdle PD, Losowsky MS: Management of patients with non-responsive coeliac disease. *Aliment Pharmacol Ther* 1996,10:671–678.
This paper provides a comprehensive review of the treatment and reasons for treatment failures in severe celiac disease.

161 Protein-Losing Enteropathy

Roy Proujansky

Protein-losing enteropathies are a diverse group of relatively uncommon pediatric disorders that have both age- and symptom-specific causes. In addition, a predominantly enteric protein-losing state occasionally can be the clinical presentation of more common gastrointestinal disorders that usually present with other clinical features. This chapter reviews the pediatric disorders that most commonly present with the symptoms and signs of excessive enteric protein loss.

DEVELOPMENTAL ANATOMY AND PHYSIOLOGY

Significant enteric protein loss usually occurs either as the result of loss of lymph from mucosal lymphatics or from leakage of interstitial fluid consequent to significant mucosal inflammation. A number of the causes of lymphatic fluid leakage result from developmental abnormalities that affect the mucosal lymphatics or lead to increased lymphatic fluid pressure.

The human lymphatic system begins to develop at approximately the fifth week of gestation. Early lymphatic structures develop into regional lymph sacs, and two of these, the retroperitoneal lymph sac and the cisterna chyli, act as the origin for lymphatic vessels, which grow along venous structures to the gut. Lacteals are the terminal portion of lymphatic channels extending into the gastrointestinal mucosa to a central location within each villus. Lymph formation is a multifaceted process that involves absorption and hydrostatic and oncotic pressures

within local capillaries and the interstitium [1•]. Abnormalities that result in altered permeability of the lining of terminal lymphatics or disorders that obstruct mucosal lymphatic drainage result in excessive loss of lymph fluid at the mucosal surface. Obstruction of major lymphatic structures early in fetal development is believed to be responsible for craniofacial, cardiac, and extremity abnormalities seen in syndromes associated with lymphatic structural defects [2•].

The gut plays an important role in metabolism of albumin. Between 6% and 10% of the plasma albumin pool is degraded daily, and rates of catabolism average 43% higher in patients with protein-losing enteropathy when compared with those of healthy controls. This albumin loss is mostly at the expense of the plasma pool, and because compensatory hepatic albumin synthesis is limited, significant sustained enteric protein loss usually becomes symptomatic.

EPIDEMIOLOGY

The patient with a clinical presentation primarily of enteric protein loss is not often seen in routine pediatric and pediatric gastroenterologic practice. Primary intestinal lymphangiectasia, Ménétrier's disease, and idiopathic eosinophilic gastroenteropathy are all relatively rare disorders. More commonly, protein-losing enteropathy may be the predominant manifestation of a disorder with varied clinical presentations. Cow's-milk protein–sensitive enteropathy is a common disorder that can present in infants with iron deficiency anemia and all the clinical features of significant gastrointestinal protein loss. Significant protein-losing enteropathy may accompany other significant symptoms and signs, as in the patient with Turner's syndrome or following the Fontan procedure for correction of congenital heart disease. Rarely, significant gastrointestinal protein loss may be observed in the course of a number of gastrointestinal infections.

ETIOLOGY AND CLINICAL FEATURES

A number of conditions have been associated with protein-losing enteropathy in infants and children (Table 161-1). These disorders can be divided into those due to lymphatic obstruction or leakage and those associated with significant mucosal inflammation, based on the pathophysiologic process resulting in gastrointestinal protein loss.

Intestinal Lymphangiectasia

Primary intestinal lymphangiectasia is a developmental disorder that results in localized or diffuse abnormalities of the intestinal mucosal lymphatics. Dilated and ectatic mucosal and submucosal lymphatics result in excessive gastrointestinal losses of albumin, immunoglobulins, and lymphocytes and may be associated with steatorrhea. The abnormal gastrointestinal lymphatics also may be associated with structural abnormalities of lymphatics in other parts of the body [3•].

Primary intestinal lymphangiectasia may present at any time during childhood. The clinical presentation usually includes edema, which may be associated with diarrhea, nausea, vomiting, failure to thrive, or abdominal pain. When there are associated lymphatic abnormalities of the extremities, asymmetric and non-pitting lymphedema may be present. Chylothorax and chylous ascites are indicative of a more diffuse disorder of lymphatic development. Primary intestinal lymphangiectasia may be familial and can also occur as one feature of several inherited malformation syndromes (Table 161-2) [2•,4].

Intestinal lymphangiectasia also may develop secondary to cardiac disease or another process that may obstruct lymphatics. Constrictive pericarditis and cardiomyopathies resulting in protein-losing enteropathy are extremely uncommon in children. However, 10% to 15% of patients who have undergone the Fontan operation for repair of congenital heart disease (*eg*, tricuspid atresia, functional single ventricle) have significant protein-losing enteropathy as a short- or long-term postoperative complication [5]. Intestinal malrotation is another potentially treatable cause of lymphatic obstruction leading to enteric protein loss.

Table 161-1. Pediatric Disorders Associated with Significant Enteric Protein Loss

Disorders with lymphatic obstruction or leakage	Disorders with mucosal disruption from inflammation or infection	Other disorders associated with enteric protein loss
Primary intestinal lymphangiectasia	Inflammatory disorders	Congenital enterocyte heparan sulphate deficiency
Isolated	Predominantly affecting the stomach	
Associated with inherited syndromes	Ménétrier's disease	
Secondary lymphangiectasia	Eosinophilic gastroenteritis	
Cardiac disease	*Helicobacter pylori* infection	
Post–Fontan procedure	Predominantly affecting the small intestine	
Congestive heart failure or cardiomyopathy	Cow's milk– and soy protein–sensitive enteropathy	
Obstructed lymphatics	Gluten-sensitive enteropathy	
Intestinal malrotation	Common variable or severe combined immunodeficiency	
Crohn's disease	Predominantly affecting the colon	
Lymphoma	Crohn's disease	
Retroperitoneal tumor	Ulcerative colitis	
	Isolated and familial juvenile polyposis coli	
	Henoch-Schölein purpura and other vasculitides	
	Necrotizing enterocolitis	
	Infection with *Clostridium difficile*	

Table 161-2. Syndromes Associated With Intestinal Lymphangiectasia

Syndrome	Major clinical features
Turner's syndrome	Females with short stature, broad chest with widely spaced nipples, low posterior hairline, webbed neck, lymphedema
Noonan's syndrome	Webbed neck, pectus excavatum, cryptorchidism, pulmonic stenosis, lymphedema
Klippel-Trenaunary-Weber syndrome	Asymmetric limb hypertrophy, hemangiomata of the extremities and viscera
Hennekam syndrome	Flat mid-face, flat nasal bridge, hypertelorism, lymphedema

Ménétrier's Disease

Ménétrier's disease is a protein-losing gastropathy characterized by hypertrophy of the gastric rugae, predominantly in the body of the stomach, and associated with foveolar hyperplasia and cystic dilation of the gastric glands. This disorder typically develops in children less than 10 years of age and presents with the abrupt onset of vomiting, abdominal pain, and edema [6]. Some children may have relatively few gastrointestinal symptoms and present with edema, hypoproteinemia, and anemia. A viral syndrome precedes the onset of symptoms in some patients, and coexistent cytomegalovirus infection has been identified in a few patients. In contrast to Ménétrier's disease in adults, Ménétrier's disease in childhood is most commonly a self-limited disorder that resolves without sequelae.

Inflammatory and Infectious Gastrointestinal Disorders

The mucosal form of idiopathic eosinophilic gastroenteritis often comes to medical attention during early childhood and is commonly associated with significant gastrointestinal protein loss [7]. Vomiting, abdominal pain, and weight loss usually are present. Some patients may have acute exacerbations of symptoms or other atopic features (*eg*, urticaria, wheezing) in association with the ingestion of specific foods. The eosinophilic mucosal inflammatory process is most consistently identified in the gastric antrum and may be present in a patchy distribution in other portions of the upper gastrointestinal tract.

Milk- and soy protein–induced enteropathy are relatively common conditions affecting infants and children less than 2 years of age [8]. An immunologic response to cow's-milk or soy protein results in mucosal inflammation that can affect any portion of the gastrointestinal tract. Although most affected children present with some combination of vomiting, diarrhea, and gastrointestinal blood loss, an occasional child has relatively few gastrointestinal symptoms and is evaluated for edema and iron deficiency anemia. A similar presentation occasionally is seen in the child with gluten-sensitive enteropathy.

Whereas most polyposis disorders have variable degrees of abdominal pain and gastrointestinal bleeding, the child with sporadic or familial juvenile polyposis coli may have a symptom complex characterized by abdominal pain, diarrhea, and edema in association with anemia and hypoproteinemia [9]. Significant erosion and inflammation of the surfaces of numerous colonic polyps is the basis for the gastrointestinal loss of blood and protein.

Vasculitic disorders affecting the gastrointestinal tract are uncommon in childhood. Henoch-Schönlein purpura is a transient disorder characterized by abdominal pain, gastrointestinal bleeding, palpable purpura of the buttocks and lower extremities, arthritis, and nephritis. It occasionally is associated with significant enteric protein loss [10].

Significant gastrointestinal protein loss (serum albumin <2.0 g/dL) can be seen in children during the course of infection with *Clostridium difficile*, and the degree of hypoproteinemia does not always correlate with the severity of other symptoms. Several children and adolescents with *Helicobacter pylori* infection have been described with hypoalbuminemia and an exuberant inflammatory response to *H. pylori* resulting in significant hypertrophy of the gastric folds and resembling Ménétrier's

disease clinically and radiographically (Fig. 161-1) [11]. Crohn's disease may result in severe enteric protein loss, not only because of weeping from the surface of intestinal ulcers, but also because of lymphatic obstruction resulting from lymphadenitis, lymphadenopathy, and mesenteric fibrosis.

Recently, severe protein-losing enteropathy and secretory diarrhea in infancy have been described in association with deficiency of enterocyte heparan sulphate [12]. Interestingly, these patients had completely normal histology of the small intestinal mucosa on repeated tissue sampling.

■ DIAGNOSTIC EVALUATION

The initial evaluation of the child with possible protein-losing enteropathy should use an age-based approach toward the identification of important historical information and physical findings. Usually this necessitates considering the differential diagnosis for a child with edema and either failure to thrive or gastrointestinal symptoms. The dietary history is an important piece of the diagnostic evaluation. The child whose protein calorie intake has been inadequate (*ie*, kwashiorkor) also may present with failure to thrive and edema. For the child less than 2 years of age, the type and quantity of formula or milk intake may be important. Children with cow's-milk protein–sensitive enteropathy often have a history of cow's milk being the major source of nutritional intake. Onset of symptoms during the second 6 months of life, at a time when a more diverse array of foods is being introduced, may suggest gluten-sensitive enteropathy. Intermittent exacerbation of symptoms with particular foods may be seen in some patients with eosinophilic gastroenteropathy. A history of a recent intercurrent viral process may be seen in childhood Ménétrier's disease.

Measurements of height, weight, and weight for height, and a generalized assessment of subcutaneous fat should be used to assess nutritional status. Physical assessment should include documentation of the location and character of edema. Asymmetric and non-pitting edema is suggestive of lymphedema caused by an underlying lymphatic abnormality. Hypoproteinemic pitting edema and lymphedema may coexist in the same patient. Deformities or dysmorphic features suggest specific syndromes. Urticaria or atopic dermatitis is consistent with protein-sensitive or eosinophilic gastroenteropathies. The

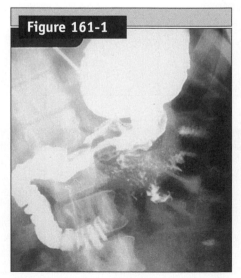

Figure 161-1

Helicobacter pylori infection simulating Ménétrier's disease in an adolescent.

detection of fecal occult blood loss by digital rectal examination may direct the evaluation toward etiologies that cause mucosal inflammation.

Initial laboratory assessment should document hypoproteinemia and exclude urinary loss of protein as a contributing factor. A complete blood count may reveal a hypochromic, microcytic anemia, suggesting chronic gastrointestinal blood loss in a patient with an inflammatory cause of protein loss. Lymphopenia, the result of the loss of lymphocytes into the stool, should raise suspicion regarding lymphangiectasia, whereas eosinophilia occurs in eosinophilic gastroenteritis, protein-sensitive enteropathies, and occasionally in Ménétrier's disease. Low levels of serum immunoglobulins also can be seen as a result of loss of intestinal protein or lymph and may simulate an underlying immunodeficiency disorder [13].

In the child with documented hypoproteinemia, adequate caloric intake, and no evidence of renal loss of protein, documentation of enteric protein loss is important for directing the subsequent evaluation. For example, the constellation of hypoproteinemia, edema, and anemia is a recognized presentation of cystic fibrosis in which the hypoalbuminemia is not related to enteric protein loss but is the result of pancreatic insufficiency and malabsorption. Documentation of enteric protein loss is most easily obtained by the evaluation of a random fecal specimen for an increased concentration of alpha$_1$-antitrypsin. Random fecal α_1-antitrypsin levels have been shown to be a reliable screening test for intestinal protein loss in children and to correlate with prolonged stool collections for the same assay or other more invasive methods for assessing enteric protein loss [14]. It should be recalled, however, that α_1-antitrypsin is sensitive to proteolytic digestion in the acid environment of the stomach, and fecal concentrations of α_1-antitrypsin in the stool, even in the setting of significant gastric loss of protein, may not be increased.

In some cases, the specific cause of protein loss is not obvious after the initial assessment. In addition, there is often a time lag until the results of a fecal α_1-antitrypsin test are available, creating inappropriate delays in the diagnostic evaluation. The next step in these situations is to consider performing a contrast study of the upper gastrointestinal tract and small intestine. Many of the causes for significant enteric protein loss in childhood involve the stomach and proximal small intestine, and contrast studies may assist in localizing the site of protein loss. Marked thickening of gastric folds also can be detected by transabdominal ultrasound examination, which may be used subsequently as a noninvasive technique to follow the clinical course. Scintigraphic techniques (*eg*, scanning following intravenous injection of Tc 99m-labeled albumin or similar agents) also are useful for localizing gastrointestinal sites of protein loss. These agents can also be injected peripherally to document enteric protein loss when it is associated with possible lymphatic abnormalities of the extremities (Fig. 161-2) [15•].

Upper or lower gastrointestinal endoscopy is used to identify and document the histologic lesion responsible for the loss of proteins across the mucosa . Diverse sites in the upper gastrointestinal tract may be responsible for protein or lymph loss, and sampling of multiple sites (*eg*, gastric body, gastric antrum, multiple sites in the proximal small intestine) may be necessary. Cow's milk– and soy protein–sensitive enteropathies, in particular, can be associated with a patchy distribution of eosinophilic inflammation (Fig. 161-3). A prolonged fast before upper gastrointestinal endoscopy is performed may reduce the prominence of dilated lacteals either visually or histologically (Fig. 161-4). This can be avoided by ensuring that the child ingests a meal containing normal quantities of dietary fat 12 to 24 hours before endoscopy.

■ TREATMENT

Treatment options for the patient with protein-losing enteropathy involve both nonspecific, palliative treatments and specific approaches for specific diagnostic entities. Cautious infusion of 5% albumin followed by furosemide (1 mg/kg/dose) may be used on occasion for the patient with pain or skin breakdown from severe edema, but should not be considered anything more than palliative. Intravenous immunoglobulin therapy may be

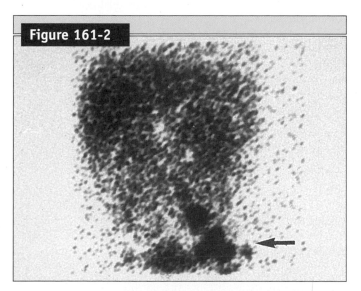

Figure 161-2

Lymphscintigram in a patient with lymphedema, chylous ascites, and lymphangiectasia. Injection into the lower extremities results in accumulation of radiolabel at the sites of lymphatic obstruction in the inguinal region (*arrow*) and in the abdomen.

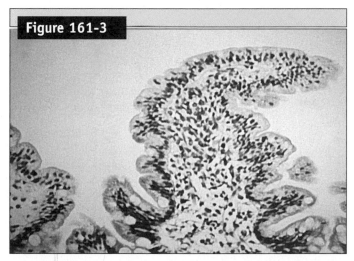

Figure 161-3

Focal collection of eosinophils in the duodenal mucosa in a patient with cow's-milk protein–sensitive enteropathy.

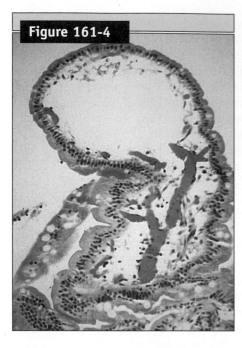

Figure 161-4

Dilated lacteals in a mucosal biopsy specimen from a patient with intestinal lymphangiectasia (see also Chapter 53).

necessary for the patient with recurrent infections. The mainstays of treatment involve a variety of nutritional alternatives and anti-inflammatory therapeutics.

Patients with cow's-milk– or soy protein–sensitive enteropathies respond to avoidance of these dietary antigens. They usually require an elemental or protein-hydrolysate formula or diet. An elemental diet also can be an effective treatment for the patient with eosinophilic gastroenteritis. Ménétrier's disease is usually a self-limited condition in childhood, but nitrogen balance may be improved with protein supplementation. A diet high in medium chain triglycerides and low in long chain fats may improve the lymphatic loss associated with lymphangiectasia [16]. Patients with severe symptoms sometimes may require total parenteral nutrition to alleviate protein loss and maintain nutritional status.

Corticosteroid therapy may be required for the patient with severe eosinophilic gastroenteritis and occasionally has been useful for patients with lymphangiectasia whose disorder has an inflammatory component or following the Fontan operation [17,18]. Specific anti-infective therapy is necessary for patients whose protein-losing state has an infectious cause. Therapy with antifibrinolytic agents and with heparin has been successful for small numbers of patients with lymphangiectasia, and octreotide has also been effective as adjunctive therapy for Ménétrier's disease [19–21]. Surgical treatments for lymphangiectasia associated with major lymphatic duct abnormalities also have had some success.

▬▬ REFERENCES

Recently published papers of particular interest have been highlighted as follows:
• Of interest
•• Of outstanding interest

1.• Benoit JN, Zawieja DC: Gastrointestinal lymphatics. In *Physiology of the Gastrointestinal Tract*, edn 3. Edited by Johnson LR. New York: Raven Press; 1994:1669–1692.
This is a comprehensive chapter that discusses the anatomy of the lymphatics and the physiology of lymph formation and lymphatic contractility.

2. Jones KL: Jugular lymphatic obstruction sequence. In *Recognizable Patterns of Human Malformation*. Philadelphia: WB Saunders; 1997:620–621.
The most recent edition of this classic text is the standard reference for evaluation of a patient with features suggesting an inherited syndrome.

3.• Levine C: Primary disorders of the lymphatic vessels—a unified concept. *J Pediatr Surg* 1989, 24:233–240.
This paper is an interesting discussion of the potential mechanisms involved in the genesis of lymphatic structural abnormalities.

4. Hennekam RCM, Geerdink RA, Hamel BCJ, *et al.*: Autosomal recessive intestinal lymphangiectasia and lymphedema, with facial anomalies and mental retardation. *Am J Med Genet* 1989, 34:593–600.

5. Driscoll DJ, Offord KP, Feldt RH, *et al.*: Five- to fifteen-year follow-up after Fontan operation. *Circulation* 1992, 85:469–496.

6. Qualman SJ, Hamoudi AB: Pediatric hypertrophic gastropathy (Ménétrier's disease). *Pediatr Pathol* 1992, 12:263–267.

7. Whitington PF, Whitington GL: Eosinophilic gastroenteropathy in childhood. *J Pediatr Gastroenterol Nutr* 1988, 7:379–385.

8. Proujansky R, Winter HS, Walker WA: Gastrointestinal syndromes associated with food sensitivity. *Adv Pediatr* 1988, 35:219–238.

9. Gourley GR, Odell GB, Selkurt J, *et al.*: Juvenile polyps associated with protein-losing enteropathy. *Dig Dis Sci* 1982, 27:941–945.

10. Reif S, Jain A, Santiago J, Rossi T: Protein-losing enteropathy as a manifestation of Henoch-Schönlein purpura. *Acta Paediatr Scand* 1991, 80:482–485.

11. Hill ID, Sinclair-Smith C, Lastovica AJ, *et al.*: Transient protein-losing enteropathy associated with acute gastritis and *Campylobacter pylori*. *Arch Dis Child* 1987, 62:1215–1219.

12. Murch SH, Winyard PJ, Koletzko S, *et al.*: Congenital enterocyte heparan sulphate deficiency with massive albumin loss, secretory diarrhea, and malnutrition. *Lancet* 1996, 347:1299–1301.

13. Garty B-Z, Levinson AI, Danon YL, *et al.*: Lymphocyte subpopulations in children with abnormal lymphatic circulation. *J Allergy Clin Immunol* 1989, 84:515–520.

14. Thomas DW, McGilligan KM, Carlson M, *et al.*: Fecal alpha 1-antitrypsin and hemoglobin excretion in healthy human milk-, formula-, or cow's milk-fed infants. *Pediatrics* 1986, 78:305–312.

15.• Mandell GA, Alexander MA, Harcke HT: A multiscintigraphic approach to imaging of lymphedema and other causes of the congenitally enlarged extremity. *Semin Nucl Med* 1993, 23:334–346.
The authors discuss a large experience with scintigraphic techniques in the diagnosis and management of disorders associated with lymphatic structural abnormalities.

16. Jensen GL, Mascioli EA, Meyer LP, *et al.*: Dietary modification of chyle composition in chylothorax. *Gastroenterology* 1989, 97:761–765.

17. Fleisher TA, Strober W, Muchmore AV, *et al.*: Corticosteroid-responsive intestinal lymphangiectasia secondary to an inflammatory process. *N Engl J Med* 1979, 300:605–606.

18. Rychik J, Piccoli DA, Barber G: Usefulness of corticosteroid therapy for protein-losing enteropathy following the Fontan procedure. *Am J Cardiol* 1991, 68:819–821.

19. Mine K, Matsubayashi S, Nakai Y, Nakagawa T: Intestinal lymphangiectasia markedly improved with antiplasmin therapy. *Gastroenterology* 1989, 96:1596–1599.

20. Donnelly JP, Rosenthal A, Castle VP, Holmes RD: Reversal of protein-losing enteropathy with heparin therapy in three patients with univentricular hearts and Fontan palliation. *J Pediatr* 1997, 130:474–478.

21. Yeaton P, Frierson HF: Octreotide reduces enteral protein losses in Ménétrier's disease. *Am J Gastroenterol* 1993, 88:95–98.

162 Intussusception
Esther Jacobowitz Israel

Intussusception, the second most common cause of intestinal obstruction in children, is characterized by telescoping of proximal bowel (the intussusceptum) into a segment of distal bowel (the intussuscipiens), usually with subsequent obstruction and vascular compromise. This chapter reviews intussusception with an emphasis on its management, which remains controversial.

EPIDEMIOLOGY

Intussusception occurs in 2.4 per 1000 children [1] and sometimes can even be seen *in utero*, in which case it results in intestinal atresia. Historically, most cases (75% to 95%) were seen in children younger than 2 years of age, with a peak incidence between 5 and 8 months of age. Recent epidemiologic studies, however, demonstrate a change in this trend, with 35% of intussusceptions now occurring in children older than 2 years of age; a bimodal age distribution exists, with peaks at 5 months and 3 years of age [2]. Males predominate by a ratio of three to two, and there is no racial predisposition. A seasonal variation has been noted, with an increased incidence in the summer months in temperate zones.

PATHOPHYSIOLOGY

Most cases of intussusception are primary and idiopathic. The site of origin in about 90% of patients is immediately proximal to the ileocecal valve. Ileoileal, colocolonic, and duodenojejunal intussusceptions are much less common. Increased intestinal lymphoid tissue in the terminal ileum has been implicated as a predisposing factor in infants. The caliber of the ileum is so much greater than that of the ileocecal valve in infants that it might also be a risk for intussusception. A lead point in the intussuscepted bowel can be identified in 5% to 10% of patients with intussusception [3]. This incidence increases in children 4 years of age or older. Potential lead points include structural abnormalities, vascular anomalies, neoplasms, inflammatory lesions, foreign bodies, and inspissated stool (Table 162-1). Studies that show an increased incidence in the summer suggest an infectious etiology, specifically rotavirus and adenovirus. Viral infection also may explain the observed increased rate of intussusception in siblings with similar illness and in children with hyperplastic Peyer's patches. Studies in dogs, however, have suggested that lymphoid hyperplasia is the result of intussusception rather than the cause. A recent report of idiopathic familial intussusception spanning several generations [5] suggests a heritable trait, perhaps an anatomic alteration, that predisposes individuals to intussusception.

PATHOLOGY

Regardless of the cause of the intussusception, injury to the bowel is secondary to compression of the invaginated bowel segment and restriction of its blood supply. Venous stasis and edema follow. Intraluminal mucus and blood from the engorged bowel mix to produce the "currant jelly" stools typical of the process. Gangrene and, finally, necrosis occur if the intussusception is not reduced promptly.

CLINICAL FEATURES

The classic clinical triad includes colicky abdominal pain, currant jelly or bloody stools, and an abdominal mass (either a sausage-shaped mass vertically along the right flank, or Dance's sign, with an absence of bowel in the right lower quadrant and a horizontal mass along the right upper quadrant). This triad is by no means pathognomonic and is present in less than 50% of affected children; however, these signs, independently or in combination with bilious emesis, diarrhea, drawing up of the legs, or dehydration with tachycardia, hypotension, and pallor, provide the necessary clues for diagnosis. Lethargy, particularly between paroxysms of pain, often is present and may be the only presenting symptom [6]. The physical examination often is nonspecific. Fever is common. Abdominal distention from

---

Table 162-1. Lead Points of Intussusception

Structural abnormalities
  Meckel's diverticulum
  Ectopic gastric mucosa
  Ectopic pancreatic mucosa
  Inflamed appendix
  Appendiceal stump
  Duplication cyst
Vascular anomalies
  Henoch-Schönlein purpura
  Hemolytic-uremic syndrome
  Abdominal trauma with hematoma formation
  Hemophilia
  Leukemia
  Idiopathic thrombocytopenic purpura
Neoplasms
  Adenomas
  Lipomas
  Hamartomas
  Hemangiomas
  Sarcomas
Inflammatory lesions
  Polyps
Foreign Bodies
  Bezoars
  Sutures
  Ascaris
  Feeding tubes
Meconium ileus equivalent (Cystic fibrosis)
Ileus

small bowel obstruction may be evident. In 1% to 2% of cases, a complete intussusception can be palpated on rectal examination or is clearly visible as it prolapses through the rectum. Chronic intussusception with partial small bowel obstruction presents with intermittent abdominal pain, anorexia, vomiting, weight loss, and dehydration. The differential diagnosis of colicky pain with or without bloody stools includes colitis (infectious, inflammatory bowel disease, Henoch-Schönlein purpura, and hemolytic-uremic syndrome), gallbladder disease, renal colic, and ureteropelvic junction obstruction.

DIAGNOSIS

The diagnosis of intussusception rests heavily on clinical suspicion after the history and physical examination. Radiographic signs of intussusception are nonspecific and include a soft tissue mass (Fig. 162-1), the target sign (crescentic lucencies associated with a soft tissue mass because mesenteric fat is sandwiched between bowel wall during the intussusception), absence of cecal gas or stool, the crescent sign (air outlining the intussusception), inability to visualize the liver tip, dilation of small bowel proximal to the obstruction, a paucity of bowel gas, or an interrupted gas column in the colon [7]. Plain abdominal radiography may miss 33% to 50% of cases of intussusception [3].

Ultrasound examination and air or contrast enema with fluoroscopy are more sensitive diagnostic tests. Sensitivity by ultrasound approaches 100% [3]. On a transverse scan, a mass with a target appearance is visible or, on longitudinal scanning, a "sandwich" appearance is noted, with the mesentery and its echogenic fat seen between the layers of the intussusceptum (Fig. 162-2). False-positive ultrasound examinations occur when thickening of the bowel wall (inflammation, edema, hematoma, or volvulus) is present, or when stool or the iliopsoas muscle is misinterpreted as a mass. For practitioners who are not comfortable with the sonographic diagnosis of intussusception, or in preparation for fluoroscopic-guided reduction, the diagnosis can be made by air insufflation or installation of contrast rectally (Fig. 162-3).

TREATMENT

Intussusception is a potential surgical emergency. The surgeon should be present to reduce an intussusception operatively if radiologic approaches are unsuccessful, and to manage any potential complication of radiologic intervention, such as bowel perforation. The patient's hydration status should be stabilized before any intervention is initiated, because 20% of deaths associated with intussusception are secondary to inadequate fluid resuscitation [1]. A nasogastric tube for decompression may be warranted. Although the risk of bacteremia associated with reduction of intussusception is as high as 20%, actual septicemia is rare [8], and antibiotics usually are not prescribed.

Nonsurgical, hydrostatic pressure reduction is done first, as long as there is no evidence of perforation and the patient has been stabilized. Reduction can be done with either air or contrast material under fluoroscopic guidance, or by ultrasound-guided saline enema. Ultrasound guidance offers enhanced visualization of the involved tissue and lead point. If the ultrasonographic thickness of the intussusception in a target configuration is greater than 8 to 10 mm in diameter, nonsurgical reduction may

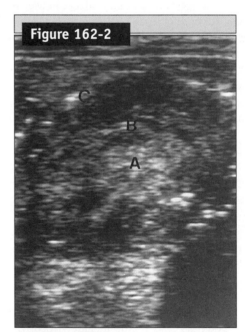

Figure 162-2

Abdominal ultrasound showing the target appearance of the intussuscepted bowel. In the middle of the target, is the mesenteric fat of the intussuscepted bowel (A). The layers around the fat include the lumen of the receiving bowel (B) and the outer wall of the receiving bowel (C).

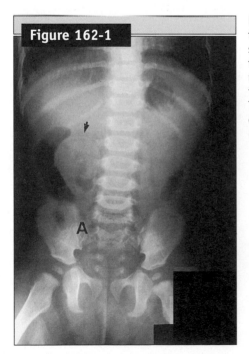

Figure 162-1

Plain radiograph of the abdomen showing a soft tissue mass (*arrow*) representing the intussusceptum. There is a paucity of air in the cecum (A) as well.

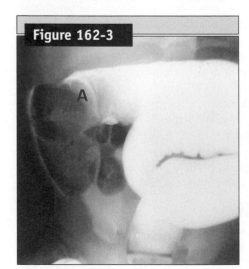

Figure 162-3

Fluoroscopic examination with water-soluble contrast material shows the interrupted column of contrast (A) with the intussuscepted bowel, represented by air, within this column.

be difficult to accomplish. When blood flow cannot be documented via ultrasound and Doppler flow study, necrotic bowel is more likely.

Reduction with liquid enemas under fluoroscopy historically has been the accepted choice. Contrast must be noted refluxing into the ileum for the study to be considered normal and the intussusception to be judged reduced. However, air insufflation is easier technically and is faster and results in less radiation exposure [10]. Reduction with air has a success rate of 75% to 95% compared with a success rate of 50% to 78% with radiopaque enemas. The risk of perforation is comparable (0.1% to 0.2%) with air and liquid [3]. When perforation does occur with air, the hole is smaller than that with contrast material, and less feculent material contaminates the peritoneal cavity. Resistance to use of the air technique comes from the difficulty of knowing whether the intussusceptum is completely reduced. The filling of the small intestine with air (*ie*, the "bunch of grapes" pattern) can be obscured if the small bowel has already been dilated with air as a result of the distal obstruction, or if the intussusceptum allowed passage of air into the small bowel before reduction was performed. When it is not clear that reduction has been successful, ultrasound may help determine whether it has been accomplished.

If radiologic reduction is unsuccessful, the patient is taken to the operating room for open surgical reduction. At surgery, the intussusception is "milked" back by progressive compression of the bowel just distal to the intussusception, pushing it proximally. If the bowel reduces easily and rapidly, there usually is no need to question the viability of the bowel. If the bowel stubbornly resists reduction, it is preferable to resect it rather than to use excessive force and risk rupturing the bowel and contaminating the peritoneal cavity. Reduced bowel often is beefy red or blue-black in color; after several minutes, however, normal color as well as peristalsis returns. Resection is necessary if a discrete lead point is identified.

PROGNOSIS

If an intussusception has been reduced successfully, the child is discharged if there is no evidence of re-intussusception, *ie*, the child is pain-free, tolerating feeds, and passing either flatus or stool. Re-intussusception occurs in 8% to 13% of patients after radiographic reduction [9] and in 5% of patients who have had surgical reduction. If re-intussusception occurs more than twice, surgery is recommended because of the increased likelihood that there is a lead point.

REFERENCES

1. Stringer MD, Pablot SM, Brereton RJ: Pediatric intussusception. *Br J Surg* 1992, 79:867–876.

2. Luks FL, Yazbeck S, Perreault G, Desjardins JG: Changes in the presentation of intussusception. *Am J Emerg Med* 1992, 10:574–576.

3. Daneman A, Alton DJ: Intussusception: issues and controversies related to diagnosis and reduction. *Radiol Clin North Am* 1996, 34:743–756.

4. Furuta GT, Bross DA, Doody D, Kleinman RE: Intussusception and leiomyosarcoma of the gastrointestinal tract in a pediatric patient: case report and review of the literature. *Dig Dis Sci* 1993, 38:1933–1937.

5. Paret G, Vardi A, Yahav J, *et al.*: Idiopathic familial intussusception. *Clin Pediatr* 1995, 34:559–560.

6. Heidrich FJ: Lethargy as a presenting symptom in patients with intussusception. *Clin Pediatr* 1986, 25:363–365.

7. Lazar L, Rathaus V, Katz S: Interrupted air column in the large bowel on plain abdominal film: a new radiological sign of intussusception. *J Pediatr Surg* 1995, 30:1551–1553.

8. Somekh E, Serour F, Goncalves D, Gorenstein A: Air enema for reduction of intussusception in children: risk for bacteremia. *Radiology* 1996, 200:217–218.

9. Champoux AN, Del Beccaro MA, Nazar-Stewart V: Recurrent intussusception: risks and features. *Arch Pediatr Adolesc Med* 1994, 148:474–478.

10. Shiels WE II: Childhood intussusception: management perspectives in 1995 [editorial]. *J Pediatr Gastroenterol Nutr* 1995, 21:15–17.

11. Lipschitz B, Patel YT, Kazlow P, *et al.*: Endoscopic pneumatic reduction of an intussusception with simultaneous polypectomy in a child. *J Pediatr Gastroenterol Nutr* 1995, 21:91–94.

163 Inflammatory Bowel Disease in Children and Adolescents

James F. Markowitz

EPIDEMIOLOGY

Children may develop Crohn's disease and ulcerative colitis at any age. Although inflammatory bowel disease (IBD) has been reported in children less than 1 year of age, 60% to 70% of affected children are diagnosed after the age of 15 years. Many studies confirm a rise in the incidence of pediatric Crohn's disease, but report a relatively stable incidence of ulcerative colitis over the past few decades [1••]. The incidence of pediatric Crohn's disease varies from less than 1 to nearly 10 per 100,000 population, with age-specific rates as high as 16 per 100,000 reported in adolescents. Prevalence rates for Crohn's disease are estimated to be between 9.5 and 12.6 per 100,000. Pediatric incidence rates for ulcerative colitis vary from 1.5 to 10 per 100,000 population, with resultant age-specific prevalence rates of 18.1 to 30 per 100,000.

GENETICS

Boys and girls are equally affected, and ethnic differences appear to be the same as in adult populations. A family history for IBD is present in 10% to 39% of affected children [2••]. Children born to a parent with Crohn's disease have a lifetime risk between 8% and 13% of developing the disease; this risk increases to 36% if both parents are affected. In families in which both a parent and child are affected, extent of disease and the frequency and type of extraintestinal manifestations are concordant in 64% and 70%, respectively.

ETIOLOGY

The causes of Crohn's disease and ulcerative colitis remain unknown. Current theories are summarized in Chapters 64, 75 and 76. Perinatal events may be important. Children with Crohn's disease appear less likely to have been breastfed and more likely to have had an infantile diarrheal illness than their healthy siblings. In ulcerative colitis, affected children are more likely than their unaffected siblings to have had diarrhea during infancy. Although other suspected risk factors such as maternal use of oral contraceptives do not appear important in pediatric patients, one report has associated passive smoking during infancy with the development of Crohn's disease in childhood. Epidemiologic studies have documented that passive smoking during childhood protects against developing ulcerative colitis as an adult, but a protective effect against the development of ulcerative colitis during childhood has not been clearly demonstrated.

CLINICAL FEATURES
Anatomic Distribution
Crohn's Disease

Studies based primarily on clinical and radiographic delineation of inflammation identify 50% to 60% of affected children as having ileocolitis; 30% to 35% as having only small bowel involvement; 10% to 15% as having only colitis; 5% as having only anorectal disease; and less than 5% as having esophageal or gastroduodenal disease. However, endoscopic and histologic examination of radiographically normal bowel often identifies evidence of inflammation. As many as 40% of children with newly diagnosed Crohn's disease have endoscopically and histologically detectable involvement of the esophagus, stomach, or duodenum despite normal contrast radiography. In addition, probably 75% of affected children have

involvement of the terminal ileum, with variable degrees of colonic involvement.

Ulcerative Colitis

Pancolitis appears less common than previously reported (Table 163-1), except in one study in the United States of children less than 10 years of age at diagnosis [1,3–5••,6]. However, the overall rates of pancolitis in children continue to be greater than those reported in adult populations.

Symptoms and Signs
Crohn's Disease

Symptoms reported at the time of diagnosis are summarized in Figure 163-1 [7–12]. Symptoms can appear suddenly or insidiously. Abdominal pain, often localized to the right lower quadrant, with or without nonbloody diarrhea, is typical of children with terminal ileal and proximal colonic involvement, and can mimic acute appendicitis. These patients often have a palpable tender fullness or mass in the right lower quadrant. In Crohn's colitis, the pain often is periumbilical, suprapubic, or localized to the left lower quadrant, and can be associated with tenesmus or bloody diarrhea, mimicking ulcerative colitis. In contrast to ulcerative colitis, however, extreme hemorrhage is rare. Children with gastroduodenal disease often have epigastric pain, anorexia, early satiety, or nausea, although many children with upper gastrointestinal tract involvement have few or no specific symptoms. Esophageal involvement usually presents with odynophagia. Adolescents may appear to have atypical eating disorders, and may be referred for gastrointestinal evaluation only after unsuccessful psychiatric and behavioral intervention has been attempted. In all patients, symptoms occur at varying times throughout the day, although nocturnal, early morning, and postprandial complaints are more common.

Systemic symptoms include fever, arthralgias, anorexia, fatigue, and weight loss, and one or more of these symptoms are present in more than 50% of children at the time of initial diagnosis. Impairment of linear growth and delay or interruption of sexual development also are common (discussed later in this chapter). It must be recognized, however, that at times there are no gastrointestinal symptoms, and that evaluation of one or more systemic symptoms may ultimately lead to a diagnosis of Crohn's disease.

Table 163-1. Extent of Ulcerative Colitis at Diagnosis

| | Older series (US and Canada) (diagnosed 1955–1979) | US series (diagnosed after 1975) | | Denmark series (diagnosed 1962–1987) | |
	Children ≤ 18 y* (n = 388)	Children ≤ 18 y† (n = 180)	Children ≤ 10 y‡ (n = 38)	Children ≤ 14 y§ (n = 77)	Children ≤ 9 y§ (n = 31)
Protosigmoiditis	67 (17%)	46 (26%)	6 (16%)	20 (26%)	11 (35%)
Left-sided colitis	87 (22%)	61 (34%)	5 (13%)	34 (44%)	16 (52%)
Pancolitis	234 (60%)	73 (41%)	27 (71%)	23 (30%)	4 (13%)

*Data combined from Michener et al. [3] and Hamilton et al. [4].
†Data from Hyams at al [5••].
‡Data from Gryboski [6].
§Data from Langholz et al. [1••].

Ulcerative Colitis

Diarrhea, rectal bleeding, and abdominal pain are almost universal. Frequent loose stools can contain either streaks of blood or clots. Children describe both tenesmus and urgency, although the former symptom is at times misinterpreted as constipation. Acute weight loss is common, but abnormalities of linear growth are unusual. When only proctitis is present, children may have stools of normal consistency, no systemic symptoms, and minimal hematochezia.

The severity of symptoms at presentation is variable. Between 40% and 50% of cases have mild symptoms, characterized by fewer than four stools per day, intermittent hematochezia, and minimal if any systemic symptoms or weight loss [1••,5••]. These children generally have normal physical examinations, or only minimal tenderness on palpation of the lower abdomen. Another third of children are moderately ill, with weight loss, more frequent diarrhea, and systemic symptoms. Physical examination demonstrates more significant abdominal tenderness. From 10% to 15% of the pediatric ulcerative colitis population have an acute, fulminant disease presentation. These patients appear moderately to severely toxic and have severe crampy abdominal pain, fever, more than six diarrheal stools per day, and, at times, copious rectal bleeding. They commonly manifest tachycardia, orthostatic hypotension, diffuse abdominal tenderness without peritoneal signs, and distention. Toxic megacolon represents the most dangerous extreme of acute, fulminant colitis, but is unusual in children.

Extraintestinal Manifestations

Apart from growth failure, the extraintestinal signs and symptoms of IBD are similar to those in adults. Any of the extraintestinal manifestations can precede gastrointestinal symptoms by months or years. Destructive perianal disease can be the first sign of Crohn's disease, and may come to attention only when a parent or physician notices the lesions and raises the suspicion of child abuse (Fig. 163-2). Perianal tags can at times be confused with hemorrhoids, but hemorrhoids are unusual in children. Perianal abscesses or fistulas occur so rarely in the general pediatric population that any child who develops one (other than an infant with a fistula in ano) should be evaluated for Crohn's disease. Among the hepatobiliary problems, sclerosing cholangitis is more common than is autoimmune hepatitis, occurring in 3.5% of children and adolescents with ulcerative colitis and less than 1% of those with Crohn's disease [13••]. Arthralgias are common, and up to 10% of children are reported to have transient, nondeforming arthritis, primarily affecting the knees or ankles.

Growth and Development

Subnormal linear growth is present at the time of diagnosis in 30% to 88% of children with Crohn's disease, but in only 10% of children with ulcerative colitis [14–16]. Inadequate growth may be the only sign of Crohn's disease in up to 10% of affected children, and growth records can demonstrate subnormal growth or growth failure for years before the initial diagnosis is made (Fig. 163-3). In addition, when growth is impaired, sexual development is delayed or halted.

After diagnosis, impaired growth continues to be a difficult problem, primarily for those with Crohn's disease. Despite medical therapy, growth failure occurs in 40% of prepubertal children during the first year after diagnosis, and in 33% in the second year [17]; 60% have at least one period of impaired growth before attaining their adult height [15]. Inadequate intake of nutrients is the most important reason for poor growth. Disease activity itself results in anorexia, but in addition, many children learn to minimize intestinal symptoms by skipping meals. Other factors that contribute to poor growth include the inflammatory process itself [18] and excessive corticosteroid exposure. Maldigestion and malabsorption of nutrients have only minor importance in the child who has not had extensive surgery. Basal metabolic rate is only modestly increased compared with healthy controls.

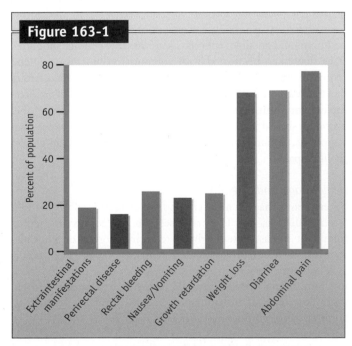

Figure 163-1

Clinical features of 426 children with Crohn's disease at initial diagnosis. (Data from Hamilton *et al.* [4], Burbige *et al.* [7], Gryboski and Spiro [8], Raine [9], Posthuma and Moroz [10], Barton and Ferguson [11] and Gryboski [12]).

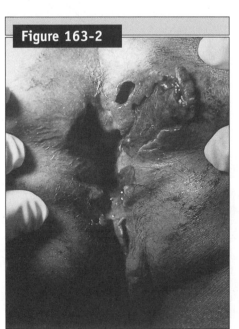

Figure 163-2

Highly destructive perianal disease in a 13-year-old girl with anorectal Crohn's disease. (*From* Markowitz *et al.* [22]; with permission.)

Although growth impairment is amenable to therapy, permanent deficits in adult stature are common in children who develop Crohn's disease before puberty. Studies in adults with childhood onset of disease from Chicago, New York, and Boston all document a skewing in the final height percentiles or height Z-scores to values below that expected for a normal population [14,15,18]. Final adult heights are less than predicted in 5% to 35% of patients whose disease began before puberty [14,15,18,19].

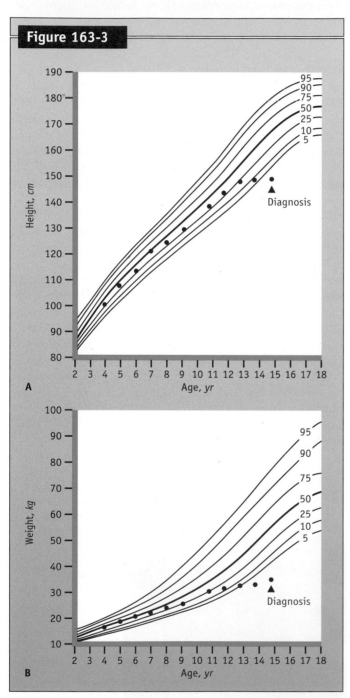

Figure 163-3

Growth chart from an adolescent presenting with gastrointestinal symptoms for the first time at age 14 years 6 months, and diagnosed with Crohn's ileocolitis at age 14 years 9 months. Despite the short duration of symptoms, growth records reveal a gradual fall in both weight for age and height for age percentiles for the years before diagnosis.

Complications

The gastrointestinal complications seen in children with IBD are similar to those described in adults. Pertinent issues related to the pediatric population are discussed in the following sections.

Obstruction

Obstruction is not seen in ulcerative colitis, and if present, should raise the possibility, even in the adolescent, of superimposed adenocarcinoma (discussed later in this chapter). In Crohn's disease, both acute high-grade and chronic partial obstruction occur. Bacterial overgrowth can develop, resulting in exacerbation of symptoms as well as varying degrees of maldigestion and malabsorption. Obstructive episodes can resolve with medical therapy, although recurrent or intractable cases require surgery. Particular attention should be given to the possibility of a previously unrecognized chronic, partial obstruction in the child whose symptoms appear resistant to medical management.

Fistula

The transmural nature of the inflammatory process in Crohn's disease results in sinus tracts and fistulas arising from areas of active inflammation. Perianal fistulas are most common [20,21], and at times can be highly destructive [22,23]. Enteroenteric, enterovesical, enterovaginal, and enterocutaneous fistulas also occur.

Perforation

In Crohn's disease, walled-off perforations, generally of the ileum, cecum, or ascending colon, occur and result in intramesenteric, interloop, or retroperitoneal abscesses. Free perforations are rare but have been described in adolescents. Free perforation of the colon is an unusual but emergent complication of ulcerative colitis, usually seen in the setting of acute, fulminant colitis or toxic megacolon (discussed later in this chapter), or after diagnostic interventions such as barium enema or colonoscopy. The resulting peritonitis and possible septic shock are life-threatening complications that must be treated with appropriate fluid resuscitation, broad-spectrum antibiotics, and surgery. Because corticosteroid therapy may mask the expected physical findings of board-like rigidity and diffuse rebound tenderness, plain radiographs of the abdomen should be done in all children who develop worsening symptoms, abdominal distention, loss of hepatic dullness, or shoulder pain.

Hemorrhage and Anemia

Severe hemorrhage is more common in ulcerative colitis than in Crohn's disease, and is usually seen in the context of acute, fulminant disease. Hemorrhage requiring urgent or multiple transfusions occurs in less than 5% of cases. Anemia can occur as a consequence of either macroscopic or microscopic blood loss resulting in iron deficiency. It can also arise because of the systemic effects of inflammation and a relative deficiency of erythropoietin production [24].

Acute Fulminant Colitis and Toxic Megacolon

Toxic megacolon has been described in up to 5% of children and adolescents with ulcerative colitis, and represents a medical and potentially surgical emergency [3]. As in adults, improper diagnosis or treatment can lead to a rapidly progressive deterioration complicated by severe electrolyte disturbances, hypoalbuminemia, hemorrhage, perforation, and sepsis, shock, or both. Precipitating factors may include the use of antidiarrheal agents such as anticholinergics or opiates, and colonic distention during barium enema or colonoscopy. Possibly as the result of recognizing and minimizing these factors, the frequency of toxic megacolon in the pediatric population appears to be decreasing, as evidenced by a recent review in which only two cases of toxic megacolon were seen in 171 children with 823 patient years of follow-up [5••]. Acute fulminant colitis represents a more common presentation, seen in both ulcerative and Crohn's colitis. These children manifest many of the signs of toxic megacolon, but marked dilation of the colon is absent. Children who continue to require blood transfusions after 14 days of intensive medical therapy are at risk for significant complications and usually require colectomy. More recent data suggest that such children can be managed with intensive medical therapy for periods longer than 2 weeks without significant morbidity or need for eventual colectomy.

Carcinoma

Children and adolescents with ulcerative colitis have a high lifetime risk of colorectal cancer, given the potential extreme duration of their illness and the high frequency of pancolitis [25••]. Patients as young as 16 years of age have been demonstrated to have colonic aneuploidy and dysplasia, although the risk for these changes does not appear to be present in the first decade of illness [26•]. In addition to duration and extent of colitis, other risk factors for colorectal cancer in patients with childhood onset disease include a defunctionalized rectal stump following previous subtotal colectomy and ileostomy, and the concomitant presence of sclerosing cholangitis. Crohn's disease may be similarly premalignant [27•], and endoscopic screening of adolescents with Crohn's colitis of more than 8 years duration has been shown to demonstrate aneuploidy and dysplasia as frequently as in a comparable group with ulcerative colitis [26•].

■ DIAGNOSIS

History

Because the symptoms and signs of IBD in children can be myriad, establishing the diagnosis often requires a high degree of suspicion. When taking the patient's history seek to elicit more than the obvious symptoms. Children and adolescents often are unwilling to discuss the frequency and consistency of their bowel movements, and parental observations often are erroneous. Nocturnal symptoms are especially important, as their occurrence often identifies the child with organic rather than functional illness. Evidence of poor growth must be sought by review of growth records obtained from primary physicians or school health offices. Similarly, the history should seek to identify signs of arrested sexual development, or in the postmenarchal girl, secondary amenorrhea. The possibility of either ulcerative colitis or Crohn's disease is heightened when family history reveals other relatives with IBD.

Physical Examination

Physical examination must include a careful abdominal examination, especially in regard to the presence or absence of abdominal tenderness, fullness, or a mass. Perianal inspection and digital rectal examination are indicated in every child, because the identification of perianal tags or circumferential fissures often allows an immediate presumptive diagnosis of Crohn's disease. General nutritional status must be evaluated, and height and weight accurately measured and compared with previous growth measurements.

Laboratory Studies

The laboratory evaluation of the child with possible IBD is similar to that for adults. Microcytic anemia, mild to moderate thrombocytosis, elevated erythrocyte sedimentation rate, and hypoalbuminemia are present in 40% to 80% of cases. Total white blood cell count is normal to only mildly elevated, unless the illness is complicated by abscess, superimposed infection, acute fulminant colitis, or toxic megacolon. Abnormal liver tests occur in 3% of children at the time of initial diagnosis, and reflect signs of potentially serious concomitant liver disease (chronic active hepatitis or sclerosing cholangitis) in about half [13••]. In a number of children, however, all laboratory studies may be normal. Appropriate studies for enteric pathogens must be performed. Given the frequency with which children are exposed to antibiotics, *Clostridium difficile*–mediated colitis must be excluded. Exposure to other potential enteric pathogens is also common in children.

Contrast Radiography

The child with suspected IBD should undergo an upper gastrointestinal series with small bowel follow-through to identify evidence of intestinal inflammation, estimate distribution and extent of disease, and help distinguish between Crohn's disease and ulcerative colitis. This study may, however, underestimate involvement of the stomach and duodenum. Although barium enema can, at times, differentiate between Crohn's and ulcerative colitis, the classic radiographic findings attributed to one form of colitis can be mimicked by the other. As subtle degrees of inflammation also are not evident on barium enema, colonoscopy is more commonly used to evaluate the colon and possibly the terminal ileum.

Abdominal ultrasound, computed tomography, and various scintigraphic techniques, including the technetium-99m-hexamethyl-propyleneamine-oxime (HMPAO)–labeled white cell scan can be used to assess the presence and extent of intestinal inflammation. The former modalities can be particularly helpful in distinguishing an intra-abdominal abscess from a phlegmon, and in directing percutaneous drainage.

Endoscopy and Biopsy

As in adults, endoscopy of the upper and lower gastrointestinal tracts allows accurate determination of the extent and distribution of IBD through direct observation and biopsy of affected and normal-appearing segments. The identification of skip lesions, aphthous ulcerations, and significant ileal inflammation helps in differentiating Crohn's disease from ulcerative colitis. Care must be taken in labeling all children with rectal sparing as having Crohn's disease, however, as young children have been described who have apparent rectal sparing at initial endoscopy but in whom ulcerative colitis is subsequently surgically confirmed. All children who undergo endoscopy should have biopsies performed, because microscopic inflammation and granulomas can be identified in specimens obtained from grossly normal-appearing mucosa. This may be especially important in the child who lacks clear-cut gastrointestinal symptoms but presents with otherwise unexplained growth failure or other systemic or extraintestinal symptoms.

Differential Diagnosis

The differential diagnosis of IBD varies with the presenting symptoms and sites of intestinal involvement (Table 163-2) [28]. Most of these conditions can be easily excluded by history, physical examination, laboratory evaluation, or endoscopy and biopsy. In contrast to adults, neoplastic disease, ischemia, and radiation-induced injury rarely are significant diagnostic concerns in the child or adolescent.

Table 163-2. Differential Diagnosis of Pediatric Inflammatory Bowel Disease

Disorders affecting the upper gastrointestinal tract

Symptoms: nausea, vomiting, dyspepsia, abdominal pain, odynophagia
Common disorders
  Gastroesophageal reflux disease
  Helicobacter pylori gastritis
  Peptic ulcer
  Feeding disorders (*eg*, anorexia nervosa, bulimia nervosa)
Uncommon disorders
  Zollinger-Ellison syndrome
  Eosinophilic gastroenteritis
  Intestinal tuberculosis
  Behçet disease
  Chronic granulomatous disease

Disorders affecting the lower gastrointestinal tract

Symptoms: abdominal cramps, loose bowel movements, bloating, weight loss, rectal bleeding
Common disorders
  Enteric infection (including amebiasis)
  Pseudomembranous (post-antibiotic) enterocolitis (*Clostridium difficile* toxin–mediated)
  Carbohydrate intolerance (*eg*, lactose, sucrose, sorbitol, xylitol)
  Acute appendicitis, appendiceal abscess
  Vasculitis (Henoch-Schönlein purpura, systemic lupus erythematosus, hemolytic-uremic syndrome)
  Celiac disease
  Allergic enteropathy, enterocolitis
  Laxative abuse
Uncommon disorders
  Neoplasms (lymphoma, adenocarcinoma, intestinal polyposis)
  Intestinal tuberculosis
  Eosinophilic gastroenteritis
  Intestinal lymphangiectasia

(From Markowitz [28]; with permission.)

TREATMENT

As in adults, treatment aims in children and adolescents include the suppression of symptoms and control of unavoidable complications. However, the treatment of children and adolescents presents the added challenge of promoting normal growth and sexual development. Current treatment options may promote one goal (*eg*, suppression of symptoms) while hindering another (*eg*, linear growth). Therapy, therefore, requires striking a balance between potentially conflicting effects. Because many of the data supporting the use of these medications have been extrapolated from adult studies, the following discussion focuses on those aspects of treatment that differ or have been shown to be particularly effective in the pediatric population.

Nutritional Therapy

Nutrition as Primary Therapy

Disease activity in Crohn's disease (but not in ulcerative colitis) appears to be amenable to nutritional intervention. Parenteral nutrition, both total and as a supplement to oral dietary intake, can suppress active disease symptoms, promote positive nitrogen balance, induce remission, and enhance growth. Enteral feedings, delivered orally or via nasogastric or gastrostomy tube, also are effective. As summarized in a recent meta-analysis that pooled results from both pediatric and adult studies, enteral feedings are inferior to corticosteroids in inducing remission (Fig. 163-4) [29••]. However, the pediatric studies analyzed actually reported comparable remission rates (75% to 90%) or decreases in disease activity scores in both the diet- and corticosteroid-treated groups. Elemental diet has no advantage compared to a polymeric formula [29••]. Once enteral feeding

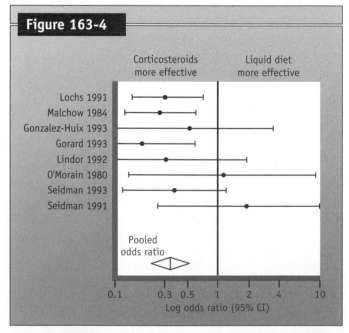

Figure 163-4

Meta-analysis of randomized controlled trials of exclusive liquid diet therapy compared to corticosteroids in the treatment of active Crohn's disease. Odds ratios (log scale) along with 95% confidence interval (CI) for induction of remission for each study are shown. Values <1 indicate a therapeutic benefit for corticosteroids compared with liquid diet therapy. The pooled odds ratio is 0.35 (95% CI, 0.23–0.53). (*From* Griffiths *et al.* [29••]; with permission.)

is discontinued, relapse rates of 43% at 6 months and 60% at 12 months are reported. However, remission can be prolonged after reintroduction of an unrestricted diet if nocturnal, supplemental enteral feedings are continued [30]. Because liquid diet therapies may promote better growth than does corticosteroid treatment (discussed later in this chapter), this approach offers advantages in children and adolescents with active Crohn's disease and growth failure.

Nutrition as Therapy for Growth Failure

Nutritional interventions can improve growth by ensuring an adequate supply of all necessary macro- and micronutrients. Oral dietary supplementation to ensure intake of the Recommended Daily Allowance of calories and protein (caloric intake of 75 to 90 kcal/kg/d for the adolescent) can result in dramatic improvement in growth, if such an intake is continued for an extended time. Unfortunately, dietary intake often is inadequate, even with high-calorie supplements, because of anorexia or discomfort resulting from eating. For such patients, continuous or intermittent nocturnal nasogastric or gastrostomy feeding of a defined liquid diet improves growth, as does parenteral nutrition.

Corticosteroids

Pediatric treatment regimens using corticosteroids have evolved through empiric use and clinical experience rather than scientific study. Oral corticosteroids are generally well absorbed, but occasionally children with apparent poor absorption or corticosteroid resistance may benefit from intravenous bolus or continuous infusion dosing. Rectal corticosteroids are particularly beneficial for severe tenesmus and urgency, but many children have difficulty retaining enema formulations, so that foam-based treatments or suppositories may be preferable in selected individuals.

The decision to use corticosteroids must be balanced by consideration of their potential adverse effects. The spectrum of complications seen in adults also occurs in children. In addition, corticosteroids interfere with linear bone growth, even in the setting of adequate dietary intake. Commonly prescribed doses of prednisone (0.3 to 1.0 mg/kg/d) taken daily for only 7 to 10 days reduce serum procollagen levels, a marker of linear bone growth. Alternate-day dosing limits these effects while still maintaining reduced disease activity. Alternate-day dosing also has been shown to have no deleterious effect on bone mineralization in adolescents with Crohn's disease [31]. However, in patients who have not completed their linear growth and whose disease activity cannot be controlled by alternate-day dosing regimes, the anti-inflammatory effects of daily corticosteroids must be weighed against the coincident suppression of linear growth.

The cosmetic side effects of corticosteroids are particularly distressing to many children and adolescents or their parents, and can be more difficult for them to accept than the symptoms of IBD. Cosmetic effects are best limited by avoiding excessive doses of corticosteroids. Poor compliance with corticosteroid treatment because of a previous experience with severe acne or a moon facies is frequent among adolescents and a common cause of "failure" to respond to an adequate dosing regimen.

The newer topically active corticosteroids (*eg*, budesonide, fluticasone propionate) have the potential to provide anti-inflammatory activity to the gut without systemic toxicity. These agents have obvious implications for the treatment of children, but studies in pediatric populations have yet to be reported.

5-Aminosalicylates

Despite extensive studies in adults, there are few pediatric studies on the use of 5-aminosalicylates (5-ASA) [32•]. Available preparations and indications for use are summarized in Table 163-3. There is extensive clinical experience with sulfasalazine in children, which, by and large, has mirrored the adult experience. The only published pediatric study comparing the efficacy of 5-ASA preparations found that, in children with mildly to moderately active ulcerative colitis, 79% of those treated with sulfasalazine, 60 mg/kg/d, demonstrated clinical improvement, compared to only 39% of those treated with olsalazine, 30 mg/kg/d. Several smaller open-label or double-blind pediatric trials, and one larger retrospective analysis of 10 years of clinical experience with Eudragit-coated 5-ASA preparations have reported therapeutic benefits in active ulcerative colitis, active Crohn's colitis, and active small-bowel Crohn's disease [32•,33]. No studies on rectal 5-ASA in children have been reported. There are no pediatric data on maintaining remission with any of the 5-ASA preparations in either ulcerative colitis or Crohn's

Table 163-3. 5-Aminosalicylates in Pediatric Inflammatory Bowel Disease

	Preparation	Dosage	Indication
Sulfasalazine	500-mg tablet (generic; Azulfidine) 500-mg enteric-coated tablet (Azulfidine Entab)	50–75 mg/kg/d ÷ bid - qid (maximum 4 g/d)	Mild to moderate colitis; maintenance of remission
Olsalazine	250-mg tablet (Dipentum)	30–50 mg/kg/d ÷ bid - qid	Mild to moderate colitis; maintenance of remission
Mesalamine	400-mg Eudragit-S tablet (Asacol)	30–50 mg/kg/d ÷ bid - tid	Mild to moderate colitis or ileocolitis; maintenance of remission
	250-mg capsule with ethylcellulose granules (Pentasa)	30–50 mg/kg/d ÷ bid - qid	Mild to moderate colitis, ileocolitis, jejunal Crohn's disease; maintenance of remission
	500-mg suppository	500 mg pr qd - bid	Proctitis
	4-g enema (Rowasa)	2–4 g pr qd - bid	Proctosigmoiditis, distal colitis

disease, or in preventing disease recurrence after surgery in Crohn's disease. Adverse reactions to all of the 5-ASA preparations have been described, requiring discontinuation in 5% to 15% of cases. The more serious complications reported in children have included pancreatitis, nephritis, exacerbation of disease, and sulfa- or salicylate-induced allergic reactions.

Antibiotics

As in adults, the use of antibiotics in children with Crohn's disease is empiric. No controlled pediatric studies have been published, but there is widespread use of a variety of antibiotics for acute and chronic therapy of inflammatory masses. Based on the adult experience, metronidazole, and, in the postpubertal adolescent, ciprofloxacin, are used for perianal disease or for the treatment of mild to moderate colitis in the 5-ASA–intolerant or allergic patient. Adverse effects are similar to those seen in adults. Ciprofloxacin must be used with caution in children because of potential toxicity to growing bone.

Immunomodulators

6-Mercaptopurine and Azathioprine

6-Mercaptopurine (6-MP) and azathioprine are increasingly being used in children with corticosteroid-dependent Crohn's disease or ulcerative colitis, and in those whose disease is unresponsive to corticosteroids [34]. Clinical experience has mirrored the results of adult studies, demonstrating that these agents induce and maintain remission in 60% to 75% of patients; act as steroid-sparing agents; and improve or close chronic draining fistulas [35,36]. The average time to onset of action is 4.5 months. At dosages of 1.0 to 1.5 mg/kg/d of 6-MP, no neutropenia, serious infection, or untoward reactions are usually seen, but adverse reactions requiring discontinuation of treatment such as allergic reaction, pancreatitis, or immunosuppression occur in up to 5% of pediatric patients.

Cyclosporine

The primary indication for cyclosporine in pediatric IBD is for the treatment of fulminant ulcerative colitis. Initial response rates, defined as avoidance of imminent surgery and discharge from the hospital, of 20% to 80% have been reported with either oral or intravenous routes of administration [37,38]. Responses generally occur within 7 to 14 days of initiation of treatment, but relapses requiring colectomy occur within 1 year in 70% to 100% of initial responders during treatment or after discontinuation of cyclosporine. However, in a recent report, four of six children with ulcerative colitis had a prolonged remission when 6-MP or azathioprine was added to the regimen once cyclosporine had induced remission [39].

There is less experience with cyclosporine in children with Crohn's disease. Two reports describe a total of 12 children with fulminant Crohn's colitis who were treated with cyclosporine and 6-mercaptopurine or azathioprine. Overall, eight initially improved within 1 to 2 weeks, but five of these, as well as the original three nonresponders, came to colectomy within 8 months [39,40]. Another small study could not demonstrate clinical improvement in a group of children with Crohn's disease in whom cyclosporine was used as the sole treatment of active disease. Although the adult literature demonstrates that

cyclosporine is effective in closing fistulas and healing pyoderma gangrenosum, comparable pediatric studies have not been reported. A recent case report has described the successful use of a related medication, tacrolimus (FK-506), in inducing remission in a child with fulminant Crohn's colitis.

Tremors, hirsutism, and systemic hypertension are the most common toxic effects of cyclosporine that have been described in pediatric IBD trials. However, isolated reports of *Pneumocystis carinii* pneumonia and serious bacterial and fungal infection in cyclosporine-treated patients merit careful monitoring in all children treated with cyclosporine, especially those whose treatment combines cyclosporine with corticosteroids, 6-MP, or azathioprine.

Other Medical Therapies

Methotrexate has been used with beneficial effects in a few children with severe Crohn's disease, but extensive experience is lacking. Short-chain fatty acid enemas have been used to treat a few children with ulcerative colitis based on the observation that children with colitis may have impaired colonic utilization of *n*-butyrate and other short-chain fatty acids. Other new and potentially revolutionary therapies for the treatment of both Crohn's disease and ulcerative colitis, such as anti-tumor necrosis factor antibodies, anti-inflammatory cytokines, and cytokine suppressive anti-inflammatory drugs, are in various stages of development. None of these treatments has yet been made available for study in children.

Surgery

Crohn's Disease

Although medical therapy can induce prolonged clinical remission, complications of Crohn's disease ultimately result in surgery during childhood or adolescence in 32% to 80% of patients. In a population-based study from the United Kingdom, 79% of patients with onset of Crohn's disease in childhood and adolescence required one or more operations for intractable disease activity or complications within 20 years of diagnosis, and 50% of those had surgery within 5 years of diagnosis [41]. Indications for surgery are similar to those in adults. Although growth failure remains an indication for surgery, long-term nutritional support and immunosuppressive therapy have made surgery solely for growth failure infrequent. Risk for surgery appears comparable among children with ileocolitis, colitis, or small intestinal Crohn's disease. Clinical recurrence after resection is seen in 50% of patients with diffuse ileocolitis within 1 year of surgery, and in 20% to 50% of those with localized disease within 5 years [42,43]. A second operation is necessary in 59% of children within 5 years of initial surgery and in 85% of children within 10 years [41]. No pediatric studies have evaluated treatments to prevent postoperative recurrence.

Given these realities, surgical management in children, as in adults, recognizes that Crohn's disease cannot be surgically cured and is directed at specific complications. Operative techniques in children are similar to those in adults. Strictureplasty surgery can be performed safely in children and adolescents, and can limit the need for resection [44•]. As a consequence of surgery, children feel better, eat better, and generally require less medication. Resting energy expenditure is reduced, and nitrogen utilization improved. Postoperatively, prepubertal and intrapubertal children with growth delay demonstrate increases in type I procollagen and linear growth as long as early clinical recurrence does not develop.

Ulcerative Colitis

Intractable or fulminant symptoms of ulcerative colitis lead to colectomy in 19% to 23% of children and adolescents within 5 years of diagnosis (see Prognosis) [1••,5••]. Given the frequent inability to distinguish definitively between ulcerative and Crohn's colitis preoperatively, many centers continue to perform subtotal colectomy and ileostomy, followed at a later date by restorative surgery if the colectomy specimen confirms a diagnosis of ulcerative colitis. An ileoanal anastomosis with an ileal J-pouch results in fewer daytime and nocturnal bowel movements and less fecal soiling than did the ileoanal anastomosis without a pouch. Anorectal function is well preserved. When growth retardation is evident preoperatively, significant increases in height velocity can be expected postoperatively. Small bowel obstruction is the most common early postoperative complication of ileal pouch anal anastomosis surgery [45•]. Pouchitis, the most common late complication described, occurs in 19% of patients and generally responds to treatment with metronidazole, ciprofloxacin, 5-ASA, or corticosteroids [45•].

Psychological Issues

As in any chronic illness, the psychosocial burden of IBD on the child or adolescent can be significant. Identifiable psychiatric disorders, most commonly depression, may be present in up to 60% of a pediatric IBD population. Children with IBD tend to be more compulsive as a group than are healthy controls, and have psychological styles characterized by depression, withdrawal, anxiety, and frequent somatizing. However, severe psychopathology is usually absent [46]. Children with IBD are less likely to report stressful life events than are controls, suggesting that they may have difficulty recognizing and reporting stressful events, or that they tend to use denial to cope with stressors. Coping styles in these patients tend to be more rigid and constricted than in healthy children. Parents can also suffer psychological disturbance as a consequence of their children's illness, and in a number of cases, mothers have manifested behaviors consistent with posttraumatic stress disorder.

▮ PROGNOSIS

Crohn's Disease

Long-term follow-up studies in patients with childhood-onset Crohn's disease reveal the chronic and at times debilitating nature of the illness. Although many children lead normal, unrestricted lives, in a sizable minority quality of life is deleteriously affected, reflected by frequent school absences, the need for home tutoring, the inability to participate in physical education classes, and the need to adapt social interactions to accommodate the need for toilet facilities [47]. Recurrent flares of disease activity or the development of fistulas or strictures leads to intermittent or daily symptoms, prompting up to 67% of patients surveyed in a long-term follow-up study from the Cleveland Clinic to report their health to be suboptimal. Periods of growth retardation occur in up to 60% of adolescents whose disease begins before

puberty, although more than half of these patients eventually experience sufficient catch-up growth to prevent permanent growth impairment [15]. In addition, one or more operations become necessary in 67% to 79% of all patients [41,42]. In those in whom surgery is avoided, many ultimately demonstrate increased risk of adenocarcinoma [26•,27•].

Ulcerative Colitis

Seventy percent of children with ulcerative colitis can be expected to enter remission within 3 months of initial diagnosis, regardless of whether their initial attack is characterized as mild, moderate, or severe, and 45% to 70% remain inactive over the first year after diagnosis [1••,5••]. However, 10% of those whose symptoms are characterized as moderate or severe remain continuously symptomatic. Over each year of the ensuing decade, approximately 55% of patients have inactive disease, 40% have chronic intermittent symptoms, and 5% to 10% have continuous symptoms. These data are similar to those reported in an adult population [48]. The colectomy rate is 5% within the first year after diagnosis and 19% to 23% by 5 years after diagnosis [1••,5••]. These rates rise to 9% and 26%, respectively, in the subgroup of children initially presenting with moderate or severe symptoms [5••]. These rates appear comparable to those reported in a Swedish pediatric population treated between 1961 and 1990 [49], and lower than those from older studies from the United States [3].

By contrast, the prognosis of those children with proctitis or proctosigmoiditis may be somewhat better. More than 90% of them are asymptomatic within 6 months of diagnosis, and in any given year of follow-up 55% remain asymptomatic and less than 5% have continuously active disease [50]. However, the likelihood of proximal extension of disease is estimated to be 25% within 3 years of initial diagnosis and 29% to 70% over the course of follow-up [1••,50]. Colectomy may eventually be required in 5% of patients. These rates of proximal extension of inflammation and colectomy appear higher than in adult populations.

▮ REFERENCES

Recently published papers of particular interest have been highlighted as follows:
- • Of interest
- •• Of outstanding interest

1.•• Langholz E, Munkholm P, Krasilnikoff PA, Binder V: Inflammatory bowel diseases with onset in childhood: clinical features, morbidity, and mortality in a regional cohort. *Scand J Gastroenterol* 1997, 32:139–147.
This paper represents a comprehensive, community-based study providing important details regarding the epidemiology and clinical course of IBD in children.

2.•• Yang H, Rotter JI. Genetics of inflammatory bowel disease. In: *Inflammatory Bowel Disease: From Bench to Bedside*. Edited by Targan SR, Shanahan F. Baltimore: Williams & Wilkins; 1994:32–64.
This remains one of the most comprehensive and up-to-date reviews of genetic studies in IBD.

3. Michener WM, Farmer RG, Mortimer EA: Long-term prognosis of ulcerative colitis with onset in childhood or adolescence. *J Clin Gastroenterol* 1979, 1:301–305.

4. Hamilton JR, Bruce GA, Abdourhaman M, Gall DG: Inflammatory bowel disease in children and adolescents. *Adv Pediatr* 1979, 26:311–341.

5.•• Hyams JS, Davis P, Grancher K, *et al.*: Clinical outcome of ulcerative colitis in children. *J Pediatr* 1996, 129:81–88.
This study details the course and prognosis of a large population of children in the United States with ulcerative colitis treated after 1975 at two tertiary care pediatric IBD centers.

6. Gryboski JD: Ulcerative colitis in children 10 years old or younger. *J Pediatr Gastroenterol Nutr* 1993, 17:24–31.

7. Burbige EJ, Huang SH, Bayless TM: Clinical manifestations of Crohn's disease in children and adolescents. *Pediatrics* 1975, 55:866–871.

8. Gryboski JD, Spiro HM: Prognosis in children with Crohn's disease. *Gastroenterol* 1978, 74:807–817.

9. Raine PAM: BAPS collective review. Chronic inflammatory bowel disease. *J Pediatr Surg* 1984, 19:18–23.

10. Posthuma R, Moroz SP: Pediatric Crohn's disease. *J Pediatr Surg* 1985, 20:478–482.

11. Barton JR, Ferguson A: Clinical features, morbidity and mortality of Scottish children with inflammatory bowel disease. *Q J Med* 1990, 75:423–439.

12. Gryboski JD: Crohn's disease in children 10 years old and younger: comparison with ulcerative colitis. *J Pediatr Gastroenterol Nutr* 1994, 18:174–182.

13.•• Hyams J, Markowitz J, Treem W, *et al.*: Characterization of hepatic abnormalities in children with inflammatory bowel disease. *Inflammatory Bowel Dis* 1995, 1:27–33.
This paper reports the largest experience in the literature characterizing the hepatic abnormalities associated with IBD in children.

14. Kirschner BS: Growth and development in chronic inflammatory bowel disease. *Acta Pediatr Scand* 1990, 366(suppl):98–104.

15. Markowitz J, Grancher K, Rosa J, *et al.*: Growth failure in pediatric inflammatory bowel disease. *J Pediatr Gastroenterol Nutr* 1993, 16:373–380.

16. Hildebrand H, Karlberg J, Kristiansson B: Longitudinal growth in children and adolescents with inflammatory bowel disease. *J Pediatr Gastroenterol Nutr* 1994, 18:165–173.

17. Griffiths AM, Nguyen P, Smith C, *et al.*: Growth and clinical course of children with Crohn's disease. *Gut* 1993, 34:939–943.

18. Motil KJ, Grand RJ, Davis-Kraft L, *et al.*: Growth failure in children with inflammatory bowel disease: a prospective study. *Gastroenterol* 1993, 105:681–691.

19. Ferguson A, Sedgwick DM: Juvenile onset inflammatory bowel disease: height and body mass index in adult life. *Br Med J* 1994, 308:1259–1263.

20. Markowitz J, Daum F, Aiges H, *et al.*: Perianal disease in children and adolescents with Crohn's disease. *Gastroenterology* 1984, 86:829–833.

21. Palder SB, Shandling B, Bilik R, *et al.*: Perianal complications of pediatric Crohn's disease. *J Pediatr Surg* 1991, 26:513–515.

22. Markowitz J, Grancher K, Rosa J, *et al.*: Highly destructive perianal disease in children with Crohn's disease. *J Pediatr Gastroenterol Nutr* 1995, 21:149–153.

23. Tolia V: Perianal Crohn's disease in children and adolescents. *Am J Gastroenterol* 1996, 91:922–926.

24. Dohil R, Hassall E, Wadsworth LD, Israel DM: Recombinant human erythropoietin for treatment of anemia of chronic disease in children with Crohn's disease. *J Pediatr* 1998, 132:155–159.

25.•• Ekbom A, Helmick C, Zack M, Adami H-O: Ulcerative colitis and colorectal cancer: a population-based study. *N Engl J Med* 1990, 323:1228–1233.
This is an important, population-based study. By highlighting data derived from patients at different ages of onset of ulcerative colitis, it details the particularly high risk of colorectal cancer found in individuals who develop colitis during childhood.

26.• Markowitz J, McKinley M, Kahn E, *et al.*: Endoscopic screening for dysplasia and mucosal aneuploidy in adolescents and young adults with childhood onset colitis. *Am J Gastroenterol* 1997, 92:2001–2006.
This study represents the only prospective study of dysplasia surveillance in children and adolescents with IBD.

27.• Ekbom A, Helmick C, Zack M, Adami H-O: Increased risk of large-bowel cancer in Crohn's disease with colonic involvement. *Lancet* 1990, 336:357–359.
This is an important population-based study.

28. Markowitz J: A primer on pediatric inflammatory bowel disease. *Contemp Pediatr* 1996, 13:25–46.

29.•• Griffiths AM, Ohlsson A, Sherman PM, Sutherland LR: Meta-analysis of enteral nutrition as primary treatment of active Crohn's disease. *Gastroenterology* 1995, 108:1056–1067.
This is an important critical evaluation of the literature.

30. Wilschanski M, Sherman P, Pencharz P, *et al.*: Supplementary enteral nutrition maintains remission in paediatric Crohn's disease. *Gut* 1996, 38:543–548.

31. Issenman RM, Atkinson SA, Radoja C, Fraher L: Longitudinal assessment of growth, mineral metabolism and bone mass in pediatric Crohn's disease. *J Pediatr Gastroenterol Nutr* 1993, 17:401–406.

32.• Leichtner AM: Aminosalicylates for the treatment of inflammatory bowel disease. *J Pediatr Gastroenterol Nutr* 1995, 21:245–252.
This paper provides a critical review of recent pediatric experience with aminosalicylate therapy in IBD.

33. D'Agata ID, Vanounou T, Seidman E: Mesalamine in pediatric inflammatory bowel disease: a 10 year experience. *Inflammatory Bowel Dis* 1996, 2:229–235.

34. Markowitz J, Grancher K, Mandel F, Daum F: Immunosuppressive therapy in pediatric inflammatory bowel disease: results of a survey of the North American Society for Gastroenterology and Nutrition. *Am J Gastroenterol* 1993, 88:44–48.

35. Markowitz J, Rosa J, Grancher K, *et al.*: Long-term 6-mercaptopurine in treatment of adolescents with Crohn's disease. *Gastroenterology* 1990, 99:1347–1351.

36. Verhave M, Winter HS, Grand RJ: Azathioprine in the treatment of children with inflammatory bowel disease. *J Pediatr* 1990, 117:809–814.

37. Benkov KJ, Rosk JR, Schwersenz AH, *et al.*: Cyclosporine as an alternative to surgery in children with inflammatory bowel disease. *J Pediatr Gastroenterol Nutr* 1994, 19:290–294.

38. Treem WR, Cohen J, Davis P, *et al.*: Cyclosporine for the treatment of fulminant ulcerative colitis in children. *Dis Colon Rectum* 1995, 38:474–479.

39. Ramakrishna J, Langhans N, Calenda K, *et al.*: Combined use of cyclosporine and azathioprine or 6-mercaptopurine in pediatric inflammatory bowel disease. *J Pediatr Gastroenterol Nutr* 1996, 32:296–302.

40. Mahdi G, Israel DM, Hassal E: Cyclosporine and 6-mercaptopurine for active, refractory Crohn's colitis in children. *Am J Gastroenterol* 1996, 91:1355–1359.

41. Sedgwick DM, Barton JR, Hamer-Dodges DW, *et al.*: Population-based study of surgery in juvenile onset Crohn's disease. *Br J Surg* 1991, 78:171–175.

42. Griffiths AM: Factors that influence the postoperative recurrence of Crohn's disease in childhood. In: *Inflammatory Bowel Disease and Coeliac Disease in Children.* Edited by Hadziselimovic F, Herzog B, Burgin-Wolff A. Boston: Kluwer Academic Publishers; 1990:131–136.

43. Davies G, Evans CM, Whand MS, Walker-Smith JA: Surgery for Crohn's disease in childhood: influence of site of disease and operative procedure on outcome. *Br J Surg* 1990, 77:891–894.

44.• Oliva L, Wyllie R, Alexander F, *et al.*: The results of strictureplasty in pediatric patients with multifocal Crohn's disease. *J Pediatr Gastroenterol Nutr* 1994, 18:306–310.

45.• Sarigol S, Caulfield M, Wyllie R, *et al.*: Ileal pouch-anal anastomosis in children with ulcerative colitis. *Inflammatory Bowel Diseases* 1996, 2:82–87.
This is a comprehensive review of pediatric surgical experience.

46. Krall V, Szajnberg NM, Hyams JS, *et al.*: Projective personality tests of children with inflammatory bowel disease. *Percept Mot Skills* 1995, 80:1341–1342.

47. Rabbett H, Elbadri R, Thwaites R, *et al.*: Quality of life in children with Crohn's disease. *J Pediatr Gastroenterol Nutr* 1996, 23:528–533.

48. Langholz E, Munkholm P, Davidsen M, Binder V: Course of ulcerative colitis: analysis of changes in disease activity over years. *Gastroenterol* 1994, 107:3–11.

49. Ahsgren L, Jonsson B, Stenling R, Rutegard J: Prognosis after early onset of ulcerative colitis. A study from an unselected patient population. *Hepatogastroenterology* 1993, 40:467–470.

50. Hyams J, Lerer T, Colletti R, *et al.*: Clinical outcome of ulcerative proctitis in children. *J Pediatr Gastroenterol Nutr* 1997, 25:149–152.

164 Short Bowel Syndrome

Jon A. Vanderhoof

Short bowel syndrome is the malabsorptive state that often follows massive resection of the small intestine. The definition is a functional one, implying the presence of significant malabsorption [1••]. The extent of resection often is independent of the degree of malabsorption, which is the reason for the functional definition. In many patients, adequate caloric and macronutrient absorption is possible despite continued significant unrecoverable loss of micronutrients and fluid [2••], whereas in other patients, panmalabsorption remains uncorrectable despite aggressive therapy.

There are many causes of short bowel syndrome in infants and children, including most of the diseases that cause problems in adults as well [3]. Most cases of short bowel syndrome in children originate in infancy, however, usually as a result of necrotizing enterocolitis or intestinal anomalies that have required significant resection [4,5].

INTESTINAL ADAPTATION

Early therapy for short bowel syndrome is directed toward stimulating intestinal adaptation, a process characterized by villus hyperplasia and resulting in an increase in the length of the villi, an increase in absorptive surface, and a gradual increase in functional absorption. Mucosal hyperplasia does not occur in the absence of enteral nutrition, despite provision of adequate calories and nutrients by parenteral alimentation. Consequently, the aggressive use of enteral feeding is key in stimulating this process. After weeks or months of aggressive enteral nutrition, it is often possible to stimulate enough growth in absorptive surface to successfully wean patients, even those with markedly reduced intestinal length, from parenteral nutrition. Nutrients function by stimulating increased work in the small intestine; this results in local stimulation of mucosal cell proliferation as well as the stimulation of a number of trophic hormones, which are secreted into the bloodstream and stimulate adaptation throughout the small bowel (Fig. 164-1).

Identification of specific growth factors has been an important focus of research in recent years. More important from a clinical standpoint is research on specific nutrients that enhance intestinal adaptation, because this information provides important direction as to what patients with short bowel syndrome should be fed. For example, lipids, long-chain fats in particular, appear to be uniquely trophic among the macronutrients and should be included in the feeding regimen of patients with short bowel syndrome [6]. There are differences among the various lipids, and highly unsaturated fish oils containing 3-omega acids appear to be the most effectively trophic; eicosapentaenoic acid probably is the predominant stimulant, perhaps because of its effect on prostaglandin metabolism. Arachidonic acid, which also acts as a precursor for prostaglandin synthesis, also may be important in permitting stimulation of gut adaptation.

Although there has been significant interest in glutamine in recent years as a means of stimulating gut adaptation, well-controlled studies in animals and humans have not demonstrated significant effects of glutamine in enhancing adaptation in short bowel syndrome, even in combination with growth hormone.

NUTRITIONAL MANAGEMENT

The management of an individual patient is a gradually evolving process. Patients are initially treated with parenteral nutrition until fluid and electrolyte loss is stabilized and the immediate postoperative state has passed. Feedings through the use of continuous enteral nutrition are subsequently initiated, usually with a chemically defined diet that contains significant quantities of long-chain fats to stimulate gut adaptation. These feedings initially are administered very slowly and are gradually advanced as tolerated based on the patient's stool output and carbohydrate loss in the stool. It is important to measure such carbohydrate loss by stool Clinitest, because malabsorption of carbohydrates has a major osmotic effect and results in increased fluid losses; lipid malabsorption, which also invariably occurs, is not as important in stimulating stool water loss [7–9]. Hydrolyzed casein appears to stimulate adaptation as well as

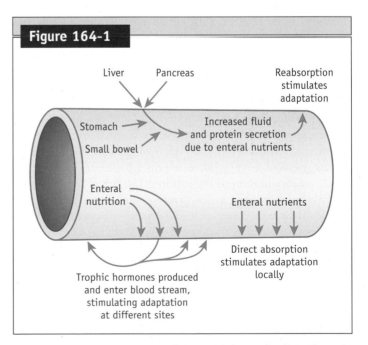

Figure 164-1

A diagrammatic representation of the multiple mechanisms through which enteral nutrients stimulate intestinal adaptation. Stimulation of enteral secretions from the stomach, the small bowel, the liver and the pancreas, enhancing the secretion of trophic hormones, and directly stimulating the absorptive process all enhance gut adaptation.

intact casein does and confers some absorptive advantage. Complex carbohydrates (*ie*, partially hydrolyized starch) probably offer some advantage over simple carbohydrates in reducing osmotic fluid losses.

Use of continuous enteral infusion has many advantages over bolus feeding: it allows for continuous stimulation of adaptation 24 hours a day; and it permits continuous saturation of transport sites in the small bowel if appropriately regulated, whereas bolus feeding invariably uses most of the absorptive surface only part of the time. Finally, as a result of enhanced absorption, continuous enteral infusion results in a reduction of parenteral nutrition requirements and, thereby, reduces many of the complications associated with parenteral nutrition, as well as its cost.

Enteral feedings may be given either through a gastrostomy tube placed surgically or endoscopically, or through a nasogastric tube. The decision as to which type of tube is used often is based on an estimate of the length of time during which continuous enteral infusion will be necessary. Obviously, in many patients enteral feedings will be used for a long time, and the gastrostomy has numerous advantages. Complications from nasogastric tubes, however, are surprisingly low, provided the parents and the child can tolerate presence of the tube.

Fluid and electrolyte management predominates in the early phases of treatment. Patients with ostomies have especially high-volume fluid losses (up to 1 to 3 L/d), often containing sodium concentrations in the range of 80 to 120 mEq/L. This fluid must be replaced to prevent dehydration. Initially, fluid replacement is conducted intravenously and is best done by measuring losses and replacing them with a solution containing comparable electrolyte concentrations. As losses stabilize, these fluids can be added to the enteral feeding solution. Using a separate replacement solution allows standard parenteral nutrition solutions to be used on a daily basis without much fluctuation in electrolyte and nutrient content. Once the patient's condition stabilizes, it may be more convenient to combine everything into one solution. Secretory diarrhea may occur in some patients with short bowel syndrome; octreotide occasionally is helpful to manage this state.

Enteral feedings are slowly advanced and parenteral calories are concomitantly and isocalorically decreased to maintain nutritional status, control fluid losses, and ensure gut adaptation. Overaggressive feeding increases fluid losses to unacceptable levels, so careful monitoring is important. Small infants should be given oral feedings at least two or three times a day so they will learn how to chew, suck, and swallow at normal levels for their ages. Otherwise, feeding refusal is likely to occur following discontinuation of continuous enteral feeding.

As enteral nutrition is increased to a level of providing 20% to 30% of the child's total caloric intake, it is usually possible to reduce the duration of parenteral nutrition infusion to 8 to 12 hours per day, thereby giving the child an opportunity to become free of parenteral nutrition and assume a somewhat more normal lifestyle. Long-term hospitalizations for children with short bowel syndrome are now fortunately uncommon, as these patients are usually cared for at home. Even in children with poor home situations, use of medical foster homes provides a significant advantage over long-term hospitalization in most cases.

Once the child is weaned free of parenteral nutrition and most of the calories are provided by continuous enteral infusion, bolus feedings are increased gradually while enteral feedings are decreased gradually. During this time, provision of most of the enteral feedings at night allows the patient to eat bolus feedings only during the daytime, helping to normalize lifestyle.

CHRONIC COMPLICATIONS

Despite the success of home parenteral nutrition, many complications confront the average patient with short bowel syndrome. Parenteral nutrition–induced liver disease, recurrent catheter sepsis, small bowel bacterial overgrowth, and, once the patient has been weaned free of parenteral nutrition, micronutrient deficiency states, all are problems that must be managed often [10•,11].

Parenteral nutrition–induced liver disease is especially common in small infants. It seems to be more of a problem in those infants in whom little or no enteral feeding can be provided; enteral nutrition appears to be somewhat protective. The injury is predominantly cholestatic, with irreversible cirrhosis developing in small infants and children. Control of bacterial overgrowth, aggressive use of enteral feedings, and prevention of catheter sepsis all seem to help avoid parenteral nutrition–induced liver disease. Specially formulated amino acid solutions such as TrophAmine (McGaw, Inc., Irvine, CA) for small infants appear to confer some advantage in the reduction of parenteral nutrition–induced liver injury. Cycling the parenteral nutrition, providing it only during part of the day or night, is considered helpful by some experts. Cholelithiasis is a common problem, and some authorities have advocated routine cholecystectomy in parenteral nutrition–dependent patients with short bowel syndrome.

Catheter sepsis is the other main parenteral nutrition–related problem confronting patients with short bowel syndrome. Although catheter sepsis often is associated with enteric organisms (which implies the organisms have seeded the catheter by translocation from the bowel), the skin of these infants is contaminated with enteric organisms, which can be introduced into the catheter externally. At the earliest sign of fever, lethargy, or other symptoms consistent with catheter sepsis, blood cultures should be drawn, prophylactic broad-spectrum antimicrobial therapy should be initiated through the catheter, and the patient should be hospitalized or monitored closely until catheter infection has been either confirmed or excluded. Bacterial infections often resolve with aggressive antibiotic therapy, whereas fungal infections invariably necessitate catheter removal.

Small bowel bacterial overgrowth is a major complicating factor in most infants and children with short bowel syndrome. Normally, the proximal small intestine contains about 10^3 bacteria per milliliter, rising to much greater levels in the ileum and colon. Gastric acid, antegrade peristalsis, and the presence of the ileocecal valve all help to reduce exposure of the small intestine to excess bacterial load. Many of these protective mechanisms are disrupted in patients with short bowel syndrome. The accumulation of more aggressive bacterial species, which can cause chronic mucosal injury [12], and degradation or deconjugation of bile acids, resulting in increased bile acid absorption and decreased bile acid availability, all contribute to worsen malabsorption.

Bacterial overgrowth should be suspected in any child who has a dilated small bowel with poor motility [12]. Screening often is done by using glucose breath hydrogen testing and looking for an early peak in breath hydrogen concentration following administration of an oral glucose load. Glucose is preferable to lactulose or lactose in looking for proximal small bowel overgrowth, because it is normally rapidly absorbed in the jejunum. Alternatively, one can measure the presence of indican in the urine or look for an elevation of D-lactate in the serum, both of which suggest the presence of bacterial overgrowth. Many intestinal bacteria produce both D- and L-lactate, but D-lactate is not metabolized by humans; consequently, its buildup in the bloodstream can result in a variety of neurologic symptoms including ataxia, disorientation, and even coma. Treatment with broad-spectrum antibiotics, either for the first 5 days of each month or continuously on a rotating basis, often is necessary.

Bacterial flora are important for the normal functioning of the intestine, and killing all of the bacteria in the small bowel by the frequent use of potent broad-spectrum antibiotics is neither realistic nor wise. Consequently, the concept of probiotics as a means of treating small bowel bacterial overgrowth is emerging. Probiotics are bacteria that do not produce mucosal inflammation, may actually stimulate gut-immune defenses against the more pathogenic bacteria, and attach to the small bowel and colonic mucosa, thereby prohibiting attachment of other more aggressive pathogenic organisms. Recent experience in the use of these organisms has been promising [13].

Nutritional deficiency states are common in patients with short bowel syndrome once they have been weaned from parenteral nutrition. During the parenteral nutrition phase, patients often are carefully monitored for nutritional deficiency states, even though they are given presumably adequate amounts of nutrients parenterally. Monitoring often ceases once the patient is off parenteral nutrition; paradoxically, this is the time most patients are likely to develop nutrition deficiency states. Such deficiencies are especially likely to occur with micronutrients, including the fat-soluble vitamins A, D, E, and K; vitamin B_{12}; and certain minerals such as zinc, calcium, and magnesium. Periodic monitoring should be routine in the first 1 to 2 years after parenteral nutrition has been stopped.

The administration of trophic hormones has been proposed as a way to enhance gut adaptation in patients with short bowel syndrome. Despite initial evidence that glutamine and growth hormone could aid gut adaptation in patients with short bowel syndrome, this combination recently has been shown to be only minimally effective in both humans and animal models [14,15]. It is unlikely that pharmacologic stimulation of adaptation will do much more than the appropriate and aggressive use of well-designed and well-constructed chemically defined enteral feeding solutions.

INTESTINAL TRANSPLANTATION

The prognosis of short bowel syndrome has improved markedly in recent years, primarily because of advances in enteral nutrition support and parenteral nutrition, and a reduction in the development of parenteral nutrition–induced liver disease through the use of aggressive enteral feedings. Nonetheless, irreversible liver disease poses a major problem for many of the infants with short bowel syndrome, and certain children are not good candidates for long-term parenteral nutrition. Intestinal transplantation has been advocated for such patients, and recent experience, although limited, has had favorable results [16•].

Two large series of patients have recently been studied in the United States. The largest reported experience is at the University of Pittsburgh and comprises 71 patients, approximately half of whom were children [17••]. After 2 years, about 50% of the patients were still alive. Patients who died generally did so because of sepsis, Eptein-Barr virus (EBV)–induced lymphoproliferative disease associated with aggressive immunosuppression, or a variety of other postoperative problems. A comparable series at the University of Nebraska containing 41 children and 8 adults has demonstrated a 1-year actuarial survival of 67% in combined liver–bowel transplant patients and 93% in patients with isolated intestinal transplant [18•]. Long-term survival in the combined group was similar to that observed in the Pittsburgh patients—slightly over 50%. However, the isolated bowel transplant patients fared much better than did the combined group, with long-term survival near 90%. The isolated bowel transplant patients were generally healthier at the time of transplantation, required shorter hospitalizations, and were off parenteral and continuous enteral nutrition faster than their combined liver–bowel counterparts. Few patients in the Nebraska series developed EBV-induced lymphoproliferative disease, and the most common cause of death was sepsis. Rejection was a common problem, occasionally occurring more than a year after transplantation, although most episodes of rejection occurred earlier, during the first year.

Currently, most active centers would advocate combined liver–bowel transplantation for patients with irreversible, progressive, parenteral nutrition–induced liver disease. Isolated intestinal transplants are offered to patients who are not able to be maintained on chronic parenteral nutrition because of recurrent catheter sepsis, early but reversible liver disease, or loss of adequate central venous access following multiple catheter removals. Three patients at the University of Nebraska have had total reversal of preoperative bilirubin levels that exceeded 10 mg/dL following isolated intestinal transplant for early parenteral nutrition–induced liver disease.

Intestinal transplantation ultimately may change our approach to patients with short bowel syndrome. A major problem with donor supply and a lack of awareness of organ donation continues to frustrate members of transplant teams. Results have continued to improve with better immunosuppression, recognition of complications, and better definition of appropriate candidates for intestinal transplantation.

REFERENCES

Recently published papers of particular interest have been highlighted as follows:
• Of interest
•• Of outstanding interest

1.•• Vanderhoof JA, Langnas AN, Pinch LW, *et al.*: Short bowel syndrome. *J Pediatr Gastroenterol Nutr* 1992, 14:359–370.

2.•• Alert J, Jeejeebhoy KN: Nutrition support and therapy in the short bowel syndrome. *Gastroenterol Clin North Am* 1989, 18:589–601.

3. Caniano DA, Starr J, Ginn-Pease ME: Extensive short bowel syndrome in neonates: outcome in the 1980s. *Surgery* 1989, 105:119–124.

4. Cooper A, Floyd TX, Rosos AJ, *et al.* : Morbidity and mortality of short bowel syndrome acquired in infancy: an update. *J Pediatr Surg* 1984, 10:711–718.

5. Lennard-Jones JE: Review article: practical management of the short bowel. *Aliment Pharmacol Ther* 1994, 8:563–577.

6. Morin CL, Grey VL, Garolfo C: Influence of lipids on intestinal adaptation after resection. In *Mechanism of Intestinal Adaptation. Proceedings of an International Congress.* Edited by Robinson JWL, Dowling RH, Reicken EO. Lancaster: NTP Press; 1982:175–185.

7. Nightingale JM, Kamm MA, van-der-sijp JR, *et al.* : Disturbed gastric emptying in the short bowel syndrome: evidence for a "colonic brake". *Gut* 1993. 34:1171–1176.

8. Gracey M: The contaminated small bowel syndrome: pathogenesis, diagnosis, and treatment. *Am J Clin Nutr* 1979, 32:234–243.

9. Nordgaard I, Hansen BS, Mortensen PB: Colonic fermentation of complex dietary carbohydrates in short bowel patients: no association with hydrogen excretion and fecal and plasma short-chain fatty acids. *Scand J Gastroenterol* 1995, 30:897–904.

10.• Moukarzel AA, Haddad I, Ament ME, *et al.*: 230 patient years of experience with home long-term parenteral nutrition in childhood: natural history and life of central venous catheters. *J Pediatr Surg* 1994, 29:1323–1327.

11. Burnes JU, O'Keefe SJD, Fleming CR, *et al.*: Home parenteral nutrition —a 3-year analysis of clinical and laboratory monitoring. *JPEN J Parenter Enteral Nutr* 1992, 16:327–332.

12. Vanderhoof JA: Diarrheal disease in infants and children. In *Pediatric GI Problems*. Edited by Hyman PE. *Gastroenterology and Hepatology: The Comprehensive Visual Reference*, vol 4. Edited by Feldman M. Philadelphia: Current Medicine; 1997:6.1–6.17.

13. Vanderhoof JA, Young RL: Use of probiotics in childhood gastrointestinal disorders. *J Pediatr Gastroenterol Nutr* 1998, in press.

14. Bryne TA, Morrissey TB, Nattakom TV, *et al.*: Growth hormone, glutamine, and a modified diet enhance nutrient absorption in patients with severe short bowel syndrome. *JPEN J Parenter Enteral Nutr* 1995, 19:296–302.

15. Vanderhoof JA, Kollman KA, Griffin SK, Adrian TE: Growth hormone and glutamine do not stimulate intestinal adaptation following massive small bowel resection in the rat. *J Pediatr Gastroenterol Nutr* 1997, 25:327–331.

16.• Vanderhoof JA: Short bowel syndrome in children and small intestinal transplantation. *Pediatric Clin North Am* 1996, 43:533–550.

17.•• Todo S, Reyes J, Furukawa H, *et al.* : Outcome analysis of 71 clinical intestinal transplantations. *Ann Surg* 1995, 222:270–282.

18.• Langnas AN, Shaw BW, Antonson DL, *et al.* : Preliminary experience with intestinal transplantation in infants and children. *Pediatrics* 1996. 97:443–448.

165 Intestinal Polyps in Childhood
Joseph F. Fitzgerald

Polyps in children, as in adults, are classified as nonneoplastic or neoplastic (Table 165-1). Nonneoplastic polyps are either inflammatory or hamartomatous, whereas neoplastic polyps are adenomatous. Most polyps in children are isolated inflammatory (juvenile) polyps, and the problem can be resolved easily. In the child from a family with a genetic predisposition for malignant polyps, however, evaluation and management pose significant problems. The gastroenterologist who usually treats adults must be aware of management concerns for the child from a family at risk. The affected parent should be urged to seek appropriate counseling from a pediatric gastroenterologist with regard to pediatric surveillance.

EPIDEMIOLOGY

Isolated inflammatory polyps (juvenile polyps) account for over 90% of polyps in children. They usually occur in the first decade of life, with a peak incidence between 3 and 4 years of age, and seldom are seen in adolescence. It is estimated that inflammatory polyps can be found in 1% of preschool- or school-aged children. There is a male predominance. Mestre has observed that 50% of children with juvenile polyps have more than one polyp identified by colonoscopy and that 60% of these polyps are located proximal to the rectosigmoid [1•].

Adenomatous polyps, whether single or multiple, have the same premalignant potential in children that they have in adults. Isolated adenomatous polyps are found in children from families with hereditary nonpolyposis colon cancer (HNPCC) and Turcot syndrome, and multiple adenomatous polyps occur in children with relatives who have familial adenomatous polyposis coli or Gardner's syndrome. With the advent of genetic screening for familial adenomatous polyposis coli and Gardner's syndrome, children at risk are becoming somewhat easier to identify. A history of a first-degree relative who developed HNPCC under the age of 50 years or a family history of a malignant polyposis syndrome is a clear indication for surveillance of a child.

PATHOGENESIS

Inflammatory polyps are composed of well-differentiated mature epithelial cells without cellular atypia. Cysts within the polyp are filled with mucin. Cellular migration from the base of the crypt is slower than normal, suggesting that polyps are formed via abnormal detachment of mature cells from the surface. In addition to the glandular proliferation there is acute and chronic inflammation.

The pathogenesis of adenomatous polyps in children is probably the same as that in adults (see Chapter 84).

Table 165-1. Pediatric Tumors of the Gastrointestinal Tract

Benign	Malignant
Polyps	—
Nonneoplastic	—
Juvenile	—
Hamartomatous	—
Inflammatory fibroid	—
Lymphoid	Lymphomas
Neoplastic	—
Adenomatous	Carcinomas
	Nonfamilial
	Familial
	Polyposis
	Nonpolyposis
Nonpolypoid	—
Mesenchymatous	—
Lipomas	—
Angiomas	—
Leiomyomas	Leiomyosarcomas
Neurogenic	—
Neurofibromas	Neurosarcomas
Ganglioneuromas	—

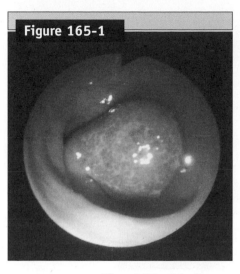

Figure 165-1

Endoscopic photograph of a large (2.5 cm) juvenile polyp encountered in a boy aged 3 years. See also **Color Plate**.

symptoms recur. The child with four or more inflammatory polyps probably should be re-endoscoped in 18 to 24 months. A family history of any type of polyposis is probably an indication to re-endoscope the patient with even one juvenile polyp in 18 to 24 months.

JUVENILE POLYPOSIS

Juvenile polyposis coli is characterized by multiple inflammatory polyps in the colon, in contrast to generalized juvenile polyposis, in which polyps may be found anywhere in the gastrointestinal tract.

Juvenile Polyposis Coli

Painless rectal bleeding and rectal prolapse (Fig. 165-3) in the first decade of life are the most common clinical features of juvenile polyposis coli. Treatment poses a significant dilemma. Although uncommon, these polyps may contain mixed juvenile adenomatous elements, creating malignant potential. There is no pharmacologic treatment. Prophylaxis against malignancy warrants subtotal colectomy (Fig. 165-4) with an ileorectal anastomosis and frequent endoscopic surveillance of the retained rectum. This disease appears to be autosomal dominant

CLINICAL FEATURES

Painless hematochezia usually is the sole presenting symptom of solitary inflammatory polyps. The blood usually is bright red, but it may be somewhat darker if the polyp is located proximally in the colon or if transit time is delayed. Bleeding seldom is significant enough to decrease the hemoglobin, and vital signs remain unchanged. When a polyp has sloughed, bleeding may become more brisk and significant.

Abdominal pain is unusual unless the colonic wall is distorted and pulled as the polyp is dragged by the colonic contents. Prolapse is most likely if the polyp is within reach of the examining finger on rectal examination, but it also may occur if the polyp is situated more proximally in the left colon. Inflammatory polyps in children almost never cause intestinal obstruction.

In situ, the inflammatory polyp is deep red in color and usually is attached to the mucosa by a stalk. The surface is either smooth or lobulated, and ulcerations with exudate are common (Fig. 165-1, see also **Color Plate**). The histologic features are shown in Figure 165-2.

TREATMENT

Isolated juvenile polyps on a stalk should be snared and excised endoscopically. Sessile polyps should be biopsied. If the tissue cannot be captured at colonoscopy, a lavage solution can be infused via nasogastric tube after colonoscopy to retrieve the specimen. If the child is discharged from the hospital before the tissue has been retrieved, the family should be given a container with formalin to preserve tissue that may be passed rectally.

Indications for recolonoscopy of the child with inflammatory polyps remain unclear. Most pediatric gastroenterologists do not reexamine a child with less than four juvenile polyps unless

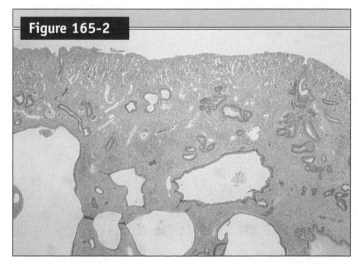

Figure 165-2

Microscopic photograph reveals the classic features of a juvenile polyp—dilated glands with a stroma densely packed with acute and chronic inflammatory cells ($\times 1$).

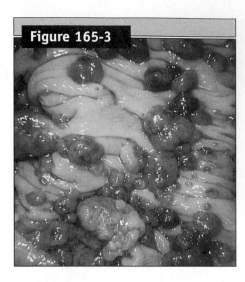

Figure 165-3
Prolapsed rectum of a girl aged 15 years with juvenile polyposis coli.

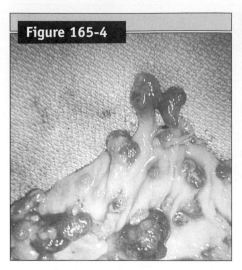

Figure 165-4
Fresh surgical specimen from the colon of a boy aged 5 years with juvenile polyposis coli.

with high penetrance. A candidate tumor suppressor gene (GP1) on the long arm of chromosome 10 (10Q22.3) has been identified [2] , but genetic testing for this abnormality is not yet available.

Generalized Juvenile Polyposis

In generalized juvenile polyposis, polyps are found throughout the gastrointestinal tract [3•]. Symptoms include hemorrhage, intussusception, hypoalbuminemia, diarrhea, electrolyte abnormalities, and failure to thrive. There is an increased risk of adenoma and adenocarcinoma. Because of the wide distribution of these lesions, surveillance and treatment are determined by the site of each lesion, and complete resolution is difficult to achieve.

Juvenile Polyposis of Infancy

Symptoms of juvenile polyposis of infancy include bloody diarrhea, anemia, failure to thrive, and increased susceptibility to infection. Several congenital anomalies, including macrocephaly and digital malformations, are associated with juvenile polyposis. This is a life-threatening condition complicated by protein-

losing enteropathy, malnutrition, and intussusception, and death has been reported in 80% of affected children.

■ OTHER CONDITIONS ASSOCIATED WITH INTESTINAL POLYPS

Cronkhite-Canada syndrome, described in Chapter 84, is exceedingly rare in children.

Recently, inflammatory cloacogenic polyps have been described at the anorectal junction in three children who presented with severe tenesmus and hematochezia [4•] (Fig. 165-5, see also **Color Plate**). The histologic characteristics are demonstrated in Figure 165-6. The pathogenesis of these polyps is unclear, but they may be due to mucosal ischemia with prolapse of the rectal mucosa.

■ HAMARTOMATOUS POLYPS

Peutz-Jeghers syndrome. Peutz-Jeghers syndrome consists of hamartomatous polyps and mucocutaneous melanotic pigmentation of the lips (Fig. 165-7, see also **Color Plate**), perioral region, and buccal mucosa [3•]. This syndrome has an autosomal dominant inheritance, and the responsible genes have not yet been identified.

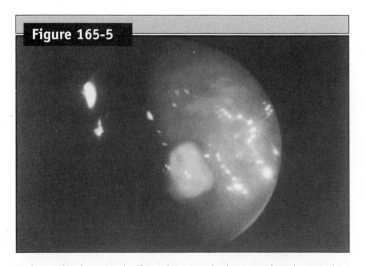

Figure 165-5

Endoscopic photograph of a pale, smooth cloacogenic polyp on the rectal floor of a girl aged 12 years with tenesmus and anorectal bleeding. See also **Color Plate**. (*Courtesy of* M.S. Murphy, MD., and the *Journal of Pediatrics.*)

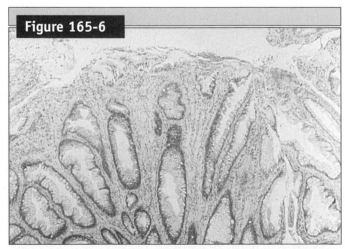

Figure 165-6

Microscopic photograph of the cloacogenic polyp shown in Figure 165-5 demonstrating disorganization of the muscularis mucosae with upward extension of muscle fibers into the lamina propria (× 10). (*Courtesy of* M.S. Murphy, M.D., and the *Journal of Pediatrics.*)

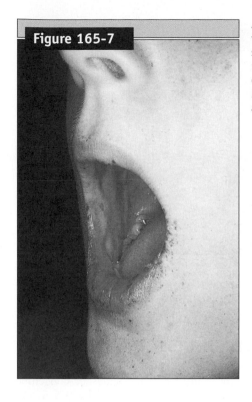

Figure 165-7

A girl aged 13 years with Peutz-Jeghers syndrome and melanotic "freckles" on her lips and buccal mucosa. See also **Color Plate**.

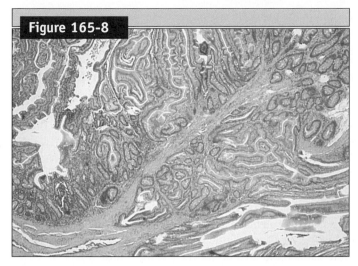

Figure 165-8

Microscopic photograph of a small bowel polyp with tall thin villi lined by tall columnar and goblet cells from a patient with Peutz-Jeghers syndrome. The underlying muscularis extends to the superficial mucosa, and glands penetrate into the stalk (× 10).

The syndrome usually is suspected following referral to a dermatologist. Imaging studies and endoscopy may reveal polyps in the stomach, small intestine, or colon.

Gastrointestinal symptoms and signs usually appear in adolescence and include abdominal pain and vomiting, with intussusception and rectal bleeding. Polypoid lesions also have been noted in the respiratory tract, gallbladder (see Chapter 181), and urinary tract.

Endoscopically, these lesions may resemble a villous adenoma. The histologic features of these polyps are illustrated in Figure 165-8. The adenomatous changes described in these polyps in adults are exceedingly rare in children. The number of polyps encountered, as well as the extensive distribution of these lesions, makes surveillance for malignant transformation exceedingly difficult. Several malignant extraintestinal tumors have been described, including malignancies of the breast, ovaries, and testes. Regular breast examination, testicular examination, and gynecologic cancer screening are recommended.

Treatment of existing polyps has not yet been well delineated. Patients with intussusception should have the responsible polyps excised either endoscopically or operatively.

Cowden's disease (Multiple Hamartoma syndrome). Cowden's disease is an autosomal dominant disorder characterized by hamartomatous polyps of the gastrointestinal tract and orocutaneous hamartomas. It usually presents between ages 10 and 30 years. There have been no reported malignancies in children, but neoplasms of the breast and thyroid occur in affected adult women.

Polypoid ganglion neuromatosis. Polypoid ganglion neuromatosis is an extremely rare, sporadic disease that results in hamartomatous polyps of the large colon and rectal bleeding. Controversy exists as to whether polypoid ganglion neuromatosis represents a subset of patients with von Recklinghausen's disease.

Ruvalcaba-Myhre-Smith disease. Ruvalcaba-Myhre-Smith disease is an autosomal dominant disease characterized by hamartomatous polyps of the small and large intestine as well as increased birth weight, mental retardation, central nervous system and facial anomalies, penile pigmentation, ophthalmologic anomalies, and a lipid storage myopathy. The polyps are associated with rectal bleeding and intussusception of the small intestine. Surgery is necessary only for intussusception.

Inflammatory fibroid polyps (Devon Family syndrome). Inflammatory fibroid polyps occur in children as young as 3 years of age but are quite rare. Polyps may occur throughout the gastrointestinal tract and small bowel and may cause intussusception.

LYMPHOID POLYPS

Lymphoid polyps represent a benign reactive process of the lymphoid tissue of the gastrointestinal tract, characterized by an increase in the size of the normal follicles of the lamina propria and submucosa. These follicles contain a polyclonal cell population and are covered by an attenuated, nonulcerated mucosa. They appear as nodules varying in size or as polypoid masses. Focal lymphoid hyperplasia without dysgammaglobulinemia commonly is found in the small and large intestines in children. Nodular lymphoid hyperplasia with dysgammaglobulinemia may be seen in late-onset hypogammaglobulinemia, characterized by diarrhea with steatorrhea, decreased serum IgG, and normal, decreased, or absent IgA and IgM in various combinations. Treatment is directed against associated complications such as infection.

Nodular lymphoid hyperplasia also may be seen with selective IgA deficiency complicated by chronic diarrhea and abdominal pain, recurrent fever, steatorrhea, *Giardia lamblia* infection, and hepatosplenomegaly.

Recently, a boy aged 11 years with a giant hyperplastic lymphoid polyp of the right colon was described. Clinically, his symptoms included intermittent crampy right lower quadrant pain and weight loss. A 4.5 cm submucosal lobular mass was noted in the proximal ascending colon and was excised. Pathology revealed normal lymphoid aggregates. The patient became asymptomatic after the polyp was excised [5].

NEOPLASTIC (ADENOMATOUS) POLYPS

Isolated adenomatous polyps are seen in children with a family history of hereditary nonpolyposis colon cancer and Turcot syndrome [6••]. Multiple adenomatous polyps are seen in familial adenomatous polyposis coli and Gardner's syndrome. Colorectal adenocarcinoma is extremely rare in the pediatric age group, with an estimated incidence of 0 to 2 per million individuals younger than 20 years of age [7]. Recently, studies have shown that familial adenomatous polyposis coli, Gardner's syndrome, and Turcot syndrome are all manifestations of the adenomatous polyposis coli (APC) gene. Data indicate that the APC gene is caused by a germ line mutation located on the long arm of chromosome 5 in band q21. Genetic testing for the APC gene is commercially available.

Hereditary nonpolyposis colon cancer. The characteristics of hereditary nonpolyposis colon cancer (HNPCC) in adults are described in Chapter 84. Although clinical diagnosis has traditionally required that three first-degree relatives be affected with colorectal cancer in two or more generations, with one of those being younger than 50 years of age, there is considerable concern among pediatric gastroenterologists that this definition may exclude children and adolescents at risk for colorectal cancer. Many pediatric gastroenterologists feel that all children with a parent younger than 50 years of age with colorectal cancer should be screened for this disease. Children with HNPCC may have adenocarcinoma of the colon by age 14 years [8]. Therefore, colonoscopy should be undertaken by at least age 10 or 11 years in the predisposed individual. In the future, genetic screening may determine which children need colonoscopic surveillance.

Turcot syndrome is a rare autosomal recessive disorder described in young adults with tumors of the brain and spinal cord. Recently, a girl aged 17 years with Turcot syndrome has been described in detail [9].

Familial adenomatous polyposis coli and Gardner's syndrome. Familial adenomatous polyposis coli and Gardner's syndrome are described in detail in Chapter 84. Children are at risk for hepatoblastoma and for adenocarcinoma of the colon by 10 to 11 years of age. The presence of mutations in the APC gene in the affected adult allows for screening of children to determine who is at risk and should undergo surveillance colonoscopies [10]. When the affected adult does not have the APC gene, children potentially at risk should be endoscopically examined starting at about age 10 years. Pigmentation of the retinal epithelium also should be considered a risk factor for Gardner's syndrome in children (Fig. 165-9). This pigmentation may be present in children even as young as 5 years of age.

In the past, treatment for adenomatous polyposis has been surgical extirpation of the colon with either an ileorectal anastomosis and subsequent surveillance or an ileal pouch anal anastomosis (IPAA). Recently, it has been observed that sulindac, a nonsteroidal anti-inflammatory medication, may cause regression of colonic adenomatous polyps [11]. Whether sulindac will prove effective in eliminating all malignant potential from these lesions

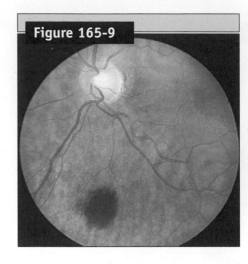

Figure 165-9 Retinoscopic photograph demonstrating congenital hypertrophy of retinal pigment epithelium (CHRPE). (*Courtesy of* F.D. Ellis, MD)

remains to be seen. Patients receiving sulindac as an alternative to total colectomy should be followed by frequent endoscopic surveillance of the retained colon with appropriate biopsies.

ACKNOWLEDGMENTS

The author expresses his deepest gratitude to Dr. Forest D. Ellis, who provided the ophthalmologic slides of congenital hypertrophy of retinal pigment epithelium (CHRPE); to Dr. Jay L. Grosfeld, who provided slides of fresh surgical specimens; to Dr. Phillip Faught, who provided the histologic photographs; and to my devoted secretary, Ms. Vicki Haviland, for her expert attention to the manuscript.

REFERENCES

Recently published papers of particular interest have been highlighted as follows:
• 	Of interest
•• 	Of outstanding interest

1.• 	Mestre JR: The changing pattern of juvenile polyps. *Am J Gastroenterol* 1986, 81:312.
In this report the author retrospectively reviewed all children managed at his institution with colon polyps between the years 1974 and 1984. There were changes in both number and location of the colon polyps during the period reviewed. This report supports a recommendation to perform complete colonoscopy in patients with painless, intermittent hematochezia.

2. 	Jacoby RF, Schlack S, Cole CE, *et al.*: A juvenile polyposis tumor suppressor locus at 10q22 is deleted from nonepithelial cells in the lamina propria. *Gastroenterol* 1997, 112:1398–1403.

3.• 	Winter HS: Intestinal polyps. In *Pediatric Gastrointestinal Disease.* Edited by Walker WA, Durie PR, Hamilton JR, *et al.* St. Louis: Mosby-Yearbook; 1996:891–907.
This is an in-depth review of intestinal polyps in children.

4.• 	Poon KKH, Mills S, Booth IW, Murphy MS: Inflammatory cloacogenic polyp: an unrecognized cause of hematochezia and tenesmus in childhood. *J Pediatr* 1997, 130:327–329.
The authors described three pediatric-age patients with cloacogenic polyps. These lesions are frequently recognized in adult patients, but they have not been diagnosed or sought in pediatric patients with severe tenesmus and bloody, mucoid stools. This study reminds all endoscopists who evaluate children to examine the rectal floor in such patients.

5. 	Mones RL, Hilfer C, Holgersen L, *et al.*: Giant hyperplastic lymphoid polyp of the intestine: a rare polypoid lesion in childhood. *J Pediatr Gastroenterol Nutr* 1995, 20:112–114.

6.•• 	Giardiello FM, Petersen GM, Piantadosi S, *et al.*: APC gene mutations and extraintestinal phenotype of familial adenomatous polyposis. *Gut* 1997, 40:521–525.

This study of 475 familial adenomatous polyposis patients from 51 families demonstrates that the classical germ line mutation of the APC gene on chromosome 5Q predisposes affected individuals to the development of the extraintestinal manifestations of APC.

7. Winawer SJ, Zauber AG, Gerdes H, *et al.*: Risk of colorectal cancer in the families of patients with adenomatous polyps. *N Engl J Med* 1996, 334:82–87.

8. Markowitz J, Aiges H, Rundles SC, *et al.*: Cancer family syndrome: marker studies. *Gastroenterol* 1986, 91:581–589.

9. Shalon L, Markowitz J, Bialer M, *et al.*: Ovarian neoplasm and endometrioid carcinoma in a patient with Turcot syndrome. *J Pediatr Gastroenterol Nutr* 1997, 25:224–227.

10. Bala S, Wunsch PH, Ballhausen WG: Childhood hepatocellular adenoma in familial adenomatous polyposis: mutations in adenomatous polyposis coli gene and p53. *Gastroenterol* 1997, 112:919–922.

11. Peleg II, Lubin MF, Cotsonis GA, *et al.*: Long-term use of nonsteroidal antiinflammatory drugs and other chemopreventors and risk of subsequent colorectal neoplasia. *Dig Dis Sci* 1996, 41:1319–1326.

166 Meckel's Diverticulum and Duplications
William J. Byrne

■ MECKEL'S DIVERTICULUM

Meckel's diverticulum is the most frequent congenital anomaly of the gastrointestinal tract, with an incidence of 0.5% to 4% in surgical and autopsy series [1,2]. Most affected people, however, remain asymptomatic, and the lifetime risk for complications is estimated to be between 4.2% and 6.4% [3,4]. Most series report the risk to be greatest in childhood, particularly in infancy, diminishing with advancing age [3,5••]. In one study of 776 patients with Meckel's diverticulum, 115 (21%) were under the age of 1 year and 270 (49%) were between the ages of 1 and 19 years [5••]. The lesion predominates in men, with male-to-female ratios of 1.6 and 1:8 to 1 reported in Europe and the United States, and 1.75:1 in Japan [6].

Anatomy

Although Fabricius Hildanus first reported the condition in 1598, it was Johann Meckel, in 1809, who described the anatomy and embryology of the diverticulum that now bears his name. In the embryo, the midgut communicates with the yolk sac through the vitelline or omphalomesenteric duct (Fig. 166-1). During the 5th to 7th embryonic week, the omphalomesenteric duct fuses with the body stalk to form the umbilical cord. Failure of the duct to obliterate along its entire course may result in a variety of anomalies (Fig. 166-2). The most common, Meckel's diverticulum (97%), forms when the intestinal end of the duct fails to close [7]. Meckel's diverticulum may be free (74%) (Fig. 166-2*A*) or attached by fibrous bands to the umbilicus (26%) (Fig. 166-2*B* and *C*). Associated anomalies, including omphalocele, diaphragmatic hernia, gastroschisis, malrotation, and duodenal atresia, are reported in 13% of patients [5••].

The blood supply to the omphalomesenteric duct is derived from the largest ventral branch of the embryonic aorta, the omphalomesenteric artery, which surrounds the gut at the junction with the duct. In its course, the artery gives rise to two paired vitelline arteries, which course along the vitelline duct and distribute over the surface of the yolk sac. During the 5th or 6th week, one of the vitelline arteries (usually the left) disap-

pears. The other persists as the superior mesenteric artery. Persistent omphalomesenteric duct remnants are supplied by remnants of the primitive vitelline artery arising from an ileal branch of the superior mesenteric artery, or, less commonly, from the ileocolic artery. Persistence of the vitelline arteries may lead to the formation of a mesodiverticular band, which can lead to intestinal obstruction.

Meckel's diverticulum is located on the antimesenteric border of the ileum 40 to 90 cm from the ileocecal valve (Fig. 166-3). In one series of 600 patients, the average distance was reported to be 50 cm [8]. The diverticulum may be up to 5 cm in length, with a diameter of up to 2 cm. Larger lesions have been

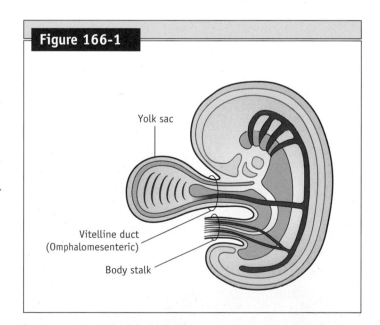

Figure 166-1

Embryo at about the 5th week of gestation. The communication between the yolk sac and the midgut narrows to become the vitelline (omphalomesenteric) duct. As the yolk sac is depleted, the omphalomesenteric duct fuses with the body stalk to form the umbilical cord.

Labels within figure: Yolk sac; Vitelline duct (Omphalomesenteric); Body stalk

Figure 166-2

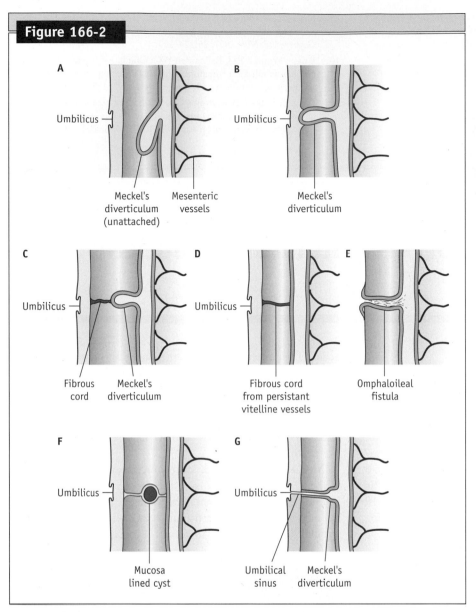

A, Unattached Meckel's diverticulum. **B**, Meckel's diverticulum persists in its entirety and is attached to the body wall. **C**, Meckel's diverticulum attached to the body wall by a fibrous cord resulting from partial involution of the omphalomesenteric duct. **D**, Complete involution of the diverticulum. Vitelline vessels persist as a fibrous cord between the ileum and umbilicus. **E**, Omphaloileal fistula resulting from a persistence of the omphalomesenteric duct. **F**, Cystic remnant of the omphalomesenteric duct. **G**, Umbilical sinus.

Figure 166-3

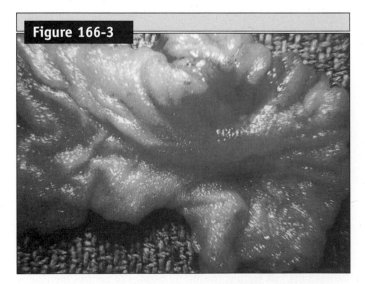

Surgical specimen revealing the typical appearance of a Meckel's diverticulum at surgery.

described and are referred to as giant Meckel's diverticula [9]. Giant Meckel's diverticulum is rare and may be either saccular or fusiform in shape. Whether the lesion is a true diverticulum or represents a segmental dilation of the ileum is unclear.

Meckel's diverticulum contains all layers of the intestinal wall. Ectopic mucosa, of gastric origin in 88% of cases, is common, with the reported incidence varying between 15% and 54% [5••,8]. Fundic glands capable of producing hydrochloric acid are present. Soderlund correlated the measured area of gastric mucosa (≥ 1.2 cm^2) with the presence of diverticular or ileal ulceration [7]. Pancreatic tissue may be found alone (in 1% to 16% of cases) or in combination with gastric mucosa (in 3% to 12% of cases). Pancreatic tissue may act as a lead point for intussusception or predispose to bowel obstruction. Rarely, colonic, duodenal, jejunal, or biliary tissue has been found in Meckel's diverticula. Because ectopic mucosa is found more frequently in symptomatic Meckel's diverticula than in those removed incidentally or discovered at autopsy, its presence is considered a risk factor for complications.

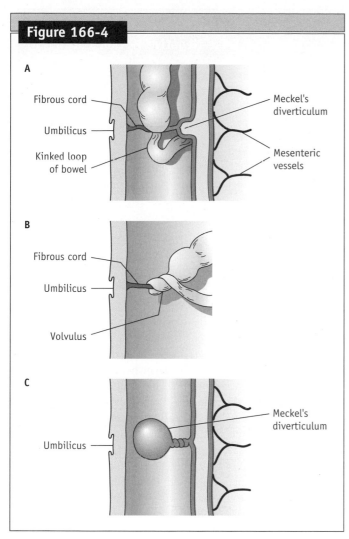

Figure 166-4

A, A loop of small bowel is kinked on a cord-like omphalomesenteric duct remnant between the umbilicus and the diverticulum. **B**, Volvulus caused by torsion of loops of bowel around the fixed point of a fibrous cord between the umbilicus and the diverticulum. **C**, The diverticulum is twisted at its base, causing obstruction and possible infarction.

Pathophysiology

Complications from the usually "silent" Meckel's diverticulum occur in three ways: obstruction (34% to 53%), hemorrhage (12% to 32%), and inflammation (13% to 31%) [5••,8,10]. Mechanisms for obstruction include kinking or volvulus due to a persistent remnant of the vitelline duct, and intussusception (Fig. 166-4). Both mechanisms are reported in children with about equal frequency [5••]. When Meckel's diverticulum inverts into the ileum, it serves as the lead point for an ileoileal intussusception.

In children under the age of 5 years, bleeding is the most common complication [11••,12]. Bleeding originates from peptic ulceration of ileal mucosa adjacent to ectopic gastric tissue in the diverticulum, or of ileal mucosa adjacent to the base of the diverticulum. *Helicobacter pylori* plays no role [13]. Bleeding may be chronic and occult, resulting in unexplained anemia. More often it is massive, resulting in maroon-colored or tarry stools. Exsanguinating hemorrhage is rare. Occasionally only

clots are passed. The hemoglobin concentration may fall by as much as 40%. In one series of children with bleeding Meckel's diverticula, the mean hemoglobin at admission was 7.5 ± 2.4 g/dL. Sixty-seven percent of patients required at least one unit of blood.

Meckel's diverticulum may become inflamed. A postulated mechanism involves peptic ulceration of the mucosa, followed by bacterial invasion. Extension of the process may lead to necrosis and perforation. As with the appendix, obstruction of the lumen may result in increased pressure with decreased tissue perfusion, tissue acidosis, and bacterial invasion of the wall. Obstruction has been reported in association with foreign bodies [5••].

When Meckel's diverticulum enters into an indirect inguinal hernia sac, it is known as Littre's hernia. Usually located on the right side, this uncommon complication (2% to 5%) can lead to strangulation [8,10]. Neoplasms within a Meckel's diverticulum are rare in children but account for up to 3% of the complications in adults [8]. Benign tumors include leiomyomas, angiomas, neuromas, and lipomas. Carcinoid tumors, the most common malignancy, tend to resemble ileal carcinoids in their biologic behavior [14]. By the time symptoms are present, 77% of these tumors have already metastasized. Crohn's disease affecting a Meckel's diverticulum has been reported in older patients.

Clinical Features

Signs and symptoms in patients under the age of 18 years include abdominal pain, gastrointestinal bleeding, or both. The anomaly predominates in males, and males also are more likely than females to become symptomatic, by a ratio of 2.7:1 [5••]. Abdominal pain that is severe, colicky, and located in the periumbilical region suggests obstruction. Bilious vomiting may not occur until late in the course. Signs of an acute abdomen, a toxic appearance, and acidosis suggest intestinal ischemia, perhaps secondary to a volvulus. Colicky pain associated with the passage of maroon-colored or "currant jelly" stool, and the finding of a mass on physical examination are consistent with intestinal obstruction caused by intussusception.

The acute onset of painless rectal bleeding of sufficient volume to decrease the hemoglobin by 2 g/dL or more warrants investigation for Meckel's diverticulum. The stools are typically maroon in color and contain more blood than fecal matter. The absence of pain, along with other symptoms such as diarrhea, fever, or weight loss, makes other causes such as infectious enteritis, inflammatory bowel disease, or peptic ulcer disease unlikely. The acute volume loss is inconsistent with juvenile polyps or formula protein intolerance in infants. Vascular lesions are rare in children. The identification or past history of hemangiomata or blue rubber bleb nevi on the skin suggests that similar lesions may be present in the gastrointestinal tract. Although Meckel's diverticulum may lead to occult blood loss, this presentation is uncommon.

Meckel's diverticulitis presents in a fashion very similar to that of appendicitis. Symptoms begin with poorly localized periumbilical pain. In younger children, localization to the right lower quadrant may not occur. Symptoms usually are progressive, but may resolve. A perforated Meckel's diverticulum is

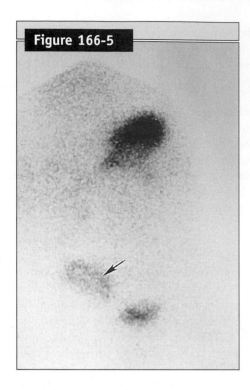

Figure 166-5

Positive Meckel's scan shows a collection of the isotope in the right lower quadrant (*arrow*).

Table 166-1. Causes for Either False-Positive or False-Negative Meckel's Scan
False-Positive Scan
Ectopic gastric tissue in other locations (*eg*, duplication, Barrett's esophagus)
Hydronephrosis, hydroureter, pelvic kidney
Inflammatory bowel disease
Abdominal abscess
Arteriovenous malformation
Tumors (lymphoma, hemangioma, sarcoma, carcinoid)
False-Negative Scan
Absence of gastric tissue
Insufficient gastric tissue
Dilution from hemorrhage
Poorly functioning gastric tissue due to ischemia or necrosis

potentially more serious than a perforated appendix because it does not "wall off." Signs of diffuse peritonitis, including pneumoperitoneum on abdominal radiographs, may prevail.

Diagnosis
Plain Abdominal Radiographs
In the patient with symptoms of obstruction, plain radiographs are not specific, and show only dilated loops of bowel and air–fluid levels. Rarely, Meckel's diverticulitis produces gas and fluid levels in the cecum.

Sonography
Ultrasound may be used to identify Meckel's diverticulum as the lead point of an intussusception. Itagaki and coworkers described the identification of two "target signs" of different sizes as a characteristic sonographic finding [15]. This finding is caused by the intussusception of the Meckel's diverticulum into the ileum, and of the ileum into the colon through the ileocecal valve.

Nuclear Medicine
For children who present with lower gastrointestinal bleeding, the most accurate test for the diagnosis of Meckel's diverticulum is ^{99m}Tc pertechnetate scintigraphy (Fig. 166-5). ^{99m}Tc pertechnetate is preferentially taken up by the mucus-secreting cells of the gastric mucosa and ectopic mucosa in the diverticulum. Stakianakis and Conway reported results of scintigraphy in 954 patients with Meckel's diverticulum, most of whom were children [16•]. Scintigraphy had a sensitivity of 85%, a specificity of 95%, and an accuracy of 90%. Cooney and coworkers reported similar results in children [17]. In contrast, adult studies show much lower sensitivity and accuracy rates. These disparities are attributed to the decreased presence of ectopic gastric tissue in patients over 30 years of age. Potential causes of false-positive and false-negative Meckel's scans are shown in Table 166-1.

Scan sensitivity may be increased by using pentagastrin, glucagon, or an H_2-blocker [18••]. Pentagastrin increases the metabolism of gastric tissue, enhancing radionuclide uptake. This technique has fallen out of favor because of the perceived risk of increasing gastrointestinal bleeding. Glucagon inhibits peristalsis and thereby reduces the dilution and washout of the intraluminal radionuclide. Cimetidine decreases peptic secretion but not radionuclide uptake, the result being a higher concentration of the isotope in the wall of the diverticulum. The dose for a child is 20 mg/kg before the study. Experience with ranitidine is less well documented. Repeating the study has been reported to increase the diagnostic yield [5••].

^{99m}Tc-labeled sulfur colloid or erythrocytes labeled with the same tracer may be used to evaluate the patient with gastrointestinal bleeding. However, the technique is no more sensitive than is pertechnetate in the diagnosis of Meckel's diverticulum and is less specific. To be visualized, the diverticulum must be actively bleeding at a rate of at least 0.1 ml/min, or must rebleed within 24 hours. False-negative pertechnetate scans may result if red cell labeling techniques using stannous-containing agents are done first. The pertechnetate Meckel's scan should be performed before labeled red cell imaging is done.

Barium Studies
Conventional small bowel studies are unreliable for the detection of Meckel's diverticulum. Enteroclysis may improve the yield, but it is a difficult examination to perform in children [18••]. The mainstay for the diagnosis on contrast study is the documentation of a diverticulum arising from the antimesenteric border of the distal ileum. Confirmation of the diagnosis rests on the visualization of its fold patterns, especially at the site of its attachment to the normal small intestine. A Meckel's diverticulum may sometimes be inverted, creating a polypoid filling defect in the intestinal lumen. Small bowel series should be performed only if Meckel's diverticulum is not the primary diagnosis, or if the ^{99m}Tc pertechnetate scan has been negative on two occasions with H_2-blocker enhancement.

Computed Tomography

Computed tomography (CT) is usually of little value in the diagnosis of Meckel's diverticulum because of the difficulty of distinguishing the diverticulum from intestinal loops.

Angiography

In the older child or adolescent, angiography is indicated when there is active bleeding at a rate greater than 0.5 ml/min or when scintigraphy and enteroclysis are normal. Selective superior mesenteric arteriography may allow visualization of an anomalous artery feeding the diverticulum, the presence of dense capillary staining, or extravasation of contrast material in the actively bleeding patient.

Treatment

Surgical intervention is indicated in patients who experience complications related to Meckel's diverticulum. Those whose diagnostic studies are normal may be followed-up. If symptoms recur, surgical exploration is warranted even if repeat diagnostic studies are inconclusive. With the exception of patients with intestinal obstruction or possible intestinal ischemia, laparotomy can be delayed until after the hemoglobin has been restored to near-normal levels. Patients with obstructive symptoms require rapid fluid and electrolyte resuscitation. Surgery should be expedited to obviate the development of bowel ischemia and the need for bowel resection.

It is often possible to resect the diverticulum without removing any of the ileum. Linear stapling at the base of the diverticulum allows complete amputation without narrowing the lumen. A V-shaped incision at the base of the remnant with transverse closure avoids ileal stenosis. When there is a large focus of ectopic mucosa, ulceration near the base of the diverticulum, or when the lesion has a wide base, ileal resection with end-to-end anastomosis is required. Obstructing lesions, such as an omphalomesenteric band, must be destroyed, and the involved intestine salvaged if possible. Meckel's diverticulitis, even with perforation, can be managed by resection and primary anastomosis. Laparoscopic resection of Meckel's diverticulum in children has been reported, but experience to date is very limited [19]. Laparoscopy does offer another means of diagnosis when scintigraphy is negative in a patient in whom there is a high index of suspicion.

The approach to the incidental Meckel's diverticulum is controversial in adults, and no clear-cut guidelines exist for children. At issue is the risk of operative morbidity relative to the risk of complication from the lesion. Soltero and Bill suggest that incidental removal is not justified unless obvious risk factors are present [3]. These include suspicion of ectopic mucosa on palpation, or the presence of fibrous bands to the umbilicus, mesodiverticular bands, or surrounding inflammation. Sex and age were not included.

Prognosis

Morbidity and mortality rates for Meckel's diverticulum are from 6% to 30% and 6% to 7.5%, respectively. In a recent series in of 164 children, overall morbidity and mortality were 7.3% and 1.8% [5••]. Morbidity resulted from postoperative bowel obstruction, wound infection, and paraumbilical hernia.

Mortality in this series occurred in the group in which Meckel's diverticulum was an incidental finding and was not directly related to the diverticulum.

◼◼ INTESTINAL DUPLICATION

Duplications of the gastrointestinal tract are rare congenital lesions that can occur throughout the alimentary tract. They are located adjacent to the duplicated structure, are composed of a muscular wall with a mucosal lining, and may communicate with the lumen. In 1937 Ladd proposed the term *duplication* in an attempt to simplify the nomenclature describing these anomalies [20]. The term is still accepted in the literature, even though very few of these lesions represent a true doubling of the alimentary tract.

Anatomy

The usual locations of gastrointestinal duplications are shown in Figure 166-6 [21]. Duplications may be cystic or tubular. Cystic lesions tend not to communicate with the lumen of the alimentary tract, and, therefore, enlarge as they accumulate secretions. Multiple mucosal types may be found in the same duplication. Gastric mucosa is present in up to one third of the duplications. Duplications may be associated with other congenital malformations, including vertebral anomalies, omphalocele, intestinal atresia, and malrotation. Because multiple duplications are found in up to 20% of cases, the finding of one duplication warrants a search for others elsewhere in the gastrointestinal tract.

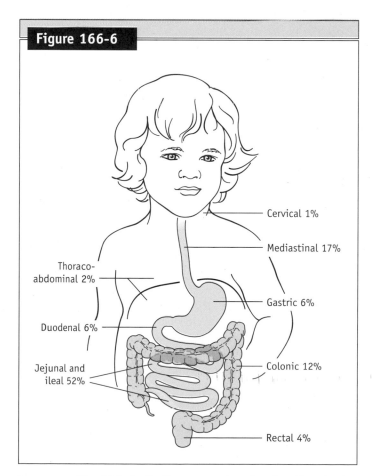

Figure 166-6

Cervical 1%
Mediastinal 17%
Thoraco-abdominal 2%
Gastric 6%
Duodenal 6%
Jejunal and ileal 52%
Colonic 12%
Rectal 4%

Frequency with which duplication occurs at various locations in the alimentary tract.

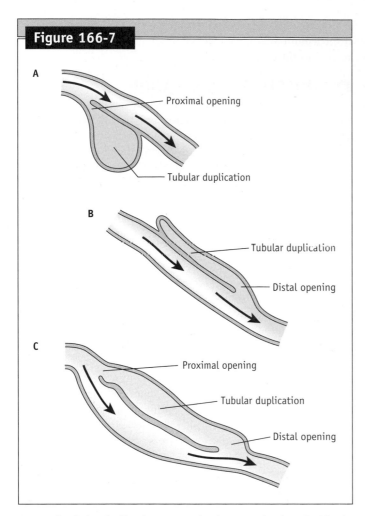

Figure 166-7

A — Proximal opening / Tubular duplication

B — Tubular duplication / Distal opening

C — Proximal opening / Tubular duplication / Distal opening

Forms of tubular duplication. **A**, Proximal communication. **B**, Distal communication. **C**, Both proximal and distal communication.

Gastric duplications usually are located along the greater curvature or on the posterior wall of the stomach. They tend to be cystic and not to communicate with the gastric lumen. Most duodenal duplications are cystic and are located posteromedial to the second or third portion of the duodenum; approximately 25% communicate with the bowel lumen. They usually contain duodenal mucosa. Fifty percent of all duplications involve the small intestine, and two thirds of these are found in the ileum. Enteric duplications are located in the mesentery. They share a common muscular wall and blood supply with the adjacent intestine. One fourth of enteric duplications are tubular. Most tubular duplications are less than 10 cm in length [22]. Communication may occur anywhere along the common wall (Fig. 166-7). If the lesion is distal, it may drain and remain asymptomatic. If the connection is proximal, the distal end of the duplication may dilate, causing obstruction or volvulus.

Colonic duplications contain normal colonic epithelium. Available evidence suggests there are three types of duplications: midline duplications, cystic remnants of the tail-gut, and bilateral duplications of the colon and rectum. Midline duplications lie posterior to the rectum and share a common wall. Tail-gut cystic remnants are located between the anus and coccyx and share no common wall with the anus or rectum. The third type of hindgut malformation, bilateral duplication, results from

a "partial twining." The duplication is located adjacent to the normal colon, rather than within the mesentery. Other hindgut structures, including the bladder, uterus, and external genitalia, may be duplicated as well. Seventy percent of these complex hindgut duplications are found in females.

No single theory adequately explains the embryologic origin of all duplications. The split notochord theory holds that very early in development a segment of the gastrointestinal endoderm herniates through the notochord and becomes an entrapped diverticulum. As the notochord migrates, it is split by the persistent neuroenteric canal, giving rise to vertebral anomalies. This mechanism may explain the 15% association of enteric duplications with vertebral defects. If the neuroenteric connection is lost, isolated mediastinal duplications result. Otherwise, a spectrum of neuroenteric pathology is possible. The median septum formation theory suggests that extrinsic compression may flatten adjacent bowel, resulting in fusion and doubling of the lumen. Failure of the complete regression of embryonic diverticula has been proposed to explain small cystic duplications. Finally, incomplete canalization of the lumen might explain the origin of submucosal duplications.

Clinical Features

Most gastric duplications present before the age of 2 years [23]. Symptoms include abdominal distention and vomiting. Weight loss is often present because of protracted vomiting. Large cysts are often palpable. Duplication should be considered in the differential diagnosis of any palpable epigastric mass. Pain may be present due to distention of the cyst or peptic ulceration. Erosion of the lesion through the diaphragm results in acute respiratory symptoms. Duplication of the pylorus presents with projectile vomiting and weight loss and is indistinguishable from pyloric stenosis.

Duodenal duplications present with symptoms of intermittent upper tract obstruction. Anemia from ulceration and bleeding may occur. Occasionally, patients present with jaundice resulting from extrinsic compression of the common bile duct.

Small bowel duplications may present either acutely in the perinatal period with signs of obstruction, or with a long indolent history of abdominal pain, abdominal distention, and, occasionally, vomiting. The lesions are difficult to palpate, with a mass noted on physical examination in less than one fourth of cases. Peptic ulceration with massive bleeding is not infrequent with small bowel duplications. Extensive evaluation often provides no apparent cause.

Colonic duplication presents with symptoms of constipation and, occasionally, obstruction. Abnormal genitalia or a mass on rectal examination should raise the index of suspicion.

Diagnosis

Ultrasound is an excellent diagnostic and screening study for enteric duplications. It allows cystic and solid abdominal masses to be distinguished and is the initial modality of choice (Fig. 166-8). The utility of a barium study depends on the size, shape, and location of the mass. When the cyst does not communicate, the barium study reveals displacement of bowel loops around a mass and possible obstruction. Tubular lesions that communicate may fill with barium, confirming the diagnosis. CT scan

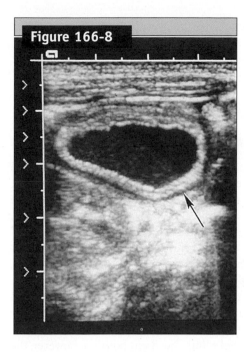

Figure 166-8

Ultrasound examination demonstrates the cystic appearance of an enteric duplication (*arrow*).

may help to clarify the displacement of the abdominal viscera and offers administration of contrast to demonstrate possible communication. CT, however, rarely provides additional information that changes the approach to therapy. Because of the high incidence of ectopic gastric tissue in duplications, technetium studies may be helpful in locating duplications in the thorax, small bowel, and hindgut.

Treatment

Most duplications are amenable to surgical repair. Correction of these anomalies should be undertaken because of the risk of bleeding or sepsis that may result from perforation. Also, malignant transformation has been reported in adults with undiagnosed duplications. The type of procedure performed depends on the size and location of the lesion. Complete excision is the procedure of choice, but when this is not possible, marsupialization or internal drainage has proven acceptable.

Prognosis

The mortality rate from duplications, independent of other anomalies, is between 8% and 10% [20,23], as reported in older series. With modern anesthetic and postoperative support techniques, mortality from this lesion should be rare.

■ REFERENCES

Recently published papers of particular interest have been highlighted as follows:
• Of interest
•• Of outstanding interest

1. Matsagas MI, Fatouros M, Koulouras B, *et al.* : Incidence, complications, and management of Meckel's diverticulum. *Arch Surg* 1995, 130:143–146.

2. Jay GD, Margulis RR, McGraw AB, *et al.*: Meckel's diverticulum: a survey of 103 cases. *Arch Surg* 1950, 61:158–169.

3. Soltero JH, Bill AH: The natural history of Meckel's diverticulum and its relation to incidental removal. *Am J Surg* 1976, 32:168–173.

4. Cullen JJ, Kelly KA, Moir CR, *et al.*: Surgical management of Meckel's diverticulum. *Ann Surg*1994, 220:565–569.

5.•• St.Vel D, Brandt ML, Panic S, *et al.*: Meckel's diverticulum in children: a 20-year review. *J Pediatr Surg* 1991, 26:1289–1292.
This is an excellent review of the topic in 164 children.

6. Hiroki K, Motofumi Y, Ikuo T, *et al.* : Complications and diagnosis of Meckel's diverticulum in 776 patients. *Am J Surg* 1992, 164:382–383.

7. Soderlund S: Meckel's diverticulum, a clinical and histologic study. *Acta Chir Scand* 1959, 248(suppl.):213–233.

8. Yamaguchi M, Takeuchi S, Awazu S: Meckel's diverticulum: investigation of 600 patients in Japanese literature. *Am J Surg* 1978, 136:247–249.

9. Koredelka J, Kralova M, Preis J: Giant Meckel's diverticulum. *J Pediatr Surg* 1992, 27:1589–1590.

10. Mackey WC, Dineen PA: A fifty year experience with Meckel's diverticulum. *Surg Gynecol Obstet* 1978, 156:56–64.

11.•• Vane DW, West KW, Grosfeld JL: Vitelline duct anomalies: experience with 217 childhood cases. *Arch Surg* 1987, 122:542–547.
This is an excellent review of the topic in 217 children.

12. Rutherford RB, Akers DR: Meckel's diverticulum: a review of 148 pediatric patients with special reference to the pattern of bleeding and to mesodiverticular bands. *Surgery* 1966, 59:618–626.

13. Bemelman WA, Bosma A, Wiersma PH, *et al.*: Role of *Helicobacter pylori* in the pathogenesis of complications of Meckel's diverticula. *Eur J Surg* 1993, 159:171–175.

14. Nies C, Zielke A, Hasse C, *et al.*: Carcinoid tumors of Meckel's diverticula. Report of two cases and review of the literature. *Dis Colon Rectum* 1992, 35:589–596.

15. Intagaki A, Uchida M, Ueki K, *et al.*: Double targets sign in ultrasonic diagnosis of intussuscepted Meckel's diverticulum. *Pediatr Radiol* 1991, 21:148–149.

16.• Stakianakis GN, Conway JJ: Detection of ectopic gastric mucosa in Meckel's diverticulum and in other aberrations by scintigraphy. *J Nucl Med* 1981, 22:647–654.
This large series reviews the utility of ^{99m}TC pertechnetate in the diagnosis of Meckel's diverticulum.

17. Cooney DR, Duszynski DO, Camboa E, *et al.* : The abdominal technetium scan (a decade of experience). *J Pediatr Surg* 1982, 17:611–619.

18.•• Rossi P, Gourtsoyiannis N, Bezzi M, *et al.* : Meckel's diverticulum: imaging diagnosis. *AJR Am J Roentgenol* 1996, 166:567–573.
This paper provides a comprehensive review of the literature regarding imaging techniques of the diagnosis of Meckel's diverticulum.

19. Teitelbaum DH, Polley TZ, Obeid F: Laparoscopic diagnosis and excision of Meckel's diverticulum. *J Pediatr Surg* 1994, 29:495–497.

20. Bower RJ, Sieber WK, Kiesewetter WB: Alimentary tract duplications in children. *Ann Surg* 1978, 188:669–674.

21. Heiss K: Intestinal duplications. In *Surgery of Infants and Children: Scientific Principles and Practice*. Edited by Oldham KT, Colombani PM, Foglia RP. Philadelphia: Lippincott-Raven; 1997:1265–1274.

22. Balen EM, Hernandez-Lizoain JL, Pardo F, *et al.*: Giant jejunoileal duplication: prenatal diagnosis and complete excision without intestinal resection. *J Pediatr Surg*1993, 28:1586–1588.

23. Grosfeld JL, O'Neill JA, Clatworthy HW: Enteric duplications in infancy and childhood: an 18-year review. *Ann Surg* 1970, 172:83–90.

167 Acute Appendicitis

Eric L. Lazar and R. Peter Altman

Acute appendicitis is the most common surgical emergency of childhood. Its presentation varies depending on the age of the child, and, accordingly, the full classic features of the history and physical examination may be absent in some children. Nonetheless, it is the features of the history and physical examination that form the basis of the clinical diagnosis. This chapter emphasizes that the diagnosis of acute appendicitis is a clinical one, and despite variations in presentation, few if any tests are required after a careful history and physical examination.

▬ ANATOMY

The classic history of acute appendicitis is that of vague periumbilical discomfort that evolves to well-localized pain and tenderness in the right lower quadrant at McBurney's point (Fig. 167-1). This progression is a consequence of the neuroanatomic pathways involved at each phase of the illness. The early, nonspecific periumbilical pain is the result of visceral afferent nerve stimulation, initiated by luminal distention of the appendix. As full-thickness mural injury develops, somatic afferents are stimulated by inflammation of the overlying parietal peritoneum. In its usual location, the appendix lies at the base of the cecum in the right lower quadrant. It is the peritoneum directly anterior to this region that becomes inflamed and defines McBurney's point. Some variations exist, however, in the location of the cecum and in the relationship of the appendix and cecum to the anterior peritoneum, that change this regional anatomy and dictate variations from the "classic" presentation. The child with malrotation and appendicitis might have pain that localizes in the right upper quadrant, where the cecum often lies in this anatomic variant (although this is a rare presentation); the child with atypical abdominal situs may have periumbilical pain that localizes to the left lower quadrant.

Even in its usual right lower quadrant position, however, the appendix may be anterior, intraperitoneal, and directed either superiorly toward the gallbladder or inferiorly into the pelvis, or may be retroileal, retrocecal, or retroperitoneal (Fig. 167-2). In the retrocecal position, the appendix is shielded from the anterior peritoneum, changing the presentation of symptoms to pain that poorly localizes to the flank region. Palpation of the right lower quadrant may not elicit guarding in this instance. Instead, irritation of the retroperitoneum overlying the psoas muscle is more likely, producing the "psoas sign", whereby extension of the right hip exacerbates the patient's pain. The appendix may lie on the ureter, with transmural inflammation accounting for the presence of white and red cells in the urine despite the absence of primary urinary pathology. Thus, the anatomic location of the appendix can alter disease presentation and result in a confusing picture in which appendicitis may masquerade as very different diagnoses (*eg*, cholecystitis or cystitis). Understanding the possible differences in regional anatomy necessarily broadens the differential diagnosis of acute abdominal pain to include appendicitis. Such an inclusive approach may lead to earlier diagnosis and the prevention of perforation and its complications [1].

Figure 167-1

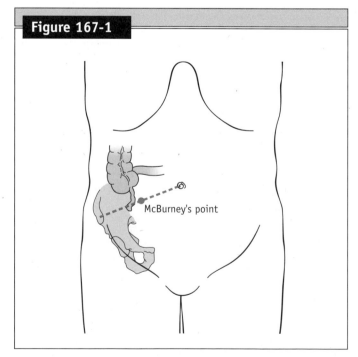

The appendix is shown here in the right lower quadrant at the cecal terminus. McBurney's point is two thirds of the way along a line drawn from the umbilicus to the anterior-superior iliac spine. This is usually the point of maximal tenderness in a patient with an anterior appendix.

Figure 167-2

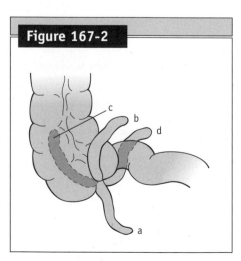

The appendix and its relationship to the cecum can vary. Two anterior positions (**a** and **b**) are demonstrated, as well as the retrocecal (**c**) and the retroileal (**d**) positions.

EPIDEMIOLOGY

The lifetime risk of appendicitis is estimated to be 7% [2], or an annual incidence of 11 cases per 10,000 persons. The pediatric age-specific incidence is 23 cases per 10,000 10- to 19-year-olds per year. Of the 200,000 appendectomies performed yearly in the United States for acute appendicitis, about half are performed in patients younger than 19 years of age.

In a recent large series of 1366 pediatric appendectomies performed in 147 hospitals, the median patient age was 12 years, with two thirds of cases falling between ages 4 and 15 years [3]. In this same series, the negative appendectomy rate was 12%, and the perforation rate was 20%. Because these figures were derived from multiple centers, they represent a standard for pediatric appendectomy.

PATHOPHYSIOLOGY

Luminal obstruction of the relatively narrow appendix by fecal material is thought to be the initiating event in the pathophysiology of acute appendicitis. The mucosal lining of the appendix continues to secrete behind the obstruction, resulting in distention and overgrowth of luminal bacteria. Eventually, luminal pressure exceeds mural pressure, causing obstruction of lymphatic and venous outflow. As venous hypertension worsens, there is progressive mural edema and transudation of fluid into the peritoneum. In this generally accepted model of uncomplicated acute appendicitis, the patient has sought medical attention, and prompt appendectomy is curative.

Unchecked, however, intraluminal pressure continues to increase and ultimately exceeds arterial inflow pressure to the appendix, resulting in ischemia and gangrene. Microscopic perforation is a common sequela. The perforated appendix may be "walled off" by nearby loops of ileum, the omentum, and the peritoneum, which contain the now-fecopurulent soilage. This abscess defines one form of complicated appendicitis. Uncontained, diffuse soilage can occur, with resulting widespread peritonitis. Perforation in this manner can progress to septicemia, multisystem organ failure, and although unusual in the uncompromised host, death.

ETIOLOGY

Although a lodged fecalith is the most common cause of obstruction, any mass or foreign body may initiate the process. Pinworms; ascaris; swallowed toothpicks, nails, screws, and pins; and tumors, including cecal or appendiceal adenocarcinoma, metastatic carcinoma, lymphoma, and carcinoid have all presented as acute appendicitis.

Luminal obstruction cannot be the only cause of appendicitis, however, because a sizable number of operative specimens do not contain an obvious offender. Local bacteriologic, viral, and inflammatory processes also must play a role in luminal obstruction, perhaps by causing hyperplasia of mucosal lymphoid tissue. The pediatric appendix is rich in lymphoid follicles, and as these become reactive, perhaps in response to a respiratory infection, mucosal congestion, edema, and obstruction ensue.

There are other causes of appendicitis as well. Cytomegalovirus infection of the appendix in the patient with human immunodeficiency virus (HIV), for example, is being diagnosed with increasing frequency. There have been reports of mild to moderate abdominal trauma leading to appendicitis [4]; the mechanism is thought to involve mesoappendiceal thrombosis. Whether the abdominal trauma is cause or coincidence is unclear. Along similar lines, there have been reports of familial appendicitis, which may reflect either polygenic transmission or a dominantly inherited anatomic variant such as a retrocecal appendix that may predispose to luminal obstruction [5].

CLINICAL FEATURES

The clinical features of acute appendicitis vary somewhat with the age of the child. Appendicitis is unusual before the age of 2 years. Early symptoms in this age group are not verbally communicated or are attributed to "the flu." Because of their poorly developed omentum, younger children do not wall off perforations, and free intraperitoneal contamination occurs more commonly than in older age groups. The young child is ill-appearing with fever and lies motionless on the examination table. In a previously well child with these features, perforated appendicitis must be considered in the differential diagnosis.

In patients over the age of 5 years, the classic features of appendicitis are seen: vague abdominal pain in the periumbilical area that localizes over a few hours to the right lower quadrant. There may be an episode or two of emesis, but this is variable. The overall appearance is that of a child who is unwell and is focused on the pain, which is constant and dull. The child will wish to remain very still, and minor movements such as bumping the examination table may intensify pain.

Of the commonly associated symptoms, anorexia (*ie*, a child refuses his or her favorite food) is a fairly reliable, albeit nonspecific, symptom for appendicitis. Nausea and vomiting, fever, and diarrhea are all well-known associated clinical features, but their presence is variable and, therefore, not reliable. Excessive vomiting should alert the clinician to gastroenteritis or, in the child with previous abdominal surgery, bowel obstruction. Low-grade fever is consistent with acute appendicitis, but patients are frequently afebrile. Diarrhea is unusual and suggests gastroenteritis, but diarrhea can also result from diffuse peritonitis or an abscess. Therefore, its presence does not exclude appendicitis from the differential diagnosis.

DIAGNOSIS

The history and physical examination are the best tools for the diagnosis. The nuances of the history and physical examination can often convey an immediate diagnosis with greater accuracy than any laboratory test or radiologic examination (Fig. 167-3).

The goal of the history is to elicit gastrointestinal complaints in the setting of abdominal pain that changes in character and location, as previously described. Further, the entire history of the illness involves only several hours to perhaps a day or two at most. Longer histories suggest that either complicated appendicitis has evolved or another diagnosis is more likely. The history begins with vague malaise and anorexia, followed by recognition of ill-defined periumbilical pain. An episode of vomiting often follows. Over four to six hours, this pain localizes, usually to the right lower quadrant. Once localized, the pain is steady and not colicky. Laughing, coughing, stairclimbing, and riding over potholes en route to the examination may all reproduce or

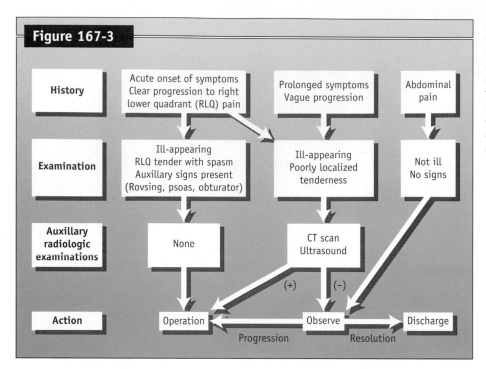

Figure 167-3

Evaluation of suspected appendicitis. The diagnosis of acute appendicitis is a clinical one. Historic and physical examination data are interpreted as either consistent with or suggestive of the diagnosis. In most cases, the need for operation can be ascertained based on the history and physical examination alone; in less clear cases, ancillary tests or continued observation is appropriate.

exacerbate the pain. If a child reports the sudden onset of right lower abdominal pain and a careful history fails to elicit any of the prodromal symptoms, appendicitis is less likely than is ovarian pathology, ureteral stone, testicular torsion, or some other explanation. It should be emphasized that appendicitis is a progressive illness and that a pattern of waxing and waning complaints usually is inconsistent with the diagnosis. Because younger children may not be able to relate an obvious, orderly progression of complaints, an extremely high index of suspicion is required. The 2- or 3-year-old, for example, may simply not feed well, appear lethargic, and wish to sleep. In older girls in the appropriate clinical setting, information about menstrual and sexual history must be obtained to exclude ectopic pregnancy or pelvic inflammatory disease.

The aim of the clinical examination is to elicit reproducible signs of right lower quadrant inflammation. Observation before examination can yield useful data. The child with appendicitis will have difficulty getting on the examination table unassisted, and once there, may lie either curled on one side or with the legs drawn up. The child will be rather still. A general physical examination should note the presence or absence of signs of upper respiratory infection. The skin should be inspected and seen to be free of hemorrhagic lesions suggestive of Henoch-Schönlein purpura or flank hemorrhages consistent with pancreatitis.

Examination of the abdomen begins with inspection for distention. Distention is unusual early in the course of appendicitis and suggests bowel obstruction or diffuse peritonitis instead. The child is asked to indicate with one finger where the pain is the greatest. If this results in prompt identification of McBurney's point, appendicitis is likely. Bowel sounds are variable but often are normal in pitch and frequency; increased bowel sounds suggest another entity, such as gastroenteritis. Palpation by gentle compression should begin away from the right lower quadrant. As the examination proceeds toward the right lower quadrant, guarding

and localized spasm will be noted. Once this is detected, the examiner should stop so as not to lose the patient's trust. Vigorous testing for peritonitis is rarely necessary—a patient lying motionless with legs drawn and localized spasm all indicate peritonitis and are sufficient to establish the diagnosis. Palpation of the left lower quadrant that produces right lower quadrant pain denotes Rovsing's sign, which is specific for right lower quadrant inflammation. The previously described psoas sign and the obturator sign (pain on external rotation of the right leg) test for an appendix that is hidden from the anterior peritoneum. In a difficult-to-diagnose appendicitis, right lower quadrant pain may be reproduced or exacerbated by having the patient jump from the examination table and repeatedly hop on the right foot. Gentle percussion of the abdomen is sufficient to elicit pain; testing for so-called "rebound peritonitis" by deep palpation and rapid release is painful and unwarranted.

Attention is then turned to the genitalia and perineum to look for a hernia, torsion, discharge, or perianal signs of inflammatory bowel disease, such as sentinel tags, an abscess, or a fistula. A pelvic examination is indicated in the adolescent or teenage girl in whom the history and physical examination strongly suggest the possibility of gynecologic infection. Rectal examination is helpful in equivocal cases but is not necessary to make the diagnosis of acute appendicitis when other clinical data suggest that this is the diagnosis. A pelvic abscess may be palpated on the right side, or presence of a fecal impaction may confirm the diagnosis of constipation. In any case, rectal examination should conclude the physical examination.

The constellation of findings from the historical and physical data usually is sufficient to render a diagnosis and warrant operation. In the vast majority of cases, complete blood counts, urine analyses, radiographs, ultrasounds, and computed tomographic (CT) scans are not needed for confirmation.

In equivocal or confusing cases, a brief period of observation is safe [6]. Within 4 to 8 hours, appendicitis usually worsens,

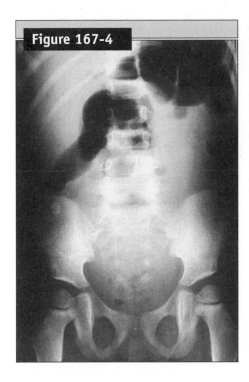

Figure 167-4

Radiograph of the abdomen shows a dense spherical opacity in the right lower quadrant overlying the iliac bone. In the setting of right lower quadrant pain, this is a significant finding. Absence of a fecalith, however, is more common.

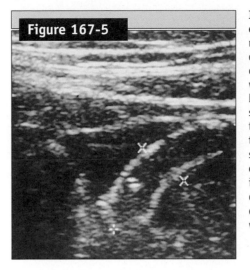

Figure 167-5

In this sonographic examination of the right lower quadrant, the layers of the abdominal wall are represented by echodense stripes at the top of the image; the thickened tubular structure with an echodense opacity in the tip clearly demonstrates a dilated appendix with a fecalith.

and the diagnosis declares itself. A demonstrably improved patient may be safely discharged. In cases that remain unclear after this period of observation, it is reasonable to perform some auxiliary tests. Each test, however, must be carefully interpreted in its own clinical context, *eg*, a urine or serum test for pregnancy is indicated in appropriate teenage patients.

Radiologic investigations can be helpful adjuncts to the history and physical examination. A plain radiograph of the abdomen might demonstrate a fecalith (Fig. 167-4). In experienced hands, graded compression ultrasound examination is 85% sensitive and 94% specific [7] and helps to delineate other causes of abdominal pain, *eg*, renal abnormalities, ovarian cysts and torsion, tubo-ovarian abscess, and ectopic pregnancy. However, the appendix cannot be localized when air-filled bowel is overlying. In the case of ultrasound, a positive study is

accurate and a negative study is inconclusive (Figs. 167-5 and 167-6). CT scan is less operator dependent, and like ultrasound, can reveal multiple other abnormalities [8•]. The scan can clearly delineate a thick-walled, obstructed appendix with inflammation of periappendiceal tissues (Fig. 167-7).

These ancillary tests, particularly CT and graded-compression ultrasound, are best employed when the diagnosis is unclear. CT scan is the diagnostic test of choice in a child whose symptom complex occurred several days prior to presentation and who now has constant, dull discomfort in the right lower quadrant and daily fevers. This child may have a walled-off abscess (Fig. 167-8).

◼◼ DIFFERENTIAL DIAGNOSIS

The differential diagnosis of acute appendicitis is straightforward—it includes virtually all causes of abdominal pain. Cope's classic monograph emphasizes that "to know acute appendicitis is to know well the diagnosis of acute abdominal pain" [9••]. Despite this seemingly daunting challenge, the diagnosis usually is apparent and, although the formal differential diagnosis is broad (Table 167-1), only a few diagnoses deserve special attention in children.

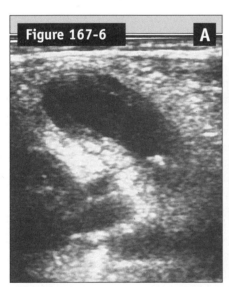

Figure 167-6   **A**

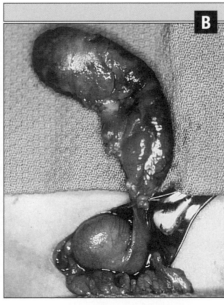

B

A, Ultrasound demonstrates a thickened, dilated appendix. **B**, The operative specimen is still attached to the cecum. The wall of the appendix is thickened and congested, and there is significant dilation at the tip of the appendix.

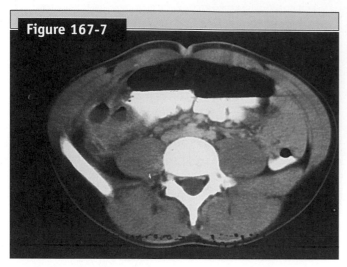

Figure 167-7

An image from a CT study clearly shows gray streaky fat in the right lower quadrant, which in the correct clinical setting is strongly suggestive of acute appendicitis. Fat is usually black on CT, but in the setting of inflammation, it becomes gray and is termed "dirty fat."

Table 167-1. Differential Diagnosis of Acute Appendicitis in Children	
Gastrointestinal	**Genitourinary**
Appendicitis	Hydronephrosis
Gastroenteritis	Pyelonephritis
Meckel's diverticulitis	Calculus
Crohn's disease	Ovarian or testicular torsion
Typhlitis (in leukemia patients)	Ovarian cyst
Tumor (carcinoid, adenocarcinoma, lymphoma)	Pelvic inflammatory disease/tubo-ovarian abscess
Cecal carcinoma	Ectopic pregnancy
Cecal or sigmoid diverticulitis	
Cholecystitis	**Miscellaneous**
Pancreatitis	Basilar pneumonia
	Sickle cell abdominal crisis
Infectious	Diabetic ketoacidosis
Tuberculosis	Rectus sheath hematoma
Cytomegalovirus	Psoas abscess
Parasitosis	
Yersinia infection	

Upper respiratory tract infections caused by *Streptococcus pneumoniae* can have an abdominal component that may be confused with an acute abdomen. More than one patient with lower lobe pneumonia has been explored by a surgeon suspecting appendicitis. Henoch-Schönlein purpura, hemolytic uremic syndrome, and sickle cell disease all cause abdominal pain, and differentiating this pain from that of appendicitis can be difficult at times. The onset of inflammatory bowel disease can mimic appendicitis. Perforated cecal cancers and right-sided diverticular disease are unusual but not unheard of in children and can present as "classic" appendicitis. Ovarian pathology can mimic appendicitis, as can an inflamed Meckel's diverticulum.

TREATMENT

The treatment of acute appendicitis is straightforward. Once the diagnosis is established by the operating surgeon, antibiotics

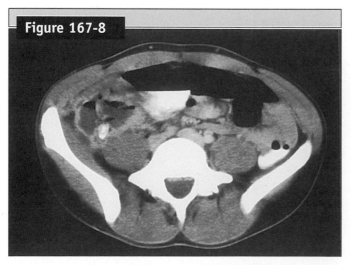

Figure 167-8

This CT shows a lucent area in the right lower quadrant with a radiodense shell that is a walled-off abscess cavity. Note the fecalith inside, which confirms the diagnosis.

and pain medication may be prescribed, but these are "points of no return" because subsequent improvements likely are due to these interventions. If it has not already been started, intravenous rehydration is begun. Appendectomy is the definitive treatment and should proceed as soon as is feasible. Operative findings of acute appendicitis characteristically include seropurulent fluid in the region and a thickened, edematous, turgid, injected appendix with a fibrous peel. A perforated appendix has either an obvious hole or deep purple or black areas suggesting gangrene; there may be diffuse fecopurulent soilage. If a normal appendix is encountered, inflammatory bowel disease, Meckel's diverticulum, mesenteric adenopathy, and ovarian pathology should be excluded by direct observation after appendectomy.

Laparoscopic appendectomy is being employed with increasing frequency. The indications are evolving, but one suggested approach is to use the laparoscope as a diagnostic tool in equivocal cases and proceed with laparoscopic appendectomy; most authorities agree that appendectomy should be performed regardless of the findings.

For the child who presents with symptoms of an abscess and has a CT scan that resembles Figure 167-8, there are several approaches to treatment. Each approach begins by starting broad-spectrum intravenous antibiotics. The traditional treatment then includes early appendectomy with debridement of the abscess cavity. Another option is to complete a course of antibiotics (*eg,* 10 days) and wait 4 to 6 weeks before an elective interval appendectomy is performed, at which time most of the inflammation will have resolved. This approach is appropriate when there is prompt resolution of fever and abdominal pain in response to the antibiotics and the child can tolerate a regular diet. A third option is prompt percutaneous drainage of the abscess under ultrasound or CT guidance, followed by a 4- to 6-week interval and appendectomy. One suggested strategy is to begin antibiotics and, for the child who responds well, to perform interval appendectomy. In the case of a child who does not respond, operation or percutaneous drainage is immediately indicated.

Recovery from acute uncomplicated appendicitis is rapid in children. They are usually able to eat the following day. Perioperative antibiotics are unnecessary, and discharge can be on the first or second postoperative day if bowel function has returned. In contrast, perforated appendicitis is treated with a course of intravenous antibiotics and careful observation in the hospital for complications of prolonged ileus, abscess, or wound infection.

PROGNOSIS

The prognosis for uncomplicated appendicitis is excellent. The complications of appendicitis usually occur in patients with perforated appendices and therefore are a direct result of delay in diagnosis. Complications are potentially worse for girls, because impaired fertility and increased risk of ectopic pregnancy are direct results of pelvic sepsis [2].

REFERENCES

Recently published papers of particular interest have been highlighted as follows:
• Of interest
•• Of outstanding interest

1. Guidry SP, Poole GV: The anatomy of appendicitis. *Am Surg* 1994, 60:68–71.

2. Kottmeir PK: Appendicitis. In *Pediatric surgery*, edn 4. Edited by Welch KJ, Randolph JG, Ravitch MM, *et al.* Chicago: Year Book Medical; 1986:989–994.

3. Pearl RH, Hale DA, Malloy M, *et al.*: Pediatric appendicitis. *J Pediatr Surg* 1995, 30:173–178.

4. Hennington MH, Tinsley EA Jr, Proctor HJ, Baker CC: Acute appendicitis following blunt trauma: incidence or coincidence? *Ann Surg* 1991, 214:61–63.

5. Budd DC, Fouty WJ: Familial retrocecal appendicitis. *Am J Surg* 1977, 133:670–671.

6. Dolgin SE, Beck AR, Tarter PI: The risk of perforation when children with possible appendicitis are observed in the hospital. *Surg Gynecol Obstet* 1992, 175:320–324.

7. Crady SK, Jones JS, Wyn T, Luttenton CR: Clinical validity of ultrasound in children with suspected appendicitis. *Ann Emerg Med* 1993, 22:1125–1129.

8.• Rao PM, Rhea JT, Novelline RA, *et al.*: Helical CT technique for the diagnosis of appendicitis: prospective evaluation of a focused appendix CT examination. *Radiology* 1997, 202:20–21.
This prospective study concludes that CT scan has a 97% positive predictive value and a 98% negative predictive value. The authors state that in every case of 100 appendix scans, the appendix was identified using both oral and rectal contrast. Nonetheless, we recommend CT scanning only in unclear cases or cases of probable abscess formation. It is not cost efficient to routinely scan every patient with right lower quadrant pain because the diagnosis usually can be reliably obtained based on clinical findings.

9.•• Silen W, ed: *Cope's Early Diagnosis of the Acute Abdomen* , edn 19. New York: Oxford University Press; 1994.
This classic paper is an important reference work for all physicians who engage the patient with abdominal pain. It is the primer for the physical diagnosis of acute abdominal surgical conditions.

168 Necrotizing Enterocolitis
William J. Klish

Necrotizing enterocolitis (NEC) is unique to the neonate. Even though it has some similarity to ischemic bowel disease in the adult, its presentation and clinical course differ sufficiently to consider it a separate disease entity. NEC is difficult to define, because its precise pathophysiology is still obscure and its clinical presentation varies widely. It is characterized by diffuse ulceration and necrosis of the distal small bowel and colon (Fig. 168-1), only occasionally involving the stomach and proximal intestine; pneumatosis intestinalis in the neonate is pathognomonic of NEC. NEC affects primarily premature infants and is the leading cause of acquired short bowel syndrome in children.

EPIDEMIOLOGY

Necrotizing enterocolitis occurs most commonly in premature babies in neonatal intensive care units [1]. The disease has an incidence of one to three cases per 1000 live births and affects 1% to 5% of all infants in intensive care units. There appears to be no seasonal, geographic, gender, or racial predilection. The risk of developing NEC is inversely proportional to birth weight and gestational age [2], even though as many as 10% to 30% of infants with this disease are full term [3,4]. Some believe that the babies most often affected are healthy "gainers and growers," but this has not been studied. The only universally accepted risk factor is prematurity [5].

ETIOLOGY

The three factors that appear to play a role in the development of NEC are intestinal ischemia, enteral feeding, and bacterial infection. Both experimental [6,7] and clinical data suggest that a combination of these risk factors in a baby with immature gastrointestinal function and immature host defense mechanisms results in NEC.

Most NEC involves the distal ileum and proximal colon, and it has been postulated that the process is caused by a diminished blood supply with resultant ischemia. The earliest pathologic lesion is superficial mucosal ulceration and submucosal edema and hemorrhage, which leads to necrosis (Fig. 168-2) and, in the most severe cases, perforation. Pneumatosis intestinalis or

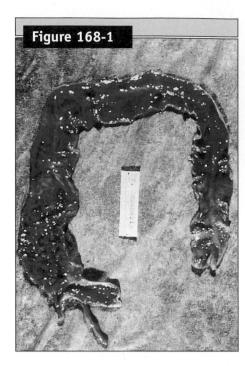

Figure 168-1

Surgically resected colon and distal ileum from an infant with necrotizing enterocolitis. Note the diffuse hemorrhagic mucosa. A large area of necrotic colonic mucosa is seen in the proximal colon. (*Courtesy of* M. J. Finegold, MD.)

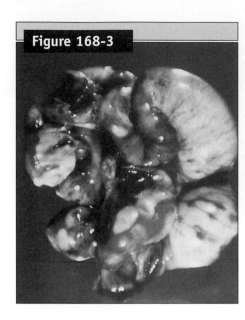

Figure 168-3

A surgically resected gross specimen of the distal ileum and proximal colon. Scattered gas-filled blebs characteristic of pneumatosis intestinalis are seen on the serosal surface of the bowel. (*Courtesy of* M.J. Finegold, MD.)

gas bubbles in the submucosa and subserosa (Fig. 168-3) are characteristic of this disease. The gas contains hydrogen, suggesting that bacterial fermentation of unabsorbed carbohydrates from the infant's diet contributes to the pathogenesis. Normal gut flora such as *E. coli*, *Klebsiella* spp., or *Staphylococcus epidermidis* [8] usually are involved, but enteropathogens such as rotavirus or clostridia occasionally have been implicated [9].

■ PATHOPHYSIOLOGY

Santulli [6] suggested in 1975 that the pathogenesis of NEC was multifactorial and involved a combination of intestinal ischemia, enteral feedings, and enteric organisms. These three factors appear to work in concert with each other to produce the disease (Fig. 168-4).

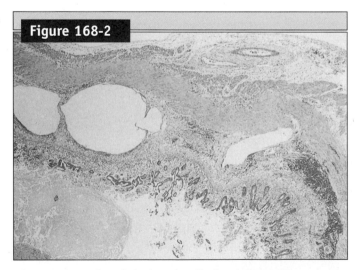

Figure 168-2

Microscopic section of the bowel wall of an infant with necrotizing enterocolitis. Note the mucosal inflammation with mucosal and submucosal necrosis. Gas-filled blebs are noted in the submucosal region of the bowel wall. (*Courtesy of* M.J. Finegold, MD.)

Ischemic Injury

Various investigators [10] have suggested that newborn infants retain a vagally-mediated reflex similar to that seen in certain aquatic animals, *eg,* seals or ducks. During periods of transient ischemia, such as the breath-holding of a diving animal, blood is shunted from the splanchnic vessels to the brain, heart, and kidneys. Infants presumably retain this reflex in utero when splanchnic blood flow is of lesser importance to them. At birth, when amniotic fluid is removed from the pharynx and lungs, this reflex is suppressed and blood flow is redistributed in the normal pattern. If ischemia occurs during the neonatal period, this reflex presumably can be reactivated. The intestine of the newborn appears to be more susceptible to tissue damage than the intestine of older animals [11], so that if blood flow decreases, the risk of ischemic mucosal damage is greater. Epinephrine [12], as well as inflammatory mediators such as nitric oxide [13], platelet-activating factor [14], tumor necrosis factor-α [14,15], endothelin-1 [16], and cachectin [17] also have been shown to play a role in perpetuating ischemic damage. Hyperviscosity associated with the polycythemia sometimes seen in newborns also has been implicated as a factor that may influence intestinal ischemia [18].

Enteral Feedings

Oral feeding with milk is closely associated with NEC in almost all patients, although the reason for this association is not well understood. Oral feeding provides substrate for the proliferation of bacteria that may play a role in the development of mucosal necrosis, and the feeding of hyperosmolar formulas may directly damage the intestinal mucosa [19]. In one study of low-birth-weight infants, 87.5% of those fed a hyperosmolar elemental formula developed NEC compared with only 25% of those fed a standard cow's milk formula [20]. The carbohydrate in formula can be maldigested and fermented, producing hydrogen gas, which is present in the wall of infants with pneumatosis intestinalis and may contribute to the further necrosis of the gut wall by decreasing capillary perfusion through increased intraluminal pressure. Breast-feeding appears to decrease the risk of NEC. In one large prospective study of newborns of

Figure 168-4

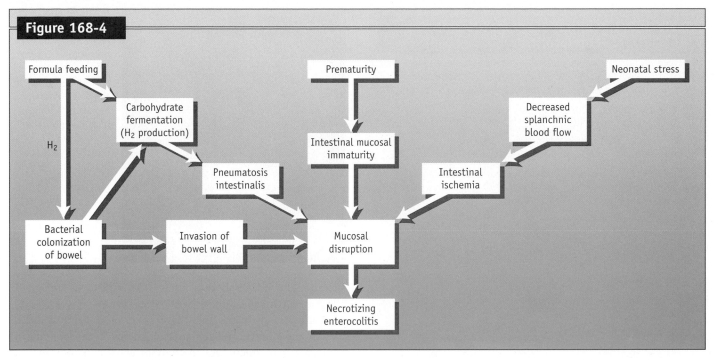

The flow diagram describes the most commonly held hypothesis for the development of necrotizing enterocolitis. As implied by this diagram, the etiology is multifactorial.

more than 30 weeks gestation, only 1% of infants fed human milk developed NEC, as compared with 8.5% of infants fed formula [21]. Protection may be afforded by human milk because of its anti-infectious and anti-inflammatory properties as well as its ability to help the developing intestine mature.

Enteric Infection

Enteric bacteria appear to play an important role in the pathogenesis of NEC. Systemic invasion of enteric organisms is associated with severe disease. Clustered outbreaks of this disease occur in most neonatal units, suggesting a role for bacteria or viruses [22]. The organisms involved in NEC usually are normal bowel flora such as *E. coli* and *Klebsiella* spp [8,23].

■ PATHOLOGY

Necrotizing enterocolitis most commonly occurs in the distal ileum and proximal colon, although lesions have been noted in the proximal bowel and stomach as well as in the descending colon. It occurs most often in the "watershed" areas of the bowel, where blood flow from the major mesenteric arteries overlaps. Early in the course of the disease, superficial mucosal ulceration, submucosal edema, and hemorrhage are present, but few acute inflammatory cells are seen [24]. As the disease progresses, coagulative transmural necrosis and bowel perforation occur. Intramural gas can be seen in the submucosa or subserosa as bubbles or gaseous clefts. If the disease does not progress to complete necrosis and perforation, healing occurs by re-epithelialization. Granulation tissue with fibroblast proliferation, which can lead to stricture formation, occurs.

■ CLINICAL FEATURES

The classic presentation of NEC includes abdominal distention, bilious vomiting, and blood in the stools. The course may

be slow and indolent, or it may be fulminant, leading to death within hours. Some infants present with only signs of sepsis, including lethargy, temperature instability, apnea, or shock. Other associated symptoms and findings include ileus, feeding intolerance, stools or vomitus positive for occult blood, stools positive for glucose, and disseminated intravascular coagulation. Complications include bowel perforation with peritonitis or pneumoperitoneum.

■ DIAGNOSIS

Radiographs of the abdomen may show pneumatosis intestinalis, air in the hepatic portal venous system (Fig. 168-5), and

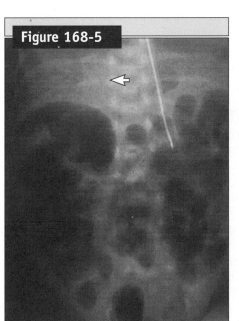

Figure 168-5

Note the fine, bubbly appearance of the pneumatosis intestinalis in this infant with necrotizing enterocolitis. Gas in the biliary tree (*arrow*) is characteristic of this disease. (*Courtesy of* R.M. Braverman, MD.)

Table 168-1. Clinical Staging of Necrotizing Enterocolitis

Stage I (suspect)

1. One or more historical factors that could produce perinatal stress
2. Systemic signs or symptoms
   a) Temperature instability
   b) Lethargy
   c) Apnea
   d) Bradycardia
3. Gastrointestinal signs or symptoms
   a) Poor feeding
   b) Increasing gastric residuals
   c) Emesis (bilious or occult blood positive)
   d) Abdominal radiographs showing distention with mild ileus

Stage II

1. All of the above
2. Persistent occult or gross gastrointestinal bleeding
3. Marked abdominal distention
4. Abdominal radiographs show:
   a) Significant distention
   b) Small bowel separation with "rigid" bowel loops
   c) Pneumatosis intestinalis or portal vein gas

Stage III

1. All of the above
2. Evidence of septic shock or marked gastrointestinal hemorrhage
3. Abdominal radiograph shows pneumoperitoneum

Data from Bell MJ et al. [25] and Walsh M, Kliegman RM [26].

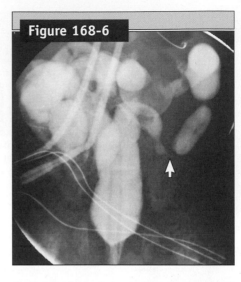

Figure 168-6

A barium enema in an infant who has recovered from necrotizing enterocolitis. The strictures (*arrow*) in the distal colon represent a long-term complication of this disease. (*Courtesy of* R.M. Braverman, MD.)

dilated loops of bowel. Pneumoperitoneum may be present and is best seen on a cross-table lateral radiograph. Intra-abdominal fluid also may be seen. Metrizamide gastrointestinal series and portal vein ultrasonography may be helpful in establishing the diagnosis of mild cases. Analyzing stool for reducing substance, occult blood, and α_1-antitrypsin may be helpful in detecting early signs of the disease. Endoscopy is not used to establish the diagnosis or to follow the course of disease, and may result in perforation.

A set of diagnostic criteria has been developed by several investigators [25,26] to help in therapeutic decision making (Table 168-1).

■ TREATMENT

The treatment of NEC is primarily supportive. As soon as the diagnosis is suspected, oral feeding is withheld. A nasogastric tube is placed to keep the stomach decompressed. Intravenous access is obtained to manage fluid and electrolytes initially and for antibiotic therapy. If patients do not progress beyond stage I, feeding by mouth can be reinstituted after 48 to 72 hours. When refeeding is started, it should be done with caution. If patients persist in stage I for longer than 1 week or advance to stage II, parenteral nutrition should be instituted. Patients who do not respond to medical management or who progress to stage III should be considered for surgery. Resection of the grossly necrotic bowel and the placing of a proximal enterostomy usually is the surgical treatment of choice [27,28].

Occasionally, infants have a lesion that is discrete enough to allow a primary anastomosis without an ostomy.

Antibiotic regimens that have been used to treat NEC include clindamycin and gentamicin; ampicillin and kanomycin; penicillin, gentamicin and metronidazole or clindamycin; and cefotaxime and vancomycin [29,30]. The routine use of an antibiotic for anaerobes does not seem to be helpful [29]. The use of vancomycin also should be restricted because of the emergence of resistant organisms such as *Enterococcus* spp.

■ PROGNOSIS

Mortality from NEC still is significant, even though it has decreased substantially, from approximately 80% in the 1960s to approximately 20% in the mid-1990s [31]. Mortality appears directly related to the presence of sepsis, cholestatic liver disease from total parenteral nutrition, and low birth weight [32]. Long-term complications include intestinal strictures (Fig. 168-6), enterocolic fistulae, anastomotic leaks or stenosis, and the short-gut syndrome resulting from extensive surgical resection of small intestine. Strictures are the most common long-term complication of NEC and occur in up to one third of survivors [33].

■ REFERENCES

1. Wilson R, Kanto WP Jr, McCarthy BJ, *et al.*: Epidemiologic characteristics of necrotizing enterocolitis: a population-based study. *Am J Epidemiol* 1981, 114:880–887.

2. Wilson R, Kanto WP Jr, McCarthy BJ, Feldman RA: Age at onset of necrotizing enterocolitis: risk factors in small infants. *Am J Dis Child* 1982, 136:814–816.

3. Cikrit D, Mastandrea J, West KW, *et al.*: Necrotizing enterocolitis: factors affecting mortality in 101 surgical cases. *Surgery* 1984, 96:648–655.

4. Kliegman RM, Fanaroff AA: Neonatal necrotizing enterocolitis: a 9-year experience. I. Epidemiology and uncommon observations. *Am J Dis Child* 1981, 135:603–607.

5. DeCurtis M, Paone C, Vetrano G, *et al.*: A case control study of necrotizing enterocolitis occurring over 8 years in a neonatal intensive care unit. *Eur J Pediatr* 1987, 146:398–400.

6. Santulli TV, Schullinger JN, Heird WC, *et al.*: Acute necrotizing enterocolitis in infancy: a review of 64 cases. *Pediatrics* 1975, 55:376–387.

7. Caplan MS, Hedlund E, Adler L, Hsueh W: Role of asphyxia and feeding in a neonatal rat model of necrotizing enterocolitis. *Pediatr Pathol* 1994, 14:1017–1028.

8. Panigrahi P, Gupta S, Gewolb IH, Morris JG, Jr: Occurrence of necrotizing enterocolitis may be dependent on patterns of bacterial adherence and intestinal colonization: studies in Caco-2 tissue culture and weanling rabbit models. *Pediatr Res* 1994, 36:115–121.

9. Rotbart HA, Nelson WL, Glode MP, *et al.*: Neonatal rotavirus-associated necrotizing enterocolitis: case-control study and prospective surveillance during an outbreak. *J Pediatr* 1988, 112:87–93.

10. Touloukian RJ, Posch JN, Spencer R: The pathogenesis of ischemic gastroenterocolitis of the neonate: selective gut mucosal ischemia in asphyxiated neonatal piglets. *J Pediatr Surg* 1972, 7:194–205.

11. Israel EJ: Neonatal necrotizing enterocolitis, a disease of the immature intestinal mucosal barrier. *Acta Paediatrica* 1994, 396(suppl):27–32.

12. Cheung PY, Barrington KJ, Pearson RJ, *et al.*: Systemic, pulmonary and mesenteric perfusion and oxygenation effects of dopamine and epinephrine. *American Journal of Respiratory and Critical Care Medicine* 1997, 155:32–37.

13. MacKendrick W, Caplan M, Hsueh W: Endogenous nitric oxide protects against platelet-activating factor-induced bowel injury in the rat. *Pediatr Res* 1993, 34:222–228.

14. Caplan M, *et al.*: Role of platelet-activating factor and tumor necrosis factor-alpha in neonatal necrotizing enterocolitis. *J Pediatr* 1990, 116:960.

15. Tan X, Hsueh W, Gonzalez-Crussi F: Cellular localization of tumor necrosis factor (TNF) -alpha transcripts in normal bowel and in necrotizing enterocolitis. TNF gene expression by Paneth cells, intestinal eosinophils, and macrophages. *Am J Pathol* 1993, 142:1858–1865.

16. Ekblad H, Arjamaa O, Vuolteenaho O, *et al.*: Plasma endothelin-1 concentrations at different ages during infancy and childhood. *Acta Pediatr* 1993, 82:302–303.

17. Tracey JK, Beutler B, Lowry SF, *et al.*: Shock and tissue injury induced by recombinant human cachectin. *Science* 1992, 234:470–474.

18. Wilson R, *et al.*: Risk factors for NEC in infants weighing more than 2,000 grams at birth: a case-control study. *Pediatrics* 1983, 71:19.

19. DeLemos RA, Roger JH, McLaughlin GW: Experimental production of necrotizing enterocolitis in newborn goats. *Pediatr Res* 1974, 8:380.

20. Book LS, Herbst JJ, Atherton SO, Jung AL: Necrotizing enterocolitis in low-birth-weight infants fed an elemental formula. *J Pediatr* 1975, 87:602–605.

21. Bunton GL, *et al.*: Necrotizing enterocolitis: a controlled study of 3 years' experience in a neonatal intensive care unit. *Arch Dis Child* 1977, 52:772.

22. Book LS, Overall JC Jr, Herbst JJ, *et al.*: Clustering of necrotizing enterocolitis: interruption by infection-control measures. *N Engl J Med* 1977, 297:984–986.

23. Virnig NL, Reynolds JW: Epidemiological aspects of neonatal necrotizing enterocolitis. *Am J Dis Child* 1974, 128:186–190.

24. Rodin AE, Nichols MM, Hsu FL: Necrotizing enterocolitis occurring in full term infants at birth. *Arch Pathol* 1973, 96:335–338.

25. Bell MJ, Ternberg JL, Feigin RD, *et al.*: Neonatal necrotizing enterocolitis: therapeutic decisions based upon clinical staging. *Ann Surg* 1978, 187:1–7.

26. Walsh M, Kliegman RM: Necrotizing enterocolitis: treatment based on staging criteria. *Pediatr Clin North Am* 1986, 33:179–201.

27. Parigi GB, Bragheri R, Minniti S, Verga G: Surgical treatment of necrotizing enterocolitis: when? how? *Acta Paediatrica* 1994, 396(suppl):58–61.

28. Luzzatto C, Previtera C, Boscolo R, *et al.*: Necrotizing enterocolitis: late surgical results after enterostomy without resection. *Eur J Pediatr Surg* 1996, 6:92–94.

29. Faix RG, Polley TZ, Grasela TH: A randomized, controlled trial of parenteral clindamycin in neonatal necrotizing enterocolitis. *J Pediatr* 1988, 112:271–277.

30. Scheifele DW, Ginter GL, Olsen E, *et al.*: Comparison of two antibiotic regimens for neonatal necrotizing enterocolitis. *J Antimicrob Chemother* 1987, 20:421–429.

31. Kliegman RM, Fanaroff AA: Neonatal necrotizing enterocolitis: a 9-year experience. II. Outcome assessment. *Am J Dis Child* 1981, 135:608–611.

32. Schullinger JN, Mollitt DL, Vinocur CD, *et al.*: Neonatal necrotizing enterocolitis: survival, management and complications. A 25-year study. *Am J Dis Child* 1981, 135:612–614.

33. Schimpl G, Hollwarth ME, Fotter R, Becker H: Late intestinal strictures following successful treatment of necrotizing enterocolitis. *Acta Paediatrica* 1994, 396(suppl):80–83.

169 Milk Protein Intolerance

Maria M. Oliva-Hemker

Since the 1950s, adverse reactions to foods have been increasingly recognized as a source of morbidity. Reactions to milk protein in particular, given its major contribution to the diet of infants and children worldwide, are extremely common in the pediatric age group. This chapter discusses issues regarding adverse reactions to cow's milk and other milk proteins, with emphasis on clinical presentation, diagnostic tests, and recommended management. Although it has been advocated that the term *cow's-milk protein allergy* (CMPA) be used specifically to indicate an immunologically-mediated intolerance objectively proven by a blinded challenge, this precise definition has not been employed routinely throughout the medical literature [1].

Thus, the broader term *cow's-milk protein intolerance* (CMPI) is used in this chapter to refer to any non-psychologically based, reproducible abnormal response to ingestion of cow's-milk protein [2].

EPIDEMIOLOGY

The incidence of CMPI, as reported in the literature, varies widely, depending on diagnostic criteria, design, and enrolled populations of each study. If primarily historical information is used, symptoms suggestive of CMPI have been reported in as many as 30% to 40% of infants. However, prospective studies performed in industrialized countries over the last 30 years have indicated a CMPI incidence of 1% to 7% [3]. In recent large, prospective studies, which have used controlled milk elimination and challenges, the incidence of CMPI has been narrowed further, to 2% to 3% in children younger than 3 years of age [4,5•]. CMPI can occur in breast-fed infants, but with a lower incidence of approximately 0.5% [3]. In most of these cases, the inadvertent use of cow's milk supplements in the nursery or cow's milk consumption by the mother with passage of cow's-milk protein into the breast milk has been implicated.

The list of foods other than cow's milk that cause allergic reactions in children in the first year of life is fairly short and includes eggs, soy, and wheat. When soy protein is introduced in the initial infant formula, adverse reactions occur almost as frequently as with cow's milk. In older children and adults, other foods, such as peanuts, nuts, fish, and shellfish, more commonly cause adverse reactions [6,7••].

Pathophysiology

Development of CMPI probably depends on multiple factors, including a genetic predisposition to atopy, early exposure to cow's-milk protein, and host handling of the protein. A history of atopic disease in at least one first- or second-degree relative is considered a risk factor for developing allergic disease in general. The fact that infants appear to be more likely than older children to develop allergic reactions to foods may result from impaired barrier function of the gut and immaturity of the localized intestinal immune system, both of which are important in determining whether tolerance or a pathologic response will occur to a particular food antigen.

Immunologic responses to cow's milk can be divided into two broad categories—immediate and delayed reactions. Immediate reactions are characterized by symptoms developing within an hour of ingestion. These are typically immunoglobulin E (IgE)–mediated and occur when there is crosslinking of two or more antigen-specific IgE molecules on the surface of mast cells and basophils following antigen ingestion in sensitive individuals. Presenting symptoms associated with early reactions include urticaria, asthma, and anaphylaxis. In delayed reactions, symptoms such as vomiting, abdominal pain, bloody stools, or atopic dermatitis may not become manifest for hours or days after the ingestion of cow's milk. The delayed reactions may be caused by cell-mediated immunity or a combination of other immune and nonimmune mechanisms. They do not necessarily exclude IgE-mediated phenomena [2,7••].

■ CLINICAL FEATURES

The spectrum of clinical signs and symptoms associated with CMPI is varied and often involves multiple organ systems (Table 169-1), most commonly the gastrointestinal, cutaneous, and respiratory systems.

Gastrointestinal Manifestations

Although gastrointestinal involvement often is noted with CMPI, the increased frequency of symptoms such as vomiting and diarrhea seen in the first year of life can make it difficult to make an appropriate diagnosis. Other disorders, such as infectious enterocolitis, Hirschsprung's colitis, cystic fibrosis, celiac

Table 169-1. Symptoms and Signs Associated with Cow's Milk Protein Intolerance

Gastrointestinal: nausea, vomiting, diarrhea, abdominal pain, bloody stools, enteric protein loss, malabsorption, failure to thrive

Nongastrointestinal:

Generalized: anaphylaxis, hypotension, shock

Cutaneous: urticaria, angioedema, lip swelling, atopic dermatitis

Respiratory: cough, wheezing, rhinorrhea/conjunctivitis, dyspnea

Behavioral: colic/irritability

disease, and intestinal obstruction, must be considered in the differential diagnoses.

Cow's-Milk Colitis

Cow's milk–induced colitis most often presents during the first 3 months of life. Despite the presence of gross or occult blood, the stools of affected infants usually are formed and are negative for pathogens. The infants are afebrile, appear healthy, and follow an appropriate pattern on their growth curves. If indicated, a rectal biopsy can be done in the outpatient setting to confirm the diagnosis. Pathologic lesions are confined to the colon and consist of mucosal edema with eosinophilic infiltration of the epithelium and lamina propria (Fig. 169-1). In severe cases, crypt destruction and neutrophils also may be observed. With restriction of cow's milk ingestion, gross bleeding rapidly resolves within 48 to 72 hours. On rare occasions occult blood in stools is noted for a longer period of time because of slower resolution of mucosal lesions. A similar picture occurs in infants fed soy formula or breast milk, in which cases soy restriction or strict elimination of cow's-milk protein from the mother's diet usually leads to a favorable response [8,9].

Cow's-Milk Enterocolitis

In the enterocolitis syndrome, the most dramatic, and the rarest, presentation is that of acute gastrointestinal symptoms with anaphylactic shock. In most cases, however, this syndrome pre-

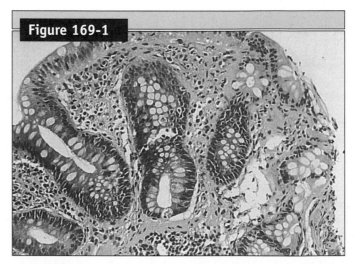

Figure 169-1

Cow's-milk colitis with eosinophilic infiltration in lamina propria. Note invasion of the crypt epithelium by eosinophils. Hematoxylin and eosin, ×100. (*Courtesy of* E. Perlman, MD.)

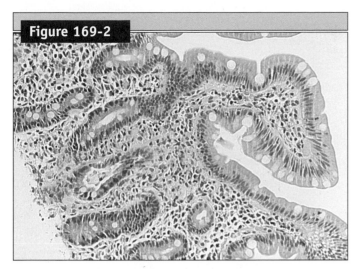

Cow's-milk enteritis with villus blunting and inflammatory infiltrate containing numerous eosinophils. Hematoxylin and eosin, ×100.

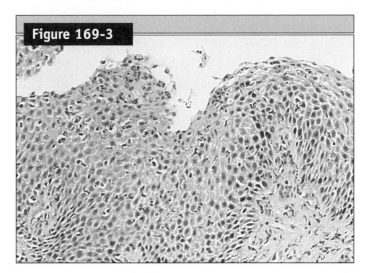

Esophageal mucosa with marked basal cell hyperplasia and eosinophilic infiltrate. Hematoxylin and eosin, ×100.

sents with protracted vomiting and diarrhea in infants up to 3 months of age. Stools can have occult blood, protein, neutrophils, and eosinophils and often are positive for reducing substances, indicating carbohydrate malabsorption. Barium radiography may demonstrate antral narrowing or mucosal thickening in the duodenum and jejunum. Histopathology of the small intestine reveals epithelial damage, with subtotal to total villous atrophy, edema, and increased numbers of lymphocytes, eosinophils, and mast cells (Fig. 169-2). The villous atrophy often is patchy, with abnormal areas interspersed among normal. It is usually not as severe as that seen with celiac disease. Colonic biopsies may show diffuse colitis with chronic inflammation and crypt abscesses. Although elimination of cow's milk leads to resolution of symptoms, usually within 72 hours, a secondary disaccharidase deficiency may persist until the small bowel mucosa regenerates. Soy allergy can present with similar symptoms and also responds to the elimination of the protein.

Postenteritis Cow's-milk Protein Intolerance

Postenteritis cow's-milk protein intolerance is a transient phenomenon that presents with persistent diarrhea in infants in whom enteric infection has resolved. It occurs most often in industrialized countries. Damage to the intestinal epithelium results from viral or bacterial infections, with a subsequent increased permeability in potential antigenic macromolecules, such as cow's-milk proteins. Small bowel biopsies may reveal an inflammatory cell infiltrate and partial villous atrophy. If significant villus blunting occurs, lactose intolerance may occur as a result of the secondary loss of the enzyme lactase-phlorizin hydrolase.

Eosinophilic Gastroenteritis

Eosinophilic gastroenteritis is a rare pediatric disorder characterized by an eosinophilic infiltrate in one or more parts of the gut. The gastric antrum is the location most commonly affected. The cause usually is unknown, but in some cases it is an allergic or immunologic reaction to a food antigen such as cow's-milk protein. Children can develop a variety of gastroin-

testinal symptoms, as well as systemic signs such as anemia and growth failure. A prominent peripheral eosinophilia has been reported in up to 80% of patients. Charcot-Leyden crystals may be found on microscopic examination of the stool. In most patients, IgE cannot be implicated in the disease process. Involvement of the mucosa, muscularis, and serosa, separately or in combination, leading to characteristic presentations has been described. With mucosal involvement the bowel mucosa can be edematous, hyperemic, nodular, or ulcerated, and presenting symptoms can include abdominal pain, diarrhea, and protein-losing enteropathy. If the muscular layers are involved, obstruction may occur and, rarely, in infants, can mimic hypertrophic pyloric stenosis. Serosal involvement can lead to hypoalbuminemia and eosinophilic ascites.

Eosinophilic Esophagitis and Gastroesophageal Reflux

Isolated esophageal eosinophilic infiltration, with or without other reactive epithelial changes, had been thought to be only a marker for the effects of acid gastroesophageal reflux (GER; Fig. 169-3). However, the possibility that esophageal mucosal eosinophilia may be related to the intake of a dietary protein, such as cow's milk, recently has been addressed. Children diagnosed with GER but unresponsive to either medical or surgical therapy, or both, have been shown to have significant symptomatic improvement and resolution of esophageal eosinophilia after their diets are changed to an elemental formula [10]. Another recent study incorporating the use of 24-hour intraesophageal pH monitoring reported a high incidence of association between GER and CMPI in infants less than 1 year of age, with symptoms responding to dietary restriction. The pH tracing of the enrolled infants with both disorders was characterized by a unique "phasic" tracing [11]. These possible adverse effects of cow's-milk protein must be further clarified by studies of larger numbers of patients.

Occult Gastrointestinal Blood Loss

Occult enteric blood loss, associated with growth failure, anemia, and gastrointestinal protein loss, has been associated with

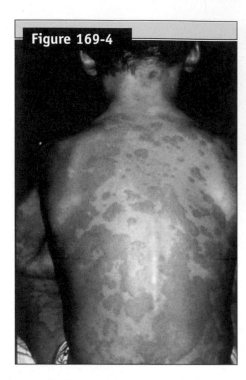

Figure 169-4

Urticaria following ingestion of cow's milk. The erythematous, well-demarcated, raised lesions are pruritic. See also **Color Plate**. (*Courtesy of* R. Wood, MD.)

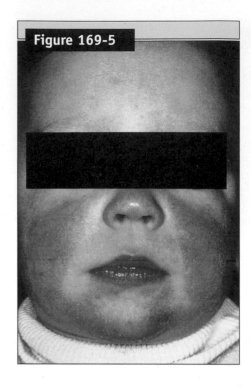

Figure 169-5

Atopic dermatitis associated with CMPI. Facial lesions are common in infancy. See also **Color Plate**. (*Courtesy of* R. Wood, MD.)

the consumption of large volumes of cow's milk. There have been very few studies of children with this syndrome.

Nongastrointestinal Manifestations

Cutaneous Symptoms

Cutaneous manifestations of CMPI are common in pediatric patients and are primarily IgE mediated. Immediate symptoms, such as angioedema, lip swelling, and urticaria, can occur. Individual urticarial lesions rarely persist longer than 24 hours, but new lesions may continue to develop and subside over days to years (Fig. 169-4, see also **Color Plate**). A more gradual presentation can be seen in children with the rash of atopic dermatitis, usually characterized by erythematous papules and vesicles and frequently with weeping and crusting; the associated pruritus can be difficult to treat and may lead to significant excoriation. Skin changes may progress to a scaly, lichenified state. In children under 12 months of age, the distribution can be diffuse or localized, but primarily involves the face, neck and scalp (Fig. 169-5, see also **Color Plate**). In older children, the classic distribution involving the extensor surfaces of the extremities becomes more common. Although the dermatitis can certainly be exacerbated by cow's-milk ingestion, it rarely remits completely with a restricted diet.

Respiratory Symptoms

Respiratory manifestations such as cough, wheezing, rhinitis, conjunctivitis, and dyspnea usually accompany gastrointestinal and cutaneous symptoms rather than occurring alone. There are no definitive data associating the ingestion of cow's milk with prolonged wheezing or coughing in the absence of an obvious viral infection or exposure to an inhalant allergen. Additionally, it is unusual for a child to present with persistent rhinorrhea, nasal congestion, or serous otitis media as the only symptoms of CMPI [12]. One rare disorder associated with cow's-milk ingestion is the syndrome of recurrent pneumonias with pulmonary infiltrates, anemia, growth failure, and hemosiderosis

(Heiner's syndrome). It has been suggested that the illness has an immunologic basis, because these children can have a positive skin-prick test to cow's milk, high serum IgE concentrations, and elevated precipitin titers to cow's-milk protein.

Anaphylaxis

Systemic anaphylaxis is an acute, potentially fatal reaction involving multiple organ systems. Symptoms include tongue swelling, throat tightness, nausea, abdominal or chest pain, dyspnea, hypotension, and shock. In most reported cases, children had ingested foods to which they had previously had adverse reactions, and in the majority of these children therapeutic intervention was delayed because patients, parents, or healthcare providers minimized early symptoms. Severe life-threatening reactions usually are not associated with cow's milk but rather with ingestion of peanuts, nuts, fish, and shellfish [7••].

Behavioral Symptoms

Some studies done with blinded challenges have suggested an association between the ingestion of cow's-milk protein and colicky symptoms (*ie*, extreme fussiness or inconsolable crying) in some infants [5•]. It is not clear whether this association has an immunologic basis. In certain situations it is probably reasonable to remove certain foods from the diet of an infant or nursing mother to see whether any change in colicky behavior occurs. However, severe restriction of the diet, with resultant caloric deprivation, or the use of expensive hydrolyzed or elemental formulas without confirmation by oral challenges is not prudent. Sleep disturbances, headaches, or other behavioral manifestations such as hyperactivity have not been shown to be secondary to CMPI.

■ DIAGNOSIS

No single test is diagnostic of CMPI. Rather, the diagnosis is a clinical one based on a complete history and physical evaluation

Table 169-2. Diagnostic Evaluation for Cow's Milk Protein Intolerance

History and physical examination: dietetic diary

Immunologic tests: skin prick test; radioallergosorbent test (RAST); serum IgE

Gastrointestinal tests: upper or lower endoscopic biopsies; carbohydrate breath hydrogen test; 72-hour fecal fat quantitation; stool analysis (blood, protein, pathogens, Charcot-Leyden crystals); D-xylose absorption test

Elimination and challenge: open; double-blind, placebo-controlled

Figure 169-6

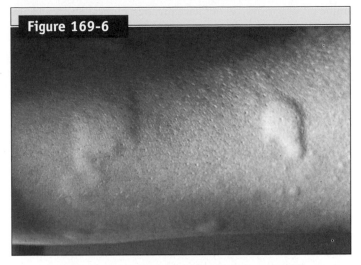

Large wheals indicate positive skin-prick tests to cow's-milk proteins (*left*) and soy protein (*right*). The small lesions surrounding wheals are negative sites. See also **Color Plate.** (*Courtesy of* R. Wood, MD.)

of the patient, the appropriate use of immunologic and gastrointestinal tests, and the response to elimination and challenge with cow's milk (Table 169-2).

History and Physical Examination

A complete and careful history can be invaluable not only for including the possibility of CMPI but also for excluding other disorders that may mimic its clinical picture. Questions regarding the quantity of cow's milk required to produce symptoms, the time between ingestion and onset of symptoms, and the type and frequency of symptoms must be asked to establish a potential association. A search for other atopic disorders and a family history for atopy also should be reviewed. It must be remembered that historical accounts can be highly subjective. In an infant who is ingesting only formula, or in the child with an immediate reaction, a historical association may be easier to obtain. When symptoms are delayed or chronic, however, histories can be quite inaccurate. Occasionally, the use of dietary diaries may help detect a previously unrecognized association between cow's milk and symptoms. Although signs of chronic atopy may be noted on the physical examination, the examination is often most useful in excluding other medical disorders.

Immunologic and Gastrointestinal Tests

Immunologic testing is not routinely done by pediatric gastroenterologists when a child's history is consistent with known gastrointestinal manifestations of CMPI. However, it is not uncommon for children suspected of having a protein allergy to undergo skin-prick tests or radioallergosorbent tests (RASTs) performed by allergists or pediatricians.

Skin-prick testing is a reliable method for demonstrating specific IgE antibodies to foods such as cow's milk and is useful in screening children with immediate reactions. Protein extracts are applied by a puncture or prick to the epidermis next to positive and negative controls. Skin sites are considered positive if they develop a wheal having a diameter at least 3 mm larger than the wheal elicited by the negative control within 15 to 20 minutes after placement (Fig. 169-6, see also **Color Plate**). Antigens also can be inoculated intradermally, but the risk of inducing a systemic reaction is greater, especially for highly sensitive children [13].

In serologic tests such as RAST, potential allergens coupled to an insoluble material are incubated with the patient's serum, which may contain allergen-specific IgE antibodies. Radioactively labeled anti-human IgE antibody is allowed to react with the antigen–antibody complexes, and the radioactivity level then is measured to quantify the specific IgE to the food allergen. Other variations of RAST using radiolabeling or enzyme-linked immunoassays (ELISAs) exist and are based on similar principles. RAST is recommended when direct skin testing is not feasible (eg, in patients with dermatoses, severe skin reactions, or anaphylaxis in response to food antigens). Although the ability of RAST to predict an immediate reaction to cow's milk is similar to that of skin testing, it is a more expensive test and results are not immediately available.

A positive skin-prick test or RAST for cow's-milk protein only indicates the presence of an antibody and does not confirm the diagnosis of CMPI. In fact, these immunologic tests have only about a 30% chance of predicting a positive response to a food challenge. Furthermore, it is not useful to obtain these tests serially to determine when to reintroduce a protein into a child's diet, because persistently positive tests often are seen even after clinical tolerance to cow's milk has developed. The tests probably are most helpful when a child is suspected of having an immediate reaction (eg, urticaria, anaphylaxis, or wheezing), to a food antigen. Although a negative skin test or RAST indicates that an immediate hypersensitivity reaction is unlikely, it does not exclude non–IgE-mediated reactions. Most gastrointestinal manifestations of CMPI in children are of the delayed type of reaction; thus, skin tests or RASTs are not helpful in making the diagnosis.

Some investigators believe that a high level of circulating IgE to cow's-milk proteins has a positive correlation with the risk of developing CMPI as well as other food allergies [3]. However, many studies have shown that measuring serum IgE levels has inadequate predictive accuracy, because many children who are nonatopic display elevated serum IgEs to various foods, and many who are highly atopic have normal IgE concentrations. The presence of circulating IgG-type antibodies to food antigens is a normal phenomenon and a sign that the child has had contact with the food—measurements of these have no clear diagnostic value in diagnosing CMPI. Other immunologic tests, such as lymphocyte stimulation tests and basophil histamine release assays, do not have practical clinical utility and are used more for research purposes [14].

In certain situations, biopsies of the gastrointestinal tract may reveal changes consistent with CMPI. Such information is particularly useful, for example, if an infant remains symptomatic even when he or she is being fed an extensively hydrolyzed formula and the use of an amino acid product is being contemplated. Histopathology is probably most beneficial in excluding other disorders, however, especially when evaluating the child with chronic symptoms such as prolonged diarrhea and failure to thrive. Other tests of gastrointestinal function, such as carbohydrate breath hydrogen tests, D-xylose absorption, 72-hour fecal fat quantitation, or examination of the stool for occult blood and protein loss should be viewed as complementary and not necessary in the routine diagnostic evaluation for CMPI. Intragastric provocation under endoscopic observation to look for morphologic changes and local mast cell desquamation is not a standard procedure in children.

Elimination and Challenge

The elimination and challenge test remains the cornerstone for making the diagnosis of CMPI. First, the child must demonstrate significant improvement or disappearance of symptoms when cow's milk is eliminated from the diet. Then, to prove that the association is not coincidental, cow's milk should be rein-

troduced into the diet to see whether symptoms recur (Fig. 169-7). Such challenging has been widely recommended to avoid unnecessary and possibly detrimental dietary manipulations in children.

Oral challenges can be performed in an open or blinded fashion. Although the original criteria by Goldman for the diagnosis of CMPI consisted of three separate elimination and challenge tests, this has proven to be too difficult and impractical to perform routinely with children [2]. In the case of an infant presenting with classic signs of cow's-milk colitis, for example, prompt resolution of symptoms on elimination of cow's milk from the diet may be sufficient evidence to make the diagnosis, and challenge is probably not necessary for at least several months. In many situations, only one open, unblinded challenge is required to confirm a cause-and-effect relationship between cow's milk and symptoms. Furthermore, because tolerance to cow's milk develops in most children by 3 years of age, oral rechallenging at recurrent intervals, such as every 6 to 12 months, is warranted until tolerance is demonstrated. The only time that oral challenging is not recommended is with an infant or child who has a convincing history of life-threatening anaphylaxis following ingestion of cow's milk.

Challenges should be done at a time when the patient is thriving and asymptomatic. In children manifesting symptoms of immediate reactions, elimination of cow's milk for 1 or 2

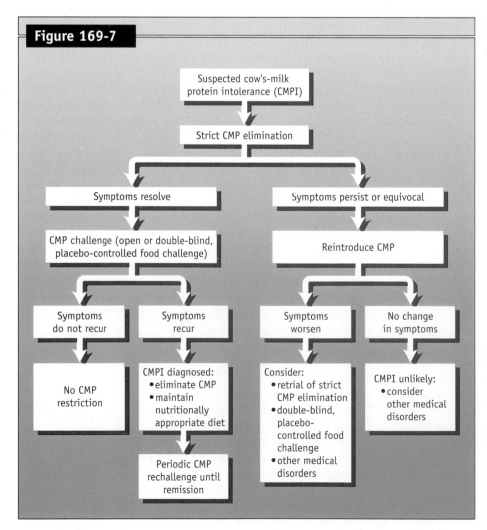

Figure 169-7

Suspected cow's-milk protein intolerance (CMPI)

↓

Strict CMP elimination

├─ Symptoms resolve
│   ↓
│   CMP challenge (open or double-blind, placebo-controlled food challenge)
│   ├─ Symptoms do not recur
│   │   ↓
│   │   No CMP restriction
│   └─ Symptoms recur
│   ↓
│   CMPI diagnosed:
│   • eliminate CMP
│   • maintain nutritionally appropriate diet
│   ↓
│   Periodic CMP rechallenge until remission
│
└─ Symptoms persist or equivocal
    ↓
    Reintroduce CMP
    ├─ Symptoms worsen
    │   ↓
    │   Consider:
    │   • retrial of strict CMP elimination
    │   • double-blind, placebo-controlled food challenge
    │   • other medical disorders
    └─ No change in symptoms
        ↓
        CMPI unlikely:
        • consider other medical disorders

Algorithm for milk protein elimination and challenge of pediatric patients with suspected cow's-milk protein intolerance.

weeks usually suffices. However, in those with enterocolitis and malabsorption, resolution of symptoms may take many months. Because oral challenges can lead to recurrence of symptoms within minutes to hours and may carry a risk of dehydration, hypotension, or anaphylaxis, they should be performed under medical supervision in a monitored inpatient or outpatient setting. Equipment must be readily available for the treatment of severe reactions and for resuscitation. A typical challenge for CMPI can begin with a few drops of milk placed on the child's skin and lips. If no reaction occurs, the oral challenge can commence with the child ingesting a small amount of cow's milk (*eg*, 5 to 10 mL), and being observed for adverse reactions. If that is tolerated, the amount can be doubled each 15 to 60 minutes until a reaction occurs or until the patient is tolerating an amount considered to be an age-appropriate portion [2].

In a child with unclear symptomatology or an equivocal response to cow's milk, or when a child's diet is being restricted, possibly unnecessarily, because of suspicion of CMPI, a double-blind, placebo-controlled food challenge (DBPCFC) may be necessary. This test is considered the "gold standard" for confirming or refuting a history of adverse food reaction and provides the safest and most definitive way to control for confounding factors [1]. DBPCFC should be performed by trained personnel—preferably an allergy specialist familiar with the technique. The endpoint of the challenge should have predefined objective observations, with the duration of the observation period depending on the type of reaction expected. Both the observer and the test subject must be blinded to which food is being given by capsule or hidden in liquid to disguise its color and flavor. Initially a quantity of food so small that it is unlikely to provoke symptoms is administered, and amounts are gradually increased as long as the child remains asymptomatic, usually until 10 g of dry food or 100 g of wet food have been ingested [7••]. DBPCFCs should be followed with open challenges to exclude the possibility of false-negative tests.

MANAGEMENT

The only definitive treatment of CMPI is avoidance of cow's milk. For infants who have been ingesting a cow's milk–based formula, extensively hydrolyzed formulas have served as replacements [15]. Such formulas have been treated with heat, enzymes, and ultrafiltration to destroy antigenic epitopes of the cow's-milk proteins and to remove residual large peptides. As a result of the way in which they are prepared, they have a bitter taste and an unpleasant smell and are more expensive than standard cow's milk–based formulations. Younger infants usually take them well in bottles, but older infants may have difficulty accepting them. These formulas have been labeled "hypoallergenic" because at least 90% of infants intolerant to cow's-milk proteins can tolerate them without symptoms. However, they are not "nonallergenic," because reactions with their ingestion have been documented in children with CMPI. Examples of extensively hydrolyzed casein formulas available in the United States are Nutramigen, Pregestimil (both Mead Johnson, Evansville, IN), and Alimentum (Ross, Columbus, OH).

Soy formulas are not recommended for the treatment of CMPI because adverse reactions to soy are common in children who are intolerant to cow's milk. Partially hydrolyzed formulas should not be used, either, because they have more antigenic products available, and the risk of allergic reactions is higher than with the extensively hydrolyzed products [16••]. Goat's-milk proteins have high cross-reactivity with cow's-milk proteins. The high solute load and composition of goat's milk also make it an unsuitable substitute for infants younger than 1 year of age.

For infants receiving primarily breast milk who develop signs of CMPI, continuation of breast-feeding should be encouraged because of its nutritional, immunologic, and psychologic advantages. However, the mother's diet must be examined, and cow's-milk protein must be eliminated from her diet. Appropriate counseling must be provided to the mother to ensure that her caloric and calcium requirements are met. If symptoms in a nursing infant are frequent or severe, or if it is difficult to alter the mother's diet, it may be necessary to discontinue breast-feeding and place the infant on a completely hydrolyzed formula. The elimination of cow's milk from the diet of older children is more difficult, because cow's-milk protein is present in the fillers and additives of many processed foods. In these cases supervision by an experienced dietitian can be invaluable in educating the family and ensuring that the child's diet includes the recommended allowance of minerals, vitamins, and calories.

Infants who demonstrate adverse reactions even to extensively hydrolyzed formulas, or children with extreme sensitivity to cow's-milk protein or with multiple food allergies, may require the use of an elemental formula. Such highly limited diets should be instituted only under the supervision of an experienced health-care provider. The most hypoallergenic, nutritionally complete elemental infant formula currently available in the United States is Neocate (SHS, Rockville, MD), which is composed of 100% synthetic amino acids [17]. For children older than 1 year of age, available elemental formulas include Neocate One + (SHS, Rockville, MD), Vivonex Pediatric (Sandoz, Minneapolis, MN), and L-Emental Pediatric (Nutrition Medical, Buffalo, MN).

No medications have been proven to be as effective as elimination of cow's milk from the diet. Although prednisone, oral disodium cromoglycate, and ketotifen have been investigated, large studies in children have not demonstrated a consistent benefit. The exception to the equivocal results of drug therapy is corticosteroid treatment of eosinophilic gastroenteritis, which has been successful. There has been no clear experimental documentation showing that oral, sublingual, or subcutaneous administration of milk protein in small doses (*ie*, immunotherapy) is beneficial in the treatment of adverse reactions to cow's milk.

PREVENTION

Dietary intervention programs aimed at reducing the incidence of CMPI have indicated that cow's-milk protein restriction should be aimed not at the general infant population, but rather at infants with a high risk for developing atopic disease (*ie*, those with first- or second-degree relatives with a history of atopy). Whether breast-feeding alone truly prevents the occurrence of future atopic disease continues to be debated. However, the incidence of CMPI in exclusively breast-fed infants has been shown to be at least five to 10 times lower than the incidence in infants receiving cow's-milk protein formulas. The best allergy-preventive effects have been reported with either 1) breast-feeding plus maternal avoid-

Table 169-3. Guidelines for Preventing Allergic Disease in Infants

Identification of the at-risk infant (positive family history for allergies)

Dietary intervention

Breast-feeding exclusively for the first 4–6 months

Eliminate cow's milk, eggs, and nuts from maternal diet during lactation

In non–breast-fed infants, use completely hydrolyzed formula for first 4–6 months

Delay introduction of solid foods until after 4–6 months

Delay introduction of cow's milk until 1 year; eggs until 2 years; nuts and fish until 3 years

Avoidance of environmental allergens: dust mites, pets, secondary smoke, mold, pollutants

ance of food allergens or 2) the use of extensively hydrolyzed formulas combined with avoidance of cow's milk and solid foods in the infant diet for at least the first 4 months of life. Studies have shown that these approaches provide preventive effects for atopic dermatitis and food allergies until approximately 2 years of age [16••]. Avoidance regimens, however, have not shown general benefit in children prospectively followed up to 7 years of age and have shown no significant decrease in inhalant allergies unless there has been concurrent elimination of aeroallergens [16••,18].

The feeding practices of most infants obviously are determined by parents, family members, and primary health-care providers. Referrals to the pediatric gastroenterologist usually are made only in cases of high parental concern or anxiety because of a strong family history of atopy. Based on dietary intervention studies, certain practical recommendations can be made for at-risk infants to reduce their potential risk for acquiring allergic disease (Table 169-3). These guidelines include 1) the promotion of breast-feeding for the first 4 to 6 months, with maternal restriction of cow's milk, eggs, and fish; 2) the use of extensively hydrolyzed formulas for the first 4 to 6 months in the non–breast-fed infant; 3) avoidance of cow's milk and eggs for the first 12 to 24 months; and 4) avoidance of respiratory allergens such as smoking, dust, pets, and environmental pollutants [16••]. Restriction of the maternal diet during pregnancy is not advocated because prenatal sensitization to foods is rare; maternal dietary restrictions during pregnancy have not had a significant impact on the prevention of food allergy in infants; and dietary restriction could harm the mother and fetus by suppressing normal weight gain [18].

PROGNOSIS

The outcome for most children with CMPI is good. Whereas allergic reactivity to peanuts, nuts, fish, and shellfish tends to persist, almost 60% of infants develop tolerance to cow's-milk protein by 1 year of age, and approximately 85% develop tolerance by their third birthday. Young children may even outgrow severe, life-threatening, anaphylactic reactions. Thus, prolonged elimination of cow's milk usually is unnecessary, and oral challenging on a regular basis is warranted until tolerance is demonstrated.

REFERENCES

Recently published papers of particular interest have been highlighted as follows:
• Of Interest
•• Of Outstanding Interest

1. Bock SA, Sampson HA: Food allergy in infancy. *Pediatr Clin N Am* 1994, 41:1047–1067.

2. Stern M: Allergic enteropathy. In *Pediatric Gastrointestinal Disease.* Edited by Walker WA, Durie PR, Hamilton JR, *et al.* St. Louis: Mosby; 1996:677–692.

3. Host A, Jacobsen HP, Halken S, Holmenlund D: The natural history of cow's milk protein allergy/intolerance. *Eur J Clin Nutr* 1995, 49:S13–S18.

4. Host A, Halken S: A prospective study of cow milk allergy in Danish infants during the first 3 years of life. *Allergy* 1990, 45:587–596.

5.• Schrander JJP, van den Bogart JPH, Forget PP, *et al.*: Cow's milk protein intolerance in infants under 1 year of age: a prospective epidemiological study. *Eur J Pediatr* 1993, 152:640–644.
In this paper, the authors report on a large prospective population study of CMPI in which more than 1100 newborn infants were followed from birth to 1 year of age. The calculated incidence of CMPI was 2.8%.

6. Moon A, Kleinman RE: Allergic gastroenteropathy in children. *Ann Allergy Asthma Immunol* 1995, 74:5–12.

7.•• Metcalf DD, Sampson HA, Simon RA, eds: *Food Allergy: Adverse Reactions to Foods and Food Additives.* St. Louis: Blackwell Scientific Publications; 1991:81–112.
This reference provides a detailed review of the etiologies, pathophysiology, and management of food allergies. It incorporates issues regarding CMPI within the larger framework of adverse reactions to foods.

8. Halpin TC, Byrne WJ, Ament ME: Colitis, persistent diarrhea, and soy protein intolerance. *J Pediatr* 1977, 91:404–407.

9. Lake AM, Whitington PF, Hamilton SR: Dietary protein-induced colitis in breast-fed infants. *J Pediatr* 1982, 101:906–910.

10. Kelly KK, Lazenby AJ, Rowe PC, *et al.*: Eosinophilic esophagitis attributed to gastroesophageal reflux: improvement with an amino-acid based formula. *Gastroenterology* 1995, 109:1503–1512.

11. Cavataio F, Iacono G, Montalto G, *et al.*: Gastroesophageal reflux associated with cow's milk allergy in infants: which diagnostic examinations are useful? *AJG* 1996, 91:1215–1220.

12. Hill DJ, Hosking CS. The cow milk allergy complex: overlapping disease profiles in infancy. *Eur J Clin Nutr* 1995, 49:S1–S12.

13. Watson WTA: Food allergy in children: diagnostic strategies. *Clin Rev Allergy Immunol* 1995, 13:347–359.

14. Burks AW, Sampson HA: Diagnostic approaches to the patient with suspected food allergies. *J Pediatr* 1992, 121:S64–S71.

15. Halken S, Jacobsen HP, Host A, Holmenlund D: The effects of hypoallergenic formulas in infants at risk of allergic disease. *Eur J Clin Nutr* 1995, 49:S77–S83.

16.•• Zeiger RS: Prevention of allergic disease in infancy. In *Asthma and Allergy in Pregnancy and Early Infancy.* Edited by Schatz M, Zeiger RS. New York: Marcel Dekker; 1993:535–574.
This reference represents a presentation of dietary intervention studies investigating the prevention of atopic disease in infants. The roles of breast-feeding, hypoallergenic formulas, solid food avoidance, and environmental allergies are addressed.

17. Sampson HA, James JM, Bernhisel-Broadbent J: Safety of an amino acid-derived infant formula in children allergic to cow milk. *Pediatrics* 1992, 90:463–465.

18. Zeiger RS, Heller S: The development and prediction of atopy in high-risk children: follow-up at age seven years in a prospective randomized study of combined maternal and infant food allergen avoidance. *J Allergy Clin Immunol* 1995, 95:1179–90.

170 Cystic Fibrosis
Harvey W. Aiges

Cystic fibrosis (CF) is the most common lethal genetic disease in white children. It is an autosomal recessive disorder that affects 1 in every 2000 live-born whites and 1 in every 15,000 live-born blacks. One of every 20 whites is a carrier for the CF gene. Cystic fibrosis is the most common cause of pancreatic insufficiency in children and adolescents, but there is enormous variation in the clinical presentation and course. Advances in the understanding and treatment of CF have led to a dramatic improvement in life expectancy, with a median survival now of more than 30 years. Men survive slightly longer than women. Cystic fibrosis should be suspected in any person with malabsorption, failure to thrive, or chronic or recurrent lung disease.

HISTORY

In 1904, Bramwell described *pancreatic infantilism* in a group of children with failure to thrive and bulky, foul-smelling stools. In 1938, Anderson defined CF of the pancreas by her description of children who had widespread pulmonary infection, destructive cystic changes of the pulmonary parenchyma, and fibrosis of the pancreas. In 1945, Farber noticed inspissated mucus secretions in the exocrine glands of such patients and characterized his findings as *mucoviscidosis*, a more apt name for the disease. In 1953, Di sant'agnese and Schwachman discovered that patients with cystic fibrosis had increased amounts of sodium and chloride in their sweat, which led to the development of the diagnostic sweat test in 1955.

PATHOPHYSIOLOGY

The clinical picture of CF is one of generalized exocrine and eccrine gland dysfunction resulting in a thick, tenacious mucus that obstructs excretory ducts and causes secondary parenchymal destruction in many organ systems. The gene responsible for CF has been located on the long arm of chromosome 7 [1•]. This gene gives rise to a protein called the cystic fibrosis transmembrane conductance regulator (CFTR), which regulates the transport of chloride and other electrolytes across epithelial cell membranes. A mutation of this gene results in an absence or malfunction of the CFTR channel, thereby preventing chloride movement out of the cell and indirectly allowing excess sodium into cells. This imbalance of electrolytes in the extracellular fluid leads to the mucus layer becoming thicker and resistant to clearance. Recent work has shown that 70% of the mutations in CF patients correspond to a loss of a phenylalanine residue at amino acid position 508 on the CF gene. The remainder of the CF mutant gene pool consists of multiple, different mutations, which may be responsible for the great clinical variation seen in the disease.

There seems to be a relationship between the percentage of normal CFTR function as determined by the different muta-tions and the presence and severity of disease in various organs (a genotype–phenotype correlation). Dramatic advances in prenatal diagnosis, genetic screening, and genetic therapies are now being made based on this new understanding of the genetics and pathophysiology of CF [2].

DIAGNOSIS

Cystic fibrosis is a multisystemic disease with a very variable course and may present at any time from birth through adulthood. Between 10% and 15% of affected patients present at birth with intestinal obstruction caused by meconium ileus. About 75% of CF patients are diagnosed by 2 years of age because of respiratory symptoms or poor growth, whereas 10% escape diagnosis until after puberty, at which time they present with cirrhosis or infertility. However, the possible initial manifestations are myriad, and the physician should be alert to the possibility of cystic fibrosis in many clinical settings (Table 170-1).

The diagnosis is established by the sweat test, preferably by the pilocarpine iontophoresis technique, in which at least 100 mg of sweat is acquired and a quantitative analysis of chloride and sodium performed. The normal value for sweat chloride is <30 mEq/L per liter; it is >60 mEq/L in more than 98% of patients with cystic fibrosis. All abnormal results must be repeated to confirm the diagnosis.

Several unusual conditions may produce elevated sweat electrolytes (Table 170-2). In cases in which the diagnosis is confusing, genotyping, use of nasal potential-difference measurements, and bronchoalveolar lavage may be helpful [3•]. Neonatal screening for cystic fibrosis using dried blood spot analysis of serum immunoreactive trypsin has demonstrated significantly increased levels in newborns with CF, even when the exocrine pancreatic function is normal. However, at present, the false-positive and false-negative rates are too high to make this assay useful.

CLINICAL FEATURES
Pulmonary Manifestations

The abnormally thick mucus secretions, abnormal cleansing activity (*ie*, impaired ciliary function and ineffective cough), and apparent hyperreactive airways (*eg*, recurrent bronchospasm) of the pulmonary tree all predispose the patient to repeated and chronic lower respiratory infections. Infections, an asthma-like picture, or a persistent cough occur frequently. Sputum is usually thick, viscid, and purulent. Early infections are viral or caused by *Staphylococcus aureus*. As the pulmonary disease progresses, however, the organism most commonly isolated from the pulmonary secretions is *Pseudomonas aeruginosa*; a subgroup of CF patients not susceptible to colonization with *P. aeruginosa* appear to have a much more benign long-term course. Patients

Table 170-1. Indications for Sweat Testing

Gastrointestinal
- Meconium ileus
- Unexplained intestinal obstruction (distal intestinal obstruction syndrome)
- Rectal prolapse
- Intussusception over the age of 2 years
- Malabsorption/failure to thrive
- Voracious appetite with poor weight gain
- Symptomatic deficiency of vitamins A, D, E, and K
- Prolonged infantile cholestasis
- Cirrhosis/portal hypertension
- Unexplained cholelithiasis
- Pancreatitis in children or adolescents

Pulmonary
- Recurrent or nonresolving pneumonia
- Staphylococcal pneumonia
- *Pseudomonas aeruginosa* in sputum
- Recurrent bronchiolitis
- Lobar atelectasis
- Chronic bronchitis/chronic cough
- Radiographic evidence of bronchiectasis
- Hemoptysis in childhood

Miscellaneous
- Family history of cystic fibrosis
- Digital clubbing
- Hyponatremic dehydration
- Metabolic alkalosis
- Salty taste of skin
- Nasal polyps
- Pansinusitis
- Unexplained hypoproteinemia/anasarca in infancy
- Azoospermia
- Unexplained delayed menarche

Table 170-2. Non–Cystic Fibrosis Causes of Abnormal Sweat Tests

Adrenal insufficiency
Glycogen storage disease, type I
Fucosidosis
Malnutrition/edema
Nephrogenic diabetes insipidus
Hypothyroidism
Ectodermal dysplasia
Prostaglandin E_1 infusion

Table 170-3. Gastrointestinal Manifestations of Cystic Fibrosis

Organ	Incidence, %
Pancreas	
Insufficiency	80–90
Chemical glucose intolerance	30–40
Clinical diabetes mellitus	1–5
Vitamin deficiency (A, D, E, and K)	Variable
Growth retardation	Variable
Liver	
Fatty liver	40–70
Focal biliary cirrhosis	25
Cirrhosis/portal hypertension	5
Neonatal cholestasis	5
Gallbladder	5–10
Intestine	
Meconium ileus	10–15
Rectal prolapse	10–20
Distal intestinal obstruction syndrome	10–35
Hypoproteinemia/edema/anasarca	5
Intussusception	1

who are colonized with *Burkholderia* (formerly *Pseudomonas*) *cepacia* (2% of all CF patients) seem to have a more stormy course. With time and recurrent respiratory infections, most CF patients develop progressive dilatation and destruction of the airways and lung parenchyma, with eventual pulmonary fibrosis, loss of pulmonary function, severe bronchiectasis (in which upper lobes are more affected than lower lobes), abscess, and bleb formation. Clinically, patients show signs of chronic obstructive pulmonary disease with ventilation-perfusion abnormalities, a barrel-shaped emphysematous chest, and digital clubbing. Finally, respiratory failure, cor pulmonale, and death occur. Respiratory complications account for more than 95% of CF deaths. Whether repeated viral infections of the respiratory tract cause progressive pulmonary damage is controversial, and it is not clear which bacteria cause progressive lung destruction. Pulmonary damage may result from an altered immune state, immune complex deposition, and subsequent lung injury. Some patients develop allergic aspergillosis, with fluffy pulmonary infiltrates, high peripheral eosinophilia, ele-

vated serum IgE levels, and a positive skin test to *Aspergillus fumigatus*. In addition, chronic pansinusitis affects almost all CF patients, and 10% to 15% of them develop significant nasal polyposis. Pneumothorax occurs in up to 10% of CF patients older than 10 years of age.

Intestinal Manifestations

The gastrointestinal manifestations of CF are listed in Table 170-3.

Meconium ileus, the most common presentation of CF in the newborn (Fig. 170-1) [4], presents as intestinal obstruction and is caused by an abnormally thick and viscid meconium plug, usually at the ileocecal valve. In two thirds of cases, Gastrografin enemas or lavage and enemas of acetylcysteine (Mucomyst) may obviate the need for surgery. The newborn with CF also may present with small intestinal obstruction from intestinal stenosis or atresia.

Rectal prolapse from large, bulky stools occurs in 20% of untreated patients (Fig. 170-2, see also **Color Plate**). These

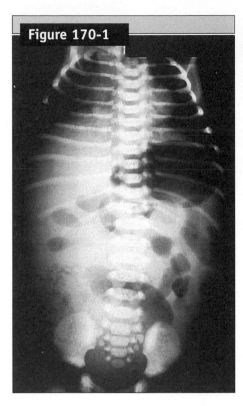

Figure 170-1

Meconium ileus. A plain radiograph of the abdomen shows numerous gas-filled loops, displaced by meconium in the right lower quadrant. Small, multiples bubbles of gas are obvious within the meconium. No air is present in the rectum. (*From* Durie [4].)

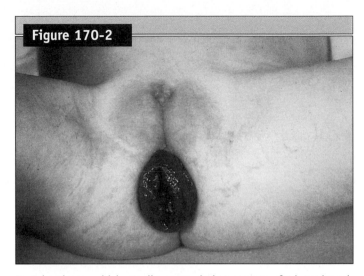

Figure 170-2

Rectal prolapse, which usually occurs during passage of a large bowel motion, can be a frightening condition for parents of young children. It is hardly ever associated with major medical complications and is easily reduced manually. See also **Color Plate**. (*From* Durie [4]).

patients usually also have a decrease in pelvic floor musculature secondary to malnutrition. Rectal prolapse is seen less frequently now than in years past because of earlier diagnosis and better treatments.

Bulky stools may cause chronic abdominal pain, recurrent intussusception, and, in older patients, the distal intestinal obstruction syndrome, formerly known as the meconium ileus equivalent. Distal intestinal obstruction syndrome consists of colicky abdominal pain, distention, and a palpable mass, usually in the right lower quadrant, which is inspissated stool causing partial obstruction. Physicians must be aware of this entity to avoid surgery for a mistaken diagnoses of appendicitis, Crohn's disease, or other causes of intestinal obstruction. Distal intestinal obstruction syndrome usually can be treated successfully with Gastrografin lavage administered by mouth, rectum, or both.

Patients with CF have small intestinal malabsorption as well as a pancreatic maldigestive disorder. Many studies have shown that this may manifest as intestinal bile acid malabsorption because the active transport mechanism is absent, resulting in increased loss of fecal bile acids; impaired absorption of vitamin B$_{12}$; impaired absorption of free fatty acids; and a decrease in intestinal disaccharidase activity, causing clinical lactose intolerance.

Some infants with CF, especially those fed with breast milk or soy-based formula, develop anemia, hypoproteinemia, and significant edema secondary to the low protein content of breast milk or the reduced usable protein in soy milk. Children with CF may be fed a formula containing medium chain triglycerides or continue to breast-feed as long as they receive adequate pancreatic enzyme supplementation.

Although there may be malabsorption of the fat-soluble vitamins (A, D, E, and K), clinical manifestations from deficien-

cies of these vitamins are uncommon. Night blindness and conjunctival xerosis from vitamin A deficiency or a neurologic disorder of ataxia, areflexia, and proprioceptive loss from vitamin E deficiency occasionally is seen in patients who fail to receive adequate vitamin supplementation.

Gastroesophageal reflux is a significant and frequent problem in patients with CF, especially as they reach adolescence and adulthood. The causes of the gastroesophageal reflux are multiple (*eg*, inappropriate relaxation of the lower esophageal sphincter, respiratory medications that decrease the lower esophageal sphincter pressure, and an increased abdominothoracic pressure gradient following coughing or wheezing). Gastroesophageal reflux may exacerbate respiratory symptoms, and vice versa.

Hepatobiliary

Liver disease is common in patients with CF. From 5% to 20% of patients have hepatomegaly, 20% to 30% have abnormal liver tests, and about 2% have portal hypertension. The CFTR is located in the bile duct epithelial cells, not the hepatocytes, and mutations may result in decreased bile flow and increased bile viscosity, leading to focal biliary obstruction. The damage is usually slowly progressive.

Prolonged neonatal cholestasis occurs in about 5% to 10% of CF infants as a result of bile duct obstruction related to inspissated bile and mucus [5]. The cholestasis usually resolves gradually. It is unclear whether neonatal cholestasis is a predictor of future biliary cirrhosis.

Focal biliary cirrhosis is the classic hepatic lesion of CF and may occur in as many as 25% of all CF patients (Fig. 170-3). As CF patients live longer, an increasing number of patients are experiencing extensive multilobular cirrhosis. About 10% of people with CF who are over the age of 25 years have cirrhosis and portal hypertension.

Liver disease (*eg*, biliary cirrhosis, portal hypertension) may be the first sign of CF, and CF should be included in the differential diagnosis of any patient with cirrhosis or hematemesis

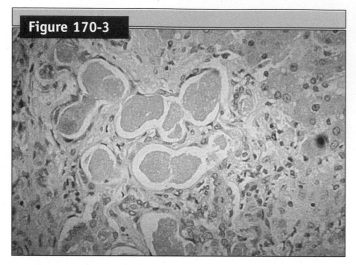

Figure 170-3

A portal area from the liver biopsy of a patient with cystic fibrosis who also has focal biliary cirrhosis. Marked eosinophilic plugging of bile ducts is present. (*From* Durie [4].)

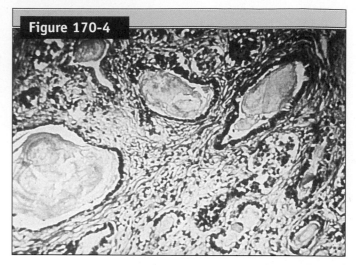

Figure 170-4

Histologic section of a pancreas from a patient with cystic fibrosis. (*From* Durie [4].)

from esophageal varices. The cirrhosis may be silent, with normal liver function tests or mildly elevated serum concentrations of alkaline phosphatase, until the patient experiences upper gastrointestinal bleeding, necessitating evaluation for portal hypertension.

Gallbladder disease (*eg*, cholecystitis, cholelithiasis) is becoming more evident as more CF patients survive into adulthood. It is seen in 40% of CF children 5 to 15 years of age and in 60% of young adult patients. The biliary disorders include gallstones, microgallbladder, and bile duct stenosis [6]. Gallbladder disease presents a particular problem for the clinician because it usually becomes apparent only after the patient has developed significant pulmonary deterioration, making anesthesia and surgery extremely risky. Laparoscopic cholecystectomy should be considered very seriously as an alternative to conventional laparotomy for gallbladder removal.

Pancreas

Eighty percent of infants with CF have total pancreatic insufficiency, and another 10% develop pancreatic achylia in the first 2 years of life. All CF patients, whether they have pancreatic insufficiency or adequate pancreatic function, show evidence of impaired pancreatic fluid secretion as a result of defective anion function within the cells of the pancreatic ducts. The insufficiency is caused by mucus obstruction of the pancreatic ducts, which prevents efflux of pancreatic enzymes and leads to ductal hypertension and autolysis of the pancreatic parenchyma, thereby producing the characteristic cystic and fibrotic changes of CF (Fig. 170-4). These infants may have voracious appetites as a compensation for the calories lost to maldigestion and malabsorption but often have progressive failure to thrive.

Individuals who have adequate pancreatic function are more susceptible to acute recurrent pancreatitis (10% of these patients) than are patients with pancreatic insufficiency.

Diabetes mellitus (usually nonketotic) is a more common problem now that patients with CF are living longer. The diabetes is probably a consequence of increasing fibrosis around the islet cells, resulting in insulinopenia. There is little of the end-organ nonresponsiveness to insulin that is seen in Type I diabetes mellitus. All CF patients should be screened for diabetes with oral glucose tolerance tests [7].

Miscellaneous

Occasionally, patients with CF may present with clinical findings unrelated to the intestinal or respiratory system. For example, they may collapse from hyponatremic dehydration following exercise on a hot day. This is caused by losses of large volumes of sodium and chloride through sweating. Men with CF are always sterile because of azoospermia and absence of the vas deferens. Most women have delayed onset of menarche [8] but can eventually become pregnant, especially with recently developed techniques that allow normal ova to be harvested and the fallopian tubes, which may be obstructed by inspissated thick mucus, to be bypassed. Pregnancy may be difficult because of respiratory embarrassment as the enlarging uterus elevates the diaphragm. Some pregnant CF patients may need respiratory support during the final stages of the third trimester. As a general rule, women who are healthy before becoming pregnant continue to do well during and after pregnancy, as do their offspring. Those whose respiratory status is significantly compromised before pregnancy tend to deteriorate during and after the pregnancy, and their infants are smaller than normal at birth.

■ TREATMENT

There is no question that early diagnosis and improved treatment of CF leads to decreased morbidity and prolonged survival. The dramatic increase in survival in the past three decades seems to be related to two developments: 1) improvements in the understanding and treatment of gastrointestinal complications, especially in the areas of nutrition and growth; and 2) a more aggressive approach to pulmonary complications, including rigorous pulmonary toileting , better antibiotics, and dramatic new medical therapies.

Pulmonary Management

The key to long-term survival is aggressive management of the bronchopulmonary disease of CF. Principles of such management include use of anti-inflammatory agents; treatment of the hyperreactive airway disease; frequent and appropriate use of antibiotics; vigorous routine chest physiotherapy and exercise; and application of newer modes of therapy based on understanding of genetics and pathophysiology (including gene vector therapy, chloride channel agonists, and sodium channel antagonists) [9].

Gastrointestinal Tract and Nutrition

Poor weight gain, linear growth retardation, and delayed sexual maturation are common in CF as results of malabsorption, poor energy intake, and increased energy expenditure [10]. More aggressive nutritional management has evolved because children with CF have genetic potential for growth similar to that of the general population and because malnutrition leads to deterioration of pulmonary function and increased mortality.

In infants, use of formulas that contain medium chain triglyceride oil (eg, Portagen, Alimentum, or Pregestimil) precludes the need for pancreatic lipase. As the child begins to eat solid foods, pancreatic enzyme supplements become necessary. Newer preparations of enteric-coated microspheres (eg, Creon, Pancrease, Cotazym S) are far more resistant to the effects of acid than are powdered enzyme, so smaller amounts are necessary than previously. Capsules are given with meals, with the dose titrated to decrease the bulk and number of stools as well as the degree of steatorrhea. For infants, capsules are opened and the microspheres sprinkled on jelly or applesauce. The toddler may require one to three capsules per meal, the school-age child three to four capsules, and the adolescent and adult four to six capsules with meals and snacks. High daily dosages of pancreatic enzyme supplements may cause fibrosing proximal colonopathy, a newly defined entity of colonic inflammation, shortening, and fibrosis [11•]. Enzyme replacement should be limited to 2500 u/kg of lipase per dose [12]. If an increasing number of capsules is required, an H_2-receptor antagonist should be added to the regimen to avoid acid deactivation of the lipase in the duodenum. Because pancreatic enzyme supplements impair iron absorption [13], iron supplements and pancreatic enzyme should be taken at least 2 hours apart.

The appropriate use of pancreatic enzyme preparations markedly diminishes the incidence of rectal prolapse and distal intestinal obstruction syndrome. To avoid the potential, albeit rare, of fat-soluble vitamin deficiencies, the patient's diet also should be supplemented with a double dose of a multivitamin preparation, along with vitamin E in a water-soluble form as liquid or capsule (50 to 100 IU/day) and a water-soluble form of vitamin K, 5 mg two times a week.

In the older child, adolescent, or adult with CF, a well-balanced, high-calorie diet is probably optimal. To achieve this goal, an increased amount of fat is necessary, a recommendation that is still somewhat controversial. Although increasing dietary fat causes increased fat loss in the stool, the total amount of fat and calories absorbed also increases. (An increase in the total number of pancreatic enzyme capsules also is needed.) When malnutrition is avoided, the CF patient remains in positive nitrogen balance and pulmonary disease progression is slowed.

In the adolescent and adult patient with respiratory exacerbations and lung deterioration, increased metabolic demands inevitably cause weight loss and malnutrition, which leads to negative nitrogen balance, wasting of muscle mass, and further progression of pulmonary disease. It is critical to reverse this process in an attempt to have fewer respiratory infections. Short-term (1 to 6 months) use of parenteral or enteral hyperalimentation increases weight gain and slows lung deterioration, but the improvements are short lived. Long-term supplemental feedings are feasible and appear to be successful in improving nutrition and stabilizing or even improving respiratory status. However, controversy continues over the optimal route for this approach. Because chronic parenteral hyperalimentation is associated with an increased incidence of sepsis and liver disease, nocturnal nasogastric or gastrostomy feedings are commonly used. Many patients with CF have motility disorders and gastroesophageal reflux, which may lead to microaspirations and worsening lung problems. Some clinicians, therefore, advocate prophylactic antireflux operations in such patients or use of jejunostomy feeding tubes [14].

Liver

Ursodeoxycholic acid, a hydrophilic bile salt, increases bile flow and thus possibly dilutes viscous bile, improves liver function tests, and appears to enhance nutritional status [15]. Sclerotherapy, variceal banding, and beta-blockade can be useful in controlling variceal bleeding. In patients with signs of hepatic failure, orthotopic liver transplantation is indicated. Results have been quite good, especially in the patient with mild to moderate pulmonary disease [16•]. Immunosuppressive therapy to prevent transplant rejection has not adversely affected the pulmonary disease of these patients.

▓▓ PROGNOSIS

The dramatic increase in life expectancy in people with CF has been truly impressive. Most patients now can be expected to survive into the third decade of life. It is clear that patients with predominantly gastrointestinal symptoms have a far better course than those with primarily respiratory manifestations, and that men survive longer than women [17]. When pulmonary function deteriorates or liver disease progresses, organ transplantation should be considered. In the future, gene vector therapy, gene replacement therapy, or both, may become the treatments of choice.

▓▓ REFERENCES

Recently published papers of particular interest have been highlighted as follows:
•   Of interest
••   Of outstanding interest

1.•   Kerem BS, Rommens JM, Buchanan JA, et al.: Identification of the cystic fibrosis gene: genetic analysis. Science 1989, 245:1073–1080.
This is a landmark paper describing the actual mutation defect on the long arm of chromosome 7 that leads to cystic fibrosis. This paper includes the classic description of the primary mutation at site 507 that is responsible for 60% to 70% of all the mutations and is associated with pancreatic insufficiency and aggressive pulmonary disease.

2.   Marino CR, Gorelick FS: Scientific advances in cystic fibrosis. Gastroenterology 1992, 103:681–693.

3.   •Stern RC: The diagnosis of cystic fibrosis. N Engl J Med 1997, 336:487–491.
This is an outstanding review of the new and sophisticated approaches to diagnosis of cystic fibrosis. Special attention is paid to the newly described cases that are clinically similar to cystic fibrosis but with normal sweat chloride testing.

4. Durie PR: Cystic fibrosis. In *Gastroenterology and hepatology: the comprehensive visual reference* , vol 4 *Pediatric GI problems*. Edited by Hyman PE. Philadelphia: Current Medicine, 1997:9.1–9.19.

5. Greenholz SK, Krishnadasan B, Marr C, *et al.*: Biliary obstruction in infants with cystic fibrosis requiring Kasai portoenterostomy. *J Ped Surg* 1997, 32:175–180.

6. O'Brien S, Keogan M, Casey M, *et al.*: Biliary complications of cystic fibrosis. *Gut* 1992, 33:387–391.

7. Hayes FJ, O'Brien C, Fitzgerald MX, *et al.*: Diabetes mellitus in an adult cystic fibrosis population. *Ir Med J* 1995, 88:102–104.

8. Johannesson M, Gottlieb C, Hjelte L: Delayed puberty in girls with cystic fibrosis despite good clinical status. *Pediatrics* 1997, 99:29–34.

9. Ramsey BW: Management of pulmonary disease in patients with cystic fibrosis. *N Engl J Med* 1996, 35:179–188.

10. Vaisman N, Pencharz PB, Corey ML, *et al.*: Energy expenditure of patients with cystic fibrosis. *J Pediatr* 1987, 111:496–500.

11.• Fitzsimmons SC, Burkhart GA, Borowitz D, *et al.*: High-dose pancreatic enzyme supplements and fibrosing colonopathy in children with cystic fibrosis. *N Engl J Med* 1997, 336:1283–1289.
The use of high doses of lipase in pancreatic supplements had become very popular and was considered safe. It is clear, however, that the higher amounts of lipase create an inflammatory reaction in the colon, possibly by causing ganglion cells to become disordered.

12. Reichard KW, Vinocur CD, Franco M, *et al.*: Fibrosing colonopathy in children with cystic fibrosis. *J Pediatr Surg* 1997, 32:237–242.

13. Zempsky WT, Rosenstein BJ, Carroll JA, Oski FA: Effect of pancreatic enzyme supplements on iron absorption. *Am J Dis Child* 1989, 143:969–972.

14. Boland MP, Stoski DS, Macdonald NE, *et al.*: Chronic jejunostomy feeding with a non-elemental formula in undernourished patients with cystic fibrosis. *Lancet* 1986, 1:232–234.

15. Colombo C, Battezzati PM, Podda M, *et al.*: Ursodeoxycholic acid for liver disease associated with cystic fibrosis: a double-blind multicenter trial. *Hepatology* 1996, 23:1484–1490.

16.• Mack DR, Traystman MD, Colombo JL, *et al.*: Clinical denouement and mutation analysis of patients with cystic fibrosis undergoing liver transplantation for biliary cirrhosis. *J Pediatrics* 1995, 127:881–887.
Liver transplantation has a definite role in the management of patients with cystic fibrosis who develop biliary cirrhosis and signs of hepatic failure. The need for immunosuppressive agents postoperatively does not seem to have a deleterious effect on pulmonary function and may actually slow the rate of pulmonary deterioration.

17. Durieu I, Bellon G, Vital Durand D, *et al.*: Cystic fibrosis in adults. *Presse Med* 1995, 24:1882–1887.

171 Constipation and Fecal Soiling
Richard B. Colletti

Constipation in children often is associated with fecal soiling. Patients may have either 1) constipation without soiling; 2) constipation and fecal soiling; or 3) fecal soiling without constipation. Constipation may be defined as infrequent bowel movements, hard stools, or pain or straining with bowel movements. There is no universal agreement on the use of the terms *fecal soiling*, *fecal incontinence*, and *encopresis*, but all signify the passage of stool into underwear or clothing at the age of 4 years or older.

The infant or young child with constipation typically has infrequent, painful defecation of hard stools. Withholding of stool because of fear of anal pain is a common feature. The school-aged child with chronic constipation often presents with fecal soiling. Pediatric constipation usually is functional in origin, and pediatric fecal soiling usually is the result of constipation.

ANATOMY, PHYSIOLOGY, AND DEVELOPMENT OF NORMAL DEFECATION

Embryologically, the hindgut is the origin of the distal transverse, descending, and sigmoid colon, the rectum, and the upper anal canal. At 7 weeks gestation the primitive perineum is formed, and the anal membrane separates from the urogenital membrane. After the 9th week, the anal membrane ruptures, and an open pathway to the rectum is formed. The upper part of the anal canal is endodermal and the lower third is ectodermal in origin. Imperforate anus and rectal fistulas can form as a result of improper hindgut development.

The mean anal diameter of the newborn is 8.6 mm for a 1.25-kg premature infant and 12.0 mm for a 3.75-kg full-term infant [1]. The normal position of the anus, defined as the ratio of the distance from the anus to the vagina or scrotum divided by the distance between the vagina or scrotum and the coccyx, is 0.39 (SD ± 0.09) in girls, and 0.56 (SD ± 0.10) in boys [2]. Anterior displacement, seen in imperforate anus with fistula, is an uncommon cause of constipation. There also are age-related changes in colonic motility. With increasing age, there are fewer high-amplitude propagated contractions before and after meals; other colonic contractions increase with age, however [3].

The sequential steps of normal defecation are distention of the rectum by stool, transient relaxation of the internal anal sphincter, sensory contact of the stool with the anus, brief contraction of the external anal sphincter, relaxation of the levator ani, Valsalva maneuver, relaxation of both the internal and external sphincters, and expulsion of stool. The ability to use the toilet for defecation requires a certain degree of neuromuscular function, such as the ability to walk, undress and dress, and sit upright. It also requires psychological readiness, including motivation and development of the cognitive skills necessary for learning and remembering. Most children have acquired such skills by 20 months of age [4••]. Fecal

Table 171-1. Normal Frequency of Bowel Movements

Age	Bowel movements per week*
0–3 mo	
Breast milk	5 to 40
Formula	5 to 28
6–12 mo	5 to 28
1–3 y	4 to 21
>3 y	3 to 14

*Approximately mean ± 2 SD
Data from Fontana M, et al. [5]

Table 171-2. Causes of Pediatric Constipation

Functional	Endocrine and metabolic
Dietary changes	Hypothyroidism
Toilet training	Hypercalcemia, hypokalemia
Febrile illness	Renal tubular acidosis
Fear	Diabetes mellitus, diabetes
Withholding	insipidus
Organic	Multiple endocrine neoplasia,
Neuromuscular disorders	type 3
Myelomeningocele	Perianal
Myotonic dystrophy	Anal fissure
Severe retardation	Streptococcal cellulitis
Diastematomyelia	Atopic dermatitis
Intestinal pseudo-	Gastrointestinal
obstruction	Gluten-sensitive enteropathy
Congenital	Cystic fibrosis
Hirschsprung's disease	Obstruction
Imperforate anus with fistula	Drugs and toxins
Anal stenosis	Pelvic tumor
Dysmorphic syndromes	Other

continence occurs on average by 28 months but may not occur until as late as 48 months of age.

EPIDEMIOLOGY

The normal frequency of bowel movements in infants and young children varies with age (Table 171-1). In the first 3 months of life, 95% of breast-fed infants have five to 40 bowel movements per week, whereas formula-fed infants have five to 28 bowel movements per week. The normal (mean ± 2 SD) frequency of bowel movements of infants 6 to 12 months of age is approximately five to 28 per week; of children 1 to 3 years of age, four to 21 per week; and of children over 3 years of age, three to 14 per week. The adult pattern (ie, three to 21 per week) usually has been established by 4 years of age [5].

Constipation occurs in about 3% to 8% of children, equally in males and females. Most parents believe that constipation is dangerous for babies, rely on personal experience to learn about constipation, and do not mention their concerns to their physicians. Approximately 3% of general pediatric outpatient visits are for constipation. Fecal soiling occurs in 3% of 4-year-olds, 2% of 6-year-olds, and 1.5% of 7- to 11-year-olds, with a male predominance of 2.5:1 to 6:1 [6].

ETIOLOGY

Constipation in children most often is functional in origin, ie, without objective evidence of a pathological state, either organic or pyschological. Organic causes of constipation are uncommon in children, and, when present, they usually are obvious (Table 171-2). Children with neurologic disorders, such as myelomeningocele, myotonic dystrophy, and disabling mental retardation, constitute the largest group of children with organic causes of constipation. Hirschsprung's disease usually is diagnosed in the newborn period, but it may present in older infants or children (see Chapter 172). Streptococcal perianal cellulitis or perianal atopic dermatitis can cause fecal retention. Other uncommon causes include hypothyroidism, celiac disease, imperforate anus with fistula, and Williams syndrome or other dysmorphic conditions [7,8].

In about 90% of children with fecal soiling, constipation is the cause. Fecal soiling in the absence of constipation often is functional, but it also may be caused by a psychological disorder, colitis, neurologic disorders, and anorectal malformation.

PATHOGENESIS

Dietary changes, such as the change to whole milk from infant formula, the addition of cereal to the infant's diet, or not eating during a febrile illness, can lead to hard stools. Anal pain from passage of a hard stool can cause fear of defecation and stool retention in preschool children. Stool retention causes further hardening and enlargement of the stool, worsens pain and fear, and establishes a cycle that perpetuates retentive behavior.

Toddlers who refuse to use a toilet for bowel movements during toilet training are more likely to develop stool retention, painful defecation, and constipation [9•]. Such toddlers tend to be temperamentally difficult but do not have an increased prevalence of behavior problems. There have been anecdotal reports of children who became frightened by an ostomy or a television commercial about a toilet and subsequently developed fecal retention. Many older children with chronic constipation have a history of withholding stool, with the development of soiling as they got older [10].

Anorectal manometry performed in children with chronic constipation and encopresis has demonstrated an increased threshold for rectal distention and decreased rectal contractility, conditions that usually persist after treatment [11•]. In some children, the external anal sphincter and pelvic floor fail to relax during defecation, and they are not able to expel a rectal balloon. Children with chronic constipation have a slowing of intestinal transit, most commonly at the level of the distal colon and rectum. This finding is consistent with outlet obstruction resulting from fecal retention.

Behavior and social competence are more likely to be abnormal in school-aged children with chronic constipation and soiling. However, prognosis and unresponsiveness to treatment do not correlate with measures of behavior or social competence. Successful treatment may result in improvement of behavior and social competence as well as of constipation, suggesting that

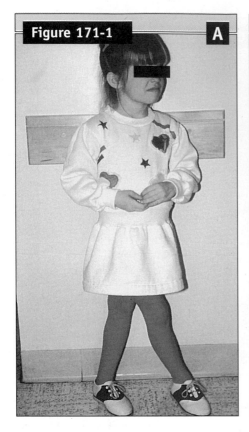
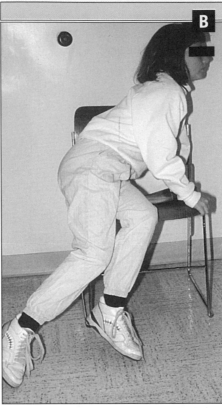

Figure 171-1

Two patients demonstrate the postures they assume during withholding of stool. **A,** The legs are extended and crossed. **B,** The patient sits on the edge of a chair with her legs squeezed together.

in many cases psychosocial abnormalities are secondary to rather than the cause of constipation and soiling [12].

CLINICAL FEATURES

The typical preschool child with constipation has decreased stool frequency, hard stools, and painful defecation. Bleeding from an anal fissure is not uncommon. A history of unusual posturing or behaviors that indicate the act of withholding stool often can be elicited: the child leans against a chair or wall with legs extended, stiff, and crossed; sits on the floor with legs extended; squats hiding in a corner; or fidgets, rocks or dances on tiptoe (Fig. 171-1). The child usually strains, reddens in the face, and appears to the parents to be trying to defecate; in fact, the posturing enhances tightening of the gluteal and anal muscles to prevent defecation. The physical examination of such a child is usually normal except for a mildly dilated rectum containing firm stool.

The school-age child with constipation has a history of chronic, infrequent, large-caliber, hard stools. Posturing to withhold stools is less common than in the younger child, but fecal soiling and mild abdominal cramps are more common, occurring daily or beginning several days after the previous bowel movement. The child denies feeling the urge to defecate or the sensation of stool seepage. Stool may be large enough to clog the toilet. Physical examination usually is normal, except for a dilated rectum filled with firm stool, and, in more severe cases, a fecaloma, a hard, stool-filled rectosigmoid mass palpable in the hypogastrium. Some children present with a chief complaint of diarrhea, which actually is overflow soiling, or with frequent passage of tiny marbles of stool because of incomplete evacuation.

The child who has soiling without constipation usually is a school-aged boy who defecates regularly on the toilet but soils frequently. He may be socially and neurodevelopmentally immature and too busy playing to take the time to defecate; attention deficit disorder may be present. Learning, motivational, and behavioral factors appear to account for the soiling. In some cases, fecal soiling is an attention-getting device, part of a power struggle between child and parent, or is associated with a psychiatric disorder.

In contrast, the child with classic Hirschsprung's disease has soft, small-caliber, painless stools, and no rectal bleeding or withholding postures. Little stool is detected in the rectum on digital examination or radiography. Poor growth, abdominal distention, or episodic febrile illness with diarrhea, indicative of enterocolitis, also suggest the diagnosis. The total colonic and short-segment forms of Hirschsprung's disease have atypical features that may result in delayed diagnosis (see Chapter 172).

Of note is the breast-fed infant who appears to be constipated but actually is not. Some healthy, thriving breast-fed infants, beginning at about 6 weeks of age, have long intervals between bowel movements, sometimes more than 7 days, followed by passage of a large, soupy, normal stool. Some of these infants appear uncomfortable after several days without a bowel movement, and are relieved after one. These infants are normal and, unless symptoms persist after weaning, they do not require investigation for Hirschsprung's disease or other disorders.

DIAGNOSIS

The diagnosis of functional constipation usually is based solely on the presence of typical historical features and absence of physical abnormalities; laboratory studies are not necessary. The absence of other symptoms, neurologic abnormalities, poor linear or ponderal growth, thyroid enlargement, abnormal deep tendon reflexes, abnormal location or appearance of

Figure 171-2

	0	1	2	3	4	5	Comments
A Stool in ascending colon	Small amount	Moderate amount	Large throughout				
B Stool in transverse colon	Little or none			Moderate amount	Large amount	Large: dilated	
C Stool in descending colon	Little or none			Moderate amount	Large amount	Large: dilated	
D Stool in rectum	Little or none		Moderate amount			Large amount: full distally	
E Rock-like stools	Few or none	Moderate amount	Large amount: transverse descending colon	Large amount: ascending colon			
F Granular stools	Little or none		Moderate amount distal*		Large amount distal*	Throughout length	

*Distal=past splenic flexure

TOTAL SCORE _____

A stool retention rating system that scores quantity, distribution, and consistency of stool. A score of 10 or greater correlates well with stool retention. (*From* Barr [14]; with permission.)

the anus, perianal cellulitis or dermatitis, a small rectum without stool, bloody diarrhea, or dysmorphic features is consistent with the diagnosis of functional constipation. A careful history and observation of parent–child interaction is performed to screen for psychological problems; further evaluation by a mental health worker may be necessary. Sexual abuse should be suspected when there is poor anal tone or a patulous anus without apparent cause. Urinary tract infections and enuresis are more common in children with constipation, particularly girls.

Fecal retention in about 85% of cases can be confirmed by finding excessive feces on the digital rectal examination. Detection of a fecaloma indicates severe fecal retention. When the presence or severity of fecal retention is uncertain, an abdominal anterior–posterior supine radiograph is useful. Interpretation of stool content on abdominal radiographs by disinterested viewers often is unreliable, but use of a methodologic scoring system can be helpful in assessing the amount and location of stool within the colon (Fig. 171-2) [13,14]. In the child with functional constipation, unless there has been a recent bowel movement, the rectum is filled with stool and dilated to the anal verge, indicative of fecal retention, incomplete evacuation, or both (Fig. 171-3). The extent of impaction is apparent from the degree of dilation and quantity of stool within the remainder of the colon.

When Hirschsprung's disease is suspected, rectal manometry and biopsy of the rectum are indicated. In functional constipation, the rectoinhibitory reflex of the internal sphincter is intact, and ganglion cells are present in the submucous and myenteric plexuses, whereas in classic Hirschsprung's disease, both are absent. Rectal biopsy is necessary for the diagnosis of gan-

gliomatosis, neuronal dysplasia, and other disorders affecting ganglion cells.

Except in early infancy, barium enema is not useful in the preliminary evaluation of pediatric constipation. The presence on abdominal plain film of a rectum filled with stool and dilated to the anal verge essentially excludes classic Hirschsprung's disease, colonic obstruction, and anorectal malformation. Because stool is radiopaque, administration of barium usually is unnecessary. The barium enema may be misleading in total colonic Hirschsprung's disease, when the colon may appear normal, or in ultra–short-segment Hirschsprung's disease, which

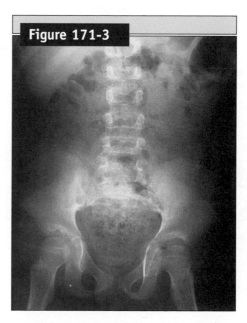

Figure 171-3

Abdominal plain film demonstrates a full rectum dilated to the anal verge and filled with granular stool. This appearance is characteristic of functional constipation associated with withholding stool. There also is a moderate amount of stool in the descending colon, for a total of 12 points according to the stool retention rating system shown in Figure 171-2.

resembles functional constipation radiologically. However, after Hirschsprung's disease has been diagnosed by rectal manometry and biopsy, the barium enema may be useful to locate the transition zone. Barium enema should be done without cleansing the colon because such preparation may abolish the transition zone between the aganglionic contracted distal segment and the normally innervated yet dilated proximal segment.

The colonic transit time test usually is not helpful; when normal, however, it does exclude a significant problem. Colonic manometry can detect gastrointestinal neuropathy and myopathy in cases of intractable constipation. Children with neuropathy have no high-amplitude propagated contractions, and the motility index does not increase after a meal; patients with myopathy have no contractions [15]. Consensus guidelines with criteria for the diagnosis of chronic intestinal pseudo-obstruction in childhood recently have been established [16].

▰▰ TREATMENT

Education is the mainstay of treatment of functional constipation. It consists of explaining 1) the pathogenesis of childhood constipation; 2) the lack of underlying disease; 3) the meaning of the child's unusual posturing; and 4) the three phases of treatment: disimpaction, laxative, and maintenance [17] (Fig. 171-4, Tables 171-3 and 171-4). For milder cases, treatment with dietary changes, dietary fiber, mineral oil, osmotic agents, or a combination of these is sufficient.

Treatment of severe impaction usually includes the use of sodium phosphate enemas (Table 171-3). A clean-out regimen consists of a 3-day cycle consisting of two enemas on the first day, two bisacodyl suppositories on the second day, and two doses of a laxative (milk of magnesia, bisacodyl tablets, or senna) on the third day. One, two, or three consecutive cycles are administered over 3 to 9 days. An alternative approach to disimpaction is high-dose mineral oil (up to 8 oz daily) [18], but seepage of oil, which may occur, is disturbing to patients and parents and damages clothes. Polyethylene glycol isotonic lavage also is effective for disimpaction, but it can require continuous infusion by nasogastric tube for 24 hours [19].

A novel approach to disimpaction and cleansing of the colon is pulsed irrigation and evacuation by a mechanical device during a 30-minute procedure. Other new approaches that are used in children with myelomeningocele include a Silastic balloon-

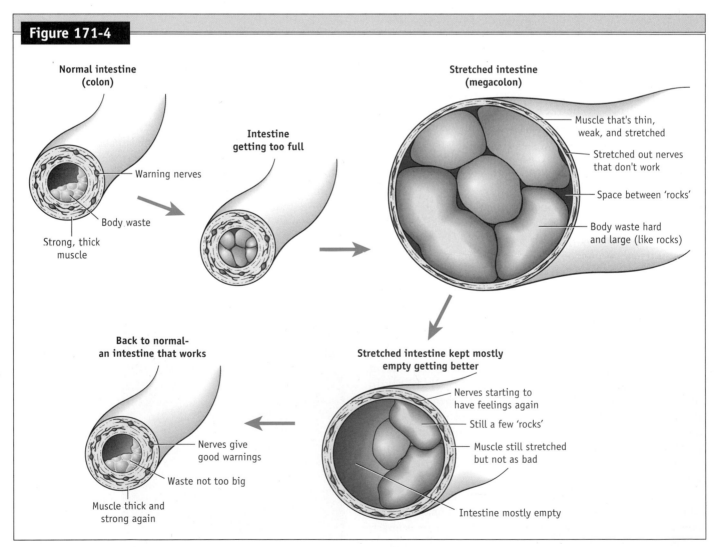

Figure 171-4

Normal intestine (colon)
Warning nerves
Body waste
Strong, thick muscle

Intestine getting too full

Stretched intestine (megacolon)
Muscle that's thin, weak, and stretched
Stretched out nerves that don't work
Space between 'rocks'
Body waste hard and large (like rocks)

Stretched intestine kept mostly empty getting better
Nerves starting to have feelings again
Still a few 'rocks'
Muscle still stretched but not as bad
Intestine mostly empty

Back to normal—an intestine that works
Nerves give good warnings
Waste not too big
Muscle thick and strong again

Diagrammatic representation of the development, consequences, and effective treatment of fecal retention and soiling. A copy of this diagram presented to the patient and family effectively reinforces the education process. (*From* Levine [17]; with permission.)

Table 171-3. Phases of Treatment: Medication Options

1. Clean-out (disimpaction)
   - Sodium phosphate enemas
   - High-dose mineral oil
   - Polyethylene glycol isotonic lavage
2. Laxative
   - Milk of magnesia
   - Senna
   - Bisacodyl
3. Maintenance
   - Dietary
   - Fiber
   - Mineral oil
   - Lactulose or sorbitol
   - Milk of magnesia
   - Barley malt extract (Maltsupex)
   - ? Polyethylene glycol isotonic lavage
   - ? Cisapride

tipped enema catheter for retrograde irrigations, and a percutaneous cecostomy tube or percutaneous placement of a skin-level button gastrostomy-type tube into an appendiceal stump or terminal ileum for antegrade irrigations.

After disimpaction, daily laxative therapy with milk of magnesia, senna, or lactulose usually is administered for 2 to 4 weeks to induce regular bowel movements. Regular bowel movements then are maintained for months or years with mineral oil, lactulose (or less expensive sorbitol), or, if necessary, milk of magnesia. More recently, daily cisapride or polyethylene glycol isotonic lavage has been proposed to maintain regular bowel movements. It may be necessary to administer an enema to prevent recurrence of impaction if there has been no bowel movement for 48 hours or if stool-withholding behaviors are evident.

Unwarranted parental anxiety about mineral oil treatment of constipation can be fueled by the lay literature. Although mineral oil therapy reduces the absorption of fat-soluble vitamins, it rarely, if ever, produces vitamin deficiency, even in patients who receive high doses. As a precaution, a multivitamin supplement can be given with chronic high-dose treatment, or mineral oil can be administered at bedtime. When effective, mineral oil (heavy, not light) is the preferred maintenance therapy because of its lack of toxicity. Mineral oil is tasteless, but it has an unpleasant greasy texture. Steps to enhance palatability include refrigerating the oil and mixing it with orange juice, chocolate milk, cola drinks, pudding, or ice cream [20].

The role of dietary fiber in the management of childhood constipation is unclear. Most healthy children eat less fiber than recommended; constipated children probably do not eat less fiber than children without constipation. Even intensive dietary counseling is not effective in increasing children's dietary fiber intake. Fiber is the basic treatment of constipation in adults, but, unlike children, adults have small stools as part of the irritable bowel syndrome.

For infants, a barley malt extract is a highly effective, although expensive, treatment of functional constipation. Mineral oil usually is not administered to children less than 1 year old, to patients with gastroesophageal reflux, or to neurologically impaired children because of the risk of aspiration pneumonia.

Rectal manometric biofeedback has been used to teach children with abnormal defecation dynamics to relax the pelvic floor during straining for defecation, with significant improvements in constipation and soiling after 1 year. However, recovery rates at long-term follow-up have not shown any advantage to biofeedback treatment compared with conventional therapy, and this treatment is still controversial [21].

Table 171-4. Medication Dosages for Pediatric Constipation

Medication	Dosage*	Comments
Hypertonic sodium phosphate/biphosphate enema	< 2 y: to be avoided ≥ 2 y: 6 mL/kg up to 135 mL	Most children dislike enemas; hypernatremia, hyperphosphatemia, and hypocalcemic tetany
Polyethylene glycol isotonic lavage	For clean-out: 25 mL/kg/h (up to 1000 mL) by nasogastric tube until clear *or* 20 mL/kg/h for 4 h/day For maintenance (older children): 5–10 mL/kg daily p.o.	Clean-out may require hospitalization and nasogastric tube; safety of long-term maintenance treatment not well established; not very palatable by mouth
Bisacodyl (tablet 5 mg, suppository 10 mg)	≥ 2 y: 0.5–1 suppository or 1–3 tablets per dose	Not recommended for long-term treatment
Senna (Senokot)†	1 to 5 y: 5–10 mL/day 5 to 15 y: 10–20 mL/day	Safety of long-term treatment is uncertain
Milk of magnesia	1–3 mL/kg/day divided into two doses	Not very palatable; cramping
Mineral oil (heavy)	< 1 y: not recommended Clean-out: 15–30 mL/year of age, up to 240 mL daily Maintenance: 1–3 mL/kg/day	Do not use if higher risk of aspiration; during maintenance, seepage indicates dose too high or need for clean-out; consider vitamin supplement.
Lactulose (10 g/15 mL) *or* Sorbitol (70%)	1–3 mL/kg/day in divided doses	Palatable, sorbitol is less expensive; cramping; not as effective as milk of magnesia.
Barley malt extract (Maltsupex)‡	5–10 mL per 240 mL of milk or juice	Unpleasant odor; suitable for infants drinking from a bottle

* Adjust dosage to induce a daily bowel movement for 1 to 2 months.

† Purdue Frederick Company, Norwalk, CT

‡ Wallace Laboratories, Cranbury, NJ

Table 171-5. Pediatric Bowel Training Program

Disimpaction is performed if necessary

Each morning the child sits on the toilet for 5–10 minutes

If there has not been a full bowel movement for 24–48 hours, then the child receives an enema to induce full evacuation

A small reward (eg, a sticker) is given for each bowel movement on the toilet; a treat is given for every three stickers; rewards are inexpensive, available, and given immediately upon success

Parent records size and consistency of stool, soiling, and when an enema is administered.

When fecal soiling is the result of constipation, treatment of the constipation effectively eliminates soiling. Soiling in the absence of constipation is treated with a bowel training program that combines medication with behavior modification (Table 171-5). The goals of the bowel training program are to establish a routine that fosters good habits and induces regular complete evacuation of rectal contents. The patient sits on the toilet for 5 to 10 minutes after one or more designated meals; if there has not been a full bowel movement for 2 consecutive days, an enema is administered to induce one. Praise and small rewards are given [4••,22].

When compliance by the patient or family is poor, when either constipation or soiling is part of a power struggle or other behavioral conflicts, or when the response to standard therapy is poor, referral for psychological evaluation and more intensive behavioral therapy is indicated. In one study, weekly therapy sessions of play with modeling clay were remarkably effective in cases of intractable soiling [23].

PROGNOSIS AND FOLLOW-UP MANAGEMENT

About 50% to 70% of children referred to a pediatric gastroenterologist for management of constipation are asymptomatic 5 to 7 years later. Factors that may predispose to persistence of constipation are early age at onset, duration of symptoms before the onset of effective therapy, presence of soiling, and a family history of constipation [24]. Three years after initiation of treatment with milk of magnesia, a high-fiber diet, and bowel training techniques, the anal resting tone and the percentage of relaxation of the rectosphincteric reflex have remained significantly lower in both recovered and nonrecovered constipated and encopretic patients compared with healthy controls.

Close monitoring by parents and the physician is a vital part of therapy, particularly at its onset. Parents are asked to record the frequency of bowel movements, stool size and consistency, and soiling, and when supplemental enemas are needed. Office visits, telephone follow-up, or both should continue until the child is having regular bowel movements on the toilet without soiling. Parents should be advised that relapses are not uncommon but are manageable. Parents dislike administering medications to their children, and premature discontinuation of medication is common. Parents should be advised that long-term administration of medication may be necessary and is preferable to persistent or worsening symptoms.

Treatment of fecal soiling with a combination of medication and behavior modification is effective in 60% to 100% of cases, with relapses in about 15% to 25% of children. Many failures are associated with noncompliance [4••,12].

REFERENCES

Recently published papers of particular interest have been highlighted as follows:
•   Of interest
••   Of outstanding interest

1. El Haddad M, Corkery JJ: The anus in the newborn. *Pediatrics* 1985, 76:927–928.

2. Bar-Maor JA, Eitan A: Determination of the normal position of the anus (with reference to idiopathic constipation). *J Pediatr Gastroenterol Nutr* 1987, 6:559–561.

3. Di Lorenzo C, Flores AF, Hyman PE: Age-related changes in colon motility. *J Pediatr* 1995, 127:593–596.

4.•• Howe AC, Walker CE: Behavioral management of toilet training, enuresis and encopresis. *Pediatr Clin North Am* 1992, 39:413–432.
This paper discusses when and how to toilet train and the assessment and treatment of encopresis (both manipulative and retentive encopresis) using medical and behavioral approaches. Conservative and more active protocols for treatment of encopresis are described in detail.

5. Fontana M, Bianchi C, Cataldo F, *et al.*: Bowel frequency in healthy children. *Acta Paediatr Scand* 1989, 78:682–684.

6. Loening-Baucke V. Encopresis and soiling. *Pediatr Clin North Am* 1996, 43:279–298.

7. Hyman PE, Fleisher DR: A classification of disorders of defecation in infants and children. *Semin Gastrointest Dis* 1994, 5:20–23.

8. Seth R, Heyman MB: Management of constipation and encopresis in infants and children. *Gastroenterol Clin North Am* 1994, 23:621–636.

9.• Taubman B: Toilet training and toileting refusal for stool only: a prospective study. *Pediatrics* 1997, 99:54–58.
This prospective study demonstrated that stool toileting refusal occurs in one in five children during toilet training. Interrupting toilet training and having the child return to diapers resulted in the child spontaneously using the toilet for bowel movements. A companion article (*Pediatrics* 1997, 99:50–53) demonstrated that children with stool toileting refusal were somewhat more difficult temperamentally, but did not have more behavior problems.

10. Partin JC, Hamill SK, Fischel JE, Partin JS: Painful defecation and fecal soiling in children. *Pediatrics* 1992, 89:1007–1009.

11.• Loening-Baucke V: Chronic constipation in children. *Gastroenterol* 1993, 105:1557–1564.
This is an overview of the clinical presentation, diagnosis, investigations, management, and outcome of childhood constipation. It contains 61 references.

12. Young MH, Brennen LC, Baker RD, Baker SS: Functional encopresis: symptom reduction and behavioral improvement. *Dev Behav Pediatr* 1995, 16:226–232.

13. Blethyn AJ, Verrier Jones K, Newcombe R, *et al.*: Radiological assessment of constipation. *Arch Dis Child* 1995, 73:532–533.

14. Barr RG, Levine MD, Wildinson RH, Mulvihill D: Chronic and occult stool retention. *Clin Pediatr* 1979, 18:674–679.

15. Di Lorenzo C, Flores AF, Reddy SN, Hyman PE: Use of colonic manometry to differentiate causes of intractable constipation in children. *J Pediatr* 1992, 120:690–695.

16. Rudolph CD, Heyman PE, Altschuler SM, *et al.*: Diagnosis and treatment of chronic intestinal pseudo-obstruction in children: report of consensus workshop. *J Pediatr Gastroenterol Nutr* 1997, 24:102–112.

17. Levine MD: Encopresis: its potentiation, evaluation and alleviation. *Pediatr Clin North Am* 1982, 29:315–330.

18. Gleghorn EE, Heyman MB, Rudolph CD: No-enema therapy for idiopathic constipation and encopresis. *Clin Pediatr* 1991, 30:669–672.

19. Tolia V, Elitsur Y, Lin CH: A prospective randomized study with mineral oil and oral lavage solution for treatment of faecal impaction in children. *Aliment Pharmacol Ther* 1993, 7:523–529.

20. McClung HJ, Boyne LJ, Linsheid T, *et al.*: Is combination therapy for encopresis nutritionally safe? *Pediatrics* 1993, 91:591–594.

21. Loening-Baucke V: Biofeedback treatment for chronic constipation and encopresis in childhood: long-term outcome. *Pediatrics*1995, 96:105–110.

22. Lowery SP, Srour JW, Whitehead, Schuster MM: Habit training as treatment of encopresis secondary to chronic constipation. *J Pediatr Gastroenterol Nutr* 1985, 4:397–401.

23. Feldman PC, Villanueva S, Lanne V, Devroede G: Use of play with clay to treat children with intractable encopresis. *J Pediatr* 1993;122:483–488.

24. Sutphen JL, Borowitz SM, Hutchison RL, Cox DJ: Long-term follow-up of medically treated childhood constipation. *Clin Pediatr* 1995, 34:576–580.

172 Hirschsprung's Disease
David A. Piccoli

Hirschsprung's disease (HD) is the most common cause of intestinal obstruction in neonates. In HD, there is a lack of normal intrinsic innervation of the bowel. Most commonly, there is aganglionosis of the rectosigmoid; however, the entire colon and even the small intestine may be aganglionic. HD also is known as *congenital aganglionosis* to distinguish it from the much rarer forms of acquired aganglionosis. HD has been called *congenital megacolon*, but this term appears inappropriate, because the presence of a megacolon at birth is unusual, and patients with long-segment aganglionosis never have megacolon. Some forms of HD are clearly heritable. Recently, animal models of aganglionosis have increased the understanding of the pathophysiology of this disorder. Complications may be fatal, and surgery is required in almost all forms of the disease. Following surgery, medical management usually is necessary to restore normal defecatory patterns.

EPIDEMIOLOGY

The incidence of HD is 1 in 5000 persons. There are important epidemiologic differences between patients with limited disease and those with total colonic aganglionosis. The male-to-female ratio for all cases is 3.8 to 1; it is 2.2 to 1 in total aganglionosis. A family history is positive in 7% of all cases, but is positive in 21% of cases of total colonic aganglionosis [1]. There is a 3.5% incidence in siblings of index cases, and the concurrence is higher in monozygotic than in dizygotic twins [2]. There does not appear to be any racial difference in incidence or severity.

GENETICS

HD is the result of a generalized defect in the normal migration of the neural crest cells in the gut and can be sporadic or familial. In different pedigrees, the inheritance pattern can be autosomal dominant or recessive and gender-related with variable penetrance. One genetic defect that leads to HD involves deletions or mutations in the RET proto-oncogene that codes for a tyrosine kinase receptor expressed in cells of neural crest lineage [3,4]. HD results from mutations that cause a decrease in the function of this gene, whereas mutations that cause increases in

its activity are responsible for multiple endocrine neoplasia type 2 (MEN-2). Mutations in the RET gene occur in 10% to 40% of patients with HD [5]. There is evidence that gene penetrance is lower in females than in males [6]. DNA testing for this gene is now available and is useful to predict persons at risk. Although 90% of persons with MEN-2 have a mutation of the RET proto-oncogene, other mutations probably account for a significant number of cases of HD.

ANATOMY

Normal embryologic development of the autonomic parasympathetic myenteric and submucosal plexuses begins in the proximal gut at about the 5th week of gestation. The neural elements gradually migrate caudally; this migration is completed by the 12th week of gestation. In HD, interruption of this process leaves an aganglionic area extending proximally for a variable length from the external anal sphincter. This results in a functional defect in the intrinsic autonomic nervous system that is comprised of three distinct plexuses of ganglion cells: the Auerbach myenteric plexus between circular and longitudinal muscle layers; the Henley submucosal plexus deep to the circular layer; and the Meissner submucosal plexus immediately beneath the muscularis mucosae. The intrinsic and enteric nervous systems operate independently of the central nervous system. In HD, the extrinsic nervous system of the gut, composed of parasympathetic and sympathetic nerve fibers, also exhibits histologic and functional abnormalities. Intrinsic reflux activity is interrupted, and propulsive peristalsis is absent. The normal relaxation of the internal anal sphincter in response to fecal distention of the rectum does not occur in HD.

Normally, there is a paucity of ganglion cells extending at least 1 to 1.5 cm above the anorectal margin. In HD, the extent of aganglionosis is variable. Rectosigmoid aganglionosis accounts for 74% of all cases of colon aganglionosis, and 89% of these cases are distal to the splenic flexure (Table 172-1). Total colonic aganglionosis occurs in 8% of children, and, in rare instances, aganglionosis extends to the ileum, jejunum, or duodenum [1]. The severity of symptoms, although influenced by the site and extent

Table 172-1. Extent of Aganglionosis

Location	%, (n=998)
Rectum–rectosigmoid	30
Sigmoid colon	44
Left colon	11
Splenic flexure	4
Transverse colon	2
Right colon	1
Total colon and above	8

Adapted from Kleinhaus et al. [1].

Figure 172-1

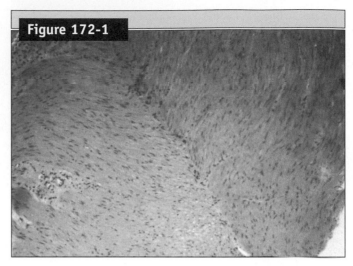

Aganglionic colon. No ganglion cells are seen, and large nerve trunks are present. (*From* Langer [25].)

of the aganglionosis, varies significantly within each specific subset of patients. Increased tone within the aganglionic segments probably is a more significant factor in causing obstructive symptoms than is the extent of the aganglionosis.

The distal aganglionic segment neither is propulsive, nor does it relax. Aganglionic bowel tends to be spastic and contracted. Proximal to the abnormal segment, the normal bowel has an appropriate number of ganglia but becomes hypertrophied and dilated because of the distal obstructive component. The bowel at the junction between the aganglionic and ganglionic segments is called the transition zone, and typically appears cone-shaped on radiopacification studies. In the newborn, the obstructed bowel often is not dilated because active colonic propulsion and defecation do not occur in utero.

Histologically, there is an absence of ganglion cells and their intrinsic nerve fibers in both the myenteric Auerbach and the submucosal Meissner plexuses, accompanied by a proliferation of hypertrophied nerve fibers from the extrinsic enteric nervous system where ganglion cells are absent (Fig. 172-1). The diagnosis of HD usually is made by light microscopic examination of rectal tissue obtained by rectal suction biopsy. The specimen must contain adequate submucosa demonstrating absence of ganglion cells. The thickened nerve fibers are more evident when the tissue is stained for acetylcholinesterase, which is released from the preganglionic nerve fibers in excessive concentrations.

■ CLINICAL FEATURES

Although the clinical manifestations of HD vary depending on the length and tone of the aganglionic segment as well as the age of the patient, normal defecation almost always is altered. In the first 24 to 48 hours of life, there usually is delay in the passage of meconium. Whereas 94% of normal full-term infants pass meconium in the first 24 hours of life and 99% by 48 hours, Swenson reported that only 6% of babies with HD defecated in the first 24 hours of life and only 43% by 48 hours [7]. Any full-term infant who has not passed meconium within 48 hours after birth must be evaluated for HD. Bilious vomiting and abdominal distention, the result of intestinal obstruction, are typical. A history that suggests that meconium was passed only after rectal stimulation, or the presence of a meconium plug in a full-term infant, also is an indication for evaluation. Babies whose abdomens are decompressed by rectal stimulation in the nursery

almost always have an abnormal pattern of defecation within several weeks after birth. Chronic abdominal distention and failure to thrive are common. In older children and adults profound constipation is common, and, although it may respond transiently to medical therapy, relapse is common. Fecal soiling, which is seen in children with fecal retention, rarely is seen in Hirschsprung's disease (Table 172-2). Swenson *et al.* [7] reported encopresis in only 3% of children with HD, although it has been reported in 13% of children with short-segment HD [8]. Unlike most malformations of the gut, other associated abnormalities are rare with HD. There is, however, an association with Down syndrome. Long-segment HD is associated with an increased incidence of cardiac anomalies, and HD occasionally has been associated with Laurence-Moon-Biedl-Bardet syndrome, Waardenburg syndrome [9], and congenital central hypoventilation syndrome (*ie*, Ondine's curse) [10].

In the patient with infrequent bowel movements and abdominal distention, HD is most likely to be the cause when fecal masses are palpable on abdominal examination and the rectal ampulla is either of normal caliber or actually contracted. In contrast, children with fecal retention have a dilated rectal ampulla. Fecal impaction in the rectum may be seen in a small number of patients with HD, especially those with ultrashort-

Table 172-2. Age at Diagnosis

Age	%, (n = 814)
0–1 mo	8
1–3 mo	32
4–6 mo	10
7–12 mo	11
1–2 y	12
2–3 y	5
3–4 y	4
5 y and older	18

Adapted from Kleinhaus et al. [1].

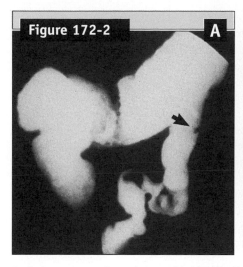
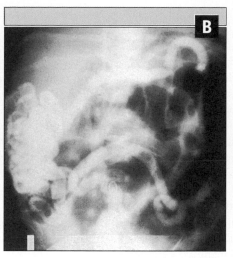
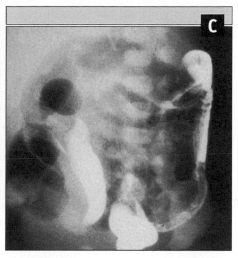

Figure 172-2

A, Contrast enema in an infant with Hirschprung's disease. Note the transition zone in the mid-descending colon (*arrow*). **B**, Contrast enema in an infant with meconium ileus. **C**, Contrast enema in an infant with small left colon syndrome. (*From* Langer [25].)

segment disease, in which aganglionosis is restricted to the last few centimeters of the rectum [7]. Rectal tone usually is normal or somewhat increased. On rectal examination, when the examining finger is withdrawn there may be a forceful explosion of fecal material that is foul-smelling and loose.

ULTRASHORT-SEGMENT HIRSCHSPRUNG'S DISEASE

The symptoms and signs of ultrashort-segment HD are different from those of classical HD. Patients with ultrashort-segment HD often present later in life with chronic constipation that is refractory to medical management. Fecal impaction in the rectum is common, and fecal soiling may occur. Rectal suction biopsy almost always results in normal ganglionic tissue above the aganglionic zone. In ultrashort-segment HD, barium enema fails to show a transition zone between aganglionic and ganglionic bowel, and a megarectum, as seen with fecal retention, usually is present. Diagnosis is by anal manometry, which demonstrates lack of relaxation of the internal sphincter. Many affected patients respond to the medical regimen prescribed for patients with fecal retention. If unresponsive to medical therapy, they may do well after a myectomy.

DIFFERENTIAL DIAGNOSIS

In the neonate, HD must be differentiated from other causes of intestinal obstruction, including volvulus, meconium plug syndrome, small left colon syndrome, cystic fibrosis, anal rectal strictures, extrinsic mass lesions that cause compression of the bowel, and intestinal atresia. In toddlers and older children, the clinician must determine whether the patient has severe fecal retention or HD. Pseudo-obstruction and neuronal dysplasia also must be considered [11]. Acquired aganglionosis from cytomegalovirus or ischemia is uncommon in childhood.

DIAGNOSIS

Eight percent of patients are diagnosed in the first month of life and 40% by 3 months of age [1] (Table 172-2). Almost all patients are identified by 5 years of age, although patients with minimal symptoms, usually from ultrashort-segment HD, may not be diagnosed until adulthood [12,13]. Diagnosis may be made radiologically, histologically, or manometrically.

Radiographic Diagnosis

The objective of radiographs is twofold: 1) to determine whether there is intestinal obstruction, and 2) to demonstrate a transition zone between ganglionic and aganglionic bowel (Fig. 172-2). A cross-table lateral or upright radiograph usually demonstrates nonspecific intestinal obstruction with dilated intestinal loops. In infancy, a barium enema is necessary to distinguish between large and small intestine.

In neonates, the transition zone commonly is absent because of the limited time that the proximal obstructed bowel has had to dilate. Total colonic aganglionosis also is difficult to diagnose in the neonate, because the entire caliber of the colon is either narrow or normal and there is no colonic transition zone.

In older infants and children, a single contrast barium enema is a reliable study as long as enemas or cathartics have been avoided for 3 to 5 days before the examination. Manipulation of the rectum may result in either decompression of the obstructed proximal bowel and loss of the transition zone or creation of a transition zone in a patient with fecal retention. A transition zone also may be missed if the enema catheter is inserted too far proximally.

The transition zone most commonly is identified on a lateral projection, particularly if the zone is in the rectosigmoid. The ratio of the sigmoid to rectal diameter is increased in HD. This is an important radiologic sign and is in contrast to the megarectum usually observed in functional constipation. The aganglionic zone also may appear spastic because of increased tone in that segment.

It is important to note that barium enema is diagnostic in only about 80% of patients, nondiagnostic in 15%, and incorrect in another 5%. False-negative rates may be even higher in neonates and in patients with disease limited to the distal anorectum.

Rectal Biopsy

Biopsy is a reliable means of identifying HD, with the exception of ultrashort-segment disease. Suction rectal biopsy, by which submucosa is obtained, is satisfactory in most cases; interpretation by a competent pediatric pathologist is crucial. In normal children and adults, there is a hypoganglionic zone that extends 1 cm proximal to the pectinate line of the anal canal [14]. Unless biopsies are taken above this zone, false-positive pathologic aganglionosis may be diagnosed. Biopsies in the hypoganglionic zone should not demonstrate hypertrophied nerve fibers, as do biopsies in the aganglionic zone in patients with HD. Rectal biopsies in children of all ages should be performed approximately 3 cm proximal to the anal verge [15]. At this distance, if perforation from the biopsy were to occur, it would be retroperitoneal rather than intraperitoneal. Biopsies should be obtained from the posterior lateral walls with the patient in the prone position. Anterior wall biopsies are more likely to result in intraperitoneal perforation because of the anatomy of the peritoneal reflection. Repeat biopsies occasionally are necessary if inadequate tissue has been obtained. A normal number of ganglion cells excludes the diagnosis of HD, whereas absence of ganglion cells in tissue with adequate submucosa and the presence of hypertrophied nerve fibers is consistent with HD. The tissue can be stained with acetylcholinesterase to delineate acetylcholinesterase-positive nerve trunks in the submucosa and coarse neural fibers in the lamina propria, which are reliable histologic signs of HD [16]. The diagnostic accuracy of this evaluation is nearly 100% when adequate samples of submucosa are evaluated by an experienced pathologist [17–19].

In those rare situations in which adequate tissue cannot be obtained by rectal suction biopsy, a full-thickness biopsy may be performed. These biopsies provide histologic evidence that is diagnostic in 98% of patients [7]; however, full-thickness biopsy requires general anesthesia, and, because of scarring, may make dissection of the rectum at surgery more difficult.

Anorectal Manometry

In normal individuals, distention of the rectum by a fecal bolus or an intrarectal balloon results in relaxation of the internal anal sphincter. This is termed the *rectoanal inhibitory reflex* (RAIR). When testing is performed correctly, this reflex is detected in only 2% of children with HD [20]. The diagnostic accuracy of anorectal manometry approaches 100% [21,22], and it is the only study that can identify the patient with ultrashort-segment HD. From a practical point of view, anorectal manometry sometimes is difficult to achieve in the uncooperative patient, and there may be technical problems with the balloons and catheters. Although anorectal manometry appears to be quite specific as well as sensitive, rectal suction biopsy still is indicated before laparotomy. Pediatric surgeons usually request a barium enema before surgery to assess the extent of aganglionosis preoperatively.

▇ SURGICAL THERAPY

Patients with HD require surgery to relieve their functional obstruction. In patients with enterocolitis, the most feared complication of HD, obstruction is alleviated by creation of a diverting ostomy proximal to the aganglionic segment. There are four operative procedures that may be used for the palliation of HD. In the *Swenson procedure*, the pentire aganglionic segment except for the distal 1 cm is resected and the proximal bowel anastomosed to the anus. This procedure has a high incidence of post-

operative enterocolitis and anastomotic disruption. The *Duhamel operation* creates a side-to-side anastomosis of normal bowel anterior to aganglionic colon to maintain peristalsis but minimizes the risk of damage to the autonomic nerves in the rectum. In the *Soave procedure*, anorectal ganglionic bowel is pulled through the muscular sleeve of the rectum and anastomosed secondarily. In the *Boley procedure*, the pull-through sleeve is anastomosed primarily to the rectal cuff. The Boley and Duhamel procedures are more commonly used than are the Swenson or Soave procedures [1].

For patients with short-segment or ultrashort-segment HD, internal sphincter myomectomy may alleviate symptoms of severe constipation [23]. This procedure also may be used following definitive repair if there are continuing problems with impaired defecation.

▇ COMPLICATIONS

Enterocolitis, the most significant complication of HD, is characterized by abdominal distention, chronic diarrhea, watery explosive stools, blood per rectum, and fever. Shock and death are common. Hospitalization is mandatory for any child with suspected enterocolitis. Intravenous fluid resuscitation, electrolyte replacement, and antibiotic administration should be initiated immediately. The bowel may be decompressed with nasogastric suction, and a soft flexible rectal tube passed proximally up the colon for purposes of irrigation with normal saline. This large bowel decompression can be done several times during a 24-hour period. At times, enterocolitis may be insidious, manifested only by chronic diarrhea and failure to thrive. Surgery should be postponed until the condition is stabilized, unless there are signs of a surgical abdomen.

The clinical symptoms and signs, as described, and the presence of normal stool cultures confirm the diagnosis of enterocolitis. Radiographically, there may be irregular mucosal folds, ulceration, air-fluid levels, and bowel obstruction. Although enterocolitis is uncommon in the presence of effective medical care, for inexplicable reasons, enterocolitis may occur even in the postoperative period [24]. The early diagnosis of HD before the development of severe enterocolitis is essential to reduce morbidity and mortality.

▇ POSTOPERATIVE THERAPY

Patients with HD often continue to have a rectal motility disorder following surgery. These individuals often have what appears to be fecal retention. On occasion, therapy such as might be used for children with functional constipation/fecal retention may be necessary. With such medical regimens, the outlook for reasonably normal defecation is favorable.

▇ REFERENCES

1. Kleinhaus S, Boley SJ, Sheran M, Sieber WK: Hirschsprung disease: a survey of the members of the surgical section of the American Academy of Pediatrics. *J Pediatr Surg* 1979, 14:588–597.
2. Passarge E: The genetics of Hirschsprung disease. Evidence for heterogeneous etiology and a study of sixty-three families. *N Engl J Med* 1967, 276:138–143.
3. Romeo G, Ronchetto P, Luo Y, *et al.*: Point mutations affecting the tyrosine kinase domain of the RET proto-oncogene in Hirschsprung disease. *Nature* 1994, 367:377–378.

4. Schuchardt A, D'Agati V, Larsson-Blomberg L, *et al.*: Defects in the kidney and enteric nervous system of mice lacking the tyrosine kinase receptor RET. *Nature* 1994, 367:380–383.

5. Eng C: The RET proto-oncogene in multiple endocrine neoplasia type 2 and Hirschsprung disease. *N Engl J Med* 1996, 335:943–951.

6. Attie T, Pelet A, Edery P, *et al.*: Diversity of RET proto-oncogene mutations in familial and sporadic Hirschsprung disease. *Human Molecular Genetics* 1995, 4:1381–1386.

7. Swenson O, Sherman JO, Fisher JH: Diagnosis of congenital megacolon: an analysis of 501 patients. *J Pediatr Surg* 1973, 85:587–594.

8. Nissan S, Bar-Maor JA: Further experience in the diagnosis and surgical treatment of short segment Hirschsprung disease and idiopathic megacolon. *J Pediatr Surg* 1971, 6:738–741.

9. Omenn GS, McKusick VA: The association of Waardenburg syndrome and Hirschsprung megacolon. *Am J Med Genet* 1979, 3:217–223.

10. Fodstad H, Ljunggren B, Shawis R: Ondine's curse with Hirschsprung disease. *Br J Neurosurg* 1990, 4:87–93.

11. Simpser E, Kahn E, Kenigsberg K, *et al.*: Neuronal intestinal dysplasia: quantitative diagnostic criteria and clinical management. *J Pediatr Gastroenterol Nutr* 1991, 12:61–64.

12. Luukkonen P, Heikkinen M, Juikuri K, Jarvinen H: Adult Hirschsprung disease: clinical features and functional outcome after surgery. *Dis Colon Rectum* 1990, 33:65–69.

13. Rich AJ, Lennard TW, Wilsdon JB: Hirschsprung disease as a cause of chronic constipation in the elderly. *Br Med J* 1983, 287:1777–1778.

14. Aldridge RT, Campbell PE: Ganglion cell distribution in the normal rectum and anal canal. A basis for the diagnosis of Hirschsprung disease by anorectal biopsy. *J Pediatr Surg* 1968, 3:475–490.

15. Campbell PE, Noblett HR: Experience with rectal suction biopsy in the diagnosis of Hirschsprung disease. *J Pediatr Surg* 1969, 4:410–415.

16. Wells FE, Addison GM: Acetylcholinesterase activity in rectal biopsies: an assessment of its diagnostic value in Hirschsprung disease. *J Pediatr Gastroenterol Nutr* 1986, 5:912–919.

17. Lake BD, Puri P, Nixon HH, Claireaux AE: Hirschsprung disease: an appraisal of histochemically demonstrated acetylcholinesterase activity in suction rectal biopsy specimens as an aid to diagnosis. *Arch Pathol Lab Med* 1978, 102:244–247.

18. Ikawa H, Kim SH, Hendren WH, Donahoe PK: Acetylcholinesterase and manometry in the diagnosis of the constipated child. *Arch Surg* 1986, 121:435–438.

19. Schofield DE, Devine W, Yunis EJ: Acetylcholinesterase-stained suction rectal biopsies in the diagnosis of Hirschsprung disease. *J Pediatr Gastroenterol Nutr* 1990, 11:221–228.

20. Faverdin C, Dornic C, Arhan P, *et al.*: Quantitative analysis of anorectal pressures in Hirschsprung disease. *Dis Colon Rectum* 1981, 24:422–427.

21. Loening-Baucke V, Pringle KC, Ekwo EE: Anorectal manometry for the exclusion of Hirschsprung disease in neonates. *J Pediatr Gastroenterol Nutr* 1985, 4:596–603.

22. Aaronson I, Nixon HH: A clinical evaluation of anorectal pressure studies in the diagnosis of Hirschsprung disease. *Gut* 1972, 13:138–146.

23. Scobie WG, Mackinlay GA: Anorectal myectomy in treatment of ultrashort segment Hirschsprung disease. *Arch Dis Child* 1977, 52:713–715.

24. Bill AH, Chapman ND: The enterocolitis of Hirschsprung disease. *Br J Neurosurg* 1990, 4:87–93.

25. Langer JC: Nenonatal surgery and the acute abdomen. In *Gastroenterology and Hepatology*, vol 4. Philadelphia: Current Medicine 1997:3.1–3.21.

173 The Infant With Cholestasis
Kathleen M. Loomes and Andrew E. Mulberg

This chapter focuses on the differential diagnosis (Table 173-1) and workup of the infant from birth to 3 months of age with cholestasis. Jaundice is very common during the first few weeks of life, because of physiologic hemolysis and the newborn's relatively immature mechanisms for excretion of bilirubin. Direct hyperbilirubinemia, however, is never physiologic. Any infant with jaundice after 2 weeks of life, or after a jaundice-free period, should be evaluated, and the serum bilirubin fractionated. A conjugated fraction greater than 2.0 mg/dL or greater than 15% of the total serum bilirubin is abnormal and requires careful evaluation. An infant with conjugated hyperbilirubinemia must have an urgent workup to identify any cause that may be amenable to medical or surgical intervention.

◼ PHYSIOLOGY AND PATHOPHYSIOLOGY
Fetal and Neonatal Bile Acid Biosynthesis and Metabolism

The biosynthesis and metabolism of bile acids in the fetus and newborn are very different from those of the adult. Bile acid biosynthesis has been reported as early as the 12th week of gestation, with a marked increase in biliary bile acid concentration from the 17th week of gestation corresponding to an increase in hepatic synthesis. In the fetus, there is a predominance of chenodeoxycholic acid synthesis. The ratios of biliary cholic acid to chenodeoxycholic acid are 0.85:1, 2.5:1, and 1.6:1 in fetal, neonatal, and adult bile, respectively. Multiple "atypical" bile acids are present in fetal bile but not in adult bile [1].

The normal bile acid profile in the fetus resembles that of the adult with cholestatic liver disease. Whether there is unmasking of fetal metabolic pathways in adults with cholestatic liver diseases remains an interesting speculation. Multiple-site hydroxylations of the bile acid nucleus at carbon-6 and carbon-1 positions (which occur only in the fetus) yield unusual derivatives: $3\alpha,6\alpha,7\alpha$-trihydroxy-5β-cholanoic acid accounts for 15% of the total fetal bile acid pool. In fetal development, there is a limitation in the percentage of secondary bile acids because of the absence of fecal flora [1].

1-, 7-, 12- and 26-Hydroxylase and sulfotransferase activities can be demonstrated in fetal liver microsomes as early as 13 weeks gestation. In adults with cholestasis, there is an increase

Table 173-1. Differential Diagnosis of Neonatal Cholestasis

Extrahepatic

Extrahepatic biliary atresia, either isolated or associated with other anomalies

Choledochal cyst

Spontaneous perforation of the bile duct

Bile duct stenosis

Inspissated bile syndrome

Obstruction by extrinsic or intrinsic mass

Cholelithiasis

Intrahepatic

1. Infectious

   Bacterial

   Sepsis, especially *E. coli*, urinary tract infection, syphilis, toxoplasmosis, Listeria, tuberculosis

   Viral

   Hepatitis B, hepatitis C, rubella, cytomegalovirus, herpes simplex virus, human immunodeficiency virus, coxsackie virus, parvovirus, echovirus

2. Metabolic

   Disorders of carbohydrate metabolism

   Galactosemia, type IV glycogen storage disease, hereditary fructose intolerance

   Disorders of amino acid metabolism

   Tyrosinemia, arginase deficiency

   Disorders of lipid metabolism

   Niemann-Pick disease, Gaucher's disease

   Peroxisomal defects—Zellweger's syndrome

   Defects of the electron transport chain

   Disorders of bile acid synthesis

   Cystic fibrosis

   α_1-Antitrypsin deficiency

   Neonatal iron storage disease

   Byler's disease, PFIC

3. Endocrine

   Panhypopituitarism (septo-optic dysplasia), congenital hypothyroidism

4. Disorders of the development of bile ducts

   Syndromic paucity of intrahepatic bile ducts (Alagille syndrome), nonsyndromic paucity of intrahepatic bile ducts, Byler's disease

5. Toxic

   TPN cholestasis, drugs—anticonvulsants, ceftriaxone

6. Ischemia or shock

7. Miscellaneous

   Langerhans' cell histocytosis (histiocytosis X), neonatal lupus

in 1-, 4-, and 6-position hydroxylation [2]. Conjugation with glycine and taurine characterizes the biochemical modification of bile acids, which facilitates their hydrophilicity. Differences in conjugation of bile acids are noted in the fetus and neonate versus the older infant and adult. The ratio of glycine to taurine in the newborn usually is about 1:4, whereas the adult ratio is 3:1. Watkins has shown that sulfated lithocholate is present in the fetal gallbladder and meconium, suggesting a priori, de novo synthesis in the fetus rather than maternal transport processes [3].

Enterohepatic Circulation and Functional Cholestasis of the Newborn

The physiologic processes of bile acid biosynthesis and secretion and intraluminal fat digestion, absorption, and reabsorption within the terminal ileum constitute the enterohepatic circulation. The enterohepatic circulation of bile acids is divided into three levels of interrelated function: hepatic events, biliary phase, and intestinal phase. In the neonate, immature development of various aspects of these individual phases may affect intraluminal bile acid concentration, serum bile acid concentration, bile acid synthesis, bile acid pool size, hepatic uptake, conjugation, and ileal transport. These altered processes lead to the development of what is known collectively as *physiologic cholestasis of the newborn* [4•]. Physiologic cholestasis originally was defined by the presence of elevated bile acid concentrations in the neonate and fetus. Early in life, infants rely predominantly on bile acid–dependent bile flow, which involves active secretion of bile acids into the canaliculus, followed by transport of water along an osmotic gradient. Inborn errors of bile acid metabolism may lead to synthesis of abnormal potentially toxic bile acids. Hepatocytes are relatively inefficient at bile acid synthesis and secretion in the neonatal period. Enterohepatic circulation is impaired by poor intestinal uptake of bile acids in the ileum and by inability of the hepatocytes to recover bile acids from the portal blood.

■ EPIDEMIOLOGY

The incidence of neonatal cholestatic liver disease has been estimated at 1 per 2500 live births and is defined as conjugated hyperbilirubinemia that lasts for more than 2 weeks in the first 4 months of life and is accompanied by evidence of biochemical abnormalities in liver function. In several series, biliary atresia and idiopathic neonatal hepatitis have each accounted for about 25% to 35% of the cases, with infectious and metabolic causes making up smaller segments of the population.

The term *neonatal hepatitis* seems to imply an infectious etiology; however, it actually defines a process of intrahepatic cholestasis, often associated with giant cell transformation and interlobular bile duct paucity on biopsy, for which a specific etiology seldom is identified. As new metabolic disorders, such as the bile acid synthetic defects, have been elucidated, the category *idiopathic liver disease* has become smaller [5–7].

■ CLINICAL FEATURES
History and Physical Examination

The differential diagnosis of neonatal cholestasis is vast, but many disorders can be excluded by a comprehensive history and physical examination. Prenatal history can provide important clues pointing to congenital infection. Mothers often relate a history of a febrile illness with or without a rash during pregnancy. Prenatal laboratory studies usually include rubella immune status and RPR for syphilis, as well as hepatitis B and HIV serologies. The mother also should be asked whether she has ever had a blood transfusion, or whether she has had previous miscarriages, which may imply infection or a genetic defect.

Birth history includes gestational age, mode of delivery, birth weight, and Apgar scores. Infants with biliary atresia are more likely to be full-term females with normal birth weights. Any history of perinatal asphyxia or sepsis is relevant. Difficulty passing meconium is common in the infant with cystic fibrosis. Cholestasis is an infrequent presentation of cystic fibrosis in the neonatal period, however, with an estimated incidence of 6 per 1000 cases of cystic fibrosis among cases of neonatal cholestasis [8] (see Chapter 170).

The history should indicate whether the child is, for example, a well-appearing jaundiced infant with acholic stools or a baby in the intensive care unit on total parenteral nutrition and extracorporeal membrane oxygenation (ECMO). It is important to ascertain the type of feedings and the infant's tolerance of feedings. Breast milk and most cow's milk formulas contain lactose, whereas soy formulas contain sucrose or a glucose polymer. The presence of reducing substances in urine suggests one of several metabolic disorders. It must be determined whether the infant has received any oral antibiotics that might contain fructose. A history of vomiting and lethargy should alert the clinician to search for an inborn error of metabolism. Acholic stools are nonspecific and can occur in neonates with severe intrahepatic or extrahepatic cholestasis. The presence of pigmented stools implies that some excretion of bilirubin is present; therefore, biliary obstruction is unlikely.

Family history may reveal sudden infant death syndrome (SIDS) or other early deaths, indicative of possible inborn error of metabolism, including the mitochondrial and respiratory chain defects, which result in lactic acidemia [9]. Other family members may have cystic fibrosis, polycystic kidney disease, or systemic lupus erythematosus. A history of jaundice in childhood may be elicited in Alagille syndrome [10•]. Other inherited disorders may be associated with Amish ancestry (eg, Byler's disease) or Ashkenazi Jewish ancestry (eg, Niemann-Pick disease).

A careful physical examination begins with an overall observation of the activity level, nutritional status, and general health of the infant (Table 173-2). A growth chart is helpful. On head, eyes, ears, nose, and throat (HEENT) examination, microcephaly is suggestive of congenital infection; a large anterior fontanelle is consistent with hypothyroidism. The triangular face of Alagille syndrome is difficult to appreciate in infancy but may become more obvious in older children (Fig. 173-1, see also **Color Plate**). The cardiac examination may reveal the murmur of peripheral pulmonic stenosis (Alagille syndrome) or patent ductus arteriosus, which can be seen in the syndromic type of biliary atresia [11]. Abdominal examination reveals hepatomegaly in many disorders, whereas splenomegaly is suggestive of congenital infection or a storage disease. An abnormal neurologic examination, with hyper- or hypotonia or failure to reach developmental milestones, may be seen in congenital infection or inborn errors of metabolism.

After taking into account any pertinent findings derived from the history or physical examination, a staged laboratory and radiographic approach may be begun to evaluate the infant with cholestasis (Table 173-3). Initial evaluation identifies any treatable conditions, determines the degree of inflammation of the hepatocytes and bile ducts, and detects any hepatocellular dysfunction. In addition, the patency of the extrahepatic biliary tree must be established early because surgical intervention is much more successful before 2 months of age (see later section

Table 173-2. Physical Examination Clues to Specific Cholestatic Disorders

Physical examination	Disease to consider
General	
Poor nutrition	Infectious or metabolic disease
Hypotonia	Metabolic disease
Appearing well or ill	Infectious or metabolic disease
Vital signs and weight	
Small for gestational age (SGA) or failure to thrive	Congenital infection, anomalies, or AAT
Microcephaly	Congenital infection
large anterior fontanelle	Hypothyroidism
Triangular facies	Alagille syndrome
Cataracts	Galactosemia
Posterior embryotoxon	Alagille syndrome
Cardiac	Alagille syndrome
Peripheral pulmonic stenosis	Alagille syndrome
Ventricular septal defect, tetralogy of fallout	
Patent ductus arteriosus	Syndromic biliary atresia
Abdominal	
Hepatomegaly	
Midline liver	Syndromic extrahepatic biliary atresia
Abdominal mass	Choledochal cyst
Splenomegaly	Storage disease
Urogenital	
Micropenis	Panhypopituitarism
Skeletal	
Butterfly vertebrae	Alagille syndrome
Lethargy, abnormal tone or abnormal reflexes	Inborn error of metabolism, congenital infection

on "Extrahepatic Biliary Atresia"). Further laboratory studies may enable specific diagnosis (Table 173-4). Disorders that more commonly present with cholestasis in the neonate include ideopathic neonatal hepatitis, extrahepatic biliary atresia, and Alagille syndrome.

Idiopathic Neonatal Hepatitis

About 30% to 35% of infants presenting with neonatal cholestasis are diagnosed with a giant cell hepatitis for which no specific etiology is identified and that is termed *idiopathic neonatal hepatitis*. Hallmarks or histology include giant cell transformation, ballooning of hepatocytes, lobular disarray, and focal necrosis. Extramedullary hematopoiesis usually is prominent. The degree of portal fibrosis is variable. Unlike biliary atresia, bile duct proliferation and bile plugging usually are not seen. Giant cell transformation and hepatocellular ballooning are relatively nonspecific responses of the immature liver to any injury and may be seen in many different processes, including viral infection, α_1-antitrypsin deficiency, and inborn errors of metabolism.

Although the causes are most likely heterogeneous, ranging from undetected viral infections to environmental factors to undiagnosed genetic or metabolic defects, some statements can be made about clinical presentation and prognosis. Typically, affected infants are male and small for gestational age at birth. Their jaundice usually becomes apparent within the first 1 to 2 weeks of life, whereas in biliary atresia there often is a jaundice-free period in the weeks after birth. Acholic stools, if they occur, may be intermittent. The majority of these infants appear otherwise healthy, although about one third may have other mani-

festations such as failure to thrive. Hepatomegaly and a moderate elevation of transaminases usually are present.

Patients with idiopathic neonatal hepatitis can be divided into two categories: sporadic and familial. In general, prognosis is better in sporadic cases, presumably because in familial cases there may be an undiagnosed genetic defect. Several long-term

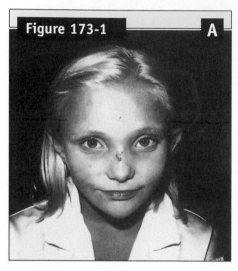

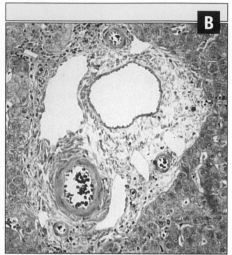

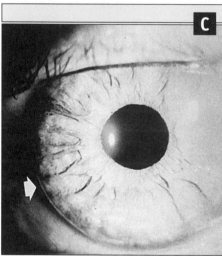

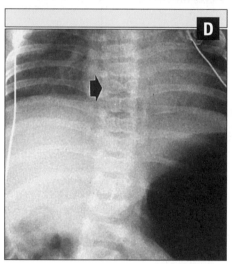

Figure 173-1

Classic features of Alagille syndrome. **A,** Facial features in an affected child. Note the triangular facies, prominent forehead, deepset eyes, and pointed chin. See also **Color Plate. B,** Large portal tract with minimal fibrosis seen on a liver biopsy. Multiple branches of the hepatic artery and portal vein are present, without bile ducts. **C,** Posterior embryotoxon. The arrow marks the prominent Schwalbe's line. **D,** Butterfly vertebra caused by abnormal clefting of the vertebral bodies. (*From* Li *et al.* [27], with permission.

Table 173-3. An Approach by Algorithm to the Infant With Cholestasis

Initial laboratory studies to assess cholestasis, extent of liver injury, and hepatocyte function

  Fractionated bilirubin (total, unconjugated, conjugated, delta)

  Hepatic enzymes

    Alkaline phosphatase, AST, ALT, γ-glutamyltranspeptidase (GGT)

Tests of liver function

  PT/PTT—In a sick infant with coagulopathy, obtain factor levels to differentiate between hepatic failure and DIC.

  Albumin, fibrinogen, ammonia, cholesterol

Laboratory studies to exclude easily treatable disorders

  Urinalysis with reducing substances

    Rule out galactosemia in an infant being fed lactose-containing formula

  Urine culture

    Catheterized specimen

T4 and TSH

  Serum bile acid assay

Ultrasound

  To look for choledochal cyst

Hepatobiliary scintigraphy

  Rule out spontaneous bile duct perforation

Liver biopsy findings

  Cholestasis, bile duct proliferation, fibrosis, and portal inflammation would be consistent with extrahepatic obstruction. Proceed with intraoperative cholangiogram and possible Kasai procedure.

  Findings of giant cell transformation and hepatocellular necrosis—continue with infectious and metabolic workup.

Table 173-4. Laboratory Studies to Make a Specific Diagnosis

Infectious

Serologies for infectious causes (mother and baby)

> Toxoplasma, rubella, cytomegalovirus (along with urine Ag), herpes simplex virus, RPR for syphilis, hepatitis B, human immunodeficiency virus

Testing for metabolic disorders

α_1 Antitrypsin with Pi typing

Serum amino acids

Urine organic acids

Bile acids (serum and urine): Byler's disease, etc

Sweat chloride (optic fibrosis)

Serum iron and ferritin (hemochromatosis)

Serum cortisol (hypopituitarism)

Eye examination—to look for signs of chorioretinitis or findings of Alagille syndrome.

Radiographs

> Long bones (syphilis)
>
> Skull (calcifications associated with congenital infection)
>
> Chest (congenital heart disease)
>
> Spine—butterfly vertebrae (Alagille syndrome)

follow-up studies have been done. In one group of five studies done between 1974 and 1987 mortality was 20% in sporadic cases and 63% in familial cases. Seventy-four percent of the sporadic hepatitis patients recovered completely, whereas only 22% of the patients with familial hepatitis recovered without evidence of ongoing liver disease [7]. Certainly, if these studies had been performed in the era of liver transplantation, mortality would be lower, but it is safe to assume that similar numbers of patients still would have developed chronic liver disease.

Since the 1950s, as understanding of viral and metabolic processes has advanced, the number of cholestatic infants fitting into the category of neonatal cholestasis has steadily declined. For instance, in recent years work has been done to elucidate several bile acid synthetic defects that were previously unknown. Until etiologies are identified and specific treatments developed, management will remain strictly supportive.

Extrahepatic Biliary Atresia

Biliary atresia is a progressive inflammation and obliteration of the extrahepatic biliary tree that can result in biliary cirrhosis. Even when the obstruction is relieved by Kasai portoenterostomy, inflammation can continue in the intrahepatic bile ducts, implying a definite intrahepatic component to the disease. Biliary atresia occurs with and without other associated anomalies (Table 173-2).

The most common form of the disease occurs in isolation, usually in a healthy full-term infant, affecting girls more often than boys by a ratio of 1.4 to 1. These babies typically have a jaundice-free period after birth and are noted to be icteric between 4 and 6 weeks of age. No etiology has been determined. About 7% to 10% of infants have a combination of anomalies (Table 173-1), including situs inversus, malrotation, preduodenal portal vein, interrupted IVC, and polysplenia.

These children also may have simple or complex congenital heart disease. Another 10% to 15% of patients have isolated cardiac, gastrointestinal (ie, jejunal atresia), and genitourinary anomalies. The presence of a constellation of other anomalies in addition to extrahepatic biliary atresia implies that the process begins during embryogenesis. Often infants with "syndromic" biliary atresia present earlier without a jaundice-free period [11].

Many theories have been proposed for the etiology of biliary atresia, including infectious, ischemic, or autoimmune causes; to date, none has been proven. Some researchers believe that biliary atresia, when it occurs in isolation, is a postnatal process that evolves over time. Viruses implicated have included reovirus, rotavirus, and hepatitis C [12]. Some recent reports indicate that these viruses cannot be recovered by PCR from patients' sera or bile duct remnants, however. Some association may exist between HLA B12 and extrahepatic biliary atresia (EHBA).

In the evaluation of neonatal cholestasis, most infants undergo biliary imaging studies (ie, diisopropyl imidodiacetic acid [DISIDA]) in an attempt to evaluate the patency of the extrahepatic biliary tree. Severe cholestasis with acholic stool from intrahepatic or extrahepatic etiologies usually results in little or no excretion of radionuclide into the intestine. Abdominal ultrasound can identify anatomic abnormalities such as choledochal cyst or cholelithiasis, but rarely is useful in diagnosing biliary atresia. Although the gallbladder usually is contracted and difficult to visualize in EHBA, its presence does not exclude the diagnosis. Hepatobiliary radiologic scans may demonstrate uptake of tracer by the hepatocytes and subsequent excretion into the bowel, obviating the need for immediate liver biopsy or surgical exploration.

Most infants with a nonexcreting hepatobiliary scan then undergo percutaneous liver biopsy. Classic pathologic features of biliary atresia are cholestasis, bile duct proliferation, and fibrosis (Figs. 173-2 [see also **Color Plate**], 173-3, and 173-4). However, if the biopsy is performed after 90 days, the process may have progressed so that bile duct paucity, not proliferation,

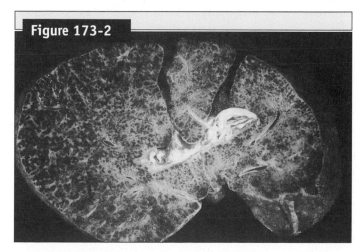

Figure 173-2

Native explanted liver exhibiting the atresia of the common bile duct and its branches from a child with biliary atresia. The liver is markedly fluorescent green from the intrahepatic cholestasis. See also **Color Plate**.

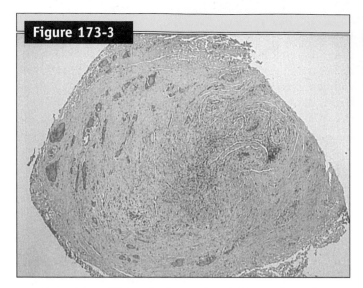

Porta hepatitis exhibiting classic scarring of the portal tract in biliary atresia (hematoxylin and eosin stain, original magnification × 10).

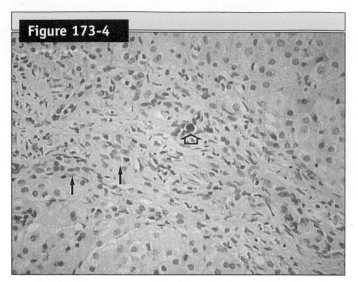

Biliary ductular proliferation in a liver biopsy from a patient with biliary atresia (*arrows*). There is a prominent amount of scarring within the portal tracts. A bile plus (*open arrowhead*) also is visible (hematoxylin and eosin stain; original magnification × 40).

is present and success of a Kasai procedure is low (about 20%). Patients with a suggestive biopsy and DISIDA scan consistent with obstruction should have a minilaparotomy and intraoperative cholangiogram. If atresia is demonstrated, a Kasai procedure is performed.

In 1955, Kasai described a procedure in which the extrahepatic biliary tree is resected (Fig. 173-5). The bile duct remnant is identified at the porta hepatis and a Roux limb of bowel is anastomosed to it. In a minority of patients, there may be a patent proximal segment of bile duct that can be attached directly to the bowel. The success of the Kasai procedure depends on the age of the patient at operation and the experience of the surgeon. Several studies quote an 80% success rate (defined as restoration of bile flow within a certain period of time postoperatively) for the Kasai procedure if the operation is performed before 60 days of life. Between 60 and 90 days, the success rate drops to 45% to 59%, and between 90 and 120 days, to 10% to 28% [13]. More recent studies have documented that most patients with biliary atresia ultimately require liver transplantation [14]. Otte and colleagues state that after Kasai portoenterostomy, 20% to 30% of children live jaundice-free into adulthood. Another third of patients have palliation of their symptoms, with the need for transplantation delayed to later childhood [14].

Indications for transplantation usually relate to the complications of cholestatic liver disease, including intractable pruritus (see section on "Treatment"), coagulopathy unresponsive to conservative therapy, portal hypertension secondary to severe biliary cirrhosis, failure to thrive, and recurrent cholangitis. The role of prophylactic antibiotics to prevent recurrent cholangitis after Kasai procedure is unclear. Unfortunately, no regimen has effectively been documented to yield a clinical difference in the care of these children or in a case-control study to reduce the need for eventual liver transplantation.

Alagille Syndrome

Alagille syndrome, or arteriohepatic dysplasia, is an autosomal dominant condition characterized by a distinct facial appear-ance, cholestasis, vertebral anomalies, cardiac defects, and ophthalmologic abnormalities (Fig. 173-1). Less frequently, mental retardation and renal or vascular anomalies, leading to development of intracranial hemorrhage or proximal renal tubular defects, are observed [15••]. Classically, liver biopsy shows a paucity of interlobular bile ducts.

▬ TREATMENT

Depending on the underlying disease process, many infants with cholestasis develop chronic liver disease (Fig. 173-2). Major concerns for the management of chronic cholestasis include nutrition and growth, deficiencies of fat-soluble vitamins, and pruritus. Chronic cholestasis leads to poor growth

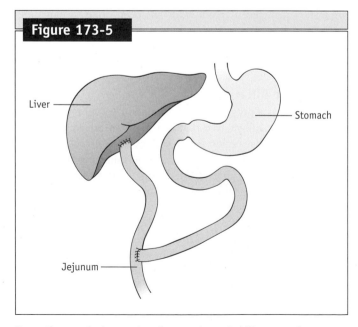

Corrective surgical procedure for extrahepatic biliary atresia.

as a result of malabsorption and increased caloric requirements. Studies have shown improved outcomes posttransplant in well-nourished patients. Because many infants require more than 150 kcal/kg/d for growth, institution of nasogastric feedings often is necessary to ensure good nutrition. The appropriate formula contains about 60% of fat calories as medium-chain triglycerides, which do not require micelle-mediated fat absorption.

Management of pruritus remains a difficult clinical challenge. Available medications include rifampin, diphenhydramine, hydroxyzine, naloxone, and ursodeoxycholic acid (Actigall). Ursodeoxycholic acid (UDCA) is a hydrophilic bile acid that has associated choleretic properties, protects the hepatocyte against hydrophobic bile acids, and enriches the bile acid pool size, displacing hydrophobic bile acids. In clinical trials UDCA has been shown to increase bile flow in patients with cystic fibrosis–dependent hepatobiliary disease [16]. It also has been shown to improve liver function tests, improve pruritus, and, ultimately, improve growth and nutrition. The accepted theory is that cystic fibrosis–related hepatobiliary disease is caused by inspissation of bile ducts with mucus, with resulting cholestasis (diminished bile flow). The mechanism of action of UDCA in improving abnormal liver function tests and cholestasis is currently unknown. Altered bile flow and cholestasis may play a role in the development of liver disease, as intimated by the beneficial effects of UDCA.

Ursodeoxycholic acid, when infused in animals, leads to a choleresis far greater than expected from bile secretion alone. This phenomenon has been termed *hypercholeresis* [17,18]. Ursodeoxycholic acid has been used safely and effectively in clinical trials of children and adults with cystic fibrosis–related hepatobiliary disease and total parenteral nutrition–related cholestasis [16–18,19••,20–23]. In biliary atresia, treatment of children with UDCA who have ongoing liver dysfunction after a Kasai procedure may increase bile flow. Improvement in liver function, growth, and nutrition may occur with therapy [24,25•,26].

◼ REFERENCES

Recently published papers of particular interest have been highlighted as follows:
• Of interest
•• Of outstanding interest

1. Colombo C, Zuliani G, Rochi M, *et al.*: Biliary bile acid composition of the human fetus in early gestation. *Pediatr Res* 1987, 21:197–200.

2. Dumaswala R, *et al.*: Identification of 3a,4b,7a-trihyhdroxy-5b-cholanoic acid in human bile: reflection of a new pathway in bile acid metabolism in humans. *J Lipid Res* 1989, 30:47–856.

3. Watkins JB, Perman JA: Bile acid metabolism in infants and children. *Clin Gastroenterol* 1977, 6:201–217.

4.• Balistreri WF, Heubi JE, Suchy FJ: Immaturity of the enterohepatic circulation in early life: factors predisposing to "physiologic" maldigestion and cholestasis. *J Pediatr Gastroenterol Nutr* 1983, 2:346–354.

5. Mieli-Vergani G, Mowat AP: Liver disease in infancy: a 20-year perspective. *Gut* 1991:S123–S128.

6. Balistreri WF: Neonatal cholestasis: lessons from the past, issues for the future. *Semin Liver Dis* 1987, 7:61–66.

7. Dick MC, Mowat AP: Hepatitis syndrome in infancy-an epidemiological survey with 10-year follow-up. *Arch Dis Child* 1985, 60:512–516.

8. Lykavieris P, Bernard O, Hadchouel M: Neonatal cholestasis as the presenting disease in cystic fibrosis. *Arch Dis Child* 1996, 75:67–70.

9. Goncalves I, *et al.*: Mitochondrial respiratory chain defect: a new etiology for neonatal cholestasis and early liver insufficiency. *J Hepatol* 1995, 23:290–294.

10.• Hoffenberg EJ, *et al.*: Outcome of syndromic paucity of interlobular bile ducts (Alagille syndrome) with onset of cholestasis in infancy. *J Pediatrics* 1995, 127:220–224.

11. Carmi R, Magee CA, Neill CA, Karrer FM: Extrahepatic biliary atresia and associated anomalies: etiologic heterogeneity suggested by distinctive patterns of associations. *Am J Med Genet* 1993, 45:683–693.

12. Steele MI, Marshall CM, Lloyd RE, Randolph VE: The association of reovirus 3 and biliary atresia: finally resolved. *Hepatology* 1995, 21:697–702.

13. Mieli-Vergani G, Howard ER, Portman B, Mowat AP: Late referral for biliary atresia: missed opportunities for elective surgery. *Lancet*, February 25, 1989:421–423.

14. Otte J-B, de Ville de Goyet, Reding R, *et al.*: Sequential treatment of biliary atresia with Kasai portoenterostomy and liver transplantation: a review. *Hepatology* 1994, 20:41S–48S.

15.•• Krantz I, Piccoli DA, Spinner NB: Alagille syndrome. *J Med Genet* 1997, 34:152–157.

16. Colombo C, Crosignani A, Assaisso M, *et al.*: Ursodeoxycholic acid therapy in cystic fibrosis-associated liver disease: a dose-response study. *Hepatology* 1992, 16:924–930.

17. Lamri Y, Erlinger S, Dumont M, *et al.*: Immunoperoxidase localization of ursodeoxycholic acid in rat biliary epithelial cells. Evidence for a cholehepatic circulation. *Liver* 1992, 12:351–354.

18. Erlinger S: Bile secretion. *Br Med Bull* 1992, 48:860–876.

19.•• Colombo C, Apostolo MG, Ferrari M, *et al.*: Analysis of risk factors for the development of liver disease associated with cystic fibrosis. *J Pediatr* 1994, 124:393–399.

20. O'Brien S, Fitzerald MX, Hegarty JE: A controlled trial of ursodeoxycholic acid treatment in cystic fibrosis-related liver disease. *Eur J Gastroenterol Hepatol* 1992, 4:857–863.

21. O'Brien CB, Senior JR, Mirchandani RA, *et al.*: Ursodeoxycholic acid for the treatment of primary sclerosing cholangitis: a 30-month pilot study. *Hepatology* 1991, 14:838–847.

22. Galabert C, Montet JC, Lengrand D, *et al.*: Effects of ursodeoxycholic acid on liver function in patients with cystic fibrosis and chronic cholestasis. *J Pediatr* 1992, 121:138–141.

23. Lindor KD, Burnes J: Ursodeoxycholic acid for the treatment of home parenteral nutrition-associated cholestasis. *Gastroenterology* 1991, 101:250–253.

24. Nittono H, Tokita A, Hayashi M, *et al.*: Ursodeoxycholic acid in biliary atresia. *Lancet* 1988, 1:528.

25.• Shah HA, Spivak W: Neonatal cholestasis: new approaches to diagnostic evaluation and therapy. *Pediatric Clin North Am* 1994, 41:943–966.

26. Ullrich D, Rating D, Shroter W, *et al.*: Treatment with ursodeoxycholic acid renders children with biliary atresia suitable for liver transplantation. *Lancet* 1987, 2:1324

27. Li L, Krantz ID, Deng Y, *et al.*: Alagille syndrome is caused by mutations in human jagged-1. *Nature Genetics* 1997, 16:245.

174 α_1-Antitrypsin Deficiency in Children

Sarah Jane Schwarzenberg and Harvey L. Sharp

The α_1-antitrypsin gene, located on chromosome 14 [1–3] encodes an approximately 55-kD serum glycoprotein of the serine protease inhibitor (SERPIN) superfamily [4]. Serum levels of α_1-antitrypsin are determined mainly by hepatic protein synthesis, whereas local tissue levels may depend on small amounts of the glycoprotein produced by monocytes and macrophages [5–8].

The primary role of α_1-antitrypsin is to protect tissues from proteolytic injury. α_1-Antitrypsin inhibits neutrophil elastase and cathepsin G [4,9]; it also may serve a role in the control of vascular thrombosis as an inhibitor of activated protein C [10]. It is a hepatic acute-phase reactant, with plasma concentrations increasing three- to five-fold during inflammation [11].

EPIDEMIOLOGY

The most common allele associated with α_1-antitrypsin deficiency is protease inhibitor or Pi*Z. In the United States the homozygous deficiency state (PiZZ) occurs in approximately 1 per 6000 to 1 per 8000 people (Tables 174-1 and 174-2) [12]. Most patients with the Z allele are white and of Northern European extraction. The incidence is much lower in Asia, Africa, and in Native American populations. Genetic epidemiologic studies suggest that the Z allele first appeared in Scandinavia several thousand years ago [13]. There is evidence that the Z allele also developed independently in another geographic location in a different genetic background; however, the number of patients in this population is very small [14].

PATHOPHYSIOLOGY

Severe deficiency of this important SERPIN is the result of mutation in the α_1-antitrypsin gene. Substitution of lysine for glutamic acid at position 342 in the peptide chain gives rise to PiZ α_1-antitrypsin [15–18], a form of α_1-antitrypsin that undergoes spontaneous polymerization in the endoplasmic reticulum of the hepatocyte, thus becoming trapped [19]. In individuals homozygous for the Z allele (PiZZ), serum α_1-antitrypsin levels are only 10% to 15% of normal levels. Although other mutations of the α_1-antitrypsin gene may result in serum deficiency, individuals with PiZZ constitute nearly all of those with liver disease.

The mechanism by which liver disease develops in PiZZ individuals is not clear. The predominant theory currently is that globules of unsecreted α_1-antitrypsin cause injury to hepatocytes (see Chapter 99). Liver disease in α_1-antitrypsin deficiency presents either soon after birth or in adulthood. There may be differences in the cause of α_1-antitrypsin–associated liver disease presenting in infancy and in adulthood, but this has not yet been systematically investigated.

PATHOLOGY

The histopathologic changes of α_1-antitrypsin deficiency liver disease are discussed in detail in Chapter 99. Specific issues unique to pediatric diagnosis are considered here.

The histopathology in the neonate is similar to that in the adult. According to Hadchouel *et al.* [20], approximately one third of children who have liver biopsies during the early (*ie*, less than 6 months of age) cholestatic period show evidence of significant portal fibrosis, often with ductular proliferation. Another third may have evidence of hepatocellular damage with cholestasis, but only small amounts of portal fibrosis. Finally, about one third of these early biopsies may reveal bile duct hypoplasia. This last group of infants may have persistent jaun-

Table 174-1. Nomenclature of α_1-Antitrypsin

Pi	Protease inhibitor
Pi*X	Designates allele, where X is the variant allele
PiXX	Genotype in which both alleles of an individual have been identified, usually through family studies
PiX	Phenotype when family studies are not available and it is unclear whether the individual is a homozygote for the X allele or a double heterozygote for X and a null allele

Table 174-2. Common α_1-Antitrypsin Alleles

Allele	Frequency	Serum deficiency	Mechanism	Liver disease	Study
M	Common (4 variants)	No	—	No	Cox
S	3%–4%	Yes	Unstable protein	No	Curiel *et al.*
Z	1%–2%	Yes	Unsecreted protein	Yes	Kidd *et al.*
Mmalton	Rare	Yes	Unsecreted protein	Yes	Cox
Mduarte	Rare	Yes	Unsecreted protein	Yes	Lieberman
Q0 (null)	Rare (many variants)	Yes	Variable	Variable	Cox

dice with pruritus, hypercholesterolemia, and malabsorption of fat-soluble vitamins. In some cases, the bile duct paucity resolves on subsequent liver biopsies.

α₁-Antitrypsin deficiency is an important diagnosis to consider in the infant with cholestatic jaundice. Portal fibrosis and proliferation of bile ductules revealed by liver biopsies may be difficult to differentiate from extrahepatic biliary atresia [20]. The periportal intrahepatic globules of α₁-antitrypsin often are smaller in neonates than are the globules seen in the older child or adult liver. Hematoxylin and eosin staining alone may make identification of the globules very difficult, particularly in the neonate. Immunoperoxidase staining of tissue using an antibody specific to α₁-antitrypsin is essential if the correct diagnosis is to be made. Periodic acid-Schiff staining after diastase digestion (to remove glycogen) improves detection of the globules.

CLINICAL FEATURES

The natural history of liver disease in children with α₁-antitrypsin deficiency is derived largely from data collected in Sweden by Dr. Tomas Sveger. Over 200,000 infants, representing 95% of births in Sweden between November 1972 and September 1974, were screened for α₁-antitrypsin deficiency. Deficient individuals were Pi typed, and clinical data were collected from their physicians. One hundred twenty-two of these patients, whose PiZ status was detected soon after birth, have been observed for 18 years, and the natural history of α₁-antitrypsin deficiency liver disease has been described in several key articles [21–25].

The PiZ newborns detected in this study often were small for gestational age. Twenty-two of the 122 infants with PiZ had clinical evidence of liver disease, and, of these, five had prolonged obstructive jaundice with mild liver disease and nine had severe liver disease. Of the 100 PiZ infants without clinical signs of liver disease, 40% had some abnormality in serum bilirubin, transaminases, or γ-glutamyl transpeptidase [21].

A second large screening study, done in Oregon in the early 1970s, identified 22 PiZZ or PiSZ children; four of their siblings also were examined. At follow-up, 22 of the original 26 children were examined, and only one patient had abnormal liver enzymes in adolescence; none had clinical liver disease [26].

Physicians who evaluate and manage large groups of children with liver disease have reported more severe liver disease in their PiZ patients than was reported by Sveger [27]. These reports likely reflect the sampling error that results from evaluating only patients referred for liver disease. The risk of liver disease for a child with PiZZ genotype is about 3% [21,22,26,28]. Thus, it is important for the physician evaluating an asymptomatic PiZZ child screened for α₁-antitrypsin deficiency because of an affected relative to exercise caution in applying information gleaned from the literature based on the experience of pediatric hepatologists.

Clinical Presentation of the PiZZ Infant With Liver Disease

Liver disease associated with α₁-antitrypsin deficiency was first described by Sharp *et al.* [29]. Infants with PiZ liver disease

usually demonstrate cholestatic jaundice and hepatomegaly in the first 4 months of life. About 50% have splenomegaly at the time of presentation. Patients often are small for gestational age. Stools are acholic, urine is dark yellow, and laboratory studies reveal elevated serum transaminases with conjugated hyperbilirubinemia [30]. Typically, normal or only minimally prolonged prothrombin and partial thromboplastin times, and normal ammonia levels suggest that significant hepatic dysfunction is rare. When there is a paucity of interlobular bile ducts, children may demonstrate hypercholesterolemia; as their motor control and ability to scratch develops, pruritus becomes evident [20, 30]. In rare cases, the initial manifestation of α₁-antitrypsin deficiency may be life-threatening hemorrhage in the neonatal period. This is associated with a prolonged prothrombin time, which usually (but not always) can be corrected with parenteral vitamin K [31]. Coagulopathy in PiZ patients often is seen in neonates whose parents refused routine supplemental vitamin K at delivery [32]. On occasion, cerebral hemorrhage with serious neurologic consequences can ensue. Rarely, PiZ infants with liver disease may present with ascites and cirrhosis without clinical or biochemical evidence of cholestatic jaundice [33].

It is controversial whether prolonged obstructive jaundice occurs more frequently in males than in females [28,30,31,34]. More boys than girls had cholestasis in Sveger's study [21].

The presentation of PiZ liver disease falls within the clinical spectrum of neonatal hepatitis syndrome and is indistinguishable from that of extrahepatic biliary atresia. The α₁-antitrypsin serum level should be measured in infants evaluated for neonatal hepatitis; Pi-type determination is indicated if the level of α₁antitrypsin is below normal. As many as 33% of infants with α₁-antitrypsin deficiency may demonstrate bile duct proliferation on liver biopsy, raising the possibility of coexisting extrahepatic biliary atresia. Although a report on one case of coexisting α₁-antitrypsin deficiency and extrahepatic biliary atresia has been published [35], laparotomy and operative cholangiopathy are not necessary to exclude extrahepatic biliary atresia in the α₁-antitrypsin deficient child unless the clinical suspicion is very high. In these very rare cases, the judgment and expertise of an experienced pediatric surgeon are essential, because α₁-antitrypsin deficient patients may have hypoplastic extrahepatic biliary ducts [36–38].

Clinical Course of Neonatal Liver Disease Associated With α₁-Antitrypsin Deficiency

Infants with α₁-antitrypsin deficiency-associated cholestatic liver disease may or may not resolve their neonatal jaundice.

In Sveger's prospective study of PiZ neonates, most of the infants with liver disease experienced resolution of their clinical and biochemical abnormalities in the first year of life [21]. Children who, as infants, had cholestatic jaundice that resolved may have recurrence of jaundice in childhood or in the teenage years. In general, such recurrences are seen in children with persistent hepatomegaly and abnormal liver enzyme tests. All PiZ individuals with neonatal liver disease may have fluctuations in biochemical markers of liver injury [30].

Infants with α₁-antitrypsin deficiency and cirrhosis whose jaundice does not resolve in the neonatal period may experience a devastating course of liver failure leading to death or the need for hepatic transplantation in the first few years of life [28,30,31,38]. α_1-Antitrypsin–deficient children with cirrhosis typically have hepatosplenomegaly without jaundice [30,31,38]. Although many of these children may thrive, they are at risk for complications of portal hypertension, including gastroesophageal varices and ascites [30]. Death in childhood from liver disease may occur [30,31,38]. Infants with a paucity of bile ducts may experience prolonged jaundice and pruritus; it is controversial whether persistent jaundice in this group suggests a poor outcome [39].

Later Childhood

The child with α_1-antitrypsin deficiency that is detected by population screening may have elevated serum levels of liver enzymes, but is unlikely to have clinical signs of liver disease [25]. A small number of children with α_1-antitrypsin deficiency develop liver disease after 1 year of age, and some of them have a history of prolonged neonatal jaundice. A few present with asymptomatic hepatosplenomegaly and abnormal liver tests in adolescence, and have cirrhosis on liver biopsy. Prognosis in these individuals is believed to be poor, but they are so few that an accurate prognosis cannot be determined. In general, prognosis is related to the degree of liver injury at the time disease is detected [31]. Children presenting with chronic liver disease at any age, particularly if the child is of northern European extraction, should have studies done for α_1-antitrypsin deficiency [34]. The presence of liver disease of unusual severity in a child with cystic fibrosis should suggest screening for a second common liver disease, α_1-antitrypsin deficiency.

Kidney Disease

Patients with α_1-antitrypsin deficiency may develop nephropathy, particularly late in the course of severe liver disease. In one study, the clinicopathologic spectrum of kidney lesions included primarily glomerular diseases (79%), the most common of which were mesangiocapillary glomerulonephritis, focal segmental mesangiocapillary glomerulonephritis, and mesangial proliferative glomerulonephritis [40]. Renal disease should be suspected in the patient with sudden onset of edema, hypertension, or both. Hypoproteinemia, proteinuria, and hematuria are common findings [41]. Proteinuria may be absent if the serum albumin concentration is less than 2.0 g/dL. The kidney disease in α_1-antitrypsin deficiency may be immune complex–mediated. PiZ protein is found in the subendothelial region of the glomerular basement membrane. The protein is likely released from the liver following hepatic parenchymal destruction [40].

◼ DIAGNOSIS

Laboratory testing for α_1-antitrypsin deficiency is discussed in detail in Chapter 99.

When a child with α_1-antitrypsin deficiency is diagnosed, parents and siblings should have Pi testing. Often, asymptomatic homozygotes or compound heterozygotes (individuals with two different deficiency alleles, *eg*, PiSZ) are detected during these screens. Family members with histories of emphysema or liver disease also should be Pi typed. Quantitation of the serum α_1-antitrypsin level is insensitive for the detection of deficient individuals.

When families are identified in which one patient has α_1-antitrypsin deficiency, counseling is advised regarding the availability of prenatal diagnosis. Pi typing is an essential first step for in utero diagnosis of α_1-antitrypsin deficiency. Prenatal diagnosis of α_1-antitrypsin deficiency is done using polymerase chain amplification and oligonucleotide hybridization on chorionic villus samples or fibroblasts from amniotic fluid to detect the Z allelic variant of α_1-antitrypsin; a second deficiency allele, S, also can be detected by this method. This test is more than 99% accurate, but it depends on prior genotyping of the parents to ensure that they are indeed heterozygotes for this allele. Patients with α_1-antitrypsin deficiency associated with some of the more rare α_1-antitrypsin variants will not be detected by these tests; and should be referred to a research laboratory willing to perform testing for these variants.

Couples desiring prenatal diagnosis should be referred to a board-certified geneticist or genetic counselor; it is preferable that counseling be done before conception. Counseling of couples considering prenatal diagnosis should include a review of the inheritance of α_1-antitrypsin deficiency, the possible risks associated with testing, and the error rates of the test being performed.

The most difficult aspect of counseling is providing information regarding the unborn child's risk of serious liver disease. Most families would be unwilling to abort a fetus because of the risk of emphysema associated with α_1-antitrypsin deficiency, because avoidance of cigarettes and other respiratory toxicities can largely mitigate that outcome. Requests for in utero testing usually come from families fearful of having another child with serious liver disease after one such birth. Studies to determine the risk of a family having a second child with severe liver disease are contradictory. Psacharopoulos *et al.* [31] found a 78% chance that parents of a PiZ child with liver disease would have a second PiZ child with similar liver disease; other studies assess the risk at 13% [42] to 21% [28]. It should be noted that these are empiric risk determinations based on small numbers of individuals in referral populations. Many families would find these percentages daunting, given the severity of liver disease in some patients. Appropriate counseling regarding the risk of liver disease may require a team approach, including a pediatric hepatologist and a geneticist.

Screening for α_1-Antitrypsin Deficiency

Asymptomatic individuals are screened for α_1-antitrypsin deficiency most frequently when a family member has been diagnosed with disease associated with α_1-antitrypsin deficiency. Some investigators have advocated universal neonatal screening for α_1-antitrypsin deficiency. They justify this recommendation by pointing out the opportunity it would provide for counseling to reduce the child's exposure to second-hand cigarette smoking and, it is hoped, to prevent smoking in the patient [26]. Neonatal screening has been associated with depression and guilt feelings, and many families fail to understand the implications of screening [23]. If instituted, neonatal screening programs must include a genetic counseling component to avoid parental and patient anxiety and depression [43].

■ TREATMENT

General Considerations

The management of cholestasis and liver disease in α_1-antitrypsin deficiency is no different than that for any other liver disease for which there is no specific therapy. Patients must be monitored to ensure good weight gain, particularly if significant hepatic impairment or cholestasis is present. In infancy, a formula high in medium-chain triglycerides may be useful. Levels of the fat-soluble vitamins (A, E, and D) and the prothrombin time and partial thromboplastin time (to assess vitamin K) should be checked every 3 to 4 months in a child with cholestasis. Failure to gain weight can be an early sign of hepatic deterioration in a child.

It is controversial whether breast-feeding is protective in children with α_1-antitrypsin deficiency [28,44]. However, with appropriate vitamin K supplementation, breast-feeding should be encouraged.

Pruritus may be a significant problem for the α_1-antitrypsin deficient child with paucity of bile ducts and cholestasis. Ursodeoxycholic acid or cholestyramine may reduce itching and improve the serum levels of hepatocellular enzyme. In some cases rifampin may be used to control itching.

Patients should receive regularly scheduled vaccinations, unless anticipated liver transplantation necessitates withholding live virus vaccines. We recommend vaccination against hepatitis B in patients with liver disease. If travel to an area with endemic hepatitis A is planned, vaccination against this virus should be considered. Acquisition of viral markers for hepatitis B and C is associated with a worse prognosis in adults with α_1-antitrypsin deficiency [45] (see Chapter 99). Proper counseling of parents and children may reduce the risk of exposure to these viruses throughout life, thus improving life expectancy.

Patients should avoid known hepatotoxins, including alcohol and some herbal remedies (*eg*, comfrey). Acetaminophen is safe to use for fever and ordinary aches and pains, if recommended doses for weight are not exceeded. Nonsteroidal anti-inflammatory agents should be avoided in patients with portal hypertension because of the increased risk of bleeding associated with their use.

If the child has portal hypertension and splenomegaly, several additional issues should be considered. Children should receive vaccination against *Streptococcus pneumoniae*, and, if not completed in childhood, vaccination against *Haemophilus influenzae*. These vaccinations may reduce the risk of infection from encapsulated bacteria in patients presumed to have deficient opsonization. Acute-onset ascites, or acute exacerbation of existing ascites, with or without fever and pain, suggests spontaneous bacterial peritonitis (see Chapter 108). Paracentesis is essential for diagnosis. After treatment and recovery, prophylaxis with penicillin should be considered.

The sudden development of hypoalbuminemia or proteinuria, especially when associated with ascites, suggests the development of glomerulonephritis. Treatment is supportive, and management of systemic hypertension usually is the major problem. Evaluation for hepatic transplantation, if not previously considered, should be entertained.

Ascites is managed in children just as it is in adults. A regular diet is prescribed, with sodium restriction limited to the avoidance of foods very high in sodium content. Fluid restriction is almost never used, because the combination of dietary and fluid restrictions is difficult to manage in children and may lead to malnutrition. Spironolactone is the initial diuretic therapy, with loop diuretics prescribed as needed.

The child without clinical liver disease should have a yearly physical examination by his or her primary care physician; serum liver enzyme concentration should be measured every other year. Patients with evidence of clinical liver disease require more frequent monitoring, and a wider spectrum of assays, including vitamin assays, urinalysis, and electrolytes.

There is no consensus in the literature as to when a liver biopsy is appropriate in patients with α_1-antitrypsin deficiency. If the diagnosis is made by Pi typing in infancy, liver biopsy adds little to clinical management. Patients with persistent hyperbilirubinemia should have a liver biopsy to determine whether paucity of bile ducts is present and to provide prognosis, particularly at 6 months to 1 year of age [46]. Once portal hypertension develops, liver biopsy is of no value.

Family Counseling

Families with a child with α_1-antitrypsin deficiency, whatever allelic variants are involved, must ensure that the child is not exposed to second-hand cigarette smoke. No family member should smoke, because even smoking at sites distant from home may cause lung injury if the toxins adhere to clothing. Smoking should not be permitted in the house, and the child should not be in homes where smoking is allowed. These restrictions are essential to preserving lung function in a child at risk of early-onset emphysema. Parents must understand the lethal nature of cigarette smoke in the α_1-antitrypsin–deficient child. Parents who smoke should be referred for counseling and nicotine patch detoxification.

Children must be counseled from an early age to avoid cigarettes as teenagers and adults. In addition, if the family can avoid living in highly congested urban areas, this may delay deterioration of lung function. The child should avoid future careers that include regular exposure to inhaled toxins.

Preadolescents and adolescents should be counseled to avoid regular or binge drinking of alcohol and to avoid intravenous illegal drug use. The power of the physician to influence young children should not be underestimated. These discussions are best carried out in a private conference with the child, without the parent.

Timing of Hepatic Transplantation

Patients with α_1-antitrypsin deficiency, particularly if they have had evidence of liver disease in the past, should be evaluated regularly for deterioration of hepatic function (Table 174-3). In general, the disease progresses rapidly once deterioration starts. In one study, patients with bilirubin elevation persisting after 1 year, or with recurrence of hyperbilirubinemia, particularly when coupled with abnormal coagulation tests unresponsive to vitamin K and low factor V levels, had a life expectancy of about 1 year [28]. Other authorities have confirmed the poor prognostic significance of recurrence of jaundice and portal hypertension with variceal hemorrhage [39]. These signals should prompt evaluation for hepatic transplantation.

Table 174-3. Factors Suggesting a Poor Prognosis in Liver Disease Associated With α_1-Antitrypsin Deficiency

Factors	Study
Cirrhosis or bridging fibrosis on hepatic biopsy obtained between 6 and 12 months of age	Mowat
Recurrence of jaundice or failure to resolve jaundice in infancy	Ibarguen et al. and Filipponi et al.
Portal hypertension	Filipponi et al.
Development of nephropathy	Ibarguen et al.
Female gender	Ibarguen et al.
Prolonged prothrombin time unresponsive to vitamin K or factor V < 65%, or both	Ibarguen et al

Unique Aspects of Hepatic Transplantation in the α_1-Antitrypsin–Deficient Patient

Although renal function is assessed in all patients evaluated for hepatic transplantation, it is particularly important in patients with α_1-antitrypsin deficiency. The membranoproliferative glomerulonephritis typical of late cirrhosis from α_1-antitrypsin deficiency may be asymptomatic, and the typical proteinuria may not be present [31], particularly in hypoalbuminemic patients. All patients should have a determination of creatinine clearance, and special attention should be paid to the α_1-antitrypsin–deficient patient with hypertension. When α_1-antitrypsin nephropathy is unrecognized before hepatic transplantation, it can lead to severe hypertension with encephalopathy, and death in the postoperative period [47]. In some cases, renal insufficiency necessitates combined liver–kidney transplantation.

Children rarely manifest the emphysematous changes common in adults with α_1-antitrypsin deficiency. However, up to 20% of children with liver disease may have reactive airway disease, and 5% may have intrapulmonary shunting, leading to varying degrees of hypoxia [28]. Patients with α_1-antitrypsin deficiency should have pulmonary function testing as part of their pretransplant evaluation. Exercise intolerance, cyanosis, or digital clubbing should prompt evaluation for intrapulmonary shunting. This complication reverses after transplantation and should not be considered a contraindication for the procedure [48]. Transplantation results in a change from recipient Pi type to donor Pi type. Theoretically, patients are protected from emphysema with normal serum α_1-antitrypsin levels; however, long-term studies of posttransplant patients are not yet available. Patients must be counseled to avoid respiratory toxins after liver transplantation.

The extrahepatic biliary system in patients with α_1-antitrypsin deficiency often is quite narrow. The transplantation team should be alert to the possible need for a Roux-en-Y anastomosis, rather than a duct-to-duct anastomosis, at the time of surgery.

PROGNOSIS

The prognosis for the child with α_1-antitrypsin deficiency diagnosed from population screening is quite good from the standpoint of liver disease. Long-term follow-up of the neonates in

Sveger's original study showed that only five of the original 122 PiZ patients died, and only two died of complications of cirrhosis. At the last follow-up report, when study subjects had reached 18 years of age, 12% had one abnormal liver test and no patient had clinical evidence of liver disease [25]. Patients do remain at risk for emphysema.

Patients with cirrhosis or complications of portal hypertension in infancy have a worse prognosis than those diagnosed from population screening, although temporary resolution of symptoms may delay the need for transplantation for many years. Although some authorities have suggested that early liver biopsy correlates well with outcome [20,30], others have disagreed [34]. In a series of 98 patients with α_1-antitrypsin deficiency followed at the University of Minnesota, only 40% were clinically asymptomatic. The remainder had received transplants, were in need of a transplant, or had died. The researchers conducting this study suggested that the degree of elevation of alanine aminotransferase and prothrombin time and the degree of depression of the trypsin inhibitory capacity correlated with poor outcome, although the overlap of values between good and poor outcome was too great for these tests to have predictive value in individuals. Recurrence of jaundice after infancy was a herald of severe disease [28]. The difference between the findings in this study and that of Sveger is that in the former, 85 of the 98 patients were referred to the institution for liver disease. Some investigators believe that cirrhosis or bridging fibrosis on hepatic biopsies obtained between the ages of 6 and 12 months suggests a poor prognosis [46]. However, without more information on the pathogenesis of liver disease in α_1-antitrypsin deficiency, it is difficult to provide precise prognostic information.

REFERENCES

Recently published papers of particular interest have been highlighted as follows:
- Of interest
- •• Of outstanding interest

1. Cox DW, Markovic VD, Teshima IE: Genes for immunoglobulin heavy chains and for α_1-antitrypsin are localized to specific regions of chromosome 14q. *Nature* 1982, 297:428–430.
2. Rabin M, Watson M, Kidd V, et al.: Regional location of α_1-antichymotrypsin and α_1-antitrypsin genes on human chromosome 14. *Somat Cell Mol Genet* 1986, 12:209–214.
3. Schroeder WT, Miller MF, Woo SLC, Saunders GF: Chromosomal localization of the human α_1-antitrypsin gene (PI) to 14q31-32. *Am J Hum Genet* 1985, 37:868–872.
4. Carrell RW, Jeppsson J-O, Laurell C-B, et al.: Structure and variation of human α_1-antitrypsin. *Nature* 1982, 298:329–334.
5. Carlson JA, Rogers BB, Sifers RN, et al.: Multiple tissues express α_1-antitrypsin in transgenic mice and men. *J Clin Invest* 1988, 82:26–36.
6. Kelsey GD, Povey S, Bygrave AE, Lovell-Badge RH: Species- and tissue-specific expression of human α_1-antitrypsin in transgenic mice. *Genes Dev* 1987, 1:161–171.
7. Perlmutter DH, Cole FS, Kilbridge P, et al.: Expression of the α_1-protease inhibitor gene in human monocytes and macrophages. *Proc Natl Acad Sci USA* 1985, 82:795–799.
8. Van Furth R, Kramps JA, Diesselhof-Den Dulk MMC: Synthesis of α_1-antitrypsin by human monocytes. *Clin Exp Immunol* 1983, 51:551–557.
9. Johnson DA, Travis J: Human α-1-proteinase inhibitor mechanism of action: evidence for activation by limited proteolysis. *Biochem Biophys Res Commun* 1976, 72:33–39.

10. Heeb MJ, Griffin JH: Physiologic inhibition of human activated protein C by α_1-antitrypsin. *J Biol Chem* 1988, 263:11613–11616.

11. Koj A: Acute phase reactants: their synthesis, turnover, and biological significance. In *Structure and Function of Plasma Proteins*. Edited by Allison AC. New York: Plenum Press; 1974: 73–131.

12. Cox DW: α_1-Antitrypsin deficiency. In *The Metabolic Basis of Inherited Disease*. Edited by Scriver CR, Beaudet AL, Sly WS, Valle D. New York: McGraw-Hill; 1989:2409–2437.

13. Cox DW, Woo SLC, Mansfield T: DNA restriction fragments associated with α_1-antitrypsin indicate a single origin for deficiency allele PI Z. *Nature* 1985, 316:79–81.

14. Whitehouse DB, Abbott CM, Lovegrove JU, et al.: Genetic studies on a new deficiency gene (PI*Ztun) at the PI locus. *J Med Genet* 1989, 26:744–749.

15. Cox DW, Billingsley GD: Restriction enzyme MaeIII for prenatal diagnosis of α_1-antitrypsin deficiency. *Lancet* 1986, 2:741–742.

16. Jeppsson J-O:Amino acid substitution Glu -> Lys in α_1-antitrypsin PiZ. *FEBS Lett* 1976, 65:195–197.

17. Kidd VJ, Wallace B, Itakura K, Woo SLC: α_1-Antitrypsin deficiency detection by direct analysis of the mutation in the gene. *Nature* 1983, 304:230–234.

18. Nukiwa T, Satoh K, Brantly ML, et al.: Identification of a second mutation in the protein-coding sequence of the Z type α_1-antitrypsin gene. *J Biol Chem* 1986, 261:15989–15994.

19. Sharp HL: α_1-antitrypsin deficiency. *Hosp Pract* 1971;6(5):83–96.

20. Hadchouel M, Gautier M: Histopathologic study of the liver in the early cholestatic phase of α_1-antitrypsin deficiency. *J Pediatrics* 1976, 89:211–215.

21. Sveger T: Liver disease in α_1-antitrypsin deficiency detected by screening of 200,000 infants. *N Engl J Med* 1976, 294:1316–1321.

22. Sveger T: α_1-Antitrypsin deficiency in early childhood. *Pediatrics* 1978, 62:22–25.

23. Sveger T, Thelin T: Four-year-old children with α_1-antitrypsin deficiency. *Acta Paediatr Scand* 1981, 70:171–177.

24. Sveger T: Prospective study of children with α_1-antitrypsin deficiency: eight-year-old follow-up. *J Pediatr* 1984, 104:91–94.

25. Sveger T, Eriksson S: The liver in adolescents with α_1-antitrypsin deficiency. *Hepatology* 1995, 22:514–517.

26. Wall M, Moe E, Eisenberg J, et al.: Long-term follow-up of a cohort of children with α_1-antitrypsin deficiency. *J Pediatr* 1990, 116:248–251.

27. Sharp HL: Wherefore art thou liver disease associated with α_1-antitrypsin deficiency? *Hepatology* 1995, 22:666–668.

28. Ibarguen E, Gross CR, Savik SK, Sharp HL: Liver disease in α_1-antitrypsin deficiency: prognostic indicators. *J Pediatr* 1990, 117:864–870.

29. Sharp HL, Bridges RA, Krivit W, Freier EF: Cirrhosis associated with α_1-antitrypsin deficiency: a case report in α_1-antitrypsin deficiency and a review of factors predisposing to hemorrhage. *J Lab Clin Med* 1969, 73:934–939.

30. Nebbia G, Hadchouel M, Odievre M, Alagille D: Early assessment of evolution of liver disease associated with α_1-antitrypsin deficiency in childhood. *J Pediatr* 1983, 102:661–665.

31. Psacharopoulos HT, Mowat AP, Cook PJL, et al.: Outcome of liver disease associated with α_1-antitrypsin deficiency (PiZ). *Arch Dis Child* 1983, 58:882–887.

32. Payne NR, Hasegawa DK: Vitamin K deficiency in newborns. *Pediatrics* 1984, 73:712–716.

33. Ghishan FK, Gray GF, Greene HL. α_1-Antitrypsin deficiency presenting with ascites and cirrhosis in the neonatal period. *Gastroenterol* 1983, 85:435–438.

34. Ghishan FK, Greene HL: Liver disease in children with PiZZ α_1-antitrypsin deficiency. *Hepatology* 1988, 8:307–310.

35. Nord KS, Saad S, Joshi VV, McLoughlin LC: Concurrence of α_1-antitrypsin deficiency and biliary atresia. *J Pediatr* 1987, 111:416–418.

36. Case records of the Massachusetts General Hospital, Case 24-1980. *N Engl J Med* 1980, 302:1405–1413.

37. Christen H, Bau J, Halsband H: Hereditary α_1-antitrypsin deficiency associated with congenital extrahepatic bile duct hypoplasia. *Klin Wochenschr* 1975, 53:90–91.

38. Odièvre M, Martin J-P, Hadchouel M, et al.: α_1-Antitrypsin deficiency and liver disease in children: phenotypes, manifestations and prognosis. *Pediatrics* 1976, 57:226–231.

39. Filipponi F, Soubrane O, Labrousse F, et al.: Liver transplantation for end-stage liver disease associated with α_1-antitrypsin deficiency in children: pretransplant natural history, timing and results of transplantation. *J Hepatology* 1994, 20:72–78.

40. Davis ID, Burke B, Freese D, et al.: The pathologic spectrum of nephropathy associated with α_1-antitrypsin deficiency. *Hum Pathol* 1992, 23:57–62.

41. Strife CF, Hug G, Chuck G, et al.: Membranoproliferative glomerulonephritis and α_1-antitrypsin deficiency in children. *Pediatrics* 1983, 71:88–92.

42. Cox DW, Mansfield T: Prenatal diagnosis of α_1-antitrypsin deficiency and estimates of fetal risk for disease. *J Med Genet* 1987, 24:52–59.

43. Sveger T: Screening for α_1-antitrypsin deficiency. *Acta Paediatr* 1994, 393(suppl):18–20.

44. Udall JJN, Dixon M, Newman AP, et al.: Liver disease in α_1-antitrypsin deficiency. A retrospective analysis of the influence of early breast- vs bottle-feeding. *JAMA* 1985, 253:2679–2682.

45. Propst A, Propst T, Ofner D, et al.: Prognosis and life expectancy in α_1-antitrypsin deficiency and chronic liver disease. *Scand J Gastroenterol* 1995, 53:1108–1112.

46. Mowat AP: α_1-Antitrypsin deficiency (PiZZ): features of liver involvement in childhood. *Acta Paediatr* 1994, 393(suppl):13–17.

47. Noble-Jamieson G, Barnes ND, Thiru S, Mowat AP: Severe hypertension after liver transplantation in $\alpha_1$antitrypsin deficiency. *Arch Dis Child* 1990, 65:1217–1221.

48. Schwarzenberg SJ, Freese DK, Regelmann W, et al.: Resolution of severe intrapulmonary shunting after liver transplantation. *Chest* 1993, 103:1271–1273.

49. Cox DW: New variants of α_1-antitrypsin: comparison of Pi typing techniques. *Am J Hum Genet* 1981, 33:354–365.

50. Curiel D, Chytil A, Courtney M, Crystal RG: Serum α_1-antitrypsin deficiency associated with the common S-type (Glu^{264}-> Val) mutation results from intracellular degradation of α_1-antitrypsin prior to secretion. *J Biol Chem* 1989, 264:10477–10486.

51. Cox DW: A new deficiency allele of α_1-antitrypsin: PiMmalton. *Protides of the biological fluids* 1975, 23:375–378.

52. Lieberman J, Gaidulis L, Klotz SD: A new deficient variant of α_1-antitrypsin (MDuarte): inability to detect the heterozygous state by antitrypsin phenotyping. *Am Rev Resp Dis* 1976, 113:31–36.

53. Cox DW, Billingsley GD: Rare deficiency types of α_1-antitrypsin: electrophoretic variation and DNA haplotypes. *Am J Hum Genet* 1989, 44:844–854

175 Hepatitis B
James E. Heubi

Although hepatitis has been recognized since the late 1800s, Krugman and colleagues demonstrated the existence of two types, MS-1 and MS-2, in 1967 in a population of mentally retarded children. The type of hepatitis that is primarily parenterally acquired and has a long incubation period, then known as MS-2, is now known as hepatitis B (HBV) [1]. Since the mid-1960s, the worldwide public health significance of HBV has been recognized, and its vertical transmission in endemic areas has been well documented. Treatment regimens and strategies to prevent the spread of HBV have been developed. This chapter focuses primarily on pediatric issues, with specific attention to treatment of chronic HBV in children and prevention of vertical transmission. The reader is also referred to two additional excellent reviews of HBV in children [2•,3].

VIROLOGY

Hepatitis B is a DNA virus of the family Hepadnaviridae. The viral particle is 42 nm in diameter, is double shelled, and contains several specific antigens. The outer viral coat is the HBV surface antigen (HB_sAg), the inner core is the HBV core antigen (HB_cAg), and a core cleavage product is called HB e antigen (HB_eAg). Located within the core is the genome of HBV, which is 3.2 kb in length and codes for HB_sAg, HBV DNA polymerase, and HBV-X (which may play a role in oncogenesis). The serologic markers of HBV are listed in Table 175-1. Hepatic injury from HBV is primarily immune mediated with direct cytotoxicity playing a minor role.

EPIDEMIOLOGY

HBV is found in all body fluids and secretions except stool. Transmission occurs via parenteral exposure or through exchange of infected secretions. After the perinatal period, transmission by sexual intercourse is probably the most common route of nonparenteral acquisition. The prevalence of HBV infection and carrier states varies in different geographic regions, with estimates ranging from a high of 18% in Southeast Asia to a low of 0.1% in Western Europe and North America. HBV infection is observed in 14% to 25% of adopted children from Korea, India, and Central and South America. Other areas of high endemicity for HBV include sub-Saharan Africa. Areas of moderate prevalence include Eastern European countries (*eg,* Bulgaria, Romania, Poland) and Saudi Arabia.

Specific situations that confer high risk for HBV infection have been observed in North American infants, children, and adolescents. Children at risk include [1] infants born to mothers who are chronic viral carriers, [4] children who have emigrated from endemic areas, [5] hemophiliacs and others who receive frequent blood transfusions, [6] adolescents who use injected street drugs, [7•] classroom contacts of mentally retarded carriers, and [8] institutionalized children and care personnel. HBV transmission in daycare centers is uncommon unless aggressive behavior or breakdown in good hygienic practices occurs.

Perinatal Transmission

All infants born to HB_sAg-positive mothers are at risk for vertical transmission of HBV. Increased risk of transmission is associated with high maternal HB_sAg titer, maternal HB_eAg positivity, HBV-DNA or DNA polymerase in maternal serum, HB_sAg-positive cord blood, and HB_sAg-positive siblings. Most transmission occurs during delivery as a result of transplacental leakage. Rarely, if ever, has breast milk been the source of HBV infection.

Few clinical manifestations of disease are present in cases of vertical transmission; however, serologic evidence of disease develops by age 1 to 3 months. Clinical hepatitis or a chronic carrier state develops in 90% of HB_sAg-positive infants. The high frequency with which a chronic carrier state is developed

Table 175-1. Definitions and Significance of Serologic Markers of Hepatitis B

HB_sAg	HBV surface antigen	Indicates acute or chronic HBV infection
HB_cAg	HBV core antigen	Not detectable in serum
HB_eAg	HBV e antigen, cleavage product of HB_cAg	Indicates active HBV infection, correlates with HBV replication, signifies high infectivity
HBV DNA	DNA of HBV	Indicates HBV replication
anti-HB_s	Antibody to surface Ag	Indicates clinical recovery from HBV and immune status
		May indicate passive immunity from HBIG
anti-HB_c	Total antibody to HB_cAg	Indicates active HBV infection (acute and chronic)
anti-HB_c IgM	IgM antibody to HB_cAg	Early index of HBV infection, not present in chronic HBV
anti-HB_e	antibody to HB_eAg	Seroconversion to anti-HB_e indicates resolution of hepatitis

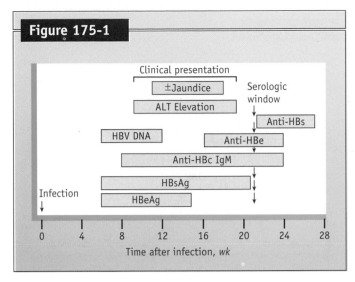

Figure 175-1

Course of acute hepatitis B. (*From* Hoofnagle JH, DiBesceglie AM [5]; with permission.)

in the perinatal period most likely is related to immaturity of the immune system. Diminished cytokine production and cytotoxic activity and a generalized suppression of the immune response may be responsible. Exposure of the fetus to maternal HBV antibodies and antigens may decrease the newborn immune response. Infants tend to have high levels of viral replication, mild to moderate liver disease, and a propensity for development of hepatocellular carcinoma. Rarely, fatal fulminant hepatitis may be precipitated by perinatal transmission. This is most likely caused by infection with precore mutants of HBV.

Infants who are born to HB$_s$Ag-positive mothers may escape vertical transmission; however, they continue to be at increased risk of acquiring infection from infected family members. As many as 46% of cases of HBV infection in children born in the United States to mothers who have immigrated from hyperendemic areas cannot be attributed to vertical transmission [4].

◼ ACUTE AND CHRONIC HEPATITIS B
Clinical Features of Acute HBV

Three phases of HBV infection acquired by parenteral or body fluid exposure are recognized: the incubation period, the symptomatic period, and convalescence. The only difference between children and adults is that children more commonly have anicteric disease. After exposure there is a prodromal phase of 50 to 180 days during which patients initially may be asympto-

matic. They then develop insidious, nonspecific complaints such as serum sickness–like illness, arthralgias, or rash. At the onset of the symptomatic phase, anorexia, nausea, vomiting, fatigue, fever, and myalgias may develop. Pruritus may accompany jaundice. The typical course and serologic markers are illustrated in Figure 175-1.

Several extrahepatic manifestations may be observed, including membranous glomerulopathy and vasculitic syndromes. Although the papular acrodermatitis of childhood is often cited as a common extrahepatic manifestation of HBV in children, it is not very common in North America and may actually be more common with other viral infections, such as Epstein-Barr virus [6].

Natural History of Acute HBV Infection

Clinical recovery is anticipated in 90% to 95% of infants and children with acute HBV acquired postnatally; fulminant hepatitis may develop in 1% to 2% of these individuals. Chronic hepatitis develops in less than 5% of children who acquire disease after infancy. Results of studies of large numbers of children with follow-up observations of up to 10 years suggest that hepatic failure is uncommon; as many as 50% of these children have active hepatitis or cirrhosis, however. Ninety percent to 95% of infants who acquire infection in the perinatal period become chronic carriers, with hepatocellular carcinoma (HCC) occurring in a small fraction of this group. In Taiwan, HCC accounts for 54% of deaths in HB$_s$Ag carriers. HCC has been seen in HB$_s$Ag-positive patients as young as age 8 months.

Diagnosis of Acute HBV Infection

The typical serologic profile for an acute self-limited HBV infection is shown in Figure 175-1 and Table 175-2. HB$_s$Ag may appear soon after exposure to HBV; more commonly it is evident at 1 to 3 months after exposure and before symptoms develop. HB$_e$Ag and HBV-DNA appear concurrently with HB$_s$Ag. Serum aminotransferases may rise 2 to 8 weeks after HB$_s$Ag is detected in serum and remain elevated for 1 to 2 months.

Initial antibody response includes the appearance of anti-HB$_c$ (IgM) and HB$_e$Ag. Anti-HB$_c$ in combination with HB$_s$Ag is characteristic of an acute HBV infection. With convalescence, anti-HB$_c$ (IgG) appears, HB$_s$Ag and HBV-DNA disappear, and anti-HB$_e$ appears. The presence of anti-HB$_s$ indicates recovery from acute HBV infection and protection against subsequent infection.

Table 175-2. Serologic Markers of Hepatitis B

HB$_s$Ag	HB$_e$Ag	Anti-HB$_e$	Anti-HB$_c$	Anti-HB$_s$	
+	+/-	-	-	-	Early acute hepatitis, carrier
+	+/-	-	+	-	Acute hepatitis (anti HB$_c$ IgM),
+	-	+/-	+	-	Late acute hepatitis, carrier
-	-	-	+	-	Recovery phase
-	-	+/-	+	+	Postinfection
-	-	-	-	+	Immune

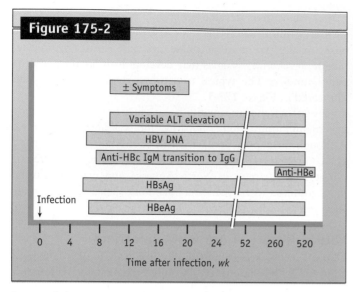

Course of chronic hepatitis B, including remission with seroconversion from HB$_e$Ag to anti-HB$_e$. (*From* Hoofnagle JH, DiBesceglie AM [5]; with permission.)

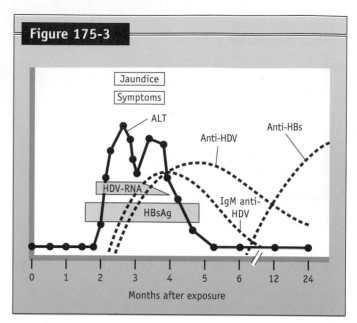

Hepatitis D coinfection with hepatitis B. (*From* Hoofnagle JH, DiBesceglie AM [5]; with permission.)

Diagnosis of Chronic HBV Infection

Two clinical patterns of chronic HBV infection are observed: 1) chronic liver disease with elevated aminotransferase and abnormal liver histology, and 2) a healthy carrier state characterized by normal aminotransferase but with persistent viral infection. Both chronic states have similar serologic findings: HB$_s$Ag is positive, HB$_e$Ag or HBV-DNA is positive or negative, and HB$_c$Ag is present in the liver (Table 175-2, Fig. 175-2).

Age at acquisition of primary HBV infection is a major determinant of chronicity. As many as 95% of infected neonates become HB$_s$Ag carriers, whereas only about 20% of acutely infected children and 10% of adults develop the carrier state. Similarly, HCC is most prevalent in areas where HBV is acquired early in life. Patients who have acquired HBV by vertical transmission have been found with HCC as early as 8 months.

■ HEPATITIS D

Hepatitis D (HDV) can produce infection and clinical illness only in the presence of active HBV infection. HDV may have a profound effect on the clinical course of coexistent HBV infection. Acute hepatitis D may be present as a coinfection (simultaneous acquisition of HBV and HDV) or as a superinfection (infection superimposed on a chronic HBV carriage). In either circumstance, the severity of hepatocellular injury may be increased by the coexistence of HDV. Figures 175-3 and 175-4 display the two possible scenarios, with attendant serologic findings, of concurrent HBV and HDV infections.

■ TREATMENT
Management of Acute HBV

Bed rest is recommended but not essential for the child with acute HBV. Dietary restrictions are of minimal value. Corticosteroids are of no proven value. School-age children may return to the classroom when they feel well. Follow-up studies of patients with acute HBV are suggested to document bio-

chemical resolution and to identify whether HB$_s$Ag has been cleared from serum, thus indicating resolution. Persistence of HB$_s$Ag is associated with the carrier state or chronic hepatitis; this has different management implications.

Management of Chronic HBV

It is essential to determine whether the patient is a chronic carrier or one who has persistent HBV infection and chronic hepatitis. Differentiating between these two conditions can be difficult. Chronic carriers typically have HB$_s$Ag in serum with normal serum aminotransferases. Anti-HB$_s$ is absent in 60% to 80% of carriers; the remainder have concurrent HB$_s$Ag and anti-HB$_s$ in the serum. Seroconversion from HB$_e$Ag-positive to anti–HB$_e$-positive occurs in 10% to 15% of carriers during their lifetime. With the disappearance of HB$_e$Ag, HBV-DNA

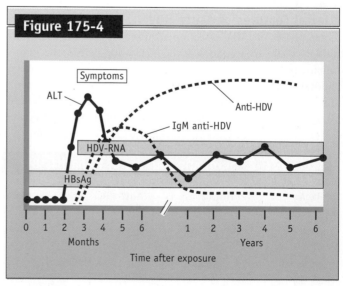

Hepatitis D superinfection with chronic hepatitis B. (*From* Hoofnagle JH, DiBesceglie AM [5]; with permission.)

also disappears from the serum. In contrast to the carrier state, patients with chronic hepatitis have increased serum aminotransferases with HB$_s$Ag, HB$_e$Ag, and HBV-DNA seropositivity.

For chronic carriers, surveillance for HCC and use of good hygienic practices to prevent viral spread should be encouraged. Household contacts should be immunized to prevent horizontal transmission of HBV. Because HBV is spread through body fluids, care regarding exposures in the household should be encouraged. Screening for HCC is encouraged because early surgical intervention favorably influences survival. Current recommendations are semiannual measurement of α-fetoprotein and hepatic ultrasonography.

Therapy for HBV-associated chronic hepatitis is directed at normalization of aminotransferase activity and suppression or clearance of HBV, with attendant loss of HB$_e$Ag, HB$_s$Ag, and HBV-DNA. Other goals of therapy include decreasing infectivity, decreasing the rate of progression of liver disease, and decreasing the incidence of HCC. In patients with HBV-associated chronic hepatitis, seroconversion from HB$_e$Ag to anti-HB$_e$ occurs at the rate of approximately 15% to 20% per year, with 50% seroconverting over time.

Although a number of anti-inflammatory or antiviral agents have been used to treat hepatitis B, only interferon (IFN) has, to date, proved useful in the treatment of chronic HBV. Interferons are naturally occurring proteins produced in response to viral infections. They have antiviral, immunomodulatory, and antiproliferative properties. IFN-α-2b, produced through recombinant DNA technology, has been approved by the FDA for treatment of HBV infection. Candidates for therapy should have had chronic HBV hepatitis, as indicated by increased serum ALT and HB$_s$Ag positivity, for at least 6 months. There should be evidence of viral replication, with HBV-DNA in serum and HB$_e$Ag positivity. The liver should be examined microsurgically to determine disease activity. IFN therapy is contraindicated in patients with decompensated cirrhosis, and caution should be exercised in treating patients with impaired hepatic synthetic function or hypersplenism, because of the potential for worsening of hepatic function and potential worsening of thrombocytopenia associated with its use. A successful response to therapy is marked by disappearance of HBV-DNA and HB$_e$Ag from serum.

Extensive clinical trials of IFN treatment for chronic hepatitis in adults have been undertaken. A 4- to 6-month course of 5 to 10 million units (MU) IFN three times weekly induced a long-term remission in 25% to 40% of patients (Fig. 175-5) [7•]. In a meta-analysis of 15 clinical trails, Wong and colleagues [9•] found that 33% of patients had persistent disappearance of HB$_s$Ag when treated with IFN compared to 12% in controls.

A smaller number of trials with IFN have been reported in children. It is essential to distinguish between the findings in children who acquired HBV infection perinatally and those who contracted it later. Asian children with normal aminotransferases who contracted HBV in the perinatal period respond poorly to IFN. Among 90 HB$_s$Ag-positive Chinese children randomized to either IFN-α (5 MU/m², 3 times per week for 16 weeks) or placebo, only 3% of the treated children

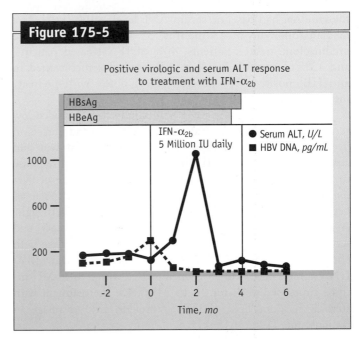

Figure 175-5

Positive virologic and serum ALT response to treatment with IFN-α$_{2b}$

Complete clinical response of chronic hepatitis B to interferon treatment. (*From* Fried M [8]; with permission.)

and none of the controls became HB$_e$Ag negative [10]. Lai and colleagues [11] performed a placebo-controlled trial in Chinese children who were HB$_s$Ag-positive chronic carriers. All 24 subjects were asymptomatic, and two had increased serum aminotransferases. Treatment consisted of 10 MU IFN/m², three times per week for 12 weeks. At the 1-year follow-up evaluation, all of the children were HB$_s$Ag positive, and at 18 months, only two patients in each group were HBV-DNA–negative. The addition of a prednisone course before IFN therapy resulted in a modest improvement in response rate. Of this prednisone-treated group, 16% had persistent absence of HBV-DNA 18 months after a 16-week course of 5 MU/m² three times weekly. These relatively poor responses are probably related to immune tolerance that develops when HBV is acquired early in life.

In contrast to the experience with chronic HBV carriers who acquire infection perinatally, children who develop chronic HBV hepatitis later in life have responses similar to those of adults treated with IFN. Two large placebo-controlled trials illustrate typical responses. Thirty-six Spanish children with persistently increased aminotransferases who were positive for HB$_s$Ag, HB$_e$Ag, and HBV-DNA for 1 year were treated with either IFN-α 10 MU/m² 3 times per week, IFN-α 5 MU/m² 3 times per week, or placebo. After 6 months of treatment 58%, 42%, and 17%, respectively, became HBV-DNA negative. Results of liver biopsies at the end of therapy showed histologic improvement in those who responded to IFN. IFN responders tended to be carriers of shorter duration, with higher ALT levels than those who did not respond [12•]. In a large multicenter trial of 95 HBV-DNA–positive, HB$_e$Ag-positive children with a mean age of 9 years, Gregorio and colleagues [13•] evaluated the effect of prednisolone followed by IFN-α, IFN-α alone, or no treatment. IFN was given three times per week at 5 MU/m² for 12 weeks. Most of the children had baseline serum AST levels ≤100 IU/L. At a median follow-up of 15 months, 35% of the IFN-positive prednisolone-treated patients, 40% of IFN-treated patients, and 13% of controls had lost HB$_e$Ag and seroconverted to anti-HB$_e$–positive. No difference was noted with pretreatment with corticosteroids.

Predictors of response to IFN in adults have included low serum HBV-DNA concentrations, active disease and fibrosis on liver biopsy, a short duration of disease before treatment, and absence of complicating HIV infections. Predictors of response to IFN in children include a higher histologic grade of liver biopsies before treatment, a lower percentage of HB$_e$Ag-stained hepatocytes, higher baseline serum ALT and AST levels, higher peak serum ALT before serum HBV-DNA clearance, and serum HBV-DNA <1 ng/mL [13•,14]. Overall, children with chronic HBV acquired after the neonatal period clear HBV-DNA at rates of 35% to 58% when treated with 5 to 10 MU/m^2 three times per week for 12 to 24 weeks. Pretreatment with steroids has not been shown to provide any advantage in response rate [12•,13•,15–17].

The side effect profile of IFN-α appears to be similar in children and adults. The most common side effect is influenza-like illness beginning 6 to 8 hours after injection and lasting up to 12 hours. With continued treatment, this reaction abates. More chronic symptoms may be observed, including malaise, fatigue, headaches, myalgias, hair loss, and bone marrow suppression. At high doses such as 10 MU/m^2, neutropenia, flu-like symptoms, and other side effects may necessitate dose reductions [12•,13•,14–17].

Other Agents

Additional therapies for HBV, including interferon-γ, thymosin, levamisole, vidarabine, acyclovir, suramin, foscarnet, zidovudine, didanosine, ribavirin, and fialuridine have been undertaken in adults without any benefit. New nucleoside analogues appear to be more promising candidates for treatment of chronic HBV hepatitis. Treatment with lamivudine for 12 weeks has resulted in clearance of HB$_e$Ag and decreases in serum aminotransferase; however, sustained response was shown in only 19% of treated patients [18]. Few trials have been undertaken in children. Ruiz-Moreno and colleagues [19] evaluated the effects of levamisole with interferon compared to interferon alone for 6 months in a group of 38 children with chronic HBV. At the 15-month follow-up evaluation, there were no differences between the groups in loss of HB$_e$Ag and HBV-DNA or normalization of serum ALT, and the combination therapy group had more severe side effects.

Orthotopic Liver Transplantation

The recurrence of HBV after liver transplantation in a high percentage of patients with active viral replication (HBV-DNA and HB$_e$Ag seropositivity) has prompted aggressive efforts at viral suppression before and after transplantation. This is particularly relevant because recurrence of HBV almost universally leads to graft and patient loss. Although controversy remains, chronic treatment with hepatitis B immune globulin (HBIG) at doses sufficient to maintain anti-HB$_s$ titers >500 IU/L prevents reinfection of the graft. When HBIG was not

given, HBV reinfection occurred in 100% of Asian children with perinatal infection, compared with 45% of non-Asians, who were presumed to have acquired HBV after infancy. When HBIG was given, 40% of Asians and no non-Asians developed recurrent HBV in the graft [20].

▬▬ PREVENTIVE STRATEGIES

Active Immunization

The first-generation vaccine for HBV was prepared from pooled plasma in 1982. It proved both safe and efficacious in producing protective titers of anti-HB$_s$ in infants, children, and adults. Because of the fear of potential transmission of other viral diseases, this vaccine was not accepted for widespread use. In 1986, the first of the recombinant DNA–derived HBV vaccines was licensed by the FDA. The recommendations for use are presented in Table 175-3 [21]. Current recommendations for administration include three intramuscular doses, at 0, 1 and 6 months of age. In 1992, the American Academy of Pediatrics (AAP) recommended HBV immunizations for all infants and high-risk adolescents and children. All children born after April 1, 1992, should be given HBV vaccine with their routine childhood immunizations. Those born before this date should be immunized as young adolescents. The recommended doses, adapted from the AAP Redbook, are shown in Table 175-4. In adults anti-HB$_s$ develops in 75% to 90% after the first dose and

---

Table 175-3. Populations for Whom Hepatitis B Vaccine is Recommended or Should Be Considered

Preexposure Vaccination

Vaccine Recommended
  Health care workers having blood or needle stick exposure
  Clients and staff of institutions for the developmentally disabled
  Hemodialysis patients
  Sexually active homosexual men
  Users of illicit drugs
  Recipients of certain blood products
  Household members and sexual contacts of HBV carriers
  Adoptees from countries of high HBV endemicity
  Population with high endemicity of HBV infection
  Universal vaccinations of infants/adolescents
Vaccine should be considered
  Inmates of long-term correctional facilities
  Heterosexually active persons with multiple sexual partners
  International travelers to HBV endemic areas
  Population with high endemicity of HBV infection

Postexposure Vaccination

Health care workers having percutaneous or per mucosal exposure to human blood
Sexual exposure to HB$_s$Ag positive partner
Infants born to HBV-positive mothers
Household exposure (infants 12 months) to HBV primary care giver

---

(Modified from Centers for Disease Control [21]; with permission.)

Table 175-4. Recommended Doses for Hepatitis B Vaccine

	Heptavax-B	Recombivax	Energix
Infants of Hepatitis B carrier mothers*	10 µg/0.5 cm³	5 µg/0.5 cm³	10 µg/0.5 cm³
Age <11 years	10 µg/0.5 cm³	2.5 µg/0.25 cm³	10 µg/0.5 cm³
Age 11–19 years	20 µg/1.0 cm³	5 µg/0.5 cm³	20 µg/1.0 cm³
Age >19 years	20 µg/1.0 cm³	10 µg/1.0 cm³	20 µg/1.0 cm³
Dialysis patients and immunocompromised	40 µg/2.0 cm³	40 µg/1.0 cm³	40 µg/2.0 cm³

Hepatitis B immune globulin should be given at time of first dose.

Table 175-5. Hepatitis B Postexposure Prophylaxis

	HBIG		Vaccine
Exposure	Dose	Recommended Timing	Recommended Timing
Perinatal	0.5mL	Within 12 hours of birth	Within 12 hours of birth*
Sexual	0.06 mL/kg	Within 14 days of contact	First dose with HBIG*

All doses intramuscular at separate site from HBIG.
HBIG–hepatitis B immune globulin.

in 95% after three doses. In infants anti-HB$_s$ appears in 95.8% after two doses and in 100% after three doses [22].

Universal immunization of infants has now been undertaken in at least 50 countries, representing 56% of the world's carriers [23•,24]. In Taiwan, the prevalence of HB$_s$Ag-positive children has decreased from 9.8% to 1.3% since immunization programs were introduced. Even in areas of low endemicity, such as the United States, this strategy appears to be cost effective [25]. Immunization should ultimately eliminate HBV and the potential long-term complications of chronic hepatitis (eg, liver failure and HCC), in the United States.

Passive Immunization

It is recommended that postexposure prophylaxis with HBIG be given after perinatal exposure of an infant born to an HB$_s$Ag-positive mother, sexual exposure to an HB$_s$Ag-positive partner, exposure to household contacts, or accidental mucosal or percutaneous exposure to materials that are HB$_s$Ag positive (Table 175-5). HBIG should be given within the first 12 hours after birth with perinatal exposure and no later than 7 days after exposure for the latter three indications. The first dose of HBV vaccine should be given at the same time at a different intramuscular site, with completion of the vaccine schedule as described earlier.

When vaccine is used as the sole means of prevention of perinatal HBV spread, efficacy is approximately 75%. This efficacy rate has been proved only when the vaccine is given within 12 hours of birth; protection is presumed but unproved when HBIG is given 12 to 48 hours after birth. Concurrent administration of HBIG and HBV vaccine has been shown to reduce the carrier rate to less than 5% in high-risk populations. It may not be possible to improve on this, because it is believed that 3% to 5% of infections may be acquired in utero. The efficacy of combined HBIG and HBV vaccination is further supported by the demonstration that it provides protection from chronic infection in 95% of infants born to HB$_s$Ag/HB$_e$Ag-positive mothers [26].

REFERENCES

Recently published papers of particular interest have been highlighted as follows:
• Of interest
•• Of outstanding interest

1. Krugman S, Giles JP, Hammond DJ: Infectious hepatitis: evidence for two distinct clinical, epidemiological, and immunologic types of infection. *JAMA* 1967, 200:365–373.

2.• Balistreri WF: Acute and chronic viral hepatitis. In *Liver Disease in Children*. Edited by Suchy FJ. St. Louis: Mosby, 1994:460–509.
This is an excellent review of hepatitis in children, with an extensive bibliography.

3. Jonas MM: Interferon-α for viral hepatitis [invited review]. *J Ped Gastroenterol Nutr* 1996, 23:93–106.

4. Franks AL, Berg CJ, Kane MA, *et al.*: Hepatitis B virus infection among children born in the United States to Southeast Asian refugees. *N Engl J Med* 1989, 321:1301–1305.

5. Hoofnagle JH, DiBisceglie AM: Serologic diagnosis of acute and chronic hepatitis. *Semin Liver Dis* 1991, 11:73–83.

6. Draelos ZK, Hansen RC, James WD: Gianotti-Crosti syndrome associated with infections other than hepatitis B. *JAMA* 1986, 256:2386–2388.

7.• Hoofnagle JH, DiBisceglie AM: The treatment of chronic viral hepatitis. *New Eng J Med* 1997, 347–356.

8. Fried M: Therapy of chronic viral hepatitis. *Med Clin North Am* 1996, 80:957–972.

9.• Wong DKH, Cheung AM, O'Rourke K, *et al.*: Effect of alpha-interferon treatment in patients with hepatitis B$_e$ antigen-positive chronic hepatitis B: a meta-analysis. *Ann Intern Med* 1993, 119:312–323.
This paper represents a meta-analysis of existing studies of the use of IFN for the treatment of chronic HBV.

10. Lai CL, Lin HJ, Lau JJN, *et al.*: Effect of recombinant alpha interferon with or without prednisone in Chinese HB$_s$Ag carrier children. *Q J Med* 1991, 78:155–163.

11. Lai CL, Lok ASF, Lin HJ *et al.*: Placebo controlled trial of recombinant α interferon in Chinese HB$_s$Ag carrier children. *Lancet* 1987, 2:877–880.

12.• Ruiz-Moreno M, Rua MJ, Molina J, *et al*: Prospective, randomized controlled trial of interferon-α in children with chronic hepatitis. *Hepatology* 1991, 13:1035–1039.
The authors present a well-designed placebo-controlled clinical trial comparing two doses of IFN-α with placebo with the endpoint of clearance of HBV-DNA.

13.• Gregoria GV, Jara P, Hierro L, *et al.*: Lymphoblastoid interferon alfa with or without steroid pretreatment in children with chronic hepatitis B: a multicenter trial. *Hepatology* 1996, 23:700–707.
The authors report here on a multicenter placebo-controlled clinical trial of IFN-α with or without prednisolone compared to placebo in 95 children from multiple centers in Europe.

14. Ruiz-Moreno M, Camps T, Jimenez J, *et al.*: Factors predictive of response to interferon therapy in children with chronic hepatitis B. *J Hepatol* 1995, 22:540–544.

15. Barbera C, Bortolotti F, Crivellaro C, *et al.*: Recombinant interferon-α 2a hastens the rate of HB$_e$Ag clearance in children with chronic hepatitis B. *Hepatology* 1994, 20:287–290.

16. Utili R, Sagnelli E, Gaeta GB, *et al.*: Treatment of chronic hepatitis B in children with prednisone followed by alfa-interferon: a controlled randomized study. *J Hepatol* 1994, 20:163–167.

17. Castaneda Guillot C, Escobar Capote MD, Garcia Bacallao E, Borbolla Bousquets E: Long term study of the treatment with recombinant alfa 2b interferon in chronic active hepatitis due to B virus in children and adolescents. *Gene* 1994, 48:219–225.

18. Dienstag JL, Perrillo RP, Schiff ER, *et al*: A preliminary trial of lamivudine for chronic hepatitis B infection. *N Engl J Med* 1995, 333:1657–1661.

19. Ruiz-Moreno M, Garcia R, Rua MJ, *et al.*: Levamisole and interferon in children with chronic hepatitis B. *Hepatology* 1993, 18:264–269.

20. Jurim O, Martin P, Shaked A, *et al*: Liver transplantation for chronic hepatitis B in Asians. *Transplantation* 1994, 57:1393–1395.

21. Centers for Disease Control. Protection against viral hepatitis: recommendations of Immunization Practices Committee (ACIP). MMWR 1990, 39(RR-2):1.

22. Lau Y-L, Tam AYC, Ng KW: Response of preterm infants to hepatitis B vaccine. *J Pediatr* 1992, 121:962–965.

23.• Chen HL, Chang MH, Ni YH, *et al.*: Seroepidemiology of hepatitis B virus infection in children: ten years of mass vaccination in Taiwan. *JAMA* 1996, 276:906–908.
This is an excellent follow-up of the results of mass immunization in a population in which hepatitis B is endemic, demonstrating the effectiveness of this public health strategy.

24. Kane M: Global programme for control of hepatitis B infection. *Vaccine* 1995, 13(suppl 1):S47–S49.

25. Margolis HS, Coleman PJ, Brown RE, *et al.*: Prevention of hepatitis B virus transmission by immunization. An economic analysis of current recommendations. *JAMA* 1995, 274:1201–1208.

26. Stevens CE, Taylor PE, Tong MJ, *et al.*: Yeast-recombinant hepatitis B vaccine. Efficacy with hepatitis B immune globin in prevention of perinatal hepatitis B transmission. *JAMA* 1987, 257:2612–2616.

27. Active and passive immunization. Edited by Peter G. *1991 Redbook: report of the Committee on Infectious Diseases*, edn 22. Elk Grove Village, Illinois: American Academy of Pediatrics;1991.

176 Pediatric Autoimmune Hepatitis

Karan E. McBride and Eric S. Maller

Two types of autoimmune hepatitis (AIH) are recognized in children, distinguished by the presence of autoantibodies: type I, with anti-actin or smooth muscle antibodies (SMA), antinuclear antibody (ANA), or both [1], and type II, with liver and kidney microsomal antibody type I (LKM-1) but no SMA or ANA [2]. Type I, the most prevalent form, is considered classic AIH. The patient is typically a young adolescent girl who presents with either an acute hepatic disorder or a more chronic illness with lethargy, arthralgia, menstrual disorders, and, possibly, slight jaundice [1].

The target of the anti–LKM-1 antibody in type II AIH is cytochrome p4502D6 (CYP2D6) [3]. Anti–LKM-1 and anti-actin antibodies are mutually exclusive. Type II AIH is less prevalent than type I. The presentation often is acute or fulminant with severe histologic features and progression to cirrhosis despite immunosuppression [2].

Antibodies to the liver-specific lipoprotein (anti-LSP), which are present in 75% of children with AIH, are a nonspecific marker of evolving autoimmune hepatitis in the patient who initially does not manifest the more typical autoantibody markers of types I and II AIH [4••].

The term *cryptogenic* is reserved for cases in which all known etiologic factors have been excluded and in which there are no detectable conventional autoantibodies [5] despite characteristic histologic changes, high serum gamma globulin, and complete response to corticosteroids.

EPIDEMIOLOGY

As in adults, there is a female preponderance in both types of AIH in children [4••]. The onset of disease in childhood can occur at any age. In Gregorio's recent review of 52 children with AIH [4••], patients with anti–liver and kidney microsomal antibody (LKM-1) had a median age at diagnosis of 7.4 years (range 0.8 to 14.2 years), whereas children with positive ANA, SMA, or both had a median age at diagnosis of 10.5 years (range 2.3 to 14.9 years).

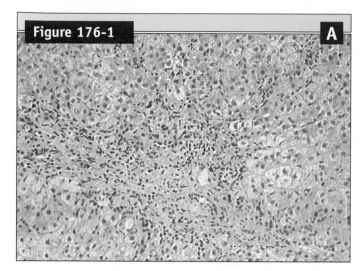

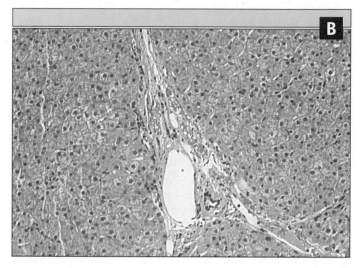

A, Classic histology of autoimmune hepatitis in a 5-year-old child presenting with elevated aminotransferases and anti-LKM antibodies. Note the mononuclear cell infiltrate in the portal triad and invading into the hepatocyte boundary of the adjacent lobule. **B,** Same patient as in *panel A* after 1 year of corticosteroid therapy. Note the resolution of the inflammation of the portal tract and healthy appearing hepatocytes at the edge of the lobule.

In Gregorio's study [4••] and in previous studies [6•,7], SMA- or ANA-positive patients make up approximately two thirds of the study population and LKM-1–positive patients make up the remaining third.

There appears to be a higher incidence of presentation with severe or fulminant liver disease among younger patients, especially with LKM-1–positive disease, whereas persons who present in later childhood or the teenage years tend to have a more chronic indolent course.

PATHOGENESIS

The current conceptual framework for the pathogenesis of the disease in children, as in adults, hypothesizes that several factors are responsible for the initiation of AIH (see Chapter 97). Environmental agents may initiate a process that leads to immunologic changes, resulting in the activation of cytotoxic T-cells as mediators of hepatic injury [2]. There is only minimal evidence implicating viral infection as a trigger mechanism.

There are considerable data supporting the role of genetic factors in the predisposition of patients to AIH. As in other autoimmune diseases, there are primary associations with major histocompatibility complexes on chromosome 6—namely, the A1, B8, and DR3 haplotypes [8•]. ANA- or SMA-positive children may have an increased frequency of the HLA haplotype A1/B8/DR3/DR52a compared with healthy controls (53% vs 14%) [4••]. This haplotype also is prevalent in pediatric patients with primary sclerosing cholangitis [5,8•].

PATHOLOGY

The characteristic histologic features of AIH in children are similar to those in adults (see Chapter 97). There is a portal mononuclear cell infiltrate that invades the hepatocyte boundary surrounding the portal triad and the surrounding lobule (Fig. 176-1) [1]. The histologic picture of AIH may vary, from minimal change to severe disruption of the hepatic architecture with widespread necrosis. In all but the mildest cases fibrosis is present at initial diagnosis.

In Gregorio's study [4••], 23% of the children had multinucleated giant hepatocytes at presentation (Fig. 176-2). Although the presence of giant cells previously had been reported to be associated with a poor prognosis, most of the patients in this study had a course similar to those without giant cells.

In previous studies of children, regardless of the type of AIH, initial liver biopsies on presentation revealed the presence of bridging hepatic fibrosis in 16 of 21 patients (80%) [7] and cirrhosis in 2 of 21 patients (10%) [6•]. In Gregorio's study [4••], which included a larger number of patients, 69% of ANA- or SMA-positive and 38% of LKM-1–positive patients were cirrhotic at presentation.

CLINICAL PRESENTATION

The clinical features of AIH in children are heterogeneous. The spectrum of clinical disease ranges from absence of symptoms (in which disease is discovered by elevated serum aminotransferases on routine screening) to severe acute hepatitis and even liver failure [9] or hematemeis from bleeding esophageal varices [4••,6•,7,10]. Hepatomegaly and splenomegaly are the most common abnormal physical findings [4••,6•,7]. Patients often present with the insidious onset of malaise, anorexia, and fatigue. Associated menstrual abnormalities (*eg*, oligomenorrhea) are common. A teenaged girl presenting with amenorrhea, with or without delayed development of sexual maturity, should be screened with autoantibodies and serum gamma globulin levels if serum aminotransferases are elevated. In many cases, these girls have other disorders of immune regulation, including Sjögren's syndrome, inflammatory bowel disease, arthritis, or autoimmune hemolytic anemia [7,11].

In general, elevations of serum aminotransferases are more striking than the elevations of bilirubin, γ glutamyl transferase, or alkaline phosphatase, although AIH occasionally can present with cholestasis. AIH sometimes is characterized by a presentation very similar to that of severe viral hepatitis. In Gregorio's series, 56% of the children presented with hepatic symptoms of acute onset indistinguishable clinically from the symptoms of

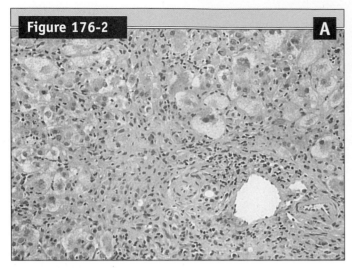
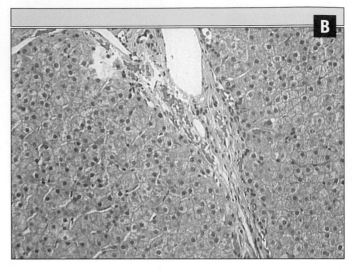

A, Multinucleated giant hepatocytes and portal inflammation in a 3-year-old child with elevated aminotransferases, antinuclear antibodies, and anti-smooth muscle antibodies. **B,** Same patient

after 1 year of corticosteroid therapy. The therapeutic response is demonstrated by resolution of the inflammation.

acute viral hepatitis, but with histologic evidence of chronic liver disease. Therefore, liver biopsy is an important part of the initial diagnostic assessment in any child suspected of having AIH.

DIAGNOSIS

As in adults, the diagnosis of AIH in children initially is a diagnosis of exclusion (Fig. 176-3). It is crucial first to exclude exposure to hepatotoxic drugs (*eg*, nitrofurantoin, isoniazid), the most common infections (particularly viral infections), and Wilson's disease (especially if hemolytic anemia is present), which may be fatal if left untreated.

The essential laboratory work-up begins with screening for hepatic synthetic dysfunction with a prothrombin time, partial thromboplastin time, serum glucose, albumin, and total protein level. If the serum globulins are elevated, serum immunoglobulin fractionation is indicated. If the IgG fraction is increased, the differential diagnosis is narrowed to AIH, HIV, and sclerosing cholangitis. Initial serologic screening for hepatitis A, B (D if patient is hepatitis B–positive), and C, Epstein-Barr virus (EBV), cytomegalovirus (CMV), and metabolic diseases such as Wilson's disease and α_1-antitrypsin deficiency also are a priority. The erythrocyte sedimentation rate (ESR) is used as a general marker for inflammation in AIH. The ESR usually is elevated at presentation in AIH and may be used as another index of inflammatory activity. If AIH is suspected, the autoantibody panel should include ANA, SMA, and anti–LKM-1 antibodies. Liver biopsy is indicated in all stable patients without coagulopathy, because the histopathology of the liver is crucial in determining the severity of the disease [11]. The pathologic features of unresolving moderate to severe chronic hepatitis discovered on liver biopsy coupled with the finding of hyperglobulinemia and autoantibodies are highly consistent with the diagnosis of AIH. The coexistence of another autoimmune disorder (*eg*, autoimmune thyroiditis, ulcerative colitis, hemolytic anemia, celiac disease, myasthenia gravis, or mixed connective tissue disorders) in these patients also supports the diagnosis.

Patients in whom AIH is the likely diagnosis who present with a coagulopathy and are unable to undergo liver biopsy safely should be treated for the coagulopathy, with a percutaneous liver biopsy performed when the coagulation studies have returned to normal. Transjugular or open liver biopsy is another option. Children may present with the classic picture of AIH but lack the definitive antibodies at the time of presentation. Several of Gregorio's patients had low or absent markers at presentation; in all such cases, the diagnosis was confirmed by a high titer of antibodies to liver specific lipoprotein (anti-LSP), histologic findings, and a prompt response to immunosuppressive therapy. Anti-LSP antibodies have been shown to react with a macromolecular antigen complex on the hepatocyte cell membrane and are present in high concentrations in patients with AIH [8•]. Testing for liver-specific lipoprotein (present in 75% of Gregorio's patients) may be recommended in patients without typical markers. These patients should have repeated testing for the other markers (*eg*, ANA, SMA, LKM-1) at several-month intervals.

Total reliance on autoantibodies (ANA, SMA and LKM-1) to make a diagnosis can be confusing. A child who presents with what appears to be SMA-positive AIH may develop a histopathologic picture more compatible with primary sclerosing cholangitis (PSC). If the child has evidence of colitis or elevated titers of perinuclear anti-neutrophil cytoplasmic antibody (p-ANCA), it is recommended that a cholangiogram be performed at presentation, by endoscopic retrograde cholangiography (ERC) or percutaneous transhepatic cholangiography (PTC), to distinguish PSC from AIH. This study also should be considered in any child who appears to have AIH but does not respond typically to treatment with corticosteroids (*ie*, does not show marked improvement in clinical and biochemical status within 2 to 3 months). PSC may mimic AIH, but usually it does not show the same dramatic response to corticosteroids. Serum aminotransferases often diminish with steroid treatment, but usually not to normal levels.

■ TREATMENT

Immunosuppressive therapy should be instituted as soon as possible. Children with mild histologic changes need not be treated immediately. However, the clinical and histologic evidence of disease must be monitored carefully. Patients with AIH rarely enter remission spontaneously. Despite the spectrum of disease severity, AIH usually is responsive to immunosuppressive therapy. The remission rate induced by initial immunosuppression is approximately 80% in adults and 85% to 90% in children [4••,6•,7,10].

Strategies for weaning from steroids include 1) decreasing the daily dose; 2) changing immediately to alternate-day therapy and then weaning; or 3) decreasing to a specific daily dose (eg, 1 mg/kg/d) and then converting to alternate-day dosing. Comparison of the different methods and outcomes reveals that as long as the weekly interval decrease in medication is not greater than 10 mg/d and the child is closely monitored for clin-

ical and biochemical changes with each weaning, no method is superior to any other.

Clinical remission has been observed in most children within 2 to 6 months after therapy is instituted [4••,6•,7]. Patients usually also have resolution of other manifestations of their disease (eg, resumption of menstruation, clearance of ascites, improvement of arthritis, and resolution of thyroiditis). There is no correlation between the duration of symptoms before clinical response and the rate of clinical response to therapy [7].

Gregorio reported that 41 of 44 patients, regardless of markers, went into remission after treatment with either prednisolone alone (6 of 44) or prednisolone in combination with azathioprine (35 of 44). Remission was defined as the absence of clinical symptoms and a normal AST (<50 IU/L) on at least two occasions at least 1 month apart. A relapse was defined as at least a two-fold increase in the AST (>100 IU/L) with or without recurrence of symptoms. At relapse, the initial dose of

Figure 176-3

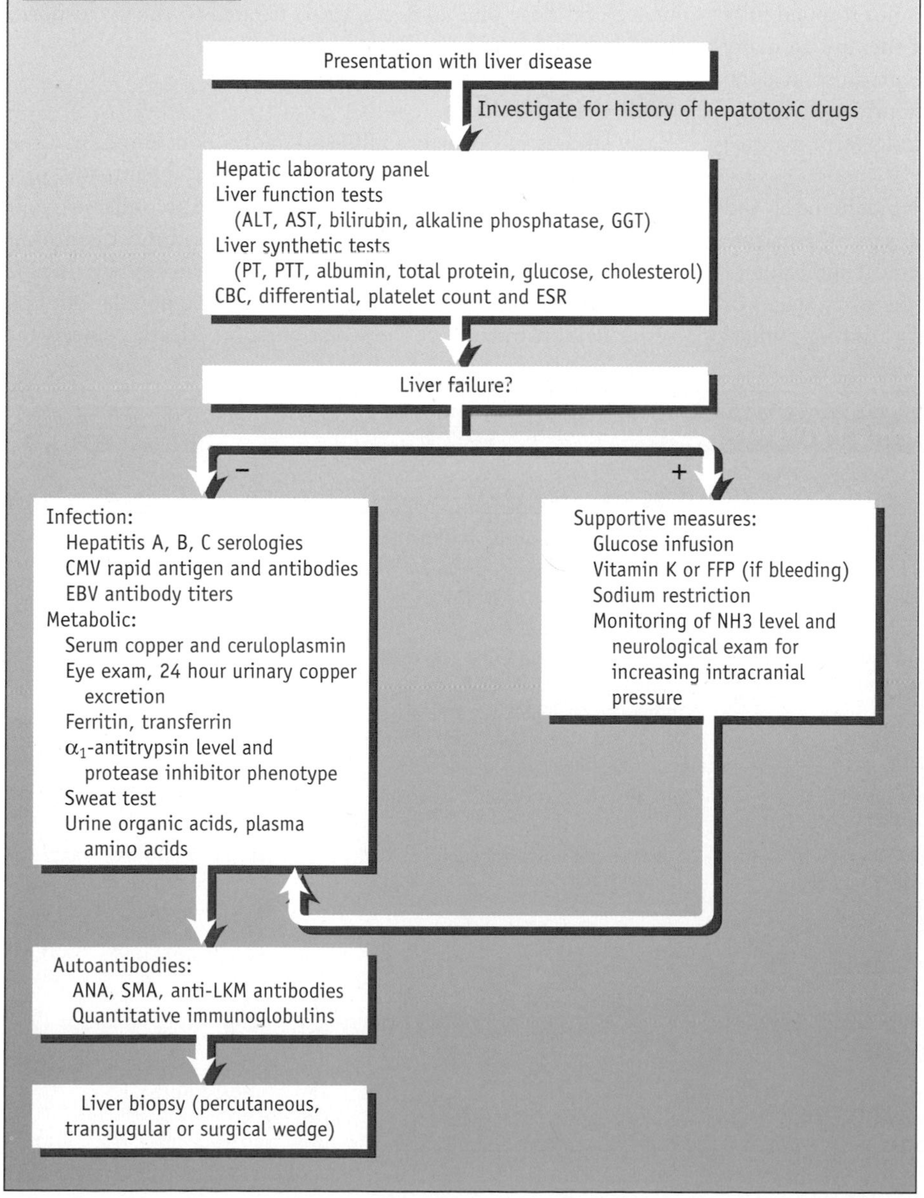

Approach to diagnosis.

prednisolone was restarted and then tapered according to the patient's response. Discontinuation of immunosuppression was considered when patients had normal aminotransferases at 3-month intervals for at least 1 year and absence of necro-inflammatory activity on liver biopsy performed just before withdrawal of therapy.

Three retrospective studies regarding therapy for AIH in children provide guidelines for the management of immunosuppression (Table 176-1). These demonstrate several strategies for the weaning of immunosuppressive medications once remission is achieved.

Patients initially are treated with prednisone (or prednisolone) with a dosage of 2 mg/kg/d to a maximum of 60 mg/d. This daily corticosteroid dose is tapered every 2 to 4 weeks by 5 to 10 mg, depending on the normalization of the serum aminotransferases and resolution of clinical symptoms. If the child is unable to tolerate the corticosteroids because of side effects (*eg*, hypertension, cataracts, or diabetes mellitus), azathioprine, 1 to 2 mg/kg/d, may be added as a steroid-sparing agent. Azathioprine also may be added if the child is unable to be weaned off the steroids, or if he or she does not respond fully to the corticosteroids after 10 to 12 weeks of therapy. In many patients, maintenance therapy with low-dose prednisone alone (5 to 15 mg/d) or in combination with azathioprine (50 to 150 mg) is successful. Some patients do well on long-term maintenance therapy with azathioprine alone.

Histologic improvement may lag behind biochemical and clinical remission. Arasu has reported that serum aspartate aminotransferase levels are a reliable biochemical indicator of disease activity in children, not only during the early stages of the disease and during exacerbations, but also during clinical

and biochemical remission as confirmed by simultaneous liver biopsies [7]. In adults, mild histologic activity or a decrease in inflammation with therapy is not predictive of long-term remission once treatment has been discontinued. In children, likewise, histologic remission manifested by resolution of interface hepatocyte necrosis (*ie*, at the "limiting plate") and decrease in portal inflammatory cells is encouraging but not predictive [13].

In most patients, immunosuppression must be continued long-term. Gregorio was able to stop treatment within 5 years in only 19% of the ANA- or SMA-positive patients and in none of the LKM-positive patients. Despite a positive response to therapy for many years, severe hepatic decompensation may develop, even after years of good control, as evidenced by four patients who required liver transplantation 8 to 14 years after diagnosis in Gregorio's series.

There have been no studies in children using immunosuppressive medications, other than corticosteroids, as a single-line initial treatment option for AIH. If treatment with prednisone and azathioprine does not induce remission, a trial of cyclosporine (1 to 2 mg/kg/d intravenously and then a maintenance oral dose of 2 to 4 mg/kg/d) titrated to the cyclosporin level in blood may be indicated [4••,12].

▄ PROGNOSIS

Early studies of AIH in adults and adolescents emphasize the serious, invariably fatal, nature of the disease. Death was primarily a consequence of hepatocellular failure secondary to cirrhosis, and variceal hemorrhage was the second most common cause [2]. Gregorio has described five statistically significant predictors for outcome of AIH in the pediatric population. His series demonstrates that the worst outcome (death or need for

Table 176-1. Treatment of Autoimmune Hepatitis in Children

	Arasu, 1979 (*n*=26)	Maggiore, 1984 (*n*=17)	Gregorio, 1997 (*n*=52)
Initial therapy	Prednisone, 2 mg/kg/d	Prednisone, 2 mg/kg/d; azathioprine 1.5–2 mg/kg/d	Prednisolone, 2 mg/kg/d
Criteria for weaning from immunosuppression	If AST < 100 IU/L, no clinical symptoms	If AST normalized; no clinical symptoms	If AST < 50 IU/L x 2, 1 mo apart and absence of clinical symptoms
Weaning protocol	Prednisone changed to every other day dosing, then weaned by 5 mg every 4 to 5 weeks	Prednisone decreased to 1 mg/kg/d daily initially and then to every other day or prednisone to every other day, then wean; azathioprine continued daily at same dose	Decrease prednisone by 5–10 mg every 2 wk
Relapse criteria	Clinical symptoms or AST > 100 IU/L	Clinical symptoms or AST > normal	Clinical symptoms or AST > 100 IU/L
If initial Rx not successful	Clinical symptoms or AST > 100 IU/L after 12 weeks or if frequent relapses, Azathioprine was added	If relapse, initial steroid dose restarted	If increase in AST with steroid weans or need to reduce steroids secondary to adverse side effects, then started azathioprine at 1–2 mg/kg/d
Outcome			
Mortality	0/26 (0%)	2/17 (11%)	6/52 (11%)
Time to achieve biochemical remission	3–9 mo	1–2 mo	Median 7 mo
Weaned off medication	19/26 (73%)	1/17 (14%)	ANA/SMA 6/32 (19%) LKM-1 0/20 (0%)

Data from [4••,6•,7].

transplantation) is associated with the following features at presentation: young age; prolonged prothrombin time; presence of anti–LKM-1 antibodies; higher total serum bilirubin levels; and a higher histologic activity index score at diagnosis [4••]. He confirmed that LKM-1 antibody–positive patients presented more commonly with acute liver failure and that none of the acute liver failure patients responded to conventional immunosuppression. When patients presenting in fulminant hepatic failure were excluded, ANA- or SMA-positive and LKM-1–positive AIH in children were equally serious conditions with similar long-term disease severity and outcome [4••].

■ REFERENCES

Recently published papers of particular interest have been highlighted as follows:
• Of interest
•• Of outstanding interest

1. Krawitt EL, Wiesner R: *Autoimmune Liver Disease.* New York: Raven Press; 1991:21–42.

2. Maddrey WC: Chronic hepatitis. *Dis Mon* Feb 1993, 57–125.

3. Duclos-Vallee JC, Hajouri O, Yamamoto A, *et al.*: Conformational epitopes on CYP2D6 are recognized by liver/kidney microsomal antibodies. *Gastroenterology* 1995, 108:470–476.

4.•• Gregorio GV, Portmann B, Reid F, *et al.*: Autoimmune hepatitis in childhood: a 20-year experience. *Hepatology* 1997, 25:541–547.
This is an extensive review from London of the pediatric experience with types I and II autoimmune hepatitis. It represents the largest pediatric series, with very complete information.

5. Johnson PJ, McFarlane IG, Eddleston AL: The natural course and heterogeneity of autoimmune-type chronic active hepatitis. *Semin Liver Dis* 1991, 11:187–194.

6.• Maggiore G, Bernard O, Hadchouel M, *et al.*: Treatment of autoimmune chronic active hepatitis in childhood. *J Pediatr* 1984, 4:839–843.
This report provided the most comprehensive series in pediatric AIH until the Gregorio article was published in 1997.

7. Arasu T, Wyllie R, Hatch T, Fitzgerald J: Management of chronic aggressive hepatitis in children and adolescents. *Pediatr* 1979, 95:514–522.

8.• Mieli-Vergani G, Vergani D: Progress in pediatric autoimmune hepatitis. *Semin Liver Dis* 1994, 14:282–287.
This paper provides a clear summary of the present knowledge of pediatric AIH.

9. Maggiore G, Porta G, Bernard O, *et al.*: Autoimmune hepatitis with presentation as acute hepatic failure in young children. *J Pediatr* 1990, 116:280–282.

10. Maggiore G, Veber F, Hadchouel M, *et al.*: Autoimmune hepatitis associated with anti-actin antibodies in children and adolescents. *J Pediatr Gastroenterol Nutr* 1993, 17:376–381.

11. Krawitt EL: Autoimmune hepatitis. *N Engl J Med* 1996, 334:897–902.

12. Hyams J, Ballow M, Leichtner A: Cyclosporine treatment of autoimmune chronic active hepatitis. *Gastroenterology* 1987, 93:890–893.

13. Vajro P, Hadchouel P, Hadchouel M, *et al.*: Incidence of cirrhosis in children with chronic hepatitis. *J Pediatr* 1990, 117:392–395.

177 Toxic Hepatitis
Parvathi Mohan

There is a lower incidence of hepatotoxicity from drugs in children than in adults, for the following reasons: 1) children are given far fewer medications such as anti-hypertensives, cardiac medications, and antidepressants; 2) children have fewer predisposing factors to drug interactions such as the use of alcohol or cigarettes [1••]; 3) children metabolize most drugs more rapidly than adolescents and adults; 4) the dosage of drugs for children is calculated per unit of body weight, whereas a set, standard dose is prescribed for adults, regardless of body weight; and 5) haphazard use of medications is less common in children because of parental supervision.

■ FACTORS PREDISPOSING TO DRUG HEPATOTOXICITY IN INFANTS AND CHILDREN

A variety of factors predispose infants and children to drug hepatotoxicity. Among them are the following:

The preterm newborn infant is uniquely susceptible to toxicity from relatively innocuous medications because of developmental immaturity of drug detoxifying or metabolizing systems [1••]. Compounding risk factors include hypoglycemia, sepsis, hyperbilirubinemia, and starvation in the sick newborn.

Children under the age of 5 years are particularly prone to accidental overdoses of drugs because they are inquisitive. They often are lured to noxious agents by color, shape, or taste. This is true for commonly used, relatively benign, over-the-counter (OTC) household medications such as acetaminophen, as well as prescription drugs.

Nonaccidental administration of drugs as a manifestation of child abuse should be considered in children at risk.

Children, like adults, who are afflicted with chronic illnesses such as cancer and AIDS, may have to be treated for prolonged periods with potentially toxic drugs. They are susceptible to serious liver injury if the drugs are not administered judiciously or their effects are not carefully monitored.

As with adults, it is difficult to identify in advance children who respond idiosyncratically to a relatively benign drug in advance. Their reactions to the drug are difficult to predict because of the nonspecificity of the symptoms, which often mimic infection or metabolic disease.

Intentional abuse of drugs by young adults with suicidal or manipulative intent is becoming more common.

The mechanisms and spectra of drug-induced toxic hepatitis are discussed in Chapter 96.

HEPATOTOXICITY OF DRUGS COMMONLY USED IN PEDIATRICS
Analgesics

Acetaminophen is the drug most often involved in drug overdoses in children under the age of 10 years. In a recent review of 73 medical records of children 10 years of age or younger with acetaminophen overdose, 28 children (39%) had severe hepatotoxicity, and six of the 28 children required liver transplantation [2•]. Delay in referral and concomitant use of other medications such as barbiturates and antituberculous drugs, associated viral or metabolic disease, and fasting contribute to the drug's toxicity.

Clinical features. Symptoms are often delayed if supratherapeutic doses are given at regular intervals rather than a single toxic dose (>150 mg/kg). If the child recovers, the clinical progression can be divided into four stages (Table 177-1).

Mechanism of injury. When an overdose of acetaminophen is taken, the sulfation and glucuronidation pathways for the usual metabolism of the drug are overwhelmed, increased oxidation by cytochrome 450 occurs, glutathione becomes depleted, and toxic metabolites, primarily N-acetyl-p-benzoquinonimine, accumulate, causing hepatocellular injury. Synergistic drug interactions have been reported from the concomitant use of enzyme inducers of the cytochrome P-450 system, such as isoniazid (INH) and phenobarbital. Administration of zidovudine with acetaminophen also may lead to hepatotoxicity.

Prevention. Acetaminophen overdose can be avoided by adherence to the following guidelines: 1) strict attention to recommended dosage based on weight; 2) recognition of the different concentrations of acetaminophen in various preparations of the medication, *ie*, drops versus syrup; 3) awareness of the cumulative dosage; 4) consideration of possible drug interactions between acetaminophen and other drugs; and 5) avoidance of overzealous attempts to decrease fever in children with self-limited illnesses [3].

Treatment. Treatment of acetaminophen overdose with N-acetylcysteine (NAC) based on the Rumack-Matthew nomogram [4] (Fig. 177-1) has significantly reduced morbidity and mortality. The nomogram predicts the potential for hepatotoxicity based on the plasma acetaminophen level measured 4 to 24 hours after ingestion. A level >300 µg/mL 4 hours and >50 µg/mL 12 hours postingestion suggests possible hepatotoxicity. Although the most favorable results are obtained when NAC is given within 10 hours after ingestion, subsequent administration of NAC also may be beneficial. Even if plasma acetaminophen levels cannot be obtained in the first 4 to 8 hours after a suspected ingestion, administration of NAC within 8 hours after ingestion of a suspected toxic dose (>150 mg/kg) is recommended, especially in the presence of the risk

Table 177-1. Clinical Progression of Acute Acetaminophen Toxicity

Stages	Clinical presentation
Stage 1	First 24 h
	Nausea, vomiting, diaphoresis, malaise
	Mean onset 6 h; complete by 14 h
	Normal liver tests*
Stage 2	Day 2
	Improvement of symptoms
	Onset of abnormal tests
	Occasional right upper quadrant pain
Stage 3	Day 3 and 4
	Overt liver failure
	Vomiting, hypoglycemia, bleeding, encephalopathy
	Hepatic tenderness, jaundice
	Transaminases > 20,000 IU/L†
	Acute renal failure, coagulopathy, shock, pancreatitis
Stage 4	Day 7 and 8
	Resolution of symptoms
	Decrease in transaminase levels
	No residual liver damage or fibrosis

If abnormal, consider other causes such as other ingestants or illnesses.

† Elevation of AST > 1000 U/L considered as pathognomonic of acetaminophen hepatotoxicity.

factors previously mentioned. Liver transplantation is the treatment of choice for irreversible fulminant hepatic failure.

Anti-Inflammatory Drugs: Acetylsalicylic Acid

Use of salicylates as analgesics or antipyretics is severely restricted in pediatric practice because salicylate may be an etiologic factor in Reye's syndrome [5]. However, acetylsalicylic acid (ASA; aspirin) remains the drug of choice for acute rheumatic fever and rheumatoid arthritis.

Clinical features. ASA toxicity may present with nonspecific features, including anorexia, nausea, vomiting, and right upper quadrant abdominal pain. Elevation of the serum transaminases (3 to 30 times the normal value) is common, whereas hyperbilirubinemia and coagulopathy are rare. Significant hyperammonemia has been described [6]. Hepatomegaly and encephalopathy distinct from Reye's syndrome are unusual [1••].

Mechanism of injury. Toxicity is primarily dose-related. Increased serum transaminase levels have been reported in 70% of children treated with high dosages of aspirin for rheumatic fever or rheumatoid arthritis [6]. Symptoms and biochemical abnormalities resolve with discontinuation of the drug. There is evidence that mitochondrial dysfunction from aspirin and viral agents, particularly varicella and influenza, plays a significant role in the pathogenesis of Reye's syndrome [5].

Prevention. In children with rheumatic fever, Hamdan *et al.* [7] have recommended reducing the dose of ASA from 100 mg/kg/d to 80 mg/kg/d if over 25 kg in weight. Maintaining ASA levels between 15 and 25 mg/dL may reduce the incidence of aspirin-related hepatotoxicity. Aspirin is contraindicated in the management of children with varicella and influenza and should be avoided in the treatment of any viral infections in infants and young children.

Antibiotics

Most courses of treatment with antibiotics in pediatrics are brief, lasting for only 7 to 14 days, and dose-related hepatic dysfunction is rare. However, drugs causing idiosyncratic hypersensitivity reactions, or those used for prolonged periods, as in patients with HIV-related infections, do have the potential for causing hepatotoxicity. Some of the antibiotics frequently used in pediatrics that may be associated with liver toxicity include erythromycin, sulfamethoxazole-trimethoprim, and amoxicillin-clavulanic acid.

Erythromycin is commonly used in children for the treatment of upper respiratory infections and *Mycoplasma pneumoniae*. It is an alternative drug for patients with known or suspected penicillin hypersensitivity. Hepatotoxicity associated with all forms of erythromycin is rare, and erythromycin-related cholestasis occurs in only about 3.6 per 100,000 users [8].

Clinical features. The clinical presentation of cholestatic liver injury may simulate extrahepatic bile duct obstruction and includes nausea, anorexia, jaundice, abdominal pain, and, less commonly, pruritus and hepatosplenomegaly. The hepatotoxic effects are mild and usually are self-limited once erythromycin is discontinued.

Mechanism of injury. The mechanism of injury is attributed to induction of the cytochrome P-450 system through which the drug is metabolized, or from production of a toxic metabolite. There is experimental evidence that erythromycin may adversely affect bile

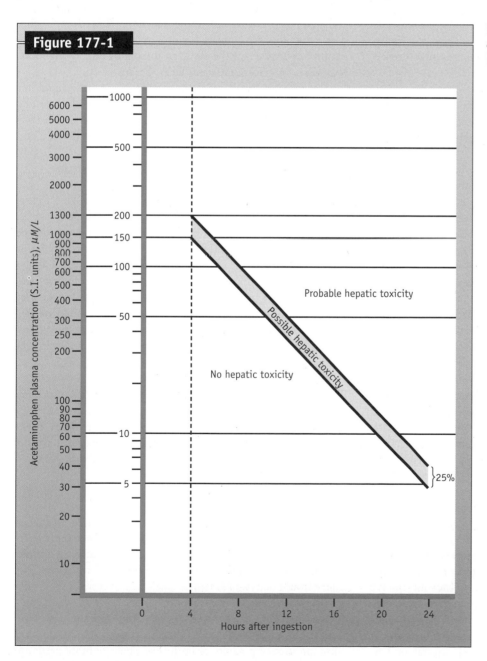

Figure 177-1

Rumack-Matthew nomogram for acetaminophen poisoning. (*From* Rumack [4]; with permission.)

flow, thereby leading to cholestasis. Progressive destruction of intrahepatic bile ducts (ductopenia) also has been described [9].

Prevention. Hepatotoxicity is idiosyncratic and, therefore, not preventable. But avoidance of the drug due to prior history of drug reaction and early withdrawal of the drug at the onset of toxic symptoms are recommended [9].

Sulfonamide
Sulfonamide preparations are used in children to treat otitis media, urinary tract infection, and inflammatory bowel disease.

Clinical presentation. Sulfonamides are well known to produce a cholestatic or hepatitic type of liver toxicity, leading infrequently to fulminant hepatic failure. The common clinical presentation is that of a hypersensitivity reaction, with fever, rash, atypical lymphocytosis, renal involvement, and lymphadenopathy [1••].

Mechanism of injury. Idiosyncratic reactions, specifically hypersensitivity, to sulfonamides lead to hepatotoxicity. Aberrant production of electrophilic metabolites may predispose certain individuals to these reactions [9].

Prevention. Hepatotoxicity is idiosyncratic and not preventable. Frequent monitoring for clinical and biochemical abnormalities may help the clinician to withdraw the drug appropriately.

Antiepileptic Drugs
Mentally handicapped children who present with seizures from birth asphyxia, metabolic diseases, or head injury often are treated with one or more antiepileptic drugs (AED) for prolonged periods of time. Biochemical abnormalities (*eg*, increased alanine aminotransferase [ALT] or aspartate aminotransferase [AST]) are common. Most AEDs cause isolated elevations of the serum transaminases or γ-glutamyltransferase by hepatic microsomal enzyme induction rather than by hepatic injury [10]. Valproic acid (VPA), phenytoin, phenobarbital, and carbamazepine also have the potential to result in significant liver damage.

Valproate
Valproic acid is commonly used, either alone or in combination, for the treatment of simple and complex seizures in children. Isolated serum transaminase elevation occurs in up to 44% of patients with an average of 11% [11]. Young children with developmental delay, especially those on polytherapy, are particularly susceptible to valproate-related fatal hepatotoxicity [12].

Clinical features. Onset of symptoms is typically within the first 6 months after initiation of therapy [13•]. The usual symptoms are lethargy, vomiting, anorexia, unexplained sudden increase in seizure frequency, and occurrence of status epilepticus. Fever is commonly a heralding symptom, but it is often underrated and mistaken for a viral infection. Increases in the serum transaminases (moderate or severe), jaundice, hyperammonemia, coagulopathy, and coma follow; death ensues unless liver transplantation is performed. Hyperammonemia or decreased serum carnitine levels, or both [14], are unique features of VPA toxicity, even in the absence of other biochemical markers of toxicity. Regular monitoring of liver function is recommended for prevention of toxic reactions, particularly in the first 6 months of therapy.

Mechanism of injury. A combination of direct dose-related and idiosyncratic reactions accounts for the variable presentations of VPA hepatotoxicity. The reversible, dose-related toxicity, mostly asymptomatic, appears shortly after the start of therapy and resolves with reduction or withdrawal of the drug.

Fatal reactions are idiosyncratic and non–dose-dependent. They occur more often in young patients, especially those under 2 years of age with underlying metabolic or developmental abnormalities augmented by multiple drug therapy. A reversal from severe liver toxicity has recently been reported in a subset of patients [13•].

Several metabolic abnormalities may be exacerbated by VPA toxicity, including urea cycle enzyme defects, α_1-antitrypsin deficiency, and primary carnitine deficiency. Therefore, in children with idiopathic mental motor retardation, it is of paramount importance for the clinician to exclude underlying metabolic diseases before initiating VPA therapy.

The primary target of VPA toxicity is the mitochondrion. Hepatotoxicity is postulated to be the result of production of a metabolite (4-ene-VPA), which inhibits β-oxidation and leads to a reduction of free coenzyme-A and carnitine [1••]. These changes, in turn, interfere with the transmitochondrial transport of carnitine conjugates of VPA and their urinary excretion.

Prevention. Because of the sudden, unpredictable onset of hepatotoxicity, awareness of clinical symptoms that suggest adverse drug reaction is most valuable in the early detection and prevention of VPA toxicity. The presence of fever may be an early warning, even when laboratory values are normal. Clinical symptoms, accompanied by an abnormal thrombin time, increased serum transaminase concentrations, and an increased serum ammonia level, are clear indications for immediate discontinuation of the drug [13•]. Discontinuation at the earliest indication of abnormal liver function reduces morbidity as well as mortality.

Treatment. L-carnitine has been recommended (100 mg/kg/d) because it may reverse certain metabolic aberrations caused by VPA [13•]. Unfortunately, consistent, clinically relevant, beneficial effects from routine carnitine supplementation have not been demonstrated in patients at high or low risk for VPA toxicity [14].

Phenytoin
Phenytoin sodium is associated with a wide range of adverse reactions, including fulminant hepatic failure. The incidence of toxicity varies from 0.01% to 0.1% [11]. Simultaneous administration of phenobarbital increases the potential for severe liver injury from phenytoin [1••].

Clinical presentation. Isolated, mild serum transaminase elevations are often encountered. Severe adverse reactions are most common in young adults of both sexes, but are more predominant among blacks. The onset of toxicity occurs primarily in the first 6 weeks of therapy. Common dose-related side effects include vomiting, anorexia, behavioral changes, drowsiness, and ataxia. The less common, idiosyncratic reaction presents with a rash, fever, lymphadenopathy, and eosinophilia, followed by moderate jaundice and elevation of the serum transaminase levels [1••]. Synthetic liver function abnormalities herald hepatic failure. The clinical picture often is confused with infections, malignancy, or collagen vascular disease. Even after the drug has been discontinued, recovery is usually prolonged, taking as long as 6 to 12 months.

Mechanism of injury. Cell-mediated hypersensitivity, production of toxic metabolites, and stimulation of the cytochrome P-450 enzyme system all contribute to toxicity [11].

Prevention and treatment. Early identification of adverse reactions is the key to prevention of hepatic failure. If possible, phenobarbital should not be prescribed in combination with phenytoin. Treatment of hepatotoxicity with high doses of corticosteroids has not shown convincing benefits [1••].

Carbamazepine
Carbamazepine hepatotoxicity is rare, but a hepatitis similar to that seen in phenytoin hypersensitivity, a mononucleosis type of presentation, and progressive liver failure have been reported in children on carbamazepine [1••].

Hepatotoxicity from phenobarbital is rare; it may present with jaundice and coagulopathy about 2 months after the start of therapy [1••].

Immunosuppressives and Antimetabolites
Patients receiving treatment for neoplasia, particularly with multiple medications, often present with asymptomatic elevation of liver enzymes. The common offending agents are azathioprine/6-mercaptopurine, methotrexate (MTX), cytosine arabinoside, and cisplatin, and, less frequently, doxorubicin and vincristine. The synergistic action of multiple drugs, *eg*, methotrexate and cisplatin, or doxorubicin and 6-mercaptopurine (6MP), may accentuate hepatotoxicity [15].

A unique type of hepatic involvement with hepatomegaly, ascites and jaundice, heralding the onset of veno-occlusive disease, is associated with azathioprine, thioguanine, busulfan, and cytosine arabinoside [1••].

Mercaptopurine and Azathioprine
Azathioprine and its metabolite 6MP are used extensively in children to treat malignancies, connective tissue disorders, inflammatory bowel disease, and autoimmune hepatitis, and to prevent transplantation rejection. Both medications, especially 6MP, are associated with hepatotoxicity, and chronic usage may lead to fibrosis and even cirrhosis [15,16].

Clinical features. Asymptomatic serum transaminase elevations are common during long-term treatment with both 6MP and azathioprine. Biochemical liver abnormalities usually resolve within 3 months after cessation of therapy, but on occasion, may last for several months.

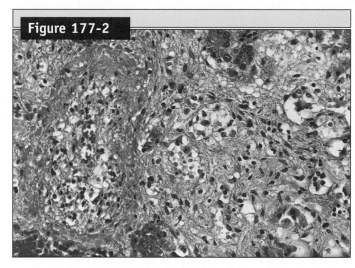

Figure 177-2

Photomicrograph showing obliteration of a vein with fibrointimal cells in veno-occlusive disease. Surrounding hepatocytes show cell drop-out, cholestasis, and early fibrosis. (*Courtesy of* R. Chandra.) See also **Color Plate**.

Acute toxicity of azathioprine may mimic the worsening of an underlying disease by an intercurrent illness or acute rejection in a posttransplant patient [17]. The onset of symptoms may vary from 2 weeks to 33 months [18]. Hepatocellular injury presents with moderate serum transaminase and alkaline phosphatase elevations.

Veno-occlusive disease (VOD) from azathioprine presents with acute hepatomegaly, jaundice, and features of portal hypertension [19] (Fig. 177-2, see also **Color Plate**). Jaundice in a posttransplant patient is confusing because of the difficulty in differentiating among its multiple etiologies—rejection, vascular or biliary complications, and infection.

Mechanism of injury. Azathioprine-induced hypersensitivity reactions can cause hepatotoxicity with involvement of other systems, *eg*, nephritis [17]. It has been suggested that hepatic involvement may be more pronounced in those who convert azathioprine to 6MP rapidly as part of an idiosyncratic metabolic reaction. Hepatic vascular and sinusoidal endothelial cell injury have been proposed as the major cause of the development of VOD [19]. A dose-related hepatotoxicity also is suggested in patients on long-term therapy with azathioprine or mercaptopurine [18].

Prevention and treatment. A prompt reduction in the dose, but not necessarily discontinuation of the medication, has been shown to reverse the abnormalities in liver function unless there is hypersensitivity, which may be life-threatening [18]. VOD may be a specific indication to discontinue the medication.

Methotrexate
Methotrexate, a folic acid analogue, is used extensively in various chemotherapy regimens, not only for treatment of cancer but also as a steroid-sparing agent in a variety of immune-mediated chronic illnesses such as psoriasis, rheumatoid arthritis, and sarcoidosis [20]. Weekly low oral-dose therapy for 3 months has been reported to be safe in treating sarcoidosis and

rheumatoid arthritis in children [20,21]. There are several reports of hepatotoxicity from low-dose MTX used for treatment of leukemia, but some of these liver function abnormalities may have resulted from concomitant viral infections [22].

Clinical features. Acute hepatitis from high doses of MTX, as reflected by a transient increase in the serum transaminase concentrations is reversible and does not result in chronic liver disease [21]. Chronic low doses may lead to mild hepatic dysfunction, but rarely lead to fulminant hepatic failure [22]. Persistent increases in serum transaminase levels and a decreasing serum albumin are indicators of hepatic fibrosis, but the severity of biochemical abnormality does not correlate with that of liver pathology [21].

Mechanism of injury. The toxicity of MTX is dose dependent. The cumulative dose rather than the duration of therapy is more likely to lead to hepatic pathology. Weekly pulse doses also have been associated with mild hepatic fibrosis and steatosis in children. A safe cumulative dose for children has not been determined. Often there are no clinical symptoms of liver involvement and periodic liver biopsies have been recommended to identify and grade the extent of liver disease. The most accepted system for grading MTX-induced abnormalities in liver histology is based on the degree of fatty change, necroinflammation, portal fibrosis, and cirrhosis (grade I–IV) [23].

Prevention. The recent recommendations of the American College of Rheumatology for monitoring MTX hepatotoxicity are geared primarily toward adult patients, but may be extended to children [21]. Unexplained elevations of the AST on five of nine AST estimations or a declining serum albumin level within a given 12-month period of treatment in otherwise well-controlled rheumatoid arthritis are clear indications for a liver biopsy. Reduction and even temporary discontinuation of MTX is advised. Persistence of hepatic biochemical abnormalities and the histologic grading of the liver biopsy should mandate decisions regarding further MTX therapy.

Cyclosporin

Cyclosporin (CYA) is an immunomodulator that is widely used in the management of organ transplantation. Mild hepatotoxicity, including conjugated hyperbilirubinemia, alone or with elevated transaminases, and an increase in serum bile acids have been described. Biliary tract involvement is characterized by gallstone and sludge formation [24]. Toxicity from CYA is rare, and in the posttransplant setting, there are other factors complicating or compromising liver function that are difficult to differentiate from pure CYA-related changes. CYA is metabolized via the cytochrome P-450 pathway, and interactions with several drugs, including phenobarbital, rifampin, and erythromycin, have been reported [1••].

Antituberculous Drugs

Isoniazid, rifampin, and pyrazinamide are associated with hepatotoxicity and a mortality rate ranging from 4% to 12% [25]. Most patients develop toxic symptoms within 1 month of starting therapy. Risk factors for the development of hepatotoxicity from antituberculous drugs (ATT) are malnutrition, hepatitis B

carrier state, hypoalbuminemia, a slow acetylator phenotype, and extensive disease, based on radiologic evidence of lung involvement [26]. Treatment of underlying tuberculosis in the face of ATT-related hepatitis often is a challenge, but reintroduction of the drugs, especially INH and rifampin, in a carefully phased manner is safe.

In children, toxic effects of ATTs are comparatively rare. Injudicious use accounts for the development of toxicity, which is dose-related. The clinical features mimic those of viral hepatitis and increase with age. Other risk factors include the concomitant use of other ATTs, especially rifampin. Children with severe disease, especially tuberculous meningitis, are more susceptible to INH toxicity [1••]. Postpubertal black and Hispanic women are at greater risk than are black men and whites of either gender. Most toxic symptoms occur within the first 2 weeks of therapy, but late-onset toxicity, with a mortality rate of 0.001% to 0.002%, has been reported [27]. The early symptoms of toxicity are often nonspecific, similar to those in viral hepatitis. Discontinuation of the drug after the onset of jaundice may be too late to prevent irreversible damage.

Clinical features. The hepatotoxicity of INH manifests itself in three forms: 1) asymptomatic, transient elevation of serum transaminase concentrations (3% to 13%); 2) reversible clinical hepatitis (0.1% to 7.1%) indistinguishable from viral hepatitis; and rarely, 3) fulminant hepatitis (0.3%) requiring liver transplantation or resulting in fatality [27].

Mechanism of injury. Two types of drug reactions are associated with INH: dose-related and idiosyncratic. Causes may include susceptibility of certain individuals to hepatotoxicity, based on polymorphism for N-acetylation, and generation of high concentrations of toxic metabolites in rapid acetylators. Induction of cytochrome P-450 pathways by drugs such as phenobarbital and rifampin also has been implicated.

Prevention. The guidelines for the safe use of INH in children established by the American Academy of Pediatrics recommend meticulous screening for a history of previous drug reactions or previous liver disease, and careful clinical monitoring for complications [27]. Routine liver function testing is not recommended unless there is clinical evidence of possible complications, *eg*, fatigue, anorexia, nausea, and vomiting. Screening of susceptible populations such as postpubertal black and Hispanic women is recommended even in the absence of symptoms.

Anesthetic Agents

Halothane

Halothane is a comparatively safe, well-tolerated anesthetic, used in children who exhibit hepatotoxicity than in adults [28]. Multiple exposures to halothane appear to be the most important risk factor in children and may lead to a fatal outcome.

Clinical features. The two presentations of halothane hepatitis are 1) a mild increase in the serum transaminase levels in the absence of symptoms, usually occurring within 2 weeks of halothane administration; and 2) a severe fulminant hepatitis leading to liver failure. Fever is a typical feature of toxicity [28].

Table 177-2. Theories Regarding the Mechanisms and Risk Factors Contributing to TPN Liver Injury in Infants and Children		
Complication	**Risk factors**	**TPN effects**
Cholestasis	Immature biliary secretory system	Amino acid excess
	Absence of oral intake	Carbohydrate/nitrogen ratio
	Prolonged duration of TPN	Deficiencies of essential fatty acids
	Hypoxia	Carnitine
	Extensive bowel surgery	Taurine
	Disturbed enterohepatic circulation	L-glutamine
		Lithocholate toxicity
	Small bowel bacterial overgrowth	Impaired drug oxygenation
Gallbladder/bile duct disease	Fasting leads to loss of enteric stimuli, bile stasis in gallbladder, impaired bile flow	Decreased bile flow
		Altered bile composition
	Ileal dysfunction	
	Drugs changing mineral balance in bile; *eg*, diuretics	

Adapted from Quigley et al. [31••]; with permission.

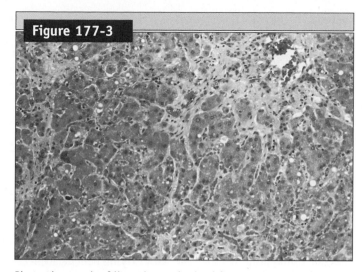

Figure 177-3

Photomicrograph of liver tissue obtained from an autopsy of an infant who died of liver failure from prolonged total parenteral nutrition. Note the perihepatocellular fibrosis, occasional multinucleated cells, and mild steatosis. See also **Color Plate**. (*Courtesy of* R. Chandra.)

Mechanism of injury. Several mechanisms for halothane hepatotoxicity have been postulated, including production of toxic metabolites, hepatic hypoxemia, hypersensitivity reactions, and a genetic predisposition [11].

Vitamins and Minerals

Vitamin A

Retinoids, including isotretinoin and etretinate, currently are used in adolescents for the treatment of cystic acne. Even a relatively low dose, *eg*, 25000 IU/day taken continuously over several years, can lead to toxicity [29]. Lower doses in over-the-counter preparations are not associated with chronic liver damage.

Clinical features. The clinical features are usually those of hepatitis, manifested by asymptomatic serum transaminase elevations and mild anicteric cholestasis; but portal hypertension secondary to chronic liver disease has been described in adults [29].

Mechanism of injury. Vitamin A is a dose-dependent hepatotoxin. The precise mechanism of toxicity is unclear. Ito cell–induced fibrogenesis and production of toxic metabolites secondary to enhanced retinol metabolism induced by cytochrome P-450 activity have been implicated.

Iron

Iron overdose occurs more commonly in children under the age of 5 years who mistake iron tablets for candy [30]. Doses of 20 to 60 mg/kg produce mild liver dysfunction; doses over 60 mg/kg produce severe hepatotoxicity.

Clinical presentation. The clinical presentation is similar to that of acetaminophen overdose. There is an initial phase of gastrointestinal symptoms such as vomiting and hematemesis followed by a quiescent period and, then, overt symptoms of hepatic damage, characterized by jaundice, coagulopathy, and serum transaminase elevations.

Total Parenteral Nutrition

The advent of total parenteral nutrition (TPN), or hyperalimentation, has enabled many infants and children to survive a variety of pathological conditions, such as short bowel syndrome, congenital or acquired malabsorption syndromes, and prematurity, despite failure of enteral nutrition. However, long-term TPN leads to well-recognized hepatic dysfunction, ranging from asymptomatic liver enzyme elevations to significant cholestasis and irreversible hepatocellular failure. TPN-related hepatic injury in infants and adults has been extensively studied and reviewed [31••] (Table 177-2).

Type of injury. In the early stages, mild to moderate centrilobular cholestasis with little steatosis or inflammation is characteristic. As the disease progresses, histologic changes include severe cholestasis, portal inflammation, and periportal fibrosis (Fig. 177-3, see also **Color Plate**). Foci of necrosis and bile duct proliferation may mimic obstructive cholangiopathies such as biliary atresia.

Clinical features. Low-birth-weight premature infants are most commonly affected by the toxicity of TPN. A 50% incidence of cholestasis has been reported in infants who weighed less than 1000 g at birth after 2 weeks of TPN. After 13 weeks of TPN, the incidence increases to 90% [32].

Elevations of the direct serum bilirubin occur within 2 weeks of onset, followed by variable changes in the serum alkaline phosphatase and transaminases within 4 to 6 weeks. There appears to be no direct correlation between the severity of enzyme abnormality and the degree of hepatic injury. The serum γ-glutamyltransferase and fasting serum bile acid levels provide the most sensitive measures of early cholestasis. Abnormalities in the serum albumin and prothrombin time are relatively late changes and herald the onset of progressive hepatic failure with a fatal outcome unless liver transplantation is performed.

Prevention. Early initiation of oral feeding, even in minimal amounts and avoidance of excessive amino acid concentrations and cyclic rather than continuous administration of TPN, can minimize the potential hepatotoxic effects. Discontinuation of TPN at the earliest clinically acceptable time is advisable [31••].

Treatment. Choleretic agents such as ursodeoxycholic acid and phenobarbital promote bile flow, with varying beneficial effects. Stasis in the biliary tract may be prevented by the use of exogenous cholecystokinin (CCK); stimulation of endogenous CCK by pulsed administration of amino acids; and, most importantly, initiation of early enteral feedings [31••]. Carnitine and glutamine supplementation and cyclical courses of antibiotics such as metronidazole are other modalities widely used in the treatment of TPN cholestasis.

■ REFERENCES

Recently published papers of particular interest have been highlighted as follows:
•   Of interest
••   Of outstanding interest

1.•• Roberts EA: Drug-induced liver disease in children. In *Liver Disease in Children*. Edited by Suchy FJ. St. Louis: Mosby-Yearbook; 1994:523–549.
This is a thorough and comprehensive review of drug-related hepatotoxicity in children including recent reports on individual drugs used in pediatrics and detailed discussion of hepatic drug metabolism.

2.• Rivera-Penera T, Gugig R, Davis J, *et al.*: Outcome of acetaminophen overdose in pediatric patients and factors contributing to hepatotoxicity. *J Pediatr* 1997, 30:300–304.
This is a detailed report of 73 cases of acetaminophen overdoses in children under 19 years of age, based on chart review from five institutions over 10 years.

3. Heubi JE, Bien JP: Acetaminophen use in children: more is *not* better [editorial]. *J Pediatr* 1997, 130:175–177.

4. Rumack BH: Acetaminophen overdose in children and adolescents. *Pediatr Clin North Am* 1986, 33:691–701.

5. Heubi JE: Reyes syndrome. In *Pediatric Gastrointestinal Disease*. Edited by Walker WA, *et al.* Philadelphia: BC Decker; 1994:1054.

6. Singh H, Chugh JC, Shembash AH, *et al.*: Hepatotoxicity of high dose salicylate therapy in acute rheumatic fever. *Ann Trop Pediatr* 1992, 12:37–40.

7. Hamdan JA, Manasra K, Ahmed M: Salicylate-induced hepatitis in rheumatic fever. *Am J Dis Child* 1985, 139:453–455.

8. Derby LE, Jick H, Henry DA, Dean AD: Erythromycin-associated cholestatic hepatitis. *Med J Aust* 1993, 158:600–602.

9. Reddy KJ, Schiff ER: Hepatoxicity of antimicrobial, antifungal and antiparasitic agents. *Gastroenterol Clin North Am* 1995, 24:923–936.

10. Aiges HW, Daum F, Olson M, *et al.*: The effects of phenobarbital and diphenylhydantoin on liver function and morphology. *J Pediatr* 1980, 97:22–26.

11. Holt C, Csete M, Martin P: Hepatotoxicity of anesthetics and other central nervous system drugs. *Gastroenterol Clin North Am* 1995, 24:853–874.

12. Bryant AE, Dreifuss FE: Valproic acid hepatic fatalities: US experience since 1986. *Neurology* 1996, 46:465–469.

13.• Konig SA, Siemes H, Blaker F, *et al.*: Severe hepatotoxicity during valproate therapy: an update and report of eight new fatalities. *Epilepsia* 1994, 35:1005–1015.
This is an excellent study of valproate-related reversible, severe hepatotoxicity in children, covering the risk factors and possible pathogenesis of the drug toxicity.

14. Kossak BD, Schmidt-Sommerfeld E, Schoeller DA, *et al.*: Impaired fatty acid oxidation in children on valproic acid and the effect of L-carnitine. *Neurology* 1993, 43:2362-2368.

15. King PD, Perry MC: Hepatotoxicity of chemotherapeutic and oncologic agents. *Gastroenterol Clin North Am* 1995, 24:969–990.

16. Bessho F, Kinumaki H, Yokota S, *et al.*: Liver function studies in children with acute lymphocytic leukemia after cessation of therapy. *Med Pediatr Oncol* 1994, 23:111–115.

17. Knowles SR, Gupta AK, Shear NH, Sauder D: Azathioprine hypersensitivity-like reactions: a case report and a review of the literature. *Clin Exp Dermatol* 1995, 20:353–356.

18. Jeurissen MEC, Boerbooms AMT, van de Putte LBA, Kruijsen MWM: Azathioprine induced fever, chills, rash and hepatotoxicity in rheumatoid arthritis. *Ann Rheum Dis* 1990, 49:25–27.

19. Sterneck M, Wiesner R, Ascher N, *et al.*: Azathioprine hepatotoxicity after liver transplantation. *Hepatology* 1991, 14:806–810.

20. Gedalia A, Molina JF, Ellis GS, *et al.*: Low-dose methotrexate therapy for childhood sarcoidosis. *J Pediatr* 1997, 130:25–29.

21. Kugathasan S, Newman AJ, Dahms BB, Boyle JT: Liver biopsy findings in patients with juvenile rheumatoid arthritis receiving long-term weekly methotrexate therapy. *J Pediatr* 1996, 128:149–151.

22. Locasiulli A, Mura R, Fraschini E, *et al.*: High-dose methotrexate administration and acute liver damage in children treated for acute lymphoblastic leukemia: a prospective study. *Haematologica* 1992, 77:49–53.

23. Kremer JM, Alarcon GS, Lightfoot RW, *et al.*: Methotrexate for rheumatoid arthritis: suggested guidelines for monitoring liver toxicity. *Arthritis Rheum* 1994, 37:316–328.

24. Kowdley KR, Keeffe EB: Hepatotoxicity of transplant immunosuppressive agents. *Gastroenterol Clin North Am* 1995, 24:991–1002.

25. Singh J, Garg PK, Tandon RK: Hepatotoxicity due to antituberculosis therapy. *J Clin Gastroenterol* 1996, 22:211–214.

26. Pande JN, Singh SPN, Khinani GC, *et al.*: Risk factors for hepatotoxicity from antituberculous drugs: a case control study. *Thorax* 1996, 51:132–136.

27. Palusci VJ, O'Hare D, Lawrence RM: Hepatotoxicity and transaminase measurement during isoniazid chemoprophylaxis in children. *Pediatr Infect Dis J* 1995, 14:144–148.

28. Hassall E, Israel DM, Gunasekaran T, Steward D: Halothane hepatitis in children. *J Pediatr Gastroenterol Nutr* 1990, 11:553–557.

29. Geubel AP, Galocsy CD, Alves N, *et al.*: Liver damage caused by therapeutic vitamin A administration: estimate of dose related toxicity in 41 cases. *Gastroenterology* 1991, 100:1701–1709.

30. Zimmerman HJ, Lewis JH: Chemical and toxin-induced hepatotoxicity. *Gastroenterol Clin North Am* 1995, 24:1027–1064.

31.•• Quigley EMM, Marsh MN, Shaffer JL, Markin RS: Hepatobiliary complications of total parenteral nutrition. *Gastroenterology* 1993, 104:286–301.
This is an extensive review of hepatobiliary complications of total parenteral nutrition in adults and children, including their pathogenesis and descriptions of pathological entities such as steatosis, cholestasis, and cholelithiasis.

32. Merritt RJ: Cholestasis associated with total parenteral nutrition. *J Pediatr Gastroenterol Nutr* 1986, 5:9–22.

178 Metabolic Liver Disease
William R. Treem

Our knowledge of metabolic diseases that cause liver dysfunction in children has expanded greatly since the mid-1970s. New techniques of analysis, including mass spectrometry, have enabled clinical investigators to pinpoint enzymatic defects and the toxic metabolites responsible for many syndromes that previously were poorly described. Knowledge of the precise enzymatic and metabolic defects has led to the development of more specific therapy, *eg*, replacement enzymes, substrates, cofactors, or special formulas and diets. Recently, liver transplantations have proven efficacious in certain disorders to replace a failing liver or prevent extrahepatic organ damage.

This chapter discusses inborn errors of metabolism that primarily damage the liver. For a more detailed discussion of the molecular genetics and pathophysiology of these complex disorders, the reader is referred to several recent excellent texts [1, 2••, 3]. Several important inborn errors of metabolism that affect the liver in children, *eg*, α_1-antitrypsin deficiency, Criglar-Najjar syndrome, Wilson's disease, and cystic fibrosis are covered separately and are not included in this chapter (see Chapters 107, 170, and 174). Other genetic defects for which the underlying metabolic derangement is just being elucidated, *eg*, Alagille's syndrome and progressive familial intrahepatic cholestasis (PFIC), are discussed in the chapter on the neonate with cholestasis (see Chapter 173).

◼ CLINICAL APPROACH TO INBORN ERRORS OF METABOLISM

Table 178-1 summarizes a diagnostic approach to the infant and child with metabolic liver disease. Conditions have been listed according to their most common form of clinical presentation.

Type I: Hepatomegaly With Cholestatic Jaundice in Infancy

Children with hepatomegaly and cholestatic jaundice present in early infancy with direct hyperbilirubinemia, and mild elevations of the serum aminotransferases. Evaluations are performed to exclude obstructive and infectious causes of neonatal cholestasis as well as the more common inherited metabolic causes such as α_1-antitrypsin deficiency, cystic fibrosis, Alagille's syndrome, and PFIC. Table 178-2 lists laboratory findings consistent with each of these disorders, and Table 178-3 summarizes the histopathologic findings seen on liver biopsy.

Defects in bile acid metabolism. Infants with autosomal recessive inborn errors of bile acid metabolism present with steatorrhea, failure to thrive, pale but not acholic stools, and signs of fat-soluble vitamin deficiencies including bleeding diathesis, pathologic fractures, and hyporeflexia [4]. In untreated patients, pruritus often becomes apparent after 6 months of age, and death from complications of cirrhosis before age 5 years is usual. On occasion, patients have survived into the second decade with chronic hepatitis. In contrast to most causes of neonatal cholestasis, infants with these disorders may have a normal or only minimally elevated γ-glutamyl transpeptidase (GGT), similar to values in PFIC. Liver biopsy shows a periportal inflammatory infiltrate, giant cells, hepatocellular and canalicu-

---

Table 178-1. Diagnostic Approach to the Infant and Child With Metabolic Liver Disease

Type I: Hepatomegaly with cholestatic jaundice
  α_1-antitrypsin deficiency
  Alagille's syndrome
  Progressive familial intrahepatic cholestasis (PFIC)
  Cystic fibrosis (CF)
  Defects in bile acid metabolism
  Peroxisomal disorders
  Niemann-Pick (type II)
Type II: Hepatomegaly, jaundice, coagulopathy, liver failure
  Galactosemia
  Hereditary fructose intolerance (HFI)
  Hereditary tyrosinemia
  Neonatal iron storage disease (NISD)
  Respiratory chain disorders

Type III: Hepatomegaly, hypoglycemia, Reyes-like presentation
  Glycogen storage disease (GSD) types I, III
  Fructose 1, 6-disphosphatase deficiency (FDP)
  Fatty acid oxidation (FAO) defects
Type IV: Hepatosplenomegaly and coarse facies, hydrops, ascites
  Gaucher's disease
  Wolman's disease
  Cholesterol-ester storage disease (CESD)
  Niemann-Pick (type I)
  Mucopolysaccharidoses
  Sialic acid storage disease
  Carbohydrate-deficient glycoprotein (CDG) syndrome
Type V: Chronic liver disease and cirrhosis
  α_1-antitrypsin deficiency
  Wilson's disease
  GSD type IV

Table 178-2. Helpful Laboratory Findings in Metabolic Diseases

Disorder	Laboratory Finding
Bile acid metabolism	Normal GGT
Peroxisomal	Increase of very long chain fatty acids
	Increase of DHCA, THCA, c_{29}-dicarboxlic bile acids
Niemann-Pick	Increase of acid phosphatase
Galactosemia	Urine reducing sugars
Hereditary fructose intolerance	Decrease of glucose, phosphate; increase of Mg^{++}, uric acid
Hereditary tyrosinemia	Increase of α-fetoprotein, tyrosine, methionine, urine δ-aminolevulinic acid
Neonatal iron storage disease	Increase of ferritin
Respiratory chain	Lactate > 2.5 mM
	Lactate: pyruvate > 20
Glycogen storage disease (type I, III)	Decrease of glucose, phosphate; increase of TG, uric acid, lactate
Fatty acid oxidation	Decrease of carnitine; increase of acyl-carnitine
	Increase of FFA; decrease of β-hydroxy-butyrate
	Increase of urine dicarboxylic acids, acylglycines
Gaucher's	Increase of acid phosphatase, angiotensin-converting enzyme
Wolman's	Bilateral adrenal calcifications
Mucopolysaccharidoses	Increase of urinary GAG
Carbohydrate deficient glycoprotein	Sialic-acid depleted transferrin

DHCA—dihydroxycholestanoic acid; FFA—free fatty acid; GAG—glycosaminoglycans; GGT—γ glutamyl transpeptidase; TG—triglyceride; THCA—trihydroxycholestanoic acid.

Table 178-3. Liver Biopsy Findings in Metabolic Disorders

Disorder	Pathologic Findings
Bile acid metabolism	Giant-cell hepatitis
Peroxisomal	Absent peroxisomes
Niemann-Pick (type II)	Foamy lipid-laden storage cells
Galactosemia	Steatosis, pseudoacini, ductular proliferation
Hereditary fructose intolerance	Hepatocyte necrosis, steatosis
Hereditary tyrosinemia	Ductular proliferation, fibrosis, cirrhosis, regenerative nodules, carcinoma
Neonatal iron storage disease	Hepatocyte necrosis, iron in hepatocytes but not in Kupffer cells
Respiratory chain	Microvesicular steatosis, abnormal mitochondria
Glycogen storage disease (type I, III)	Pale glycogen-filled hepatocytes, steatosis, adenomas, fibrosis (type III)
Fructose 1,6-diphosphatase deficiency	Steatosis
Fatty acid oxidation	Micro- and macrovesicular steatosis, fibrosis (LCHAD-deficiency)
Gaucher's	Multinucleated storage cells; tubular lysosomal inclusions
Wolman's	Foamy histocytes; fibrosis, cirrhosis, cholesterol-ester crystals
Niemann-Pick (type I)	Foam cells, "sea-blue" histocytes, membrane-bound lamellar inclusions
Mucopolysaccharidoses	Granular lysosomal inclusions
Glycogen storage disease (type IV)	Micronodular cirrhosis, periodic acid Schiff-positive, diastase-resistant "glycogen"

LCHAD—long-chain 3-hydroxyacyl CoA dehydrogenase.

lar bile stasis, mild hepatocellular necrosis, and, at times, bridging fibrosis (Fig. 178-1, see also **Color Plate**). Serum bile acids (glycocholate), which are expected to be elevated in conditions associated with neonatal direct hyperbilirubinemia, are often reported as normal. The diagnosis is made by analyzing urine or plasma via fast atom bombardment mass-spectrometry (FAB-MS), which detects abnormal unsaturated dihydroxy- and trihydroxy-cholestanoic bile acid metabolites [5•]. Deficiency in the enzyme 3β-dehydrogenase leads to a block in the synthesis of both primary bile acids, cholate and chenodeoxycholate, and accumulation of metabolites produced from 7α-hydroxycholesterol. These metabolites may be hepatotoxic. Alternatively, failure of bile acid–dependent bile flow may lead to hepatocyte damage, possibly as a result of the accumulation of toxic compounds normally eliminated in the bile.

Peroxisomal disorders. The peroxisome packages enzymes required for the beta-oxidation of bile acids as well as the conjugating enzymes for bile acid synthesis. Thus, generalized peroxisomal defects disrupt bile acid synthesis and often present with neonatal cholestasis. Zellweger's (cerebrohepatore-

nal) syndrome is the most common of the peroxisomal disorders, occurring in 1 per 25,000 to 50,000 live births. In Zellweger's syndrome, peroxisomes are absent, and patients exhibit a multisystem disorder with profound abnormalities of neuronal migration and brain structure, hepatic malfunction, renal cortical cysts, abnormal calcifications, retinal degeneration, and dysmorphic features, including a prominent forehead, shallow orbital ridges, epicanthal folds, a broad nasal bridge, micrognathia, and abnormal external ears [6]. Hepatomegaly is present at birth in about 50% of the cases, but develops in the first month in 80%. Approximately 60% of infants are jaundiced after the first week, and cirrhosis is present early in the first year in about 40% of the reported cases. The diagnosis is suggested by the demonstration of high levels of very-long-chain fatty acids (VLCFA) in the serum and elevated levels of dihydroxycholestanoic acid (DHCA), trihydroxycholestanoic acid (THCA), and a C$_{29}$dicarboxylic bile acid in urine analyzed by FAB-MS. These metabolites are characteristic of all the other generalized peroxisomal disorders, including neonatal adrenoleukodystrophy and infantile Refsum's disease. Electron microscopic examination of liver

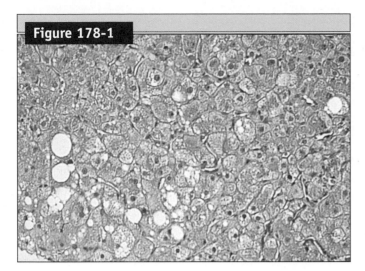

A boy 9 years of age with 3-β-hydroxysteroid dehydrogenase isomerase deficiency. The liver biopsy shows marked hepatocyte giant cell transformation and canicular and hepatocyte bile stasis. See also **Color Plate**. (*Courtesy of* D. Piccoli, MD.)

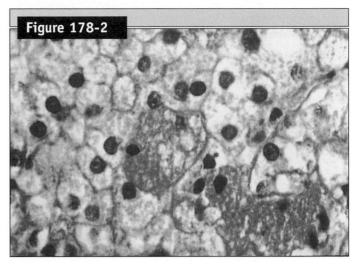

Characteristic large, pale foamy Kuppfer cells (Niemann-Pick cells) containing deposits of sphingomyelin (Masson stain, original magnification x 589). See also **Color Plate**. (*From* Klatskin and Conn [27].)

biopsy tissue from patients with Zellweger's syndrome reveals the absence of peroxisomes.

Sphingolipidoses. Sphingolipids are complex membrane lipids, including cerebrosides, sphingomyelins, and gangliosides. The catabolism of the sphingolipids requires lysosomal hydrolases. Deficiency of these hydrolases results in sphingolipidoses, which are classified according to the compound stored, and include three main storage diseases affecting the liver: Niemann-Pick disease, Gaucher disease, and GM_1 gangliosidosis. Only Niemann-Pick type II (formerly type C) presents with neonatal conjugated hyperbilirubinemia, and only in about half the cases [7]. Type II actually is a defect in intracellular cholesterol transport, and the sphingomyelinase that is deficient in type I is normal in type II [8]. These patients may initially be categorized as having "neonatal hepatitis," with biopsies in infancy characterized by giant cells, pseudoacinar formation, expansion of the portal areas by predominantly mononuclear cells, stellate fibrosis, and cholestasis. Early clues to the diagnosis before obvious neurologic deterioration include progressive splenomegaly more impressive than hepatomegaly, persistently abnormal liver enzymes, elevated acid phosphatase levels, subtle delays in developmental milestones, and a family history of consanguinity. Biopsy specimens must be carefully reviewed for the presence of foamy lipid-laden cells (Fig. 178-2, see also **Color Plate**). These hepatic storage cells may be difficult to differentiate from Kuppfer cells in babies with neonatal hepatitis. The diagnosis is confirmed by the detection of foamy storage cells in bone marrow and by measuring cholesterol esterification in skin fibroblast culture.

Type II: Hepatomegaly, Jaundice, Coagulopathy, and Liver Failure in Infancy

Type II liver disease includes inborn errors of intermediary metabolism that lead to an acute or progressive intoxication from accumulation of toxic compounds proximal to the meta-

bolic block. All the conditions in this group present with a symptom-free interval; then clinical signs of intoxication, including vomiting, lethargy, and coma; and ultimately signs of liver failure, including coagulopathy, hypoglycemia, hyperammonemia, bleeding, ascites, peritonitis, and sepsis.

Galactosemia. Galactose-1-phosphate uridyltransferase catalyzes the metabolism of galactose-1- phosphate to uridine diphosphate (UDP)-galactose, and its absence leads to the rapid accumulation of galactose-1-phosphate, galactose, and galactitol as soon as milk or lactose-containing formula is ingested in infancy. This autosomal recessive defect occurs in 1 per 40,000 to 50,000 live births. Symptoms appear in the first week of life and include irritability, refusal to feed, vomiting, diarrhea, jaundice, lethargy, variable hypoglycemia, hepatomegaly, edema, ascites, and renal tubular dysfunction. Galactose-1-phosphate uridyltransferase deficiency causes hypoglycemia by decreasing glucose release from glycogen and inhibiting enzymes involved in gluconeogenesis. Nuclear cataracts appear within days or weeks secondary to galactitol accumulation and become irreversible within weeks of their appearance. If untreated, patients often die undiagnosed with gram-negative sepsis (particularly *Escherichia coli*) within weeks. Early in the course of disease, liver histology is marked by macrovesicular steatosis, pseudoacinar transformation of hepatic plates, and periportal bile ductular proliferation (Fig. 178-3, see also **Color Plate**). Later, increasing fibrosis is evident, leading to cirrhosis by 3 to 6 months if the infant survives.

Newborns with galactosemia often are discovered by mass screening of neonatal blood spots for elevated galactose, provided they have been fed lactose-containing nutrients prior to the test. Reducing sugars, including galactose and galactitol, may be found in the urine. An unequivocal diagnosis is made by assaying enzyme activity in heparinized blood or erythrocyte lysates, or by measuring abnormally high levels of galactose-1-phosphate in red blood cells. If an infant is to receive an exchange transfusion, which is not unusual in these critically ill infants, a

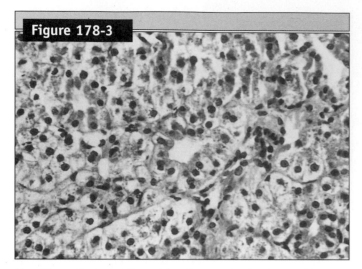

Figure 178-3

Liver biopsy from an infant with galactosemia showing marked pseudoacinar transformation of hepatic plates. See also **Color Plate**.

blood specimen should be collected before the procedure is performed, because diagnostic assays in blood must be postponed for 3 to 4 months after the transfusion. Antenatal diagnosis is possible by measuring enzyme activity in cultured amniotic fluid cells or biopsied chorionic villi, or galactitol in amniotic fluid.

Hereditary fructose intolerance. The specialized metabolism of fructose is facilitated by three enzymes that are found only in liver, kidney, cortex, and small intestinal mucosa. Aldolase B is the isozyme of the second enzyme in the pathway and is found primarily in the liver, where it catalyzes the splitting of fructose-1-phosphate into intermediates of the gluconeogenic pathway [9]. Patients with hereditary fructose intolerance (HFI) have a profound deficiency of aldolase B as the result of least 21 different genetic mutations. The disease is autosomal recessive and occurs in approximately 1 in 20,000 live births. One manifestation of the metabolic toxicity of the intrahepatic accumulation of fructose-1-phosphate in patients with HFI is hypoglycemia due to inhibition of gluconeogenesis and a block in glycogenolysis. The latter effect probably is the result of a combination of a depletion of ATP and inorganic phosphate that decreases the liver's capacity to form cyclic AMP and leads to an inhibition of phosphorylase a, a key enzyme in glycogenolysis. By depleting ATP and inorganic phosphate, fructose-1-phosphate accumulation also causes marked effects on purine metabolism, inhibition of RNA and protein synthesis, and hyperuricemia.

Infants do well during breast-feeding or while ingesting lactose-containing formulas. Symptoms appear when fructose, sorbitol, and sucrose-containing formulas, juices, or baby foods are introduced. The first signs usually are nausea, vomiting, pallor, sweating, trembling, lethargy, and eventually convulsions, with hypoglycemia following meals containing fructose. If the condition is not recognized, failure to thrive, hepatomegaly, jaundice, coagulopathy, edema, ascites, and proximal renal tubular disease appear. Hypoglycemia, lactic acidemia, hypophosphatemia, hypermagnesemia, and hyperuricemia are characteristic laboratory findings. The liver is characteristically enlarged, and liver histology shows scattered hepatocyte necrosis, periportal fibro-

sis, and diffuse macrovesicular steatosis. Traditionally, direct measurement of fructose-1-phosphate aldolase in hepatic tissue has been used to diagnose HFI; however, the recent isolation and sequencing of the human aldolase B gene on chromosome 9, and the recognition of multiple mutations, has led to the diagnosis of more than 95% of cases by amplification of DNA with a limited number of allele-specific oligonucleotides, thereby circumventing the need for tissue biopsy [10].

Hereditary tyrosinemia. Hereditary tyrosinemia (type 1) is an autosomal recessive disorder caused by deficiency of fumarylacetoacetate hydrolase (FAH), which is the last enzyme in the tyrosine degradation pathway [11••]. The enzyme block results in accumulation of fumaryl- and, possibly, maleylacetoacetate, which are alkylating agents thought to be responsible for hepatorenal damage. These metabolites are converted to succinylacetone (SA), which accumulates in the plasma and urine. SA is a potent inhibitor of the porphyrin biosynthetic pathway, and high concentrations result in elevations of δ-amino levulinic acid, which may explain the porphyria-like symptoms that occur in some patients.

Recent studies have shown that the spectrum of disease severity is wider than previously appreciated, ranging from acute liver failure with a bleeding diathesis in the first weeks of life to asymptomatic hepatomegaly or rickets in the second decade. In infants who present early with coagulopathy, epistaxis, gastrointestinal bleeding, and liver failure, sepsis is common, as is hypophosphatemic bone disease secondary to renal tubular dysfunction. The first laboratory evidence of an impending liver crisis may be a disproportionate prolongation of the prothrombin time in spite of normal or near-normal aminotransferases. Jaundice is present in approximately 33% of patients. In a more chronic form that presents later in infancy and childhood, cirrhosis, portal hypertension, and hepatocellular carcinoma may develop, even in those with few early symptoms of liver disease. Hepatocellular carcinoma is a common complication that may occur as early as 1 year of age but more often occurs in late childhood or adolescence. Occasionally, episodes of abdominal pain, polyneuropathy, and hypertension supervene, resembling acute intermittent porphyria. Hepatosplenomegaly, nephromegaly, and even nephrocalcinosis are common in the more chronic forms. In addition to standard laboratory indications of liver synthetic failure and renal tubular disease, there is a striking elevation of serum α-fetoprotein, especially in patients presenting early with the acute form. Plasma tyrosine, phenylalanine, and methionine often are increased, as is urinary excretion of δ-aminolevulinic acid, p-hydroxyphenylpyruvic acid, lactic acid, and catecholamines.

In the acute stage, liver histopathologic findings often are nonspecific, with fatty infiltration, pseudoacinar formation, hepatocellular necrosis, some giant-cell transformation, and prominent bile duct proliferation within portal tracts and fibrotic septa. Micronodular cirrhosis may be present very early and has even been reported to be present in utero. In the older child with a more chronic course, there is gradually increasing evidence of macronodular cirrhosis with coarse nodularity and regenerative nodules. The hallmark of the disease is elevated levels of succinylacetone (SA) in the urine. However, some

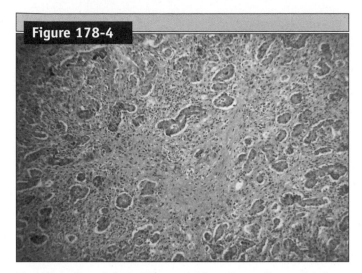

Figure 178-4

Liver biopsy in an infant with neonatal iron storage disease showing marked dropout of hepatocytes with hepatocellular necrosis and collapse, and prominent replacement with dense connective tissue. See also **Color Plate**. (*Courtesy of* D. Piccoli, MD.)

patients excrete only low levels of SA, and in these, the diagnosis should be confirmed by assay of FAH in lymphocytes or fibroblasts. Enzyme diagnosis in liver tissue may be misleading because of a peculiar phenomenon: in some areas of the liver the genetic defect may have "corrected," and high FAH activity is present in these areas. The human gene for FAH is localized on chromosome 15, and more than a dozen mutations have now been recognized, indicating a high degree of molecular heterogeneity in this disease.

Neonatal iron storage disease. Neonatal iron storage disease (NISD), sometimes called neonatal hemochromatosis, is a poorly understood congenital disorder, unrelated to classic hemochromatosis and characterized by extensive antenatal hepatocellular destruction [12]. Although the pathogenesis of this disorder is controversial, the clinical presentation is stereotypic. A family history of pregnancy loss or early neonatal deaths is common. Intrauterine growth retardation and oligohydramnios are noted almost universally, beginning early in the third trimester. Jaundice and direct hyperbilirubinemia usually are present immediately at birth, and ascites and edema develop soon after. Nonspecific symptoms of irritability, feeding intolerance, and lethargy often are mistaken for neonatal sepsis.

The most striking findings in this disorder are indications of liver failure in the first days of life and long-standing hepatocellular necrosis. Typical laboratory findings include hypoglycemia, marked coagulopathy, hypoalbuminemia, and conjugated hyperbilirubinemia, with only minimal elevation of aminotransferases and the absence of hepatomegaly. Often associated, but not diagnostic, is the significant elevation of serum ferritin, often exceeding 4000 mg/L. Serum iron levels often are normal for age, and transferrin levels may be low, reflecting hepatic insufficiency. Liver histologic examination shows extensive hepatocellular necrosis and collapse, with prominent pericellular fibrosis, giant cell transformation, and even cirrhosis (Fig. 178-4, see also **Color Plate**). The most

characteristic histologic feature is the extensive deposition of iron within residual hepatocytes but not in the Kupffer cells or other reticuloendothelial elements, as is commonly seen in other iron overload states. Iron deposition also is noted in the pancreas, heart, kidney, thyroid, Brunner's glands, and salivary glands, but not in the spleen, bone marrow, or lymph nodes. These distributions should prompt MRI examinations and biopsies of the lip salivary glands to confirm the diagnosis.

Few disorders present with liver failure at birth, but when they do, infectious etiologies (*eg*, enteroviral infections, herpesvirus, parvovirus B19, or adenovirus) and other inborn errors of metabolism that present with increased hepatic iron must be excluded. These include the previously discussed tyrosinemia type I, peroxisomal defects, and disorders of bile acid synthesis.

Respiratory chain disorders. Although often considered disorders of the central nervous system, muscle, or heart, mitochondrial disorders of the respiratory chain can present in the neonatal period with hepatic failure and lethargy, hypotonia, and proximal renal tubulopathy. The mitochondrial respiratory chain catalyzes oxidation of fuel molecules by oxygen and the concomitant energy transduction into ATP. During the oxidation process, electrons are transferred to oxygen via the energy-transducing complexes of the respiratory chain. The five functional units or complexes that form the respiratory chain are embedded in the inner mitochondrial membrane, and four of the five contain proteins encoded by nuclear DNA and mitochondrial DNA inherited from the mother. Disorders of the respiratory chain (also known as disorders of oxidative phosphorylation) would be expected to result in increased concentrations of reducing equivalents, NADH, $FADH_2$, and reduced levels of ATP. This imbalance affects multiple intramitochondrial pathways, including the citric acid cycle, and results in an increase in the intramitochondrial ratios of 3-hydroxybutyrate to acetoacetate and of lactate to pyruvate. The secondary elevation of blood lactate and the elevated blood and urine molar ratios of lactate:pyruvate (>20) and 3-hydroxy butyrate:acetoacetate (>2) are diagnostic hallmarks of these disorders. The observation of a persistent hyperlactatemia (>2.5 mM), particularly in the postabsorptive period, is highly suggestive of a respiratory chain deficiency.

Several cases of fatal neonatal liver failure have been reported in infants found to have defects of the mitochondrial respiratory chain because of decreased activity of complex III (cytochrome c reductase), complex IV (cytochrome c oxidase), or to actual depletion of mitochondrial DNA [13••,14,15]. Clinically, these infants have been characterized as hypotonic, with a poor suck, weak cry, apnea, lethargy, or coma in the neonatal period. Hepatomegaly or ascites can be present in the first days or weeks of life, and accompanying evidence of severe hepatic dysfunction includes moderate elevations of aminotransferases, marked direct hyperbilirubinemia, coagulopathy, hypoalbuminemia, hypoglycemia, hyperammonemia, and lactic acidosis. Hepatic histology shows microvesicular and macrovesicular steatosis, cholestasis, and glycogen depletion, but often is devoid of fibrosis or cirrhosis. Electron microscopy of the liver is reminiscent of that associated with Reye's syn-

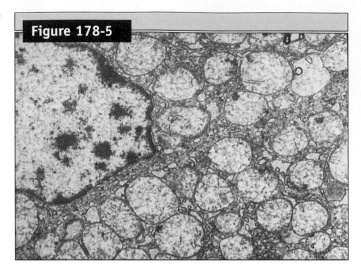

Figure 178-5

Electron microscopy of liver biopsy in an infant with a mito-chondrial respiratory chain disorder showing swollen pleomorphic mitochondria with a loss of cristae and a flocculent matrix. (*Courtesy of* M. Narkowitz, MD.)

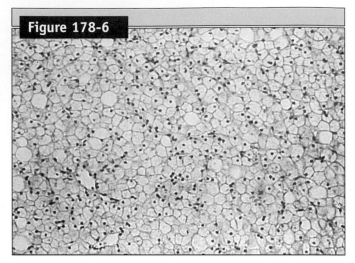

Figure 178-6

Liver biopsy in type I glycogen storage disease showing large, pale vacuolated hepatocytes with small dark nuclei. Macrovesicular steatosis is also present.

drome, revealing pleomorphic and swollen mitochondria with decreased numbers of cristae and variable inclusions (Fig. 178-5). Most reported patients with these disorders have died of liver failure or sepsis within the first few months of life.

An exception may be infants with complex I deficiency, which appears to be responsible for Alper's disease. These infants present later in the first 2 years of life with failure to thrive, vomiting, hypotonia, and elevated blood and CSF lactate, soon followed by seizures [16]. Neurologic deterioration is the rule, with death usually occurring by 4 to 5 years of age. Hepatic involvement with prolongation of the prothrombin time, hyperbilirubinemia, and mildly elevated aminotransferases often is a late event. It signals micronodular cirrhosis, hepatic microvesicular steatosis, massive neoductular proliferation, and lobular collapse, often seen on postmortem examination of the liver.

Type III: Hypoglycemia, Hepatomegaly, and Reye's Syndrome–Like Presentation

The presentation of type III disorders often is dominated by fasting-induced hypoglycemia and hepatomegaly, but usually not by true signs of hepatic failure. Although these patients may be encephalopathic and hyperammonemic, their degree of aminotransferase elevation and coagulopathy is mild; jaundice is rare; and hepatic necrosis, fibrosis, or cirrhosis is distinctly unusual. Liver size can be used to separate this group into those with disorders provoking permanent hepatomegaly and those with waxing and waning liver size.

Glycogen storage disease. Hepatic glycogen storage disease (GSD) encompasses mainly types I, III, and IV [17]. Type IV usually is not associated with hypoglycemia but presents with a more silent progression to cirrhosis; it is considered later in this chapter. GSD types I and III are associated with fasting-induced hypoglycemia and permanent hepatomegaly. Deficiency of glucose-6-phosphatase (type Ia) is the most common form of GSD. It is associated with profound hypo-glycemia, growth failure, and massive hepatomegaly. A less common form of this disorder results from a defect in the microsomal transport of glucose-6- phosphatase (type Ib) and is associated with impaired neutrophil function, neutropenia, recurrent infections, and, occasionally, inflammatory bowel disease. Hydrolysis of glucose-6-phosphate to glucose is the final common enzymatic event in the hepatic release of glucose from both the gluconeogenic and glycogenolytic pathways. Therefore, deficiency of glucose-6-phosphatase results in severe hypoglycemia, occurring within 3 to 6 hours of beginning a fast, and is associated with ketosis and lactic acidosis in infancy as the duration between feedings increases. The lactic acidemia is the direct result of the block in gluconeogenesis, and the ketosis is derived from exaggerated lipolysis and low basal insulin levels. Hypertriglyceridemia, hypophosphatemia, and hyperuricemia also are characteristic.

If hypoglycemia is severe, seizures may complicate the initial presentation. Virtually all patients present with abdominal distention caused by the markedly enlarged but soft, smooth liver. Splenomegaly may occur but is uncommon. Striking features include excessive adiposity with particularly fat cheeks and trunk but with poor muscle bulk in the limbs. The patient may bruise easily and have recurrent nosebleeds because of impaired platelet function. Later, xanthoma may develop in association with hypercholesterolemia and hypertriglyceridemia, and gouty tophi may occur because of chronic hyperuricemia. Serum aminotransferases are only modestly elevated (2 to 12 times normal). Other clinical manifestations seen in older patients (by the second decade) include hepatic adenomas, which occasionally undergo malignant change; proteinuria; renal stones; renal failure; pancreatitis; osteoporosis; and pulmonary hypertension. Hepatic histology shows pale hepatocytes distended by glycogen, with some fatty infiltration (Fig. 178-6). There is rarely increased fibrosis. Glycogen levels are markedly elevated in the liver, usually reaching 6 to 10 g per 100 g of liver tissue. A biochemical assay of glucose-6-phosphatase activity in a liver biopsy is indicated to confirm the diagnosis. The inheritance of GSD type Ia is autosomal recessive. The gene has been cloned and localized to chromosome 17, but a genetic screening test is not yet readily available.

Glycogen storage disease type III is a deficiency of the debrancher enzyme that results in an inability to degrade the 1,6- glucose linkages that form the branch points in glycogen. The clinical presentation of type III is similar to that of type I, with some notable differences. Because there is no block in gluconeogenesis and there is no problem with glycogen degradation until the terminal 1,4 glucose linkages have been cleaved, hypoglycemia develops later, usually 6 to 12 hours after a fasting period begins. Other differences include the prominence of hepatic fibrosis and the development of cirrhosis, portal hypertension, and splenomegaly by 4 to 6 years of age. This most likely is the result of the formation of limit dextrins (glycogen with short side chains ending in 1-6 glucose linkages), which act as foreign bodies in the liver, stimulating an inflammatory response. Cardiomyopathy and muscle weakness commonly develop during the second and third decades of life. Blood lactate levels are normal during fasting because there is no defect in gluconeogenesis.

Fructose 1,6-diphosphatase deficiency. Hepatic fructose-1,6-diphosphatase deficiency (FDD) results in a defect in the conversion of fructose-1,6-diphosphate to fructose-6-phosphate, which is then converted to glucose-6-phosphate. Thus, this enzyme deficiency prevents the formation of glucose from all gluconeogenic substrates including glycerol, lactate, and alanine. Maintenance of normoglycemia depends exclusively on glucose intake and on degradation of hepatic glycogen. When glycogen reserves are limited, as in newborns, or exhausted after a prolonged fast, hypoglycemia is likely to occur, accompanied by an elevation of the main gluconeogenic precursors. Patients with this rare enzyme defect usually present during the first year (even the first weeks) with life-threatening episodes of hypoglycemia, acidosis, ketosis, and coma provoked by ingestion of fructose or sucrose or simply by fasting or catabolic stress (eg, infections or fever). Other signs, symptoms, and laboratory findings are similar to those of GSD type I. However, hypoglycemia occurs later in a fast, and excessive hepatic glycogen accumulation does not occur because the glycogenolytic pathway is intact. The moderate hepatomegaly is secondary to hepatic steatosis, and aminotransferases are either normal or only mildly deranged. Between crises of hypoglycemia and metabolic acidosis, the liver remains enlarged, and the most frequent findings are hyperventilation, mild lactic acidosis, and hypotonia and muscle weakness. The diagnosis is confirmed by demonstrating the specific enzyme deficiency in a fresh, snap-frozen liver biopsy specimen.

Defects in fatty acid oxidation. In contrast to metabolic defects presenting with hypoglycemia and fixed hepatomegaly, the disorders of long- and medium-chain fatty acid oxidation (FAO) can present with serious episodes of hypoglycemia, lethargy, coma, and marked hepatomegaly after a prolonged fast, with complete disappearance of signs of liver dysfunction and hepatomegaly between episodes. As seen in Figure 178-7, these enzyme defects include disorders affecting the carnitine cycle, which facilitates the entry of long-chain fatty acids into the

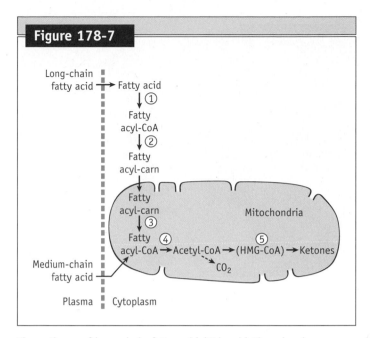

Figure 178-7

The pathway of long-chain fatty acid (FA) oxidation showing: conversion in the cytosol of the FA to a FA ester of coenzyme A (acyl-CoA); conversion in the cytosol to a FA ester of carnitine (acylcarnitine) and transport of the acylcarnitine across the mitochondrial membranes into the mitochondria; conversion of the acylcarnitine back to an acyl-CoA inside the mitochondria; oxidation of the long-chain acyl-CoA to acetyl-CoA fragments with each turn of the intramitochondrial β-oxidation cycle; and conversion of the acetyl-CoA fragments to ketone bodies.

mitochondria; disorders of intramitochondrial beta-oxidation of fatty acids; and disorders of intramitochondrial ketone body synthesis.

Fatty acid oxidation does not play a major role in energy production until late in fasting, when it becomes the essential source of energy production in the heart and skeletal muscle, and the precursor of ketone body synthesis in the liver. Thus, afflicted individuals may remain asymptomatic until provoked beyond the usual overnight period of 12 hours, or until the need for FAO is accelerated by catabolic stress. In general, disorders that affect the most proximal steps in FAO result in more profound reductions in ketogenesis, more severe hypoglycemia, and a more precipitous presentation after a shorter period of fasting. Thus, defects affecting the carnitine cycle (eg, carnitine palmityl transferase deficiency and carnitine transport deficiency) and those affecting the oxidation of long-chain fatty acids (eg, long-chain acyl-CoA dehydrogenase deficiency and long-chain 3-hydroxyacyl-CoA dehydrogenase [LCHAD] deficiency) are most likely to present in the first few months of life with potentially life-threatening episodes of hypoketotic hypoglycemia and coma, marked hepatomegaly, liver dysfunction, hypotonia, or cardiomyopathy. Although the heart, skeletal muscle, and liver are the organs most affected by the energy deficiency created, other organ systems may be affected in specific disorders. Peripheral neuropathy and retinal degeneration are seen in older patients with LCHAD-deficiency. Deficiencies in the pathway for transferring electrons from the first step in beta-oxidation to the electron transport system, also known as glu-

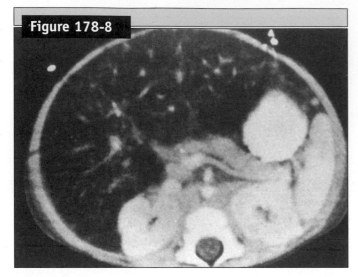

Figure 178-8

Hepatic computed tomography scan with intravenous contrast in an infant with a defect in long-chain fatty acid oxidation showing massive hepatomegaly with marked intrahepatic steatosis and a very low attenuation signal compared to spleen.

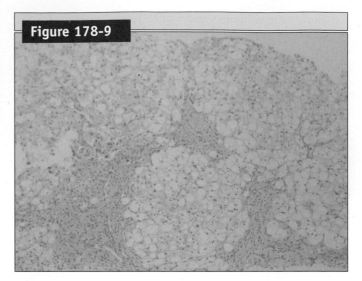

Figure 178-9

Marked hepatic fibrosis and macrovesicular steatosis in an infant with long-chain 3-hydroxyacyl-CoA dehydrogenase deficiency. Portal fibrosis and nodule formation are already present in this 4-month-old infant. See also **Color Plate**.

taric aciduria type 2 or multiple acyl-CoA dehydrogenation deficiency, may result in facial dysmorphism, rocker-bottom feet, and large polycystic kidneys.

Liver involvement in these disorders usually consists of marked increases in hepatic size during critical metabolic episodes of hypoketotic hypoglycemic coma, with mild elevations in aminotransferases (usually without hyperbilirubinemia), mild prolongation of the prothrombin time, and normal or mildly elevated serum ammonia [18•]. The encephalopathy associated with these crises often precedes overt hypoglycemia and probably is caused by the accumulation of toxic intermediate metabolites, which precipitate mitochondrial damage, uncouple oxidative phosphorylation, and result in increased intracranial pressure. Accompanying laboratory perturbations include moderate to marked hyperuricemia, elevated levels of creatinine phosphokinase (CPK), mild acidosis, marked elevations of free fatty acids (FFA), and levels of beta-hydroxybutyrate that are inappropriately low for the degree of fasting and hypoglycemia. Serum carnitine levels usually are depressed, with a higher ratio of acylcarnitines to free carnitine, especially in the non-fasted state. Abdominal ultrasound, CT scan, and MRI may show dramatic changes consistent with profound hepatic steatosis (Fig. 178-8). Light microscopic examination of liver biopsies shows microvesicular or mixed microvesicular and macrovesicular steatosis but little or no fibrosis or inflammation. An exception is sometimes seen in patients with LCHAD deficiency, in whom prominent fibrosis, and even jaundice and cirrhosis, may be present within the first few years of life (Fig. 178-9, see also **Color Plate**).

The diagnosis of disorders of FAO may be suggested by the finding of accumulating abnormal metabolites such as dicarboxylic acids, 3-hydroxydicarboxylic acids, and acylglycines in the urine. Plasma profiles of fatty acid esters of carnitine (acylcarnitines) determined by mass spectrometry often are diagnostic. Cultured skin fibroblasts or cultured lymphocytes have become the preferred material in which to measure the in vitro activities of specific

enzymes in the FAO pathway by using specific isotope-labeled precursors. All of the known defects are expressed in these cells, and results of assays in cells from both control and affected patients have been reported. All of the genetic disorders of FAO are inherited in autosomal recessive fashion. Heterozygote carriers are clinically normal, with the possible exception of the occurrence of acute fatty liver of pregnancy in LCHAD- heterozygote mothers carrying an affected fetus [19]. In some defects, notably medium-chain acyl-CoA dehydrogenase deficiency (MCAD) and LCHAD, common mutations in the cloned human genes have been identified. Simple polymerase chain reaction-based assays have been developed to detect these mutations from newborn blood spot cards.

Type IV: Early Hepatosplenomegaly Without Liver Dysfunction, and Occasional Coarse Facies, Hydrops Fetalis, and Ascites

The presentation of these storage disorders is dominated by marked hepatosplenomegaly, coarse facies, and, in some cases, hydrops fetalis, or the early onset of ascites. Table 178-4 lists the

Table 178-4. Inborn Errors of Metabolism Presenting With Hydrops or Congenital Ascites

Niemann-Pick (type II)
Hereditary tyrosinemia
Gaucher's disease
Wolman's disease
Mucopolysaccharidosis VII
Infantile free sialic acid storage disease
Carbohydrate-deficient glycoprotein syndrome
α_1–Antitrypsin deficiency
Neonatal hemochromatosis

metabolic causes of fetal or neonatal ascites. Although the visceromegaly associated with these disorders can be impressive, signs of liver failure usually are absent, and intrahepatic and intramitochondrial metabolic pathways are not immediately compromised. Within the first year of life, progressive neurologic deterioration with dementia, movement disorders, ataxia, spasticity, and myoclonic seizures become the dominant concerns in some of these disorders. Bony abnormalities, hirsutism, and corneal opacities also may be prominent features. An early clue to the presence of these disorders may be vacuolated lymphocytes in the peripheral blood. Rarely, significant liver injury and even cirrhosis can develop.

Most of these defects are classified as lysosomal storage diseases because they involve deficiency of a lysosomal acid hydrolase; inability to cleave sulfates, fatty acids, and sugar moieties from larger macromolecules; and the accumulation of an undegraded macromolecule within the lysosome. Most of the lysosomal enzymes act in sequence, such that substrates are degraded by a stepwise removal of terminal residues. Failure to remove a terminal residue makes the substrate inaccessible for further hydrolysis by other lysosomal enzymes. Macrophages and cells of the reticuloendothelial system are particularly rich in lysosomes, and it is swelling of lysosomes stuffed with undegraded substrate in these organs that is responsible for the prominent visceromegaly. Only those disorders with marked early signs of visceromegaly and hepatic involvement or potential progression to significant liver dysfunction or cirrhosis are mentioned in this chapter.

Lipid storage disorders. Among the lipidoses, Gaucher's disease, Wolman's disease, and Niemann-Pick disease are the most important causes of visceromegaly and hepatic dysfunction. Gaucher's disease is the most common lipid storage disorder known, occurring in 1 per 40,000 people in the general population and in about 1 per 450 to 865 people of Eastern European (Ashkenazi) Jewish descent [20]. It results from at least 34 different mutations to a gene mapped to chromosome 1. These mutations cause a deficiency of the enzyme glucocerebrosidase, which catalyzes the cleavage of glucose from glucocerebroside. This compound contains sphingosine, fatty acids, and glucose, and is produced in the central nervous system and by the turnover of red and white blood cells. Type I (adult chronic nonneuropathic form) is the most common form and often presents with hepatomegaly and more prominent splenomegaly within the first few years of life. Anemia, thrombocytopenia, and leukopenia resulting from hypersplenism, and osteopenia, bone pain, pathologic fractures, or avascular necrosis of the femoral or humoral heads secondary to marrow expansion by storage cells are common later findings. Patients with type I disease have no neurologic findings; children with the rare type II disease, however, present earlier and are severely affected with the triad of trismus, strabismus, and retroflexion of the head, as well as spasticity and seizures in the first year of life. Hepatic morphology is characterized by Gaucher's cells—large multinucleated cells with eccentric nuclei and fibrillar cytoplasm surrounding the central hepatic veins and within and obstructing the sinusoids. The liver architecture often is deranged, and, although uncommon, hepatic fibrosis may be severe, leading to

cirrhosis. Electron microscopy reveals long tubular inclusions in lysosomes. The diagnosis of all types of Gaucher's disease is established by determination of beta- glucocerebrosidase activity in leukocytes or in cultured fibroblasts. Serum acid phosphatase and angiotensin-converting enzyme levels may be elevated but are not specific.

Wolman's disease (WD) and cholesterol ester storage disease (CESD) are caused by a deficiency of the lysosomal enzyme acid lipase, which results in failure to degrade endogenous cholesterol esters and triglyceride [21]. Patients with WD typically present in infancy with vomiting, diarrhea, malabsorption, hepatosplenomegaly, severe anemia, and vacuolated lymphocytes, and normal serum triglycerides and cholesterol. Fifty percent die before reaching 3 months of age, and over 90% die by the age of 6 months. In some cases, jaundice and severe liver involvement occur before death. In contrast, infants with CESD may be asymptomatic apart from hepatomegaly and elevated triglycerides and cholesterol but may progress slowly over years to hepatic fibrosis, cirrhosis, and portal hypertension. In WD, the liver is greasy and yellow with enlarged vacuolated hepatocytes and Kupffer cells. The portal and periportal areas are filled with foamy histiocytes; fibrosis and frank cirrhosis are commonly seen; and large amounts of birefringent cholesterol ester crystals are found in the cytoplasm of hepatocytes. Bilateral enlargement and calcification of the adrenal glands are seen on abdominal radiographs and are pathognomonic of this disorder. Lipid accumulation also is marked in histiocytes stuffing the intestinal mucosa, making the mucosal surface velvety and bright yellow and causing severe malabsorption. Involvement of the myenteric plexus also may account for the abdominal distention. The definitive diagnosis is made by the demonstration of deficient acid lipase activity in fibroblasts, leukocytes, or liver using radiolabeled triglycerides or cholesterol.

Niemann-Pick disease is caused by a deficiency of the enzyme sphingomyelinase (type I), or a defect in the intracellular esterification and transport of cholesterol (type II). Fifty percent of type II patients present in infancy with a neonatal hepatitis syndrome; they are discussed earlier in this chapter with those disorders presenting with predominant neonatal cholestasis and jaundice. These patients also may present with nonimmune hydrops fetalis and neonatal or congenital ascites. Neonatal conjugated hyperbilirubinemia may be an important marker for the severe form of the disease because the onset of neurologic signs has occurred earlier in type II patients with jaundice compared to those without cholestasis. However, in type I patients the onset often is insidious, with feeding difficulties, poor visual contact, and neurologic deterioration during the first year of life. Hepatosplenomegaly without jaundice and failure to thrive may predate obvious neurologic impairment. In contrast to Gaucher's disease, hepatomegaly predominates over splenomegaly. Corneal opacifications may be present, and a cherry-red spot may be noted on the macula in approximately 50% of patients. Widening of the medullary cavities and cortical thinning are seen in long bones. Vacuolated lymphocytes appear in the peripheral blood, and foam cells appear in the liver, spleen, bone marrow, lungs, lymph nodes, and brain. "Sea-blue" histiocytes also may be demonstrated with Romanowsky

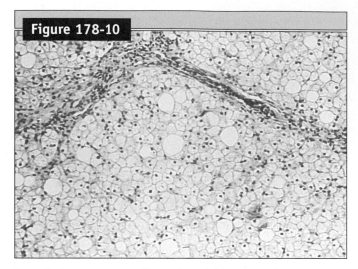

Figure 178-10

Type IV glycogen storage disease in a child 3 years of age with enlarged fibrotic portal tracts and portal fibrosis. Pale hepatocytes are arranged in a mosaic pattern.

staining. The ultrastructural features include large pleomorphic membrane-bound lamellar inclusions, which distend the cytoplasm of macrophages or are found in the pericanalicular region of hepatocytes. Deficient activity of sphingomyelinase may be demonstrated in leukocytes or cultured skin fibroblasts.

Mucopolysaccharidoses and glycoprotein storage disorders. The mucopolysaccharidoses are characterized by a progressive accumulation of mucopolysaccharides (*eg*, glycosaminoglycans [GAG]) within lysosomes of mesenchymal and parenchymal tissues and by an excessive excretion of GAG in the urine. Affected patients suffer from single or combined deficiencies of lysosomal enzymes involved in the degradation of dermatan sulfate, keratan sulfate, or heparin sulfate. Most affected children are normal at birth, although types IVb (Morquio disease) and VII (Sly disease) have been associated with non-immune hydrops and congenital ascites. After the first 6 months of life, gradual coarsening of facial features, including flattening of the midface and widening of the nasal bridge, takes place. Macrocephaly, macroglossia, thickening of the skin, and corneal clouding may develop, and hepatosplenomegaly is variably present. Hypersplenism may develop, but liver enzymes and function usually are normal. Bone dysplasia is prominent, leading to growth retardation and deformities of the trunk and extremities. Mental retardation is common but is not invariably present. Liver biopsies in type I (Hurler's syndrome), type II (Hunter's syndrome), and type III (Sanfillipo's syndrome) often show marked vacuolization and swelling of hepatocytes and Kupffer cells. Liver fibrosis has been described. Electron microscopy demonstrates finely granular or flocculent material housed in single membrane-bound (lysosomal) vacuoles. Elevations of urinary heparin-, dermatan-, keratan-, or chondroitin-sulfate are characteristic of these disorders, and specific enzymatic diagnosis can be performed in leukocytes or skin fibroblasts.

Glycoprotein storage disorders are caused by a defect of a proton-driven carrier that is responsible for the efflux of sialic acid (and other acidic monosaccharides) from the lysoso-mal compartment. Clinically, they resemble the mucopolysaccharidoses, but urinary mucopolysaccharide excretion is normal. An infantile form of sialic acid storage disease presents with nonimmune hydrops, congenital ascites, severe hepatosplenomegaly, severe skeletal dysplasia, psychomotor retardation, and, usually, death by 4 years of age [22]. Other associated findings include coarse facial features, generalized hypotonia, bony dysplasia, gingival hyperplasia, pulmonary hypoplasia, and anemia. Enlarged clear lysosomal vacuoles are prominent in the liver and other tissues. The routine diagnostic test is demonstration of free sialic acid in the urine, generally done by thin-layer chromatography.

Carbohydrate-deficient glycoprotein (CDG) syndromes are characterized by the presence of multiple secretory glycoproteins that are deficient in terminal carbohydrate moieties. The most helpful diagnostic marker is an abnormal transferrin in serum (deficient in sialic acid moieties), measurable by the carbohydrate-deficient transferrin assay. Clinically, these disorders are recognizable in early infancy by strabismus, axial hypotonia, psychomotor retardation, hyporeflexia, and variable dysmorphic features, including large ears and an abnormal adipose tissue distribution. Hepatomegaly, ascites, edema with a low serum albumin, and mildly raised aminotransferases are common. Liver biopsy shows hepatic steatosis and fibrosis and ultrastructural evidence of granular lysosomal inclusions. During the first year, vomiting and diarrhea develop with severe failure to thrive. If the infant survives, retinitis pigmentosa, stroke-like episodes, and epilepsy may supervene. Although clinically and pathologically CDG syndromes share features of lysosomal degradation defects, recent evidence suggests that deficiencies in specific synthetic enzymes localized to the endoplasmic reticulum and Golgi apparatus may be responsible.

Type V: Chronic Liver Disease and Late Development of Cirrhosis

Most of the disorders described earlier present with significant and dramatic extrahepatic findings and metabolic derangements that bring the patient to immediate medical attention in the newborn or infant period. However, some inborn errors of metabolism affecting the liver may be relatively silent until later, presenting with manifestations of severe chronic liver disease and cirrhosis. Examples include α_1- antitrypsin deficiency, Wilson's disease, and cystic fibrosis, which are covered in other chapters. Several defects related to those previously described in this chapter also can present in this fashion. Chief among them is GSD type IV (branching enzyme deficiency, glucose-6-glycosyltransferase deficiency). This rare form of GSD typically presents later than types I or III and is not characterized by episodes of hypoglycemia, but by failure to thrive, abdominal distention, hepatosplenomegaly, progressive liver dysfunction, and complications of cirrhosis, usually between 15 months and 4 years of age. The other striking metabolic abnormalities of uric acid, lactate, triglycerides, and phosphate characteristic of GSD types I and III are conspicuously absent in type IV. Biopsy of the liver shows micronodular cirrhosis and periodic acid Schiff-positive, diastase-resistant deposits in hepatocyte cytoplasm (Fig. 178-10). Ultrastructural studies show glycogen particles with fewer branch points, accumulating cytoplasmic fib-

Table 178-5. Emergency Investigations of Suspected Inborn Errors of Metabolism

Immediate
  Urine
    Smell (special odor)
    Acetone, reducing substances
    Urinalysis, pH
    Organic acids
  Blood
    CBC
    Electrolytes, BUN, creatinine
    Glucose, free fatty acids, β-hydroxybutyrate
    Blood gas
    Uric acid, phosphate, calcium, magnesium
    Triglycerides, cholesterol
    AST, ALT, GGT, bilirubin, alkaline phosphatase, amylase

    PT, PTT, total protein, albumin
    Ammonia
    Lactate, pyruvate
  Miscellaneous
    Chest radiograph
    Echocardiogram
    Head ultrasound (CT scan)
    EEG
  Stored (Frozen)
    Urine
    Heparinized plasma
    Blood spot on filter paper
    Whole blood (10 mL on EDTA-DNA studies)
    Skin biopsy—cultured fibroblasts

ALT—alanine aminotransferase; AST—aspartate aminotransferase; BUN—blood urea nitrogen; CBC—complete blood count; EEG—electroencephalogram; GGT—γ glutanyl transpeptidase; PT—prothrombin time; PTT—partial thromboplastin time.

Table 178-6. Specific Diagnostic Tests in Inborn Errors of Metabolism

Disorder	Material	Test	Findings
Bile acid metabolism	Urine, plasma	FAB-MS	Unsaturated
			Dihydroxy-, trihydroxy- cholestanoic bile acids
Niemann-Pick (type II)	Skin fibroblasts	Cholesterol esterification	Decreased
Galactosemia	RBC	Galactose-1-phosphate	Increased and decreased activity
	Blood, RBC	Galactose-1-uridyltransferase	
Hereditary fructose intolerance	Liver	Fructose-1-aldolase	Decreased activity + mutation
	DNA	Human aldolase	
		B gene	
Hereditary tyrosinemia	Urine	Succinyl acetone	Increased
	Lymphocyte	Fumarylacetoacetate hydrolase (FAH)	Decreased activity + mutation
	Skin fibroblasts	Human FAH gene	
	DNA		
Respiratory chain	Liver, muscle	Cytochrome c oxidase	Decreased activity
		Cytochrome c reductase	
Glycogen storage disease type I	Liver	Glucose-6-phosphatase	Decreased activity
Glycogen storage disease type III	Liver	Debrancher enzyme	Decreased activity
Fructose 1,6-diphosphatase	Liver	Fructose 1,6-diphosphatase	Decreased activity
Fatty acid oxidation	Plasma	FAB-MS	Specific acylcarnitine profile
	Leukocytes	Specific step in FAO pathway	Low activity + common mutation
	Skin fibroblasts	PCR; MCAD, LCHAD gene	
	DNA		
Gaucher's	Leukocytes	β-glucocerebrosidase	Decreased activity
	Skin fibroblasts		
Wolman's	Leukocytes	Acid lipase	Decreased activity
	Skin fibroblasts		
Niemann-Pick (type I)	Leukocytes	Sphingomyelinase	Decreased activity
	Skin fibroblasts		
Mucopolysaccharidases	Leukocytes	Specific enzyme analysis	—
	Skin fibroblasts		
Glycogen storage disease type IV	Leukocytes	Branching-enzyme	Decreased activity
	Skin fibroblasts		

FAB-MS—fast atom bombardment-mass spectrometry; FAO—fatty acid oxidation; MCAD—medium-chain acyl CoA dehydrogenase; LCHAD—long-chain 3 hydroxyacyl CoA dehydrogenase; RBC—red blood cell.

Table 178-7. Specific Therapy for Inborn Errors of Metabolism

Disorder	Diet	Medical	Transplantation
Bile acid metabolism	—	Cholic acid, chenodeoxycholic acid Ursodeoxycholic acid	—
Peroxisomal	—	Docosahexanoic acid Cholic, chenodeoxycholic acid	—
Niemann-Pick (type II)	—	—	Liver
Galactosemia	Lactose-, galactose-free	—	—
Hereditary fructose intolerance	Fructose-, sorbitol-, sucrose-free	—	—
Hereditary tyrosinemia	Low tyrosine, phenylalanine	2-(2-nitro-4-trifluoromethyl benzoyl) -1,3 cyclohexanedione (NTBC)	Liver
Neonatal iron storage disease	—	Tocopherol polyethylene glycol succinate (vitamin E), n-acetylcysteine, selenium, prostaglandin E-1, desferrioxamine	Liver
Respiratory chain	Low carbohydrate	Coenzyme Q 10, menadione (vitamin K_3), riboflavin, carnitine, ascorbic acid	—
Glycogen storage disease (type I)	Nocturnal continuous feeds, q-2–3 h daytime feeds, uncooked cornstarch, low lactose, sucrose-free high carbohydrate	—	Liver
Glycogen storage disease (type III)	Nocturnal continuous feeds, high protein	—	—
Fructose 1,6-diphosphatase deficiency	Sucrose-, fructose-, sorbitol-free, low fat, low protein	Bicarbonate	—
Fatty acid oxidation	Frequent feeds, overnight drip feeds, low-fat, MCT oil (in long-chain FAO disorders), uncooked cornstarch	Carnitine, riboflavin	—
Gaucher's	—	Alglucerase, Imiglucerase (glucocerebrosidase, enzyme replacement)	Liver, bone-marrow
Wolman's	Fat-free TPN	Safflower oil to skin	Liver, bone-marrow
Cholesterol-ester storage disease	Low-fat	HMG-CoA, reductase inhibitors (lovastatin) cholestyramine	Liver
Niemann-Pick (type I)	—	—	Liver, bone-marrow
Mucopolysaccharidoses	—	—	Bone-marrow
Glycogen storage disease (type IV)	—	—	Liver

FAO—fatty acid oxidation; HMG—hydroxymethylglutaryl; MCT—medium chain triglycerides; TPN—total parenteral nutrition.

rils, and finely granular material. Branching-enzyme deficiency can be verified in leukocytes and cultured skin fibroblasts.

THERAPY OF INBORN ERRORS OF METABOLISM

In many of the disorders described, it is imperative that a rapid diagnosis be made and therapy be instituted as soon as possible to prevent irreversible multi–organ system damage. The key to diagnosing many of these disorders is first to entertain them in the differential diagnosis of common symptoms such as poor feeding, lethargy, and failure to thrive. Many physicians think that because individual inborn errors are rare, they should be considered only after more common conditions such as sepsis have been excluded. It is essential, however, to obtain the appropriate samples at the time of metabolic decompensation. These data, obtained before therapeutic intervention has masked the metabolic abnormalities, direct the clinician toward the proper metabolic pathway (Table 178-5). Obtaining an extra urine and plasma sample and freezing them before the institution of intra-venous dextrose or other therapy in the emergency room is critical in making the diagnosis. Obtaining a family history is also important to uncover the presence of stillbirths, early infant deaths, unexplained neurologic, cardiac, muscle, or liver disease, or consanguinity. It must be remembered, however, that although most genetic metabolic errors are hereditary and transmitted as recessive disorders, most cases appear only sporadically because of the small size of most sibships in developed countries. Another misconception is to associate all inborn errors of metabolism with mental-motor retardation, seizures, or both, dating back to infancy. Many of these disorders occur in neurologically normal infants and children, and some present beyond the infant age group with late-onset forms in childhood or adolescence.

Table 178-6 summarizes the methods currently available for diagnosing these disorders. Sophisticated techniques of gas chromatography and mass spectrometry that can detect minute amounts of accumulating metabolites now are available in many reference laboratories. The detection of abnormal urinary and plasma organic acids, fatty acids, mucopolysaccharides, bile acids, and amino acid metabolites allows the clinician to choose a specific enzymatic defect to investigate. Fortunately, most enzymatic defects can be detected using in vitro assays performed on peripheral blood cells or cultured skin fibroblasts, avoiding the need for a potentially dangerous liver biopsy. Genetic testing for common mutations in the gene responsible for the enzymatic defect recently has become available in several of these disorders, confirming the biochemical/enzymatic diagnosis and opening the way for family and neonatal screening tests.

Until recently, specific therapy was not available for most of these disorders. The recent marked increase in our understanding of the specific enzyme deficiencies has allowed intervention with more specific dietary and biochemical therapy. A discussion of these therapies is beyond the scope of this chapter, but Table 178-7 highlights some of these new vitamin, drug, and enzyme replacement therapies [23•,24,25••,26]. In addition, Table 178-7 lists those disorders for which liver or bone-marrow transplant has been successfully used.

REFERENCES

Recently published papers of particular interest have been highlighted as follows:
* Of interest
** Of outstanding interest

1. Scriver CR, Beaudet AL, Sly WS, Valle D, eds: *The Metabolic and Molecular Basis of Inherited Disease.* New York: McGraw-Hill; 1995.
2.•• Fernandes J, Saudubray JM, Van den Berghe G, eds: *Inborn Metabolic Disease: Diagnosis and Treatment.* Berlin: Springer-Verlag; 1995.
This book provides an excellent, succinct summary of inborn errors of metabolism with a focus on diagnosis and treatment.
3. Suchy FJ, ed: *Liver Disease in Children.* St. Louis: Mosby; 1994.
4. Setchell KDR, O'Connell NC: Inborn errors of bile acid biosynthesis: update on biochemical aspects. In *Bile Acids in Gastroenterology: Basic and Clinical Advances.* Edited by Hofmann AF, Paumgartner G, Stiehl A. London: Kluwer Academic Publishers; 1995:129–136.
5.• Balistreri WF: Inborn errors of bile acid metabolism clinical and therapeutic aspects. In *Bile Acids in Gastroenterology: Basic and Clinical Advances.* Edited by Hofmann AF, Paumgartner G, Stiehl A. London: Kluwer Academic Publishers; 1995:333–353.
This article provides a good summary of clinical aspects of this new class of hepatic metabolic disorders.
6. Wanders RJA, van Roermund CWT, Schutgens RBH, *et al.*: The inborn errors of peroxisomal beta-oxidation: a review. *J Inherit Metab Dis* 1990, 13:4–36.
7. Sereraro L, Riely C, Kolodny E, *et al.*: Niemann- Pick variant lipidosis presenting as "neonatal hepatitis." *J Pediatr Gastroenterol Nutr* 1986, 5:492–500.
8. Gieselmann V: Lysosomal storage disease: a review. *Biochim Biophys Acta* 1995, 1270:103–136.
9. Van den Berghe G: Inborn errors of fructose metabolism. *Annu Rev Nutr* 1994, 14:41–58.
10. Tolan D Molecular basis of hereditary fructose intolerance: mutations and polymorphisms in human aldolase B gene. *Human Mutation* 1995, 6:210–218.

11.•• Holme E, Lindstedt S: Diagnosis and management of tyrosinemia type I. *Curr Opin Pediatr* 1995, 7:726–732.
This article offers an excellent summary of new medical treatment modalities for hereditary tyrosinemia.
12. Knisely AS: Neonatal hemochromatosis. *Adv Pediatrics* 1992:383–398.
13.•• Cormier V, Rustin P, Bonnefont JP, *et al.*: Hepatic failure disorders of oxidative phosphorylation with neonatal onset. *J Pediatr* 1996, 119:951–954.
This is the largest series of mitochondrial respiratory chain disorders affecting the liver in infants and children.
14. Vilaseca MA, Briones P, Ribes A, *et al.*: Fatal hepatic failure with lactic acidaemia, Fanconi syndrome and defective activity of succinate: cytochrome c reductase. *J Inherit Metab Dis* 1991, 14:285–288.
15. Mazziota MRM, Ricci E, Bertini E, *et al.*: Fatal infantile liver failure associated with mitochondrial DNA depletion. *J Pediatr* 1992, 121:896–901.
16. Narkewicz MR, Sokol RJ, Beckwith B, *et al.*: Liver involvement in Alpers' disease. *J Pediatr* 1991, 119:260–267.
17. Moses S: Pathophysiology and dietary treatment of the glycogen storage disease. *J Pediatr Gastroenterol Nutr* 1990, 11:155–174.
18.• Treem WR, Witzleben CA, Piccoli DA, *et al.*: Medium-chain and long-chain acyl-CoA dehydrogenase deficiency: clinical, pathological, and ultrastructural differentiation from Reyes syndrome. *Hepatology* 1986, 6:1270–1278.
A good summary of clinical and pathologic features of typical disorders of fatty acid oxidation is detailed in this article.
19. Treem WR, Shoup M, Hale D, *et al.*: Acute fatty liver of pregnancy, hemolysis, elevated liver enzymes, and low platelets syndrome, and long chain 3-hydroxyacyl-coenzyme A dehydrogenase deficiency. *Am J Gastroenterol* 1996, 91:2293–2300.
20. Morales L: Gaucher's disease: a review. *Annals of Pharmacotherapy* 1996, 30:381–387.
21. Wolman M: Wolman disease and its treatment. *Clin Pediatr* 1995:207–212.
22. Hale L, van de Ven C, Wenger D, *et al.*: Infantile sialic acid storage disease: a rare cause of cytoplasmic vacuolation in pediatric patients. *Pediatric Pathology & Laboratory Medicine* 1995, 15:443–453.
23.• Daugherty C, Setchell K, Heubi J, Balistreri W: Resolution of liver biopsy alterations in three siblings with bile acid treatment of an inborn error of bile acid metabolism (δ^4-3-oxosteroid 5beta-reductase deficiency). *Hepatology* 1993, 18:1096–1101.
This is the first report of the use of comprehensive primary bile acid therapy to treat inborn errors of bile acid metabolism.
24. Martinez M: Docosahexaenoic acid therapy in docosahexaenoic acid-deficient patients with disorders of peroxisomal biogenesis. *Lipids* 1996, 31(suppl):145–152.
25.•• Lindstedt S, Holme E, Lock E, *et al.*: Treatment of hereditary tyrosinaemia type I by inhibition of 4-hydroxyphenylpyruvate dioxygenase. *Lancet* 1992, 340: 813–817.
This study was the first report of 2-(2-nitro-4-trifluoromethyl benzoyl)-1,3 cyclohexanedione treatment of hereditary typosinemia.
26. Elstein D, Zimran A: Recent advances in diagnosis and therapy in Gaucher's disease. *Isr J Med Sci* 1995, 31:505–509.
27. Klatskin G, Conn HO, eds: *Histopathology of the Liver.* New York: Oxford University Press; 1993:66.

179 Portal Hypertension

Philip Rosenthal

Portal hypertension is uncommon in childhood, but when it does occur morbidity and mortality are significant. Its clinical hallmark is the development of gastrointestinal bleeding. Portal hypertension is associated with an increased risk for bacteremia, impaired hepatic function, and hepatic encephalopathy.

ANATOMY

The portal vein is formed from the confluence of the superior mesenteric, inferior mesenteric, and splenic veins. In healthy children, the portal venous system is a low-resistance system with a normal flow pressure of only 2 to 8 mm Hg [1]. Portal hypertension is defined as a portal pressure elevated above 10 to 12 mm Hg.

Because the portal vein lacks endothelial flaps, reverse flow in the portal venous system may occur if resistance is increased. With portal vein obstruction, collateral vessels for drainage may develop, resulting in cavernous transformation of the portal vein.

The increased pressure and the shunting of blood that result from portal hypertension occur in an orderly progression. An increase in splenic vein pressure causes splenomegaly. Increased flow to the coronary vein of the stomach dilates the gastroesophageal venous plexus, resulting in esophageal varices. Distal intestinal veins also may be affected, and hemorrhoids and anal rectal varices may be seen [2•]. Symptomatic distal intestinal varices are much less common in children than in adults.

The distal one third of the esophagus and the proximal stomach are the most common sites for upper gastrointestinal bleeding from portal hypertension in children. Varices form when the intrinsic veins that penetrate the circular and longitudinal muscle layers of the esophagus become engorged and displace the superficial veins [3](Fig. 179-1, see also **Color Plate**). Bleeding from varices was thought to be the result of vessel wall erosion, but recently it has been recognized that as veins dilate, tension in the vessel wall increases until tensile strength is surpassed, and rupture ensues.

Bleeding from the stomach is associated with portal hypertensive gastropathy, a congestive vasculopathy that is related to gastric mucosal blood flow [3] (Fig. 179-2, see also **Color Plate**) and is characterized by dilation of the mucosal and submucosal vessels without accompanying inflammation [4].

PATHOPHYSIOLOGY

Studies of the pathophysiology of portal hypertension have been done predominantly in adults. Caution should be used when extrapolating these data to children.

CLINICAL FEATURES

Portal hypertension may be classified as extrahepatic or intrahepatic, according to its cause. Portal hypertension in adults is usually intrahepatic, whereas in children extrahepatic portal hypertension predominates [5••,6,7•,8]. The main cause is portal vein thrombosis. Portal hypertension resulting from extrahepatic vein thrombosis causes gastrointestinal bleeding (particularly from esophageal varices), but hepatic function is preserved.

Umbilical vein catheterization in the newborn period, omphalitis, and trauma can cause portal vein obstruction and cavernous transformation (the recanalization of a thrombosed portal vein). Deficiencies of the anticoagulant proteins protein C, protein S, and antithrombin III also can lead to vascular thrombosis, with resultant portal hypertension. Congenital malformations of the cardiac and urinary tracts also have been associated with portal vein obstruction. Partial or complete obstruction of the suprahepatic vena cava or hepatic veins by congenital membranes or by thrombosis can lead to the development of the Budd-Chiari syndrome.

Figure 179-1

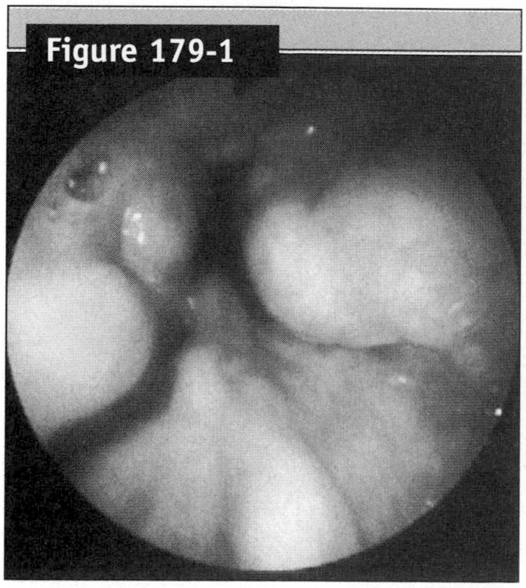

Endoscopy shows esophageal varices as tortuous prominences at the distal esophagus. See also **Color Plate**. (*From* Tolia V [3]; with permission.)

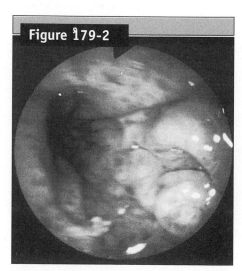

Figure 179-2

Portal hypertensive gastropathy as seen at endoscopy. See also **Color Plate**. (*From* Tolia V [3]; with permission.)

The many intrahepatic causes of portal hypertension are classified based on whether the insult is to the biliary tract or the hepatic cell. Among the biliary tract causes are biliary atresia, paucity of bile ducts, choledochal cysts, Caroli's disease, and cystic fibrosis. Hepatocellular causes include metabolic diseases, *eg*, Wilson's disease, α_1-antitrypsin deficiency, glycogen storage diseases, viral hepatitis (*ie*, hepatitis B virus, hepatitis C virus), and autoimmune hepatitis.

Portal hypertension often presents with hematemesis or melena in a child in whom there was no previous indication of an underlying problem. Growth and development may be perfectly normal, especially in the child with extrahepatic portal hypertension. Bleeding may result from rupture of an esophageal varix, from portal hypertensive gastropathy [9], or from gastric, duodenal, or anorectal varices. There is often a concomitant upper respiratory illness with coughing that results in increased intra-abdominal pressure or fever, causing tachycardia and an increase in cardiac output and leading to bleeding as a result of increased portal hypertension.

Careful history may reveal that the child has a chronic sensation of a vague fullness in the left upper quadrant; physical examination may reveal incidental splenomegaly. However, hypersplenism (*ie*, thrombocytopenia with petechiae and ecchymoses), leukopenia, and anemia are unusual presenting signs. Whereas splenomegaly correlates with the presence of portal hypertension, the size of the spleen is not a good indicator of the severity of increased portal pressure.

Cutaneous manifestations of portal hypertension, *eg*, prominent vascular markings on the abdomen caused by portocollateral shunting via superficial subcutaneous vessels, often are observed in children. In contrast, a caput medusae, *ie*, prominent paraumbilical collateral veins caused by decompressing portal hypertension via the umbilical vein, is rare, probably because of the high incidence of obstruction of the portal and umbilical veins seen in childhood.

Other manifestations of portal hypertension include ascites and hyponatremia. Growth and development may be significantly retarded in children with severe liver disease and portal hypertension.

DIAGNOSIS

Portal hypertension must be considered as a possible cause of splenomegaly or unexplained gastrointestinal bleeding in a child. Improvements in diagnostic ultrasonography and endoscopy have been useful in its detection. Doppler ultrasonography allows evaluation of vessel patency, vessel diameter, and direction of flow [10] (Fig. 179-3). In children, portal flow is normally hepatopedal at a rate of 10 to 30 cm/sec. Hepatofugal flow, particularly in the left gastric, paraduodenal, or paraumbilical veins, is highly suggestive of portal hypertension. Esophageal varices may be detected using ultrasound to examine blood flow through the lesser omentum. Ultrasound examination of the abdomen also may provide important information regarding the size of the spleen and the size and echogenicity of the liver, with hyperechoic areas suggesting cirrhosis. Bile duct dilation indicates extrahepatic obstruction. The presence of ascites can be readily appreciated by ultrasound examination. Renal abnormalities often associated with portal vein thrombosis also are evident. Doppler ultrasonography is

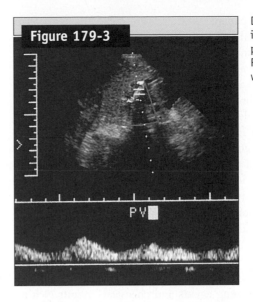

Figure 179-3

Doppler ultrasound investigation of the portal vein. (*From* Rosenthal P [10]; with permission.)

more cost effective and efficient than is magnetic resonance imaging with angiographic sequencing (MRA).

Flexible fiberoptic endoscopy has been invaluable in the definitive diagnosis of esophageal varices. In the child with upper gastrointestinal bleeding, endoscopic evaluation can localize the source of bleeding. Recent investigations in adults have used endoscopic ultrasonography to evaluate submucosal vessel dilation and shunting and to determine the effectiveness of therapy [11] to reduce portal hypertension and obliterate varices. Recently, endosonographic evaluation of the rectum in children with extrahepatic portal venous obstruction has been successful [12].

Selective angiography of the celiac axis, superior mesenteric artery, and splenic vein may be necessary to demonstrate extrahepatic vascular anatomy, especially if there is portal vein thrombosis. Measurement of portal pressure by determining the splenic pulp pressure via splenoportography is rarely performed because of the potential complications (*ie*, significant incidence of splenic bleeding intraperitoneally and a high incidence of false-positive results for portal vein thrombosis). Although hepatic venous pressure often is measured in adults to help in the evaluation of portal hypertension, there are limited data with regard to hepatic venous pressure gradients in children.

TREATMENT

Acute Variceal Bleeding

The management of portal hypertension is directed primarily toward controlling variceal bleeding. The caretaker of a child with portal hypertension should be instructed to seek immediate medical attention if there is hematemesis or a change in stool quality that is consistent with internal bleeding.

Children with variceal bleeding should be admitted to a pediatric intensive care unit or its equivalent, and their vital signs should be monitored closely. Tachycardia and hypotension are good clinical indicators of the severity of blood loss. Replacement of intravascular volume with intravenous administration of saline or lactated Ringer's solution if blood is not readily available should be instituted promptly. Resuscitation with blood and blood products and placement of a large-bore nasogastric or orogastric tube to aid in evacuation of blood and clots and assessment of upper gastrointestinal bleeding is essential. However, once the bleeding has stopped and the patient's vital signs are stable, the nasogastric tube may be removed and monitoring performed using only the patient's vital signs and sequential hematocrits. In small children, fluid replacement must be done carefully to avoid increasing intravascular volume and inadvertently increasing the portal pressure as a result. If thrombocytopenia and coagulation defects are present with active bleeding, platelet transfusions should be given if the platelet count is below 50 X 10⁹/L . Vitamin K and fresh frozen plasma also should be administered.

In children, bleeding from esophageal varices usually subsides spontaneously, and supportive therapy is all that is required. If bleeding persists for more than 6 to 12 hours, or if multiple blood transfusions are required, additional intervention is warranted. Upper esophageal endoscopy can be performed to document the site of bleeding, and sclerotherapy or variceal band ligation can be performed to control esophageal varices [13–16]. Emergency sclerotherapy is technically challenging in a child with significant and active bleeding. Sclerosing agents and chemical irritants such as ethanolamine and tetradecyl sulfate injected intravariceally or paravariceally are used in a fashion similar to that used in adults. In children, 1 mL of sclerosant is injected per varix, not to exceed 10 mL as the upper limit for one sclerotherapy session. Potential major complications of sclerotherapy include uncontrollable bleeding, esophageal ulceration, stricture formation, dysphagia, pleural effusion, and sepsis.

In elastic band ligation, the varix is suctioned into a plastic fitting attached to the endoscope tip, and an elastic band is discharged over the varix [15]. Accessories are available that allow five or six bandings before the endoscope has to be withdrawn and reloaded (*eg*, Six-shooter; Wilson-Cook, Winston Salem, NC). Caution must be used with this technique, especially in small children, because the esophagus is thinner than in adults and there is the risk of completely banding the entire wall of the esophagus, with necrosis and perforation of the esophagus as a result. General anesthesia often is necessary to perform these procedures safely in children.

Numerous medications have been used alone or in combination in an attempt to control portal hypertensive bleeding [17••,18•]. Vasopressin, which has a half-life of only 30 minutes, increases splanchnic vascular tone and thereby decreases portal blood flow. It is administered as an intravenous bolus of 0.33 U/kg over 20 to 30 minutes followed by a continuous infusion of 0.33 U/kg/h. If necessary, the concentration of the continuous infusion can be increased up to three times its initial rate.

Octreotide, a long-acting synthetic octapeptide of naturally occurring somatostatin, reduces portal pressure by reducing azygous and collateral blood flow. Octreotide has a longer half-life than vasopressin and is an effective splanchnic vasoconstrictor. In adults, octreotide and somatostatin appear to be equal to vasopressin in efficacy, but patients experience fewer side effects with them than with vasopressin. There are no published controlled trials of octreotide in children. Anecdotally, octreotide appears to be well tolerated by children and is moderately effective in controlling variceal bleeding. Octreotide is administered initially as an intravenous bolus of 1 to 2 μg/kg over 2 to 5 minutes followed by a continuous infusion of 1 to 2 μg/kg/h. Since the advent of sclerotherapy and other pharmacotherapeutic

options, balloon tamponade [18•], usually with a Sengstaken-Blakemore tube, is seldom used in children.

Transjugular Intrahepatic Portosystemic Shunt

Transjugular Intrahepatic Portosystemic Shunts (TIPS) are a non-operative method used to create a portosystemic shunt. Although experience in adults has been increasing rapidly, use of TIPS in children has been limited [19–21]. The small size of the liver and the caliber of the portal vein and hepatic vein make the procedure technically more demanding and the potential for shunt thrombosis is greater. Preliminary data from our own program [21] demonstrate successful placement of TIPS in seven of nine children. Shunt thrombosis developed in four patients, and variceal bleeding was controlled in four out of five children who underwent TIPS for variceal bleeding. Encephalopathy following TIPS was not a significant problem. TIPS appears to be useful for short-term management of portal hypertension and gastrointestinal bleeding in children, especially as a bridge to liver transplantation.

Surgery

Surgical intervention, including shunt therapy and liver transplantation, is the last alternative for acute variceal bleeding from portal hypertension and is rarely warranted.

Prophylactic Therapy

Several studies have demonstrated the benefit of propanolol therapy in adults with varices and portal hypertension when there is at least a 25% reduction in resting heart rate. There are no reported controlled trials of beta blockade therapy for children. Further, the cost effectiveness of indefinite primary prophylaxis with nonselective beta blockade has not been determined.

In children, parents are always concerned about whether physical activities should be limited, especially in the child who has splenomegaly with thrombocytopenia and leukopenia. Whereas contact sports (*eg*, boxing, football) and activities that cause increased intra-abdominal pressure (*eg*, weight lifting) should be avoided, other activities such as swimming and jogging are encouraged to maintain muscle mass. Children who insist on continued participation in team sports may benefit from the use of specially designed spleen guards to protect the enlarged spleen from direct trauma. I have not observed an increased number of infections in these children, even with leukopenia associated with hypersplenism. Although many physicians recommend pneumococcal vaccine for these children, vaccination may not produce sufficiently protective titers.

■ REFERENCES

Recently published papers of particular interest have been highlighted as follows:
•   Of interest
••   Of outstanding interest

1.   Watanabe FD, Rosenthal P: Portal hypertension in children. *Curr Opin Pediatr* 1995, 7:533–538.

2.•   Heaton ND, Davenport M, Howard ER: Incidence of haemorrhoids and anorectal varices in children with portal hypertension. *Br J Surg* 1993, 80:616–618.
This study is one of the few to address this problem in children

3.   Tolia V: Peptic ulcer disease and *Helicobacter pylori*-related gastroduodenal disease in pediatrics. In *Pediatric GI Problems*, vol 4. Edited by Hyman PE. Philadelphia: Current Medicine; 1997:5.1–5.21.

4.   Hyman JS, Treem WR: Portal hypertensive gastropathy in children. *J Pediatr Gastroenterol Nutr* 1993, 17:13–18.

5.•• Groszmann RJ: Hyperdynamic circulation of liver disease 40 years later: pathophysiology and clinical consequences. *Hepatology* 1994, 20:1359–1363.

Thoughts on pathophysiology and subsequent clinical consequences by an acknowledged expert in the field are provided in this article.

6.   Michielsen PP, Pelckmans PA: Hemodynamic changes in portal hypertension: new insights in the pathogenesis and clinical implications. *Acta Gastroenterol Belg* 1994, 57:194–205.

7.• Hassall E: Nonsurgical treatments for portal hypertension in children. *Gastrointest Endosc Clin North Am* 1994, 4:233–258.

This article discusses therapeutic options available for children with portal hypertension.

8.   Goh DW, Myers NA: Portal hypertension in children: the changing spectrum. *J Pediatr Surg* 1994, 29:688–691.

9.   Pak JM, Lee SS: Glucagon in portal hypertension. *J Hepatol* 1994, 20:825–832.

10. Rosenthal P: Pediatric liver disease. In *Pediatric GI Problems*, vol 4. Edited by Hyman PE. Philadelphia: Current Medicine; 1997:11.1–11.25.

11. Van Dam J: Endosonography of the esophagus. *Gastrointest Endosc Clin North Am* 1994, 4:803–826.

12. Yachha SK, Dhiman RK, Gupta R, Ghoshal UC: Endosonographic evaluation of the rectum in children with extrahepatic portal venous obstruction. *J Pediatr Gastroenterol Nutr* 1996, 23:438–441.

13. Hassall E, Treem WR: To stab or strangle: how best to kill a varix? [editorial] *J Pediatr Gastroenterol Nutr* 1995, 20:121.

14. Yachha SK, Ghoshal UC, Gupta R, *et al.*: Portal hypertensive gastropathy in children with extrahepatic portal venous obstruction: role of variceal obliteration by endoscopic sclerotherapy and *Helicobacter pylori* infection. *J Pediatr Gastroenterol Nutr* 1996, 23:20–23.

15. Fox VL, Carr-Locke DL, Connors PJ, Leichtner AM: Endoscopic ligation of esophageal varices in children. *J Pediatr Gastroenterol Nutr* 1995, 20:202–208.

16. Yachha SK, Sharma BC, Kumar M, Khanduri A: Endoscopic sclerotherapy for esophageal varices in children with extrahepatic portal venous obstruction: a follow-up study. *J Pediatr Gastroenterol Nutr* 1997, 24:49–52.

17.•• Lebrec D: Pharmacologic treatment of portal hypertension: hemodynamic effects and prevention of rebleeding. *Pharmacol Ther* 1994, 61:65–107.

This article provides an excellent survey comparing trials of pharmacologic control of portal hypertension.

18.• Carey WD, Grace ND, Reddy KR, Shiffman ML: *Managing Variceal Hemorrhage in the Cirrhotic: A Primer*. Arlington: American College of Gastroenterology; 1996:1–12.

This paper details recent recommendations for adults from the American College of Gastroenterology.

19. Kerns SR, Hawkins IF: Transjugular intrahepatic portosystemic shunt in a child with cystic fibrosis. *Am J Roentgenol* 1992, 159:1277–1278.

20. Berger KJ, Schreiber RA, Tchervenkov J, *et al.*: Decompression of portal hypertension in a child with cystic fibrosis after transjugular intrahepatic portosystemic shunt placement. *J Pediatr Gastroenterol Nutr* 1994, 18:785–789.

21. Heyman MB, LaBerge JM, Somberg KA, *et al.*: Transjugular intrahepatic portosystemic shunts (TIPS) in children. *J Pediatr* 1997, 131:914–919.

180 Liver Transplantation in Children
Estella M. Alonso

Approximately 350 children per year in the United States undergo liver transplantation as a life-saving therapy for otherwise fatal liver disease. With innovations in surgical technique, improved postoperative care, and newer immunosuppressive regimens, posttransplantation survival in children has increased steadily over the past 10 years [1•,2•]; 2-year survival in most established programs approaches 85% [2•]. This chapter summarizes the aspects of liver transplantation that are unique to children.

▣ PRETRANSPLANT EVALUATION

The common diagnoses leading to liver transplantation in children are listed in Table 180-1. Most pediatric liver transplants are performed in children with biliary atresia. Metabolic liver diseases that result in cirrhosis, such as α_1-antitrypsin deficiency and Wilson's disease, also are common indications. Approximately 5% of the children who receive transplants have fulminant hepatitis, most of which is sporadic. Transplantation

Table 180-1. Common Indications for Liver Transplantation in Children

	Frequency of transplants, %
Biliary Atresia	50
α_1-Antitrypsin deficiency	10
Familial cholestasis	9
Chronic active hepatitis	6
Fulminant hepatic failure	5
Neonatal hepatitis and perinatal hemochromatosis	4
Wilson's disease	3
Tyrosinemia	2
Glycogen storage disease	2
Primary sclerosing cholangitis	2
Other	7

Table 180-2. Medical Complications Indicating the Need for Liver Transplantation in Pediatric Patients

Biliary atresia
  Failed Kasai procedure
  Recurrent ascending cholangitis
  Complications of cirrhosis as listed below
Cirrhosis of any etiology with the following complications
  Growth failure
  Refractory ascites
  Refractory episodes of variceal bleeding
  Hypersplenism causing thrombocytopenia
  Liver synthetic failure
  Other major systemic complications
Fulminant hepatic failure
Neonatal liver failure
Inborn errors of metabolism
  Tyrosinemia
  Glycogen storage disease
  Crigler-Najjar syndrome
  Ornithine transcarbamylase deficiency
  Other defects with the potential to cause neurologic or other
    major systemic complications
Unresectable hepatic tumors without extension

is performed uncommonly in those with inborn errors of metabolism without cirrhosis, such as Crigler-Najjar syndrome or ornithine transcarbamylase deficiencies.

Children with chronic liver disease are not actively listed for transplantation unless they are judged to have a life expectancy of less than 6 months [3]. Predicting life expectancy depends on the form of liver disease. Biliary atresia, for example, has a very predictable progression, and patients who do not have successful biliary drainage following a Kasai procedure invariably develop end-stage liver disease with hepatic insufficiency by 2 years of age. Transplantation is actively pursued when these children begin to experience linear growth failure and the first complications of portal hypertension. Patients with familial cholestatic syndromes, which ultimately lead to cirrhosis, may have a less predictable course. Growth failure is characteristic of these syndromes, even when liver function is preserved. Signs of advancing portal hypertension and liver synthetic failure are the earliest indications for transplant in this group.

Children with metabolic defects that can be corrected by transplantation are approached using a different strategy. In such a setting, the goal should be to perform the transplant before the patient develops significant complications from the metabolic defect. The child with fulminant hepatic failure should undergo transplantation as soon as a suitable organ is available, because fewer than 25% of these patients survive without it [4]. Table 180-2 summarizes the medical complications that indicate the need to proceed with transplantation.

The preoperative evaluation of a child awaiting liver transplantation includes establishing the etiology of the liver disease, predicting the timing of the need for transplant, and identifying anatomic abnormalities or other organ system impairment that would complicate the surgical procedure. For liver transplantation to be indicated, children with cirrhosis should show signs of hepatic insufficiency, such as growth failure or coagulopathy, or have significant complications of portal hypertension, such as ascites or variceal bleeding. A child who has not developed these complications may have many years of quality life before liver transplantation is needed [3].

CONTRAINDICATIONS

The most important contraindication is availability of an acceptable alternative therapy. If a surgical procedure or alteration in medication can improve the quality of life in the patient who has not reached hepatic insufficiency, this option should be pursued actively. A second important contraindication to liver transplantation is the expectation of suboptimal quality of life after the transplant. This is important with regard to children who already have significant irreversible neurologic damage at the time of transplant referral. The third contraindication is impairment of other organ systems, either primary or secondary to liver disease, which would preclude successful transplantation, *eg*, congenital heart disease and pulmonary failure. Renal failure secondary to hepatorenal syndrome is quickly reversed after successful liver transplantation, and, when secondary to primary renal disease, can be corrected with combined liver–kidney transplant. Liver transplantation should be avoided in patients who have a disease that is expected to recur after transplant, such as malignancy or viral infection. Transplantation during a major systemic infection, however, is only a relative contraindication. For example, if a patient has persistent ascending cholangitis as a complication of Biliary Atresia, liver transplantation is the only successful treatment method. In this situation, the patient may proceed to transplantation even with repeated positive blood cultures.

SURGICAL PROCEDURE

The shortage of size-matched organs for pediatric candidates is a continuing and difficult problem. When a whole liver is transplanted, the donor should be within 15% to 20% of the recipient's size. The median age at transplantation at most large centers is 1 to 2 years of age, reflecting the large proportion of patients transplanted in infancy for biliary atresia. Because most pediatric organ donors are school-aged children who are accident victims, most pediatric liver donors are too large for the younger and smaller pediatric liver recipients; such donor-to-recipient mismatches cause excessively long waiting times and high pretransplant mortality among small children.

Reduced-size liver transplantation is a technique in which the liver is divided along anatomic segments to provide a hepatic allograft for a smaller recipient (Fig. 180-1) [5,6]. Using this technique, grafts can be obtained from a donor up to eight times the weight of the recipient. This allows an adult donor to provide a liver for a child who weighs less than 10 kg. The most recent application of reduced-sized liver grafting is the use of living related donors [7•]. A portion of the left lobe of a healthy donor is resected to provide a liver graft for an infant. Because the resection must be limited to prevent vascular and bile duct complications in the donor, the vessels of the resulting liver

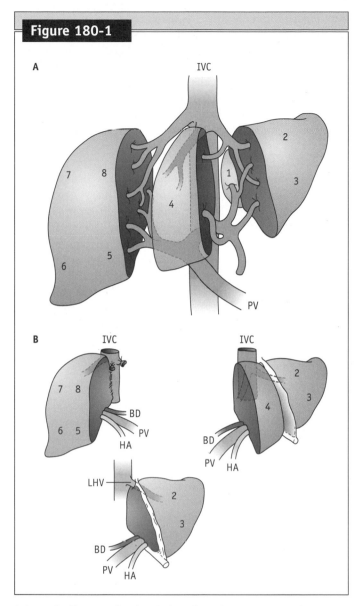

Figure 180-1

A

IVC

7 8 1 2 3

4

6 5

PV

B

IVC   IVC

7 8   2

4   3

6 5

BD   BD

PV

HA   PV HA

LHV

2

3

BD

PV HA

Schematic diagram of reduced size allografts. **A,** Segmental anatomy of the liver. **B,** Right lobe, left lobe, and left lateral segment grafts. BD—bile duct; HA—hepatic artery; IVC—inferior vena cava; LHV—left hepatic vein; PV—portal vein.

graft must be reconstructed for extension and anastomosis with the native portal vein and hepatic artery. The bile duct is reconstructed using a typical Roux-en-Y biliary enterostomy. Living, related donor liver transplantation provides children with several clear-cut advantages: 1) the earlier and more elective transplantation of smaller infants provides a major advantage, mitigating malnutrition and pretransplant complications and resulting in improved survival rates, shorter hospitalizations, and a reduced overall cost of care; 2) living-related-donation provides a good quality graft, reducing the incidence of primary nonfunction to less than 1%; and 3) patients with living-related-donor grafts are less likely to develop steroid-resistant rejection. Fewer lose their grafts to chronic rejection than do recipients of cadaveric allografts, and overall, in long-term follow-up, these patients appear to need less immunosuppression than do recipients of cadaveric grafts [8].

IMMUNOSUPPRESSION

The challenge when choosing an immunosuppressive regimen for a child is to balance the need to prevent rejection against the infectious complications of these therapeutic agents. Cyclosporine, which was introduced in the mid-1980s, is a potent lymphocyte-specific immunosuppressive. Its development was essential to successful liver transplantation, and it has been the cornerstone of therapy of most immunosuppressive regimens. A new oral formulation, Neoral, has better intestinal absorption than previous compounds, even in the setting of poor bile flow. Neoral is of particular advantage in small infants, who typically require large doses of cyclosporine secondary to poor intestinal absorption [9•,10•].

Tacrolimus, which shares many characteristics with cyclosporine, is a more potent immunosuppressant. It has gained general acceptance as a preferred alternative to cyclosporine in most adult liver transplant centers. Because it is more potent, children treated with tacrolimus are less dependent on steroid administration, and may avoid steroid-related complications, such as growth failure and hypertension [11••]. Unfortunately, tacrolimus can be difficult to administer to smaller children because it is not available in an oral suspension. It does not cause gingival hyperplasia and hirsutism, as cyclosporine does, but it can cause anorexia and chronic gastrointestinal symptoms. Blood levels of tacrolimus in children are less predictable than those in adults, sometimes resulting in unexpected values within the toxic range. There is also a growing concern that posttransplant lymphoproliferative disease is more common in children who have received tacrolimus [12]. At this time, although opinions are mixed as to which drug is better for infants and children, cyclosporine appears preferable because of its ease of administration and predictable blood levels.

In addition to cyclosporine and tacrolimus, most regimens include an anti-metabolite such as Imuran or micophenolic acid and a corticosteroid regimen (Table 180-3). Some centers use induction with antilymphocyte antibodies, such as OKT3, before initiation of their immunosuppressive regimen.

Acute rejection is common following transplantation in children, with as many as 60% to 80% of children developing at least one episode of rejection. Rejection occurs most commonly within 2 to 6 weeks after transplantation. The common signs and symptoms of rejection in children include fever, tachypnea, abdominal pain, pleural effusion, and jaundice. Frequent moni-

Table 180-3. Standard Immunosuppression Regimens

Cyclosporine A	Whole blood HPLC 200–300 ng/mL	First 12 mo
	100–200 ng/mL	Second 12 mo
	50–100 ng/mL	Long-term
Methylprednisolone	2 mg/kg/d to 0.3 mg/kg/d at 1 mo	—
Azathioprine	1 mg/kg/d for 6 mo	—

It is standard to wean corticosteroids to an alternative day schedule at 18 months posttransplant.

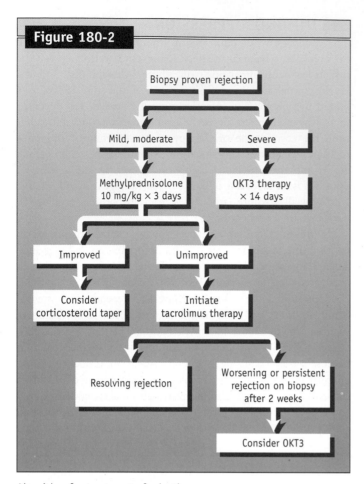

Figure 180-2

Algorithm for treatment of rejection.

toring of biochemical indicators of cholestasis allow the clinician to suspect rejection before physical signs become evident. Because the laboratory and physical signs are not specific for rejection, however, rejection always must be confirmed by histologic diagnosis. Rejection is treated in a step-wise fashion, with the first step being an intensified corticosteroid regimen. Most centers use boluses of 10 to 20 mg/kg/d of methylprednisolone followed by tapering doses of corticosteroids during the following week. If the intensified corticosteroid regimen does not result in improvement in the biochemical parameters and in the liver histology, the next step might be administration of an antilymphocyte preparation such as OKT3, or conversion from cyclosporine to tacrolimus. Figure 180-2 provides an algorithm for the treatment of rejection in the pediatric patient.

Many programs are attempting to avoid OKT3 therapy by conversion to tacrolimus for steroid-resistant rejection. Recent publications suggest a very high incidence of posttransplant lymphoproliferative disease in children who have been treated with both OKT3 and tacrolimus, and, therefore, many physicians are attempting to avoid antilymphocyte preparations completely. Although approximately 70% of children develop an episode of rejection, less than 10% eventually lose their liver to chronic or ongoing rejection.

Chronic rejection can occur either following an episode of refractory acute rejection or de novo, weeks to months after transplantation. Chronic rejection is characterized by slow progression of the clinical signs of cholestasis without many con-

stitutional symptoms. Liver biopsies rarely show much acute inflammation, except around intralobular bile ducts. Treatment of chronic rejection is controversial. Whereas tacrolimus has been shown to be effective in reversing chronic rejection in children, many children with chronic rejection improve even without alteration in their therapy. In this situation, however, the risks and problems involved with tacrolimus therapy seem to be acceptable compared with the potential for graft loss.

GRAFT SURVIVAL

Although 85% to 90% of children survive the first year after transplant, only 60% do so with the primary graft [13•]. Vascular complications are the most common cause (15%) of graft loss following transplantation in children. Many of the biliary complications that cause graft loss in long-term follow-up can be traced back to hepatic vascular problems in the initial posttransplant period. Although it seems obvious that anastomosis of very small vessels would result in a high vascular complication rate, what might be less obvious is the increased risk related to vascular extension grafts used in reduced-size and living related donor liver transplants [14].

POSTTRANSPLANT LYMPHOPROLIFERATIVE DISEASE

Posttransplant lymphoproliferative disease (PTLD) is an uncommon but serious event in children following liver transplantation [15••]. It is estimated to occur in approximately 5% of children treated with cyclosporine-based primary immunosuppression. With the use of newer drugs, such as tacrolimus, the incidence of this problem appears to be increasing, and it may approach 30% in children who are treated with combinations of tacrolimus and antilymphocyte preparations for refractory rejection. The spectrum of posttransplant lymphoproliferative disease ranges from a generally reversible polyclonal expansion of B cells to lymphoma. One of the more common presentation sites is in the head and neck region. Children should be assessed carefully for tonsillar hypertrophy and cervical lymphadenopathy. Children with a history of sinusitis are carefully followed for its resolution, because sinusitis can be the presenting sign of a PTLD in the maxillary sinuses. PTLD often presents with high fever and can be associated with hepatic allograft dysfunction and intestinal perforation from small bowel involvement; it can explode into multisystem disease over a period of days. The disease is caused by a clonal expansion of B cells, which are stimulated by the Epstein-Barr virus. Serologic investigation usually reveals high titers of IgG antibodies against the Epstein-Barr viral capsid antigen. Some of these cases, especially when polyclonal, respond to cessation or reduction of immunosuppression, whereas others require the addition of therapy with α-interferon or treatment with standard chemotherapy. Overall survival after PTLD is approximately 30%–50%. Survival appears to be improving, however, as clinicians are becoming more aggressive in treating monoclonal tumors with chemotherapy.

OUTPATIENT MANAGEMENT

The routine length of hospitalization after liver transplantation is approximately 3 weeks. After discharge, patients are monitored frequently to allow the clinician to recognize early signs and symptoms of rejection and infection. After the first month to 6 weeks, follow-up is weekly, and then, ultimately, monthly. Following the first year after transplant, laboratory tests are obtained quarterly, and children are examined twice a year to monitor growth and look for signs of chronic graft dysfunction. The immunosuppressive regimen is tapered slowly during the first year to 18 months after liver transplant. At that time, most children can be switched to alternate-day corticosteroids. Children receiving primary therapy with tacrolimus may tolerate complete corticosteroid withdrawal 6 months after transplant. Cyclosporine and tacrolimus doses also are weaned to approximately 50% of the initial values after the first year following transplant. Unfortunately, it is nearly impossible to predict which children will tolerate complete withdrawal of immunosuppressive therapy; some children who have had to be taken off all immunosuppressive therapy because of serious complications have not developed graft rejection, even in long-term follow-up. Future research will focus on ways in which the clinician can determine which children have developed graft tolerance and, therefore, are no longer in need of chronic immunosuppression.

Once the immunosuppressive regimen has been decreased somewhat, children can resume a routine schedule of immunizations (Table 180-4). At our program, immunizations are resumed at 6 months posttransplantation when azathioprine is discontinued and cyclosporine doses are tapered by 25%–30%. The intramuscular polio vaccine preparation should be substituted for the live attenuated vaccine. A very poor response rate may be seen to measles vaccine and varicella vaccine, but no serious consequences of immunization have been observed, even in children on standard levels of immunosuppression. Because both of these viruses are common community-acquired infections that pose a real threat to this population of children, immunization with follow-up titers to determine the protective effect of the immunization program is strongly recommended. In addition, most liver transplant recipients receive hepatitis B vaccine and yearly influenza vaccine. Children who have a history of asplenia or splenectomy also are immunized with Pneumovax.

Outpatient management also focuses on patient education. As children mature, they begin to assume more responsibility for administration of their own medications and become more concerned with their physical appearance. Because cyclosporine frequently causes hirsutism and gingival hyperplasia, these two issues are intimately related. Although the cosmetic complications become less problematic as cyclosporine doses are tapered, many children begin to experiment with noncompliance in an attempt to improve their physical appearance. The clinician must continue to emphasize the importance and necessity of these medications, even years after transplantation. Even children who are allowed to supervise their own schoolwork and social schedules should be carefully monitored by their parents to ensure that they are taking their medications. Adolescents and teenagers are particularly notorious for skipping medications, and noncompliance should be assumed whenever an older child presents with a late-onset rejection. The final objective of the outpatient visit is to evaluate chronic medical disabilities secondary to the trans-

Table 180-4. Recommended Immunization Schedule for Liver Transplant Recipients

Begin the following schedule **6 months after** the transplant

Hepatitis B	Month 7, month 9, month 12
DTP	Resume standard schedule
H. influenza type b	Resume standard schedule
Polio	Resume standard schedule Patient and siblings must receive IPV*
Measles, Mumps, Rubella	Month 7 if not previously protected; confirm vaccine response with titers†
Varicella	Month 7 if not previously protected; confirm vaccine response with titers+
Pneumovax	Required for patients with splenectomy or asplenia‡
Hepatitis A	Newly recommended vaccine for immunocompromised patients, including organ transplant recipients
Influenza	Yearly

* Inactivated polio vaccine

† Patients may experience low grade fever and vesicles at injection site.

‡ Penicillin prophylaxis also is recommended for these patients

plant. Most children have minimal medical complaints. A few children are plagued by chronic minor infections, such as otitis media, thrush, or *Clostridium difficile* colitis. Persistence of these infections occasionally warrants a decrease in immunosuppression to allow the patient to clear the pathogen naturally.

■ REFERENCES

Recently published papers of particular interest have been highlighted as follows:
* •   Of interest
* •• Of outstanding interest

1.• Ryckman FC, Ziegle MM, Pedersen SH, *et al.*: Liver transplantation in children. In *Liver Disease in Children.* Edited by Suchy FJ. St. Louis: CV Mosby; 1994:930–950
This recent book chapter reviews details of patient selection, pre- and postoperative management, and common posttransplant complications. It provides an excellent review and summary of the literature and also includes specifics of pediatric liver transplant experiences at the University of Cincinnati.

2.• Esquivel CO: Results: survival and quality of life after orthotopic liver transplantation in children. In *Transplantation of the Liver.* Edited by Busuttil RW, Klintmalm GB. Philadelphia: WB Saunders; 1996:236–249.
This book chapter reviews survival and outcomes after pediatric liver transplantation. This review compares survival by type of transplant, living related versus cadaveric, and includes recent patient survival data from international programs.

3.   Whitington PF, Balistreri WF: Pediatric OLT: indications, contraindications, and pretransplant management. *J Pediatr* 1991, 118:169–177.

4.   Whitington PF: Fulminant hepatic failure in children. In *Liver Disease in Children.* Edited by Suchy FJ. St. Louis:CV Mosby; 1994:180–213.

5.   Emond JC, Whitington PF, Thistlethwaite JR, *et al.*: Reduced-size OLT: use in management of children with chronic liver disease. *Hepatology* 1989, 10:867–872.

6.   Otte JB, De Ville de Goyet J, Sokal E, *et al.*: Size reduction of the donor liver is a safe way to alleviate the shortage of size-matched organs in pediatric liver transplantation. *Ann Surg* 1990, 211:146–157.

7.• Broelsch CE, Whitington PF, Emond JC, *et al.*: OLT in children from living related donors: surgical techniques and results. *Ann Surg* 1991, 214:428–439.
This article offers a summary of the original living related transplant (LRT) experience at the University of Chicago. The authors describe the surgical procedure for the donor and recipient and the results of the first 20 LRT operations performed in this country. Overall graft survival was 75% with short-term follow-up, and patient survival approached 85%. This publication led to acceptance and general application of LRT at most pediatric transplant centers.

8.   Alonso EM, Piper JB, Echols G, *et al.*: Allograft rejection in pediatric recipients of living related liver transplantation. *Hepatology* 1996, 23:40–43.

9.• Superina RA, Strong DK, Acal LA, *et al.*: Relative bioavailability of Sandimmune and Sandimmune Neoral in pediatric liver recipients. *Transplant Proc* 1994, 26:2979–2980.
This article provides a review of the bioavailability of Neoral in pediatric patients.

10.• Whitington PF, Alonso AM, Millis JM: Potential role of Neoral in pediatric liver transplantation. *Transplant Proc* 1996, 28:2267–2269.
Poor oral bioavailability is an obstacle to cyclosporine A use in small children. This paper summarizes the results of conversion from Sandimmune to Neoral in 14 stable pediatric OLT recipients. The data emphasize that, although many studies show improved bioavailability with Neoral, in this small series, trough levels were not significantly elevated when patients were converted at the same dose.

11.•• McDiarmid SV, Busuttil RW, Ascher NL, *et al.*: FK506 (tacrolimus) compared with cyclosporine for primary immunosuppression after pediatric liver transplantation. Results from the US Multicenter trial. *Transplantation* 1995, 59:530–536.
This paper summarizes the pediatric data from the multicenter US randomized trial of FK506 use in pediatric OLT recipients. Thirty patients received FK506 for primary immunosuppression. Graft survival was 70% in both the FK and cyclosporine groups. A total of 48% of the FK-treated patients were rejection-free versus 21% of the patients treated with cyclosporine. Drug toxicity was similar in both groups.

12. Cox KL, Lawrence-Miyasaki LS, Garcia-Kennedy R, *et al.*: An increased incidence of Epstein-Barr infection and lymphoproliferative disorder in young children on FK506 after liver transplantation. *Transplantation* 1995, 59:524–529.

13.• Langnas AN, Inagaki M, Bynon JS, *et al.*: Hepatic retransplantation in children. *Transplant Proc* 1993, 25:1921–1922.
This study reviews the results of liver transplantation performed in 191 children at the University of Nebraska. Retransplantation was required in 14 % for the indications of rejection (8%), vascular thrombosis (5%), and primary nonfunction (3%). Fifty-five percent of retransplants occurred within the first 30 days of the original transplant, and 1-year actuarial survival for retransplantation was 73%.

14. Millis JM, Seaman DS, Piper JB, *et al.*: Portal vein thrombosis and stenosis in pediatric liver transplantation. *Transplantation* 1996, 62:748–754.

15.•• Newell KA, Alonso EM, Whitington PF, *et al.*: Posttransplant lymphoproliferative disease in pediatric liver transplantation. *Transplantation* 1996, 62:370–375.
Eight percent of pediatric OLT recipients at the University of Chicago developed PTLD. Intensity of immunosuppression was found to be a major risk factor, with the combination of OKT3 and FK506 leading to an incidence of PTLD of 28%.

181 The Pancreas and the Gallbladder
Linda Shalon

Diseases of the pancreas and gallbladder are relatively uncommon in children. Symptoms often are nonspecific. Recognition of pancreatic and gallbladder disease, therefore, requires a high index of suspicion. This chapter supplies the clinical information necessary to identify and manage pancreatic and gallbladder conditions in childhood.

■ THE PANCREAS
Congenital Abnormalities of the Exocrine Pancreas
Annular Pancreas
Annular pancreas may become symptomatic at any age. The age of presentation is determined largely by the severity of duodenal obstruction and symptoms from coexistent anomalies [1]. In the Mayo Clinic experience with a review of the literature in English, 143 of 281 (51%) symptomatic patients with annular pancreas presented in childhood, 123 (86%) of them as neonates [2]. In affected newborns, feeding intolerance, emesis, and abdominal distention are common. In Kopelman's description of a study involving 138 neonates with congenital duodenal obstruction, annular pancreas was found either alone or in combination with other lesions

in 21 (15%) of the children [1]. The "double bubble" sign is a typical radiographic finding, and an upper gastrointestinal series (Fig. 181-1) may suggest partial or complete duodenal obstruction.

In older children, complete obstruction is uncommon. Milder symptoms of partial obstruction include nausea, recurrent vomiting, postprandial fullness, weight loss, and gastrointestinal bleeding [1,3•]. The presence of congenital anomalies, seen in 18 of 24 (75%) of patients in one series, may suggest the diagnosis of annular pancreas in patients with milder, more subtle symptoms [4]. The treatment of choice for symptomatic annular pancreas is a duodenoduodenostomy. Division of the annular ring is not recommended.

Ectopic Pancreas
Ectopic pancreas (pancreatic rest) usually is an incidental finding, and complications are uncommon (Fig. 181-2).

Agenesis, Hypoplasia, and Dysplasia
Clinical features. Complete pancreatic agenesis usually is fatal within the neonatal period. Partial pancreatic agenesis rarely is sympto-

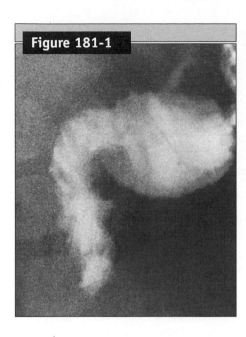

Figure 181-1

Barium study shows a fixed filling defect of the duodenum with proximal dilation resulting from annular pancreas in a 21-month-old child. (*From* Kopelman [1]; with permission.)

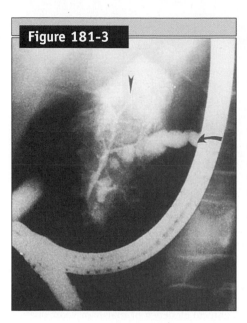

Figure 181-3

Pancreas divisum is seen in a 12-year-old patient with recurrent pancreatitis. The ventral pancreas is shown on actinogram (*straight arrow*). The dorsal pancreas is dilated, and there are multiple strictures (*curved arrow*). (*From* Guelrud *et al.* [5•]; with permission.)

matic, because patients have sufficient pancreatic tissue to maintain normal function. In contrast, children with pancreatic hypoplasia and dysplasia may present with malabsorption. Severely affected children require insulin. Congenital disorders associated with hypoplasia and dysplasia include Shwachman syndrome, sideroblastic bone marrow dysfunction, Johanson-Blizzard syndrome, hepatic and renal dysplasia, and chromosomal anomalies [1].

Diagnosis. A reduction in pancreatic size characteristic of complete or partial pancreatic agenesis can be determined by abdominal sonography, computed tomography (CT), or magnetic resonance imaging (MRI). In pancreatic hypoplasia, altered pancreatic tissue density resulting from replacement of exocrine structures by fat is evident on abdominal CT. Definitive diagnosis is made at surgery.

Pancreas Divisum

Pancreas divisum is the most common congenital abnormality of the pancreas, resulting from failure of the dorsal and ventral pancreatic ducts to join during embryogenesis; as a result, the main pancreatic duct drains through the accessory ampulla. Endoscopic

retrograde cholangiopancreatography (ERCP) demonstrates pancreas divisum by delineating the pancreatic ductal anatomy (Fig. 181-3) [5•]. Typical findings include a short duct of Wirsung, which ends in fine terminal branches, and lack of filling of the main pancreatic duct. Pancreas divisum was identified in two of 147 neonates or young infants who underwent an ERCP for evaluation of neonatal cholestasis—one with neonatal hepatitis, the other with biliary atresia [6]. Of 125 children older than 1 year of age who underwent ERCP for pancreatic or biliary symptoms, seven had pancreas divisum [6].

Symptoms include epigastric pain radiating through to the back. Although an association between pancreatitis and pancreas divisum has not been clearly established, six of 51 (12%) children undergoing ERCP for evaluation of recurrent pancreatitis had pancreas divisum [6]. In the rare child with pancreas divisum and disabling symptoms from recurrent acute pancreatitis, good results have been reported following endoscopic sphincterotomy of the minor papilla, with [7] or without [6] temporary stent placement in the dorsal pancreatic duct.

Hereditary Disorders of the Exocrine Pancreas
Shwachman Syndrome
Shwachman syndrome is the second most common inherited disorder of exocrine pancreatic dysfunction, following cystic fibrosis. Shwachman syndrome is an autosomal recessive disease with an incidence of one per 20,000 live births. In contrast to cystic fibrosis, which is caused by a defect in the pancreatic duct cells, the defect in Shwachman syndrome is acinar cell hypoplasia, which develops in utero. Universal features of Shwachman syndrome include exocrine pancreatic dysfunction and hematologic manifestations, including cyclic neutropenia (95%), anemia (50%), thrombocytopenia (50%), and pancytopenia [8••]. Additional characteristics include short stature, skeletal abnormalities (*eg*, metaphyseal dysostosis of the long bones or ribcage abnormalities; Fig. 181-4), life-threatening infections, and hepatomegaly. Leukemia is more common than in the general population. Most patients are diagnosed in infancy because of steatorrhea and growth failure, with or without hematologic abnormalities. Sonography often demon-

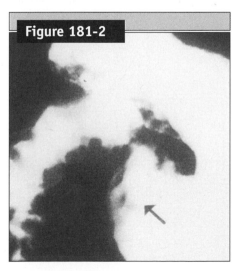

Figure 181-2

Typical radiographic appearance of ectopic pancreas (*arrow*) in the antrum of the stomach. Note the surrounding halo and central umbilication, which contains barium. (*From* Kopelman [1]; with permission.)

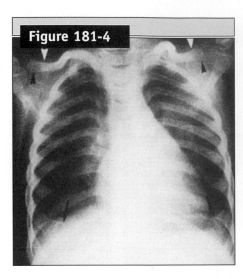

Figure 181-4

In this patient with Schwachman syndrome, a cup deformity of the ribs, which are widened, especially at the anterior ends (*arrows*), and widened clavicles (*arrowheads*) are seen. The humeral epiphyses are widened, with metaphyseal herniation. (*From* Berrocal *et al.* [9]; with permission.)

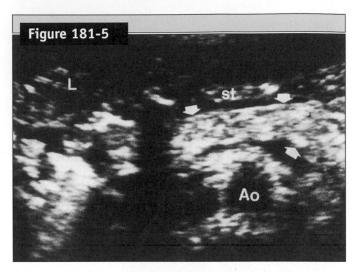

Figure 181-5

Sonogram of a patient with Schwachman syndrome shows a pancreas of normal size (*arrows*) with increased echogenicity, similar to that of the retroperitoneal fat. Ao—aorta; L—liver; st—stomach. (*From* Berrocal *et al.* [9]; with permission.)

strates a hyperechoic pancreas (Fig. 181-5) [9]. Although some patients may not have clinical evidence of malabsorption, quantitative pancreatic stimulation testing is abnormal in all patients. Despite persistent defects in enzyme secretion, 11 of 25 (45%) patients in one series showed moderate age-related improvements that resulted in pancreatic sufficiency [8••].

Johanson-Blizzard syndrome

Johanson-Blizzard syndrome (JBS) is a rare cause of pancreatic insufficiency. Affected children have a characteristic facial appearance (Fig. 181-6) [10]; other somatic features include short stature, congenital deafness, microcephaly, ectodermal scalp defects, hypothyroidism, dental abnormalities, imperforate anus, rectourogenital malformations, and psychomotor retardation. Like Shwachman syndrome, JBS is a primary defect in acinar cell function.

Pearson Syndrome

Pearson syndrome is characterized by pancreatic insufficiency and sideroblastic anemia. Additional features include muscle weakness and encephalopathy caused by muscle and liver involvement,

respectively. The defect on a molecular level appears to be the result of deletions in the mitochondrial genes that code for components of the mitochondrial respiratory chain [11].

Isolated Enzyme Deficiencies

Although uncommon, deficiencies in lipase, colipase, and combined lipase–colipase all have been described, as has amylase deficiency. Steatorrhea is the predominant clinical feature. In trypsinogen and enterokinase deficiency, severe hypoalbuminemia and edema are common. Therapeutic options include pancreatic enzyme replacement therapy and dietary modification. The diagnostic work-up for each deficiency has been described in an excellent review by Lerner *et al.* [3•].

Pancreatic Tumors

Pancreatic tumors are classified by the pancreatic cell of origin (Table 181-1).

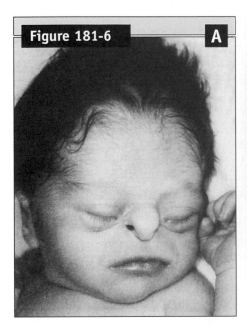
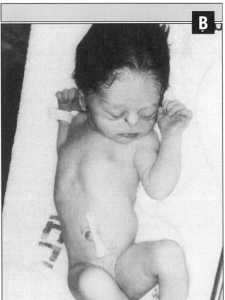

Figure 181-6 **A** **B**

Facial manifestations (*panel A*) and general appearance (*panel B*) characteristic of Johanson-Blizzard syndrome. (*From* Gershoni-Baruch *et al.* [10]; with permission.)

Table 181-1. Classification of Pancreatic Tumors

Location	Benign	Malignant
Exocrine pancreas	Duct adenoma	Acinar cell carcinoma
	Intraductal papilloma	Duct cell adenocarcinoma
	Mucinous cystadenoma	
		Pancreatoblastoma
Connective tissue	Hemangioendothelioma	Histiocytoma
	Histiocytoma	Leiomyosarcoma
	Lymphangioma	Lymphoma
	Neurilemoma	Neurilemoma
		Sarcoma
Secretory/endocrine	Gastrinoma (40%)	Gastrinoma (60%)
	Insulinoma (90%)	Insulinoma (10%)
	Islet cell adenoma	
	Islet cell hyperplasia	
	VIPoma	

From Kopelman [1]; with permission.

Tumors of the Exocrine Pancreas

Malignant tumors. In adults, pancreatic carcinoma has a poor prognosis, because 90% of cases are the result of a highly malignant, well-differentiated duct cell adenocarcinoma [12]. In children, however, less than 50% of pancreatic tumors result from pancreatic duct carcinoma. Half of the cases occur in children younger than 6 years of age. The remaining 50% of tumors are less aggressive and more easily treated. Jaundice caused by obstruction of the common bile duct is less common in children than in adults. The serum amylase, alkaline phosphatase, AST, ALT, and bilirubin may be abnormal, and anemia and hypoalbuminemia are not uncommon.

Techniques for diagnosis in children are similar to those for adults. Fine-needle aspiration biopsy under ultrasound guidance has been used successfully. However, laparotomy often is required to obtain adequate specimens for definitive histologic diagnosis.

Pancreatoblastoma occurs in children as young as 3 weeks of age. In contrast to the survival rates in patients with duct cell adenocarcinoma and acinar cell carcinoma, the prognosis for patients with pancreatoblastoma is very favorable. Aggressive surgical resection is the treatment of choice in children. The average survival time for nonresected patients is about 4 months, whereas that for resected patients is about 12 years [12].

Benign tumors. Serous (microcystic) cystadenomas, dermoid cysts, and intraductal papillomas are benign tumors of the exocrine pancreas. The evaluation, treatment, and management of these lesions in children are similar to that in adults. Mucinous cystadenomas are considered premalignant because of their capacity to undergo malignant transformation to mucinous cystadenocarcinoma. Pancreatic neoplasms can be distinguished from pancreatic pseudocyst by histologic examination: pancreatic neoplasms are encapsulated by an epithelial lining, whereas pancreatic pseudocysts are encapsulated by nonepithelial fibrous tissue.

Secretory and endocrine tumors. Endocrine pancreatic neoplasia includes both benign and malignant lesions, which may be either secretory or nonsecretory. These tumors account for a higher percentage of pancreatic tumors in children (20%) than in adults (5%) [12]. The most common pancreatic secretory symptom in children is hypoglycemia from hyperinsulinism associated with beta-cell adenoma or hyperplasia. In infants, diffuse adenomatosis is the most common cause of hyperinsulinism. These tumors usually are benign, but malignant transformation is possible. When medical management in infants fails, an aggressive surgical approach is justified because severe damage to the developing brain may result from hypoglycemia. Clinical features and treatments of other secretory and endocrine syndromes in children are similar to those in the adult population (see Chapter 140).

Nonexocrine and nonendocrine tumors. Nonexocrine and nonendocrine tumors of the pancreas are discussed in Chapter 140.

Pancreatitis

Acute Pancreatitis

Specific Etiologies. Acute pancreatitis occurs much less frequently in children than in adults, but it is not rare. Weizman *et al.* reported treating 61 children with pancreatitis over a 7-year period [13]. A history of abdominal trauma should be carefully considered, because minor injuries may be forgotten by the time of presentation (Fig. 181-7). Child abuse also should be considered. Children with recurrent attacks of pancreatitis require evaluation of pancreatic ductal anatomy. Guelrud *et al.* [5•] reported that anatomic abnormalities were found in most pediatric patients with recurrent episodes of pancreatitis. Other causes of pancreatitis in childhood include hemolytic uremic syndrome, Henoch-Schönlein purpura, Kawasaki syndrome, Reye's syndrome, mumps, rubella and other childhood viruses, and various metabolic disorders such as organic acidemias (Table 181-2).

Clinical presentation. The presentation in childhood often is more subtle than that in adults. The predominant symptoms are

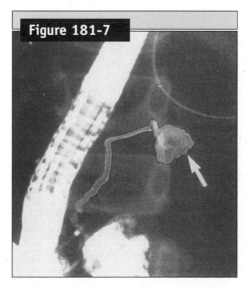

Figure 181-7

Transection of the main pancreatic duct is shown by endoscopic retrograde cholangiopancreatography, with extravasation of contrast into the lesser sac (*arrow*). (*From* Rescorla *et al.* [16]; with permission.)

Table 181-2. Causes of Acute Pancreatitis in Children

Obstruction/anatomic
 Choledocholithiasis, tumor, worms or foreign bodies, pancreas divisum with accessory duct obstruction, anomalous union of the pancreaticobiliary ducts, choledochal cyst, periampullary duodenal diverticula, hypertensive sphincter of Oddi

Toxins
 Ethanol, methanol, scorpion venom, organophosphorus insecticides

Drugs
 Azathioprine and mercaptopurine, didanosine, valproic acid, estrogens, tetracycline, metronidazole, nitrofurantoin, pentamidine, furosemide, sulfonamides, methyldopa, cimetidine, ranitidine, sulindac, acetaminophen, erythromycin, salicylates, L-asparaginase

Trauma
 Blunt abdominal injury, iatrogenic surgery, ERCP with or without sphincterotomy or sphincter manometry

Metabolic abnormalities
 Hypertriglyceridemia, hypercalcemia, organic acidemia, refeeding syndrome, malnutrition: juvenile tropical pancreatitis, cystic fibrosis

Infection
 Parasitic: ascariasis; clonorchiasis; malaria
 Viral: Mumps, rubella, hepatitis A, B, C; coxsackievirus B; echovirus; adenovirus; cytomegalovirus; varicella; Epstein-Barr virus; HIV
 Bacterial: mycoplasma, *Campylobacter jejuni; Mycobacterium tuberculosis; Mycobacterium avium–intracellulare; Legionella;* leptospirosis

Vascular abnormalities
 Ischemia, Kawasaki syndrome, systemic lupus erythematosus, polyarteritis nodosa, malignant hypertension
 Vasculitis: hemolytic uremic syndrome, Henoch-Schönlein purpura

Miscellaneous abnormalities
 Penetrating peptic ulcer, Crohn's disease, Reye's syndrome, hypothermia, familial pancreatitis

ERCP—endoscopic retrograde cholangiopancreatography.
Adapted from Fox [13].

---

nonspecific. Abdominal pain often is absent or nonepigastric in location. Pain radiating to the back is uncommon in children.

Diagnosis. The laboratory evaluation in children is similar to that in adults. The evaluation should include a sweat test for cystic fibrosis and a variety of urine and blood studies for metabolic disorders. The most useful imaging modality in children is abdominal sonography (Fig. 181-8). If interposed bowel gas obscures visualization of the pancreas on sonographic examination, abdominal computed tomography (CT) is indicated. CT with intravenous contrast can detect pancreatic necrosis. Conventional magnetic resonance imaging (MRI) offers the advantages of CT without exposure to ionizing radiation, but usually requires sedation. In children, as in adults, ERCP provides the most accurate delineation of pancreatic and biliary duct anatomy [15•,16,17•]. Pediatric indications for diagnostic ERCP with pancreatitis include the following: 1) pancreatitis that does not resolve after 1 month; 2) recurrent pancreatitis; 3) persistent elevation of pancreatic enzymes; 4) the first episode of pancreatitis in a child with a family history of hereditary pancreatitis; 5) pancreatitis following liver transplantation; 6) pancreatitis associated with cystic fibrosis; 7) pancreatic duct dilatation; and 8) pancreatitis in association with gallstones, pancreatic or biliary duct obstruction, or trauma [16]. The development of pediatric duodenoscopes has made it possible to use ERCP in children of all ages. The Olympus (Olympus Corporation of America, Melville, NY) duodenoscope with an outside diameter of 8.0 mm has been used successfully in infants younger than 1 year of age. The standard duodenoscope (11.0 mm) is appropriate for children older than 1 year of age.

Management. Adequate fluid replacement is essential. Requirements are based on body weight, surface area, or both in the pediatric patient. In small children, correction of intravas-

cular fluid and electrolyte losses, as well as the estimation of ongoing requirements, must be made on an individual basis, with frequent adjustments. Like adults, pediatric patients often require albumin infusions, total parenteral nutrition, and appropriate pain medication, which may be best achieved through patient-controlled analgesia (PCA).

Nutritional therapy is of primary importance in children with pancreatitis because of added requirements based on growth. Despite the widely recommended strategy of "putting the pancreas to rest," there is no conclusive evidence that inter-

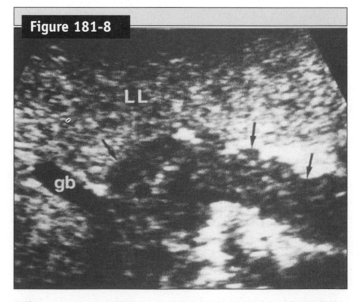

Figure 181-8

Diffuse acute pancreatitis is seen in a 5-year-old girl with AIDS. A globally enlarged pancreas with diffuse decreased echogenicity and irregular borders (*arrows*) is visualized by ultrasound. Definition of the splenic vein is poor. gb—gallbladder; LL—left lobe of the liver. (*From* Berrocal *et al.* [9]; with permission.)

rupting enteral feeding has a positive effect on the clinical outcome of pancreatitis. Both enteral feedings and total parenteral nutrition may be required [18].

The principles of management in children are the same as those in adults. Currently, there are insufficient data in children to recommend peritoneal lavage in severe pancreatitis or early surgical debridement for necrotizing pancreatitis [13•].

Children with acute pancreatitis are at risk for developing the same complications as adults. Although no prognostic scoring system has been developed specifically for children, hemorrhagic or necrotic pancreatitis is associated with a poor outcome. In children, mortality usually is limited to patients with a multisystem disorder, and rarely occurs in those with isolated acute pancreatitis. If no complications are encountered, the pancreatitis usually resolves in less than 1 week.

Chronic Pancreatitis

Etiology. The etiology of chronic pancreatitis in children often is unclear. Calcific and obstructive chronic pancreatitis are distinct entities. Calcific pancreatitis is relatively uncommon in childhood, whereas in adults it is the most common form of chronic pancreatitis, often associated with ethanol ingestion. Causes of calcific pancreatitis in children include juvenile tropical pancreatitis, hereditary pancreatitis, hypercalcemia, hyperlipidemia, and cystic fibrosis. Chronic obstructive pancreatitis usually is caused by trauma, congenital anomalies, sphincter of Oddi dysfunction, renal disease, sclerosing cholangitis, and idiopathic fibrosing pancreatitis. About one third of cases of chronic pancreatitis in children are idiopathic [18]. Hereditary pancreatitis, which leads to chronic pancreatitis, is associated with an increased incidence of pancreatic adenocarcinoma.

Clinical features. Recurrent bouts of abdominal pain may be severe or insidious. Self-restriction of food to decrease abdominal pain or malabsorption resulting from pancreatic exocrine insufficiency may result in weight loss and growth failure. Diabetes mellitus also may complicate chronic pancreatitis because of the destruction of islet cells.

Diagnosis. The diagnostic tools for children are similar to those used in adults. However, normal laboratory values in children may be different from those in adults. Abdominal sonography is useful in determining the presence of a pseudocyst (Fig. 181-9), and ERCP may demonstrate abnormalities of the ductal system.

Management. The treatment rationale for children with chronic pancreatitis is similar to that for adults. Controlling pain, minimizing nutrient malabsorption, providing adequate nutritional support, replacing pancreatic enzymes, and using insulin when necessary must all be considered. A low-fat diet should be avoided in the underweight or malnourished child, especially in light of the unproven efficacy of low-fat diets in controlling pain. There are only sporadic reports of the use of the somatostatin analogue octreotide in children [19]. Endoscopic sphincterotomy or biliary stent placement may provide relief of pain or biliary duct obstruction. Treatment is indicated for pancreatic pseudocysts that remain present for more than 6 weeks, are

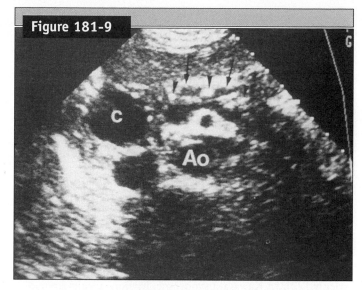

Figure 181-9

In this patient with chronic pancreatitis, the sonogram shows a small pancreas (*arrows*) with calcium deposition (*arrowheads*) and a pseudocyst (c) at the level of the pancreatic head. Ao—aorta. (*From* Berrocal *et al.* [9]; with permission.)

symptomatic, or exceed 4 cm in diameter. Therapeutic options include operative drainage procedures or ultrasound-guided percutaneous endoscopic approaches. When medical treatment fails, surgical intervention is an option for patients with pancreatic ductal dilatation or for those with severe debilitating pain.

Clinical course. The clinical course of chronic pancreatitis in children is extremely variable and is influenced largely by its cause. Even in patients with hereditary pancreatitis, pain may resolve spontaneously, without surgical intervention. Moir *et al.* reported that surgery for hereditary pancreatitis resulted in complete symptomatic relief in 43% of patients. Between 75% and 90% of patients reported excellent to good health at long-term follow-up, whether or not they underwent surgery [20••,21].

■ GALLBLADDER
Congenital Anomalies of the Gallbladder

Agenesis of the gallbladder occurs in 1 per 7500 to 10,000 individuals and may be associated with the formation of biliary tract calculi [22]. Agenesis occurs as an isolated anomaly or with bicuspid aortic valves, anencephaly, cerebral aneurysms, genitourinary anomalies, and imperforate anus. Hypoplasia of the gallbladder is associated with cystic fibrosis, trisomy 18, and Alagille's syndrome. Ectopic gastric mucosa in the gallbladder may cause inflammation and abdominal pain. The floating gallbladder is suspended from the undersurface of the liver by mesentery and carries a risk of torsion. Double or triple gallbladders, multiple-chamber gallbladders, and malpositioned gallbladders have been described.

Acalculous Gallbladder Disease
Hydrops of the Gallbladder

Gallbladder hydrops is associated with a variety of conditions, but most commonly occurs in children with Kawasaki syndrome, in whom the incidence ranges from 5% to 20% of

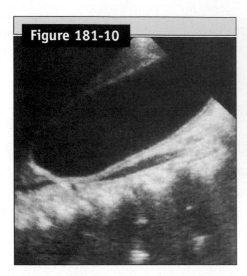

Figure 181-10

This child with Kawasaki disease has gallbladder hydrops. A longitudinal sonogram with the child supine shows a markedly distended gallbladder. (*From* Haller [24]; with permission.)

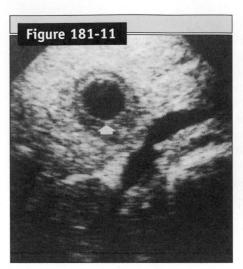

Figure 181-11

Ultrasound shows a distended gallbladder and a markedly thickened gallbladder wall (*arrow*). When a patient presents with right upper quadrant abdominal pain, acute acalculous cholecystitis should be strongly suspected. (*From* Heubi and Lewis [23]; with permission.)

patients [22]. In Kawasaki syndrome, hydrops results from cystic duct obstruction caused by vasculitis of the gallbladder wall. Pathologic examination has demonstrated perivascular leukocytic infiltration with vascular congestion in the gallbladder wall and sterile bile. In neonates, conditions associated with gallbladder hydrops include sepsis, α_1-antitrypsin deficiency, and fasting. Patients receiving total parenteral nutrition also develop hydrops. In infants and older children, mesenteric adenitis, viral hepatitis, streptococcal pharyngitis, staphylococcal infection, Henoch-Schönlein purpura, hypokalemia, Sjögren's syndrome, and nephrotic syndrome have been described in association with hydrops.

In children, hydrops typically causes abdominal pain and a right upper quadrant mass. Vomiting and fever are common. Sonography shows a markedly distended anechoic gallbladder and a normal biliary tree (Fig. 181-10) [23]. Management is supportive, because perforation of the gallbladder is extremely rare. Gallbladder function usually returns to normal after the distention resolves. Failure to resolve or clinical deterioration suggests the possibility of acalculous cholecystitis.

Acute Acalculous Cholecystitis

Acute acalculous cholecystitis may occur at any time during childhood, including the neonatal period. Predisposing factors are found in 50% of pediatric cases [24••]. Contributing factors include gallbladder stasis, cystic duct obstruction, sphincter of Oddi dysfunction, and gallbladder hypoperfusion. The clinical presentation is similar to that of calculous cholecystitis. Recognition of acute acalculous cholecystitis may be delayed if the patient is otherwise well.

Sonographic features include distention of the gallbladder, thickening of the gallbladder wall, and echogenic intraluminal debris (Fig. 181-11). Cholescintigraphy typically demonstrates nonvisualization of the gallbladder. Cholecystectomy is recommended.

Tumors of the Gallbladder

Gallbladder neoplasms are rare in children. Adenomatous polyps of the gallbladder have been reported, sometimes in association with Peutz-Jeghers syndrome. Resection is required because of the potential for malignant transforma-

tion. Rhabdomyosarcoma arising from the gallbladder and biliary tree also has been reported; it is the most common biliary tract malignancy in childhood and has a very poor prognosis [25•]. Obstructive jaundice is unusual in the pediatric age group.

Calculous Gallbladder Disease [22]

Incidence of Cholelithiasis

The incidence of gallstones increases with age in the pediatric population [26]. Gallstones have been detected in utero, and they are not uncommon in infancy. The incidence of cholelithiasis in infancy and childhood has not been documented. Among 1500 Italian children aged 6 to 19 years screened with ultrasound, gallstones were discovered in two (0.13%). In infancy, boys are affected more often than girls, whereas the incidence is negligible in adolescent males. In females, the incidence increases significantly during puberty (Fig. 181-12).

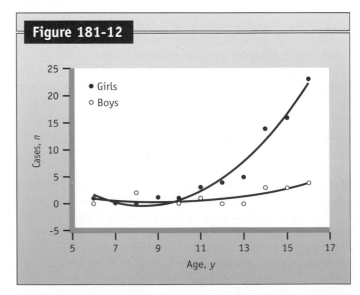

Figure 181-12

Incidence of gallstones illustrated by age and sex in 89 hospitalized Swedish patients under 16 years of age. Boys showed a slow increase with age. Girls had a similar slow increase until the age of 10 to 11 years, after which the rise became exponential. (*From* Shaffer [27]; with permission.)

Figure 181-13

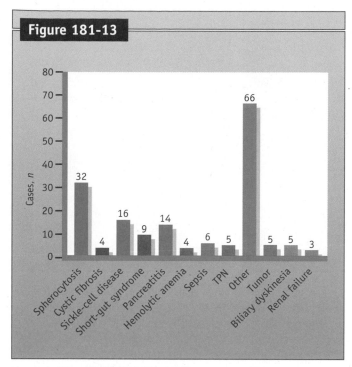

The underlying disorders and conditions associated with gallstones in infants and children (*n*=169). TPN—total parenteral nutrition. (*From* Grosfeld *et al.* [30]; with permission.)

Table 181-3. Associated Conditions of Cholelithiasis by Age*

0–12 mo, *n*=54	1–5 y, *n*=19	6–21 y, *n*=358
None (36%)	Hepatobiliary disease (29%)	Pregnancy (37%)
TPN (29%)	Abdominal surgery (21%)	Hemolytic disease (23%)
Abdominal surgery (29%)	Artificial heart valve (14%)	Obesity (8%)
Sepsis (15%)	None (14%)	Abdominal surgery (5%)
Bronchopulmonary dysplasia (13%)	Malabsorption (7%)	None (3%)
Hemolytic disease (6%)		Hepatobiliary disease (3%)
Malabsorption (6%)		TPN (3%)
Necrotizing enterocolitis (6%)		Malabsorption (3%)
Hepatobiliary disease (4%)		

*A total of 693 patients, 262 of unknown age.

TPN—total parental nutrition.

Data from Friesen and Roberts [28].

Gallstone Composition

Friesen *et al.* [27] reported that 66% of their patients with gall-stones had pigmented stones, and 17% had cholesterol stones. In 11%, the composition was unknown. Conditions associated with pigment stone formation include hemolytic disease, ileal resection, parenteral nutrition, cirrhosis with cholestasis, and *Ascaris lumbricoides* infection [28]. Cholesterol gallstones are associated with obesity, ileal resection, jejunoileal bypass, ileal Crohn's disease, cystic fibrosis, and pregnancy.

Etiology of Gallstone Formation

In children, gallstone disease usually is associated with a predisposing condition (Fig. 181-13) [29]. The causes of pediatric gallstone disease are related to the age of the patient (Table 181-3). Additional associations of interest in pediatric patients include urinary tract infection, cyclosporin therapy, and pseudo-hypoaldosteronism. Idiopathic cholelithiasis is more common in younger children, with a frequency as high as 54% in affected neonates and children [30].

Clinical Features

Clinical symptoms vary according to the age of the child. The biliary colic typical of cholelithiasis in adult patients is seen in pediatric patients over 15 years of age, but not necessarily in younger patients. In children younger than 5 years of age, symptoms tend to be nonspecific, pain is not well localized, and there often is no association between painful episodes and ingestion of fatty foods. Moreover, chronic cholecystitis, which is more common than acute cholecystitis in children, may present with vague recurrent right upper quadrant or epigastric pain [28]. In young children, irritability after eating suggests the possibility of gallstones. Whereas acute cholecystitis may cause signs in

children similar to those in adults, in chronic cholecystitis, the physical examination in children often is normal.

Diagnosis of Cholelithiasis

Laboratory tests often are normal, but there may be a leukocytosis and a left shift. In children with choledocholithiasis, liver tests may be abnormal. Gallstone pancreatitis results in elevations of the serum amylase and lipase concentrations.

The incidence of radiopaque gallstones is much higher in children (35% to 50%) than in adults (15%) [27]. Radiopaque stones occur in only 15% of adolescents with cholesterol stones, but they are present in 50% of patients with pigmented stones from hemolytic disorders [30••].

In children and adolescents, ultrasonography is the procedure of choice for diagnosing cholelithiasis [31]. In children, a thickened gallbladder wall is defined as one that is thicker than 3 mm. Cholescintigraphy is the preferred method for diagnosing acute cholecystitis.

Therapy

Indications for treatment. The natural history of asymptomatic gallstones in the pediatric populations has not been described. Each patient should, therefore, be considered individually. In neonates and infants, there appears to be a high rate of spontaneous resolution of asymptomatic gallstones (Fig. 181-14). McEvoy *et al.* found that none of the children in whom cholelithiasis had been detected prenatally (Fig. 181-15) developed symptoms during follow-up after birth [32]. Morad *et al.* noticed spontaneous resolution of gallstones in 13 of 14 patients in whom gallstones were diagnosed incidentally in the neonatal period [33•]. Calcified gallstones are unlikely to resolve spontaneously. Interventional management is reserved for neonates and infants with calcified or symptomatic stones or those with underlying lithogenic disorders. In neonates and infants with noncalcified or asymptomatic gall-

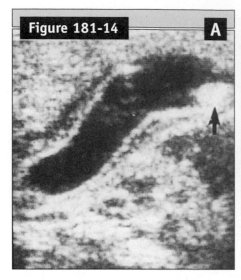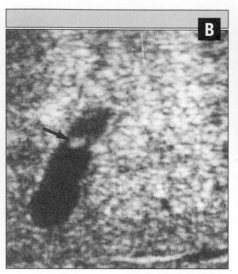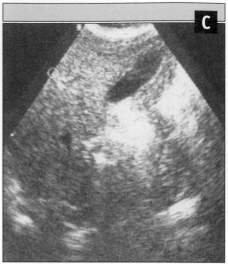

Ultrasonographic findings of right abdomen in an infant with gallstones. (**A**) At the age of 60 hours, a mobile stone (*arrow*) is observed in the gallbladder. (**B**) At 6 weeks, the gallbladder stone (*arrow*) still is present but is significantly smaller. (**C**) Examination at the age of 3 months shows complete disappearance of the gallstone. (*From* Morad *et al.* [34]; with permission.)

stones, expectant management for at least 12 months appears warranted.

Because most patients with sickle cell anemia and gallstones develop symptoms if the gallstones are left untreated, elective cholecystectomy has been recommended to avoid complications [28]. Cholecystectomy for asymptomatic gallstones also is usually recommended for patients with thalassemia major or hereditary spherocytosis who undergo therapeutic splenectomy. Elective cholecystectomy in otherwise healthy children also may be reasonable for the treatment of larger stones (>2 cm in diameter), because these stones are less likely to pass spontaneously and may carry a greater risk of carcinoma of the gallbladder.

Elective cholecystectomy should be encouraged for children with symptomatic gallstones. Surgery for neonates and infants with symptomatic gallstones, however, must be considered on an individual basis, because even infants with bile duct obstruction have a high rate (29%) of spontaneous resolution of gallstones [30].

Therapeutic modalities. Laparoscopic cholecystectomy has been performed successfully in many pediatric patients [28,34,35]. In the rare poor-surgical-risk patient (*eg*, a patient with cystic fibrosis with severe pulmonary compromise), alternatives to cholecystectomy include cholecystotomy for obstructive gallstone disease and gallstone dissolution with ursodeoxycholic acid. Lithotripsy is not approved for use in children.

Clinically stable patients with choledocholithiasis (common duct stones) are treated initially with antibiotics. As in adults, therapeutic options include ERCP or bile duct exploration with removal of the stone and the gallbladder. Combined endoscopic sphincterotomy and common stone extraction followed by laparoscopic cholecystectomy have been performed successfully even in infants [16].

■ REFERENCES

Recently published papers of particular interest have been highlighted as follows:
- • Of interest
- •• Of outstanding interest

1. Kopelman HR: The pancreas: congenital anomalies. In *Pediatric Gastrointestinal Disease*, edn 2. Edited by Walker WA, Durie PR, Hamilton JR, *et al.* St. Louis: Mosby; 1996:1427–1436.

2. Kiernan PD, ReMine SG, Kiernan PC, *et al.*: Annular pancreas: Mayo Clinic experience from 1957 to 1976 with review of the literature. *Arch Surg* 1980, 115:46–50.

3.• Lerner A, Branski D, Lebenthal E: Pancreatic diseases in children. *Pediatr Clin North Am* 1996, 43:125–157.
A recent, broad overview of various pancreatic conditions that occur in children, including congenital abnormalities, hereditary disorders, acute pancreatitis, and hereditary pancreatitis, and treatment of pancreatic insufficiency.

4. Merrill JR, Raffensperger JG: Pediatric annular pancreas: twenty years experience. *J Pediatr Surg* 1976, 11:921–925.

5.• Guelrud M, Mujica C, Jaen D, *et al.*: The role of ERCP in the diagnosis and treatment of idiopathic recurrent pancreatitis in children and adolescents. *Gastrointest Endosc* 1994, 40:428–436.
Endoscopic retrograde cholangiopancreatography was successfully performed in 98% of 51 pediatric patients, ages 1 to 18 years, for evaluation of recurrent pancreatitis. Thirty-four (68%) patients had anatomic findings that con-

Figure 181-15

In this fetus with a gallstone, a prenatal sonogram of the fetal abdomen shows an echogenic shadowing focus in the gallbladder (*arrow*). This child was followed up postnatally until the stone ultimately resolved. The child had no associated risk factors for cholelithiasis. (*From* Haller [24]; with permission.)

tributed to the pancreatitis, and three (6%) had findings suggestive of sphincter of Oddi dysfunction. Eighteen of the 37 (49%) patients with ductal abnormalities underwent endoscopic therapy. The results of the endoscopic therapy are discussed in detail.

6. Guelrud M: The incidence of pancreas divisum in children. *Gastrointest Endosc* 1996, 43:83–84.

7. Lemmel T, Hawes R, Sherman S, *et al.*: Endoscopic evaluation and therapy of recurrent pancreatitis and pancreatobiliary pain in the pediatric population [abstract]. *Gastrointest Endosc* 1994, 40:A54.

8.•• Mack DR, Forstner GG, Wilschanski M, *et al.*: Shwachman syndrome: exocrine pancreatic dysfunction and variable phenotypic expression. *Gastroenterology* 1996, 111:1593–1602.
The phenotypes of 25 patients with Shwachman syndrome is described. Pancreatic acinar dysfunction was an invariable abnormality, but 45% of patients developed pancreatic sufficiency over time. Neutropenia was the most common hematologic abnormality (88%), but leukopenia, thrombocytopenia, and anemia also occurred frequently. Prognosis with respect to phenotypic features is discussed.

9. Berrocal T, Prieto C, Pastor I, *et al.*: Sonography of pancreatic disease in infants and children. *Radiographics* 1995, 15:301–313.

10. Gershoni-Baruch R, Lerner A, Braun J, *et al.*: Johanson-Blizzard syndrome: clinical spectrum and further delineation of the syndrome. *Am J Med Genet* 1990, 35:546–551.

11. Sano T, Ban K, Kobayshi, *et al.*: Molecular and genetic analyses of two patients with Pearson's marrow-pancreas syndrome. *Pediatr Res* 1993, 34:105–110.

12. Kopelman HR: Tumors of the pancreas. In *Pediatric Gastrointestinal Disease*, edn 2. Edited by Walker WA, Durie PR, Hamilton JR, *et al.* St. Louis: Mosby; 1996:1494–1501.

13. Weizman Z, Durie P: Acute pancreatitis in childhood. *J Pediatr* 1988, 113:24–29.

14. Fox V: Acute pancreatitis. *International Seminars in Paediatric Gastroenterology and Nutrition* 1995, 4:2–7.

15. Steinberg W, Tenner S: Acute pancreatitis. *N Engl J Med* 1994, 330:1198–1210.

16. Rescorla FJ, Plumley DA, Sherman S, *et al.*: The efficacy of early ERCP in pediatric pancreatic trauma. *J Pediatr Surg* 1995, 30:336–340.

17. Werlin S: Endoscopic retrograde cholangiopancreatography in children. *Gastrointest Endosc Clin North Am* 1994, 4:161–178.

18. Guelrud M: Endoscopic retrograde cholangiopancreatography in children. *The Gastroenterologist* 1996, 4:81–97.

19.• Freeman KB, Adelson JW: Chronic pancreatitis. *International Seminars in Paediatric Gastroenterology and Nutrition* 1995, 4:8–15.
This recent, in-depth review of chronic pancreatitis in children discusses pathology and histology, specific disorders, clinical features, radiologic studies, treatment, and indications for surgery and general types of surgery.

20. Mulligan C, Howell C, Hatley R, *et al.*: Conservative management of pediatric pancreatic pseudocyst using octreotide acetate. *Am Surg* 1995, 61:206–209.

21.• Konzen KM, Perrault J, Moir C, *et al.*: Long-term follow-up of young patients with chronic hereditary or idiopathic pancreatitis. *Mayo Clin Proc* 1993, 68:449–453.
The clinical courses of 42 patients with hereditary pancreatitis and 28 patients with idiopathic pancreatitis were compared. Initial clinical symptoms were similar for both groups, except that vomiting was more frequent in patients with hereditary pancreatitis. Complications, including pseudocysts, steatorrhea, ascites, portal hypertension, unrelenting pain, and diabetes occurred more often and required surgical intervention more often in patients with hereditary pancreatitis.

22. Moir CR, Konzen KM, Perrault J: Surgical therapy and long-term follow-up of childhood hereditary pancreatitis. *J Pediatr Surg* 1992, 27:282–287.

23. Heubi JE, Lewis LC: Diseases of the gallbladder in infancy, childhood, and adolescence. In *Liver Disease in Children*. Edited by Suchy FJ. St. Louis: Mosby; 1994:605–621.

24. Haller JO: Sonography of the biliary tract in infants and children. *AJR Am J Roentgenol* 1991,157:1051–1058.

25.•• Tsakayannis DE, Kozakewich HPW, Lillehei CW: Acalculous cholecystitis in children. *J Pediatr Surg* 1996, 31:127–131.
In this paper 25 children (ages 2 months to 20 years) with acalculous cholecystitis are described. All of the children presented with fever, and a right upper quadrant mass was present in six (23%). Two distinct forms were identified: acute (duration of symptoms <1 month) and chronic (duration > 3 months). The differences in clinical settings and presentations between the two groups are described.

26. Ruyman FB, Raney RB, Crist WM, *et al.*: Rhabdomyosarcoma of the biliary tree in childhood: a report from the Intergroup Rhabdomyosarcoma Study. *Cancer* 1985, 56:575.

27. Shaffer EA: Gallbladder disease. In *Pediatric Gastrointestinal Disease*, edn 2. Edited by Walker WA, Durie PR, Hamilton JR, *et al.* St. Louis: Mosby; 1996:1399–1421.

28. Friesen CA, Roberts CC: Cholelithiasis: clinical characteristics in children. *Clin Pediatr* 1989, 28:294–298.

29. Rescoria FJ, Grosfeld JL: Cholecystitis and cholelithiasis in children. *Semin Pediatr Surg* 1992,1:98–106.

30. Grosfeld JL, Rescorla FJ, Skinner MA, *et al.*: The spectrum of biliary tract disorders in infants and children. *Arch Surg* 1994, 129:513–520.

31.•• Debray D, Parente D, Gauthier F, *et al.*: Cholelithiasis in infancy: a study of 40 cases. *J Pediatr* 1993, 122:385–391.
Experience with 40 infants less than 1 year of age with cholelithiasis was reported. Based on the observed outcomes, management suggestions included 1) conservative management, if no clinical, biochemical, or radiologic signs of common bile duct obstruction are present; 2) urgent treatment in infants with common bile duct obstruction and signs of sepsis; 3) a period of observation if no signs of infection are present; and 4) surgical repair when lithiasis is associated with strictures or congenital anatomic abnormalities of the common bile duct.

32. Stephens CG, Scott RB: Cholelithiasis in sickle cell anemia. *Arch Intern Med* 1980, 140:648–651.

33.• McEvoy CF, Suchy FJ: Biliary tract disease in children. *Pediatr Clin North Am* 1996, 43:75–99.
A recent review of the more common neonatal cholangiopathies and unique aspects of biliary disorders in older children.

34. Morad Y, Ziv N, Merlob P: Incidental diagnosis of asymptomatic neonatal cholelithiasis: case report and literature review. *J Perinatol* 1995, 15:314–317.

35.• Holcomb GW: Laparoscopic cholecystectomy. *Semin Pediatr Surg* 1993, 2:159–167.
Laparoscopic cholecystectomy was performed in 25 children without intraoperative or postoperative complications. The technical approach and the essential modifications made for the pediatric patient are described; numerous illustrations are included.

36. Tagge EP, Othersen HB Jr, Jackson SM, *et al.*: Impact of laparoscopic cholecystectomy on the management of cholelithiasis in children with sickle cell disease. *J Pediatr Surg* 1994, 29:209–213.

182 Failure to Thrive
Anupama Chawla

Failure to thrive is common in infancy. It accounts for an estimated 1% to 5% of pediatric tertiary care hospital admissions [1], and more affected children are managed on an outpatient basis [2]. Nonorganic failure to thrive accounts for 50% of all cases, organic diseases for 25%, and mixed causes for approximately 25% [3]. Organic diseases often are compounded by psychosocial factors [4].

No single definition exists for failure to thrive, reflecting the complexity and diversity of its presentations. In most infants, the term *failure to thrive* describes infants with weight lower than the expected weight for measured length [5]; use of this criterion alone, however, could lead to the inclusion of healthy infants. For a child to be labeled as having failure to thrive, the assessment must be based on several growth points plotted on the standard age- and sex-appropriate growth charts (Fig. 182-1). To be characterized as having failure to thrive, a child must meet at least two of the following criteria:

1. Weight progressing in a downward deviation across at least two major percentile lines on the standard chart
2. Weight less than 90% of the expected weight for measured length
3. Weight below the third percentile of expected weight for age
4. Actual weight loss.

ORGANIC FAILURE TO THRIVE

The differential diagnosis of organic failure to thrive encompasses almost every pediatric subspecialty. The most common organ systems involved are the cardiac, endocrine, gastrointestinal, and renal tracts (Table 182-1).

NONORGANIC FAILURE TO THRIVE

Nonorganic failure to thrive, also described as *environmental failure to thrive*, is the result of psychosocial factors, most commonly impaired interaction between the caregiver and infant or parental deprivation [6]. The infant as well as the caregiver appears to contribute significantly to this dysfunctional relationship. Parental issues (*eg*, postpartum depression, a physically or emotionally absent father, marital stress), characteristics of the child (*eg*, temperament, neurologic integrity), and environmental conditions (*eg*, inadequate support network, poverty) [7] all contribute to failure to thrive.

ERRONEOUS DIAGNOSIS OF FAILURE TO THRIVE

The size of an infant at birth is related more to maternal and intrauterine influences than to genetic factors. Growth patterns erroneously labeled as failure to thrive include growth characteristics of infants born with intrauterine growth retardation, constitutional growth delay, familial short stature, and the pattern noted in infants who are breast fed [8•,9••].

In the first years of life, there often is a change in growth velocity, in both weight and height, as the result of genetic patterns. Some of this change also may result from changes in feeding. For instance, it is not uncommon to see a decrease in weight velocity and height velocity once an infant is weaned from the bottle. Caloric intake tends to diminish at this time because milk intake from a cup is less than that from a bottle. Variations in growth patterns of otherwise healthy children whose caloric intake is appropriate do not require laboratory evaluation or nutritional rehabilitation.

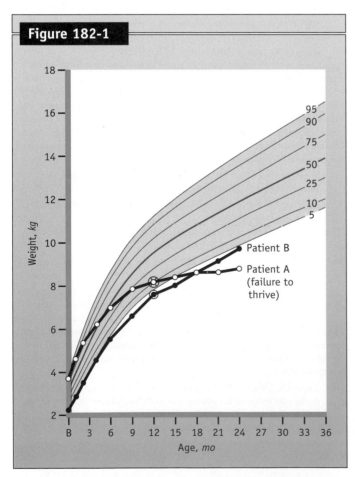

Figure 182-1

A standard growth chart specific for age and sex illustrates the importance of evaluating the growth trend rather than weight measurement at a single point. At 12 months, patient A weighs more than patient B but is falling off the growth curve and is failing to thrive. Patient B is gaining weight steadily and is most likely normal.

Table 182-1. Organic Causes of Failure to Thrive

Oropharyngeal
  Palatal anomaly
  Pierre Robin syndrome
Central nervous system
  Cerebral palsy
  Fetal alcohol syndrome
  Intracranial tumors, cysts,
    hematoma
Cardiac
  Congenital heart defects
Pulmonary
  Bronchopulmonary dysplasia
  Chronic infection (eg, secondary
    to cystic fibrosis)
Gastrointestinal
  Decreased intake
    Oropharyngeal disorders
    Cerebral palsy
  Chronic vomiting
    Gastroesophageal reflux
    Malrotation
    Pseudo-obstruction
    Increased intracranial pressure
  Chronic diarrhea
    Celiac disease
    Cystic fibrosis
    Giardiasis
    Microvillus inclusion disease
    Abetalipoproteinemia
    Inflammatory bowel disease
    Short bowel syndrome
  Chronic liver disease
  Selective enzyme deficiency
    Enterokinase
    Isomaltase
    Sucrase

Genitourinary
  Renal tubular acidosis
  Fanconi syndrome
Endocrine
  Hypothyroidism
  Hypopituitarism
  Diabetes mellitus
  Diabetes insipidus
  Congenital adrenal hyperplasia
  Growth hormone deficiency
Congenital infections
  Syphilis
  Cytomegalic inclusion virus
  Rubella
  Toxoplasmosis
  HIV infection
Metabolic disorders
Malignancies
Iatrogenic
  Prolonged use of steroids
Chromosomal disorders
  Turner's syndrome
Immunodeficiency disease
  Severe combined immunodefi-
    ciency
  DiGeorge syndrome
  HIV infection

Intrauterine Growth Retardation

Infants with intrauterine growth retardation (IUGR) fail to grow in utero and weigh less than 2500 g at term. Intrauterine growth retardation is classified as a separate entity distinct from failure to thrive. The different outcomes observed in the growth patterns of IUGR infants most likely reflect multiple factors and variations in the duration of the intrauterine insults. Although infants with intrauterine growth retardation do have an accelerated growth phase during the first 3 to 6 months after birth, they continue to be small when compared with other infants of the same age.

Constitutional Growth Delay

Children with constitutional growth delay typically are "slow growers" and "late bloomers" [9••]. These children usually have a deceleration of growth in the first 2 years of life that can be confused with failure to thrive. Affected children subsequently grow steadily along a curve that parallels the normal curve until well beyond the age at which the usual adolescent growth spurt occurs. Often they are 17 to 18 years of age when their growth spurt occurs during pubertal development [10]. When the initial deceleration phase of growth occurs, it is reasonable to consider a variety of organic abnormalities. If a decrease in height velocity is the prominent feature, growth hormone deficiency should be excluded. If a decrease in weight velocity precedes a decrease in height velocity, or if the two occur simultaneously, inadequate caloric intake, possibly associated with an organic cause, should be considered.

Familial Short Stature

Familial short stature is defined as genetic short stature. Affected patients remain short throughout life. They also readjust their growth percentiles to their genetic potential by 2 to 3 years of age. These children differ from infants with constitutional growth delay because their bone age is not delayed as it is in constitutional growth delay. Children with familial short stature maintain their own growth curve, which tends to be appropriate when compared to the heights of their first-degree relatives.

Breast-fed Infants

Infants who are breast fed exclusively may gain weight at a slower rate than infants who are formula fed. In a study by Darling and colleagues [11] the mean weight of breast-fed infants dropped below the median in infants 6 to 8 months of age and was significantly lower than that of the formula-fed group between 6 and 18 months of age. Despite their slow weight gain, these infants double their birth weight by 4 to 6 months of age and triple their birth weight by 1 year. They do not require nutritional supplementation.

■ EVALUATION

History

The assessment of a child with failure to thrive requires a careful history with special emphasis on nutritional intake, particularly caloric intake. Every child with failure to thrive has incurred malnutrition for one of the following reasons: 1) not being offered adequate calories; 2) inability to consume adequate calories; 3) difficulty retaining adequate calories; or 4) an energy expenditure rate in which caloric demands have exceeded caloric intake.

In infants less than 5 or 6 months of age in whom formula is the only source of calories, it is easy to ascertain a daily caloric intake. Because errors in formula preparation are common, specific questions should be asked about how the parent or caregiver prepares the formula. McJunkin and colleagues [12] have demonstrated that 11% of infants with failure to thrive were fed improperly prepared formula. Although it seems that ready-to-feed formulas should have diminished such errors, parents often add extra water, thus diluting the formula, especially in babies who are constipated or if the parents are concerned about dehydration because of hot summer weather. Dilution of the formula obviously results in decreased calories per ounce and may result in failure to gain weight. Diluted formulas also have been given, often by doctors orders to children with gastrointestinal disorders, obesity, and hypercholesterolemia [13,14].

The perinatal history must be reviewed in great detail. Maternal illnesses (*eg*, infections such as rubella or cytomegalovirus [CMV]), alcohol ingestion, use of illicit drugs, or cigarette smoking during pregnancy can result in intrauterine growth retardation.

The medical history should include a review of organ systems. Delay in achieving developmental milestones, especially in the first year of life, suggests an underlying neurologic pathology. However, malnourished children without primary neurologic abnormalities also may have some delay in achieving their milestones because of poor nutritional status. Vomiting may be secondary not to gastrointestinal disease but rather to increased intracranial pressure. A neurologic cause may be suspected if there has been developmental delay, loss of achieved developmental milestones, or deviation of head circumference across two percentile lines. Shortness of breath, pallor, and sweating during feedings suggest underlying cardiac disease. Cystic fibrosis is of concern in the child with repeated episodes of bronchitis or pneumonia and failure to thrive. Children with cystic fibrosis also may have maldigestion or malabsorption, reflected by the presence of large, oily, foul-smelling stools. Defects in metabolism of amino acids or fatty acids may present with failure to thrive and chronic vomiting. These children often are quite ill.

Unexplained fevers and the need for repeated courses of antibiotics may indicate an immune deficiency such as severe combined immunodeficiency (SCID) or AIDS.

The social history should be reviewed carefully. It is important to ascertain who the child's specific caretakers are, a situation that has changed significantly over the last decade as more families have needed to have two working parents or, in single-parent families, that parent working full-time to provide for the children. Children often have multiple caretakers or are cared for in daycare centers. Inadequate food in the house, as a result of financial hardship is another significant contributing factor to nonorganic failure to thrive.

Examination

The child's general appearance must be evaluated for signs of neglect. The neglected, malnourished child often appears apathetic and lacks interest in his or her environment [15]. Congenital malformations must be searched for and noted. Even minor congenital anomalies such as body asymmetry, low-set ears, and extra digits may be associated with developmental delay, mental retardation, and consequent poor caloric intake with failure to gain weight. Congenital heart disease, especially cyanotic heart disease, is a common cause of organic failure to thrive in infancy. Anthropometric measurements must be obtained from previous health records and carefully plotted. Weight usually declines before height. Weight loss in the presence of normal height and head circumference suggests the recent onset of malnutrition or dehydration, if the situation is acute, whereas an absolute decline in weight or in weight velocity associated with a decline in height velocity indicates a more chronic nutritional deprivation. Height velocity usually begins to decline 4 to 6 months after a decline in weight gain [16]. A decrease in the growth velocity of the head circumference usu-

ally is seen in severe nutritional deprivation, and is more likely to reflect a primary disturbance in brain growth.

Laboratory Evaluation

The history and physical examination are the most sensitive indicators of an underlying organic disease and should determine which laboratory studies are ordered. Table 182-2 outlines certain guidelines to assist in the evaluation of children with failure to thrive. In children with specific abnormalities, the evaluation should be organ specific. Several basic screening tests may be helpful. A complete blood count with a white blood cell differential, red cell indices, and erythrocyte sedimentation rate should be obtained to screen for hematologic and inflammatory diseases. Anemia may be the result of malnutrition, malabsorption, chronic blood loss, or deficient utilization of iron in chronic disease states. In the anemic child, a lead level should be obtained, because lead toxicity may result in anemia and failure to thrive. Children with malnutrition and iron deficiency also have increased lead absorption [17].

A simultaneous urine pH and serum bicarbonate concentration should be requested to rule out renal tubular acidosis. Urine should be analyzed for specific gravity, glucose and protein concentrations, and microscopic examination to screen for diabetes insipidus, diabetes mellitus, urinary tract infection, and renal tubular defects.

Liver tests to screen for chronic liver disease and antibodies (*ie*, antigliadin IgA and endomysium antibodies) for celiac sprue also should be obtained. Serum immunoglobulins should be evaluated to rule out IgA deficiency. Patients with serum IgA deficiency who also have celiac sprue cannot mount an IgA antibody response to gliadin or monkey-esophagus smooth muscle (endomysium antibody). In children who are not IgA deficient, the antigliadin IgA and endomysium antibodies currently appear to be the most sensitive and specific means of screening for celiac disease [18] (see Chapter 54).

A sweat chloride test should be performed if failure to thrive is associated with symptoms and signs of pulmonary or gastrointestinal disease. In addition to the sweat chloride test and celiac antibodies, if there is a history of diarrhea, stool should be tested for pH, reducing substances, and fat to screen for malabsorption. A 72-hour fecal fat study may be necessary to quantitate fecal fat loses. If the patient has been in an area endemic for parasites or has been in contact with an individual with a parasitic infestation, stools also should be obtained to check for ova and parasites. The giardia-specific stool antigen test [19] is more specific and sensitive for *Giardia lamblia* infection than is a routine ova and parasite study. *G. lamblia* infection can result in significant malabsorption and failure to thrive.

An upper gastrointestinal study with barium should be obtained to rule out anatomic abnormalities such as an antral web or malrotation in the child with chronic vomiting and failure to thrive. An intracranial space–occupying lesion also should be considered, blood pressure determined, and a neurologic and funduscopic examination performed in such patients. A magnetic resonance imaging study of the brain may reveal a tumor located in the floor of the fourth ventricle that is responsible for the chronic vomiting.

If the child's height is more significantly affected than his or her weight, an endocrine abnormality is more likely than is failure to thrive. If nonorganic failure to thrive is suspected, confirmation of the diagnosis is based on exclusion of an underlying organic condition and a positive growth response to better nutrition and caloric intake.

MANAGEMENT

For a child with organic failure to thrive, specific measures are directed at controlling the major medical problem. At the same time, attempts are made to correct the infant's nutritional status by providing a disease-appropriate modified diet with increased calories. Intervention in the child with nonorganic failure to thrive may be much more complex and require a multidisciplinary approach. Nutritional management is the keystone of therapy for these infants. However, management also must focus on improving interaction between the infant and mother (or caregiver) and establishing a social, emotional, and financial support system for the family.

Previously, hospitalization was routinely recommended as part of the initial management for failure to thrive, especially for children with nonorganic failure to thrive. Today, hospitalization is reserved for children with severe malnutrition or dehydration or in cases of suspected child abuse. Hospitalization for short periods of time can be justified to confirm the diagnosis of nonorganic failure to thrive by documenting weight gain with improved nutrition, especially if outpatient therapy has failed. However, studies have shown that hospitalization should be avoided, if possible, because it may disrupt the child–parent relationship and communicate to the parents that they are incompetent [20].

Home Intervention

Home intervention is much preferred for the long-term management of children suffering from failure to thrive resulting from deprivation. In a recent study by Block and colleagues, children with nonorganic failure to thrive were divided into two groups. One group was followed only in the clinic, whereas the second group was followed in the clinic and also received home intervention. With weekly home visits, maternal support and parenting techniques improved, and parent advocacy became evident. Height and weight parameters did not differ in the two groups, but children in the home intervention group had less developmental delay [21•].

Nutritional Intervention

The goal of nutritional treatment is to promote compensatory catch-up growth to restore deficits in weight and height [22]. *Catch-up growth* is defined as acceleration of growth that occurs when a period of growth retardation ends and measured parameters begin to climb across percentile lines toward the expected height and weight percentiles. Farrell [16] has suggested the following formula to calculate the calories needed for catch-up growth:

$$\text{Energy requirement for catch-up (kcal/kg/day)} = \frac{\text{calories required for weight age} \times \text{ideal weight for age (kg)}}{\text{actual weight in kg}}$$

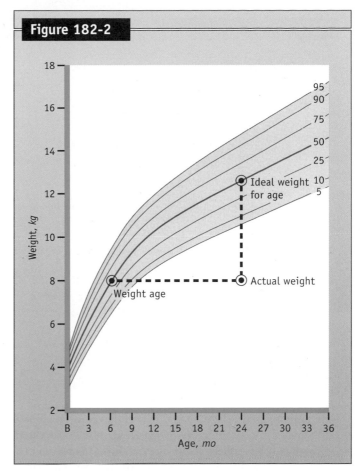

Figure 182-2

How to calculate the ideal weight for age and weight age based on the child's actual weight.

Ideal weight for age is the 50th percentile weight for that age. Weight age is the age at which the child's current weight would be at the 50th percentile. Therefore, if one considers a boy 2 years of age and weighing 8 kg, his ideal weight for his age would be 12.5 kg, making his weight age 6.5 months (Fig. 182-2). Calories per kilogram required at a particular age are noted in Table 182-3.

Malnourished infants often require 110% to 200% percent of the normal daily calorie dietary intake for catch-up growth. In children with severe malnutrition, caloric intake should be advanced slowly to avoid the refeeding syndrome [23]. Severely malnourished children, if fed too rapidly, may develop life-threatening hypocalcemia and hypophosphatemia. Cardiac failure also can be induced. Caloric intake should be advanced slowly, achieving the required daily caloric intake for catch-up growth by the end of 2 weeks. This usually can be achieved most successfully through the use of a modified infant formula. The number of calories per ounce of formula can be increased by supplementing the available infant formulas. Carbohydrate can be added in the form of glucose polymer (3.8 kcal/g). Medium chain triglycerides or corn oil also are appropriate additives to increase the caloric density of the formulas (7.7 kcal/mL). Protein supplementation usually is not needed and may prove dangerous (*eg*, by inducing increased intracranial pressure, fever, or metabolic acidemia) if the protein intake exceeds 4 g/kg.

Table 182-2. Assessment of Infants With Failure to Thrive

Document failure to gain weight
Obtain history and perform physical examination
Note any specific abnormality:
  Oropharyngeal disorder
  Cardiac defect
  Hepatomegaly
  Cerebral palsy
  Chronic vomiting
  Chronic diarrhea

If suspicious of nonorganic failure to thrive:
  3-Day calorie counts
  Consider hospitalization to document weight gain with
    adequate nutrition

If suspicious of organic failure to thrive

Perform laboratory studies	To screen for
Complete blood count, leukocyte differential, platelet count, erythrocyte sedimentation rate	Anemia, inflammatory causes
Serum electrolytes, bicarbonate, arterial blood pH, liver profile	Renal and hepatic disease
Urine pH, specific gravity, glucose, protein, microscopic examination	Tubular acidosis, diabetes mellitus, diabetes insipidus, urinary tract infection
Serum immunoglobulins	Immunodeficiency
Sweat chloride test	Cystic fibrosis
Antigliadin and antiendomysial antibodies	Celiac disease
Somatomedin C/bone age, thyroid function tests	Endocrine disease
Serum amino acids/urine organic acids	Metabolic defects

A multivitamin preparation that includes iron and zinc is recommended for all undernourished children, because catch-up growth may be reduced if the diet is deficient in these nutrients. Caution should be taken to preserve the desired ratio of calories derived from protein, fat, and carbohydrate: approximately 30% from protein, 30% from fat, and 40% from carbohydrates. If adequate amounts of calories cannot be delivered by mouth, enteral feedings by nasogastric tube or endoscopically placed gastrostomy tube should be considered. Nasogastric feedings are the preferred method, especially if short-term therapy is expected. Both Talia and Corwin have demonstrated significant improvement in height and weight percentiles following the use of nasogastric and gastrostomy tube feedings. Unfortunately, neither study commented on the eventual reestablishment of oral feedings in children with failure to thrive, an essential goal for normal psychosocial development [24,25]. Parenteral nutrition is rarely required unless there is severe gastrointestinal compromise and other techniques are not feasible.

LONG-TERM EFFECTS OF FAILURE TO THRIVE

There are few long-term follow-up studies on the growth and development of infants with nonorganic failure to thrive. Catch-up growth in children with nonorganic failure to thrive seems to be greatest among those who are treated with an intensive multidisciplinary approach. Despite extended intervention, these children still may manifest persistent intellectual delay, even with maintenance of adequate weight gain. In a recent study [26••], 61 children with nonorganic failure to thrive during infancy were evaluated 5 years after initial presentation and compared to age-, sex-, and social status–matched controls. The children with a history of failure to thrive had gained less weight and were shorter. They also had more learning difficulties and significant developmental delay than did children in the control group. When different parameters were studied within the failure-to-thrive group, birth weight, maternal height, and social status were good predictors of the catch-up capabilities of these infants in terms of weight and height. Children with adequate birth weights, with mothers whose height was above average, and from families of higher socioeconomic status showed significantly better catch-up growth. Children who caught up faster had better school performance.

Despite all efforts, an optimal outcome often is not obtained in children with nonorganic failure to thrive. The question remains whether these infants could have a yet unidentified organic explanation for their condition and a poorer prognosis than infants with organic failure to thrive.

Table 182-3. Caloric Requirements/kg Body Weight

Age	kcal
0–6 mo	108
6–11 mo	98
1–3 y	102
4–6 y	90
7–10 y	70
11–14 y	55

▓▓ REFERENCES

Recently published papers of particular interest have been highlighted as follows:
• Of interest
•• Of outstanding interest

1. Powell GF, Low JF, Speer MA: Behavior as a diagnostic aid in failure to thrive. *J Dev Behav Pediatr* 1987, 8:18–24.

2. Mitchell WG, Gorrell RW, Greenberg RA: Failure to thrive: a study in a primary care setting. *Pediatrics* 1980, 65:971–977.

3. Homer C, Ludwig S: Categorization of etiology of FTT. *Am J Dis Child* 1981, 135:848–851.

4. Casey PH: FTT: a re-conceptualization. *J Dev Behav Pediatr* 1983, 4:63–66.

5. Powell GF: Failure to thrive. In *Pediatric Endocrinology* . Edited by Lifshitz F. New York: Marcel Dekker; 1996:121–130.

6. Loco MI, Bernard KE, Combs JB: Failure to thrive: parent-infant interaction perspective. *J Pediatr Nurs* 1992, 7:251–261.

7. Skuse DH: Non-organic failure to thrive: a reappraisal. *Arch Dis Child* 1985, 60:173–178.

8.• Lifshitz F, Moses-Finch N, Ziffer-Lifshitz J: Failure to thrive. In *Children's Nutrition*. Edited by Lifshitz F. Boston: Jones and Barlett; 1991:253–270

This chapter reviews the psychosocial aspects of nonorganic failure to thrive. Maternal attitudes and beliefs and infant behaviors that predispose the infants not to thrive are discussed in depth.

9.•• Maggioni A, Lifshitz F: Nutritional management of failure to thrive. *Pediatr Clin North Am* 1995, 42:791–810.

This paper presents an in-depth review of the psychosocial and nutritional management of infants with nonorganic failure to thrive.

10. Bierich JR: Constitutional delay of growth and development. *Growth Genet Horm* 1987, 3:9–12.

11. Dewey KG, Heining MJ, Nommsem LA, *et al.*: Growth of breast fed infants from 0–18 months: the Darling study. *Pediatrics* 1992, 89:1035.

12. McJunkin JE, Bithoney WJ, McCormic MC: Errors in formula concentration in an outpatient population. *J Pediatr* 1987, 111:848–850.

13. Pugliese MT, Lifshitz F, Grad G, *et al.*: Fear of obesity, the cause of short stature and delayed puberty. *N Engl J Med* 1993, 309:513 518.

14. Pugliese MT, Weyman-Daum M, Moses N, *et al.*: Parental health beliefs as a cause of unknown organic failure to thrive. *Pediatrics* 1978, 80:175–182.

15. Powell GF, Low J: Behavior in non-organic failure to thrive. *J Dev Behav Pediatr* 1983, 4:26–33.

16. Farrell MK: Failure to thrive. In *Pediatric Gastrointestinal Diseases*. Edited by Wyllie R, Hyams JS. Philadelphia: WB Saunders; 1993:271–280.

17. Bithoney WG: Elevated lead levels in children with non-organic failure to thrive. *Pediatrics* 1986, 78:891–895.

18. Bottaro G, Volta U, Spina M, *et al.*: Antibody pattern in childhood celiac disease. *J Pediatr Gastroenterol Nutr* 1997, 24:559–562.

19. Aldeen WE, Hale D, Robinson AJ, Carroll K: Evaluation of a commercially available ELISA assay for detection of *Giardia lamblia* in fecal specimens. *Diagn Microbiol Infect Dis* Feb 21, 1995, 2:77–79.

20. Yoos L: Taking another look at failure to thrive. *MCN: Am J Matern Child Nurs* 1984, 9:32–36.

21.• Black MM, Doubowitz H, Hutcheson J, *et al.*: A randomized clinical trial of home intervention for children with failure to thrive. *Pediatrics* 1995, 95:807–814.

This article prospectively compares infants with nonorganic failure to thrive receiving home intervention and clinic support with children receiving only clinic support. Early in-house intervention, a relatively new concept in the management of these children is covered in depth and illustrated to be beneficial for the child's development.

22. Pipes PL, Trahms CM: Nutrition: growth and development. In: *Nutrition in Infancy and Childhood* , edn 5. Edited by Pipes PL, Trahms CM. St. Louis: Mosby; 1993:1–29.

23. Mezoff AG, Gremse DA, Farrell MK: Hypophosphatemia in the nutritional recovery syndrome. *Am J Dis Child* 1989, 1992:111–112.

24. Tolia V: Very early onset non-organic failure to thrive in infants. *J Pediatr Gastroenterol Nutr* 1995, 20:73–80.

25. Corwin DS, Isaacs JS, Georgeson KE, *et al.*: Weight and length increases in children after gastrostomy placement. *J Am Diet Assoc* 1996, 9:874–879.

26.•• Reis S, Beller B, Villa Y, Spirer Z: Long-term follow-up and outcome of infants with non-organic failure to thrive. *Isr J Med Sci* 1995, 8:483–489.

This paper presents an overview and controlled matched evaluation of children with nonorganic failure to thrive who were followed over a period of 5 years. Factors that may predict a better outcome are highlighted.

183 Munchausen Syndrome By Proxy

Robert H. Squires, Jr

That a parent, usually the mother, would intentionally inflict injury or illness on a child, deceive the treating physician with fictitious information, and perpetuate such trickery for months or years seems unimaginable. However, in 1977, Morrow described two such cases [1]. One involved the mother's deliberate contamination of her daughter's urine, which prompted numerous unnecessary invasive procedures; the second resulted in the tragic death of a toddler by salt poisoning. The author likened these maternal fabrications to those of Baron K.F.H. von Munchausen, who invented or embellished elaborate tales of his mercenary activities with the Russian troops as they fought the Turks in the 18th century [2••].

Whereas Munchausen syndrome involves children or adults who falsify their own disease [3], Morrow reasoned these children served as "proxy" for the parent's fabrication.

As a result of Morrow's observation, the evaluation of children with ill-explained recurrent or persistent afflictions now must include a certain skepticism about the child's medical his-

Table 183-1. Definition of Munchausen Syndrome by Proxy

Adult parent or caretaker, usually the mother, fabricates symptoms or induces illness in a child

Perpetrator denies any knowledge of etiology of illness or reported symptoms

Symptoms disappear or significantly improve when child is removed from abusive environment

Physician and health care system are instruments for the abuse of the child

tory. The physician's natural trust and faith in a mother's testimony concerning her child's illness must be balanced with independent observation and assessment. This is especially true when signs or symptoms cannot be explained by known diagnoses or pathophysiologic principles.

DEFINITION

Munchausen syndrome by proxy (MSBP) is a unique form of child abuse in which a parent or caretaker, usually the mother, deliberately fabricates symptoms or induces an illness in a child (Table 183-1) [1,2••,4,5]. The perpetrator often is familiar with medical terminology. This knowledge allows her to contrive a believable story of a child with a serious or chronic medical condition such as chronic diarrhea, apnea, or gastroesophageal reflux. For example, signs and symptoms can be simulated by adding fluid or exogenous blood to stool, thus creating the appearance of diarrhea or colitis. A more ominous form of MSBP involves the induction of symptoms in the child—the mother can cause apnea or seizures by suffocation, diarrhea by oral cathartics, and anemia by exsanguination.

The nature of the feigned clinical condition compels the physician to respond with tests to evaluate and treat the patient. The perpetrator does not disclose and usually denies any knowledge of the cause of the child's complaints. Rosenberg coined the phrase *a web of deceit* to describe the intricate entrapment of the well-intentioned but unsuspecting physician by the perpetrator [2••]. Symptoms disappear or improve dramatically only if the child is removed from the abusive environment.

The physician's involvement as an instrument of abuse distinguishes MSBP from other forms of abuse [6]. Fabrication alone does not identify the abuse as MSBP. History or physical circumstances typically are altered by a parent or adult supervisor who injures a child. As with sexual abuse, MSBP continues for months or years, because the perpetrator's emotional desires can be played out only by harming the child. The physician is led to inflict injury on the child through the tests and invasive procedures that are ordered to evaluate the informant's complaints. Thus, the physician is both victim and perpetrator.

DEMOGRAPHICS
The Victim

For the typical victim, abuse begins within the first year of life [2••,7]. The mean age at diagnosis is 40 months (range 1 to 252 months). The mean interval between the onset of symptoms and diagnosis is 15 months [2••,8]. Bools and colleagues [9]

identified multiple fabricated illnesses in 35 of 54 (65%) children diagnosed with MSBP. Cases are distributed evenly between boys and girls. In contrast to physical or sexual abuse [10], the perpetrator is almost always the mother.

The child usually appears to have a legitimate illness (*eg*, gastroesophageal reflux, chronic diarrhea, vomiting, seizures, or apnea). The evaluation process evokes considerable short-term morbidity with multiple painful laboratory tests, invasive diagnostic procedures, prolonged hospitalizations, and, on rare occasions, surgery (*eg*, central line placement for total parenteral nutrition [TPN] or exploratory laparotomy). The combined actions of the mother and medical personnel account for 75% of the inflicted injuries, whereas medical personnel alone cause 25% of the injuries [2••]. Long-term permanent disfigurement or impairment of function (*eg*, gastrointestinal dysfunction, psychiatric problems, and mental retardation) occur in at least 8% of patients. Death is reported in 10% of patients, a figure that probably underestimates the severity of the problem [8]. Causes of death include suffocation, salt poisoning, and other poisonings [2••].

Psychological morbidity can be particularly devastating. Adverse effects include immaturity, separation anxiety, aggressiveness, and a peculiar symbiotic relationship with the mother. Some older children adopt the mythic symptoms as genuine even after the abuse has been uncovered [2••,11••,12]. Careful long-term follow-up care for these patients is achieved only rarely.

The Perpetrator

The perpetrator typically is a friendly, caring, attentive, concerned biologic mother described as the "perfect mother." This caregiver appears emotionally strong and calm despite the uncertainties of her child's condition. She may even provide emotional support and encouragement to discouraged medical and nursing staff.

Less commonly, the mother is aggressive, demanding, intimidating, or threatening. Perpetrators other than the mother are rare, but include adoptive mothers (2%), fathers (1.5%), and babysitters and grandmothers (<1%) [2••,7]. As many as 34% of perpetrators have a connection with the medical professions. For instance, they may be nurses, social workers, medical assistants, or students in a health care field [2••].

The perpetrator's motive for committing the deceitful act remains unclear; these mothers are unable to explain their behavior [2••]. A desire for secondary gain (*eg*, custody, insurance payments) is surprisingly absent in most cases. Although few mothers experienced physical or sexual abuse as children or young adults, many felt unwanted or undervalued in a home with absent fathers and favored brothers [4]. The perpetrator may have a history of Munchausen syndrome, self-harm, alcohol or substance abuse, previous suspicion of child abuse, or a personality disorder [13].

Family Dynamics

Although little is known of the father's role in MSBP, he is often described as emotionally distant, despite the perceived seriousness of the child's condition [4]. The father rarely accompanies the child during outpatient visits or visits the child in the hospital. He passively accepts the mother's explanation of the need for tests and hospitalizations. Marital dysfunction and substance abuse are present in some families [7].

Siblings provide a window into an unsettling home environment. As many as 40% suffer from fabricated illnesses, and others experience neglect, failure to thrive, or nonaccidental injury [9]. Studies by Rosenberg [2••] and Bools [9] noted that about 10% of siblings died under "unusual circumstances" before identification of the index MSBP patient. Death among the siblings most commonly was attributed to sudden infant death syndrome (SIDS).

The Doctor as Victim and Perpetrator

A typical profile of the doctor misled by MSBP shows a subspecialist physician eager to identify the cause or at least develop a treatment plan for the child's complex and persistent symptoms. The drive to find a rare or unusual diagnosis blinds the physician to the totality of the child's problem [4]. For the physician, failure to diagnose and treat the child accurately questions his or her credibility, honor, and empathy. Tests and procedures are eagerly used to search for the missing data that will condense the child's symptoms and laboratory findings into a singular diagnosis [6]. Lacking an answer, the physician has his or her shaken confidence restored after conversations with the mother, who may express appreciation of and confidence in the physician's sometimes heroic, but still unsuccessful, efforts. Diagnostic tests beget further tests and procedures, which raise more questions and lead to longer intricate discussions with the mother. *Folie à deux* develops between the mother and physician that is difficult for the physician to recognize and overcome [11••]. The physician is a victim of the mother's "web of deceit" and, at the same time, a perpetrator of abuse [2••,6].

■ RECOGNITION

For MSBP to be recognized, it must be included in the differential diagnosis. Unfortunately, the condition often simply is not considered when the physician's mission is to find "real disease." The most common fabricated or induced illness are listed in Table 183-2.

A genuine illness also may hide within a fabricated illness. Therefore, the presence of established diagnoses such as gastroesophageal reflux, poor weight gain (*ie*, failure to thrive), protracted diarrhea, and intestinal pseudo-obstruction should not exclude consideration of MSBP. The physician must strike a healthy balance between trust of the family's story and pursuit of the truth. Identification of warning signs for MSBP affords the physician an opportunity to prevent the disorder (Table 183-3) [14].

MSBP should be considered in any child when medical problems are not as responsive as expected to treatment or follow an unusual course; when physical or laboratory findings are unusual; when a disproportionate number of physicians are involved in the case; or when a discrepancy exists between the history and the physical examination [4,11••,15••]. A mother eager to stay in the hospital "as long as it takes" to find the correct diagnosis for her child may be either the child's advocate or adversary. The physician should be cautious if the mother is surprisingly calm despite the apparent seriousness of her child's

Table 183-2. Common Presentations of Munchausen Syndrome by Proxy

Vomiting	Bleeding
Ipecac poisoning	Anticoagulant poisoning
Fabrication	Exsanguination
Diarrhea	Nonhuman blood
Laxative poisoning	Stool mixed with dye or paint
Alteration of stools	Seizures
Fabrication	Poisoning
Apnea	Suffocation
Suffocation	Fabrication
Fabrication	Altered level of consciousness
	Poisoning
	Suffocation

problems. The child life and nursing specialists may be seduced by the mother who eagerly attends to her child's every need and never leaves the patient's bedside, only to find later that she altered bedside records. On the other hand, some mothers are aggressive, abusive, demanding, and quick to put medical personnel on the defensive. They may divert attention to unimportant details of the case. A higher incidence of MSBP occurs in patients who leave the hospital against medical advice [4].

Three subsets of MSBP deserve particular attention. The first is the child with apnea induced by suffocation [16]. Multiple apnea episodes that required the mother to provide mouth-to-mouth resuscitation to the child at home are reported. Episodes also may occur in the hospital setting. Deaths are mistakenly attributed to sudden infant death syndrome [17,18]. A second group involves older patients whose families use the child as a proxy to "doctor shop" throughout the country [19•]. Fathers, in this setting, support the mother's concerns. Medical records are said to be "lost" or "in the mail," but are never forthcoming. Despite the child's normal growth, maturation, and absent or minimal physical findings, complaints are long-standing and involve multiple organ systems. Over the course of an

Table 183-3. Warning Signs of Munchausen Syndrome by Proxy

Mother's complaints defy a recognized condition

Symptoms are unusual or serious but not verified

Symptoms disappear in mother's absence

History and physical examination are incongruous

Previous medical records are incomplete or difficult to obtain

Medical condition does not respond to treatment as expected

Medical condition follows unusual course

Multiple physicians are involved and confused by child's condition

Mother is calm and confident amidst confusion of child's complex symptoms

Mother is eager to stay in the hospital

Child is removed from the hospital against medical advice

Father is detached

alleged illness, school absenteeism can range from 40 to 200 days and may involve multiple physicians in many states. Negative results are the outcome of numerous extensive and sometimes invasive diagnostic studies. In the third category, Meadow [20] reported a series of children aged 3 to 9 years who had been indoctrinated by their mothers to report realistic stories of sexual abuse. These allegations resulted in extensive and repeated examinations by medical personnel before the accusations were proved false. The mothers in these cases were eager to repeat the story and insisted on multiple examinations and second opinions from physicians, social workers, and others. Mothers appear callous to the feelings of the child in such instances.

Recognition of the persistent mother may identify a mother–child pair at risk for MSBP. The appropriateness of the mother's persistence in pursuing the cause of her child's symptoms should be assessed carefully. At the extremes, absent or excessive persistence constitutes neglect or MSBP, respectively. Waring [21•] described a tool that requires the answer to two questions to assess the appropriateness of the mother's persistence. The first is "What is wrong with the patient?" and the second is "Why did you bring the child to see me today?" The mother's reply to the first question will address whether the child is seriously ill, and, if so, whether treatment is available. Her answer to the second may reveal hidden anxieties, fears, or a cry for reassurance and support. Revealing answers to the second question include: "The daycare keeps calling me and I cannot take off from work;" "My niece had symptoms like this before they found the cancer;" or "He gets like this after a weekend at his father's house." If the mother cannot answer the second question satisfactorily, ignores the physician's effort to reassure her, or jumps quickly to another area of concern, or if her answer is incongruent with the presenting complaint, then the history should be reviewed in more detail.

Exaggeration and mild deception are encountered daily in the practice of medicine. These tactics are part of a continuum of behavior a mother adopts to expresses her anxiety toward and perception of her child's symptoms [15••]. Most commonly, a reasonable balance exists between the mother's anxiety and her acceptance of the child's illness [22••]. Difficulties arise if her behavior deviates far from that balance. On the one hand, the mother's acceptance may drift to indifference, carelessness, and neglect. On the other, her insatiable anxiety may keep her from being able to separate her needs from those of the child and can lead to reporting signs and symptoms that are exaggerated, invented, or induced to meet the mother's level of anxiety (ie, MSBP).

DIAGNOSIS

The diagnosis of MSBP is hastened when objective evidence is present (eg, phenolphthalein in the stool, or nonhuman blood in stool or vomitus). Unfortunately, the diagnosis is often missed or delayed, for reasons listed in Table 183-4. A meticulous history and physical examination are the keys to the diagnosis.

A detailed history obtained not only from the mother, but also from the father, siblings, in-laws, and others, will identify moment-to-moment details that are needed to provide an independent assessment of the mother's story. Even with established

Table 183-4. Factors That Delay Diagnosis of Munchausen Syndrome by Proxy
Not considered in differential diagnosis
Past medical history not adequately scrutinized
Disarmingly attentive and involved mother
Physician insecurity that a rare diagnosis is being overlooked
Trivial abnormalities not recognized as trivial
Few patients exhibit all the symptoms

patients within a medical practice it is necessary to review their family history and past medical history carefully to identify self-referral patterns, empiric therapies, and interval changes in the family structure or dynamics. Medical records should be carefully reviewed to verify that certain studies were done and therefore need not be repeated. Review of original or copied radiographs can confirm or be at odds with written reports. Clear communication among all treating physicians must be established. The physician must be cautious of the family bearing incomplete medical records or records that never quite seem to be available for review. The physical examination should be complete and detailed to avoid unnecessary repetition. Particular care must be taken to secure the child's dignity and comfort.

If the child is asymptomatic, a coordinated plan is necessary to examine the child at a time when symptoms are present to verify the nature of the illness. Such a plan must include the primary care physician, all subspecialists, including those who share call schedules with the involved physicians, and local emergency room personnel. The family can develop clever reasons to avoid contact with the medical system at the times when they report that the child is ill.

Admission to the hospital is necessary in some cases. Consultative services are carefully coordinated. Documentation of symptoms and findings is critical to establish the diagnosis of MSBP. Because the mother can produce the symptoms in the hospital or alter bedside medical records, 24-hour visual or video surveillance may be necessary to document or deter maternal transgressions [7,23].

MANAGEMENT STRATEGIES

If MSBP is suspected, the physician has a moral and legal responsibility to report the case to Child Protective Services and to inform the family [2••]. The facts should be presented to the family in laymen's terms. Attempts to convince the mother of the diagnosis are best avoided. The physician should be prepared for a range of responses, including acceptance, denial, or accusations that the medical caregivers created the symptoms and framed the mother. The mother may challenge the diagnosis by referring to the child's real illnesses or results that are irrelevant and meaningless. It is important to be confident, secure, honest, and supportive with the mother. A full range of supportive services should be readily available to the mother and the family. The mother should be informed that the case has been referred to the state's child protective services, who will evaluate the situation and decide whether the child should be removed from her care. Arrangements should be in place to take custody of the child by court order if the family threatens to flee with the child.

Management strategies must also include nursing and support services, social services, police, and the courts [2••]. Everyone who encounters the child and family must understand the diagnosis, dangers to the child, and proposed interventions. Ignorance of the complexity of MSBP within the medical and legal professions, compounded by the assumption that every mother has the best interests of her child at heart, creates an atmosphere of disbelief and ambivalence that hampers intervention and management.

Removal of the child from the home and placement into foster care is the proper strategy. (The state's protective services agency will decide if the siblings are at risk. If so, they also will be placed into foster care.) The risk for further abuse is great if the child remains with the mother [2••,12]. While the child is in foster care, the mother and family are encouraged to seek counseling and psychiatric evaluation.

PROGNOSIS

The safety of the child is the first priority and takes precedence over parental rights. Extreme caution must be exercised if the child remains in custody of the offending parent [12]. Deaths occur most often in children younger than 3 years, and 20% of fatalities reported in one study occurred after the child had been returned to the home after the parents had been confronted with the diagnosis [2••].

A study by Bools and colleagues [24] of 54 victims with a mean follow-up of 5.6 years identified further fabrications in 30% of children returned to live with their biologic mothers compared with none in those who went to foster care. No deaths occurred in either group, although there were 11 unexplained deaths of siblings before the diagnosis of the index case. Forty-nine percent of the patients were determined to have unacceptable outcomes, characterized by conduct and emotional disorders and school-related problems such as decreased attention and concentration. Persistent problems after foster placement were attributed to a continuation of the disturbance that prompted removal from the home: children who were smothered exhibited sleep disturbances, and others had fears and avoidance of specific places or situations and post-traumatic stress disorder. Features that may predict outcomes for victims of MSBP are listed in Table 183-5.

Libow [25•] interviewed 10 adults who identified themselves as victims of MSBP. These adults describe themselves as being insecure, avoiding medical treatment, suffering from symptoms of post-traumatic stress disorder, and having difficulty maintaining relationships. Many have sought psychiatric help for depression, anxiety, and suicidal feelings. Although they remain angry toward their mothers, there is surprising sympathy toward their fathers. There appeared to be no difference in outcome whether symptoms were fabricated or induced.

CONCLUSION

MSBP is a serious form of child abuse associated with high morbidity and mortality and is probably more common than previously suspected. In contrast to other forms of abuse, in

---

Table 183-5. Features that Predict Outcomes for Victims of Munchausen Syndrome by Proxy

Good outcomes
  Positive, dependable paternal involvement
  Long-term relationship with a counselor
  Early adoption after diagnosis
  Successful short-term foster care before returning to mother
  Long-term placement with the same foster family
Poor Outcomes
  Victim older at time MSBP was discovered
  Siblings experienced abuse or neglect

MSBP—Munchausen syndrome by proxy.

MSBP the physician serves as an agent of the abuse. An evidence-based history and physical examination along with a high index of suspicion will minimize or prevent unnecessary trauma to the child.

REFERENCES

Recently published papers of particular interest have been highlighted as follows:
•   Of interest
••   Of particular interest

1. Meadow SR: Munchausen syndrome by proxy: the hinterland of child abuse. *Lancet* 1977, ii:343–345.

2.•• Rosenberg DA: Web of deceit: a literature review of Munchausen syndrome by proxy. *Child Abuse Negl* 1987, 11:547–563.

3. Sneed RC, Bell RF: The dauphin of Munchausen: factitious passage of renal stones in a child. *Pediatrics* 1976, 58:127–130.

4. Schreier HA, Libow JA: Munchausen by proxy syndrome: a modern pediatric challenge. *J Pediatr* 1994, 125:S110–115.

5. Jones DP: Editorial: the syndrome of Munchausen by proxy. *Child Abuse Negl* 1994, 18:769–771.

6. Donald T, Jureidini J: Munchausen syndrome by proxy: child abuse in the medical system. *Arch Pediatr Adolesc Med* 1996, 150:753–758.

7. Skau K, Mouridsen SE: Munchausen syndrome by proxy: a review. *Acta Paediatr* 1995, 84:977–982.

8. Schreier HA, Libow JA: Munchausen syndrome by proxy: diagnosis and prevalence. *Am J Orthopsychiatry* 1993, 63:318–321.

9. Bools CN, Neale BA, Meadow SR: Co-morbidity associated with fabricated illness (Munchausen syndrome by proxy). *Arch Dis Child* 1992, 67:77–79.

10. Berkowitz CD: Pediatric abuse: new patterns of injury. *Emerg Med Clin North Am* 1995, 13:321–341.

11.•• Meadow SR: Management of Munchausen syndrome by proxy. *Arch Dis Child* 1985, 60:385–393.

12. McGuire TL, Feldman KW: Psychologic morbidity of children subjected to Munchausen syndrome by proxy. *Pediatrics* 1989, 83:289–292.

13. Bools CN, Neale BA, Meadow SR: Munchausen syndrome by proxy: a study of psychopathology. *Child Abuse Negl* 1994, 18:773–788.

14. Kaufman KL, Coury D, Pickrel E, McCleery J: Munchausen syndrome by proxy: a survey of professionals' knowledge. *Child Abuse Negl* 1989, 13:141–147.

15.•• Eminson DM, Postlethwaite RJ: Factitious illness: recognition and management. *Arch Dis Child* 1992, 67:1510–1516.

16. Light MJ, Sheridan MS: Munchausen syndrome by proxy and apnea (MBPA). *Clin Pediatr* 1990, 29:162–168.

17. Every JL: Child abuse, sudden infant death syndrome, and unexpected infant death. *Am J Dis Child* 1993, 147:1097–1100.

18. Rosen CL, Frost JD, Glaze DG: Child abuse and recurrent infant apnea. *J Pediatr* 1986, 109:1065–1067.

19.• Woollcott P, Aceto T, Rutt C, *et al.*: Doctor shopping with the child as proxy patient: a variant of child abuse. *J Pediatr* 1982, 101:297–301.

20. Meadow SR: False allegations of abuse and Munchausen syndrome by proxy. *Arch Dis Child* 1993, 68:444–447.

21.• Waring WW: The persistent parent. *Am J Dis Child* 1992, 146:753–756.

22.•• Boyce WT: The vulnerable child: new evidence, new approaches. *Adv Pediatr* 1992, 39:1–33.

23. Epstein MA, Markowitz RL, Gallo DM, *et al.*: Munchausen syndrome by proxy: considerations in diagnosis and confirmation by video surveillance. *Pediatrics* 1987, 80:220–224.

24. Bools CN, Neale BA, Meadow SR: Follow up of victims of fabricated illness (Munchausen syndrome by proxy). *Arch Dis Child* 1993, 69:625–630.

25.• Libow JA: Munchausen by proxy victims in adulthood: a first look. *Child Abuse Negl* 1995, 19:1131–1142.

184 Pediatric AIDS

Edwin Simpser and Ellen Kahn

Despite ongoing research, vigorous educational programs, preventive programs, and a variety of new therapies, the incidence of childhood infection with the human immunodeficiency virus (HIV) and the acquired immunodeficiency syndrome (AIDS) has continued to increase. By the fall of 1996, almost 7500 cases of AIDS in children under 13 years of age had been reported to the Centers for Disease Control and Prevention (CDC) [1]. Infection with HIV and the subsequent development of AIDS leads to gastrointestinal and nutritional problems with significant morbidity.

■ PATHOPHYSIOLOGY
Transmission
In the past, most children with HIV infection acquired it either from infected blood products or perinatally (*ie*, via vertical transmission from an infected mother). With the advent of appropriate screening of donors and blood products, transfusion- and blood product–related infection have diminished markedly. Almost all newly diagnosed HIV-infected children currently acquire their disease through vertical transmission. Antiretroviral treatment of the HIV-infected mother has been shown to reduce the transmission of HIV substantially, but the number of children exposed and infected remains high.

Because antiretroviral therapies also have allowed infected children to survive longer, gastroenterologists caring for children with AIDS see a broad age range of patients with a wide spectrum of gastrointestinal, hepatobiliary, pancreatic, and nutritional problems.

Pathogenesis of Gastrointestinal Involvement
The human immunodeficiency virus primarily targets CD4-positive T-lymphocytes, monocytes, or macrophages. There is disagreement as to whether HIV infection in the gastrointestinal tract is limited to the lymphoid elements of the lamina propria or whether there is epithelial cell infection as well. Unfortunately, because mucosal immune function has not been studied in HIV-infected children, it is not known whether observations of mucosal immune function in the adult AIDS population are relevant [2]. HIV-infected cells have been demonstrated in the macrophages and lymphocytes in the lamina propria of the gastrointestinal tract in HIV-infected adults. Bacterial overgrowth, endotoxin production, enteric infection, cytokine production, and probably, epithelial cell dysfunction, occur; further immune dysfunction leads to malabsorption and malnutrition and an ensuing vicious cycle (Fig. 184-1). In the growing child, who has relatively high energy needs, even minimal diminution of mucosal immunity can be significant, induc-

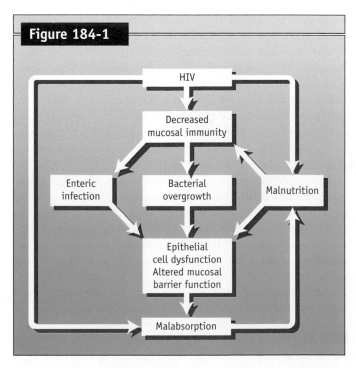

Figure 184-1

Interrelationship of HIV infection, immune dysfunction, gastrointestinal dysfunction, and malnutrition.

Table 184-1. Gastrointestinal and Nutritional Presentations of AIDS

Failure to thrive
Chronic diarrhea
Gastrointestinal bleeding
Hepatobiliary disease
Dysphagia or thrush
Associations
  Lymphadenopathy
  Fever
  Increased serum IgG

Table 184-2. Morphologic Changes of the Gastrointestinal Tract

	Infection	LPL	Tumors	Other
Oral cavity	+	—	—	+
Esophagus	+	—	—	+
Stomach	+	+	+	—
Intestine	+	+	+	+
Anus	—	—	—	+

+—present.
LPL—lymphoproliferative lesions.

ing this vicious cycle at a much earlier stage of HIV infection than in older children and adults.

CLINICAL FEATURES

Gastrointestinal and Nutritional Manifestations as Initial Presentation of AIDS

The gastroenterologist may see children, especially infants, in whom gastrointestinal or nutritional sequelae, or both, are the first manifestation of HIV infection. Evaluation of the child with chronic diarrhea, failure to thrive, gastrointestinal bleeding (more commonly in the lower gastrointestinal tract), and liver disease must include the possibility of HIV infection. The classic presentation of an infant with HIV infection includes failure to thrive (ie, poor weight gain on a pediatric growth curve), diarrhea, hepatomegaly, diffuse lymphadenopathy, and fever (Table 184-1). In such patients, obtaining a parental history for risk factors for HIV disease and testing of the child for HIV are essential. Stool tests, as described later in this chapter, for unusual pathogens should be requested. Most children with HIV infection have increased serum IgG concentrations. Infants with hepatomegaly, hepatitis, and/or cholestasis associated with increased serum IgG levels are more likely to have HIV infec-

tion than they are to have immune hepatitis or primary sclerosing cholangitis.

Upper Gastrointestinal Tract: Oral Cavity, Esophagus, and Stomach

Lesions of the upper gastrointestinal tract can cause significant symptoms in children with AIDS. These include odynophagia, dysphagia, hematemesis, anorexia, nausea, vomiting, and abdominal pain. Poor intake, undernutrition, and failure to thrive are commonly seen in children with upper gastrointestinal tract symptoms even in the absence of malabsorption [3]. Table 184-2 summarizes the types of lesions found in the gastrointestinal tract of children with AIDS, and Table 184-3 lists the infectious pathogens that affect the gastrointestinal tract.

Oral lesions from candidiasis are a frequent presenting feature in children with AIDS. Less commonly, children with AIDS may have herpes gingivostomatitis, idiopathic ulcers, and hairy leukoplakia (Fig. 184-2), the last being much more common in adults than in children and associated with herpes simplex and Epstein-Barr virus (EBV) infection. Kaposi's sarcoma, which can occur anywhere in the gastrointestinal tract, is rare in children but can originate in the mouth.

Table 184-3. Common Gastrointestinal Infections in Pediatric AIDS

Bacterial
  Salmonella spp
  Shigella spp
  Campylobacter jejuni and *C. lari*
  Clostridium difficile
  Enteroadherent *Escheria coli*
  Mycobacterium avium intracellulare
Viral
  Rotavirus
  Cytomegalovirus
  Adenovirus
  Herpes simplex virus
  HIV
  Human papilloma virus

Protozoan
  Giardia lamblia
  Cryptosporidia
  Microsporidia
  Blastocystis hominis
  Entamoeba histolytica
  Leishmania spp
Fungal
  Candida albicans
  Pneumocystis carinii

Figure 184-2

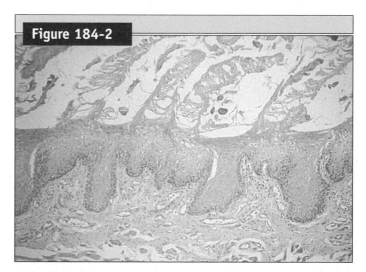

Leukoplakia of oral mucosa characterized by epithelial hyperplasia with spike-like projection of hyper- and parakeratosis. (Hematoxylin and eosin stain, original magnification × 250.)

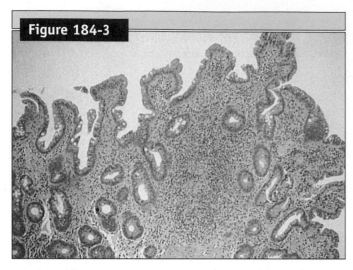

Figure 184-3

Lymphoproliferative process of the duodenal mucosa composed of a lymphoplasmacytic infiltration with focal crypt destruction. (Hematoxylin and eosin stain, original magnification × 250.)

Esophageal involvement is common in AIDS, with as many as one third of adult patients suffering from esophageal symptoms [4]. In a recent review of autopsy and surgical pathologic findings from 58 children with AIDS, 35% of the esophageal specimens were found to be diseased, including one with a severe esophageal stricture [5••]. Infectious causes include Candida spp., cytomegalovirus (CMV), *Mycobacterium avium intracellulare* (MAI), and herpes simplex virus (HSV). Candidal esophagitis is by far the most common esophageal disease and is seen with or without oral candidiasis. Although the literature on adult patients suggests that infection with two simultaneous pathogens is common [4], there are no pediatric data to corroborate this. Esophageal ulcers can cause significant symptoms. Whether these ulcers are caused by HIV, prior esophagitis, zidovudine, AIDS-associated vasculopathy, or unknown pathogens is not known [5••,6].

There are no reliable studies on the incidence of gastroesophageal reflux in patients with AIDS. Children with upper gastrointestinal symptoms consistent with gastroesophageal reflux often respond to antireflux therapy alone. Certain medications used in the treatment of AIDS and its complications may themselves cause esophagitis, specifically zidovudine (Retrovir; AZT, Zidorudin; Glaxo Wellcome Oncology/HIV, Research Triangle Park, NC) and dideoxycytidine (Hivid; ddC-dideoxycytidine; Roche Pharmaceuticals, Nutley, NJ).

Gastric lesions are somewhat less common than are esophageal lesions in children and adults with AIDS. Also as in adults, *Helicobacter pylori* appears to have a lower prevalence in HIV-positive than in HIV-negative children [7]. Candida, MAI, and CMV of the stomach have been described in children with AIDS, and CMV may cause gastric outlet obstruction [8]. Polyclonal lymphoplasmacytic infiltrations of the stomach, small intestine, and large intestine were found in 5% of pediatric AIDS patients at autopsy (Fig. 184-3) [5••]. It is postulated that this lymphoplasmacytic process results from HIV, EBV, or other viral infections [9]. These lesions may be associated with lymphoid interstitial pneumonia, may progress to a B-cell lymphoma, or may resolve on their own [5••].

Gastric involvement by smooth muscle tumors, Kaposi's sarcomas, and lymphoma has been reported [5••].

Diagnosis and Treatment

The approach to a child with upper gastrointestinal symptoms of AIDS should be similar to that for adults [4]. In patients with odynophagia or dysphagia, pill ingestion, gastroesophageal reflux, or infectious processes should be considered as possible causes and physical examination performed to look for oropharyngeal lesions. If the cause of the symptoms is not clear, an empiric trial of oral antifungal therapy (*eg*, fluconazole) is warranted, with upper intestinal endoscopy reserved for patients refractory to the therapeutic trial. Acid-suppressive and/or antireflux medications often are prescribed before proceeding to diagnostic endoscopy.

If a diagnostic procedure is necessary, endoscopy with biopsies are more sensitive and specific than is barium esophagram. Biopsies can reveal a variety of pathogens, and brushings, cytology, culture, immunohistochemistry, and in situ DNA studies increase diagnostic yield.

In addition to oral antifungal agents, a variety of symptomatic treatments can be used. Complaints of early satiety or gastroesophageal reflux–related symptoms can be treated with prokinetics such as metoclopramide or cisapride. Acid-suppressive agents may be helpful, but, by inhibiting gastric acid, may potentiate the risk of bacterial overgrowth. Pediatricians occasionally use phenothiazines such as prochlorperazine or promethazine as well as hydroxyzine and trimethobenzamide hydrochloride to control nausea. Sucralfate, available in a suspension, may be beneficial for children with acid-induced esophageal or gastric lesions. Candida may respond to fluconazole or ketoconazole, but sometimes intravenous amphotericin-B is required. CMV and herpes simplex may be treated with intravenous ganciclovir and intravenous acyclovir, respectively.

Intestine

Abdominal pain and diarrhea, the hallmarks of small intestinal disease, are seen in as many as two thirds of children with AIDS. Diarrhea usually is caused by infections, malabsorption, or a combination of both. Medications such as didanosine (Videx; ddi; Bristol-Myers Squibb, Princeton, NJ) and lamivudine (Epivir; 3-TC) also may contribute to diarrhea [10].

Symptoms of large intestine involvement of children and adults with AIDS consist of bloody or mucoid stools, small volume diarrhea, tenesmus, abdominal pain, distention, and fever. They usually are secondary to the variety of infectious agents. Cryptosporidia causes a more secretory small bowel diarrhea and less colitic-type symptoms. Because many children with AIDS receive frequent courses of antibiotics, *Clostridia difficile* toxin–induced pseudomembranous colitis also must be considered [3]. Necrotizing infection can lead to pneumatosis coli, which can be self-limited or can cause severe disease [11].

Enteric pathogens often cannot be identified even after an exhaustive search. The infections of the gastrointestinal tract clinically seen in children with AIDS are listed in Table 184-3. MAI, cryptosporidia, and CMV are the most common opportunistic organisms, and in an autopsy study accounted for 75% of the organisms identified [5••]. Patients with low CD4 counts

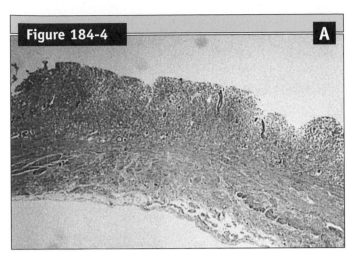

Figure 184-4 **A**

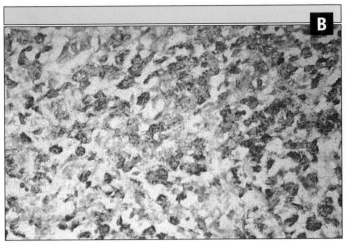

B

Mycobacterium avium intracellulare infection of the small intestine. **A**, Widened mucosa with loss of villi and an infiltrate of numerous enlarged macrophages. Hematoxylin and eosin, × 250.

B, The enlarged macrophages are filled with acid-fast microorganisms. (Ziehl-Neelsen stain, original magnification × 500.)

(<100) are at highest risk for serious infection with certain pathogens (*eg*, MAI and Cryptosporidium spp.).

MAI infection can be diffuse, involving the entire gastrointestinal tract and causing abdominal pain, diarrhea, and malabsorption. Velvety yellow plaques noted on endoscopy result from infiltration of the lamina propria by macrophages with a large number of bacilli, mimicking Whipple disease, and villous atrophy (Fig. 184-4). MAI-associated appendicitis with perforation and intestinal intussusception each have been reported [12,13]. CMV commonly causes ulcerations, transmural inflammation, vasculitis, and ganglioneuritis (*ie*, mononuclear infiltration of the myenteric plexus) of the gastrointestinal tract [5••]. CMV-related ulcers in the gastrointestinal tract may be large and numerous, resulting in life-threatening gastrointestinal bleeding as well as small bowel obstruction, intestinal perforation, and stricture formation (Fig. 184-5, see also **Color Plate**) [14,15]. Radiologically, CMV can simulate typhlitis [16]. Organisms of Cryptosporidium spp. can be seen in as many as 10% of children with AIDS. Cryptosporidia may affect the entire gastrointestinal

tract, the large and small intestine, or the small intestine only (Fig. 184-6). Infection restricted to the appendix and involvement of the bile ducts [17] and pancreatic duct [18] also have been reported. Massive secretory diarrhea from cryptosporidia often is unresponsive to therapy.

HIV enteropathy is another gastrointestinal lesion reported in children with AIDS [19]. HIV enteropathy is characterized by weight loss and diarrhea, friable mucosa, and a variable degree of villous blunting and active inflammation of the intestinal mucosa on microscopic examination. These changes may represent an immune reaction of the gastrointestinal mucosa to HIV-positive cells [20]; may be the result of a yet unidentified infectious agent, or HIV, EBV, herpes simplex, CMV, adenovirus or enterovirus [21]; or may be the result of absorption of noninfectious luminal antigens. Whereas in situ hybridization studies have failed to demonstrate HIV in the intestinal epithelium or lymphoid aggregates in children [22], the virus has been identified in these tissues in adults with AIDS.

Noninfectious ulcers and tumors occur in the gastrointestinal tract of children with AIDS. Intestinal ulceration resulting

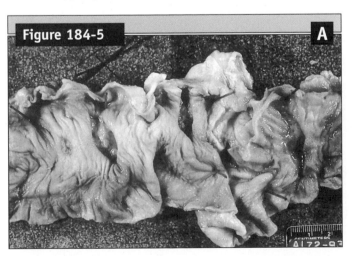

Figure 184-5 **A**

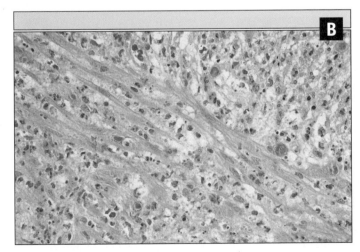

B

Cytomegalovirus infection of the colon. **A**, Macroscopic appearance with large, deep, and well-defined ulcerations undermining the adjacent colonic mucosa. **B**, Polymorphic inflammatory infiltration

of the muscularis propria. Intranuclear viral inclusions are seen in macrophages and smooth muscle cells. (Hematoxylin and eosin stain, original magnification × 250.) See also **Color Plate.**

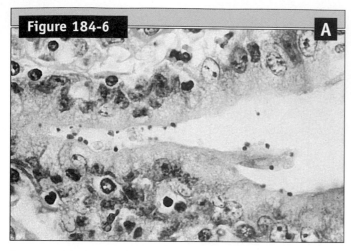

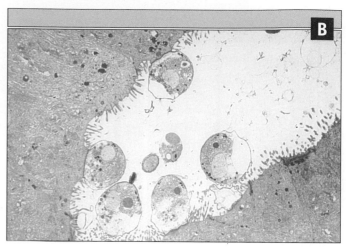

Cryptosporidiosis of the colon. **A,** Cryptosporidia appear as round bodies adherent to the luminal pole of the crypt cells. Giemsa stain, original magnification × 500. **B,** Electron microscopic characterization of cryptosporidia. Each microorganisms is contained in a parasitophorous vacuole. The outer membrane is in continuity with the membrane of the absorptive cell. × 7000. (*Courtesy of* S. Teichberg, PhD).

from AIDS-associated vasculopathy of the mesenteric and mesocolic arteries may be superficial and subclinical, or may be complicated by perforation (Fig. 184-7) [5••]. This process is characterized by intimal fibrosis, fragmentation of the internal elastic lamina, and vascular luminal narrowing and has been attributed to viral, bacterial, or other infections or to an altered immune response, all resulting in elastic tissue damage [23]. Nonvascular and noninfectious ulcerations, involving the ileum, the cecum, or both with perforation and alteration of the submucosal vessels, also have been described [5].

Smooth muscle tumors, Kaposi's sarcoma, and lymphoma affect the gastrointestinal tract of children with AIDS (*see* Table 184-2).

Both leiomyomas and leiomyosarcomas have been described [24]. The tumors may be numerous, affecting the stomach, duodenum , small bowel, appendix, colon, and rectum in the same patient and causing abdominal pain, gastrointestinal bleeding, and intestinal obstruction. Leiomyomas and leiomyosarcomas of the gastrointestinal tract also occur in HIV-negative

immunosuppressed children, after liver transplantation [25], renal transplantation, and chemotherapy for leukemia. The identification of EBV genomes in tumor cells by in situ hybridization and a high copy number of EBV by quantitative polymerase chain reaction (PCR) suggest an etiologic role of EBV in these smooth muscle tumors [26]. Decreased immuno-surveillance, increased expression of EBV receptors, and high levels of EBV in the plasma may contribute to the pathogenesis of these smooth muscle tumors.

Kaposi's sarcoma involves the gastrointestinal tract as part of disseminated disease.

AIDS-associated lymphomas are B-lineage, non-Hodgkin's lymphomas, and often are fatal despite initial response to chemotherapy. These lymphomas are commonly multifocal, are of the Burkitt's or lymphoblastic type, and have been reported to involve the stomach, duodenum, and small bowel [27]. Both HIV and EBV have been implicated in the development of lymphomas [28]. The etiologic role of EBV is strengthened by the frequent association of EBV-related interstitial lymphoid

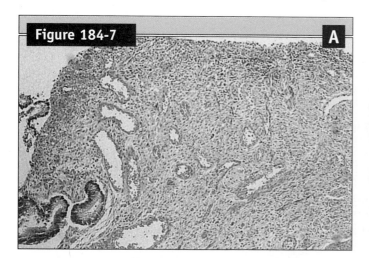

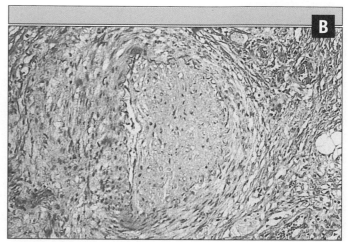

AIDS-associated vasculopathy of the colon. **A,** Nonspecific ulceration of the mucosa associated with granulation tissue. Hematoxylin and eosin stain, original magnification × 250.

B, Intimal fibrosis of a corresponding mesocolic artery with marked luminal narrowing. (Hematoxylin and eosin stain, original magnification × 250.)

pneumonia and lymphoma, seropositivity for EBV, and the presence of EBV DNA in lymphoma tissue.

Malabsorption

Malabsorption must be considered in children with AIDS who have diarrhea and weight loss. Lactose malabsorption occurs in approximately 40% to 60% of studied children with AIDS [29]. Lactose malabsorption often, but not invariably, correlates with intestinal symptoms [29]. Many patients with lactose malabsorption also have identifiable pathogens [29]. In children, abnormalities of d-xylose absorption correlate with lactose malabsorption [29].

Diagnosis and Treatment

The evaluation of a child with AIDS and diarrhea is similar to that of an adult [30]. Although a stepwise approach (Fig. 184-8) is preferred, multiple tests often are performed simultaneously because of the difficulty in obtaining samples and performing invasive procedures in children. For example, sequential upper

and lower endoscopic examinations may be done in a single session to obtain stool, and duodenal fluid for analysis and tissue for histology and measure of mucosal disaccharidase activity.

In patients with pure colitic symptoms or symptoms of left-sided colonic disease, flexible sigmoidoscopy and biopsy usually are diagnostic [31]. When sigmoidoscopy yields normal findings or proximal colonic disease is suspected based on the patient's symptoms (eg, severe gastrointestinal hemorrhage associated with CMV colitis may involve only the ileum and right colon), colonoscopy should be performed and biopsy samples obtained [5••,14].

Treatment is directed toward whatever pathogens have been isolated.

Pathogens such as MAI and *Cryptosporidium* organisms are as difficult to eradicate in children as they are in adults. Multidrug therapies recommended for MAI often are ineffective in eradicating the organism but do ameliorate symptoms. Given the lack of effective specific anti-infectious therapies for cryptosporidia, the mainstays of therapy remain supportive care,

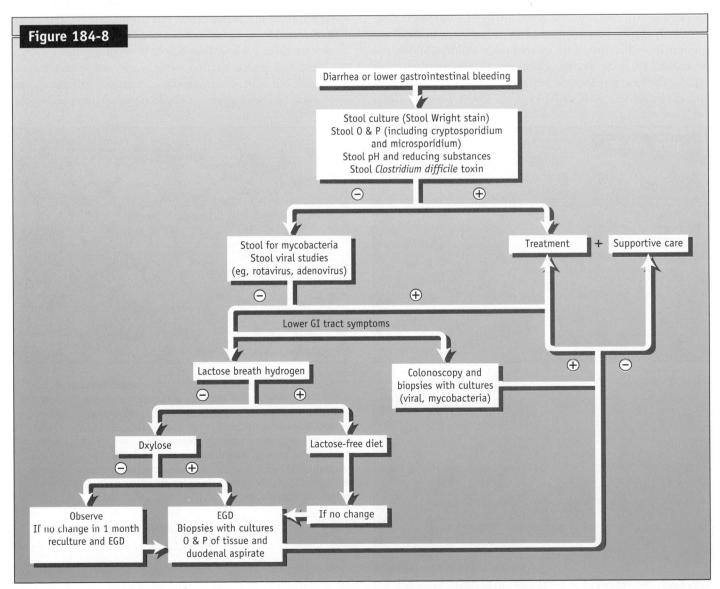

Figure 184-8

Algorithm for evaluation of an HIV-infected child with diarrhea, lower gastrointestinal (GI) bleeding, or both. EGD— esophagogastroduodenoscopy; O & P—ova and parasites. (*Adapted from* Lewis and Winter [30].)

including fluid and electrolyte replacement, and nutritional support. Despite the ineffectiveness of intravenous somatostatin in adults with diarrhea, most pediatric gastroenterologists still use somatostatin for the most severely affected patients. Dietary modifications (*eg*, a lactose-free diet, MCT oil–containing formula) are used to minimize the symptoms of malabsorption and improve nutritional status. Occasionally, loperamide hydrochloride is given in an attempt to slow intestinal transport, decrease the frequency of stools, and increase water absorption.

Anus
Anogenital warts and perianal condylomata caused by human papillomavirus (HPV) have been observed in children with AIDS.

HEPATOBILIARY AND PANCREATIC DISEASE
Most children infected with HIV have hepatomegaly and biochemical evidence of hepatic dysfunction, but few develop severe hepatocellular dysfunction or hepatic failure [2]. Elevated serum transaminase levels are quite common in children with AIDS and are caused by infections, medications, and nutritional factors. Tumors are rare in children and do not contribute to their deaths. Common pathogens that cause hepatic dysfunction include hepatitis B and C virus, opportunistic infections such as MAI (Fig. 184-9, see also **Color**

Plate), CMV, cryptococcus, cryptosporidia, and adenovirus [32]. Liver failure resulting from confluent or massive hepatic necrosis has been described with adenovirus infection [33]. Symptoms and signs of chronic hepatitis also can have an immune cause related to EBV, HIV, or both [32]. Such an immune pattern of chronic hepatitis, noted only in tissue obtained by liver biopsy, is not apparent at autopsy, perhaps because of the pronounced lymphocytic depletion in the terminal stage of AIDS (Fig. 184-10).

Although children occasionally develop hepatobiliary obstruction, it is most commonly related to parenteral nutrition and caused by sludge and stones. CMV and cryptosporidia, thought to cause acalculous cholecystitis in adults, have not been documented to do this in children. Whereas cryptosporidial involvement of the biliary tract and pancreatic duct can lead to suppurative cholangitis, hepatic abscess, dilatation of the extrahepatic biliary tract, and acute pancreatitis, infection with *Cryptococcus* spp. can cause suppurative cholangitis. Concomitant infection with *Cryptosporidium* and *Cryptococcus* organisms may occur [17]. AIDS-related sclerosing cholangitis, described in adults, is not often seen in children. Nevertheless, ERCP should be considered in the child with persistent cholestatic disease whose liver biopsy is nondiagnostic.

Giant cell transformation, with signs and symptoms of cholestasis but without demonstrable infectious pathogens, has been noted in liver biopsies of children with AIDS [32,34]. At

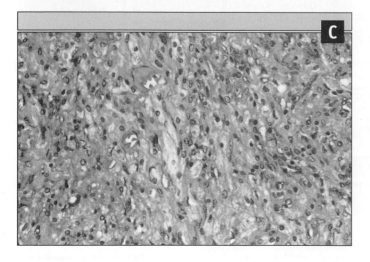

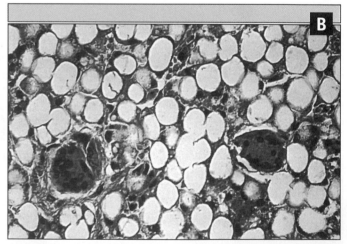

Figure 184-9

Different morphologic expressions of *Mycobacterium avium intracellulare* (MAI) infection of the liver. **A,** Loose granuloma composed of epithelioid cells with abundant cytoplasm. Hematoxylin and eosin, × 400. **B,** Multinucleated foreign body giant cells (special stains show MAI organism in the cytoplasm, not shown). Hematoxylin and eosin stain, original magnification × 250. **C,** Pseudosarcomatous variant of MAI with fascicle of densely packed spindle cells, some with abundant pale cytoplasm. (Hematoxylin and eosin stain, original magnification × 500.) See also **Color Plate.**

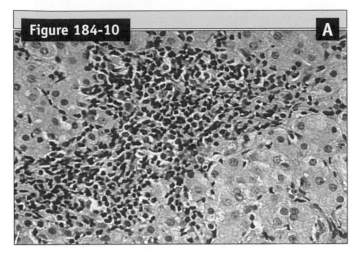

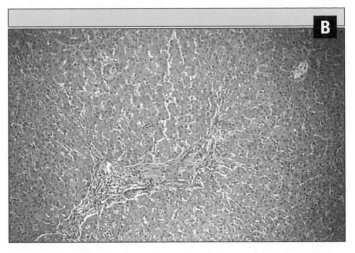

Chronic hepatitis. **A,** Biopsy specimen with a patchy lobular infiltrate and portal inflammation with piecemeal necrosis. Hematoxylin and eosin stain, original magnification × 250.

B, Tissue from same patient obtained at autopsy. The lobular and portal infiltrate is no longer seen. Mild portal fibrosis persists. (Hematoxylin and eosin stain, original magnification × 125.)

autopsy, giant cell transformation of periportal hepatocytes was the only significant hepatic change (Fig. 184-11). No microorganisms were discernible within these cells by special stains, and viral inclusions or excessive amounts of hemosiderin were not noted. In addition, no other disease states were found that might cause giant cell transformation, specifically CMV and herpes virus [32]. Therefore, it is possible that giant cell formation in the liver may reflect a reaction to the HIV similar to the reaction that occurs in other organs.

Many of the medications used in children with AIDS cause hepatocellular injury as well as cholestasis. These include zidovudine (AZT), erythromycin, amphotericin-B, ketoconazole, pentamidine, rifampin, dapsone, and ddi. The effects of therapeutic drugs and malnutrition associated with liver dysfunction are noted at autopsy as steatosis, cholestasis, and hepatocellular necrosis [32]. Confluent necrosis secondary to shock, sepsis, or both may manifest itself as liver failure.

Smooth muscle tumors, Kaposi's sarcoma, and lymphoma occur in the liver of children with AIDS.

Primary leiomyomas and leiomyosarcomas of the liver reported in five children with AIDS may express the increased incidence of smooth muscle tumors in these children [35–38]. Kaposi's sarcoma of the liver is associated with tumor infiltration of extrahepatic organs [34]. Lymphoma of the liver either is seen as primary disease [34] or occurs in the setting of systemic involvement [32].

There are no studies in children with AIDS to ascertain the value of liver biopsy in elucidating the cause of hepatocellular dysfunction or cholestasis, although liver biopsy provides significant information in approximately 50% of adults with AIDS. Liver biopsies with appropriate culture technique may be helpful in elucidating the source of persistent fever in a child with AIDS.

Treatment of hepatobiliary dysfunction in AIDS is diagnosis specific. No information is yet available regarding the use of interferon in the treatment of hepatitis B or C in children with AIDS.

Pancreatic involvement has been reported in 17% of children with AIDS [39]. The frequent use of ddi appears to have increased the incidence of pancreatitis in adults and children.

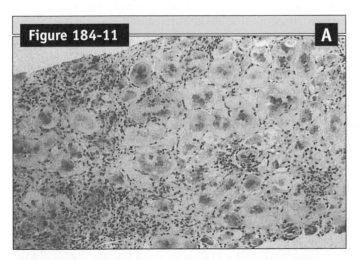

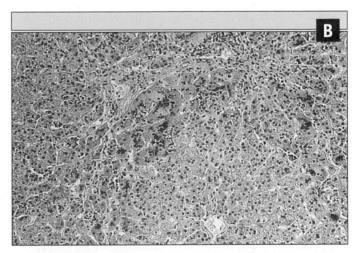

Giant cell transformation of hepatocytes. **A,** The liver biopsy specimen shows disorganization of the cell plates, cholestasis, extramedullary hematopoiesis, and multinucleated hepatic giant cells. **B,** Specimen obtained from same patient at autopsy.

Multinucleated hepatocytes are restricted to the periportal area. No other changes are noted. (Hematoxylin and eosin stain, original magnification × 250.)

Figure 184-12

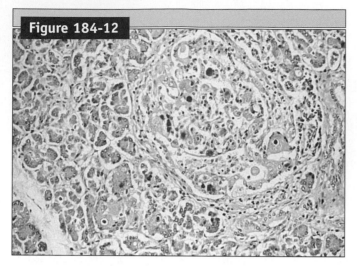

Cytomegalovirus infection of the pancreas with numerous intranuclear inclusions in acinar (*curved arrow*) and endocrine (*straight arrow*) cells. (Hematoxylin and eosin stain, original magnification × 500.)

Pancreatic changes noted at autopsy in 83% of children with AIDS usually are mild, reflect systemic disease states, and usually are not life threatening [40]. These changes may be nonspecific or may be the result of CMV (Fig. 184-12), MAI, or *Mycobacterium tuberculosis* infection. Only one report describes pancreatic involvement by systemic Burkitt's lymphoma [41].

Subclinical acute pancreatitis has been noted following *Pneumocystitis carinii* pneumonia in patients treated with pentamidine, and in children with MAI infection given rifampin [40]; one child had clinical symptoms and signs of acute fatal pancreatitis following treatment with ddi (Fig. 184-13, see also **Color Plate**) [40].

Symptomatic acute pancreatitis in children with AIDS has been ascribed to opportunistic infections such as CMV, cryptosporidia, MAI and *Pneumocystis carinii* [39], and to therapeutic drugs, such as pentamidine and ddi [42,43]. Pancreatitis following pentamidine administration developed 7 days to 4.5 months after onset of treatment [39]. Five of nine children reported by Miller *et al.* [39] who had developed pentamidine-associated acute pancreatitis had also received zidovudine.

Clinically, the children had vague periumbilical pain, decreased bowel sounds, elevation of the serum amylase and lipase concentrations, and an enlarged echogenic pancreas. Of eight patients followed, seven died between 0.5–13 days (mean 5 days), all of whom had an absolute CD4 T-lymphocyte count less than 100 cells/mm^3. Therefore, in this group of patients, pancreatitis was a poor prognostic sign and was responsible for death in 27% of the total patient population. These observations differ from those of Kahn *et al.* [40], who (based on autopsy findings) noted that of 11 children with AIDS and pancreatitis, only one died as the result of pancreatic disease.

Butler *et al.* [43] described ddi-associated acute pancreatitis in 7% of children with AIDS 12 to 16 weeks after initiation of therapy. The pancreatitis resolved with discontinuation of the drug and recurred after rechallenge [43]. Whereas the initial episode of pancreatitis developed only in patients treated with the highest daily dose levels of at least 360 mg/mm^2, recurrences occurred at lower doses. It was thought that pancreatitis was related to the daily dosage of ddi, not to the duration of therapy or a cumulative dose effect. These authors found no correlation between the development of pancreatitis and the patients' absolute CD4 counts or pentamidine therapy, although one third of the patients had received pentamidine. Although pancreatitis recurred in some patients after rechallenge, it did not constitute a contraindication to the use of ddi in the absence of other therapeutic options [43]. The fatal case of ddi-associated acute pancreatitis [40] dictates extreme caution and close surveillance of children treated with ddi.

Symptomatic chronic pancreatitis has been reported in a child with AIDS with malabsorption, foul-smelling stools, and failure to thrive. At autopsy, the pancreas was fibrotic. Severe malnutrition may result in chronic pancreatitis. Chronic pancreatitis also can result from repeated episodes of acute pancreatitis from adenovirus infection or during treatment with pentamidine and ddi for PCP [40].

Children who present with moderate to severe abdominal pain or vomiting, or both, associated with a high serum amylase level should have serum lipase concentrations measured and ultrasound or CT scans performed (as needed) to diagnose pancreatitis. Stool studies, blood cultures, and possibly even tissue analysis (either liver or intestine) should be considered if an

Figure 184-13   **A**   **B**

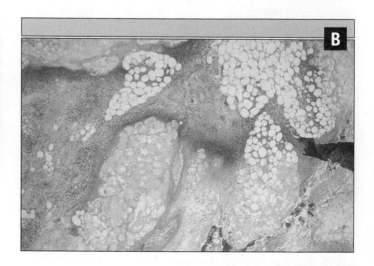

A case of ddi-associated acute hemorrhagic fatal pancreatitis associated with ddi. **A,** Macroscopic appearance of the pancreas with focal dark red areas of discoloration. **B,** Recent necrosis of the pancreas, with fat necrosis and neutrophilic infiltrate. (Hematoxylin and eosin stain, original magnification × 125.) See also **Color Plate**.

infectious agent is suspected. Treatment is supportive and also directed toward any diagnosed infection.

Malnutrition and Failure to Thrive

Significant tissue wasting and malnutrition are major clinical consequences of HIV infection. Both contribute to the progression, morbidity, and mortality of HIV disease. Indeed, growth failure itself may be a subtle prognostic indicator for progression to active AIDS in the HIV-seropositive child. In adults, death from AIDS may be related to the magnitude of tissue depletion [44]. Likewise, in children, failure to thrive has been associated with a shorter survival time [45]. In addition to these direct effects on morbidity and mortality, malnutrition adversely affects the integrity of the mucosal barrier, the ability to mount an acute phase response, and cellular immune function.

Although there are many studies in the literature that address the nutritional issues of adults with AIDS, there are few comparable studies in HIV-infected children. It is clear, however, that malnutrition, as evidenced by weight loss and decreased height velocity, is a common feature in pediatric HIV infection. Studies suggest that more than 80% of HIV-infected children have growth abnormalities. HIV-infected children appear to become stunted early in life, and have lower weight-for-age and lower length-for-age z-scores than do uninfected controls born to HIV-infected mothers [46]. Despite these decreases in weight-for-age and length-for-age measurements, linear growth and weight appear to be decreased proportionally; thus, acceptable weight-for-height measurements are preserved, often delaying referral for nutritional care until severe malnutrition and wasting have occurred. Adolescent boys with HIV infection have been shown to have decreased growth and pubertal delay even in the absence of severe nutritional wasting [47].

Specific nutrient deficiencies vary among HIV-infected individuals. Losses of specific macronutrients, such as carbohydrates or fats, often are related to the degree of gastrointestinal disturbances. However, malabsorption of all macronutrients—carbohydrates, fats, and proteins—can be found in a large percentage of children with HIV infection, even in the absence of gastrointestinal symptoms, malnutrition, or enteric infection [48].

Although deficiencies of many micronutrients, including selenium, vitamin B_6, vitamin A, vitamin B_{12}, and vitamin D, have been described in adults with AIDS, minimal information about such deficiencies in children is available. It is unclear whether micronutrient supplementation to prevent or correct micronutrient deficiencies slows the progression of HIV disease.

Similarly, although there are numerous studies of body composition changes in adults with AIDS, there are few such studies in children. Skinfold measurements suggest that HIV-infected children have an early decrease in lean body mass [49••].

The pathogenesis of undernutrition in children with AIDS is multifactorial and includes impaired nutrient absorption, increased energy requirements and metabolic derangements, and reduced food intake.

Table 184-4. Etiology of Nutritional Deficiencies in AIDS

Reduced food intake
  Primary anorexia
  Gastroesophageal reflux, delayed gastric emptying, or dysmotility
  Oral or esophageal lesions/infections
  Psychological (depression)
  AIDS-related encephalopathy
  Medications
  Environmental or socioeconomic factors
Impaired nutrient absorption
Increased energy expenditure or metabolic derangements

Impaired nutrient absorption obviously is related to gastrointestinal dysfunctions caused by enteric infections, disaccharidase deficiency, and small bowel bacterial overgrowth. Resting energy expenditure has not been studied in children with AIDS. The role of cytokines, such as TNF, IL-1, and IL-6, with regard to increased energy expenditure and futile cycling of substrates, well-known in adults, is beginning to emerge in pediatric patients with AIDS as well.

By far the most common feature associated with undernutrition in children with AIDS is reduced food intake (Table 184-4). Although not well-documented in the literature, symptoms of gastrointestinal dysmotility, sometimes associated with gastroesophageal reflux and esophagitis, appear to be common in these children. Complaints such as heartburn, early satiety, nausea, and abdominal pain often accompany poor intake. The socioeconomic situation of many families with HIV-infected children often diminishes the availability of food. In addition, in many instances the caretakers of these children also are suffering from AIDS and may be physically unable to purchase or prepare appropriate meals for their children.

Nutritional Assessment

A nutritional history, in addition to assessing caloric intake, also includes specific questions about the availability and preparation of infant formulas and foods for older children. Pediatric growth curves should be assessed to ascertain the nutritional status of the patient over time. Symptoms of gastrointestinal disturbances such as anorexia, nausea, vomiting, diarrhea, early satiety, heartburn, and fever should be elicited. Appropriate laboratory tests to determine significant gastrointestinal complications can then be undertaken.

Nutritional Interventions

Because of the risk of viral transmission, infants born to HIV-infected mothers should not be breast-fed, but, rather, should be given standard infant formulas. Modifications of formulas, either to increase caloric density or to provide more easily absorbed nutrients, can be undertaken. In older infants, the caloric density of their favorite foods should be increased using carbohydrate or fat supplements. Nutritional supplements specifically designed for children are now available. Their expense may preclude availability for some children, although certain agencies may provide them if need can be documented. Newer elemental and semi-elemental formulas for children with malabsorption have been developed; these can be made relatively palatable with the flavor packet provided by the manufacturer, or delivered via feeding tube.

Treatment of underlying gastrointestinal infections, especially those causing esophagitis, can be helpful in improving oral intake. For patients with early satiety or gastroesophageal reflux, nutrient intake may be improved by use of gastrointestinal motility agents. Appetite stimulants (*eg,* megestrol acetate [Megace] and dronabinol [Marinol]; Roxane Laboratories, Columbus, OH) have been used with some success in adult patients. Although some centers are using these agents in children, there are as yet no published data on efficacy. Dronabinol has significant side effects such as lethargy and mental status changes that may preclude long-term use in children (unpublished data). Cyproheptadine (Periactin; Merck & Co. West Point, PA) may be useful as an appetite stimulant.

All interventions in children with HIV require the evaluation of environmental and psychosocial factors, including assessment of the availability of food. Enlisting the assistance of the social service department is crucial, and healthcare providers must work hand-in-hand with social workers in implementing their plans.

The feasibility, safety, and efficacy of enteral and parenteral nutrition in HIV-infected adults has been documented [50]. In children, enteral nutritional support has been shown to be safe and efficacious whether delivered via nasogastric tube, percutaneous endoscopic gastrostomy (PEG), or surgical gastrostomy [51•]. Because of better wound healing, PEGs appear to be slightly better tolerated than operative gastrostomies. Use of continuous infusions instead of intermittent bolus feedings also can be helpful, especially in patients with GE reflux or malabsorption or maldigestion [51•].

Parenteral nutrition is an appropriate option for the child with gastrointestinal dysfunction that precludes enteral feedings. At times, because these children already have venous access devices for frequent intravenous medications, there may be a psychological benefit to providing parenteral nutrition instead of tube feedings. However, because of the increased costs, the significant increase in workload for the child's caretaker, and the risk of infection, most clinicians defer parenteral nutrition for the child with significant gastrointestinal problems. Parenteral nutrition can be safely provided in various stages of HIV infection, and, at least in adults, significant improvement has been demonstrated in healing, weight gain, and quality of life. Social and environmental issues also must influence the choice of modality for nutrition support.

PROGNOSIS

Gastrointestinal and nutritional problems in children with AIDS can be a significant cause of morbidity. Aggressive diagnostic evaluation and support, especially in treating gastrointestinal infections and providing adequate nutrition, can improve outcome and quality of life. Certain gastrointestinal complications, especially infection with agents such as

Cryptosporidium spp., still are not easily managed and contribute to the mortality of this disease.

Quality-of-life issues are paramount in any discussion of the management of gastrointestinal and nutritional problems in children with AIDS. The goals of childhood include both physical and emotional growth and development and the acquisition of educational and practical skills for adult life. With the possibility that newer antiretroviral agents will help lengthen the lifespan of these children, it is incumbent upon all physicians caring for these children to provide optimal medical as well as psychological and social support. For example, children with AIDS-related enteropathy and diarrhea should be encouraged to go to school and partake in activities with other children of their own age. The physician must be an advocate for children with AIDS, in the school and in the community, and the gastroenterologist must be an integral part of the healthcare team.

REFERENCES

Recently published papers of particular interest have been highlighted as:

• Of interest
•• Of outstanding interest

1. Centers for Disease Control: AIDS Among Children: United States, 1996. *MMWR Morb Mortal Wkly Rep* 1996, 45:1005–1010.

2. Winter H, Chang T: Gastrointestinal and nutritional problems in children with immunodeficiency and AIDS. *Pediatr Clin North Am* 1996, 43:573–590.

3. Benkov KJ: Gastrointestinal aspects of acquired immunodeficiency syndrome in children. In *Pediatric Gastrointestinal Disease. Pathophysiology, Diagnosis, Management.* Edited by Wyllie R, Hyams JS. Philadelphia; WB Saunders, 1993:712–723.

4. Dieterich DT, Wilcox M, *et al.*: Diagnosis and treatment of esophageal disease associated with HIV infection. *Am J Gastroenterol* 1996, 91:2265–2269.

5.•• Kahn E. Gastrointestinal manifestations in pediatric AIDS. *Pediatr Pathol Lab Med* 1997, 17:171–208.
A recent comprehensive review of pathologic findings from specimens obtained after surgery or autopsies in children with AIDS. This paper reviews the infectious and neoplastic processes as well as lymphoproliferative and miscellaneous lesions of the gastrointestinal tract.

6. Kotler DP, Wilson CS, Harutounian G, *et al.*: Detection of human immunodeficiency virus I by 35S-RNA in situ hybridization in solitary esophageal ulcers in two patients with acquired immunodeficiency syndrome. *Am J Gastroenterol* 1989, 84:313–317.

7. Blecker U, Keymolen K, Lanciers S, *et al.*: The prevalence of *Helicobacter pylori* positivity in human immunodeficiency virus-infected children. *J Pediatr Gastroenterol Nutr* 1994, 19:417–420.

8. Victoria MS, Nangia BS, Gindrack K: Cytomegalovirus, pyloric obstruction in a child with acquired immunodeficiency syndrome. *Pediatr Infect Dis* 1985, 4:550–552.

9. Joshi VV, Kauffman S, Oleske JM, *et al.*: Polyclonal polymorphic B-cell lymphoproliferative disorder with prominent pulmonary involvement in children with acquired immune deficiency syndrome. *Cancer* 1987, 59:1455–1462.

10. Schindzielorz A, Pike I, Daniels M, *et al.*: Rates and risk factors for adverse events associated with didanosine in the expanded access program. *Clin Infect Dis* 1994, 19:1076–1083.

11. Sivit CJ, Josephs SH, Taylor GA, Kushner DC: Pneumatosis intestinalis in children with AIDS. *Am J Roentgenol* 1990, 155:133–134.

12. Patrick CC, Hawkins EP, Guerra C, Taber LH: A patient with leukemia in remission and abdominal pain. *J Pediatr* 1987, 111:624–629.

13. Cappell MS, Hassan T, Rosenthal S, Mascarenhas M: Gastrointestinal obstruction due to *Mycobacterium avium intracellulare* associated with the acquired immunodeficiency syndrome. *Am J Gastroenterol* 1992, 87:1823–1827.

14. Schwartz DL, So HB, Bungarz WR, *et al.*: A case of life threatening gastrointestinal hemorrhage in an infant with AIDS. *J Pediatr Surg* 1989, 24:313–315.

15. Dolgin SE, Larsen JG, Shah KD, David E: CMV enteritis causing hemorrhage and obstruction in an infant with AIDS. *J Pediatr Surg* 1990, 25:696–698.

16. Haller JO, Cohen JL: Gastrointestinal manifestations of AIDS in children. *Am J Roentgenol* 1994, 162:387–393.

17. Rusin JA, Sivit CJ, Rakusan TA, Chandra RS: AIDS-related cholangitis in children: Sonographic findings. *Am J Roentgenol* 1992, 159:626–627.

18. Beeg T, Linde R, Mentzer O, *et al.*: Acute pancreatitis in HIV infected child with chronic cryptosporidiosis [abstract PUB 7030]. *Int Conf AIDS* 1992; 8:54.

19. McLoughlin LC, Nord KS, Joshi VV, *et al.*: Severe gastrointestinal involvement in children with the acquired immunodeficiency syndrome. *J Pediatr Gastroenterol Nutr* 1987, 6:517–523.

20. Batman PA, Miller ARO, Forster SM, *et al.*: Jejunal enteropathy associated with human immunodeficiency virus infection: quantitative histology. *J Clin Pathol* 1989, 42:275–281.

21. Lewin KJ, Riddel RH, Weinstein WM: Immunodeficiency disorders. In *Gastrointestinal Pathology and Its Clinical Implications.* New York: Igaku-Shoin; l992:104–150.

22. Winter HS, Miller TL, Hobson CD: Enteropathy in congenital HIV infection: histologic and molecular evaluation. *Gastroenterology* 1991,100(suppl A):626A.

23. Joshi VV: Pathology of acquired immunodeficiency syndrome (AIDS) in children. In *Pathology of AIDS and Other Manifestations of HIV Infection.* Edited by Joshi VV. New York: Igaku-Shoin; 1990:239–269.

24. Chadwick EG, Connor EJ, Guerra Hanson IC, *et al.*: Tumors of smooth-muscle origin in HIV infected children. *JAMA* 1990, 263:3182–3184.

25. Timmons CF, Dawson DB, Richards CS, *et al.*: Epstein-Barr virus-associated leiomyosarcomas in liver transplantation recipients. *Cancer* 1995, 76:1481–1489.

26. McLain KL, Leach CT, Jenson HB, *et al.*: Association of Epstein-Barr virus with leiomyosarcomas in young people with AIDS. *N Engl J Med* 1995, 332:12–18.

27. Serraino D, Salamina G, Franceschi S, *et al.*: The epidemiology of AIDS-associated non-Hodgkin's lymphoma in the World Health Organization European Region. *Br J Cancer* 1992, 66:912–916.

28. Laurence J, Astrin SM: Human immunodeficiency virus induction of malignant transformation in human B lymphocytes. *Proc Natl Acad Sci U S A* 1991, 88:7635–7639.

29. Yolken RH, Hart W, Oung I, *et al.*: Gastrointestinal dysfunction and disaccharidase intolerance in children infected with human immunodeficiency virus. *J Pediatr* 1991, 118:359–363.

30. Lewis J, Winter H: Intestinal and hepatobiliary diseases in HIV infected children. *Gastroenterol Clin North Am* 1995, 24:119–132.

31. Wilcox CM, Rabeneck L, Friedman S: American Gastroenterologic Association medical position statement: guidelines for the management of malnutrition and cachexia, chronic diarrhea, and hepatobiliary disease in patients with human immunodeficiency virus infection. *Gastroenterology* 1996, 111:1722–1752.

32. Kahn E, Greco MA, Daum F, *et al.*: Hepatic pathology in pediatric AIDS. *Hum Pathol* 1991, 22:1111–1119.

33. Janner D, Petru AM, Belchis D, Azimi PH: Fatal adenovirus infection in a child with acquired immunodeficiency syndrome. *Pediatr Inf Dis J* 1990, 9:434–436.

34. Jonas NM, Roldan EO, Lyons HJ, *et al.*: Histopathologic features of the liver in pediatric acquired immune deficiency syndrome. *J Pediatr Gastroenterol Nutr* 1989, 9:73–81.

35. Mueller BU, Butler KM, Higham MC, *et al.*: Smooth muscle tumors in children with human immunodeficiency virus infection. *Pediatrics* 1992, 90:460–463.

36. van Hoeven KH, Factor SM, Kress Y, Woodruff JM: Visceral myogenic tumors: a manifestation of HIV infection in children. *Am J Surg Pathol* 1993, 17:1176–1181.

37. Ross JS, Del Rosario A, Bui HX, *et al.*: Primary hepatic leiomyosarcoma in a child with acquired immunodeficiency syndrome. *Hum Pathol* 1992, 23:69–72.

38. Ninane J, Moulin D, Latinne D, *et al.*: AIDS in two African children—one with fibrosarcoma of the liver. *Eur J Pediatr* 1985, 144:385–390.

39. Miller TL, Winter HS, Luginbuhl LM, *et al.*: Pancreatitis in pediatric human immunodeficiency virus infection. *J Pediatr* 1992, 120:223–227.

40. Kahn E, Anderson VM, Greco MA, Magid M: Pancreatic disorders in pediatric acquired immune deficiency syndrome. *Hum Pathol* 1995, 26:765–770.

41. Graif M, Kessler A, Newman T, *et al.*: Pancreatic Burkitts lymphoma in AIDS: sonographic appearance. *Am J Radiol* 1987, 149:1290–1291.

42. Butler KM, Husson RN, Balis FM, *et al.*: Dideoxyinosine in children with symptomatic human deficiency virus infection. *N Engl J Med* 1991, 324:137–144.

43. Butler KM, Venzon D, Henry N, *et al.*: Pancreatitis in human immunodeficiency virus-infected children receiving dideoxyinosine. *Pediatrics* 1993, 91:747–751.

44. Kotler DP, Tierney AR, Wang J, Pierson RN: Magnitude of body cell mass depletion and the timing of death from wasting in AIDS. *Am J Clin Nutr* 1989, 50:444–447.

45. Tovo PA, DeMartino M, Gabiano C, *et al.*: Prognostic factors in survival in children with perinatal HIV-1 infection. *Lancet* 1992, 339:1249–1253.

46. Saavedra JM, Henderson RA, Perman JA, *et al.*: Longitudinal assessment of growth in children born to HIV infected mothers. *Arch Pediatr Adolesc Med* 1995, 149:497– 502.

47. Gertner JM, Kaufman FR, Donfield SM, *et al.*: Delayed somatic growth and pubertal development in HIV infected hemophiliac boys: hemophilia, growth and development study. *J Pediatr* 1994, 124:896–902.

48. Italian Pediatric Intestinal HIV Study Group: Intestinal malabsorption of HIV infected children: relationships to diarrhea, failure to thrive, enteric micro-organisms and immune impairment. *AIDS* 1993, 7:1435–1440.

49.•• Miller TL, Evans SJ, Orav EJ, *et al.*: Growth and body composition in children infected with the human immunodeficiency virus. *Am J Clin Nutr* 1993, 57:588–592.

This paper was one of the first to suggest decreased growth and body mass in HIV-infected infants, even prior to overt signs of AIDS. It has spawned interest in studies of early nutritional intervention in these children.

50. Kotler DP, Tierney AR, Ferraro R, *et al.*: Enteral alimentation in repletion of body cell mass in malnourished patients with AIDS. *Am J Clin Nutr* 1991, 53:149–154.

51.• Henderson RA, Saavedra JM, Perman JA, *et al.*: Effective enteral tube feeding on growth of children with symptomatic human immunodeficiency virus syndrome. *J Pediatr Gastroenterol Nutr* 1994, 18:429–434.

A recent study of the efficacy of tube feedings in children with AIDS. It is pointed out that gastrostomy tubes can be safe and useful to provide nutrition support. As with most pediatric studies in AIDS, the number of patients was small and only skinfold measurements were used to assess body composition.

9

Special Topics

Edited by Lawrence S. Friedman

Contributors

Lawrence J. Brandt

Carolyn C. Compton

Mark H. DeLegge

Rebecca Copenhaver
 DeLegge

Anthony J. DiMarino, Jr

Gary W. Falk

M. Brian Fennerty

Christopher J. Gostout

David A. Greenwald

Ian Grimm

Ronald J. Hapke

Aminah Jatoi

Kris V. Kowdley

Howard S. Kroop

Anne M. Larson

Joel B. Mason

Kevin W. Olden

Hugo R. Rosen

Mark W. Russo

Rebecca G. Wells

Gary J. Whitman

C. Mel Wilcox

Jacqueline L. Wolf

Steven Zacks

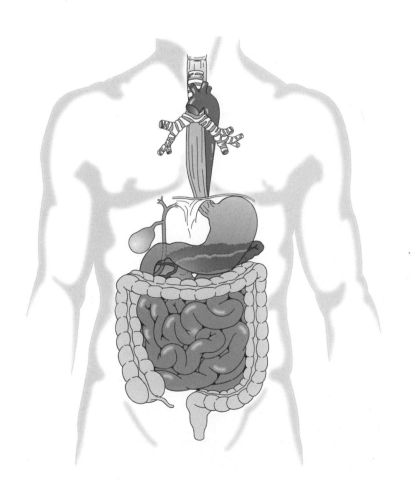

185 Gastrointestinal Manifestations of AIDS

C. Mel Wilcox

Human immunodeficiency virus (HIV) infection is an important cause of morbidity and mortality throughout the world. Although the incidence of HIV infection in developed countries has stabilized or decreased, the epidemic continues unabated in developing countries. Gastrointestinal complications associated with the acquired immunodeficiency syndrome (AIDS) are important because of their high incidence, associated morbidity, and impact on health care systems [1]. During the past decade, the spectrum of diseases involving the gastrointestinal tract has evolved as a result of improvements in diagnostic testing, the increased use of prophylactic therapy to prevent HIV-related complications such as *Pneumocystis carinii* pneumonia (PCP), and the development of potent antiretroviral therapy. As the incidence of PCP has fallen, however, an increase in other complications, including cytomegalovirus (CMV) infection, has been observed [2,3•]. This chapter focuses on the major organ systems involved in AIDS-related gastrointestinal disease and reviews the etiologies, manifestations, evaluation, and treatment of gastrointestinal disease in patients with AIDS.

GENERAL PRINCIPLES

A number of important principles, many of which are unique to patients with AIDS, guide the evaluation of the HIV-infected patient with gastrointestinal complaints:

1. In patients with AIDS, multiple diseases frequently coexist.
2. Opportunistic infections occur when immunodeficiency is severe. Therefore, the CD4 lymphocyte count helps to determine the likelihood of an opportunistic process (Fig. 185-1).
3. Opportunistic disorders are often systemic. Identification of a pathogen in other tissues (*eg*, blood) may establish a presumptive cause of gastrointestinal disease.
4. Demonstration of a pathogen in tissue is the most specific means of establishing an etiologic diagnosis.
5. A nihilistic approach to evaluation is inappropriate because many therapies are effective in decreasing morbidity and improving the quality of life.
6. Despite effective therapy, recurrence is common for all opportunistic infections because of persistence of immunodeficiency.

OROPHARYNGEAL DISEASES

Disease of the oropharynx may be the initial manifestation of HIV infection; in particular, oropharyngeal candidiasis (thrush) is a common presentation [4•]. Patients with oropharyngeal disease may not have symptoms or may present with taste disturbances or pain. Oropharyngeal or hypopharyngeal pain is

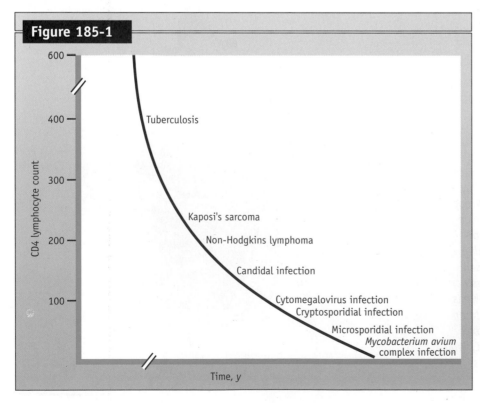

Figure 185-1

Graphic relation between the occurrence of opportunistic infections and the CD4 lymphocyte count in the natural history of human immunodeficiency virus infection.

usually a manifestation of ulceration. Aphthous ulcers are the most commonly seen single or multiple well-circumscribed ulcers (Fig. 185-2; see also *Color Plate*), but the causes of these lesions are undetermined in most cases. Identifiable causes of oropharyngeal ulcers include CMV, herpes simplex virus (HSV), and rare infections and malignancies (*eg*, squamous cell carcinoma). Other neoplasms that involve the oropharynx include lymphoma, which usually presents as an ulcerating mass, and Kaposi's sarcoma (KS), which presents as characteristic purple plaques or nodules. Oral hairy leukoplakia, which is caused by Epstein-Barr virus infection, appears as a white plaque that coats the lateral aspect of the tongue, giving it a slightly furrowed appearance.

Given the high frequency of aphthous ulcers, biopsy of all oropharyngeal ulcers is unnecessary. Rather, empiric therapy should be instituted based on the appearance of the lesion, with close follow-up of the patient. Biopsy should be performed when lymphoma is suspected, when the appearance of the lesion is nondiagnostic, or when empiric therapy is ineffective.

Treatment of most oropharyngeal diseases is similar to that of the corresponding esophageal disease (discussed later). Although systemic therapy is highly effective, thrush can be treated with locally acting agents, such as clotrimazole troches (1 tablet dissolved in the mouth 3 to 5 times a day) [5]. Similarly, for aphthous ulcers, corticosteroid mouth rinses or intralesional injection of corticosteroids may provide symptomatic relief and clinical cure; if these approaches are ineffective, oral prednisone is indicated (20 to 40 mg/d tapered over 2 to 4 weeks). Although not widely available in the United States, thalidomide also appears to be highly effective. Like most opportunistic infections in patients with AIDS, recurrence is common once therapy is discontinued.

■ ESOPHAGEAL DISEASES

Disorders of the esophagus occur frequently in patients with AIDS and are found in as many as 40% of patients at some point during the course of the disease. The most common disease is candidal esophagitis, which occurs in 40% to 70% of patients [5,6••]. Next in importance are viral diseases. In con-

trast to its occurrence in non–HIV-infected immunocompromised patients, CMV is a much more frequent esophageal pathogen in HIV-infected patients than is HSV [7••]. Another important cause of esophageal disease is the HIV-associated idiopathic esophageal ulcer (IEU), the pathogenesis of which is poorly understood. Multiple, coexistent esophageal disorders may be identified in 10% or more of patients with symptoms [7••]. Gastroesophageal reflux disease may be seen at any stage of HIV-associated immunodeficiency. Pill-induced esophagitis and neoplasms (*eg*, KS, lymphoma, carcinoma) occur infrequently.

Esophageal disease is manifested by dysphagia (difficulty in the transit of a food bolus, usually described as food sticking in the throat) or odynophagia (painful swallowing). Symptoms localized to the neck or throat generally implicate hypopharyngeal rather than esophageal disease. In HIV-infected patients, odynophagia is highly suggestive of esophageal ulceration, usually caused by an opportunistic pathogen, whereas dysphagia is more commonly due to candidal esophagitis or to a benign or malignant stricture. Substernal chest pain or back pain also may be reported with severe ulcerative esophagitis. True "heartburn" suggests a diagnosis of gastroesophageal reflux disease rather than an opportunistic infection. Because symptoms alone are rarely diagnostic, however, further testing is often required.

Examination of the oropharynx may provide a clue to the cause of esophageal complaints. Most patients (about 66%) with candidal esophagitis have concomitant thrush. Oropharyngeal ulcerations are frequently associated with HSV esophagitis but rarely are present with CMV esophagitis and IEU.

Because of the high frequency of candidal esophagitis, empiric antifungal therapy is commonly prescribed to HIV-infected patients with the new onset of esophageal symptoms [7••]. The clinical response to therapy is usually rapid, with most patients improving within days. If no symptomatic response is seen within 1 week of initiating empiric therapy, especially in a patient with severe symptoms, additional diagnostic testing is required, rather than initiation of further empiric trials such as acid suppressive or antiviral therapy. Upper endoscopy is the preferred diagnostic approach. Cytology devices passed through the nares or mouth have been shown to detect candidal and HSV esophagitis but are not sensitive for the cytologic detection of CMV disease and do not identify IEU. Radiographic studies of the esophagus may suggest a specific etiology but are rarely diagnostic. Candidal esophagitis manifests radiographically as single or multiple plaque-like lesions that, when severe, may mimic ulcerations. Single or multiple well-circumscribed, large (>2 cm), deep ulcers are typical of CMV and IEU, whereas HSV presents radiographically as single or multiple shallow ulcers or as diffuse esophagitis (see Chapter 198).

Endoscopy is the definitive diagnostic test for esophageal disease in patients with AIDS. At the time of endoscopic evaluation, the appearance of some lesions, such as candidal plaques, may be diagnostic, but ulcerative lesions should be biopsied. Candidal infection appears endoscopically as multiple yellow plaque-like lesions, which may be isolated or become circumferential, coating the esophageal wall. The clinical, radiographic, and endoscopic features of CMV and

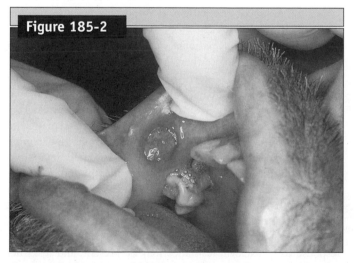

Figure 185-2

Photograph of a large oropharyngeal aphthous ulcer of the buccal mucosa. See also **Color Plate**.

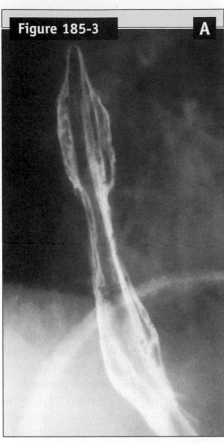

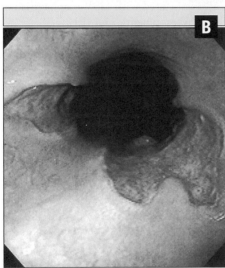

Idiopathic esophageal ulcers. **A**, Barium swallow demonstrating several large ulcers. **B**, Endoscopic photograph of two large, well-circumscribed ulcers in the midesophagus. The intervening mucosa is normal. Cytomegalovirus lesions can have a similar appearance. See also **Color Plate**.

IEU are similar (Fig. 185-3; see also *Color Plate*). HSV esophagitis usually results in multiple shallow ulcers or diffuse esophagitis, whereas deep, well-circumscribed lesions are typically caused by CMV or IEU. CMV or CMV and HSV coinfection may result in a patchy, superficial esophagitis.

Cytologic brushing is more sensitive than biopsy in diagnosing candidal infection. Cytologic brushings from ulcerative lesions (particularly those caused by CMV) are less sensitive and specific than is microscopic evaluation in detecting viral pathogens and are unnecessary if biopsy material is adequate. Viral culture of mucosal biopsy specimens is often diagnostic but rarely adds information to that obtained by multiple biopsy specimens and histologic evaluation. Multiple biopsy specimens

(at least 10) of all ulcerative lesions should be obtained to maximize sensitivity. Biopsy of the ulcer base is essential in detecting CMV, whereas HSV is best identified in squamous epithelium obtained from biopsy of the ulcer edge. Immunohistochemical stains for viral pathogens improve the diagnostic yield and specificity (see Chapter 198). Additional histologic examination for other fungi or mycobacteria should not be performed routinely, but rather should be performed on the basis of the clinical, endoscopic, and histologic findings. An ulcer can be considered idiopathic (IEU) if it is seen endoscopically and histologically, if infections are excluded by histologic studies, and if neither pill-induced esophagitis nor reflux disease is suggested by the clinical presentation or endoscopic findings.

Treatment of most esophageal diseases in patients with AIDS is highly effective. Candidal esophagitis can be cured with systemic antifungal therapy in 80% or more of patients. Fluconazole (100 mg/d) is the drug of choice because of its excellent absorption, minimal drug interactions and side effects, and superior efficacy [8•]. Although slightly less effective, itraconazole (200 mg/d) may be an alternative to fluconazole [9•]; ketoconazole is inferior to these two agents [8•]. In addition, ketoconazole has a number of potential drug interactions, and both ketoconazole and itraconazole have reduced bioavailability in an alkaline gastric pH. Seven to 14 days of antifungal therapy is adequate for most patients. A longer course of therapy may be required if the response is poor. Close follow-up of the patient is important because the relapse rate of candidal esophagitis is high; long-term antifungal prophylaxis may be required if relapses are frequent.

Long-term azole therapy and severe immunodeficiency are both associated with the development of azole resistance [10]. When clinical resistance to azole therapy occurs, increasing the dose of the drug, switching to another azole, or using intravenous amphotericin B may be required.

Herpes simplex virus esophagitis is treated effectively with acyclovir (400 mg five times a day) [11•], valacyclovir (1 g three times a day), or famciclovir (500 mg three times a day). Acyclovir should be administered intravenously in cases of severe disease. Rare cases of acyclovir resistance have been documented; in this situation, foscarnet is the drug of choice. Close follow-up of the patient is important because relapses may occur.

In about 80% of patients, CMV esophagitis responds to administration of either ganciclovir (5 mg/kg given intravenously twice a day) or foscarnet (90 mg/kg given intravenously twice a day), which often effect clinical and endoscopic cure [12••]. The main side effect of ganciclovir is myelosuppression, whereas foscarnet is nephrotoxic and may cause electrolyte disturbances (*eg*, hypocalcemia, hypophosphatemia). Renal insufficiency due to foscarnet may be prevented by vigorous hydration of the patient before and during therapy and by adjustment of the drug dose based on creatinine clearance. Combination therapy with both ganciclovir and foscarnet also has been used. At most medical centers, ganciclovir is the drug of choice, because of its relative tolerability and lower cost. If the patient has a poor response to ganciclovir, resistance may be present, and foscarnet should be used. CMV retinitis should be excluded at the time of diagnosis because long-term therapy is required in patients with this disease. About 40% to 50% of patients relapse after therapy. Maintenance ganciclovir is not routinely given for isolated gastrointestinal disease. Oral ganciclovir has not been evaluated for the primary or secondary treatment or prophylaxis of gastrointestinal CMV disease in patients with AIDS.

In more than 90% of patients, IEU responds to oral prednisone both symptomatically and endoscopically [13•]. This drug can be administered for 1 month, beginning with a dose of 40 mg/d and tapering by 10 mg/d each week. This regimen is well-tolerated and does not appear to predispose to other infections. Relapse occurs in many patients and can be treated similarly to the initial episode. Like oropharyngeal aphthous ulcers, IEU also responds well to thalidomide.

GASTRIC DISEASES

Disorders of the stomach are relatively uncommon in HIV-infected patients. Recent studies suggest that HIV-infected patients are less likely than those without HIV to have *Helicobacter pylori* infection, which may explain the low incidence of ulcer disease in these patients [14]. In addition, hypochlorhydria occurs in about 10% to 25% of patients with AIDS [15], a finding that has implications not only for the incidence of ulcer disease but also for the intestinal absorption of certain drugs, such as ketoconazole.

Epigastric pain, nausea, and vomiting are the most common symptoms of gastric diseases; these symptoms may mimic acute pancreatitis. Rarely, upper gastrointestinal hemorrhage is the initial presentation of gastric disease, suggesting ulceration. Nausea and vomiting are particularly common symptoms in HIV-infected patients, although usually not an indication of gastroduodenal mucosal disease. The most frequently occurring opportunistic infection involving the stomach in AIDS patients is CMV, which appears endoscopically as a patchy gastritis or as single or multiple ulcers. Infrequently seen gastric infections include cryptosporidiosis, cryptococcosis, and other parasitic disorders, such as toxoplasmosis and PCP. KS frequently involves the stomach, and although usually asymptomatic, it may result in pyloric obstruction, bleeding, or abdominal pain (Fig. 185-4). In contrast, gastric lymphoma is almost always symptomatic and manifests with epigastric pain; fever and peripheral adenopathy are rare associated findings.

Nonopportunistic disease, such as nonsteroidal anti-inflammatory–induced gastropathy, should be considered in the appropriate setting.

Evaluation of patients for possible gastric disease may be accomplished by a variety of methods. Upper endoscopy or upper gastrointestinal series may identify inflammatory changes, ulcerations, or mass lesions. Computed tomography (CT) may reveal thickening of the gastric wall or mass lesions. CT also may disclose hepatic, pancreatic, or splenic diseases as well as adenopathy, which suggests a widely disseminated process such as lymphoma. In light of the broad differential diagnosis in patients with AIDS and abdominal complaints, endoscopy and mucosal biopsy are generally required for definitive diagnosis.

SMALL BOWEL DISEASES

Infections of the small intestine are not unexpected in HIV-infected patients, in part because of altered gut immune function. A reduction in the number of CD4 lymphocytes in the lamina propria parallels the decrease in the systemic CD4 lymphocyte count. The reduced number of CD4 lymphocytes in small bowel may account for alterations in small intestinal morphology and function (discussed later). In addition, decreased local production of IgA may further predispose to intestinal infection.

Diseases of the small bowel in patients with AIDS are usually caused by opportunistic infections. Worldwide, *Cryptosporidium parvum*, a coccidian parasite, is the most common infection involving the small bowel. This infection causes a self-limited illness in normal hosts, but in HIV-infected patients, the prevalence and severity of disease parallel the degree of immunodeficiency. Patients with CD4 lymphocyte counts of more than 200/mm^3 may have self-limited disease, whereas in patients with CD4 lymphocyte counts less than 50/mm^3, the disease is chronic, can be life-threatening, and is associated with poor survival [16]. The severity of disease, both clinically and morphologically, also is related to the parasite burden (Fig. 185-5).

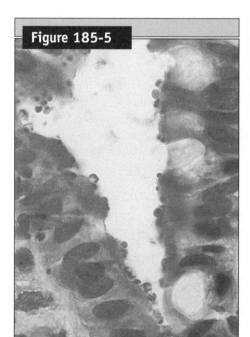

Figure 185-5

Microscopic view of duodenal cryptosporidiosis. Note the multiple round spherical structures on the epithelial surface.

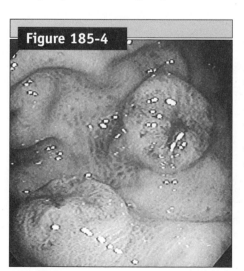

Figure 185-4

Gastric Kaposi's sarcoma. Endoscopic photograph showing multiple raised lesions with central umbilication and subepithelial hemorrhage involving the gastric body.

Diarrhea caused by *C. parvum* infection is characteristically secretory and, when severe, results in dehydration and electrolyte disturbances. Weight loss is common and results from fluid loss, malabsorption, or reduced caloric intake from associated nausea and vomiting. Periumbilical crampy abdominal pain and gaseousness are frequent complaints. The diagnosis can be established by modified acid-fast staining of fresh stool, although the sensitivity of this technique may be as low as 50%. Direct fluorescent antibody staining of stool samples is more sensitive than standard stool staining but also is more expensive. Because intestinal shedding of the organism may be sporadic, evaluation of multiple stool specimens may be required to establish the diagnosis. When the stool test results are negative but the disease is suspected clinically, upper endoscopy and small bowel biopsy usually establish the diagnosis. Colonic biopsies occasionally are diagnostic, and ileal biopsies obtained at the time of colonoscopy appear to have a high diagnostic yield [17••].

Many medications have been used to treat cryptosporidiosis. Paromomycin, a nonabsorbable aminoglycoside, results in clinical improvement in about half of patients [18]. Eradication of the organism rarely is achieved, however, and patients with the most severe infections tend to have the poorest response. The use of orally administered bovine immunoglobulin has shown some promise in open-label trials [19].

Microsporidiosis has emerged as one of the most common gastrointestinal infections in patients with AIDS. *Microsporida* species have been identified in 10% to 20% of HIV-infected patients with diarrhea worldwide [20]. One prospective study from New York identified small bowel microsporidiosis in 39% of HIV-infected patients undergoing small bowel biopsy for diarrhea [21]. Gastrointestinal disease is caused by two species, *Enterocytozoon bienusi* and *Encephalitozoon intestinalis*; *E. bienusi* accounts for more than 80% of cases of gastrointestinal disease caused by *Microsporida* species. Infection occurs when immunodeficiency is severe; most patients have CD4 lymphocyte counts of less than 100/mm³. Diarrhea is the most common presenting symptom. The true pathogenicity of the organisms remains controversial, however, because these parasites may be found in patients without symptoms and because the clinical illness is much less severe than cryptosporidiosis; dehydration and electrolyte disturbances are rare. Weight loss, if present, is usually mild, although D-xylose and fat malabsorption can often be detected. On small bowel biopsy, organisms appear as small round structures in the supranuclear portion of the enterocyte cytoplasm (Fig. 185-6). Colonic involvement is rare. Unlike *E. bienusi*, *E. intestinalis* can be identified in the lamina propria and can result in disseminated disease. As with cryptosporidial infection, a high parasite burden is associated with greater inflammation and small bowel morphologic changes. These small intracellular parasites may be difficult to recognize on hematoxylin and eosin staining, and additional staining methods are often required; electron microscopy has been considered the gold standard for diagnosis and permits a species-specific diagnosis. It is now possible to detect the organism in stool, which should reduce the need for diagnostic small bowel biopsy.

The treatment options are limited. Despite initial promising reports, metronidazole has been shown to be largely ineffective. *E. intestinalis* infection responds to albendazole, and some patients achieve clinical and microbiologic cure; but *E. bienusi* responds poorly to this agent [22].

Other small bowel parasitic diseases seen in AIDS patients are isosporiasis and cyclosporiasis. *Isospora* species is a common diarrheal pathogen in developing countries. *Cyclospora* species has been identified as a small bowel pathogen in both developed and developing countries. It has a number of microbiologic and clinical similarities to *Cryptosporidium* species. Trimethoprim-sulfamethoxazole (double-strength tablet given twice a day for 10 to 14 days) is effective therapy for both pathogens [23]. The incidence and clinical expression of giardiasis and amebiasis appear to be the same in HIV-infected and healthy persons.

Mycobacteria are important intestinal pathogens in patients with AIDS. Infection can be caused by *Mycobacterium avium* complex (MAC; previously termed *Mycobacterium avium-intracellulare*) and, less commonly, by *Mycobacterium tuberculosis*. MAC is the most common mycobacterial infection complicating AIDS, and its incidence may be increasing as a result of the widespread use of PCP prophylaxis [2,3•]. Although diarrhea and abdominal pain may be observed in disseminated MAC, fever and wasting tend to dominate the clinical presentation. Diarrhea is usually mild or moderate but may be associated with significant weight loss when small bowel disease is severe. Common associated laboratory findings include anemia and elevated serum alkaline phosphatase level, which are present in about 75% of affected patients [24•]. MAC is seen only when the CD4 lymphocyte count is less than 100/mm³; the median CD4 lymphocyte count in infected patients in most series is less than 60/mm³. Positive stool culture results for MAC may not be predictive of gastrointestinal disease but are associated with a high frequency of subsequent disseminated disease. Acid-fast staining of stool is less sensitive than is culture for detection of MAC. In the appropriate clinical setting, MAC may be considered the likely cause of diarrhea when results of blood cultures are positive; however, small bowel biopsy is the definitive diagnostic test (Fig. 185-7; see also *Color Plate*). When the index of suspicion for MAC infection is high, empiric therapy often is initiated pending blood culture results. In contrast to past experience, current multidrug

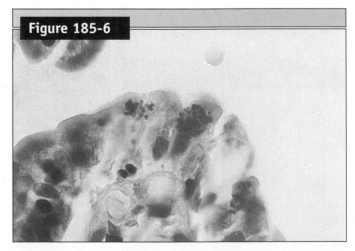

Figure 185-6

Microscopic view of small bowel microsporidiosis. Multiple small, round gram-positive organisms are present in clusters in epithelial cells. Electron microscopy confirmed the presence of *Enterocytozoon bienusi* infection.

regimens against MAC are clinically effective because of the high in vitro efficacy of clarithromycin, azithromycin, and ethambutol [25]. Nevertheless, treatment is not considered curative and must be administered indefinitely. Combination therapy with clarithromycin (500 mg twice a day) plus ethambutol (15 mg/kg/d) is recommended. Prophylaxis for MAC with clarithromycin or rifabutin (300 mg/d) appears effective and should be considered when the CD4 lymphocyte count is less than $50/mm^3$.

Tuberculosis can involve any portion of the gastrointestinal tract. In contrast to MAC, tuberculosis can occur at any stage of immunodeficiency and is usually cured by 9 to 12 months of multidrug therapy (isoniazid, 5 mg/kg/d; rifampin, 10 mg/kg/d; and pyrazinamide, 25 mg/kg/d for the first 2 months), provided resistance is not present. The recurrence rate after successful therapy, even for extrapulmonary disease, is low.

Viral diseases of the small bowel are uncommon causes of chronic diarrhea in patients with AIDS. CMV disease of the small bowel presents as abdominal pain or bleeding due to mucosal ulceration, rather than as diarrhea. Therapy of small intestinal CMV disease is similar to that for esophageal and colonic CMV disease. The roles of adenovirus and coronavirus are not well-defined in AIDS, but both viruses have been associated with diarrhea, often in association with other pathogens. The importance of HIV-1 as a cause of intestinal disease remains controversial (see later discussion).

Neoplasms, including KS and lymphoma, may involve the small bowel and result in abdominal pain, intussusception, or bleeding. The diagnosis of intestinal neoplasm in a patient with AIDS may be suspected by the presence of cutaneous disease (as in KS), by documented extraintestinal neoplastic disease, or by the appearance of the lesion on a small bowel radiograph or CT scan. When a tumor is observed in the duodenum or proximal jejunum on imaging studies, endoscopy and biopsy may be diagnostic.

HIV Enteropathy

The term *HIV enteropathy* has been applied to diarrhea in the AIDS patient for which no cause can be found despite extensive evaluation. However, there is no consensus on the precise definition of this entity. A variety of pathologic and functional abnormalities of the small intestine have been identified in HIV-infected patients, many of which are independent of opportunistic infections. These changes are usually seen when immunodeficiency is advanced. Chronic inflammation of both the small and large bowel is common in HIV-infected patients. Small bowel atrophy resembling celiac disease also has been observed. Functional abnormalities of the small intestine described in these patients include reduced enzyme levels (*eg*, lactase), malabsorption of sugars (D-xylose), and vitamins (*eg*, vitamin B_{12}), and increased small bowel permeability. The cause of these abnormalities has not been clearly delineated but does not appear to be HIV infection of the enterocyte. Loss of CD4 lymphocytes in the lamina propria paralleling declines in the systemic circulation have been considered the likely cause of some of these mucosal changes, in part because these cells appear to have a trophic effect on the intestinal mucosa [26].

■ COLONIC DISEASES

In contrast to the protozoan infections of the small intestine, bacteria and CMV are the most important colonic pathogens in patients with AIDS. The spectrum of bacterial pathogens is similar to that in normal hosts and includes *Campylobacter*, *Shigella*, and *Salmonella* species. More recently, enteroadherent bacteria have been identified in the stools and colonic biopsy specimens of patients with AIDS, although the precise role of these organisms in causing diarrhea remains undefined. *Clostridium difficile* colitis occurs commonly in patients with AIDS because frequent hospitalization and use of antibiotics are both risk factors for this infection.

Bacterial colitis typically presents acutely with fever, abdominal pain, and watery or bloody diarrhea. Fecal leukocytes are often present. Bacteremia occurs frequently in AIDS patients, and in the ill-appearing patient with fever, blood cultures as well as stool cultures should be obtained. The clinical presentation, response to therapy, and relapse rate of *C. difficile* colitis are no different in HIV-infected patients than in other patients.

One of the more common causes of chronic diarrhea in late-stage AIDS patients is CMV colitis; most of these patients have CD4 lymphocyte counts of less than $70/mm^3$. As in patients with CMV esophageal disease, coexistent retinitis may be present in 10% to 20% of AIDS patients with CMV colitis. Although the presentation of CMV colitis is variable, watery diarrhea is the most common symptom. When the distal colon

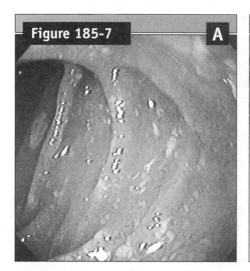
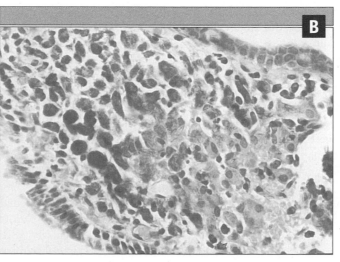

Figure 185-7

*Mycobacterium avium complex (MAC) infection of the small bowel. See also **Color Plate**. **A**, Endoscopic photograph of multiple yellow plaques in the duodenum, which are characteristic of MAC. **B**, Microscopic view of acid-fast bacillus stain of small bowel biopsy showing multiple bacteria in macrophages, mimicking the appearance of Whipple's disease.*

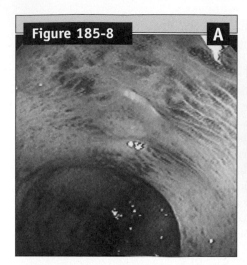

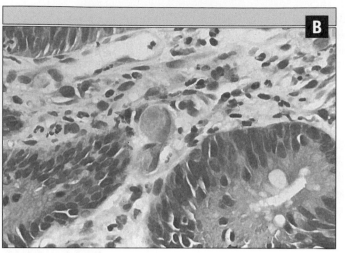

Cytomegalovirus colitis. **A**, Endoscopic photograph of small ulcer with surrounding subepithelial hemorrhage in the distal colon. See also **Color Plate**. **B**, Microscopic view of two endothelial cells with large intranuclear inclusions characteristic of cytomegalovirus infection.

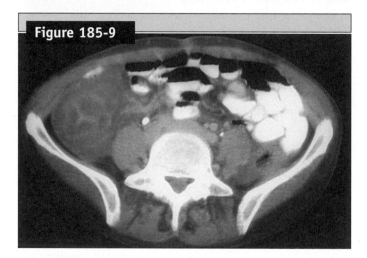

Cytomegalovirus colitis. Abdominal computed tomographic scan of a patient with diarrhea and severe abdominal pain showing a markedly thickened colonic wall in the cecum, which is typical of cytomegaloviral or bacterial colitis.

is involved, symptoms of proctitis are prominent. Abdominal pain is seen in at least half of patients, may be severe, and can occur in the absence of diarrhea. Fever is inconsistent, whereas weight loss is almost universal. Infrequent manifestations include gastrointestinal bleeding or perforation. CMV colitis should be suspected in any HIV-infected patient with severe immunodeficiency who has abdominal pain, chronic diarrhea, weight loss, and repeatedly negative stool culture and ova and parasite examination results.

The endoscopic appearance of CMV colitis includes isolated ulcerations, patchy hemorrhage, or findings resembling ulcerative colitis or Crohn's disease (Fig. 185-8; see also *Color Plate*). In some patients, the disease may be limited to the right colon, and colonoscopy is necessary for diagnosis [27•]. In patients who present with severe abdominal pain, CT often is performed initially and may suggest the diagnosis when the colon is markedly thickened, although this finding is not specific (Fig. 185-9). The diagnosis of CMV colitis is best established by identification of the pathognomonic viral cytopathic effect in colonic biopsy specimens. Treatment with ganciclovir or foscarnet usually results in clinical and endoscopic improvements [12••], although a longer course of

therapy (4 to 6 weeks) may be required than is indicated for esophageal disease.

A number of other opportunistic infections have been reported to involve the colon in patients with AIDS. These include histoplasmosis, bartonellosis, PCP, toxoplasmosis, and mycobacteriosis. KS and non-Hodgkin's lymphoma may also involve the colon. As for other segments of the gastrointestinal tract, colonic KS usually is asymptomatic, whereas colonic lymphoma usually presents with abdominal pain, obstruction, or both. Diarrhea rarely is a manifestation of a colonic neoplasm.

In most patients presenting with advanced immunodeficiency and colorectal symptoms, stool testing and colonoscopic evaluation (in patients with diarrhea) are most appropriate. Barium enema examination may demonstrate colitis, ulcers, or mass lesions, but endoscopic examination and tissue sampling is often required for determination of the cause of the abnormality. Barium studies should not be used in the evaluation of diarrhea because barium interferes with stool testing for parasites and endoscopy. Furthermore, diagnosis of opportunistic disorders is best established by mucosal biopsy because the clinical presentation and radiographic findings are nonspecific.

Approach to the AIDS Patient With Diarrhea

Given the many etiologic agents that can cause diarrhea and the possibility of either small or large bowel involvement, a systematic approach to diagnosis is essential (Fig. 185-10). Three important features should be considered:

1. The likelihood of the cause of diarrhea being in the colon or small intestine should be assessed on the basis of a careful history and physical examination.
2. The differential diagnosis should be based on the peripheral CD4 lymphocyte count. When the CD4 lymphocyte count is less than $100/mm^3$, opportunistic processes are most likely.
3. Stool tests are often diagnostic and should be performed initially.

Symptoms of small bowel disease include crampy periumbilical abdominal pain, flatulence, borborygmi, large stool volume (particularly with fasting), nausea, and vomiting. Lower abdominal pain and symptoms of proctitis indicate inflammatory disease of the distal colon. Fever suggests an infectious cause of diarrhea, and when fever is present, blood cultures should be obtained to exclude bacteria as the cause of colitis in patients with acute diarrhea or disseminated MAC.

The presence of fecal leukocytes indicates colitis and warrants evaluation for bacterial causes (*eg, C. difficile)* and CMV colitis. If, when testing for *C. difficile* toxin, routine bacterial stool culture results are negative and symptoms of proctitis are present, evaluation of the distal colon with sigmoidoscopy is appropriate. In the setting of severe immunodeficiency, if multiple stool tests are negative and fecal leukocytes are absent, evaluation of the distal colon should be performed to exclude CMV colitis [28•]. The appropriate number of stool samples for bacterial culture, ova and parasites examination, and *C. difficile* toxin that should be evaluated before proceeding to endoscopic evaluation is unknown. Most investigators suggest three samples, although evaluation of up to six samples increases the diagnostic yield further for parasitic causes. Colonoscopy may be required when the patient complains of right-sided abdominal pain because CMV may be confined to the right colon [27•]. Empiric therapy with antimicrobials is not routinely recommended, given the broad etiologic spectrum of infectious causes.

Weight loss and severe immunodeficiency in a patient with chronic diarrhea strongly suggest an opportunistic infection. Upper endoscopy with small bowel biopsy has a better diagnostic yield than stool tests alone for microsporidiosis and cryptosporidiosis. Nevertheless, the use of small bowel biopsy should be individualized because therapies for these parasitic diseases are neither uniformly effective nor widely available.

If no cause of diarrhea is found, symptomatic therapy is indicated. Antimotility drugs may be safely administered while obtaining additional stool studies if fecal leukocytes are absent. When diarrhea is mild, a bulking agent and an antimotility drug such as loperamide can be helpful. When diarrhea is more severe, tincture of opium can be effective. Although there was initial enthusiasm for octreotide acetate (Sandostatin; Sandoz Pharmaceuticals, East Hanover, NJ), a randomized, double-blind, placebo-controlled trial failed to document its effectiveness [29].

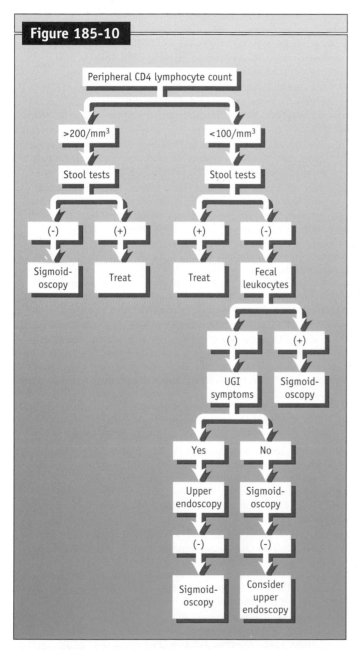

Figure 185-10

Suggested approach to the evaluation of diarrhea in human immunodeficiency virus–infected patients. Stool tests include culture for enteric pathogens, assay for *Clostridium difficile* toxin, and examinations for ova and parasites. Colonoscopy should be considered when sigmoidoscopy results are negative and when colonic disease is highly suspected. UGI—upper gastrointestinal.

ANORECTAL DISEASES

The frequency of acute anorectal disorders has decreased in the homosexual population as a result of increased condom use. Infectious disorders related to unprotected anal intercourse include acute gonorrheal, syphilitic, and chlamydial proctitis. Human papillomavirus infection has been implicated as the main etiologic factor in squamous cell carcinoma of the anus in homosexual men. Traumatic disease of the anorectum including fissures should be considered in the appropriate clinical setting. Idiopathic ulcers involving the anorectum also have been described. Non-Hodgkin's lymphoma and KS also can involve the anorectum.

As with all anorectal diseases, the usual manifestations are anorectal pain, dyschezia, bleeding, urgency, tenesmus, and frequent, low-volume stools. Dyschezia (painful evacuation) is usually a manifestation of ulceration of the anal canal (fissure, infection). In the patient with symptoms, careful inspection of the anorectum should be performed with attention to the presence of vesicles, ulcers, fissures, fistulas, hemorrhoids, or mass lesions. Digital examination also should assess sphincter tone, which may be reduced in HSV infection. Culture of perianal ulcers is the best method for diagnosing HSV. Confirmation of suspected CMV infection requires biopsy of lesions, if cultures are negative. Visualization of the anorectum is best performed with anoscopy and proctoscopy or with sigmoidoscopy. If severe anorectal pain precludes a thorough evaluation, evaluation with conscious sedation or general anesthesia may be required. All mucosal abnormalities should be sampled. Treatment of these disorders is no different from that for the same disease elsewhere in the gastrointestinal tract.

PANCREATIC DISEASES

Diseases involving the pancreas usually manifest as acute pancreatitis in AIDS patients and can arise from a variety of causes [30]. The clinical presentation is similar to that in patients without HIV-related disease, and prognosis correlates with the APACHE (Acute Physiology and Chronic Health Evaluation) II score [31]. Affected patients usually have elevated serum amylase and lipase levels, unless acute pancreatitis occurs in a patient with pre-existing chronic pancreatitis. Mild increases in serum amylase are seen frequently and are clinically unimportant in the patient without symptoms. Amylase elevations in the absence of pancreatic disease suggest macroamylasemia, which has also been observed in patients with AIDS. Macrolipasemia has also been described.

The most common cause of acute pancreatitis in patients with AIDS is drug-induced disease caused by pentamidine or dideoxyinosine. Occasional cases of drug-induced pancreatitis also have followed the use of trimethoprim-sulfamethoxazole. Pancreatitis may develop after either inhaled or parenterally administered pentamidine and is associated with the typical clinical features of acute pancreatitis. The clinical course may be mild, severe, or even fatal and is often accompanied by hyperglycemia. A 10% incidence of symptomatic pancreatitis has been reported in early trials of dideoxyinosine.

Infectious causes of pancreatitis in patients with AIDS are multiple, although their diagnosis is usually difficult because pancreatic biopsy is rarely performed. Reported causes include CMV, HSV, and mycobacterial and cryptococcal infection. Infectious causes of pancreatitis may not be obvious clinically but should be suspected when immunodeficiency is severe. Most cases of infectious pancreatitis are diagnosed at autopsy, with pancreatic involvement being part of a widespread, disseminated infection. In addition, autopsy studies have identified infections and neoplasms involving the pancreas in the absence of antemortem clinical disease. When suspected antemortem, these disorders may be detected by fine-needle aspiration, although this approach has not been formally tested and is rarely used clinically.

Endoscopic retrograde cholangiopancreatography (ERCP) may be helpful when gallstone pancreatitis is suspected clinically. ERCP may also demonstrate changes of chronic pancreatitis. Changes in the pancreatic ducts suggestive of chronic pancreatitis have also been demonstrated in patients with coexistent AIDS cholangiopathy. It is likely that infections involving the biliary tree also involve the pancreatic ductular epithelium. Pancreatic infiltration by lymphoma and KS occurs occasionally and is manifested by acute pancreatitis, a mass effect on the adjacent duodenum with gastric outlet obstruction, or pancreatic exocrine insufficiency if the pancreatic duct is obstructed.

CONCLUSION

Gastrointestinal complications occur frequently in patients with AIDS. Given the wide spectrum of potential causes, a thoughtful evaluation that takes into account patient history, physical examination, and routine laboratory tests, including CD4 lymphocyte counts, can help to tailor the differential diagnosis considerably. Optimism should be maintained when evaluating these patients, because of the high diagnostic yield of available tests and the efficacy of available medical therapy.

REFERENCES

Recently published papers of particular interest have been highlighted as follows:
- •   Of interest
- •• Of outstanding interest

1. May GR, Gill MJ, Church DL, et al.: Gastrointestinal symptoms in ambulatory HIV-infected patients. *Dig Dis Sci* 1993, 38:1388–1394.

2. Bacellar H, Munoz A, Hoover DR, et al.: Incidence of clinical AIDS conditions in a cohort of homosexual men with CD4+ cell counts <100/mm³: multicenter AIDS Cohort Study. *J Infect Dis* 1994, 170:1284–1287.

3.• Selik RM, Chu SY, Ward JW: Trends in infectious diseases and cancers among persons dying of HIV infection in the United States from 1987 to 1992. *Ann Intern Med* 1995, 123:933–936.
This study documents the changing spectrum of opportunistic infections caused by the use of prophylactic therapies such as trimethoprim-sulfamethoxazole for the prevention of PCP. As the incidence of PCP has decreased, other opportunistic processes have increased, including CMV infection, MAC infection, and lymphoma.

4.• Weinert M, Grimes RM, Lynch DP: Oral manifestations of HIV infection. *Ann Intern Med* 1996, 125:485–496.
This article provides an excellent pictorial review of the oral manifestations of HIV infection.

5. Bonacini M, Young T, Laine L: The causes of esophageal symptoms in human immunodeficiency virus infection: a prospective study of 110 patients. *Arch Intern Med* 1991, 151:1567–1572.

6.•• Wilcox CM, Alexander LN, Clark WS, et al.: Fluconazole compared with endoscopy for human immunodeficiency virus-infected patients with esophageal symptoms. *Gastroenterology* 1996, 110:1803–1809.
This prospective randomized study compares use of empiric fluconazole to use of endoscopy to treat HIV-infected patients who have esophageal symptoms. These investigators found that the use of empiric fluconazole, regardless of the presence of oropharyngeal candidiasis, was the most cost-effective management strategy. In patients whose condition did not improve within 1 week of initiation of fluconazole therapy, the endoscopy results were almost uniformly abnormal, demonstrating esophageal ulcers.

7.•• Wilcox CM, Schwartz DA, Clark WS: Causes, response to therapy, and long-term outcome of esophageal ulcer in patients with human immunodeficiency virus infection. *Ann Intern Med* 1995, 122:143–149.
This prospective trial documented the spectrum of causes of esophageal ulceration in 100 patients with HIV infection. CMV infection or idiopathic esophageal ulceration constituted more than 80% of cases of esophageal ulceration in these patients. HSV was an uncommon cause of esophagitis in these HIV-infected patients, even though it was a common cause of esophagitis in patients with other immunosuppression disorders.

8.• Laine L, Dretler RH, Conteas CN, et al.: Fluconazole compared with ketoconazole for the treatment of candida esophagitis in AIDS: a randomized trial. *Ann Intern Med* 1992, 117:655–660.
This prospective randomized trial demonstrated the clinically significant superiority of fluconazole over ketoconazole in the treatment of candidal esophagitis.

9.• Barbaro G, Barbarini G, Caladeron W, et al.: Fluconazole versus itraconazole for *Candida* esophagitis in acquired immunodeficiency syndrome. *Gastroenterology* 1996, 111:1169–1177.
This prospective randomized multicenter study of more than 2000 patients performed in Europe demonstrated that fluconazole is superior to itraconazole in the treatment of candidal esophagitis.

10. Maenza JR, Keruly JC, Moore RD, et al.: Risk factors for fluconazole-resistant candidiasis in human immunodeficiency virus-infected patients. *J Infect Dis* 1996, 173:219–225.

11.• Genereau T, Lortholary O, Bouchaud O, et al.: Herpes simplex esophagitis in patients with AIDS: report of 34 cases. *Clin Infect Dis* 1996, 22:926–931.
This article describes the largest study to date reporting the clinical characteristics, response to therapy, and outcome of HSV esophagitis in patients with AIDS.

12.•• Blanshard C, Benhamou Y, Dohin E, *et al.*: Treatment of AIDS-associated gastrointestinal cytomegalovirus infection with foscarnet and ganciclovir: a randomized comparison. *J Infect Dis* 1995, 172:622–628.
This is the only randomized study published to date comparing ganciclovir to foscarnet for the treatment of gastrointestinal CMV infection. The response rates were about 80% in each treatment group, and the difference between the responses to the two medications was not statistically significant.

13.• Wilcox CM, Schwartz DA: Comparison of two corticosteroid regimens for the treatment of idiopathic esophageal ulcerations associated with HIV infection. *Am J Gastroenterol* 1994, 89:2163–2167.
This trial compared short-course treatment with corticosteroids to a 1-month tapered treatment course in patients with IEUs. More than 90% of patients responded to corticosteroids in both groups. The relapse rate appeared to be slightly higher with a shorter course of therapy.

14. Vaira D, Miglioli M, Menegatti M, *et al.*: *Helicobacter pylori* status, endoscopic findings, and serology in HIV-1-positive patients. *Dig Dis Sci* 1995, 40:1622–1626.

15. Welage LS, Carver PL, Revankar S, *et al.*: Alterations in gastric acidity in patients infected with human immunodeficiency virus. *Clin Infect Dis* 1995, 21:1431–1438.

16. McGowan I, Hawkins AS, Weller IVD: The natural history of cryptosporidia diarrhea in HIV-infected patients. *AIDS* 1993, 7:349–354.

17.•• Greenberg PD, Koch J, Cello JP: Diagnosis of *Cryptosporidium parvum* in patients with severe diarrhea and AIDS. *Dig Dis Sci* 1996, 41:2286–2290.
This trial demonstrated that duodenal biopsy could miss cryptosporidial enteritis. The technique with the highest diagnostic yield appeared to be ileal biopsy.

18. White AC, Chappell CL, Hayat CS, *et al.*: Paromomycin for cryptosporidiosis in AIDS: a prospective, double-blind trial. *J Infect Dis* 1994, 170:419–424.

19. Greenberg PD, Cello JP: Treatment of severe diarrhea caused by *Cryptosporidium parvum* with oral bovine immunoglobulin concentrate in patients with AIDS. *J Acquir Immune Defic Syndr Hum Retrovirol* 1996, 13:348–354.

20. Weber R, Bryan RT, Schwartz DA, *et al.*: Human microsporidial infections. *Clin Microbiol Rev* 1994, 7:426–461.

21. Kotler DP, Orenstein JM: Prevalence of intestinal microsporidiosis in HIV-infected patients referred for gastroenterological evaluation. *Am J Gastroenterol* 1994, 89:1998–2002.

22. Dore GJ, Marriott DJ, Hing MC, *et al.*: Disseminated microsporidiosis due to *Septata intestinalis* in nine patients infected with the human immunodeficiency virus: response to therapy with albendazole. *Clin Infect Dis* 1995, 21:70–76.

23. Pape JW, Verdier R-I, Boncy M, *et al.*: Cyclospora infection in adults infected with HIV: clinical manifestations, treatment, and prophylaxis. *Ann Intern Med* 1994, 121:654–657.

24.• Havlik JA, Horsburgh CR, Metchock B, *et al.*: Disseminated *Mycobacterium avium* complex infection: clinical identification and epidemiologic trends. *J Infect Dis* 1992, 165:577–580.
This article reports on a large study demonstrating the clinical presentation and laboratory features associated with this infection in patients with AIDS.

25. Shafran SD, Singer J, Zarowny DP, *et al.*: A comparison of two regimens for the treatment of Mycobacterium avium complex bacteremia in AIDS: rifabutin, ethambutol, and clarithromycin versus rifampin, ethambutol, clofazimine, and ciprofloxacin. *N Engl J Med* 1996, 335:377–383.

26. Keating J, Bjarnason I, Somasundaram S, *et al.*: Intestinal absorptive capacity, intestinal permeability and jejunal histology in HIV and their relation to diarrhoea. *Gut* 1995, 37:623–629.
This study demonstrated the unique intestinal abnormalities in HIV-infected patients. Some patients with HIV disease had intestinal abnormalities mimicking celiac sprue.

27.• Dieterich DT, Rahmin M: Cytomegalovirus colitis in AIDS: presentation in 44 patients and a review of the literature. *J Acquir Immune Defic Syndr Hum Retrovirol* 1991, 4(suppl 1):29–35.

28.• Wilcox CM, Schwartz DA, Cotsonis GA, *et al.*: Evaluation of chronic unexplained diarrhea in human immunodeficiency virus infection: determination of the best diagnostic approach. *Gastroenterology* 1996, 110:30–37.

29. Simon DM, Cello JP, Valenzuela J, *et al.*: Multicenter trial of octreotide in patients with refractory acquired immunodeficiency syndrome-associated diarrhea. *Gastroenterology* 1995, 108:1753–1760.

30. Bonacini M: Pancreatic involvement in human immunodeficiency virus infection. *J Clin Gastroenterol* 1991, 13:58.

31. Cappell MS, Marks M: Acute pancreatitis in HIV-seropositive patients: a case control study of 44 patients. *Am J Med* 1995, 3:243.

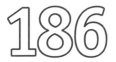

Gastrointestinal Tract and Hepatobiliary Involvement in Systemic Diseases

Anne M. Larson and Kris V. Kowdley

Gastrointestinal and hepatobiliary involvement occur during the course of many systemic illnesses. In fact, gastrointestinal symptoms often are the presenting feature of many of these illnesses (Table 186-1).

■ VASCULITIDES

The vasculitides are a group of disorders characterized by inflammation and necrosis of the blood vessels. Any type or size of vessel in any organ system may be affected (Table 186-2).

Vasculitides may be associated with rheumatologic disorders or can occur as isolated syndromes.

Behçet's Disease

Behçet's disease is a rare, chronic, recurring disorder characterized by a necrotizing vasculitis of the mucocutaneous, intestinal, articular, vascular, pulmonary, ocular, urogenital, and neurologic systems. The classic triad consists of aphthous stomatitis, genital ulcers, and relapsing uveitis. The disorder primarily affects adults between 25 and 35 years of age, and men are affected more frequently and severely; persons of HLA-B51 type are at greater risk. This disease is most common in Japan, Korea, and the eastern Mediterranean countries. Arteries and veins of all sizes may be involved, although venulitis is the primary disorder. Its cause is unknown, although circulating immune complexes have been found within vessel walls. The diagnosis is made on clinical grounds, and because there are no pathognomic serologic or pathologic features, diagnostic criteria have been developed.

Gastrointestinal lesions are uncommon in Behçet's disease, occurring in fewer than 10% of patients, although the frequency varies geographically, with the greatest incidence in Japan [1••]. Patients with a predominance of gastrointestinal symptoms are said to have "entero-Behçet's disease." Oral aphthous ulcerations may be seen and are a major criterion for diagnosis [2] (Fig. 186-1; see also *Color Plate*). Esophageal ulceration has been described and can lead to bleeding, stricture, or perforation. Intestinal ulcers occur in fewer than 1% of cases, predominantly in the terminal ileum or cecum [1••], and may lead to bleeding, fistulas, and tumor-like constriction. Perforation has been described in up to 40% to 50% of patients with colonic Behçet's disease. A colitis resembling Crohn's disease also is described.

Table 186-1. Gastrointestinal Manifestations of Systemic Diseases

Vasculitides	Connective tissue disorders	Endocrinologic disorders	Genetic/metabolic disorders	Hematologic disorders
Behçet's disease	Ehlers-Danlos syndrome	Acromegaly	α_1-Antitrypsin deficiency*	Hemolytic-uremic syndrome*
Buerger's disease	Felty's syndrome	Adrenal disease	Amyloidosis	Hypercoagulability*
Churg-Strauss disease	Mixed connective tissue disorders	Diabetes mellitus*	Anderson-Fabry disease	Plummer-Vinson syndrome*
Cryoglobulinemia		Parathyroid disease	Cholesterol ester storage diseases*	
Drug-related vasculitides	Polymyositis and dermatomyositis	Thyroid disease	Cystic fibrosis*	Sickle cell anemia
Giant cell arteritis		Pregnancy*	Down syndrome	Hemoglobin C
Henoch-Schönlein purpura	Pseudoxanthoma elasticum	Endocrine tumors*	Gaucher's disease*	
Kawasaki disease	Rheumatoid arthritis		Hemochromatosis*	
Köhlmeier-Degos disease	Scleroderma		Hereditary angioedema*	
Polyarteritis nodosa	Sjögren's syndrome		Hyperlipidemias*	
Takayasu's arteritis	Systemic lupus erythematosus		Niemann-Pick disease*	
Wegener's granulomatosis			Porphyria*	
			Turner's syndrome*	
			Wilson's disease*	

Covered elsewhere in this book.

Table 186-2. Causes of Vasculitis

Vasculitis	Vessel involved	Type of destruction
Systemic necrotizing vasculitis		
Polyarteritis nodosa	Small to medium arteries	Fibrinoid necrosis
Churg-Strauss disease (allergic granulomatosis)	Small to medium arteries	Fibrinoid necrosis
Hepatitis B virus–associated vasculitis	Small to medium arteries	Fibrinoid necrosis
Köhlmeier-Degos syndrome	Small to medium arteries	Lymphocyte-mediated necrosis
Leukocytoclastic (hypersensitivity) vasculitis		
Henoch-Schönlein purpura	Small vessels	Leukocytoclastic angiitis
Drug-related vasculitis	Small vessels	Leukocytoclastic angiitis
Vasculitis associated with		
Neoplasms	Small vessels	Leukocytoclastic angiitis
Infectious diseases	Small vessels	Leukocytoclastic angiitis
Connective tissue disease	Small vessels	Leukocytoclastic angiitis
Wegener's granulomatosis	Small arteries and veins	Necrotizing, granulomatous
Giant cell arteritis		
Temporal arteritis	Medium to large arteries	Necrotizing, granulomatous
Takayasu's arteritis	Medium to large arteries	Necrotizing, granulomatous
Buerger's disease (thromboangiitis obliterans)	Small to medium arteries	Occlusive inflammation
Kawasaki disease (mucocutaneous lymph node syndrome)	Small to medium arteries	Fibrinoid necrosis
Behçet's disease	Small vessels	Leukocytoclastic angiitis
Cryoglobulinemia	Small to medium vessels	Fibrinoid necrosis

There is no effective medical treatment for Behçet's disease, and therapy remains empiric. Corticosteroids may suppress some symptoms but are ineffective in up to half of cases. Other immunosuppressive agents (chlorambucil, cyclosporine) have been used with variable results. A recent randomized, controlled trial describes successful treatment of mucocutaneous lesions with thalidomide [2]. Surgical resection of severely diseased segments of the intestine may be necessary in patients with refractory symptoms.

Giant Cell Arteritis

Giant cell arteritis, also known as *cranial arteritis* or *temporal arteritis*, is a focal granulomatous disease involving the large and medium-sized arteries [3•]. It generally affects persons older than 50 years with a female predominance (2:1), and a prevalence ranging from 20 to 133 per 100,000. The disorder affects arteries originating from the aortic arch, although smaller vessels are involved in about 13% of cases. The classic presentation is with headache, jaw claudication, and pain over the temporal artery. Gastrointestinal complications are less common, although involvement of splanchnic (small) arteries may lead to visceral ischemia with abdominal pain, nausea, anorexia, weight loss, bleeding, mesenteric infarction, and intestinal perforation [3•]. Primary aortoduodenal fistula has been reported rarely. Results of serum laboratory tests are nonspecific. Hepatobiliary abnormalities are even less common and include liver test results abnormalities associated with hepatic steatosis, granulomas, and nonspecific portal inflammation [4••]. Treatment with corticosteroids is highly effective, with most symptoms remitting within 1 month.

Henoch-Schönlein Purpura

Henoch-Schönlein purpura, characterized by a leukocytoclastic or hypersensitivity vasculitis, is a multisystem immuno–complex-mediated vasculitis that involves the skin, kidneys, gastrointestinal tract, and joints; it affects children primarily. The cause may be related to a deficiency in the regulation of immunoglobulin A (IgA) synthesis in response to mucosal antigenic stimulation; about 30% to 50% of affected persons have a preceding history of upper respiratory tract infection [5]. Entrapment of IgA immune complexes in the postcapillary venules of the target organs leads to an inflammatory reaction mediated by macrophage infiltration and fibrin deposition. The disease usually runs a benign course in children, with the prognosis related primarily to the severity of renal involvement. The estimated mortality rate is between 1% and 5%.

The classic presentation of Henoch-Schönlein purpura is with palpable purpura (Fig. 186-2; see also *Color Plate*), arthritis, abdominal pain, and renal manifestations. Gastrointestinal manifestations may be the presenting feature and are observed in 35% to 85% of patients, although they may be more common in patients younger than 16 years and in patients with concomitant renal involvement [6]. The small intestine, particularly the distal ileum, is the most commonly involved gastrointestinal organ, although esophageal, gastroduodenal, and colorectal involvement has been reported.

Symptoms of gastrointestinal tract involvement include colicky abdominal pain, nausea, vomiting, diarrhea, rectal bleeding, bloody diarrhea, and melena. Abdominal pain occurs in more than half of patients and in more than 80% of those with other gastrointestinal complaints [6]. About one fourth of patients present with features suggestive of an acute abdomen requiring surgical evaluation, and 2% to 6% have significant surgical lesions requiring laparotomy [7]. Evidence of gastrointestinal bleeding, from a positive fecal occult blood test or melena, may be seen in 25% to 50% of patients [6]. Bleeding is attributed to vasculitis, with resulting ischemia, submucosal edema, and hemorrhage (Fig. 186-3). Other gastrointestinal abnormalities include ileus, protein-losing enteropathy, intussusception (rare in adults), intestinal perforation, terminal ileitis, total bowel infarction, and massive gastrointestinal hemorrhage. Radiologic findings are generally nonspecific and include "thumbprinting" caused by submucosal edema or hemorrhage, bowel wall thickening, or, rarely, pseudotumors (Fig. 186-4). Late complications of gastrointestinal ischemia, such as intestinal or esophageal obstruction secondary to strictures, have been described. Vascular disease of the gallbladder and pancreas may lead to gallbladder infarction, hemorrhagic pancreatitis, pancreatic insufficiency, or steatorrhea.

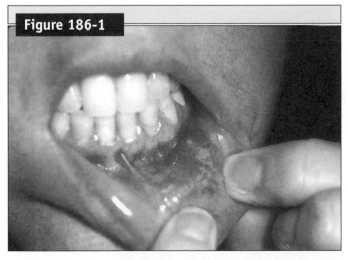

Figure 186-1

Oral lesions seen in a patient with Behçet's disease. See also **Color Plate**. (*From* Pandya [50]; with permission.)

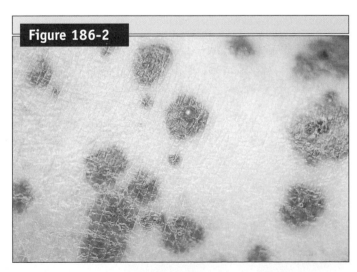

Figure 186-2

Palpable purpura on the lower extremities of a patient with Henoch-Schönlein purpura. See also **Color Plate**. (*From* Pandya [50]; with permission.)

The prognosis of Henoch-Schönlein purpura generally is good; most long-term morbidity and mortality are from renal complications. Gastrointestinal symptoms often respond to treatment with corticosteroids, but controversy remains about whether the more severe manifestations, such as intussusception and perforation, can be prevented.

Polyarteritis Nodosa

Polyarteritis nodosa is an uncommon syndrome of unknown cause that afflicts predominantly middle-aged men (mean age, 45 years; 2:1 male-to-female ratio). The disorder affects about 6 of every 100,000 persons. The classic, or macroscopic, form is a necrotizing vasculitis that involves medium-sized muscular arteries [8•]. The microscopic form involves small arterioles, venules, and capillaries. Nearly any organ system can be involved; furthermore, polyarteritis nodosa may be a secondary manifestation of rheumatoid arthritis, Sjögren's syndrome, mixed cryoglobulinemia, hairy cell leukemia, or chronic infection with hepatitis B virus. Fever, anorexia, weight loss, malaise, arthralgia, subcutaneous nodules, hypertension, and peripheral neuritis are common.

Gastrointestinal involvement is a common cause of morbidity and mortality and occurs in at least 50% to 70% of patients [8•]. Abdominal pain is the most common gastrointestinal complaint (25% to 50% of patients), but intestinal angina is distinctly unusual. Other gastrointestinal symptoms include epigastric pain, nausea, and diarrhea. Mucosal ulceration may occur, especially of the small intestine. Rare complications include gastrointestinal hemorrhage, intestinal obstruction, peritonitis, intestinal infarction, and perforation. Mortality rates range from 75% to 100% when infarction or perforation occur. Appendicitis, cholecystitis, and pancreatitis have been reported rarely. Systemic disease does not always occur coincident with gastrointestinal involvement [9•]. Laboratory abnormalities are nonspecific. Angiography may be useful in delineating the extent of vascular involvement. Aneurysm formation in the mesenteric, renal, and hepatic vasculature is characteristic but nonspecific (Figs. 186-5 and 186-6).

Polyarteritis nodosa involves the liver in up to 65% of cases in autopsy series [4••]. Although hepatomegaly and jaundice are

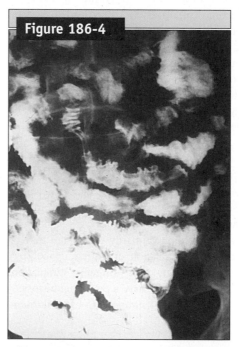

Figure 186-4

Barium study showing multiple small bowel (jejunal) loops with thickened mucosal folds (thumbprinting) and thickened bowel wall in a patient with Henoch-Schönlein purpura. (*Courtesy of* C. A. Rohrmann, Jr., MD.)

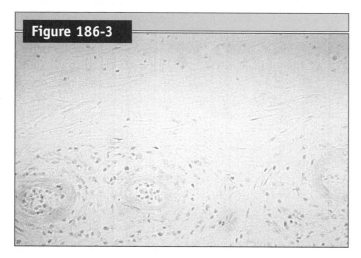

Figure 186-3

Microscopic view of small vessel vasculitis in a patient with Henoch-Schönlein purpura. Note the characteristic fibrinoid necrosis of the vessel walls, surrounding edema, and mononuclear cells. (*From* Friedman *et al.* [51]; with permission.)

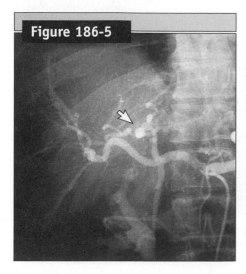

Figure 186-5

Arteriogram revealing peri-arteritis with a single aneurysm (*arrow*) in a patient with polyarteritis nodosa. (*Courtesy of* C. A. Rohrmann, Jr., MD.)

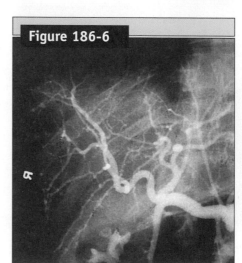

Figure 186-6

Arteriogram revealing distal arterial involvement with multiple small aneurysms in a patient with polyarteritis nodosa. (*Courtesy of* C. A. Rohrmann, Jr., MD.)

common, other symptoms resulting from liver disease are not. Hepatic arteritis with secondary rupture of an aneurysm or hepatic infarction may present as acute abdominal pain. Patients also may present with fever of unknown origin, leukocytosis, and abnormal liver tests (particularly elevation of the serum alkaline phosphatase level). Causing some confusion is the vasculitis associated with hepatitis B virus infection. Almost half of patients with classic polyarteritis nodosa are hepatitis B surface antigen seropositive. Angiography may demonstrate characteristic fusiform aneurysms of the hepatic arteries.

Prognosis in untreated patients with polyarteritis nodosa is poor. The prognosis in patients with gastrointestinal involvement is not statistically different from that in patients without gastrointestinal involvement, unless such involvement is severe [8•]. Although treatment with corticosteroids is effective in some patients, cyclophosphamide and azathioprine improve overall survival dramatically.

Churg-Strauss Syndrome

Churg-Strauss syndrome is an uncommon disorder characterized by allergic granulomatosis and angiitis of small vessels. Men are afflicted more commonly than women. Typical features include asthma, allergic rhinitis, peripheral eosinophilia, extravascular granulomas, and systemic necrotizing vasculitis [10]. Pulmonary vasculitis is the hallmark of Churg-Strauss syndrome and differentiates it from polyarteritis nodosa. The disease has three phases. The prodromal phase generally is associated with allergic symptoms, such as asthma and rhinitis. A second phase is marked by eosinophilia and eosinophilic tissue infiltrates (Löffler's syndrome, chronic eosinophilic pneumonia, eosinophilic gastroenteritis). The third phase is characterized by systemic vasculitis involving the skin (nodules, erythema, palpable purpura), cardiovascular system, kidneys, and central nervous system (mononeuritis multiplex).

The gastrointestinal tract is involved in 30% to 40% of cases, with symptoms including abdominal pain, bloody stool, diarrhea, and nausea. Multiple gastrointestinal tract ulcerations may develop, are most common in the small intestine, and may be complicated by perforation.

Peripheral eosinophilia is seen on laboratory evaluation. An elevated erythrocyte sedimentation rate, elevated serum IgE level, and normochromic anemia are also common. Angiography reveals findings similar to those of polyarteritis nodosa, with involvement of the mesenteric arteries, although

aneurysm formation is not so common as in polyarteritis nodosa. Treatment consists of high-dose corticosteroids and, in refractory cases, either azathioprine or cyclophosphamide.

Wegener's Granulomatosis

Wegener's granulomatosis is characterized by respiratory tract disease associated with segmental necrotizing glomerulonephritis and vasculitis of other organs. As in Churg-Strauss syndrome, Wegener's granulomatosis is associated with necrotizing granulomatous vasculitis of small blood vessels. Middle-aged men are most commonly afflicted, and initial manifestations usually involve the respiratory tract. Fever, anorexia, and weight loss may be present. Involvement of the gastrointestinal tract is uncommon [11•], although both esophageal and colonic involvement have been described. Laboratory studies commonly are nonspecific, and the diagnosis is based on clinical and histologic findings. Treatment with cyclophosphamide is highly effective, especially when combined with corticosteroids early in the course of therapy; azathioprine is effective as maintenance treatment.

Cryoglobulinemia

Cryoglobulins are immunoglobulins that reversibly precipitate in serum at low temperatures [12]. They are divided into three major groups as outlined in Table 186-3.

The most common clinical complaint in patients with cryoglobulinemia is recurrent palpable purpura (present in nearly 100% of cases), and the most serious complication is renal involvement. Gastrointestinal manifestations of mixed cryoglobulinemia are related to vasculitis, which results in ischemia and intramural hemorrhage of the gastrointestinal tract. Symptoms are nonspecific, and patients may complain of abdominal pain. Recurrent acute abdominal crises are uncommon (2.3% of cases). Rare complications include enteritis or colitis, intestinal infarction, or perforation. Gastrointestinal lesions may resemble those seen in Crohn's disease.

Hepatosplenomegaly and liver function abnormalities can be seen. Mixed cryoglobulins have been found in association with hepatitis C virus infection; more than half of patients infected with hepatitis C virus have measurable cryoglobulins, but only about 2% of patients with chronic hepatitis C have symptomatic cryoglobulinemia [13]. Patients with chronic hepatitis C and a rash, renal disease, or joint symptoms should be evaluated for cryoglobulinemia. Diagnosis is based on laboratory identification of cryoglobulins in serum.

Table 186-3. Cryoglobulinemia

Type	Cases, %	Clonality	Class of immunoglobulin	Associations
I	25–40	Monoclonal	IgG or IgM (without antibody activity)	Multiple myeloma Waldenström's macroglobulinemia Lymphoproliferative disorders
II	15–25	Mixed	Two or more classes; one monoclonal IgM with rheumatoid factor activity	Inflammatory processes Infectious diseases (*eg*, hepatitis C virus) Connective tissue disorders
III	~50	Polyclonal	Two or more classes; the polyclonal IgM component has rheumatoid factor activity	Inflammatory processes Infectious diseases Connective tissue disorders

Köhlmeier-Degos Syndrome

Köhlmeier-Degos syndrome, also called *malignant atrophic papulosis*, is a fatal cutaneointestinal obliterative arteritis of unknown cause that affects mainly young men [14]. Systemic involvement follows several weeks to years after onset of the characteristic atrophic skin lesions. Gastrointestinal involvement is seen in 50% to 60% of cases (Table 186-4); the most common cause of death is fulminant peritonitis secondary to intestinal perforation. Abdominal pain is an ominous sign. Diagnosis is based on detection of the characteristic skin lesions. About 60% of patients die within 2 years of onset of systemic disease. No proven effective treatment exists.

Takayasu's Arteritis

Takayasu's arteritis is an inflammatory, obliterative disorder of the large and medium-sized arteries, especially the aorta and its major branches, predominantly affecting young women. Presentation is variable, but the classic presentation is lack of pulse in the extremities, hypertension, and cardiac and neurologic involvement. Gastrointestinal symptoms occur in about 15% of patients [15] and include nausea, vomiting, and weight loss. An association with inflammatory bowel disease also has been documented. Systemic corticosteroids are the best available treatment.

Kawasaki Disease

Kawasaki disease, or *mucocutaneous lymph node syndrome*, is an acute febrile illness of young children with erythema multiforme–like skin lesions. Gastrointestinal involvement is limited to stomatitis (fissuring, erythema, and crusting of the lips) and oropharyngeal lesions (diffuse oropharyngeal erythema and strawberry tongue). Mortality is related to cardiac manifestations. Treatment is with aspirin, 50 to 100 mg/kg/d. Aspirin is used for its anti-inflammatory and antiplatelet effects.

■ CONNECTIVE TISSUE DISORDERS

Ehlers-Danlos Syndrome

Ehlers-Danlos syndrome encompasses a group of connective tissue disorders defined by the triad of skin hyperextensibility, articular hypermobility, and tissue fragility [16••]. Each of the eleven subtypes has a distinctive presentation (Table 186-5). Oral complications are most severe in the periodontal type (type VIII), leading to fragile, maldeveloped teeth, significant blood loss after tooth extractions, and premature tooth loss. These patients also may experience temporomandibular joint laxity.

Table 186-4. Gastrointestinal Manifestations of Köhlmeier-Degos Syndrome

Dyspepsia
Altered bowel habits
  Alternating constipation and diarrhea
Abdominal distention
Abdominal pain
Acute surgical abdomen with signs and symptoms of
Gastrointestinal hemorrhage
Acute pancreatitis
Intestinal obstruction
Peritonitis with or without intestinal perforation

Table 186-5. Ehlers-Danlos Syndrome

Type	Form	Cases, %	Genetics	Clinical presentation	Gastrointestinal involvement
I	Gravis type	~40	AD	Skin hyperextensibility, articular laxity, tissue fragility	Standard*
II	Mittis type	~40	AD	Milder form of type I	Standard*; less severe than type I
III	Familial hypermobile type	~10	AD	Gross laxity of large and small joints	Standard*
IV	Arterial and ecchymotic type	—	AD, AR	Thin face, pinched nose, large eyes, pale skin with prominent venous network, prematurely aged limbs	Standard*; life threatening gastrointestinal complications: bowel rupture, catastrophic hemorrhage; paraesophageal hernia; colonic ileus
V	X-linked type	—	X-linked	Similar to type II	Standard*
VI	Ocular-scoliotic type	—	AR	Similar to type I; kyphoscoliosis, marfanoid habitus, ocular complications	Standard*
VII	Arthrochalasis multiplex congenita type	—	AD, AR	Marked joint laxity (multiple dislocations), stunted growth, micrognathia, midface hypoplasia	Standard*
VIII	Periodontal type	—	AD	Mild cutaneous and joint laxity, premature tooth loss, maldeveloped teeth	Gum breakdown; hypermobility of tongue; standard*
IX†	Vacant	—	—	—	—
X	—	—	AR	Similar to type I	Standard*
XI‡	Vacant	—	—	—	—

*Hiatal hernia, epiphrenic diverticula, megaesophagus, gastric diverticula, intestinal intramural hematomas, and rectal prolapse have been described in all forms.
†No longer designated as part of the Ehlers-Danlos syndrome; reclassified as a disorder of copper metabolism (cutis laxa).
‡No longer designated as part of the Ehlers-Danlos syndrome; reclassified as a disorder of joint instability.
AD—autosomal dominant; AR—autosomal recessive.

Gastrointestinal complications may occur in all subtypes but are most common in the arterial-ecchymotic type (type IV). Esophageal structural defects, such as epiphrenic diverticula and megaesophagus, have been described. Hiatal hernia and asymptomatic gastric diverticula are common; gastroparesis is known. Patients also are predisposed to gastric volvulus secondary to structural abnormalities, such as diaphragmatic eventration, hiatal hernia, kyphoscoliosis, and adhesions. Diverticula in the colon, most commonly located in the sigmoid, may perforate spontaneously. Diverticula also may occur in the small bowel, predominantly on the mesenteric border.

Other rare large and small bowel complications of Ehlers-Danlos syndrome include intramural hematomas, which may lead to focal necrosis; megaduodenum (with subsequent bacterial overgrowth and malabsorption); and rectal prolapse. Symptoms may include vomiting, hematemesis, abdominal pain, peritonitis, and hematochezia [16••]. Severe constipation may predispose to colonic perforation as the firm stool tears the walls of the colon; therefore, stool softeners should be prescribed routinely.

In general, treatment is difficult in this group of patients because of tissue fragility. Endoscopy may result in perforation or tearing. Surgical intervention can be complicated by bleeding, difficulty placing sutures, and slow wound healing. Postsurgical mortality rates range from 23% to 70%.

Scleroderma

Scleroderma, also known as *systemic sclerosis* or *progressive systemic sclerosis*, is a multisystem disorder of unknown cause characterized by mononuclear cell infiltration, widespread vascular damage, and enhanced production and deposition of collagen in the skin and various internal organs [17••]. Gastrointestinal tract involvement is common (50% to 90% of cases). The major clinical gastrointestinal manifestation of scleroderma is gut dysmotility as a result of impaired gut neurologic function; this leads to atrophy of smooth muscle followed by development of fibrosis (Fig. 186-7), the characteristic histologic lesion. The gastrointestinal mucosa generally is normal in appearance and function.

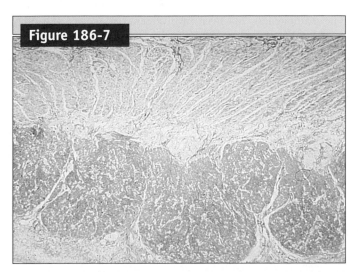

Figure 186-7

Microscopic view of smooth muscle atrophy with fibrosis characteristic of progressive systemic sclerosis (scleroderma). (*From* Greenson [52]; with permission.)

Esophageal abnormalities occur in up to 90% of patients and manifest as dilation and impaired peristalsis of the lower two thirds of the esophageal body and incompetence of the lower esophageal sphincter (Fig. 186-8). The first symptom of scleroderma often is dysphagia resulting from gastroesophageal reflux disease caused by esophageal dysmotility. Patients may experience chronic sore throat, laryngitis, aspiration pneumonia, and impaired lung diffusion secondary to chronic gastroesophageal reflux. More than 75% of patients develop erosive esophagitis, Barrett's metaplasia, or esophageal stricture. Candidal overgrowth is a frequent problem, especially in patients on antireflux therapy with H_2-receptor antagonists or proton pump inhibitors. Esophageal manometry is the diagnostic procedure for detection of esophageal dysmotility. Management is the same as in any patient with chronic gastroesophageal reflux. Lifestyle changes alone usually are insufficient, however, and patients often require intensive pharmacologic therapy. Proton pump inhibitors provide rapid and complete resolution of symptoms in more than 90% of patients, although high doses (*eg*, up to 120 mg/d of omeprazole) may be required. Treatment with cisapride appears to improve gastric motility and may be a useful adjunct. Symptomatic strictures may require dilation.

Abnormal gastric motility can be seen in 5% to 10% of patients and may manifest as abdominal distention (especially postprandial bloating), esophageal reflux, nausea, vomiting, early satiety, and weight loss. Patients are predisposed to developing gastric bezoars. The migrating myoelectric complex, which is

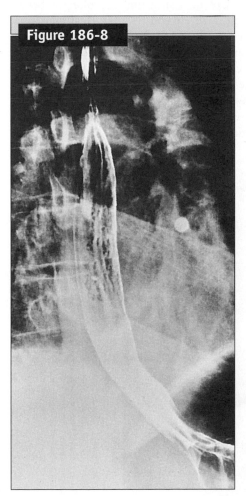

Figure 186-8

Radiographic view of scleroderma of the esophagus with candidal esophagitis. (*From* Mittal [53]; with permission.)

considered important in the generation of peristalsis, is absent in patients with scleroderma. Treatment with prokinetic agents, such as cisapride, often is useful, especially early in the disease.

Small bowel involvement may be seen in up to half of patients (Fig. 186-9), with the frequency decreasing distally in the intestine (duodenum, 40%; jejunum, 20%; ileum, 10%) [18]. Manifestations include dysmotility, diverticula, strictures, and malabsorption. Bacterial overgrowth results from stasis of the intraluminal contents, leading to diarrhea, abdominal pain, and bloating. Malabsorption due to bacterial overgrowth is common. Pancreatic exocrine dysfunction and abnormalities of the intestinal absorptive surface also may cause malabsorption. Both acute and chronic intestinal pseudo-obstruction have been described. Rare complications include pneumatosis cystoides intestinalis and gastric and small intestine telangiectasias, which may lead to gastrointestinal blood loss. Strictures occur and are considered part of the fibroproliferative process. Management is primarily medical. Bacterial overgrowth in the absence of pseudo-obstruction responds well to intermittent cyclic oral antibiotic therapy. Prokinetic drugs (eg, metoclopramide, cisapride, erythromycin) are central to the treatment of pseudo-obstruction. Patients report improvement in nausea, bloating, and abdominal pain with the use of octreotide. Correction of nutritional deficiencies may be necessary.

The reported frequency of colonic involvement varies from 10% to 50% [18]. Wide-mouth diverticula, which are true diverticula (involving all layers of the bowel wall), are considered pathognomonic. Colonic transit time is prolonged. Severe dysmotility may result in severe constipation, fecal impaction, and bowel obstruction.

Anorectal involvement is seen in 50% to 70% of patients and occurs early in the course of the disease [17••,18]. Functional disturbances of the rectum and anus include reduced anal sphincter resting pressure, disruption of the rectoanal inhibitory reflex, and reduced rectal compliance. The result may be fecal impaction or incontinence.

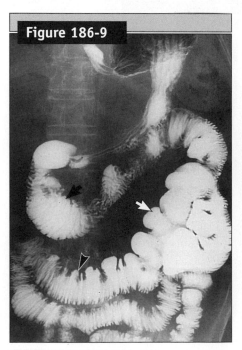

Figure 186-9

Barium study revealing multiple abnormalities in a patient with scleroderma, including dilated duodenum (*black arrow*), multiple wide-mouthed diverticula of the jejunum (*white arrow*), and packed ("hide-bound") valvuli (*arrowhead*). (*Courtesy of* C. A. Rohrmann, Jr., MD.)

Liver involvement is uncommon in patients with scleroderma [4••]. Autopsy series have shown no increased prevalence of hepatic abnormalities in patients with scleroderma when compared with controls. Primary biliary cirrhosis, however, occurs with increased frequency in patients with scleroderma. Idiopathic or noncirrhotic portal hypertension also has been reported.

Rheumatoid Arthritis

Rheumatoid arthritis is a chronic, progressive, destructive disorder of the joints. Extra-articular or systemic manifestations are common and include rheumatoid nodules, scleritis, pleuritis, pericarditis, splenomegaly, neuropathy, and vasculitis [19]. Vasculitis of the gastrointestinal tract is uncommon and may lead to serious complications, such as ulcers or ischemia. Esophageal dysmotility has been described in about 30% of patients and may lead to heartburn, dysphagia, and esophagitis. Diffuse dysmotility of the entire gastrointestinal tract has been described and treated successfully with octreotide and cisapride. Fasting hypergastrinemia has been found in 23% to 41% of patients, usually in combination with decreased gastric acid output, and does not appear to correlate with the inflammatory activity of the underlying arthritis [19]. The pathogenesis has not been established, although gastric mucosal atrophy with hypochlorhydria or achlorhydria is suspected. Mesenteric arteritis with end-organ ischemia can lead to intestinal ulceration or necrosis, perforation, stricture, gangrene, and pancolitis. Rarely, mesenteric artery aneurysmal rupture has resulted in hemoperitoneum. No therapy has been proved effective for the gastrointestinal vasculitis of rheumatoid arthritis.

Asymptomatic hepatomegaly is common in patients with rheumatoid arthritis, and liver size has been shown to correlate with the titer of rheumatoid factor in serum. Liver enlargement also is common in Felty's syndrome and Still's disease [4••]. Elevated serum levels of γ-glutamyl transpeptidase (GGTP) and alkaline phosphatase have been observed in up to 40% of patients with rheumatoid arthritis. Serum aminotransferase levels generally are not elevated. There is a direct correlation between disease activity and the alkaline phosphatase and GGTP levels. The pathogenesis of liver involvement is unclear but may involve biliary capillary inflammation. Liver histologic findings are nonspecific and generally include Kupffer's cell hyperplasia and fatty infiltration (in up to 80% of cases).

The acute systemic form of rheumatoid arthritis (Still's disease) is characterized by high fever, arthralgias, rash, lymphadenopathy, splenomegaly, and pleuropericarditis. Hepatomegaly and abnormal liver tests also have been described in this disease; improvement in overall clinical status is associated with improvement in liver function tests.

Felty's Syndrome

Felty's syndrome is characterized by the triad of rheumatoid arthritis, leukopenia, and splenomegaly. Liver disease is common in Felty's syndrome [4••]; up to 56% of patients have abnormal liver tests, and 60% to 70% reveal abnormal liver histology. Nodular regenerative hyperplasia commonly is associated with Felty's syndrome, and such patients often have anemia, leukopenia, and thrombocytopenia as a result of hypersplenism, but normal liver test results. Patients may present with complications of portal hypertension, including variceal bleeding. There is controversy about the optimal management of nodular regenerative hyperplasia. Because liver function is preserved, patients with bleeding from portal hypertension may benefit from splenectomy or a portosystemic decompression procedure.

Polymyositis and Dermatomyositis

Polymyositis and dermatomyositis involve the skeletal muscle primarily. Both disorders may be associated with motor dysfunction of the entire gastrointestinal tract, indicating that smooth muscle dysfunction also occurs [20]. Esophageal motor dysfunction is well recognized, and small and large bowel involvement also has been documented. Associated symptoms include dysphagia, heartburn, acid regurgitation, anorexia, nausea, early satiety, upper abdominal discomfort or distention, vomiting, and abdominal pain [20].

Primary biliary cirrhosis has been reported in association with polymyositis and as part of a syndrome with scleroderma and polymyositis [4••,21]. There also are case reports in the literature of polymyositis associated with chronic hepatitis. Dermatomyositis commonly is associated with malignancy, including lymphoma, melanoma, breast carcinoma, ovarian carcinoma, nasopharyngeal carcinoma, and hepatocellular carcinoma. Most instances of liver dysfunction in patients with dermatomyositis, however, are caused by metastatic disease. Hepatosplenomegaly has been reported in some cases, which included nonspecific portal inflammation and steatosis.

Sjögren's Syndrome

Sjögren's syndrome is a chronic inflammatory disorder associated with autoimmune destruction of the exocrine glands (autoimmune exocrinopathy) that leads to diminished or absent glandular secretions [22••]. Women are affected predominantly (90% of cases), with an average age at onset of symptoms of 45 years [23]. The classic findings of xerostomia (dry mouth), keratoconjunctivitis sicca (dry eyes), and chronic arthritis were described by Sjögren in 1933. Lymphocytic inflammation of the lacrimal and salivary glands is a cardinal feature. Serum autoantibodies are found commonly and include rheumatoid factor, Ro/SSA, and La/SSB, which are associated with increased activity of polyclonal B lymphocytes. Sjögren's syndrome is associated with the histocompatibility antigens HLA-B8 and HLA-Dw3 and may be either primary or secondary [23].

Sjögren's syndrome may affect any part of the gastrointestinal tract. Lymphocytic infiltration of the salivary glands leads to their irreversible destruction with markedly diminished or absent secretion of saliva [24]. This leads to difficulty in chewing, swallowing, and phonation; adherence of food to the buccal surfaces; abnormalities of taste and smell; mucosal erythema and fissures; increased frequency of dental caries; and frequent ingestion of fluids in an attempt to alleviate the symptoms. Management is directed toward improving patient comfort and preserving dentition. Use of sugarless mints or gum and frequent intake of fluids may be beneficial. Treatment with the muscarinic-cholinergic agonist pilocarpine may help to stimulate salivary flow.

Dysphagia is one of the most common complaints in patients with Sjögren's syndrome and usually is attributed to the lack of saliva and subsequent failure to neutralize and clear refluxed gastric secretions [22••,23]. There is conflicting evidence of the role that esophageal dysmotility may play in dysphagia. Esophageal webs are seen in as many at 10% of patients.

Sjögren's syndrome may involve the stomach, and patients may complain of epigastric pain and nausea. Atrophy of the gastric glands in association with chronic inflammation is seen. Chronic atrophic gastritis with achlorhydria is much more prevalent in Sjögren's syndrome than in other rheumatologic diseases, but pernicious anemia is rare. There are only a few case reports of small or large intestinal involvement in Sjögren's syndrome.

Although the salivary glands and pancreas are similar exocrine glands, pancreatic insufficiency in Sjögren's syndrome has not been reported frequently. Asymptomatic, defective pancreatic exocrine function (based on secretin stimulation testing) has been observed in up to 37% of cases. Acute pancreatitis is less common in this syndrome than is chronic pancreatitis. A rare complex of chronic pancreatitis, sclerosing cholangitis, and Sjögren's syndrome has been described.

Hepatomegaly and abnormal liver tests are found in up to 25% of patients, and Sjögren's syndrome commonly is associated with primary biliary cirrhosis, autoimmune hepatitis, chronic hepatitis, and cryptogenic cirrhosis [4••]. It has been suggested that the sicca complex and autoimmune hepatic disease may be part of an immunologically mediated systemic disorder. Up to 11% of patients with Sjögren's syndrome may have concurrent antimitochondrial and anti–smooth muscle antibodies. Antimitochondrial antibody and abnormalities of liver chemistries are more common in patients with Sjögren's syndrome and rheumatoid arthritis than in those with rheumatoid arthritis alone. Non–organ-specific autoantibodies and hypergammaglobulinemia often are seen in patients with both primary biliary cirrhosis and Sjögren's syndrome, and Sjögren's syndrome is one of the most common extrahepatic diseases associated with primary biliary cirrhosis (69% to 81% of cases) [4••]. Hepatitis C virus infection has been associated with lymphocytic sialadenitis, similar to that seen in Sjögren's syndrome. Therefore, abnormal liver chemistries in a patient with Sjögren's syndrome should be evaluated thoroughly.

Systemic Lupus Erythematosus

Systemic lupus erythematosus (SLE) is a multisystem disease characterized by exacerbations and remissions [25]. It is more common in women than men and is relatively more prevalent among persons of African, Hispanic, Native American, and Polynesian descent. SLE generally presents between the first and fourth decades of life, although in about 10% of cases, the age of onset is beyond 60 years. There is evidence to support a genetic influence, and an association is seen with HLA class II alleles DR3 and DR2. The presentation of SLE is varied, with skin, musculoskeletal system, cardiovascular, renal, pulmonary, central nervous system, hematologic, and gastrointestinal tract involvement.

Gastrointestinal symptoms are common in patients with SLE. About half of patients experience anorexia, nausea, vomiting, diarrhea, or abdominal pain [26]. Abdominal pain is the most common gastrointestinal complaint (34%). Lupus enteritis caused by small vessel arteritis may lead to local ischemia, vascular insufficiency, and possibly necrosis of the bowel wall with perforation, infarction, or focal stricture formation. Frank or occult rectal bleeding may be seen. Laboratory features are nonspecific, although roentgenographic changes may suggest bowel vasculitis. Patients may respond to high-dose corticosteroids early in the course of disease, but management is difficult in patients with advanced ischemic disease of the gastrointestinal tract.

Ulcerations may occur on the oral, vaginal, or nasal mucosa and usually are painless (Fig. 186-10; see also *Color Plate*). The incidence of gastrointestinal hemorrhage is about 5% but is 20% to 50% in patients with prior or coexisting gastrointestinal tract disease [27]. Gastrointestinal bleeding also may result from aspirin or nonsteroidal anti-inflammatory agents used in the treatment of SLE.

Esophageal dysmotility has been reported in up to 30% of patients with SLE, and the lower third of the esophagus is affected most commonly. Esophagitis and esophageal ulcerations may result from arteritis. Patients may complain of dysphagia or odynophagia. Motor dysfunction of the stomach and small bowel also has been reported and may lead to gastric outlet obstruction and intestinal pseudo-obstruction. Malabsorption and protein-losing enteropathy have been described. Acute pancreatitis has been reported in patients with SLE, possibly caused by vasculitis with resulting ischemia.

Hepatomegaly is noted in about one third of patients; however, there are conflicting reports on the prevalence of clinically significant liver disease [4••,27]. Abnormalities in serum liver enzymes have been observed in 20% to 60% of patients. Antimitochondrial antibodies have been detected in up to 40% of patients, but the presence of these antibodies often is not associated with other liver biochemical abnormalities. Histologic abnormalities of the liver may be present in up to 20% of patients; the most common are steatosis and portal inflammation. Hepatic cell necrosis is rare. Vascular diseases associated with the presence of "lupus anticoagulant" in serum (in patients

with and without SLE) include Budd-Chiari syndrome, hepatic veno-occlusive disease, and hepatic arteritis. There is no direct relation between SLE and "lupoid (autoimmune) hepatitis," although chronic hepatitis may occur in these patients.

Mixed Connective Tissue Disorder

Mixed connective tissue disorder is a syndrome characterized by overlapping features of progressive systemic sclerosis, SLE, and polymyositis and is associated with high titers of antibodies directed against the ribonucleoprotein fraction of extractable nuclear antigen. Overall, gastrointestinal symptoms occur in about 75% of patients with mixed connective tissue disorder and most closely resemble those seen in scleroderma. Heartburn (48%), dysphagia (38%), and dyspepsia (20%) are most common [28••]. Esophageal dysmotility has been reported; most affected patients demonstrate a hypotensive upper esophageal sphincter and esophageal hypomotility. Some studies have suggested that corticosteroids may improve this esophageal motor dysfunction. Vomiting, diarrhea, and constipation are less common manifestations. Other gastrointestinal tract abnormalities include duodenal and jejunal dilation, intestinal pseudo-obstruction, wide-mouth colonic diverticula, pneumatosis cystoides intestinalis, gastrointestinal bleeding, and malabsorption. Pancreatitis has been reported, but liver involvement is rare.

Pseudoxanthoma Elasticum

Pseudoxanthoma elasticum is a rare hereditary disease of connective tissue synthesis characterized by skin, eye, and vascular involvement. Degeneration of the elastic fibers in the visceral blood vessels leads to gastrointestinal bleeding in about 13% of patients. Recurrent hematemesis is more common than melena [29]. Conservative medical treatment often is unsuccessful, and selective angiography or surgical intervention may be required to control the bleeding.

◼◼ ENDOCRINE DISORDERS
Acromegaly

Acromegaly is a clinical syndrome resulting from long-standing growth hormone excess, usually secondary to a pituitary adenoma [30•]. Sustained elevations of growth hormone lead to increased hepatic and tissue production of insulin-like growth factor-1 (formerly somatomedin C), which mediates the somatic and mitogenic effects of growth hormone. Increased longevity appears to be associated with an increasing risk of complications.

Visceromegaly is a common finding on autopsy examination; however, clinical hepatosplenomegaly is noted much less frequently and often is associated with a secondary condition, such as congestive heart failure or alcoholism [30•]. Liver chemistries generally are normal despite hepatomegaly, and there is poor correlation between the degree of organ enlargement and the extent of growth hormone excess.

Cancer is the second leading cause of death in patients with acromegaly; most tumors are neoplasms of the gastrointestinal tract, estimated to occur in up to 10% of patients with acromegaly [30•,31]. The overall incidence of colonic adenomas is about 40%, and patients with acromegaly appear to develop colonic polyps with greater frequency (three- to eightfold) and at a younger age than do persons in the normal control group.

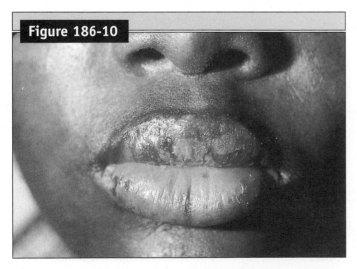

Figure 186-10

Oral erosions associated with systemic lupus erythematosus. See also **Color Plate**. (*From* Pandya [50]; with permission.)

Increased expression of the c-*myc* proto-oncogene has been implicated in the pathogenesis. There does not appear to be a correlation between serum levels of growth hormone or insulin-like growth factor-1 and the frequency of polyps, but skin tags are seen more commonly in patients with adenomatous colonic polyps than in controls. Risk factors for colon cancer include male gender, age older than 50 years, more than three skin tags, family history of colon cancer, and a history of polyps. It is recommended that patients with acromegaly undergo colonoscopy every 5 to 7 years, or every 3 to 5 years if multiple risk factors for polyps are present.

Adrenal Disease

Addison's Disease

Addison's disease is an uncommon disorder in which adrenal cortical destruction results in adrenocortical insufficiency. It may be primary and result from an autoimmune (80%) or granulomatous (about 20%) process or secondary, resulting from pituitary disease. Patients present with anorexia (90%), nausea and vomiting (90%), weight loss (97%), abdominal pain (30% to 40%), watery diarrhea (20% to 30%), and malabsorption [32•]. Symptoms generally resolve completely with glucocorticoid and mineralocorticoid replacement therapy. Acute adrenal insufficiency (adrenal crisis) often presents with gastrointestinal symptoms, including nausea, vomiting, abdominal pain, and diarrhea, and may be associated with headache, fever, hypotension, confusion, or coma. It is a clinical emergency and is treated with intravenous hydrocortisone. In patients with acquired immunodeficiency syndrome, adrenal insufficiency is seen with cytomegalovirus, mycobacterium avium complex, and other infections.

Liver dysfunction is observed commonly and generally is characterized by an increase in the serum levels of aspartate aminotransferase and lactate dehydrogenase [33], although the pathogenesis remains unclear. Lymphocytic portal infiltrates and mild centrilobular fibrosis have been described on liver biopsy. Liver enzymes return to normal with cortisol replacement.

Cushing's Disease

Hyperadrenocorticism, the ectopic production of adrenocorticotropin, can result from a pituitary tumor (60%), adrenal neoplasm (10% to 20%), ectopic neoplasm (15%), or exogenous glucocorticoids. Few symptoms are referable to the gastrointestinal tract, but patients often are obese and may develop hepatic microvesicular steatosis. Serum aminotransferase levels usually are below normal values secondary to the excess of circulating glucocorticoids.

Parathyroid Disease

Primary hyperparathyroidism may result from hyperplasia or adenomatous proliferation of the parathyroid glands, whereas secondary hyperparathyroidism results when nonparathyroid malignancies produce parathyroid hormone. The most common complications of hyperparathyroidism are renal and bone disease, but gastrointestinal symptoms may result from hypercalcemia [34•]. Constipation, at times severe, is the most common gastrointestinal symptom and is likely related to colonic inertia. Nausea and vomiting, often associated with

severe anorexia, may be present, probably secondary to a decrease in gastric tone and possibly gastroparesis. Epigastric or diffuse abdominal pain is seen in up to one third of patients with hyperparathyroidism, and the cause in most cases is obscure. Duodenal ulcer occurs with increased frequency in patients with hyperparathyroidism, with a prevalence of 5% to 30%. The frequency of acute pancreatitis also is increased, presumably because of the hypercalcemia. Pancreatic calcifications are usually evident, small, and distributed throughout the gland, as in alcoholic pancreatitis. Primary hyperparathyroidism may be associated with gastrointestinal neoplasms.

Thyroid Disease

Hyperthyroidism

Gastrointestinal complaints often accompany hyperthyroidism. Gastritis occurs in nearly 80% of patients and is associated with decreased gastric acid secretion. Other symptoms include diarrhea, malabsorption, and steatorrhea, presumably the result of abnormal intestinal motility. Significantly shortened gastrointestinal transit times have been demonstrated in hyperthyroid patients and normalize after correction of hyperthyroidism [35].

Forty-five to 90% of patients with hyperthyroidism have one or more abnormal liver tests, including elevations in serum aminotransferase and alkaline phosphatase levels, and hypoalbuminemia. On physical examination, hepatomegaly, gynecomastia, and jaundice may be noted. During episodes of thyrotoxicosis (thyroid storm), the liver may be subjected to relative hypoxia, which may be complicated by high-output cardiac failure. Excess thyroid hormone also may have a direct effect on the hepatic metabolism of bilirubin.

Hypothyroidism

Hypothyroid patients may present with constipation, obstipation, and colonic gas retention. The mechanism is believed to be abnormal gut motility. In contrast to patients with hyperthyroidism, those with hypothyroidism have a prolonged gastrointestinal transit time [36]. Studies of the bowel wall in hypothyroid patients reveal myxedematous infiltration of the stroma, atrophy of the mucosa, and diffuse infiltration of the submucosa with lymphocytes and plasma cells. Symptoms resolve when a euthyroid state is attained.

Hypothyroidism may cause a profound decrease in exocrine pancreatic function, with resulting malabsorption [37]. A marked decrease in acinar cell function reverses completely with thyroid replacement therapy. The precise cause of pancreatic insufficiency in these patients is not well understood.

Slightly abnormal liver tests and hepatomegaly are observed commonly in patients with hypothyroidism. In severe myxedema, marked elevations of serum aminotransferase and bilirubin levels may be seen. Ascites is uncommon in patients with myxedema. Its pathogenesis is poorly understood, but it usually is associated with peripheral edema and may result from congestive heart failure due to myxedema [38]. Pathologic examination of the liver discloses central "congestive" fibrosis. Elevated serum cholesterol and triglyceride levels are common in advanced hypothyroidism, and an increased frequency of gallstones is seen.

GENETIC AND METABOLIC DISORDERS

Amyloidosis

Amyloidosis is characterized by the deposition of an amorphous, insoluble proteinaceous material in the extracellular spaces of various organs [39•]. Many organs may be involved, and the initial presentation depends on which organ is affected most severely. Several forms of amyloidosis are recognized and differ with regard to the underlying cause and nature of the deposited protein. Amyloidosis resulting from deposition of immunoglobulin light chains is called *AL* or *primary amyloidosis*. AL, AF (familial), AA (secondary), and AH (hemodialysis-related) amyloid account for 90% of all cases associated with gastrointestinal symptoms. Most patients with amyloidosis have gastrointestinal involvement on postmortem examination.

Common clinical gastrointestinal symptoms in patients with amyloidosis include anorexia, diarrhea, macroglossia, and intestinal pseudo-obstruction. Amyloid-associated dysmotility may be the cause of intestinal pseudo-obstruction, diarrhea, constipation, or achalasia. Treatment with prokinetic agents may be helpful, and surgery is not indicated in patients with intestinal pseudo-obstruction. Macroglossia is seen in 20% of patients, leading to respiratory compromise, malnutrition, and cachexia because the large tongue prevents the patient from breathing and eating. Tracheostomy may be required if breathing is compromised. Other oral symptoms include salivary gland swelling and xerostomia. Small bowel biopsy for amyloid protein has the highest sensitivity rate (86% to 100%) for diagnosis of gastrointestinal involvement, followed by rectal biopsy (75% to 85%) and abdominal fat aspiration (75% to 85%) [40].

Whereas the frequency of liver involvement ranges from 70% to 90% in autopsy series, detectable hepatomegaly occurs in only 30% to 50% of patients, and symptomatic liver disease is rare [39•]. Most patients with hepatic amyloidosis also have involvement of other organs. Amyloid protein is deposited in the hepatic parenchyma, usually within Disse's space, as well as within hepatic blood vessel walls. Ascites may occur, but jaundice is unusual and portal hypertension uncommon. Elevated serum alkaline phosphatase levels are seen most commonly, and coagulopathy and elevated serum aminotransferase levels may occur. Reports have not been confirmed that liver biopsy in patients with amyloid liver disease should be avoided because of the risk of hepatic fracture. Patients with hepatomegaly but without cholestasis have a much better prognosis than those with cholestasis. Death from amyloidosis usually is related to cardiac or renal involvement.

Anderson-Fabry Disease

Anderson-Fabry disease is a rare, X-linked recessive disorder of glycolipid metabolism. The basic defect is absence of the enzyme α-galactosidase A, leading to deposition of ceramide trihexoside in endothelial and smooth muscle cells of small blood vessels as well as in ganglion cells [41,42]. The incidence is about 1 in 40,000. Glycosphingolipid deposition within endothelial cells leads to thrombotic and embolic sequelae. The most common presentation is with painful crises and constant burning paresthesias in association with characteristic angiokeratomas of the skin. Gastrointestinal manifestations are seen in 62% of afflicted men and in 29% of female carriers and

are thought to result primarily from vascular and neurologic involvement. The most common gastrointestinal symptom is mild episodic diarrhea, but patients also may have intermittent constipation, anorexia, nausea, vomiting, crampy abdominal pain, and weight loss and rarely develop intestinal ischemia and perforation [43]. Gastrointestinal dysmotility with jejunal diverticulosis and small bowel bacterial overgrowth also has been reported (Fig. 186-11). Diagnosis is suspected on the basis of history and confirmed by renal or skin biopsy. Jejunal or rectal biopsy samples show foamy, electron-dense deposits in the vascular endothelium and accumulation of ceramide trihexoside in the myenteric nervous plexus of the gut [41]. Treatment is unsatisfactory. Antiplatelet therapy may help prevent thrombotic and embolic sequelae, and antiseizure medications, such as carbamazepine, may alleviate painful crises.

Down Syndrome

Down syndrome is a major cause of mental retardation, congenital heart disease, and gastrointestinal tract anomalies. Affected persons have an extra chromosome 21 (trisomy 21). Mental retardation and neonatal hypotonia occur in nearly 100% of patients. There is a wide variation in phenotypic expression. Gastrointestinal symptoms typically present in infancy, often are life-threatening, and may require surgical intervention [44•]. Duodenal stenosis or atresia is the most common gastrointestinal anomaly seen. Affected infants present with vomiting, abdominal distention, and a "double-bubble" sign (distention of both the stomach and duodenum) on abdominal radiographs (Fig. 186-12). The overall mortality rate is 13% to 55%, primarily from pneumonia and heart failure. Annular pancreas and intestinal malrotation also are common and may be associated with duodenal stenosis, contributing to symptoms. Common esophageal anomalies include stenosis or atresia, hiatal hernia, tracheoesophageal fistula, gastroesophageal reflux disease often with Barrett's mucosa and stricture, and primary motility disorders. Symptoms related to these anomalies usually do not respond to standard medical management, and surgical intervention may be required. Hirschsprung's disease also is common. Imperforate anus generally requires surgical repair. Uncommon intestinal

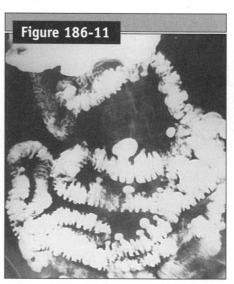

Figure 186-11

Barium study showing multiple jejunal diverticula associated with Anderson-Fabry disease. (*Courtesy of* C. A. Rohrmann, Jr., MD.)

disorders include small bowel hypoplasia and Meckel's diverticulum. The incidence of hepatitis B virus infection is increased in patients with Down syndrome, but primary hepatobiliary abnormalities (other than biliary atresia) are not generally seen.

Hereditary Angioedema

Hereditary angioedema, a disorder of the complement system, is inherited in an autosomal dominant fashion. The gene for the disorder is located on chromosome 11 and leads to a decrease in the quantity or activity of the C1 inhibitor, which is a serine protease inhibitor [45]. The incidence of the disorder is about 1 in 10,000 to 1 in 50,000. Type I hereditary angioedema accounts for 85% of cases and manifests as low or undetectable levels of normal C1 inhibitor. Type II accounts for the remaining 15% of cases and is associated with normal or increased levels of dysfunctional C1 inhibitor. C1 inhibitor regulates the complement, coagulation, and kinin systems, and deficiency of the enzyme leads to unopposed activation of the complement cascade and decreased modulation of the kinin pathway.

Patients present with recurrent episodes of self-limited, soft tissue swelling involving the face, extremities, upper airway, and gastrointestinal tract. Attacks may be spontaneous or precipitated by trauma, emotion, or stress. Gastrointestinal symptoms include nausea, vomiting, and diarrhea. Severe colicky abdominal pain results from bowel wall edema and transient luminal obstruction and may be the only symptom in up to half of patients. Ascites has been reported. Acute pancreatitis may occur if edema involves the pancreatic duct. The mortality rate can be as high as 30% if the larynx is involved and the patient remains untreated. Treatment in the acute setting consists of intravenous C1 inhibitor concentrates and fresh frozen plasma. The most widely used oral agents for prophylaxis are the attenuated androgens, such as danazol and stanozolol, which are highly effective in preventing attacks. Analgesics, antiemetics, and epinephrine may be useful for symptomatic relief.

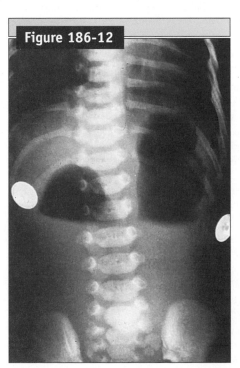

Figure 186-12   Upright abdominal radiograph revealing the classic "double-bubble" sign of Down syndrome, with dilation of the stomach and proximal duodenum. (*Courtesy of* C. A. Rohrmann, Jr., MD.)

Turner's Syndrome

Turner's syndrome is the most common sex-linked chromosomal abnormality in females and is characterized by a 45,X karyotype (X chromosome monosomy). The disease is associated with gonadal dysgenesis, webbed neck, and cubitus valgus (elbows twisted outward). The frequency is 1 in 1500 to 2500 live births [46]. Although cardiovascular disorders are the major cause of increased mortality in patients with Turner's syndrome, gastrointestinal hemorrhage has been described. Abnormal mesenteric vascular development may lead to intestinal vascular malformations, particularly in the small intestine. Most affected patients present with melena, hematochezia, or frank anemia; hematemesis is uncommon. Patients may have an increased incidence of lymphagiectasia, Crohn's disease, and ulcerative colitis.

■ HEMATOLOGIC DISORDERS
Hemolytic-Uremic Syndrome

The classic triad of hemolytic-uremic syndrome (HUS) is microangiopathic hemolytic anemia, thrombocytopenia, and acute renal failure [47]. The most common antecedent precipitating factor is gram-negative enteric infection, especially with *Escherichia coli* O157:H7, but also with *Salmonella, Shigella, Campylobacter,* and *Yersinia* species and with *Streptococcus pneumoniae*. The pathophysiology of HUS is poorly understood. Gastrointestinal symptoms are common in children with the disorder, particularly during the prodrome, and are usually self-limited. Diarrhea (100%), vomiting (80%), hemorrhagic colitis (79%), and abdominal discomfort or tenderness (59%) are the most common gastrointestinal symptoms. Mild and transient elevations of serum aminotransferase (58%) and indirect bilirubin levels (49%) result from hemolytic anemia. Pancreatitis has been reported in up to 21% of patients with HUS. Uncommon complications include rectal prolapse (13%), colonic stricture (3%), colonic perforation (1%), and intussusception (1%). Management consists of supportive care, antibiotics, and dialysis.

Hypercoagulability

The hypercoagulable states are a poorly defined group of conditions that predispose to thromboembolism. Primary hypercoagulable states result from congenital or familial defects in the proteins of the coagulation or fibrinolytic systems and include antithrombin III deficiency, protein C deficiency, protein S deficiency, factor XII (Hageman) deficiency, factor V (Leiden) mutation, and antiphospholipid syndromes. The disorders are characterized by recurrent deep venous thrombosis and pulmonary embolism. Thrombosis usually is venous and can involve any organ system, including the gastrointestinal and hepatobiliary tracts. Intestinal ischemia or portal vein thrombosis secondary to mesenteric involvement and Budd-Chiari syndrome may be seen.

Sickle Cell Anemia

Sickle cell anemia, an autosomal recessive disorder of hemoglobin synthesis, is characterized by intermittent acute painful crises ("sickle cell crisis"), which may be precipitated by stress, infection, dehydration, or other events [48]. The erythrocytes "sickle" under conditions of low oxygen tension and lodge in capillary beds, leading to venous congestion, thrombosis, and microinfarction. As patients age, irreversible damage of the spleen, brain, kidneys, lungs, eyes, bones, skin, and gastrointestinal tract occurs.

The spleen is the most common abdominal organ involved, and autosplenectomy occurs in nearly 90% of patients by 6 years of age [49]. Painful abdominal crises are attributed to small infarcts of the mesentery and abdominal viscera and are characterized by severe abdominal pain and signs of peritoneal irritation. Ileus may be present. Mucosal ulceration is less common. With age, the frequency of hepatomegaly increases. Abnormal serum liver tests reflect vascular and biliary damage, and some patients develop jaundice, which usually is accompanied by abdominal pain and is caused by sickling of erythrocytes in the hepatic sinusoids. Hemosiderosis is seen as a consequence of frequent blood transfusions. Hepatic infarction is rare, and some patients ultimately develop cirrhosis. The frequency of gallstones in affected patients increases with age, although the true prevalence is unclear. Although gallstones often are found in the common bile duct, biliary obstruction as a cause of jaundice is exceedingly rare and most often caused by sludging of sickled red blood cells in the hepatic sinusoids. Treatment of painful crises is supportive with hydration, blood transfusions as needed, and analgesia. Hemoglobin C is a less severe variant of sickle cell anemia in which the spleen is involved less commonly.

■ REFERENCES

Recently published papers of particular interest have been highlighted as follows:
• Of interest
•• Of outstanding interest

1.•• Yurdakul S, Tüzüner W, Yurdakul I, et al.: Gastrointestinal involvement in Behçet's syndrome: A controlled study. *Ann Rheum Dis* 1996, 55:208–210.
This well-organized article covers the gastrointestinal manifestations of Behçet's disease. In a review of the records of 1000 patients, the authors found 147 patients with gastrointestinal symptoms; these 147 patients were then followed prospectively.

2.   Hamuryudan V, Mat C, Saip S, et al.:Thalidomide in the treatment of the mucocutaneous lesions of the Behçet syndrome. *Ann Intern Med* 1998, 128:443.

3.•   Nordborg E, Nordborg C, Malmvall BE, et al.: Giant cell arteritis. *Rheum Dis Clin North Am* 1995, 21:1013–1026.
This is an excellent review of the varied manifestations of giant cell arteritis.

4.•• Kowdley KV, Kaplan MM: The liver in collagen-vascular diseases. In *The Liver in Systemic Disease*. Edited by Rustgi VK, Van Thiel DH. New York: Raven; 1997:43–63.
This well-referenced chapter addresses hepatobiliary manifestations of the collagen vascular diseases.

5.   White RHR: Henoch-Schönlein purpura. In *Systemic Vasculitides*. Edited by Churg A, Churg J. New York: Igaku-Shoin; 1991:203–218.

6.   Park SH, Kim CJ, Chi JG, et al.: Gastrointestinal manifestations of Henoch-Schönlein purpura. *J Korean Med Sci* 1990, 5:101–104.

7.   Katz S, Borst M, Seekri I, et al.: Surgical evaluation of Henoch-Schönlein purpura: experience with 110 children. *Arch Surg* 1991, 126:849–854.

8.•   Guillevin L, Lhote F, Gallais V, et al.: Gastrointestinal tract involvement in polyarteritis nodosa and Churg-Strauss syndrome. *Ann Med Interne* (Paris) 1995, 146:260–267.
The authors provide an up-to-date and well-referenced overview of gastrointestinal involvement in both polyarteritis nodosa and Churg-Strauss syndrome.

9.•   Burke AP, Sobin LH, Viramani R: Localized vasculitis of the gastrointestinal tract. *Am J Surg Pathol* 1995, 19:338–349.
In this study, 63 patients with localized gastrointestinal tract vasculitis were followed for a mean of 5 years. Patients without serum autoantibodies appeared to have a low short-term risk for development of systemic disease.

10.   Manganelli P, Troise Rioda W, Buzio C, et al.: Churg-Strauss syndrome: personal caseload and review of the literature. *Minerva Med* 1994, 85:387–393.

11.• Leavitt RY, Fauci AS: Less common manifestations and presentations of Wegener's granulomatosis. *Curr Opin Rheumatol* 1992, 41:16–22.
This well-referenced article presents the less common manifestations of the disease, including gastrointestinal involvement.

12.   Iwasaki T, Kakishita E: Cryoglobulinemia. *Nippon Rinsho* 1994, 53:736–740.

13.   DeBandt M, Ribard P, Meyer O, et al.: Type II IgM monoclonal cryoglobulinemia and hepatitis C virus infection. *Clin Exp Rheumatol* 1991, 9:659–660.

14.   Snow JL, Muller SA: Degos syndrome: malignant atrophic papulosis. *Semin Dermatol* 1995, 14:99–105.

15.   Sharma BK, Jain S, Sagar S: Systemic manifestations of Takayasu arteritis: the expanding spectrum. *Int J Cardiol* 1996, 54(suppl):149–154.

16.•• Solomon JA, Abrams L, Lichtenstein GR: GI manifestations of Ehlers-Danlos syndrome. *Am J Gastroenterol* 1996, 91:2282–2288.
This is an excellent, up-to-date review of the gastrointestinal manifestations of Ehlers-Danlos syndrome and of the therapeutic options. It is well referenced, easy to read, and informative, including information on collagen physiology.

17.•• Abu-Shakra M, Guillemin F, Lee P: Gastrointestinal manifestations of systemic sclerosis. *Semin Arthritis Rheum* 1994, 24:29–39.
This prospective study followed 262 patients with scleroderma between 1978 and 1992, detailing all of the gastrointestinal manifestations encountered. Complete and well referenced, this article details all aspects of gastrointestinal disease in scleroderma.

18.   Hendel L: Esophageal and small intestinal manifestations of progressive systemic sclerosis: a clinical and experimental study. *Dan Med Bull* 1994, 41:371–385.

19.   Janssen M, Dijkmans BAC, Lamers CBHW: Upper gastrointestinal manifestations in rheumatoid arthritis patients: intrinsic or extrinsic pathogenesis. *Scand J Gastroenterol* 1990, 25(suppl 178):79–84.

20.   Plotz PH, Rider LG, Targoff IN, et al.: Myositis: immunologic contributions to understanding cause, pathogenesis, and therapy. *Ann Intern Med* 1995, 122:715–724.

21.   Milosevic M, Adams P: Primary biliary cirrhosis and polymyositis. *J Clin Gastroenterol* 1990, 12:332–335.

22.•• Sheikh SH, Shaw-Stiffel TA: The gastrointestinal manifestations of Sjögren's syndrome. *Am J Gastroenterol* 1995, 90:9–14.
This is an excellent, concise, and well-researched clinical review of the gastrointestinal manifestations of Sjögren's syndrome that covers the complete gastrointestinal and hepatobiliary systems.

23.   Constantopoulos SH, Tsianos EV, Moutsopoulos HM: Pulmonary and gastrointestinal manifestations of Sjögren's syndrome. *Rheum Dis Clin North Am* 1992, 18:617–635.

24.   Daniels TE, Fox PC: Salivary and oral components of Sjögren's syndrome. *Rheum Dis Clin North Am* 1992, 18:571–589.

25.   von Feldt JM: Systemic lupus erythematosus: recognizing its various presentations. *Postgrad Med* 1995, 97:79, 83, 86, 89–90, 92–94.

26.   Pisetsky DS, Gilkeson G, St Clair EW: Systemic lupus erythematosus: diagnosis and treatment. *Med Clin North Am* 1997, 81:113–128.

27.   Jaspersen D: Gastrointestinal manifestations of systemic lupus erythematosus: symptoms, diagnosis, and differential diagnosis. *Fortschr Med* 1992, 110:167–169.

28.•• Marshall JB, Kretschmar JM, Gerhardt DC, *et al.*: Gastrointestinal manifestations of mixed connective tissue disease. *Gastroenterology* 1990, 98:1232–1238.
The authors describe their prospective longitudinal study of esophageal motility in 34 patients with mixed connective tissue disease, including manometric and radiographic evaluation. Medical charts were reviewed in these 34 patients, plus an additional 27 patients, with regard to extraesophageal gastrointestinal tract abnormalities.

29. Spinzi G, Strocchi E, Imperiali G, *et al.*: Pseudoxanthoma elasticum: a rare cause of gastrointestinal bleeding. *Am J Gastroenterol* 1996, 91:1631–1634.

30.• Ezzat S: Hepatobiliary and gastrointestinal manifestations of acromegaly. *Dig Dis* 1992, 10:173–180.
The authors present a complete overview of the clinical gastrointestinal manifestations seen in acromegaly, with particular emphasis on gastrointestinal tract neoplasms.

31. Molitch ME: Clinical manifestations of acromegaly. *Endocrinol Metab Clin North Am* 1992, 21:597–613.

32.• Oelkers W: Adrenal insufficiency. *N Engl J Med* 1996, 335:1206–1212.
This well-organized overview of adrenal insufficiency addresses the causes, clinical manifestations, diagnosis, and treatment options.

33. Olsson RG, Lindgren A, Zettergren L: Liver involvement in Addison's disease. *Am J Gastroenterol* 1990, 85:435–438.

34.• Gardner EC, Herse T: Primary hyperparathyroidism and the gastrointestinal tract. *South Med J* 1981, 74:197–199.
The authors undertook a retrospective review of 100 patients to determine the frequency of gastrointestinal symptoms in primary hyperparathyroidism. This article remains a good review of the overall frequency of gastrointestinal complaints among various studies.

35. Wegener M, Wedmann B, Langhoff T, *et al.*: Effect of hyperthyroidism on the transit of a caloric solid-liquid meal through the stomach, the small intestine, and the colon in man. *J Clin Endocrinol Metab* 1992, 75:745–749.

36. Rahman Q, Haboubi NY, Hudson PP, *et al.*: The effect of thyroxine on small intestinal motility in the elderly. *Clin Endocrinol Oxf* 1991, 35:443–446.

37. Gullo L, Pezzilli R, Bellanova B, *et al.*: Influence of the thyroid on exocrine pancreatic function. *Gastroenterology* 1991, 100:1392–1396.

38. Tsutsu N, Okumura M: Gross ascites as a first manifestation of primary hypothyroidism due to post-treatment of radioiodine therapy for Graves' disease. *Intern Med* 1992, 31:256–259.

39.• Lee JG, Wilson JAP, Gottfried MR: Gastrointestinal manifestations of amyloidosis. *South Med J* 1994, 87:243–247.
The authors reviewed the medical records of 40 patients admitted to Duke University Medical Center with amyloidosis, specifically their gastrointestinal manifestations, laboratory data, endoscopic data, and follow-up reports when available.

40. Tada S, Iida M, Iwashita A, *et al.*: Endoscopic and biopsy findings of the upper digestive tract in patients with amyloidosis. *Gastrointest Endosc* 1990, 36:10–14.

41. Morgan SH, Crawfurd MA: Anderson-Fabry disease. *Br Med J* 1988, 297:872–873.

42. Radcliff KW, Evans BA: Anderson-Fabry disease (angiokeratoma corporis diffusum universale). *Genitourin Med* 1990, 66:399–400.

43. Jardine DL, Fitzpatrick MA, Troughton WD, *et al.*: Small bowel ischaemia in Fabry's disease. *J Gastroenterol Hepatol* 1994, 9:201–204.

44.• Buchin PJ, Levy JS, Schullinger JN: Down's syndrome and the gastrointestinal tract. *J Clin Gastroenterol* 1986; 8:111–114.
The authors undertook a 12-year retrospective review of the gastrointestinal involvement in 187 Down syndrome patients admitted to a tertiary care referral center. The overall incidence of GI involvement was 14%. A small comparative review of other reports of gastrointestinal involvement is included.

45. Cicardi M, Agostoni A: Hereditary angioedema. *N Engl J Med* 1996, 334:1666–1667.

46. Saenger P: Turner's syndrome. *N Engl J Med* 1996, 335:1749–1754.

47. Grodinsky S, Telmesani T, Robson WLM, *et al.*: Gastrointestinal manifestations of hemolytic uremic syndrome: recognition of pancreatitis. *J Pediatr Gastroenterol Nutr* 1990, 11:518–524.

48. Rao VM, Mapp EM, Wechsler RJ: Radiology of the gastrointestinal tract in sickle cell anemia. *Semin Roentgenol* 1987, 22:195–204.

49. Powars DR: Sickle cell anemia and major organ failure. *Hemoglobin* 1990, 14:573–598.

50. Pandya AG: The skin and gastrointestinal system. In *Gastroenterology and Hepatology: The Comprehensive Visual Reference*, vol 3: *Stomach and Duodenum*. Edited by Feldman M. Philadelphia: Current Medicine; 1996:12.1–12.16.

51. Friedman LS, Graeme-Cook F, Schapiro RH: Inflammatory colitides. In *Gastroenterology and Hepatology: The Comprehensive Visual Reference*, vol 2: *Colon, Rectum, and Anus*. Edited by Boland CR. Philadelphia: Current Medicine; 1996:4.1–4.17.

52. Greenson JK: Pathology of the colon and rectum. In *Gastroenterology and Hepatology: The Comprehensive Visual Reference*, vol 2: *Colon, Rectum, and Anus*. Edited by Boland CR. Philadelphia: Current Medicine; 1996:11.1–11.19.

53. Mittal RK: Esophageal motor disorders. In *Gastroenterology and Hepatology: The Comprehensive Visual Reference*, vol 5: *Esophagus and Pharynx*. Edited by Orlando RC. Philadelphia: Current Medicine; 1997:6.1–6.14.

187 Evaluation and Management of Acute Upper Gastrointestinal Bleeding

Christopher J. Gostout

The successful management of acute upper gastrointestinal (UGI) bleeding requires recognition of key features of the patient's history, physical examination, and hemodynamic status on presentation and during the course of management. Successful management of acute UGI bleeding requires accurate assessment of the severity of bleeding; a relevant differential diagnosis; triage into inpatient, observational, or outpatient care; effective therapy; and efforts to minimize the length of hospitalization or intensive care unit (ICU) stay, morbidity, and mortality.

Mortality rates associated with acute UGI bleeding have been stable for years and remain below 10% [1••,2•,3•]. The clinician can have a significant impact on patient care by reducing costly complications through preventive measures and early recognition of complications, such as myocardial ischemia and aspiration pneumonia.

The information reviewed in this chapter focuses on nonvariceal bleeding and is derived from personal experience, the literature, and the ongoing experience of the Mayo Clinic Gastrointestinal Bleeding Team. The Bleeding Team, which was conceived in 1988, is a highly specialized urgent management effort to improve patient care and provide a quality educational experience for trainees and paramedical personnel [1••].

Upper gastrointestinal bleeding accounts for 75% to 80% of all acute gastrointestinal bleeding [1••]. As many as 90% of cases of acute UGI bleeding occur in outpatients [1••,4]. Acute UGI bleeding is defined as the abrupt onset of arterial, capillary, or venous hemorrhage from the esophagus, stomach, or duodenum, sufficient in amount to cause symptoms or a decline in hemoglobin and hematocrit values. Torrential bleeding is massive bleeding that is accompanied by hemodynamic instability and prevents endoscopic intervention.

Bleeding from the small intestine has emerged as a distinct subcategory of acute gastrointestinal bleeding. Small intestinal bleeding may emanate anywhere from the distal duodenum and ligament of Treitz to the terminal ileum. This new classification of bleeding location relegates lower gastrointestinal bleeding to originate in the colon and rectum.

HISTORY AND PHYSICAL EXAMINATION

History

Elements of the patient history and physical examination can provide an estimate of the duration and severity of bleeding and can help to identify patients at risk for complications from bleeding. History taking typically occurs simultaneously with resuscitation efforts in the patient presenting with symptoms and signs of major bleeding.

Advanced age (older than 70 years) and concurrent major (vital) organ system disease affect both mortality and morbidity [2•,3•]. Elderly patients and those with known cardiovascular disease, especially ischemic heart disease, are at risk of unstable angina, myocardial infarction, and ischemia-related cardiac dysrhythmia. These complications usually have occurred by the time of presentation. The onset of bleeding during hospitalization for a major illness, especially sepsis and renal failure, also is thought to increase the risk of complications and mortality [3•].

Patients with major bleeding demonstrate overt manifestations, visceral discomfort, and orthostatic symptoms within a few hours of presentation. Large-volume, repeated emesis of bright red blood and clots is associated with greater morbidity and mortality than is emesis of coffee grounds–like material. Bleeding from the esophagus and stomach presents as hematemesis more often than does bleeding from the duodenum. Major bleeding from a duodenal source often presents as hematochezia [1••,5].

Visceral symptoms include generalized or periumbilical cramping and gaseousness and indicate rapid intestinal transit of blood. Melena accompanied by crampy abdominal discomfort suggests severe bleeding, whereas melena without abdominal cramping does not provide an estimate of the severity of bleeding. Hematochezia from a UGI source is a reliable indicator of major blood loss, either arterial or variceal, and is typically associated with visceral discomfort.

Additional historical information that should be sought is a prior history of bleeding, the cause of previous bleeding episodes, the presence or absence of liver disease, and recent medication use. About half of patients with acute UGI bleeding have been using nonsteroidal anti-inflammatory drugs (NSAIDs), even as little as a single baby aspirin per day [1••,6•,7]. Adequate questioning of the patient often requires reciting a list of common aspirin-containing and other NSAID preparations (Table 187-1). Identifying anticoagulation use or a history of a bleeding disorder is of obvious importance. A review of the patient's surgical history should include inquiry regarding repair of an abdominal aortic aneurysm; a positive response should raise immediate concern about an aortoenteric fistula.

Key Aspects of the Physical Examination

Pallor in the setting of overt bleeding within a short period of time (*ie*, less than 24 hours) indicates significant volume loss that can arise only from arterial or variceal bleeding. Vital signs should be taken with the patient in both the supine and sitting positions, unless the patient is hypotensive. A fall in systolic blood pressure of more than 20 mm Hg or a rise in pulse rate of more than 20 bpm after the patient sits up indicates at least a 20% loss of intravascular blood volume. Hypotension indicates at least a 40% loss of blood volume and is associated with an increased risk of rebleeding [8,9,10••,11•]. Isolated tachycardia with a rate greater than 100 bpm also may connote an increased risk of rebleeding.

The patient with continuing hematemesis or with hematochezia on presentation is considered to be actively bleeding. A nasogastric tube can be placed if there is uncertainty about the presence, severity, or general location of bleeding. Aspiration of a large and sustained volume of bright red blood from the nasogastric tube indicates significant recent, if not active, bleeding and a high risk of rebleeding. Nasogastric tube suction is otherwise not routinely needed, nor is gastric lavage. A rectal examination to assess stool color may be useful. Stool color guides have been used to reduce uncertainty regarding the presence or absence of melena and hematochezia (see Figure 73-5 elsewhere in this book), but occult blood testing of stool or a nasogastric sample is unnecessary.

The physical examination should include a search for findings of liver disease or portal hypertension, including cirrhotic body habitus, cutaneous spider telangiectases, and splenomegaly. Evidence of coagulopathy or a bleeding disorder (purpura, ecchymoses, petechiae) should be sought because these problems can interfere with control of bleeding.

Table 187-1. Prescription and Nonprescription Products Containing Nonsteroidal Anti-inflammatory Drugs

Nonprescription products containing aspirin or aspirin-like compounds

Alka-Seltzer antacid and pain reliever effervescent tablets
Alka-Seltzer Plus Cold tablets
Anacin caplets and tablets
Anacin Maximum Strength tablets
Arthritis Pain Formula tablets
Arthritis Strength Bufferin tablets
Ascriptin caplets and tablets
Ascriptin A/D caplets
Aspergum
Bayer aspirin caplets and tablets
Bayer Children's Aspirin chewable tablets
Bayer Plus tablets
Maximum Bayer caplets and tablets
8-Hour Bayer Extended-Release tablets
BC Powder
BC Cold Powder
Buffaprin caplets and tablets
Bufferin Arthritis Strength caplets
Bufferin caplets and tablets
Cama Arthritis Pain Reliever tablets
Doan's Pills caplets
Ecotrin caplets and tablets
Empirin tablets
Excedrin Extra-Strength caplets and tablets
Midol caplets
Mobigesic Analgesic tablets
Norwich tablets
P-A-C Analgesic tablets
Pepto-Bismol liquid and tablets
Sine-Off tablets, aspirin formula
St. Joseph Adult Chewable aspirin
Therapy Bayer caplets
Trigesic tablets
Ursinus Inlay-Tabs
Vanquish Analgesic caplets

Nonprescription products containing ibuprofen

Advil caplets and tablets
Advil Cold/Sinus caplets
Bayer Select Ibuprofen Pain Relief Formula caplets
Dristan Sinus caplets
Haltran tablets
Ibuprohm Ibuprofen caplets and tablets
Midol IB tablets
Motrin IB caplets and tablets
Nuprin Ibuprofen caplets and tablets
Sine-Aid IB

Nonprescription products containing naproxen sodium

Aleve caplets and tablets

Prescription products containing aspirin or aspirin-like compounds

Darvon Compound-65
Disalcid capsules and tablets
Easprin tablets
Empirin With Codeine tablets
Equagesic tablets
Fiorinal capsules and tablets
Fiorinal With Codeine capsules and tablets
Lortab ASA tablets
Magsal tablets
Mono-Gesic tablets
Norgesic; Norgesic Forte tablets
Percodan; Percodan-Demi tablets
Robaxisal tablets
Salflex tablets
Soma Compound tablets
Soma Compound With Codeine tablets
Synalgos-DC capsules
Talwin Compound tablets
Trilisate tablets and liquid

Prescription products containing ibuprofen

Children's Motrin Suspension
Children's Advil Suspension
Motrin tablets

Prescription products containing naproxen or naproxen sodium

Anaprox; Anaprox DS tablets
Naprosyn Suspension tablets

Data from the American College of Gastroenterology, Gastrointestinal Bleeding Registry.

Assessment of the patient should be performed promptly. At the completion of the initial encounter, it should be possible to estimate the patient's relative risk (high or low) for continued bleeding or rebleeding. Table 187-2 summarizes high-risk screening criteria used by the Mayo Clinic Gastrointestinal Bleeding Team [1••].

CRITICAL LABORATORY TESTS

The most important laboratory tests used to assess the severity of the initial bleeding episode and to monitor the patient for rebleeding are the hemoglobin and hematocrit values. Profound anemia (hemoglobin value less than 8 g/dL) may predict recurrent bleeding. A hemoglobin value below 7.5 g/dL has critical physiologic consequences; it forces the resting cardiac output to increase significantly, with increases in both heart rate and stroke volume. The oxygen-carrying capacity of the blood also becomes compromised, potentially impairing perfusion and oxygenation of major organs and tissues.

Measurement of serum electrolytes, calcium, glucose, prothrombin time, activated partial thromboplastin time, and platelet count are needed to guide intravenous fluid therapy and blood transfusions, especially after intravenous resuscitation. Coagulation studies are needed in patients on anticoagulation therapy and in those with little or no oral intake while taking antibiotics. Efforts should be made to correct coagulation abnormalities with the immediate administration of fresh frozen plasma and, in patients with prolonged prothrombin times, with administration of vitamin K. Liver biochemical tests are useful in identifying otherwise occult liver disease. Moreover, elevated serum aminotransferase, creatinine, and blood urea nitrogen levels have all been reported to predict mortality in hospitalized patients with acute UGI bleeding [2•,3•]. An elevation in the blood urea nitrogen to creatinine ratio of greater than 25 strongly suggests a UGI source of bleeding. An arterial blood gas determination provides information about the patient's metabolic and respiratory status and is especially useful in elderly patients with known cardiac or respiratory disease and with hemodynamic instability.

An electrocardiogram is essential in a patient with profound anemia, hemodynamic instability, cardiovascular disease, and accompanying chest pain (in whom cardiac enzymes are also indicated) and in the elderly patient. In some cases, emergency echocardiography may help to identify a patient with acute myocardial infarction complicating bleeding. Myocardial ischemia and resulting congestive heart failure or cardiac dysrhythmias are the most common vital organ complications related to acute UGI bleeding [1••].

RESUSCITATION: RESPIRATORY AND CARDIAC PREVENTIVE MEASURES

Placement of a central venous line allows hemodynamic monitoring in a patient with massive bleeding in the setting of marginally compensated major organ system disease or evidence of myocardial ischemia (Table 187-3). Transfusion of packed red blood cells is adequate for blood replacement and is indicated in patients with active bleeding, hemodynamic instability, a history of cardiac ischemia, and a hemoglobin value of less than 10 g/dL. Patients who receive 4 U or more of blood during the first 24 hours are usually bleeding from an exposed artery or a varix and are at high risk of rebleeding. Fresh frozen plasma is given to prevent clotting derangements in patients who have received at least 4 U of packed red blood cells. Platelet transfusions may be needed in patients with platelet counts of less than 20,000/mm³. In patients with higher platelet counts, the decision to transfuse platelets should be individualized. As a general rule, therapeutic anticoagulation should be reversed; in selected patients in whom continued anticoagulation is desired, the degree of anticoagulation may be carefully controlled by continuous intravenous infusion of heparin [12•].

One of the most important measures to reduce morbidity is protection of the patient's airway from aspiration of vomitus and blood. Endotracheal intubation is indicated in patients with torrential bleeding and repeated hematemesis and in obtunded or combative patients with active bleeding and pooling of blood in the stomach. For less severe bleeding, an esophageal variceal band ligation overtube can be used to divert blood away from the airway, minimizing the potential for aspiration. If gastric lavage is performed, it should be done with the patient in the left lateral decubitus position. Airway suction should be readily available during lavage and endoscopy.

Supplemental oxygen is routinely delivered to elderly patients and to patients with hemodynamic instability,

---

Table 187-2. Early Assessment: High-Risk* Patient Criteria for Screening Upper Gastrointestinal Bleeding

History
Age ≥ 70 y
Concurrent major organ system disease
History of cancer
Currently hospitalized

Symptoms
Repeated hematemesis—fresh blood, large volume
Bright red blood through nasogastric tube
Hematochezia
Abdominal cramping
Rapid development of orthostatic changes or syncope
Overt bleeding symptoms of < 24 hours' duration

Physical findings
Pallor
Blood pressure
Hypotension (systolic < 100 mm Hg)
Orthostasis (systolic drop ≥ 20 mm Hg)
Heart rate
Tachycardia > 100 bpm
Orthostatic change > 20 bpm
Bright red blood through nasogastric tube

Transfusion requirement
First 24 hours: ≥ 4 U
With rebleeding event: > 2 U
Total: 6–8 U

*High risk for rebleeding and mortality.
BPM—beats per minute.

hemoglobin values of less than 10 g/dL, and known cardiac or respiratory disease. Prophylactic administration of nitrates may be necessary in a patient with cardiac ischemia. A myocardial ischemic event should be suspected in a patient who has hypotension that does not respond to fluid administration and who has no overt evidence of torrential bleeding or rebleeding.

◼ PATIENT TRIAGE

The skilled clinician extracts essential information from the patient's history, physical examination, and laboratory data to arrive at a global assessment of the severity of bleeding and the patient's risk of continued bleeding and complications (Table 187-2). Resuscitative efforts are performed to stabilize the patient and to prevent potential complications resulting from compromise of vital organ systems.

The initial triage of the patient involves two critical management decisions (Table 187-4). The first is whether to proceed to inpatient, intensive care, or outpatient management. The second is whether to proceed to endoscopy. All the information obtained can be distilled into a practical decision-making process. Validated scoring systems have also been developed to permit confident management decisions [10••,13••,14•].

Minor Bleeding

Patients with minor bleeding can usually be managed as outpatients. They do not need to be transferred to an ICU if they are already hospitalized and do not need urgent endoscopy. These patients have normal hemoglobin and hematocrit levels, little or no change from previous values (*ie*, a drop in hemoglobin of 1.0 g/dL or less), no evidence of severe active bleeding (stable vital signs, no hematemesis or only coffee grounds–like emesis, and no hematochezia), normal clotting parameters, and no compromise of vital organs, especially the cardiorespiratory system. If there is uncertainty about the stability of the patient or the severity of bleeding, an extended period of observation in the emergency room or in a short-admission unit can be arranged in most hospitals. Patients who have advanced liver disease, varices, a history of variceal bleeding, or a history of endoscopic hemostatic therapy are ideal candidates for this approach. Subsequent endoscopy is useful to assess these patients further and to complete the triage process.

Moderate Bleeding

Patients with bleeding of intermediate severity require hospitalization to monitor rebleeding. These patients may be elderly or

---

Table 187-3. Resuscitative Measures for the Patient With Upper Gastrointestinal Bleeding

Measure	Rationale	Specific action
Hemodynamic monitoring	Precise organ perfusion; shock and existing vital organ system disease	Central venous line; Swan-Ganz catheter
Transfusion	Replacement of blood volume	Intravenous packed red blood cells
	Replacement of clotting factors After massive transfusions Abnormal prothrombin time	Intravenous fresh frozen plasma (2-U doses)
Airway protection	Correction of thrombocytopenia (<20,000/mm³ platelet count)	Intravenous platelets (6-U doses)
	Prevention of aspiration; hematemesis; obtundation; active bleeding with large gastric pool, and in patients who are combative	Endotracheal intubation Esophageal (variceal band ligation) overtube
Supplemental oxygen	Prevention of myocardial ischemia; maintenance of vital organ oxygenation	Oxygen by nasal cannula Combination oxygen port and bite block during endoscopy
Systemic nitrates	Correction of ischemia; prevention of myocardial infarction	Transdermal nitrates; intravenous nitroglycerin

---

Table 187-4. Initial Triage Decisions for Upper Gastrointestinal Bleeding

Triage decision	Severity of bleeding	Common clinical situation
Extended outpatient observation *Elective* endoscopy	Minor	Stable patient and laboratory; coffee ground-like emesis; melena only
Prompt endoscopy		Cirrhosis; varices
Admission Transfer to intensive care unit *Prompt* endoscopy	Severe	Fresh hematemesis; hematochezia; altered hemodynamics; immediate transfusion needs (≥ 4 U) Hemoglobin < 10 g/dL or decrease of ≥ 2 g/dL
Admission *Prompt* endoscopy	Minor or severe	Clotting derangement
Transfer to intensive care unit *Prompt* endoscopy	Severe	Mandatory anticoagulation requirement for life-threatening problem; profound thrombocytopenia; cirrhosis with nonreversible clotting derangement

have comorbid illnesses that are stable but that put them at risk of complications (*eg*, myocardial infarction, congestive heart failure). Other features of this group include the need for only minimal or readily accomplished resuscitation and rapid reversal of mild hemodynamic changes, including tachycardia and orthostatic blood pressure changes, a hemoglobin value of more than 10 g/dL, a drop in the hemoglobin of 2 g/dL or less, and transfusion of 2 U or less of blood.

Severe Bleeding

Outpatients with severe bleeding require hospital admission and urgent endoscopy. Severe UGI bleeding is accompanied by fresh hematemesis, hematochezia, hemodynamic instability, compromise of vital organ systems, a hemoglobin value of less than 10 g/dL (or a decrease of >2 g/dL), and immediate transfusion needs of 4 U or more. A critical decision is whether management in the ICU is required. The outcome of prompt diagnostic and therapeutic endoscopy in these patients influences the decision to admit such patients for ICU monitoring.

Clotting Abnormalities

Outpatients with clotting derangements or profound thrombocytopenia are best admitted to the hospital for correction, either by complete reversal with vitamin K or by supplemental infusion of blood products (fresh frozen plasma, platelets). Subsequent intravenous infusion of heparin may be required, depending on the underlying clinical problem (*eg*, an artificial heart valve). Inpatients with clotting derangements require individualized decision-making regarding transfer to an ICU, based on the cause of the derangements and the cause and severity of bleeding. This decision may require input from a hematologist or the results of additional diagnostic testing, such as a transesophageal echocardiogram in a high-risk patient with an artificial heart valve, especially aortic. High-risk patients with clotting abnormalities who have experienced major bleeding are best served by urgent endoscopy to identify the cause of bleeding and to determine the appropriate management pathway.

■ COMMON CAUSES OF NONVARICEAL BLEEDING

In most cases, acute gastrointestinal bleeding is due to a UGI source. In the experience of the Mayo Clinic Gastrointestinal Bleeding Team, a UGI source accounts for 75% to 80% of all cases of acute bleeding [1••]. About 40% of patients with UGI bleeding have peptic ulcer disease, usually gastric or duodenal ulcers and rarely esophageal ulcers [1••,15]. NSAIDs are an important cause of ulcer disease and can be implicated in up to half of bleeding events. Hemorrhagic stress gastritis is encountered less often; risk factors for this condition have been well characterized, and prophylactic therapy is used commonly (Table 187-5).

Severe bleeding with the potential for major complications and continued bleeding arises from an exposed artery. The location and size of the artery are important determinants of the severity of bleeding and risk of rebleeding. The two critical locations for bleeding from peptic ulcers are the posterior wall of the duodenal bulb and the proximal lesser curve of the stomach. In these locations, the gastroduodenal artery and left gastric artery are in direct contact with duodenum and stomach, respectively. In patients with a Mallory-Weiss tear, the esophageal branch of the left gastric artery can be compromised. In other locations in the stomach and duodenum, a greater depth of ulceration increases the likelihood that a larger penetrating artery arising from the serosa will be exposed, thereby increasing the potential for severe bleeding and rebleeding. Exposed vessels arising in neoplasms also may be large, with a neovascular structure that responds poorly to therapeutic interventions.

The most common conditions associated with an exposed artery, or "visible" vessel as seen on endoscopy, are as follows:
- Ulcer
- Dieulafoy lesion
- Mallory-Weiss tear
- Early postoperative anastomosis (before 10 days)
- Polypectomy site
- Abdominal aortic graft
- Ulcerated benign neoplasm (*eg*, leiomyoma)
- Primary or metastatic malignant ulcer

Ulcers account for more than 90% of cases of severe bleeding from an exposed artery. The Mayo Clinic Gastrointestinal Bleeding Team encounters about 700 such patients yearly, of which an average of only 12 are bleeding from a Dieulafoy lesion in a UGI location. Although Mallory-Weiss tears may occur with some regularity, most of these are associated with minor, self-limited bleeding, unless the patient has a coagulopathy [16].

Dieulafoy Lesion

Bleeding from a Dieulafoy lesion is typically acute and recurrent, with intervals between episodes spanning days to years. The lesion usually occurs within 6 cm of the esophagogastric junction [17] but may be encountered throughout the gut; the duodenal bulb and proximal jejunum are the next most common locations, followed by the proximal colon [18].

Table 187-5. Risk Factors for Hemorrhagic Stress Gastritis

Age > 65 y

Extensive burns (Curling's stress ulcer)

Head injury (Cushing's stress ulcer)

Coma

Trauma

Major surgery (aortic, pancreatic, transplantation)

Multiple operative procedures

Hypotension

Sepsis

Renal failure

Respiratory failure and mechanical ventilation*

Hepatic failure

Acidosis

Transfusion > 5 U

Coagulopathy*

Associated with highest risk in patients in a medical intensive care unit.

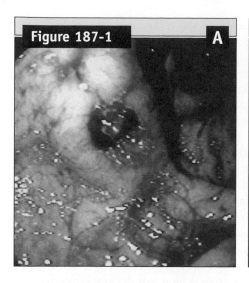 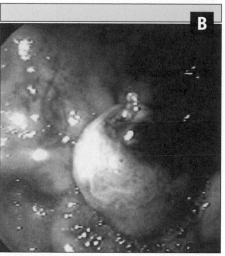

Endoscopic photographs of a Dieulafoy lesion in the proximal body of the stomach. **A,** A translucent artery can be seen projecting above the mucosa. **B,** The artery has been banded. See also **Color Plate.**

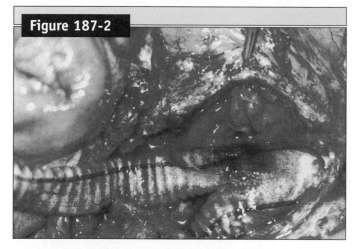

Surgical photograph of an aortoduodenal fistula. The bile-stained, eroded portion of graft is readily apparent adjacent to the duodenal defect. See also **Color Plate.**

A Dieulafoy lesion results from failure of transmural arterial ramifications to progress into smaller vessels that end with the mucosal microvasculature. Failure of the ramification process results in a persistently large-caliber muscular artery situated beneath the mucosa. The artery subsequently becomes tortuous, ruptures through the mucosa, and results in severe bleeding. The mechanism by which the disruption of both artery and mucosa occurs remains unexplained; NSAIDs have not been implicated [17]. The lesions are encountered most often in elderly men but can be seen in teenagers as well as women [17].

Dieulafoy lesion is best diagnosed by endoscopy timed to an acute bleeding episode (Fig. 187-1, see also **Color Plate**). Often, multiple endoscopy procedures must be performed before the lesion can be identified. The lesion should be suspected when a careful and thorough endoscopy performed close in time to a major UGI bleed is negative. Once a Dieulafoy lesion is identified and localized, endoscopic therapy is the treatment of choice and results in a gratifying end to episodic severe bleeding.

Abdominal Aortic Graft

Any patient with an abdominal aortic graft and acute UGI bleeding should be suspected of having an aortoenteric fistula

(Fig. 187-2, see also **Color Plate**). These can be readily diagnosed during endoscopy of the distal duodenum. The lesion also should be suspected when a CT scan fails to demonstrate a tissue plane between the aortic graft and duodenum and discloses air in the surrounding area.

DIAGNOSTIC AND THERAPEUTIC APPROACHES

Endoscopy

Endoscopy plays a pivotal role in the diagnosis and therapy of acute UGI bleeding and should be performed promptly in all patients with major bleeding (see Chapter 34). The purposes of the examination are to establish a diagnosis, administer specific therapy, and provide an estimate of the likelihood of rebleeding to guide critical patient management decisions affecting hospitalization, ICU stay, pharmacotherapy, angiography, and surgery. Endoscopy should follow hemodynamic stabilization of the patient and a deliberate decision regarding airway protection. The endoscopist must choose the type of instrumentation needed, *eg,* a standard upper endoscope, a therapeutic instrument, or a longer instrument when bleeding is thought to arise from the distal duodenum or proximal jejunum (as in an aortoenteric fistula or Dieulafoy lesion). Early endoscopy guides management of patients with clotting derangements by establishing an estimate of the risk of rebleeding and of the need for complete reversal of anticoagulation.

Urgent endoscopy may be thwarted by torrential bleeding or a large retained organized clot. In the former situation, endoscopy may be repeated after several hours, during a nonbleeding period, if the patient can be stabilized. On occasion, excessive amounts of blood and clot must be cleared to complete the diagnostic examination; this usually requires lavage of the stomach with a large-bore tube. Jumbo-channel therapeutic endoscopes also evacuate blood and clots effectively [19]. Torrential bleeding and the presence of copious blood and clot within the stomach are indications for endotracheal intubation or placement of an esophageal variceal band ligation overtube to prevent aspiration [1••].

Focal bleeding from an exposed or visible vessel is the only indication for endoscopic therapy in patients with bleeding ulcers or a Dieulafoy lesion because the visible vessel is associated with severe bleeding and is at high risk of rebleeding. A variety of effective endoscopic treatment modalities can be used alone or in combination, including the following:

- Injection with epinephrine solution (in a concentration of 1:10,000)
- Injection with sclerosants or alcohol
- Injection with cyanoacrylate glue
- Injection with fibrin glue
- Monopolar electrocautery
- Bipolar electrocautery
- Heater probe unit coagulation
- Argon plasma coagulation
- Microwave coagulation
- Laser photocoagulation
- Hemoclip ligation

Visual criteria for endoscopic therapy include active bleeding and nonbleeding stigmata of a high risk of bleeding. Unfortunately, there is significant interobserver variability in the interpretation of these findings (Fig. 187-3, see also **Color Plate**; Table 187-6) [11•, 20].

Rebleeding rates after endoscopic therapy average 20%; after a second course of therapy for rebleeding, the overall success rate is more than 90%. Most rebleeding occurs within 48 to 72 hours of initial therapy, but in some patients, rebleeding occurs up to 96 hours later [8]. The success of endoscopic therapy depends on the skill and experience of the endoscopist, the endoscopist's familiarity with the therapeutic modality selected, accessibility of the exposed vessel, the size of the vessel (2 mm or less in diameter), and absence of abnormal clotting parameters.

The rate of rebleeding from low-risk clean-based ulcers is about 4%. A small number of ulcers that rebleed are subsequently found to have visible vessels not seen during the index endoscopy. Indeed, whether a finding represents a visible vessel may be unclear. Newer technology, such as Doppler probes, is available to identify and localize surface or subsurface vessels and to confirm ablation of the target vessel [21]. Alternative methods of imaging, such as infrared and optical coherence tomography, also hold promise but are in experimental stages of development [22].

Patients with bleeding peptic ulcers should be assessed for the presence of *Helicobacter pylori* infection; those with gastric ulcers should be evaluated for gastric malignancy [23,24,25]. One way to detect *H. pylori* infection is biopsy of the antral mucosa during the endoscopic procedure. Samples also may be taken safely from the margins of a gastric ulcer to exclude a malignancy during the index endoscopy (see Chapters 28 and 29).

Angiography

The need for selective visceral angiography in acute nonvariceal UGI bleeding is infrequent and generally restricted to torrential bleeding when surgery is not desirable. Angiography should be

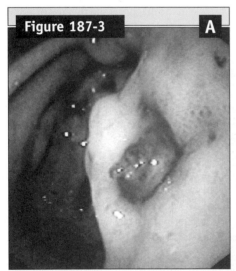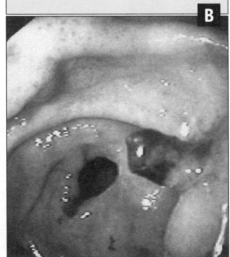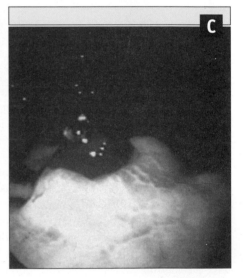

Figure 187-3

Endoscopic photographs of nonbleeding visible vessel stigmata. **A,** A small translucent artery protruding above a small gastric ulcer. **B,** A large arterial pigmented protuberance. **C,** Fresh clot that is densely adherent to gastric ulcer. See also **Color Plate**.

Table 187-6. Bleeding and Nonbleeding Endoscopic Findings Associated With Severe Bleeding, High Risk for Rebleeding, and Indicators for Endoscopic Therapy

Primary endoscopic finding	Secondary endoscopic finding	Estimated risk of rebleeding, %
Active bleeding	Arterial spurting	100
	Micropulsatile streaming (focal vigorous oozing)	60
Nonbleeding stigmata	Frankly protruding vessel	60
	Pigmented protuberance	20
	Fresh densely adherent clot	34

performed to establish the site of bleeding and to provide control of bleeding. Timing is critical for both diagnostic and therapeutic success. The procedure should be performed when active bleeding is suspected. Angiography is also used to control refractory bleeding after endoscopic sphincterotomy and for recurrent bleeding from a visible vessel within an ulcerated neoplasm resistant to endoscopic therapy.

Complete arteriographic evaluation of UGI bleeding entails study of the left gastric, gastroduodenal, pancreaticoduodenal, and splenic arteries. If there is suspicion of an aortoduodenal fistula, biplane aortography should be performed. The sensitivity of arteriography for identifying active bleeding depends on the selectivity of the injection and quality of the imaging technique (rapid digital angiography is preferable).

Intra-arterial infusion of vasopressin on arteriography is associated with a 70% rate of bleeding control and an 18% rate of rebleeding. With selective infusion of the left gastric artery or celiac axis, the rate of bleeding control is closer to 80%. The rate of controlling bleeding is lower (42%) and the rebleeding rate is higher (25%) with infusions into the gastroduodenal, hepatic, or splenic arteries [26,27]. Intra-arterial infusion of vasopressin is not effective in controlling bleeding from lesions in the pyloroduodenal, hepatic, or pancreatic regions, largely because of the dual blood supply from the celiac axis and superior mesenteric artery. In addition, infusion of vasopressin is ineffective when bleeding arises from large arteries or their branches (eg, gastroduodenal artery), which do not constrict in response to vasopressin, and in the presence of inflammation, such as results from a peptic ulcer.

Embolization therapy at arteriography is another option that demands careful subselective catheterization to avoid misplacement of the embolic material, inadvertent distal reflux of the embolic agent, and excessive devascularization of an organ. Embolization is effective in controlling pyloroduodenal bleeding (96%). Superselective embolization of the gastroduodenal artery, however, carries a 25% risk of eventual duodenal stenosis [26,27]. Embolization with autologous blood clot is preferred for initial control of refractory bleeding from duodenal ulcers; superselective embolization with a more permanent occlusive agent is used if embolization with an autologous clot fails.

The left gastric artery accounts for up to 80% of all cases of gastric bleeding and may be the source of gastric and distal esophageal bleeding. Embolization of the left gastric artery has been advocated in patients who have endoscopic evidence of bleeding within its distribution, are at high risk of rebleeding, and are at high-risk of multiorgan failure if bleeding continues. In contrast, "blind" embolization in the absence of an identified bleeding site is not advocated. Patients with coagulopathies are at greatest risk of rebleeding (2.9-fold) and eventual death (9.6-fold) after embolization [26,27]. In patients with hemobilia, selective hepatic arteriography with superselective embolization is the preferred approach. It is important to demonstrate that the portal venous system is patent to ensure viability of the liver after embolization. In a patient with continued bleeding and an indwelling transhepatic catheter, use of a larger-bore catheter may control the bleeding.

Surgery

Despite the overall success of endoscopic therapy in controlling bleeding in a variety of situations, there remains a need for surgical intervention in some cases [28]. In relation to angiography, the timing of surgery is critical. In contrast to angiography, however, early surgical intervention appears to reduce mortality and morbidity as well as the rate of rebleeding and the transfusion requirement. Advanced age, comorbid illness, shock, and extent of transfusion are key determinants of postoperative outcome [9,28].

Surgery should be considered in the following situations:
- Torrential bleeding from the duodenal bulb, particularly the posterior bulb (although it is often difficult to assess the location of bleeding within the duodenal bulb accurately) [28]
- Torrential bleeding from a penetrating ulcer in other locations
- A large penetrating ulcer with a nonbleeding visible vessel that exceeds 2 mm in estimated diameter
- Rebleeding after repeated endoscopic therapy
- Rebleeding with frank shock
- A blood transfusion requirement for resuscitation of 4 U or more for an index or rebleeding event

The choice of operation (vagotomy, oversewing, wedge excision, or resection) depends on the urgency of the operation, the presence of comorbid illnesses, technical demands, and the cause of the bleeding. Intraoperative endoscopy may be useful when the bleeding is obscured by torrential bleeding during initial endoscopy. Rebleeding may occur in the postoperative period, especially from duodenal ulcers that have been oversewn, and may require endoscopic therapy or reoperation to be controlled.

Pharmacotherapy

Drug therapy for nonvariceal UGI bleeding is of limited value and directed predominantly at prophylaxis, treatment of ulcerative and erosive conditions, and eradication of H. pylori infection. Vigorous suppression of gastric acid secretion and intensive antireflux measures are needed in the hospitalized patient with refractory bleeding from severe ulcerative esophagitis.

Many pharmacologic studies have examined the possibility of stabilizing the macroscopic or microscopic thrombus plugging the defect in a bleeding vessel. Measures studied include control of the local acid environment surrounding an ulcer with H_2-receptor antagonists or proton-pump inhibitors and inhibition of fibrinolysis with antifibrinolytic drugs, such as tranexamic acid. There is little evidence that the risk of rebleeding (eg, from a peptic ulcer) can be reduced significantly with acute interventional pharmacotherapy [29]. Omeprazole, administered in doses that induce anacidity, has been demonstrated to reduce rebleeding and the need for surgery in patients with peptic ulcers harboring nonbleeding visible vessels [30••]. There is no convincing evidence to suggest that reduction of splanchnic blood flow by intravenous vasopressin, somatostatin, or octreotide can control refractory bleeding from nonvariceal sources [31,32].

Adjunctive acid suppressive therapy is employed regularly to reduce potential complications (including pain and bleeding) from treatment-site ulceration, which occurs predictably after thermal or tissue-destructive injection sclerotherapy. Although this practice is common, it incurs added expense and is of no proven benefit.

OVERALL APPROACH TO THE HOSPITALIZED PATIENT

Reducing the length of hospital stay and the cost of care are driving forces behind decision-making in a clinical management pathway for acute UGI bleeding. Expeditious and accurate diagnosis and therapy of high-risk bleeding lesions and appropriate resource use for low-risk patients reduce the rates of complications and mortality as well as the length of stay and costs.

The use of intravenous medications, prolonged fasting, and the ICU add expense and length to a hospitalization, and their necessity should be evaluated in each case. The use of intravenous medications should be restricted to the drugs required by this route because of comorbid illness or proven efficacy. Fasting is the most common reason for the intravenous delivery of many drugs, especially H_2-receptor antagonists, but the need for fasting is infrequent and generally does not influence outcome [33]. Fasting should be restricted to hemodynamically unstable patients and those who require repeat endoscopic intervention within a short interval of time because of

uncertainty regarding the effectiveness of endoscopic therapy or a possible complication of initial therapy. Examples include patients with torrential bleeding in whom a second endoscopic procedure is desirable for diagnosis and an attempt at therapy, and patients for whom access to a bleeding vessel was suboptimal on initial endoscopy. In these settings, the patient should fast until the second endoscopy is attempted, either within 12 hours or sooner if bleeding recurs.

The ICU should be used only for critically ill or unstable patients, including the following:

- Hospitalized patients with severe bleeding and serious comorbid illness
- Outpatients of advanced age or with a suspected (or at high risk of) cardiac or respiratory complications
- Patients with hemodynamic instability and significant immediate transfusion needs (more than 4 U) in whom endoscopic therapy of a large exposed vessel has been attempted; a penetrating ulcer was incompletely examined because of anatomy, blood, or clots; or endoscopic

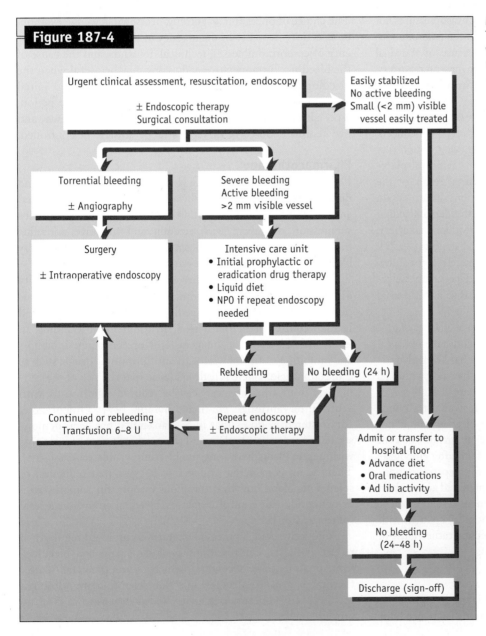

Figure 187-4

Management scheme for high-risk patients. The initial endoscopy should be performed within 1 to 2 hours of presentation. NPO—nothing by mouth.

therapy was suboptimal because of lack of access to the bleeding point

- Patients in whom angiographic control of bleeding was attempted to monitor for complications or during perfusion therapy with thrombolytic medication or vasopressin
- Patients with severe variceal bleeding and advanced cirrhosis

ICU care also may be indicated in infirm, confused, or mentally impaired patients.

The period during which the risk of rebleeding is greatest (48 to 72 hours) influences the length and location (*eg,* ICU) of hospitalization. In most instances, rebleeding after endoscopic therapy is not severe and can be handled by prompt reintervention with endoscopic therapy and without transfer to the ICU. There is little evidence to support routine second-look endoscopy to minimize the risk of rebleeding [34]. Most complications arising from the stress of hemorrhage also develop by 72 hours and influence the period of hospitalized observation [10••].

Two algorithms are provided that outline the critical management pathways for patients at high and low risk of rebleeding and of complications resulting from severe bleeding and rebleeding (Figs. 187-4 and 187-5). It is important to establish criteria for rebleeding that can be applied consistently, such as the following:

- Fall in hemoglobin level of 1.5 g/dL or more, alone or in combination with symptoms
- Overt symptoms of melena, hematochezia, or hematemesis (recurrent or at an increased rate)
- Bright red blood through the nasogastric tube
- Hemodynamic instability indicated by tachycardia and a decrease in blood pressure

Rebleeding events, especially more than two, may be regarded as an independent risk factor for mortality [2•,13••].

Patients admitted for extended outpatient observation typically have minor bleeding, do not have high-risk lesions on endoscopy, or have small exposed vessels readily amenable to endoscopic therapy. These patients may be very old (older than 90 years) and may have underlying cardiac disease, mild anemia, or other comorbid conditions warranting close observation. These patients need not fast, and most can be discharged within 24 hours.

CONCLUSION

Acute UGI bleeding remains a common problem, with a stable yearly incidence of about 100 hospitalizations per 100,000 population [4]. The traditional goals of patient management are to establish a diagnosis, stop bleeding, prevent rebleeding, and reduce both mortality and morbidity. Additional contemporary goals are to establish a confident prognosis on which to base management decisions, triage patients effectively into the appropriate care setting, expedite the hospitalization, and contain costs. Using an organized approach (critical pathway) to the care of patients with acute UGI bleeding will help to achieve both the traditional and newer goals.

REFERENCES

Recently published papers of particular interest have been highlighted as follows:
- • Of interest
- •• Of outstanding interest

1.•• Gostout CJ, Ahlquist DA, Wang KK, *et al.*: Acute gastrointestinal bleeding: Experience of a specialized management team. *J Clin Gastroenterol* 1992, 14:260–267.
This article presents a thorough review of the spectrum of acute gastrointestinal bleeding from the perspective of an organized approach to care and use of a comprehensive database.

2.• Zimmerman J, Siguencia J, Tsvand E, *et al.*: Predictors of mortality in patients admitted to hospital for acute upper gastrointestinal hemorrhage. *Scand J Gastroenterol* 1995, 30:327–331.
This article is a useful analysis of high-risk factors in outpatients presenting with acute UGI bleeding. Malignancy, elevated serum creatinine level, and elevated serum aminotransferase level were among the predictors of mortality.

3.• Zimmerman J, Meroz Y, Arnon R, *et al.*: Predictors of mortality in hospitalized patients with secondary upper gastrointestinal haemorrhage. *J Intern Med* 1995, 237:331–337.
This is a focused review of the predictors of mortality in hospitalized patients who developed acute UGI bleeding. Predictors include sepsis, hypoalbuminemia, and elevated serum aminotransferase levels.

4. Longstreth GF: Epidemiology of hospitalization for acute upper gastrointestinal hemorrhage: a population-based study. *Am J Gastroenterol* 1995, 90:206–210.

5. Wilcox CM, Alexander LN, Cotsonis G: A prospective characterization of upper gastrointestinal hemorrhage presenting with hematochezia. *Am J Gastroenterol* 1997, 92:231–235.

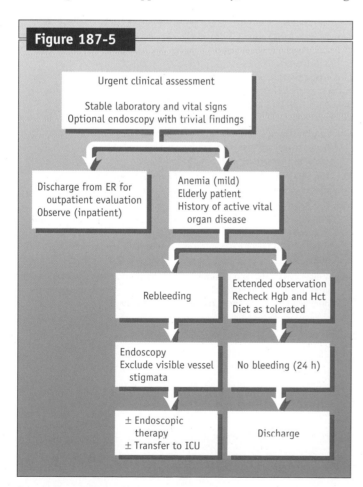

Figure 187-5

Urgent clinical assessment

Stable laboratory and vital signs
Optional endoscopy with trivial findings

Discharge from ER for outpatient evaluation Observe (inpatient)

Anemia (mild)
Elderly patient
History of active vital organ disease

Rebleeding

Extended observation Recheck Hgb and Hct Diet as tolerated

Endoscopy Exclude visible vessel stigmata

No bleeding (24 h)

± Endoscopic therapy ± Transfer to ICU

Discharge

Management scheme for low-risk patients. The endoscopy should be performed within 12 hours of presentation. ER—emergency room; Hbg—hemoglobin; Hct—hematocrit; ICU—intensive care unit.

6.• Peura DA, Lanza FL, Gostout CJ, *et al.*: The American College of Gastroenterology Bleeding Registry: preliminary findings. *Am J Gastroenterol* 1998, in press.

This professional society membership-based study nicely identifies the major bleeding issues.

7. Weil J, Colin-Jones D, Langman M, *et al.*: Prophylactic aspirin and risk of peptic ulcer bleeding. *Br Med J* 1995, 310:827–830.

8. Hsu PI, Lin XZ, Chan SH, *et al.*: Bleeding peptic ulcer: risk factors for re-bleeding and sequential changes in endoscopic findings. *Gut* 1994, 35:746–769.

9. Mueller X, Rothenbuehler JM, Amery A, *et al.*: Factors predisposing to further hemorrhage and mortality after peptic ulcer bleeding. *J Am Coll Surg* 1994, 179:457–461.

10.•• Hay JA, Lyubashevsky E, Elashoff J, *et al.*: Upper gastrointestinal hemorrhage clinical guideline: determining the optimal hospital length of stay. *Am J Med* 1996, 100:312–322.

This paper proposes a clinical practice guideline that may safely reduce the length of hospital stays for low-risk patients and avoid premature discharge of high-risk patients with acute UGI bleeding.

11.• Jaramillo JL, Glavaz C, Carmona C, *et al.*: Prediction of further hemorrhage in bleeding peptic ulcer. *Am J Gastroenterol* 1994, 89:2135–2138.

This study identified bleeding stigmata (active bleeding, visible vessel, adherent clot) and altered hemodynamics as the most relevant predictors of further hemorrhage in peptic ulcers, exclusive of age, concurrent disease, and laboratory abnormalities.

12.• Kuwada SK, Balm RK, Gostout CJ: The risk of withdrawing chronic anticoagulation due to acute gastrointestinal bleeding. *Am J Gastroenterol* 1996, 91:1116–1119.

This is the only study available that examines management of anticoagulation in high-risk patients. The authors identify a safe window of time during which anticoagulation may be withheld.

13.•• Rockall TA, Logan RFA, Devlin HB, *et al.*: Risk assessment after acute upper gastrointestinal haemorrhage. *Gut* 1996, 38:316–321.

This article presents a prospective evaluation of a scoring system that can be used to identify patient groups at low risk of rebleeding and death due to acute UGI bleeding.

14.• Saeed ZA, Ramirez FC, Hepps KS, *et al.*: Prospective validation of the Baylor bleeding score for predicting the likelihood of rebleeding after endoscopic hemostasis of peptic ulcers. *Gastrointest Endosc* 1995, 41:561–565.

This prospective study validates the Baylor scoring system based on a pre-endoscopy and endoscopy score.

15. Wolfsen HC, Wang KK: Etiology and course of acute bleeding esophageal ulcers. *J Clin Gastroenterol* 1992, 14:342–346.

16. Bharucha A, Gostout CJ, Balm RK: Acute gastrointestinal bleeding due to a Mallory-Weiss tear. *Am J Gastroenterol* 1997, 92:805–808.

17. Stark ME, Gostout CJ, Balm RK: Clinical features and endoscopic management of Dieulafoy's disease. *Gastrointest Endosc* 1992, 38:545–550.

18. Dy NM, Gostout CJ, Balm RK: Bleeding from the endoscopically identified Dieulafoy lesion of the proximal small intestine and colon. *Am J Gastroenterol* 1995, 90:108–111.

19. Kodali VP, Petersen BT, Miller CA, *et al.*: A new jumbo-channel therapeutic gastroscope for acute upper gastrointestinal bleeding. *Gastrointest Endosc* 1997, 45:409–411.

20. Laine L, Freeman M, Cohen H: Lack of uniformity in evaluation of endoscopic prognostic features of bleeding ulcers. *Gastrointest Endosc* 1994, 40:411–417.

21. Kohler B, Rieman JF: Does Doppler ultrasound improve the prognosis of acute ulcer bleeding? *Hepatogastroenterology* 1994, 41:51–53.

22. Gostout CJ, Jacques SL: Infrared video imaging of buried vessels: a feasibility study for the endoscopic management of gastrointestinal bleeding. *Gastrointest Endosc* 1995, 41:218–224.

23. Labenz J, Brosch G: Role of *Helicobacter pylori* eradication in the prevention of peptic ulcer bleeding relapse. *Digestion* 1994, 55:19–23.

24. Powell KU, Bell GD, Bolton GH, *et al.*: *Helicobacter pylori* eradication in patients with peptic ulcer disease: clinical consequences and financial implications. *Q J Med* 1994, 87:284–290.

25. Laine L: The long-term management of patients with bleeding ulcers: *Helicobacter pylori* eradication instead of maintenance antisecretory therapy. *Gastrointest Endosc* 1995, 41:77–79.

26. Rosen RJ, Sanchez G: Angiographic diagnosis and management of gastrointestinal hemorrhage: current concepts. *Radiol Clin North Am* 1994, 32:951–967.

27. Shapiro MJ: The role of the radiologist in the management of gastrointestinal bleeding. *Gastroenterol Clin North Am* 1994, 23:123–181.

28. Miller AR, Farnell MB, Kelly KA, *et al.*: Impact of therapeutic endoscopy on the treatment of bleeding duodenal ulcers: 1980–1990. *World J Surg* 1995, 19:89–95.

29. Villanueva C, Balanzo J, Torras X, *et al.*: Omeprazole versus ranitidine as adjunct therapy to endoscopic injection in actively bleeding ulcers: a prospective and randomized study. *Endoscopy* 1995, 27:308–312.

30.•• Khuroo MS, Yattoo GN, Javid G, *et al.*: A comparison of omeprazole and placebo for bleeding peptic ulcer. *N Engl J Med* 1997, 336:1054–1058.

This article provides a long overdue evaluation of a proton pump inhibitor in the setting of bleeding peptic ulcers. Patient groups were stratified by endoscopic criteria (spurting, oozing, nonbleeding visible vessels, and adherent clots).

31. Lin HJ, Perng CL, Wang K, *et al.*: Octreotide for arrest of peptic ulcer hemorrhage: a prospective, randomized controlled trial. *Hepatogastroenterology* 1995, 42:856–860.

32. Lin HJ, Wang K, Perng CL, *et al.*: Octreotide and heater probe thermocoagulation for arrest of peptic ulcer hemorrhage. *J Clin Gastroenterol* 1995, 21:95–98.

33. Laine L, Cohen H, Brodhead J, *et al.*: Prospective evaluation of immediate versus delayed refeeding and prognostic value of endoscopy in patients with upper gastrointestinal hemorrhage. *Gastroenterology* 1992, 102:314–316.

34. Villanueva C, Balazno J, Torras X, *et al.*: Value of second-look endoscopy after injection therapy for bleeding peptic ulcer: a prospective and randomized trial. *Gastrointest Endosc* 1992, 40:34–39.

188 Principles of Endoscopy

Gary W. Falk

Endoscopy is a powerful tool that provides precise diagnostic information regarding the gastrointestinal tract and permits interventions that save lives and improve the quality of life. The rapid rise in the number of endoscopic procedures performed and associated costs has raised many questions about its appropriate role in health care today. This chapter considers the technique of endoscopy, the training required for its performance, and indications for the various endoscopic procedures available. The subsequent chapter (Chapter 189) reviews risks and complications associated with endoscopy.

GENERAL CONSIDERATIONS

Informed Consent

Before all endoscopic procedures, the risks and benefits of the proposed study must be discussed with the patient. Risks include bleeding, perforation, infection, and adverse effects of sedation. Elective endoscopic procedures generally are safe, although the risk is increased in emergency settings as well as with endoscopic retrograde cholangiopancreatography (ERCP). Cardiopulmonary complications caused by oversedation, aspiration, airway obstruction, or vasovagal episodes account for most endoscopic complications (see Chapter 189).

Antibiotic and Endocarditis Prophylaxis

The overall risk of bacterial endocarditis is low in patients undergoing gastrointestinal endoscopy, and there are no trials to show that antibiotic prophylaxis prevents endocarditis. Endoscopic procedures also have the potential to cause noncardiac infectious complications, such as ERCP-induced cholangitis and cellulitis from the insertion of percutaneous gastrostomy tubes. The decision to prescribe antibiotic prophylaxis for endocarditis should take into account the risk of bacteremia associated with the endoscopic procedure and the risk that endocarditis will occur with a specific cardiac lesion [1,2]. Endoscopic procedures associated with a higher risk of bacteremia and for which antibiotic prophylaxis is recommended are sclerotherapy of esophageal varices (but not band ligation of varices), dilation of esophageal strictures, and ERCP performed in the setting of an obstructed biliary tree. All other diagnostic and therapeutic endoscopic procedures are associated with a minimal risk of bacteremia. Cardiac conditions at highest risk for the development of endocarditis are prosthetic heart valves of any type, surgically constructed systemic and pulmonary shunts, a prior history of endocarditis, and complex cyanotic congenital heart disease. Cardiac conditions of intermediate risk include other congenital malformations, rheumatic valvular disease, hypertrophic cardiomyopathy, and mitral valve prolapse with regurgitation. All other cardiac conditions are considered to be of low risk (see Chapter 189).

For endoscopic procedures associated with minimal risk of bacteremia, current guidelines recommend no antibiotic prophylaxis for low- and moderate-risk cardiac lesions. Although a case-by-case approach is suggested for antibiotic prophylaxis in patients with high-risk cardiac lesions undergoing endoscopic procedures [1], it would be prudent to err on the side of prophylaxis, given the devastating consequences of endocarditis [2].

For patients undergoing procedures associated with increased rates of bacteremia, a different approach is recommended. Routine prophylaxis should take place in all patients with high-risk cardiac lesions, whereas no prophylaxis is warranted in patients with low-risk cardiac conditions. For patients with intermediate risk conditions, a case-by-case approach is again recommended [1], although prophylaxis would again seem prudent. Antibiotic prophylaxis regimens are shown in Table 188-1 [2]. Antibiotic prophylaxis also is recommended in patients undergoing endoscopic procedures, who are at increased risk of developing bacteremia during the first year after placement of synthetic vascular grafts. No antibiotic prophylaxis is recommended for patients with prosthetic joints.

Antibiotic prophylaxis is recommended before instrumentation of an obstructed biliary system and in patients with pancreatic pseudocysts. It also should be administered before placement of percutaneous feeding tubes. Finally, prophylaxis should be considered in patients with cirrhosis and ascites and in immunocompromised patients before the high-risk endoscopic procedures of stricture dilation, variceal sclerosis, and ERCP.

Anticoagulant and Antiplatelet Therapy

The approach to the patient on anticoagulant or antiplatelet therapy should take into account the risk of bleeding associated

Table 188-1. Antibiotic Prophylaxis Regimens for Gastrointestinal Endoscopy

Esophageal procedures	Nonesophageal procedures
Ampicillin 2 gm IV or IM within 30 minutes prior to the procedure	Ampicillin 2 gm IM or IV within 30 minutes prior to the procedure *plus*
If penicillin allergic:	gentamicin 1.5 mg/kg not to exceed 80 mg
Clindamycin 600 mg IV within 30 minutes prior to the procedure	*If penicillin allergic:*
or	Substitute vancomycin 1 gm IV over 1 to 2 hours for ampicillin
Cefazolin 1 gm IV within 30 minutes prior to the procedure	

IM—intramuscularly; IV—intravenously.

with the particular endoscopic procedure and the risk of a thromboembolic event related to interruption of anticoagulant therapy [3], as summarized in Table 188-2. For deep venous thrombosis, in which case anticoagulation therapy is temporary, elective endoscopy should be delayed, if possible, until anticoagulation is discontinued. For low-risk endoscopic procedures, no adjustment of anticoagulation therapy is necessary, unless the level of anticoagulation is above therapeutic levels.

For high-risk procedures in patients with low-risk conditions, warfarin therapy should be discontinued for 3 to 5 days before the procedure (Table 188-3). In patients with high-risk conditions, warfarin also should be discontinued 3 to 5 days before to the procedure, and heparin should be administered based on the judgment of the physician after the prothrombin time falls below the therapeutic range. If used, heparin should be discontinued 4 to 6 hours before the procedure and resumed 2 to 6 hours after the procedure. Warfarin can be restarted immediately after the procedure.

Administration of aspirin and other nonsteroidal anti-inflammatory drugs (NSAIDs) does not increase the risk of significant

bleeding after either high- or low-risk procedures and need not be discontinued before endoscopy.

Conscious Sedation

Sedation is defined as a decrease in the level of consciousness induced by medications used to facilitate the performance of endoscopic procedures. The term *conscious sedation* means that sedation is attained without the loss of protective airway reflexes. During endoscopy, patients should be able to respond to verbal stimuli and maintain their airways and ventilatory drive. Although administration of conscious sedation alleviates pain, anxiety, and agitation during endoscopy, it also accounts for much of the risk associated with the performance of endoscopy (see Chapter 189).

Appropriate and safe conscious sedation requires adequate assessment of the patient's risk and knowledge of the pharmacology of drugs used commonly in the endoscopy suite. The guiding principle of conscious sedation is to use the smallest amount of medication necessary to make the patient comfortable. Administration of conscious sedation improves patient

---

Table 188-2. Endoscopy in Patients on Antiplatelet or Anticoagulation Therapy

Low risk endoscopic procedures	Low risk conditions	High risk endoscopic procedures	High risk conditions
EGD + biopsy	Deep venous thrombosis	Colonoscopy + polypectomy	Any mechanical valve with prior thromboembolic event
Colonoscopy + biopsy	Paroxysmal atrial fibrillation	Endoscopic sphincterotomy	Mitral valve replacement
Sigmoidoscopy + biopsy	Bioprosthetic valve	Percutaneous gastrostomy	Atrial fibrillation + dilated cardiomyopathy
Enteroscopy	Mechanical aortic valve replacement	EGD + polypectomy	Atrial fibrillation + valvular disease
Endosonography	—	Laser therapy	Sustained atrial fibrillation
ERCP	—	Pneumatic dilation	Atrial fibrillation + recent thromboembolic event
ERCP + stent change	—	Bougie dilation	
		Endosonography + fine needle aspiration	

EGD—esophagogastroduodenoscopy; ERCP—endoscopic retrograde cholangiopancreatography.

Table 188-3. Recommendations for the Management of Anticoagulation and Antiplatelet Therapy in Patients Undergoing Endoscopic Procedures

Procedure risk	Condition risk for thromboembolism	
	High	**Low**
High	Discontinue warfarin 3–5 days prior to procedure; consider heparin while INR is subtherapeutic	Discontinue warfarin 3–5 days prior to procedure; restart warfarin after procedure
Low	No change in anticoagulation; elective procedures should be delayed while INR is in supratherapeutic range	—

Aspirin and other NSAIDS

In absence of bleeding disorder, elective procedures may be performed; urgent procedures should not be delayed	

INR—international normalized ratio; NSAIDs—nonsteroidal anti-inflammatory drugs.

acceptance of endoscopic procedures. In general, pain is prevented by analgesics, whereas anxiety is prevented by anxiolytics, although some overlap exists. Topical anesthesia with either lidocaine or benzocaine may improve patient tolerance of upper endoscopy. Benzodiazepines are the principal agents used and induce relaxation, cooperation, and, at times, amnesia (Table 188-4). They are given alone or in conjunction with opiate analgesics. The major side effect is respiratory depression. The most commonly used agent is midazolam (Versed), which has several advantages over diazepam (Valium). Because midazolam is water soluble, it does not cause phlebitis. Also, it has a more rapid onset of action than diazepam and is cleared rapidly; it is 1.5 to 2 times as potent as diazepam. The optimal dose of midazolam is 0.01 to 0.04 mg/kg administered intravenously by slow titration [4•]. The dose should be decreased by 25% to 30% if midazolam is coadministered with narcotic analgesics. Opiate analgesics provide both analgesia and sedation. The most commonly used opiate is meperidine. at doses of 0.5 to 1 mg/kg given intravenously by slow titration.

The goal of conscious sedation is to have the patient cooperative, oriented, and tranquil or drowsy but still responsive to commands. This is best assessed by talking to the patient to assess for slurred speech, loss of spontaneous eye opening, and depressed consciousness.

Antagonists of both opiate analgesics and benzodiazepines are available and should be used in patients who are oversedated. Naloxone in a dose of 0.1 to 0.4 mg given intravenously (much lower than the typical emergency room dose) is used to reverse opiate analgesics. Flumazenil in a dose of 0.2 to 0.5 mg given intravenously reverses benzodiazepine-induced sedation by competitively inhibiting central nervous system benzodiazepine-binding sites. The duration of action of this agent is less than that of the benzodiazepines, however, and sedation may recur after the initial reversal. Caution also should be observed in administering flumazenil to patients who use benzodiazepines on a chronic basis because of the risk of seizures.

One of the most common pitfalls of conscious sedation is the failure to recognize hypoxemia. Any patient who becomes restless and agitated during a procedure should be considered to be hypoxemic until proved otherwise. Individual variability and inadequate analgesia is handled best by slow titration of agents.

Monitoring

Patients should be monitored before, during, and after endoscopy to detect changes in the pulse rate, blood pressure, ventilatory status, oxygen saturation, and level of consciousness. Before the procedure, a brief history, including drug allergies, and an assessment of cardiopulmonary status allow assessment of the patient's relative risk. Older age, particularly associated with underlying cardiopulmonary disease, may increase the risk associated with endoscopy.

The most important component of patient monitoring during endoscopy is a well-trained gastrointestinal assistant. In addition, automatic blood pressure and heart rate monitoring and continuous determination of oxygen saturation by pulse oximetry are helpful. Continuous intravenous access is maintained throughout the course of endoscopy with an indwelling catheter.

Infection Control

Infection rarely is caused by endoscopy. Nevertheless, patients are concerned about the possibility of acquiring infection during endoscopy. Those performing endoscopy should be familiar with the principles of infection control, which include mechanical cleaning, high-level disinfection, and, rarely, sterilization (see Chapter 195).

■ ESOPHAGOGASTRODUODENOSCOPY

Upper endoscopy enables inspection of the mucosal surfaces of the esophagus, stomach, and duodenum as well as additional diagnostic maneuvers, such as biopsy and cytologic brushings, and therapeutic interventions, such as dilation of strictures, measures to control bleeding, removal of foreign bodies, polypectomy, and treatment of tumors.

Technique

In the United States, virtually all upper endoscopic procedures are done with video technology, which processes and transmits images electronically. Fiberoptic technology is still used but is less popular because of lower image quality and operator fatigue associated with use of these instruments.

Patients should be prepared for upper endoscopy by having nothing to eat or drink for at least 4 to 6 hours before the procedure. Topical anesthesia is optional but improves patient tolerance [5]. After administration of conscious sedation, the patient is turned on the left side, the neck is slightly flexed, and a mouthpiece is inserted (even in edentulous patients) to

Table 188-4. Agents Commonly Used in Conscious Sedation

Generic and trade name	Intravenous dose	Comments
Benzodiazepines		
Diazepam (Valium)	0.02–0.05 mg/kg	Affected by age, liver function; usual duration of action 2–4 h; elimination half-life 20–70 h.
Midazolam (Versed)	0.01–0.04 mg/kg	Elimination half-life 1–4 h
Benzodiazepam reversal agent		
Flumazenil (Romazicon)	0.2–0.5 mg	Repeat dose to 1 mg maximum; elimination half-life 0.6–1.3 h.
Opiates		
Meperidine (Demerol)	0.5–1 mg/kg	—
Fentanyl (Sublimaze)	0.8–1.2 µg/kg	Typical adult dose 50–100 µg
Opiate reversal agent		
Naloxone (Narcan)	0.1–0.4 mg	—

Adapted from Higgins [4•]; with permission.

prevent damage to the insertion tube. The instrument should be inserted under direct vision to provide precise orientation and to decrease discomfort and the risk of complications. The epiglottis, vocal cords, and piriform sinuses are identified, and the scope is inserted either midline or via the right or left piriform sinus, after which gentle pressure enables it to traverse the cricopharyngeus. To minimize the risk of perforation, the instrument should not be forced blindly. Difficult intubation may be caused by poor patient cooperation, a Zenker's diverticulum, osteophytes, or tumors.

The esophagus is viewed on insertion by maintaining a central luminal view. The squamous epithelium is characterized by a pearly-white appearance. The gastroesophageal junction is marked by the ora serrata or Z line, a jagged confluence of reddish gastric columnar epithelium and the whitish esophageal squamous epithelium (Fig. 188-1). This landmark typically is at the diaphragmatic impression but may be difficult to identify in patients with a hiatal hernia. The size of a hiatal hernia should be estimated, in part because antireflux surgical techniques may vary accordingly.

When the tip of the endoscope enters the stomach, the endoscopist should remove retained gastric contents to decrease the risk of subsequent aspiration. If residual food cannot be cleared, it is best to halt the examination entirely or remove the endoscope and place a large-diameter orogastric tube into the stomach and lavage the material out. When the stomach is clear (Fig. 188-2), the instrument is advanced to the pylorus. To visualize the lesser curvature, fundus, and cardia of the stomach adequately, a retroflexed view should be obtained routinely, either before the duodenum is entered or after completion of the duodenal portion of the examination (Fig. 188-3).

The pylorus is passed, and the duodenal bulb is examined on entry to avoid misinterpretation of any artifacts caused by instrument trauma seen on withdrawal of the scope. The duodenal mucosa typically is paler than the gastric mucosa and often has small, slightly raised nodules, which are visible Brunner's glands (Fig. 188-4). Once past the bulb, the instrument is inserted into the second part of the duodenum, which has characteristic circumferential folds (Fig. 188-5). Examination is complete when the instrument is inserted to the distal second part of the duodenum, although on occasion (eg, to exclude an aortoenteric fistula), the third part of the duodenum should be inspected. The instrument is then withdrawn.

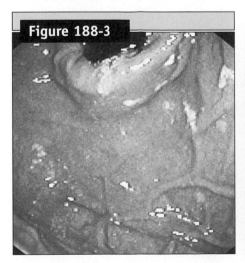

Figure 188-1

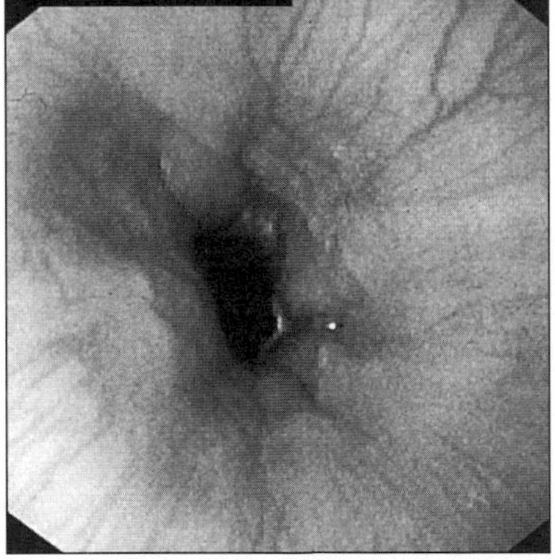

Normal endoscopic appearance of the gastroesophageal junction. Note the pearly white appearance of the esophagus and the salmon red appearance of the cardia of the stomach.

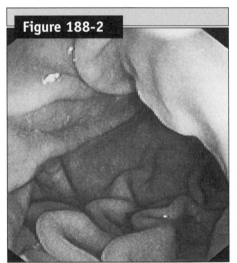

Figure 188-2

Normal endoscopic appearance of the gastric corpus, characterized by gastric folds.

Figure 188-3

Retroflexed endoscopic view of the gastric cardia and fundus.

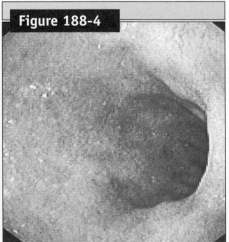

Figure 188-4

Normal endoscopic appearance of the duodenal bulb.

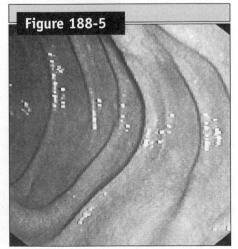

Figure 188-5

Normal endoscopic appearance of the descending duodenum, characterized by circular folds.

Training

The American Society for Gastrointestinal Endoscopy (ASGE) recommends performing a minimum of 100 upper endoscopy procedures as a threshold before clinical competence is assessed [6]. This recommendation was based on expert opinion. In a landmark study, Cass and colleagues [7••] examined the number of supervised upper endoscopy procedures needed before trainees achieved competence in both the technical and cognitive components of the procedure. When trainees were presented with a case mix representative of clinical practice, the success rate of esophageal intubation did not reach 90% until more than 100 procedures were performed. Therefore, the threshold number of 100 upper endoscopy procedures may be lower than needed for clinical competence.

Indications

Indications for upper endoscopy are shown in Table 188-5. Most of these indications are based on expert opinion, not randomized clinical trials. Nevertheless, compared with barium radiography, endoscopy has the advantage of permitting mucosal biopsy and therapeutic intervention.

Perhaps no indication for endoscopy is more controversial than dyspepsia (see Chapter 25). Currently, there are four possible diagnostic approaches to the patient with dyspepsia: 1) a short trial of empiric antisecretory therapy; 2) immediate endoscopy; 3) empiric antibiotic therapy for *Helicobacter pylori* (without initial testing for *H. pylori* infection) and; 4) noninvasive testing for *H. pylori* followed by antibiotic treatment of positive patients. At least two decision-analysis models have found that,

---

Table 188-5. Indications for Esophagogastroduodenoscopy

Dyspepsia
  Unresponsive to medical therapy; new onset in patients over age 45–50 y; associated with alarm signs (nausea, vomiting, weight loss, gastrointestinal bleeding)
Dysphagia or odynophagia
GERD symptoms despite medical therapy or recurrent after medical therapy
Persistent vomiting
Cancer surveillance
  Barrett's esophagus; prior adenomatous polyps; familial adenomatous polyposis; gastric ulcer to exclude cancer
Gastric polyps
Gastrointestinal bleeding
  Acute; recent; chronic blood loss/iron deficiency, obscure etiology
Assess for varices in patients with portal hypertension
Small bowel biopsy
Assess injury after caustic ingestion
Modification of patient management of other diseases
  Potential organ transplantation and prior ulcer disease; head and neck cancer
Treatment
  Stricture dilation; gastrointestinal bleeding; polypectomy; esophageal cancer (laser ablation, photodynamic therapy, stent insertion); foreign body removal; food impaction
Confirmation of radiographic abnormality

GERD—gastroesophageal reflux disease.

---

in patients with uncomplicated dyspepsia, a strategy of initial noninvasive testing for *H. pylori* followed by antimicrobial therapy in positive patients (the so-called test-and-treat approach) is most cost-effective [8,9]. Immediate endoscopy in the management of dyspepsia in the pre–*H. pylori* era resulted in less physician visits, less antisecretory drug use, a decrease in the number of sick days, and greater patient satisfaction than did empiric treatment with H_2-receptor antagonists [10]. Finally, another recent decision-analysis study found that the choice between empiric antisecretory therapy and initial endoscopy was essentially a "toss-up" [11]. There are no randomized controlled clinical trials that allow the physician to make evidence-based decisions on the optimal role of endoscopy in patients with dyspepsia.

Another controversial issue is the role of endoscopy in patients with gastroesophageal reflux disease (GERD; see Chapter 4). Symptoms of GERD are common in the United States, and endoscopy of all affected patients would be prohibitively expensive. Furthermore, excellent symptom control is achievable with H_2-receptor antagonists and proton pump inhibitors. The incidence of esophageal adenocarcinoma is increasing rapidly, however, and Barrett's esophagus, a diagnosis that can be made with only endoscopy and biopsy, is the only known risk factor for this cancer. Moreover, endoscopic assessment of the severity of GERD permits estimation of prognosis; patients with erosive esophagitis generally are unable to discontinue aggressive antisecretory drug therapy and may be candidates for antireflux surgery.

In this era of cost containment, it is important to recognize inappropriate reasons to perform upper endoscopy. These include follow-up of benign lesions, such as duodenal ulcers; evaluation of metastatic carcinoma of an unknown primary tumor, especially when results will not influence subsequent therapy; and radiographic evidence of a hiatal hernia, deformed duodenal bulb, or duodenal ulcer. Cancer surveillance is not indicated for patients with achalasia, gastric atrophy, pernicious anemia, or prior gastric surgery.

There are few absolute contraindications to the performance of upper endoscopy. These include an uncooperative patient, suspected peritonitis or perforation, cardiopulmonary instability, and any setting for which the apparent risk outweighs the perceived benefit of the procedure. Relative contraindications include the presence of a Zenker's diverticulum, coagulopathy, decompensated cardiopulmonary disease, recent myocardial infarction, and respiratory insufficiency.

Risks and Complications

Complications of upper endoscopy are rare and include perforation, bleeding, and oversedation, in about 0.08% to 0.13% of cases. Cass and colleagues [7••], however, reported a complication rate of 0.4% in their study assessing thresholds of competence. The mortality rate of the procedure is 0.5 to 3 per 10,000.

■ SMALL BOWEL ENTEROSCOPY

The purpose of small bowel enteroscopy is to inspect the small intestine distal to the reach of a standard upper endoscope. This can be accomplished by three different techniques: push enteroscopy, sonde enteroscopy, and intraoperative enteroscopy.

Technique

Push enteroscopy, the simplest and most commonly used technique, can be accomplished with a pediatric or adult colonoscope or a special dedicated instrument. When performed with a colonoscope, the technique used is identical to that of routine upper endoscopy. The instruments can be inserted 50 to 60 cm beyond the ligament of Treitz.

Newer dedicated instruments are available that use either video or fiberoptic technology. They vary in length from 200 to 250 cm and can reach about 100 cm beyond the ligament of Treitz. The length of these instruments, however, typically results in formation of a loop in the stomach. Therefore, after the tip of the enteroscope reaches the distal duodenum, an overtube is passed through the patient's mouth and over the instrument into the proximal duodenum to facilitate advancement of the scope. Fluoroscopic confirmation of the position of the overtube is advocated by some authorities. After the overtube is passed, principles of colonoscopy (see later), such as loop removal, abdominal counterpressure, and a combination of pushing and pulling, are used to advance the enteroscope. Once the enteroscope is advanced to its full length, the patient is given glucagon, and the instrument is withdrawn. The advantages of push enteroscopy over sonde enteroscopy (see later) are tip deflection controls and a channel that permits both biopsy and therapeutic interventions.

Sonde enteroscopy offers the potential to inspect the small intestine. The instruments used are 5 to 8 mm in diameter and are passed transnasally or orally. The transnasal technique requires simultaneous oral passage of a conventional endoscope, which then is used to move the sonde device through the pylorus. When the tip is in the duodenum, a balloon surrounding the distal portion of the instrument is inflated, and intestinal peristalsis facilitates passage of the scope to the terminal ileum. The peroral technique relies on a weighted tip instead of a balloon to facilitate passage to the distal small bowel. Tip deflection is not possible with any of the available sonde instruments, and reinsertion to inspect more carefully a given sequence of intestine is impossible once the withdrawal process begins. Sonde enteroscopy requires fluoroscopy to confirm the position of the scope and is time-consuming, requiring up to 7 hours to complete.

Finally, enteroscopy can be performed in the operating room in conjunction with laparoscopy or laparotomy, and 6 inches to 1 foot of small bowel is inspected before the subsequent "telescoping" or pleating. Inspection precedes pleating because of the damage done to the intestine during the process. A surgeon then "telescopes" the small bowel over a conventional colonoscope while the endoscopist evaluates the bowel. This technique permits therapeutic interventions but has the disadvantages associated with surgical exploration.

Indications

The major indication for small bowel enteroscopy is evaluation of gastrointestinal bleeding of obscure origin (see Chapters 34 and 197). The yield of enteroscopy ranges from 34% to 80% in various reports and is related to the depth of instrument insertion. Most lesions detected are vascular (eg, telangiectasias or arteriovenous malformations), although other abnormalities may be encountered. Additional indications include evaluation of small

bowel radiographic abnormalities, percutaneous jejunostomy placement, and access to the papilla in patients with Roux-en-Y surgical reconstruction. Enteroscopy may be of use in selected patients with suspected malabsorption and in the management of inherited polyposis syndromes.

Risks and Complications

The complication rate of enteroscopy is similar to that encountered with diagnostic upper and lower endoscopy. Insertion of overtubes is associated with mucosal stripping and may increase the risk of perforation.

▄▄ PERCUTANEOUS GASTROSTOMY

Percutaneous gastrostomy is the technique of choice for long-term enteral nutrition (see Chapter 192). It has largely replaced surgical gastrostomy based on cost considerations and is an ideal method of feeding patients with persistent swallowing difficulties. Percutaneous gastrostomy should not be used if the patient's anticipated survival is less than 30 days.

Technique

Several different techniques of percutaneous gastrostomy are available. All offer comparable results, and the choice of technique depends on the training and experience of the endoscopist. Prophylactic antibiotics (cefazolin, 1 g given intravenously) should be given 30 minutes before the procedure to decrease the risk of postprocedural infectious complications; patients already on systemic antibiotics do not need additional antibiotics.

The "pull" technique involves pulling the proximal part of the gastrostomy tube through the mouth into the stomach and through the abdominal wall. First, the upper endoscope is passed into the stomach, which is inflated with air to allow the anterior wall to meet the abdominal wall. The abdominal wall is then transilluminated with the endoscope in the stomach, and the site of tube insertion is selected where transillumination is maximal. The site is marked, the abdomen is cleaned and draped in a sterile fashion, and local anesthesia is applied so that a small incision can be made in the skin over the site. A cannula is then passed percutaneously into the stomach and a suture is threaded through the cannula and grasped by either a snare or forceps through the endoscope and drawn back through the mouth. The percutaneous gastrostomy tube is attached to the thread and pulled through the mouth down the esophagus, into the stomach, and through the abdominal wall, after which it is secured. Finally, the endoscope may be reinserted to check for positioning and to be certain that the tension on the catheter is not excessive. Feeding commences the following day.

The "push" technique involves the same techniques of preparation, endoscope insertion, and abdominal wall puncture. Instead of a suture, however, a guidewire is passed into the stomach, grasped using a forceps passed through the endoscope, and pulled out of the mouth. The gastrostomy tube is pushed over the guidewire through the mouth and into the stomach. The long tapered end of the tube dilates the tract through the abdominal wall and is grasped and pulled out. Final position is assessed by a second passage of the endoscope.

The final technique, the "introducer" method, involves only a single passage of the endoscope. The abdominal wall is prepared as for the previously described techniques, the endoscope inserted, and the abdominal wall transilluminated. A needle is then placed through the abdominal wall into the stomach. A guidewire is passed through the needle, and after removal of the needle, an introducer with a pull-away sheath is passed over the guidewire into the stomach. The wire is pulled out with the introducer, and the sheath is left in place. The gastrostomy tube is then inserted through the sheath.

Percutaneous jejunostomy feeding tubes sometimes are placed after placement of a percutaneous endoscopic gastrostomy tube. This can be done by grasping the jejunal tube with the endoscope and dragging it distally or by placing a guidewire into the duodenum, sometimes with a steerable catheter, and passing the jejunostomy tube over the guidewire. It is essential to place the tube at or beyond the ligament of Treitz to ensure its optimal functioning.

Training

The ASGE recommends performing 10 percutaneous endoscopic gastrostomy procedures before clinical competence is assessed [6].

Indications

Percutaneous endoscopic gastrostomy is indicated in patients with an intact and functioning gastrointestinal tract who cannot or will not consume adequate calories to meet their metabolic demands, as long as access can be obtained safely [12]. The standard indication for the procedure is dysphagia related to a neurologic abnormality or head and neck malignancy. The procedure also may be used palliatively for gastric decompression in patients with chronic intestinal pseudo-obstruction, diabetic gastroparesis, or malignant obstruction [13].

The role of percutaneous jejunostomy remains controversial. The procedure may be considered instead of percutaneous endoscopic gastrostomy in the following settings: tracheal aspiration of tube feedings; reflux esophagitis; delayed gastric emptying, especially after head injury; insufficient gastric remnant as a result of prior surgery, and obstruction from unresectable gastric or pancreatic cancer [14]. Percutaneous jejunostomy does not decrease the risk of aspiration of oropharyngeal contents.

Percutaneous gastrostomy is contraindicated if the endoscope cannot be passed into the stomach or the abdominal wall cannot be transilluminated. Other contraindications are massive ascites, intra-abdominal sepsis, correctable intestinal obstruction, sepsis, and multiorgan failure. The latter two situations are best handled by nasoenteric feedings until the patient stabilizes. Relative contraindications include lesser amounts of ascites, morbid obesity, hepatomegaly, gastric varices, and prior subtotal gastrectomy. There is no role for percutaneous gastrostomy in patients with rapidly progressive, incurable illness and an anticipated survival of less than 30 days [15].

Risks and Complications

The overall complication rate of percutaneous endoscopic gastrostomy is about 3% to 10%, with a mortality rate approaching 1%. The most common complication is infection of the gastrostomy site. A rare but more serious infectious complication is necrotizing fasciitis, which requires surgical débridement. Peristomal leak may cause minor skin irritation or

peritonitis. Less common complications include bleeding, tube dislodgment or clogging, aspiration, bowel perforation, gastrocolic fistula, and peritonitis from spillage of tube feedings into the peritoneal cavity.

Percutaneous jejunostomy may be complicated by tube dislodgment, kinking, or clogging, all of which necessitate tube replacement or repositioning.

■ COLONOSCOPY

The goal of colonoscopy is to examine the mucosal detail of the colon from the rectum to the cecum and, if necessary, the terminal ileum. Colonoscopy permits biopsy of normal and abnormal mucosa, polyp removal, and treatment of gastrointestinal bleeding.

Preparation

Iron-containing compounds should be discontinued at least 1 week before the procedure because iron makes colonic contents difficult to clear. There are two options for colonic cleansing: a polyethylene glycol–based balanced electrolyte lavage solution or an oral sodium phosphate laxative [16•]. Clear liquids should be given for 24 hours and solid food should be avoided for 3 to 4 hours immediately before the preparation is begun.

Polyethylene glycol–based balanced electrolyte solutions have been the mainstay of colonoscopy preparation for years. These are available as unflavored or flavored formulations (GoLYTELY, Colyte, and NuLYTELY). The only difference among the preparations is that the sodium content is lower and sulfate is absent in NuLYTELY (Table 188-6). Four liters of the oral lavage solution should be taken by mouth over 2 to 4 hours. Oral ingestion may be facilitated by having the patient take metoclopramide, 10 mg, 30 minutes before commencing the preparation. These preparations result in minimal fluid and electrolyte shifts and a clear view of the colonic mucosa at colonoscopy, with no distortion of the mucosal architecture. These preparations, however, may not be tolerated by patients because of the large volume that must be ingested, their salty taste, and ensuing nausea and vomiting. Contraindications to administration of balanced electrolyte lavage include ileus or suspected bowel obstruction, swallowing disorders, gastric retention, and severe colitis.

Table 188-6. Composition of Oral Lavage Solutions

	Golytely	Nulytely	Colyte
Na^+ (mEq/L)	125	65	125
K^+ (mEq/L)	10	5	10
Cl^- (mEq/L)	35	53	35
HCO_3^- (mEq/L)	20	17	20
SO_4^- (mEq/L)	40	0	80
Polyethylene glycol (g/L)	60	105	60
Osmolality	280	288	280

Cl—chloride; HCO_3^-—bicarbonate; K^+—potassium; Na—sodium; SO_4^-—sulfate.
From Keeffe [16•]; with permission.

Oral sodium phosphate laxatives are an excellent alternative to balanced electrolyte solutions. The preparation involves administration of 1.5 oz of oral sodium phosphate in 4 oz of water, followed by three 8-oz glasses of water the evening before the examination and an additional 1.5 oz of oral sodium phosphate in 4 oz of water on the morning of the procedure. This preparation requires consumption of a much smaller volume than balanced electrolyte solutions, is inexpensive, and is just as effective. It may, however, cause a variety of electrolyte disturbances, such as elevation of phosphate and sodium levels and decreases in potassium and calcium levels. Therefore, the preparation is contraindicated in patients with congestive heart failure, chronic renal failure, and cirrhosis accompanied by ascites.

Technique

After administration of conscious sedation and with the patient in the left lateral decubitus position, a digital rectal examination is performed. The tip of the colonoscope is lubricated and introduced into the rectum.

To advance the instrument to the cecum safely and comfortably, the endoscopist uses a variety of maneuvers to avoid loop formation. Loops occur because the sigmoid and trans-

verse colon is attached simply to the mesentery and is freely mobile, in contrast to the cecum, descending and ascending colon, which are retroperitoneal in 85% of persons. Numerous techniques are used to navigate the twists and bends of the colon, including instrument insertion and withdrawal, tip deflection, application of torque to the instrument shaft, repositioning of the patient, and application of abdominal counterpressure by the gastrointestinal assistant to stent mobile colonic segments.

After passing through the rectum (Fig. 188-6, see also **Color Plate**), the sigmoid colon is characterized by frequent circular haustral folds that tend to become more prominent when there is diverticular disease. The descending colon(Fig. 188-7, see also **Color Plate**) typically is short and straight and ends in an acute angle at the splenic flexure. At that point, shifting the patient to either the supine or right lateral decubitus position facilitates entering the transverse colon, which is triangular as a result of the three longitudinal muscles of the colon (Fig. 188-8, see also **Color Plate**). The hepatic flexure may be identified by mucosal darkening caused by the adjacent liver. At this point, the instrument should be fully shortened by pulling back with clockwise torque as the colon is deflated to facilitate entry into the ascending colon, which is identified by the characteristic bulge of the ileocecal valve on the first haustral fold and by the concentric or circular appearanceof the appendix (Fig. 188-9, see also **Color Plate**). The terminal ileum may be entered by removing as much air as possible from the cecum and withdrawing the instrument with 90° angulation toward the ileocecal valve fold. The instrument will catch the valve and then can be inserted into the ileum, which is characterized by a granular mucosa (Fig. 188-10, see also **Color Plate**), in contrast to the smooth, glistening mucosaand lacy pattern of blood vessels of the colon. Skilled colonoscopists should reach the cecum in at least 95% of cases. Extensive diverticular disease, pelvic surgery (especially hysterectomy), stricturing, and previous irradiation may hamper success of the procedure. In those situations, us of

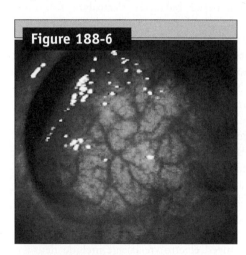

Figure 188-6

Normal colonoscopic appearance of the rectum, characterized by prominent vascular detail of the mucosa. See also **Color Plate**. (*From* Nostrant [40].)

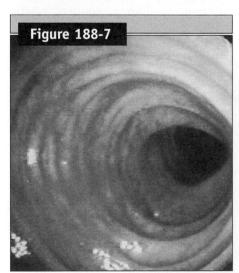

Figure 188-7

Normal colonoscopic appearance of the descending colon, characterized by a tubular appearance of the lumen. See also **Color Plate**. (*From* Nostrant [40].)

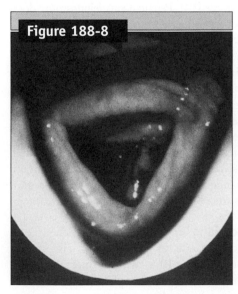

Figure 188-8

The normal transverse colon has characteristic triangular folds seen at colonoscopy. See also **Color Plate**. (*From* Nostrant [40].)

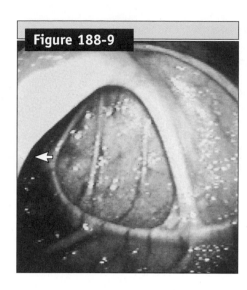

Figure 188-9

The normal cecum is characterized by fusing of the three taeniae coli and the bulge of the ileocecal valve fold seen at colonoscopy. See also **Color Plate**. (*From* Nostrant [40].)

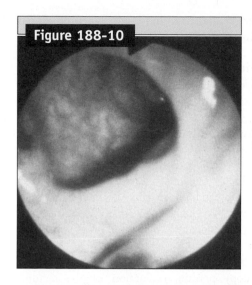

Figure 188-10

The normal terminal ileum, as seen at colonoscopy, has a more granular appearance, smaller lumen, and less prominent vascular pattern than does the colon. See also **Color Plate**. (*From* Nostrant [40].)

the more flexible and smaller-diameter pediatric colonoscope often permits successful intubation.

Training

The ASGE recommends performing a minimum of 100 diagnostic colonoscopies and 20 snare polypectomies as a threshold for assessing clinical competence [6]. This recommendation was based on expert opinion. Cass and colleagues [7••] examined the number of supervised colonoscopies needed before a group of trainees achieved competence in both the technical and cognitive components of the procedure. When presented with a case mix representative of clinical practice, the success rate for reaching the cecum did not exceed 90% until more than 200 procedures had been performed. Other authorities have confirmed that competence in performing colonoscopy increases with experience over time and that the threshold number of 100 procedures is below that needed for clinical competence [17].

Indications

The indications for colonoscopy are listed in Table 188-7. Guidelines for colorectal cancer screening have recently been revised [18••]. For persons at average risk of developing colon cancer, screening colonoscopy beginning at 50 years of age and done at 10-year intervals is now considered a reasonable option. For individuals with a single first-degree relative with either colon cancer or adenomatous polyps, it is recommended that screening colonoscopy commence at age 40. Patients in families characterized by hereditary nonpolyposis colon cancer should begin screening colonoscopy at age 20 to 30, yearly or every other year, increasing to yearly after age 40. For patients with a history of adenomatous polyps, colonoscopy should be repeated at 3 years and, if negative or if one small adenoma is encountered, every 5 years thereafter. Patients diagnosed with colorectal cancer should undergo a "clearing" examination within 1 year of surgery and, if negative, should be examined 3 years later and then every 5 years. Finally, patients with ulcerative colitis involving the entire colon should begin surveillance

Table 188-7. Indications for Colonoscopy

Abnormalities on barium enema
   Filling defect; polyp/mass; stricture
Gastrointestinal bleeding
   Unexplained iron deficiency anemia; occult blood in stool;
     hematochezia in absence of convincing anorectal etiology;
     melena (after upper gastrointestinal source excluded)
Surveillance of colon neoplasia
   Complete examination in patients with known colorectal cancer or
     adenomatous polyp
   Follow-up of patients with history of colorectal cancer or
     adenomatous polyp
   Family history of adenomatous polyps
   Family history of colon cancer: multiple relatives (hereditary
     nonpolyposis colon cancer); one first-degree relative
Ulcerative colitis
   Pancolitis > 8 years; left-sided colitis > 15 years
Inflammatory bowel disease
   Determine extent of disease
Unexplained chronic diarrhea
Therapeutic interventions
   Polyp removal; foreign body removal; gastrointestinal bleeding
   Decompression: nonobstructive colonic dilation; sigmoid volvulus
   Cancer palliation; dilate stenosis (anastomotic strictures)

colonoscopy after 8 years of disease and continue every 1 to 2 years thereafter. Patients with left-sided disease should begin surveillance examinations after 15 years of disease.

In the evaluation of patients with chronic abdominal pain, the yield of colonoscopy generally is low, and the risk-to-benefit ratio does not favor routine colonoscopy. Absolute contraindications to colonoscopy are the same as for upper endoscopy. In addition, colonoscopy should not be performed in patients with suspected colonic perforation, peritonitis, fulminant colitis, acute diverticulitis, or an inadequate preparation. Colonoscopy is not indicated for the evaluation of metastatic adenocarcinoma of unknown primary when the results of the examination will not alter management, irritable bowel syndrome, acute diarrhea, and upper gastrointestinal bleeding after documentation of an obvious source.

Risks and Complications

The overall complication rate of colonoscopy is 0.6% to 0.7%. There are several risks and complications unique to colonoscopy. Perforation occurs in 0.14% to 0.17% of cases, typically as a result of looping or pressure in the sigmoid colon, and after polypectomy. Bleeding occurs in 0.7% to 2.5% of patients and may be seen 7 to 10 days after polypectomy. Polypectomy also may cause a transmural thermal injury known as *postpolypectomy syndrome*, which is characterized by abdominal pain, peritoneal irritation, leukocytosis, and fever. Although conservative management often suffices, surgery occasionally is warranted in this situation.

■ FLEXIBLE SIGMOIDOSCOPY

Flexible sigmoidoscopy permits evaluation of the rectum, sigmoid, and a variable length of the descending colon. The examination is brief and can be performed after less intensive preparation of the colon than colonoscopy. Sigmoidoscopy is used to screen average-risk persons for colorectal cancer and to evaluate distal colonic disease.

Preparation

Patients are prepared for flexible sigmoidoscopy with one or two enemas just before the procedure. Enemas usually consist of hypertonic phosphate, but saline or tap water may be used instead.

Technique

The technique of sigmoidoscopy is similar to the initial part of colonoscopy; however, conscious sedation typically is not administered. Mucosal detail may be examined during insertion and withdrawal of the instrument; the area under each fold should be carefully checked. Insertion of the scope should be terminated when an adequate examination is obtained or the patient experiences discomfort.

Training

Twenty-five supervised procedures are the minimum necessary before competence can be assessed [6], although no formal studies of training in flexible sigmoidoscopy have been reported.

Indications

The major role of flexible sigmoidoscopy is in screening asymptomatic, average-risk persons for colorectal cancer. Screening should begin at age 50 and, if negative, is repeated every 5 years thereafter. Sigmoidoscopy also has a role in screening persons with a family history of familial adenomatous polyposis, beginning at puberty and annually thereafter. Flexible sigmoidoscopy is an appropriate diagnostic test in younger patients with minor disturbances in bowel habits or apparent hemorrhoidal bleeding and is used to evaluate the distal colon, often in conjunction with a barium enema.

Flexible sigmoidoscopy is not indicated in acute diverticulitis, fulminant colitis, toxic megacolon, and suspected peritonitis or when the findings will not influence future management

decisions, including need for subsequent colonoscopy. The examination should be terminated in patients who are poorly prepared or uncooperative.

Risks and Complications

Perforation has been described in 0.1% of subjects undergoing flexible sigmoidoscopy.

■ ENDOSCOPIC RETROGRADE CHOLANGIOPANCREATOGRAPHY

Endoscopic retrograde cholangiopancreatography is the most technically demanding gastrointestinal procedure and carries the highest risk of complications, including death. It is a powerful tool that permits visualization of the papilla, provides diagnostic information about the biliary and pancreatic ductal systems, and allows for a variety of therapeutic interventions.

Technique

As for all endoscopic procedures, the patient must be counseled about the risks of the procedure, which are substantially higher than those for any other endoscopic procedure. In the initial assessment, it is essential to ascertain if the patient has dysphagia because the duodenoscope used for the procedure is passed blindly down the esophagus, and structural abnormalities of the esophagus may create unforeseen difficulty and risk.

Routine antibiotic prophylaxis is not indicated before ERCP. In one study, a single dose of piperacillin was not associated with a reduction in the frequency of cholangitis after ERCP in patients suspected of having biliary tract stones or a distal common bile duct stricture [19]. Antibiotics should be used in high-risk patients, however, such as those in whom complete drainage of the bile duct is not obtained, and should be strongly considered in patients in whom incomplete drainage can be anticipated, such as those with suspected primary sclerosing cholangitis or cholangiocarcinoma.

ERCP is a combined endoscopic and radiographic procedure, and the procedure room requires high-quality fluoroscopic and radiographic equipment. ERCP is accomplished with a side-viewing duodenoscope that may have a smaller diameter for diagnostic studies or a larger diameter for therapeutic use. The instruments also have an elevator at the end of the channel to facilitate manipulation of a cannula into the ductal system.

The patient is placed in the left lateral decubitus position during instrument insertion. After blind passage through the esophagus, the tip is angled down to obtain a view of the stomach as the pylorus is approached. When through the pylorus, the instrument is advanced into the duodenum, and the papilla is observed (Fig. 188-11). The pancreatic duct orifice and the bile duct orifice can be selectively cannulated, after which radiolucent material is injected into the ductal systems to produce a pancreatogram and a cholangiogram. Either high or low osmolality contrast media may be used during ERCP, and studies to date do not support the routine use of the more expensive low-osmolality contrast solutions. In patients who have had a previous anaphylactic reaction to intravascular contrast media, however, low-osmolality contrast media should be used after premedication with corticosteroids [20]. Low-osmolality contrast media do not clearly decrease the risk of ERCP-induced pancreatitis.

Endoscopic sphincterotomy can be done safely as an out-patient procedure and is indicated for removal of bile duct stones, placement of stents, and treatment of suspected sphincter of Oddi dysfunction. The standard technique requires free cannulation of the biliary system, which is confirmed by injection of contrast material. Access to the duct is then secured with a guidewire, and the sphincter is incised using electrocautery applied by a papillotome bowed against the papilla (Fig. 188-12). An alternative technique involves use of a precut sphincterotomy if the bile duct cannot be cannulated easily. This technique involves endoscopic dissection of the papilla with a "needle knife" or a fine cutting wire to unroof the papilla gradually in increments until the bile duct is exposed.

Training

In 1988, the Health and Public Policy Committee of the American College of Physicians recommended only 35 supervised ERCP procedures for attaining minimum competence [21]. The ASGE, based on expert opinion, later recommended a minimum of 100 diagnostic procedures and 25 therapeutic procedures to attain clinical competence [6]. Subsequent work by Watkins and colleagues [22] suggested that at least 100 procedures were necessary to obtain an 85% success rate for cannulation of both the biliary and pancreatic ducts. In a recent rigorous study, trainees were observed prospectively while learning ERCP, and procedural competence was defined as a success rate of 80% for cannulation of the desired duct [23••]. The threshold numbers of ERCPs performed to achieve that success rate were 160 for cholangiography, 140 for pancreatography, 120 for stone extraction, and 60 for stent insertion. Trainees achieved overall competence as defined above only after performing 180 to 200 procedures, numbers clearly greater than those suggested in earlier guidelines. Because of the high risk of ERCP, rigorous standards are necessary for attaining clinical competence in this procedure.

Indications

Indications for ERCP are listed in Table 188-8 [24]. The role of diagnostic ERCP presently is limited, and the test is generally undertaken as a prelude to endoscopic therapeutic intervention as outlined in Table 188-8. In fact, magnetic resonance cholangiopancreatography may replace diagnostic ERCP in the future (see Chapter 196). Currently, diagnostic ERCP is

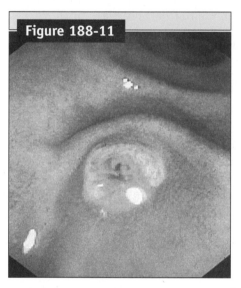

Figure 188-11

Normal endoscopic appearance of the papilla in the second part of the duodenum.

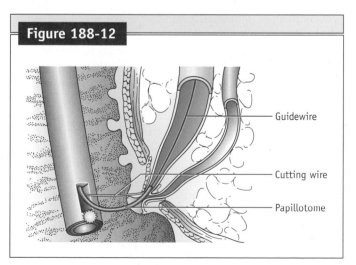

Figure 188-12

Guidewire

Cutting wire

Papillotome

Schematic view of conventional endoscopic sphincterotomy with the cutting wire of papillotome bowed against the papilla. (*From* Freeman *et al.* [27••]; with permission.)

Table 188-8. Indications for Endoscopic Retrograde Cholangiopancreatography

Diagnostic
  Jaundice when biliary obstruction is suspected if therapeutic maneuvers can be performed
  Patients without jaundice with clinical, biochemical, or imaging data suggestive of pancreatic or biliary tract disease
  Evaluation of pancreatic cancer when other imaging tests are equivocal or nondiagnostic
  Pancreatitis of uncertain etiology
  Preoperative planning for patients with chronic pancreatitis or pancreatic pseudocyst
  Suspected dysfunction of the sphincter of Oddi
Therapeutic
  Endoscopic sphincterotomy
    Choledocholithiasis
      Complicated by ascending cholangitis or pancreatitis
      In selected individuals with intact gallbladder who are deemed to be too high an operative risk
    Facilitate stent insertion
    Facilitate balloon dilation of biliary stricture
    Sump syndrome
    Choledochocele involving major papilla
    Ampullary carcinoma in patients that are not surgical candidates
    Selected individuals with sphincter of Oddi dysfunction
  Stent insertion
    Palliation of malignant jaundice
    Biliary fistula
    Postoperative bile duct injury
    Dominant stricture in primary sclerosing cholangitis
    High risk patients with large unremovable common bile duct stones
  Balloon dilation of biliary strictures
  Nasobiliary drainage
    Prevention or treatment of cholangitis or retained stones for decompression of obstructed common bile duct

used to evaluate unexplained pancreatitis or suspected pancreatic cancer when clinical, laboratory, and imaging data are inconclusive (see Chapter 142). ERCP is a central tool in the approach to obstructive jaundice. It defines the anatomy of the biliary and pancreatic ducts, permits biopsy and cytologic brushings of suspicious lesions, and facilitates therapeutic interventions such as stone extraction and stent insertion. ERCP is useful in patients with suspected biliary pancreatitis, although there is controversy about the optimal timing of the procedure in this setting (see Chapters 134 and 142). Early ERCP within 24 to 72 hours is appropriate in patients with cholangitis and progressive jaundice [25]. Early ERCP, however, is no more beneficial than conventional conservative therapy and may be associated with more complications in patients presenting without jaundice or cholangitis [26]. ERCP appears to have no role in the management of severe or worsening acute pancreatitis if there is no evidence of biliary obstruction. Suspected sphincter of Oddi dysfunction is perhaps the most controversial indication for ERCP, in part because of the inconsistent definition of the syndrome, the high complication rate of endoscopic sphincterotomy in affected patients, and the possibility that the disorder may be a manifestation of brain–gut dysfunction rather than a structural abnormality (see Chapter 128).

Endoscopic retrograde cholangiopancreatography should not be used in patients with chronic abdominal pain of unknown cause in the absence of other objective findings suggestive of pancreaticobiliary tract disease. It also has no role in suspected gallbladder disease or in the diagnosis of pancreatic cancer when the diagnosis has already been made by radiographic imaging with percutaneous biopsy or cytology. Contraindications to ERCP are otherwise the same as for upper endoscopy. ERCP should not be done when there is an obstruction or suspected perforation of the gastrointestinal tract. ERCP generally should not be performed in the setting of acute pancreatitis, except under select circumstances as outlined previously. Coagulopathy and contrast allergy are relative contraindications to the procedure.

Risks and Complications

The risks associated with ERCP and endoscopic sphincterotomy are higher than those of any other endoscopic procedure. The complication rate is about 10% [23••,27••,28] and includes pancreatitis, cholangitis, perforation, and bleeding. About 1% of patients undergoing ERCP and endoscopic sphincterotomy die [27••]. Pancreatitis is the most common complication of ERCP and sphincterotomy. With sphincter of Oddi dysfunction, the complication rate soars to 19% [27••]. Procedural risk factors for the development of pancreatitis are a difficult cannulation, higher number of injections of contrast media into the pancreatic duct, and use of precut sphincterotomy [27••]. Bleeding, often late, occurs in 1% to 3% of patients [28]. Bleeding occurs primarily after ERCP for stone removal. Patient risk factors for bleeding include coagulopathy, acute cholangitis, and anticoagulation therapy within 3 days [27••]. Procedural risk factors for bleeding include any observed bleeding during the procedure and a case volume of one or less sphincterotomies weekly [27••]. Cholangitis occurs in 1% to 3% of patients [29]. The risk for this increases in patients with per-

sistent obstruction in whom there is failure to achieve adequate drainage at the time of the procedure [29]. Finally, perforation, primarily retroperitoneal, occurs in less than 1% of cases [29].

ENDOSCOPIC ULTRASONOGRAPHY

Endoscopic ultrasonography (EUS) combines features of endoscopy and ultrasonography and provides information not available by either technique alone on the structure of the gastrointestinal tract and its surrounding tissues. The major application of EUS is in staging of gastrointestinal malignancies, but a number of exciting new applications are under development.

Instrumentation

Two types of dedicated echoendoscopes are available. One device uses a built-in mechanical transducer that is rotated in a 360° arc by a motor mounted in the proximal part of the endoscope. The image obtained is a radial sector scan in a plane perpendicular to the long axis of the endoscope. Endoscopic images can be obtained simultaneously, but the angle of view is 80°, oblique to the image obtained with a standard forward-viewing endoscope. The other instrument uses an electronic curved array transducer mounted in front of the optical lens of an oblique-viewing endoscope. This instrument obtains a 100° linear sector scan in a plane parallel to the long axis of the endoscope. This echoendoscope also is capable of Doppler studies and other interventions, such as fine-needle aspiration and neurolysis.

Both types of instruments use frequencies of 5 to 12 MHz to obtain ultrasonographic images of the gastrointestinal tract. Higher frequencies are associated with decreased depth of visualization. To eliminate air artifacts, acoustic coupling with the target structure is obtained by filling a small latex balloon covering the transducer with deaerated water or by placing 300 to 500 mL of water into the intestinal lumen. In addition, small probes devoid of optical views are available that can be placed into structures such as stenotic tumors and the pancreaticobiliary tree.

Technique

Preparation for EUS is the same as that for routine endoscopic procedures. Because direct visualization of anatomy with echoendoscopes is limited, a standard endoscopic examination should be carried out first to identify areas of potential interest for the subsequent endosonographic examination. A satisfactory interface with the esophagus requires that the balloon surrounding the transducer be filled with water, whereas interface with the stomach requires that the stomach be filled with 300 to 500 mL of water. Proper imaging typically requires a perpendicular orientation of the scanning plane to the target organ. The pancreas is visualized from several positions: the body and tail are viewed best from the gastric antrum, whereas the head and papilla are viewed best from the duodenum with balloon insufflation. The intrahepatic biliary tree and porta hepatis are examined best from the lesser curvature, and the common bile duct is viewed best from the duodenum.

The normal gastrointestinal wall typically is imaged as a five-layered structure of alternating hyperechogenicity and hypoechogenicity (Fig. 188-13). The first hyperechoic layer represents the superficial mucosa; the second hypoechoic layer represents the deep mucosa and muscularis mucosa; the third hyperechoic layer represents submucosa and muscularis propria interface; the fourth hypoechoic layer represents the muscularis propria; and the fifth hyperechoic layer represents the serosa or adventitia. The total wall thickness depicted by EUS does not correlate with histologic thickness of the structure imaged. Neoplasms typically cause disruption in the continuity of a layer.

Training

Endoscopic ultrasonography is one of the most technically demanding endoscopic procedures. Facility with the side-viewing duodenoscope is essential, so that the examiner can orient the oblique views obtained. In addition, training is required in the principles of gastrointestinal anatomy, ultrasonography, image interpretation, and artifacts, especially those related to tangential wall imaging. Expert opinion suggests that a minimum of 50 examinations is necessary to master EUS of the esophagus and stomach, whereas 100 to 150 examinations are necessary to achieve proficiency in the pancreaticobiliary region [30]. Proficiency in esophageal EUS, however, may require far more

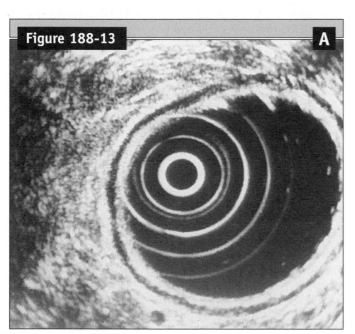

Figure 188-13   **A**

than 50 examinations. Fockens and associates [31] demonstrated a clear learning curve for EUS in esophageal cancer, with an overall accuracy of only 58% for T staging in the first 100 examinations, compared with 83% in the subsequent 100 examinations. Interobserver variation also is a problem, especially in the interpretation of stage T2 lesions and lymph nodes [32].

Indications

The major role of EUS is in the staging of gastrointestinal neoplasms, for which it routinely is superior to computed tomographic (CT) scanning and conventional ultrasonography in assessing depth of tumor invasion and regional lymph node involvement. EUS has an accuracy of about 90% for T staging of esophageal, gastric, rectal, and pancreatic carcinoma and of 80% for nodal staging [33]. EUS also may help to delineate subepithelial masses, such as varices, leiomyomas, and adjacent structures, by providing information on the size and location of the lesion relative to the bowel wall and its characteristics, such as whether it is intrinsic or extrinsic to the wall, cystic, solid, or vascular.

In the stomach, EUS may be useful in the evaluation of enlarged gastric folds. Infiltrating gastric carcinoma, lymphoma, and Ménétrier's disease may otherwise be difficult to distinguish on routine endoscopy with biopsy.

In the pancreas, EUS may be especially helpful in detecting invasion of splenic and portal veins in patients with pancreatic cancer and is more accurate than CT scanning [34•]. EUS also is useful for detecting small islet cell tumors of the pancreas [35], although this application has been eclipsed by somatostatin receptor scintigraphy, which is now considered the single best imaging test for pancreatic endocrine tumors. EUS may provide useful information in patients with suspected chronic pancreatitis and help to guide puncture of a pseudocyst before endoscopic cystenterostomy drainage, so as to avoid vascular structures.

Endoscopic ultrasonography has emerged as an excellent imaging option in patients with suspected choledocholithiasis and is more accurate than CT and ultrasonography. It is as accurate as ERCP, but without some of the associated risks [36].

In the anorectum, EUS provides information complementary to physiologic studies in the preoperative assessment of patients

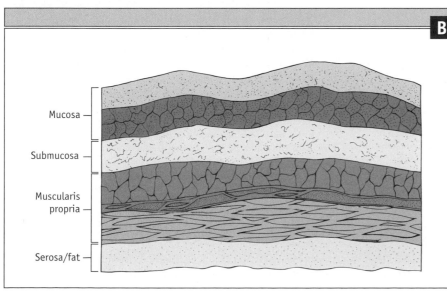

B

Endosonographic appearance of a normal esophagus (**A**) and the various layers of the esophagus to which it corresponds (**B**). The first hyperechoic layer represents the superficial mucosa; the second hypoechoic layer represents the deep mucosa and muscularis mucosa; the third hyperechoic layer represents the submucosa and muscularis propria interface; the fourth hypoechoic layer represents the muscularis propria; and the fifth hyperechoic layer represents the serosa or adventitia. (*From* Wu [41].)

with incontinence. This permits better selection of patients with sphincter damage who may benefit from surgery.

Fine-needle cytologic aspiration of lesions detected by EUS may further enhance its applicability [37]. In addition, EUS may be used for directed injection of the celiac plexus for pain control in patients with intra-abdominal malignancy and chronic pain [38].

Endoscopic ultrasonography has a number of limitations. The technique is operator dependent with a definite learning curve and interobserver variation, especially for stage T2 tumors, as described previously. The depth of tumor invasion may be overestimated if there is a concomitant inflammatory reaction. Malignant strictures pose an increased risk of perforation and inaccurate staging. Small lymph nodes with microscopic metastases generally are not detected by EUS, and criteria for lymph node abnormalities are still uncertain. Leiomyomas may be difficult to distinguish from leiomyosarcomas.

Risks and Complications

Contraindications and risks of EUS are comparable to those for standard upper and lower endoscopy. Esophageal perforation is the most common complication, occurring in 0.17% to 0.035% of cases [39].

■ REFERENCES

Recently published papers of particular interest have been highlighted as follows:
- •   Of interest
- ••   Of outstanding interest

1. The ASGE Standard of Practice Committee: Antibiotic prophylaxis for gastrointestinal endoscopy. *Gastrointest Endosc* 1995, 42:615–617.

2. Dajani AS, Taubert KA, Wilson W, *et al.*: Prevention of bacterial endocarditis: recommendations by the American Heart Association. *JAMA* 1997, 277:1794–1801.

3. The ASGE Standard of Practice Committee: Management of anticoagulation and antiplatelet therapy for endoscopic procedures. *Gastrointest Endosc* (In press)

4.• Higgins TL, Hearn CJ, Maurer WG: Conscious sedation: what an internist needs to know. *Cleve Clin J Med* 1996, 63:355–361.
This excellent review of the principles of conscious sedation includes appropriate dosing of anxiolytics and analgesics, and potential pitfalls.

5. Froelich F, Schwizer W, Thorens J, *et al.*: Conscious sedation for gastroscopy. *Gastroenterology* 1995, 108:697–704.

6. The ASGE Standards of Training Committee: Principles of training in gastrointestinal endoscopy. *Gastrointest Endosc* 1992, 38:743–746.

7.•• Cass OW, Freeman ML, Peine CJ, *et al.*: Objective evaluation of endoscopy skills during training. *Ann Intern Med* 1993, 118:40–44.
Using a mix of patients typical of clinical practice, trainees did not achieve esophageal intubation on endoscopy with a success rate of 90% until more than 100 procedures had been performed. After 100 colonoscopies, the success rate for cecal intubation was 84%, whereas it was more than 90% when more than 200 procedures had been performed. This study calls into question the ASGE thresholds for clinical competence.

8. Fendrick AM, Chernew ME, Hirth RA, *et al.*: Alternative management strategies for patients with suspected peptic ulcer disease. *Ann Intern Med* 1995, 123:260–268.

9. Ofman JJ, Etchason J, Fullerton S, *et al.*: Management strategies for *Helicobacter pylori*-seropositive patients with dyspepsia: clinical and economic consequences. *Ann Intern Med* 1997, 126:280–291.

10. Bytzer P, Hansen JM, Schaffalitzky de Muckadell OB: Empirical H_2-blocker therapy or prompt endoscopy in management of dyspepsia. *Lancet* 1994, 343:811–816.

11. Silverstein MD, Petterson T, Talley NJ: Initial endoscopy or empirical therapy with and without testing for *Helicobacter pylori* for dyspepsia: a decision analysis. *Gastroenterology* 1996, 110:72–83.

12. American Gastroenterological Association Medical Position Statement: Guidelines for the use of enteral nutrition. *Gastroenterology* 1995, 108:1280–1281.

13. Herman LL, Hoskins WJ, Shike M: Percutaneous endoscopic gastrostomy for decompression of the stomach and small bowel. *Gastrointest Endosc* 1992, 38:314–318.

14. Kirby DF, Delegge MH, Fleming CR: American Gastroenterological Association technical review on tube feedings for enteral nutrition. *Gastroenterology* 1995, 108:1282–1301.

15. Taylor CA, Larson DE, Ballard DJ, *et al.*: Predictors of outcome after percutaneous endoscopic gastrostomy: a community-based study. *Mayo Clin Proc* 1992, 67:1042–1049.

16.• Keffe EB: Colonoscopy preps: what's best [Editorial]. *Gastrointest Endosc* 1996, 43:524–528.
In this report, the author provides a summary of the composition of different colonoscopy preparations as well as problems associated with them.

17. Marshall JB: Technical proficiency of trainees performing colonoscopy: a learning curve. *Gastrointest Endosc* 1995, 42:287–291.

18.•• Winawer SJ, Fletcher RH, Miller L, *et al.*: Colorectal cancer screening: guidelines and rationale. *Gastroenterology* 1997, 112:594–642.
In this report current recommendations for colorectal cancer screening are justified by a thorough literature review.

19. van den Hazel SJ, Speelman P, Dankert J, *et al.*: Piperacillin to prevent cholangitis after endoscopic retrograde cholangiopancreatography: a randomized, controlled trial. *Ann Intern Med* 1996, 125:442–447.

20. The ASGE Technical Assessment Committee: Radiographic contrast media used in ERCP. *Gastrointest Endosc* 1996, 43:647–651.

21. Health and Public Policy Committee, American College of Physicians: Clinical competence in endoscopic retrograde cholangiopancreatography. *Ann Intern Med* 1988, 108:142–144.

22. Watkins JL, Etzkorn KP, Wiley TE, *et al.*: Assessment of technical competence during ERCP training. *Gastrointest Endosc* 1996, 44:411–415.

23.•• Jowell PS, Baillie J, Branch MS, *et al.*: Quantitative assessment of procedural competence: a prospective study of training in endoscopic retrograde cholangiopancreatography. *Ann Intern Med* 1996, 125:983–989.
The authors report here, that the number of ERCPs done by a group of trainees before competency was attained was 140 for pancreatography, 160 for cholangiography, 120 for stone extraction, and 60 for stent insertion. Overall competence was achieved only after completing 200 ERCPs, a number much greater than previous recommendations.

24. The ASGE Standards of Practice Committee: The role of endoscopy in diseases of the biliary tract and pancreas: guidelines for clinical application. *Gastrointestin Endosc* 1989, 35:598–599

25. Baillie J: Treatment of acute biliary pancreatitis [Editorial]. *N Engl J Med* 1997, 336:286–287.

26. Folsch UR, Nitsche R, Ludtke R, *et al.*: Early ERCP and papillotomy compared with conservative treatment for acute biliary pancreatitis. *N Engl J Med* 1997, 336:237–242.

27.•• Freeman ML, Nelson DB, Sherman S, *et al.*: Complications of endoscopic biliary sphincterotomy. *N Engl J Med* 1996, 335:909–919.
This multicenter study of 2347 patients demonstrated an overall complication rate of 9.8%. Five significant risk factors for complications were identified on multivariate analysis: suspected sphincter of Oddi dysfunction, cirrhosis, difficulty cannulating the bile duct, precut sphincterotomy, and combined percutaneous and endoscopic procedures. Endoscopists who performed less than one sphincterotomy per week had a higher complication rate.

28. Huibregtse K: Complications of endoscopic sphincterotomy and their prevention [Editorial]. *N Engl J Med* 1996, 335:961–963.

29. Bjorkman DJ, Van Dam J: Outpatient therapeutic ERCP: cutting sphincters and cutting costs [Editorial]. *Am J Gastroenterol* 1996, 91:1485–1486.

30. Caletti G, Odegaard S, Rosch T, *et al.*: Endoscopic ultrasonography (EUS): a summary of the conclusions of the working party for the Tenth World Congress of Gastroenterology, Los Angeles, California, October 1994. *Am J Gastroenterol* 1994, 89(suppl):5138–5143.

31. Fockens P, Van den Brande JHM, van Dullemen HM, *et al.*: Endosonographic T-staging of esophageal carcinoma: a learning curve. *Gastrointest Endosc* 1996, 44:58–62.

32. Catalano MF, Sivak MV, Bedford R, *et al.*: Observer variation and reproducibility of endoscopic ultrasonography. *Gastrointest Endosc* 1995, 41:115–120.

33. Chang KJ: Endoscopic ultrasound: moving toward permanence [Editorial]. *Gastrointest Endosc* 1996, 44:502–504.

34.• Tenner S, Banks PA, Wiersma MJ, *et al.*: Evaluation of pancreatic disease by endoscopic ultrasonography. *Am J Gastroenterol* 1997, 92:18–26.
The authors present a comprehensive review of the current role of EUS in pancreatic diseases.

35. Rosch T, Lightdale CJ, Botet JF, *et al.*: Localization of pancreatic endocrine tumors by endoscopic ultrasonography. *N Engl J Med* 1992, 326:1721–1726.

36. Sugiyama M, Atomi Y: Endoscopic ultrasonography for diagnosing choledocholithiasis: a prospective comparative study with ultrasonography and computed tomography. *Gastrointest Endosc* 1997, 45:143–146.

37. Wiersema MJ, Wiersema LM, Khusro Q, *et al.*: Combined endosonography and fine-needle aspiration cytology in the evaluation of gastrointestinal lesions. *Gastrointest Endosc* 1994, 40:199–206.

38. Wiersema MJ, Wiersema LM: Endosonography-guided celiac plexus neurolysis. *Gastrointest Endosc* 1996, 44:656–672.

39. ASGE technology assessment status evaluation: endoscopic ultrasonography. *Gastrointest Endosc* 1994,40:796–797.

40. Nostrant TT: Colonoscopy of the anus, rectum, and normal colon. In *Gastroenterology and Hepatology: The Comprehensive Visual Reference*, vol 2: *Colon, Rectum, and Anus*. Edited by Boland CR. Philadelphia: Current Medicine; 1996:2.1–2.16

41. Wu WC: Diagnostic esophageal endoscopy. In *Gastroenterology and Hepatology: The Comprehensive Visual Reference*, vol 5: *Esophagus and Pharynx*. Edited by Orlando RC. Philadelphia: Current Medicine; 1997:2.1–2.11.

189 Complications of Endoscopy
M. Brian Fennerty

Gastrointestinal endoscopy is a remarkably safe procedure, and complications occur infrequently. However, given the millions of endoscopic procedures performed each year in the United States, physicians may encounter procedure-related complications. Furthermore, certain procedures, such as colonoscopy with polypectomy and endoscopic retrograde cholangiopancreatography (ERCP), are associated with substantially increased incidence and severity of complications. Perforation at the time of endoscopy is the most frequent cause of malpractice litigation against gastroenterologists. The endoscopist must be aware of the risks associated with the procedure and with ways to avoid, recognize, and treat complications. This chapter covers the global complications of endoscopy, including those related to patient sedation and monitoring; the risks and complications specific to each procedure; and the prevention, recognition, and treatment of those complications.

EPIDEMIOLOGY OF ENDOSCOPIC COMPLICATIONS
Overall, endoscopy is a remarkably safe procedure. The morbidity rate associated with endoscopic procedures is about 0.5%, and the overall mortality rate is 0.05% (Table 189-1). When considering all endoscopic procedures, most complications are cardiopulmonary, often associated with sedation. In patients undergoing specific procedures, however, cardiopulmonary complications are less common than other serious complications; for example, hemorrhage can occur after colonoscopic polypectomy and pancreatitis can occur after ERCP. Cardiopulmonary complications often are related to other med-

ical illnesses and not to the procedure itself, whereas perforation and bleeding are related to technical aspects of the procedure.

RISKS OF SEDATION AND CARDIOVASCULAR COMPLICATIONS
The most common endoscopic complications of diagnostic examinations are cardiopulmonary; in therapeutic procedures, however, bleeding and perforation are more common than cardiopulmonary complications. Most cardiopulmonary complications are related to

Table 189-1. Frequency of Complications of Endoscopy

Procedure	Morbidity Rate, %	Mortality Rate, %
All	0.5	0.05
EGD		
Diagnostic	0.1	0.02
Dilation	2.0	1.00
PEG	10.0	1.00
Colonoscopy		
Diagnostic	0.5	0.01
Polypectomy	2.0	0.10
ERCP		
Diagnostic	5.0	0.10
Sphincterotomy	10.0	0.40

EGD—esophagogastroduodenoscopy; ERCP—endoscopic retrograde cholangiopancreatography; PEG—percutaneous endoscopic gastrostomy.

patient sedation, which can induce hypoxia, decrease blood pressure, and incite hemodynamic events:

Dysrhythmia
Myocardial ischemia
Hypotension
Cerebrovascular accident
Aspiration
Respiratory arrest or apnea
Bronchospasm
Hypoxia
Hypercarbia
Laryngospasm

Cardiac ischemia can occur during endoscopic procedures as a result of increases in heart rate and blood pressure caused by anxiety or discomfort in an unsedated or undersedated patient. Thus, cardiopulmonary complications are not always directly related to sedation.

The incidence of cardiopulmonary complications during endoscopy is particularly low, ranging from 0.2% to 0.54% in database reviews and prospective surveys [1••,2]. Mortality from a cardiopulmonary complication during endoscopy is even less common, occurring in 0.03% to 0.05% of cases [1••,2].

Who is at risk of endoscopic cardiopulmonary complications, and what are the precipitating factors? Oxygen desaturation occurs frequently during upper endoscopy, colonoscopy, and ERCP. Between 20% and 50% of patients undergoing sedation for endoscopic procedures demonstrate desaturation to less than 90% during the procedure [3]. The incidence of oxygen desaturation is greatest in patients who are given narcotic sedatives and in those who undergo colonoscopy or ERCP. The greater frequency of hypoxia seen with colonoscopy and ERCP is related, in part, to the deeper degree of sedation and to the more frequent use of both narcotics and sedatives in these procedures. Severe desaturation (to less than 85%) occurs in about 15% of sedated patients undergoing endoscopy. During upper endoscopy, oxygen desaturation may be more frequent with use of a large endoscope. Hypoxia also occurs in about 10% of unsedated patients and, in this situation, is probably secondary to endoscopic obstruction of the airway, abdominal distention caused by insufflation of air, or decreased ventilatory excursion. Thus, avoidance of sedation does not necessarily prevent oxygen desaturation, nor does it prevent cardiopulmonary complications during endoscopy.

Abnormalities in blood pressure also are observed frequently during endoscopy [3]. Hypotension occurs in as many as one third of patients undergoing colonoscopy, although it is less common with upper endoscopy. Whether this is because of a vagal response or a physiologic response to bowel distention or stretching is unknown. Hypertension is more frequent in patients who are undersedated and uncomfortable during the procedure and probably represents a physiologic response to pain and anxiety.

Abnormalities in cardiac rhythm, especially bradycardia or tachycardia, also are common during endoscopic procedures, usually occurring in response to discomfort, anxiety, or distention and stretching of the bowel. Abnormalities of the pulse have been reported in as many as 10% to 20% of patients and are more common in patients undergoing colonoscopy [3].

Although these physiologic changes in oxygen saturation, blood pressure, and cardiac rhythm are not actually complications, they may contribute to cardiac ischemia, which can result in dysrhythmia or myocardial infarction. Furthermore, oversedation decreases the ventilatory drive and pharyngeal protective mechanisms, which may result in respiratory arrest or aspiration if the patient's airway is not protected.

Given the frequency of physiologic perturbations in patients undergoing endoscopy and the possibility of cardiopulmonary complications, can patients at increased risk of these complications be identified? Some clinicians assume that patients with coronary artery disease have an increased incidence of adverse cardiopulmonary events during endoscopic procedures. Evidence shows, however, that only 15% of patients with unstable angina pectoris have ischemia before, during, or immediately after endoscopy, and only 2% suffer myocardial infarction after the examination [4]. These findings highlight the infrequent occurrence of cardiopulmonary complications, even in high-risk patients.

In the United States, patients undergoing endoscopic procedures are monitored physiologically. Monitoring usually consists of measurement of oxygen saturation, respiratory and pulse rates, blood pressure, and often cardiac rhythm. No data, however, have shown that monitoring decreases the frequency of cardiopulmonary complications or improves clinical outcome. Monitoring may lead the endoscopist to a false sense of security. Although a patient's oxygen saturation may remain adequate during a procedure, hypercarbia may develop. This is most likely to occur in patients receiving supplemental oxygen during deep sedation for ERCP or colonoscopy [5]. Furthermore, peripheral oxygen saturation correlates poorly with actual tissue ischemia. Nonetheless, monitoring of oxygen saturation, blood pressure, and pulse appears to be prudent, despite the lack of proven efficacy, because it is safe and may prevent serious morbidity. There are substantial costs associated with such physiologic monitoring during endoscopy, however, and its cost-effectiveness is unknown but probably low.

How best to prevent physiologic perturbations and to minimize cardiopulmonary complications is uncertain. Use of prophylactic supplemental oxygen decreases the incidence of oxygen desaturation from about 40% to less than 10% during procedures performed with the patient sedated [6]. Despite these data, no prospective trial has shown an improvement in overall outcome or a reduction in the frequency of concomitant dysrhythmia or cardiac ischemia with the use of supplemental oxygen.

The incidence of hypoxia can be decreased by minimizing the degree of sedation, the amount of air insufflated, and hence the severity of bowel distention. Whether a reduction in hypoxia is clinically relevant or improves overall outcome is unknown.

Narcotic and sedative agents with a quicker onset of action and shorter duration of effect were initially considered safer than longer-acting agents. Prospective trials have shown, however, that the various types of narcotics and sedatives affect oxygen saturation, blood pressure, and heart rate similarly. Newer anesthetic agents, such as propofol, although effective, do not appear to be safer than standard agents and have narrow therapeutic ranges with potential to cause severe hypoventilation. They should be used only by trained personnel. The widespread practice of using general anesthesia during pediatric endoscopy is, for the most part, unnecessary and associated with a higher incidence of cardiopulmonary complications and greater cost than is the use of conscious sedation.

When oxygen desaturation occurs during an endoscopic procedure, it is prudent to treat the patient with supplemental oxygen. This nearly always corrects desaturation, although it may not correct hypercarbia (and hypoventilation). If oxygen desaturation is not reversed with oxygen, the procedure should be discontinued. In patients who continue to manifest desaturation or other physiologic abnormalities, reversal of sedation with the benzodiazepine antagonist flumazenil, the opiate antagonist naloxone (when narcotics have been used), or both reverses the sedation within minutes. When narcotics have been used, hypoventilation may persist or recur for 1 hour or longer despite the appearance of an awake patient, and continued monitoring is required.

Although part of the standard of care during endoscopy, monitoring has not been shown to decrease the incidence of cardiopulmonary complications, and it is incumbent on the endoscopist not to develop a false sense of security regarding endoscopic safety simply because the patient is being monitored.

Rarer complications of endoscopy related at least in part to the use of sedation include phlebitis at the intravenous needle or catheter insertion site and toxic reactions to topical pharyngeal anesthetics used to facilitate upper endoscopy.

■ INFECTIOUS COMPLICATIONS

Infectious complications of invasive procedures, including endoscopy, have received increased scrutiny since the emergence of the human immunodeficiency virus epidemic (see Chapter 195). Transmission of infection during endoscopy is extremely rare, however, with an incidence of only four to five infectious complications per 1 million endoscopic procedures. Therefore, it is unlikely that efforts designed to avoid these rare complications will prove cost-effective, nor is it likely that efficacy can be demonstrated in clinical studies.

Most infectious complications of endoscopy are iatrogenic, with the infectious agents transmitted by contaminated endoscopes. *Mycobacterium* and *Pseudomonas* species, *Helicobacter pylori*, and other pathogens have been shown to be transmitted iatrogenically during endoscopic procedures, almost always as a result of insufficient decontamination of the endoscope. In addition, *Mycobacterium* and *Pseudomonas* species have been cultured from automated washers, representing another possible source of contamination. Viral contamination of endoscopes and washers probably also occurs but has not been demonstrated. There has not been a single documented case of human immunodeficiency virus transmission during an endoscopic procedure.

Another infectious complication is endocarditis secondary to bacteremia, which occurs frequently during endoscopic procedures. There is no evidence, however, that endoscopy has ever directly caused a case of endocarditis, nor is there evidence that prophylactic administration of antibiotics prevents endocarditis after endoscopy.

Only two endoscopic procedures, variceal sclerotherapy and dilation of esophageal strictures, are considered high-risk procedures for bacteremia and presumably endocarditis. These procedures are associated with a significantly higher incidence of bacteremia than are other endoscopic procedures. The frequency of bacteremia during routine endoscopy is no greater than that associated with teeth brushing.

Antibiotic prophylaxis for endocarditis should be prescribed only to patients with prosthetic valves, systemic pulmonary shunts, or a prior history of bacterial endocarditis (Table 189-2). Even in this higher-risk group, prophylaxis is indicated only for patients undergoing either variceal sclerotherapy or dilation of an esophageal stricture.

It is unknown whether mitral valve prolapse confers an increased risk of endocarditis after endoscopy, or whether prophylactic treatment of patients with mitral valve prolapse is warranted. This cardiac lesion is found in as many as 5% of patients undergoing endoscopy [7] and could account for more than half of patients receiving prophylactic antibiotics. Even if the risk of endocarditis were confined to patients with mitral valve prolapse accompanied by mitral regurgitation, this disease would still account for 28% of all patients who have a possible indication for prophylactic antibiotics and for 1.4% of all patients undergoing endoscopy. Given the rare occurrence of endocarditis after endoscopy, it is apparent that mitral regurgitation secondary to mitral valve prolapse is not an appropriate indication for endocarditis prophylaxis during endoscopic procedures.

Despite clearly defined recommendations, only half of patients receive the correct antibiotic regimen and doses (Table 189-3) [7].

Table 189-2. Indications for Antibiotic Prophylaxis for Endoscopy

High-risk procedure indications—prophylaxis indicated
  Sclerotherapy
  Esophageal dilation
High-risk clinical conditions—prophylaxis indicated
  Prosthetic heart valve
  Prior history of endocarditis
  Surgically constructed systemic-pulmonary shunt
Lower-risk clinical conditions—prophylaxis optional
  Congenital malformations
  Acquired valvular dysfunction
  Mitral valve prolapse with regurgitation
  Hypertrophic cardiomyopathy

Table 189-3. Regimens for Endocarditis Prophylaxis in Endoscopy

Low-risk patients
  Amoxicillin, 3000 mg PO 60 min before procedure, then 1500 mg
    6 h later
High-risk patients
  Ampicillin, 2000 mg IV or IM and gentamicin, 1.5 mg/kg IV or IM
    30–60 min before procedure, then repeat doses 8 h later, or give
    amoxicillin, 1500 mg PO 6 h later
Penicillin-allergic patients
  Vancomycin, 1000 mg IV, and gentamicin, 1.5 mg/kg IV
    or IM 60 min before procedure; may repeat 8 h later

IM—intramuscularly; IV—intravenously; PO—by mouth.

Furthermore, endocarditis prophylaxis is widely overused and often prescribed when not indicated [8]. Because the estimated risk of endocarditis is only 1 in 5 to 10 million endoscopic procedures, prophylaxis is probably not cost-effective unless the patient falls into a high-risk category and is undergoing either variceal sclerotherapy or dilation of an esophageal stricture. Even in these patients, however, cost-effectiveness has not been proved.

Another infectious complication of endoscopy is bacterial contamination of ascites (bacterascites), which can result in bacterial peritonitis. The risk of bacterascites is increased in patients undergoing endoscopy for upper gastrointestinal hemorrhage, especially in those undergoing variceal sclerotherapy. The incidence of bacteremia during sclerotherapy can be decreased from 30% to 5% with the prophylactic use of an antimicrobial agent, such as cefotaxime. Antimicrobial therapy, however, has not been shown to reduce the frequency of clinically relevant infectious outcomes, such as bacterial peritonitis.

■ COMPLICATIONS OF UPPER ENDOSCOPY

Two additional risks of upper endoscopic procedures are perforation and bleeding (Table 189-4). The overall complication rate from upper endoscopy is about 0.1%, with death occurring in 0.01% to 0.03% of patients [9].

During diagnostic upper endoscopic examinations, perforation occurs in about 0.02% to 0.4% of patients, with a mortality rate secondary to perforation of 0.8% or less. In patients undergoing endoscopy with dilation, perforation can occur in up to 3%, with mortality rates of 1% or more [10]. Perforation during upper endoscopy most commonly occurs in the thoracic esophagus and is usually related to underlying esophageal pathology, such as a stricture. Less commonly, perforation occurs in the cervical esophagus, usually as a result of trauma during passage of the endoscope. The clinical syndromes resulting from perforation of these two esophageal sites are distinct, as are the subsequent morbidity and mortality rates. The mortality rate associated with cervical perforation is 0% to 15%, and that associated with thoracic perforation is 50% to 65% [9]. This difference in mortality rates reflects comorbidity in patients who experience thoracic perforations as well as the more serious nature of the thoracic perforation.

The risk of perforation of the cervical esophagus is associated with the presence of anterior cervical osteophytes, Zenker's diverticula, rings, webs, and strictures at this site. In many cases, perforation occurs during blind esophageal intubation and usually can be avoided by intubation of the esophagus under direct vision.

Perforation of the thoracic esophagus usually occurs at benign or malignant strictures. The rate of perforation of malignant strictures is substantially higher than that of benign strictures.

Table 189-4. Complications of Esophagogastroduodenoscopy*	
Cardiopulmonary	Infections
Perforation	Mallory-Weiss tear
Bleeding	Hematoma

In estimated order of frequency.

Perforation of a stricture occurs either during advancement of the instrument tip through the stricture or during dilation of the stricture (with a wire-guided bougie, perioral passage of a bougie, or through-the-scope balloon dilators). The increased mortality rate of thoracic esophageal perforations as compared with cervical esophageal perforations reflects in part the higher incidence of malignant strictures.

Esophageal perforation usually manifests clinically within minutes or hours, although a delay in presentation of as long as 1 week has been reported. Patients with perforation of the thoracic esophagus usually develop substernal chest pain, whereas those with cervical perforation usually complain of neck or jaw pain. Crepitus may accompany both types of perforation. Radiographs of the chest or neck usually reveal evidence of subcutaneous or intrapleural gas as well as fluid collections in the neck or chest, depending on the site of perforation.

When esophageal perforation is suspected, radiographic imaging can help localize the site (Fig. 189-1). Initial imaging with a water-soluble contrast agent is appropriate, followed if necessary by imaging with barium (which is more sensitive) to demonstrate the disruption. The presence of a free perforation usually indicates that the disruption is large and that surgical repair is necessary, whereas small, contained perforations can sometimes be managed conservatively. Computed tomographic (CT) scanning also can be used to stage the perforation and may help in determining whether surgical or medical therapy is indicated.

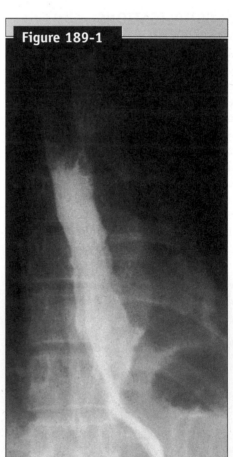

Figure 189-1

Contrast study of the esophagus showing a distal esophageal perforation after balloon dilation for achalasia.

Treatment of esophageal perforation depends on the underlying disease process, extent of delay in recognizing the perforation, and presence of comorbid medical factors. Clinical management includes nasogastric suction, broad-spectrum antibiotics, intravenous nutrition, and in most cases, surgical repair. In clinically stable patients with small, contained perforations, medical therapy alone may suffice; in patients with large leaks, surgical drainage of the infected surrounding tissue and repair of the perforation almost always are required.

Endoscopic perforation at the stomach or duodenum is rare and is usually related to underlying pathology (usually strictures) at the perforation site. The rate of perforation during dilation of pyloric stenosis may be 5% or more [11]. Recognition, diagnostic evaluation, and management of gastric or duodenal perforations are similar to those of esophageal perforations.

Bleeding is a rare complication of diagnostic upper endoscopy, even with ancillary procedures such as biopsy and dilation. Use of nonsteroidal anti-inflammatory drugs by the patient does not appear to increase the risk of clinically important bleeding during endoscopy [12•]. Bleeding can occur secondary to mucosal trauma induced by the instrument tip, at the site of a biopsy or polypectomy, from a stricture that has been dilated, or in unusual circumstances, from a Mallory-Weiss tear caused by retching during the procedure. In almost all cases, bleeding is rarely of arterial origin and follows a clinically benign course.

The clinical presentation of bleeding as a complication of endoscopy is identical to that of gastrointestinal bleeding from other causes, namely hematemesis, melena, and altered vital signs. Therapy is supportive, unless severe hemorrhage results in altered hemodynamics. In this unusual circumstance, attempts at endoscopic thermal ablation or injection therapy, followed, if necessary, by angiography, surgery, or both, may be warranted.

Complications of Dilation

As mentioned previously, dilation accompanying upper intestinal endoscopy significantly increases the risk of perforation, which may be as high as 1% to 3%, with a mortality rate of up to 1%. Perforation, as well as mortality, is increased when the stricture is malignant (Fig. 189-2) [13].

Dilation also results in an increased incidence of bacteremia. The rate of bacteremia with dilation is as high as 50%, which is

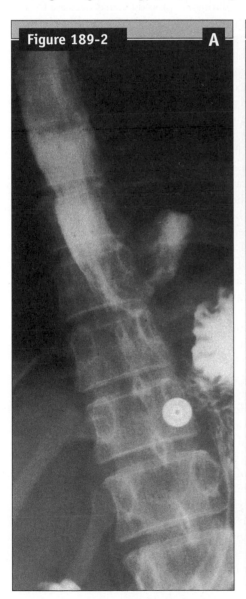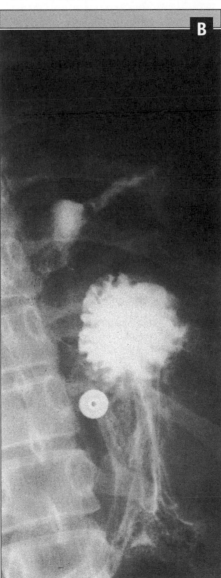

Figure 189-2   **A**   **B**

Contrast study of the esophagus showing free perforation of the distal esophagus after dilation of a malignant distal stricture. The left panel (**A**) reveals contrast outside the esophageal lumen, whereas the right panel (**B**) shows contrast tracking into the mediastinum.

10-fold higher than that with endoscopy alone. This high rate of bacteremia is the rationale for preprocedure antibiotic prophylaxis in patients at high risk of endocarditis.

The relative risk of perforation after dilation is 1% or less for benign stricture, 10% for malignant strictures; 3% to 10% for radiation-induced stricture, and 1% or less for anastomotic strictures [13]. Perforation occurs in up to 5% of patients undergoing forceful balloon dilation for achalasia. The risk of perforation during balloon dilation for achalasia has been associated with malnutrition, higher balloon pressures, and prior dilations [14].

It has been assumed that the risk of perforation during endoscopic dilation of strictures can be minimized by dilating to no more than 2 mm (6F) greater than the initial diameter of the stricture at the start of the dilation session. Although this conservative approach is of unproven efficacy, prudence dictates that tight strictures be dilated gradually over a few sessions. The maximal safe increase in diameter per session is not known. It also is assumed that a guide wire adds to the safety of dilation, but this has not been proved. The widespread use of fluoroscopy during dilation procedures is not justified because it does not decrease the incidence of perforation and adds substantially to the cost of the procedure. Fluoroscopy is a useful safety technique, however, in patients with complex or difficult-to-dilate strictures.

COMPLICATIONS OF PERCUTANEOUS ENDOSCOPIC GASTROSTOMY

Complications during percutaneous endoscopic gastrostomy (PEG) placement occur in about 10% of patients, with a mortality rate of less than 1%. The most common complication related to placement of a PEG is peristomal wound infection. The incidence of wound infection is generally between 5% and 10% but has been reported to be as high as 30% or 40% (most of these infections were minor). Infection usually manifests as erythema, pain, and warmth around the gastrostomy site. Rarely, necrotizing fasciitis occurs, with substantial tissue destruction and much higher morbidity and mortality rates.

Periprocedural administration of antibiotics decreases the incidence of wound infections after PEG from between 30% and 40% to about 15%. Therefore, prophylactic antibiotic coverage with an agent active against staphylococci and streptococci, such as a cephalosporin, is indicated. A single dose given 1 hour before the procedure is adequate. It is unnecessary to perform the procedure, which is not sterile, in an operating room because this approach does not decrease the incidence of post-PEG infections but does increase substantially the cost of the procedure.

Bleeding is rare after PEG placement, as is perforation of adjacent organs, both of which occur in less than 1% of cases. Perforation or fistulization usually occurs when small bowel or colon is trapped between the anterior gastric wall and the abdominal wall during PEG placement. This anatomic phenomenon can sometimes be detected by using a safe-tract approach, in which the local anesthetic needle is continuously aspirated as it is introduced into the abdominal cavity. This technique allows detection of air if a luminal organ is traversed before visualization of the needle as it enters the stomach. No data, however, have shown that this technique decreases the incidence of this unusual complication.

The second most common complication of PEG placement is aspiration pneumonia. This usually occurs as a result of compromised airway protection and the supine positioning of the patient during the procedure. Aspiration can be minimized by keeping the chest of the patient elevated relative to the abdomen during the procedure and by meticulously suctioning the oropharynx and monitoring the airway throughout the procedure.

Unusual complications of PEG include postprocedure ileus and seeding of the stomal tract with cancer in patients with head and neck malignancies. The overall mortality rate of PEG placement is low (1%), but the morbidity rate is high (40%) as a result of the high degree of comorbidity in these patients.

COMPLICATIONS OF THE TREATMENT OF BLEEDING LESIONS

The most common complication of therapeutic endoscopy for upper gastrointestinal bleeding is aspiration (see Chapter 34). Patients who are bleeding typically have large amounts of clotted and liquid blood in their stomachs and are therefore at increased risk of aspiration during upper endoscopy. Intubation of the airway and lavage of gastric contents before endoscopy, as well as meticulous suctioning during the procedure, may decrease the risk of aspiration. In patients with severe bleeding and in obtunded patients who have lost protective reflexes, intubation of the airway before endoscopy also may decrease the risk of aspiration.

Less common complications during therapeutic endoscopy for gastrointestinal bleeding include intramural hematomas at the site of injection and hypertensive emergencies or dysrhythmias related to the use of epinephrine as a therapeutic agent. Perforation during thermal treatment of bleeding lesions is unusual, occurring in less than 1% of cases, and is presumably related to both pressure and thermal injury of the bowel wall where it is thin because of disease, such as an ulcer.

Variceal sclerotherapy is associated with a much higher complication rate than is endoscopic treatment of other upper gastrointestinal bleeding lesions. Necrosis of tissue occurs with all sclerosants used for endoscopic variceal sclerotherapy, and complication rates for this procedure range from 20% to 40% [15]. Peritonitis has been reported in 1% to 3% or cases, pulmonary complications in 20% to 50%, stricture formation in 15% to 20%, and bleeding from ulceration in 10% to 15%. These complications are associated with a periprocedure mortality rate of 1% to 2%. Endoscopic variceal ligation (EVL) is associated with a much lower rate of complications, with strictures occurring in only 0% to 5% of cases and bleeding in less than 5%. The use of an overtube with EVL has been associated with perforation of the cervical esophagus as a result of avulsion injury during insertion of the overtube. The availability of multiband ligators obviates the need for an overtube and therefore rarely is associated with this complication.

The prevention of complications during therapy for esophageal varices is best achieved by EVL rather than sclerotherapy. Strictures caused by sclerotherapy or ligation are treated with dilation. Bleeding from sclerotherapy or EVL-induced ulcers can be severe, and therapy is supportive; transjugular intrahepatic portosystemic shunting is of questionable effectiveness in this setting. Further injection or banding of the ulcer site to control bleeding actually may increase bleeding, precipitating clinical deterioration.

■ COMPLICATIONS OF COLONOSCOPY

The mortality rate associated with colonoscopy is about 0.006%; perforations occur in 0.17% of diagnostic procedures and in 0.41% of procedures that include polypectomy, and hemorrhage occurs in 0.2% of diagnostic procedures and in up to 3% of procedures that include polypectomy [16]. In estimated order of frequency, complications of colonoscopy include the following:

    Cardiopulmonary
    Bleeding
    Postpolypectomy syndrome
    Perforation
    Infection
    Ileus
    Chemical colitis
    Electrolyte abnormalities
    Lacerated solid organ
    Appendicitis

As discussed previously, up to 40% of patients demonstrate transient oxygen desaturation during colonoscopy, and as many as 25% experience oxygen desaturation during the recovery period. Some investigators have shown that colonoscopy can be performed safely and effectively without sedation and with fewer adverse physiologic events. Whether unsedated colonoscopy is safer than colonoscopy with sedation is not known.

An uncommon complication of colonoscopy is disinfectant colitis secondary to inadequate rinsing of the endoscope. This chemical colitis has been reported in association with both glutaraldehyde and hydrogen peroxide [17,18]. The incubation period for disinfectant colitis is 0 to 24 hours, and symptoms last between 6 hours and 1 week. Fever is unusual, but bloody diarrhea and crampy abdominal pain are common. Spontaneous resolution is the rule. CT scanning shows circumferential thickening of the bowel wall, usually greater on the left side than the on right, with heterogeneous mural enhancement that may mimic ischemic, inflammatory, or infectious colitis (the so-called target sign) [19]. Other unusual complications of colonoscopy include acute appendicitis and incarceration of the endoscope within a hernia sac.

The risks of colonoscopy have been considered to be higher in certain patients. Data indicate, however, that colonoscopy is as safe in the elderly as in younger patients, is safe to perform within 3 weeks of bowel surgery, and in selected, stable patients, is safe immediately after myocardial infarction.

Other complications of colonoscopy include those related to bowel preparation. For example, Mallory-Weiss tears have been reported secondary to vomiting during ingestion of the polyethylene glycol bowel preparation, as has fecal incontinence in elderly patients [20]. Adverse reactions to oral sodium phosphate solutions also have been described [21,22]. Although generally better tolerated than polyethylene glycol solutions, oral sodium phosphate solutions may cause increases in serum phosphate levels and decreases in serum calcium and ionized calcium levels. These electrolyte disturbances are rarely of clinical consequence but can be substantial, resulting in symptoms and rarely in death. Therefore, sodium phosphate preparations should be avoided in patients with heart failure, renal disease, or hepatic disease.

Colonoscopic Perforation

The incidence of colonoscopic perforation is less than 0.1% in patients undergoing diagnostic procedures. Perforation rates as low as 0.2% have been reported in those undergoing therapeutic procedures. The incidence of perforation is increased when polypectomy (mainly for large sessile or submucosal lesions), dilation, or thermal ablation of tumors is performed.

The recognition of colonoscopic perforation can be difficult at times. The diagnosis is delayed in as many as 60% of patients, which may explain the associated operative mortality rate of 10% or more and the morbidity rate of 40%. Operative morbidity and mortality are related to the size of the perforation and to comorbidity in the patient. The sigmoid colon is the site of the perforation in 70% of cases, and gross peritonitis is present in more than half of perforations, despite prior bowel preparation.

The mechanism of cecal perforation is different from that of rectosigmoid perforation. Although most perforations in the rectosigmoid colon are secondary to pressure from the tip or the shaft of the endoscope, cecal perforations are usually related to ancillary procedures, such as biopsy or cautery [23]. In addition, many cecal perforations occur at the sites of epithelial pathology, such as an inflammatory or ulcerative disease. Finally, some cecal perforations occur because of excessive air insufflation with consequent colon dilation.

Perforation is most often diagnosed by observing the peritoneum during the procedure or by the detection of free air in the abdominal cavity on plain abdominal radiographs after the procedure. In patients in whom perforation is suspected but plain abdominal films are negative, the diagnosis can be confirmed by a CT scan, which usually shows an extracolonic fluid collection or small amounts of air not recognized on the plain film. Sometimes the only diagnostic sign of colonic perforation is localized peritonitis on physical examination. Benign pneumatosis intestinalis can be observed by endoscopic examination of the colon. This is easily differentiated from a perforation based on the benign clinical course.

Therapy for colonoscopic perforation includes decompression of the bowel by nasogastric suction, prevention or treatment of infection with broad-spectrum antibiotic coverage against both aerobic and anaerobic organisms, bowel rest with intravenous alimentation, and in most cases, operative repair. Nonoperative management can be attempted in some patients, such as those in whom perforation occurred during a therapeutic procedure (perforation small and localized at polypectomy site), in whom the perforation is small, or in whom the perforation is well tolerated [24]. In some cases, exploratory laparoscopy can help determine whether an operative or nonoperative approach is appropriate, and laparoscopic repair of the perforation can be undertaken if clinically necessary.

Bleeding as a Result of Colonoscopy

Bleeding after colonoscopy is most often a result of polypectomy and occurs in 0.1% to 1.5% of patients. Delayed hemorrhage can occur up to 30 days after the procedure but usually is seen within 10 to 14 days [25]. The risk of bleeding does not appear to be increased in patients taking nonsteroidal anti-inflammatory drugs or in those undergoing endoscopic mucosal resections or saline-assisted polypectomy and is not related to the size of the polyp. Bleeding immediately after polypectomy reflects inadequate coagulation, whereas delayed bleeding is a result of erosion of the thermal-induced ulcer into a blood vessel. Bleeding that appears 7 to 10 days after polypectomy is a result of clot or eschar sloughage.

Three fourths of postpolypectomy bleeding episodes can be managed conservatively; the other one fourth of patients require endoscopic electrocauterization, angiography, or rarely, surgery. Bleeding immediately after polypectomy can often be controlled by regrasping the polypectomy site with a snare if some residuum of stalk remains.

Bleeding also can occur from use of a hot biopsy forceps and, in this situation, is more common in the right colon than in the left colon [26]. For reasons that are unclear, the incidence of hot biopsy forceps–induced bleeding in the cecum is about 1.5%, compared with an incidence of 1% in the ascending colon and of 0.25% in the remainder of the bowel. These data suggest that use of this instrument should be reserved for lesions distal to the hepatic flexure. Whether using a cold or bipolar snare or forceps is safer than conventional monopolar techniques is unknown.

■ ENDOSCOPIC RETROGRADE CHOLANGIOPANCREATOGRAPHY

First described in 1974, ERCP has become a commonly performed endoscopic procedure. About 150,000 ERCP procedures are performed in the United States each year, and half or more of these are for therapeutic interventions, such as stone removal, sphincterotomy, or stent placement. This technically complex endoscopic procedure is associated with a high incidence of severe complications, including, in estimated order of frequency, pancreatitis, bleeding, cholangitis or sepsis, cardiopulmonary, perforation, lacerated solid organ, and cholecystitis. In addition, cardiopulmonary complications may occur, as for other endoscopic procedures in which the patient is sedated.

Although many factors have been associated with an increased risk of ERCP-related complications, little prospective information is available on conditions that predispose to complications or technical risks of the procedure. Although sphincterotomy is associated with the highest frequency of complications (10%), the complication rate for diagnostic ERCP is also substantial (2% to 5%). In a large, multicenter, prospective study, 2347 patients underwent endoscopic biliary sphincterotomy, with a complication rate of 9.8% that included pancreatitis in 5.4% and bleeding in 2% of patients [27••]. Ten deaths were directly or indirectly related to ERCP, representing a mortality rate of 0.4%. By multivariate analysis, five risk factors for complications related to sphincterotomy were identified. Two of these were patient related (suspected sphincter of Oddi dysfunction and cirrhosis) and three were endoscopy-related (difficulty in cannulating the bile duct, precut sphincterotomy, and a "rendezvous" procedure involving a combined transhepatic and endoscopic approach). Complication rates ranged from 5% to 22%, depending on the indication for the procedure. The study results suggested that both patient-related and procedure-related factors can be identified for ERCP and permit risk stratification. The study confirmed that an overall complication rate of 10% makes sphincterotomy the most hazardous of all endoscopic procedures.

Pancreatitis

Pancreatitis is the most common complication of diagnostic and therapeutic ERCP. Efforts to identify factors associated with post-ERCP pancreatitis, such as the type of contrast agent used, acinarization of the gland during pancreatography, and difficulty in cannulation, have identified only the latter as being associated with an increased risk of post-ERCP pancreatitis. Prospective double-blind studies comparing low-osmolality, nonionic contrast agents with high-osmolality agents have shown no differences between the two in the incidence or severity of post-ERCP pancreatitis [28,29]. Therefore, the use of more expensive nonionic contrast agents is not justified. Similarly, prophylactic use of the somatostatin analog octreotide does not decrease the incidence of post-ERCP pancreatitis [30]. Data from a retrospective study suggest that preprocedure administration of corticosteroids may decrease the incidence of post-ERCP pancreatitis [31]. These data require confirmation in a prospective trial, and no intervention has been proved to reduce the risk of post-ERCP pancreatitis.

Pancreatitis occurring after ERCP is usually easy to recognize. Most patients exhibit typical epigastric abdominal pain radiating through to the back within hours of the procedure and before discharge from the recovery unit. In 10% to 15% of patients, however, symptoms of pancreatitis do not appear until after discharge from the procedure unit. Therefore, all patients need to be informed of the possibility of delayed complications.

In suspected post-ERCP pancreatitis, elevation of the serum amylase level is not usually diagnostically helpful because half or more of all patients have a transient elevation of the serum amylase level after the procedure. The absence of an elevated serum amylase level, however, suggests that the patient's pain is from a source other than the pancreas.

The treatment of post-ERCP pancreatitis is no different from that of pancreatitis of other causes (see Chapter 134). Most patients have a mild course, and many can be managed in an outpatient setting. The cornerstones of therapy include intravenous hydration, resting the pancreas by avoiding oral feeding, and control of pain with narcotic analgesics. About 10% to 15% of patients with acute pancreatitis develop additional complications, including formation of pseudocysts and infected pancreatic necrosis.

Bleeding

Bleeding is rare after diagnostic ERCP but is the second most common complication of sphincterotomy and occurs in about 2% of patients. In most cases, bleeding is mild or moderate, ceases spontaneously, and requires only observation, supportive care, and possibly blood transfusions. Severe bleeding occurs in about 0.5% of patients undergoing sphincterotomy and usually can be managed by endoscopic means, surgery, or in rare cases, angiography. In about half of cases, bleeding occurs at the time of sphincterotomy and is readily apparent during the procedure. In the other half of cases, however, bleeding is delayed from 1 to 10 days. These patients present with melena or hematemesis.

The management of bleeding from sphincterotomy is identical to that for other causes of upper gastrointestinal bleeding and includes hemodynamic support and blood transfusions with attempts at endoscopic control, angiography, and surgery if necessary. Endoscopic control of postsphincterotomy bleeding usually can be achieved by injection of epinephrine into the apex of the sphincterotomy site. Other techniques include impaction of a cannula into the bleeding site and injection of contrast to tamponade the vessel.

Cholangitis

Infections are the third most common complication of ERCP. Of these, cholangitis is the most common, occurring in about 1% of cases. Cholangitis usually occurs in the setting of biliary obstruction with inability to drain an unobstructed bile duct; however, cholangitis also can occur after cholangiography of an unobstructed duct or despite successful drainage of an obstructed duct.

In patients undergoing therapeutic ERCP, prophylactic administration of broad-spectrum antibiotics has been shown to reduce the incidence of bacteremia and sepsis [32,33,34•]. The best antibiotic for prophylaxis has not been identified, but third-generation cephalosporins, ciprofloxacin, and piperacillin are all efficacious.

Other septic complications of ERCP include acute cholecystitis, which may occur in up to 0.5% of patients, and infected pseudocysts related to pancreatography in patients with preexisting pseudocysts that communicate with the pancreatic duct.

Other Complications

Complications related to sedation are uncommon in patients undergoing ERCP. Although sedation is generally deeper in patients undergoing ERCP than in those undergoing esophagogastroduodenoscopy or colonoscopy, recognition of the potential for sedation-associated complications and a commensurate increased attentiveness to physiologic monitoring of these patients may account for the lack of an appreciably increased risk of adverse outcomes. Nevertheless, even though patients monitored with oximetry can be well oxygenated, hypercarbia, indicating reduced ventilation, is surprisingly common in patients undergoing ERCP [5]. Monitoring of carbon dioxide levels in patients undergoing ERCP has been suggested but requires additional study.

Intestinal perforation rarely occurs with diagnostic ERCP and occurs in less than 1% of those undergoing sphincterectomy. Perforation at sphincterotomy is usually recognized during the procedure because extravasation of contrast can be seen on fluoroscopy. Most patients can be managed conservatively with antibiotics, bowel rest, and biliary drainage to prevent chemical peritonitis. Perforations caused by the duodenoscope are usually large and require surgical repair.

◼ CONCLUSION

Although endoscopy is remarkably safe, complications are not infrequent given the substantial number of procedures performed. Medical professionals performing endoscopic procedures should understand the associated risks, be practiced in techniques that help to avoid complications, and be able to recognize and treat associated complications. This expertise can be obtained only through formal extensive training and development of a thorough understanding of gastrointestinal disease processes.

◼ REFERENCES

Recently published papers of particular interest have been highlighted as follows:
•   Of interest
••   Of outstanding interest

1.•• Arrowsmith J, Gertman S, Fleischer D, *et al.*: Results from the ASGE/US FDA collaborative study on complication rates and drug use during gastrointestinal endoscopy. *Gastrointest Endosc* 1991, 37:421–427.
These authors have developed the best database for estimating cardiorespiratory complications of endoscopy and their association with sedation.

2. Quine M, Bell G, McCloy R, *et al.*: Prospective audit of upper gastrointestinal endoscopy in two regions of England: safety, staffing, and sedation methods. *Gut* 1995, 36:452–457.

3. Fennerty M, Earnest A, Hudson P, *et al.*: Physiologic changes during colonoscopy. *Gastrointest Endosc* 1990, 36:22–25.

4. Lee J, Krucoff M, Brazer S: Periprocedural myocardial ischemia in patients with severe symptomatic coronary artery disease undergoing endoscopy: prevalence and risk factors. *Am J Med* 1995, 99:270–275.

5. Nelson D, Silvis S, Yakshe P, *et al.*: Inaccuracy of clinical assessment in detecting hypoxemia and hypoventilation during ERCP. *Gastrointest Endosc* 1992, 38:227.

6. Jurell K, O'Connor K, Slack J, *et al.*: Effect of supplemental oxygen on cardiopulmonary changes during gastrointestinal endoscopy. *Gastrointest Endosc* 1994, 40:665–670.

7. Zuckerman G, O'Brien J, Halsted R: Antibiotic prophylaxis in patients with infectious risk factors undergoing gastrointestinal endoscopic procedures. *Gastrointest Endosc* 1994, 40:538–543.

8. Mogadam M, Malhotra S, Jackson R: Pre-endoscopic antibiotics for the prevention of bacterial endocarditis: do we use them appropriately? *Am J Gastroenterol* 1994, 89:832–834.

9. Chan M: Complications of upper gastrointestinal endoscopy. *Gastrointest Endosc Clin N Am* 1995, 6:287–303.

10. Quine M, Bell G, McCloy R, *et al.*: Prospective audit of perforation rates following upper gastrointestinal endoscopy in two regions of England. *Br J Surg* 1995,82:530–533.

11. Disario J, Fennerty M, Tietze C, *et al.*: Endoscopic balloon dilatation for peptic ulcer induced gastric outlet obstruction. *Am J Gastroenterol* 1994, 89:868–871.

12.• Shiffman M, Farrel M, Yee Y: Risk of bleeding after endoscopic biopsy or polypectomy in patients taking aspirin or other NSAIDs. *Gastrointest Endosc* 1994, 40:458–462.
This study indicates that the risk of clinically significant hemorrhage is not increased in patients undergoing polypectomy or biopsy while on nonsteroidal anti-inflammatory drug (NSAID) therapy.

13. Clouse R: Complications of endoscopic gastrointestinal dilation techniques. *Gastrointest Endosc Clin N Am* 1996, 6:323–341.

14. Fennerty M: Esophageal perforation during pneumatic dilatation for achalasia: a possible association with malnutrition. *Dysphagia* 1990, 5:227–228.

15. Lee J, Lieberman D: Complications related to endoscopic hemostasis techniques. *Gastrointest Endosc Clin N Am* 1996, 6:305–321.

16. Waye J, Kahn O, Auerbach M: Complications of colonoscopy and flexible sigmoidoscopy. *Gastrointest Endosc Clin N Am* 1996, 6:343–377.

17. Ryan C, Potter G: Disinfectant colitis: rinse as well as you wash. *J Clin Gastroenterol* 1995, 21:6–9.

18. Dolce P, Gourdeau M, April N, *et al.*: Outbreak of glutaraldehyde-induced proctocolitis. *Am J Infect Control* 1995, 23:34–39.

19. Birnbaum B, Gordon R, Jacobs J: Glutaraldehyde colitis: radiologic findings. *Radiology* 1995, 195:131–134.

20. Thomson A, Naidoo P, Crotty B: Bowel preparation for colonoscopy: a randomized prospective trial comparing sodium phosphate and polyethylene glycol in a predominantly elderly population. *Gastroenterol Hepatol* 1996, 11:103–107.

21. DiPalma J, Buckley S, Warner B, *et al.*: Biochemical effects of oral sodium phosphate. *Dig Dis Sci* 1996, 41:749–753.

22. Huynh T, Vanner S, Paterson W: Safety profile of 5-h oral sodium phosphate regimen for colonoscopy cleansing: lack of clinically significant hypocalcemia or hypovolemia. *Am J Gastroenterol* 1995, 90:104–107.

23. Foliente R, Chang A, Youssef A, *et al.*: Endoscopic cecal perforation: mechanisms of injury. *Am J Gastroenterol* 1996, 91:705–708.

24. Damore L, Rantis P, Vernava A, *et al.*: Colonoscopic perforations: etiology, diagnosis and management. *Dis Colon Rectum* 1996, 39:1308–1314.

25. Gibbs D, Opelka F, Beck D, *et al.*: Postpolypectomy colonic hemorrhage. *Dis Colon Rectum* 1996;39:806–810.

26. Weston A, Campbell D: Diminutive colonic polyps: histopathology, spatial distribution, concomitant significant lesions, and treatment complications. *Am J Gastroenterol* 1995, 90:24–28.

27.•• Freeman M, Nelson D, Sherman S, *et al.*: Complications of endoscopic biliary sphincterotomy. *N Engl J Med* 1996, 335:909–918.
This article describing a large, multicenter, prospective trial outlines the risk factors associated with sphincterotomy-induced complications.

28. Sherman S, Hawes R, Rathgaber S, *et al.*: Post-ERCP pancreatitis: randomized, prospective study comparing a low- and high-osmolality contrast agent. *Gastrointest Endosc* 1994, 40:422–427.

29. Johnson G, Geenen J, Bedford R, *et al.*: A comparison of nonionic versus ionic contrast media: results of a prospective, multicenter study. Midwest Pancreaticobiliary Study Group. *Gastrointest Endosc* 1995, 42:312–316.

30. Arcidiacono R, Gambitta P, Rossi A, *et al.*: The use of a long-acting somatostatin analogue (octreotide) for prophylaxis of acute pancreatitis after endoscopic sphincterectomy. *Endoscopy* 1994, 26:715–718.

31. Weiner G, Geenen J, Hogan W, *et al.*: Use of corticosteroids in the prevention of post-ERCP pancreatitis. *Gastrointest Endosc* 1995, 42:579–583.

32. van den Hazel S, Speelman P, Dankert J, *et al.*: Piperacillin to prevent cholangitis after endoscopic retrograde cholangiopancreatography: a randomized, controlled trial. *Ann Intern Med* 1996, 125:442–447.

33. Mehal W, Culshaw K, Tillotson G, *et al.*: Antibiotic prophylaxis for ERCP: a randomized clinical trial comparing ciprofloxacin and cefuroxime in 200 patients at high risk of cholangitis. *Eur J Gastroenterol Hepatol* 1995, 7:841–845.

34.• Niederau C, Pohlmann U, Lubke H, *et al.*: Prophylactic antibiotic treatment in therapeutic or complicated diagnostic ERCP: results of a randomized controlled clinical study. *Gastrointest Endosc* 1994, 40:533–537.
This study found that prophylactic antibiotics in ERCP are only indicated in patients with an obstructed biliary system.

190 Eating Disorders
Ronald J. Hapke and Hugo R. Rosen

Eating disorders, defined as "deviations in alimentary behavior that lead to disease" [1], include anorexia nervosa, bulimia nervosa, and rumination disorder. Pica is no longer considered a distinct eating disorder. Eating disorders have been described for several centuries in the form of case reports and studies of small series. Our understanding of the pathogenesis, clinical manifestations, and optimal management of eating disorders has evolved considerably in the past two decades.

Although not common, eating disorders can seriously influence the lives of patients and their families, especially when a young patient is first stricken. The illnesses do not appear to be either entirely physiologic or psychological in origin but instead probably represent an intricate interplay between the two.

ANOREXIA NERVOSA

Anorexia nervosa, first named in 1868 by Sir William Gull, has received increasing attention in the medical literature, in part because of Western society's perception of the ideal body habitus. For instance, half of the students in the third to sixth grade express a desire to be thinner, and up to a third have tried to lose weight [2]. More than half of all women have dieted by the age of 14 years. Two-thirds of girls and young women, aged 12 to 23, are not satisfied with their weight, and up to 60% of women who have never been overweight have dieted [3]. Thinness is believed to reflect a person's self-discipline, self-control, assertiveness, competitiveness, and worth. It is not surprising

that, with all of these pressures, the susceptible person exhibits abnormal eating habits to achieve the weight and body image perceived as necessary for acceptance.

Anorexia nervosa affects between 0.2% and 1.3% of the population, [RJH1] with an incidence of 5 to 10 per 100,000 population [4••]. The incidence among women is considerably greater; only 5% to 10% of patients with anorexia nervosa are men. The mean age of onset is 17 years, but anorexia nervosa has also been described in grade-school children and in middle-aged adults. About 50% of women with anorexia nervosa are seen before age 20 and 75% before age 25. Lifetime prevalence has been calculated as 0.3% for women and 0.02% for men in the United States [5•]. Studies have demonstrated that up to 17% of college-aged women show some evidence of disordered eating patterns, and as many as 1.2 million women in the United States are thought to have anorexia [6].

Over the years, the definition of anorexia nervosa has changed, culminating in the diagnostic criteria listed in the American Psychiatric Association's *Diagnostic and Statistical Manual of Mental Disorders, 4th Edition*, (DSM-IV) shown in Table 190-1. The most significant change in DSM-IV criteria from DSM-III-R diagnostic criteria is the inclusion of two specific subtypes of anorexia nervosa: the *restricting* type (patients avoid caloric intake but do not binge or purge) and the *bulimic* type (patients binge and purge and are less than 85% of their ideal body weight). This distinction has therapeutic and prognostic significance.

The most distinctive characterization of anorexia nervosa is that affected persons have a distorted perception of their weight and body shape. They may believe that their entire body is overweight or that a specific body part is oversized for their physique. Patients with anorexia nervosa have an intense fear of gaining weight and go to great lengths to avoid caloric intake, even to the point of counting the calories in chewing gum, postage stamps, and medications. They do not acknowledge that they are grossly underweight and are not satisfied with any weight loss they achieve. Amenorrhea in women and diminished libido in men are requirements of the DSM-IV diagnostic criteria, but their inclusion as prerequisites has been questioned by some authorities.

Etiology

The etiology of anorexia nervosa has not been fully elucidated and is likely multifactorial (Table 190-2). The following factors may be involved:

Genetic predisposition. Studies of monozygotic twins have shown concordance rates of anorexia nervosa of 56% to 65%, compared with 7% to 10% for dizygotic twins [7].

Sociocultural setting. The adolescent responds to the external pressure to be thin and sees her prepubertal body as idealizing this goal. She diets to prevent the insecurity she feels from the pubertal changes her body is undergoing. She may pursue thinness even to the point of death.

The disorder is less common in blacks than in whites, but few data are available regarding anorexia nervosa in Asian, Hispanic, and Native American populations. Studies in Japan suggest that the frequency of anorexia nervosa increases as the culture becomes more exposed to Western thought and mores.

Personality disorders. Personality disorders are found in a substantial proportion of patients with anorexia nervosa: a coexistent personality defect of any type is seen in 27% to 93%, and up to 60% have an avoidant personality type [8]. Affected persons may demonstrate increased risk avoidance, less emotional expression, and higher conformity to authority than controls. When compared with siblings, patients with anorexia nervosa show increased control of self and impulse, higher interpersonal insecurity, and greater regimentation of behavior [9].

Patients with a predisposing personality disorder may shift their concerns about life into categories related to weight in an attempt to make their problems more manageable. Patients with anorexia nervosa often show evidence of obsessive/compulsive disorder (OCD). They may rearrange food on the plate, cut it into progressively smaller pieces, and conceal it; exercise to exhaustion; ritualize body habitus assessment (*ie*, weighing themselves, bathing, homework, and occupational activities); and count the calories of any and all items placed in their mouths [10••].

Family factors. Family studies have shown an increased risk of depression and affective disorders in relatives of patients with anorexia nervosa. The affected person often is not able to resolve conflicts within the family because of parental overinvolvement, and may turn to diet and weight loss as a means of exercising self-control when she cannot exert control over the family situation.

Sexual abuse. Sexual abuse and anorexia nervosa are frequently found in association. In a study of 200 patients, 44 (22%) were victims of childhood sexual abuse [11•]. Childhood sexual abuse probably takes place in family situations that may independently foster the development of anorexia nervosa.

Psychiatric illnesses. Depression, the degree of which is usually mild to moderate, may be found in up to 50% of patients with anorexia nervosa. One study demonstrated that the lifetime prevalence of major depression in patients with anorexia nervosa is greater than 60% even up to 10 years after therapy for anorexia nervosa [12]. A starvation state predisposes to symptoms of depression. Depression is, however, often found in

Table 190-1. Criteria for Anorexia Nervosa from Diagnostic and Statistical Manual for Mental Disorders, Edn. 4

1. Refusal to maintain body weight at or above a minimally normal weight for age and height, (*eg*. weight loss leading to maintenance of body weight less than 85% of that expected); or failure to make expected weight gain during a period of growth, leading to body weight less than 85% of that expected
2. Intense fear of gaining weight or becoming fat, even though underweight
3. Disturbance in the way in which one's body weight or shape is experienced, denial of the seriousness of current low body weight, or undue influence of body shape and weight on self-evaluation
4. In post-menarchal females, amenorrhea (*ie*, absence of at least three consecutive menstrual cycles)

Binge-eating/purging type: During the current episode of anorexia nervosa, the person has regularly engaged in binging-or-purging behavior

Restricting type: During the current episode of anorexia nervosa, the person has *not* regularly engaged in binging-or-purging behavior.

Adapted from American Psychiatric Association [7]; with permission.

Table 190-2. Proposed Etiologies of Anorexia Nervosa (see text)

Factor	Comments
Genetic	Higher concordance in monozygotic rather than dizygotic twins
Sociocultural	Societal pressures to be attractive
Personality	Disorders such as obsessive compulsive disorder may commonly occur in the patient with anorexia nervosa
Family	Parental overinvolvement may lead to control issues
Sexual abuse	May occur in up to 20% of patients with anorexia nervosa
Psychiatric illness	Depression common and substance abuse less common
Physiologic disturbances	Possible disorder in hypothalamus-pituitary-adrenal axis

patients with anorexia nervosa even before weight loss begins. Substance abuse may occur in patients with anorexia nervosa, but not as frequently as in patients with bulimia nervosa. In one study of calls to a cocaine hot line, 22% of the callers met criteria diagnostic for bulimia nervosa, whereas only 2% met the criteria for anorexia nervosa [13]. Drug abuse may be seen as a loss of self-control; anorexia nervosa likely represents the need for extreme self-control.

Physiologic disturbances. Much research has centered on the role of the hypothalamus-pituitary-adrenal axis in anorexia nervosa. However, the function of starvation in the observed abnormalities of the hypothalamic axis remains unclear. Abnormal serum levels of growth hormone, vasopressin, serotonin, norepinephrine, cholecystokinin (CCK), corticotropin-releasing hormone (CRH), neuropeptide Y, dopamine, endogenous opiates, and substance P are findings characteristic of anorexia nervosa.

Clinical Features

Clinical manifestations of anorexia nervosa are related to the states of semistarvation and starvation. Presentation may be acute, subacute, or chronic; each presentation, moreover may occur as phases in the same patient. Acute presentation with marked weight loss and increased activity occurs after a period of intermittent fasting and often is associated with hypothermia and amenorrhea. A subacute phase follows 3 to 6 months of weight loss and is often manifested by mood swings and irritability. Physical findings may include dry skin, sallow appearance, hair loss, constipation, dehydration, edema, the development of lanugo, and hypercarotenemia (Fig. 190-1). Signs include hypotension, bradycardia, hypothermia, and insomnia. This phase can begin weeks after initiation of dieting and can persist for months to years. The chronic phase occurs after 1 to 2 years of semistarvation. Marked muscle wasting, loss of body fat, and numerous medical complications are present.

In the patient with anorexia nervosa in whom there are marked distortions of body habitus and altered food intake, a "binge" may be characterized by ingestion of a single piece of candy or other forbidden item. Patients often become preoccupied with food and with the preparation of meals for others, especially elaborate gourmet meals. Excessive exercise, to the point of exhaustion or bone fractures, can be a significant part of the life of the patient with anorexia nervosa. As the disease progresses, apathy and psychosocial withdrawal often worsen.

Delayed Psychosexual and Psychosocial Development

The adult patient with anorexia nervosa often lives alone, remains single, and, if she does marry, has few, if any, children. These adult patterns stem from the adolescent's goal of avoiding the physical changes associated with puberty. Beyond concerns over changes in body habitus, the considerations of parental separation, dating, and other social interactions may be frightening.

Diagnosis and Differential Diagnosis

Unfortunately, no single tool is best for the diagnosis of anorexia nervosa. A significant proportion of patients with anorexia nervosa deny that their eating habits and body perception *are* abnormal. Anorexia nervosa should be considered in any young, otherwise healthy girl or woman with weight loss. Because anorexia nervosa is often a diagnosis of exclusion, other disorders should first be considered. The differential diagnosis includes malignant disease, metabolic disorders (hyperthyroidism, hypothyroidism, diabetes mellitus, hypercalcemia, and hyperparathyroidism), central nervous system disorders (*eg*, hypothalamic tumors), infectious disorders associated with human immunodeficiency virus (HIV), and gastrointestinal diseases including celiac sprue, pancreatic insufficiency, Crohn's disease, ulcerative colitis, and partial small-bowel or gastric outlet obstruction.

A careful history, physical examination, nutritional assessment, and laboratory evaluation (complete blood count, chemistry panel, tests for liver function, serum amylase and albumin levels,

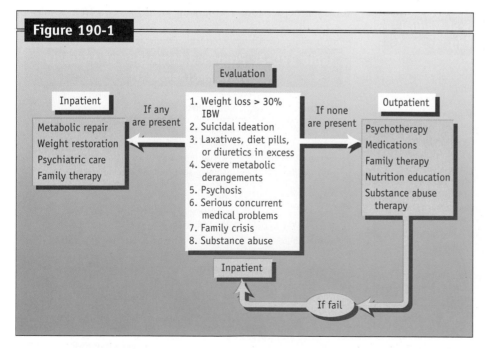

Figure 190-1

Algorithm for the treatment of anorexia nervosa or bulimia nervosa. Note that substance abuse is most often associated with bulimia nervosa. IBW—ideal body weight.

erythrocyte sedimentation rate, urinalysis, thyroid function, and measurement of fasting plasma cortisol level) are essential in the exclusion of other diagnoses. In selected patients, electrocardiography, radiography of the chest, upper and lower gastrointestinal barium series, stool examinations for blood, fat, and infectious agents, and computed tomographic (CT) scan of the head also may be considered.

Steatorrhea, fever, elevation of the erythrocyte sedimentation rate, or marked elevation of the leukocyte count are uncommon in patients with anorexia nervosa. Rectal bleeding may result from anal fissures in patients with anorexia nervosa because of constipation, but inflammatory bowel disease as a diagnosis must always be excluded in such persons.

Multiple psychological disorders also may mimic anorexia nervosa or present with weight loss. These include depression, conversion reactions, schizophrenia (particularly in severely starved patients), anxiety reaction, adjustment disorders, and substance abuse. Use of several tests to diagnose anorexia nervosa, including the Goldberg Anorectic Attitude Scale and the Eating Attitudes Test, may be limited by concomitant physical effects of semistarvation and starvation.

Medical Complications
Medical complications are usually related to the starvation state (Table 190-3).

Cardiovascular Findings
Cardiovascular disturbances can be found in up to 87% of anorexia nervosa patients. The most common is bradycardia, probably caused by a decrease in the basal metabolic rate secondary to starvation and conservation of energy. Other electrocardiographic findings include ST depression, ventricular arrhythmias, and U waves. Sudden death may occur. Blood pressure should be measured frequently and electrocardiograms should be performed regularly in patients with anorexia nervosa.

Renal and Metabolic Findings
Renal dysfunction may occur in up to 70% of patients and is more pronounced in patients who use laxatives or diuretics to increase weight loss. Decreased glomerular filtration rate, elevated blood urea nitrogen level, hypokalemia, hyponatremia, hypochloremia, and metabolic alkalosis are often observed. Because of increased intake of dietary oxalate, dehydration, and decreased output of urine, there is also an increased frequency of renal stones.

Because of lowered basal metabolic rate, temperature regulation may be impaired, resulting in inappropriate loss of body heat. Hypoglycemia is likely related to decreased intestinal absorption of glucose and to impaired gluconeogenesis and glycogenolysis. Hypercholesterolemia, is seen in up to 50% of patients and may relate to ineffective androgen metabolism. Refeeding syndrome may occur in patients in a starvation state. Whole body depletion of potassium, phosphorous, and magnesium plays an integral role in this potentially fatal complication of protracted starvation. As food is provided to patients who have been in a catabolic state, anabolism ensues, accompanied by an intracellular shift of electrolytes with a resulting decrease in serum concentrations. Electrolyte abnormalities can lead to cardiac dysrhythmias, seizures, respiratory distress, and hemolytic anemia. Large shifts in volume, which may accompany the shifts in electrolytes, can result in congestive heart failure and cardiac arrest.

Hematologic Findings
Marked starvation may be associated with pancytopenia, and up to one third of patients with anorexia nervosa have mild anemia and a slight decrease in the leukocyte count. Bone marrow biopsy typically demonstrates relative hypoplasia, especially of the erythrocyte line. Refeeding returns most parameters to normal.

Skeletal Findings
Osteoporosis and bone fractures may occur in patients with anorexia nervosa. If the patient is physically active, bone density may be maintained, but pathologic fractures can occur in patients who pursue too rigorous an exercise program. A positive correlation exists between the frequency of these complications and the duration of illness, as well as amenorrhea and an inverse correlation with the body mass index. Calcium homeostasis may be deranged, resulting in loss of bone; bone resorption is greater

Table 190-3. Medical Complications of Anorexia Nervosa and Bulimia Nervosa

System	Anorexia nervosa	Bulimia nervosa
Oral	—	Caries, parotid enlargement, and gum disease
Cardiovascular	Hypotension, bradycardia, and arrhythmias	Pneumopericardium, and cardiomyopathy (syrup of ipecac abuse)
Renal	Nephrolithiasis, decreased glomerular filtration rate, dehydration, and electrolyte disturbances	Electrolyte disturbances, and metabolic alkalosis
Endocrine	Amenorrhea, impaired temperature regulation, hypoglycemia, hypercholesterolemia, diabetes insipidus, and euthyroid sick syndrome	Menstrual irregularities
Hematologic	Anemia, and pancytopenia	—
Musculoskeletal	Osteoporosis, and stress fractures	Myopathy (syrup of ipecac abuse)
Gastrointestinal	Esophagitis, esophageal rupture, delayed gastric emptying, pancreatitis, constipation, protein-losing enteropathy, hepatomegaly, and early satiety	Esophagitis, Mallory-Weiss tears, esophageal rupture, pancreatitis, constipation, acute gastric dilation, cathartic colon, and hemorrhoids
Dermatologic	Dry, pale skin, hair loss, lanugo, and hypercarotenemia	Finger lacerations, facial ecchymoses, conjunctival hemorrhages, and self-mutilation

than bone formation. These complications are also thought to be related to decreased levels of follicular stimulating hormone (FSH) and luteinizing hormone (LH) in a patient with anorexia nervosa. Unfortunately, hormone replacement therapy has not been proven to protect against bone disease in patients with anorexia nervosa [14].

Endocrine Findings

Amenorrhea is a diagnostic criterion for anorexia nervosa and may precede weight loss in up to 16% of patients. Up to one half of patients with anorexia nervosa remain amenorrheic despite a return to a normal weight. Amenorrhea is thought to result from a starvation-induced increase in serum cortisol levels, which then decreases the hypothalamic secretion of adrenocorticotropin (ACTH) and gonadotropin-releasing hormone (GnRH). This secretion, in turn, leads to decreased circulating concentrations of FSH and LH, culminating in amenorrhea. The release of vasopressin may be significantly diminished but is reversible with weight gain. Diabetes insipidus may be found in up to 40% of patients with anorexia nervosa and may contribute to dehydration. Levels of thyroxine (T4) are typically in the low to normal range, and free triiodothyronine (T3) levels are approximately half those found in normal persons, most likely because of decreased peripheral conversion of T4 to T3. Decreased T4 levels are a response to starvation; most authorities do not recommend thyroid hormone replacement. Cortisol can inhibit bone production, and elevated serum cortisol levels are often found in the serum of patients with anorexia nervosa.

Gastrointestinal Findings

Most gastrointestinal organs are affected to some extent in patients with anorexia nervosa. Dental caries and erosion of dental enamel may result from a diet high in carbohydrates and purging, respectively. Benign parotid gland enlargement with elevated serum amylase levels is often seen in patients with eating disorders (up to 25%); this likely relates to purging episodes. Esophagitis with erosions and ulcers is the most common esophageal complication; esophageal rupture also has been described. Delayed gastric emptying resulting from muscle atrophy, endocrine disturbances, and electrolyte imbalances may occur. Patients often describe early satiety, fullness, and bloating after eating. Gastric dilation is rare and may necessitate urgent decompression. Duodenal dilation, however, is found in up to 50% of patients. In some patients, this complication is secondary to refeeding pancreatitis and a resulting ileus. Constipation resulting from long-term abuse of stimulant laxatives, electrolyte disturbances, and dehydration are also common. Alternatively, patients who use stimulant laxatives frequently and over a long period may experience steatorrhea, malabsorption, and enteropathy, leading to protein loss. Hepatomegaly resulting from fatty infiltration can occur in anorexia nervosa as it can in other starvation states. Low serum protein and elevated lactate dehydrogenase (LDH) and alkaline phosphatase levels may be seen in up to 33% of patients [15••].

Dermatologic Findings

Dry, thin scaly skin is present in up to 25% of patients with anorexia nervosa and is thought to be secondary to a decrease in the collagen content of skin. Loss of scalp hair and growth of lanugo (especially on the arms, legs, face, and back) occur in up to one third of patients. Up to 80% of patients have hypercarotenemia with a characteristic orange discoloration of the soles and palms; this is not usually seen in other starvation states. Self-induced emesis can lead to purpura, bruising, and calluses on the dorsum of the hands. Rarely, scurvy or pellagra may develop.

Miscellaneous Findings

Deficiency of selected essential fatty acids may be seen in patients with anorexia nervosa and require supplementation. Surprisingly, however, patients with anorexia nervosa are usually able to avoid deficiencies of most vitamins and minerals. Brain weight is decreased but returns to normal with restoration of normal body weight [16,17].

Therapy

Approach

The first goal of any therapeutic plan for patients with anorexia nervosa is correction of the starvation state. Comorbid medical and psychiatric conditions may preclude the ability of the anorexia nervosa patient to take an active part in therapy. The severely malnourished patient may require hospitalization and careful management to avoid refeeding syndrome. Criteria for inpatient therapy are outlined in Figure 190-1.

If the patient is admitted to a care facility, enteral feedings should be initiated first to limit the potential complications associated with parenteral nutrition. Medical staff must supervise refeeding, because life-threatening hypophosphatemia can result when glucose is provided, as phosphorus is transported intracellularly with glucose. After the acute phase, the goal should be to gain 1 to 3 pounds per week. Mealtimes should be supervised and should occur in social settings, not with the patient alone in the room. The patient should not be given access to areas where purging may be possible.

Most patients with anorexia nervosa require 10 to 12 weeks of hospitalization if inpatient therapy is undertaken [18]. After appropriate weight gain, more diverse therapies may be undertaken incorporating medical management, psychiatric medications, dietary training, and psychotherapy for the patient and her family [19•].

Psychoactive Medications

Medications have little efficacy in the patient with anorexia nervosa, except in treating associated depression, OCD, or adjustment disorder. However, even these psychiatric disturbances may resolve with adequate weight restoration. Neuroleptics, tricyclic antidepressants, and lithium have shown some efficacy, but the potential risks of these medications usually outweigh their potential benefits, and most authorities recommend their use only with extreme caution. Serotonin reuptake inhibitors (eg, fluoxetine) are beneficial in treating patients with anorexia nervosa and are well tolerated, although they are most helpful in relieving the depression associated with anorexia nervosa. More studies are needed before their routine use can be recommended.

Psychosocial Therapy

Most attention should focus on psychosocial therapies. Behavioral therapy can be quite effective and usually requires fewer inpatient days than psychotherapy. Goals of behavioral therapy include setting expectations for weight gain, rewarding "good eating," keeping a food diary, and positive and negative reinforcements.

Strict behavioral programs are no more effective than lenient ones [20]. Cognitive therapy, also useful, employs education regarding the disease and feedback about the patient's weight, caloric intake, and changes in general health status. Helping the patient identify negative concepts and develop problem-solving skills, and alternative methods of coping are important in the application of cognitive therapy [19•]. Family therapy is most useful for patients younger than 18 years, who still live at home with a relatively supportive family. All patients with anorexia nervosa may need long-term psychiatric support to help them deal with lifelong symptoms.

Prognosis

Of all the most common psychiatric illnesses, anorexia nervosa leads most frequently to death. Some authorities report mortality rates between 5% to 20%, depending on the population studied. In a meta-analysis of 42 studies, the aggregate mortality rate for patients with anorexia nervosa was 0.56% per year, or 5.6% per decade [21••]. This rate is twice the death rate of the general psychiatric population of women and 12 times that of all women. Patients with anorexia nervosa have a suicide rate 200 times higher than that of the entire population of women. Mortality is primarily related to starvation and electrolyte disturbances, which lead to sudden death as well as suicide.

For survivors, the prognosis for cure is poor. In one study of 76 patients with a 10-year follow-up, 6.6% died, 25% recovered fully, 25% had normal weight and return of menses (but still had disordered eating habits), and 45% had significant weight or menstrual disturbances [22]. Increased rates of morbidity and mortality were associated with extremely low weight, long duration of illness, poor family support, purging behaviors, and multiple relapses.

The patient with anorexia nervosa has a severe, debilitating, and chronic illness that encompasses both physical and psychological realms. Long-term management requires a sustained commitment by the patient, health care-provider, and family.

■ BULIMIA NERVOSA

Bulimia nervosa has been defined as an abnormal increase in hunger and a craving for food. Bulimia nervosa was first described as a syndrome by Russell in 1979, although it had been recognized long before that time. In contrast to anorexia nervosa, with which bulimia nervosa shares some features, patients with bulimia nervosa may be underweight, of normal weight, or even overweight. The main similarity with anorexia nervosa is an undue emphasis by the patient on body weight and shape. Investigators have postulated that bulimia nervosa occurs along a continuum: in some studies, up to 17% of college-aged women and up to 13% of teenagers exhibited bulimic behaviors but lacked other criteria necessary for diagnosis of bulimia nervosa [23] Although onset is typically before age 25, the mean age of onset is higher than that of patients with anorexia nervosa.

Estimating the incidence and prevalence of bulimia nervosa is more difficult than for anorexia nervosa because the typical patient does not reveal that she (or he) "binges" and purges. In a study from Minnesota, the mean age of presentation of women with bulimia nervosa was 23±26 years, with an incidence of 7.4 per 100,000 in 1980 and 30 per 100,000 after 1983 [24]. Whether this trend represents a true increase in incidence or recognition of bulimia nervosa as a distinct disorder is unclear. The overall age- and sex-adjusted annual incidence rates for the total population were 13.5 per 100,000 (0.8 per 100,000 for men and 26.5 per 100,000 for women). Bulimia nervosa may affect up to 1.3% of the women in the United States and is probably increasing in some patient subpopulations, such as in homosexual men [25]. Patients most likely afflicted are white women between ages 14 and 40. In 1991, Kendler and colleagues concluded that 1 in 25 women is at risk of developing the full syndrome of bulimia nervosa over her lifetime [26].

The typical patient with bulimia nervosa is preoccupied with food and eating but uses laxatives, diuretics, and self-induced emesis rather than starvation to prevent weight gain. Because of feelings of guilt, shame, and loss of self-control associated with the binge-purge cycle, the bulimia nervosa patient typically does not present to a health-care provider until age 25; presentation can be delayed for up to two decades. Anxiety, tension, frustration, or depression are common precipitants of binge-eating behavior; other impulsive behaviors often coexist with bulimia nervosa. Unlike patients with anorexia nervosa, those with bulimia nervosa are usually distressed by their symptoms, and if confronted, are less likely to deny their symptoms or problems.

The physical complications of bulimia nervosa are not related to a starvation state but rather to the act of purging or to the use of laxatives, diuretics, and diet pills. Patients with bulimia nervosa are more likely than patients with anorexia nervosa to seek help and to be cared for on an outpatient basis with a greater use of medications. They experience a lower lifetime risk of mortality.

The criteria for bulimia nervosa as given in DSM-IV include both *purging* and *nonpurging* subtypes (Table 190-4). The purging subtype of bulimia nervosa includes patients who self-induce emesis or who use laxatives, diuretics, and diet pills in an attempt to reverse the loss of self-control during a period of binge eating. Patients with the nonpurging subtype of bulimia nervosa rely on fasting or excessive exercise and do not use emesis or medications to regain their sense of self-control after a binge.

Binge-eating is a prerequisite to allow the diagnosis of bulimia nervosa. A *binge* is defined as eating an amount of food most people would consider excessive in a given time period. Some patients consume up to 20,000 kilocalories in a sitting. The foods consumed are usually high in fat and carbohydrates—typically "forbidden foods," which are usually also easily ingested, for example, ice cream and breads. The food is usually consumed quickly when the patient is alone. The binge is usually halted by abdominal discomfort or by interruption, that is, when the patient is almost "caught in the act." For a diagnosis of bulimia nervosa, it is imperative that during the binge period the patient feel a lack of self-control and an inability to stop eating on his or her own. Episodes must occur at least twice each week for at least 3 months before a diagnosis of bulimia nervosa can be made. Depending on the subtype—purging or nonpurging—

comorbid behaviors (*ie*, excessive exercise, fasting, self-induced emesis, and use of laxatives, diet pills, or diuretics) may help prevent a change in body weight or shape after a binge. The binge period represents the impulsive lack of self-control. The purge period represents the response to guilt and shame as well as fear of a gain in weight or a distortion in body shape. The patient with bulimia nervosa is more likely to partake in impulsive behaviors, including substance abuse, than her counterpart with anorexia nervosa.

Etiology

Compared with anorexia nervosa, less research has been conducted on the pathogenic mechanisms of bulimia nervosa than for anorexia nervosa, but several theories have been proposed:

Genetic predisposition. Limited data suggest an increased concordance rate in monozygotic versus dizygotic twins of patients with bulimia nervosa [26].

Sociocultural setting. Sociocultural pressures on young people include those related to body weight, size, and shape. If a person does not conform to society's standards—whether real or perceived—she or he is made to feel less equipped to cope with life's expectations and changes. A substantial proportion of college-aged women and men engage in some degree of bulimic behaviors. It is possible that bulimia nervosa represents an end-point along the continuum of binge-and-purge behavior induced by social pressures.

Psychological factors. Persons with bulimia nervosa often demonstrate other impulsive behaviors that stem from a lack of self-control. These may include alcoholism, illicit drug use, stealing, self-mutilation, and sexual promiscuity. About 50% of patients with bulimia nervosa have a history of substance abuse [27]. Moreover, first-degree relatives of patients with bulimia nervosa are more likely than relatives of nonbulimic persons to have affective disorders, eating disorders, and alcoholism. In contrast to anorexia nervosa, patients with bulimia nervosa appear more likely to have an affective disorder (65% vs 41%) and to demonstrate hostility, isolation, lack of empathy, and lack of nurturing [28]. Most patients with bulimia nervosa are thought to have personality trait disturbances, and a history of sexual abuse appears to be more prevalent in persons with bulimia nervosa than in those with anorexia nervosa, although not more prevalent than in the general psychiatric population of women [29]. Up to one third of patients with anorexia nervosa and up to 60% of patients with bulimia nervosa have reported sexual abuse in their past.

Physiology

Several lines of evidence support physiologic aberrations as possible contributors to the development of bulimia nervosa. In one study, persons with bulimia nervosa were found to have decreased plasma cholecystokinin (CCK) levels following a meal, when compared with controls. Such a response may allow for large quantities of food to be consumed during a binge because CCK produces satiety; with lower levels of CCK, normal satiation is not reached during a binge. It is not clear, however, whether this abnormality is a cause of bulimia nervosa or an adaptive response to bingeing and purging. Similarly, serotonin release is associated with satiety, and women with bulimia nervosa have a diminished release of serotonin after meals when compared with normal women.

Clinical Features

Clinical findings are usually not as striking as those found in patients with anorexia nervosa (Table 190-2). In fact, many patients with bulimia nervosa are of normal weight or even overweight. Whereas disease manifestations usually relate to the starvation state in patients with anorexia nervosa, clinical manifestations in those with bulimia nervosa relate to bingeing-and-purging behavior as well as concurrent impulsive behaviors.

Oral Findings

Gum disease and dental caries may be secondary to self-induced emesis. If these abnormalities are noted on dental examination in an otherwise healthy young woman, bulimia nervosa needs to be considered. Parotid gland enlargement may occur, is usually painless, and typically resolves once the disorder has been controlled.

Gastrointestinal Findings

Symptomatically, the patient with bulimia nervosa may complain of abdominal bloating, flatulence, constipation, lack of appetite, abdominal pain, borborygmi, and nausea. Esophagitis, Mallory-Weiss tears, and, more rarely, esophageal rupture can result from forced emesis. Acute gastric dilation and rupture may occur as a result of a vicious cycle of altered gut motility, excessive food intake, and forced emesis. Diminished gut motility is usually related to electrolyte abnormalities from diuretic use

---

Table 190-4. Criteria for Bulimia Nervosa

Recurrent episodes of binge eating. An episode of binge eating is characterized by both of the following:

1. Eating, in a discreet period of time (*eg*, within any 2-hour period), an amount of food that is definitely larger than most people would eat during a similar period of time and under similar circumstances, and,
2. A sense of lack of control over eating during the episode (*eg*, a feeling that one cannot stop eating or control what or how much one is eating).

Recurrent inappropriate compensatory behavior to prevent weight gain, such as: self-induced vomiting; misuse of laxatives; diuretics, or other medications; fasting; or excessive exercise

The binge eating and inappropriate compensatory behaviors both occur, on average, at least twice a week for 3 months

Self-evaluation is unduly influenced by body shape and weight

The disturbance does not occur exclusively during episodes of anorexia nervosa

Purging type: During the current episode of bulimia nervosa, the person has regularly engaged in self-compensatory behaviors, such as fasting or exercise, but has not regularly engaged in self-induced vomiting or the misuse of laxatives, diuretics, or enemas.

Nonpurging type: During the current episode of bulimia nervosa, the person has used other inappropriate compensatory behaviors, such as fasting or exercise, but has not regularly engaged in self-induced vomiting or the misuse of laxatives, diuretics, or enemas.

Adapted from American Psychiatric Association [7]; with permission.

and is reversible. Ileus or "cathartic colon" (misuse of laxatives to the point of dependence on them for bowel movements) may result from the long-term use of laxatives. Rectal prolapse and hemorrhoids are usually secondary to the constipation experienced between periods of laxative use. Elevated serum amylase levels (from parotid gland enlargement) can occur; these should be differentiated from acute pancreatitis, which also can occur during a purge period.

Cardiovascular and Pulmonary Findings

Whereas cardiac symptoms can occur in patients with anorexia nervosa because of complications of starvation, in patients with bulimia nervosa, cardiac manifestations are generally related to syrup of ipecac–induced cardiomyopathy. Bradycardia and hypotension are much less frequently seen than in anorexia nervosa. Pneumopericardium and pneumomediastinum have been described as resulting from forced self-emesis. Pneumonia from aspiration of gastric contents may occur.

Endocrine Findings

Amenorrhea is not a requirement for the diagnosis of bulimia nervosa, but menstrual irregularities are not infrequent. Patients with the nonpurging subtype of bulimia nervosa often exercise excessively, which may lead in turn to amenorrhea.

Renal Findings

Hypokalemia, hypochloremia, hypophosphatemia, and metabolic alkalosis can all be found in patients who routinely take diuretics to control their weight. These abnormalities may become life-threatening and are frequently the reason for inpatient therapy of bulimia nervosa.

Musculoskeletal and Dermatologic Findings

Use of syrup of ipecac has been associated with drug-induced myopathy, which can be devastating. Self-mutilation, contusions, erosions over the knuckles, and lacerations of fingers can occur with repetitive contact of those areas with the teeth during purges. Forceful emesis can cause ecchymoses of the face and neck, as well as conjunctival hemorrhages.

Therapy

As in anorexia nervosa, nutritional repletion may be indicated before any other form of treatment is undertaken. Patients should undergo a complete assessment, including evaluation of their understanding of the disorder, a psychiatric history and assessment of the family situation, a physical (including dental) examination, and laboratory studies. Most patients requiring therapy are able to undergo only outpatient care. Inpatient care is indicated if the patient has suicidal or homicidal ideations, severe drug or alcohol abuse, electrolyte imbalance, or has experienced a failure of outpatient management [30••] (Fig. 190-1).

In the patient for whom outpatient care is reasonable, early goals of management focus on nutritional counseling, education about the disorder, and individual or group psychotherapy. One study showed that in mild cases, a full course of cognitive behavioral therapy, partial cognitive behavioral therapy, and self-care recommendations were equally effective [31]. In highly motivated patients, a response to therapy may be seen in 2 to 4 months.

Psychosocial Therapies

Cognitive behavioral therapy appears to be most effective at modifying the attitudes of the patient with bulimia nervosa regarding body shape and weight. It is also useful in educating the patient that purging behaviors are, in fact, maladaptive. Other forms of psychotherapy (eg, interpersonal psychotherapy and group psychotherapy) are successful to varying degrees.

Psychoactive Medications

Psychoactive medicotherapy may be of benefit if there is concomitant depression, obsessive behavior, or impulse disorder syndromes. It may also be a reasonable adjunct to psychotherapy in patients who have failed psychotherapy alone. Several studies have suggested that fluoxetine, especially at higher doses, may aid in the management of the binge-and-purge cycle, but these studies involved patients who exhibited some degree of depression [32]. Other studies have demonstrated that other antidepressants (monoamine oxidase inhibitors, lithium, tricyclic antidepressants) may be effective, but most authorities caution against their widespread use in impulsive patients because of the narrow therapeutic range of these drugs. The most effective approach has been a combination of cognitive behavioral therapy and desipramine, which has rendered 78% of patients symptom-free. When prescribed, antidepressants are generally recommended for 6 months to 2 years or more.

Prognosis

Overall, treatment success rates for bulimia nervosa range from 50% to 90%. If the presenting medical or psychiatric symptoms are mild, a better chance exists for long-term sustained recovery. Natural history evaluations reveal a 25% to 30% decrease in overall levels of bingeing and purging, as well as of laxative abuse between 1 to 2 years after presentation to a health-care provider.

Patients with bulimia nervosa may respond to standard therapies more rapidly than those with anorexia nervosa. Starvation is not usually a problem in most subjects with bulimia nervosa, and the number of medical complications is usually lower. Prognosis is less certain, but persons with bulimia nervosa generally achieve more long-term benefit from treatment than do those with anorexia nervosa.

■ RUMINATION DISORDER

Rumination was first described in adults in 1618 by Aquapendente. The term *rumination* reflects its similarity to cud chewing by herbivores. It differs from vomiting in that it is an act of effortless regurgitation of chewed food from the stomach into the mouth where the food is rechewed and reswallowed. This process usually is continued until the food tastes acidic. Sometimes, the act is performed more than 20 times. The amount of food brought back into the mouth from the stomach is usually limited, often no more than a single mouthful. At times, however, a full meal will be rechewed. The patient experiences no discomfort from the act and may even gain pleasure from it. Persons with the rumination syndrome may feel that the food is at least as tasteful on rechewing as it was on the initial swallow; some patients believe it gives even greater taste pleasure. The timing of the act is variable, usually soon after completion of a meal and continuing for up to 5 hours after the meal is completed. There are usually no associated reflux symptoms, chest pain, or other esophageal or abdominal complaints.

Most cases of the syndrome have been described in infants and adults of limited mental capacity, but a few cases have been described in intellectually intact adults. Among the latter group, it is difficult to discern any adverse consequences of this activity. Socially, the action is not acceptable, but the patient typically finds pleasure in it. For infants, rumination may be a source of comfort from anxiety or lack of maternal bonding, as the infant attempts to recreate the pleasurable act of eating. Adults with mental handicaps likely ruminate for many of the same reasons as infants; psychological factors including depression and anxiety seem to play a role.

The etiology of rumination is unclear, but some familial tendencies may exist [33]. Manometric studies may demonstrate a characteristic pattern of synchronous pressure spikes diffusely in the esophagus and stomach upon rumination.

Therapy in infants involves either maternal surrogating or aversive therapy, including electric shock [34•]. In mentally handicapped adults, behavioral therapy is used, including differential reinforcement and extinction procedures. In intellectually intact adults, regulation of eating habits with reminders not to ruminate have been successful. Biofeedback therapy may help.

Long-term consequences in infants can include failure to thrive and even death from malnutrition. In adults, whether adverse outcomes occur is not clear and, if present, they most likely relate to the underlying psychiatric abnormality.

■ SUMMARY

Both anorexia nervosa and bulimia nervosa are poorly understood and potentially fatal disorders that predominantly affect young people. A complex interplay between psychological and physiologic abnormalities may lead to these disorders. Therapy is initially directed toward careful stabilization of the medical state of the patient and prevention of metabolic catastrophes, such as severe electrolyte abnormalities that could lead to death. Once this is achieved, psychiatric intervention, possibly including use of antidepressants, is undertaken. The patient with an eating disorder has a chronic condition and a potentially poor prognosis. Successful therapy may require a life-long commitment.

■ REFERENCES

Recently published papers of particular interest have been highlighted as follows:
• Of interest
•• Of outstanding interest

1. Lucas AR, McAlpine DE: Eating disorders: anorexia nervosa, bulimia nervosa, pica and rumination. In *Gastroenterology*. Edited by Haubrich WS and Schaffner F. Philadelphia: WB Saunders; 1995:3254–3270.

2. Maloney MJ, McGuire J, Daniels SR, *et al.*: Psychiatric disorders in the first-degree relatives of probands with bulimia nervosa. *Am J Psychiatry* 1989, 146:1468–1471.

3. Moore DC: Body image and eating behavior in adolescent girls. *Am J Dis Child* 1988, 142:1114–1118.

4.•• Woodside DB: A review of anorexia nervosa and bulimia nervosa. *Curr Probl Pediatr* 1995, 25(2):67–89.
The authors present here, an overall review of both anorexia nervosa and bulimia nervosa, with excellent descriptions of etiology and therapeutic interventions. It is especially geared toward the younger patient (adolescents).

5.• Lucas AR, Beard CM, O'Fallon WM, *et al.*: 50 year trends in the incidence of anorexia nervosa in Rochester, MN: a population based study. *Am J Psychiatry* 1991, 148:917–922.
The authors use a somewhat limited study population, but provide one of the most comprehensive descriptions of long term longitudinal follow-up available.

6. Zerbe KJ: *The Body Betrayed: Women, Eating Disorders, and Treatment.* Washington, DC: American Psychiatric Press, 1993:321–372.

7. Holland AJ, Sicotte N, Treasure J: Anorexia nervosa: evidence for a genetic basis. *Psychosom Res* 1988, 32:561–571.

8. Herzog DB, Keller MB, Lavori PW, *et al.*: The prevalence of personality disorders in 210 women with eating disorders. *J Clin Psychiatry* 1992, 53:147–152.

9. Casper RG: Personality features in women with good outcome from restricting anorexia nervosa. *Psycholsom Med* 1990, 52:156–170.

10.•• Hobbs WL, Johnson CA: Anorexia nervosa: an overview. *Am Fam Physician* 1996, 54:1273–1279.
This is a brief, very readable, yet thorough review. It provides helpful and copious tables, and multiple useful references. It also provides a quick review of all the basics of diagnosis and therapy.

11.• Kinzl JF, Traweger C, Guenther V, Biebl W: Family background and sexual abuse associated with eating disorders. *Am J Psychiatry* 1994, 151:1127–1131.
This intriguing study helps to answer the question of whether sexual abuse is more likely to lead to anorexia nervosa or bulimia nervosa than to any other psychiatric disorder.

12. Toner BB, Garfinkel PE, Garner DM: Long term follow-up of anorexia nervosa. *Psychosom Med* 1986, 48:520–529.

13. Jonas JM, Gold MS, Sweeney D: Eating disorders and cocaine abuse: a survey of 259 cocaine abusers. *J Clin Psychiatry* 1987, 48:47–50.

14. La Ban MM, Wilkins JC, Sackeyfio AH, *et al.*: Osteoporotic stress fractures in anorexia nervosa: etiology, diagnosis, and review of four cases. *Arch Phys Med Rehabil* 1995, 76:884–887.

15.•• Hall RC, Beresford TP: Medical complications of anorexia and bulimia. *Psychiatric Medicine* 1989, 7:165–192.
This is an extremely thorough review of the potential complications of patients with either anorexia nervosa or bulimia nervosa. It provides very helpful references, and detail of text which is appropriate for most health care providers.

16. Golden NH, Ashtari M, *et al.*: Reversibility of cerebral ventricular enlargement in anorexia nervosa, demonstrated by quantitative magnetic resonance imaging. *J Pediatrics* 1996, 128:296–301.

17. Swayze VW, Anderson A, Arndt S, *et al.*: Reversibility of brain tissue loss in anorexia nervosa assessed with a computerized Talairach 3-D proportional grid. *Psychol Med* 1996, 26:381–390.

18. Giannini AJ, Newman M, Gold M: Anorexia and bulimia. *Am Fam Physician* 1990, 41:1169–1176.

19.• Yager J: Psychosocial treatments for eating disorders. *Psychiatry* 1994, 57:153–164.
This is a thorough and useful descriptive guide of multiple psychological therapies for both anorexia nervosa and bulimia nervosa. The information provided is particularly helpful after the medical complications of the disorders are managed. Good references are provided.

20. Tuoyz SW, Beumont PJ, Glaun D, *et al.*: A comparison of lenient and strict operant conditioning programs in refeeding patients with anorexia nervosa. *Br J Psychiatry* 1984, 144:517–520.

21.•• Sullivan PF: Mortality in anorexia nervosa. *Am J Psychiatry* 1995, 152:1073–1074.
This is a quick overview of the observation that female patients with anorexia nervosa are at a markedly greater risk of mortality than their counterparts with other psychiatric disorders.

22. Eckert ED, Halmi KA, Marchi P, *et al.*: Ten year follow up of anorexia nervosa: clinical course and outcome. *Psychol Med* 1995, 25:143–156.

23. Killen JD, Taylor CB, Telch MJ, *et al.*: Self-induced vomiting and laxative and diuretic use among teenagers: precursors of the binge-purge syndrome? *JAMA* 1986, 255:1447–1452.

24. Soundy TJ, Lucas AR, Suman VJ, Melton LJ: Bulimia nervosa in Rochester, MN from 1980 to 1990. *Psychol Med* 1995, 25:1065–1071.

25. Andersen AE: *Males with Eating Disorders.* New York: Brunner/Mazel, 1990:133–162.

26. Kendler KS, MacLean C, Neale M, *et al.*: The genetic epidemiology of bulimia nervosa. *Am J Psychiatry* 1991, 148:1627–1637.

27. Shisslak CM, Perse T, Crago M: Coexistence of bulimia nervosa and mania: a literature review and case report. *Compr Psychiatry* 1991, 32:181–184.

28. Braun KL, Sunday SR, Halmi KA: Psychiatric comorbidity in patients with eating disorders. *Psychol Med* 1994, 24:859–867.

29. Bulik CM, Sullivan PF, Rorty M: Childhood sexual abuse in women with bulimia. *J Clin Psychiatry* 1989, 50:460–464.

30.•• American Psychiatric Association: Practice guideline for eating disorders. *Am J Psychiatry* 1993, 150(2):212–228.

This definitive position statement of the American Psychiatric Association, in regards to therapy of eating disorders, provides detailed rationale for treatment as well as helpful information concerning etiology.

31. Treasure J, Schmidt U, Troop N, *et al.*: Sequential treatment for bulimia nervosa incorporating a self-care manual. *Br J Psychiatry* 1996, 168:94–98.

32. Goldstein DJ, Wilson MG, Thompson VI, *et al.*: Long-term fluoxetine treatment of bulimia nervosa. *Br J Psychiatry* 1995, 166:660–666.

33. Levine DF, Wingate DL, Pfeffer JM, Butcher P: Habitual rumination: a benign disorder. *Br Med Journal* 1983, 287:255–256.

34.• Amarnath RP, Abell TL, Malagelada JR: The rumination syndrome in adults. *Ann Intern Med* 1986, 105:513–518.

This paper combines a good manometric study with a review of rumination syndrome. It contains excellent references for both adult and pediatric cases.

191 An Approach to Nutritional Assessment

Aminah Jatoi and Joel B. Mason

Starvation typically leads to death within 70 days in healthy, nonobese adults. Catabolism from illness potentiates the starvation process, worsens morbidity, and hastens mortality associated with malnutrition. Diligent attention to nutritional assessment and, when appropriate, initiation of nutritional support therefore are as important as drug therapy, ventilatory support, or any other medical or surgical intervention in the care of patients. Yet several studies have demonstrated that nutritional needs among hospitalized patients often are neglected. In a landmark paper entitled, "The Skeleton in the Hospital Closet," published in 1974, Butterworth described a high prevalence of malnutrition, much of which was iatrogenic, in patients in a tertiary care center. In a follow-up study, he and his colleagues observed that 62% of all hospitalized patients had protein-calorie, or protein-energy, malnutrition (PEM).

Subsequent studies have confirmed that malnutrition is present in 30% to 60% of all hospitalized patients [1]; it affects both young and old medical and surgical patients, generally worsens during hospitalization, and, during the past decade, has become only somewhat less pervasive, with a decline in frequency from 62% to 46%. In short, evidence of malnutrition still can be found in many hospitalized patients.

Malnutrition is not restricted to the hospital setting. A recent study that evaluated malnutrition in 109 outpatients who presented for the first time to a geriatric clinic found that 21% had evidence of PEM. PEM also has been found in a substantial percentage of outpatients with renal failure, cirrhosis, and other chronic medical problems.

The high prevalence of PEM underscores the importance of nutritional assessment and intervention. Clinical outcomes improve in many malnourished patients as a result of aggressive nutritional intervention in the form of nutritional counseling, oral liquid nutritional supplements, enteral tube feedings, or parenteral nutrition [2•]. Prompt identification of malnourished patients and initiation of appropriate nutritional interventions require an appreciation of the importance of nutrition and a willingness to

develop and carry out a therapeutic plan. On the other hand, not every hospitalized or ambulatory patient with malnutrition benefits from nutritional interventions. For example, most malnourished patients with metastatic cancer are unlikely to benefit from nutritional therapy. All patients should, however, undergo an initial nutritional assessment and periodic reassessments, and deliberate decisions about whether to initiate nutritional support or formal nutritional counseling should follow.

▄▄▄ DEFINITIONS

Nutrients are classified into two categories: macronutrients and micronutrients. *Macronutrients* consist of carbohydrates, proteins, lipids, calcium, magnesium, and phosphate, all of which are required in gram quantities to meet daily requirements. In contrast, *micronutrients* consist of other minerals, trace elements, and vitamins. These substances serve a variety of metabolic functions and are required in milligram quantities or less. In the broadest sense, malnutrition can be considered a consequence of either too little or too much of a nutrient. It also can exist when the amount of a particular nutrient is out of proportion to that of other nutrients.

In practice, however, the term *malnutrition* usually refers to PEM, a pathologic condition that manifests after a sustained period of inadequate intake of protein or nonprotein caloric sources, such as carbohydrate and fat, and which subsequently results in impairment of normal physiologic functioning. PEM has been subclassified into *primary* and *secondary* types. Primary PEM results from the intake of food of insufficient quantity or quality to meet metabolic demands. Secondary PEM occurs when illness or other factors lead to impaired uptake or use of nutrients, an increase in protein or energy requirements, or an increase in metabolic losses that exceeds the availability of nutrients. Secondary PEM most commonly is the result of illness that incites a systemic inflammatory response, leading to increased energy demands, depletion of energy stores, and drastic alteration of the patterns of nutrient use observed in health. Because no storage form of protein exists in humans, the increase in protein catabolism associated with such illness is particularly damaging.

Primary PEM is uncommon in the United States, except in select subpopulations. In contrast, secondary PEM is seen commonly in hospitalized patients and often coexists with primary PEM. An illness that leads to secondary PEM often drives a cascade of inflammatory responses, including release of tumor necrosis factor and interleukin-1. These two cytokines induce anorexia independently and synergistically, in part through direct effects on the hypothalamus [3].

Protein-energy malnutrition also can be subtyped into *kwashiorkor* or *marasmus*. Although these terms are used less commonly today than in the past, the distinctions they evoke have both etiologic and prognostic value. Marasmus, a term derived from the Greek word *maramos*, meaning "a dying away," denotes a condition that results from a prolonged period of inadequate intake of both protein and calories, usually in the absence of acute catabolic illness. With time and with depletion of skeletal muscle mass, the affected person develops a wasted appearance, with relative sparing of protein contained within the visceral organs and plasma. Marasmus rarely is fatal unless it is severe or associated with an underlying medical illness.

In contrast, kwashiorkor results when protein intake is disproportionately low relative to caloric intake. The term is derived from the Ga language of Ghana and was first used to describe a precipitously lethal affliction in Gold Coast children who were eating a protein-deficient, maize diet. Kwashiorkor is fatal far more commonly than is marasmus and can develop in a matter of weeks. In the parlance of modern-day hospitals, the term kwashiorkor has been replaced by *hypoproteinemic PEM*, reflecting the disproportionate loss of visceral and serum proteins in the body, a phenomenon that contributes to the prominent edema characteristic of the condition. Transformation from marasmus to kwashiorkor often is precipitated by an acute illness, most commonly an infection. In fact, most hospitalized patients with PEM have marasmic kwashiorkor, a combination of marasmus and kwashiorkor.

Semistarvation leads to a loss of not only body fat but also muscle mass [4••]. Attrition of muscle mass in starvation is directly proportional to total weight loss. In contrast, the wasting of body fat is out of proportion to total weight loss and exceeds that of muscle mass. Thus, fat is expended more readily than muscle in pure starvation. Basal metabolic rate also decreases with ongoing semistarvation and eventually plateaus. From a teleologic standpoint, the metabolic effects of starvation are an attempt by the body to preserve the tissues that are most critical for immediate survival.

Weight loss occurs with both primary and secondary PEM but affects different body compartments. Lean body mass is depleted at a much faster rate in secondary PEM than in primary PEM. Therefore, prolonged secondary PEM is particularly detrimental because lean body mass contains essentially all the metabolic machinery in the body. Figure 191-1 illustrates the disproportionate loss of body cell mass (the major component of lean body mass) as a result of acute illness [5••].

Although micronutrient deficiencies commonly accompany PEM, their effects often are less notable in the face of the overwhelming effects of macronutrient deficiency. Nonetheless, the consequences of micronutrient deficiencies can be substantial,

and detecting such deficiencies is important. Although all micronutrients (except vitamin B_{12}) are absorbed primarily in the upper small intestine, ileal disease or resection may lead to bile salt malabsorption, resulting in malabsorption of fat-soluble vitamins. Similarly, chronic cholestatic liver disease (serum bilirubin chronically more than 5 mg/dL) is associated with inadequate bile secretion into the intestinal lumen and often results in malabsorption and depletion of fat-soluble vitamins. Other specific micronutrient deficiencies may occur either in the absence of PEM or in association with mild PEM. Table 191-1 provides a brief overview of some vitamins and their functions. For a complete table of vitamins and nutritional trace elements and their functions, the reader is referred to the following source: Mason [46].

▉ NUTRITIONAL ASSESSMENT
Overview

The purpose of nutritional assessment is to identify PEM and other nutritional deficiencies even when they are not readily discernible. Malnutrition can be detected when a nutritional assessment is carried out systematically. It can be subtle, as in patients with Child's class A alcoholic cirrhosis. Although these patients appear well nourished (and, by the Child-Turcotte classification, are considered to be "well nourished"), careful nutritional assessment by body composition analysis reveals that the actual frequency of substantial PEM in this population exceeds 50% [6].

There is no gold standard to define and measure PEM in the ill patient, in part because many of the parameters used to assess malnutrition in otherwise healthy persons are altered artifactually by illness. Although the accuracy of identifying malnourished patients is limited, the utility of nutritional assessment has been demonstrated repeatedly: malnourished patients sustain higher rates of malnutrition-related morbidity, and, more important, nutritional intervention in such patients is likely to improve clinical outcome (7,8,9••,10,11–14). Therefore, the primary aim of nutritional assessment is to identify patients who are likely to derive clinical benefit from nutritional intervention.

A comprehensive nutritional assessment consists of a history, physical examination, evaluation of certain anthropometric or functional measures, and, if warranted, laboratory blood tests. Typically, the assessment can be tailored to the clinical circumstances of the patient. In most cases, a brief history and physical

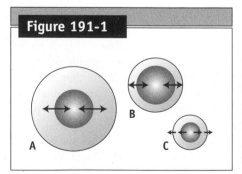

Figure 191-1

The disproportionate loss of body cell mass as a result of acute illness. **A**, Well-nourished state. **B**, Primary malnutrition, with contraction of the fat compartment (*outer circle*). **C**, Secondary malnutrition, with contraction of the fat compartment as well as body cell mass (*inner circle*). (*From* Hoffer [44]; with permission.)

Table 191-1. Vitamins and Their Functions

Fat-Soluble Vitamins

	Biochemistry and Physiology	Deficiency	Toxicity	Assessment of Status
Vitamin A	A subset of the retinoid compounds with biologic activity qualitatively similar to retinol. Carotenoids are structurally related to retinoids. Some carotenoids, most notably β-carotene, are metabolized into compounds with vitamin A activity and are considered to be provitamin A compounds. Vitamin A is an integral component of rhodopsin and iodopsins, light-sensitive proteins in retinal rod and cone cells.	Follicular hyperkeratosis and night blindness are early indicators. Conjunctival xerosis, degeneration of the cornea (keratomalacia), and de-differentiation of rapidly proliferating epithelia indicate more severe deficiency. Bitot spots (focal areas of the conjunctiva or cornea with foamy appearance) are an indication of xerosis. Blindness and retinal dysfunction ensues if left uncorrected. Increased susceptibility to infection also a consequence.	≥ 500 000 IU may cause *acute* toxicity, intracranial hypertension, skin exfoliation and hepatocellullar necrosis. *Chronic* toxicity may occur with habitual daily intake of >33,000 IU: alopecia, ataxia, dermatitis, cheilitis, pseudotumor cerebri, hepatocellullar necrosis and hyperlipidemia. Daily ingestion of >15,000 IU during early pregnancy can be teratogenic. Excessive intake of most carotenoids causes a benign, yellowish discoloration of the skin.	Retinol concentration in the plasma as well as vitamin A concentrations in the milk and tears are reasonably accurate measures. Toxicity best assessed by elevated levels of retinyl esters in plasma. A quantitative measure of dark adaptation for night vision or an electroretinograph are useful functional tests.
Vitamin D	A group of sterol compounds whose parent structure is cholecalciferol (vitamin D_3). Cholecalciferol is formed in the skin from 7-dehydrocholesterol by exposure to UV-B radiation. A plant sterol, ergocalciferol, can be similarly converted into vitamin D_2, and has similar vitamin D activity. Maintains intracellular and extracellular concentrations of calcium and phosphate by enhancing intestinal absorption of the two ions and, in conjunction with parathormone, promoting their mobilization from bone mineral.	Deficiency results in rickets in childhood and *osteomalacia* in adults. Expansion of the epiphyseal growth plates and replacement of normal bone with unmineralized bone matrix are the cardinal features. Deformity of bone and pathologic fractures occurs. Serum concentrations of calcium and phosphate may decline.	Excess amounts result in abnormally high serum concentrations of calcium and phosphate: metastatic calcifications, renal damage, and altered mentation may ensue.	The serum concentration of the major circulating metabolite, 25-hydroxy vitamin D indicates systemic status except in chronic renal failure, in which the impairment of renal 1-hydroxylation results in disassociation of the monohydroxy and dihydroxy vitamin concentrations. Measuring the serum concentration of 1.25-dihydroxy vitamin D is then necessary.
Vitamin E	A group of at least 8 naturally occurring compounds that share a spectrum of biologic activities. Some are tocopherols and some tocotrienols. The most biologically active of the vitameric forms is α-tocopherol. Acts as an antioxidant and free radical scavenger in lipophilic environments, most notably in cell membranes. Acts in conjunction with other antioxidants such as selenium.	Deficiency due to dietary inadequacy rare in developed countries. Usually effects premature infants, individuals with fat malabsorption, and persons with abetalipoproteinemia. Red blood cell fragility can produce hemolytic anemia. Neuronal degeneration produces peripheral neuropathies, ophthalmoplegia. and destruction of posterior columns of spinal cord. May contribute to hemolytic anemia and retrolental fibroplasia in premature infants.	Depressed levels of viamin K dependent procoagulants and potentiation of oral anticoagulants have been reported, as has impaired leukocyte function. Doses of 50 mg/d of α-tocopherol may increase the incidence of hemorrhagic stroke.	Plasma or serum concentration of a-tocopherol is most commonly used. Additional accuracy is obtained by expressing this value per mg of total plasma lipid. Red blood cell peroxide hemolysis test is not entirely specific, but is a useful functional measure of antioxidant potential of cell membranes.
Vitamin K	Phylloquinone (vitamin K_1) is derived from plants: a variety of menaquinones (vitamin K_7) is derived from bacterial sources. Serves as an essential cofactor in the post-translational α- or γ-carboxylation of glutamic acid residues in many proteins. These proteins include several circulating procoagulants and anticoagulants as well as proteins in the bone matrix and renal epithelium.	Deficiency syndrome uncommon except in (1) breast-fed newborns, in whom it may cause "hemorrhagic disease of the newborn": (2) adults with fat malabsorption or who are taking drugs that interfere with vitamin K metabolism (eg, coumarin, phenytoin, broad-spectrum antibiotics), and (3) individuals taking large doses of vitamin E. Excessive hemorrhage is usual manifestation.	Rapid intravenous infusion of K_1 has been associated with dyspnea, flushing, and cardiovascular collapse, probably related to dispersing agents in the solution. Supplementation may interfere with coumarin-based anticoagulation. Pregnant women taking large amounts of the provitamin menadione may deliver infants with hemolytic anemia, hyperbilirubinemia, and kernicterus.	The prothrombin time is typically used as a measure of functional K status; it is neither sensitive nor specific for vitamin K deficiency. Determination of undercarboxylated prothrombin in the plasma is more accurate but less widely available.

Water-Soluble Vitamins

Thiamine (vitamin B_1)	The coenzyme form is thiamine pyrophosphate (TPP). Serves as a coenzyme in many -keto acid decarboxylation and transketolation reactions. Inadequate thiamine availability leads to impairment of above reactions, resulting in inadequate ATP synthesis and abnormal carbohydrate metabolism. May have an additional role in neuronal conduction independent of above mentioned actions.	Classic deficiency syndrome ("beriberi") described in Asian populations consuming polished rice diet. Alcoholism and chronic renal dialysis are also common precipitants. High carbohydrate intake increases need for B_t. Deficiency produces various combinations of peripheral neuropathy, cardiovascular and cerebral dysfunction. Cardiovascular involvement ("wet beriberi") includes congestive heart failure and low peripheral vascular resistance.	Excess intake is largely excreted in the urine although parenteral doses of > 400 mg/d are reported to cause lethargy, ataxia, and reduced tone of the gastrointestinal tract.	The most effective measure of B_1 status is the erythrocyte transketolase activity coefficient, which measures enzyme activity before and after addition of exogenous TPP. Red cells from a deficient individual express a substantial increase in enzyme activity with addition of TPP. Thiamine concentrations in the blood or urine are also used.
Riboflavin (vitamin B_2)	Serves as a coenzyme for diverse biochemical reactions. The primary coenzymatic forms are flavin mononucleotide (FMN) and flavin adenine dinucleotide (FAD). Riboflavin holoenzymes participate in oxidation-reduction reactions in myriad metabolic pathways.	Deficiency is usually found in conjunction with deficiencies of other B vitamins. Isolated deficiency of riboflavin produces hyperemia and edema of nasopharyngeal mucosa, cheilosis, angular stomatitis, glossitis, seborrheic dermatitis and a normochromic, normocytic anemia.	Toxicity not known in humans.	The most common assessment is determining the activity coefficient of glutathione reductase in red blood cells (the test is invalid for individuals with glucose-6-phosphate dehydrogenase deficiency). Measurements of blood and urine concentrations are less desirable methods.

For a complete list of vitamins and nutritional and trace elements and their functions, the reader is referred to reference 46.

Adapted from Mason [46]; with permission.

examination suffice. A complete list of the patient's medications should be obtained because several drugs can induce nutrient deficiencies (Table 191-2).

Specific Tools

A variety of parameters have been used in the assessment of protein-energy status. Some of the more commonly used assessment tools include weight and height; other anthropometric measures, including skinfold thickness and mean arm circumference; functional measures, such as hand-grip strength and skin testing for evidence of anergy; assessment of specific serum protein concentrations, such as albumin, prealbumin, transferrin, and retinol-binding protein; complete blood count, including determination of the absolute lymphocyte count; and 24-hour urinary creatinine and urea nitrogen determinations. Less readily available tests to examine body composition, such as bioelectrical impedance and total-body potassium measurement, can be helpful in the appropriate setting. Although none of these tests has great specificity, they all continue to be used in practice, primarily because of their prognostic significance in both hospitalized and ambulatory patients.

Of these assessment tools, four stand out because of their ease of use and wide acceptance: a history of unintentional weight loss, measurement of weight, serum albumin level, and anthropometry. Because no single parameter is sufficiently sensitive or specific, these tools are used best in combination. Nevertheless, a history of unintentional weight loss is probably the best single indicator of PEM and can be used to grade PEM. Unintentional weight loss of 10% or more of premorbid weight indicates a diagnosis of PEM of substantial enough severity to predict a high likelihood of adverse clinical outcomes [15••]. For example, hospitalized patients with this degree of weight loss have an increased risk of developing pneumonia during their hospital stay [12]. Because of the disproportionate loss of lean body mass in acute illness, a 10% loss of premorbid weight translates into a 15% to 20% loss of total-body protein, a level of depletion that leads to impairment of many physiologic functions and to adverse clinical outcomes [15••]. Weight loss in excess of 20% indicates severe PEM with marked physiologic and clinical debility. Basing prognosis on an unintentional weight loss of 10% or more has limitations, however, because weight loss can be masked by excessive extracellular fluid accumulation. Furthermore, patients and family members often are unsure about recent changes in weight.

When a patient is unable to provide accurate information about recent weight changes, an alternative approach is to compare actual and ideal weight using normative weight-for-height tables. A weight substantially below the ideal suggests a diagnosis of PEM, and the severity of PEM can be assessed by a grading system analogous to that used for a history of weight loss. A weight of less than 85% of ideal indicates moderate to severe PEM [16]. Use of the Metropolitan Height-Weight Charts of 1959 is preferred because more recent weight standards are biased by the growing prevalence of obesity in the United States (Table 191-3). Interindividual variability in the population, however, limits the accuracy of this method in predicting PEM. As an alternative to height and weight tables, the body mass index (BMI), widely used to assess obesity, can be used to detect PEM. The BMI is the patient's weight in

Table 191-2. Drug-Nutrient Interactions*

Drug	Nutrient effect
Anti-infective agents	
Amikacin, gentamicin, sisomicin, and tobramycin	Hypokalemia, hypomagnesemia, and hypocalcemia; increased urinary potassium and magnesium loss
Aminosalicyclic acid	Decreased vitamin B_{12} and fat absorption
Amphotericin B	Increased urinary excretion of potassium and decreased serum potassium and magnesium levels
Capreomycin	Hypokalemia, hypomagnesemia, and hypocalcemia
Cycloserine	Decreased serum folate
Isoniazid	Pyridoxine deficiency
Neomycin	Decreased absorption of carotene, iron, vitamin B_{12}, and cholesterol
Rifampin	Decreased serum 25-hydroxy-cholecalciferol level
Sulfasalazine	Folate deficiency
Anticoagulants	
Warfarin, indanedione derivatives	Decreased vitamin K–dependent coagulation factors
Cardiovascular drugs	
Hydralazine	Pyridoxine deficiency
Sodium nitroprusside	Decreased total serum vitamin B_{12}
Central nervous system drugs	
Aspirin	Decreased serum folate
Monamine oxidase inhibitors	
Isocarboxazid	Decreased leukocyte and platelet ascorbic acid levels
Pargyline	Increased sensitivity to tyramine-containing foods; possible development of hypertensive crisis
Phenelzine	
Tranylcypromine	
Phenelzine	Pyridoxine deficiency
Tranylcypromine	
Phenobarbital	Decreased serum vitamin K_1
Phenytoin	Decreased serum folate, calcium, and 25-hydroxycholecalciferol levels
Electrolyte drugs	
Potassium chloride, slow release	Decreased vitamin B_{12} absorption
Gastrointestinal drugs	
Aluminum hydroxide	Decreased absorption of iron, phosphate, and vitamin B_{12}
Cholestyramine	Decreased absorption of vitamins A, D, E, K, B_{12} and folate along with decreased absorption of inorganic phosphate and fat
Cimetidine,	Decreased absorption of protein-bound vitamin B_{12}
Omeprazole	Decreased B_{12} absorption
Mineral oil	Decreased absorption of vitamins A, D, E, and K
Hormones	
Oral contraceptives	Decreased serum folate; pyridoxine deficiency; riboflavin deficiency
Other agents	
Colchicine	Decreased absorption of vitamin B_{12}, sodium, potassium, fat, and nitrogen
Penicillamine	Pyridoxine deficiency

Adapted from Weisner and Morgan [47]; with permission.

kilograms divided by the square of the height in meters. A BMI of less than 20 may indicate the presence of PEM.

Although serum albumin is a reasonable marker of PEM in undernourished but otherwise healthy persons, its usefulness in detecting PEM is limited in ill patients [17•]. Unlike unintentional weight loss, the serum albumin level cannot be used as the sole criterion for PEM. Values below 2.8 g/dL raise a suspicion of severe PEM, but such a low serum albumin level is not necessarily a direct reflection of malnutrition. Other serum proteins, such as transferrin, prealbumin, and retinol-binding protein, also are synthesized by the liver and may substitute for serum albumin as a marker for PEM. The half-lives of transferrin (8 to 9 days), prealbumin (2 to 3 days), and retinol-binding protein (0.5 days) are shorter than the half-life of albumin (14 to 20 days) and, therefore, theoretically reflect changes in nutritional status sooner. None of these other serum proteins, however, has been found to be more useful than serum albumin in detecting PEM.

The limitation of serum albumin is its lack of specificity for PEM, especially among severely ill hospitalized patients. Both interleukin-1 and tumor necrosis factor, cytokines involved in inflammation, lower serum albumin levels by down-regulation of the albumin gene [18]. The serum albumin level reflects the severity of illness rather than the severity of malnutrition.

Although serum albumin is neither a reliable physiologic marker of nutritional status nor an accurate marker of response to

Table 191-3. Weight and Height Reference Chart (Adults)*

| Height (without shoes) | | Reference weight | | | |
Feet and inches	Centimeters	Women lb	kg	Men lb	kg
4'10"	147	101	46	—	—
4'11"	150	104	47	—	—
5'0"	152	107	49	—	—
5'1"	155	110	50	—	—
5'2"	157	113	51	124	56
5'3"	160	116	53	127	58
5'4"	162	120	54	130	59
5'5"	165	123	56	133	60
5'6"	167	128	58	137	62
5'7"	170	132	60	141	64
5'8"	172	136	62	145	66
5'9"	175	140	63	149	68
5'10"	178	144	65	153	69
5'11"	180	148	67	158	71
6'0"	183	152	69	162	74
6'1"	185	—	—	167	76
6'2"	188	—	—	171	78
6'3"	190	—	—	176	80
6'4"	193	—	—	181	82

Adapted from Weisner et al [50]; with permission.

nutritional intervention, it is a good indicator of clinical prognosis. Because the serum albumin level reflects the severity of illness, it identifies patients who are undergoing the greatest protein catabolism and, therefore, are most likely to derive clinical benefit from nutritional support. For instance, in the Veterans Affairs Total Parenteral Nutrition Cooperative Study [9••], low serum albumin, in conjunction with other simple measures of PEM, was a predictor of postoperative complication.

Anthropometry is another useful tool for nutritional assessment. The term *anthropometry*, as used here, refers specifically to triceps skinfold thickness and upper arm circumference; the former provides an estimate of total-body fat and the latter of skeletal muscle mass. Anthropometry can be particularly helpful in patients with peripheral edema that spares the upper body, in whom weight measurements are likely to be spurious, or in patients with cirrhosis, in whom body weight can be grossly altered by ascites [6]. There are good correlations between triceps skinfold thickness and total-body fat and between upper arm circumference and lean body mass, and comparing results with those of age- and sex-matched controls provides a reasonable indication of body composition and nutritional status. The reader is referred to tables on *normal values for midarm muscle area* and *triceps skinfold thickness* found in the following reference: Mason and Rosenberg [48].

The limited sensitivity and specificity of any single nutritional parameter has prompted development of several nutritional indices that combine parameters in a weighted fashion. Several such indices have been studied and shown to predict clinical outcomes, such as duration of hospitalization, occurrence of postoperative complications, and mortality [19,20]. In addition, functional measures, such as fist-grip strength and forced expiratory volume in 1 second, have been used with some success to assess nutritional status and predict complication rates [15••].

The Decision to Initiate Nutritional Support

A diagnosis of PEM should not necessarily prompt initiation of nutritional support, particularly if the degree of malnutrition is mild. Large studies and meta-analyses have demonstrated repeatedly that aggressive nutritional support does not benefit well-nourished or mildly malnourished hospitalized patients [9••,21]. Instead, the decision to initiate nutritional support in such patients should be made only in the context of clinical trials.

Some groups of patients have been shown in prospective randomized interventional trials to benefit from nutritional support, with lower morbidity and mortality rates. These patients merit complete and careful nutritional assessment. Patients who derive benefit include those who have just undergone bone marrow transplantation [22]; have sustained significant weight loss and are about to undergo major abdominal or thoracic surgery [23]; have experienced severe trauma [24]; are unable to ingest or absorb nutrients for more than 10 days [25,26]; have decompensated alcoholic liver disease [27,28]; and are older than 65 years and hospitalized with a femoral neck fracture [10]. These patients should be monitored closely for evidence of PEM. If the patient has lost weight or has evidence of PEM, aggressive nutritional support in the form of oral liquid nutritional supplements, enteral tube feedings, or total parenteral nutrition should be considered (see Chapter 192). Other patients with moderate malnutrition also should be considered for nutritional interventions, particularly if the patient is expected to experience a prolonged period (>7 to 10 days) of reduced oral intake.

DETERMINING NUTRITIONAL REQUIREMENTS

Recommended Dietary Allowances, which are guidelines designed for healthy individuals, are not reliable estimates of nutritional needs in ill patients and are particularly unreliable in predicting macronutrient needs.

Direct measurement of energy requirements or regression equations derived from direct measurements are reasonable approaches to estimating energy needs in ill patients. Doubly-labeled water and indirect calorimetry are used commonly to determine caloric needs directly, with the former now considered the gold standard. Regression equations derived from these standards are readily available and accurate. One set of equations, the Harris Benedict equations, has gained great popularity in clinical nutrition support.

Although the Harris Benedict equations have been criticized for overestimating or underestimating energy needs and for a predilection for being transcribed incorrectly into textbooks, they nonetheless provide suitable estimates of caloric requirements. The following are acceptable versions of the equations:

For women: BEE = 655/day + 9.6W + 1.8H − 4.7A
For men: BEE = 66/day + 13.8W + 5H − 6.8A

where BEE denotes basal energy expenditure; W denotes weight in kilograms; H denotes height in centimeters; and A denotes age in years.

Basal energy expenditure must be multiplied by a stress factor and activity factor to estimate total caloric needs accurately in hospitalized patients. That is, total caloric needs = (BEE) (activity factor)(stress factor). Stress factors can range from a doubling of the BEE in patients with burn injuries, depending on the extent of the burn, to 1.7 for ventilator-dependent patients with multiple trauma, to 1.5 for patients in septic shock (Fig. 191-2). Activity factors usually range from 0.9 to 1.1 in ill, hospitalized patients but increase to about 2 in healthy, ambulatory persons performing light activity.

An alternative method of estimating energy needs is use of the World Health Organization (WHO) equations. These equations differ from the Harris Benedict equations in that a different regression equation has been derived for different decades of life and for each sex. Although the WHO equations are more accurate than the Harris Benedict equations, they also are more tedious to calculate because they require the use of six different equations for adults [29•]. Moreover, both sets of equations are less reliable in ill patients than they are in healthy persons. Overall, the Harris Benedict equations are preferable in the setting of severe illness.

Obesity presents a special problem in determining energy needs. Because adipose tissue is not metabolically active to a significant degree, the use of the Harris Benedict equations without modification can result in overestimation of energy needs. A more appropriate approach is to estimate the BEE based on the sum of ideal body weight plus 20% of weight in excess of ideal weight. This adjustment is useful in patients whose BMI exceeds 28. Other modifications should be made in patients whose body weight has been increased artifactually by peripheral edema or ascites; under these circumstances, use of either an estimated "dry" weight or the ideal body weight is preferable.

Although the hypercatabolism of illness depletes the body's protein compartment, the process can be attenuated by protein supplementation in conjunction with other needed nutrients [30]. Whereas the normal, unstressed person requires about 0.8 g/kg/d of protein [30], requirements increase with stress. Moderate stress should lead to empiric protein administration of 1 to 1.5 g/kg/d, and severe stress to 1.5 to 2 g/kg/d [30,31].

Although dietary protein requirements in cirrhotic patients with or at immediate risk of hepatic encephalopathy are comparable to those of someone without liver disease, patients with cirrhosis may be less able to tolerate protein. Restriction of protein intake to as little as 0.4 to 0.6 g/kg/d may be necessary to avoid exacerbation of encephalopathy. Routine protein restriction should be discouraged, however, and usually is unnecessary when other medical approaches for treating encephalopathy are adequately administered. Moreover, use of branched-chain amino acid–enriched, aromatic amino acid–depleted sources of protein in selected settings enables patients with liver disease to consume larger quantities of protein without exacerbating encephalopathy [32,33].

Renal insufficiency also is not necessarily an indication for dietary protein restriction because the protein needs of ill patients with kidney disease are just as great as (and sometimes

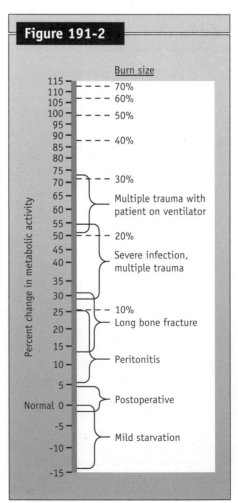

Figure 191-2

Percent change in metabolic activity

Burn size
115 — ---- 70%
110 — ---- 60%
105 —
100 — ---- 50%
95 —
90 — ---- 40%
85 —
80 —
75 —
70 — ---- 30%
65 —
60 — Multiple trauma with patient on ventilator
55 —
50 — --- 20%
45 —
40 — Severe infection, multiple trauma
35 —
30 —
25 — --- 10%
            Long bone fracture
20 —
15 —
10 — Peritonitis
5 —
Normal 0 — Postoperative
-5 —
-10 — Mild starvation
-15 —

Metabolic rate alterations by disease. (*Adapted from* Wilmore [45]; with permission.)

greater than) those of persons without kidney disease, and protein restriction only places the patient at risk for further wasting of lean body mass and debility. Instead, the physician must assess the body's protein needs in comparison with the body's ability to handle the greater urea generation that results from increased protein administration [34]. Sometimes, short-term dialysis is part of the compromise between these two considerations. When dialysis is used, protein losses increase further: 4 hours of hemodialysis results in protein losses of 5 to 10 g, and a session of peritoneal dialysis results in losses of 10 to 14 g. These losses must be compensated by nutritional repletion. Hemodialysis patients require 1.2 g/kg/d of protein, and patients on peritoneal dialysis require 1.2 to 1.5 g/kg/d plus repletion of protein needs, which arise secondary to illness. In short, protein needs must be balanced against protein tolerance when determining the appropriate amount of protein to prescribe to patients with renal insufficiency.

Whereas determination of the initial amount of protein to be administered can be empiric, the consequences of catabolic illness dictate that the decision be reassessed periodically. Two days after a patient reaches the targeted nutritional goals, nitrogen balance should be assessed by a 12- or 24-hour urinary collection. For a 24-hour collection, the following formula is used:

Nitrogen balance = [protein intake (g/d) ÷ (6.25 g of protein per 1 g of nitrogen)] − [(24-hour urine urea nitrogen + 4 g)]

This equation is invalid in patients who are undergoing hemodialysis or peritoneal dialysis. Similarly, the nitrogen balance of patients whose renal function is changing rapidly cannot be assessed accurately by this equation. Other, more complex equations have been formulated for these special circumstances [35]. In prescribing nutritional support in the form of tube feedings or total parenteral nutrition, the aim should be to maintain either a neutral or positive nitrogen balance. Note that amino acids or protein cannot be used adequately if insufficient calories are administered [30]. A persistently negative nitrogen balance may require an increase not only in protein delivery but also in nonprotein calorie sources.

■ AN APPROACH TO NUTRITIONAL ASSESSMENT: INFLAMMATORY BOWEL DISEASE—A CASE IN POINT

Adequate ingestion and assimilation of nutrients is dependent on a normally functioning gastrointestinal tract. Therefore, many gastrointestinal illnesses are complicated by nutritional problems, and the evaluation and care of patients with such disorders warrants careful attention to nutritional issues. Inflammatory bowel disease (IBD) is a case in point. Important issues pertaining to both macronutrients and micronutrients are common in IBD. This discussion complements the comprehensive discussion of IBD in Chapter 68 and elsewhere in this textbook.

Protein-energy malnutrition is common at the time of diagnosis of IBD and usually is the most conspicuous component of inadequate nutrition in patients with IBD. Clinically significant depletion of a variety of vitamins and minerals also is common. Many factors conspire to create nutritional deficiencies in patients with IBD [36]. Table 191-4 presents a collation of data from several nutritional surveys of hospitalized

(and, therefore, particularly ill) IBD patients; the high frequency of nutritional deficiencies underscores the importance of these issues in IBD.

Dietary Modifications

The major principle of dietary management in patients with IBD is to set nutritional goals. As for many gastrointestinal disorders, it is helpful to administer frequent, small meals to decrease the amount of food and secretions that the bowel must accommodate at any one time. If dietary restrictions are imposed, it is important to replenish the diet with other foods that will provide sufficient nutrients to restore and maintain desirable body weight and nutritional status. In some patients, this goal is achievable only with liquid nutritional supplements (see Chapter 192). A multivitamin and mineral supplement benefits all patients in a cost-effective manner, with no significant side effects [36]. In many instances, patients with IBD require vitamin or mineral supplements in quantities that exceed the amounts typically found in multinutrient supplements. Supplementation with large, supraphysiologic dosages should be prescribed on an individual basis and with caution because some vitamins and minerals can cause serious side effects when administered in high doses.

Dairy foods provide an important source of protein, calcium, and vitamin D. They should not be eliminated routinely from the diet because of concerns about lactose intolerance. Instead, lactose intolerance should be diagnosed in an objective manner by either a therapeutic trial of lactose withdrawal or a lactose breath test. Studies suggest that the prevalence of lactose intolerance in IBD corresponds to the prevalence observed in the patient's eth-

Table 191-4. Frequency of Diminished Nutritional Status in Patients With Inflammatory Bowel Disease*

Nutritional Status	Frequency, %
Protein-energy malnutrition	
<80% of ideal body weight	30
<80% of standard for upper arm muscle area	50–60
Growth retardation in children	40
Micronutrient deficiency	
Vitamins	
Low serum folate	3–64
Low plasma vitamin B_{12}	5–60[†]
Low vitamin 25OH vitamin D	25–65
Low serum retinol	21
Low serum vitamin C	12
Minerals	
Iron deficiency	40
Low serum Zn^{2+}	40–50
Low serum Mg^{2+}	14–33
Low serum K^+	6–20

*Adapted from Mason and Rosenberg [49].
†Reported figures for Crohn's disease; rarely reported in ulcerative colitis.

nic group, although lactose intolerance is nearly universal in those Crohn's disease patients who have small bowel disease extending proximal to the ileum. As an alternative to eliminating dairy products, the use of lactase-treated milk or exogenously administered lactase can be helpful to patients with mild to moderate symptoms of lactose intolerance.

In patients with narrowed segments of bowel, restriction of dietary fiber can help to minimize symptoms of obstruction. Otherwise, the results of adjusting dietary fiber content are highly variable; one study observed that gastrointestinal symptoms could be reduced with a high fiber diet. Soluble fibers, such as guars and pectins, retain water and occasionally are useful in patients with frequent watery bowel movements.

Dietary fat should be restricted when ileal disease or resection has resulted in steatorrhea; otherwise, excessive loss of fluid and important minerals will occur. Similarly, IBD complicated by primary sclerosing cholangitis and chronic elevation of serum bilirubin levels above 5 mg/dL can lead to low intraluminal concentrations of bile salts, which leads to malabsorption of fat-soluble nutrients. Disease involving less than 100 cm of ileum usually produces choleic, not steatorrheic, diarrhea, in which case a bile acid–binding resin, such as cholestyramine, and not fat restriction, is the preferred treatment. In patients with an ileostomy and steatorrhea, the unabsorbed fatty acids cannot stimulate colonic water and electrolyte secretion, and ostomy output is not altered substantially by the amount of fat in the diet. Nevertheless, modest fat restriction to 70 g/d is warranted in such patients because unabsorbed fatty acids bind and thereby enhance the excretion of calcium and magnesium. Because dietary fat restriction reduces the most calorically dense component of the diet, medium-chain triglyceride products can be used to replace these calories. The caloric density of medium-chain triglycerides is the same as that of conventional fat, but the absorption does not require a micellar phase in the intestine.

Symptomatic nephrolithiasis from calcium oxalate stones is a common complication in patients with ileal disease or prior ileal resection. In such patients, steatorrhea increases the colonic absorption of dietary oxalate. Free fatty acids bind to calcium and thereby allow increased mucosal permeability of oxalate. Dietary fat restriction reduces urinary supersaturation with oxalate. Alternative, or adjunctive, forms of dietary therapy include use of calcium supplementation with meals, which diminishes the proportion of free oxalate in the colon, and liberal intake of water, which decreases the urinary concentration of oxalate. Recent evidence suggests that use of calcium-rich foods is more effective in this regard than use of calcium supplements. Reducing dietary sources of oxalate is feasible but, because of the wide distribution of oxalate, often imposes unreasonable dietary restrictions. Lists of high oxalate foods are available.

Drug–Nutrient Interactions

Special attention must be paid to patients who are taking drugs that interfere with the absorption and metabolism of certain nutrients. Cholestyramine binds vitamins such as folic acid and vitamin D, reducing their bioavailability. Sulfasalazine inhibits both the intestinal absorption of folate and the activity of folate-dependent enzymes. Corticosteroids inhibit bone formation and

intestinal absorption of calcium and increase urinary excretion of calcium. Even modest doses of prednisone administered for a few months may lead to an impressive decrease in bone density.

Vitamins and Minerals

Vitamin B_{12} deficiency usually is seen in patients with Crohn's disease but not in those with ulcerative colitis. Among Crohn's disease patients, however, the prevalence of low plasma vitamin B_{12} levels is highly variable (5% to 60%). The length of the terminal ileum that is diseased or resected determines whether vitamin B_{12} malabsorption will occur: patients with disease or resection of less than 60 cm usually have normal vitamin B_{12} absorption, whereas those with a resection length of more than 90 cm do not. Another factor that plays an important role in determining whether vitamin B_{12} absorption is abnormal is bacterial overgrowth of the small intestine; the frequency of vitamin B_{12} malabsorption in patients with this condition is twice that associated with Crohn's disease in the absence of overgrowth. Small bowel bacterial overgrowth has classically been described with "blind loops" of intestine, intestinal strictures, bowel dysmotility, enteroenteric fistulas between proximal an distal loops of bowel, and loss of the ileocecal valve. Recently, subtle states of small bowel bacterial overgrowth, which do not produce overt steatorrhea, have been identified in patients with marked reduction in gastric secretion, including those with atrophic gastritis and those taking proton pump inhibitors. Both conditions result in substantial inhibition of vitamin B_{12} absorption and, at least in the case of atrophic gastritis, may lead to vitamin B_{12} deficiency. Whether long-term treatment with proton pump inhibitors leads to clinically significant vitamin B_{12} depletion remains a matter of debate.

Formerly, it was believed that of vitamin B_{12} deficiency was excluded by serum of vitamin B_{12} levels of more than 200 pg/mL. It is now clear, however, that neuropsychiatric complications of vitamin B_{12} deficiency develop in 7% to 10% of patients who have serum of vitamin B_{12} levels in the low-normal range (ie, 150 to 400 pg/mL) and that administration of vitamin B_{12} to these persons can improve their condition. The diagnosis of covert vitamin B_{12} deficiency can be made by means of a therapeutic trial of vitamin B_{12}, although a more objective approach is to measure serum levels of methylmalonic acid, which is a commercially available, highly sensitive indicator of early of vitamin B_{12} deficiency.

Patients with Crohn's disease and ulcerative colitis are prone to folate depletion for a variety of reasons, including inhibition of folate absorption by sulfasalazine and cholestyramine. Up to 63% of IBD patients present with serum folate levels below 3.5 ng/mL, although in only about 3% to 10% of these patients are stores sufficiently depleted to result in megaloblastic anemia. Mild degrees of folate depletion that are insufficient to produce megaloblastic anemia may still produce adverse clinical effects. Low folate intake at the time of conception leads to an increased incidence of congenital neural tube defects, and habitually low dietary intake of folate or blood levels of folate in the low-normal range have been implicated as risk factors for colonic mucosal dysplasia and cancer in ulcerative colitis [37,38]. Daily supplementation with at least 400 µg of folic acid has been reported to reduce the risk of colorectal neoplasia.

Inflammatory bowel disease perturbs the homeostasis of vitamin D and other minerals essential for bone health. A few small surveys suggested that 7% to 15% of patients with IBD have significant loss of bone mass; the frequency is 40% to 60% among those with low blood vitamin D levels [39]. Impairment of vitamin D absorption often is an important factor. The absorption of vitamin D is directly proportional to the concentration of bile salts in the intestine. Patients with ileal Crohn's disease or a prior ileal resection and IBD patients with a serum bilirubin level of more than 5 mg/dL caused by sclerosing cholangitis are particularly prone to low 25-OH vitamin D levels in the blood. In one large survey, 65% of patients with Crohn's disease had blood 25-OH vitamin D levels of less than 15 ng/mL, a level associated with accelerated bone loss. As mentioned previously, two drugs commonly used in IBD, prednisone and cholestyramine, inhibit the actions of vitamin D. In a recent placebo-controlled trial, a prednisone dose of 10 mg/d for 20 weeks led to a decrease in lumbar bone density of nearly 10%.

Although many laboratories report normal 25-OH vitamin D levels to be 10 to 50 ng/mL, levels between 35 and 50 ng/mL maintain bone mass better than lower levels. Maintenance of adequate vitamin D levels usually is achieved with a daily dose that is 1 to 2 times the RDA (ie, 200 to 400 IU/d). In IBD patients with ileal disease or cholestatic liver disease, however, the maintenance of adequate vitamin D levels may require a dose that is 5 to 10 times the RDA (ie, 1000 to 2000 IU/d). Liquid drops of vitamin D_2 often are the easiest method for administering large doses of vitamin D. Alternatively, the 25-OH and 1,25-dihydroxy metabolites of vitamin D are considerably more polar and therefore better absorbed in patients with fat malabsorption. Because these metabolites are extremely bioactive, serum total and ionized calcium should be monitored to prevent vitamin D toxicity until a steady-state vitamin D level is achieved. Hydroxylated forms of the vitamin also are considerably more expensive.

Steatorrhea also increases fecal losses of the divalent cations calcium and magnesium. Magnesium is intimately associated with the structure of bone mineral, and magnesium depletion impairs the secretion and, possibly, the action of parathyroid hormone. In turn, hypocalcemia and renal wasting of phosphate contribute to bone loss. Magnesium deficiency is common in patients with IBD, even though serum magnesium levels may be normal. The serum level, however, is a poor indicator of total-body magnesium status; urinary excretion of magnesium is a more sensitive indicator of body stores. Preliminary results of a study of 16 patients with short bowel syndrome demonstrated that most had normal serum magnesium levels but low urinary magnesium levels.

On a practical level, the homeostasis of calcium, magnesium, and phosphate is handled best by measures that minimize steatorrhea and by prescribing 1000 mg of supplemental calcium for any IBD patient who habitually consumes less than 600 mg/d of calcium or who is on long-term corticosteroid therapy. In addition, 200 to 400 IU/d of vitamin D_2 or D_3 should be taken in a multivitamin. If this regimen is adequate, the 24-hour urinary excretion of calcium should be between 200 and 300 mg. If calcium excretion is less than 200 mg/d, the patient is absorbing calcium inadequately; if the excretion exceeds 300 mg/d, the patient is inappropriately excreting calcium in the urine, in which case a thiazide diuretic may be prescribed to reduce renal loss of calcium.

Zinc deficiency is well described in patients with IBD, particularly those with Crohn's disease. Some studies suggest that up to 40% to 50% of all IBD patients have low serum zinc levels. Normally, about 50% of zinc is excreted in stool, and patients with diarrhea may require two to three times the normal zinc requirement. Furthermore, upper intestinal secretions are rich in zinc, and large quantities of the mineral can be lost through small bowel enterocutaneous fistulas. Because serum and red blood cell zinc levels are not accurate measures of zinc status, particularly in the setting of acute illness, zinc should be administered empirically when deficiency is suspected or impending. During acute exacerbations of IBD and in patients with high-output diarrhea or fistula drainage, parenteral administration of zinc, 10 to 15 mg/d, is the best means of preventing deficiency. Parenteral supplementation is preferable to aggressive oral supplementation, which may cause nausea and vomiting. During remission of IBD, the zinc contained in a multimineral supplement suffices.

Anemia in patients with IBD usually is due to the "anemia of chronic disease," iron deficiency, or both. Serum ferritin measurements can often distinguish these two causes: a level below 18 ng/mL confirms iron deficiency, whereas a level higher than 54 ng/mL excludes iron deficiency. Intermediate ferritin values have little diagnostic value in this setting. In addition to hemoglobin, myoglobin and other muscle proteins are iron dependent, and iron deficiency can lead to muscle fatigue, lassitude, and exercise intolerance in the absence of anemia. Because anemia appears only in the later stages of iron depletion, it is important to consider iron deficiency in any patient with IBD who complains of chronic fatigue and weakness.

During acute exacerbations of IBD, patients can become profoundly iron deficient. Oral iron supplementation often exacerbates gastrointestinal symptoms and may not replete the iron deficit. Therefore, parenteral iron supplementation should be considered in this setting. Up to 100 mg/d of iron dextran can be administered safely. Anaphylactoid reactions to parenteral iron occur with less than 3% of infusions when doses of less than 100 mg/d are administered. Rare "serum-sickness" reactions also have been reported. The total dose of iron needed is based on the calculated iron deficit. If more than 2 mg/d of iron is to be administered, an initial test dose of 25 mg given intravenously over 15 to 30 minutes should be administered in a setting where an anaphylactic reaction can be treated promptly.

Intensive Nutritional Support

In patients with severe intestinal disease or acute flares of disease, nutritional requirements often are not met by oral intake. Poor palatability of liquid supplements can limit the patient's ability to meet caloric requirements. In these situations, nutrients may be administered through either a nasoenteric or enterostomy tube (see Chapter 192). The latter option must be approached with caution, however, because intestinal inflammation can complicate the placement and maintenance of a gastrostomy or jejunostomy tube.

Only occasionally is parenteral nutrition necessary. Enteral feeding is safer and less expensive than parenteral nutrition and should be used first when tolerated. In the hospital setting, enterally fed patients sustain far fewer morbid events than those who are fed parenterally. A prospective randomized multicenter trial in hospitalized IBD patients demonstrated no significant advantage of parenteral over enteral nutrition with regard to symptoms, rate of recovery, or risk of relapse [40]. In general, parenteral nutrition should be instituted only when the enteral route causes exacerbation of symptoms despite adequate pharmacologic therapy, is precluded by disease activity, or cannot supply nutritional needs. Prolonged courses of total parenteral nutrition and bowel rest also are used often to heal enteric fistulas in Crohn's disease. Whether such an approach is truly effective has yet to be tested in a rigorous fashion; nevertheless, experience to date suggests that about half fistulas heal in the short-term with this approach, and about half of these remain closed for an extended period.

Two exciting advances in nutritional therapy have been proposed for the treatment of patients with IBD. The first is use of omega-3 fatty acids. A recent prospective, controlled trial in patients at high risk of relapse of Crohn's disease demonstrated that daily administration of an enteric-coated fish oil capsule led to more than a 50% reduction in the relapse rate at 1 year [41]. A similar study demonstrated marginal clinical improvements in patients with ulcerative colitis [42]. The second advance relates to use of enteral or parenteral glutamine to enhance recovery of damaged gastrointestinal mucosa. Whereas animal studies have demonstrated faster recovery of damaged small bowel mucosa with glutamine supplementation, human trials demonstrating improved clinical outcomes have been confined to patients undergoing bone marrow transplantation [43]. Nevertheless, use of glutamine in patients with severe IBD holds theoretical promise.

■ REFERENCES

Recently published papers of particular interest have been highlighted as follows:
- • Of interest
- •• Of outstanding interest

1. Coats KG, Morgan SL, Bartolucci AA, et al.: Hospital-associated malnutrition: a re-evaluation 12 years later. *J Am Diet Assoc* 1993, 93:27–33.

2.• Mason JB: A clinical nutritionist's search for meaning: why should we bother feeding the acutely ill, hospitalized patient [editorial]? *Nutrition* 1996, 12:279–281.
This well-referenced editorial emphasizes the importance of assessing outcomes when deciding to provide nutrition support to hospitalized patients.

3. Dinarello CA, Endres S, Meydani SN, et al.: Interleukin-1, anorexia, dietary fatty acids. *Ann N Y Acad Sci* 1990, 587:332–338.

4.•• Keys A, Brozek J, Henschel A, et al.: *The Biology of Human Starvation.* Minneapolis: University of Minnesota Press; 1950.
This landmark study describes the metabolic and body composition changes that occur with starvation.

5.•• Wilmore DW: Catabolic illness: strategies for enhancing recovery. *N Engl J Med* 1991, 325:695–702.
The authors provide a succinct review of the pathophysiology of catabolic illness.

6. Prijatmoko DWI, Strauss BJG, Lambert JR: Early detection of protein depletion in alcoholic cirrhosis: role of body composition analysis. *Gastroenterology* 1993, 105:1839–1845.

7. Sullivan DH, Walls RC: Impact of nutritional status on morbidity in a population of geriatric rehabilitation patients. *J Am Geriatr Soc* 1994, 42:471–477.

8. Detsky AS, Baker JP, O'Rourke K, et al.: Predicting nutrition-associated complications for patients undergoing gastrointestinal surgery. *JPEN* 1987, 11:440–446.

9.•• The VA Total Parenteral Nutrition Cooperative Study Group: Perioperative total parenteral nutrition in surgical patients. *N Engl J Med* 1991, 325:525–532.
This well-designed randomized study demonstrates that total parenteral nutrition benefits severely malnourished patients.

10. Delmi M, Rapin CH, Bengoa JM, et al.: Dietary supplementation in elderly patients with fractured neck of the femur. *Lancet* 1990, 335:1013–1016.

11. Kearns PJ, Young H, Garcia G, et al.: Accelerated improvement of alcoholic liver disease with enteral nutrition. *Gastroenterology* 1992, 102:200–205.

12. Windsor JA, Hill GL: Risk factors of postoperative pneumonia: the importance of protein depletion. *Ann Surg* 1988, 208:209–214.

13. Hermann FR, Safran C, Levkoff SE, et al.: Serum albumin level on admission as a predictor of death, length of stay, and readmission. *Arch Intern Med* 1992, 152:125–130.

14. Windsor JA, Hill GL: Weight loss with physiologic impairment: a basic indicator of surgical risk. *Ann Surg* 1988, 207:290–296.

15.•• Hill GL: Body composition research: clinical implications for the practice of clinical nutrition. *JPEN* 1992, 16:197–218.
The author presents an excellent review of the implications of nutritional assessment.

16. Stack JA, Babieau TJ, Bistrian BR: Assessment of nutritional status in clinical practice. *Gastroenterologist* 1996, 1(suppl):8–15.

17.• Klein S: The myth of serum albumin as a measure of nutritional status. *Gastroenterology* 1990, 99:1845–1846.
This is a well-written review of the limitations of serum albumin as a nutritional assessment tool.

18. Perlmutter DH, Dinarello CA, Punsal PI, et al.: Cachectin/tumor necrosis factor regulates hepatic acute-phase gene expression. *J Clin Invest* 1986, 78:1349–1354.

19. Smale BF, Mullen JL, Buzby GP, et al.: The efficacy of nutritional assessment and support in cancer surgery. *Cancer* 1981, 47:2375–2381.

20. Harvey KB, Moldawer LL, Bistrian BR, et al.: Biological measures for the formulation of a hospital prognostic index. *Am J Clin Nutr* 1981, 34:2013–2022.

21. Detsky AS, Baker JP, O'Rourke K, et al.: Perioperative parenteral nutrition: a meta-analysis. *Ann Intern Med* 1987, 107:195–203.

22. Weisdorf SA, Lysne J, Wind D, et al.: Positive effect of prophylactic total parenteral nutrition on long-term outcome of bone marrow transplantation. *Transplantation* 1987, 43:833–838.

23. Fan ST, Lo CM, Lai ECS, et al.: Perioperative nutritional support in patients undergoing hepatectomy for hepatocellular carcinoma. *N Engl J Med* 1994, 331:1547–1552.

24. Grahm TW, Zadrozny DB, Harrington T: The benefits of early jejunal hyperalimentation in the head-injured patient. *Neurosurgery* 1989, 25:729–735.

25. Gouttebel MC, Saint-Aubert B, Astre C, et al.: Total parenteral nutrition needs in different types of short bowel syndrome. *Dig Dis Sci* 1986, 31:718–723.

26. Messing B, Lemann M, Landais P, et al.: Prognosis of patients with nonmalignant chronic intestinal failure receiving long-term home parenteral nutrition. *Gastroenterology* 1995, 108:1005–1010.

27. Cerra FB, Cheung NK, Fischer JE, et al.: Disease-specific amino acid infusion in hepatic encephalopathy: a prospective, randomized double-blind, controlled trial. *JPEN* 1985, 9:288–295.

28. Nasrallah SM, Galambos JT: Amino acid therapy of alcoholic hepatitis. *Lancet* 1980, ii:1276–1277.

29.• *The Recommended Dietary Allowances*, edn 10. Washington, DC: National Academy Press; 1989.
This is a good reference source.

30. Young VR, Yu Y-M, Fukagawa NK: Protein and energy interactions throughout life: metabolic basis and nutritional implications. *Acta Paediatr Scand* 1991, 80(suppl):373–324.

31. Campbell WW, Crim MC, Dallal GE, *et al.*: Increased protein requirements in elderly people: new data and retrospective reassessments. *Am J Clin Nutr* 1994, 60:501–509.

32. Egberts E-H, Schomerus H, Hamster W, *et al.*: Branched chain amino acids in the treatment of latent portosystemic encephalopathy. *Gastroenterology* 1985, 88:887–895.

33. Horst D, Grace ND, Conn HO, *et al.*: Comparison of dietary protein with an oral, branched chain-enriched amino acid supplement in chronic portal-systemic encephalopathy: a randomized controlled trial. *Hepatology* 1984, 4:279–287.

34. Bergstrom J: Why are dialysis patients malnourished? *Am J Kidney Dis* 1995, 26:229–241.

35. Murray RL: Protein and energy requirements. In *Dynamics of Nutrition Support*. Edited by Krey SH, Murray RL. CT: Appleton-Century-Crofts; 1986:188–189.

36. Mason J: Vitamin and mineral supplementation in inflammatory bowel disease. *Practical Gastroenterology* 1995, 18:18A–18H.

37. Mason JB, Levesque T: Folate: effects on carcinogenesis and the potential for cancer prevention. *Oncology* 1996, 10:1727–1743.

38. Lashner BA, Provencher KS, Seidner DL, *et al.*: The effect of folic acid supplementation on the risk for cancer or dysplasia in ulcerative colitis. *Gastroenterology* 1997, 112:29–32.

39. Clements D, Motley R, Evans A, *et al.*: Longitudinal study of cortical bone loss in patients with IBD. *Scand J Gastroenterol* 1992, 27:1055–1060.

40. Greenberg GR, Fleming CR, Jeejeebhoy KN, *et al.*: Controlled trial of bowel rest and nutritional support in the management of Crohn's disease. *Gut* 1988, 29:1309–1315.

41. Belluzzi A, Brignola C, Campieri M, *et al.*: Effect of enteric-coated fish-oil preparation on relapses in Crohn's disease. *N Engl J Med* 1996, 334:1557–1560.

42. Stenson WF, Cort D, Rodgers J, *et al.*: Dietary supplementation with fish oil in ulcerative colitis. *Ann Intern Med* 1992, 116:609–614.

43. Ziegler TR, Young LS, Benfell K: Clinical and metabolic efficacy of glutamine-supplemented parenteral nutrition after bone marrow transplantation: a randomized, double-blind, controlled study. *Ann Intern Med* 1992, 116:821–828.

44. Hoffer LJ: Starvation. In *Modern Nutrition in Health and Disease*, vol 2. Edited by Shils ME, Olson JA, Shike M. Philadelphia: Lea & Febiger; 1994:937.

45. Wilmore WD: The metabolic management of the critically ill. New York: Plenum Medical; 1977:36.

46. Mason JB: Consequences of altered micronutrient status. In *Cecil Textbook of Medicine*, edn 20. Edited by Bennett JC, Plum F. Philadelphia: WB Saunders; 1996:1145–1150.

47. Weisner RL, Morgan SL: *Fundamentals of Clinical Nutrition*. St Louis: Mosby-Year Book; 1993.

48. Mason JB, Rosenberg IH: Protein-energy malnutrition. In *Harrison's Principles of Internal Medicine*, edn 13. Edited by Isselbacher KJ, Braunwald E, Wilson JD, *et al*. New York: McGraw-Hill; 1994:442.

49. Mason JB, Rosenberg IH: Nutritional therapy of inflammatory bowel disease. In *Inflammatory Bowel Diseases*, edn 2. Edited by Allan RN, Keighley MRB, Alexander-Williams J, *et al*. Edinburgh: Churchill Livingstone; 1993:412.

50. Weisner RL, Heimburger DC, Butterworth CE: *Handbook of Clinical Nutrition*, edn 2. St. Louis: Mosby-Year Book, 1989.

192 Enteral and Parenteral Nutrition
Mark H. DeLegge and Rebecca Copenhaver DeLegge

No condition or disease process is improved by prolonged starvation. In adults of normal weight, death from protein-energy malnutrition occurs after 60 to 70 days of total starvation. Consequences of malnutrition can develop rapidly, however, in the presence of acute stress without adequate nutrient intake. Epidemiologic studies suggest that weight loss, a clinical sign of negative energy and protein balance, is associated with adverse outcomes in hospitalized adults [1] (see Chapter 191). Functional consequences of starvation occur more rapidly in stressed and catabolic patients than in healthy persons. When malnutrition persists, weakness, compromised immunity, decreased wound healing, and other complications are likely to occur and influence the patient's response to medical and surgical treatment. Recent data have shown that addressing a patient's nutritional needs within the first 48 hours of hospitalization can impact positively on the length of stay and overall cost of care [2].

ENTERAL VERSUS PARENTERAL NUTRITION

Nutritional support is a major factor in the successful treatment of critically ill patients. Increased safety and efficacy of enteral access devices and procedures have shifted nutritional therapy away from parenteral nutrition as the first approach to re-establishing nutritional stability. Enteral nutrition has proved to be less costly and to carry less risk of complications [3]. Early enteral intervention has been shown to reduce the frequency of septic complications and to shorten the length of hospital stays, perhaps because of prevention of bacterial translocation from the intestinal tract [4]. Currently, candidates for enteral nutrition are patients who will not, should not, or cannot eat, but who have a functional gastrointestinal (GI) tract. Candidates for parenteral nutrition are patients for whom enteral feeding techniques have failed to provide some or all of the nutritional requirements or those for whom enteral nutrition is contraindicated [5].

ENTERAL NUTRITION

Enteral nutrition includes both the oral ingestion of food and the delivery of nutrients by a tube into the GI tract. In this chapter, the term *enteral nutrition* refers to food entering the GI tract by means other than oral ingestion.

Contraindications to enteral feeding include diffuse peritonitis, intestinal obstruction, intractable vomiting, paralytic ileus, and severe diarrhea. Other possible contraindications include severe pancreatitis, enterocutaneous fistula, GI ischemia, and severe malabsorptive disorders.

Route and Destination

After deciding to use the GI tract for the delivery of nutrition, two key decisions must follow: the route of enteral access and the destination of tube feedings. Each route and destination has its own efficacy, drawbacks, and risks.

Route Considerations: Longevity and Risk Assessment

The first factor to consider is the number of days before oral feeding can be resumed. Current guidelines recommend a nasoenteric delivery route if the patient is thought to be able to resume oral feedings within 30 days [6]. The average life span for most nasoenteric tubes is 10 to 12 days [7]. Complications associated with the use of nasoenteric tubes include clogging, accidental removal, and lack of acceptance by the patient or patient's family (Table 192-1). If after multiple attempts, a patient cannot maintain nor tolerate a nasoenteric tube, a percutaneous route should be considered. Percutaneous tubes are less cosmetically distracting and generally are larger in diameter than nasoenteric tubes and therefore are less likely to clog. Although placement of percutaneous enteral access tubes may be more technically challenging and costly than placement of nasoenteric tubes, the reliability of the percutaneous tubes allows uninterrupted delivery of nutrients and medications.

The second factor in choosing an enteral access route is assessing the patient's risk of gastric aspiration. A nasoenteric tube must pass through the upper and lower esophageal sphincters, thereby potentially compromising their ability to protect against gastroesophageal reflux and gastric aspiration. In addition, nasoenteric tubes, by stimulating the pharynx, increase the frequency of lower esophageal sphincter (LES) relaxation, thereby contributing to reflux of gastric contents into the esophagus and ultimately into the lungs. The combination of compromised esophageal sphincter function and increased frequency of LES relaxation may place a patient at high risk of gastric aspiration [8], making the percutaneous access route potentially safer.

Destination

Determination of tube-feeding destination hinges on three concepts: appropriate gastric anatomy, tolerance of gastric feedings, and risk of gastric aspiration. Gastric access rarely is limited by gastric anatomy, except in the cases of major gastric resection or gastric outlet obstruction. More commonly, determination of the appropriateness of gastric feeding is based on gastric feeding tolerance and the risk of gastric aspiration. A patient's tolerance for gastric feeding usually is determined by the gastric emptying rate. Patients with reduced gastric emptying rates, such as diabetic or critically ill patients, often do not tolerate feedings delivered to the stomach because of the presence of high gastric residuals (> 200 mL) [9]. Such patients are more appropriately fed through the small bowel [10]. A patient's calculated risk of gastric aspiration also influences the destination of tube feedings. Patients with a prior histories of gastric aspiration or those at risk for gastric aspiration, such as critically ill, ventilated patients or neurologically impaired patients in whom the upper airway cannot be protected from gastric aspiration, may be candidates for small bowel feedings [11].

Short-Term Enteral Access

Short-term enteral access placement with a nasogastric, nasoduodenal, or nasojejunal tube is performed routinely in most intensive care units. Nasogastric tubes are technically easier to place than are nasoduodenal or nasojejunal feeding tubes because of the tendency of the latter two to coil within the stomach rather than to pass through the pylorus into the small bowel. Nasoenteric feeding tubes depend on gastric motility to carry the tube tip through the pylorus and into the small bowel. Some nasoenteric feeding tubes have distal weights to aid passage through the pylorus; however, these tips are of no proven benefit and have been shown in some studies actually to inhibit passage through the pylorus [12]. Studies also have shown that if bedside attempts at nasoenteric feeding tube placement do not result in proper positioning within 24 hours, success is unlikely with further attempts [13]. At this point, it is appropriate to call an endoscopist or radiologist for endoscopic or fluoroscopic tube placement.

Nasoenteric Access

Endoscopic placement of nasoenteric feeding tubes requires familiarity with at least several placement techniques (see Chapter 188). Nasoduodenal and nasojejunal tubes range in length from 105 to 200 cm and in diameter from 8F to 14F and are made of polyurethane or polyvinyl chloride. Some nasoenteric tubes can be placed over a guidewire under direct endoscopic observation, whereas others are passed through the biopsy channel of an endoscope. An alternative, although generally ineffective, endoscopic technique requires attaching a suture loop to the end of a feeding tube and dragging the tube into place beyond the pylorus. Although studies have touted placement times of less than 15 minutes, it is not uncommon for placement procedures to last up to 1 hour. Frustration with nasoenteric tube placement is compounded by the knowledge that the life span of the tube is less than 10 days, usually because of displacement by the patient or staff. Nevertheless, they are effective tools for providing immediate enteral access to medicate, feed, or monitor hospitalized patients.

Percutaneous Enteral Access

Percutaneous tube enterostomy provides access to the stomach or intestine through surgical, endoscopic, or radiologic means. Generally accepted contraindications to endoscopic tube

Table 192-1. Complications Associated With Nasoenteric Tubes	
Otitis media	Reflux esophagitis
Pharyngitis	Aspiration pneumonia
Sinusitis	Tube migration
Nasal mucosa ulceration	Displacement and clogging

enterostomy include ascites, coagulopathy, inability to transilluminate through the abdominal wall with an endoscope, marked hepatomegaly, previous gastrectomy, morbid obesity, peritoneal dialysis, peritoneal metastases, portal hypertension, or marked esophageal obstruction prohibiting the passage of the endoscope. Preprocedure administration of antibiotics is standard [14].

Endoscopic techniques generally are the first-line procedures for gaining access percutaneously [15]. Placement may be by either the Sacks-Vinc ("push") or Ponsky ("pull") technique, depending on the physician's preference, as discussed in Chapter 188.

Percutaneous Endoscopic Gastrojejunostomy Versus Percutaneous Endoscopic Jejunostomy

Endoscopic placement of a distal duodenal or jejunal feeding tube for enteral access may be accomplished by one of two techniques, each of which is capable of delivering nutrients directly into the small bowel, thereby bypassing the stomach.

In the first technique, percutaneous endoscopic gastrojejunostomy, a percutaneous endoscopic gastrostomy (PEG) is performed with subsequent passage of a second feeding tube, or J tube, through the existing PEG tube. This technique requires pulling a guidewire through the PEG down into the small bowel with a grasping forceps (Fig. 192-1, see also **Color Plate**) [16]. While maintaining tension on the guidewire, the J tube is passed through the PEG over the guidewire until it is positioned in either the distal duodenum or jejunum. This tube system allows concurrent feeding into the small bowel through the J tube and decompression of the stomach through the PEG, which may be important in patients at high risk of gastric aspiration.

In the percutaneous endoscopic jejunostomy technique, the jejunum is accessed directly using a standard PEG insertion technique. A longer endoscope is required to reach the jejunum. Procedural failure often is a result of inability to transilluminate an appropriate jejunal access site. Medications, such as atropine or glucagon, often are administered to paralyze the small intestine temporarily so that needle catheter puncture can be performed. Because the small bowel is thin walled, as compared with the stomach, direct percutaneous small bowel feeding tubes may be more prone to wound infection and tract breakdown.

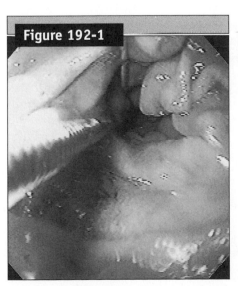

Figure 192-1

Endoscopic view of forceps dragging a guidewire into the distal duodenum during PEG/J placement. See also **Color Plate**.

Tube Complications

Although percutaneous placement techniques have evolved to a state of low risk, wound care complications still are relatively common (see Chapter 189). Silicone, the predominant material in the implant, is inert and rarely the cause of tissue reactions. Attention to cleaning, handling, and proper medication use reduces the risk of complications and may increase the longevity of the feeding tube.

The overall complication rate for a percutaneously placed gastrostomy tube is about 4% to 10%. Minor complications include bleeding and infection at the placement site and are easily treated medically. Tube clogging is a common complication and may necessitate PEG replacement. Home remedies for maintaining tube patency include flushing with at least 60 mL of water after each feeding to remove residual food particles. Medications should be crushed thoroughly or given in a liquid form. Nonliquid bulk-forming agents should be avoided.

Major complications, although rare, can be debilitating and may result in tube removal, surgical intervention, and even death from septic complications (see Chapter 189). Major complications include procedure-related aspiration pneumonia, pneumoperitoneum (usually transient), colocutaneous fistula, peritonitis, and necrotizing fasciitis in addition to buried bumper syndrome, tube clogging, and early accidental removal.

Intra-procedure aspiration has been shown to occur during placement of gastrostomy tubes, is associated with postprocedure pneumonia, and can be minimized by reducing the time of procedure, elevating the patient's head to 30 degrees during the procedure, and aggressively aspirating the posterior pharynx [17].

Pneumoperitoneum is common after PEG placement, but generally is not a problem unless it persists longer than 2 weeks or is associated with a small bowel ileus or clinical signs of peritonitis [18].

Colocutaneous fistula occurs when the colon is trapped between the abdominal wall and the stomach during PEG placement. Often, this complication is not noticed during initial PEG placement but is discovered when attempts are made to replace the initial PEG [19]. This complication may disappear by simply removing the PEG and allowing the fistula tract to heal. Occasionally, surgical intervention is required.

If the initial PEG incision was made too small to pull the gastrostomy tube through comfortably and without compromising adjacent tissues, tissue ischemia may occur, resulting in wound breakdown [20]. Treatment includes antibiotics, aggressive wound care, and, frequently PEG removal. Buried bumper syndrome results when the external PEG bolster is pushed tight against the external abdominal wall and, concurrently, the internal bolster of the PEG is pulled tight against the gastric mucosa. Continued external bolster pressure may pull the internal bumper completely into the gastric or abdominal wall (Fig. 192-2, see also **Color Plate**). The internal bolster is not seen on endoscopy, which may reveal only a dimple on the gastric mucosa as a sign that the internal bolster bumper has migrated into the gastric wall. Treatment may range from external removal of the tube to surgical intervention.

Early accidental removal before tract formation, which usually occurs within 2 to 3 weeks after PEG placement, can be treated with antibiotics and tube replacement or may require surgical intervention. Often, a new tube can be placed through or near the site of the removed PEG so as to pull the tissues containing the previous stoma site against the abdominal wall, thereby creating a seal [21]. Antibiotics should be administered.

Enteral Formulas

Once an appropriate enteral access device has been inserted, a decision is required regarding the type of enteral nutrition the patient should receive. This determination requires attention to a patient's overall caloric and protein needs (Table 192-2), the cost of various enteral products, and the presence of comorbid diseases such as diabetes or pancreatitis. Most enteral nutrition used today is in the form of commercial formulas. Enteral formulas can be categorized as blenderized, lactose-containing, lactose-free, elemental, modular, and specialty formulas, each with its own potential benefits and disadvantages.

Blenderized formulas are combinations of table food with added vitamins and minerals. They tend to be viscous and are not appropriate for small-bore feeding tubes. Because of their high osmolarity, they may cause diarrhea and nausea if infused directly into the small bowel. Lactose-containing enteral formulas are used only rarely because they may induce diarrhea, bloating, and nausea. Most commercial formulas are lactose free. Lactose-free formulas are moderately osmotic and contain 1 to 2 kcal/mL. Their protein content typically is 12% to 20% but may be higher. Protein-fortified formulas are designated by the initials HN ("high nitrogen"). Carbohydrates, fats, and proteins in them are in complex forms and require the patient to have normal digestive and absorptive capacities. Some of these formulas are flavored for oral consumption.

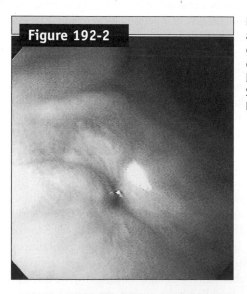

Figure 192-2

Endoscopic view of a dimple in the gastric mucosa caused by buried bumper syndrome. See also **Color Plate.**

Elemental formulas are used in patients who may have a problem with digestion or absorption of complex proteins, carbohydrates, and fats [22]. They are delivered as easily absorbed free amino acids, dipeptides and tripeptides, simple carbohydrates (maltodextrins) and simple fats (medium-chain triglyceride oil). The small particle size of these formulas makes them highly osmotic. They have a bad taste and therefore must be administered by a feeding tube.

Specialty enteral formulations have been developed to meet presumed special nutritional needs of patients with specific diseases (Table 192-3). Laboratory and animal data often are used in the development of these formulas. For example, special formulas for patient with diabetes contain the sugar fructose to reduce the demand for insulin production; hepatic failure formulations contain a large amount of branched-chain amino acids, believed to prevent the development of hepatic encephalopathy; immune system–enhancing formulas contain arginine, an immune system–stimulating amino acid; and pulmonary failure formulations contain a reduced amount of carbohydrates so as to decrease CO_2 production. Many of these formulas are costly, and their efficacy is often not supported by human clinical data [23–27].

Modular formulas are individual nutrient components (proteins, carbohydrates, and fats) that are mixed to create a custom enteral formula. They rarely are required in view of the abundance of products available commercially.

Water

All commercial enteral formulas contain a certain amount of free water. The more calorie-concentrated a formula is, the less free water contained within the formula. Additional free water may be administered as bolus injections through the feeding tube.

Enteral Formula Delivery

Enteral formulas may be delivered by bolus, gravity, or pump systems. Bolus feedings usually are administered through a syringe over a course of 5 to 20 minutes. Volumes in the range of 240 to 400 mL are delivered in one setting. This is the method of choice for active patients who are alert and do not want to be hooked to delivery equipment. The technique is easily taught to patients and caregivers. Bolus feedings almost always are deliv-

Table 192-3. Abbreviated Specialty Enteral Formula

Type	Disease state	Special formula
Pulmocare	Respiratory failure	Low carbohydrate
Impact	Immune deficiency	Arginine fortified
Hepatic-Aid II	Liver failure	Branched chain amino acid
Nepro	Renal failure	Low potassium and phosphate
Glucerna	Diabetes	Low glucose and high fructose
Lipisorb	Fat malabsorption	Medium-chain triglycerides
Alitrac	Malabsorption	Glutamine fortified

Table 192-2. Common Daily Calorie and Protein Needs

Disease state severity	Calories, *kcal/kg*	Protein, *g/kg*
Mild	25	0.8–1.0
Moderate	30	1.2–1.4
Severe	33–35	1.5–1.8

ered into the stomach. Small bowel bolus feedings may result in abdominal pain, nausea, and diarrhea.

Gravity feedings are delivered with the use of a bedside pole. There is no mechanical pump involved, thereby reducing the cost of enteral formula delivery. Gravity feedings may be delivered either intermittently as a set amount of formula over a period of time or continuously. Intermittent feedings are preferred for patients who cannot tolerate bolus feedings. Gravity is used most often for gastric feedings. This delivery method does not permit precise control of the amount of formula delivered per minute and therefore is not appropriate for patients who are at risk of gastric aspiration or who have demonstrated intolerance to tube feedings.

Pump feedings require the use of a bedside mechanical device and permit greatest accuracy in the delivery of formula. Feeding may be delivered either intermittently or continuously. This is the preferred modality for small bowel feedings and for patients at risk of gastric aspiration. It is the delivery method of choice in the intensive care unit because of a reduced frequency of abdominal distention and gastric aspiration, compared with other delivery methods [28].

Assessment of Feeding Tolerance

Assessment of feeding tolerance is important. Stool frequency and consistency, abdominal distention, bowel sounds, and urinary output should be monitored. Enteral formulas can be colored with methylene blue to monitor for the presence of gastroesophageal reflux and gastric aspiration. Suctioning of blue secretions from the patient's posterior pharynx or endotracheal tube indicates that the patient is at high risk of aspiration.

Regardless of the tube-feeding delivery system used, the most critical factor in the safe delivery of tube feeding is bedside nursing care. All patients should be fed with the head of their bed at 30 degrees [29]. With gastric feedings, gastric residuals should be checked every 6 hours. Residuals greater than 200 mL require that the tube feeding be stopped and the residual placed back into the stomach. The residual should be checked again in 2 hours. If it remains greater than 200 mL, small bowel feedings should be considered.

Advancement of Tube Feedings

Advancement of tube feedings, once initiated, is an imperfect science. In our center, continuous tube feedings are initiated at 30 mL/h and advanced by 10 mL every 6 hours, until the goal rate of infusion is reached. Any sign of tube-feeding intolerance results in temporary cessation of tube feeding or a reduction in the tube-feeding rate. Once a patient has reached the goal rate, he or she may be maintained on continuous 24-hour tube feedings or changed to 18- or 12-hour continuous tube feedings, intermittent tube feedings, or bolus tube feedings. It is common for hospitalized patients to receive their tube feedings in a 12-hour time period overnight. This is accomplished by doubling the infusion rate of the tube feeding that the patient had been receiving over 24 hours. Tube-feeding delivery methods and rates are individualized for the patient's comfort and safety.

Enteral Feeding Complications

Gastrointestinal side effects of tube feeding are reported in 15% to 30% of patients and include nausea, vomiting, abdominal

distention, abdominal cramping, and diarrhea. Nausea, vomiting, and abdominal distention often resolve by slowing the rate of delivery. Concomitant gastroesophageal reflux disease, peptic ulcer disease, gastric outlet obstruction, or small bowel ileus should be treated.

Diarrhea is the most common enteral feeding complication and may result from numerous causes [30] (Table 192-4). The most common cause is *Clostridium difficile* colitis resulting from antibiotic use. Treatment is with oral metronidazole or vancomycin.

In many patients, medications are changed from tablet to liquid form for easy instillation through the feeding tube. These liquid medications often contain sorbitol, a known cathartic. Magnesium-containing medications, hypertonic medications, and promotility agents also may promote diarrhea. High osmolar tube feedings often are cited as a cause of diarrhea, but studies have demonstrated tolerance for tube feedings as concentrated as 600 mOsm/kg. It does not make sense to dilute commercial enteral formulations in an attempt to improve the patient's tolerance. Often, changing a patient's feeding delivery from bolus or intermittent feedings to continuous delivery reduces the effects of tube-feeding osmolarity and improves patient tolerance.

For patients with true intestinal malabsorption, the use of an elemental formula may improve absorption and reduce the severity of diarrhea. This also may be true in patients with hypoalbuminemia. Such patients often develop small bowel wall edema secondary to fluid shifts resulting from the low plasma oncotic pressure. Small bowel wall edema may hinder absorption.

Rarely, stool impaction results in flow of liquid stool around the impaction. This problem can be suspected by the presence of abdominal distention and an abdominal radiograph demonstrating colonic dilation. Fiber supplementation may improve diarrhea in such patients once the obstructing impaction is relieved. A number of fiber-supplemented commercial enteral formulas are available.

Metabolic complications are less common with enteral feedings than with parenteral feedings (see later discussion). Dehydration and fluid shifts may occur with high osmotic

Table 192-4. Causes and Treatment of Tube-Feeding–Associated Diarrhea

Cause	Treatment
Clostridium difficile colitis	Antibiotics
Liquid medication with sorbitol	Avoid sorbitol-containing medications
Magnesium-containing medications	Avoid magnesium-containing medications
Promotility medications	Discontinue
High osmolar tube feedings	Slow rate and increase delivery time
Malabsorption	Slow rate, administer anticholinergics, consider elemental feedings
Hypoalbuminemia	Slow rate, administer anticholinergics, consider elemental feedings

feedings, especially if sufficient free water is not administered. Hyperglycemia may occur with delivery of a concentration of high carbohydrates in patients with glucose intolerance. Careful monitoring of serum glucose, especially at initiation of tube feedings, avoids this complication. In patients with renal failure, strict attention must be paid to the potassium, magnesium, and phosphorous content of the enteral formula. Many enteral formulas in a concentration of 2 cal/mL are appropriate for renal failure patients who do not require use of the more costly specialty renal failure formulations.

Drug levels also may be affected by tube feeding. Delivery of phenytoin is reduced because of binding of this drug to feeding tubes when concurrent enteral formula is delivered [31]. A precipitate in the tubing has been reported with the use of over-the-counter cold medications in conjunction with enteral feedings. Vitamin K present in many enteral formulas may make a patient more resistant to the effects of warfarin. If there are any questions regarding the interaction between tube feeding and medications, the hospital pharmacist or dietitian should be consulted.

■ PARENTERAL NUTRITION

For patients with nonfunctioning GI tracts, nutrients can be delivered into the venous system; this is referred to as *total parenteral nutrition* (TPN). Nutrients may be delivered into a central vein, referred to as *central parenteral nutrition*, or into a peripheral vein, referred to as *peripheral parenteral nutrition* (PPN).

Total parenteral nutrition solutions consist of water, electrolytes, amino acids, carbohydrates, fats, proteins, vitamins, and trace elements. These compounds are mixed and delivered over a period of time, generally 12 to 24 hours. Table 192-5 demonstrates a typical TPN feeding formula. The wide variety of indications for TPN have in common the presence of a nonfunctional or nonaccessible GI tract that precludes the enteral delivery of nutrition. Common indications include small bowel obstruction, short bowel syndrome, and small bowel malabsorption [32].

Total parenteral nutrition solutions are six times more concentrated than blood (1800 to 2400 mOsm/L) and generally consist of about 30 to 50 g of protein and 800 to 1200 cal/L [33].

Table 192-5. Common Total Parenteral Nutrition Solutions

70% Dextrose	350–500 g
10%–15% Amino acid	50–100 g
10%–20% Fat	50–100 g
NaCL Na acetate	50–150 mEq/L
Kcl or K acetate	15–30 mEq/L
Mg sulfate	10–20 mEq/L
Ca gluconate	4–12 mEq/L
Multivitamins and trace elements	

Common elective additives: insulin, heparin, H₂ receptor antagonists, vitamin K.

Determination of caloric and protein needs requires a nutritional assessment (see Chapter 191). The dietitian often is helpful in determining a patient's protein and calorie needs. Table 192-2 provides an approximation of a patient's daily protein and caloric needs based on the severity of the underlying disease. Overall daily water requirements can be estimated at 20 to 30 mL/kg.

Total Parenteral Nutrition Compounding

In prescribing a TPN formula, determination is first made of its protein, carbohydrate, and fat content. A step-wise approach is effective. The caloric content of protein is 4 kcal/g, that of carbohydrate is 3.4 kcal/g, and that of fat is about 10 kcal/g. A patient's overall protein and caloric needs also must be determined. The protein component (that which meets the patient's daily protein requirements) is compounded into the formula first, and the total calories from the protein component are then subtracted from the patient's total caloric needs. The patient's carbohydrate needs (5 to 7g/kg/d) are then added to the formula, and the total calories of this component are subtracted from the remaining daily caloric needs. Finally, the remaining caloric needs are compounded from the fat component, generally in the range of 0.5 to 1.5 g/kg/d. Figure 192-3 gives an example of such a calculation.

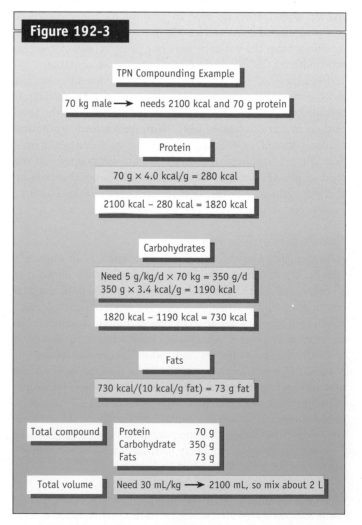

Figure 192-3

TPN Compounding Example

70 kg male ⟶ needs 2100 kcal and 70 g protein

Protein

70 g × 4.0 kcal/g = 280 kcal

2100 kcal − 280 kcal = 1820 kcal

Carbohydrates

Need 5 g/kg/d × 70 kg = 350 g/d
350 g × 3.4 kcal/g = 1190 kcal

1820 kcal − 1190 kcal = 730 kcal

Fats

730 kcal/(10 kcal/g fat) = 73 g fat

Total compound	Protein	70 g
	Carbohydrate	350 g
	Fats	73 g

| Total volume | Need 30 mL/kg ⟶ 2100 mL, so mix about 2 L |

Calculation of a patient's overall protein and caloric needs.

Once a base TPN formula has been designed, electrolytes, trace elements, multivitamins, and elective additives are placed into the solution, as shown in Table 192-5. The amount of any of the additives may be increased or decreased depending on the patient's laboratory values and comorbid diseases. It is important to monitor the patient's serum electrolyte, blood urea nitrogen, creatinine, calcium, magnesium, and phosphate levels while on TPN, especially in the initials days or when the patient's clinical status has changed dramatically. In addition, serum glucose levels should be maintained below 200 mg/dL by the addition of insulin to the solution. For patients who will remain on long-term TPN, the addition of 3000 to 5000 U of heparin per liter of TPN will help prevent catheter thrombus formation.

Peripheral Parenteral Nutrition Compounding

Formulation of PPN requires attention to serum osmolarity. A hyperosmolar solution may cause thrombophlebitis, resulting in loss of peripheral venous access and in patient discomfort. The addition of heparin and hydrocortisone to the PPN solution may reduce the incidence of such chemical thrombophlebitis. It also is recommended that the osmolarity of the PPN solution be maintained at less than 1200 mOsm/L [34]. (Osmolarity of a solution can be calculated using the formula in Table 192-6.) A rule of thumb is to maintain the final dextrose concentration of the PPN solution at less than 10% and the final protein concentration at less than 5%. Fats can be added because they do not contribute significantly to the overall osmolarity of the final solution. Electrolytes and other appropriate additives are listed in Table 192-5.

Vascular Access Devices

Central venous catheters may be categorized as tunneled catheters, implanted catheters (ports), and short-term catheters. Tunneled and short-term catheters may be single or multiple lumen. Ports also are available as single or multiple lumen.

The subclavian and internal jugular veins provide the safest and easiest anatomic access. The femoral vein also is available but is easily contaminated. Nonsurgical catheters may be placed at the bedside with the patient in the Trendelenburg position. The neck and chest are cleansed and draped. The skin is anesthetized, and catheters are inserted over a guidewire. The subclavian vein often is chosen for long-term access, as for parenteral nutrition, because of the reduced incidence of complications at this site [35]. Multiple-lumen catheters allow the ability to infuse a number of fluids and medications at the same time. Multiple lumens also allow blood drawing in patients with poor venous access. Generally, the risk of central venous catheter infection increases with the number of catheter lumens.

Catheter composition materials vary among manufacturers. They may be constructed of Teflon (DuPont, Wilmington, DE), polyurethane, silicone, or Silastic material. Teflon and polyurethane are stiff and prone to scarring and thrombosis. Silastic and silicone catheters are softer and more prone to kinking and displacement. Tunneled Silastic catheters (Hickman, Broviac) are the most common types used for long-term vascular access. They have a Dacron (DuPont, Wilmington, DE) cuff for fibrotic tissue adherence, which is believed important in preventing bacterial migration up the catheter. Another common central venous access device is a peripherally inserted venous catheter; the catheter is inserted in a peripheral vein, and the tip of the catheter is positioned in the superior vena cava. These catheters are available with single or double lumens. They are associated with a lower risk of complications than are central venous catheters but are, more prone to thrombophlebitis. The addition of heparin and hydrocortisone to infused TPN solutions is believed to reduce the incidence of chemical thrombophlebitis.

Central Venous Catheter Complications

Central venous catheter complications occur with a reported incidence of 1% to 10% [36]. Complications of subclavian vein catheterization include hemothorax, pneumothorax, brachial plexus injury, hematoma, and subcutaneous emphysema. Common long-term catheter complications include sepsis, thrombosis, and catheter occlusion.

Catheter infection generally occurs from touch contamination and often involves coagulase-negative staphylococci. The major mechanism of contamination is tracking of organisms from the skin to the subcutaneous tissues and catheter tip. Construction of the catheter with a silver-impregnated collagen cuff and antibiotic binding is designed to prevent this complication, but such catheters are not widely used.

Diagnosing catheter infections can be difficult. Peripheral blood cultures often are negative. Culture of the catheter tip is more sensitive in documenting catheter infection. Generally, bacterial infections of catheters can be treated with the catheter in place. Fungal catheter infections and tunnel infections of the catheter tract, however, require removal of the catheter for effective treatment [37].

Catheter-induced thrombosis results from irritation of the vessel wall by the catheter. The thrombus usually is composed of fibrin; precipitation of medication is less common. Catheter occlusion may result in inability to infuse solutions or draw blood. Symptoms of central vein thrombus formation include neck pain and swelling, anterior chest wall venous distention, and reduced catheter function.

Treatment of fibrin thrombus formation is with a thrombolytic agent such as urokinase given by bolus or continuous

Table 192-6. Calculation of Osmolarity in Peripheral Parenteral Nutrition Solutions

Step 1:		
Amino acid, *g*	× 10.0 =	_____
Dextrose, *g*	× 5.0 =	_____
Fat, *g*	× 1.3 =	_____
Na, *mEq*	× 2.0 =	_____
K, *mEq*	× 2.0 =	_____
Ca, *mEq*	× 2.0 =	_____
Mg, *mEq*	× 2.0 =	_____
Phosphorous, *mmol*	× 4.0 =	_____
Step 2:		
Total from Step 1	=	_____
Step 3:		
Total from Step 2 ÷ volume of peripheral hyperalimentation in liters	= mOsm/L	_____

infusion. Agitation of the thrombolytic agent using a syringe and a push-and-pull method may assist in thrombus dissolution. Medication-precipitate occlusions may be treated with instillation of hydrochloric acid.

Administration of Total Parenteral Nutrition

The typical TPN solution is about 25% to 30% solute. Initial infusion should be over 24 hours. Patients with glucose intolerance or those at risk of refeeding syndrome (see later discussion) should receive only half their daily caloric needs during the first 24 hours. The amount may be increased to the full caloric requirement over the next 24 to 72 hours with monitoring of serum glucose, electrolytes, magnesium, and phosphate levels and fluid tolerance [38].

Central parenteral nutrition is infused through a large central vein, whereas less hypertonic PPN may be infused through a peripheral vein. In either case, the port or lumen of the catheter used for TPN must be used solely for TPN infusion. Use of the TPN port or lumen for drawing blood or infusing other solutions dramatically increases the risk of catheter infection.

Monitoring Laboratory Tests

In the first few days after insertion of the catheter and initiation of TPN, serum levels of electrolytes, magnesium, phosphorus, calcium, and blood urea nitrogen should be monitored closely. After stabilization, these blood tests may be checked weekly. If indicated, serum levels of zinc, selenium, copper, chromium, and vitamins B_{12} and B_6 may be monitored.

In most hospitals, TPN solutions are mixed in the pharmacy. Orders for a patient's TPN solution should be at the pharmacy by 2:00 to 3:00 PM so that the new solution can be compounded and ready for infusion by 6:00 PM. Morning laboratory values can guide changes in the solution that will be infused that evening. More emergent abnormalities, such as severe hypokalemia, hyperkalemia, or hyperphosphatemia, may require infusion of additional solute while the current TPN solution is infused. Discontinuation of TPN may be necessary until blood tests are corrected.

Metabolic Complications

Metabolic complications may be classified according to the glucose, amino acid, lipid, vitamin, electrolyte, and mineral content of the TPN solution [39] (Table 192-7). Hyperglycemia is the most common complication and is related directly to the dextrose content of the TPN solution and its rate of infusion. Critically ill patients and those with pre-existing glucose intolerance require the most aggressive monitoring of serum glucose levels. Serum glucose levels should be maintained at less than 200 mg/dL. If hyperglycemia develops, the patient should first be maintained on a sliding scale of regular insulin. Two thirds of the total amount of sliding-scale insulin required over 24 hours should be added to the next day's TPN formula. Further adjustments in daily insulin dosing may be required.

Refeeding syndrome is a common metabolic consequence of TPN. This is a consequence of the sudden provision of calories to a patient who previously was malnourished. With TPN infusion, these patients attempt to become anabolic with movement of potassium, phosphorus, and magnesium into cells, which

results in a risk of hypokalemia, hypophosphatemia, and hypomagnesemia. Large fluid shifts also may occur, and the patient may develop congestive heart failure.

Other common metabolic abnormalities are hypercarbia that results in respiratory acidosis, hyperlipidemia, elevated liver function tests, and bleeding. Hypercarbia usually is related to the infusion of excess carbohydrate or total calories and may precipitate respiratory acidosis by the formation of excess CO_2. It responds to a reduction in the amount of carbohydrate or calories infused. Hyperlipidemia is related to the total dose or rate of infusion of lipids and may resolve after the infusion time or total daily dose of infused lipids is adjusted. Elevated liver function tests are common after initiation of TPN; elevations in serum aminotransferase levels up to twice normal are most common and generally resolve in 10 to 15 days. Further elevations in aminotransferase levels, particularly when associated with hyperbilirubinemia, warrant investigation. Liver diseases, such as viral hepatitis, sclerosing cholangitis, primary biliary cirrhosis, autoimmune hepatitis, and hemochromatosis, should be excluded. A right upper quadrant ultrasound examination can exclude the diagnosis of cholelithiasis or biliary sludge. Acalculous cholecystitis should be excluded because normal stimulation of gallbladder contraction is absent when a patient has no enteral intake. Liver biopsy may be necessary to make a diagnosis of TPN-induced liver disease, which generally presents as fatty infiltration of the liver, especially prominent in the periportal areas; TPN-induced fatty liver may respond to a reduction in the patient's total daily carbohydrate or caloric infusion [40]. Bleeding is an uncommon event that may result

Table 192-7. Total Parenteral Nutrition Troubleshooting

Abnormality	Treatment
Hypokalemia	Monitor diuretic therapy, check renal function, add potasium to solution
Hyperkalemia	Check renal function, reduce potassium or stop TPN infusion, give insulin or calcium gluconate if severe
Hypomagnesemia	Increase magnesium administration, monitor diuretic therapy
Hypermagnesemia	Check renal function, decrease or stop magnesium administration, initiate dialysis for renal failure, delete magnesium-containing medications
Hypophosphatemia	Administer IV phosphorous immediately, add phosphorous to TPN
Hyperphosphatemia	Check renal function, reduce phosphate in TPN
Hypocalcemia	Increase calcium dose in TPN, check and correct laboratory value for serum albumin level
Hypercalcemia	Decrease calcium, administer vitamin D
Hyponatremia	Reduce free water infusion, monitor diuretic therapy, add sodium to TPN solution
Hypernatremia	Increase free water infusion, reduce sodium in TPN solution

IV—intravenous; TPN—total parenteral nutrition.

from vitamin K deficiency. Addition of vitamin K to the TPN solution reverses this complication.

CONCLUSION

Nutritional therapy supports all other therapies in the treatment of complex disease processes. Adequately assessing a patient's nutritional status and addressing his or her nutritional needs is the foundation of nutritional therapy. The delivery of enteral or parenteral nutrition requires adequate access. Enteral nutrition may be delivered orally, or via a nasoenteric or percutaneous tube. Parenteral nutrition requires placement of a venous catheter. Each delivery system has its own advantages and disadvantages, although enteral nutrition often is less costly and is associated with fewer complications.

REFERENCES

1. ASPEN Board of Directors: Guidelines for the use of parenteral and enteral nutrition in adult and pediatric patients. *JPEN* 1993, 17(II):5sa–6sa.

2. Tucker HN: Shortened length of stay is an outcome benefit of early nutritional intervention. In *Physiology, Stress and Malnutrition*. Edited by Kinney JM, Tucker HN. New York: Lippincott-Raven; 1997:1–21.

3. Kudsk KA, Croce MA, Fabian TC, *et al.*: Enteral versus parenteral feeding: effects on septic morbidity after blunt and penetrating abdominal trauma. *Ann Surg* 1992, 215:503–511.

4. Moore FA, Feliciano DV, Andrassy RJ, *et al.*: Early enteral feeding, compared with parenteral, reduces postoperative septic complications: the results of a meta-analysis. *Ann Surg* 1992, 216:172–183.

5. ASPEN Board of Directors: Guidelines for the use of parenteral and enteral nutrition in adults and pediatric patients. *JPEN* 1993, 17(III):5sa–6sa.

6. AGA Patient Care Committee: AGA technical review on tube feedings and enteral nutrition. *Gastroenterology* 1995, 108:1282–1301.

7. Baskin WN: Advances in enteral nutrition techniques. *Am J Gastroenterol* 1992, 87:1547–1553.

8. Mittal RK, Stewart WR, Schirmer BD: Effect of a catheter in the pharynx on the frequency of lower esophageal sphincter relaxations. *Gastroenterology* 1992, 103:1236–1240.

9. McClave SA, Snider HL, Lowen CC, *et al.*: Use of residual volume as a marker for enteral feeding intolerance: prospective blinded comparison with physical examination and radiographic findings. *JPEN* 1992, 16:99–105.

10. DeLegge MH, Duckworth PF Jr, McHenry L Jr, *et al.*: Percutaneous endoscopic gastrojejunostomy (PEG/J) made easy: a new over-the-wire technique. *Gastrointest Endosc* 1994, 40:350–353.

11. Weltz CR, Morris JB, Mullen JL: Surgical jejunostomy in aspiration risk patients. *Ann Surg* 1992, 215:140–145.

12. Lord LM, Weiser-Maimone A, Pulhamus M, *et al.*: Comparison of weighted vs unweighted enteral feeding tubes for efficacy of transpyloric intubation. *JPEN* 1993, 17:271–273.

13. Ugo PJ, Mohler PA, Wilson GL: Bedside postpyloric placement of weighted feeding tubes. *Nutr Clin Pract* 1992, 7:284–287.

14. Jain NH, Larson DE, Schroder KW, *et al.*: Antibiotic prophylaxis for percutaneous endoscopic gastrostomy: a prospective randomized trial. *Ann Intern Med* 1987, 107:824–828.

15. Grant JP: Comparison of percutaneous endoscopic gastrostomy and Stamm gastrostomy. *Ann Surg* 1988, 207:598–603.

16. DeLegge MH, Patrick P, Gibbs R: Percutaneous endoscopic gastrojejunostomy with a tapered tip, nonweighted jejunal feeding tube: improved placement success. *Am J Gastroenterol* 1996, 91:1130–1134.

17. Patel PH, Thomas E: Factors predisposing to aspiration in patients with percutaneous endoscopic gastrostomy. *Am J Gastroenterol* 1987, 82:937.

18. Schnall HA, Falkenstein DB, Raicht RF: Persistent pneumoperitoneum after percutaneous endoscopic gastrostomy. *Gastrointestinal Endosc* 1987, 33:248–250.

19. Fernadez ET, Hollabaugh R, Hixon SD, *et al.*: Late presentation of gastrocolic fistula after percutaneous gastrostomy. *Gastrointest Endosc* 1988, 34:368–369.

20. Martindale R, Witte M, Hodges G, *et al.*: Necrotising fasciitis as a complication of percutaneous endoscopic gastrostomy. *JPEN* 1987, 11:583–585.

21. Galat SA, Gerig KD, Porter JA, *et al.*: Management of premature removal of percutaneous gastrostomy. *Am Surg* 1990, 56:733–736.

22. Grimble GK, Rees RG, Keohane PP, *et al.*: Effect of peptide chain length on absorption of egg protein hydrolysates in normal human jejunum. *Gastroenterology* 1987, 92:135–142.

23. Lieberman MD, Shou J, Torres AS, *et al.*: Effects of nutrient substrate on immune function. *Nutrition* 1990, 6:88–91.

24. Hwang O'Dwyer ST, Smith RJ, Wilmore DW: Preservation of small bowel mucosa utilizing glutamine-enriched parenteral nutrition. *Surg Forum* 1986, 37:56–58.

25. Benya R, Mobarhan S: Enteral alimentation: administration and complications. *J Am Coll Nutr* 1992, 10:209–212.

26. Erikson LS, Conn HO: Branched chain amino acids in the treatment of encephalopathy: an analysis of variants. *Hepatology* 1989, 10:228–246.

27. Peters AL, Davidson MB, Isaac RM: Lack of glucose elevation after simulated tube feeding with a low-carbohydrate, high-fat enteral formulation in patients with type 1 diabetes. *Am J Med* 1989, 87:178–182.

28. Ciocon JO, Galindo-Ciocon DJ, Tiessen C, *et al.*: Continuous compared with intermittent feeding in the elderly. *JPEN* 1992, 16:525–528.

29. Torres A, Serra-Battles J, Ros E, *et al.*: Pulmonary aspiration of gastric contents in patients receiving mechanical ventilation: the effect of body position. *Ann Intern Med* 1992, 116:540–543.

30. Edes TE, Walk BE, Austin JL: Diarrhea in tube-fed patients: feeding formula not necessarily the cause. *Am J Med* 1990, 88:91–93.

31. Fleisher D, Sheth N, Kou J: Phenytoin interaction with enteral feeding administration with nasogastric tubes. *JPEN* 1989, 14:513–516.

32. Dudrick SJ, Rhodes JE: New horizons for intravenous feedings. *JAMA* 1971, 215:939–951.

33. Dudrick SJ, Latifi R, Forsnocht D: Management of short bowel syndrome. *Surg Clin North Am* 1991, 71:1–51.

34. Hardaway LC: An overview of vascular access devices inserted via the anteriolateral vein. *J Intravenous Nurs* 1990, 13:297–306.

35. Benotti PN, Bothe P, Miller JD, *et al.*: Safe cannulation of the internal jugular vein for long-term hyperalimentation. *Surg Gynecol Obstet* 1977, 144:574–576.

36. Herbst CA: Indication, management and complications of percutaneous subclavian catheters: an audit. *Surgery* 1978, 113:1421–1425.

37. Buchman AL, Moukarzel A, Goodson B, *et al.*: Catheter related infection associated with home parenteral nutrition and predictive factors for the need for catheter removal in their treatment. *JPEN* 1994, 18:297–302.

38. Soloman SW, Kirby DF: The refeeding syndrome: a review. *JPEN* 1990, 14:90–97.

39. Dudrick SJ, Latifi R: Total parenteral nutrition. II. Administration, monitoring, and complications. *Pract Gastr* 1992, 7:29–38.

40. Meguid M, Akahoshi MP, Jeffers S: Amelioration of metabolic complications of conventional TPN. *Arch Surg* 1984, 119:1294–1301.

193 Gastrointestinal Diseases in the Elderly

Lawrence J. Brandt and David A. Greenwald

Symptoms of gastrointestinal (GI) disorders account for a large portion of the reasons that elderly persons visit their physicians. The number of Americans older than 65 years of age has been growing steadily, and physicians who treat patients with GI diseases are seeing an increasing share of disease in the elderly. Thus, it is important for physicians to be knowledgeable about the normal physiologic changes associated with aging, the varied presentations of GI diseases in the elderly, and the alterations in patient management required by the aging process.

AN APPROACH TO GASTROINTESTINAL DISEASE IN THE ELDERLY

Most of the GI disorders seen in the aged also occur in younger persons, although some occur more commonly with aging. For example, cancer is more prevalent with advancing age, as is diverticulitis, and most deaths from peptic ulcer disease occur in the elderly. The morbidity associated with common problems, such as swallowing disorders, fecal incontinence, and constipation, is considerably greater in the older population (Table 193-1).

Symptoms of digestive diseases may be misinterpreted or atypical in the aged [1]. For example, chest pain indicative of gastroesophageal reflux disease or esophageal dysmotility initially may be perceived as angina, and iron-deficiency anemia

or bone fractures may be the only manifestations of celiac sprue. Comorbid illness, including depression and dementia, may impair adequate communication, leading to difficulties in obtaining a complete and accurate history. What appears to be the same disease in the aged and the young may have different causes (Table 193-2). Ischemic colitis in the elderly may mimic inflammatory bowel disease and not respond to conventional therapy with sulfasalazine or corticosteroids. Physical examination and some laboratory tests similarly may not disclose expected abnormalities and can lead, on occasion, to a delay in diagnosis. Most laboratory tests, however, including tests of liver function, are unaffected by aging, and any abnormality should be evaluated for the presence of a disease state and not dismissed as an age-related change (Table 193-3).

Objective testing often plays an important diagnostic role in the evaluation of GI complaints in the elderly. Numerous studies support the notion that GI endoscopy is safe and efficacious in the elderly [2]. Although some physicians may be hesitant to perform upper or lower endoscopy in the elderly for fear that the risks of complications are greater than in the young, there is no evidence to support this concern. The doses of sedating and analgesic medicines must be monitored closely in the elderly, but endoscopy has been demonstrated to be safe in both

Table 193-1. Influence of Age on Diagnosis of Gastrointestinal Symptoms

Symptom	Young patient	Elderly patient
Dysphagia	Peptic stricture Primary achalasia	Malignant stricture Secondary achalasia
Odynophagia	Acquired immunode- ficiency syndrome	Pill-induced esophagitis
Chest pain	Motility disorder	Angina
Eructation	Aerophagia (gum)	Aerophagia (candy)
Hematemesis	Duodenal ulcer	Gastric cancer
Rectal bleeding	Hemorrhoids Inflammatory bowel disease Colonic polyp	Diverticulosis Vascular ectasia Colon cancer
Constipation	Irritable bowel syndrome	Obstructing lesion
Anal stricture	Inflammatory bowel disease	Neoplasm Radiation-induced injury
Jaundice (intrahepatic)	Viral hepatitis	Drug-induced hepatitis
Jaundice (extrahepatic)	Gallstones	Neoplasm

Table 193-2. Influence of Age on Interpretation of Radiographic Findings

Finding	Young patient	Elderly patient
Achalasia	Primary	Secondary
Gastric outlet obstruction	Peptic ulcer	Malignant neoplasm
Malabsorption	Sprue	Lymphoma
Segmental colitis	Crohn's disease	Ischemia

Table 193-3. Long-term Sequelae of Gastrointestinal Disorders in the Elderly

Disorder	Sequelae
Barrett's esophagus	Gastroesophageal adenocarcinoma
Gastrectomy	Vitamin B_{12} and iron deficiency Osteopenia Gastric adenocarcinoma
Celiac sprue	Esophageal and gastric cancer Intestinal lymphoma
Ulcerative colitis	Malignancy

inpatient and outpatient settings as well as in routine and emergency circumstances. Accompanying this relatively low risk of endoscopy is a high yield of diagnostic findings. Upper endoscopy has a diagnostic yield as high as 77% to 89%, and management often is altered in patients in whom an important abnormality is detected. Colonoscopy has been shown to detect abnormalities with a similarly high frequency. The yield depends on its indication; for example, the diagnostic yield is greater when the indication for the procedure is anemia as opposed to a change in bowel habits [3•].

Finally, close attention must be paid to drug effects and interactions in the elderly. Polypharmacy is common; in one report, 80% of elderly Americans living independently were written for 20 or more prescriptions every year [4]. In another study, nursing home patients were found to receive an average of 8 to 10 medications daily [5]. At the same time, noncompliance is common, visual and cognitive impairment may lead the elderly to take the wrong medicines, and the aged often share medications on the advice of well-intentioned friends. The frequency of adverse drug effects increases with age and the number of drugs prescribed, so the possibility of drug reactions always should be considered when assessing GI complaints in the elderly [6]. It has been estimated that drug reactions are responsible for approximately 3% of total hospital admissions and contribute to the admission of about another 10% of elderly patients.

ORAL CAVITY

The mouth is a commonly forgotten portion of the GI tract, but knowledge of oral cavity dysfunction is important not only for the dentist but also for the gastroenterologist, to whom it may give hints about the nature of disease elsewhere.

Aging has an effect on the oral cavity. Age-related changes in the structures of the oral cavity are summarized in Table 193-4. The decrease in lean body mass that accompanies aging can lead to impaired functioning of the muscles of mastication. In addition, eating may become more difficult because of tooth loss, largely caused by periodontal disease. Indeed, 50% of the American population is edentulous by 65 years of age, and the

percentage increases to 85% only one decade later [7]. Taste sensation, particularly for sweet and salty foods, changes as a result of a decrease in the number of taste buds. Dysgeusia, or abnormal taste perception, may be an unpleasant side effect of many medications, including metronidazole, sulfasalazine, clofibrate, levodopa, gold salts, lithium, and tricyclic antidepressants. Certain nutritional deficiencies also may lead to dysgeusia, glossitis, or angular stomatitis. Examples include vitamin B_{12} and niacin deficiency, which are associated with a "bald" and magenta-colored tongue, respectively.

Xerostomia is found in up to 30% of elderly persons and most often is caused by salivary dysfunction that accompanies other diseases or their treatments [8]. Salivary flow does not appear to decrease solely as a result of the aging process. Many medications, including antihypertensives, psychotropics, antidepressants, and antihistamines, particularly those with anticholinergic properties, can lead to decreased salivary gland secretion and xerostomia. Dryness of the mouth may accompany systemic diseases, such as Sjögren's syndrome, and autoimmune disorders, such as systemic lupus erythematosus and rheumatoid arthritis. Depression is common in the elderly, and xerostomia in patients with depression may result from a combination of poor fluid intake and the side effects of therapy with antidepressants that have anticholinergic properties.

Oral mucosal lesions in the elderly may be an unwanted side effect of medical therapy for other conditions, an indicator of systemic disease, or a premalignant change. Thrush (oral candidiasis), with its characteristic soft whitish plaque-like lesions, may develop in association with diabetes mellitus, especially in denture wearers, after use of systemic antibiotics or immunosuppressive chemotherapy. Stomatitis, or painful inflammation and erosions of the oropharyngeal mucosa, commonly occurs in cancer patients treated with radiation or chemotherapy. Patients who have had extensive radiotherapy to the head and neck may develop "hairy tongue," which is typified by hypertrophy of the filiform papillae and a lack of normal desquamation. The condition may be asymptomatic or may cause patients to complain of dysgeusia and halitosis. Leukoplakia refers to a white plaque that is commonly found in the buccal mucosa, tongue, or floor of the mouth of persons in their sixth and seventh decades. Some authorities use the term to connote malignant dyskeratosis and epithelial atypia, whereas others use the term more broadly to describe areas of hyperkeratosis and chronic inflammation. Although the terminology is controversial, the persistent presence of a white lesion in the oral mucosa, especially when it contains areas of red (erythroleukoplakia) is an indication for biopsy; in about 10% of such cases, invasive carcinoma is present or will develop.

Between 3% and 5% of all new cancers arise in the oral cavity, the bulk of which are epidermoid carcinomas. Carcinoma of the lip is seen almost exclusively in elderly men and appears to be related to lengthy sun exposure and related actinic damage as well as prolonged tobacco use, particularly pipe smoking. Intraoral tumors originate in the tongue in about half of cases, with the balance arising from the palate, buccal mucosa, floor of the mouth, and gingiva. Intraoral cancers are found predominantly in older men. Factors thought to contribute to their development include tobacco and alcohol use, nutritional

Table 193-4. Senescence of the Oral Cavity in the Elderly		
Organ	**Change**	**Consequence**
Tooth	Increased density of enamel	Decreased frequency of surface caries
	Increased cementum	Forensic value
	Increased dentin	Difficult extraction
		Decreased pain sensitivity
Gingiva	Recession	Increased frequency of periodontal disease
		Cemental (root) caries
Tongue	Decreased number of taste buds	Altered taste perception
Salivary glands	?Reduced secretion	Xerostomia

deficiencies, syphilis, and irritation from pipe stems and dentures. Symptoms of oral malignancy may include a mass in the oral cavity, dysphagia, pain, lump in the neck, limitation in the movement of the tongue, or change in the fit of dentures. Prompt biopsy of any suspicious lesion is essential because early detection is crucial if patients are to survive more than 1 year after diagnosis.

■ OROPHARYNX

The oropharyngeal phase of swallowing is exceedingly complex, involving many distinct structures in the mouth, pharynx, and esophagus and requiring coordination by six cranial nerves and the swallowing center of the central nervous system (see Chapter 7). Numerous physiologic changes in the oropharynx have been noted with aging (Table 193-5).

With the decrease in lean body mass seen with aging, striated muscle function crucial to the oropharyngeal phase of swallowing may become impaired. Pharyngeal muscle weakness and abnormal cricopharyngeal relaxation are reported commonly in studies examining oropharyngeal changes in the elderly, but often affected subjects do not have symptoms. Thus, although functional changes in the oropharyngeal phase of swallowing appear to occur with aging, the significance of these changes is unclear.

Oropharyngeal, or transfer, dysphagia often occurs as a result of disorders affecting the nerves or muscles of the oropharynx and may be accompanied by signs of neuromuscular dysfunction elsewhere, such as nasal speech, dysarthria, weakness, or sensory abnormalities. This topic is discussed fully in Chapter 8.

Cricopharyngeal achalasia actually is a misnomer because the cricopharyngeus muscle of patients with this disorder is able to relax. The defect in cricopharyngeal achalasia is inability of the muscle to function in synchrony with the other parts of the swallowing mechanism [9]. The result is that the pharyngeal muscles propel the contents of the mouth against a contracted cricopharyngeus muscle, and food is unable to pass. Such "cervical" dysphagia generally is caused by disease of the central nervous system, and oropharyngeal dysphagia is the predominant symptom. Many elderly persons with this disorder have more difficulty swallowing liquids than solids, as is characteristic of many neuromuscular swallowing disorders.

Cervical dysphagia also may result from trauma occurring at the time of endotracheal intubation, which may be complicated by unilateral vocal cord weakness. Patients with vocal cord weakness may develop coughing and aspiration with swallowing because the vocal cords are critical to the formation of a tight laryngeal seal during the oropharyngeal phase of swallowing.

Hypopharyngeal diverticula are found almost exclusively in the elderly, with about 85% of cases occurring in persons older than 50 years. A Zenker's diverticulum (Fig. 193-1) is a posterior herniation of the hypopharynx through the weak triangular area (Killian's triangle) just above the upper esophageal sphincter, where the transverse and oblique fibers of the cricopharyngeus muscle join. Lateral pharyngeal diverticula, or pharyngoceles, develop in the gap between the superior and middle pharyngeal constrictors.

Incomplete or uncoordinated relaxation of the upper esophageal sphincter during swallowing has been described in association with Zenker's diverticulum. The diverticulum is thought to occur because high pharyngeal pressures exert increased force over time on the muscles of the hypopharynx. Many patients with Zenker's diverticulum, however, have normal or even reduced upper esophageal sphincter pressures, so the association between high esophageal pressure and Zenker's diverticulum is uncertain. Nevertheless, high pharyngeal pressure

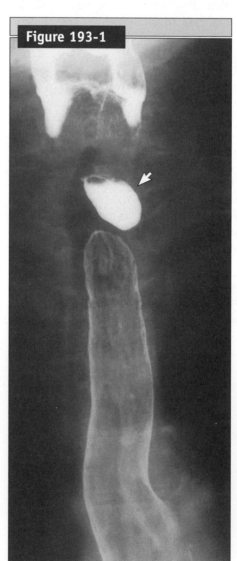

Figure 193-1

Barium esophagogram demonstrating a Zenker's diverticulum (*arrow*). The triangular area where the oblique and transverse muscles of the cricopharyngeus join is an area of potential weakness through which a posterior diverticulum may protrude.

Table 193-5. Oropharyngeal Changes that Accompany Aging

Parameter	Change
Oropharyngeal transit	Prolonged
UES opening	Delayed
UES cross-sectional area	Decreased
UES resistance	Increased
UES resting pressure	Decreased
UES compliance	Decreased
Pharyngoesophageal–UES reflex	Abnormal

UES—upper esophageal sphincter.

can be demonstrated and may be caused by progressive age-related fibrosis of the hypopharyngeal muscles with loss of compliance.

ESOPHAGUS

Senescent changes in the musculature of the esophagus have been described and include reduction in the number of myenteric ganglion cells, thickening of the smooth muscle layer, and decrease in the number of slow-acting type I muscle fibers in the distal esophagus. Esophageal motility abnormalities in the elderly were first described in 1964 by Soergel and colleagues, who referred to such disturbances of motility as *presbyesophagus* [10]. Most of the patients they described, however, had comorbid diseases subsequently shown to affect esophageal motility adversely. Although esophageal motility may be abnormal in elderly persons, the only consistently demonstrated manometric abnormality is a reduction in the amplitude of muscle contractions after swallowing [11], the significance of which is unclear.

Although alterations in esophageal structure have been described with aging, they have not been correlated with symptomatic esophageal muscle dysfunction or manometric abnormalities. Barium esophagography often reveals disordered motility, or *tertiary contractions* (Fig. 193-2); however, these findings also rarely are associated with symptoms. Because the motility changes seen with aging do not appear to have any clinical importance, elderly patients with complaints of dysphagia must be evaluated for the presence of esophageal diseases, and complaints should not be ascribed to the aging process alone.

Dysphagia in the elderly also may be due to mechanical compression on the esophagus. Dysphagia aortica (Fig. 193-3) refers to compression of the esophagus by the thoracic aorta, which may undergo degeneration and become increasingly tortuous in the elderly. Similar compression on the esophagus also may result from mediastinal adhesions after surgery,

Figure 193-2

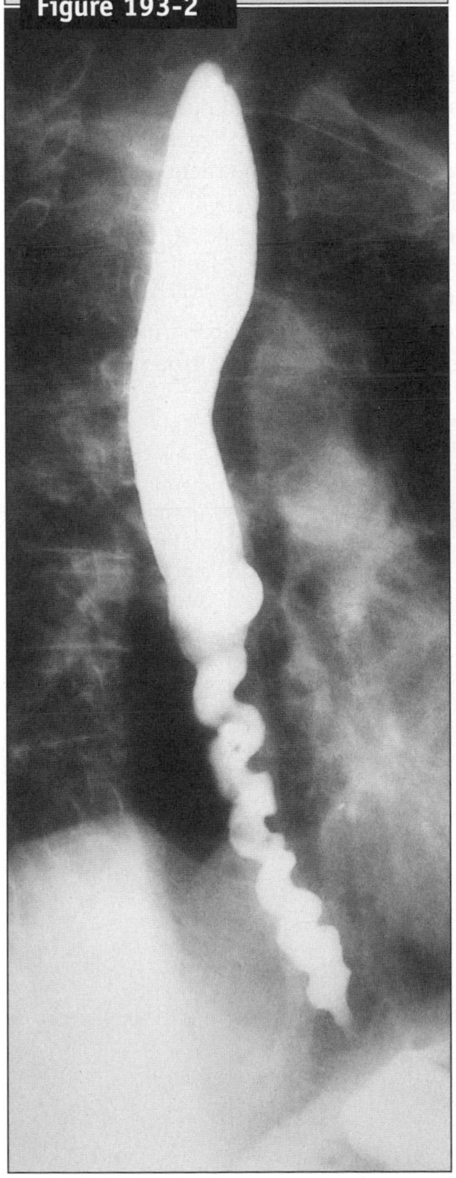

Tertiary contractions are multiple, irregular, ringlike, nonpropulsive contractions that occur in the lower two thirds of the esophagus. This barium esophagogram demonstrates a pronounced corkscrew pattern in a patient with diffuse esophageal spasm.

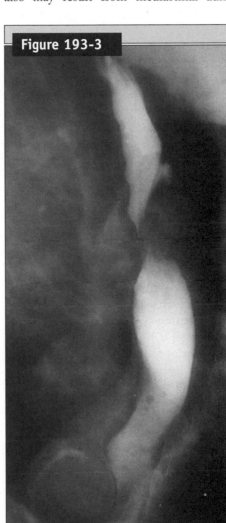

Figure 193-3

Dysphagia aortica. Note the impression of the calcified aorta on the esophagus at the level of both the aortic arch and the gastroesophageal junction. Calcifications are seen in the aorta.

profound left atrial enlargement, or a thoracic aneurysm, in which case the distal esophagus may be squeezed between an atherosclerotic aorta posteriorly and the heart or esophageal hiatus anteriorly.

Elderly patients often use numerous medications and are at increased risk of medication-induced esophageal injury [12]. Most patients with pill-induced esophageal injury do not have underlying esophageal disorders. Factors that contribute to the occurrence of pill-induced esophagitis in the elderly include the number and kind of pills taken, a relative decrease in production of saliva, and a tendency to take pills while in the recumbent position. Pills often are taken with insufficient liquid and before bedtime. Quinidine, potassium chloride, emepronium bromide (not available in the United States), antibiotics (particularly tetracycline), nonsteroidal anti-inflammatory drugs (NSAIDs) and alendronate are the medications most commonly implicated. Pills become lodged at the level of the aortic knob or the lower esophageal sphincter and cause local damage. Most cases of pill-induced esophageal injury resolve, in many cases without ever being recognized clinically, but stricture formation, hemorrhage, and perforation all have been reported.

Gastroesophageal reflux disease (GERD) is more common in the elderly than in younger persons [13,14•]. With aging, lower esophageal sphincter (LES) contraction amplitude is decreased; however, this decrease is counterbalanced by increased secretion of gastrin, which potentiates contraction of the LES, and, in elderly persons with comorbid illness, by decreased gastric acid secretion. Overall, the new onset of reflux esophagitis in the elderly is unusual. Elderly patients with GERD, however, may have more severe disease than their younger counterparts as well as an increased prevalence of mucosal abnormalities, such as esophagitis, esophageal ulcers, and Barrett's esophagus, albeit with minimal symptoms [15••]. Because symptoms do not accurately predict whether patients will have esophagitis, endoscopic examination is required to confirm its presence. In light of the disparity between symptoms and mucosal abnormalities, upper endoscopy is indicated in the elderly with new onset "heartburn."

An uncommon diaphragmatic defect found most often in persons between the ages of 60 and 70 years is a paraesophageal hernia (Fig. 193-4). Frequently asymptomatic or causing only mild discomfort until mechanical entrapment of the stomach in the diaphragmatic defect occurs, paraesophageal hernias may be the cause of significant morbidity. Left uncorrected, these hernias tend to enlarge and ultimately the bulk of the stomach may lie in the thorax, where the stomach may rotate around its long axis, forming an organoaxial volvulus. When strangulation occurs, hemorrhage, gangrene, and perforation may ensue. Therefore, the presence of a paraesophageal hernia is an indication for surgical repair. Such intrathoracic catastrophes manifest with chest pain and commonly are confused with angina, leading to delay in appropriate care.

Intramural esophageal pseudodiverticulosis is another disorder associated with dysphagia, is seen almost exclusively in the elderly, and usually is diagnosed during the seventh decade of life. In this condition of unknown cause, multiple small (1- to 3-mm) invaginations of the esophageal wall occur, probably as a result of dilation of the ducts of the submucosal secretory glands. These changes may involve the entire esophagus or portions of it; affected segments typically are involved in a circumferential fashion. A coexistent malignant neoplasm, GERD, or a motility disorder is found in at least 20% of cases, and in about half of patients, smears or cultures of the esophageal mucosa reveal *Candida albicans*. Stenoses or areas of reduced distensibility, particularly in the upper esophagus, are found in up to 90% of patients with pseudodiverticulosis; however, no clear relation exists between the stenotic segments and the portion of esophagus with pseudodiverticulosis.

■ STOMACH

Both the motor and secretory functions of the stomach are affected by aging; just as with the esophagus, however, alterations in gastric physiology attributable to age alone rarely are responsible for symptoms. Gastric emptying of liquids, as demonstrated by studies employing radioactive isotopes, is prolonged in the elderly; however, the emptying of solids appears to be unchanged with advancing age [16]. Slowed transit may lead to functional obstruction of the stomach, which can result in decreased bioavailability of medications and formation of a bezoar.

Gastric acid secretion changes as people age, although, in general, gastric acid production is preserved with aging if health is preserved. Older studies of gastric acid production showed that both basal and stimulated gastric acid output decline with advancing age, but more recent work suggests that, in the absence of *Helicobacter pylori* infection, there actually is an increase in gastric acid secretion with age [17]. Pepsin secretion is either normal or decreased in elderly persons. The belief that aging is responsible for a reduction in gastric acid secretion probably was related to the high prevalence of *H. pylori* infection and associated chronic atrophic gastritis with secondary achlorhydria in older persons, rather than a true senescence of

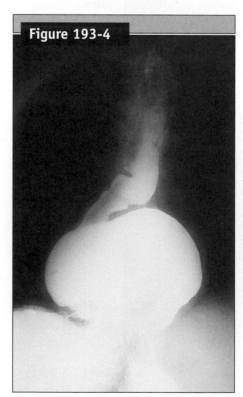

Figure 193-4

Large paraesophageal hernia. If left untreated, this type of hernia typically enlarges until most of the stomach lies in the thorax.

the gastric secretory apparatus. Potential consequences of achlorhydria are shown in Table 193-6.

The term *gastritis* implies the presence of inflammation seen on histologic examination and should not be used unless examination of the gastric biopsy specimen reveals typical mucosal inflammatory changes, such as infiltration of the lamina propria with polymorphonuclear leukocytes and mononuclear cells (see Chapter 19). Common in the elderly is type A (autoimmune) gastritis, in which a diffuse inflammatory process of the fundus and proximal portions of the stomach leads to pernicious anemia (see Chapter 19). This type of gastritis is characterized by destruction of parietal cells, leading to a deficiency of intrinsic factor; decreased acid secretion and secondary hypergastrinemia result. Type B (bacterial) gastritis most often is caused by *H. pylori* infection. The prevalence of type B gastritis rises with age. The inflammatory process typically begins in the antrum and gradually spreads proximally into the body and fundus of the stomach [18•]. Inflammation ultimately extends to the deeper glandular portion of the epithelium; normal glands are destroyed and replaced by metaplastic glands (intestinal metaplasia) or by atrophic gastric mucosa (chronic atrophic gastritis). Intestinal metaplasia is a precursor lesion to gastric carcinoma (Fig. 193-5).

Peptic ulcer disease is associated with colonization with *H. pylori* and the presence of type B gastritis (see Chapters 27 to 33); the other common cause of ulcer disease in the elderly is ingestion of NSAIDs. Peptic ulcer disease is a more serious disorder in the elderly than in younger persons; it often presents in an atypical manner and commonly with a serious complication as its first manifestation [19•]. Although peptic ulcer disease affects about 10% of the population at some time in their lives, the incidence of both gastric ulcer and duodenal ulcer increases with advancing age in both sexes, especially women. The elderly are more likely to have perforation, hemorrhage, and mortality from peptic ulcer disease; the complication rate of peptic ulcer disease rises progressively from 31% of patients between 60 and 64 years of age to 76% of those 75 to 79 years of age [20]. The increased incidence of complications in the elderly reflects the increased incidence and severity of ulcer disease and also the relatively high number of comorbid conditions found in the elderly.

Much of the increased frequency of peptic ulcer disease in the aged, particularly gastric ulcer, is attributed to the use of NSAIDs [21]. About 3 million persons in the United States, or 1.2% of the population, take at least one NSAID daily, and because many NSAIDs are available "over the counter," the extent of their use probably is underestimated. NSAID-related ulcers, with their associated morbidity and mortality, are more prevalent in the elderly than in younger persons; each year, 2% to 4% of chronic NSAID users have a significant drug-induced complication involving the GI tract. The elderly take more NSAIDs than do the young, in large part because of age-related increased prevalence of arthritis; about half of the NSAID prescriptions are written for patients older than 60 years of age. At the same time, the elderly appear particularly vulnerable to the deleterious effects of NSAIDs; in one study, almost 30% of the ulcers diagnosed in persons older than 65 years may have been caused by NSAIDs [22••].

Use of NSAIDs leads to mucosal damage and peptic ulceration by a direct toxic effect on the mucosa and, more important, by a dose-dependent systemic inhibition of prostaglandin synthesis (see Chapter 32). The analgesic properties of NSAIDs may mask the symptoms of the ulcers they produce, and often the first presentation of an NSAID-induced ulcer is a serious complication, such as hemorrhage or perforation. NSAIDs have been shown to increase the probability that existing ulcers will bleed and also have been shown to increase the chance of mortality related to upper GI bleeding [22••].

Several features of ulcer disease may be unique to the elderly. In general, the ulcers tend to be large and located proximally. The so-called geriatric ulcer (Fig. 193-6), often several centimeters in diameter, is found high in the cardia and may cause complaints, such as dysphagia, which may mimic symptoms of an esophageal neoplasm, or chest pain, which may suggest angina. Giant (over 2 cm in diameter) duodenal ulcers typically occur in men over aged 70 years and may be mistaken for the duodenal bulb on upper GI series (Fig. 193-7). In the past, these ulcers commonly were fatal; today, however, most ulcers heal with acid suppressive therapy and treatment of *H. pylori* infection, if indicated. Giant gastric ulcers over 3 cm in diameter usually are seen in persons older than aged 65 years and are more common in men than in women [23]. Although these ulcers typically are benign, hemorrhage may be a frequent and serious complication, and morbidity and mortality rates are high.

Ligamentous laxity, resulting from age-related degeneration and stretching of the gastric ligaments, results in an increased

Table 193-6. Potential Consequences of Achlorhydria in the Elderly

Esophageal candidiasis

Iron and vitamin B_{12} malabsorption

Infection (*Salmonella* and *Shigella* species, and tuberculosis)

Hypergastrinemia

Decreased gastric emptying

Bacterial overgrowth

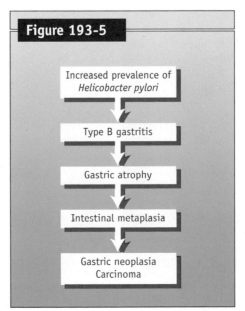

Figure 193-5

Increased prevalence of *Helicobacter pylori*

Type B gastritis

Gastric atrophy

Intestinal metaplasia

Gastric neoplasia Carcinoma

Gastric consequences of *H. pylori* infection over time. The final stages of this sequence usually occur in the elderly.

frequency of gastric volvulus in the elderly (see Chapter 42) (Fig. 193-8). Gastric volvulus may lead to chronic abdominal symptoms or may present acutely with a "complete twist," leading to severely impaired gastric blood flow and gangrene. Most patients (60%) with volvulus have rotation around the long axis (organoaxial type); 30% have rotation around the short axis (mesenteroaxial type); and 10% have a combined form. Although fixing the stomach into the correct position using dual percutaneous endoscopic gastrostomies has been used to treat gastric volvulus, corrective surgery usually is necessary [24].

■ SMALL BOWEL

The structure of the small bowel does not appear to change significantly with age, and overall, histologic features appear to be preserved. Some older studies demonstrated that villi are more likely to be broad and flat in a geriatric population than in younger persons, whereas others have demonstrated that the jejunum in older subjects has a smaller mucosal surface area but the same villous height as in younger persons [25]. There are data to suggest that there may be impairment of jejunal epithelial function with aging and compensatory hypertrophy of the ileal mucosa, although there is no clear evidence that loss of jejunal absorptive area occurs. The concentration of bacterial flora of the proximal small bowel may be increased in the elderly, probably as a result of a reduction in gastric acid secretion, although bacterial overgrowth may be caused by other conditions commonly seen in the elderly, such as small bowel diverticulosis, with or without a motility disorder, and adhesions [26].

Although there have been reports of prolonged intestinal transit time in aged mice, intestinal motility in humans appears to be unaffected by advancing age, unless the person has an underlying illness known to affect motor function, such as diabetes mellitus, or is taking a medication known to alter intestinal motility, such as a tricyclic antidepressant [27]. The presence of jejunal diverticulosis has been found to be associated with a primary disorder of small bowel motility.

Absorption of some nutrients has been reported to be abnormal in the elderly, although intestinal permeability does not decline as a result of aging. There is a progressive decrease in human jejunal lactase with aging, and lactose intolerance is prevalent among the elderly [28•]. D-xylose absorption has been reported to decline with advancing age, but this apparent decrease could be explained on the basis of impaired renal function and a resulting decrease in the urinary excretion of D-xylose. The body preserves its ability to absorb fat and fat-soluble vitamins with age; absorption of two fat-soluble vitamins, vitamins A and K, appears to increase in the elderly [29]. Protein absorption has not been well studied in the elderly.

In general, vitamin and mineral absorption appears to be unchanged with aging. Intestinal calcium absorption is reduced with increasing age, although the factors that mediate this reduction are unclear. Reduced absorption of calcium may result from decreased intestinal absorption of cholecalciferol or from decreased renal metabolism of vitamin D, which leads to lower serum levels of 1,25-dihydroxycholecalciferol. Vitamin D has been reported to be less well absorbed in the elderly, but findings of reduced serum vitamin D levels may be caused as much by decreased exposure to sunlight as by lessened intestinal absorption. Zinc is less well absorbed in older persons than younger persons, but losses also are less, so zinc balance does not change appreciably in older persons as compared with the young.

Acute and chronic mesenteric ischemia result from inadequate circulation to the intestinal tract. Their prevention, diagnosis, and management are discussed in detail in Chapter 65.

■ COLON AND RECTUM

Age-associated anatomic changes in the colon and rectum have been reported rarely and include atrophy of the mucosa,

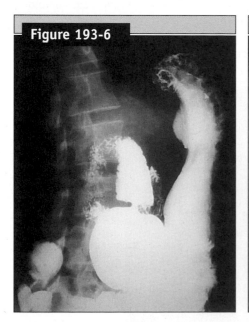

Figure 193-6

An upper gastrointestinal series showing a large ulcer in the proximal stomach, typical for a "geriatric ulcer."

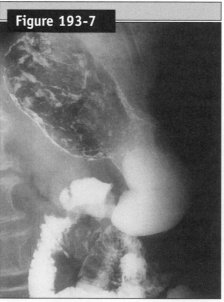

Figure 193-7

Upper gastrointestinal series demonstrating a giant duodenal ulcer. These ulcers may be misinterpreted in radiographic studies as the duodenal bulb or as a diverticulum.

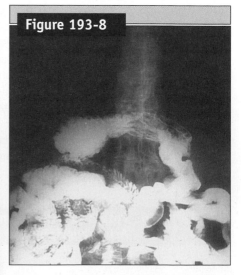

Figure 193-8

Gastric volvulus. This is an example of an organoaxial volvulus, in which the stomach rotates on its longitudinal axis, *ie*, the line connecting the cardia and the pylorus.

morphologic abnormalities in the intestinal glands, and an increase in connective tissue with atrophy of the muscular layer. The significance of these changes is unclear. Colonic transit does not differ between healthy elderly and young subjects. Colonic diverticulosis is known to increase with age. Anorectal function, in contrast to colonic function, does appear to change with age. The elderly have decreased resting and maximal anal sphincter pressures as well as decreased rectal elasticity [30]. Anal sensation has been shown to be decreased in two thirds of elderly subjects [31]. A larger volume of rectal distention is needed to signal the sensation of impending defecation. Possible explanations for the changes in anorectal function in the elderly include decreased muscle mass in the involved structures and nerve damage. No difference has been found between the young and the old in the anorectal angle.

Fecal incontinence is a prevalent condition among the elderly and is estimated to occur in 3% to 4% of those living in the community and in 32% to 62% of patients in geriatric extended-care facilities. Among the most common causes of fecal incontinence in the elderly is overflow of liquid stool around a fecal impaction, so-called overflow incontinence. Constipation leading to fecal incontinence is associated with a more obtuse anorectal angle, decreased resting anal pressure, decreased maximal squeeze pressure, impairment of anorectal sensation, and an overall decrease in mobility. Fecal incontinence also may result from impairment of one or more of the factors that ordinarily maintain continence and may indicate the presence of an underlying acute or chronic medical problem. For example, causes of fecal incontinence in the elderly include impaired anal sphincter function resulting from weakening of the muscles of the pelvic floor, decreased rectal sensation caused by diabetes, functional impairment resulting from generalized weakness or dementia, and a physiologic decline in the reservoir capacity of the rectum.

Constipation implies a relative lack or difficulty of bowel movements as compared with a person's prior bowel function; the term means different things to different people. Elderly patients commonly complain about moving their bowels, but constipation is not seen more commonly in the healthy elderly, despite changes in their mobility and diets [32]. With ill health, and often because of side effects of medications, some elderly persons experience a change in their bowel habits. Laxatives are used more often by the elderly than by the young, in part because many of the current generation of elders believe that a daily bowel movement is essential for maintenance of good health. Because bowel transit is not altered in the elderly, their constipation generally is attributed to a decrease in fecal water content. Factors contributing to constipation in the elderly include immobilization, physical weakness, depression, hypothyroidism, and long-standing laxative abuse, resulting in "cathartic colon." Medication use is increased markedly in the elderly, and many drugs have constipation as an unpleasant side effect. Examples of constipating medications include iron preparations, antidepressants, antacids, and bismuth-containing compounds.

Colonic ischemia is the most common vascular disorder of the GI tract and is discussed in detail in Chapter 79.

Colonic diverticula are a common cause of lower intestinal hemorrhage, although endoscopic documentation of the actual bleeding diverticulum is unusual. Diverticulosis is present in about half of persons older than 80 years. Despite the prevalence of diverticulosis in the elderly, complications such as bleeding, infection, perforation, or stricture develop in only about 20% of affected persons. Whereas most diverticula are found on the left side of the colon, most bleeding proved by angiography emanates from diverticula on the right side of the colon. Colonic diverticula are thought to arise as a result of increased intraluminal pressure secondary to sustained large bowel contraction, probably as a result of lack of adequate dietary fiber. In addition, deposition of elastin or collagen in the colonic wall may cause narrowing and stiffening of the large bowel, ultimately contributing to the formation of diverticula by further decreasing wall compliance and raising intraluminal pressure.

Vascular ectasias typically occur in the cecum and proximal ascending colon and probably arise from an age-related degeneration of previously normal blood vessels (Fig. 193-9, see also **Color Plate**). They, too, are an important cause of lower GI bleeding and, together with diverticula, are responsible for most significant lower GI bleeding episodes in the elderly [33]. Ectasias are found in up to 25% of persons older than 60 years who do not have symptoms; they typically are multiple and less than 5 mm in diameter. Colonic vascular ectasias are not associated with other vascular lesions of the mucous membranes or skin. Despite a long-standing belief to the contrary, there is no etiologic connection between vascular ectasias and aortic stenosis [34]. Vascular ectasias probably arise as a result of repeated episodes of incomplete, low-grade obstruction of submucosal veins caused by increased tension in the colonic wall (Fig. 193-10). The ultimate result is tortuosity and dilation of the venules and the arteriolar–capillary unit that feeds it, resulting in a small arteriovenous communication. This connection leads to the characteristic "early filling vein" seen on angiography. Whereas the nature of ectasias was established by angiographic studies, today most are found by colonoscopy and treated adequately using a variety of transcolonoscopic methods, including heater probe, bicap, and laser.

LIVER AND BILIARY TRACT

The liver achieves its maximum size in early adult life and thereafter decreases progressively in size, both in terms of

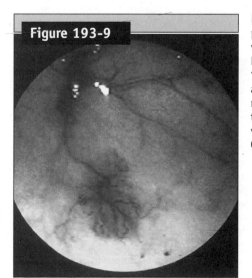

Figure 193-9

Endoscopic photograph of a vascular ectasia. Note the prominent "submucosal" vein and the coral reef–like pattern of the surrounding vessels. See also **Color Plate**.

absolute mass and its percentage of total body weight [35]. This reduction has been estimated to be 37% in persons aged 24 to 90 years and is more pronounced in women than in men. Liver blood flow also declines with advancing age, possibly because of decreased cardiac function. When measured by indocyanine green clearance, liver blood flow is reduced by as much as 35% between the third and tenth decades, and liver perfusion also

decreases by 10% in persons 20 to 90 years of age [36]. The number of hepatocytes decreases as liver size decreases; however, there appears to be no clinical significance to either of these findings, probably because of the substantial metabolic reserves of the liver. With advancing age, the liver turns a darker brown, so-called brown atrophy, as a result of deposition of lipofuscin pigment in hepatocytes. The space of Disse between hepatocytes enlarges with aging, and an associated increase occurs in the amount of collagen and fibrosis, but no change in the type of collagen.

Although liver size declines with age, human hepatocytes become larger. This change is associated with polyploidy and increased nuclear size and DNA, but not with impairment in liver function. Most studies indicate that results of liver function tests do not vary with age; any alteration in liver chemistry should be evaluated, not accepted as a consequence of aging. Enzymes responsible for the conjugation of metabolites in preparation for biliary excretion appear to be well preserved with age, but the activity of microsomal mono-oxygenase enzymes declines by 5% to 30% with age [37]. Drug clearance in the elderly is variable, in light of many disparate contributing factors, including uneven absorption of drugs, differing sensitivity of drug receptors, changes in liver function, and differences in the overall state of health (Table 193-7).

Drug-induced liver disease is a common cause of jaundice in the elderly as a result of cholestasis and hepatitis (see Chapter 96). The apparent high incidence of drug-induced liver disease in the elderly simply may reflect greater prescription drug use in this population. Drugs taken by older patients and commonly associated with hepatitis include antibiotics, antidepressants, anesthetics (*eg,* halothane), isoniazid, antihypertensives (*eg,* methyldopa) and acetaminophen. The effects of alcohol on the liver are similar in older and younger patients. Alcoholic liver disease, which often is overlooked or misdiagnosed in the elderly, actually is common in this age group [38]. In a British series, 28% of patients with alcoholic liver disease were older than 60 years, and 7% were older than 70 years, when they first sought attention for this problem. Older patients with alcoholic liver disease tend to have more severe clinical features, are more likely to have cirrhosis, and tend to have a worse prognosis than do their younger counterparts.

The presence of gallstones increases with advancing age, and about 30% of the population older than 65 years has gallstones. Gallbladder disease is the most common condition necessitating abdominal surgery in the elderly [39]. The size of the gallbladder remains unchanged with aging, as do the kinetics of gallbladder

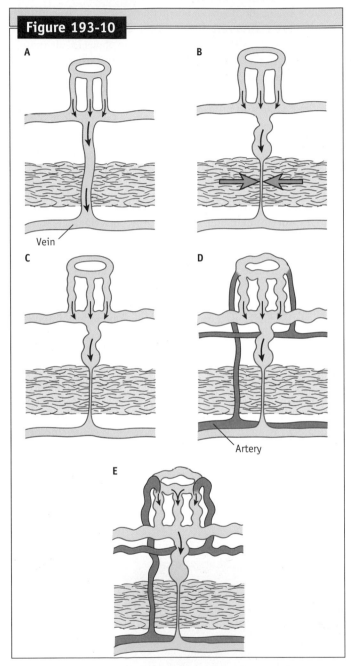

Figure 193-10

Proposed concept of the development of cecal vascular ectasias. **A,** Normal state of vein perforating muscular layers. **B,** With muscle contraction or increased intraluminal pressure, the vein is partially obstructed. **C,** After repeated episodes over many years, the submucosal vein becomes dilated and tortuous. **D,** Later, the veins and venules draining into the abnormal submucosal vein become similarly dilated and tortuous. **E,** Ultimately, the capillary ring becomes dilated, the precapillary sphincter becomes incompetent, and a small arteriovenous communication is present through the ectasia. (*From* Boley and coworkers [41]; with permission.)

Table 193-7. Alterations in Drug Metabolism in the Elderly

Change	Examples of affected drug
Decreased first pass metabolism	Propranolol, nitrates, lidocaine
Decreased phase I metabolism	Diazepam, quinidine, theophylline
Unaltered phase 2 metabolism	Oxazepam, lorazepam, tamazepam
Reduced binding capacity of albumin and transferrin	Salicylates, phenytoin, indomethacin

emptying. The lithogenic index of bile, a measure of cholesterol solubility, increases with advancing age, probably because of increased hepatic secretion of cholesterol and decreased bile salt synthesis, which lead to an increased prevalence of cholelithiasis in the elderly. The proximal common bile duct dilates slightly with age, at a rate of about 1 mm per decade after the sixth decade of life, whereas the preampullary portion becomes progressively narrowed.

Complications of cholelithiasis, such as acute cholecystitis, cholangitis, biliary-enteric fistulas, ischemic necrosis of the gallbladder, and gallstone ileus, are more common in the elderly than in the young. Gallbladder or biliary tract disease may be subtle in presentation in the elderly, in whom gallbladder necrosis and perforation have been reported to occur without peritoneal signs or leukocytosis.

Elderly men are at particular risk of acute acalculous cholecystitis, which often is seen in critically ill or postoperative patients; complications such as gangrene, empyema, and perforation are seen more commonly in patients with acalculous cholecystitis than in those with cholecystitis caused by gallstones. A rare cause of acalculous cholecystitis is torsion of the gallbladder. This is seen especially in elderly women and most likely is the result of compromised blood flow to the gallbladder caused by a lax or prominent mesentery, which allows the gallbladder to twist.

▮▮ PANCREAS

The pancreas atrophies after 70 years of age, decreasing from about 60 to 40 g or less by 85 years of age. Profound histologic changes occur as well, including lipofuscin and lactoferrin deposition, parenchymal fibrosis, fat deposition, and degeneration of acinar cells. Progressive dilation of the main pancreatic duct has been demonstrated by ultrasonography and endoscopic retrograde cholangiopancreatography; the caliber of the duct increases with age at a rate of about 0.8% per year. Dilation of the main pancreatic duct is accompanied by a patchy proliferation of the ductal epithelium in about 10% of persons older than 60 years.

In healthy persons older than 70 years, the volume and output of pancreatic bicarbonate and amylase are normal, although many have a moderate reduction in the capacity to secrete lipase. When secretin is used to stimulate production of bicarbonate and amylase, the output of the aged pancreas is no different than that of a younger pancreas. On repeated stimulation, however, the pancreas appears to fatigue, and secretory volume and bicarbonate and amylase output decrease. Perhaps because the human pancreatic gland appears to have a large functional reserve, structural and physiologic changes in the pancreas that occur with aging do not have any adverse clinical consequences [40].

▮▮ REFERENCES

Recently published papers of particular interest have been highlighted as follows:
• Of interest
•• Of outstanding interest

1. Brandt LJ: *Gastrointestinal Disorders in the Elderly.* New York: Raven Press; 1984.

2. Greenwald DA, Brandt LJ: Endoscopy in the elderly patient. In *Problems in General Surgery: Gastrointestinal Surgery in the Elderly,* Vol 13. Edited by Zenilman ME. Philadelphia: Lippincott-Raven; 1996:32–43.

3.• Ure T, Dehghan K, Vernava AM, *et al.*: Colonoscopy in the elderly: low risk, high yield. *Surg Endosc* 1995, 9:505–508.

This is a retrospective study comparing 354 elderly patients (defined as greater than or equal to 70 years) with 302 controls aged 50 to 70 years. The authors examined the utility, morbidity, and patient tolerance of colonoscopy in the two groups. They found that colonoscopy in the elderly was safe and had a low incidence of complications. Moreover, the yield was high; elderly patients were significantly more likely to have an abnormality detected by colonoscopy than were younger patients.

4. Jernigan JH: Update on drugs and the elderly. *Am Fam Phys* 1984, 29:238–247.

5. Beller SA, Evans ER: Drug therapy in the elderly: effects on mental status. 1987, 36:149–152.

6. Gurwitz J, Avorn J: The ambiguous relationship between aging and adverse drug reactions. *Ann Intern Med* 1991, 114:956–966.

7. Levitan R: GI problems in the elderly, part I: Age related considerations. *Geriatrics* 1989, 44:53–56.

8. Wu AJ, Ship JA: A characterization of major salivary gland flow rates in the presence of medications and systemic diseases. *Oral Surg Oral Med Oral Pathol Oral Radiol Endod* 1993, 76:301–306.

9. Castell JA, Castell DO: Upper esophageal sphincter and pharyngeal function and oropharyngeal (transfer) dysphagia. *Gastroenterol Clin North Am* 1996, 25:35–50.

10. Soergel KH, Zboralski F, Amberg JR: Presbyesophagus: esophageal motility in nonagenarians. *J Clin Invest* 1964, 43:1472–1479.

11. Richter JE, Wu WC, Johns DN, *et al.*: Esophageal manometry in 95 healthy adult volunteers: variability of pressures with age and frequency of "abnormal" contraction. *Dig Dis Sci* 1987, 32:583–592.

12. Eng J, Sabanathan S: Drug-induced esophagitis. *Am J Gastroenterol* 1991, 86:1127–1133.

13. Mold JW, Reed LE, Davis AB, *et al.*: Prevalence of gastroesophageal reflux in elderly patients in a primary care setting. *Am J Gastroenterol* 1991, 86:965–970.

14.• Zhu H, Pace F, Sangaletti O, *et al.*: Features of symptomatic gastroesophageal reflux in elderly patients. *Scand J Gastroenterol* 1993, 28:235–238.

In this study, patterns of gastroesophageal reflux and reflux-related esophageal lesions were compared in elderly patients and their younger counterparts. The elderly had pathologic reflux and reflux esophagitis more frequently than the young. The study demonstrated that older subjects with reflux esophagitis, as compared with a similar group of younger patients, had more severe reflux (ie, a greater percentage of time that the esophagus was exposed to a pH<4) on 24-hour pH testing. The elderly also were more likely to have higher grades of esophagitis detected by endoscopic examination.

15.•• Collen MJ, Abdulian JD, Chen YK: Gastroesophageal reflux disease in the elderly: more severe disease that requires aggressive therapy. *Am J Gastroenterol* 1995, 90:1053–1057.

Patients with GERD who were older than 60 years and had pyrosis symptoms severe enough to require upper GI endoscopy were found to have significantly more esophageal mucosal disease (erosive esophagitis, Barrett's) than those who were younger. Aggressive therapy using relatively high doses of acid-blocking agents, similar to those employed for younger patients, was found to be necessary to heal esophageal mucosal lesions in elderly patients.

16. Altman DF: Changes in gastrointestinal, pancreatic, biliary, and hepatic function with aging. *Gastroenterol Clin North Am* 1990, 19:227–234.

17. Goldschmiedt M, Barnett CC, Schwarz BE, *et al.*: Effect of age on gastric acid secretion and serum gastrin concentration in healthy men and women. *Gastroenterology* 1991, 101:977–990.

18.• Green LK, Graham DY: Gastritis in the elderly. *Gastroenterol Clin North Am* 1990, 19:273–292.

This article contains a thorough discussion of both acute and chronic gastritis as it pertains to the elderly patient. The text focuses on Type A and B gastritis, chronic erosive gastritis, and the relationship of gastritis to gastric carcinoma.

19.• McCarthy DM: Acid peptic disease in the elderly. *Clin Geriatr Med* 1991, 7:231–254.

This review examines peptic ulcer disease in the elderly, initially covering the epidemiology, clinical features, and diagnosis of acid-peptic disorders. The authors go on to look at specific problems related to acid-peptic disease in the elderly, namely gastric ulcer, duodenal ulcer, NSAID-associated ulcers, complications of ulcers, nonulcer dyspepsia, and side effects of therapy.

20. Issacs, KL: Severe gastrointestinal bleeding. *Clin Geriatr Med* 1994, 10:1–17.

21. Scheiman JM: NSAIDs, gastrointestinal injury, and cytoprotection. *Gastroenterol Clin North Am* 1996, 25:279–298.

22.•• Griffin MR, Piper JM, Daugherty JR, *et al.*: Nonsteroidal anti-inflammatory drug use and increased risk for peptic ulcer disease in elderly persons. *Ann Intern Med* 1991, 114:257–263.

This nested case-control study of an elderly population (older than 65 years) demonstrated that users of prescription nonaspirin NSAIDs were four times more likely to be hospitalized for ulcer disease or upper GI bleeding than were nonusers. The risk of ulcer formation and bleeding increased with use of higher doses of NSAIDs. New users of NSAIDs at a high dose had a 10 times greater likelihood of developing ulcers compared with nonusers.

23. Yii MK, Hunt PS: Bleeding giant gastric ulcer. *Aust NZ J Surg* 1996, 66:540–542.

24. Schaefer DC, Nikoomenesh P, Moore C: Gastric volvulus: an old disease process with some new twists. *Gastroenterologist* 1997, 5:41–45.

25. Webster SG, Leeming JT: The appearance of the small bowel mucosa in old age. *Age Aging* 1975, 4:168–174.

26. Montgomery RD, Haboubi NY, Chesner IM, *et al.*: Causes of malabsorption in the elderly. *Age Aging* 1986, 15:235–240.

27. Kupfer RM, Heppell M, Haggith JW, *et al.*: Gastric emptying and small bowel transit rate in the elderly. *J Am Geriatr Soc* 1985, 33:340–343.

28.• Holt PR: Diarrhea and malabsorption in the elderly. *Gastroenterol Clin North Am* 1990, 19:345–359.

Neither diarrhea nor malabsorption is commonly thought of when discussing gastrointestinal diseases in the elderly. However, this review focuses first on diarrhea in the elderly, looking at intestinal infections, fecal impaction, drug-induced diarrhea, and diabetic diarrhea. The author goes on to discuss intestinal malabsorption in the elderly, specifically detailing chronic pancreatitis, celiac disease, mesenteric ischemia, and bacterial overgrowth.

29. Arora S, Kassarjian Z, Krazinski SD, *et al.*: Effect of age on tests of intestinal and hepatic function in healthy humans. *Gastroenterology* 1989, 96:1560–1565.

30. McHugh SM, Diamant NE: Effect of age, gender and parity on anal canal pressures. *Dig Dis Sci* 1987, 32:726–736.

31. Wald A: Constipation and fecal incontinence in the elderly. *Semin Gastrointest Dis* 1994, 5:179–188.

32. O'Brien MD, Phillips SF: Colonic motility in health and disease. *Gastroenterol Clin North Am* 1996, 25:147–162.

33. Reinus JF, Brandt LJ: Vascular ectasias and diverticulosis: common causes of lower intestinal bleeding. *Gastroenterol Clin North Am* 1994, 23:1–20.

34.•• Bhutani MS, Gupta SC, Markert RJ, *et al.*: A prospective controlled evaluation of endoscopic detection of angiodysplasia and its association with aortic valve disease. *Gastrointest Endosc* 1995, 42:398–402.

This prospective, controlled study demonstrated no relationship between the endoscopic detection of angiodysplasia and the presence of aortic valvular disease. These data support other authors' critiques of the previously published and widely held association between aortic stenosis, angiodysplasia, and gastrointestinal bleeding.

35. Van Dam J, Zeldis JB: Hepatic diseases in the elderly. *Gastroenterol Clin North Am* 1990, 19;459–472.

36. Wynne HA, Cope E, Mutch E, *et al.*: The effect of age upon liver volume and apparent liver blood flow in healthy man. *Hepatology* 1989, 9:297–301.

37. Vestal RE: Aging and determinants of hepatic drug clearance. *Hepatology* 1989, 9:331–334.

38. Potter JR, James OF: Clinical features and prognosis of alcoholic liver disease in respect of advancing age. *Gerontology* 1987, 33:380–387.

39.• Magnuson TH: Surgery of the biliary tree in the aging patient. In *Problems in General Surgery: Gastrointestinal Surgery in the Elderly*, Vol 13. 1996:75–83.

40. Lillemoe KD: Pancreatic disease in the elderly patient. *Surg Clin North Am* 1994, 74:317–344.

41. Boley SJ, Sammartano R, Adams A, *et al.*: On the nature and etiology of vascular ectasias of the colon: degenerative lesions of aging. *Gastroenterology* 1977, 72:650–660.

194 Gastrointestinal Disease in Pregnancy

Rebecca G. Wells and Jacqueline L. Wolf

Even during normal pregnancy, pregnant women have significant gastroenterologic complaints. They also may present with chronic illnesses that require special consideration during pregnancy or with disorders unique to or especially common in pregnancy. The care that a pregnant woman requires, although generally similar to that of a nonpregnant woman, must take into account the sensitivity of the fetus to maternal pathophysiologic changes and to medications and diagnostic procedures. In many cases, however, the instinct to delay or withhold treatment out of concern for the pregnancy is unfounded and potentially dangerous.

This chapter focuses on the most common gastrointestinal (GI) symptoms, including nausea, vomiting, heartburn, and constipation; on the common GI diseases that pose special problems in pregnancy, namely inflammatory bowel disease (IBD) and biliary disease; and on the common disorders with the most potential for catastrophe, including intestinal obstruction and appendicitis.

■ DISORDERS OF THE UPPER GASTROINTESTINAL TRACT

Nausea and Vomiting of Pregnancy

Nausea and vomiting of pregnancy and hyperemesis gravidarum represent different degrees of the same symptom complex. The incidence of nausea and vomiting, although variable in different populations, ranges from 50% to 90%, with a prospective multicenter study of 9098 patients reporting a frequency of 56% [1•,2,3]. Risk factors include first pregnancy, obesity, younger age, and nonsmoking status [1•]. Symptoms tend to recur in subsequent pregnancies, although they are usually shorter in duration [1•,3].

Nausea and vomiting are characteristic of early pregnancy, with 91% of patients developing symptoms in the first trimester, generally in the first 6 to 8 weeks [3]. Only 3% of patients develop symptoms in the third trimester [3]. Symptoms almost always resolve, often abruptly, by week 20 [1•]. Although the disorder is classically termed *morning sickness,* symptoms are episodic and confined to the morning in only a minority of patients [2,3], leading one authority to suggest that *episodic daytime pregnancy sickness* is a more accurate name [2].

The pathophysiology of this disorder continues to be debated. Symptoms have been attributed to hormonal fluctuations, although recent data suggest that human chorionic gonadotropin (hCG) is not involved, and the roles of progesterone and estradiol remain unclear [4]. It has also been speculated that psychological factors are important.

Treatment usually is limited to changes in diet (*ie,* smaller, more frequent meals and increased carbohydrate intake). The outcome for mother and fetus is excellent, with no evidence of an increased frequency of congenital malformations. In fact, first-trimester nausea and vomiting bode well for pregnancy outcome, with decreased rates of miscarriage and preterm labor in affected patients [1•,3].

Hyperemesis Gravidarum

Hyperemesis gravidarum refers to intractable nausea and vomiting in pregnancy, often associated with dehydration, electrolyte abnormalities, and weight loss. It affects 0.3% to 1% of pregnant women and, like nausea and vomiting, is more common in Western countries than elsewhere [5•]. Risk factors are similar to those for nausea and vomiting and include obesity, first pregnancy, and twin pregnancies; also, like nausea and vomiting of pregnancy, hyperemesis gravidarum tends to recur in subsequent pregnancies and does not correlate with the occurrence of other pregnancy complications [1•,5•]. In one study of 12 patients, however, half of affected patients had elevated serum aminotransferase levels, up to 20 times the upper limit of normal, and 2 patients who underwent liver biopsy were found to have central zone vacuolization with cell dropout [5•].

Hyperemesis gravidarum occurs primarily in the first trimester, with an onset between weeks 4 and 10; in some women, symptoms begin before the first missed menstrual period. Symptoms resolve by 20 weeks and rarely persist into the second half of pregnancy. The diagnosis should be made with extreme caution if symptoms begin after the first trimester or are accompanied by severe abdominal pain; in such cases, the alternative diagnoses of peptic ulcer, bowel obstruction, and liver disease should be entertained.

There are multiple theories concerning the cause of hyperemesis gravidarum. Abell and Riely [5•] have divided the possible causes into the following categories: psychological and behavioral factors, hyperthyroidism, increased hormone levels (hCG or

progesterone), delayed gastric emptying, and abnormal autonomic nervous system response. Thus far, however, none of these has been convincingly demonstrated to have a pathophysiologic role.

Treatment is primarily supportive, including fluid and electrolyte repletion, attention to adequate nutrition, and, in patients with particularly severe and long-lasting symptoms, parenteral hyperalimentation. Drug treatment should be avoided, if possible, although metoclopramide or prochlorperazine are often needed. The outcome for mother and fetus is good, and there is no evidence that hyperemesis leads to congenital anomalies, prematurity, or low birth weight [1•,6].

Gastroesophageal Reflux Disease

Between 45% and 80% of women have symptomatic gastroesophageal reflux disease (GERD) during pregnancy. Although it is often perceived as a disorder of late pregnancy, GERD begins in the first (52%) or second (40%) trimester in most women and persists throughout pregnancy [7•]. Resolution occurs almost immediately postpartum in 98% of women [4], a phenomenon illustrated by a study of 25 women in whom 24-hour esophageal pH monitoring probes showed a significant decrease in the number of reflux episodes by 2 days after delivery [8].

Proposed causes of GERD during pregnancy include abnormal esophageal motility and decreased esophageal and increased gastric pressures [7•]. The hormonal milieu of pregnancy is probably the most important factor, with increased serum progesterone levels, alone or in combination with estrogen, causing decreased lower esophageal sphincter pressure [9] (Fig. 194-1).

Symptoms, precipitants, and potential complications of GERD are similar in affected pregnant and nonpregnant women. Symptoms tend to recur in subsequent pregnancies [7•]. The diagnosis is usually clinical, and initial treatment consists of conservative measures, such as elevating the head of the bed at night, minimizing food intake within 4 hours of bedtime, and avoiding foods that exacerbate symptoms. There are no published, controlled trials of therapy for GERD in

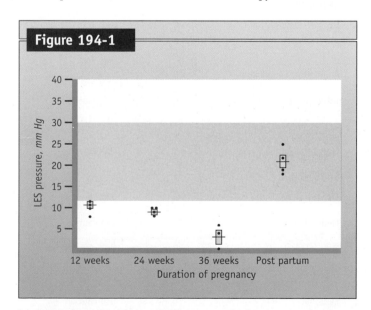

Figure 194-1

Lower esophageal sphincter (LES) pressure in four women during pregnancy and postpartum. (*From* van Thiel *et al.* [9].)

pregnancy. Antacids, thought to be safe, generally are prescribed as first-line medical therapy when conservative measures fail (Table 194-1). Because it is not absorbed from the intestine, sucralfate suspension is an appropriate second-line therapy, particularly in women with esophagitis, although its efficacy is unproved in this situation. In women with severe symptoms, cimetidine, ranitidine, and famotidine are acceptable because of their extensive safety history in pregnant women. If symptoms persist and a proton pump inhibitor is required, lansoprazole (Food and Drug Administration category B) is preferred over omeprazole (category C). Cisapride (category C) is not recommended during pregnancy.

Table 194-1. Common Gastrointestinal Drugs in Pregnancy and Lactation

Drug name	FDA category	Safety in breastfeeding	Comments
Peptic ulcer disease and GERD			
Antacids (calcium, magnesium, aluminum)	—	Safe	No controlled trials, but widely used and believed to be safe
Sodium bicarbonate	—	Safe	Avoid in pregnancy due to potential metabolic alkalosis and fluid overload in mother and fetus
Cimetidine	B	Likely safe	No association with congenital defects, excreted into breast milk
Ranitidine	B	Likely safe	No association with congenital defects, excreted into breast milk
Famotidine	B	Likely safe	No evidence of adverse effects, less excretion in breast milk than cimetidine or ranitidine
Nizatidine	B	Unknown	No studies in humans; congenital malformations seen in rabbits, the three H_2 blockers above are preferred in pregnancy, minimal excretion in breast milk although growth suppression seen in rat pups
Omeprazole	C	Unknown	Dose-related fetotoxicity in rodent studies, no adequate studies in women, use not recommended, excretion in breast milk unknown
Lansoprazole	B	Use caution	No studies in women; no teratogenicity in animal studies, unknown if excreted in breast milk but tumorigenicity unknown, should use caution
Cisapride	C	Use caution	Fetotoxic in rats and rabbits, decreased birth weight in rats, no studies in women, not recommended in pregnancy, excreted in breast milk, effects unknown
Metoclopramide	B	Use caution	No evidence of adverse effects, effects of long-term use in pregnancy unknown, excreted into breast milk: no adverse effects reported, but use caution due to potential CNS effects
Sucralfate	B	Safe	No association with congenital defects, minimal absorption, no evidence for elevated aluminum levels in women with normal renal function, breast feeding likely safe due to minimal absorption
Misoprostol	X	Contraindicated	Abortifacient, possible teratogen, contraindicated in pregnancy, excretion of drug into breast milk unknown but potential severe diarrhea in nursing infant
Treatment of *Helicobacter pylori*			
Bismuth subsalicylate	C	Not recommended	Significant amounts of salicylate absorbed with potential for congenital defects, risk of bismuth unknown, salicylate excreted in breast milk, no indication for treatment of *H. pylori* with this medication in pregnant or nursing women
Ampicillin, amoxicillin	B	Safe	Extensive experience, no evidence for teratogenicity, excreted into breast milk but no reported adverse effects
Tetracycline	D	Use caution	Adverse effects on fetal bones and teeth, can cause liver disease in pregnant women, possible cause of minor congenital malformations, theoretical danger in breastfeeding but no adverse effects reported
Clarithromycin	C	Unknown	Teratogenic rats and mice, growth retardation in monkeys, no adequate studies in women, avoid use in pregnant or nursing women
Endoscopy			
Lidocaine (topical)	C†	Safe	Widely and safely used as a local anesthetic in labor and delivery, safe for short-term topical use
Meperidine	B	Use caution	Safe if used short term, avoid use near term, excreted into breast milk but no adverse effects reported
Midazolam	D	Not recommended	No teratogenicity in limited animal studies but congenital malformations reported with other benzodiazepines, excreted in breast milk
Diazepam	D	Not recommended	Likely teratogenic, can cause prolonged CNS depression in neonates, excreted in breast milk, avoid use in pregnant or nursing women
Fentanyl	C	Use caution	No known teratogenicity, no studies in women, short-term use (not at term) safe, excreted into breast milk

Table 194-1. Common Gastrointestinal Drugs in Pregnancy and Lactation (*continued*)

Drug name	FDA category	Safety in breastfeeding	Comments
Flumazenil	C	Unknown	No adequate studies in women, no teratogenicity in animals, increased fetal loss in rabbits at high doses, use only if clearly indicated
Naloxone	B	Use caution	No evidence for adverse effects but minimal information available
Inflammatory bowel disease			
Sulfasalazine	B	Use caution	Widely used and considered safe, should supplement with folate, excreted in breast milk, one possible case of bloody diarrhea in breast fed infant
Mesalamine	B	Use caution	Considered safe, excreted in breast milk, possible diarrhea in breastfed neonate
Olsalazine	C	Use caution	Rat studies show reduced weight, retarded ossifications, and immature viscera; excreted in breast milk, observe breastfed neonate for diarrhea
Steroids (prednisone, prednisolone)	B	Safe	Extensive experience, considered safe, supplemental steroids should be given during labor
Azathioprine	D	Unknown Not recommended	Most data from organ transplant recipients; teratogenic in animals; no defects seen in humans; may cause intrauterine growth retardation, bone marrow suppression, and prematurity; risk/benefit ratio may be acceptable (with patient consent) if necessary to control disease
6-mercaptopurine	D	Unknown Not recommended	As for azathioprine, minimal experience in IBD in pregnancy, but no anomalies seen; risk/benefit ratio may be acceptable, with patient consent, if necessary to control disease
Cyclosporin	C	Contraindicated	Fetotoxic in rats, no evidence of teratogenicity although neonates may be growth retarded or premature
Methotrexate	X	Contraindicated	Data from use as antineoplastic agent, causes congenital anomalies and possible myelosuppression and low birth weight, may persist in tissue after discontinuation of treatment
Metronidazole	B	Unknown	Studies offer conflicting conclusions about teratogenicity and overall safety; contraindicated in first trimester but probably safe in third, excreted in breast milk, use caution with breast feeding if needed for disease control
Ciprofloxacin	C	Not recommended	Cartilage defects in experimental animals, no abnormalities seen in human infants but experience is limited, not recommended in pregnancy
Loperamide	B	Likely safe	No known adverse effects
Diphenoxylate	C	Unknown Use caution	No known teratogenicity
Constipation			
Fiber	B	Safe	Not absorbed, preferred treatment
Hyperosmotic agents (lactulose)	B	Likely safe	No reports available but likely safe, approximately 3% absorbed
Mineral Oil	C	Unknown	Chronic use may lead to decreased absorption of fat-soluble vitamins and neonatal hypoprothrombinemia may occur, not absorbed
Senna	C	Safe	Not teratogenic in animals, human data limited, not excreted into breast milk
Docusate sodium	C	Safe	No evidence of teratogenicity, observe breastfed neonate for diarrhea
Saline laxatives (milk of magnesia, phospho-soda)	—	Unknown	May cause volume overload or electrolyte disturbances
Castor oil	—	Unknown	May cause premature contractions
Cascara sagrada	C	Unknown	No evidence for adverse effects, excreted into breast milk, possible increased diarrhea in breastfed infants
Bisacodyl	B	Unknown	No evidence for teratogenicity, low level of systemic absorption
Phenolphthalein	C	No adverse effects reported	No evidence of teratogenicity, metabolites excreted into breast-milk although no diarrhea seen in breastfed infants

*FDA categories are from reference 43 and from medication package inserts. Categories are: A—Controlled studies show no risk to the fetus. B—No evidence of risk in humans. Either animal findings negative but human studies not done, or risk seen in animal studies not confirmed in humans. C—Risk cannot be ruled out. Human studies lacking; animal studies either lacking or show risk. D—Positive evidence of risk to the fetus. Benefits may outweigh risk. X—Contraindicated in pregnancy. Risk outweighs any possible benefit.

†No rating for topical use.

CNS—central nervous system; GERD—gastroesophageal reflux disease; IBD—inflammatory bowel disease.

Data from ——— [7•,35,37,38,48].

Empiric treatment is appropriate, with a more extensive evaluation limited to patients whose symptoms fail to respond. Barium studies are contraindicated because of radiation exposure, but endoscopy is safe and is the diagnostic procedure of choice. If necessary, ambulatory pH monitoring or esophageal manometry may be done.

Peptic Ulcer Disease

Peptic ulcer disease is rare in pregnancy. Although there is a paucity of data on its incidence, older literature reviews suggest an incidence of 0.005% [10]. It is commonly believed that peptic ulcer disease improves in pregnancy. This notion derives in part from older retrospective studies, the most recent of which was published in 1953 by Clark [11]. Clark interviewed 118 women with surgically or radiologically confirmed peptic ulcer disease and found that 88% reported a remission in symptoms starting early in pregnancy, with a postpartum recurrence, generally within 3 to 6 months of parturition. The improvement in symptoms was attributed to a decrease in gastric acid output in pregnancy, coupled with increased mucus production and mucosal protection from progesterone. None of the studies in the literature, however, is prospective or from the era of H_2-receptor antagonists, proton pump inhibitors, or *Helicobacter pylori* identification. It is not clear whether the incidence and prevalence of peptic ulcer disease in pregnant women are in fact lower than the already low incidence and prevalence in women of childbearing age. The incidence of peptic ulcer disease in pregnancy is almost certainly underestimated, in part because symptoms overlap with those of a normal pregnancy.

Symptoms of peptic ulcer disease are the same in pregnant and nonpregnant women. Complications, most notably upper GI bleeding and perforation, are managed similarly in both populations, with the caveat that maternal hypovolemia is particularly dangerous to the fetus, and patients with bleeding should be resuscitated aggressively and transfused if necessary. Complications are more likely to occur in the third trimester or early puerperium than at other times [4]. Diagnosis is by endoscopy. Although empiric treatment is acceptable, patients with refractory symptoms should undergo diagnostic evaluation because gastric cancer, although rare, does occur in pregnancy.

The H_2-receptor antagonists cimetidine, ranitidine, and famotidine are the first choice for treatment (Table 194-1). Lansoprazole is the proton pump inhibitor of choice because of its safety in animal studies. Treatment of *H. pylori* infection is not urgently required and should be postponed until pregnancy and breast-feeding are completed because several of the recommended medications (including bismuth subsalicylate, metronidazole, and tetracycline) are relatively contraindicated.

Endoscopy

Endoscopy is the diagnostic procedure of choice in the pregnant woman with complicated or refractory upper GI symptoms or upper GI bleeding. Although there has never been a controlled study, retrospective analyses of endoscopy in pregnant women suggest that it is safe [12,13•]. Cappell and Sidhom [13•], in a review of more than 29,000 deliveries in three teaching hospitals over seven and a half years, found that 0.06% of women (20 patients) underwent endoscopy, all without changes in maternal

vital signs, induction of labor, an increased rate of congenital malformations, or other complications. The most common indications for endoscopy in these studies were vomiting, upper GI bleeding, and epigastric or abdominal pain. Esophagitis (32% to 35%), gastritis (15% to 24%), and ulcers (10% to 12%) were the most common findings, with a significant number of studies (30%) being normal [12,13•]. A lesion was diagnosed by endoscopy in 70% of cases, and treatment was changed as a result of endoscopy in 50% [13•].

Endoscopy should be performed only in stable patients, with monitoring of vital signs and pulse oximetry. There are no clear recommendations for fetal monitoring. Although preprocedure and postprocedure fetal heart rate determination is advisable, the utility of continuous fetal monitoring is uncertain. The standard medications for conscious sedation are safe in pregnant women (Table 194-1). Midazolam (Versed) is preferable to, although less well studied than, diazepam (Valium), and both are category D drugs. Meperidine (Demerol) and fentanyl appear safe for short-term use during endoscopy and are the narcotic agents of choice.

■ GALLSTONES AND GALLBLADDER DISEASE

Gallstones are twice as common in women as in men. The increased frequency in women is explained in part by the high rate of gallstone and sludge formation in pregnancy. Gallstones are an important cause of abdominal pain in pregnancy and are the most common cause of acute pancreatitis; cholecystectomy is the second most common nonobstetric operation (after appendectomy) performed during pregnancy.

Epidemiology and Pathophysiology

Prospective studies have shown that biliary sludge develops in up to 31% of women during pregnancy, and new gallstones develop in 2% [14••,15]. The risk is most pronounced during the second and third trimesters and first month postpartum. The risk of gallstones increases with each pregnancy, particularly in younger women who have had several children, and is independent of breast-feeding [16]. In a substantial percentage of affected women, stones and sludge regress or pass after delivery; in one study, sludge and stones seen at the time of delivery had disappeared in 61% and 28% of patients, respectively, after a mean of 5 months [14••].

By altering biliary physiology, the hormonal changes of pregnancy are primarily responsible for the increased incidence of stone and sludge formation. Estrogen mediates increased cholesterol saturation in bile, whereas progesterone promotes bile stasis by increasing the residual volume (to more than twice the prepartum size [15]) and decreasing emptying of the gallbladder.

Symptoms and Diagnosis

Pregnant women with gallstones have a strikingly high frequency of symptoms compared with nonpregnant women with gallstones; several studies have shown that up to one third of affected pregnant women have biliary colic during their pregnancies [14••,17], a rate about 10 times that in nonpregnant women. Although the symptoms are identical in affected pregnant and nonpregnant women, making the correct diagnosis may be difficult because of the expanded differential diagnosis of abdominal pain (see below and Table 194-2). In particular, acute appendicitis needs to be considered because it may cause pain localized to the right upper quadrant in a pregnant patient.

Ultrasound is the major tool for the diagnosis of sludge and gallstones during pregnancy, although, as in the nonpregnant population, its ability to detect common bile duct stones is limited. Oral cholecystography and computed tomography should be avoided because of possible radiation exposure to the fetus. Nuclear medicine scans also should be avoided, although they are probably safe in late pregnancy if required for diagnosis.

Treatment

Treatment of pregnant women with biliary disease should be undertaken with the understanding that the major risks to the fetus are not from treatment but rather from poor health and complications in the mother. Women with evidence of biliary obstruction, cholangitis, or pancreatitis should undergo immediate endoscopic retrograde cholangiopancreatography, with appropriate fetal shielding. Acute pancreatitis is a particularly dangerous complication in pregnant women, with rates of fetal loss of 10% to 20%, and maternal mortality of more than 3% in some studies [18•].

In women with severe biliary colic, conservative management with intravenous hydration, narcotics, antibiotics, and dietary restriction is the first line of treatment. Nevertheless, 70% of women treated successfully still suffer relapse; the earlier the presentation, the higher this risk [19] (Fig. 194-2). Cholecystectomy is indicated in women with persistent (longer than 4 days) or recurrent symptoms, significant nutritional compromise, or weight loss, but is required in less than 0.1% of pregnancies. Surgery is safest during the second trimester. Many older reports suggested increased fetal loss with surgery in the first trimester, but a more recent study has questioned the validity of these reports [20]. In the third trimester, cholecystectomy leads to an increased incidence of preterm labor,

although it generally can be treated successfully with tocolytic agents [20,21•]. Intraoperative cholangiography can be undertaken after shielding of the fetus. Laparoscopic cholecystectomy is being performed increasingly, although most experience has been in women in the first and second trimesters; there have been case reports of successful laparoscopic cholecystectomy in the early third trimester [22].

In symptomatic women who deliver without having had a cholecystectomy and who have small (<5 mm) stones, it may be appropriate to consider a trial of ursodeoxycholic acid. There is no justification for a prophylactic cholecystectomy in an asymptomatic woman planning pregnancy; silent stones should be followed expectantly, as in the general population.

ABDOMINAL PAIN

The pregnant patient with abdominal pain can be challenging both diagnostically and therapeutically (Table 194-2). The gravid uterus and the nausea, vomiting, and anorexia associated with many normal pregnancies combine to confound diagnosis even as the potential harm to mother and fetus from misdiagnosis or inappropriate management is increased. The single most important consideration in the care of a pregnant patient with abdominal pain is to avoid a delay in diagnosis and treatment.

Physiology

An understanding of the physiologic changes of pregnancy is a prerequisite to an understanding of abdominal pain in pregnancy. The uterus undergoes a tremendous change in size during pregnancy, increasing from 70 g to greater than 1100 g and developing an internal volume of greater than 5 L [23]. By the end of the second trimester, the adnexa have moved from the pelvis into the abdomen, and the intestine and omentum have been displaced superiorly and laterally, making the diagnosis of acute appendicitis difficult because the appendix is in the right upper quadrant (Fig. 194-3). Moreover, the omentum is less able than usual to contain peritonitis if it occurs. Rapid shifts in

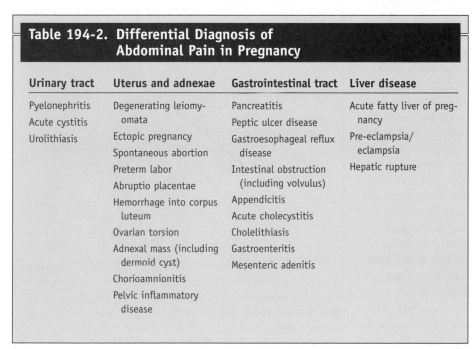

Urinary tract	Uterus and adnexae	Gastrointestinal tract	Liver disease
Pyelonephritis	Degenerating leiomyomata	Pancreatitis	Acute fatty liver of pregnancy
Acute cystitis		Peptic ulcer disease	
Urolithiasis	Ectopic pregnancy	Gastroesophageal reflux disease	Pre-eclampsia/eclampsia
	Spontaneous abortion		Hepatic rupture
	Preterm labor	Intestinal obstruction (including volvulus)	
	Abruptio placentae	Appendicitis	
	Hemorrhage into corpus luteum	Acute cholecystitis	
	Ovarian torsion	Cholelithiasis	
	Adnexal mass (including dermoid cyst)	Gastroenteritis	
	Chorioamnionitis	Mesenteric adenitis	
	Pelvic inflammatory disease		

Table 194-2. Differential Diagnosis of Abdominal Pain in Pregnancy

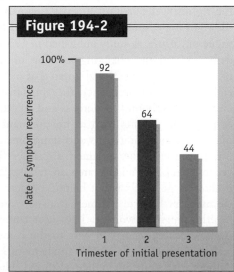

Figure 194-2

The risk by trimester of recurrent biliary colic in pregnancy after initially successful conservative therapy, from a study of 72 pregnant women with biliary disease. (*From* Swisher *et al.* [19].)

the location of the uterus, which occur at weeks 16 to 20, at term when the head descends, and in the puerperium, predispose pregnant patients to volvulus of the colon [24•]. Elevation of the anterior abdominal wall may result in masking of the signs of peritoneal irritation.

Differential Diagnosis

The differential diagnosis of abdominal pain in a pregnant woman includes both gynecologic and nongynecologic causes (Table 194-2). Early in pregnancy, spontaneous abortion and ectopic pregnancy are frequent causes, whereas later in pregnancy, abruptio placentae and preterm labor are seen. Uterine leiomyomas and adnexal pathology also should be considered in the evaluation. Acute pyelonephritis occurs in 1% to 2% and urolithiasis in up to 0.5% of pregnancies [23].

The GI tract is the source of abdominal pain in a substantial percentage of pregnant women. Gallbladder pathology, acute pancreatitis, peptic ulcer disease, GERD, and liver disease (see Chapter 110) always should be considered in the pregnant patient with abdominal pain, particularly because the symptoms can be both nonspecific and atypical. Acute appendicitis and intestinal obstruction are important causes of abdominal pain that require special consideration in pregnancy.

Appendicitis

Acute appendicitis occurs in about 1 in 1500 pregnancies and is the most common indication for nonobstetric surgery during pregnancy, with a rate four to five times higher than that for cholecystectomy [25,26]. The incidence of appendicitis is not increased in the pregnant patient compared with the nonpregnant patient, but the risks of misdiagnosis and delayed surgery are substantially greater for the pregnant patient.

Making a diagnosis of acute appendicitis may be difficult and requires a high index of suspicion. The decision to perform surgery usually is made on clinical grounds. Typical symptoms include anorexia, nausea, and vomiting, all of which are common in normal pregnancies. Pain localizes most often to the right lower quadrant in early pregnancy but commonly to the right upper quadrant during the third trimester and may be vague or diffuse. A study published in 1932 using barium meals demonstrated the changing location of the appendix during pregnancy (Fig. 194-3) and noted that in 93% of women in the eighth month of pregnancy, the appendix was above the iliac crest [27•]. Rebound tenderness and guarding are less common in pregnant patients than in nonpregnant patients, and there may be no localizing signs and symptoms at all if the enlarged uterus prevents the inflamed appendix from contacting the peritoneum [25]. Patients rarely are febrile [25,26], and laboratory evaluation generally is not helpful because leukocytosis and an elevated erythrocyte sedimentation rate are seen commonly in healthy pregnant women. The most common misdiagnosis is pyelonephritis, related in part to the coincidental presence of pyuria and bacteriuria in 22% and hematuria in 12% of pregnant women with acute appendicitis [25,26]. The presence of abnormalities on urinalysis does not exclude acute appendicitis.

Maternal mortality from appendicitis is rare, but fetal mortality remains high, particularly in cases of appendiceal perforation. In patients with nonperforated appendices, the fetal

mortality rate is less than 1.5%, but it is greater than 30% in those with perforation [25,28]. About 70% of appendiceal perforations occur in the third trimester, when diagnosis is most difficult [25]; overall, appendiceal perforation is two to three times more common in pregnant women than in nonpregnant women [28]. Perforation is particularly likely to occur after a delay in diagnosis; in one study, a perforation rate of 34% (12 of 35 patients) was reported in patients in whom diagnosis and surgery were delayed for more than 24 hours [26]. For these reasons, conservative management is not an option, timely diagnosis is essential, and a higher rate of negative laparotomies (25% to 30% in most studies) is tolerated than in nonpregnant patients [25,26,28]. In a retrospective Swedish Registry study of 778 patients with presumed acute appendicitis, the diagnosis was confirmed at laparotomy in only 64%. The absence of an inflamed appendix, however, does not exclude abdominal pathology, and it is important to search for other causes of abdominal pain if the appendix is normal at surgery (Table 194-2).

Intestinal Obstruction

Intestinal obstruction occurs in 1 in 2500 to 3500 pregnancies and appears to be increasing in frequency [23,25]. As in nonpregnant patients, 55% to 60% of intestinal obstructions are caused by adhesions, and the frequency approaches 77% in patients with a history of abdominal surgery [24•,29]. The incidence of intestinal obstruction from adhesions increases as pregnancy progresses, probably as a result of increasing displacement of abdominal viscera by the enlarging uterus. Overall, 6% of obstructions occur in the first trimester, 27% in the second, 44% in the third, and 21% in the puerperium [24•].

Other causes of intestinal obstruction are the same in pregnant and nonpregnant women, with the significant exception of

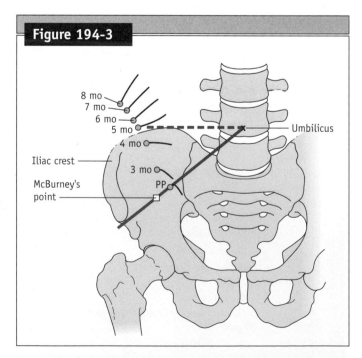

Figure 194-3

Changes in the location of the appendix during pregnancy, as determined by sequential barium meals. The position of the appendix postpartum (pp) correlates with its position in nonpregnant patients. (*From* Baer *et al.* [27••].)

volvulus, which accounts for only 3% to 5% of cases of obstruction in nonpregnant patients but for 25% in pregnant patients (Fig. 194-4). Rapid shifts in uterine location in pregnant patients are the most likely explanation because half of cases occur in the third trimester at the time of engagement of the fetal head, and 26% occur in the puerperium, when the uterus shrinks rapidly [24•]. Volvulus can involve all regions of the small and large intestine but is particularly common in the sigmoid colon, and, to a lesser extent, in the cecum [24•].

Intussusception is a less common cause of intestinal obstruction in pregnancy, accounting for 5% of cases in most series. The intussusception usually involves the ileocecal valve (eg, from a Meckel's diverticulum or, rarely, a malignant neoplasm). Hernias and cancer are rare causes of intestinal obstruction in pregnant women. Acute colonic pseudo-obstruction (Ogilvie's syndrome) may be seen in the postpartum period, particularly after cesarean section.

Symptoms of intestinal obstruction differ little between pregnant and nonpregnant patients. Abdominal discomfort, obstipation, and vomiting are common but nonspecific and often are seen in uncomplicated pregnancies as well. Feculent vomitus is a more specific finding of intestinal obstruction, as is vomiting without nausea. Hyperemesis gravidarum is a common misdiagnosis, and particular care should be used in making this diagnosis in a patient beyond the first trimester. In one series, four of nine cases of small bowel obstruction were initially diagnosed incorrectly [30]. Laboratory evaluation is not helpful because chemical abnormalities, when they occur, reflect dehydration and fluid shifts dangerous to the fetus, not the specific cause of obstruction. Ideally, intervention should occur long before this point is reached. Radiologic evaluation can be helpful, and its benefits in establishing a diagnosis far outweigh the risks of a subsequent malignancy in the fetus [24•,30], particularly when the fetus is shielded appropriately. About 80% of patients with intestinal obstruction have diagnostic plain abdominal films [29,30], although sequential studies may be required. Ultrasound, which is thought to be completely safe in pregnancy, also may be useful in showing dilated loops of bowel, as can magnetic resonance imaging, also thought to be safe.

There is no role for conservative management in a pregnant patient suspected of having intestinal obstruction. The condition is a surgical emergency for mother and fetus. Maternal mortality rates are higher than in affected nonpregnant patients, about 6% in one series [29], and the fetal mortality rate is 20% to 26%, increasing dramatically later in pregnancy [24•,29] (Fig. 194-5). As for acute appendicitis, a delay in surgery is responsible for significant morbidity and mortality. About 23% of obstructed patients reported in the literature have required resection of infarcted bowel; the mean time from hospital admission to surgery was 48 to 60 hours [24•,29]. Overall, proper management of patients with intestinal obstruction requires a high index of suspicion because 20% of radiographs (when taken) are negative.

After the diagnosis of intestinal obstruction is made, fluid and electrolyte repletion and nasogastric suction are indicated to stabilize the patient in preparation for immediate surgery. Induction of labor to relieve obstruction is not indicated.

Surgery

Abdominal surgery generally is safe in pregnant women, and the benefits, particularly for those indications discussed in this section, far outweigh the risks. Maternal morbidity and mortality are not increased because of the pregnancy. For the fetus, the second trimester is the safest time for surgery. The major complication is preterm labor. In a review of 90 pregnant patients undergoing nonobstetric surgery, Allen and colleagues [31] observed that preterm labor occurred in 21%, although tocolytic therapy was effective in all 16 patients in whom it was tried. In a study of 78 patients, Kort and associates [32] showed that preterm labor is more common in the third trimester than in the second (25.7 versus 8.2%); these investigators found that tocolytic therapy was effective in 11 of 15 patients in the third trimester. Preterm labor occurred up to 2 weeks after surgery. To minimize the risk of preterm labor, uterine manipulation should be avoided, and the patient should be positioned so as to optimize blood flow to the fetus. The utility of prophylactic tocolytic agents during surgery is controversial because these medications can cause maternal pulmonary edema. Cesarean section should be performed only for standard obstetric indications.

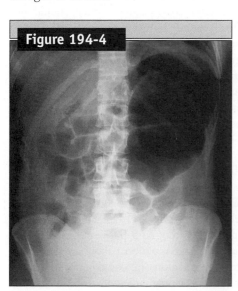

Figure 194-4

Volvulus in a primagravida patient, 31 years of age, at 14 weeks gestation. Note the gravid uterus at the bottom of the figure. (*Courtesy of* J. Braver, MD.)

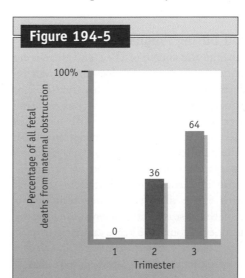

Figure 194-5

Fetal death rates from maternal intestinal obstruction, by trimester, summarized from the literature. (*From* Connolly *et al.* [24•].)

■ INFLAMMATORY BOWEL DISEASE

Because the peak incidence of IBD occurs during the child-bearing years, the care of pregnant women with IBD is of importance to internists, gastroenterologists, and general surgeons. The chance of a successful pregnancy correlates directly with the activity of IBD at conception and during gestation; therefore, preconception counseling as well as aggressive disease management before and during pregnancy are priorities in caring for affected patients.

Fertility and Pregnancy Outcome

Fertility in patients with IBD is considered normal, although some studies suggest a decrease in fertility in patients with Crohn's disease, possibly related to severe malnutrition [33,34]. Older studies that showed decreased fertility did not control for the frequency of sexual intercourse, which may be reduced for psychological or physical reasons, including perianal disease and lack of continence. With the exception of methotrexate, none of the drugs typically used for treatment of IBD interferes with fertility in women, although sulfasalazine (but not the newer 5-aminosalicylate preparations) causes reversible infertility in men because of oligospermia and reduced sperm motility [35••].

The effect of IBD on the outcome of pregnancy is a function of disease activity both at the time of conception and during the pregnancy. In patients with quiescent disease (Crohn's disease or ulcerative colitis), the outcome of pregnancy is similar to that of women without IBD, although there may be a slightly increased frequency of preterm labor. Women with active disease, in contrast, have a two- to three-fold increased frequency of preterm births as well as a significantly increased rate of spontaneous abortion and low birth-weight infants [33,34,36]. In one study, only 50% of women with active Crohn's disease had uncomplicated live births, compared with 79% of those with inactive disease at conception; the difference was unrelated to the site of disease [36]. Not surprisingly, women in whom active disease develops during pregnancy have worse outcomes than those in whom the disease remains inactive, whereas women with active Crohn's disease at conception in whom the activity improves during pregnancy have relatively improved outcomes [36]. The risk of congenital anomalies is not increased in infants born to women with IBD.

Disease Progression During Pregnancy

Pregnancy does not change the course of IBD, and there is no evidence that termination of a pregnancy has any impact on disease activity. Similarly, there is no evidence that the course of IBD during one pregnancy is predictive of its course during subsequent pregnancies. One third of women with ulcerative colitis in whom the disease is in remission at conception relapse during pregnancy or the puerperium; this relapse rate is similar to that seen in nonpregnant women followed for a similar length of time. Relapse is particularly common in the first trimester. Women with active disease at conception have a roughly 45% chance of the disease activity worsening during pregnancy, although in one fourth, disease activity actually improves [33].

About one fourth of women with Crohn's disease that is quiescent at conception relapse during pregnancy [33,36], and,

as for ulcerative colitis, this rate is similar to that of nonpregnant patients followed for a similar length of time. Relapses most commonly occur in the first trimester or puerperium. In patients with active disease at conception, the disease improves in one third, worsens in one third, and is unchanged in one third during pregnancy; these figures are similar to those for the general population of patients with Crohn's disease followed for a comparable length of time.

Diagnosis and Treatment

Nearly three fourths of women with active ulcerative colitis and two thirds of women with active Crohn's disease at the time of conception continue to have active disease during pregnancy. Because of the implications for the outcome of the pregnancy, these women should be counseled about the importance of aggressive disease management before conception. Similarly, every effort should be made to control disease activity in women with active disease during pregnancy. Women in remission who are not dependent on medications should not start medications in anticipation of pregnancy; women who are dependent on medications, however, should continue the drugs but attempt to minimize the dosages needed to maintain remission.

Most medications used to treat IBD are safe in pregnant and nursing women (Table 194-1). Pregnant and nursing women can be safely treated with sulfasalazine or the newer 5-aminosalicylate compounds. Similarly, women who require corticosteroids for disease control can be treated safely during pregnancy and lactation. Metronidazole is probably safe in the third trimester, but ciprofloxacin causes arthropathy in dogs and should be avoided. Most experience with the immunosuppressants azathioprine and 6-mercaptopurine comes from the organ transplant population [35••]. These drugs are rated category D by the Food and Drug Administration and have been associated with congenital malformations, fetotoxicity, prematurity, and fetal growth restriction. Nevertheless, there are reports of their safe use in IBD [37], and if the medications are needed to control disease activity and the patient understands the potential risks, they may be continued through pregnancy. Methotrexate is an abortifacient and teratogen and is contraindicated during pregnancy; the drug is particularly dangerous if taken during the first 6 to 8 weeks after conception. Women should not become pregnant for several months after discontinuing methotrexate because of concern that the drug persists in the body [35••,38]. Elemental and parenteral diets can provide effective nutritional repletion during pregnancy, are safe, and, in case of severe maternal disease, may reduce disease activity and prevent maternal and hence fetal malnutrition. Most of the common medications are safe in women who breast-feed (Table 194-1), and the presence of IBD is not a contraindication to breast-feeding.

Sigmoidoscopy during pregnancy is safe and indicated if necessary to manage the mother's disease. Colonoscopy also is safe but may be more difficult than in nonpregnant women, and sedatives must be selected carefully [39] (see above and Table 194-1). A single abdominal radiograph poses minimal risk to the fetus and is indicated if there is concern about an abdominal catastrophe such as toxic megacolon or colonic perforation. The safety of surgery for IBD in a pregnant woman is difficult to evaluate because surgery often is performed only for emergencies; in this setting in general, elective surgery should be performed before a woman becomes pregnant (at least 1 year before pregnancy in the case of an ileostomy, to permit healing) or in the postpartum period. Operative intervention in pregnancy should be reserved for emergencies such as toxic megacolon, bleeding, intestinal obstruction, or perforation. Surgery should not be postponed in these cases because the fetal mortality rates have approached 50% in some series when appropriate treatment was delayed [40].

Women with ileostomies or ileoanal pouch anastomoses do well during pregnancy except for a slightly increased rate of stomal prolapse and obstruction in patients with ostomies [41]. Pregnancy does not permanently affect pouch or ostomy function, and the presence of a pouch or ostomy should not influence a woman's decision to conceive or continue a pregnancy. Patients may have slightly increased daytime (mean increase, 5.5 to 6.6 stools) and nocturnal (mean increase, 0.9 to 1.4 stools) stool frequencies and incontinence persisting up to 3 months postpartum [41]. A women with a pouch or ostomy can deliver vaginally unless there are obstetric contraindications.

Patients with active IBD, particularly Crohn's disease, require individualized management at delivery. There are no firm recommendations regarding the advisability of cesarean section versus vaginal delivery in this population. One retrospective and methodologically limited study reported an 18% rate of new perianal disease after vaginal delivery [42]. Although a cesarean section in a women with anal or perineal Crohn's disease may prevent local complications, disease activity may develop at the site of the incision, and vaginal delivery avoids the risk of small bowel adhesions in the future. Episiotomies should be performed carefully and away from fissures and fistulas. Vaginal delivery should be avoided in women with rigid perineums as a result of prior surgery.

▆ CONSTIPATION
Incidence

Constipation and symptoms of bloating and abdominal distention are considered anecdotally and in most textbooks to be a common complaint of pregnancy. The literature on the topic is surprisingly scant, however, and there are few studies (none prospective) which document convincingly an increased frequency of these symptoms in pregnant women. The largest study, by Levy and colleagues [43], failed to show an increase in the frequency of constipation during pregnancy: only 11% of 1000 healthy pregnant Israeli women interviewed reported a decrease in stool frequency, and only 1.5% required laxatives. These patients may not be typical, however, because women who took iron preparations regularly were excluded from the study. In contrast, 38% of 200 British women studied by Anderson and Whichelow [44] in the third trimester of pregnancy were constipated at some point during the pregnancy, and 18% reported ongoing symptoms [44]. Greenhalf and Leonard [45], who also studied British women, found that 31% of 350 had pregnancy-associated constipation. The differences between the Israeli and British studies may reflect regional differences in diet and medication use. In two studies, the onset of symptoms generally occurred in the first or third trimester [43,45].

Etiology

The etiology of constipation in pregnancy probably is multifactorial. Several investigators have shown that GI transit time (stomach or duodenum to cecum) is slowed, thereby increasing the potential for small bowel reabsorption of liquid. This effect is most marked in the third trimester (Fig. 194-6) and parallels the rise in serum progesterone levels to at least 80 ng/mL; progesterone levels and transit time return to normal in the postpartum period [46,47]. An increase in transit time, however, does not clearly correlate with symptoms. Animal studies suggest that slowed intestinal transit may result from decreased colonic contractility or from disorganized small intestine myoelectric activity [48]. Other potential causes include increased colonic absorption of water and sodium, uterine (or fetal head) pressure on the abdominal or back muscles and rectum, decreased physical activity, hemorrhoids or other painful anal lesions, use of aluminum-containing antacids for heartburn, use of iron supplements, and reduced levels of motilin, a stimulatory GI hormone [48,49].

Management

As in the nonpregnant population, fiber is the mainstay of treatment. In a study of 40 women in the third trimester of pregnancy, increasing dietary fiber intake from 20 to 27 g/d led to an increase in stool frequency and a softer stool consistency [44]. Bulk-forming fiber preparations (*eg*, psyllium, calcium polycarbophil, or methylcellulose) in doses up to 30 to 40 g/d are safe; no systemic absorption occurs. Stool softeners (*eg*, sodium docusate) and hyperosmotic agents (*eg*, lactulose, glycerine, or sorbitol) also are safe. Other laxatives should be used judiciously because of the risk of dependence in the mother and possible side effects in mother and fetus (Table 194-1). Drugs that have adverse effects in pregnancy include saline laxatives (*eg*, milk of magnesia and Fleet Phospho-Soda), which potentially can cause sodium retention, and castor oil, which can lead to premature uterine contractions. Mineral oil should be avoided in women with a risk of aspiration and should only be used in others for short periods of time, because of maternal

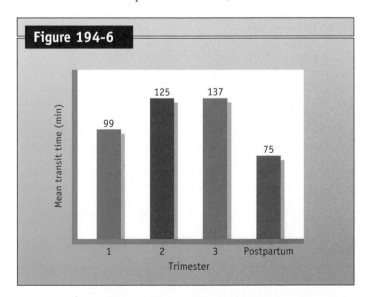

Figure 194-6

Variation in gastrointestinal transit time by trimester, as measured by the lactulose hydrogen breath test. A total of 59 studies were performed in 27 women. (*From* Lawson *et al.* [46].)

malabsorption of fat-soluble vitamins and neonatal hypoprothrombinemia. Enemas should be used with care in pregnant women if necessary to relieve a fecal impaction.

▓▓ CONCLUSION

The pregnant woman with GI complaints often is a diagnostic or management challenge. Some of the more common complaints—nausea and vomiting of pregnancy, GERD, and constipation—are benign and require the physician to remember that to "do no harm" is one of the first directives of medicine. Management consists of maximizing patient comfort and nutrition while avoiding potentially toxic medications and therapies. Other problems, including IBD and abdominal pain, require a more proactive approach because overly cautious treatment in deference to the pregnancy can have catastrophic results.

▓▓ REFERENCES

Recently published papers of particular interest have been highlighted as follows:
- • Of interest
- •• Of outstanding interest

1.• Klebanoff MA, Koslowe PA, Kaslow R, *et al.*: Epidemiology of vomiting in early pregnancy. *Obstet Gynecol* 1985, 66:612–616.
This prospective, multicenter study of more than 9000 pregnant women evaluated the frequency and characteristics of nausea and vomiting of pregnancy.

2. Gadsby R, Barnie-Adshead AM, Jagger C: A prospective study of nausea and vomiting during pregnancy. *Br J Gen Pract* 1993, 43:245–248.

3. Jarnfelt-Samsioe A, Samsioe G, Velinder G-M: Nausea and vomiting in pregnancy: a contribution to its epidemiology. *Gynecol Obstet Invest* 1983, 16:221–229.

4. Singer AJ, Brandt LJ: Pathophysiology of the gastrointestinal tract during pregnancy. *Am J Gastroenterol* 1991, 86:1695–1712.

5.• Abell TL, Riely CA: Hyperemesis gravidarum. *Gastroenterol Clin N Am* 1992, 21:835–849.
The authors provide a concise review of hyperemesis gravidarum, paying particular attention to theories of pathophysiology.

6. Hallack M, Tsalamandris K, Dombrowski MP, *et al.*: Hyperemesis gravidarum: effects on fetal outcome. *J Reprod Med* 1996, 41:871–874.

7.• Olans LB, Wolf JL: Gastroesophageal reflux in pregnancy. *Gastrointest Endosc Clin North Am* 1994, 4:699–711.
The authors review GERD in pregnancy, with particular attention to the possible pathophysiology.

8. Vanner RG, Goodman NW: Gastro-oesophageal reflux in pregnancy at term and after delivery. *Anaesthesia* 1989, 44:808–811.

9. van Thiel DH, Gavaler JS, Joshi SN, *et al.*: Heartburn of pregnancy. *Gastroenterology* 1977, 72:666–668.

10. Baird RM: Peptic ulcer in pregnancy: report of a case with perforation. *Can Med Assoc J* 1966, 94:861–862.

11. Clark DH: Peptic ulcer in women. *Br Med J* 1953, 1:1254–1257.

12. Rustgi VK, Cooper JN, Colcher H: Endoscopy in the pregnant patient. In *Gastrointestinal and Hepatic Complications of Pregnancy*. Edited by Rustgi VK, Cooper JN. New York: Churchill Livingstone; 1986:104–123.

13.• Cappell MS, Sidhom O: A multicenter, multiyear study of the safety and clinical utility of esophagogastroduodenoscopy in 20 consecutive pregnant females with follow-up of fetal outcome. *Am J Gastroenterol* 1993, 88:1900–1905.
This retrospective study showed the safety of upper endoscopic procedures in pregnancy.

14.•• Maringhini A, Ciambra M, Baccelliere P, *et al.*: Biliary sludge and gallstones in pregnancy: incidence, risk factors, and natural history. *Ann Intern Med* 1993, 119:116–120.
This prospective study of 272 pregnant Italian women demonstrated the incidence of development of biliary stones and sludge during pregnancy as well as the degree of spontaneous disappearance postpartum.

15. Tsimoyiannis EC, Antoniou NC, Tsaboulas C, *et al.*: Cholelithiasis during pregnancy and lactation: a prospective study. *Eur J Surg* 1994, 160:627–631.

16. Jorgensen T: Gall stones in a Danish population: fertility period, pregnancies, and exogenous female hormones. *Gut* 1988, 29:433–439.

17. Valdivieso V, Covarrubias C, Siegal F, *et al.*: Pregnancy and cholelithiasis: pathogenesis and natural course of gallstones diagnosed in early puerperium. *Hepatology* 1993, 17:1–4.

18.• Scott LD: Gallstone disease and pancreatitis in pregnancy. *Gastroenterol Clin North Am* 1992, 21:803–815.
The authors provide an extensive review of the literature on gallstones in pregnancy, with a discussion of pathophysiology. Some treatment recommendations are outdated.

19. Swisher SG, Schmit PJ, Hunt KK, *et al.*: Biliary disease during pregnancy. *Am J Surg* 1994, 168:576–581.

20. McKellar DP, Anderson CT, Boynton CJ, *et al.*: Cholecystectomy during pregnancy without fetal loss. *Surg Gynecol Obstet* 1992, 174:465–468.

21.• Davis A, Katz VL, Cox R: Gallbladder disease in pregnancy. *J Reprod Med* 1995, 40:759–762.
The authors review cholecystectomy in pregnant women in three hospitals over 10 years, demonstrating the safety of the procedure as well as the recurrent nature of the symptoms in this population. It is, however, not a prospective study.

22. Eichenberg BJ, Vanderlinden J, Miguel C, *et al.*: Laparoscopic cholecystectomy in the third trimester of pregnancy. *Am Surg* 1996, 62:874–877.

23. Nathan L, Huddleston JF: Acute abdominal pain in pregnancy. *Obstet Gynecol Clin North Am* 1995, 22:55–68.

24.• Connolly MM, Unti JA, Nora PF: Bowel obstruction in pregnancy. *Surg Clin North Am* 1995, 75:101–113.
The authors review all cases of bowel obstruction in the literature since 1945.

25. Sharp HT: Gastrointestinal surgical conditions during pregnancy. *Clin Obstet Gynecol* 1994, 37:306–315.

26. Tamir IL, Bongard FS, Klein SR: Acute appendicitis in the pregnant patient. *Am J Surg* 1990, 160:571–576.

27.•• Baer JL, Reis RA, Arens RA: Appendicitis in pregnancy: with changes in position and axis of the normal appendix in pregnancy. *JAMA* 1932, 98:1359–1364.
In this classic study of changes in location of the appendix in pregnancy, 78 healthy patients were given barium meals and studied fluoroscopically and with plain films at regular intervals from 2 months of gestation to 10 days postpartum.

28. Al-Mulhim AA: Acute appendicitis in pregnancy: a review of 52 cases. *Int Surg* 1996, 81:295–297.

29. Perdue PW, Johnson HW, Stafford PW: Intestinal obstruction complicating pregnancy. *Am J Surg* 1992, 164:384–388.

30. Myerson S, Holtz T, Ehrinpreis M, *et al.*: Small bowel obstruction in pregnancy. *Am J Gastroenterol* 1995, 90:299–302.

31. Allen JR, Helling TS, Langenfeld M: Intraabdominal surgery during pregnancy. *Am J Surg* 1989, 158:567–569.

32. Kort B, Katz VL, Watson WJ: The effect of nonobstetric operation during pregnancy. *Surg Obstet Gynecol* 1993, 177:371–376.

33. Miller JP: Inflammatory bowel disease in pregnancy: a review. *J Roy Soc Med* 1986, 79:221–225.

34. Baird DD, Narendranathan M, Sandler RS: Increased risk of preterm birth for women with inflammatory bowel disease. *Gastroenterology* 1990, 99:987–994.

35.•• Connell WR: Safety of drug therapy for inflammatory bowel disease in pregnant and nursing women. *Inflammatory Bowel Dis* 1996, 2:33–47.
This up-to-date review of the safety in pregnant and nursing women of drugs used for IBD includes discussions of teratogenicity, fetal growth and prematurity, chromosomal effects of drugs, and transfer of drugs through the placenta and breast milk.

36. Woolfson K, Cohen Z, McLeod RS: Crohn's disease and pregnancy. *Dis Colon Rectum* 1990, 33:869–873.

37. Alstead EM, Ritchie JK, Lennard-Jones JE, *et al*.: Safety of azathioprine in pregnancy in inflammatory bowel disease. *Gastroenterology* 1990, 99:443–446.

38. Briggs GG, Freeman RK, Yaffe SJ: *Drugs in pregnancy and lactation*. Baltimore: Williams & Wilkins; 1994.

39. Cappell MS, Colon VJ, Sidhom OA: A study at 10 medical centers of the safety and efficacy of 48 flexible sigmoidoscopies and 8 colonoscopies during pregnancy with follow-up of fetal outcome and with comparison to control groups. *Dig Dis Sci* 1996, 41:2353–2361.

40. Anderson JB, Turner GM, Williamson RCN: Fulminant ulcerative colitis in late pregnancy and the puerperium. *J Roy Soc Med* 1987, 80:492–494.

41. Juhasz ES, Fozard B, Dozois RR, *et al*.: Ileal pouch-anal anastomosis function following childbirth: an extended evaluation. *Dis Colon Rectum* 1995, 38:159–165.

42. Brandt LJ, Estabrook SG, Reinus JF: Results of a survey to evaluate whether vaginal delivery and episiotomy lead to perineal involvement in women with Crohn's disease. *Am J Gastroenterol* 1995, 90:1918–1922.

43. Levy N, Lemberg E, Sharf M: Bowel habit in pregnancy. *Digestion* 1971, 4:216–222.

44. Anderson AS, Whichelow MJ: Constipation during pregnancy: Dietary fibre intake and the effect of fibre supplementation. *Hum Nutr Appl Nutr* 1985, 39A:202–207.

45. Greenhalf JO, Leonard HSD: Laxatives in the treatment of constipation in pregnant and breast-feeding mothers. *Practitioner* 1973, 210:259–263.

46. Lawson M, Kern FJ, Everson GT: Gastrointestinal transit time in human pregnancy: prolongation in the second and third trimesters followed by postpartum normalization. *Gastroenterology* 1985, 89:996–999.

47. Everson GT: Gastrointestinal motility in pregnancy. *Gastroenterol Clin North Am* 1992, 21:751–776.

48. Baron TH, Ramirez B, Richter JE: Gastrointestinal motility disorders during pregnancy. *Ann Intern Med* 1993, 118:366–375.

49. West L, Warren J, Cutts T: Diagnosis and management of irritable bowel syndrome, constipation, and diarrhea in pregnancy. *Gastroenterol Clin North Am* 1992, 21:793–801.

195 Nosocomial Infections: Risks to Health Care Workers

Howard S. Kroop and Anthony J. DiMarino, Jr

Health care workers, as well as their patients, are at risk of nosocomial infection. All health care employees, from physicians and nurses to housekeepers, place their health and even their lives at risk on a daily basis. In addition to their personal health, medical workers jeopardize their employment and standing in the community if they acquire an infectious disease and become a potential source of illness to others. The acquired immunodeficiency syndrome (AIDS) epidemic has highlighted how quickly physicians can be shunned by patients, colleagues, and hospitals once they become infected in the line of duty.

Despite the risks to health and career, medical personnel often pay too little attention to basic steps in preventing nosocomial infection (Table 195-1). Hand washing is an essential measure for preventing the spread of infection, yet few physicians and nurses wash their hands regularly after examining patients with known or suspected infectious diseases. Semmelweis, in 1847, observed a higher incidence of puerperal fever in patients tended by medical students than in those cared for by midwives and was able to reduce the rate of infection by having the students wash their hands in chlorinated lime. He had a difficult time, however, convincing his colleagues in Vienna to adopt these preventative measures [1]. Numerous studies continue to document the persistent problem of poor compliance with hand-washing recommendations. Even in intensive care units, physicians and nurses often do not follow recommended guidelines. The spread of antibiotic-resistant organisms, such as vancomycin-resistant enterococci, by the hands of health care workers is a costly problem, particularly for very ill patients, and can even pose personal risk if caregivers infect themselves with these organisms. Implementation of universal precautions and use of gloves have helped to reduce the rate of nosocomial infections, but these measures often are viewed as a barrier to patient access.

Another key factor in disease prevention is immunization, yet health care workers at risk generally have had a poor track record of receiving proper immunization. For instance, less than half of health care workers are immunized with the influenza vaccine on a regular basis.

A third basic tenet of preventing nosocomial infection is rapid identification and appropriate isolation of infected patients. The recent spread of resistant tuberculosis has increased awareness of the importance of complying with isolation measures. Rising health care costs and the speed with which patients move through the health care system are factors that place a high priority on the need to identify highly contagious

Table 195-1. Basic Steps to Prevent Infections in Health Care Workers

Hand washing

Vaccination

Identification of infected patients

patients rapidly. Paradoxically, these factors may also make it difficult to implement necessary measures. For example, patients are now cared for in settings that are not accustomed to dealing with acutely ill patients, who may pose a risk to personnel. Home care aides, medical office workers, and ambulatory endoscopy employees must now be cognizant of infection control measures that traditionally have been practiced and monitored in acute care hospital settings [2•].

In this chapter, nosocomial infections that pose a risk to health care workers are discussed and can be classified as bloodborne, airborne, and enteric. Clinical features, preventive measures, and postexposure prophylaxis are reviewed. Finally, the particular risks to health care workers who disinfect instruments for reuse are discussed.

■ BLOODBORNE INFECTIONS

Needlesticks remain a common hazard for health care personnel even though new equipment designs have improved safety. Needles should not be recapped, and appropriate containers for disposal of sharp objects must be available in all patient care settings. Human immunodeficiency virus (HIV), hepatitis B virus (HBV), and hepatitis C virus (HCV) are potentially lethal bloodborne organisms that can be transmitted by needlestick. In addition, body fluid splashes with eye contact, mucosal exposure, and cutaneous contact with broken skin are sources of occupational infection (Table 195-2).

HIV

The risk of HIV infection from a needlestick exposure is estimated to be 0.32%. Infectivity depends in large part on the viral titer in the source patient. The titer of HIV in the serum of patients with AIDS is estimated to be 100 to 1000 times higher than that in HIV-positive persons without symptoms. The stage of disease and the use of antiretroviral therapy also affect viral titers. Additionally, the volume of blood inoculated during a percutaneous injury is important in determining the risks of viral transmission. The amount of blood delivered depends on the size of the needle, whether it is hollow-bore (higher risk) or solid (lower risk), the presence or absence of visible blood on the needle, depth of penetration, and whether the needle is used in the patient's artery or vein [3]. As of June 1996, the Centers for Disease Control had received reports of 51 documented and 108 possible health care workers who had been infected with HIV as a result of occupational exposure. A recent case report documented simultaneous transmission of HIV and HCV to a health care worker during a phlebotomy with an ultimately fatal outcome [4].

Postexposure treatment with zidovudine has been shown to reduce the rate of HIV infection by 79%. Serious morbidity from short-term use of this drug has not been reported, but about one third of patients discontinue zidovudine because of side effects. Moreover, the rising rate of resistance to zidovudine in HIV-infected patients has made single drug therapy inadequate.

Table 195-2. Risk Assessment after Occupational Exposure to Bloodborne Pathogens

| Virus | Risk of transmission | | | Infectious material | | |
	Percutaneous Injury, %†	Mucosal contact or contact with injured (broken skin)‡	Bite wound§	Documented	Possible¶	Unlikely
HBV	2–40	Not quantified (transmission by this route has been documented; the magnitude of risk probably is high relative to that for HCV and HIV)	Not quantified (transmission by this route has been documented)	Blood, blood products	Semen, vaginal fluid, bloody fluids, saliva	Urine, feces
HCV	3–10	Not quantified (transmission by this route has not been documented but is plausible)	Not quantified (transmission by this route has not been documented)	Blood	Blood products, bloody fluids, semen, vaginal fluid	Saliva, urine, feces
HIV	0.2–0.5	Not quantified (transmission by this route has been documented; pooled risk estimate, 0.1%)	Not quantified (possible route of transmission in two cases of nonoccupational exposure)	Blood, blood products, bloody fluids	Semen, vaginal fluid, cerebrospinal fluid, breast milk, exudates, serosal fluids, amniotic fluid, saliva (during dental procedures)	Saliva, urine, feces

†The risk estimates are based on pooled data evaluating percutaneous exposures to blood through needle punctures and other injuries inflicted by contaminated sharp objects.

‡Contact with intact skin is not a proven route of transmission of bloodborne viruses. However, small breaks in the skin may escape detection, and many experts consider contact with skin a potential route of transmission, especially when the surface area is large or the duration of contact prolonged.

§The person inflicting the bite may be at risk of mucosal contact with blood if the bite causes bleeding.

¶These fluids have not yet been implicated in occupational transmission but are considered potential sources because they are likely to contain virus or have been implicated in other modes of transmission.

From Gerberding [6]; with permission.

Combined used of lamivudine with zidovudine for postexposure treatment probably is more efficacious, and addition of a protease inhibitor, such as indinavir, should maximize antiviral activity; trials of combination therapy after needlestick exposure to HIV have not yet been reported. Nevertheless, based on current evidence and experience, the US Public Health Service has released new guidelines for postexposure therapy (Table 195-3).

Counseling must be available for exposed persons, so that decisions can be made within hours of exposure to maximize benefits of treatment. Obtaining information on the status of the source patient is useful in deciding the optimal approach to the needlestick victim. If the source patient is unknown, unavailable for testing, or refuses serologic testing, then decisions must be based on the best available clinical information (Table 195-4).

Hepatitis B Virus

It is estimated there are 1.2 million HBV carriers in the United States (see Chapters 93 and 94). Although HBV can be found

---

Table 195-3. Summary Protocol from the Multicenter Trial of Postexposure Prophylaxis for Health Care Providers Exposed to HIV†

Zidovudine dosage
   200 mg orally, three times per day

Lamivudine dosage
   150 mg orally, twice per day

Indinavir dosage
   800 mg orally, three times per day‡

Initiation
   As soon as possible after known or possible exposure to HIV, but within 72 hours

Treatment duration
   4 weeks

Toxicity monitoring
   Symptoms
   Focused physical examination
   Complete blood count
   Liver function tests
   Amylase tests
   Renal function tests
   Urinalysis

Monitoring frequency
   Every 2 weeks while receiving treatment
   At 6 weeks, 3 months, 6 months, and 12 months

HIV monitoring
   HIV antibody test at baseline, 6 months, and 12 months (required)
   HIV antibody test at 6 weeks and 3 months (optional)
   HIV antigen test, HIV polymerase chain reaction, and culture if symptoms of acute retrovirus illness occur in a seronegative health care worker

---

†*Principal investigators for this are Al Gerberding (University of California, San Francisco and San Francisco General Hospital, San Francisco, California) and DK Henderson (Clinical Center National Institutes of Health, Bethesda, Maryland). Complete study protocol is available form http://epi-center.ucsf.edu.*

‡*If the source patient has experience with zidovudine and lamivudine or when the exposure is to a large volume of material with a high titer of virus.*

---

in saliva and transmission has been reported after bites by HBV-infected patients, the usual mode of infection in the health care setting is by inoculation with infected blood. The risk of transmission correlates with the viral load HBV DNA in the serum of the source patient and by the presence or absence of the hepatitis B early antigen (HBeAg) in serum. The risk from a single needlestick varies from 1% to 6% for HBeAg-negative blood and from 22% to 40% for HBeAg-positive blood [5].

In contrast to HIV, there is an effective vaccine to prevent infection with HBV, yet it is estimated that about 20% of health care workers remain unvaccinated. An estimated 6500 to 9000 health care employees were infected with HBV in 1990 [5]. If chronic hepatitis develops in 10% of them, up to almost 1000 of these persons will be at risk of developing cirrhosis and possibly hepatocellular carcinoma.

The original HBV vaccine Heptavax-B (Merck and Co., West Point, PA) was licensed in 1981. It was derived from plasma collected from chronic HBV carriers and subsequently inactivated. This vaccine has been replaced with vaccines in which hepatitis B surface antigen (HBsAg) is produced by recombinant DNA in yeast (Recombivax-HB and Engerix-B; both by Smith-Kline Beecham Pharmaceuticals, Philadelphia, PA). These recombinant vaccines are equally immunogenic and effective. Protective antibody titers develop in 95% to 99% of healthy recipients after three intramuscular injections. Higher-than-standard doses are recommended in immunocompromised patients or those on hemodialysis (Table 195-5). Immunogenicity is not altered by simultaneous administration with hepatitis B immune globulin (HBIG) when administered in a separate intramuscular site for postexposure prophylaxis.

Development of symptomatic HBV is rare in vaccine recipients with titers of antibody to anti-HBsAg of 10 mIU/mL or higher. By 5 to 10 years after immunization, antibody levels become undetectable in up to half of vaccinated persons. It appears, however, that the lengthy incubation period for HBV allows a previously vaccinated person to mount an anamnestic antibody response on re-exposure despite low or absent anti-HBsAg titers. Therefore, routine postvaccination measurement of anti-HBsAg titers or a booster injection years after initial vaccination is not currently recommended. If a person experiences parenteral exposure to HBV, however, and the anti-HBsAg titer is found to be less than 10 mIU/mL at that time, it is reasonable to give both a booster dose of the vaccine and HBIG at a different site within 24 hours of the exposure. Persons who had been vaccinated but never responded with detectable anti-HBsAg levels cannot be distinguished from those who did respond but whose titers subsequently declined to less than 10 mIU/mL [6••]. For postexposure prophylaxis, the combination of vaccination and administration of HBIG is more effective than either the vaccine alone or the HBIG alone.

Hepatitis C Virus

Although there are nearly 4 million persons infected with HCV in the United States, the risks of HCV infection in health care workers is less than that of HBV infection, and occupational exposure accounts for only about 2% of all cases of HCV infection (see Chapters 93 and 94). The seroprevalence of HCV infection among health care professionals is about the same as that of the general population (1%) and lower than that of dentists and oral surgeons (9%). Seroconversion has been reported in 1.2% to 10% of vulnerable health care workers who are stuck with needles from HCV-infected patients [5]. There is no vaccine to prevent HCV infection, and postexposure prophylaxis with immune globulin is not effective. In general, prophylactic treatment with interferon-α therapy is not recommended after a needlestick exposure, but the exposed person should be tested immediately for antibody to HCV (anti-HCV), as up to 5% of infections may be missed unless HCV RNA testing has been included or HCV RNA with repeat testing 6 to 9 months later.

Cytomegalovirus

The prevalence of cytomegalovirus (CMV) infection is high in the general population. CMV may be transmitted by blood contact, sexual contact, respiratory secretions, saliva, and urine. Nevertheless, recent studies have shown that the risk of transmission to health care workers is low [5].

Ebola Virus

Ebola virus and other viral hemorrhagic diseases are highly contagious. With the explosive rise of rapid worldwide travel, universal precautions must be used in caring for all travelers from endemic areas who are suspected of having viral hemorrhagic fevers.

Creutzfeldt-Jakob Disease

Creutzfeldt-Jakob disease is a fatal neurodegenerative disorder transmitted by prions. Cases have been reported in two neurosurgeons, two histology technicians, and a pathologist [5]. Although sterilization of equipment used in patients lessens the risk of transmission, gastrointestinal endoscopes cannot withstand the recommended steam sterilization method. Chemical disinfection with glutaraldehyde is not adequate to prevent infection in these cases.

■ AIRBORNE INFECTIONS
Tuberculosis

During outbreaks of tuberculosis, 20% to 50% of susceptible health care workers may become infected. In the United States, 5% of the general population, but up to 40% of urban health care workers, have a positive tuberculin skin test [7]. Several health professionals have died of tuberculosis during recent outbreaks of drug-resistant tuberculosis. Susceptible employees include housekeeping, laundry, and dietary workers, as well as physicians and nurses. Early identification and isolation of cases and rapid treatment are essential. Skin testing of all health care workers for tuberculosis and prompt initiation of isoniazid therapy for recent converters are important. After exposure to resistant tuberculosis, use of two drugs to which the source case was susceptible should probably be prescribed for prophylaxis.

Varicella-Zoster Virus

Although chicken pox is a common infection in the United States, about 2% to 5% of health care workers still are susceptible to varicella-zoster virus [7]. A vaccine against varicella-zoster became available in 1994, but the logistical problems and costs of identifying and vaccinating susceptible employees are considerable.

Measles

Since 1963, vaccination has sharply reduced the incidence of measles infection. Periodic outbreaks still occur, however, and health care workers are believed to be the source in 5% to 10%

Table 195-4. Advice about Prophylaxis after Exposure to HIV at San Francisco General Hospital*

Attributes of the Exposure	Attributes of the Source Patient		
	Asymptomatic known low titer	AIDS, symptomatic infection	Preterminal AIDS, acute infection, known high titer
Percutaneous injuries			
Superficial injury	Offer	Recommend	Strongly encourage
Visibly bloody device used in artery or vein	Recommend	Recommend	Strongly encourage
Deep intramuscular injury or actual injection	Recommend	Strongly encourage	Strongly encourage
Mucosal contacts			
Small volume and brief contact	Offer	Offer	Offer
Large volume or prolonged contact	Offer	Recommend	Recommend
Large volume and prolonged contact	Recommend	Recommend	Strongly encourage
Cutaneous contacts			
Small volume and brief contact	Offer if obvious portal of entry	Offer if obvious portal of entry	Offer if obvious portal of entry
Large volume or prolonged contact	Offer (recommend if obvious portal of entry)	Offer (recommend if obvious portal of entry)	Offer (recommend if obvious portal of entry)
Large volume and prolonged contact	Offer (recommend if obvious portal of entry)	Recommend (especially with portal of entry)	Recommend (especially with portal of entry)

*From Gerberding [5]; with permission.

of all cases [7]. Susceptible workers should be vaccinated. Persons born after 1957 are probably at greatest risk and are prime candidates for vaccination.

Influenza

Vaccine failures and poor compliance with recommendations for vaccination have impeded efforts to prevent illness caused by influenza, with its associated absenteeism during winter outbreaks. The current guidelines for vaccination have emphasized the importance of vaccinating the elderly and the chronically ill. Health care employees have underestimated their vulnerability and potential role in transmitting influenza in hospitals and nursing homes. Even in a year without a major epidemic, it is estimated that over 20,000 deaths can be attributed to influenza.

Rubella

Susceptible health care workers should be vaccinated against rubella because 10% to 20% of hospital employees are at risk [7]. The risk to the fetus makes this a particularly important issue for female personnel.

Mumps

Vaccination is decreasing the incidence of mumps in the United States, but 6.8% of medical students are reported to be susceptible [7]. Pediatricians and dentists are particularly vulnerable to nosocomial infection.

Pertussis

The incidence of pertussis has increased in the past decade. Up to 25% of vaccinated persons may remain susceptible [7]. Effective prophylaxis for exposed employees includes erythromycin, clarithromycin, and trimethoprim-sulfamethoxazole.

Other Airborne Infections

The list of other airborne infections transmitted to health care employees includes parvovirus B-19, respiratory syncytial virus, adenovirus, hand-foot-and-mouth disease, mycoplasmosis, parainfluenza, and rhinovirus. Legionnaire's disease is not a common risk to health care workers [7].

■ INFECTIONS TRANSMITTED BY THE ORAL–FECAL ROUTE

See Chapters 60, 62, and 72 for further discussion of diarrhea and food-borne diseases.

Clostridium difficile

Clostridium difficile is the most common cause of nosocomial diarrhea in the United States. Index cases cause widespread environmental contamination in the hospital, especially if the patient is incontinent. Floors, commodes, window sills, toilets, bed rails, buzzers, and sheets may become contaminated. In one study, hand cultures were positive in 14% of personnel caring for patients and correlated with the degree of environmental contamination [8]. Despite this high figure, symptomatic *C. difficile* infection is rare in health care workers. In our community hospital, there is an average of three cases of *C. difficile* colitis each month, but no personnel yet have been reported to develop symptomatic infection. Health care workers, therefore, act as vectors to patients rather than to themselves.

195-5. Typical Intramuscular Dosages and Administration Schedules for Hepatitis Vaccines*†

Group	Hepatitis B vaccines		
	Schedule	Recombivax, µg/mL	Engerix-B, µg/mL
Infants			
HBsAg-negative mother	0–2, 1–4, and 6–18 mo	2.5	10
HBsAg-positive mother	At birth (<12 h) with HBIG, 1–2, and 6 mo	5.0	10
Children (1–10 y)	0, 1–2, and 4–6 mo	2.5	10
Adolescents (11–19 y)	0, 1–2, and 4–6 mo	5.0	10
Adults (≥20 y)	0, 1–2, and 4–6 mo	10	20
Immunocompromised adults (hemodialysis)	0, 1 and 6 mo	40	40

	Hepatitis A vaccine‡			
	Havrix	Schedule	Vaqta	Schedule
Children	(2–18 y)		(2–17 y)	
	720/0.5 mL	0 and 6–12 mo§	25/0.5 mL	0 and 6–18§
	or			
	360/0.5 mL	0, 1 and 6–12 mo§		
Adults (>18 y)	1440/1 mL	0 and 6–12 mo	50/0.5 mL	0 and 6–12

*From Lemon and Thomas [9•]; with permission.

†For details, consult the recommendations of the Advisory Committee for Immunization Practices or the American Academy of Pediatrics Committee on Infectious Diseases.

‡Enzyme-linked immunosorbent assay (ELISA) units of Havrix and units of Vaqta are different proprietary measures of antigen content.

§The schedule depends on the specific formulation.

HBIG—hepatitis B immune globulin.

It is entirely possible in the managed care setting, where patients are discharged quickly from the hospital, that a patient may be seen in an outpatient office for acute diarrhea caused by *C. difficile* shortly after discharge. If such a patient undergoes flexible sigmoidoscopy in the office or in an ambulatory endoscopy center, employees must know that the office facilities and equipment may become contaminated. Therefore, appropriate measures to disinfect the environment must be carried out. Vegetative forms of *C. difficile* and spores on fomites, instruments, and contaminated surfaces can be destroyed by alkaline glutaraldehyde, sodium hypochlorite, or ethylene oxide. These solutions, however, are not appropriate for hand washing, which should be done using ordinary disinfectant soaps [9•].

Hepatitis A Virus

Outbreaks of hepatitis A virus (HAV) have occurred in neonatal intensive care units and burn units. Staff who care for adults with diarrhea also may be infected. Eating on the hospital ward, poor hand-washing techniques, and ingestion of previously contaminated foods are the most common risk factors.

Two vaccines against HAV are available: Havrix (Smith-Kline Beecham, Philadelphia, PA) and Vaqta (Merck and Co., West Point, PA) (Table 195-5). They both contain formalin-inactivated viral particles. Both are effective and require a booster dose 6 months after an initial injection. Antibody to HAV develops in 95% of healthy adults within 1 month of receiving a single dose of Havrix [10]. Nevertheless, an unvaccinated person exposed to HAV should receive immediate prophylaxis with standard immune globulin.

Salmonellosis

Person-to-person transmission and food-related outbreaks of salmonellosis make this infection a common problem. In hospital cafeterias and nursing homes, prepared foods, such as mashed potatoes, egg nog, and mayonnaise made with raw eggs, may be the source of an outbreak [11]. Laundry workers handling contaminated linens also are at risk.

Shigellosis

Considering the small inoculum needed for transmission, shigellosis is a relatively uncommon nosocomial infection.

Escherichia coli O157:H7

Infection caused by *Escherichia coli* O157:H7 most often is associated with eating undercooked beef; however, person-to-person transmission has been reported. In one nursing home outbreak of hemorrhagic colitis, 13% of staff members developed symptoms [5]. *E. coli* O157:H7 may be responsible for up to 10% of cases of acute diarrhea and for one third of those cases associated with acute bloody diarrhea. The infection usually is self-limited but may be fatal, especially when associated with hemolytic-uremic syndrome or thrombotic thrombocytopenic purpura, especially in the elderly and very young. The role of antibiotic therapy is uncertain.

Helicobacter pylori Infection

A number of studies have shown a higher seroprevalence of *Helicobacter pylori* in physicians and nurses who work in

endoscopy suites than in the general population or in internists used as controls (see Chapter 27). In one study, 53% of endoscopy personnel were seropositive, compared with 14% of a control group of blood donors [12]. Seroprevalence rates in endoscopy suite nurses and physicians were equal. The rate was higher in foreign-born personnel but did not correlate with the number of procedures done nor the years of endoscopic practice. Spread may be by the fecal–oral or oral–oral route. Whether all endoscopy personnel should be tested for *H. pylori* and treated if positive is uncertain at this time.

◼ GUIDELINES FOR REPROCESSING GASTROINTESTINAL ENDOSCOPIC INSTRUMENTS TO MINIMIZE THE RISK OF INFECTION

To protect patients from infections potentially transmitted by reusable endoscopy equipment, guidelines have been issued for the disinfection of equipment. Although the primary focus of these guidelines is to prevent transmission of pathogens from one patient to another undergoing a gastrointestinal procedure, health care workers involved in the procedure also are at risk. Proper handling of infected instruments is important, and the guidelines stress not only the importance of adequate cleaning of the instruments but also the protection of health care workers who handle the equipment.

An extensive review has been published of the issues involved in prevention of infection after gastrointestinal endoscopy [13]. The ad hoc Committee on Disinfection of the American Society for Gastrointestinal Endoscopy, in conjunction with the Society of Gastroenterology Nurses and Associates (SGNA), also published guidelines for the reprocessing of gastrointestinal instrumentation, with emphasis on the appropriate manual cleaning of these instruments before disinfection. Adherence to Occupation Safety and Health Administration (OSHA) guidelines in handling infected instruments immediately after withdrawal from the patient and subsequently during the cleaning and disinfection process is critical to avoiding infection [14••]. Inherent to the reprocessing guidelines are certain principles, including development of a *written* quality assurance program for the cleaning and disinfection of fiberoptic and video gastrointestinal endoscopic equipment. The cleaning and disinfection protocol should include methods to identify and train specialists in cleaning the instruments. Persons who are designated as endoscopic cleaners should take a written and practical examination, during which they should demonstrate competence in the cleaning and disinfection technique. Handling of the instruments should be strictly limited to individuals who have proven competence in these techniques; therefore, temporary nursing or technical assistants are precluded from serving this function.

After an endoscopic procedure, the flexible gastrointestinal instrument should be taken immediately from the patient and carried in a container that will not allow infected material to be dislodged and thereby to contaminate surrounding areas before delivery of the instrument to a cleaning and disinfecting station. Once the instrument is clean, it should be exposed for at least 20 minutes at 20°C to a 2% glutaraldehyde solution or to a suitable substitute, such as hydrogen peroxide, peracetic acid, or other chemical disinfectants or sterilants that can achieve high-level disinfection when the manufacturer's guidelines are followed. A test of the efficacy of reused disinfectant solutions, particularly glutaraldehyde or peracetic acid solutions, should be performed on a daily basis to guarantee that potency levels are sufficient to achieve high-level disinfection. Automated reprocessing devices may be used to save time during the disinfection portion of gastrointestinal instrument reprocessing. However, reprocessing machines cannot substitute for effective manual cleaning with removal of particulate debris before exposure to the disinfecting solution.

By adhering to these reprocessing guidelines, the risk of infection to the patient is estimated to be less than 1 in 1.8 million [14••]. Risks to health care workers also should be negligible.

EFFECT OF EXPOSURE TO DISINFECTANTS AND STERILANTS ON GASTROINTESTINAL HEALTH CARE WORKERS

Flexible gastrointestinal endoscopic instruments are heat labile and should be disinfected only by chemical sterilants or disinfectants. Therefore, health care personnel who are involved in reprocessing instruments or who work with these instruments need to be protected from exposure to these solutions by adhering closely to OSHA regulations. Because most gastrointestinal endoscopic units use 2% glutaraldehyde solutions for reprocessing gastrointestinal flexible endoscopes, it is essential that ambient air concentrations of glutaraldehyde be monitored. OSHA guidelines permit a maximal concentration of glutaraldehyde in air of 0.2 ppm. Because glutaraldehyde is heavier than air, lateral or downdraft ventilation may be used in well-ventilated areas to protect health care personnel from exposure to high ambient air glutaraldehyde concentrations.

The effects of glutaraldehyde on health care personnel may result from its potential to act as an irritant, toxin, or allergen. Generally, irritation of the skin and mucous membrane occurs with concentrations of glutaraldehyde exceeding 0.3 ppm. Allergic symptoms, including rhinitis, dermatitis, conjunctivitis, nausea, asthma, and headaches, have been reported after exposure to glutaraldehyde vapors [15]. In 1993, SGNA issued a questionnaire to 6131 members, mostly nurses involved in reprocessing gastrointestinal instruments. About two thirds of the surveys were returned. The results showed that the frequency of allergic symptoms among respondents had increased by about 60% after exposure to glutaraldehyde. Eye irritation, dermatitis, rhinitis, and headaches were the most commonly reported symptoms. Many of the respondents thought that there was inadequate monitoring of the glutaraldehyde ambient air concentrations in their gastrointestinal units.

Although glutaraldehyde most commonly is potentially toxic to the health care personnel in the endoscopy suite, usually as a result of recurrent exposure to its vapors, it also is potentially toxic to the patient, and instances have been reported of severe glutaraldehyde proctitis and colitis caused by mucosal irritation from residual glutaraldehyde on the inserted endoscope. Minimal irritation has been reported after the use of hydrogen peroxide or peracetic acid solutions, but direct skin contact with these agents is potentially irritating, and proper handling of all chemical sterilants and disinfectants is recommended. Close adherence to OSHA guidelines is necessary to minimize direct exposure to these chemical irritants. After accidental exposure, proper procedure, including prompt eye washing and skin cleansing, is critical.

REFERENCES

Recently published papers of particular interest have been highlighted as follows:
• Of interest
•• Of outstanding interest

1. Chong J, Marshall BJ, Barkin JS, *et al.*: Occupational exposure to *Helicobacter pylori* for the endoscopy professional: a sera epidemiological study. *Am J Gastroenterol* 1994, 89:1987–1992.

2.• DiMarino AJ: The prevention of infection following gastro-intestinal endoscopy: the importance of prophylaxis and reprocessing. In *Gastrointestinal Disease: An Endoscopic Approach*, vol 1. Edited by DiMarino AJ, Benjamin S. Cambridge: Blackwell Scientific; 1997:93–104.
An updated approach to maintaining endoscopy equipment to prevent the spread of infections to patients is given.

3. DiMarino AJ, Gage T, Leung J, *et al.*: American Society for Gastrointestinal Endoscopy Position Statement: reprocessing of flexible gastrointestinal endoscopes. *Gastrointest Endosc* 1996, 43:451.

4. Fekety R: Guidelines for the diagnosis and management of *Clostridium difficile*–associated diarrhea and colitis. *Am J Gastroenterol* 1997, 92:739–750.

5. Gerberding JL: Prophylaxis for occupational exposure to HIV. *Ann Intern Med* 1996, 125:497–501.

6.•• Gerberding JL: Management of occupational exposures to blood-borne viruses. *N Engl J Med* 1995, 332:444–451.
A concise review of hepatitis B and C and HIV risks and postexposure prophylaxis and treatment is provided.

7. Goodman RA, Solomon SL: Transmission of infectious diseases in outpatient health care settings. *JAMA* 1991, 265:2377–2381.

8. Jarvis WR: Handwashing: the Semmelweis lesson forgotten? *Lancet* 1994, 344:1311–1312.

9.• Lemon SM, Thomas DL: Vaccines to prevent viral hepatitis. *N Engl J Med* 1997, 336:196–204.
A thorough discussion of the types of vaccines available and the indications for their use are given.

10. Lynch DA, Parnell P, Porter C, *et al.*: Patient and staff exposure to glutaraldehyde from KeyMed autodisinfector endoscopy washing machine. *Endoscopy* 1994, 22(4):359–361.

11. Ridzon R, Gallagher K, Ciesielski C, *et al.*: Simultaneous transmission of human immunodeficiency virus and hepatitis C virus from a needle-stick injury. *N Engl J Med* 1997, 336:919–922.

12. Samore MH, Venkataraman L, Degirolami PC, *et al.*: Clinical and molecular epidemiology of sporadic and clustered cases of nosocomial *Clostridium difficile* diarrhea. *Am J Med* 1996, 100:32–40.

13. Sepkowitz KA: Occupationally acquired infections in health care workers, part I. *Ann Intern Med* 1996, 125:826–834.

14.•• Sepkowitz KA: Occupationally acquired infections in health care workers, part II. *Ann Intern Med* 1996, 125:917–928.
An encyclopedic two-part review of infections that can be transmitted to health care workers is provided. The first article covers airborne infections and the second details bloodborne diseases.

15. Telzak EE, Budnick LD, Greenberg MS, *et al.*: A nosocomial outbreak of *Salmonella enteritidis* infection due to the consumption of raw eggs.

Radiologic Techniques
Gary J. Whitman

Many techniques are available for imaging known or suspected gastrointestinal disease. Selection of the appropriate examination depends on the specific clinical problem as well as an understanding of the benefits and limitations of each technique. For practical purposes, imaging of gastrointestinal disease can be divided into two categories: imaging of the gastrointestinal tract (esophagus, stomach, small bowel, and large bowel) and imaging of the upper abdominal solid organs (liver, gallbladder, and pancreas). Entities that affect the gastrointestinal tract are best visualized with barium studies. Processes that affect the solid organs are optimally imaged with cross-sectional techniques (*eg*, computed tomography [CT], ultrasound, magnetic resonance imaging [MRI]) and nuclear medicine studies.

PLAIN RADIOGRAPHS OF THE ABDOMEN

Plain radiographs of the abdomen are useful in detecting free intraperitoneal gas, bowel obstruction, and abdominal or pelvic calcifications. In critically ill patients, plain radiographs are usually the first and often the only examination obtained to image the abdomen.

The best views for detecting free intraperitoneal gas are the upright posteroanterior chest radiograph and the left-side-down decubitus view of the abdomen. On the upright chest radiograph, free gas is seen under the hemidiaphragms (Fig. 196-1). On the left-side-down decubitus view of the abdomen, free gas accumulates under the diaphragm or adjacent to the lateral liver margin.

Plain radiographic findings characteristic of small bowel obstruction include disproportionately dilated (luminal diameter greater than 3 cm) small bowel loops with gas–fluid levels on upright or decubitus views and a paucity of gas in the large bowel (Fig. 196-2). In large bowel obstruction, stool, fluid, and gas are identified proximal to the point of obstruction, and little gas is noted distal to the obstruction. Sigmoid volvulus is

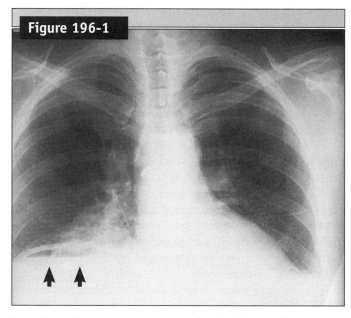

Figure 196-1

Free intraperitoneal gas is present under the right hemidiaphragm (*arrows*) on an upright posteroanterior chest radiograph in a patient who underwent recent abdominal surgery.

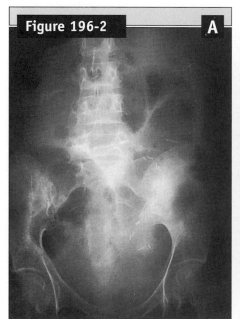
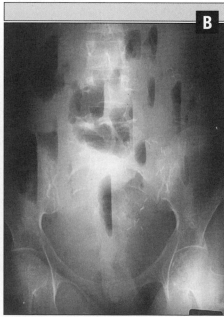

Figure 196-2

Small bowel obstruction is present on plain radiographs. **A,** The supine view shows dilated central small bowel loops. **B,** The left lateral decubitus view demonstrates multiple gas–fluid levels.

characterized by a large, distended loop of colon arising out of the pelvis into the lower abdomen. In cecal volvulus, there is gas in dilated small bowel loops and a dilated cecum and little or no gas in the remainder of the colon. Pneumatosis intestinalis, seen as linear or cystic gas collections tangential and circumferential to the colon, may result from bowel infarction or obstruction or may occur in association with long-standing conditions, such as chronic obstructive pulmonary disease, acquired immunodeficiency syndrome (AIDS) [1], leukemia, or lymphoma.

Abdominal plain radiographs can play a major role in detecting portal venous gas and gas in the biliary tree. Portal venous gas usually demonstrates a peripheral distribution, whereas gas in the bile ducts usually is seen centrally. Plain radiographs are also sensitive for detecting intra-abdominal calcifications, including gallstones and pancreatic calcifications.

■ BARIUM STUDIES

Despite the advent of CT, ultrasound, and MRI as valuable modalities for imaging the abdomen, barium contrast studies remain the gold standard for imaging the gastrointestinal tract, especially the mucosa. Barium studies can be performed with single-contrast, double-contrast, or mucosal relief views. The radiologist's role is to perform and interpret the studies, which include diagnostic fluoroscopy, spot radiographs, and larger "overhead" radiographs.

Techniques

Single-contrast barium studies are performed with a large volume of low-density barium. Single-contrast (or barium-filling) views are particularly valuable for demonstrating contour abnormalities, strictures, and large polypoid filling defects. Single-contrast examinations also are helpful in showing extravasation and extraluminal contrast collections. Single-contrast techniques may be used in uncooperative patients and in patients in poor physical condition.

Mucosal relief studies use a small amount of barium, to image the mucosal folds. Mucosal relief views, for example, may demonstrate mucosal ulcerations in patients with inflammatory bowel disease.

Double-contrast studies are obtained after the mucosa has been coated with a thin layer of high-density barium and the viscus has been distended with gas. Double-contrast views are helpful in demonstrating subtle, early mucosal neoplastic or inflammatory lesions. To maximize the yield of double-contrast barium studies, care is needed to obtain adequate mucosal coating and distention. Inadequate distention may hide subtle lesions, and overdistention may obscure some findings, such as shallow ulcers. Several views should be obtained to project each bowel loop free of overlapping loops. Efforts should be made to demonstrate each segment in profile (especially in the colon).

Esophagus

When performing contrast studies of the esophagus, barium is the appropriate contrast material for nearly all applications. If esophageal perforation is suspected, the use of water-soluble contrast material is recommended because leakage of barium into the mediastinum may lead to mediastinitis (see Chapter 13). If no perforation is seen with the water-soluble agent, then a repeat study with barium should be performed because a small leak may be difficult to image with water-soluble contrast material.

Squamous cell carcinomas or adenocarcinomas of the esophagus often are seen as solitary filling defects on barium studies (see Chapter 16). Esophagograms reveal plaque-like ulcerating lesions or regions of rigid narrowing in the early stages (Fig. 196-3) and circumferential narrowing with overhanging margins in advanced tumors. The most common metastatic tumor in the esophagus is gastric adenocarcinoma, which often extends from the cardia to involve the distal esophagus.

Leiomyomas are the most common benign esophageal neoplasms. On barium studies, leiomyomas characteristically appear as round, smooth-walled submucosal lesions. They usually are solitary, and some may be calcified. Other less common benign esophageal tumors, such as fibromas, hemangiomas, lipomas, and neurofibromas, have a similar radiographic appearance. Inflammatory polyps arise in the distal esophagus as smooth, polypoid masses and often are seen in patients with chronic gastroesophageal reflux disease.

Extrinsic processes may simulate esophageal filling defects. Mediastinal lymphadenopathy may cause extrinsic impressions on the esophagus. Duplication cysts (usually diagnosed in childhood) and vascular structures (such as an aberrant right subclavian artery, an ectatic aorta, or an enlarged left atrium) may exert mass effect on the esophagus.

Enlarged esophageal folds are seen in esophagitis, varices, lymphoma, and, rarely, varicoid carcinoma. In esophagitis, thickened folds may be associated with ulceration, nodularity, and luminal narrowing. Other causes of esophageal narrowing include malignant neoplasms, motility disorders, and extrinsic compressions. Barium studies do not reliably distinguish benign from malignant causes of esophageal narrowing. In esophagitis, acute inflammatory changes, characterized by ulceration, thickened folds, and nodularity, may progress to fibrosis and stricture formation (see Chapter 6). Peptic and reflux strictures have a variable radiographic appearance, ranging from smooth and

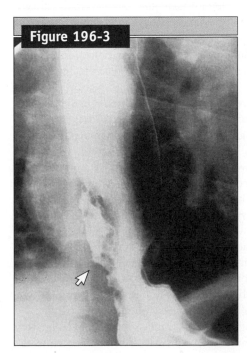

Figure 196-3

A large ulcerated lesion, representing squamous cell carcinoma, is present in the distal esophagus (*arrow*) on the esophagram.

circumferential to asymmetric and irregular. On barium studies, Barrett's esophagus usually is identified as an area of narrowing in the middle or distal esophagus. There may be associated mucosal nodularity, a reticular mucosal pattern, or focal ulceration.

Scleroderma is characterized by abnormal esophageal motility secondary to smooth muscle atrophy and fibrosis in the lower esophagus (see Chapter 15). Incompetence of the lower esophageal sphincter results in free gastroesophageal reflux and often secondary stricture formation. Achalasia, in which there is decreased or absent esophageal motility and failure of the lower esophageal sphincter to relax, appears as distal esophageal narrowing, resembling a bird's beak, on barium contrast studies (see Chapter 7). A fixed smooth and symmetric narrowing in the distal esophagus is characteristic of a lower esophageal, or Schatzki's, ring, which may best be demonstrated by having the patient swallow barium in solid form (eg, a barium tablet) (see Chapter 9).

In addition to detecting abnormal morphology, esophagography may provide information regarding altered esophageal motility and the presence of gastroesophageal reflux. On fluoroscopy, normal esophageal peristalsis is characterized by continuous, smooth, wavelike esophageal contractions. The primary wave is initiated by swallowing, whereas a secondary wave is produced in response to a bolus in the esophagus. Tertiary contractions are disordered and nonpropulsive and may be found in patients with esophageal motility disorders; however, tertiary contractions do not necessarily correlate with symptoms.

Stomach

Barium studies of the stomach, performed with a single- or double-contrast technique, permit evaluation of gastric morphology and peristalsis. Discrete gastric filling defects may be due to benign or malignant lesions. Gastric filling defects are classified by size and location (greater or lesser curvature and mucosal or submucosal). Large, ulcerated gastric masses may represent malignancies such as adenocarcinoma or lymphoma and, less commonly, leiomyosarcoma or metastatic disease (see Chapters 38 and 39). Metastatic lesions also may present as gastric filling defects; primary tumors that commonly metastasize to the stomach include breast cancer, lung cancer, melanoma, and Kaposi's sarcoma. Metastatic foci may ulcerate, resulting in target lesions.

Submucosal lesions in the stomach are often caused by benign mesenchymal tumors, such as leiomyomas. Less common submucosal tumors are neurofibromas and lipomas. On barium studies, leiomyomas and other submucosal masses usually are smooth walled and well circumscribed. They may grow to a large size and demonstrate central umbilication. Gastric varices may present as localized submucosal masses in the fundus of the stomach.

Hyperplastic polyps are common gastric mucosal lesions that are often multiple, with a predilection for the antrum and the body of the stomach. They have no significant malignant potential. In contrast, adenomatous polyps usually are single and have a malignant potential. Hamartomatous polyps, which have little or no malignant potential, may be seen in the stomach in patients with Peutz-Jeghers syndrome (see Chapter 37).

Gastric narrowing may result from neoplasms, inflammatory conditions, and granulomatous disease. Fixed narrowing of the

stomach, also called *linitis plastica*, may be seen in patients with primary gastric adenocarcinoma, gastric lymphoma, metastatic cancer (especially from breast carcinoma) and benign conditions such as tuberculosis. Inflammatory and infectious causes of gastric narrowing include peptic ulcer disease, corrosives, eosinophilic gastroenteritis, radiotherapy, Crohn's disease, and syphilis. Peptic ulcer disease may be associated with thickened gastric folds and erosions as well as with one or more ulcers (see Chapters 29 and 30).

Evaluation of gastric fold thickness is an important component of the upper gastrointestinal examination. Folds thicker than 1 cm are considered abnormal and may result from inflammatory conditions, tumors, and infiltrative processes. Gastritis and peptic ulcer disease are leading causes of gastric fold thickening. Other inflammatory causes include Zollinger-Ellison syndrome and acute pancreatitis. Neoplastic diseases, such as lymphoma of the stomach and gastric adenocarcinoma as well as hypertrophic gastropathy (Ménétrier's disease) often result in fold thickening.

Traditionally, barium studies have played a major role in the detection of gastric ulcers (see Chapter 29). The role of the upper gastrointestinal study also includes monitoring ulcers on follow-up studies to document healing, although upper endoscopy has been used increasingly for this purpose. On barium studies, ulcers are identified as contour defects. Although the radiologic findings in benign and malignant gastric ulcers overlap, some features can help to distinguish a benign from a malignant ulcer. Benign gastric ulcers demonstrate extension of the ulcer crater beyond the lumen, with folds radiating into the crater (Fig. 196-4). The crater of a benign ulcer often is sharply defined, and the mucosa may be undermined by edema, resulting in Hampton's line. In malignant gastric ulcers, the crater usually does not project beyond the lumen, and the folds do not radiate into the crater (see Chapter 38). Gastric erosions, which are usually small, superficial, and

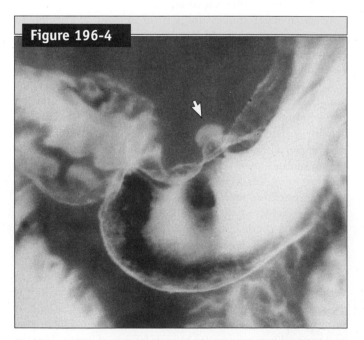

Figure 196-4

Double-contrast upper gastrointestinal study showing an antral ulcer along the lesser curvature. The ulcer (*arrow*) extends beyond the lumen. Endoscopic biopsy revealed a benign ulcer.

confined to the mucosa, may be difficult to detect on upper gastrointestinal studies, and double-contrast techniques usually are required to demonstrate them.

Barium studies continue to play a major role in the evaluation of the postoperative stomach to detect obstruction, intussusception, ulceration, or tumor (see Chapter 45). It often is easier to perform the postoperative barium study with the patient standing, especially when the exact postoperative anatomy is not known.

Small Bowel

The small bowel may be studied by a small bowel followthrough (after an upper gastrointestinal series) or by a small bowel series, in which the examination is focused on evaluating the small bowel loops. A more invasive method of evaluating the small bowel is enteroclysis, in which a nasoenteric tube is placed at the level of the ligament of Treitz and thick barium and methyl cellulose are administered, followed by compression, fluoroscopy, spot radiographs, and overhead views.

Duodenum

Evaluation of the duodenum, especially the bulb, is challenging. If duodenal bulb distention is suboptimal on supine views, examining the patient in the upright position, with compression, may be helpful. Abnormalities noted in the proximal duodenum usually are benign, whereas those in the distal duodenum usually are malignant. Nonneoplastic duodenal lesions include prolapsed antral mucosa, ectopic pancreas, Brunner's gland hyperplasia, and lymphoid hyperplasia. Brunner's gland hyperplasia, which involves the proximal duodenum, is characterized by multiple small filling defects. In benign duodenal lymphoid hyperplasia, small (1- to 3-mm) nodules are seen in the duodenum. Duplication cysts, pancreatic pseudocysts, and hematomas may displace the duodenum.

Barium studies can be helpful in identifying benign and malignant duodenal tumors (see Chapters 37 and 39). Adenomas and leiomyomas are the most common benign duodenal tumors. Adenomas usually are less than 1 cm in size and may be smoothly lobulated or pedunculated. Leiomyomas are submucosal masses and may demonstrate ulceration. Duodenal adenocarcinomas account for 80% to 90% of primary duodenal malignancies and usually arise distal to the ampulla of Vater.

Duodenal fold thickening usually is secondary to an inflammatory process, such as duodenitis. Pancreatitis may result in duodenal fold thickening and often is accompanied by a masslike impression on the duodenal C sweep. Crohn's disease and tuberculosis may cause duodenal fold thickening. Zollinger-Ellison syndrome is characterized by thickening of the duodenal folds, ulcerations, and excessive fluid in the duodenum (see Chapter 35).

There are many intrinsic and extrinsic causes of duodenal narrowing. A common intrinsic lesion is duodenal stenosis secondary to postbulbar ulceration (Fig. 196-5). Chronic duodenitis also can result in narrowing of the duodenum. Other causes of duodenal narrowing include primary duodenal adenocarcinoma, lymphoma, and metastatic disease. Adenocarcinoma often is seen as an annular, constricting lesion with overhanging margins.

Less common causes of duodenal narrowing include annular pancreas, duodenal duplication cysts, and intraluminal diaphragms. Annular pancreas usually presents as a defect in the lateral duodenal wall, resulting in a short segment of eccentric narrowing. Duodenal duplication cysts may be intramural or extrinsic and usually are asymptomatic. On barium studies, an intraluminal diaphragm or web may be seen as a thin line traversing the lumen, usually in the second portion of the duodenum. Extrinsic processes, including inflammatory and metastatic processes which can cause duodenal narrowing include enlarged lymph nodes from lymphoma or other tumors of the gastrointestinal tract.

Jejunum and Ileum

In the jejunum and the ileum, inflammatory conditions are more common than neoplasms. Crohn's disease is the most common inflammatory disease of the small bowel (see Chapter 64). Although Crohn's disease may involve the entire gastrointestinal tract, the most common site of involvement is the terminal ileum. Radiographic features include discrete, linear ulcers, and "cobblestoning" (Fig. 196-6). Involvement may be discontinuous, with "skip areas." The inflammation is transmural,

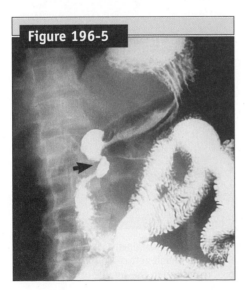

Figure 196-5

Upper gastrointestinal study revealing postbulbar ulceration (*arrow*), resulting in a distorted duodenal C sweep.

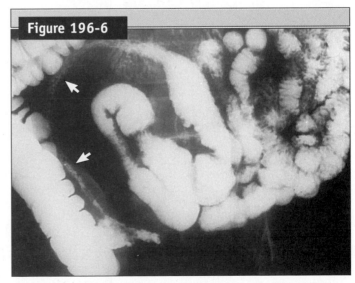

Figure 196-6

Small bowel follow-through demonstrating a markedly narrowed segment of terminal ileum (*arrows*) with irregular mucosa in a patient with Crohn's disease. There is significant separation between the diseased loop of ileum and the remaining small bowel loops.

and there may be associated mesenteric masses (often best seen on CT), fistulas, and sinus tracts.

Eighty percent of benign small bowel neoplasms are discovered incidentally on imaging studies (see Chapter 55). The most common benign tumors of the jejunum and ileum are adenomatous polyps, leiomyomas, lipomas, and hamartomas (especially in patients with Peutz-Jeghers syndrome). In contrast, only 20% of malignant small bowel tumors are discovered incidentally. Adenocarcinoma of the small bowel, which has a predilection for the duodenum and the proximal jejunum, often is identified as a short, annular, ulcerated lesion. Sarcomas (including leiomyosarcomas) often are large, ulcerating lesions. Lymphomas most commonly involve the terminal ileum and may have variable radiographic appearances, including large, excavating tumors, polypoid masses, masses that extend from the bowel wall to infiltrate the mesentery, and aneurysmal dilation of small bowel loops. Carcinoids usually are identified as small submucosal lesions, often arising in the ileum.

Secondary malignancies of the jejunum and ileum are more common than primary tumors. Tumors arising from the kidneys or pancreas may involve the small bowel by direct extension. Melanoma, breast cancer, and lung cancer may disseminate hematogenously to the jejunum and ileum, and tumors of the ovary, colon, and pancreas may involve the small bowel by serosal spread.

A large number of diseases may affect the small bowel in a diffuse manner. In celiac sprue, small bowel radiographs often show dilution of barium and dilated small bowel loops (see Chapter 187). Whipple's disease demonstrates coarsely nodular and irregular mucosa (see Chapter 59). Bacterial overgrowth caused by stasis may occur secondary to postsurgical blind loops, scleroderma, or small bowel diverticula (see Chapter 58).

Zollinger-Ellison syndrome often demonstrates a coarse small intestinal mucosal pattern in addition to multiple ulcers in the duodenum. Small bowel hemorrhage and edema are manifested as thickened folds, often with a characteristic "stack-of-coins" appearance. Hemorrhage resulting from trauma usually affects the duodenum, whereas hemorrhage from other causes (including bleeding dyscrasias) has no site of predilection. Mesenteric ischemia, resulting from emboli, atherosclerosis, or hypotension, usually is associated with thickened intestinal mucosal folds (see Chapter 65). In the reparative phase, ischemia may result in stricture formation. Infections of the small intestine, especially *Yersinia* species and tuberculosis, often involve the terminal ileum (see Chapter 60).

Colon

The barium enema examination plays a significant role in identifying colonic polyps and carcinomas (Fig. 196-7; see Chapters 80 and 81). Although colonoscopy detects more small polyps that are less than 1 cm in size and allows for tissue sampling at the time of the diagnostic examination, the cost of a barium enema is about one third the cost of a colonoscopic examination, and the accuracy rates are comparable for detection of polyps 1 cm and larger in size. Relative disadvantages of colonoscopy include the need for sedation, pain, risk of perforation, and inability to reach the cecum in 5% of cases [2]. Similar to colonoscopy, optimal performance and interpretation of barium enemas is highly dependent on proper technique and experience [3].

Most colonic malignancies are thought to arise from preexisting adenomatous polyps, and barium enemas are sensitive for the detection of large polyps. Small hyperplastic and adenomatous polyps can be detected by barium enemas in well-cleansed colons. On barium enema examination, colonic carcinomas are characterized by mucosal destruction; usually, an abrupt transition between the tumor and normal colon is present (Fig. 196-8). Certain features may suggest that a lesion is a villous adenoma,

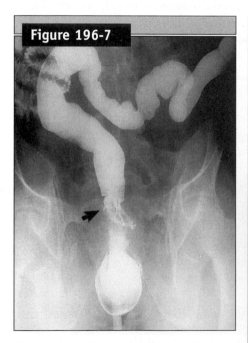

Figure 196-7

Single-contrast barium enema showing an irregular constricting lesion in the lower sigmoid (*arrow*), which represents a colonic carcinoma.

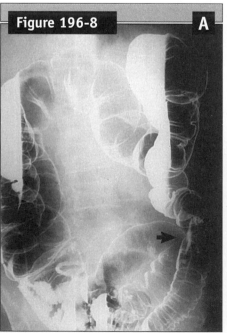

Figure 196-8 **A**

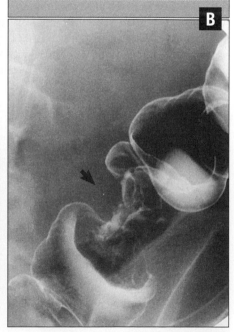

B

Carcinoma is identified in the left colon on a double-contrast barium enema. **A**, The radiograph of the entire colon reveals irregularity and narrowing in the middle left colon (*arrow*). **B**, Spot view shows a constricting "apple-core" lesion (*arrow*), representing the colonic carcinoma.

such as when barium fills its interstices. Lipomas are demonstrated as smooth-walled, fatty submucosal lesions. Barium enema is an effective examination for the detection of colonic lymphoma, which may range in appearance from a single smooth tumor to multiple polypoid nodules.

Barium enema is a sensitive technique for detecting colonic diverticula and evidence of diverticulitis (see Chapter 83). Diverticulitis is the most common cause of extravasation of barium (*ie.*, fistulas, sinus tracts, and free perforations). Although barium studies are useful for detecting mucosal inflammation, CT has a well-defined role in diverticulitis, especially in identifying drainable collections (see pages 21 and 35).

Ulcerative colitis can be demonstrated on barium enema as a mucosal disorder that affects the colon in a continuous manner (see Chapter 83). The rectum almost invariably is involved, and there are no skip areas. The findings may be accompanied by a dilated ileum, with granular mucosa, characteristic of back-wash ileitis. In patients with Crohn's disease of the colon, the terminal ileum is commonly involved (see Chapter 74). Discrete ulcers may be seen, and the distribution in the colon often is asymmetric, with frequent skip areas. Double-contrast barium enema is a useful examination for diagnosing and monitoring both ulcerative colitis and Crohn's disease of the colon, and barium enema complements colonoscopy. Barium enema is the better modality for detecting fistulas, strictures, and perforations and for estimating the depth of ulcerations [4].

Findings on barium enema may suggest a diagnosis of pseudomembranous colitis, which is characterized by thickening of the bowel wall with prominent haustra and occasionally plaquelike lesions (see Chapter 60). Colonic ischemia may mimic inflammatory disease; thumbprinting, ulceration, and stricturing may be seen on barium enema examinations (see Chapter 65). The most common region affected by ischemia is the splenic flexure. In addition to detecting intrinsic colonic abnormalities, barium enemas may be employed to detect extrinsic processes, such as endometriosis, abscesses, and metastatic disease (*eg*, from gastric or ovarian primary tumors).

Barium enema should be the first examination for evaluation of a suspected structural abnormality in patients with constipation (see Chapter 69). A colonic transit study after ingestion of radiopaque markers may provide additional data regarding the colonic transit time. Defecography, a radiographic study of the distal colon and rectum as the patient evacuates thick barium, can be a useful examination in identifying rectal prolapse, enterocele, rectocele, dyskinetic puborectalis, and descending perineum syndrome [5].

▉▉▉ DIRECT OPACIFICATION STUDIES OF THE BILIARY TRACT

Percutaneous transhepatic cholangiography, endoscopic retrograde cholangiopancreatography (ERCP), and T-tube contrast studies are helpful in defining biliary anatomy and in delineating filling defects in the biliary tree and the level of biliary obstruction. Once access is established, additional procedures may be performed (*eg*, biopsy or cytologic brushing, stone extraction, papillotomy, stricture dilation, or biliary stent placement). ERCP is preferred when an ampullary, pancreatic, or distal bile duct lesion is suspected (see Chapter 142). ERCP is particularly useful in the diagnosis and simultaneous treatment of biliary calculus disease.

▉▉▉ ANGIOGRAPHY

Angiography may be performed to evaluate and control a site of gastrointestinal bleeding, determine the presence of bowel ischemia and infuse vasodilating agents, evaluate the resectability of lesions, identify vascular tumors (*eg*, islet cell tumors), and deliver chemotherapeutic agents. To diagnose a gastrointestinal bleed by angiography, the rate of bleeding should be at least 0.5 mL/min. In patients with active gastrointestinal hemorrhage, vasopressin may be administered or transcatheter embolization may be performed to attempt to arrest the bleeding (see Chapter 187). Angiography provides a preoperative vascular "road map" for hepatic surgeons, and angiographic findings may be valuable in assessing surgical resectability of liver lesions. Hemangiomas may be characterized accurately on angiography as small vascular lakes, in which there is contrast pooling, with small feeding vessels. Other vascular lesions, such as adenomas, focal nodular hyperplasia, hemangioendotheliomas, and hepatocellular carcinomas may be characterized by angiography (see Chapters 92, 101, and 102).

▉▉ CT

CT is the preferred modality for imaging the solid organs of the upper abdomen. Recent advances in helical CT have allowed for quicker, more detailed scans, with less volume averaging, and an increased ability to detect small lesions. With conventional CT scanners, the CT table remains in a stationary position, whereas the x-ray tube rotates 360 degrees. With helical scanners, the table moves and the tube rotates continuously. Helical techniques result in a CT scan of the liver in about 30 seconds, as opposed to 5 minutes with conventional CT [6•,7••]. CT is the best modality for detecting hepatic as well as extrahepatic disease and for staging patients with known or suspected malignancies. In patients with abdominal trauma, CT is the most efficacious imaging technique; current protocols allow for quick scanning of the entire abdomen and pelvis. CT has a well-established role in identifying hepatic and splenic lacerations, fractures, and subcapsular hematomas as well as pelvic fluid collections.

Abdominal Cavity and Gastrointestinal Tract

CT has a well-defined role in characterizing abdominal and pelvic fluid collections in patients with diverticulitis (see Chapter 83). Inflammatory changes in the pericolonic fat are seen in almost all patients with diverticulitis. Colonic wall thickening and complications such as pericolonic abscesses, sinus tracts, and fistulas also may be detected. In patients with Crohn's disease, mesenteric involvement and abscess formation are best seen on CT. CT is more sensitive than MRI but less sensitive than transrectal ultrasound for local staging of colorectal carcinoma and for determining local recurrence [8,9]. CT plays a major role in assessing more advanced tumors and in determining the presence of lymphadenopathy and distant metastatic disease. Findings that favor metastatic involvement of lymph nodes include large size (those greater than 14 mm usually are malignant), high attenuation after intravenous infusion of contrast, and large "short-to-long" axis ratios [10••].

CT of the abdomen requires adequate bowel opacification with 1% to 2% barium or a 2% to 3% water-soluble contrast agent administered orally. Some radiologists have advocated the use of dilute rectal contrast material to opacify the rectosigmoid. Failure to opacify the gastrointestinal tract adequately results in difficulty in distinguishing lesions from unopacified bowel loops.

Liver

CT is accurate for detecting focal liver lesions (see Chapter 92). The sensitivity of CT in detecting liver lesions is highest using CT arterial portography (CTAP), followed in order by helical contrast-enhanced CT, conventional contrast-enhanced dynamic incremental CT, and noncontrast CT. CTAP, which requires a superior mesenteric or a splenic artery injection, has a sensitivity of 81% to 91% in detecting hepatic neoplasms and is the most sensitive technique to detect the site and number of hepatic tumors [11]. In general, CTAP is reserved for patients being considered for segmental hepatic resection, hepatic arterial chemotherapy, or chemoembolization. The sensitivity of intravenous contrast-enhanced helical CT in detecting hepatic tumors has been reported to be 81%, which compares favorably with CTAP [11]. On CT, most metastases are hypodense to iso-

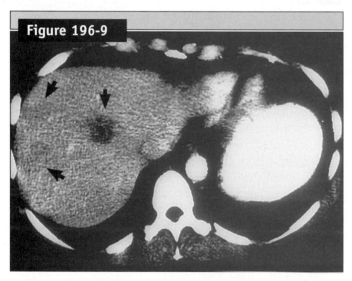

Figure 196-9

CT after intravenous contrast showing three hypodense lesions (*arrows*) in the dome of the liver, representing metastases in a patient with breast cancer.

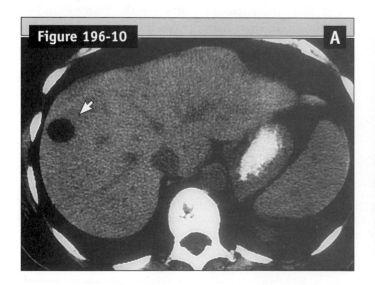

Figure 196-10   **A**

dense on precontrast studies and heterogeneous and hypodense on postcontrast examinations (Fig. 196-9). Noncontrast CT may be used to detect calcifications and hypervascular malignancies (including hepatocellular carcinomas and metastases from breast, carcinoid, islet cell, renal cell, and thyroid tumors as well as pheochromocytomas and choriocarcinomas).

CT can be helpful in diagnosing fatty infiltration of the liver as low density, nonspherical, geographic lesions without mass effect and with no displacement of vessels. On CT, hepatocellular carcinoma in noncirrhotic patients usually is a well-defined, heterogeneous mass. In patients with cirrhosis, hepatocellular carcinoma often is seen as one or multiple poorly defined masses. Early cirrhosis often appears as fatty change on CT. More advanced disease is characterized by a small, nodular liver, with hypertrophy of the caudate lobe, heterogeneous density, and portosystemic collateral vessels.

Cysts, which demonstrate the attenuation characteristics of water, are well demonstrated on CT (Fig. 196-10). Hepatic abscesses often are low in attenuation, and a few contain gas. Some abscesses may demonstrate rim enhancement after intravenous contrast infusion. Hemangiomas may be diagnosed accurately by CT, although only half of all hemangiomas demonstrate the "classic" features: a hypodense mass on precontrast images, which, with dynamic contrast enhancement, shows early, intense peripheral enhancement; the enhancement progresses to the center of the mass, leading to centripetal fill-in, with delayed isodensity. Focal nodular hyperplasia demonstrates low attenuation on precontrast CT scans. After the infusion of contrast the attenuation is variable, due to the presence of a central scar. Adenomas are low in attenuation on precontrast studies and heterogeneous on postcontrast scans.

Gallbladder and Biliary Tract

CT is a reliable technique for defining the level and cause of obstruction of the intrahepatic and extrahepatic biliary ducts, especially in patients with biliary calculi. Thin sections and helical techniques permit identification of small biliary calculi.

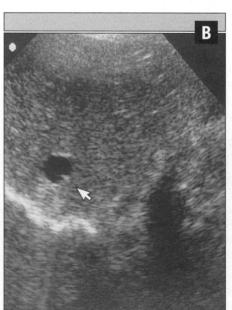

B

Hepatic cyst demonstrated on CT and ultrasound. **A**, CT without intravenous contrast showing a low attenuation mass (*arrow*) in the dome of the liver. **B**, Sagittal sonogram showing a cyst with a single incomplete septation (*arrow*).

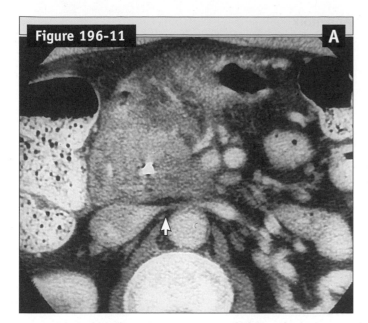

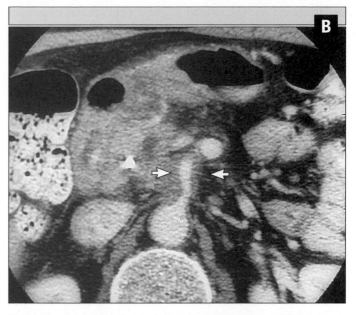

Pancreatic carcinoma detected on contrast-enhanced helical CT.
A, A 2-cm low attenuation mass is present in the uncinate process of the pancreas (*arrow*) in a patient with pancreatic adenocarcinoma.

B, The tumor involves the superior mesenteric artery (SMA) at its origin, and there is anterior tumor extension with encasement of the SMA (*arrows*). (*Courtesy of* C. Charnsangavej, MD.)

CT is less sensitive than ultrasound in detecting gallstones but superior to ultrasound in identifying common bile duct calculi and masses in the pancreatic head.

Pancreas

In acute pancreatitis, CT plays a role in detecting a focal low attenuation mass in the pancreas, a poorly marginated pancreas, and extrapancreatic fluid collections, phlegmon, and abscesses (see Chapter 134). CT also can identify fluid collections containing necrotic material and gas. CT is the major imaging modality for diagnosis and staging of pancreatic adenocarcinoma, with an overall accuracy of more than 90% [12] (see Chapter 139). On CT, pancreatic adenocarcinomas usually are low in attenuation after intravenous contrast; there may be associated necrosis, pancreatic duct dilation, and associated peripancreatic lymphadenopathy. Helical CT permits accurate staging of pancreatic adenocarcinomas by demonstrating adjacent small peripancreatic vessels and liver metastases (Fig. 196-11) [12].

▆▆ CT COLOGRAPHY

CT colography (also called *virtual colonoscopy*) was introduced recently. This technique combines helical CT and specialized two-dimensional and three-dimensional software to produce a computer-rendered intraluminal view of the colon, simulating a colonoscopic view. CT colography can provide a complete intraluminal colorectal examination with minimal use of bowel instrumentation [13]. One study showed excellent colographic detection of polyps 1 cm or larger [14] (Fig. 196-12, see also **Color Plate**), but the role of CT colography in clinical practice remains to be defined.

▆▆ ULTRASOUND

Ultrasound traditionally has played a prominent role in assessing patients with suspected cholecystitis or cholelithiasis. Recently, ultrasound has gained an expanded role in the evalu-

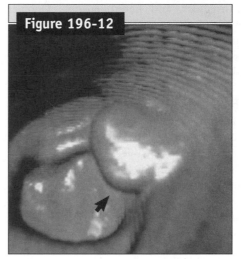

Three-dimensional perspective volume-rendered CT colographic image of a 1-cm sigmoid polyp (*arrow*) obtained with Voxel View software, Vital Images, Inc., Minneapolis, MN. (*Courtesy of* E. McFarland, MD.)

ation of gastrointestinal disease, especially with advances in intraoperative and intraluminal techniques. The sensitivity of intraoperative ultrasound (IOUS) for detecting hepatic tumors is greater than 95%, and IOUS can guide surgical decision making in patients thought to be candidates for resection of hepatocellular carcinomas or hepatic metastases [11,15]. Endosonography, in which an ultrasound transducer is attached to the tip of an endoscope, permits precise determination of the depth of stomach and small bowel tumors as well as identification of gastroesophageal varices and small pancreatic neoplasms.

The portability of transabdominal ultrasound is particularly valuable for imaging patients in an intensive care unit. At most institutions, ultrasound has become the technique of choice for guiding most percutaneous biopsy procedures. Nevertheless, ultrasound is operator dependent, and there are some ultrasonographic "blind spots" (including the dome of the liver and the left lobe) that may not be imaged adequately. Also, the value of ultrasound may be limited in obese patients and in patients with diffuse liver disease.

Liver

In general, focal hepatic lesions are better identified on ultrasound than are diffuse processes such as fatty infiltration, hepatitis, and cirrhosis (see Chapter 92). Simple hepatic cysts appear anechoic with smooth walls on ultrasound (Fig. 196-10). Some cysts are complicated with internal septations. Ultrasound plays a useful role in detecting hemangiomas, which usually are round or oval echogenic masses. Ultrasonographic features of most focal noncystic hepatic lesions, however, are nonspecific, limiting the ability of ultrasound to characterize lesions precisely. Ultrasound lacks specificity in diagnosing hepatocellular carcinoma (which usually is heterogeneous and may be discrete or diffuse), hepatic abscesses (which may be poorly marginated), and focal nodular hyperplasia (which often demonstrates a central scar). On ultrasound, metastases exhibit a variable appearance.

Fatty infiltration of the liver is seen on ultrasound as a diffuse increase in echogenicity compared with the kidneys, decreased echo transmission, and obscured portal venous walls. In early cirrhosis, ultrasound demonstrates a normal to enlarged liver, with heterogeneous echogenicity. In advanced cirrhosis, the liver is small, irregular, and heterogeneous. Doppler ultrasound may reveal portosystemic collaterals. In Budd-Chiari syndrome, ultrasound typically reveals caudate lobe enlargement, venous clots, hepatic veins that are decreased in size or not visualized, ascites, and hepatomegaly.

Gallbladder and Biliary Tract

Ultrasound is the primary modality for assessment of the gallbladder and bile ducts in patients with right upper quadrant pain. Ultrasound is quick and noninvasive, providing excellent visualization of the gallbladder, major intrahepatic bile ducts, and proximal common bile duct. Often, however, there is difficulty in demonstrating the distal common bile duct because of overlying gas in the duodenum or hepatic flexure. Ultrasound is more than 95% sensitive in identifying gallstones [6•] and is associated with a high positive predictive value for the diagnosis of acute cholecystitis when gallstones, a thickened gallbladder wall, and a positive ultrasonographic Murphy's sign are present. In complicated cholecystitis, ultrasound may be valuable in detecting adjacent abscesses. In a dilated biliary tract, ultrasound reveals multiple parallel, hypoechoic tubular structures, extending to the periphery of the liver. Ultrasound is variable in identifying the level and cause of biliary obstruction and demonstrates choledocholithiasis with a sensitivity ranging from 20% to 80% [16] (see Chapter 123).

Pancreas

In cases of acute pancreatitis, ultrasound may show a hypoechoic mass and pancreatic ductal dilation. Ultrasound demonstrates most well-defined intrapancreatic and extrapancreatic fluid collections but may miss small collections and collections containing gas. Pancreatic adenocarcinoma usually appears as a hypoechoic mass with irregular margins and dilated ducts. IOUS and endosonography play a role in identifying small pancreatic neoplasms, especially pancreatic islet cell tumors.

Appendix

Ultrasound has an established role in the investigation of suspected acute appendicitis (see Chapter 78). Ultrasound may detect acute appendicitis with high sensitivity and specificity; an inflamed appendix usually has a diameter of 6 mm or more. Often, an associated abscess or fluid collection is seen.

■■■ MAGNETIC RESONANCE IMAGING

Magnetic resonance imaging offers direct multiplanar imaging capability superior to that of conventional CT, with excellent soft tissue contrast and no ionizing radiation. Also, MRI is an excellent technique for detecting blood flow. MRI is a useful modality in patients who cannot be given iodinated contrast material. Although limited in detecting calcifications, MRI is very sensitive in detecting hemorrhage and iron. MRI is often used as a first-line modality in patients with known or suspected focal or diffuse liver lesions, and MRI plays an important role in clarifying CT findings.

Liver

The sensitivity of MRI in detecting hepatic lesions is greater than that of CT. MRI is the best technique for detecting focal masses in cirrhotic livers, such as hepatocellular carcinomas, regenerating nodules, and malignant degeneration in regenerating nodules. MRI cannot, however, always distinguish primary from metastatic tumors. Magnetic resonance contrast agents have been developed to increase specificity. For example, MRI with the superparamagnetic iron oxide AMI-25, an agent taken up by the reticuloendothelial system, is superior to unenhanced and gadolinium-enhanced MRI in diagnosing focal liver lesions [17] (Fig. 196-13). Another hepatic magnetic resonance contrast agent, mangafodipir trisodium (Mn-DPDP), has been shown to enhance hepatocellular carcinomas but not other tumors (Fig. 196-14). Murakami and colleagues also showed that the use of MRI after Mn-DPDP can detect hepatocellular carcinomas not identified on unenhanced studies [18].

Magnetic resonance imaging of the liver is the technique of choice for diagnosing hemangiomas, which usually are low in signal on T1-weighted images and high in signal on T2-weighted studies. On MRI performed with gadolinium, hemangiomas usually exhibit peripheral, globular enhancement (Fig. 196-15). MRI can identify more than 90% of hemangiomas and most areas of focal nodular hyperplasia [6•]. On MRI, hepatic metastases are heterogeneous and poorly marginated; they exhibit low signal on T1-weighted images (Fig. 196-16) and high signal on T2-weighted images. MRI is the study of choice to confirm fatty infiltration of the liver and to detect metastases in fatty livers. In patients with Budd-Chiari syndrome, MRI shows slow flow or thrombosis in the hepatic veins. MRI is the most sensitive imaging test for identification of iron overload.

■■■ MAGNETIC RESONANCE CHOLANGIOPANCREATOGRAPHY

Magnetic resonance cholangiopancreatography (MRCP) is a useful, noninvasive modality for imaging the gallbladder, biliary tree, and the pancreatic ductal system. MRCP requires no contrast material; the high signal of bile and pancreatic secretions on T2-weighted images permits depiction of the gallbladder, common duct, cystic duct, intrahepatic ducts, and the pancreat-

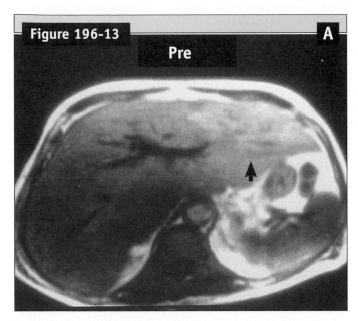

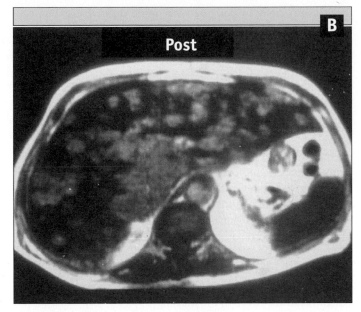

Hepatic MRI with the superparamagnetic iron oxide AMI-25. **A**, T1-weighted spin-echo image without contrast material showing heterogeneous signal in the left lobe (*arrow*) in a patient with metastatic adenocarcinoma. **B**, T1-weighted spin-echo image with AMI-25 demonstrating multiple metastases, hyperintense to normal liver parenchyma. (*Courtesy of* R. Weissleder, MD.)

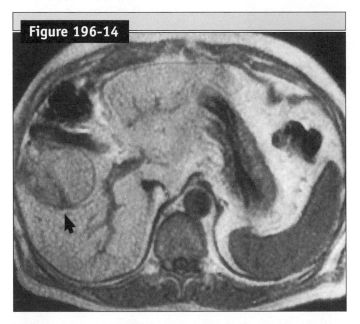

MRI with manganese DPDP showing uptake in the round, encapsulated hepatocellular carcinoma in the right lobe (*arrow*). Manganese DPDP uptake is consistent with hepatocyte origin of the tumor. (*Courtesy of* M. Fenstermacher, MD.)

ic duct. Although small stones may be missed, MRCP has been reported to detect choledocholithiasis with a sensitivity of 95% [16,19]. MRCP is accurate in delineating the presence of malignant bile duct obstruction, especially in cases of cholangiocarcinoma [20•] (Fig. 196-17).

NUCLEAR MEDICINE

In many centers, scintigraphy of the biliary tree is performed in patients with suspected cholecystitis. Other common applications of nuclear medicine techniques include liver imaging and gastrointestinal bleeding studies. Tumor imaging with anti–carcinoembryonic antigen antibody (for colorectal carcinomas) and somatostatin analogues (for neuroendocrine tumors) has shown great promise.

Abdominal Cavity and Gastrointestinal Tract

Gastroesophageal reflux and gastric emptying may be quantified by technetium-99m sulfur colloid or indium-111 diethylenetriaminepentaacetic acid (DTPA) scans (see Chapter 22). Radionuclide scans with technetium-99m sodium pertechnetate are useful in identifying Meckel's diverticula. Indium-111–labeled leukocyte scans and gallium-67 citrate scans may help to localize infectious processes in the abdomen. Gallium scans also may be useful in imaging hepatocellular carcinoma, Hodgkin's disease, and non-Hodgkin's lymphomas. In the diagnosis of lower gastrointestinal bleeding, technetium-99m sulfur colloid scans and technetium-99m red blood cell scans are often helpful (see Chapter 86).

Liver

The most commonly used radiopharmaceutical for anatomic evaluation of the liver is technetium-99m sulfur colloid, which is taken up by the reticuloendothelial (Kupffer) cells of the liver. Technetium-99m–labeled red blood cell studies may be useful in diagnosing hemangiomas. Single-photon emission computed tomography techniques increase the accuracy of red blood cell imaging, especially in characterizing smaller (less than 2 cm) lesions. On technetium-99m sulfur colloid scans, focal nodular hyperplasia is isointense to hyperintense, whereas metastases usually demonstrate no radiopharmaceutical uptake.

Gallbladder and Biliary Tract

A number of radiopharmaceuticals are cleared by hepatocytes and excreted in the bile, thus permitting scintigraphic examination of the biliary tract. Diisopropyl iminodiacetic acid and related agents are more than 95% accurate in diagnosing acute cholecystitis, especially in patients with cystic duct obstruction (see Chapter 120). False-positive studies may occur in patients receiving parenteral nutrition or narcotics. Biliary scintigraphy also may be helpful in evaluating patients with cholestasis, acute and chronic biliary obstruction, bile leaks, and choledochal cysts.

SOMATOSTATIN IMAGING

Somatostatin receptor scintigraphy (with iodine-123 octreotide or indium-111-DTPA-D-PHE1-octreotide) has shown great promise in the detection and staging of gastroenteropancreatic neuroendocrine tumors, such as carcinoid tumors, islet cell tumors, and Zollinger-Ellison syndrome [21] (Fig. 196-18; see Chapter 140). In a study of 160 patients with neuroendocrine tumors, somatostatin imaging modified patient staging in 24% of cases and altered surgical strategies in 25% of cases [22].

CONCLUSION

With multiple modalities available to image known or suspected gastrointestinal diseases, the most appropriate technique should be selected to answer a specific question or to delineate a specific pathophysiologic feature. Barium studies remain the gold standard for evaluation of the gastrointestinal tract. However, there are some disease entities for which there is no single best examination. For example, in suspected diverticulitis, barium enema may be employed to show mucosal irregularity, but CT is required to show infiltration of the pericolonic fat or a drainable fluid collection. In patients with metastatic colon cancer, it is common for lesions to be detected initially on helical CT scans with intravenous contrast. If the patient is then considered a candidate for hepatic resection, CTAP, IOUS, or both are performed at most institutions. Algorithms for evaluation of lesions in the liver, pancreas, and gallbladder are evolving, and a tailored approach is suggested. For example, calcification may be identified on plain radiographs or CT. Whether a lesion is cystic or solid is easily determined by ultrasound. Tumor vascularity and vessel patency may be demonstrated by color Doppler ultrasound, contrast-enhanced CT or MRI, CT or magnetic resonance angiography, or conventional angiography.

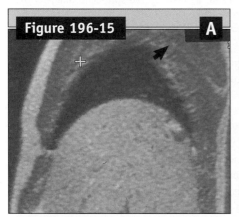
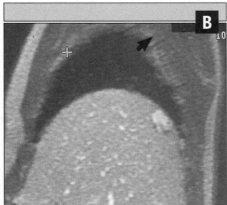

Liver hemangioma demonstrated on sagittal T1-weighted MRI with dynamic gadolinium enhancement. **A**, Thirty seconds after contrast infusion, there is nodular peripheral enhancement (*arrow*). **B**, Ninety seconds after contrast infusion, there is nearly complete, intense fill-in with contrast (*arrow*). (*Courtesy of* M. Fenstermacher, MD.)

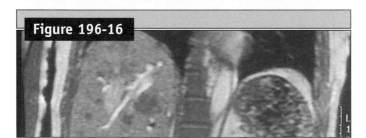

Coronal T1-weighted MRI showing multiple low-signal hepatic lesions in a patient with a metastatic islet cell tumor. (*Courtesy of* A. Delpassand, MD.)

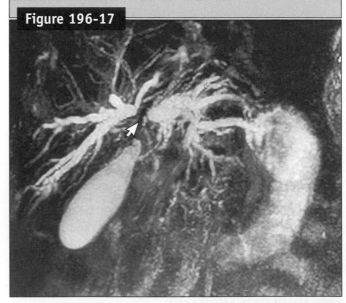

Magnetic resonance cholangiopancreatography demonstrating intrahepatic bile ducts dilated to the origin of the common hepatic duct (*arrow*) and nearly complete absence of signal in the common duct in a patient with a Klatskin tumor. (*Courtesy of* M. Fenstermacher, MD.)

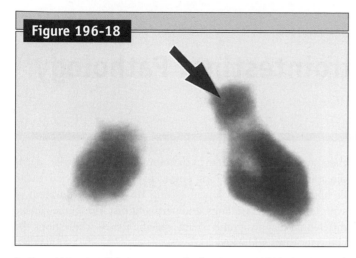

Figure 196-18

Indium-111 octreotide transverse single-photon emission computed tomography scan at 24 hours demonstrating intense uptake in the pancreatic tail (*arrow*) in a patient with an insulinoma. Normal renal activity is noted bilaterally. (*Courtesy of* A. Delpassand, MD.)

As imaging techniques continue to evolve, more comprehensive information may be gained with one modality. For example, it is not inconceivable that, in the near future, a patient with bloody stools will be scheduled first for CT colography. After the virtual colonoscopic images of the colon are obtained, the remainder of the abdomen and pelvis can be scanned, if necessary, to evaluate the liver and to assess for lymphadenopathy. Similar protocols may be developed for MRI. For example, MRCP could be used to image the biliary tree in a patient with cholangiocarcinoma; thereafter, the patient could undergo conventional liver MRI to assess for focal hepatic lesions.

■ REFERENCES

Recently published papers of particular interest have been highlighted as follows:
- Of interest
- • Of outstanding interest

1. Wood BJ, Kumar PN, Cooper C, *et al*.: Pneumatosis intestinalis in adults with AIDS: clinical significance and imaging findings. *AJR* 1995, 165:1387–1390.

2. Waye JD, Bashkoff E: Total colonoscopy: is it always possible? *Gastrointest Endosc* 1991, 37:152–154.

3. Johnson CD, Ilstrup DM, Fish NM, *et al*.: Barium enema: detection of colonic lesions in a community population. *AJR* 1996, 167:39–43.

4. Dijkstra J, Reeders JWAJ, Tytgat GNJ: Idiopathic inflammatory bowel disease: endoscopic-radiologic correlation. *Radiology* 1995, 197:369–375.

5. Karasick S, Ehrlich SM: Is constipation a disorder of defecation or impaired motility? Distinction based on defecography and colonic transit studies. *AJR* 1996, 166:63–66.

6.• Saini S: Imaging of the hepatobiliary tract. *N Engl J Med* 1997, 336:1889–1894.
This concise review article covers imaging of the hepatobiliary system with an emphasis on CT and MRI.

7.•• Brink JA, McFarland EG, Heiken JP: Helical/spiral computed body tomography. *Clin Radiol* 1997, 52:489–503.
This comprehensive review article encompasses all facets of helical CT, including CT angiography and CT colography. Considerable attention is devoted to the technical aspects of scanning, including methods of reconstruction and reformatting.

8. Zerhouni EA, Rutter C, Hamilton SR, *et al*.: CT and MR imaging in the staging of colorectal carcinoma: report of the Radiology Diagnostic Oncology Group II. *Radiology* 1996, 200:443–451.

9. Rotondano G, Esposito P, Pellecchia L, *et al*.: Early detection of locally recurrent rectal cancer by endosonography. *Br J Radiol* 1997, 70:567–571.

10.•• Fukuya T, Honda H, Hayashi T, *et al*.: Lymph-node metastases: efficacy of detection with helical CT in patients with gastric cancer. *Radiology* 1995, 197:705–711.
Helical CT was performed in 58 patients with gastric cancer before lymph node resection. A total of 1082 lymph nodes were surgically resected, and CT findings were compared with histopathology. The sensitivity for detecting metastasis-positive lymph nodes was higher than that for detecting metastasis-negative nodes. CT attenuation and lymph node configuration aided in the diagnosis of malignant lymphadenopathy.

11. Kuszyk BS, Bluemke DA, Urban BA, *et al*.: Portal-phase contrast-enhanced helical CT for the detection of malignant hepatic tumors: sensitivity based on comparison with intraoperative and pathological findings. *AJR* 1996, 166:91–95.

12. Bluemke DA, Cameron JL, Hruban RH, *et al*.: Potentially resectable pancreatic adenocarcinoma: spiral CT assessment with surgical and pathologic correlation. *Radiology* 1995, 197:381–385.

13. Hara AK, Johnson CD, Reed JE, *et al*.: Colorectal polyp detection with CT colography: two- versus three-dimensional techniques. Work in progress. *Radiology* 1996, 200:49–54.

14. Hara AK, Johnson CD, Reed JE, *et al*.: Detection of colorectal polyps by computed tomographic colography: feasibility of a novel technique. *Gastroenterology* 1996, 110:284–290.

15. Fuhrman GM, Curley SA, Hohn DC, *et al*.: Improved survival after resection of colorectal liver metastases. *Ann Surg Oncol* 1995, 2:537–541.

16. Chan Y-l, Chan ACW, Lam WWM, *et al*.: Choledocholithiasis: comparison of MR cholangiography and endoscopic retrograde cholangiography. *Radiology* 1996, 200:85–89.

17. Vogl TJ, Hammerstingl R, Schwarz W, *et al*.: Superparamagnetic iron oxide-enhanced versus gadolinium-enhanced MR imaging for differential diagnosis of focal liver lesions. *Radiology* 1996, 198:881–887.

18. Murakami T, Baron RL, Peterson MS: Hepatocellular carcinoma: MR imaging with mangafodipir trisodium (Mn-DPDP). *Radiology* 1996, 200:69–77.

19. Reuther G, Kiefer B, Tuchmann A: Cholangiography before biliary surgery: single-shot MR cholangiography versus intravenous cholangiography. *Radiology* 1996, 198:561–566.

20.• Reinhold C, Bret PM: Current status of MR cholangiopancreatography. *AJR* 1996, 166:1285–1295.
This comprehensive review of MR cholangiopancreatography encompasses both technical and clinical aspects. Potential roles and limitations of MRCP are discussed, and comparison is made with CT, ultrasound, and ERCP.

21. Kvols LK, Brown ML, O'Connor MK, *et al*.: Evaluation of a radiolabeled somatostatin analog (I-123 octreotide) in the detection and localization of carcinoid and islet cell tumors. *Radiology* 1993, 187:129–133.

22. Lebtahi R, Cadiot G, Sarda L, *et al*.: Clinical impact of somatostatin receptor scintigraphy in the management of patients with neuroendocrine gastroenteropancreatic tumors. *J Nucl Med* 1997, 38:853–858.

197 Principles of Gastrointestinal Pathology

Carolyn C. Compton

ROLE OF THE PATHOLOGIST IN THE DIAGNOSIS AND MANAGEMENT OF GASTROINTESTINAL DISEASE

The pathologist plays a key role in the diagnosis and treatment of many gastrointestinal diseases. The scope and accuracy of any pathology consultation, however, hinge on three important factors that are under the clinician's control: 1) the type of specimen provided, 2) the quality of the specimen provided, and 3) the clinical information communicated.

The type of specimen provided largely determines the kind of information the pathologist is able to provide. In general, endoscopic biopsies can provide answers to one or more of the following questions:

Is an abnormality present?

If abnormal, what is the disease process or differential diagnosis?

Is more than one disease process present?

Is the disease acute or chronic?

What is the severity of the disease?

What are the distribution and extent of the disease?

Are any dysplastic or neoplastic changes present?

If dysplastic or neoplastic, what is the grade of the process?

If the diagnosis is known and treatment has already been instituted, biopsy can help to evaluate the effectiveness of therapy and to detect therapeutic complications.

Resection specimens may provide additional information and are often the only means of providing tissue diagnosis of deep processes, such as mural tumors or large-vessel vasculitis. Tumor resections provide the definitive information necessary to stage neoplastic disease accurately, determine the presence of modulating prognostic factors, and assess the completeness of excision.

The quality of the submitted specimen may determine the pathologist's degree of certainty about the diagnosis. Small or superficial specimens, large amounts of biopsy trauma with hemorrhage and crush artifact, tissue autolysis or bacterial overgrowth from delayed fixation, or air drying of the specimen after acquisition all can severely limit and even preclude definitive interpretation of the biopsy (see next section).

One of the most widespread myths about pathology is that diagnostic answers "reside" in affected tissues and can be "extracted" by competent pathologists without the need for clinical information. Although some disease processes have pathognomonic histologic findings, tissue pathology more often presents its own differential diagnosis and requires clinico-pathologic correlation. Unfortunately, pathology is a service whereby the consultant rarely sees or speaks directly to the patient or reviews the patient's medical record. Perhaps more than any other consultant, therefore, the pathologist needs direct input from the treating physician and should, in particular, be apprised of 1) the clinical setting (*ie*, type and duration of symptoms, clinical findings, and pertinent history); 2) the clinical differential diagnosis; and 3) any specific issues or questions the clinician wants addressed.

In most settings, the pathology specimen submission form is the only vehicle for this interchange. The information provided may alter the way the pathologist processes, cuts, or stains the tissue. Urgent cases may require special handling of the specimen.

SPECIMEN ACQUISITION AND HANDLING

Mucosal Biopsy

As a rule, biopsy specimens obtained with endoscopic forceps contain only mucosa and muscularis propria (Fig. 197-1). Small amounts of superficial submucosa may also be present. Thus, pathologic processes that involve primarily the submucosa (*eg*, vasculitis, lymphoma) may be difficult to evaluate by endoscopic biopsy unless deeper tissue is obtained. This may be accomplished by repeated biopsy sampling at the same site or by using "jumbo" forceps. Sometimes tissue samples are superficial or scanty and thus nondiagnostic or insufficient for diagnosis. Occasionally, however, even scant specimens yield important diagnostic information (*eg*, the presence of *Giardia* species on the surface of the duodenum or *Helicobacter pylori* on the surface of the stomach) or may be sufficient for diagnosing malignancy by cytology alone. Therefore, all specimens should be submitted to the pathologist, even if the endoscopist doubts the adequacy of the sample obtained.

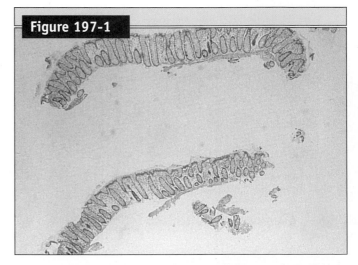

Figure 197-1

Colonoscopic biopsy specimen showing that endoscopic forceps biopsies usually include only the mucosa and muscularis mucosae and little or no submucosa (original magnification × 10).

Technically inadequate handling of the specimen may contribute to difficulties in endoscopic biopsy interpretation. Problems may be generated by the endoscopist or in the histology laboratory. Even with expert technique, artifacts produced during biopsy acquisition are relatively difficult to avoid. The most common among these include the following:

Crush artifact produced by the forceps

Burn artifact from the use of electrocautery

Tissue desiccation produced when the biopsy sample is allowed to air dry before being immersed in formalin (the thinner the biopsy, the more susceptible it is to desiccation; therefore, this is particularly common with needle biopsies)

Autolytic artifact produced when the biopsy sample sits unfixed at room temperature (or warmer) before being immersed in formalin

Crush and burn artifacts may cause such severe distortion that the histologic characteristics of the tissue are completely effaced and the biopsy is rendered uninterpretable. In these cases, repeat biopsy may be necessary. Cautery causes streaming (marked elongation) of cell nuclei, nuclear hyperchromatism, and architectural distortion of the tissue, resulting in a pseudoadenomatous appearance. If cautery is severe and the artifact extends throughout the tissue, it may be impossible to differentiate an adenomatous from a nonadenomatous polyp. In contrast, tissue desiccation and autolysis both produce changes mimicking cell necrosis and may result in misdiagnosis of a necrotizing pathologic process. This problem is obviated if all biopsy samples are placed immediately into 10% buffered formalin (the best all-purpose tissue fixative) after acquisition. If fresh tissue is required for analysis (as for certain types of immunohistochemical or histochemical stains), the biopsy should be snap-frozen immediately in a glycerol-based mounting medium to prevent desiccation and ice crystal formation. If a fresh specimen must be transported before freezing, it should be placed on a piece of saline-soaked filter paper in an air-tight container, kept cool, and snap-frozen as soon as possible.

Technical problems generated in tissue processing that may interfere with biopsy interpretation or (rarely) preclude diagnosis are less common and include the following:

•Improper orientation of the specimen during embedding in paraffin

•Loss of diagnostic tissue during slide preparation by overtrimming of the paraffin block

•Loss of surface epithelium with repeated handling of the tissue

Improper orientation of the tissue leads to tangential rather than transverse sectioning; under the microscope, tissue architectural features cannot be seen optimally in tangentially cut sections. If enough tissue remains in the paraffin block, this problem can be rectified by melting the block and reorienting the tissue. Inadvertent overtrimming of the block during slide preparation is a relatively rare occurrence that can lead to irrevocable tissue loss. Loss of surface epithelium from repeated surface abrasion by biopsy forceps creates "bald" patches on the mucosa, a potentially serious problem in some settings (*eg*, assessment of dysplasia in Barrett's esophagus or ulcerative colitis). Denudation of the surface seldom is universal throughout the biopsy, however, and additional tissue levels may reveal intact epithelium.

Polypectomy

The reader is referred to Chapter 80 for additional information on polypectomy. The three most important issues surrounding pathologic examination of polypectomy specimens are 1) determination of histologic type; 2) evaluation for dysplasia and malignancy; and 3) assessment of the completeness of excision. The latter two pose the most problems. Diagnosis of polyp type is usually straightforward, except, as discussed in the previous section, in cases of severe crush or burn artifact. In contrast, evaluation of polyps for dysplasia or malignancy frequently can be difficult, even with optimal specimens, because definitive assessment may be rendered impossible by the presence of artifact, especially that caused by electrocautery. Many types of nonadenomatous polyps require evaluation for dysplasia because of their potential to undergo malignant transformation; examples are the hamartomatous polyps of Peutz-Jeghers syndrome and juvenile polyposis, esophageal papillomas, and anal condylomas. Hyperplastic polyps of the colon with adenomatous foci (mixed hyperplastic–adenomatous polyps) also are common but may be impossible to recognize in the presence of significant artifact. Assessment of dysplasia also is complicated by the fact that reversible cytologic atypia induced in epithelium by inflammatory injury and proliferative reparative responses cannot be reliably differentiated from the irreversible premalignant changes of true dysplasia. If severe cytologic atypia is seen in the presence of ongoing inflammation or repair (*eg*, in response to infarction), a diagnosis of *indefinite* or *highly suspicious* for dysplasia may be justifiable.

Adenomatous polyps are by definition composed entirely of dysplastic epithelium and must be evaluated for malignancy. If present, the extent of invasion of the malignancy within the polyp should be assessed. Crush and burn artifacts may complicate this evaluation, as may infarction of the polyp head. Infarction and ulceration caused by twisting of the stalk and intermittent vascular occlusion produce scarring and glandular entrapment within the polyp stalk or head that resembles invasive malignancy with stromal sclerosis. This has been called *pseudoinvasion* and may be misdiagnosed as invasive tumor.

In evaluating adenomatous polyps, it often is difficult to assess the completeness of excision. Such assessment is possible only if the base or stalk of the polyp can be identified and bisected transversely in a coronal plane through the center of the polyp head. The base can first be marked with India ink to aid in its subsequent identification under the microscope. If the polyp is small and lacks a stalk, the base usually is not apparent on macroscopic examination, and orientation on embedding may be random. If the base of the polyp is not seen on histologic section, completeness of the excision cannot be assessed. For larger polyps, the major problem is fragmentation. Large polyps may be removed in chunks or, if excised whole, may fragment after excision. The true base of a fragmented polypectomy specimen usually is impossible to identify on gross examination. In fact, it is impossible to be certain that all fragments are from the same polyp, unless the endoscopist conveys this information. Ironically, burn artifact may help in some cases by permitting microscopic identification of the resection margin (Fig. 197-2).

Special Stains and Studies

Special stains (*ie*, dyes other than hematoxylin and eosin used to enhance particular structures in tissue), immunohistochemistry (*ie*, localization and visualization of specific antigens in tissue using antibodies), and electron microscopy are all part of the surgical pathologist's armamentarium. These techniques can increase diagnostic yield and certainty and may even be essential for diagnosis. Because they are labor intensive and add significantly to the time delay and cost of a pathologic examination, these special stains and studies rarely are used routinely. Use of special studies is usually dictated by the histologic or clinical differential diagnosis. The clinician should communicate specific concerns to the pathologist at the time the specimen is submitted. For electron microscopic examination, which requires fixation in glutaraldehyde, or immunohistochemical stains which require frozen tissue, additional biopsy samples and special processing may be necessary. Special stains commonly used in the pathologic diagnosis of gastrointestinal diseases are shown in Table 197-1.

◼ THE PATHOLOGY REPORT
Key Words: The Lexicon of the Pathologist

In a pathology report, the diagnostic impression is stated as succinctly as possible using standard pathologic and clinical diagnostic terms. Unfortunately, many biopsies are not completely diagnostic, and even fewer are pathognomonic. Thus, in many cases, the major findings are described, followed by the pathologist's best interpretation. Alternative diagnoses "excluded" or "ruled out" may also be listed.

The vocabulary used by pathologists to report findings is idiosyncratic and may be cryptic to nonpathologists. For example, an unwritten rule in pathology is that tissue is never interpreted

as "normal." Rather, it is described as "lacking pathology," and a mutually agreed on or historically based catch phrase is used, such as "no significant pathologic changes present" or "no diagnostic abnormality recognized." This virtually universal

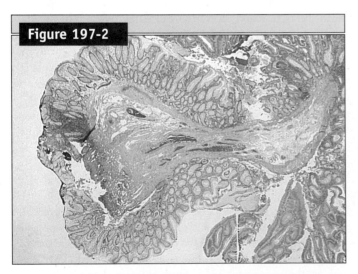

Figure 197-2

Burn artifact at the base of this adenoma marks the surgical resection margin, which is encompassed by normal colonic mucosa and is free of adenomatous epithelium, demonstrating that the resection is complete (original magnification × 10).

Table 197-1. Special Stains Commonly Used in Gastrointestinal Pathology

Periodic Acid–Schiff (PAS) stain

Whipple's disease bacilli (*Tropheryma whippelii*)
Fungi
Neutral mucin (goblet cells, adenocarcinoma cells)
Glycogen (PAS positivity disappears after digestion with diastase)
Cryptosporidia

Methenamine silver stain
Fungi
Pneumocystis carinii

Thiazine stain
Helicobacter pylori or *H. heilmanni*

Warthin-starry stain
H. pylori or *H. heilmanni*
Spirochetes

Giemsa stain
H. pylori or *H. helimanni*
Toxoplasma gondii

Tissue Gram's stain
(*eg*, Brown and Brenn or Brown and Hopps)
Bacterial pathogens (*eg*, *Yersinia enterocolitica*)
Microsporidia

Acid-fast stain
Mycobacterium tuberculosis
M. avium complex
Microsporidia
Schistosome eggs

Modified acid-fast stain
Nocardia

Trichrome stain
Fibrosis (scarring)
Thickening of subepithelial collagen table (*eg*, collagenous colitis)
Fibromuscular stromal replacement (*eg*, mucosal prolapse)
Fibrin thrombi

Alcian blue stain
Acid mucins (in upper gastrointestinal tract, seen only in metaplastic cells)

Mucicarmine stain
Neutral mucin (goblet cells, adenocarcinoma cells)
Cryptococcus neoformans

Iron stain (Prussian blue)
Hemochromatosis (*eg*, affected gastric mucosa)
Hemosiderin deposition (*eg*, mucosal ischemia or hemorrhage)

Amyloid stain (Congo red)
Primary or secondary amyloidosis

Argentaffin stain (Fontana-Masson)
Melanin or melanin-like pigment (melanosis coli)

custom is based, at least in part, on the fact that some diseases may produce no histopathologic changes in the tissue (as is the case for the small bowel mucosa in cholera). Other commonly used terms and their definitions follow:

Phlegmonous—dramatically inflamed (purulent, suppurative) and forming an inflammatory mass

Atypical—abnormal looking, but not definitively dysplastic (*ie,* neoplastic)

Dysplastic—transformed (*ie,* neoplastic) and not reactive

Focal—spotty in distribution; opposite of diffuse

Active—containing ongoing inflammation of uncertain duration

Chronic—containing inflammation of sufficient duration to cause architectural abnormalities, metaplastic changes, or scarring in the tissue (may be active or inactive but not acute in a temporal sense)

Reading Between the Lines

Although pathologists function as consultants, they usually offer no therapeutic advice in the pathology report, primarily because they rarely know the full clinical scenario. Nevertheless, based on the biopsy features, the pathologist may recommend actions to confirm the diagnosis or to narrow the differential diagnosis, usually qualified by a phrase such as "if clinically warranted."

Excisional biopsies are seen by the pathologist in an altogether different perspective. These are usually therapeutic resections rather than diagnostic procedures, and the pathologist is often in a unique position to determine whether further therapy is required. In such cases, therapeutic suggestions are more readily offered. For example, in the case of a completely excised adenoma with infiltrating carcinoma but no features associated with an adverse outcome, the pathologist may reassure the clinician that no further therapy is required. Conversely, wide excision may be recommended in cases of incompletely excised tumors with a potentially aggressive biologic behavior predicted by histopathologic features.

■ UPPER GASTROINTESTINAL DISEASE
The Normal and the Pathologic

It is not always possible to recognize mucosal pathology, either because it so closely mimics normal (*eg,* well-differentiated metaplasia) or because the deviation from ideal textbook histology is within the normal range of acceptability.

Esophagus

The reader is referred to Chapters 4, 6, 11, 12, and 14 for additional information on the esophagus. Normal esophageal mucosa is not keratinized and has neither granular nor cornified layers. These features, often in association with parakeratosis (retention of nuclei in the abnormal keratotic layer), indicate chronic inflammation, irritation, or both. The epithelium normally is devoid of granulocytes, the presence of which is diagnostic of an active inflammatory process. Intraepithelial lymphocytes and Langerhans' cells are normal, and although these cells may increase in number dramatically with chronic inflammation, their presence in the epithelium is not a diagnostic criterion for esophagitis. Mucous glands and their tubular excretory ducts are normally present in the submucosa and lamina propria of the

lower third of the esophagus and may be an important anatomic landmark for the pathologist in deciding whether or not the gastroesophageal junctional mucosa is metaplastic (Fig. 197-3). The presence of these glands within gastric-type mucosa that would be interpreted otherwise as gastric cardia establishes definitively that the mucosa is metaplastic. Unfortunately, these structures are present infrequently in esophageal biopsy specimens. In general, the pathologist must rely on mucosal architectural atypicality or on the presence of intestinal goblet or Paneth's cells to help confirm the diagnosis of metaplasia. The definitive diagnosis of dysplasia, whether or not it is metaplastic, can be extremely difficult in the presence of ongoing inflammation.

Knowledge of the exact site of the biopsy can be an important element in the diagnosis of esophageal disease. A diagnosis of an inlet patch (gastric heterotopia), for example, can be made only if the pathologist knows the sample came from the proximal esophagus.

In addition to metaplasia of esophageal epithelium (Barrett's esophagus), other common types of esophageal pathology are marked by distinctive epithelial changes. Inflammation, including reflux, other chemical injury, viral or fungal infection, and malignant tumors are usually easily diagnosed on representative biopsy specimens.

Stomach

The reader is referred to Chapters 18, 19, and 27 to 29 for additional information on the stomach. Normal gastric mucosa has little or no stromal lymphoid tissue and contains no granulocytes (Fig. 197-4). The absence of stromal lymphoid tissue sets the stomach apart from all other segments of the gastrointestinal tract and represents a paradox because the stomach is the most common site of extranodal lymphomas. The presence of lymphoid and plasma cells in the gastric mucosa is a hallmark of chronic gastritis, both autoimmune and nonautoimmune. Other diagnostic signs of chronic gastric inflammatory disease are intestinal metaplasia and glandular atrophy (shortening, cystic dilation, and scarcity of glands). The gastric epithelium contains no granulocytes, and the presence of intraepithelial granulocytes in the stomach is diagnostic of active inflammation.

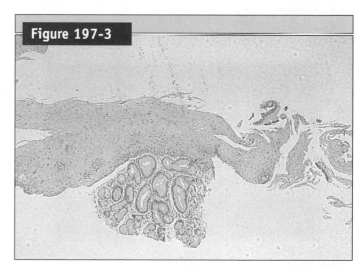

Figure 197-3

Esophageal submucosal glands are seen beneath the squamous mucosa (original magnification × 16).

Intraepithelial lymphocytes, however, are normal unless markedly increased in number. Normally, there are 4 to 7 intraepithelial lymphocytes per 100 epithelial cells in the stomach. The presence of more than 25 intraepithelial lymphocytes per 100 epithelial cells is considered diagnostic of lymphocytic gastritis, a unique pattern of chronic gastritis that is most often seen in patients with sprue or as an atypical response to *H. pylori* infection (see later discussion of gastritis).

The most common abnormal findings on gastric biopsy are inflammatory injuries and their sequelae, including metaplasia, with or without dysplasia, and malignant tumors. The nomenclature for gastritis has undergone revision, and histologic definitions of the most common forms of gastritis have been established. Thus, pathology reports should no longer read "chronic antral" or "type B" gastritis; rather, specific etiologies should be given in most cases. Nevertheless, problems in interpretation arise in cases with indeterminate histopathologic appearance or with more than one cause of gastritis.

Duodenum

In the normal duodenum, the villi are about four times longer than the crypts are deep. Only perfectly oriented biopsy samples (a rarity) allow the pathologist to judge this ratio with certainty. Stromal inflammatory cells in varying amounts are a normal finding, but lymphoid follicles are considered abnormal. Commonly, the amount of stromal cellularity appears increased above the normal range, and if no other abnormal features are present, the pathologist diagnoses "chronic nonspecific duodenitis." Some pathologists are reluctant to make this diagnosis, however, because the range of normal duodenal stromal cell content is undefined. Brunner's glands can normally be present in the lamina propria of the first and second part of the duodenum; however, they are considered hyperplastic if they fill the mucosa and push crypts aside, correlating with polypoid projections seen endoscopically.

Findings encountered on duodenal biopsy include inflammation (peptic disease), immune-mediated injury (*eg*, celiac sprue), infection (*eg*, giardiasis, Whipple's disease, strongyloidiasis),

adenomas, and malignant tumors. Unfortunately, noninfectious inflammatory and immune-mediated diseases are the most common and have the least specific pathologic features.

Incisional and Excisional Biopsy
Esophagitis

The only inflammatory disorders of the esophagus with pathognomonic histologic pictures are the infectious esophagitides, acute graft-versus-host disease, and some of the bullous diseases. All other disorders of the esophagus have a differential diagnosis that requires clinicopathologic correlation. Histologic diagnosis of fungal esophagitis is based on demonstration of fungal forms invading esophageal tissue (Fig. 197-5). Isolated or detached organisms may represent contamination from the oropharynx rather than esophageal infection. Biopsy samples from both the center and edges of a fungal ulcer improve the diagnostic yield; however, the biopsies must be taken from deep enough to include the underlying tissue as well as the overlying pseudomembrane of fungal organisms, fibrin, inflammatory cells, and necrotic epithelial cells.

The typically small, punched-out ulcers of viral esophagitis also must be sampled at the edges and center to ensure acquisition of diagnostic tissue. In herpetic esophagitis, only the epithelium at the ulcer edge shows diagnostic intranuclear viral inclusions, whereas in cytomegalovirus infection, the endothelial cells and fibroblasts from the ulcer bed are more likely than are the epithelial cells to display diagnostic intranuclear and intracytoplasmic inclusions. When viral inclusions are absent in histologic preparations, the diagnosis of viral esophagitis can be made only if immunohistochemical staining reveals the presence of viral antigens. Communication of the gastroenterologist's clinical suspicion of viral disease often contributes to the pathologist's decision to perform immunohistochemical stains. Immunohistochemical staining also may be used to confirm or exclude viral infection when observed cytologic changes, such as enlarged inclusion-like nucleoli, resemble viral inclusions.

Gastroesophageal reflux produces mucosal inflammatory changes that are highly characteristic but not pathognomonic:

Figure 197-4

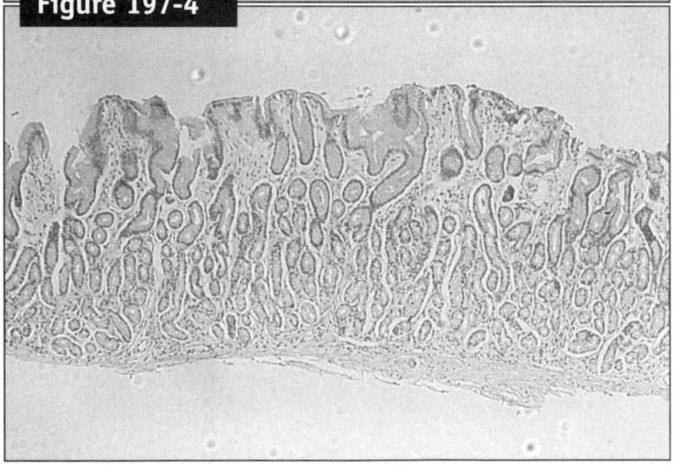

Normal gastric antrum contains neither inflammatory cells nor lymphocytes (original magnification × 35).

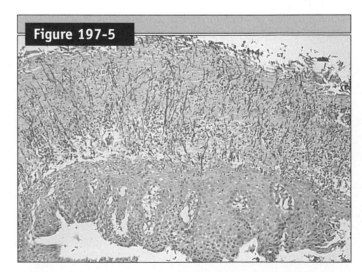

Figure 197-5

Pseudohyphal and yeast forms invading the esophageal squamous mucosa are diagnostic of candidal esophagitis (original magnification × 16).

eosinophilic infiltration of the epithelium and varying degrees of mucosal injury, from edema (spongiosis; Fig. 197-6) to frank ulceration. Similar changes result from eosinophilic or allergic gastroenteritis, chemical or drug reactions (*eg*, "pill esophagitis"), certain infections (*eg*, candidiasis), underlying malignancy, and vasculitis. Of all causes of these changes, reflux is by far the most common, and the pathologist often designates epithelial eosinophilia and injury seen on biopsy specimens as "consistent with" esophageal reflux disorder.

Barrett's Esophagus

The reader is referred to Chapter 6 for additional information on Barrett's esophagus. In the assessment of biopsy specimens for Barrett's esophagus, it can be difficult to determine both whether the tissue is metaplastic and whether it is dysplastic. These issues are also the most critical to clinical management [1••,2•,3–5]. Goblet cells, absorptive cells, or Paneth's cells typify metaplastic mucosa. Their absence, however, may make it impossible to differentiate metaplastic mucosa from true gastric mucosa, especially inflamed cardia or fundus in a sliding hiatal hernia. Even if intestinal metaplasia is seen, a diagnosis of Barrett's esophagus cannot be made unless the tissue has been shown to originate from the esophagus. As mentioned previously, esophageal submucosal glands or their ducts are a histopathologic marker of the esophagus but are not always present in random biopsy samples. Thus, if the mucosa is metaplastic and lacks these anatomic markers, the possibility of chronic carditis or pangastritis (with or without *H. pylori* infection) extending to the gastroesophageal junction cannot be excluded [6]. It may be helpful for the gastroenterologist to submit samples of the gastric antrum and corpus along with samples of the gastroesophageal junction to permit a clearer picture of the overall distribution of disease.

In patients with known Barrett's esophagus in whom surveillance for dysplasia is undertaken, ongoing inflammation and reactive epithelial atypia are frequently seen. As discussed previously, active inflammation accompanied by cytologic atypia often precludes definitive assessment for dysplasia. Therefore, surveillance biopsies should be performed, if possible, during asymptomatic periods or after aggressive antireflux therapy when the mucosa is less likely to be inflamed. When the mucosa is inflamed and significant epithelial atypia is seen, a diagnosis of "indefinite for dysplasia" may be made, signifying both uncertainty about the correct interpretation of the cytologic atypicality and concern that the tissue might truly be dysplastic. In such cases, repeat biopsy after an additional 3 to 6 months of antireflux therapy is appropriate. In the absence of active inflammation, dysplasia may be diagnosed more confidently and graded as either mild, moderate, or severe; more commonly, a two-grade system of high-grade and low-grade dysplasia is used, similar to that used for inflammatory bowel disease (Fig. 197-7).

Because the natural history of dysplasia in Barrett's esophagus is not yet fully understood, management decisions based on biopsy assessment of dysplasia are controversial. With a diagnosis of "negative for dysplasia," follow-up at regular intervals (*eg*, every 1 or 2 years) is continued. A diagnosis of low-grade dysplasia in the absence of a grossly identifiable mass on endoscopy generally leads to follow-up surveillance at shorter intervals (*eg*, every 3 to 6 months) because low-grade dysplasia has a high degree of interobserver variability. In contrast, a biopsy diagnosis of high-grade dysplasia in the absence of a visible mass usually prompts either repeat biopsy, with wider sampling in search of concomitant carcinoma, or surgical resection because high-grade dysplasia is associated with concomitant carcinoma in 30% of cases. In contrast to low-grade dysplasia, high-grade dysplasia has a low degree of interobserver variability. For either low-grade or high-grade dysplasia in the presence of a mass lesion, surgical resection of Barrett's esophagus is appropriate.

Esophageal Carcinoma

The reader is referred to Chapter 16 for additional information on esophageal carcinoma. Squamous cell carcinoma emerges through a sequence of progressive dysplasia to carcinoma *in situ* and finally to invasive carcinoma. Differentiation of squamous cell carcinoma from florid proliferation of regenerating immature

Figure 197-6

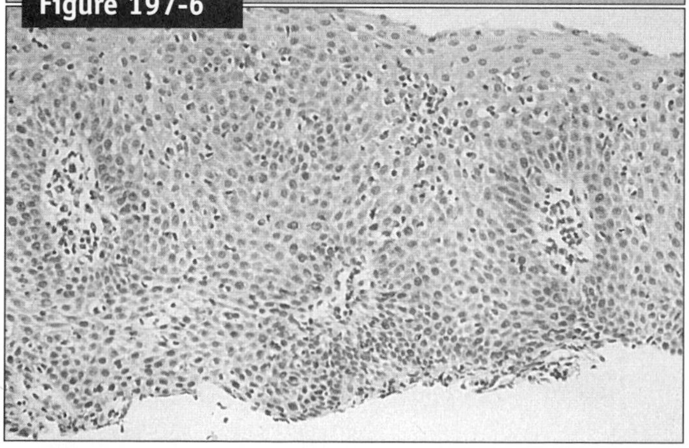

Esophageal squamous mucosa with intercellular edema and large numbers of intraepithelial eosinophils, changes that are characteristic of reflux esophagitis (original magnification × 35).

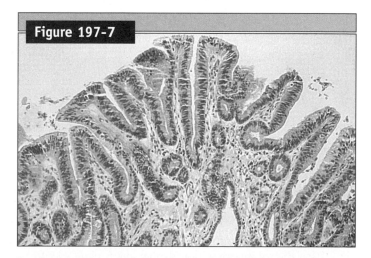

Figure 197-7

Esophageal biopsy specimen showing glandular mucosa with hyperchromatic enlarged epithelial nuclei that stratify to the surface of the cells in most foci, which is diagnostic of Barrett's esophagus with high-grade dysplasia (original magnification × 35).

squamous cells in severe esophagitis may be difficult, especially when active inflammation and necrosis are present. The effects of combined chemotherapy and radiation therapy also may mimic squamous dysplasia.

Early squamous cell carcinoma of the esophagus may present insidiously, and the mucosa may look normal at endoscopy. More commonly, flat, granular, plaquelike, or slightly depressed tumors are seen. Pathologically, superficial squamous cell carcinomas include not only *in situ* malignancies but also those that invade the submucosa and, therefore, that may be associated with lymph node metastasis. Deep giopsies to sample submucosal tissue may help to determine whether submucosal invasion is present. Because about 20% of superficial squamous carcinomas are multifocal, wide sampling with mapping may be appropriate in patients at risk or in those known to have squamous dysplasia. The prognosis of superficial squamous carcinoma is related primarily to the depth of invasion and the presence of lymph node metastasis rather than to tumor grade.

Adenocarcinomas almost always arise in patients with Barrett's esophagus and usually are associated with glandular dysplasia in the surrounding epithelium. The combination of adequate cytologic preparations and at least two endoscopic mucosal biopsy specimens from the edge and center of an ulcerating lesion confirms the diagnosis in nearly all cases. Biopsies may also be useful in mapping the extent of malignant epithelium.

For either squamous cell carcinoma or adenocarcinoma, endoscopic biopsy also may be useful after therapy to monitor for recurrent disease or to detect therapy-related complications.

Gastritis

The reader is referred to Chapters 18, 19, 27, 28, 31, 32, and 40 for additional information on gastritis. The endoscope is the diagnostic tool of choice for gastric mucosal disease and has replaced traditional radiologic procedures in most settings. Unfortunately, the diagnostic accuracy of endoscopic examination is limited. Correlations between endoscopic and histopathologic findings in the assessment of gastritis are particularly poor. The endoscopic appearance of the gastric mucosa may be highly deceptive: what appears to be normal gastric mucosa on endoscopy may be severe gastritis on biopsy, or vice versa. For this reason, it has been proposed that all gastroscopies be accompanied by biopsy sampling [7].

In the past, histopathologic assessment of chronic gastritis was of limited value because the features of specific etiologic types of gastritis were unknown. Autoimmune (type A) gastritis was recognized, with its microscopically distinctive histopathology and geographic distribution within the stomach; all other types of chronic gastritis, however, were lumped together as type B, or antral, gastritis. With the discovery that chronic gastritis usually is caused by *H. pylori* infection, pathologists have been able to recognize the distinctive microscopic features of this form of gastritis and to define the histopathology of the remaining forms of chronic gastritis more precisely [8•,9,10•]. Biopsy interpretation is now much more specific to cause and gives the gastroenterologist additional valuable information regarding complicating features, such as metaplasia, dysplasia, and malignancy.

Acute gastritis. The term *acute gastritis* is usually reserved for acute erosive conditions that typically result in mucosal necrosis and hemorrhage, with relatively little inflammation. Causes include alcohol, aspirin, other nonsteroidal anti-inflammatory drugs (NSAIDs), and shock, all of which produce identical histologic changes.

Chronic gastritis. Several distinct types of chronic gastritis can be differentiated histologically. Multiple gastritides may coexist. For example, coexistence of *H. pylori* gastritis and chemical gastritis may become obvious only after successful treatment of *H. pylori* infection. Most forms of chronic gastritis can produce long-term sequelae, such as intestinal or pyloric metaplasia, glandular atrophy, dysplasia, and neoplasia.

Helicobacter pylori **gastritis.** *H. pylori* gastritis involves the antrum, and biopsies of this area are usually diagnostic (Fig. 197-8); with severe long-standing disease, the body and fundus may also be involved. Organisms may be visible with a hematoxylin and eosin stain or may require special stains, such as a Warthin-Starry or thiazine stain (Fig. 197-9, see also **Color Plate**). Additional features include intestinal metaplasia, atrophic changes, G-cell hyperplasia, ulceration, and dysplasia.

Pitfalls in the biopsy diagnosis of *H. pylori* gastritis include previously treated disease and long-standing disease with widespread metaplasia. Treated *H. pylori* gastritis may be difficult to diagnose histopathologically because the neutrophilic inflammation resolves quickly but the chronic inflammation and lymphoid follicles may persist for more than 1 year. Also, the morphology of *H. pylori* may change after treatment. The diagnosis may also be difficult to establish if the patient is being treated with other drugs that reduce the load of organisms or change their distribution in the stomach, such as proton pump inhibitors or antibiotics for other infections. Diagnosis also may be difficult in severe disease with widespread intestinal metaplasia because the organisms do not attach readily to metaplastic cells. Biopsies of the proximal stomach are more likely to be diagnostic in these cases.

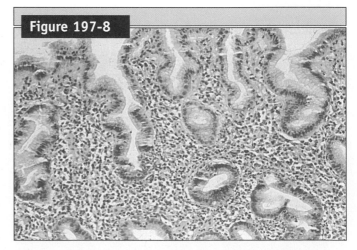

Figure 197-8

Gastric antral biopsy specimen shows the typical appearance of *Helicobacter pylori* gastritis characterized primarily by a dense lymphoplasmacytic cellular infiltrate in the lamina propria (original magnification × 16).

Bacterial gastritis that is similar to but typically more mild than *H. pylori* gastritis can be caused by *Helicobacter heilmannii* (formerly known as *Gastrospirillum hominis*) [11]. This organism can be identified by the same techniques used for *H. pylori*.

Autoimmune gastritis. Autoimmune gastritis typically involves the gastric body and fundus. For the pathologist to be certain of this distribution, biopsy samples of both the body and the antrum must be provided for comparison. If pernicious anemia is present, cellular atypia (macrocytosis) secondary to the metabolic defect may be difficult to differentiate from true dysplasia. Neuroendocrine (G-cell and enterochromaffin-like cell) hyperplasia is more common and severe in autoimmune gastritis than in other forms of chronic gastritis and may evolve into carcinoid tumors as a consequence of chronic hypergastrinemia. Therefore, samples should be taken from the antrum as well as the body and fundus in these patients.

Chemical gastritis. Chemical gastritis may be caused by a wide variety of injurious substances, including NSAIDs, bile, and alcohol and usually involves the antrum; antral biopsies are diagnostic in most cases (Fig. 197-10). When the antrum has been surgically removed, chronic reflux commonly involves the gastric body and fundic remnant, causing hyperplastic polypoid mucosa at the anastomotic site (chronic gastritis cystica polyposa). Endoscopic biopsy may be required to differentiate this form of severe, chronic chemical gastritis from carcinoma or to evaluate possible dysplastic changes in this condition because it predisposes to carcinoma.

Environmental gastritis (metaplastic atrophic gastritis, type B). Environmental gastritis is typically multifocal and can affect any part of the stomach; most commonly, it involves the junction of the antrum and body along the lesser curvature. Associated lesions include gastric ulcers, hyperplastic polyps, carcinoid tumors, and gastric carcinoma. The cause of this form of gastritis is not well defined and is thought to be related to the interplay of *H. pylori* infection either with ingested substances, such as nitrates, or with a lack of a protective substances, such as are found in fresh fruits and vegetables. The histologic picture is identical to that of *H. pylori* gastritis, except that no organisms are seen. For the pathologist, it is a diagnosis of exclusion, and the possibility of false-negative biopsy results for *H. pylori* makes it virtually impossible to diagnose this type with certainty.

Lymphocytic gastritis. Lymphocytic gastritis usually is clinically silent but produces an endoscopic appearance of varioloform gastritis, or thickened folds, most commonly in the gastric body, topped by small bumps or nodules with central depressions that may look like tiny erosions. The lesion is histopathologically distinctive and characterized by intense lymphocytic infiltration of the surface and foveolar epithelium, accompanied by surface and foveolar epithelial injury and lymphoplasmacytosis of the lamina propria (Fig. 197-11). Neutrophils and erosions are variable features. The intraepithelial lymphocytes are small mature T cells, most of which are CD8+ suppressor cells. This pattern of gastritis may be seen in association with *H. pylori*

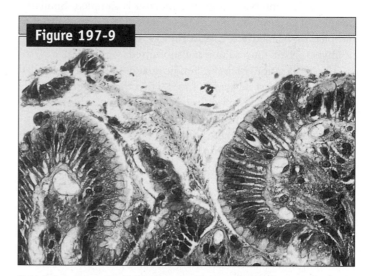

Figure 197-9

Thiazine staining for *Helicobacter pylori* reveals large numbers of short, plump, curved rods at the surface of the gastric antral mucosa (original magnification × 65). See also **Color Plate**.

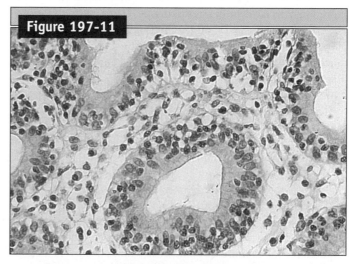

Figure 197-10

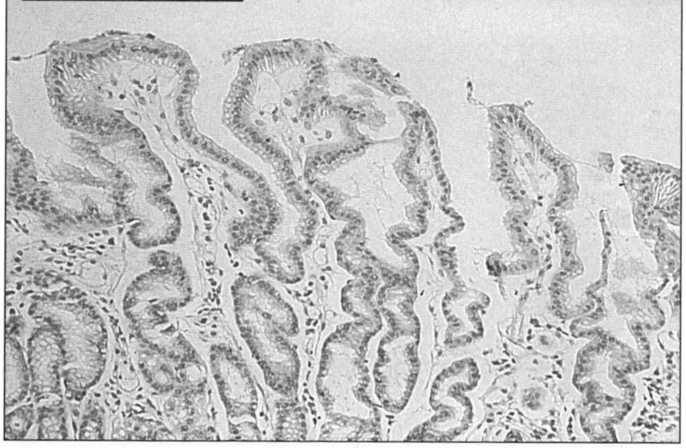

Chemical gastritis characteristically shows marked edema and epithelial injury with elongation and tortuosity of the gastric pits but little or no inflammatory cellular infiltration (original magnification × 16).

Figure 197-11

A marked increase in intraepithelial lymphocytes in the surface and foveolar epithelium is diagnostic of lymphocytic gastritis in this patient with celiac sprue (original magnification × 50).

infection, celiac disease, or gastric lymphoma, or as a precursor to Ménétrier's disease [12•,13,14,15•,16•].

Gastric Polyps

The reader is referred to Chapters 37 to 39 for additional information on gastric polyps. Most polyps in the stomach are focal mucosal hyperplasias (*eg*, hyperplastic polyps) or hamartomas (fundic gland polyps) and have little, if any, malignant potential. Exceptions are the relatively rare gastric adenomas and even rarer polypoid carcinomas. Because gastric hyperplastic polyps, adenomas, and carcinomas all typically occur in a background of chronic gastritis and may be difficult to differentiate endoscopically, diagnostic biopsy or endoscopic polypectomy is justified. Biopsy specimens of the intervening gastric mucosa can be as important as the polypectomy specimen for accurate interpretation of the overall process. For example, the pathologist cannot differentiate fragments of a gastric adenoma (a focal lesion) from chronic gastritis with high-grade dysplasia (a patchy or diffuse lesion) unless intervening gastric mucosa is sampled. Similarly, samples of hyperplastic polyps (focal lesions) appear identical to samples of Ménétrier's disease unless samples of intervening nonhyperplastic mucosa also are submitted.

The association between fundic gland polyps and familial polyposis coli must be kept in mind when this diagnosis is made by the pathologist; however, in most cases, these polyps are sporadic and incidental. In contrast, other hamartomas, such as juvenile polyps or Peutz-Jeghers polyps, usually occur in the stomach as part of a multiple hamartomatous polyposis syndrome.

Gastric Malignancy

The reader is referred to Chapters 38 and 39 for additional information on gastric malignancy. The ease with which gastric malignancy can be diagnosed by endoscopic biopsy may depend, in part, on the configuration and growth pattern of the tumor. Ulcerating malignancies are most common, and the probability of obtaining diagnostic tissue is greatly enhanced if all four quadrants of the ulcer edge, as well as the ulcer base, are sampled. If the lesion is a carcinoma, the peripheral biopsy specimens are more likely to be diagnostic; if it is a lymphoma, the ulcer base is more likely to contain diagnostic tissue. If the malignancy produces a pattern of rugal enlargement (giant folds), multiple, deep biopsy samples through the full thickness of the expanded mucosa in the most markedly affected area are most likely to be diagnostic. Among the various histologic types of gastric carcinoma, signet-ring cell carcinoma is by far the easiest to miss or misdiagnose on endoscopic biopsy. The infiltrating tumor cells may lack significant cytologic atypicality and masquerade as mucosal macrophages. Special stains for intestinal mucins or immunohistochemical stains for keratins or other epithelial markers may be needed to identify signet cells definitively, especially when they are few in number, widely scattered in the biopsy tissue, or masked by associated inflammation or fibrosis.

Diagnosis of gastric lymphoma typically poses more problems than that of gastric carcinoma because fresh tumor tissue may be required for the immunohistochemical studies needed to demonstrate clonality and to define the lymphoma subtype. Because gastric lymphomas often display prominent submucosal infiltration, repeated biopsies at a single site may facilitate diagnosis. The

tissue should be kept moist and cool and delivered for processing as quickly as possible after acquisition; placement on a piece of saline-soaked filter paper in an enclosed container works well.

The prognosis of gastric carcinoma depends primarily on the stage of the disease at diagnosis; histologic type is of secondary prognostic importance. For gastric lymphoma, however, both histologic type and stage are major prognostic factors.

Duodenitis

The reader is referred to Chapters 18 and 19 for additional information on duodenitis. The first portion of the duodenum commonly shows nonspecific inflammatory changes thought to relate to the effect of gastric acid. Severe inflammation of the duodenal bulb or active inflammation of more distal segments of the duodenum commonly indicate peptic disease related to *H. pylori* gastritis or chemical injury related to NSAIDs. The pathologist cannot accurately evaluate these possibilities without an accompanying antral biopsy. Thus, it is prudent to sample both the gastric antrum and duodenum if duodenitis is suspected.

In many cases of enteric parasitic infection, duodenal biopsy specimens are diagnostic. Although the appearance of the underlying mucosa may vary from essentially normal to sprue-like, the specific diagnosis is based on the presence of organisms. The duodenum is the tissue of choice for the diagnosis of giardiasis (Fig. 197-12) and strongyloidiasis and often yields diagnostic biopsies in immunosuppressed patients infected with *Mycobacterium avium* complex, cytomegalovirus, cryptosporidia, microsporidia (either *Enterocytozoon bieneusi* or *Encephalitozoon intestinalis*), *Isospora belli*, or *Pneumocystis carinii*.

Celiac Disease (Sprue)

The reader is referred to Chapter 54 for additional information on celiac disease. The most common indication for duodenal biopsy is the clinical suspicion of celiac disease. Although the biopsy appearance of the mucosa in celiac disease is distinctive (*ie*, complete flattening of villi, crypt hyperplasia, dense stromal lymphoplasmacytic infiltrates, and markedly increased intraepithelial lymphocytes; Fig. 197-13), it is not pathognomonic.

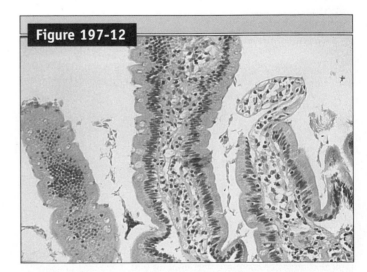

Figure 197-12

Duodenal biopsy specimen from a patient with giardiasis shows small collections of crescent-shaped organisms, about the size of an epithelial cell, between mucosal villi (original magnification × 35).

The same appearance may be produced by infections or chemical injuries of various types; however, the distribution of the mucosal changes in these disorders is seldom as diffuse and confluent as it is in celiac disease. Thus, in establishing the diagnosis of celiac disease, it is extremely helpful to sample the duodenum widely. If any of the biopsy specimens is uninvolved, celiac disease is virtually excluded. Because of the association between celiac disease and lymphocytic gastritis, biopsy of the antrum should not be overlooked in patients under evaluation for sprue.

Tumors

The reader is referred to Chapter 55 for additional information on tumors. Small intestinal adenomas and carcinomas occur more commonly in the duodenum than in any other region of the small intestine. The periampullary region is a common site of duodenal epithelial tumors, including neuroendocrine neoplasms such as carcinoids. Adequate endoscopic sampling establishes the histologic type of tumor in most cases; with tumors in the periampullary region, however, establishing the origin of the malignancy may be difficult. Precise diagnosis is important because duodenal and ampullary carcinomas are staged differently. Neuroendocrine tumors tend to grow submucosally and may require deep biopsy samples for diagnosis.

◼◼◼◼ LOWER GASTROINTESTINAL DISEASE
The Normal and the Pathologic
Ileum

In contrast to other parts of the gastrointestinal tract, the normal ileum is characterized by dense cellularity of the lamina propria with lymphoid follicle formation (Peyer's patches). The same mucosal appearance in any other small bowel segment would raise the suspicion of Crohn's disease, infection, or even lymphoma. Large numbers of granulocytes are abnormal, however, and granulocytic infiltration of the epithelium of villi or crypts suggests active inflammatory, infectious, or hypersensitivity disease.

Ileal biopsies are most useful in patients with thickening of the terminal ileum and a clinical differential diagnosis that includes Crohn's disease, *Yersinia enterocolitica* infection, intestinal tuberculosis, and lymphoma. Ileal biopsies also may help to differentiate ulcerative colitis from Crohn's disease. There are limitations, however, to the degree of assistance that the pathologist can provide because Crohn's ileitis and the back-wash ileitis of ulcerative colitis cannot be distinguished easily when active inflammation is present but ulceration and granulomas are absent. Moreover, architectural distortion, which is a marker of chronic inflammation, is difficult to judge in the ileum. Peyer's patches, which may vary markedly in size, cause varying degrees of displacement of mucosal crypts that can mimic crypt atrophy. The most reliable marker of chronic inflammatory injury of the ileum is pseudopyloric metaplasia, which is uncommon.

Colon and Rectum

The normal colonic mucosa has low stromal cellularity, scattered small lymphoid aggregates between colonic glands, and tubular, straight-sided glands that extend to the muscularis mucosae. Alterations of the colonic glandular architecture caused by repeated injury and repair, such as bifurcation, tortuosity, and shortening, are relied on to differentiate chronic from acute colonic disease (Fig. 197-14). The same is true of epithelial metaplasia, which is most commonly represented by the abnormal occurence of Paneth's cells in glands of the transverse or distal colon. Paneth's cells are normally found only in the cecal and proximal right colonic mucosa and are considered metaplastic elsewhere. The presence of these alterations, especially when marked, is diagnostic of chronicity but is nonspecific as to etiology. Any chronic inflammatory process may mimic inflammatory bowel disease histologically.

Acute Inflammatory and Ischemic Diseases
Maximizing the Odds of Making the Diagnosis

The reader is referred to Chapters 64, 65, and 73 to 80 for additional information on acute inflammatory and ischemic diseases. Most acute inflammatory and ischemic disorders of the colon produce lesions that are unevenly distributed throughout the colon. Typically, the histopathologic appearance also varies

Figure 197-13

Duodenal biopsy specimen in a patient with celiac sprue shows the typical changes of complete flattening of villi, increased lymphoplasmacytic cellular infiltration of the lamina propria, diffuse epithelial injury, and increased numbers of intraepithelial lymphocytes (original magnification × 16).

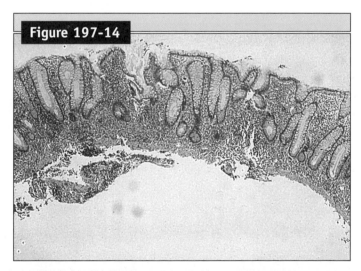

Figure 197-14

Colonic mucosa in a patient with ulcerative colitis shows the typical glandular architectural changes of chronic colitis, including gland branching, shortening, and tortuosity (original magnification × 16).

markedly with the temporal stage of the disease and many disorders are diagnostic only at an early stage of evolution (Figs. 197-15 and 197-16). Thus, strategic targeting of biopsies is essential if diagnostic tissue is to be acquired, as shown in Table 197-2. In general, obtaining five or more biopsy samples minimizes sampling error and maximizes the odds of acquiring diagnostic tissue.

Chronic Inflammation: Features Mimicking Inflammatory Bowel Disease

In the patient with diarrhea who undergoes colonoscopy, biopsy is an essential adjunct regardless of the appearance of the mucosa. At one end of the spectrum, the colon may look normal endoscopically, but microscopic colitis (ie, lymphocytic or collagenous colitis) may be present. At the other extreme, obvious colitis may be seen endoscopically, but differentiation between acute self-limited colitis and chronic inflammatory bowel disease may be possible only on microscopic examination.

A pathologic diagnosis of chronic colitis is made when glandular architectural distortion, metaplasia, or both are seen, although these features cannot be interpreted as definitive evidence of inflammatory bowel disease. A number of other conditions may produce identical changes in the colonic mucosa (Table 197-3), mimicking inflammatory bowel disease. In contrast, in some cases of early, quiescent, or successfully treated inflammatory bowel disease, chronic architectural changes may be lacking. In these cases, the pathologist can neither confirm nor exclude a diagnosis of inflammatory bowel disease and can comment only on the degree of ongoing inflammatory activity (Table 197-4); the presence or absence of special features, such as erosions, giant cells, and granulomas; and possibly, the distri-

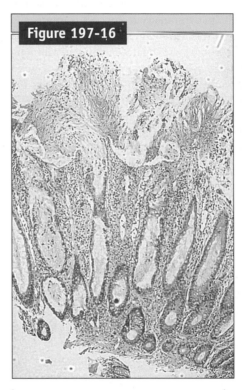

Figure 197-16

Colonic mucosa showing the early and most diagnostic phase of *Clostridium difficile* pseudomembranous colitis, in which "volcanic" lesions (fanlike streaming of fibrin, neutrophils, and necrotic epithelial cells from the mucosal surface) are present (original magnification × 35).

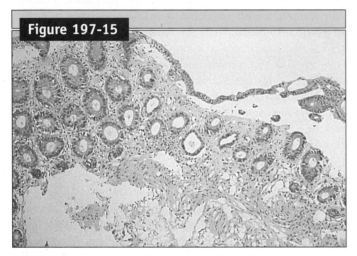

Figure 197-15

Colonic mucosal biopsy specimen showing the typical changes of the early phase of ischemic colitis, including marked fibrin deposition in the lamina propria and marked gland injury with focal dropout but little or no inflammation (original magnification × 16).

Table 197-2. Biopsy Guide to Colonic Inflammatory and Ischemic Disease

Disease	Usual location in colon	Characteristic legion to target
Microscopic colitis	Throughout*	No visible lesions
Collagenous colitis	Throughout*	No visible lesions
Pseudomembranous colitis	Right colon* Left colon	Small pustule (stage 2); avoid biopsy of pseudomembranes
Ischemic colitis	Right to transverse colon Sigmoid colon	Early erosion (avoid biopsy of pseudomembranes only)
Tuberculous colitis	Ileocecal valve	Most abnormal-appearing area
Yersinia enterocolitica infection	Ileocecal valve	Aphthous ulcers
Amebic colitis	Cecum (sigmoid)	Exudate from ulcer
Amyloidosis	Rectum	Submucosa
Acute self-limited colitis	Throughout	Nonulcerated but inflamed mucosa
Enterohemorrhagic *Escherichia coli* infection	Throughout Mainly right to transverse colon	Early erosion (avoid biopsy of pseudomembranes only)

*Lesions may be present only in the right colon.

bution of disease, if specimens from different colonic segments are submitted. Thus, a definitive diagnosis of inflammatory bowel disease cannot be made on endoscopic biopsy alone, and clinicopathologic correlation is required.

Dysplasia in Inflammatory Bowel Disease

The reader is referred to Chapters 73 and 74 for additional information on dysplasia in inflammatory bowel disease. Colonoscopic surveillance is common practice in patients with long-standing ulcerative colitis [17,18] and has been shown to reduce mortality from colorectal cancer [19]. Increasingly, surveillance is also being undertaken in patients with Crohn's disease. The problems associated with the assessment of mucosal dysplasia in inflammatory bowel disease are identical to those for Barrett's esophagus (discussed previously), although recommendations for management based on surveillance biopsy results are perhaps better defined in inflammatory bowel disease.

Colorectal Polyps

The reader is referred to Chapter 80 for additional information on colorectal polyps. Endoscopically resected or sampled colorectal polyps are among the most common specimens encountered in gastrointestinal pathology and present the pathologist with some unique problems.

Colonic Adenomas

Terminology. In general, pathologists reserve the term *tubular adenoma* for adenomas composed entirely of tubular structures or less than 5% villous structures (Fig. 197-17). *Tubulovillous adenomas* are intermediate between tubular and villous

adenomas; however, definitions of the proportions of the components vary, and no universal definition has been accepted among pathologists. Some regard tubular adenomas with any villous components as tubulovillous. Thus, villous adenomas have been variably defined as more than 50% villous, more than 75% villous, more than 80% villous, or 100% villous. This lack of uniformity in terminology can be frustrating for both the pathologist and clinician. However, the histologic subclassification of the adenoma is of relatively little importance. Rather, the size of the adenoma is far more predictive of malignancy than is its histologic type, and an adenoma of any type that is more than 2 cm in diameter has a high likelihood (about 35% to 50%) of harboring invasive carcinoma. Any type of adenoma may be either *sessile* or *stalked*.

A unique histologic type of adenoma usually classified separately from tubular, tubulovillous, or villous adenomas is the *serrated adenoma*. This lesion has the cytologic features of an adenoma but the architectural features of a hyperplastic polyp. Serrated adenomas are true adenomas, with the same propensity for malignant transformation as other types of adenomas.

Table 197-3. Histologic Features Mimicking Inflammatory Bowel Disease

Chronic ischemic bowel disease

Vasculitis

Radiation colitis

Diverticular disease–associated segmental colitis

Enterocolonic endometriosis

Nonsteroidal anti-inflammatory drug–associated enterocolitis

Chronic laxative abuse

Pneumatosis intestinalis

Colitis in Behçet's disease

Chronic infection without granulomas
    Amebic colitis
    Chronic salmonellosis

Granulomatous diseases
    Chronic granulomatous disease of childhood
    Enteric tuberculosis
    Enteric histoplasmosis
    Yersinia enterocolitica infection
    Chronic salmonellosis
    Cytomegalovirus colitis

Enterohemorrhagic *Escherichia coli* infection

Rectal prolapse (solitary rectal ulcer syndrom) chronic graft
    vs. host disease

Diversion loop colitis

Table 197-4. Pathologic Grading of Activity in Acute or Chronic Colitis

Minimal	A few scattered glands show infiltration by sparse numbers of granulocytes (eosinophils or neutrophils); usually unaccompanied by significant stromal inflammatory infiltrates.
Mild	Cryptitis (glandular epithelial infiltration by granulocytes) is present multifocally, but no crypt abscesses are present; with or without inflammatory infiltrates in the lamina propria.
Moderate	Cryptitis and crypt abscesses are present along with increased stromal cellularity (inflammatory infiltrates in the lamina propria); no erosion or ulceration.
Severe	Marked cryptitis and numerous crypt abscesses with focal erosion or ulceration; stromal cellularity that typically is dense.

Figure 197-17

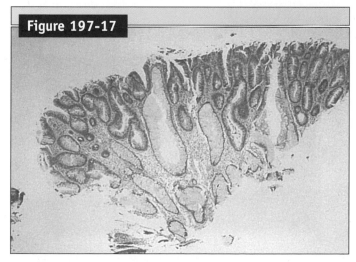

Tubular adenoma composed entirely of adenomatous glands and containing no villous projections (original magnification × 16).

Evaluation of adenomas for malignancy. The histopathologic term *carcinoma in situ* is synonymous with severe epithelial dysplasia and intraepithelial carcinoma. It refers to cytologically and histologically defined malignancy that is confined to the epithelium; that is, the malignant cells do not penetrate the glandular basement membrane to invade the surrounding lamina propria. The Tumor-Node-Metastasis (TNM) Staging System for colon cancer of the American Joint Committee on Cancer and the International Union Against Cancer define carcinoma *in situ* differently [20]. The primary tumor category, designated as Tis (carcinoma *in situ*), includes both intraepithelial carcinomas and carcinomas that invade the lamina propria up to and including the muscularis mucosae. These tumors are also known as *intramucosal carcinomas*. Thus, the definition of pTis (*p* stands for pathologic, as opposed to clinically determined, T category) is a pathophysiologic rather than structural one and is based on the observation that intramucosal tumors have virtually no metastatic potential because of the lack of lymphatics in the colonic mucosa. If a polyp with pTis is completely removed, no further therapy is required.

It may be extremely difficult to determine whether invasive malignancy is present. Carcinoma invading the submucosa of the head or stalk of an adenoma is usually recognized most easily by the irregular shapes of the infiltrating glands and the reactive, fibrotic nature of the periglandular stroma. Occasionally, however, no stromal reaction is discernible, and the invasive glands are well formed, making the diagnosis of invasion difficult. More commonly, the changes produced by ischemic injury and repair in the polyp head, known as pseudoinvasion (discussed previously), lead to diagnostic uncertainty and interobserver variability. Unfortunately, pseudoinvasion or glandular entrapment occurs in 2.5% to 10% of adenomas, about the same frequency as invasive carcinoma. If uncertainty exists even after consultation has been sought, it is wisest to assume that carcinoma is present and treat accordingly.

Even when invasive carcinoma is easily recognized in an adenomatous polyp, problems may arise in the assessment of microscopic features associated with adverse outcome (eg, metastasis, local recurrence, or both). Accurate evaluation of these features is essential and constitutes a key element in deciding whether segmental surgical resection should be performed. The risk of metastatic disease in polyps with invasive carcinoma correlates with high tumor grade, cancer involving the entire polyp head, angiolymphatic invasion or invasion to the level of the submucosa (particularly in polyps lacking stalks), and positive resection margins. Local recurrence has also been shown to correlate with positive resection margins. In short, endoscopically removed malignant polyps with a negative margin (cancer more than 1 mm from the margin), grade I or II cancer, and absence of lymphatic or venous invasion probably are curable with polypectomy alone. The most common difficulties lie in diagnosing angiolymphatic invasion (because interobserver variability is high) and in identifying the surgical margin. The latter may be precluded by fragmentation of the polyp on removal.

Hyperplastic Polyps

Many pathologists believe that hyperplastic polyps are not precursors of neoplasms. Others believe that a small proportion (estimates vary from 1% to 10%) may undergo adenomatous transformation and that hyperplastic lesions more than 1 cm in diameter should be examined with multiple sections to exclude adenomatous foci. Polyps composed partly of adenomatous epithelium and partly of hyperplastic epithelium (in separate, distinct glands) are called *mixed* polyps. They should be regarded as adenomas for purposes of treatment, follow-up, and assessment of colorectal cancer risk.

Hamartomatous Polyps

Among the hamartomatous polyps, juvenile polyps are the only type that commonly occurs sporadically and singly, outside of a multiple hamartomatous polyposis syndrome. Solitary, sporadic juvenile polyps typically occur in children younger than 10 years and are usually located in the rectosigmoid colon (Fig. 197-18). However, they may occur at any age, be of any size, and arise anywhere in the colon.

Once thought to be benign lesions, harmartomatous polyps are now considered to have malignant potential because of increasing reports of dysplastic and adenomatous transformation and the demonstrated increased risk of colorectal carcinoma in patients with familial juvenile polyposis, nonfamilial juvenile polyposis, and Peutz-Jegher polyposis. The frequency of adenomatous and carcinomatous transformation of these lesions is unknown. Foci of dysplasia or adenomatous change should be sought in all hamartomatous polyps, and care must be taken to differentiate true dysplasia and adenomatous transformation from reactive changes in glands located near an eroded surface or involved by inflammation.

Mucosal Prolapse Polyps

Mucosal prolapse polyps encompass a group of lesions with a common etiology, namely, prolapse of a polypoid excrescence of mucosa into the gut lumen, with secondary ischemic injury and repair (Fig. 197-19, see also **Color Plate**) [21–23,24•, 25,26•,27]. This family of polyps includes the polypoid phase of solitary rectal ulcers, inflammatory cloacogenic polyps at the anorectal junction, prolapsing mucosal folds in diverticular

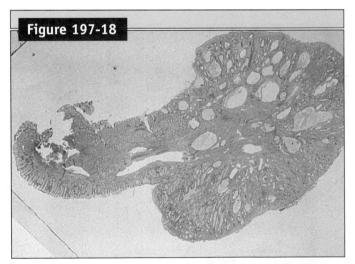

Figure 197-18

Juvenile polyp, characteristically composed of cystically dilated, cytologically normal glands separated by abundant edematous and inflamed lamina propria (original magnification × 10).

disease, fibrin cap or inflammatory cap polyps, and inflammatory myogenic polyps. Mucosal prolapse polyps also occur occasionally in the gastric antrum and the small bowel. Prolapse polyps are usually solitary; however, as many as 30 polyps in a single colonic region have been described in patients.

Although prolapse polyps may be incidental findings, they may have underlying conditions as follows:
- Adjacent to colonic adenomas or carcinomas
- In colostomies or ileostomies
- In ileoanal pouches
- In diverticular disease (in mucosa between diverticular openings)
- In ulcerative colitis
- With endometriosis

The histology of mucosal prolapse polyps in all of these settings is similar; however, polyps associated with diverticular disease are often distinctive, with a broad and somewhat flattened tonguelike appearance. Mucosal prolapse polyps have no known malignant potential.

Colorectal Malignancy

The reader is referred to Chapter 81 for additional information on colorectal malignancy. The diagnosis of colorectal malignancy by endoscopic biopsy is often complicated by procedural difficulties and sampling errors that produce false-negative or nondiagnostic results. Diagnostic yield is improved by multiple biopsies and sampling sites. At least five samples, taken from both the edges and the center of an ulcerated mass, should be acquired. Even when invasive malignancy is seen, the depth of invasion cannot be assessed accurately by endoscopic biopsy alone. Invasion into muscle should be noted; however, distinguishing invasion of muscularis mucosae from invasion of muscularis propria is not possible. Additional features of prognostic importance that may be assessed by endoscopic biopsy include the following:
- The histologic type of tumor (*eg*, signet-ring cell adenocarcinoma or mucinous adenocarcinoma)

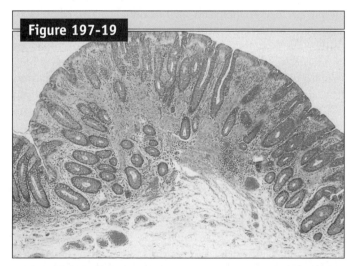

Figure 197-19

Marked fibromuscular proliferation of the lamina propria, characteristic of a mucosal prolapse polyp (original magnification × 16). See also **Color Plate**.

- The histologic grade of tumor (grades 1 through 4, corresponding to well, moderately, poorly, and undifferentiated carcinoma, respectively)
- Angiolymphatic invasion (an independent indicator of unfavorable outcome)

▨ REFERENCES

Recently published papers of particular interest have been highlighted as follows:
- •   Of interest
- ••   Of outstanding interest

1.•• Haggitt R: Barrett's esophagus, dysplasia and adenocarcinoma. *Hum Pathol* 1994, 25:982–993.
The pathologic analysis and biologic significance of Barrett's esophagus are discussed thoroughly and clearly in this reference.

2.• Levine DS, Haggitt RC, Blount PL,*et al.*: An endoscopic biopsy protocol can differentiate high-grade dysplasia from early adenocarcinoma in Barrett's esophagus. *Gastroenterology* 1993, 105:40–50.
A rigorous protocol is presented here for surveillance of patients with Barrett's esophagus and high-grade dysplasia that may save some patients from having surgical resection.

3. McArdle JE, Lewin KJ, Randall G, *et al.*: Distribution of dysplasias and early invasive carcinoma in Barrett's esophagus. *Hum Pathol* 1992, 23:479–482.

4. Pera M, Trastek VF, Carpenter HA, *et al.*: Barrett's esophagus with high-grade dysplasia: an indication for esophagectomy? *Ann Thorac Surg* 1992, 54:199–204.

5. Streitz JM, Andrews CW, Ellis FH: Endoscopic surveillance of Barrett's esophagus. *J Thorac Surg* 1993, 105:383–388.

6. Genta RM, Huberman RM, Graham DY: The gastric cardia in *Helicobacter pylori* infection. *Hum Pathol* 1994, 25:915–919.

7. Carpenter HA, Talley NJ: Gastroscopy is incomplete without biopsy: clinical relevance of distinguishing gastropathy from gastritis. *Gastroenterology* 1995, 108:917–924.

8.• Appelman HD: Gastritis: terminology, etiology, and clinicopathological correlations: another biased view. *Hum Pathol* 1994, 25:1006–1019.
In this article the histologic classification and clinicopathologic correlations of the recognized forms of gastritis are discussed from a pathologist's point of view and beautifully depicted.

9. Correa P, Yardley JH: Grading and classification of chronic gastritis: one American response to the Sydney system. *Gastroenterology* 1992, 102:353–359.

10.• Dixon MF: Recent advances in gastritis. *Curr Diagn Pathol* 1994, 1:80–89.
This article presents the British point of view on the current pathologic classifications of gastritis.

11. Yeomans ND, Kolt SD: *Helicobacter heilmannii* (formerly *Gastrospirillum*): association with pig and human gastric pathology. *Gastroenterology* 1996, 111:244–259.

12.• Niemelä S, Karttunen T, Kerola T, *et al.*: Ten year follow-up of lymphocytic gastritis: further evidence on *Helicobacter pylori* as a cause of lymphocytic gastritis and corpus gastritis. *J Clin Pathol* 1995, 48:1111–1116.
In this article the authors present compelling evidence linking *H. pylori* infection to lymphocytic gastritis.

13. De Giacomo C, Gianatti A, Negrini R, *et al.*: Lymphocytic gastritis: a positive relationship with celiac disease. *J Pediatr* 1994, 124:57–62.

14. Groisman GM, George J, Berman D, *et al.*: Resolution of protein-losing lymphocytic gastritis with therapeutic eradication of *Helicobacter pylori*. *Am J Gastroenterol* 1994, 89:1548–1551.

15.• Lynch DAF, Sobala GM, Dixon MF, *et al.*: Lymphocytic gastritis and associated small bowel disease: a diffuse lymphocytic gastroenteropathy? *J Clin Pathol* 1995, 48:939–945.
The authors present compelling evidence linking gluten sensitivity to lymphocytic gastritis.

16.• Miettinen A, Karttunen TJ, Alavaikko M: Lymphocytic gastritis and *Helicobacter pylori* infection in gastric lymphoma. *Gut* 1995, 37:471–476.
This paper describes evidence suggesting a possible association between gastric lymphoma and lymphocytic gastritis, perhaps with *H. pylori* infection as the common denominator.

17. Levin B: Inflammatory bowel disease and colon cancer. *Cancer* 1992, 70:1313–1316.

18. Levin B: Ulcerative colitis and colon cancer: biology and surveillance. *J Cell Biochem Suppl* 1992, 16G:47–50.

19. Choi PM, Nugent FW, Schoetz DJ, *et al.*: Colonoscopic surveillance reduces mortality from colorectal cancer in ulcerative colitis. *Gastroenterology* 1993, 105:418–424.

20. Fleming ID, Cooper JS, Henson DE, *et al.*: *AJCC Manual for Staging of Cancer*, edn 5. Philadelphia: Lippincott-Raven Publishers; 1997.

21. Chetty R, Bhathal PS, Slavin JL: Prolapse-induced inflammatory polyps of the colorectum and anal transitional zone. *Histopathology* 1993, 23:63–67.

22. Campbell AP, Cobb CA, Chapman RWG, *et al.*: Cap polyposis: an unusual cause of diarrhoea. *Gut* 1993, 34:562–564.

23. Kang YS, Kamm MA, Engel AF, *et al.*: Pathology of the rectal wall in solitary rectal ulcer syndrome and complete rectal prolapse. *Gut* 1996, 38:587–590.

24.• Kelly JK: Polypoid prolapsing mucosal folds in diverticular disease. *Am J Surg Pathol* 1991, 15:871–878.
This article is the definitive pathologic publication on this topic, with beautiful macroscopic and microscopic depiction.

25. Tjandra JJ, Fazio VW, Church JM, *et al.*: Clinical conundrum of solitary rectal ulcer. *Dis Colon Rectum* 1992, 35:227–234.

26.• Tjandra JJ, Fazio VW, Petras RE, *et al.*: Clinical and pathologic factors associated with delayed diagnosis in solitary rectal ulcer syndrome. *Dis Colon Rectum* 1993, 36:146–153.
This article provides a thorough clinicopathologic analysis of solitary rectal ulcer syndrome in 25 patients.

27. Washington K, Rourk MH, McDonagh, *et al.*: Inflammatory cloacogenic polyp in a child: part of the spectrum of solitary rectal ulcer syndrome. *Pediatr Pathol* 1993, 13:409–414.

198 Surgery in Patients with Gastrointestinal and Liver Disease

Mark W. Russo, Steven Zacks, and Ian Grimm

Many people have gastrointestinal and liver diseases, and people with these disorders may require surgery for unrelated reasons. This chapter discusses the perioperative management of patients with a variety of gastrointestinal and hepatic disorders who require surgery.

■ MANAGEMENT OF THE SURGICAL PATIENT WITH ESOPHAGEAL DISEASE

Gastroesophageal Reflux Disease

Gastroesophageal reflux disease (GERD) is common in many people undergoing surgery (see Chapter 3). Approximately one third of the population complains of heartburn, with 7% experiencing symptoms daily [1]. Although reflux symptoms are reported equally by men and women, extensive esophagitis is more likely to occur in men. Complications of GERD, such as stricture formation, are more common in older people.

If occasional retrosternal burning or discomfort is the patient's only complaint, additional investigation is unnecessary before surgery. Atypical symptoms, such as wheezing or nocturnal cough, may reflect aspiration and not underlying asthma or chronic obstructive pulmonary disease. Thus, it may be better to postpone elective surgery until after such respiratory symptoms have been evaluated and treated. Symptoms of GERD and esophageal motility disorders occasionally can mimic those of coronary artery disease. Retrosternal discomfort can represent underlying coronary artery disease, especially in people with a family history of heart disease or other risk factors, such as diabetes or hypercholesterolemia. Symptomatic coronary artery disease may need to be excluded by exercise tolerance testing or nuclear imaging in high-risk patients who are scheduled for elective surgery.

Assessment for GERD may include upper endoscopy and an ambulatory esophageal pH study (Fig. 198-1). Esophageal manometry is performed if a motility disorder is suspected. Once the diagnosis of esophageal disease is established, consideration should be given to the possible presence of complications.

Preoperative findings that merit investigation include dysphagia, regurgitation, and anemia. Dysphagia or regurgitation may indicate the presence of a stricture or Zenker's diverticulum. Either of these entities increases the risk of postoperative aspiration and could lead to esophageal perforation when blind esophageal intubation is required intra- or postoperatively. Patients with these symptoms should undergo preoperative assessment, either by careful upper endoscopy or a barium esophagogram. A history of hoarseness and wheezing may indicate the presence of pulmonary complications of reflux disease. A chest roentgenogram and additional evaluation of pulmonary function may be indicated. Persons with GERD who have a positive result of a fecal occult blood test or anemia should also be evaluated by upper endoscopy to determine if esophagitis is the source of bleeding. Preoperative assessment of anemia in those with GERD is especially important if postoperative anticoagulation is anticipated.

Few physical findings are associated with GERD unless there is an underlying systemic disorder, such as obesity, diabetes mellitus, smoking, scleroderma, polymyositis, dermatomyositis, CREST (calcinosis, Raynaud's phenomenon, esophageal dysmotility, sclerodactyly, telangiectasia) syndrome, and hereditary hollow visceral myopathy, neuropathy. Some patients with GERD develop erosion of the enamel of the posterior molars, canine teeth, and incisors. Specific questions in the history and a focused physical examination should identify these conditions, which may require management postoperatively.

The risk of aspiration in patients with uncomplicated GERD who undergo elective surgery is minimal [2]; however, strictures and erosive esophagitis with bleeding are complications of reflux disease that could affect postoperative care. Because agents with anticholinergic properties decrease the pressure of the lower esophageal sphincter (LES) and impede saliva production, these drugs should be used judiciously. Antisecretory therapy with either H_2-receptor antagonists or proton pump inhibitors should be reinstituted as soon as possible in patients who were taking these medications before surgery. Prokinetic agents to increase LES pressure (*eg*, cisapride, 10 mg orally with meals and at bedtime) can be added to the antireflux regimen in patients who respond only partially to antisecretory therapy. Antireflux precautions, specifically elevation of the head of the bed, should be instituted. Whether placement of a nasogastric tube promotes reflux has been a matter of debate. In a study of normal persons with an indwelling nasogastric tube for a 6-hour period, no difference was seen in the number of reflux episodes or the duration of time that esophageal pH was lower than 4 compared with persons without a nasogastric tube in place [3]. Thus, contrary to popular belief, the presence of a tube across the esophagogastric junction may not promote reflux.

Achalasia

Patients who complain of chronic dysphagia to solids and liquids and regurgitation may have achalasia. Achalasia is important to recognize preoperatively because of the increased risk of aspiration during induction of anesthesia or postoperatively. Assessment for achalasia ideally should take place before surgery. If endoscopic or surgical therapy is not performed preoperatively, then efforts should focus on preventing aspiration, primarily by elevating the head of the bed. In patients with a tortuous enlarged "sigmoid" esophagus, consideration should be given to preoperative evacuation of esophageal contents using a large bore tube or endoscopic lavage.

▬ MANAGEMENT OF PATIENTS UNDERGOING SURGERY WITH PEPTIC ULCER DISEASE

Peptic ulcer disease is common, and many patients undergoing surgery may have unrecognized ulcers or develop them in the perioperative period (see Chapter 30). Patients with active peptic ulcers who undergo unrelated surgery do not appear to be at increased risk of postoperative hemorrhage [4,5]. However, preoperative assessment may uncover reasons to postpone surgery in patients with symptoms of ulcers. If complications such as recent bleeding or gastric outlet obstruction are present, then elective surgical procedures should be deferred, and the patient should undergo definitive treatment of the ulcer complication. Patients with dyspepsia and positive test results for fecal occult blood should undergo upper endoscopy. If gastric outlet obstruction is suspected, nasogastric suctioning should be instituted and upper endoscopy performed to confirm the presence and determine the cause of the obstruction. Signs

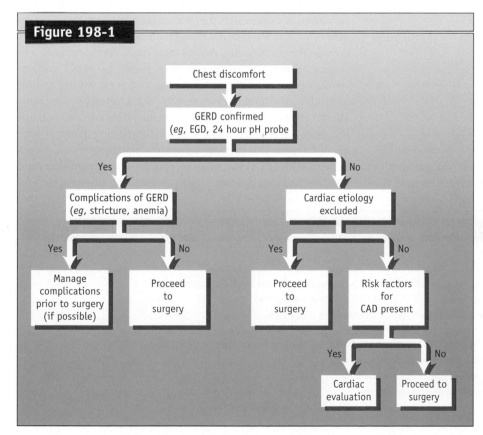

Figure 198-1

Chest discomfort

↓

GERD confirmed
(*eg*, EGD, 24 hour pH probe

Yes ← → No

Complications of GERD
(*eg*, stricture, anemia)   Cardiac etiology excluded

Yes → No   Yes → No

Manage complications prior to surgery (if possible)   Proceed to surgery   Proceed to surgery   Risk factors for CAD present

Yes → No

Cardiac evaluation   Proceed to surgery

Algorithm for preoperative assessment of patients with reflux symptoms. GERD—gastroesophageal reflux disease; EGD—esophagogastroduodenoscopy; CAD—coronary artery disease.

of free perforation into the peritoneal cavity usually are obvious, easy to document by plain radiographic film of the abdomen, and contraindicate endoscopy. Posterior penetrating ulcers can be more subtle in their presentation. A history of recurrent ulcers with intractable pain and diarrhea necessitates evaluation for gastrinoma.

Patients with documented peptic ulcer ideally should complete a course of antisecretory therapy before undergoing elective surgery. For patients with *Helicobacter pylori* infection, including virtually all patients with duodenal ulcers, antimicrobial regimens that include a proton pump inhibitor and two antibiotics can be completed in 7 days (*eg*, omeprazole, 20 mg orally twice daily; clarithromycin, 500 mg orally twice daily; and metronidazole, 500 mg orally three times daily). Patients with nonulcer dyspepsia can proceed to surgery without delay.

In the postoperative period, potential complications of peptic ulcers and ulcer treatment should be stressed. Acid suppression may increase the risk of aspiration pneumonia by promoting gastric bacterial overgrowth [6,7]. Precautions against aspiration should be taken, including elevation of the head of the bed, nasogastric decompression, and in special circumstances endotracheal intubation. Ulcer surgery may be complicated by gastroparesis, partial mechanical obstruction, or pseudo-obstruction, all of which can cause vomiting and aspiration. Pseudo-obstruction may result from electrolyte disturbances or narcotics. Nasogastric decompression, early mobilization, and treatment with prokinetic agents are important therapeutic approaches. Acid-base status should be monitored carefully in patients requiring prolonged nasogastric suction because of the possibility of hypochloremic alkalosis.

Stress ulceration can be a cause of gastrointestinal hemorrhage in the postoperative period (see Chapter 31). Risk factors for this complication include the following:

Ulceration
Respiratory failure
Coagulopathy
Sepsis
Renal failure
Hypotension
Pancreatitis
Liver failure

Coagulopathy and mechanical ventilation have been identified as two major independent risk factors; however, the presence of only one of these conditions may not significantly increase the postoperative risk of bleeding in patients with ulcers [5,8••]. Mortality rates may be as high as 40% in patients who bleed from stress ulceration [6]. Prophylactic administration of H_2-receptor antagonists or proton pump inhibitors and elimination of the underlying predisposing factors may prevent bleeding in 88% to 97% of patients [9]. Compared with H_2 blockers, prophylaxis with sucralfate has been associated with a lower risk of aspiration pneumonia and less bleeding [7].

■ MANAGEMENT OF THE SURGICAL PATIENT WITH INFLAMMATORY BOWEL DISEASE

Inflammatory bowel disease (IBD) is uncommon compared with ulcer disease and GERD; however, patients with IBD may require special care during the pre- and postoperative periods.

Complications of ulcerative colitis and Crohn's disease that may affect the operative course are listed in Table 198-1. Preoperative evaluation of any patient with IBD undergoing surgery should include assessment of intravascular volume and electrolyte status, as well as evaluation of extraintestinal manifestations of IBD. Persons with active disease and diarrhea may be dehydrated or have electrolyte abnormalities. Potassium, magnesium, and bicarbonate deficits should be replaced when necessary. Up to 5% of patients with ulcerative colitis can have coexisting ankylosing spondylitis, and rarely the cervical spine may be involved. Before airway intubation, films of the cervical spine may be necessary in those with severe erosive disease and poor cervical mobility. When liver test values are elevated and biliary surgery is planned, evaluation for primary sclerosing cholangitis and other liver diseases is prudent before anesthesia is given.

A thorough medication history is essential, particularly with regard to corticosteroid use. Stress doses of corticosteroids (*eg*, hydrocortisone, 100 mg intravenously every 8 hours) should be prescribed postoperatively for patients taking corticosteroids at the time of surgery. Patients not taking corticosteroids who have taken them in the past also may require stress doses postoperatively. The surgical team understandably may prefer to avoid corticosteroids because of the associated risk of poor wound healing and infection. In this case, results of a Cortrosyn (Organon, West Orange, NJ) adrenocorticotropic hormone stimulation test may help guide therapy by distinguishing patients with adrenal suppression from those with adequate adrenal reserves. Patients with IBD, especially those with ongoing gastrointestinal bleeding and iron deficiency or those receiving myelosuppressive

---

Table 198-1. Conditions Associated with Inflammatory Bowel Disease That May Affect Perioperative Care

Perioperative Assessment	Perioperative management
Diarrhea	Intravenous hydration, electrolyte replacement, exclude infectious etiology
Recent steroid use	Stress-dose steroids (hydrocortisone, 100 mg every 8 h)
Elevated liver function tests	Review medications, assess for sclerosing cholangitis
Abdominal pain or distention	Exclude toxic megacolon, serial abdominal films, give nothing by mouth, surgical consultation, intravenous hydration and intravenous antibiotics, discontinue narcotics
Hypercoagulable state	Compression boots, subcutaneous heparin
Erythema nodosum	Exclude infectious causes, analgesia
Pyoderma gangrenosum	Steroids, aggressive wound care
Erosive arthritis	If cervical involvement, check cervical spine films to assess upper airway

drugs such as azathioprine or 6-mercaptopurine, require close monitoring of blood counts. Once gastrointestinal function has returned to normal, oral medications can be resumed when oral intake is permitted.

A worrisome complication of IBD is toxic megacolon. Thus, if possible, narcotics and agents with anticholinergic properties should be avoided. Repeated abdominal examinations are indicated, and early mobility to help stimulate gut motility is encouraged. If abdominal distention or pain develops, abdominal plain films should be obtained. Early surgical consultation is appropriate. Prolonged bedrest also may have a deleterious effect on patients with severe osteoporosis and should be avoided.

■ MANAGEMENT OF THE SURGICAL PATIENT WITH A HISTORY OF INTESTINAL OBSTRUCTION OR PSEUDO-OBSTRUCTION

A history of medical conditions or medications that impair gastric or intestinal motility should be ascertained before surgery (Table 198-2) (see Chapters 26 and 51). For example, patients with diabetes mellitus or hypothyroidism and those taking anticholinergic medication may be at increased risk of gastroparesis and pulmonary aspiration. If the risk of aspirating gastric contents is increased, nasogastric suctioning should be instituted preoperatively. Patients with a history of abdominal surgery, such as those with IBD, are at increased risk of intestinal obstruction from adhesions. Therefore, patients at increased risk of obstruction who complain of abdominal pain, nausea, and vomiting in the presence of abdominal distention warrant a prompt evaluation with abdominal plain films.

Mechanical obstruction must be distinguished from ileus or pseudo-obstruction, and this usually can be determined with abdominal plain films. Features suggestive of mechanical obstruction include lack of gas distal to the obstruction, dilated loops of bowel proximal to the obstruction, and multiple air-fluid levels, often described as a "stepladder" pattern. In pseudo-obstruction, there are fewer air fluid levels, and gas is present distal to the site of obstruction. Intestinal obstruction can prolong postoperative recovery by causing abdominal distention, which impairs diaphragmatic mobility and ventilation. Atelectasis or aspiration pneumonia may result. Fever and sepsis may result from bacterial translocation through the bowel wall.

Small-bowel obstruction should be treated with nasogastric decompression and intravenous fluid and electrolyte replacement. If conservative therapy fails, surgery may be necessary. Pseudo-obstruction usually can be managed by correction of electrolyte disturbances and discontinuation of offending medications and by treatment of underlying infections. Narcotics and other agents that decrease intestinal motility should be discontinued, if possible.

The effect of narcotics on postoperative intestinal function and recovery was evaluated in a study of 90 patients who were randomly assigned to intramuscular morphine, patient-controlled analgesia (PCA) with morphine, or intramuscular ketorolac. Those assigned to ketorolac were least likely to develop an ileus and had the shortest hospital stay [10]. However, the group receiving ketorolac required additional analgesia compared with the group receiving morphine, whereas the group using PCA was the most satisfied with pain control. These results raise the possibility that a combination of ketorolac and PCA morphine would adequately relieve postoperative pain and minimize the adverse effects associated with narcotics.

■ MANAGEMENT OF THE SURGICAL PATIENT WITH DIARRHEA

Acute diarrhea has many causes but most commonly results from medications or an infection (Table 198-3). Infectious diarrhea is often viral and self-limiting, whereas drug-induced diarrhea stops quickly after discontinuation of the offending medication. Thus, routine postoperative stool cultures on patients with diarrhea have a low yield and incur unnecessary costs [11]. Today, any persisting or recurrent diarrheal illness is an indication to exclude HIV-related disease (see Chapter 60). Tests for *Clostridium difficile* toxin, enteric bacterial pathogens, and fecal leukocytes are indicated if diarrhea is severe and in patients presenting with a suspected exacerbation of IBD. Prompt exclusion of *C. difficile* infection is critical in any patient who develops diarrhea on or after a course of antibiotics. Continuation of the offending medication in the presence of symptoms increases the risk of an adverse outcome.

Postoperative diarrhea often can be treated effectively. Medications such as magnesium-containing compounds and products containing osmotically active agents (*eg*, sorbitol) are

Table 198-2. Conditions Associated with Obstruction or Pseudo-obstruction	
Small intestine	**Large intestine**
Medications (narcotics, anticholinergics)	Medications (narcotics, anticholinergics)
Hypokalemia, hypocalcemia	Hypokalemia, hypocalcemia
Immobility	Immobility
Diabetes mellitus	Fecal impaction*
Hypothyroidism	Volvulus*
Hypoparathyroidism	Rectocele*
Adhesions	
Incarcerated hernia	

These conditions affect mainly the large intestine.

Table 198-3. Causes of Diarrhea in the Postoperative Patient
Magnesium-containing compounds, sorbitol, lactulose, serotonin reuptake inhibitors
Lactose intolerance
Antibiotic-associated colitis
Clostridium difficile colitis
Sepsis, infection
Ischemic colitis
Truncal vagotomy
Cholecystectomy
Ileal Resection
Pancreatic resection

frequent offenders and should be discontinued. Pseudomembranous colitis usually is associated with recent antibiotic use. In the appropriate setting, a positive assay for *C. difficile* toxin in the stool is diagnostic; the sensitivity of this test is 94% to 100% [12•]. Flexible sigmoidoscopy also is diagnostic if yellow-white plaquelike membranes are identified; however, occasionally, patients have only proximal colonic involvement. The treatment of choice is oral metronidazole, 250 mg every 8 hours for 10 to 14 days. Patients who fail to respond to metronidazole can be treated with oral vancomycin 125 mg four times daily for 7 to 10 days. Patients unable to take oral medication should be treated with intravenous metronidazole; parenteral vancomycin is ineffective for this condition.

Ischemic colitis may cause bloody diarrhea in the postoperative period, particularly after acute or prolonged hypovolemia or if the inferior mesenteric artery is ligated during aortic surgery. Evaluation should include abdominal films, which characteristically show "thumbprinting," resulting from submucosal hemorrhage and edema of the bowel wall. Management includes nasogastric suction, bowel rest, volume resuscitation, intravenous antibiotics, and surgical consultation.

Diarrhea that develops in the postoperative period occasionally may be the first presentation of a previously silent medical condition, such as celiac disease or IBD, that has been unmasked by gastric or small bowel resection.

MANAGEMENT OF THE SURGICAL PATIENT WITH CONSTIPATION

Constipation is common postoperatively in patients and can lead to abdominal bloating, distention, or abdominal pain (see Chapter 70). Medications, metabolic disorders, intestinal obstruction, and anorectal disease are possible causes. Narcotics, pain medications, anticholinergic agents, and antipsychotics frequently are associated with constipation. Mechanical obstruction from adhesions, hernia, or strictures also can cause constipation. Hemorrhoids, fissures, and perirectal abscess may make defecation painful. Fecal impaction can cause constipation in elderly or bedridden patients. If mechanical obstruction is suspected, abdominal radiographs should be obtained. A barium study may be necessary to delineate an intestinal stricture or narrowing from adhesions.

In our experience, patients usually require medical therapy postoperatively in addition to a high-fiber diet to prevent constipation. This is especially true of patients who are prone to constipation, such as the elderly, the obese, or those with diabetes. Because constipation may become more difficult to treat the longer it persists without a bowel movement, we use an aggressive approach. In addition to encouraging early mobilization, we recommend initially using a stool softener (docusate sodium, 200 mg orally at bedtime) and an osmotic agent (sorbitol or lactulose, 15 mL orally every 6 to 8 hours). If the patient has not had a bowel movement while on this regimen for 24 hours, then we suggest proceeding to suppositories (bisacodyl, 10 mg per rectum as needed) and enemas (sodium biphosphate per rectum as needed). Polyethylene glycol mixture, 8 oz every 15 to 30 minutes until evacuation, is useful in refractory cases.

MANAGEMENT OF THE SURGICAL PATIENT WITH PANCREATIC DISEASE

Acute Pancreatitis

Surgery in patients with acute pancreatitis is best avoided. In patients undergoing emergency surgery for acute pancreatitis or other disorders, potential complications (*eg*, shock, sepsis, and multiorgan failure) are major concerns. Maintenance of fluid and electrolyte homeostasis is crucial. Frequent monitoring of electrolytes (particularly calcium), urine output, and central venous pressure is recommended. Intravenous colloidal solutions can usually be given without causing pulmonary edema, in contrast to large volumes of crystalloid, which may have a detrimental effect on oxygen extraction by tissues [13,14]. In seriously ill patients with acute necrotizing pancreatitis and unstable hemodynamics, use of low doses of volatile anesthetics is the preferred approach to anesthesia. It may not be possible to extubate a patient in the setting of sepsis or multiorgan dysfunction because of compromised oxygenation due to acute respiratory distress syndrome (ARDS) [14].

Chronic Pancreatitis

The principal concern for the patient with chronic pancreatitis who undergoes surgery is pancreatic insufficiency, which may result in maldigestion and diabetes mellitus. Maldigestion may lead to fluid and electrolyte abnormalities; of special concern is hypocalcemia, which can precipitate cardiac arrhythmias. Nutritional depletion increases the likelihood of adverse outcomes, such as poor wound healing. Perioperatively, electrolyte abnormalities should be corrected and calcium gluconate should be administered to correct hypocalcemia. A combination of balanced anesthesia (an inhalational agent with an intravenous neuromuscular agent) and epidural anesthesia may lighten the depth of anesthesia and permit faster recovery [14]. Careful attention to blood glucose levels is mandatory. Patients with diabetes mellitus secondary to chronic pancreatitis are very "brittle" because they lack the normal counterregulatory mechanisms. Hence, tight control of glucose levels with its attendant risk of hypoglycemia should be avoided.

Insulinoma

The potential for intraoperative hypoglycemia during resection of an insulinoma is of utmost concern; hypoglycemia may go undetected intraoperatively. Preoperative intravenous administration of glucose solutions and frequent intraoperative serum glucose measurements are advised. Some authorities have advocated preoperative administration of corticosteroids because of their ability to cause hyperglycemia. Because halothane may produce a relative, though mild, hyperglycemia, it may be the anesthetic agent of choice in these patients.

Postoperative Analgesia in Pancreatitis

After pancreatic surgery, epidural analgesia has been advocated, because it may improve splanchnic perfusion and encourage early return of gut motility.

Nutrition and Enzyme Supplementation

In alcoholics, deficiencies of vitamin B_1, vitamin B_6, folic acid, nicotinic acid, magnesium, and zinc are frequent. Repletion may reduce the risk of adverse surgical outcomes such as poor wound healing. Enteral nutrition is the preferred postoperative method of feeding, provided that intestinal motility has returned and feeding does not exacerbate pancreatic disease. Although about 90% of a healthy pancreas may be removed without causing pancreatic insufficiency, removal of lesser amounts can be detrimental in patients with pre-existing pancreatic disease. Patients most likely to be in need of pancreatic enzyme supplementation include those undergoing a total pancreatectomy or a subtotal pancreatectomy for chronic pancreatitis. Enzyme supplements have not been advocated as a matter of routine in other types of pancreatic (eg, resection of proximal pancreatic malignancies) or gastric surgery [15].

Cystic Fibrosis and Surgery

Management of surgical patients with cystic fibrosis often focuses on pulmonary complications of the disorder; however, pancreatic insufficiency often also is present in these patients (see Chapter 170). Malnutrition associated with chronic lung and pancreatic disease in cystic fibrosis is compounded by a marked increase in resting energy expenditure. Perioperative management includes supplementation of fat-soluble vitamins, especially vitamin K [16]. Patients with cystic fibrosis are susceptible to hyponatremia because of abnormally active sodium pumps [17] and may develop the adult equivalent of meconium ileus–distal ileal obstruction syndrome. Treatment is conservative and consists of nasogastric suction and oral polyethylene glycol solutions. Although few data discuss how to prevent the condition, adequate hydration, prompt treatment of infection, and the prophylactic use of cisapride and avoidance of medications that slow motility have been advocated [18].

■ MANAGEMENT OF THE SURGICAL PATIENT WITH LIVER DISEASE

Pathophysiology

Many factors account for the increased mortality and morbidity rates seen in patients with liver disease who undergo surgery (Table 198-4). Baseline cardiac output is often elevated, whereas systemic vascular resistance is typically low. High serum levels of bilirubin are believed to have negative inotropic and chronotropic effects. Most inhalational, spinal, and epidural anesthetics reduce hepatic blood flow by 30% to 50% during induction. Among the inhalational anesthetics, halothane and

Table 198-4. Pathophysiologic Derangements in Surgical Patients with Liver Disease	
Increased cardiac output	Hyperbilirubinemia
Decreased systemic vascular resistance	Coagulopathy
	Thrombocytopenia
Reduced hepatic perfusion	Immunocompromise
Increased extracellular volume	Reticuloendothelial dysfunction
Portosystemic shunting	Malnutrition
Altered hepatic metabolism of drugs	Endotoxemia

enflurane decrease portal and hepatic arterial flow. In contrast, isoflorane, although reducing portal venous blood flow, increases hepatic arterial flow. Splanchnic vascular resistance increases during surgery because of increased sympathetic tone, further diminishing hepatic blood flow. This is particularly true if traction on the abdominal viscera is present. Intermittent positive-pressure ventilation may precipitate hypotension, which, in combination with splanchnic vasoconstriction, further compromises hepatic blood flow. Because oxygen extraction is independent of hepatic perfusion, progressive oxygen desaturation may occur as blood flows through the hepatic sinusoids, thereby leading to hypoxic damage in the centrilobular zones.

Drug Metabolism

Hepatic disease predictably alters the metabolism of certain drugs. Drugs used perioperatively, such as benzodiazepines, induce hepatic mixed-function oxidases. Drugs that are highly extracted by the liver, such as morphine and meperidine, may have prolonged half-lives in patients with liver disease and thus precipitate or worsen encephalopathy. Drugs with low extraction ratios, such as antibiotics and benzodiazepines, are bound to plasma proteins, and their levels may be affected by changes in these proteins and in hepatic blood flow. Increased extracellular fluid volume in cirrhosis increases the volume of distribution of some drugs, whereas portosystemic shunting may increase the bioavailability of orally administered drugs by reducing their first-pass metabolism by the liver.

Anesthetic Agents

The halogenated hydrophobic inhalational anesthetics (eg, halothane, enflurane, and isoflurane) are metabolized by the liver into hydrophilic compounds that are excreted in bile. Although generally thought to be safe, these agents can cause liver dysfunction. The degrees of hepatic metabolism of halothane, enflurane, and isoflurane are 20%, 2.0%, and 0.2%, respectively. In part, therefore, halothane is the most likely of the three to cause hepatotoxicity, with an incidence of 1 in 7000. This is because hepatotoxicity results from oxidative metabolism of halothane to toxic metabolites and centrilobular hepatic necrosis mediated by antibodies against hepatocyte proteins bound to trifluroacetate, a metabolite of halothane. Isoflurane and enflurane undergo less biotransformation to trifluroacetate. Drugs that induce the cytochrome P-450 system (eg, alcohol, phenytoin, and phenobarbital) increase the formation of trifluroacetate, and thus potentiate the hepatotoxicity of these anesthetics [19]. Other factors believed to play a role in halothane hepatitis include multiple exposures to halothane, a family history of similar reactions, female gender, and obesity.

Hemostasis

Vitamin K deficiency in patients with cholestasis or malnutrition leads to impaired production of vitamin K–dependent coagulation factors (factors II, VII, IX, and X). Reduced hepatic clearance of proteases can worsen the coagulopathy by increasing plasma proteolysis of coagulation factors. Thrombocytopenia, owing to splenic sequestration in patients with portal hypertension, may be worsened by folate deficiency or bone marrow suppression by alcohol. Endotoxemia arising from impairment of the reticuloendothelial system and a lack of bile salts in the lumen of the gut may also contribute to the coagulopathy by causing disseminated intravascular coagulation (DIC). Impairment of the reticuloendothelial system increases susceptibility to postoperative infection. This susceptibility can be worsened by hyperbilirubinemia, diminished Kupffer cell function, impaired delayed hypersensitivity, and abnormal neutrophil function [20•,21•,22,23••].

Other Effects of Liver Disease

Postoperative renal failure occurs with increased frequency in surgical patients with liver disease or obstructive jaundice; hypotension, hypovolemia, and increased levels of circulating bile salts may be contributory. DIC from circulating endotoxins may lead to glomerular and peritubular fibrin deposition and acute tubular necrosis [24]. Endotoxemia also may play a role in impaired wound healing and gastric stress ulceration. Protein and caloric malnutrition in the setting of cirrhosis also increases the risk of an adverse outcome after surgery.

Predictors of Perioperative Mortality

Levels of conventional liver tests (*eg*, aminotransferases, alkaline phosphatase) correlate poorly with degree of liver dysfunction. Overall liver function may be better estimated using the serum albumin level and prothrombin time. Various additional quantitative tests of hepatic function have been advocated in the preoperative assessment of patients with chronic liver disease. These include the indocyanine green test, galactose elimination capacity, and aminopyrine breath test. At this time, however, these tests are not routinely used. Moreover, they have not been shown to add information to the prediction of risk beyond that learned from the Pugh modification of the Child's class (see discussion later in this chapter).

The Child-Turcotte classification (CTC) originally was developed to estimate the prognosis of patients with cirrhosis undergoing portosystemic shunting (see Chapter 112). Over time this classification system has been used to guide decision-making in other types of surgery. One of the most commonly used variants of the CTC is the Pugh modification (Table 198-5). Although the

CTC was developed for shunt surgery, others have demonstrated a correlation between the CTC or many of the factors in the CTC and mortality after nonshunt surgery [25]. Furthermore, the CTC correlates with postoperative morbidity rates and is a good predictor of overall survival in various types of liver disease.

Jaundice appears to increase the risk of postoperative renal failure. The probability of azotemia is directly related to the degree of hyperbilirubinemia. Clinical renal failure occurs in 9% of patients with jaundice undergoing surgery, with an associated mortality rate of 50% [24]. In the setting of obstructive jaundice, three factors have been associated with increased operative mortality: a hematocrit value of less than 30%; an initial serum bilirubin level of greater than 11 mg/dL; and a malignant cause for the obstruction [26]. Another study has shown that a combination of elevated serum bilirubin (>3 mg/dL) and creatinine levels and a decreased serum albumin level was associated with an increased risk of death [27].

Preoperative Assessment

A thorough history and physical examination are necessary to establish the presence of liver disease, clinical variables of the CTC, and need for additional liver tests (Fig. 198-2). A history of postoperative jaundice or other complications should be sought; if present, a careful review of previous perioperative records including drug exposure is necessary to determine the causes of the complication and which drugs to avoid.

Unsuspected Liver Test Abnormalities

Ordering routine preoperative liver tests in patients without a history or physical findings of liver disease is not advised. In patients in whom unsuspected liver test abnormalities are detected, however, a careful search for the cause is indicated. It is best to postpone elective surgery until the cause has been discovered and the severity of the liver disease assessed. A liver biopsy may be required for both the evaluation and management of the particular liver disease and clarification of surgical risk. If emergency surgery is required, the most important consideration is whether test results of hepatic synthetic and excretory function (prothrombin time, serum bilirubin, and serum albumin) are abnormal. If these test results are normal and no overt clinical signs of hepatic decompensation are present, patients are not likely to be at increased risk of surgical mortality.

Acute and Chronic Liver Disease

In patients with acute viral hepatitis, it is best to avoid elective surgery. It has been suggested that surgery should wait at least 1 month after liver tests return to normal [28]. In the setting of alcoholic hepatitis, elective surgery is contraindicated. It has been shown that finding alcoholic hyaline (Mallory bodies) on preoperative biopsies before portosystemic shunt surgery correlates with increased mortality [29]. Thus, a liver biopsy would seem reasonable in the preoperative assessment of patients in whom alcoholic liver disease is possible. In such cases, the patient should abstain from alcohol and surgery should be postponed until laboratory test results have improved. Histologic resolution of alcoholic hepatitis may take up to 6 months.

Some chronic liver diseases do not increase the risk of perioperative complications. Asymptomatic carriers of hepatitis B virus (those who have the hepatitis B surface antigen in the

Table 198-5. The Child-Turcotte Classification*

	Points†		
	1	**2**	**3**
Serum albumin, *g/dL*	>3.5	3.0–3.5	<3.0
Prothrombin time, *s prolonged*	<4.0	4.0–6.0	>6.0
Serum bilirubin, *mg/dL*	<2.0	2.0–3.0	>3.0
Ascites	Absent	Slight–moderate	Tense
Encephalopathy†	None	Grades I–II	Grades III–IV

*As modified by Pugh et al. [40].
†Class A, 5—6 points; class B, 7—9 points; class C, 10—15 points. According to the grading of Trey, et al. [41].

serum and normal liver function) are not at increased risk. Similarly, in patients with fatty liver from whatever cause, as long as liver function is intact and nutritional status is good, surgery need not be delayed. An isolated, elevated, unconjugated serum bilirubin level as seen in Gilbert's syndrome does not increase perioperative risk.

In patients with chronic liver disease and significant liver dysfunction, the challenge is to optimize the patient's status before surgery. Emphasis should be placed on the management of coagulopathy, ascites, encephalopathy, azotemia, and susceptibility to infection. Nonoperative or less invasive alternatives to surgery should be considered. Laparoscopic surgery may be preferable to traditional laparotomy; portal hypertension and coagulopathy are considered relative contraindications to laparoscopic cholecystectomy. Some authors believe that laparoscopic cholecystectomy is preferable to the open approach in patients with Child's class A or B cirrhosis [30]. Management of choledocholithiasis by endoscopic retrograde cholangiopancreatography (ERCP) generally is preferable to choledochotomy. The average risk of clinically significant hemorrhage after endoscopic sphincterotomy is 2%; however, the risk increases by threefold in patients with cirrhosis [31]. Subtotal cholecystectomy or cholecystostomy may be an alternative in a patient with decompensated liver disease and cholecystitis. Herniorrhaphies can be tolerated without significant risk; however, ascites must be controlled. Good postoperative outcomes have been reported in patients with liver disease undergoing a wide range of procedures [27].

Patients with autoimmune hepatitis on corticosteroid therapy should receive "stress doses" on the day of surgery (*eg*, hydrocortisone, 100 mg intravenously every 8 hours) followed by a quick taper, if they have been taking corticosteroids for more than several weeks (see Chapter 97). Azathioprine may be held in the perioperative period until the patient is able to take oral medications. In patients with Wilson's disease, the dose of D-penicillamine should be reduced during the first 2 weeks of postoperative recovery because the drug impairs wound healing (see Chapter 107). D-penicillamine also carries the risk of inducing a hypercoagulable state, which is a concern in patients who are immobile after surgery.

Hepatic Resection

Hepatic resection in a patient with cirrhosis represents a particular challenge. The risk of postoperative liver failure correlates with the size of resection and the function of the remaining liver. Because morbidity and mortality rates can be quite high, careful selection of the appropriate surgical candidate is called for. With improvement in care, reported mortality rates have been decreasing but morbidity rates remain as high as 60%. Some authors have advised that only patients with Child's class A cirrhosis should undergo surgery; however, others have suggested that objective measurements such as the indocyanine green test, wedged hepatic venous pressure gradient, or estimated volume of the remaining liver may be better than Child's classification to predict postoperative complications [32,34]. Considering the risks and complexity of treating these patients, this type of surgery is best handled in centers with extensive experience [34].

Coagulopathy

A single dose of vitamin K_1, 10 mg intramuscularly, should be sufficient to correct vitamin K deficiency caused by poor nutrition or malabsorption arising from cholestasis. However, this dose will not correct coagulopathy caused by hepatocellular dysfunction. In such cases, up to 8 U of fresh frozen plasma should be given "on call" during surgery. Because it may be difficult to determine which is the predominant cause of hypoprothrombinemia (vitamin K deficiency or hepatocellular dysfunction), both fresh frozen plasma and vitamin K may be given. If the prothrombin time does not correct to within 3 seconds of the control value,

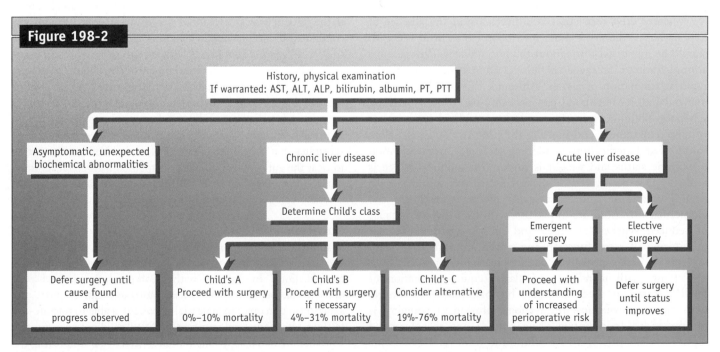

Figure 198-2

Algorithm for preoperative assessment of patients with liver disease. AST—aspartate aminotransferase; ALT—alanine aminotransferase; PT—prothrombin time; PTT—partial thromboplastin time.

other measures should be considered. Cryoprecipitate (10 U intravenously preoperatively) contains von Willebrand factor (vWF) and large amounts of fibrinogen, whereas desmopressin (DDAVP, 0.3 μg/kg intravenously preoperatively) causes release of endogenous vWF [35]. In patients with refractory coagulopathy, plasma exchange may be beneficial [36]. Prophylactic platelet transfusions should be considered when the platelet count is below 50,000/mm^3.

Ascites

In patients with ascites preoperatively, consideration should be given to a diagnostic paracentesis to exclude spontaneous bacterial peritonitis, which may be asymptomatic (see Chapters 113 and 114). Although spontaneous bacterial peritonitis can be managed with a third-generation cephalosporin (eg, cefotaxime, 2 g intravenously every 8 hours for 5 days), secondary bacterial peritonitis requires surgical management. Spontaneous bacterial peritonitis often is caused by a single species of bacterium, whereas in bowel perforation and contamination of ascites, multiple species are typically found. Ideally, ascites should be controlled before surgery to improve respiratory mechanics and, in the case of abdominal surgery, to prevent wound dehiscence. Careful diuresis can be instituted with combinations of spironolactone and furosemide; more aggressive diuresis is possible when ascites is associated with peripheral edema. Typically, spironolactone and furosemide are started at daily doses of 100 and 40 mg, respectively, both orally. This fixed ratio, which may be slowly increased to 400 mg of spironolactone and 160 mg of furosemide), usually maintains normokalemia. The effects of changes in spironolactone dosing may not be apparent for 5 days. Amiloride (10 to 40 mg by mouth daily) can be substituted for spironolactone and has the advantage of a more rapid onset of action. Large-volume paracentesis is a safe rapid alternative to diuretic therapy, particularly in patients with tense ascites and even in the absence of peripheral edema.

Whereas fluid restriction is unnecessary in the absence of hyponatremia, dietary sodium restriction (to as little as 1 g/d) should be instituted throughout the hospital stay. Perioperative administration of intravenous fluids is often associated with the rapid accumulation of ascites. Although this problem is often unavoidable, its likelihood can probably be reduced by using salt-poor albumin, fresh frozen plasma, or blood products for volume replacement and limiting the use of intravenous saline solutions and medications containing sodium. Careful attention to volume status and weight is important; sodium balance is probably best monitored by measuring urinary sodium levels. Serum creatinine and urea levels often overestimate the glomerular filtration rate in patients with liver disease, because of reduced synthesis of urea and muscle wasting. Regular monitoring of renal function and potassium and magnesium levels is advised, especially in patients receiving diuretics.

Patients with jaundice particularly require prevention of renal dysfunction. Anemia should be corrected preoperatively with blood transfusions. Intravenous infusion of mannitol is recommended to maintain urine output; one recommended regimen is 500 mL of a 10% solution to run over 1 to 2 hours preoperatively, then a 5% solution postoperatively to maintain a urine output of 60 mL/h [24]. Careful attention to volume

status is important. By reducing endotoxemia, lactulose, 30 mL by mouth every 6 hours for 3 days before surgery, may help preserve renal function. Some authors have advocated use of low-dose dopamine 2 μg/kg/h to dilate the splanchnic bed and improve renal perfusion [22]. These measures have been recommended for patients with significant liver disease, even without jaundice. Whether or not the patient has jaundice, aminoglycoside antibiotics and nonsteroidal anti-inflammatory drugs should be avoided. Third-generation cephalosporins (eg, cefotaxime), some of the antipseudomonal penicillins (eg, ticarcillin/clavulanate or piperacillin tazobactam), aztreonam, and imipenem are better choices for gram-negative infections.

Encephalopathy

There are many potential causes of worsening encephalopathy in the perioperative period:

Hypoxia
Hypotension
Infection
Dehydration
High protein load, including gastrointestinal bleeding
Constipation
Central nervous system depressant drugs
Renal failure
Hypokalemic metabolic alkalosis
Portosystemic shunts
Hepatic resection
Progression in underlying liver disease

If encephalopathy is present preoperatively, elective surgery should be avoided. In the absence of encephalopathy, dietary protein restriction is not routinely advised, especially because patients facing the catabolic stress of surgery may be malnourished. No evidence suggests that perioperative prophylactic lactulose is of value if the patient was not on the drug before admission; however, if the patient was on lactulose before admission, it should be continued. If encephalopathy develops, dietary protein restriction of 30 to 40 g/d and lactulose, 30 mL every 6 hours daily and titrated to two or three soft bowel movements daily, should be started. If the patient cannot tolerate oral lactulose, it may be given with a nasogastric tube or as a suspension enema (300 mL in 700 mL of tap water up to 3 times daily). Oral or rectal neomycin (up to 4 g/d) has been used to sterilize the gut and reduce production of substrates that contribute to encephalopathy. Nasogastric suction to clear the gut of blood should be combined with rectal administration of lactulose (or neomycin) if the patient is unable to take enteral preparations, as after bowel surgery.

Nutrition

Malnutrition is common in patients with either acute or chronic liver disease and may increase the frequency of perioperative complications. In patients with alcoholic hepatitis and poor oral intake, supplemental enteral nutrition can improve the short-term outcome. In general, if a patient is able to tolerate oral feeding, total parenteral nutrition (TPN) should not be instituted. Enteral nutritional supplementation is effective in improving the serum albumin level and Child's class and reducing the mortality rate in patients with cirrhosis complicated by malnutrition [38].

A polymeric enteral diet, which includes medium-chain triglycerides and branched-chain amino acids, may be delivered through a fine-bore nasogastric tube, if recommended. If TPN is required, formulations containing standard amino acid solutions may be used safely without worsening encephalopathy [39]. The patient should receive sufficient calories to provide 1.2 times the estimated resting energy expenditure (30% to 35% as fat, the balance as carbohydrate) and 1 g/kg/d of protein. Special attention should be paid to supplementing fat-soluble vitamins, especially vitamin K.

Anesthetic Agents

Premedication may provoke encephalopathy and is probably best avoided in patients with Child's class B and C cirrhosis. Short-acting benzodiazepines, such as temazepam, are good choices when premedication is required. Among longer acting benzodiazepines, oxazepam and lorazepam are preferred in patients with liver disease. The effect of induction agents may be enhanced in patients with cirrhosis because of reduced protein binding. Even though etomidate and thiopentone are metabolized by the liver, their action is terminated by redistribution. Thus, their durations of activity should remain normal unless large or repeated doses are given [20•].

As noted previously, isoflurane is the preferred inhalational anesthetic agent in patients with liver disease because it undergoes little hepatic metabolism and, thus, rarely causes hepatitis [19]. In addition, isoflurane produces a relatively smaller decrease in hepatic arterial blood flow than do other anesthetics. Fentanyl and alfentanil are appropriate opioid analgesic agents because they have short half-lives and produce inactive metabolites [20•]. The metabolism of sufentanil also is unaffected by liver disease.

Larger doses of nondepolarizing muscle relaxants, such as pancuronium and vecuronium, may be required because they have an increased volume of distribution in patients with liver disease. However, because these agents are metabolized by the liver and excreted in bile, their durations of action may be prolonged. Furthermore, plasma cholinesterase, which is synthesized by the liver, is required for the metabolism of agents such as succinylcholine, and smaller maintenance doses are required in patients with liver disease. In patients with coexisting renal and liver disease, the metabolism of these agents can be unpredictable; therefore, frequent monitoring of the degree of neuromuscular blockade is helpful. Because atracurium is not metabolized by the liver nor dependent on plasma cholinesterase or the kidney for elimination, it may be considered the agent of choice for routine surgery [20•,40]. Doxacurium, a long-acting nondepolarizing muscle relaxant, is excreted unchanged in the urine and bile and is suggested for long procedures, such as liver transplantation [40].

Postoperative pain management requires balancing the need for analgesia with the side effects of the agents and their potential to precipitate encephalopathy. Coexisting renal disease can affect the metabolism of analgesics in patients with liver disease. Intermittent bolus doses of analgesics are safe [20•].

Prognosis

Most of the published experience regarding the outcome of surgery in patients with liver disease pertains to alcoholic cirrhosis. Whether the information from these studies can be applied to other types of liver disease is not known. Much of the literature is relatively old and often reflects the mortality and morbidity associated with laparotomy performed to distinguish intrahepatic from extrahepatic cholestasis, a situation that rarely occurs today. It is reasonable to assume that mortality and morbidity rates have declined for many patients with liver disease undergoing surgery, as a result of improved perioperative care and operative techniques.

In patients with acute viral hepatitis, perioperative mortality has been reported to range from 10% to 100%. One series found that the mortality rate was five times higher in patients with alcoholic hepatitis diagnosed by open biopsy (60%) than in those diagnosed by percutaneous biopsy. Other series report mortality rates as high as 100%. Given the risks of surgery in the presence of alcoholic hepatitis, nonoperative approaches to biliary tract diseases (*eg*, cholecystostomy, endoscopic papillotomy) are advisable until clinical improvement occurs or an alternative diagnosis is made.

Risks pertaining to perioperative complications in patients with cirrhosis have been better characterized than have those in patients with acute hepatitis. Operative mortality for portosystemic shunt surgery in the setting of cirrhosis has been reported as 0% to 10% for patients in Child's class A, 4% to 31% for class B, and 19% to 76% for class C [21]. As mentioned previously, it has been widely assumed that these percentages apply to nonshunt surgery as well. Not surprisingly, emergency surgery carries a higher risk than does elective surgery. Abdominal surgery, and biliary tract surgery in particular, is associated with higher perioperative morbidity and mortality rates. Obviously, more extensive surgery of whatever type increases the risk of an adverse outcome.

■ REFERENCES

Recently published papers of particular interest have been highlighted as follows:
•   Of interest
••   Of Outstanding interest

1. Nebel OT, Fornes MF, Castell DO: Symptomatic gastroesophageal reflux: incidence and precipitating factors. *Am J Dig Dis* 1976, 21:953–956.

2. Olsson GL, Hallen B, Hambraeus-Jonzon K: Aspiration during anaesthesia: a computer-aided study of 185,358 anaesthetics. *Acta Anaesthesiol Scand* 1986, 30:84–92.

3. Kuo B, Castell DO: The effect of nasogastric intubation on gastroesophageal reflux: a comparison of different tube sizes. *Am J Gastroenterol* 1995, 90:1804–1807.

4. Kurata J: Ulcer epidemiology: an overview and proposed research framework. *Gastroenterology* 1989, 96:569–580.

5. Della Ratta RK, Corapi MJ, Horowitz BR, Calio AJ: Risk of postoperative upper gastrointestinal tract hemorrhage in patients with active ulcer disease undergoing nonulcer surgery. *Arch Intern Med* 1993, 153:2141–2144.

6. Silverstein FE, Gilbert DA, Tedesco JF, *et al.*: The national ASGE survey on upper gastrointestinal bleeding: I. Study design and baseline data. *Gastrointest Endosc* 1981, 27:73–79.

7. Cook DJ, Reeve BK, Guyatt GH, *et al.*: Stress ulcer prophylaxis in critically ill patients: resolving discordant meta-analyses. *JAMA* 1996, 275:308–314.

8.•• Cook DJ, Fuller HD, Guyatt GH, *et al.*: Risk factors for gastrointestinal bleeding in critically ill patients: Canadian Critical Care Trials Group. *N Engl J Med* 1994, 330:377–381.
A critical analysis of risk factors for bleeding from stress ulceration is given.

9. Zuckerman GR, Shuman R: Therapeutic goals and treatment options for prevention of stress ulcer syndrome. *Am J Med* 1987, 83:29.

10. Nitschke LF, Schlosser CT, Berg RL, *et al.*: Does patient-controlled analgesia achieve better control of pain and fewer adverse effects than intramuscular analgesia? A prospective randomized controlled trial. *Arch Surg* 1996, 131:417–423.

11. Siegel DL, Edelstein PH, Nachamkin I: Inappropriate testing for diarrheal diseases in the hospital. *JAMA* 1990, 263:979–982.

12.• Kelly CP, Pothoulakis C, Lamont JT: *Clostridium difficile* colitis. *N Engl J Med* 1994, 330:257–262.
This article reviews the diagnosis and treatment of *C. difficile* colitis.

13. Albrecht DM, Dworschak M, Frey L, *et al.*: Does the resuscitation modality influence lung water after canine traumatic hemorrhagic shock? *Eur Surg Res* 1986, 18(suppl 1):12.

14. Van Ackern K, Albrecht DM: Anaesthesia in pancreatic surgery. In *Surgery of the Pancreas.* Edited by Trede M, Canter DC. New York: Churchill Livingstone; 1993:623–627.

15. Freiss H, Bohm J, Ebert M, Buchler M: Enzyme treatment after gastrointestinal surgery. *Digestion*1993, 54(suppl 2):48–53.

16. Bruno MJ, Haverkort EB, Tytgat GNJ, van Leeuwen DJ: Maldigestion associated with exocrine pancreatic insufficiency: implications of gastrointestinal physiology and properties of enzyme preparations for a cause-related and patient-tailored treatment. *Am J Gastroenterol* 1995, 90:1383–1393.

17. Bursztein-DeMyttenaere S, Askanazi J: Gastrointestinal disorders. In *Anesthesia and Uncommon Diseases,* edn 3. Edited by Katz J, Benumof JL, Kadis LB. Philadelphia: WB Saunders; 1990:437–494.

18. Khoshoo V, Udall JN: Meconium ileus equivalent in children and adults. *Am J Gastroenterol* 1994, 89:153–157.

19. Sinha A, Clatch RJ, Stuck G, *et al.*: Isoflurane hepatotoxicity: a case report and review of the literature. *Am J Gastroenterol* 1996, 91:2406–2409.

20.• McEvedy BA, Shelly MP, Park GR: Anaesthesia and liver disease. *Br J Hosp Med* 1986, 36: 26–28, 30–32, 34.
This article is of value to the anesthetist in the perioperative management of the patient with liver disease.

21.• Gholson CF, Provenza JM, Bacon BR: Hepatologic considerations in patients with parenchymal liver disease undergoing surgery. *Am J Gastroenterol* 1990, 85:487–496.
This reference remains one of the most complete reviews of this topic.

22. Siefkin AD, Bolt R: Preoperative evaluation of the patient with gastro-intestinal or liver disease. *Med Clin North Am* 1979, 63:1309–1320.

23.•• Friedman LS, Maddrey WC: Surgery in the patient with liver disease. *Med Clin North Am* 1987, 71:453–476.
This article remains one of the definitive reviews of this topic.

24. Pain JA, Cahill CJ, Bailey ME: Perioperative complications in obstruc-tive jaundice: therapeutic considerations. *Br J Surg* 1985, 72:942–945.

25. Garrison RN, Cryer HM, Howard DA, Polk HC: Clarification of risk factors for abdominal operations in patients with hepatic cirrhosis. *Ann Surg* 1984, 199:648–655.

26. Dixon JM, Armstrong CP, Duffy SW, *et al.*: Factors affecting morbidity and mortality after surgery for obstructive jaundice: a review of 373 patients. *Gut* 1983, 24:845–852.

27. Runyon BA: Surgical procedures are well tolerated by patients with asymptomatic chronic hepatitis. *J Clin Gastroenterol* 1986, 8:542–544.

28. Lamont JT: The liver. In *To Make the Patient Ready for Anesthesia: Medical Care of the Surgical Patient.* Edited by Vandam LD. Menlo Park: Addison-Wesley; 1984:47–66.

29. Mikkelsen WP, Kern WH: The influence of acute hyaline necrosis on survival after a emergency and elective portocaval shunt. *Major Probl Clin Surg* 1974, 14:233–242.

30. D'Albuquerque LAC, de Miranda MP, Genzini T, *et al.*: Laparoscopic cholecystectomy in cirrhotic patients. *Surg Laparosc Endosc* 1995, 5:272–276.

31. Freeman ML, Nelson DB, Sherman S, *et al.*: Complications of endo-scopic biliary sphincterotomy. *N Engl J Med* 1996, 335:909–918.

32. Fan S, Lai ECS, Lo C, *et al.*: Hospital mortality of major hepatectomy for hepatocellular carcinoma associated with cirrhosis. *Arch Surg* 1995, 130:198–203.

33. Yamanaka N, Okamoto E, Kuwata K, Tanaka N: A multiple regression equation for prediction of posthepatectomy liver failure. *Ann Surg* 1984, 200:658–663.

34. Burroughs AK, Matthews K, Qadiri M, *et al.*: Desmopressin and bleeding time in patients with cirrhosis. *Br Med J Clin Res* 1985, 291:1377–1381.

35. Munoz SJ, Balls SK, Mortiz M, *et al.*: Perioperative management of fulminant and subfulminant hepatic failure with therapeutic plasma-pheresis. *Transplant Proc* 1989, 31:3535–3536.

36. Cabre E, Gonzalez-Huix F, Abad-Lacruz A, *et al.*: Effect of total enteral nutrition on short-term outcome of severely malnourished cirrhotics. *Gastroenterology* 1990, 98:715–720.

37. Hurst RD, Butler BN, Soybel DI, Wrighy HK: Management of groin hernias in patients with ascites. *Ann Surg* 1992, 216:696.

38. Nompleggi DJ, Bonkovsky HL: Nutritional supplementation in chronic liver disease: an analytical review. *Hepatology* 1994, 19:518–533.

39. Hunter JM: New neuromuscular blocking agents. *N Engl J Med* 1995, 332:1691–1699.

40. Pugh RNH, Murray-Lyon IM, Dawson JL, *et al.*: Transection of the esophagus for bleeding esophageal varices. *Br J Surg*1973, 60, 646–649.

41. Trey C, Burns DG, Saunders SJ: Treatment of hepatic coma by exchange blood transfusion. *N Engl J Med* 1966, 274:473–481.

199 Psychosocial Aspects of Gastroenterology: Doctor–Patient Interactions

Kevin W. Olden

During the past 25 years, tremendous progress has been made in the diagnosis and treatment of gastrointestinal disorders, predominantly through technologic advances, such as fiberoptic endoscopy, and the development of a wide spectrum of highly effective medications, such as the H_2-receptor antagonists and proton pump inhibitors. The revolution in the treatment of chronic liver disease as a result of orthotopic liver transplantation has allowed gastroenterologists to mitigate suffering and save lives as never before. Because of these and other advances, gastroenterologists more commonly are requested to perform highly technical interventions in a narrow consultative role. One potential casualty of this role is the doctor–patient relationship [1]. The medical interview can be as incisive a diagnostic instrument as the endoscope, but practicing clinicians often take for granted interviewing skills. Like endoscopy, the interview can elicit important information if performed properly. Like endoscopy, interviewing techniques require training and practice.

From the physician's perspective, the goal of the medical interview is to obtain information necessary to make a diagnosis and formulate recommendations for treatment. The patient's perspective is much broader, with a wider spectrum of issues, and is likely to be accompanied by anxiety or other emotions. That varying issues can occur in the context of the medical interview is demonstrated by the fact that physicians interrupt a patient's initial statement within an average of 16 seconds after the patient begins to report his or her chief concern. The tendency of physicians to dominate the physician–patient interaction is further elucidated by a study that found the physician's contribution to the medical dialogue is 60% on average, whereas the patient's contribution is only 40% [2••]. Two models traditionally have characterized the medical interview. In the "cure model," emphasis is placed on information exchange that results in specific treatment recommendations. In the "care model," the emphasis is on conveying understanding and support for the patient [3] (Table 199-1). Both these models are associated with characteristic behaviors and goals. Two other terms that respectively reflect these models are *doctor centered* and *patient centered*. The cure model can best be described operationally as a "need to understand," mainly on the part of the physician, whereas the care model is best described as the "need to feel known and understood" on the part of both patient and physician.

The differing issues that occur in the course of the doctor–patient interaction can be divided into task-oriented interactions, which reflect the cure model, or an affective style of interaction, with attention paid to the social and emotional elements that focus on the care model. Physicians often enter the interaction well prepared for cure-oriented task completion.

This style depends heavily on cognitive and technical skills, the foundation of a physician's training. The affective component of care is much less tangible. It is difficult to qualify specific behaviors associated with an affective style. One study showed that physicians who attended, in a meaningful way, to the patient's needs were more likely to address the patient by name; 72% of interactions were characterized by highly affective behavior, with the physician often addressing the patient by name. At first glance, it would appear obvious that a physician would address a patient by name during a medical interaction. More often than not, however, physicians ignore this most basic form of respect. Other physician behaviors associated with an affective style are laughing with and reassuring the patient, showing approval and empathy, and engaging in small talk.

Traditionally, physicians have tended to dominate doctor–patient interactions. Stewart and colleagues characterized doctors' interactive style as high to low in "physician control." In this model, the interactions of high-control physicians are characterized by intense questioning, frequent interruption of the patient, and dispensing information and instructions without monitoring whether patients really understand what is presented (Table 199-2). The high-control style is still the most common approach used in clinical medicine and exemplifies doctor-centered interactions. The alternative, low-control style allows patients unlimited opportunity to speak and contribute information. Most physicians would agree that the latter style, if unstructured, can be nonproductive.

Kaplan developed a conceptual model that divides the doctor–patient interaction into three phases [4•]. The first is phase is "physician-directed," characterized by questions and interruptions initiated by the doctor. In the second, "patient-directed," phase, the patient is allowed to ask questions and interrupt the doctor. In the final, "emotional/opinion exchange," phase, the discussion between doctor and patient is summarized, the physician gives emotional support to the patient, and clarification of instructions and recommendations is attended to by both parties. Physicians who organize their interactions with patients according to Kaplan's model are more likely to have a productive and satisfying interaction with their patients.

The same can be said of patient satisfaction. The emphasis on patient satisfaction by health maintenance organizations and

Table 199-1. Cure versus Care Interview Models: Attitudes and Behaviors

Cure model	Care model
Focus is on specific symptoms	Focus is on the patient's concerns about the illness
Emphasis is on closed-ended (yes or no) questions	Emphasis is on exploratory questions
Physician is formal and impersonal	Physician and patient are egalitarian; physician refers to patient by name and engages in small talk
Physician is less likely to offer emotional support	Physician is supportive and empathic
Little information is given to the patient	Diagnosis, prognosis, results of tests, and treatment recommendations are offered
Emphasis is on the treatment plan	Emphasis is on the patient "feeling cared for"

Table 199-2. Styles of Physician Interaction

High control	Low control
Frequently interrupts the patient	Allows patient to talk without interruptions
Asks closed-ended (yes or no) questions	Asks open-ended questions
Asks symptom-oriented questions	Asks patient-oriented questions
Ignores expressions of emotion	Acknowledges and supports the patient's feelings
Presents unemotionally	Projects own persona with jokes, compliments

From Ong and coworkers [2••]; with permission.

other managed care organizations has made this topic increasingly important. One study found that nearly 40% of patients are dissatisfied after a physician visit. The basis for this dissatisfaction was attributed most often to poor communication between the physicians and patient [5]. Physicians also tend to underestimate the patient's desire for information during an office visit. In another study, the physician's expectations about the information conveyed and the patient's satisfaction with the information received coincided in only 29% of interviews [6]. Other studies have found that information provided by the physician was related significantly to patient satisfaction. In general, physicians who have a more affective style (*ie*, are less controlling) garner higher patient satisfaction ratings than those who have a dominant, task-oriented, and controlling style.

For a doctor–patient interaction to be successful, patients must understand how to comply with treatment recommendations. The quality of the doctor–patient interaction can influence a patient's understanding and subsequent behavior profoundly. Ley found that 7% to 47% of patients in a primary care setting left the doctor's office without understanding the diagnosis or treatment plan [7•]. Similarly, 13% to 52% of these patients did not understand the prognosis of their conditions. In addition, when a physician referred to the medical chart frequently rather than looking at the patient, or when a physician touched the patient frequently, the patient was less likely to remember the information given. Conversely, when a physician stood close to but did not touch the patient, maintained frequent eye contact, referred less to the medical chart, and spent more time on providing information, the patient's retention of information increased [8]. If information is retained, then patient compliance with treatment recommendations should increase. Other studies have demonstrated a positive correlation between "sharing opinions" and "patient knowledge about illness" on the one hand and subsequent compliance with medical recommendations on the other. Similarly, compliance tends to be associated with a high frequency of patient-centered, as opposed to doctor-centered, behaviors. Factors affecting patient comliance include the following:

Shared opinions between physician and patient

Patient's knowledge about illness

Patient-centered physician communication

Physician information giving

An additional important finding was that the quality of physician– patient communications ultimately can affect health status. Kaplan and colleagues found that interactions characterized by controlling behaviors resulted in poor outcome, assessed by disease measures, such as improvement in vital signs and laboratory studies, as well as by subjective reports of improvement given by the patient [9]. Conversely, interactions characterized by frequent expression of emotion, a tendency of the physician to give information, and a willingness of the patient to seek information were related to better health outcomes.

These data support the contention that the doctor–patient interaction is not a trivial matter; rather, it is a medical procedure that has a profound effect on medical outcomes, patient satisfaction, and promotion of health. Effective doctor–patient communication goes beyond having a satisfied, as opposed to unsatisfied, patient. There also are implications for medical risk management and prevention of medical malpractice suits. One review of depositions of plaintiffs in medical malpractice suits found that poor doctor–patient communication was the most common factor prompting initiation of a lawsuit [10]. Improvement in patient satisfaction, compliance, and outcomes, as well as the potential for reducing exposure of the physician to liability, make the study of the psychosocial dimensions of doctor–patient interactions a worthy endeavor.

IMPEDIMENTS TO DOCTOR–PATIENT COMMUNICATION

Physicians operate almost universally in an environment characterized by pressure from crammed schedules and other time constraints. The demands of medical practice and frequent reprioritization of physician schedules as a result of medical emergencies can affect the quality of doctor–patient interactions adversely. Moreover, the trend of some managed care organizations toward emphasizing physician productivity in terms of the number of patients seen per unit of time exerts additional pressure on physician–patient interactions. Consequently, it is a challenge for the physician to use a supportive and noncontrolling style in the face of a practice environment that all too often promotes high-control behaviors, such as asking closed-ended questions, interrupting the patient frequently, and failing to allow time for the patient to ask questions.

GENDER AND CULTURAL ISSUES

The variety of patients encountered in daily practice is almost limitless. Patients present with a wide spectrum of personality styles and issues. In addition, gender, socioeconomic, and cultural differences between the physician and patient can greatly influence the interaction. No one set of physician behaviors is equally effective for all patients. The anxiety that a physician may feel because of these differences can lead to a high degree of controlling behavior and to a less-than-optimal interaction. Cultural sensitivity and language skills can contribute enormously toward mitigating these differences. Having a patient's family members and others assist in communicating and interpreting the patient's concerns and behavior can be an invaluable asset for both patient and physician. Developing some fluency in the native languages spoken by patients seen frequently in the physician's practice is enormously beneficial. Also, taking time to learn cultural concepts of illness, such as the yin–yang and hot–cold theories found in Asian and Hispanic cultures, respectively, can be an aid to more effective communication. Learning the colloquial terms for symptoms in a patient's native language can greatly improve history taking. For example, a Hispanic patient is more likely to respond correctly to an inquiry about *agrudas en pecho* (burning in the chest) than to a question referring to heartburn. Knowledge of even only a few key words and phrases in a patient's native language can pay enormous dividends both for effective history taking and establishing rapport with the patient.

Physicians also need to be aware of circumstances in their own lives that can affect the doctor–patient interaction adversely. An endoscopy or office schedule running increasingly behind, a sick family member, and the physician's own physical exhaustion can contribute to internal stress. At first glance, this may seem like a difficult concept to identify, but strategies have been developed to address this problem. The concept of *autognosis*, proposed by Messner, is defined as "all knowledge of the self which might be relevant to the clinician's professional activities" [11]. Pragmatically, this concept means that the physician needs to evaluate (or take pause to recognize) all the circumstances occurring both inside and outside the examination room that can affect his or her communication style with the patient. The use of autognosis allows the physician to "get in touch" with his or her countertransference feelings for the patient. Transference is the emotional reaction of a patient to the physician. Countertransference, in turn, is the emotional reaction of the physician to the patient. Although these terms originally were developed for use in psychotherapy, they have great usefulness in all types of medical practice. If not identified, negative countertransference can lead to poor doctor–patient interactions as well as unnecessary stress for the physician. Some clues associated with negative countertransference that can be identified easily using autognosis are listed in Table 199-3.

▆▆ PSYCHOSOCIAL DIMENSIONS OF GASTROENTEROLOGIC PRACTICE

The history of gastroenterology is filled with accounts of the influence of stress and physiologic factors on gastrointestinal function. Beaumount's work in 1833 was a milestone for its use of the scientific method in demonstrating changes in gastric acid secretion provoked by alterations in mood. Further, the work of Wolf, Alverez, and Alexander contributed to an understanding of psychosocial and emotional dimensions of gastrointestinal disease. These and numerous other studies provide a historical context for current investigations into the brain–gut interface.

The relation between emotional distress and gastrointestinal illness has been studied in two major contexts. The first comprises gastrointestinal disorders commonly associated with psychiatric comorbidity that may or may not be etiologic (Table 199-4). Examples include esophageal motility disorders, nonulcer dyspepsia, irritable bowel syndrome (IBS), and other functional gastrointestinal disorders (Table 199-5). Each of these disorders is discussed in this chapter separately. The second context is consideration of the emotional consequences of gastrointestinal diseases such as inflammatory bowel disease (IBD) and chronic viral hepatitis.

Gastrointestinal Disorders With Psychiatric Comorbidity

Irritable Bowel Syndrome

DaCosta, in 1871, first postulated a relation between IBS-like symptoms and the post-traumatic stress–like syndromes he observed in Civil War veterans [12]. Osler and Bockus, early in the 20th century, made similar observations. A number of contemporary investigators have refined and confirmed these early observations. Psychiatric comorbidity of IBS has been described in studies that have found associations between panic disorder, depressive disorders, somatoform disorders, disorders of sexual function, and IBS. Panic disorder is characterized by attacks of intense paroxysmal anxiety, commonly accompanied by somatic symptoms such as shortness of breath, chest pain, abdominal pain, and diarrhea in the absence of any obvious environmental stimulus that would precipitate such levels of anxiety. Lydiard and colleagues found that the lifetime prevalence of panic disorder in patients with IBS is 31%, and 26% have panic disorder at the time they present for treatment of gastrointestinal symptoms [13]. Similar findings were reported by Walker and colleagues [14]. The

---

Table 199-3. Autognosis: Clues that the Physician has Countertransference to the Patient

An unreasonable dislike of the patient

Overemotional response to the patient's troubles

Excessive fondness for the patient

Daydreaming in the patient's presence

Frequent lateness on the part of the physician for the patient's appointments

Intense or frequent arguments with the patient

Derogatory criticism of the patient

Appearance of the patient in the clinician's dreams

Forgetfulness regarding clinical material

Persistent thoughts of the patient outside the clinical setting

Undue pessimism or optimism

Thoughts of discharging the patient

Emotional withdrawal

Regression to orthodoxy

Feelings of inadequacy

Unusual handling of fees

Table 199-4. Psychiatric Disorders Often Seen in Difficult Patients

Multisomatiform disorder	Generalized anxiety disorder
Panic disorder	Major depressive disorder
Dysthymia	Alcohol abuse or dependence

From Hahn and coworkers [33●]; with permission.

Table 199-5. Psychiatric Comorbidity and Gastrointestinal Disorders

Gastrointestinal disorder	Comorbid psychiatric disorders
Esophageal motility disorder	Generalized anxiety disorder, major depressive disorder, panic disorder, somatization disorder
Irritable bowel syndrome	Major depressive disorder, panic disorder, obsessive compulsive disorder, somatization disorder
Nonulcer dyspepsia	Panic disorder, somatization disorder
Normal transit constipation	Major depressive disorder; somatization disorder

importance of recognizing comorbid mood and anxiety disorders in patients with IBS is supported by the observation that when properly identified and treated, the patient's gastrointestinal, as well as psychological, symptoms tend to improve [15]. Panic disorder can be treated with benzodiazepines, tricyclic antidepressants, and selective serotonin reuptake inhibitors; however, the gastrointestinal side effects of the latter two classes of agents include anticholinergic-induced constipation and reduction of lower esophageal sphincter pressure associated with the tricyclic antidepressants and nausea, vomiting, and diarrhea in up to 25% of patients treated with selective serotonin reuptake inhibitors.

Functional Dyspepsia

Discomfort of the upper gastrointestinal tract without evidence of ulcer disease is a common gastrointestinal complaint (see Chapter 25). In one community-based sample, 26% of respondents reported dyspepsia, for an age- and sex-adjusted prevalence rate of 26 per 100. The Rome Working Teams have divided functional dyspepsia into three subtypes: ulcerlike dyspepsia, dysmotility-like dyspepsia, and refluxlike dyspepsia [16••]. In studying the prevalence of the various subtypes of dyspepsia, Talley and colleagues found that 64%, 31%, and 38% of dyspeptic persons were classified into each of these three categories, respectively [17].

The relation among anxiety, neuroticism, and depression in patients with functional dyspepsia was investigated by Talley and colleagues [17]. According to a variety of psychological screening instruments, patients with non–ulcerlike dyspepsia were more neurotic, anxious, and depressed when compared with community controls who had no symptoms [18]. In a similar study, Magni and colleagues found that patients with functional (non–ulcerlike) dyspepsia were significantly more likely to have an Axis I psychiatric disorder by DSM-III criteria than were patients with ulcerlike dyspepsia [19]. The reason for this relation is not clear. One proposed hypothesis is that stress-induced changes can affect vagal tone. Haug and colleagues investigated this possibility and found that patients presenting with functional dyspepsia who had high levels of anxiety, depression, and neuroticism, as measured by standard psychological instruments, also had lower levels of vagal tone as well as lower gastrointestinal motility indices [20]. In addition, they found that changes in vagal tone and motility indices correlated with the abnormalities measured on psychometric testing. These psychosocial correlates affect the success of treatment because purely medical approaches, such as the use of H_2-receptor antagonists or eradication of *Helicobacter pylori* infection, have not been shown to be effective in treating nonulcer dyspepsia [21].

Esophageal Motility Disorders

The relation between psychosocial stress and esophageal symptoms, particularly chest pain, pyrosis, and dysphagia, has been well documented (see Chapter 7). A number of studies using psychometic testing have shown that patients with nonspecific esophageal motility disorders have significantly elevated levels of depression, somatization, and anxiety when compared with controls. These patients also have psychological profiles similar to those of patients with IBS. Bradley found that patients who were psychologically vulnerable, as measured by the Millon Behavioral Health Inventory, were more likely to report reflux

symptoms under experimentally induced stressful conditions, even though simultaneous pH monitoring could not detect increased levels of acid reflux during these stressful periods [22]. Moreover, patients who presented for treatment of gastroesophageal reflux disease experienced more phobia, somatization, and obsessional thoughts when compared with controls who did not seek health care who had documented gastroesophageal reflux disease [23••].

These findings suggest a role for psychopharmacologic and psychotherapeutic modalities in the treatment of upper functional gastrointestinal disorders. To test this hypothesis, North and colleagues studied 29 patients with contraction abnormalities of the esophagus [24••]. Patients were treated with trazodone, an antidepressant void of anticholinergic properties, in doses of 100 to 150 mg/d or placebo. The patients treated with trazodone had a significant improvement in overall well-being and level of gastrointestinal distress compared with those treated with placebo. The observed improvement in well-being and symptoms was unaccompanied by changes in esophageal motility.

Emotional Consequences of Gastrointestinal Disease

The IBDs ulcerative colitis and Crohn's disease have long been observed to be associated with psychiatric distress (see Chapters 64 and 75). During the 1930s and 1940s, Franz Alexander suggested a "psychosomatic" hypothesis for the causes of these disorders based on "specificity theory." This theory stated that various forms of intrapsychic conflicts resulted in "specific" types of gastrointestinal dysfunction. For example, the theory postulated that bleeding seen with ulcerative colitis was caused by unresolved mourning and depression. Studies undertaken to demonstrate the validity of the specificity hypothesis suffered from a number of methodologic shortcomings, including the lack of control groups, unsystematic collection of data, and absence of standardized diagnostic criteria. Studies that were based on the early work of Alexander have been the subject of a recent meta-analysis. In a review of 138 studies in the English medical literature, North and colleagues found that all the studies reporting some relation between psychiatric disorder and subsequent development of IBD had serious flaws in methodology [24••]. The seven studies that, in their opinion, represented solid methodology failed to show any such association.

Recent experimental studies also have failed to show an etiologic relation between psychiatric factors and subsequent development of IBD. In a retrospective case-control study of 50 patients with ulcerative colitis who were screened psychiatrically for a lifetime prevalence of psychiatric diagnosis, Helzer and colleagues found no greater frequency of diagnosable psychiatric disorder in the patients with ulcerative colitis than in control patients with nongastrointestinal chronic medical illnesses [25]. In the patients with ulcerative colitis found to have psychiatric illness, there was no correlation between the nature of the psychiatric illness and severity of gastrointestinal symptoms or intestinal inflammation. The severity of the ulcerative colitis did not predict the frequency or seriousness of a psychiatric disorder, when present. No correlation was found between the frequency of potentially stressful life events in the 6 months before evaluation and the severity of ulcerative colitis at the time of the psychiatric interview. One other important finding was that, in 26% of the patients with ulcerative colitis and a concomitant psychiatric disorder, the psychiatric disorder was documented in the medical charts or treated only rarely [25].

In a study using the same methodology, Helzer and colleagues found an increased prevalence of psychiatric disorders in 50 patients with Crohn's disease who were compared with non-IBD medical controls. This difference was statistically significant for depression (36% in patients with Crohn's disease compared with 18% in controls); but as in the previous study of patients with ulcerative colitis, there was no association between the presence or absence of a psychiatric disorder and the severity of Crohn's disease or extent of intestinal involvement [26].

The possibility that major depression could exacerbate pre-existing IBD was studied by North and Alpers [27]. Their prospective study of 32 consecutive patients with IBD followed for 2 years found no association between intestinal symptoms and life events. When the effect of mood was studied using the Beck Depression Inventory, a significant association between intestinal symptoms and the presence of depression was demonstrated. The authors concluded there was no evidence that stressful life events or the presence of depressed mood precipitate exacerbations of disease activity in patients with IBD [27].

The conclusion that can be drawn from the literature is that there is no causal nor predictive relation between IBD and the presence of psychiatric disorders. The challenge for the clinician is to correct the common misconception that IBD patients are suffering from a stress-induced disease and to focus instead on the biologic basis of the disease. Asking a patient about his or her understanding of the cause of IBD can lead to clarification of misconceptions that the patient may have about the disease but often is afraid to discuss. The clinician also should explain to the patient that the physical and economic toll taken by IBD can induce emotional distress, which should be addressed as part of a comprehensive management strategy.

An important aspect of treating patients with IBD is attention to emotional sequelae of surgery. Colectomy often is performed in patients with ulcerative colitis for intractability and for the risk of colorectal cancer, whereas patients with Crohn's disease require surgery for persistent intestinal strictures, abscesses, fistulas, or intractable disease activity despite medical management. Tremendous progress has been made in the surgical treatment of IBD during the past 20 years. In particular, conventional total colectomy with ileostomy has been superseded, when feasible, by the ileal pouch and anal anastomosis and, less commonly, by the Kock pouch, or continent ileostomy. McLeod and colleagues studied the impact of surgery on overall quality of life in 93 patients who underwent a Kock continent ileostomy or ileal pouch and anal anastomosis [28]. Surgery significantly improved both psychological status and overall quality of life in addition to reducing disease activity. Other studies have confirmed the negligible emotional impact of surgery on patients with IBD. Investigators have found no evidence to support the contention that serious psychopathology itself results in poor adaptation to colectomy, and evidence suggests that no diagnosable depression or anxiety results from the surgery for IBD. Some patients with discrepancies between perception of body image and perceived body ideal, however, may adapt poorly to postoperative symptoms. Also, patients who have difficulty expressing emotions may have more postoperative adaptive difficulties, and patients with a history of

participating in intensive physical exercise had poor psychological coping after colectomy. Thus, patients should be informed of all the implications of surgery, including changes in body image and physical and sexual functioning, to achieve better postoperative adjustment.

Psychological Aspects of Chronic Liver Disease and Liver Transplantation

Chronic hepatitis C infection has been associated with depression. In addition, antiviral therapy with interferon-alpha has a wide range of side effects, which can produce anxiety and depression (see Chapter 93). Myalgias, arthralgias, fevers, chills, and other systemic side effects of antiviral therapy may have significant emotional sequelae in patients. Indeed, there is some suggestion that interferon itself is capable of inducing depression in patients with chronic hepatitis.

The advent of orthotopic liver transplantation has revolutionized the treatment of end-stage liver disease (see Chapter 116). This technologic advance has been accompanied by new psychosocial challenges for both physicians and patients. The selection process can produce anxiety in patients and their families, particularly during the often long wait for a donor liver. The intraoperative and postoperative periods and ongoing concerns about possible rejection in the late postoperative period can exact a profound emotional toll.

One psychosocial aspect of gastroenterology that is only now being studied is the emotional effect of endoscopy on patients (see Chapter 188). What has become a routine part of gastroenterologic practice for physicians remains, all too often, a mysterious and threatening experience for patients. Two recent studies have shown that patients have significant concerns about endoscopy [29,30]. All too often these concerns are not addressed before the procedure. Dealing with a patient's specific concerns about a procedure before the procedure reduces the patient's level of distress, improves patient cooperation during the procedure, and has implications for risk management.

■ THE DIFFICULT PATIENT

No discussion of doctor–patient interactions would be complete without addressing the issue of the difficult patient. All physicians in the course of their practice have encountered patients who are angry, intimidating, demanding, or in other ways unpleasant. These patients often generate a whole spectrum of negative reactions (countertransference) from the physician and staff. All too often, these interactions end abruptly, which is unsatisfying for the patient and physician.

Groves has categorized difficult patients into four general types: dependent clingers, entitled demanders, manipulative help-rejecters, and self-destructive deniers [31•]. The characteristics of each of these patient types are described in Table 199-6. Groves believes that the key to dealing with a difficult patient is to identify the emotions generated by the behavior. Once the physician identifies these feelings, he or she can muster appropriate responses to the patient's difficult style. The clinger responds to limits on expectations for an intense and overly close doctor–patient relationship. The demander needs to have his or her feelings of entitlement rechanneled into a partnership based not on grandiose demands but on reasonable improvement in medical care. The help-rejecter is best approached by sharing his or her pessimism and by breaking the connection whereby the patient feels he or she only can maintain the interest and support of the physician by being hopelessly pessimistic. The self-destructive denier in many ways is the most difficult type of patient because of the intense anger he or she often generates in the physician. The physician should convey expectations of a reasonable outcome. Some patients, however, simply cannot be helped and have a particularly poor prognosis. Adopting the approach of Groves allows the physician to pay a lower emotional toll when dealing with these difficult patients [31•].

The concept of the difficult patient has been studied extensively. Hahn and colleagues developed a screening instrument to identify a difficult patient [32]. Using five factors that measure self-destructiveness, seductiveness, compliance, communication, and level of irritation induced in the physician by the patient, they were able to predict in advance which patients would be difficult. In a subsequent study, Hahn and colleagues demonstrated that the difficult patient usually had at least one of six psychiatric disorders [33•]. They also tended to have a higher use of health care, lower satisfaction with care, and greater functional impairment (as opposed to disease activity) than did other patients. Demographic characteristics and the type of physical illness were not associated with difficulty. Hahn and colleagues concluded that the presence of a psychiatric disorder can contribute disproportionately to functional impairment in difficult patients [33•].

These data show that early detection of a psychiatric disorder can help identify a patient who otherwise would be classified as difficult to treat. These patients do not respond to interventions based only on a cure model. Considering psychosocial dimensions in the care of such patients, the biopsychosocial model can pay significant dividends. The difficult patient, as described by Hahn and others, is much more likely than others to be suffering from a comorbid psychiatric disorder, and all physicians should understand that psychiatric disorders are treatable, often with anxiolytics or antidepressants. In addition, a number of studies published in the past 10 years have demonstrated the efficacy of psychotherapy for "refractory" functional gastrointestinal patients [34]. There are a number of rating scales available for the diagnosis of depression and anxiety disorders that are easy to use and score and generally are well accepted by patients [35•]. Somatization and hypochondriasis also can be treated but tend to respond better to a behavioral rather than pharmacologic approach [36•,37].

Care of the difficult patient must be holistic, integrating physiologic, psychological, and sociocultural dimensions. Clinicians who incorporate all these dimensions into their medical practices stand to gain significant benefits in terms of patient outcomes, satisfaction, and self-satisfaction and ultimately in terms of their own satisfaction and empowerment.

■■■ REFERENCES

Recently published papers of particular interest have been highlighted as follows:
• Of interest
•• Of outstanding interest

1. Brandt LJ: Holding a hand is often as important as examining one. *Am J Gastroenterol* 1993, 88:1817–1821.

2.•• Ong LML, DeHaes JCJM, Hoos AM, *et al.*: Doctor-patient communication: A review of the literature. *Soc Sci Med* 1995, 40:903–918.
The authors provide an excellent contemporary review of all aspects of doctor–patient communications that is well referenced and authoritative.

3. Bensing JM: Doctor-patient communication and the quality of care: An observation study into affective and instrumental behavior in general practice. Dissertation. NIVEL, Utrecht, 1991.

4.• Kaplan SH, Greenfield S, Ware JE: Assessing the effects of physician-patient interactions on the outcomes of chronic disease. In *Communicating With Medical Patients*. Edited by Stewart MM, Roter DL. Newbury Park, CA: Sage; 1989.
The authors report on their study of the impact of doctor–patient communications on patients with chronic illness.

5. Cuisinier MCJ, Van Eijk JTM, Jonkers R, *et al.*: Psychosocial care and education of the cancer patient: Strengthening the physician's role. *Patient Educ Counseling* 1986, 8:5.(AU: Please provide page range.)

6. Waitzkin H: Doctor-patient communication: Clinical implications of social scientific research. *JAMA* 1984, 252:2441. (AU: Please provide page range.)

7.• Ley P: *Communicating With Patients: Improving Communication, Satisfaction and Compliance*. London: Chapman and Hall; 1988.
The authors provide a good "how to" text on improving communication with patients.

8. Brock DW, Wartman SA: When competent patients make irrational choices. *N Engl J Med* 1990, 322:1595. (AU: Please provide page range.)

9. Kaplan SH, Greenfield S, Ware JE: Assessing the effects of physician-patient interactions on the outcomes of chronic disease. *Med Care* 1989, 27:S110. (AU: Please provide page range.)

10. Beckman HB, Markakis KM, Suchman AL, *et al.*: The doctor-patient relationship and malpractice: Lessons from plaintiffs' depositions. *Arch Intern Med* 1994, 154:1365–1370.

11. Messner E: Autognosis: diagnosis by the use of the self. In *Outpatient Psychiatry: Diagnosis and Treatment*. Edited by Lazare A. Boston: Williams & Wilkins; 1988.

12. DaCosta J: Mucous enteritis. *Medicine & Medical Science* 1871, 83:321–335.

13. Lydiard RB, Fossey MD, Marsh W, *et al.*: Prevalence of psychiatric disorders in patients with irritable bowel syndrome. *Psychosomatics* 1993, 34:229–234.

14. Walker EA, Katon WJ, Jemelka RP, *et al.*: Comorbidity of gastrointestinal complaints, depression and anxiety in the epidemiologic catchment area (ECA) study. *Am J Med* 1992, 92:26S–30S.

15. Tollefson GD, Luxenberg M, Valentine R, *et al.*: An open label trial of alprazolam in comorbid irritable bowel syndrome and generalized anxiety disorder. *J Clin Psychiatry* 1991, 52:502–508.

16.•• Drossman DA: *Functional Gastrointestinal Disorders: Diagnosis and Treatment*. Boston: Little Brown; 1994.
This is the standard textbook on nosology, diagnostic criteria, and epidemiology of the functional gastrointestinal disorders.

Table 199-6. Types of Difficult Patients

Patient type	Behavior
Dependent clinger	Makes repeated requests for attention, analgesics, and telephone calls
Entitled demander	Intimidates the physician, induces a sense of guilt, and devalues the physician's opinion
Help-rejecter	Appears hopeless and pessimistic about outcome ("medicine makes me worse")
Self-destructive denier	Is noncompliant, minimizes severity or impact, may be a substance abuser

From Groves [31•]; with permission.

17. Talley NJ, Zinsmeister AR, Schleck CD, *et al.*: Dyspepsia and dyspepsia subgroups: A population-based study. *Gastroenterology* 1992, 102:1259–1268.

18. Talley NJ, Fung LH, Gilligan I, *et al.*: Association of anxiety, neuroticism and depression with dyspepsia of unknown cause: A case-control study. *Gastroenterology* 1986, 90:886–892.

19. Magni G, DiMario F, Bernasconi G, *et al.*: DSM-III diagnoses associated with dyspepsia of unknown cause. *Am J Psychiatry* 1987, 144:1222–1223.

20. Haug TT, Svebak S, Hausken T, *et al.*: Low vagal activity as mediating mechanism for the relationship between personality factors and gastric symptoms in functional dyspepsia. *Psychosom Med* 1994, 56:181–186.

21. Talley NJ: A critique of therapeutic trials in *Helicobacter pylori*–positive functional dyspepsia. *Gastroenterology* 1994, 106:1174–1183.

22. Bradley LA, Richter JE, Pulliam TJ, *et al.*: The relationship between stress and symptoms of gastroesophageal reflux: The influence of psychological factors. *Am J Gastroenterol* 1993, 88:11–19.

23.•• Johnston BT, Gunning J, Lewis SA: Health care seeking by heartburn sufferers is associated with psychosocial factors. *Am J Gastroenterol* 1996, 91:2500–2504.
This study was well done and shows clearly the disparity between patient's complaints and their actual physiologic findings.

24.•• North CS, Clouse RE, Sptznagel EL, *et al.*: The relation of ulcerative colitis to psychiatric factors: A review of findings and methods. *Am J Psychiatry* 1990, 147:974–981.
This definitive review article refutes a psychiatric cause of inflammatory bowel disease.

25. Helzer JE, Stillings W, Chammas S, *et al.*: A controlled study of the association between ulcerative colitis and psychiatric diagnoses. *Dig Dis Sci* 1982, 27:513–518.

26. Helzer JE, Chammas S, Norland CC, *et al.*: A study of the association between Crohn's disease and psychiatric illness. *Gastroenterology* 1984, 86:324–330.

27. North CS, Alpers DH, Helzer JE, *et al.*: Do life events or depression exacerbate inflammatory bowel disease? *Ann Intern Med* 1991, 114:381–386.

28. McLeod RS, Cohen Z, Churchill DA, *et al.*: Measurement of quality of life of patients with ulcerative colitis undergoing surgery. *Gastroenterology* 1991, 101:1307–1313.

29. Drossman DA, Brandt LJ, Sears CL, *et al.*: A preliminary study of patients' concerns related to GI endoscopy. *Am J Gastroenterol* 1996, 91:287–291.

30. Lin M, Kearney D, Olden KW, *et al.*: Patient concerns about endoscopy: a preliminary report. [Abstract] *Gastroenterology* 1996, 110:A26.

31.• Groves JE: Taking care of the hateful patient. *N Engl J Med* 1978, 298:883–887.
This classic article covers the styles of difficult patients and provides specific recommendations on how to deal with each style.

32. Hahn SR, Thompson KS, Wills TA, *et al.*: The difficult doctor-patient relationship: Somatization, personality and psychopathology. *J Clin Epidemiol* 1994, 47:647–657.

33.• Hahn SR, Kroenke K, Spitzer R, *et al.*: The difficult patient: Prevalence, psychopathology and functional impairment. *J Gen Intern Med* 1996, 11:1–8.
This thoughtful study covers what constitutes the "difficult" patient and how to intervene medically and psychiatrically.

34. Guthrie E, Creed FH, Dawson D, *et al.*: A randomised controlled trial of psychotherapy in patients with refractory irritable bowel syndrome. *Br J Psychiatry* 1993, 163:315–321.

35.• Naifeh K: Psychometric testing in functional GI disorders. In *Handbook of Functional Gastrointestinal Disorders*. Edited by Olden KW. New York: Marcel Dekker; 1996:79–126.
The authors provide an excellent review of the wide spectrum of psychiatric screening instruments available in medical practice and how to use them.

36.• Barsky A: Hypochondriasis: medical management and psychiatric treatment. *Psychosomatics* 1996, 37:48–56.
The author provides an excellent review of the contemporary management of hypochondriasis.

37. Warwick HC, Clark DM, Cobb AW, *et al.*: A controlled trial of cognitive-behavioral treatment of hypochondriasis. *Br J Psychiatry* 1996, 169:189–195.

Index

Page numbers followed by *f* indicate figures, those followed by *t* indicate tabular material.

Nutritional therapy (*continued*)
  for surgical patient with pancreatic disease, 1634–1635
  in ulcerative colitis, 681
Nystatin, for esophageal candidiasis, 122

O

Obesity, energy needs in, determination of, 1562
Obstetric trauma, and fecal incontinence in women, 639, 639*f*, 644
Obstructive jaundice. *See* Jaundice, obstructive
Obstructive pancreatitis, 1185, 1185*f*
Occult blood test. *See* Fecal occult blood test
Occupational agents, hepatotoxicity of, 861*t*
OCG. *See* Oral cholecystography
OctreoScan, 194
Octreotide (Sandostatin)
  antineoplastic effects of, 498
  for bacterial overgrowth, 521*t*, 522, 522*f*
  for dumping syndrome, 408
  for endocrine pancreatic neoplasms, 1217
  for esophageal variceal bleeding, 194
  for gastrointestinal manifestations of amyloidosis, 474
  for gastrointestinal neuroendocrine tumors, 499
  for graft-versus-host disease, 471
  for intestinal pseudo-obstruction, 460
  for metastatic gastrinoma in Zollinger-Ellison syndrome, 322
  for pancreatic ascites, 1174
  for pancreatic cyst, 1167
  for pancreatic fistulas, 1174, 1178–1180
  for pancreatitis, 194
    acute, 1165
    chronic, 1192
    hereditary, 1240
  as pre-ERCP medication, 1160
  for secretory diarrhea, 194
  for short-bowel syndrome, 512
  for small bowel carcinoids, 498
  structure of, 193, 193*f*
  for upper gastrointestinal bleeding in children, 1307
  for variceal bleeding, 311, 983–984
    in children, 1450
Ocular larva migrans, 917
Ocular-vestibular circuit, and motion sickness, 218*f*, 218–219
Oddi, Rugero, 1096
Odynophagia
  with *Candida* esophagitis, 18–19
  clinical significance of, 18–19
  in elderly, 1576*t*
  with esophageal foreign bodies, 85
  in esophageal infection, 117
  with esophageal ulcer, 18, 45
  in HIV-infected (AIDS) patients, 18–19, 1491
  in immunocompromised patients, 18–19, 19*t*
  with infectious esophagitis, 18–19
  with pill-induced esophagitis, 91, 94
Ogilvie's syndrome, constipation in, 628
Oil red O stain, for gastrointestinal tract uses, 157*t*
OKT3, for immunosuppression
  in liver transplantation, 1024
  in pediatric liver transplantation, 1453–1454
Olsalazine
  for Crohn's disease, 564–565
  hepatotoxicity of, 859*t*
  for pediatric inflammatory bowel disease, 1351*t*, 1351–1352

for proctitis, 721, 721*t*
OLT (orthotopic liver transplantation). *See* Liver, transplantation
Omega fatty acids, antiemetic effect of, 225
Omega-3 fatty acids, therapeutic use of, in inflammatory bowel disease, 1566
Omeprazole (Prilosec). *See also* Proton pump inhibitors
  acid hyposecretion induced by, 326–327
  for duodenal ulcer, 278, 278*t*, 279*f*
  for gastric ulcer, 270–271
  for gastroesophageal reflux disease, 28*t*, 28–29, 29*f*, 35, 41–42, 62
    in asthmatic patients, 38–39, 40*f*
    with cisapride, in combination, 30
    contraindications to, 28*t*
    dosage and administration of, 28*t*, 35
    maintenance therapy, 30
  for *Helicobacter pylori* infection, 262*t*, 262–263, 263*t*
  hepatotoxicity of, 859*t*
  for initial nonurgent control of acid hypersecretion, 319–320
  for reflux esophagitis, in children, 1259–1260
  safety of, 278, 328
  for short-bowel syndrome, 511
  for ulcer-related hemorrhage, 308
  and vitamin B12 deficiency, 329, 368
Omphalitis, and pediatric portal hypertension, 1448
Omphalomesenteric duct, 1363, 1363*f*
  persistence of, 1363, 1364*f*
  remnant of, 1363, 1364*f*–1365*f*
Ondansetron (Zofran)
  for cyclic vomiting, in infants and children, 1289–1290
  hepatotoxicity of, 859*t*
  for nausea and vomiting, 223
  for pediatric patients, 1289*t*, 1289–1290
  for primary sclerosing cholangitis, 1112
Ondine's curse, 1400
Oophorectomy, in colorectal cancer, 768
OPD (oropharyngeal dysphagia). *See* Dysphagia, oropharyngeal
Opiate agonists, for intestinal pseudo-obstruction, 460
Opiate antagonists, 1527, 1527*t*
  for intestinal pseudo-obstruction, 460
Opiates, in conscious sedation for endoscopy, 1527, 1527*t*
Opisthorchiasis, 915
  and cholangiocarcinoma, 1123
Opium, tincture of, for short-bowel syndrome, 512
Opportunistic infections
  hepatic, in pediatric AIDS, 1482
  in HIV-infected (AIDS) patients, 1490, 1490*f*
    gastric, 1493
    liver involvement in, 969, 970*f*
  pancreatitis caused by, in pediatric AIDS, 1483
Oral cancer, in elderly, 1577–1578
Oral cavity
  age-related changes in, 1577, 1577*t*
  caustic injury to. *See* Caustic injury, to upper gastrointestinal tract
Oral cholecystography, 1046–1047, 1047*f*
Oral contraceptives
  esophageal injury due to, 92*t*
  hepatotoxicity of, 858*t*, 861, 863*t*–864*t*, 866*t*, 897–899
  ischemic colonic injury due to, 713
Oral dissolution therapy, for gallstones, 1051, 1051*f*, 1051*t*

Oral hypoglycemics, hepatotoxicity of, 858*t*
Organophosphorus compounds, and acute pancreatitis, 1160
Organ transplantation, infectious complications of, 115–116
Oriental cholangiohepatitis, 1085
Oriental hepatolithiasis, 1123
Oropharyngeal dysphagia. *See* Dysphagia, oropharyngeal
Oropharynx
  age-related changes in, 1578, 1578*t*
  innervation of, 66, 66*t*
  muscular components of, 66, 66*t*
Orthotopic liver transplantation. *See* Liver, transplantation
Osler-Weber-Rendu disease, 336
  small bowel bleeding with, 433*t*
Osmotic gap, 615, 616*t*
Osteomalacia
  in bacterial overgrowth syndrome, 521
  after gastric surgery, 412
Osteomyelitis, *Salmonella*, 533
Osteopenia
  with chronic cholestasis, 930, 932
  in Crohn's disease, 560
Osteoporosis
  in inflammatory bowel disease, 683
  in ulcerative colitis, 683
Oxacillin, hepatotoxicity of, 859*t*, 863*t*
Oxaprozin, hepatotoxicity of, 858*t*
Oxycodone (Percocet), for recurrent attacks of pancreatitis, 1168
Oxyntic cells, 159
  in gastric acid secretion, 180
Oxyntic mucosa, *Color Plate*, 158–160, 159*f*–160*f*
Oxyntomodulin, 196, 196*t*
Oxyphenbutazone, hepatotoxicity of, 863*t*
Oxyphenisatin, hepatotoxicity of, 856*t*, 859*t*, 860
Oxyphil, definition of, 159
Oxytetracycline, esophageal injury due to, 91*t*
Oxytocin, 217, 217*f*

P

Pacemaker
  gastric, 152
  gastroduodenal, 200, 200*f*, 201
    aberrant, and nausea and vomiting, 218*f*, 219–220
Pain
  abdominal. *See* Abdominal pain
  anorectal, chronic idiopathic, 780
  in anorectal examination, 775
  biliary. *See* Biliary pain
  chest. *See* Chest pain
  in chronic pancreatitis, 1185–1186, 1186*t*
  with esophageal perforation, 108
  with esophageal tumors, 131
  with pancreatic cancer, 1205
  parietal, neuroanatomic characteristics of, 210
  with pill-induced esophagitis, 92
  radiation, with acute abdominal pain, 448, 449*f*
  referred. *See* Referred pain
    neuroanatomic characteristics of, 210
    patterns of, 212, 446–467, 466*f*
  with small bowel malignancy, 496
  on swallowing. *See* Odynophagia
  visceral, neuroanatomic characteristics of, 210
Palpation, with abdominal examination, 451
Pamidronate, esophageal injury due to, 92*t*, 95

Color Plates

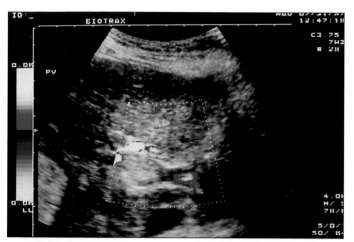

Chapter 92, Figure 1.

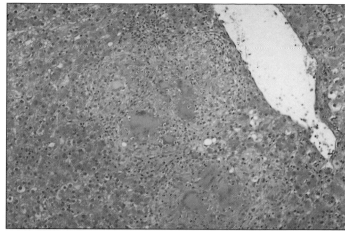

Chapter 98, Figure 3.

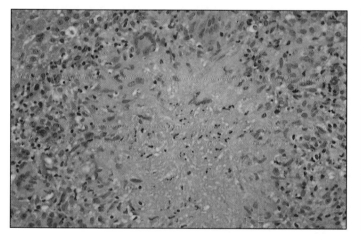

Chapter 98, Figure 6.

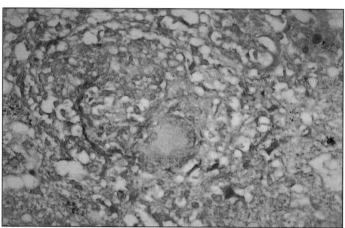

Chapter 98, Figure 10A.

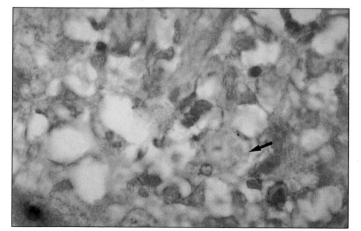

Chapter 98, Figure 10B.

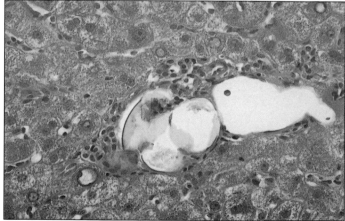

Chapter 98, Figure 11A.

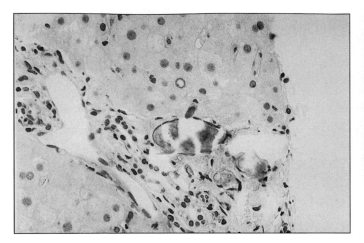

Chapter 98, Figure 11B.

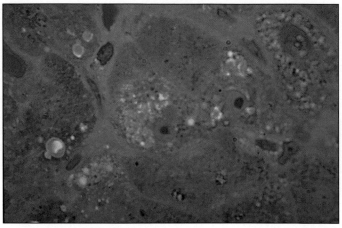

Chapter 99, Figure 1.

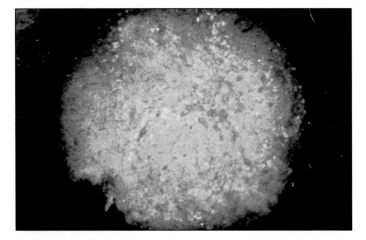

Chapter 99, Figure 6.

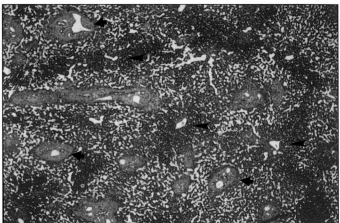

Chapter 100, Figure 8.

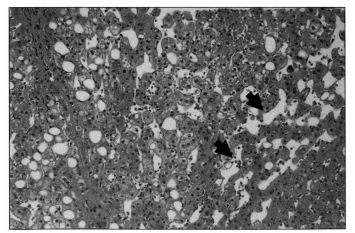

Chapter 100, Figure 9.

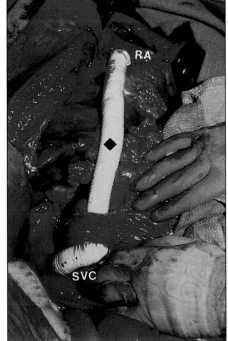

Chapter 100, Figure 16.

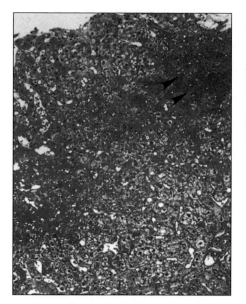

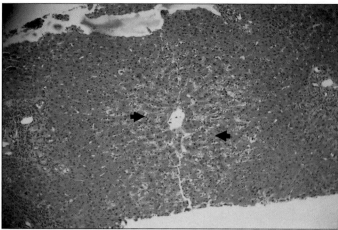

Chapter 100, Figure 20.

Chapter 100, Figure 17.

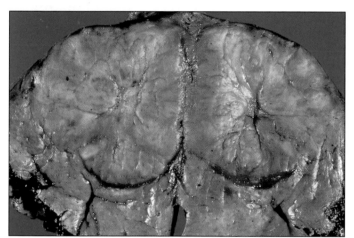

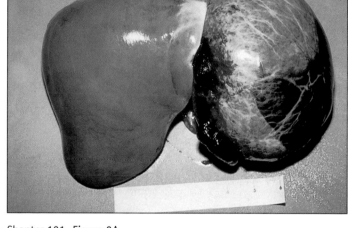

Chapter 101, Figure 4.

Chapter 101, Figure 9A.

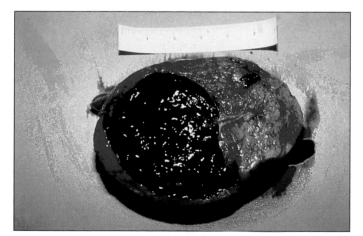

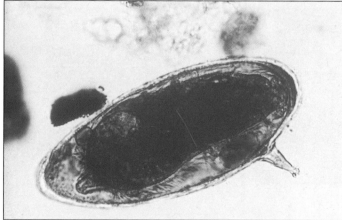

Chapter 101, Figure 9B.

Chapter 104, Figure 4.

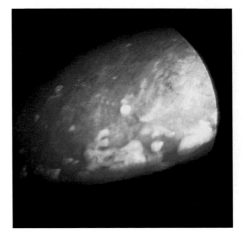

Chapter 104, Figure 6.

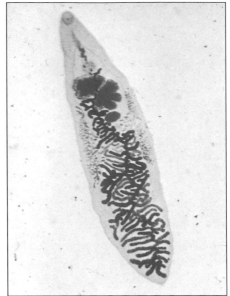

Chapter 104, Figure 10.

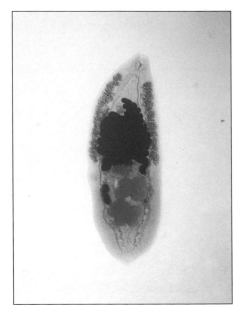

Chapter 104, Figure 14A.

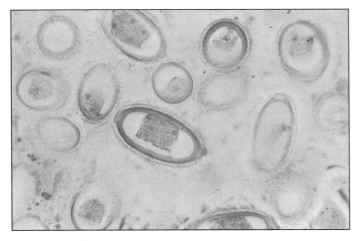

Chapter 104, Figure 16.

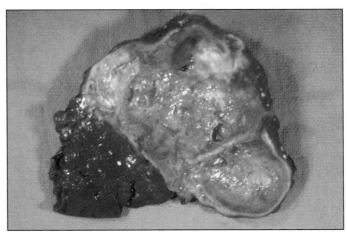

Chapter 104, Figure 19C.

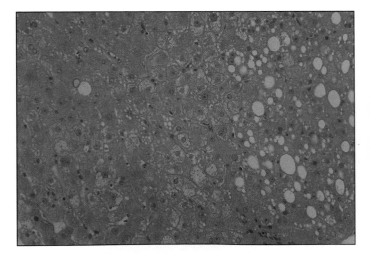

Chapter 107, Figure 2A.

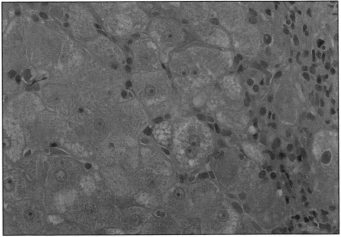

Chapter 107, Figure 2B.

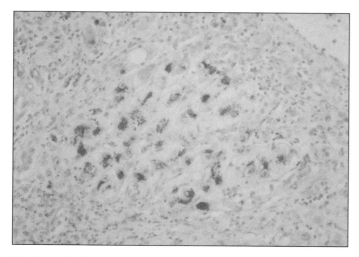

Chapter 107, Figure 2C.

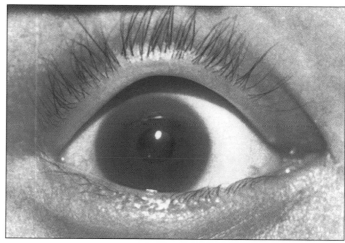

Chapter 107, Figure 3.

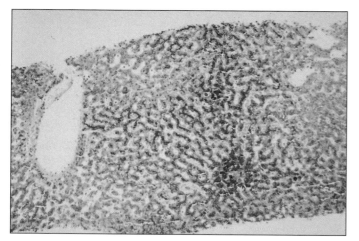

Chapter 108, Figure 1A.

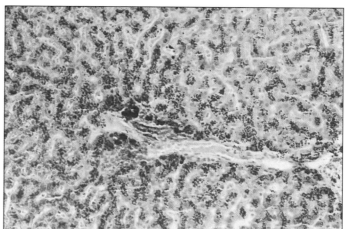

Chapter 108, Figure 1B.

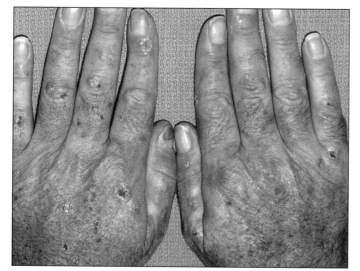

Chapter 109, Figure 7A.

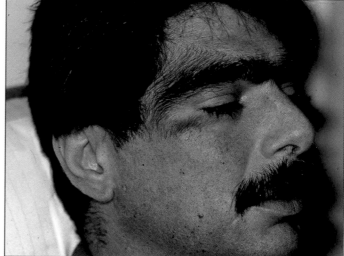

Chapter 109, Figure 7B.

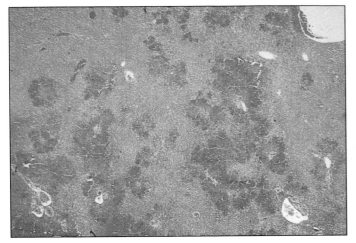

Chapter 110, Figure 1.

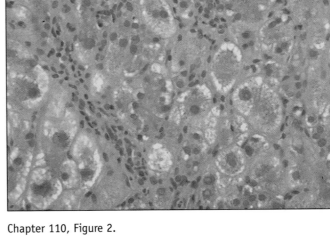

Chapter 110, Figure 2.

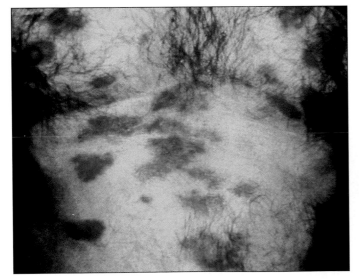

Chapter 111, Figure 8A.

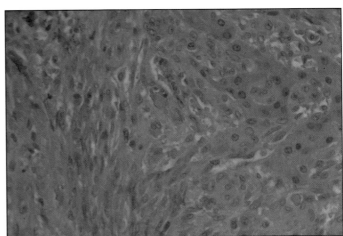

Chapter 111, Figure 8B.

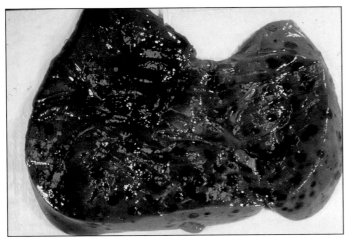

Chapter 111, Figure 9A.

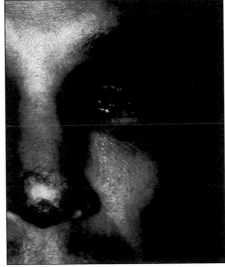

Chapter 111, Figure 9B.

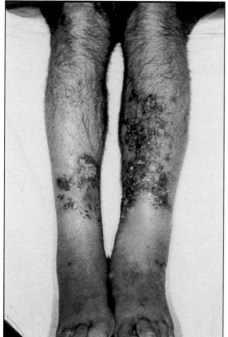

Chapter 111, Figure 9C.

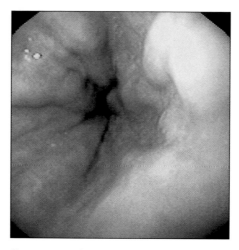

Chapter 112, Figure 2A.

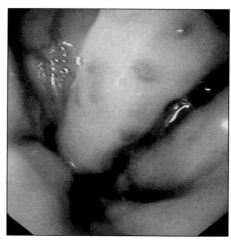

Chapter 112, Figure 2B.

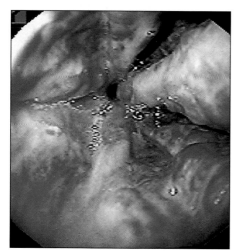

Chapter 112, Figure 2C.

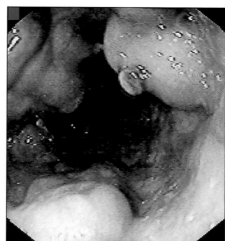

Chapter 112, Figure 3A.

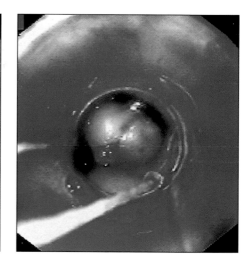

Chapter 112, Figure 3B.

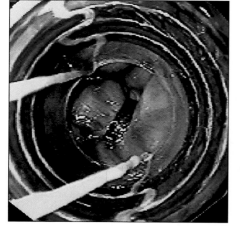

Chapter 112, Figure 3C.

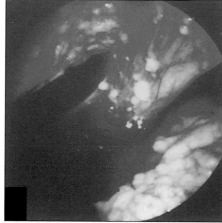

Chapter 113, Figure 1.

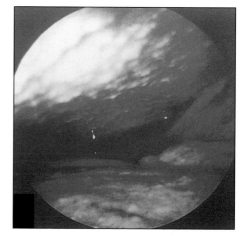

Chapter 113, Figure 2.

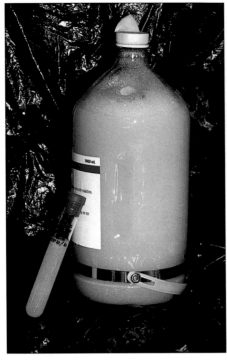

Chapter 113, Figure 3.

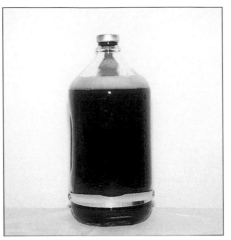

Chapter 113, Figure 4.

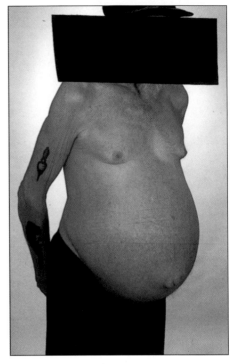

Chapter 113, Figure 5.

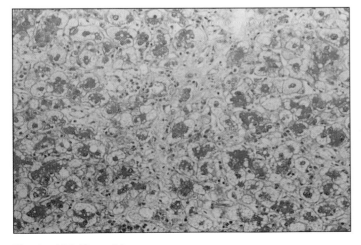

Chapter 113, Figure 6.

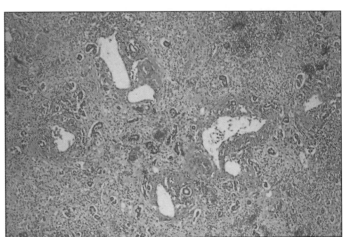

Chapter 116, Figure 2.

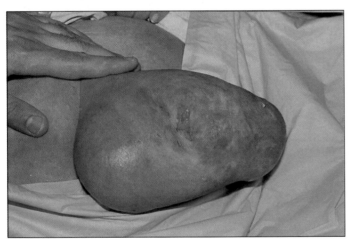

Chapter 116, Figure 3A.

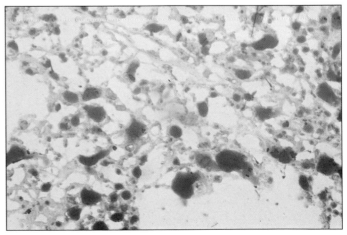

Chapter 116, Figure 3B.

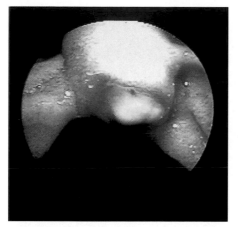

Chapter 119, Figure 8A.

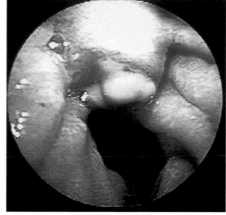

Chapter 119, Figure 8B.

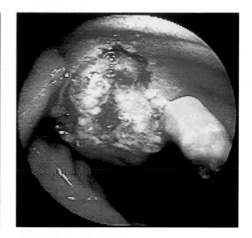

Chapter 119, Figure 8C.

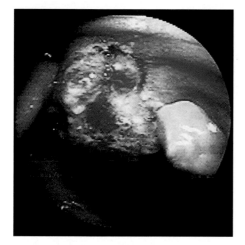

Chapter 119, Figure 8D.

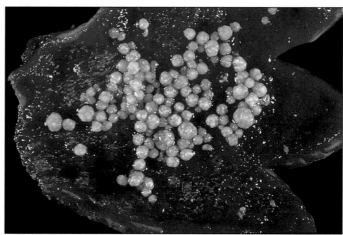

Chapter 120, Figure 1.

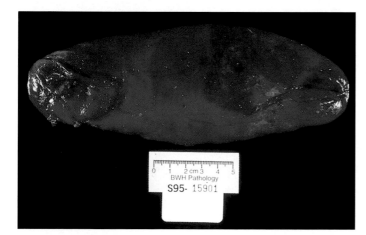

Chapter 120, Figure 4.

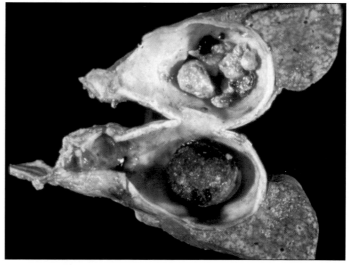

Chapter 120, Figure 15.

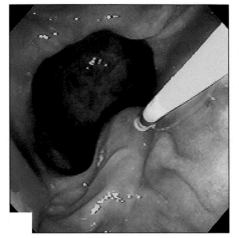

Chapter 123, Figure 4.

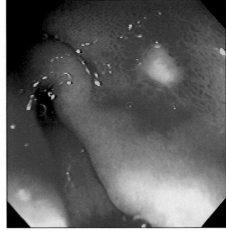

Chapter 123, Figure 5.

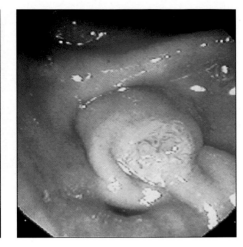

Chapter 127, Figure 3A.

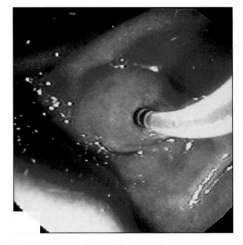

Chapter 127, Figure 3B.

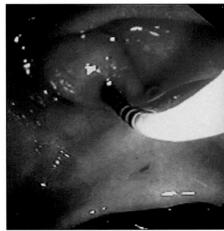

Chapter 127, Figure 3C.

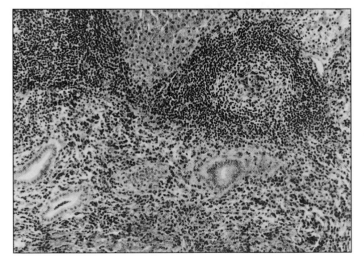

Chapter 128, Figure 1.

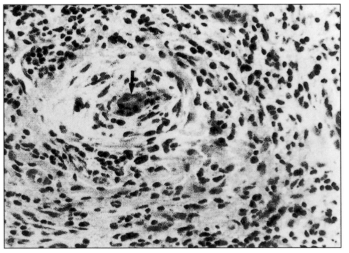

Chapter 128, Figure 2.

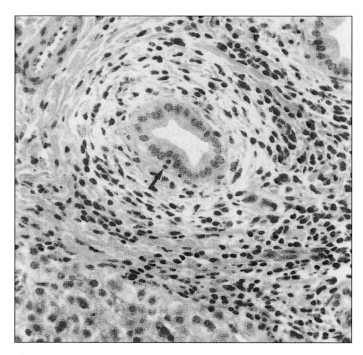

Chapter 128, Figure 3.

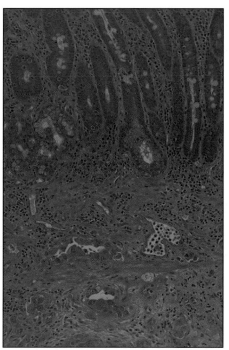

Chapter 128, Figure 4.

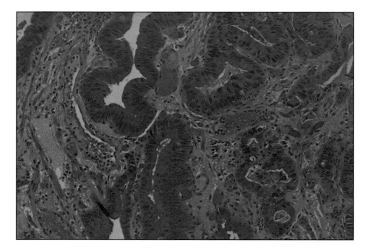

Chapter 129, Figure 1.

Chapter 129, Figure 2.

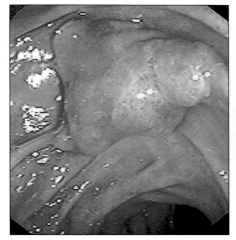

Chapter 129, Figure 3A.

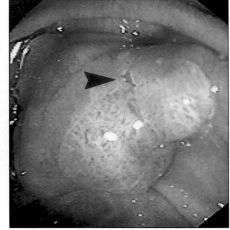

Chapter 129, Figure 3B.

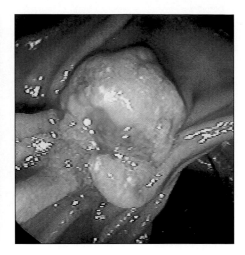

Chapter 129, Figure 3C.

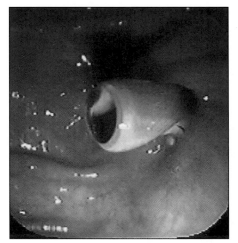

Chapter 131, Figure 10.

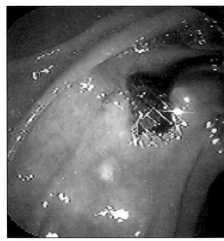

Chapter 131, Figure 13.

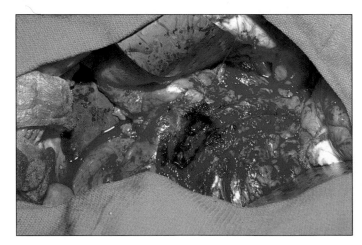

Chapter 138, Figure 4.

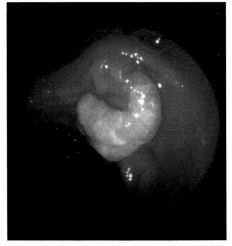

Chapter 142, Figure 7.

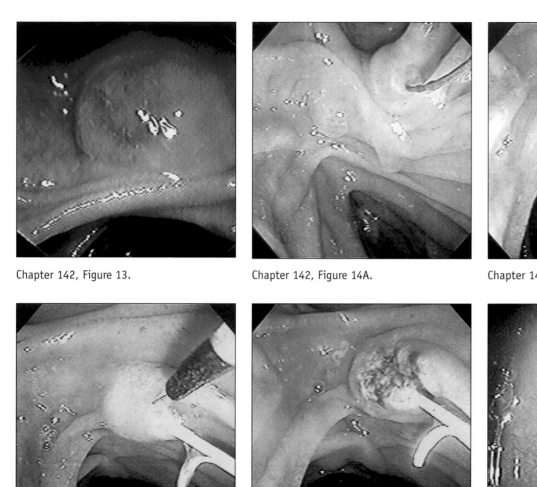

Chapter 142, Figure 13.

Chapter 142, Figure 14A.

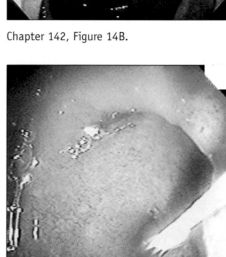

Chapter 142, Figure 14B.

Chapter 142, Figure 14C.

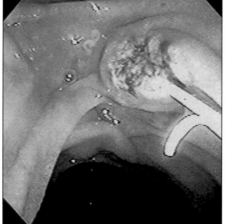

Chapter 142, Figure 14D.

Chapter 142, Figure 18A.

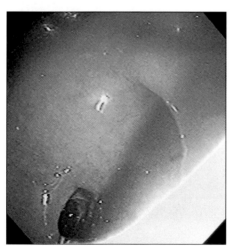

Chapter 142, Figure 18B.

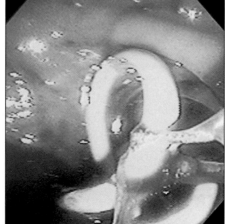

Chapter 142, Figure 18C.

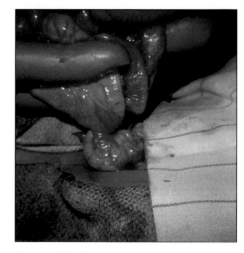

Chapter 150, Figure 6.

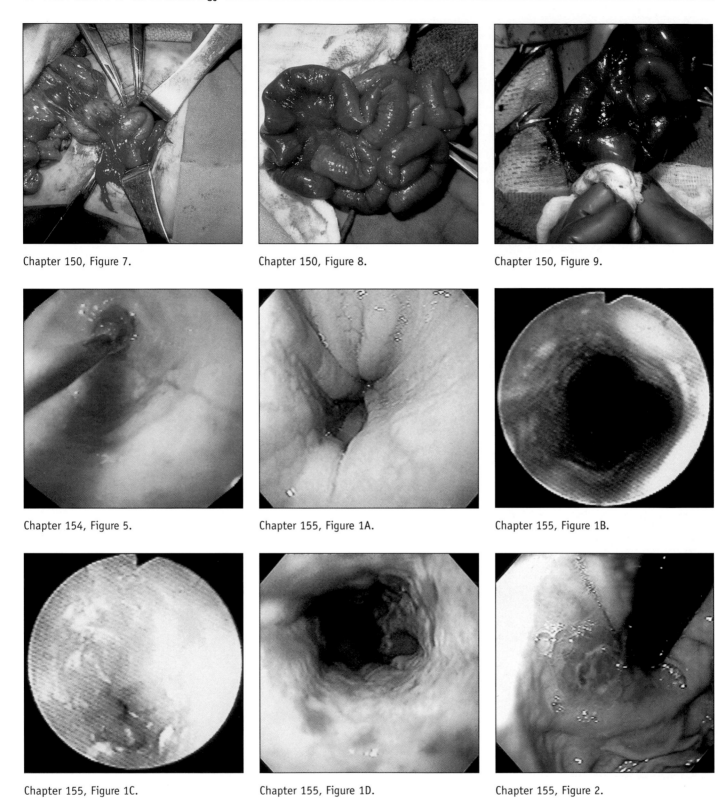

Chapter 150, Figure 7.

Chapter 150, Figure 8.

Chapter 150, Figure 9.

Chapter 154, Figure 5.

Chapter 155, Figure 1A.

Chapter 155, Figure 1B.

Chapter 155, Figure 1C.

Chapter 155, Figure 1D.

Chapter 155, Figure 2.

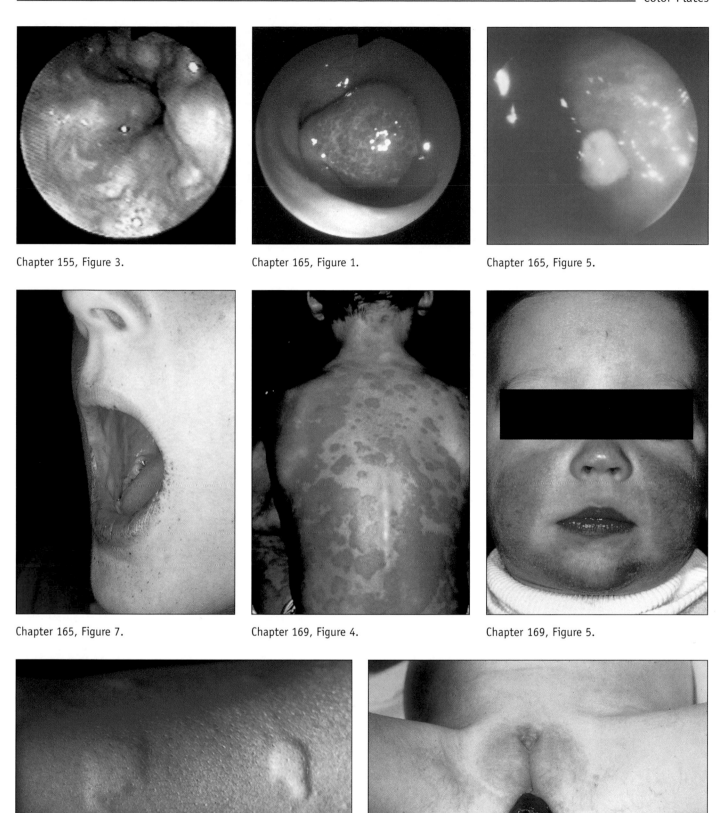

Chapter 155, Figure 3.

Chapter 165, Figure 1.

Chapter 165, Figure 5.

Chapter 165, Figure 7.

Chapter 169, Figure 4.

Chapter 169, Figure 5.

Chapter 169, Figure 6.

Chapter 170, Figure 2.

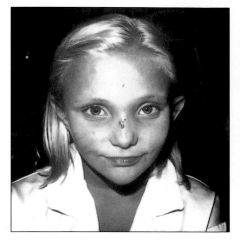

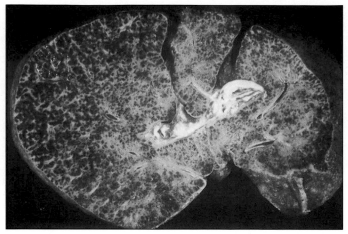

Chapter 173, Figure 1A.

Chapter 173, Figure 2.

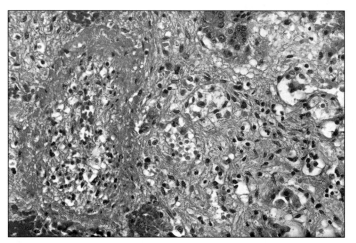

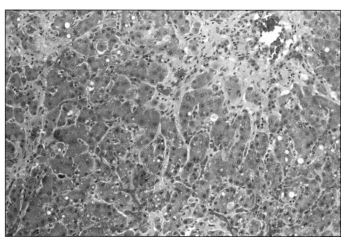

Chapter 177, Figure 2.

Chapter 177, Figure 3.

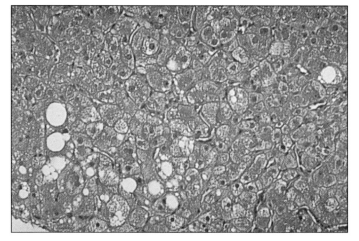

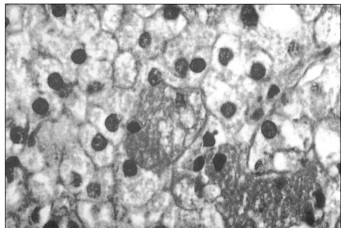

Chapter 178, Figure 1.

Chapter 178, Figure 2.

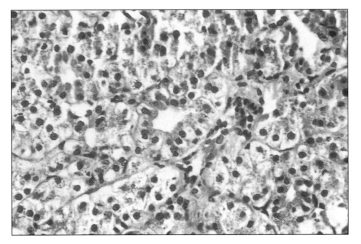

Chapter 178, Figure 3.

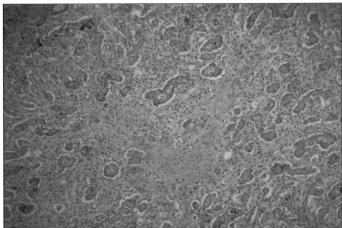

Chapter 178, Figure 4.

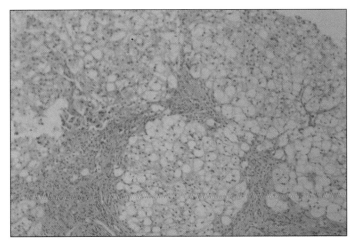

Chapter 178, Figure 9.

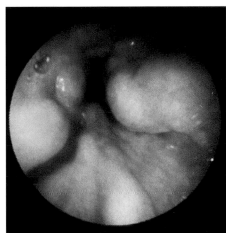

Chapter 179, Figure 1.

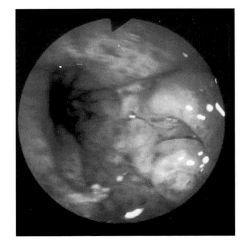

Chapter 179, Figure 2.

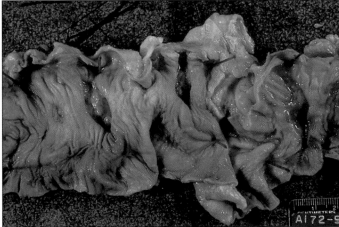

Chapter 184, Figure 5A.

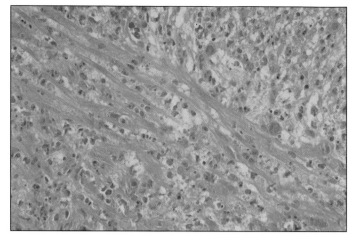

Chapter 184, Figure 5B.

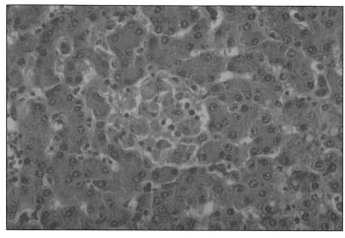

Chapter 184, Figure 9A.

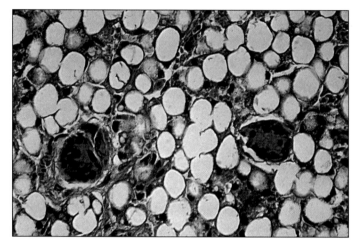

Chapter 184, Figure 9B.

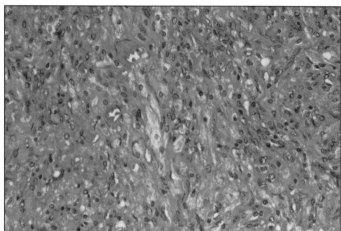

Chapter 184, Figure 9C.

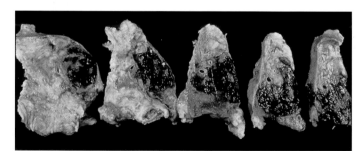

Chapter 184, Figure 13A.

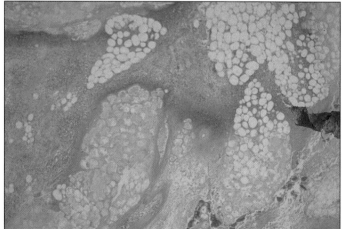

Chapter 184, Figure 13B.

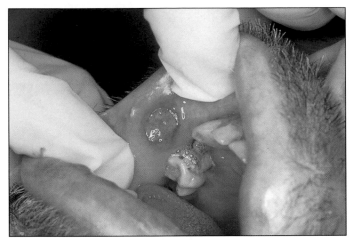

Chapter 185, Figure 2.

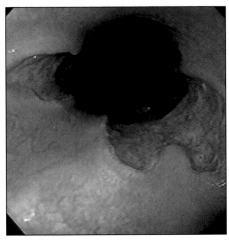

Chapter 185, Figure 3B.

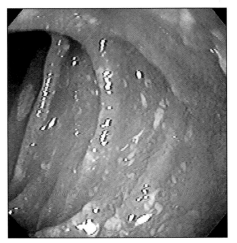

Chapter 185, Figure 7A.

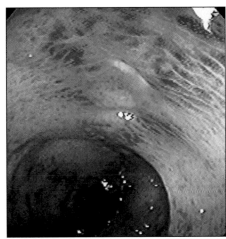

Chapter 185, Figure 8A.

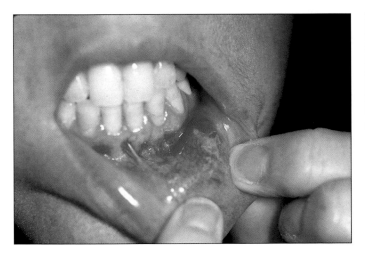

Chapter 186, Figure 1.

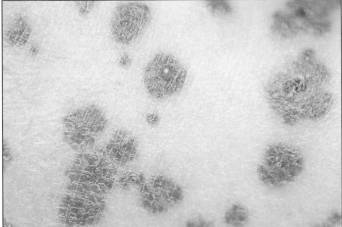

Chapter 186, Figure 2.

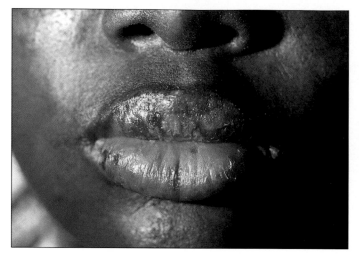

Chapter 186, Figure 10.

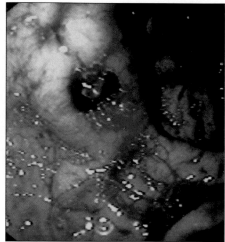

Chapter 187, Figure 1A.

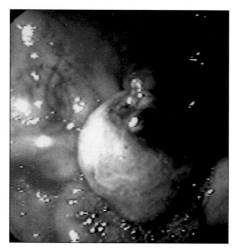

Chapter 187, Figure 1B.

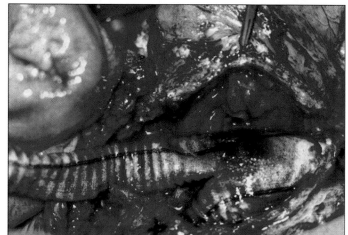

Chapter 187, Figure 2.

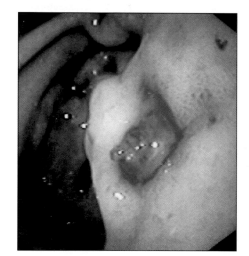

Chapter 187, Figure 3A.

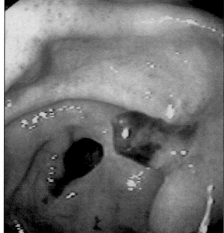

Chapter 187, Figure 3B.

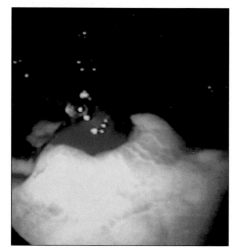

Chapter 187, Figure 3C.

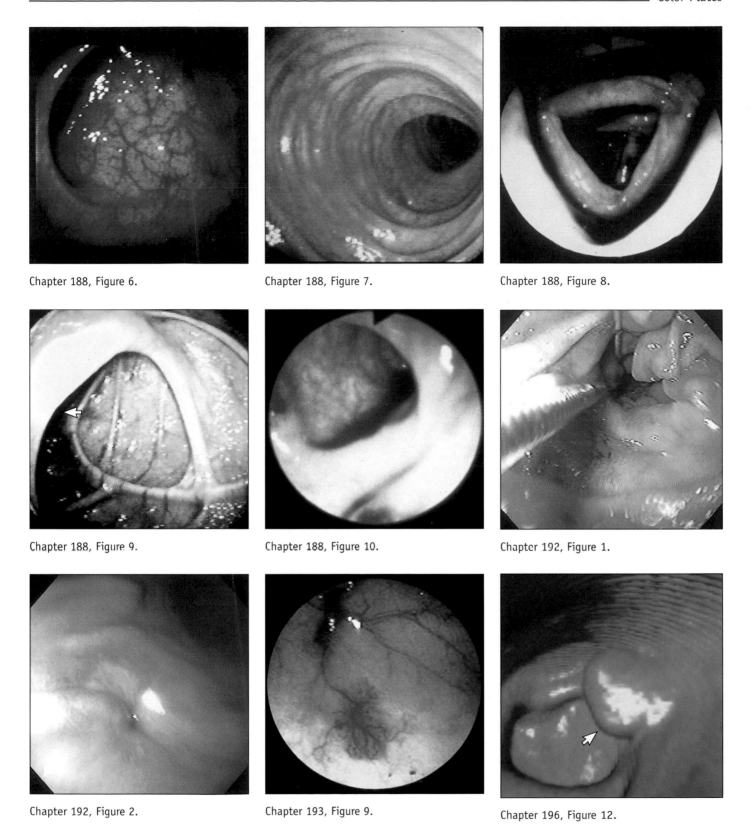

Chapter 188, Figure 6.

Chapter 188, Figure 7.

Chapter 188, Figure 8.

Chapter 188, Figure 9.

Chapter 188, Figure 10.

Chapter 192, Figure 1.

Chapter 192, Figure 2.

Chapter 193, Figure 9.

Chapter 196, Figure 12.

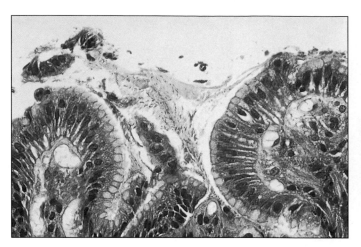

Chapter 197, Figure 9.

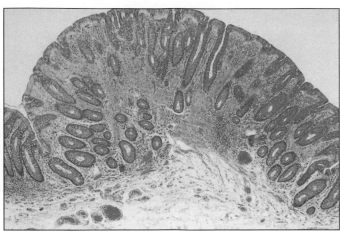

Chapter 197, Figure 19.